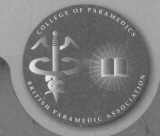

AAOS

Nancy Caroline's
Emergency
Care in the Streets

Sixth Edition

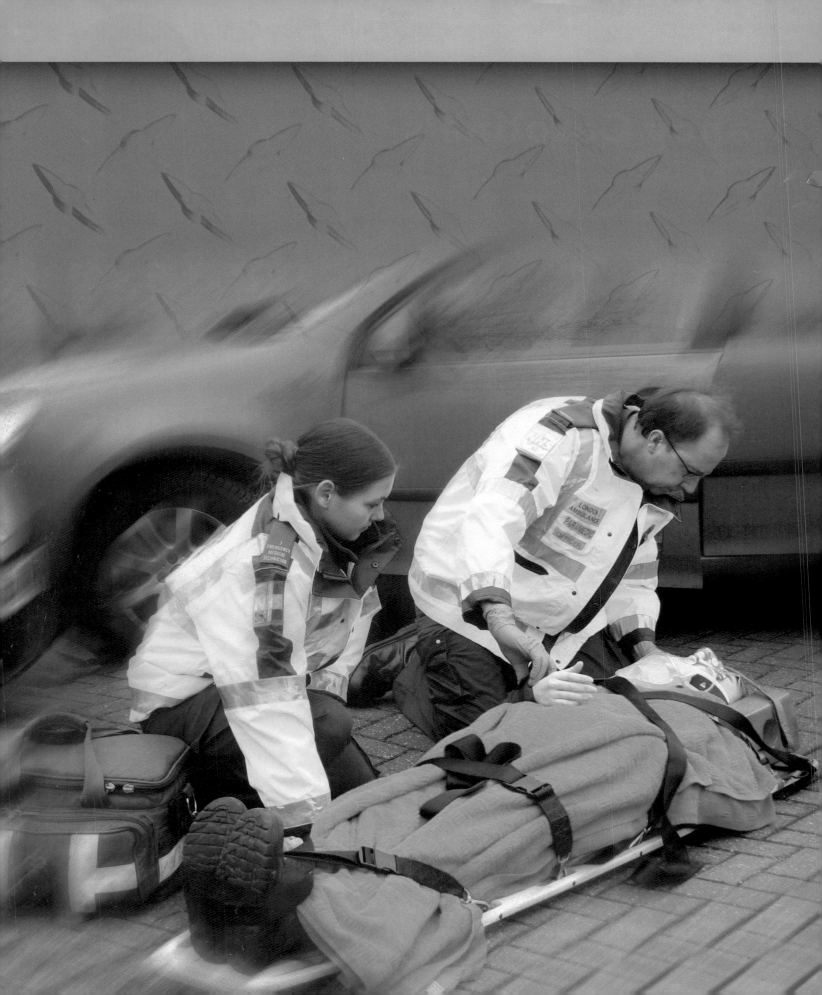

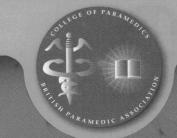

AAOS

Nancy Caroline's
Emergency
Care in the Streets

Sixth Edition

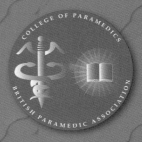

Author:
Nancy L. Caroline, MD

Series Editor:
Andrew N. Pollak, MD, FAAOS

Editors:
Bob Fellows, BSc, Paramedic, PGCE   Mark Woolcock, Paramedic

JONES AND BARTLETT PUBLISHERS
Sudbury, Massachusetts
BOSTON   TORONTO   LONDON   SINGAPORE

Jones and Bartlett Publishers

World Headquarters
Jones and Bartlett Publishers
40 Tall Pine Drive
Sudbury, MA 01776
info@jbpub.com
www.EMSzone.com

Jones and Bartlett Publishers Canada
6339 Ormindale Way
Mississauga, ON L5V 1J2
Canada

Jones and Bartlett Publishers International
Barb House, Barb Mews
London W6 7PA
United Kingdom

Jones and Bartlett's books and products are available through most bookstores and online booksellers. To contact Jones and Bartlett Publishers directly, call +44 (0) 1278 723553, fax +44 (0) 1278 723554, or visit our website, www.jbpub.com.

AAOS
AMERICAN ACADEMY OF ORTHOPAEDIC SURGEONS

Editorial Credits
Chief Executive Officer: Mark W. Wieting
Director, Department of Publications: Marilyn L. Fox, PhD
Managing Editor: Barbara A. Scotese

Production Credits

Chief Executive Officer: Clayton Jones
Chief Operating Officer: Donald W. Jones, Jr
President, Higher Education and Professional Publishing: Robert Holland
V.P., Sales and Marketing: William J. Kane
V.P., Production and Design: Anne Spencer
V.P., Manufacturing and Inventory Control: Therese Connell
Publisher, Public Safety: Kimberly Brophy
Acquisitions Editor, EMS: Christine Emerton
Managing Editor: Carol Guerrero

Editor: Jennifer S. Kling
Associate Managing Editor: Amanda Green
Editorial Assistant: Amanda Brandt
Editorial Assistant: Justin Keogh
Senior Production Editor: Susan Schultz
Production Editor: Karen Ferreira
Associate Production Editor: Jamie Chase
Photo Research Manager/Photographer: Kimberly Potvin
Director of Marketing: Alisha Weisman
Product Manager: Lorna Downing

Interior Design: Anne Spencer and Kristin Ohlin
Cover Design: Kristin Ohlin
Cartoons: Nick Bertozzi
Composition: Shepherd, Inc.
Text Printing and Binding: Replika Press
Cover Printing: Replika Press
Cover Photograph: © Jones and Bartlett Publishers, Inc. Photographed by Kimberly Potvin
Photos of Nancy L. Caroline provided in loving memory by her mother, Zelda Caroline.

The procedures and protocols in this book are based on the most current recommendations of responsible medical sources. The British Paramedic Association, the American Academy of Orthopaedic Surgeons, and the publisher, however, make no guarantee as to, and assume no responsibility for, the correctness, sufficiency, or completeness of such information or recommendations. Other or additional safety measures may be required under particular circumstances.

This textbook is intended solely as a guide to the appropriate procedures to be employed when rendering emergency care to the sick and injured. It is not intended as a statement of the standards of care required in any particular situation, because circumstances and the patient's physical condition can vary widely from one emergency to another. Nor is it intended that this textbook shall in any way advise emergency personnel concerning legal authority to perform the activities or procedures discussed. Such local determinations should be made only with the aid of legal counsel.

Notice: The patients described in "You are the Paramedic," "Assessment in Action," and "Points to Ponder" throughout this text are fictitious.

ISBN: 978-0-7637-7539-1

Library of Congress Cataloging-in-Publication Data
Caroline, Nancy L.
  Nancy Caroline's emergency care in the streets / American Academy of Orthopaedic Surgeons, British Paramedic Association. -- 6th ed. / [edited by] Bob Elling, Andrew N. Pollak.
    p. ; cm.
  Includes index.
  Rev. ed. of: Emergency care in the streets / Nancy L. Caroline. 5th ed. c1995.
  Adapted for use in the U.K.
  ISBN-13: 978-0-7637-5057-2 (casebound)
1. Medical emergencies. 2. Emergency medical technicians. I. Elling, Bob. II. Pollak, Andrew N. III. Caroline, Nancy L. Emergency care in the streets.
  IV. American Academy of Orthopaedic Surgeons. V. British Paramedic Association. VI. Title. VII. Title: Emergency care in the streets.
  [DNLM: 1. Emergency Treatment. 2. Emergency Medical Services. 3. Emergency Medical Technicians. WB 105 C292e 2007]
  RC86.7.C38 2007
  616.02'--dc22
6048   2007019381

Printed in India
13 12 11 10 09   10 9 8 7 6 5 4 3 2

Additional illustration and photo credits appear on page C.1, which constitutes a continuation of the copyright page.

Brief Contents

Contents

Paramedic Skill Drills

Resource Preview

CAROLINE'S BACK!

The textbook synonymous with ambulance education on both sides of the Atlantic is back! In the United States, this textbook has been central to paramedic training since the 1970s. Its reputation travelled to the United Kingdom (UK) where *Emergency Care in the Streets* was adopted by front line ambulance staff. Much loved and greatly respected, this textbook is still unrivalled in its ability to speak directly to the paramedic through humour and wisdom. Now for the first time, this ground breaking text has been adapted by a team of UK paramedics. The British Paramedic Association and the American Academy of Orthopaedic Surgeons are proud to continue Dr Caroline's legacy. At last, the UK and Ireland ambulance services have the text they deserve.

Join us in welcoming back Dr Caroline's legacy, *Emergency Care in the Streets*! The *Sixth Edition* honours Dr Caroline's work with a clear, empathetic, and understandable writing style full of the humour for which she was known.

Chapter Resources

A multitude of innovative, dynamic features have been incorporated to make learning more engaging, in the spirit of Dr Caroline's approach. The following pages show you the features to help you learn—from case studies to skill drills to an interactive website. On Dr Caroline's behalf, the British Paramedic Association and American Academy of Orthopaedic Surgeons wishes you a successful and rewarding paramedic career!

Chapter Objectives

Learning objectives are provided for each chapter.

You are the Paramedic

Each chapter contains a progressive case study to start students thinking about what they would do if they encounter a similar case at the scene. This feature is a valuable learning tool that encourages critical thinking skills.

The case study introduces patients and follows their progress from dispatch to delivery at the accident and emergency department.
The case becomes gradually more detailed as new medical information is presented.

A summary of the case study concludes the chapter.

At the Scene

Discuss practical applications of material for use in the context of an ambulance call.

Notes from Nancy

Provide words of wisdom from Dr. Nancy Caroline.

Special Considerations

Discuss the specific needs and emergency care of special populations, including paediatric patients, older patients, and special needs patients.

Vital Vocabulary

Terms are easily identified and defined within the text. A comprehensive vocabulary list follows each chapter.

Controversies

Highlight issues that may be under debate in the prehospital community.

Documentation and Communication

Provide advice on how to document patient care and tips on how to communicate with other health care professionals.

Skill Drills

Provide written step-by-step explanations and visual summaries of important skills and procedures.

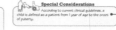

Prep Kit

End-of-chapter activities reinforce important concepts and improve students' comprehension.

Ready for Review

Summarise chapter content in a comprehensive bulleted list.

Assessment in Action

Promote critical thinking with case studies and provide discussion points for classroom presentation.

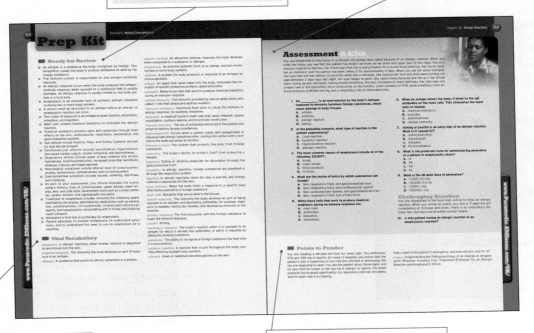

Vital Vocabulary

Provide key terms and definitions from the chapter.

Points to Ponder

Tackle cultural, ethical, and legal issues through case studies.

Technology Resources

www.Paramedic.EMSzone.com/UK/

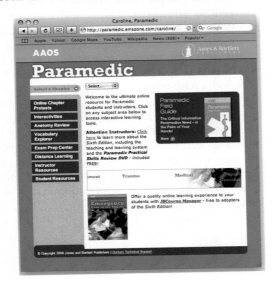

This site has been specifically designed to complement *Nancy Caroline's Emergency Care in the Streets, Sixth Edition* with interactivities and simulations to help students become great paramedics. Some of the resources available include:

- **Chapter pretests** prepare students for training. Each chapter has a pretest and provides instant results, feedback on incorrect answers, and page references for further study.
- **Interactivities** allow your students to experiment with the most important skills and procedures in the safety of a virtual environment.
- **Anatomy review** provides interactive anatomical figure labeling exercises to reinforce students' knowledge of human anatomy.
- **Vocabulary explorer** is a virtual dictionary. Here, students can review key terms, test their knowledge of key terms through flashcards, and complete exercises.
- **Skill sheets** provide skill evaluation sheets from the text.
- **Enhancement chapters** offering *Irish Perspectives*, *The Private Ambulance Service*, and *Further Readings*.

Instructor Resources

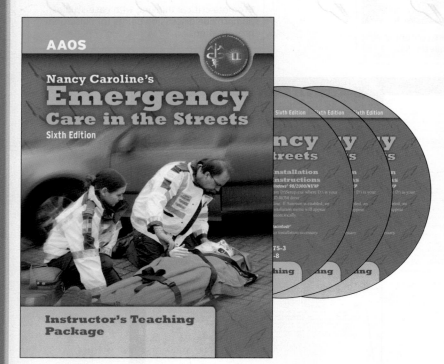

ISBN-13: 978-0-7637-5486-0

This robust package contains everything needed to support the delivery of a dynamic paramedic programme. The CD-ROMs in the package contain:

- **Instructor's manual**, providing you with creative ideas and tools to enhance your teaching. For each chapter, this indispensable manual contains:
  - Objectives
  - Support materials
  - Enhancements
  - Teaching tips
  - Readings and preparation
  - Presentation overview with suggested teaching times
  - Lesson plans and corresponding PowerPoint slide text
  - Skill drill evaluation sheets
  - Answers to all end-of-chapter student questions found in the text
  - Activities and assignments
- **PowerPoint presentations**, providing you with educational and engaging presentations. Following the content of the chapter, the slides also contain case studies and images throughout. The presentations can be modified and edited to meet your needs.
- **Lecture outlines**, providing you with complete, ready-to-use lesson plans that outline all of the topics covered in the chapter. The lesson plans can be modified and edited to fit your course.
- **Image and table bank**, providing you with many of the images and tables found in the text. You can use them to incorporate more images into the PowerPoint presentations, make handouts, or enlarge a specific image for further discussion.
- **Test bank**, providing you with multiple-choice general knowledge and critical thinking questions. With the test bank, you can originate tailor-made mock exams and quizzes quickly and easily by selecting, editing, organizing, and printing a question paper along with an answer key, that includes page references to the text.
- **Skill sheets**, allowing you to track students' skills and conduct skill proficiency assessments.

The resources found in the *Instructor's Teaching Package* have been formatted so that you can seamlessly integrate them into the most popular course administration tools. Please contact Jones and Bartlett Publishers technical support at www.jbpub.com at any time with questions.

Acknowledgements

Editorial Board

Bob Fellows, BSc, Paramedic, PGCE

Mark Woolcock, Paramedic
British Paramedic Association

Editors and Authors

SECTION 1

Section Editor: Dave Halliwell, MSc, Paramedic
Head of Education
South Western Ambulance NHS Trust

Authors

Chapter 1: Bob Fellows, BSc, Paramedic, PGCE

Chapter 1: Jim Petter, Paramedic
Great Western Ambulance NHS Trust

Chapter 1: Sam Weekes, Paramedic
South Western Ambulance NHS Trust

Chapter 2: Paul Burke
Senior Lecturer in Emergency Care
Course Director Fd Paramedic Science
Faculty of Health and Social Care Sciences
Kingston University/St. George's University of London

Chapter 3: Matthew Davis, BSc (Hons), PG Dip, Cert Ed
Paramedic, Clinical Facilitator in Emergency Care
University of Plymouth

Chapter 4: Rose Ann O'Shea, MN, FFEN, Paramedic
Consultant Nurse Emergency Care and Immediate Care Practitioner

Chapter 5: John Donaghy
Sector Training Officer
City and Hackney Complex
London Ambulance Service NHS Trust

Chapter 6: Paul Jones, Paramedic
South Western Ambulance NHS Trust

Chapter 7: Robbie Cameron, BSc Biochemistry, Paramedic
Emergency Care Practitioner
North West Ambulance NHS Trust

Chapter 7: Ann Richards, MSc, RN, RNT
Senior Lecturer
University of Hertfordshire

Chapter 8: Simon Standen, RN, Dip HE (Nursing), Paramedic
Emergency Care Practitioner, Clinical Field Trainer
East of England Ambulance Service NHS Trust

Chapter 9: Tracy Nicholls, PGC (TLHE)
Paramedic General Manager, Clinical Operations
East of England Ambulance Service NHS Trust

Chapter 10: Paul Fayers, BSc (Hons), Paramedic
Training Officer, University of Hertfordshire
London Ambulance Services NHS Trust

SECTION 2

Section Editor: Bob Fellows, BSc, Paramedic, PGCE

Author
Chapter 11: Bob Fellows, BSc, Paramedic, PGCE

SECTION 3

Section Editor: Richard Pilbery, BMedSc, PG Cert, Paramedic
Paramedic Lecturer
Sheffield Hallam University
Yorkshire Ambulance Service NHS Trust

Authors

Chapter 12: Richard Pilbery, BMedSc, PG Cert, Paramedic
Paramedic Lecturer
Sheffield Hallam University
Yorkshire Ambulance Service NHS Trust

Chapter 13: Steve Hatton, BSc (Hons), PG Cert Paramedic
Emergency Care Practitioner
Yorkshire Ambulance Service NHS Trust

Chapter 14: Kelly Lyng, BMedSc, PG Dip, Paramedic
South East Coast Ambulance Service NHS Trust

Chapter 15: Richard Pilbery, BMedSc, PG Cert, Paramedic
Paramedic Lecturer
Sheffield Hallam University
Yorkshire Ambulance Service NHS Trust

Chapter 16: Mike Parker
Operations Manager A&E
Yorkshire Ambulance Service NHS Trust

Chapter 16: Richard Pilbery, BMedSc, PG Cert, Paramedic
Paramedic Lecturer
Sheffield Hallam University
Yorkshire Ambulance Service NHS Trust

SECTION 4

Section Editor: Stephen Hines, BSc (Hons), Dip IMC RCS Ed
Department of Education and Development
London Ambulance Service NHS Trust

Authors

Chapter 17: Archie Morson
Head of Clinical Quality and Development
East of England Ambulance Service NHS Trust

Chapter 18: Graham Chalk, BSc (Hons), Paramedic
Lead Flight Paramedic and Specialist Response Coordinator
London Ambulance Service NHS Trust

Chapter 19: Gil Taylor, Dip (HE), Cert Ed (HE), Paramedic
Clinical Skills Instructor
University of Surrey

Chapter 20: Bob Fellows, BSc, Paramedic, PGCE

Chapter 21: John William Martin, BSc (Hons), Paramedic, PG Cert (TLHE)
Assistant Clinical Services Manager
East of England Ambulance Service NHS Trust

Chapter 22: Stephen Hines, BSc (Hons), Dip IMC RCS Ed
Department of Education and Development
London Ambulance Service NHS Trust

Chapter 22: Russell Thornhill
Assistant Chief Ambulance Officer
Head of Clinical Development
Isle of Man Ambulance and Paramedic Service

Chapter 23: Shane Knox, Advanced Paramedic, AASI
Training and Development Officer
National Ambulance Service, Ireland

Chapter 24: Bob Willis, BSc (Hons), Paramedic
Senior Lecturer Paramedic Science
The University of Northampton

Chapter 25: Jeremy Cowen, Paramedic
Assistant Emergency Planning Officer
Northern Ireland Ambulance Service

SECTION 5

Section Editor: David Whitmore, Paramedic
Senior Clinical Advisor to the Medical Director
London Ambulance Service NHS Trust

Authors

Chapter 26: Ian Wilmer, BSc (Hons) Paramedic Science, Paramedic
Emergency Care Practitioner and Instructor
London Ambulance Service NHS Trust

Chapter 27: Joanne Smith, Paramedic
Community Defibrillation Officer
London Ambulance Service NHS Trust

Chapter 27: Mark Whitbread, MSc, Paramedic
Clinical Practice Manager
Medical Directorate
London Ambulance Service NHS Trust

Chapter 28: John William Martin, BSc (Hons), Paramedic, PG Cert (TLHE)
Assistant Clinical Services Manager
East of England Ambulance Service NHS Trust

Chapter 29: Tim Jones, BSc (Hons) Prehospital Care, PG Dip (Advanced Clinical Practice), Paramedic
Senior Advanced Paramedic Practitioner
Welsh Ambulance Services NHS Trust

Chapter 30: Andy Freeman May
Principal Lecturer
Programme Lead Paramedic Emergency Care
Oxford Brookes University School of Health and Social Care

Chapter 31: Vince Clarke, BSc (Hons), Paramedic, PGCE
Training Officer, University of Hertfordshire
London Ambulance Service NHS Trust

Chapter 32: Caryll Overy, BSc (Hons) Physiology, Paramedic
Clinical Education Manager
South East Coast Ambulance Service NHS Trust

Chapter 33: David Haigh, Paramedic
Clinical Education Development Specialist
East Midlands Ambulance Service NHS Trust

Chapter 34: Paul Cassford, BA (Hons), Paramedic, Cert Ed (FE/HE)
Education & Development Manager
Isle of Wight Ambulance Service NHS Trust

Chapter 35: Paul Bates, BSc (Hons), PGCE, ODP
University Programme Manager
London Ambulance Service NHS Trust

Chapter 36: Caryll Overy, BSc (Hons) Physiology, Paramedic
Clinical Education Manager
South East Coast Ambulance Service NHS Trust

Chapter 37: Steve Murray, BSc, PGCE, AASI
Trainee Consultant Practitioner
Winchester and Eastleigh Healthcare NHS Trust

Chapter 38: Paul Down, BSc (Hons), Paramedic, Cert Ed (PCET)
Emergency Care Practitioner
South Western Ambulance Service NHS Trust

Chapter 39: Ron Webster, Paramedic, Cert Ed
Education Centre Manager
London Ambulance Service NHS Trust

Chapter 39: Mark Woolcock, Paramedic
British Paramedic Association

SECTION 6

Section Editor: Mark Woolcock, Paramedic
British Paramedic Association

Authors

Chapter 40: Michael Page, BSc (Hons), Paramedic, Cert Ed
Emergency Care Practitioner and IHCD Clinical Tutor
Great Western Ambulance Service NHS Trust

Chapter 41: Mark Woolcock, Paramedic
British Paramedic Association

Chapter 42: Chris Buscombe, Paramedic, Cert Ed
Emergency Care Practitioner
South Western Ambulance Services NHS Trust

Chapter 43: Paul Down, BSc (Hons), Paramedic, Cert Ed (PCET)
Emergency Care Practitioner
South Western Ambulance Service NHS Trust

Chapter 44: Carrie Stevenson, Paramedic
South Western Ambulance Service NHS Trust

Chapter 45: Simon Williams, BSc (Hons), Paramedic
Emergency Care Practitioner
TLC Solutions Ltd

SECTION 7

Section Editor: David G. Jones, PG Dip Risk Crisis and
    Disaster Management, Paramedic
Regional Staff Officer, Emergency Planning and Special Projects
Welsh Ambulance Services NHS Trust

Section Editor: Tim Jones, BSc (Hons) Prehospital Care, PG
    Dip (Advanced Clinical
Practice), Paramedic
Senior Advanced Paramedic Practitioner
Welsh Ambulance Services NHS Trust

Authors

Chapter 46: Steve Irving, BSc (Hons) Paramedic Science
Executive Officer
London Ambulance Service NHS Trust

Chapter 46: Mark Woolcock, Paramedic
British Paramedic Association

Chapter 47: David G. Jones, PG Dip Risk Crisis and Disaster
    Management, Paramedic
Regional Staff Officer, Emergency Planning and Special Projects
Welsh Ambulance Services NHS Trust

Chapter 47: Mark Woolcock, Paramedic
British Paramedic Association

Chapter 48: David G. Jones, PG Dip Risk Crisis and Disaster
    Management, Paramedic
Regional Staff Officer, Emergency Planning and Special Projects
Welsh Ambulance Services NHS Trust

Chapter 48: Mark Woolcock, Paramedic
British Paramedic Association

Chapter 49: David W. Brown, MSc, BEd, Paramedic
Senior Lecturer, University of Hertfordshire
Team Leader, East of England Ambulance Service NHS Trust

Chapter 50: Gary Hardacre
Head of Resilience
Scottish Ambulance Service

Chapter 50: David G. Jones, PG Dip Risk Crisis and Disaster
    Management, Paramedic
Regional Staff Officer, Emergency Planning and Special Projects
Welsh Ambulance Services NHS Trust

Chapter 50: Gerry Kelly, DMS, Paramedic
Head of Education and Training
Scottish Ambulance Service

Chapter 50: George Miller, Paramedic, AASI
Divisional Training Officer
Scottish Ambulance Service

Chapter 51: Phil Grieve, BSc (Hons), Paramedic
Clinical Team Leader
London Ambulance Service NHS Trust

Reviewers

Paul Abdey, Dip IMC RCS (Ed), Paramedic
Kent Police Tactical Medicine Unit

Stephanie Adams, Cert Mgmt (HSC),
    Paramedic
Ambulance Operations Manager
London Ambulance Service NHS Trust

Hafez Ahmed, PhD, MSc, Dip RCPath
    (Chemical Pathology)
Senior Lecturer, Faculty of Health and Social
    Care Sciences
Kingston University St George's Medical
    School, University of London

Marilena Antonopoulou, MSc
    Immunology, BSc (Hons) Medical
    Microbiology, FHEA
School of Health Sciences and Social Work

Andrew Ashman, Paramedic
Clinical Paramedic and Driving Training
    Officer-Fulham
London Ambulance Service NHS Trust

Michael Asquith, Paramedic, Cert Ed
Clinical Training Co-ordinator
Education and Development Centre (south)
Yorkshire Ambulance Service NHS Trust

Chris Baker, BSc (Hons)
Emergency Care Practitioner
Bromley Department of Education and
    Development
London Ambulance Service NHS Trust

Matthew Baker, BSc (Hons), REMT-A
    (EMTP AEu), R-ICA-M (EMTP AEu)
Training and Contracts Manager
Thames Ambulance Service Limited

Thomas David Barton, PhD, Dip N RGN,
    RNT, Head of Studies BSc (Hons) Pre-
    hospital Care, MSc Advanced Clinical
    Practice
Coordinator of Advanced Clinical Studies,
    School of Health Science
University of Wales Swansea

Marcia L Baxter, RGN, RM, Cert Ed HDU
Matron, Labour Ward, The Jessop Wing,
    Sheffield
Health and Wellbeing, Sheffield Hallam
    University

Christine Bearne, PG Cert (Paramedic);
    Dip HE; MA (Ed and Professional
    Development)
Senior Lecturer in Paramedic Science
Faculty of Health and Life Science
Coventry University

Reviewers, continued

Amanda Blaber, RGN, MSc, BSc (Hons)
Teaching Fellow
School of Health and Social Care
University of Greenwich

Anthony Bleetman, PhD, FRCS Ed, FCEM
Consultant in Emergency Medicine
Heart of England NHS Foundation Trust
Clinical Director Helicopter Emergency
 Medicine
West Midlands Ambulance Service NHS Trust

David Blowers, BSc, Paramedic
Community Paramedic
North East Ambulance Service NHS Trust

Susan Boardman, Paramedic, PG Dip
 (Adult Ed) FHEA
Paramedic Course Leader
Sheffield Hallam University

David Bradley
Senior Lecturer
Liverpool John Moores University

A. J. Brind, BSc (Hons), Paramedic
Emergency Care Practitioner
South Western Ambulance Service NHS Trust

Bob Brotchie
Paramedic Clinical Team Leader
East of England Ambulance NHS Trust

Graham Brown, MSc, Paramedic
Clinical Services Manager
South Western Ambulance Service NHS Trust

Dominic Browne, BSc (Hons), PGCE
Paramedic Training Officer
London Ambulance Service NHS Trust

Paul Burke
Senior Lecturer in Emergency Care
Course Director Fd Paramedic Science
Faculty of Health and Social Care Sciences
Kingston University/St. George's University
 of London

Simon Butler, BSc (Hons), PG Cert,
 Paramedic
Soham Village College Faculty of Science
University of East Anglia & British
 Paramedic Association

Dr Vic Calland, OStJ, FIMC, RCS Ed
Honorary Treasurer, British Association for
 Immediate Care

Robbie Cameron, BSc Biochemistry,
 Paramedic
Emergency Care Practitioner
North West Ambulance NHS Trust

Jon Careless, BSc (Hons), PG Cert,
 Paramedic
Senior Lecturer and Paramedic Practitioner
University of Northampton

Jason Challen, Paramedic
Senior Training Officer
London Ambulance Service NHS Trust

Helen Charman, BEng (Hons), PG Cert
 (FE), Paramedic
Staff Development Officer
Yorkshire Ambulance Service NHS Trust

Richard Chilton, BMedSci (Hons),
 Paramedic
Emergency Care Practitioner
Yorkshire Ambulance Service NHS Trust

Val Cochrane, BSc (Hons), PGCTLCP,
 Paramedic
Senior Paramedic
North West Ambulance Service NHS Trust

Mark E. Cooke, MSc, BMedSc (Hons)
National Clinical Effectiveness Manager
Ambulance Service Association (UK)

Anne Copson, Dip Management Studies,
 Paramedic
Clinical Operations Manager
South East Coast Ambulance Service NHS
 Trust

Mark Cutler, Paramedic, QTS
Paramedic Practioner and Associate Lecturer
Sheffield Hallam University

Kay Dark
Training Officer
London Ambulance Service NHS Trust

Kevin Dark, BSc (Hons), Paramedic
Bromley Education Centre
London Ambulance Service NHS Trust

Matthew Davis, BSc (Hons), PG Dip,
 Cert Ed
Paramedic Clinical Facilitator in Emergency
 Care
University of Plymouth

Jonathan Dermott, Dip HE (Paramedic
 Science), Paramedic
Emergency Medical Paramedic and IHCD
 Instructor
East of England Ambulance Service NHS
 Trust

Simon Doble, RN, BSc (Emergency Care),
 Paramedic
Charge Nurse and Emergency Care
 Practitioner
Emergency Department, Treliske Hospital
Royal Cornwall Hospitals Trust

Stephen Dolphin
Emergency Care Practitioner
East of England Ambulance Service NHS
 Trust

Maggie Doman, RN, RSCN, MSc
Lecturer in Nursing (Child)
Faculty of Health and Social Work
University of Plymouth

Paul Down, BSc (Hons), Paramedic, Cert
 Ed (PCET)
Emergency Care Practitioner
South Western Ambulance Service NHS Trust

Rosie Doy, MA, Cert Ed, RN
Director of Post Registration Studies and
 Team Leader Primary and Pre-Hospital
 Care
School of Nursing and Midwifery, University
 of East Anglia

Ricky Ellis, H Dip (EMT)
Advanced Paramedic, Clinical Tutor, EMS
 Development
Dublin Fire Brigade/Royal College of
 Surgeons

Dianna Evans, Cert Ed
Tactical Medicine and Specialist First Aid
 Trainer
Bedfordshire Police

Professor Philip Fennell, BA (Hons)
 (Law), MPhil (Law), PhD (Law)
Professor of Medical Law and Human Rights
Cardiff Law School, Cardiff University

Dave Facer, Paramedic
Clinical Support Officer
South Western Ambulance Service NHS Trust

Gary Malcolm Flack, BSc (Hons)
Paramedic Training Officer
London Ambulance Service NHS Trust

Paul Gibson, Cert HE (Para Sc),
 Paramedic, AASI
Ambulance Operations Manager
London Ambulance Service NHS Trust

Jacqui Gladwin, MA, Dip N, PG Cert
Senior Lecturer in Nursing and Emergency
 Care
Manchester Metropolitan University

Sue Greenwood, BN, BEd, Dip
 Management
Emergency Care Practitioner
Hull Teaching Primary Care Trust

Gina Grumke, PhD, Anthropology
Senior Research Scientist
Intel Corporation

Karen D. Gubbins, Paramedic, Cert FE
 HE, Cert Nat Sc
Lecturer, Worcester University
West Midlands Ambulance Service NHS Trust

Dr Henry Guly, FRCP, FCEM
Consultant in Emergency Medicine
Derriford Hospital, Plymouth

David Haigh, Paramedic
Clinical Education Development Specialist
East Midlands Ambulance Service NHS Trust

Gary Hardacre
Head of Resilience
Scottish Ambulance Service

Adam Harding, Paramedic
Sector Training Officer
London Ambulance Service NHS Trust

Fundamentals

Section Editor: Dave Halliwell

Emergency Medical Services

Objectives

Cognitive

- Define the following terms:
  - Ambulance Services
  - Registration
  - Profession
  - Professionalism
  - Guidelines
  - Health care professional
  - Ethics
  - Peer review
  - Medical direction
- Describe key historical events that influenced the development of the British Ambulance Services.
- Identify national groups important to the development, education, and implementation of ambulance service.
- Differentiate among the four nationally recognised levels of ambulance service training/education, leading to registration.
- Describe the attributes of a paramedic as a health care professional.
- Describe the recognised levels of ambulance service training/education, leading to registration in his or her region.
- Explain paramedic registration and renewal of registration requirements.
- Evaluate the importance of maintaining one's paramedic registration.
- Describe the benefits of paramedic continuing education.
- List current requirements for paramedic education in his/her region.
- Discuss the role of a national professional association and of a national registration.
- Discuss current issues in his/her region impacting the ambulance service.
- Discuss the roles of the professional body in setting curriculum standards.
- Identify the key components of an ambulance service.
- Describe how professionalism applies to the paramedic while on and off duty.
- Describe examples of professional behaviours in the following areas: integrity, empathy, self-motivation, appearance and personal hygiene, self-confidence, communication, time management, teamwork and diplomacy, respect, patient advocacy, and careful delivery of service.
- Provide examples of activities that constitute appropriate professional behaviour for a paramedic.
- Describe the importance of quality ambulance service research to the future of the ambulance service.
- Identify the benefits of paramedics teaching in their community.
- Describe what is meant by "community involvement in the ambulance service".
- Analyse how the paramedic can benefit the health care system by supporting primary care to patients in the out-of-hospital setting.
- List the primary and additional responsibilities of paramedics.
- Describe the role of the ambulance service medical director in providing clinical and medical direction.
- Describe the benefits of clinical and medical direction, during and after calls.
- Describe the process for the development and application of local policies and guidelines.
- Provide examples of locally supported clinical guidelines.
- Discuss prehospital and out-of-hospital care as an extension of the doctor or medical director of your service.
- Describe the relationship between a doctor on the scene, the paramedic on the scene, and the doctor providing on-line clinical and medical direction.
- Describe the components of continuous quality improvement.
- Analyse the role of continuous quality improvement with respect to continuing medical education and research.
- Define the role of the paramedic relative to the safety of the crew, the patient, and bystanders.
- Identify local health care agencies and transportation resources for patients with special needs.
- Describe the role of the paramedic in health education activities related to illness and injury prevention.
- Describe the importance and benefits of research.

Affective

- Assess personal practices relative to the responsibility for personal safety, the safety of the crew, the patient, and bystanders.
- Serve as a role model for others relative to professionalism in the ambulance service.
- Value the need to serve as the patient advocate inclusive of those with special needs, alternate life styles, and cultural diversity.
- Defend the importance of continuing medical education and skills retention.
- Advocate the need for supporting and participating in research efforts aimed at improving ambulance services.
- Assess personal attitudes and demeanour that may distract from professionalism.
- Value the role that family dynamics plays in the total care of patients.
- Advocate the need for injury prevention, including abusive situations.
- Exhibit professional behaviours in the following areas: integrity, empathy, self-motivation, appearance and personal hygiene, self-confidence, communications, time management, teamwork and diplomacy, respect, patient advocacy, and careful delivery of service.

Psychomotor

None

Introduction

Early in the ambulance service development, the role of a responder was to identify an individual who was ill or injured and rapidly transport the person to a medical facility, often called "scoop and run". Today that has changed dramatically because of the expectations of communities and findings in research. As a paramedic you will encounter many different situations, from life threatening to simply lending an ear to a person who just needs someone to listen. People you meet in the prehospital environment may evaluate you based on what they see on television or read in published articles, or on how you treat a loved one of theirs.

Ambulance Service Development

Pre-20th Century

The modern-day ambulance service is a relatively new profession when compared with many other professions **Figure 1-1 ▶**. Way back in the Babylon of 1700 BC, the medical care professional went to the patient's home, and the Code of Hammurabi (the king who invented rule by law in Mesopotamia) spelled out protocols and reimbursements for medical care—including punishment for malpractice **Figure 1-2 ▶**.

Sending the care provider to the patient was the way it was done until Napoleon's time. In the 1790s Jean Larrey, a French doctor, developed *ambulances volantes,* or flying travellers. Care was brought to patients in the prehospital environment as quickly as possible to take patients to hospital.

The first documented ambulance services were started in the 1860s in major UK cities such as Liverpool and London, whilst developments also started to prepare medics for working underground in mining communities.

The 20th Century and Modern Technology

Lessons had been learnt from major conflicts such as European Naval Battles, the Crimean War, the US Civil War, and the Boer War. Many of these lessons were able to be utilised in the war-torn Europe of World War I and II, with an urgent need to care for and remove injured persons from the battlefields and take them to hospitals far from the front. During the 1950s and the Korean War, military medical researchers recognised that bringing the hospital closer to the scene would give patients a better chance of surviving **Figure 1-3 ▶**.

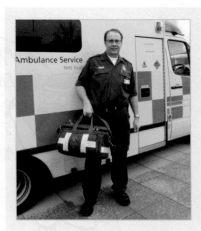

Figure 1-1 Today's prehospital care professionals are highly trained to provide a wide variety of medical services to the public.

Helicopters, another new technology, brought patients to Mobile Army Surgical Hospitals (M*A*S*H units). This helped thousands survive and recover more quickly, allowing them to return to the front line. In the late 1950s and early 1960s, the focus moved back to bringing the hospital to the patient with cardiac ambulances in Northern Ireland (Pantridge), Germany, and Eastern European countries.

Mobile intensive care units (MICUs) were staffed by specially trained doctors. The idea quickly spread to the United

You are the Paramedic Part 1

You are dispatched to an episode of syncope at a local church. En route to the scene, ambulance control informs you that your patient is an older woman who was reported by family members to have fainted during a wedding service. She is now conscious and complaining of shortness of breath and light-headedness. Because the location of this call is 15 minutes from your station, first responders who are closer to the scene have also been dispatched.

First responders quickly arrive on the scene to find a 70-year-old woman surrounded by members of her family, including her grandchildren, the eldest of whom was getting married. Her family members believe she is "just worn out", and think that she should go home and rest. The mobile data terminal (MDT) provides you with this updated information. Shortly after arriving at the scene, you introduce yourself to the patient and perform an intial assessment.

Initial Assessment	Recording Time: 0 Minutes
Appearance	Noticeably perspiring and pale
Level of consciousness	Conscious but confused
Airway	Patent
Breathing	Increased respirations; adequate depth
Circulation	Very weak radial pulse

1. How is patient care initiated for this or any call?
2. What role does ambulance control play in patient care?

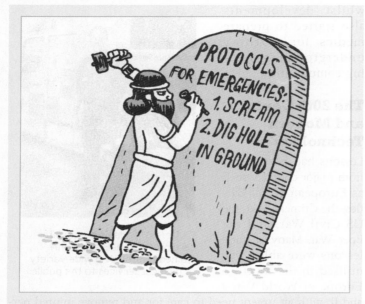

Figure 1-2

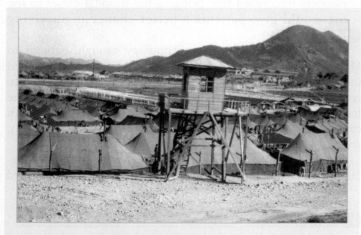

Figure 1-3 Temporary hospitals, such as this one in use during the Korean War, were set up to provide more rapid care for the injured.

Table 1-1	Critical Points

- Develop collaborative strategies to identify and address community health and safety issues.
- Align the financial incentives of ambulance services and other health care providers and payers.
- Participate in community-based prevention efforts.
- Develop and pursue a national ambulance service research agenda.
- Allocate adequate resources for clinical and medical direction.
- Develop information systems that link ambulance services across the country.
- Determine the costs and benefits of the ambulance service to the community.
- Ensure that all calls for emergency help are automatically accompanied by location-identifying information on the screen to assist with ambulance control.

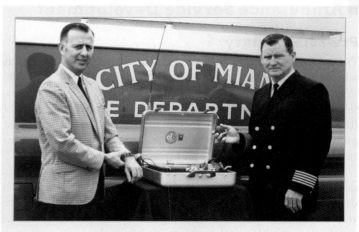

Figure 1-4 Dr Eugene Nagel, widely considered the father of paramedicine, provided much-needed leadership to the developing field of EMT training. Here he is shown (on left) in 1967 with Chief Larry Kenney of the Miami Fire Department, with the first telemetry package to be used by US paramedics.

States, but US trained doctors were in short supply, and those doctors who were interested had minimal expertise to venture into the prehospital area. So the question was asked: "Can a non-doctor be trained to perform advanced medical skills"? The answer was "Yes".

In 1966 the National Academy of Science and the National Research Council released a "White Paper" entitled "Accidental Death and Disability: The Neglected Disease of Modern Society", in which they outlined 10 critical points ⟨ Table 1-1 ▸ ⟩. From these points the National Highway Safety Act was instituted in 1966. In this act the US Department of Transportation (US DOT) was created, providing authority and financial support for the development of basic and advanced life support programs. The first EMT textbook, *Emergency Care and Trans-*

portation of the Sick and Injured, was published by the American Academy of Orthopaedic Surgeons (AAOS) in 1971.

In 1969, the same year the basic training course for EMTs was released, Dr Eugene Nagel, then of Miami, Florida, USA, began training fire fighters from the Miami Fire Department with advanced emergency skills ⟨ Figure 1-4 ▲ ⟩. Dr Nagel took the use of advanced emergency treatment one step further. He developed a telemetry system that enabled fire fighters to transmit a patient's electrocardiogram to doctors at Jackson Memorial Hospital and to receive radio instructions from the doctors regarding what measures to take. Dr Nagel is often called the "Father of Paramedicine".

In 1973 the Emergency Medical Services System Act defined 15 required components of an ambulance service in the US ⟨ Table 1-2 ▸ ⟩, with emphasis on regional development and trauma care. The act provided a structure and uniformity to the ambulance service that came out of pioneering programs in Miami, Seattle, and Pittsburgh, and the Illinois Trauma System (Dr David Boyd).

Table 1-2	Required Components

- Integration of health services
- Ambulance service research
- Legislation and regulation
- Ambulance service system finance
- Human resource directorate
- Clinical and medical direction
- Education systems
- Public and community education
- Public access defibrillation
- Health communication systems
- Advanced critical care
- Management of information systems
- Clinical audit research and evaluation

Many US cities set up individual advanced ambulance service training, and regions added their own spin to what they thought was the essential standard of care; however, it wasn't until 1977 that the first National Standard Curriculum for paramedics was developed by the US DOT. This first paramedic curriculum was based on the work of Dr Nancy Caroline.

In the UK, the enthusiasm for training ambulance men and women to carry out advance resuscitation procedures occurred slightly later than in the United States. The first UK paramedic scheme started in Brighton in the summer of 1971 under the stewardship of Dr (now Professor) Douglas Chamberlain, a cardiologist. Dr Peter Baskett, an anaesthetist, followed with another widely acclaimed scheme in Bristol the following year. In 1972, other pilot sites such as Dorset and London became operational, although generally low numbers were trained. The focus and content of these schemes and the many others that followed often differed, reflecting local medical opinion; but the original intubation and infusion (I&I) projects shared the essential features of strong medical direction and absolute commitment from the ambulance staff that were recruited to the schemes. Enthusiasm and a pioneering spirit characterised these early projects and proved to be important ingredients to the considerable local success that followed. In 1973 the

National Health Service Reorganisation Act, implemented on 1 April 1974, transferred all ambulance services, including those services with experimental paramedic schemes, from local authority control to the National Health Service (NHS).

Following this transition there was considerable discussion regarding the training of paramedics or, as it was referred to at the time, extended trained ambulance staff. The Department of Health commissioned an analysis as to the potential benefits of such training. This research, conducted by University of York's Institute for Research in the Social Sciences, was published in 1984 and proved extremely positive, providing a compelling and economically sound vision for extended (paramedic) training. Despite some resistance, acceptance of the need for more highly trained ambulance crews grew rapidly and led to the Department of Health introducing a national scheme in 1985 that was ultimately adopted by all UK ambulance services. This initiative brought together the many disparate schemes in operation into a standardised National Health Service Training Directorate (NHSTD) package of training taught within regional ambulance training schools and in local hospitals.

During the mid 1990s a small number of educational establishments formed partnerships with ambulance services to develop degree schemes in paramedic science, setting the future pattern of development that will see a much wider role of Higher Education Institutes in the preparation of paramedics. After the registration of paramedics in 2000 with the Council of Professions Supplementary to Medicine (CPSM), which was shortly thereafter succeeded by the Health Professions Council (HPC), paramedics became the 12th group of health workers to become registered Allied Health Professionals (AHPs). This important evolutionary step had the effect of accelerating the professionalising process, setting national minimum standards for education and training that complied with established academic levels.

In 2001, the British Paramedic Association (BPA) became the professional body for paramedics and soon became engaged in collaborative work with the HPC, the Joint Royal Colleges Ambulance Liaison Committee (JRCALC), the QAA

You are the Paramedic Part 2

As you perform a focused history and physical examination, your colleague takes the patient's vital signs. Her pulse rate and blood pressure concern you, and you apply the cardiac monitor. As you question the patient and her family about her medical history and events that have occurred during today's festivities, you immediately note an arrhythmia.

Vital Signs	Recording Time: 5 Minutes
Level of consciousness	Conscious but confused
Skin	Perspiring, pale, and cool
Pulse	180 beats/min, regular and weak
Blood pressure	80/42 mm Hg
Respirations	24 breaths/min; adequate depth
S_PO_2	95% on 15 l/min using a nonrebreathing mask
ECG	Ventricular tachycardia

3. What care can first responders provide for this patient?

and others to help develop the instruments and reference points that would enable the profession to move forward, including the curriculum guidance document.

In just 34 years, paramedic services have been developed in the UK from an experimental idea initiated by a few leading authorities and a few enthusiastic ambulance staff to the situation today where paramedics are well established within the health care landscape. During most of this short history, their primary purpose has been firmly rooted in providing emergency care. This role is now growing to incorporate the assessment and management of undifferentiated cases, traditionally within the province of primary care. Paramedics are now found in the majority of industrialised countries, and the United Kingdom can be rightly proud of producing personnel who have the knowledge, skills, attitudes, and aptitudes to play an increasingly important part in the delivery of health care in the 21st century.

Controversies

Many communities initially fought against ambulance drivers "playing doctor", or in other words, becoming paramedics. Now, even the smallest communities expect access to advanced life support (ALS)-trained personnel.

The Ambulance Service

The modern-day ambulance service is a complex network of coordinated services that provide various levels of care to a community. These services work in unison to meet both the growing and standing needs of the general public in the community in which they reside. You as a paramedic are part of this network; therefore, you must stay active in your community to be able to meet the ever-changing needs.

The ambulance service network generally begins with citizen involvement in the complex ambulance service. The public needs to be taught how to recognise that an emergency exists, how to activate the ambulance service, and how basic care can be provided before the ambulance service arrives Figure 1-5 ▸ . Remember that the public's idea of an emergency may be drastically different from yours.

At the Scene

A patient may only experience once what a paramedic may experience hundreds of times. Try to understand the patient's anxiety.

When you are called to a "sick person" at 02:00 hrs who only has a common cold and can't sleep, there is no reason to become angry at the patient or your ambulance service. Instead, use this time to educate the public by offering sympathy and insight on cold treatment, and, perhaps tactfully discuss why a cold is not an emergency. Remember, a paramedic is a public servant. You will often respond to nonemergency calls.

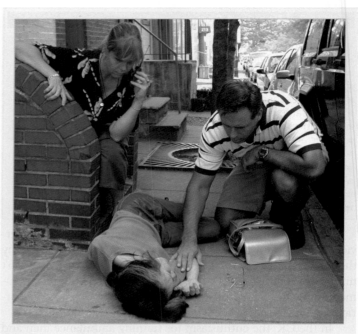

Figure 1-5 One of your roles as a paramedic is educating the public about how to first respond to an emergency, before medical help has arrived.

When the public calls for an ambulance, their first contact is usually ambulance control via the 999 operator network. Requirements for ambulance control training vary greatly from area to area, although the Department of Health is coordinating new control training as part of the ambulance workforce review. Controllers are limited in interpreting an emergency and in extracting appropriate information from a stressed caller. Once on scene, you have to determine what is really going on, which in many cases is a far cry from what control told you. Despite this or limited information, you will develop your care plan for the patient and decide on the appropriate transport method and receiving facility for your patient.

Good local knowledge will keep you on top of the best local resources. When you are drawing up a potential care plan, you will ask yourself, "Does the receiving hospital have the appropriate facilities to treat this patient"? When you have good local knowledge, you will know the answer. If the answer is no, the next question, "Is there an appropriate facility within a reasonable distance"? will also be a part of your community knowledge. Of course, it may be appropriate to transport the patient to a hospital that has treated them before.

Special Considerations

Your ambulance service must be capable of handling many different situations, including obstetric, paediatric, and older person emergencies. Proper procedures, drug dosages, and even assessment techniques are often different in children, adults, and older people.

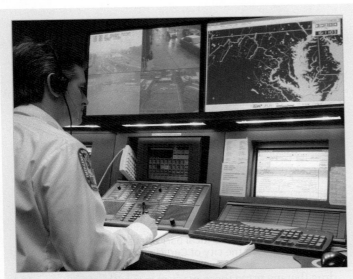

Figure 1-6 The ambulance controller coordinates the entire rescue effort. He or she interprets a caller's information and then sends appropriate personnel and resources to the scene.

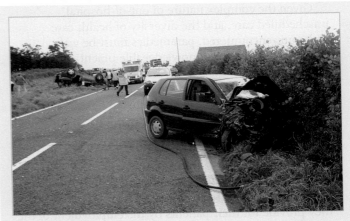

Figure 1-7 The first responder is critical for providing the initial emergency patient care, particularly when medical personnel must travel long distances to a scene.

There are currently several levels of providers in the ambulance service. Each level has a scope of practice, as outlined by the HPC and the BPA. The scope of practice is reevaluated from time to time and may change as a result. Let's take a look at these various levels.

The Ambulance Controller

The ambulance controller plays a key role in a 999 call. He or she must receive and enter all information on the call, interpret the information, and then relay it to the appropriate resources **Figure 1-6 ▲**. In some locations the ambulance controller may be trained as an emergency medical dispatcher (EMD), which charges these individuals with the added task of giving simple medical direction (eg, CPR, bleeding control) to a caller in the hope that this care may benefit the patient until ambulance service personnel are on scene.

First Responder

The ambulance services in the UK utilise a number of approaches to dealing with first responders. Several use local training schemes to prepare volunteers and equip them with a pager, mobile phone, and response kit including safety equipment. Others have taken on board more formal training such as First Person on Scene (FPOS, Edexcel). It is also an increasing and welcome development to see fire fighters and police personnel being dispatched to life-threatening calls when they can be released between other more specific professional duties **Figure 1-7 ▶**.

The Emergency Care Assistant

This role provides support to and is guided clinically by a qualified ambulance practitioner. The emergency care assistant may occasionally be required to provide immediate resuscitative measures in cases of acute, immediately life-threatening conditions until more qualified help arrives. This new role was launched in 2007 to replace the technician as the second crew member working with the paramedic.

The Ambulance Technician

For many years the preparation to becoming a paramedic has been via the emergency medical technician route. The training programme initially was born out of the Millar report from 1966, which standardised the Civil Defence Training that existed at that time into a 6-week programme that has remained as the core curriculum for the past 40 years. Since the Agenda for Change bandings in 2006 giving many technicians band 5, it has now caused many ambulance services to review the makeup of their workforce. The emergency care assistant is expected to be the resulting support worker for paramedics and some qualified ambulance technicians.

Controversies

The role of the technician is back under the spotlight since the Agenda for Change pay awards gave many technicians band 5. It is widely believed that the role will be replaced with an emergency care assistant to work alongside the paramedic.

The Paramedic

The British Paramedic Association curriculum guidance states:

Paramedics are independent practitioners working, to their specified level of competence, with patients of all ages, with individuals and in groups, and are essential members of interdisciplinary and inter-agency teams. Effective practice requires the recognition and understanding of the social and economic context of their patients in assessing, planning, delivering, and evaluating care.

Given the complex nature of out-of-hospital, unscheduled care, and the diversity of health care situations encountered, paramedics must be well-educated, skilled, and knowledgeable practitioners in a range of subjects and be able to appraise and adopt an enquiry-based approach to the delivery of care.

Paramedic practice is evidence based health care that applies vocational and academic disciplines that are often practised in a variety of complex situations across the health-illness continuum. They are able to act as first contact practitioners, and patients usually seek direct care without referral from another health care professional. They are responsible for the quality of care they provide for their patients by the employment of the principles and practice of clinical governance.

Higher Education Institutions (HEI) providers and their ambulance service partners will need to embrace changing and developing roles which will affect the scope of practice for staff at all grades, for example the transition from the storage and administration of drugs to their independent and supplementary prescribing.

A defining feature of paramedic practice is that it is always available, 24 hours a day, 365 days a year, with a focus on meeting people's immediate care needs Figure 1-8 ▸.

Each paramedic will have a sound understanding of the principles of paramedic practice, and will be able to apply those principles more widely, through vocational training and academic education, having completed a further programme supported by the employing organisation in collaboration with their HEI partners. Staff at this level will be clinically safe and accurate when working alone or as part of a team.

They will be able to utilise their advanced knowledge and skills to act independently to best meet the patients' individual needs. These skills will include advanced airway adjuncts and procedures, intravenous fluid therapy and

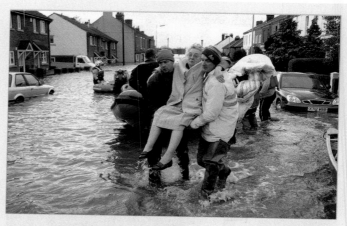

Figure 1-8 EMTs were a critical part of evacuation efforts following flooding in the city of Carlisle in 2005.

drug therapy using those medicines available to registered paramedics, and other invasive procedures. They will be able to use their knowledge and experience to determine the extent of the patients' presenting condition and to decide on the appropriate receiving facility based on clinical need.

On award of the diploma/degree they will be proficient, co-ordinated and confident in the delivery of care. They will be able to apply their own professional judgement and experience to make clinical decisions to best suit the patients' individual needs and be able to accept, explain, and justify these decisions when challenged.

With the advantage of preceptorship, they will be able to take the leadership role in care delivery within a team. Through reflection, mentorship, preceptorship, and review, they will be able to continually evaluate their own performance and recognise their personal strengths and areas for development, demonstrating a commitment to lifelong learning. They will also be able to evaluate the performance of others by embracing the role of supervisor, mentor, and preceptor.

You are the Paramedic Part 3

Your paramedic colleague asks the patient whether she has any allergies to medication and then administers an appropriate dose of lignocaine. You explain the actions and possible side effects of the drug to your patient and what you must do and what she should expect. You advise your crewmate to be prepared for deterioration of the patient's condition and you pre-alert the receiving accident and emergency (A&E) department of her condition and the treatment she has received. Having successfully converted your patient's heart rhythm, you take another set of vital signs.

Reassessment	Recording Time: 10 Minutes
Level of consciousness	A (Alert to person, place, and day)
Skin	Pink, warm, and dry
Pulse	88 beats/min, regular and strong
Blood pressure	130/60 mm Hg
Respirations	16 breaths/min and unlaboured
S_PO_2	99% on 15 l/min using a nonrebreathing mask
ECG	Sinus rhythm

4. Is there one team member who is more important than another?

At the Scene

Paramedics have a clear duty to keep up-to-date on basic life support skills as well as advanced life support skills.

At the Scene

The number of calls you go on isn't the deciding factor on how much more training you need.

Education for Paramedics

Preregistration Education and Training

Today's paramedics are now established health care professionals in their own right, with all the attendant responsibilities that such status brings. The provision of training has, until recently, rested with ambulance services and stood apart from the further and higher education sector both in its planning and delivery. A broader input to the curriculum was made from other professions including medical, nursing, midwifery, and mental health professionals. Nevertheless, preparation was short, dominated by a training rather than educational ethos, and was focused at the basic life support level of care provision. This situation changed with the advent of advanced life support training schemes for ambulance staff in the 1970s, ultimately leading to the development of today's registered paramedic.

The profession has now made its clear choice at the crossroads in its journey to develop the very best in provision of care to patients. The transition from a training paradigm to the world of higher education has taken us to the next era of preparing the profession to fulfil its role in the modern health service.

Curriculum guidance alone will not ensure that paramedics are suitably and fully prepared for the role expected of them. Closely linked to this work and to the process of approvals for HEIs are three other important documents that influence strongly the standards and quality of paramedic services:

- Health Professions Council (HPC) Standards of Proficiency
- HPC Standards of Education and Training
- Quality Assurance Agency (QAA) Benchmarking statements

The Standards of Proficiency (SoP) and the Standards of Education and Training (SET) are established by the HPC to define the requirements in these two important areas. The QAA benchmarks are an external reference used for the design and development of new programmes. These documents, along with the British Paramedic Association Curriculum Guidance, will provide HEIs with a complete framework within which to operate.

Improving the delivery and standards of education through the use of this curriculum guidance will be inclusive for the whole profession, whatever level of care or from wherever the service is being provided. The wealth of experience and good practice that has been developed throughout the current training-based model will need to be moulded into the HEI model by establishing very strong yet flexible partnerships between HEIs and ambulance services for the effective delivery of high standards of appropriate education and training.

Post-education and Development

The delivery of any paramedic curriculum leading to qualification and registration will need to be supported by taking up the personal responsibility for continuous professional development (CPD).

The Scope of Practice in curriculum guidance from the British Paramedic Association and the HPC Paramedic Standards of Proficiency statements define what is expected from paramedics at each level of their career development. These documents also acknowledge that, while clinical knowledge and skills remain central to good practice, these aspects must be complemented by appropriate attitudes. They recognise that student paramedics need to develop the interpersonal and interdisciplinary behaviours characterised by good communication with patients, staff, and others—including the ability to work as a member of a team **Figure 1-9 ▶**. It will also be essential to ensure that the important issues of patient safety, leadership, and the other factors, such as clinical governance, each have an effect on patient outcome and are fully considered and internalised.

The Paramedic Professional Body

Soon after the HPC was formed and the Orders in Council were approved by the Privy Council, the HPC was required to liaise with professional bodies for all the professions for which the registrar was responsible. At that time the only profession not to have a professional body was the ambulance profession. Two paramedics from the Essex Ambulance Service were persuaded to undertake the necessary work to set up a professional body in order to ensure that the profession would be represented and fulfil the self-regulation responsibilities for standards and education. The name of British Paramedic Association was agreed at an inaugural meeting held at the Annual Conference and Exhibition for all Professionals working in Prehospital, Urgent, and Emergency Care (AMBEX) in 2001, and the development of the association began. A formal business plan was prepared for the BPA to provide some firm direction and structure.

What are the benefits of a professional body? The main areas for benefit to members lie in the philosophy that as a profession they shall work towards undertaking responsibility for their own professional future. Having a professional body provides an opportunity to change the way that education, training, and associated awards are established.

Within this work the main objectives are:

- To strengthen and develop the profession and represent the interests of its practitioners

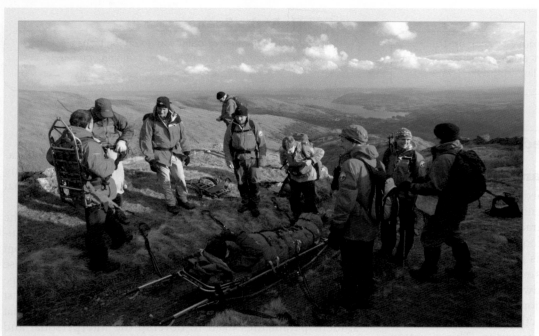

Figure 1-9 Continuing professional education and development can keep you up-to-date on technological improvements that are continually made available to paramedics.

Professionalism

During your paramedic education and training process, you learn a vast amount of information designed to make you a health care professional, practising at the paramedic level. A profession is a field of endeavour that requires a specialised set of knowledge, skills, and expertise, often gained after lengthy training.

As a paramedic, you will be trained at length for registration with standards, competencies, and continuing education requirements.

A paramedic is considered a health care professional. The following are attributes of a health care professional:

- Conforms to the same standards as other health care professions
- Provides quality patient care
- Instills pride in the profession
- Strives continuously for high standards
- Earns respect from others in the profession
- Meets societal expectations of the profession whether on or off duty

The paramedic profession has developed standards and performance parameters as well as a code of ethics. Collectively, these are the standards by which you will be measured as a paramedic.

As a paramedic you are in a highly visible role in your community **Figure 1-10 ▸**. Professional image and behaviour must be a top priority. You are a representative of the locality you work in. Sometimes, people will make a positive or negative judgement within the first 10 seconds of meeting you. As a paramedic you will be meeting new people as an everyday part of your career. To provide the best possible care, you must establish and maintain credibility and instill confidence. As you walk into a situation, never forget that a big part of your job is to continually show that you are truly concerned for the well-being of your patients and their families **Figure 1-11 ▸**. Your appearance is also of utmost importance—it has more impact than you may think. It is not appropriate to arrive at a call in dirty clothes, with dirty hands, and smelling offensively. You must look and act like a professional at all times.

Also, you must keep high standards of professionalism, performance, and ethical behaviour. You must always:

1. Act in the best interests of your patients, clients, and service users.
2. Respect the confidentiality of your patients, clients, and service users.

- To raise the general awareness of the existing and potential contribution of the profession to patient care
- To encourage and share good clinical practice and high standards of care
- To develop and expand the potential of the profession for contributing to patient care in a modern health service
- To represent the views of the profession to government, employers, and other external bodies
- To encourage higher standards of initial and continuing professional education and development
- To commission, report, and analyse research in out-of-hospital patient care

For the first time in the history of the ambulance service, the profession is taking responsibility for its own educational and clinical development. A good example of this is the production of the curriculum guidance for higher education institutes and their partner ambulance service. The document was prepared completely by registered paramedics who were also professional body members with advice from universities and other specialists. The constitution of the CoP is set to fulfil the professional development for its members and not to act in relation employment matters, contracts or pay. In essence, the College was never established to be a trade union.

The requirement for CPD is the responsibility of every individual paramedic professional registered with the HPC and is linked to renewal of registration which occurs bi-annually. As a direct and tangible benefit to the CoP members, they have invested in an on-line CPD scheme that is suitable for all in the ambulance profession and fully fits the HPC requirements.

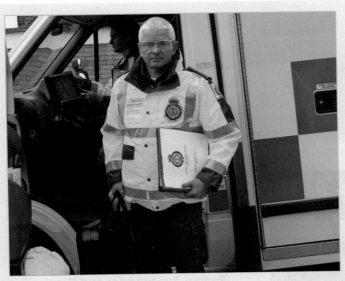

Figure 1-10 Adopting a professional attitude and appearance is a critical part of working with the public and earning their trust.

3. Maintain high standards of personal conduct.
4. Provide any important information about conduct, competence, or health.
5. Keep your professional knowledge and skills up-to-date.
6. Act within the limits of your knowledge, skills, and experience and, if necessary, refer on to another professional.
7. Maintain proper and effective communications with patients, clients, service users, carers, and professionals.
8. Effectively supervise tasks you have asked others to carry out for you.
9. Get informed consent to give treatment (except in an emergency).
10. Keep accurate patient, client, and service user records.
11. Deal fairly and safely with the risks of infection.
12. Limit your work or stop practising if your performance or judgement is affected by your health.
13. Carry out your duties in a professional and ethical way.
14. Behave with integrity and honesty.

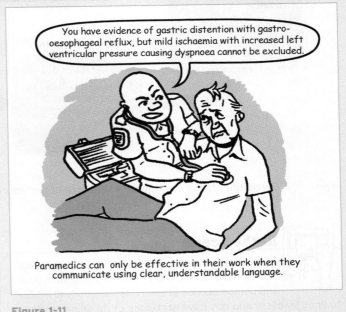

Paramedics can only be effective in their work when they communicate using clear, understandable language.

Figure 1-11

15. Make sure that your behaviour does not damage the reputation of your profession.

You are the Paramedic Part 4

Your patient's pulse has decreased, blood pressure has increased, and she no longer feels short of breath or light-headed. Her skin signs are much improved, with colour returning to her cheeks. Your patient and her entire family thank you. You feel gratified to know that all of your hard work has paid off.

5. Why is it important to keep skills and knowledge current?
6. Why is it important to practise these skills as a team?

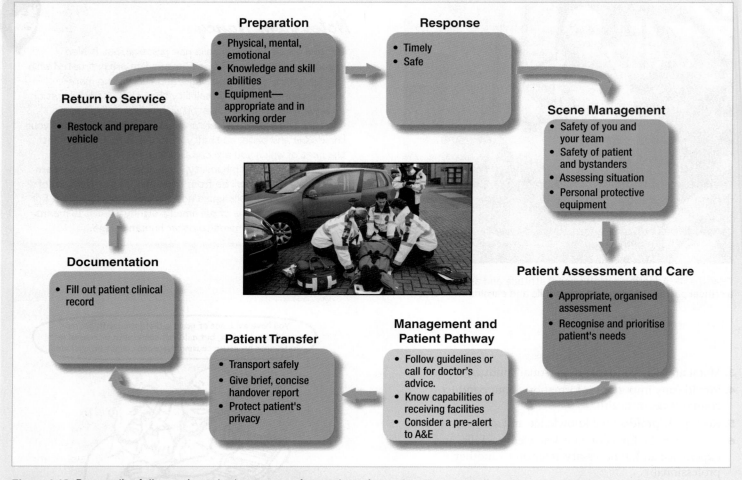

Figure 1-12 Paramedics follow an important sequence of procedures for each emergency call.

Roles and Responsibilities

So what does it actually mean to be a paramedic? What are my roles? What am I responsible for? These are questions that you should ask yourself throughout your career. The ambulance service continues to grow and mature, and with those changes will come new roles and additional responsibilities. Some of the primary responsibilities are shown in **Figure 1-12** and include:

- **Preparation.** Be prepared physically, mentally, and emotionally. Keep up your knowledge and skill abilities. Be sure you have the appropriate equipment for your call and that it is in good working order.

- **Response.** Responding to the event in a timely, safe manner is very important, with due regard to your own safety, that of your colleagues, your patient, and people on the road.

- **Scene management.** Ensuring your own safety and the safety of your team is the first priority. You must also ensure the patient's safety and the safety of any bystanders. Part of your preparation before you reach the scene should include assessing the situation; the nature of the call will give valuable information. Preparing for scene safety starts with the use of personal protective equipment such as gloves and high visibility clothing.

- **Patient assessment and care.** An appropriate organised assessment based on the principles you will learn in the classroom and this book should be performed on all patients. You will need to recognise and prioritise the patient's needs on the basis of the injuries he or she has sustained or the illness that most urgently needs treatment.

- **Management and patient pathway.** A paramedic usually follows guidelines and protocols signed off by the Joint Royal Colleges Ambulance Liaison Committee (JRCALC). Sometimes, however, when you are in the prehospital

Prep Kit

■ Ready for Review

■ World Wars I and II saw the development of ambulance corps to rapidly care for and remove those injured from the battlefields.

■ During the Korean and Vietnam Wars, wounded soldiers could be saved by using helicopters to rapidly remove them from the battlefields to a medical unit.

■ In 1966 the National Academy of Science and the National Research Council in the USA released a "White Paper" outlining 10 critical points.
  - From these points the National Highway Safety Act was instituted in 1966.
  - The US Department of Transportation was also created.

■ In 1971, the first paramedic schemes started in the UK.

■ In 1974, the UK ambulance service moved from local authority to NHS management.

■ The public needs to be taught how to recognise when an emergency exists, how to activate the ambulance service, and how to perform basic care until the ambulance service arrives.

■ The highest level of ambulance service training is the paramedic practitioner level. At this level, personnel may perform invasive procedures under the direction of medical control.

■ Continuing education programmes expose paramedics to new research findings and refresh their skills and knowledge.

■ Paramedics are required to be registered.

■ The paramedic profession sets expected standards and performance parameters as well as a code of ethics.

■ Some of the primary paramedic responsibilities include:
  - Preparation
  - Response
  - Scene management
  - Patient assessment and care

  - Management and disposition
  - Patient transfer
  - Documentation
  - Return to service

■ The medical director provides advice on patient treatment.

■ Research helps bring together the findings of many professionals involved in ambulance service and brings forth a consensus of what ambulance service personnel should or should not do.

■ Vital Vocabulary

British Paramedic Association (BPA) The professional body for paramedics.

health care professional A person who follows specific professional standards that are outlined in the health profession.

Health Professions Council (HPC) The registrant body for health professionals and paramedics.

medical direction Direction given to an ambulance service or provider by a medical director.

mobile intensive care units (MICUs) An early title given to an ambulance-style unit.

preceptorship A period of practical experience, training, and development that is structured to facilitate learning for a trainee, whilst being overseen by an educator/trainer/coach or mentor.

profession A specialised set of knowledge, skills, and/or expertise.

professional A person who follows expected standards and performance parameters in a specific profession.

protocol A treatment plan developed for a specific illness or injury.

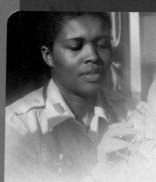

Assessment in Action

You plan to become a qualified and registered paramedic one day. At present you work as an ambulance technician and you volunteer as a first responder in the rural area where you live.

You come upon a road traffic collision near your home. No ambulance or police are on scene yet. You have your own personal "response bag" with rescue supplies in your vehicle, including advanced life support supplies you would use as a paramedic. There are two patients, both with significant injuries. They were both unrestrained in the vehicle. One patient is having noticeable trouble breathing.

1. **Even though you are not "on duty", what should you do first in this situation, assuming a bystander has already called for help?**
   A. Call 999.
   B. Put on gloves and any other personal protective equipment you may need.
   C. Call control and get permission to treat the patient.
   D. Assess the ABCs.

2. **Which of the following are you *allowed* to do based on the training you already have?**
   A. C-spine stabilisation, pressure to stop bleeding, talk to victims to calm them and let them know what to expect.
   B. Put a c-collar in place, bandage bleeding wounds, use a bag-valve-mask if necessary to help the patient who is having trouble breathing.
   C. Help stop bleeding, and intubate if necessary.
   D. Gain IV access and administer fluid replacement therapy.

3. **If a doctor arrives and offers to help, is it appropriate to turn over care to that doctor?**
   A. Yes, a doctor is a higher authority than you are.
   B. Yes, but only if the doctor is willing to take responsibility for the patients, including riding with them to hospital and signing paperwork.
   C. No, you are not authorised to turn over care until an emergency ambulance arrives.
   D. It is the option of the ambulance crew that arrives on scene.

4. **When the ambulance arrives on scene, it is your responsibility to:**
   A. explain quickly and accurately your assessments and any treatment or intervention you have administered.
   B. help prepare the patient(s) for transport in any way you can under the direction of the paramedic on scene.
   C. maintain patient care unless the person on scene has the same authority as you or higher.
   D. all of the above.

5. **Are you legally allowed to perform ANY paramedic treatments in this situation?**
   A. Yes
   B. No

6. **Because you are not on duty, is it appropriate to tell the patient "everything will be fine", or do anything else you would not be allowed to do in uniform while working with your ambulance service?**
   A. Yes, you're not on duty, so those sets of rules do not apply. You are acting as a Good Samaritan.
   B. No, you are a health professional whether on duty or off duty, which means being professional at all times.

Challenging Questions

7. **Being a paramedic is not just a job you work at during a shift. You are always a paramedic, being a role model for the public at all times. With the increase in television programmes that do not always accurately depict the roles of health care providers, do you feel it is your responsibility to educate the public in every situation possible as to what the ambulance service field is truly like, correct misconceptions, and give an accurate portrayal of what you are responsible for and capable of as a paramedic?**

8. **You are called to the scene of a two-car crash with serious injuries to the drivers and passengers of both vehicles. You call for additional assistance, but know it will be several minutes until more help arrives. Someone stops, and offers his assistance. He does seem to be knowledgeable in what needs to be done for the victims of the collision. Should you enlist his help in stabilising your patients? Why or why not?**

▬ Points to Ponder

You and your crew are called to a scene in which a car has hit an electrical pylon. Live power lines have fallen around the vehicle, and the driver seems to be unconscious.

Is your first priority the injured patient, or the safety of yourself and your crew?

Issues: Scene Safety, Patient Care, Patient Access.

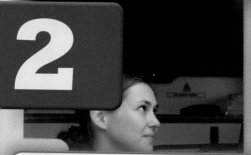

2 Health, Safety, and Welfare of the Paramedic

Objectives

Cognitive

- Discuss the concept of wellness and its benefits.
- Define the components of wellness.
- Describe the role of the paramedic in promoting wellness.
- Discuss the components of wellness associated with proper nutrition.
- List principles of weight control.
- Discuss how cardiovascular endurance, muscle strength, and flexibility contribute to physical fitness.
- Describe the impact of shift work on circadian rhythms.
- Discuss how periodic risk assessments and knowledge of warning signs contribute to cancer and cardiovascular disease prevention.
- Differentiate appropriate from inappropriate body mechanics for lifting and moving patients in emergency and nonemergency situations.
- Describe the problems that a paramedic might encounter in a hostile situation and the techniques used to manage the situation.
- Given a scenario involving arrival at the scene of a road traffic collision, assess the safety of the scene and propose ways to make the scene safer.
- List factors that contribute to safe vehicle operations.
- Describe the considerations that should be given to:
  - Using medical escorts
  - Adverse environmental conditions
  - Using lights and siren
  - Proceeding through junctions
  - Parking at an emergency scene
- Discuss the concept of "due regard for the safety of all others" while operating an emergency vehicle.
- Describe the equipment available for self-protection when confronted with a variety of adverse situations.
- Describe the benefits and methods of smoking cessation.
- Describe the three phases of the stress response.
- List factors that trigger the stress response.
- Differentiate between normal/healthy and detrimental reactions to anxiety and stress.
- Describe the common physiological and psychological effects of stress.
- Identify causes of stress in the ambulance service.
- Describe behaviour that is a manifestation of stress in patients and those close to them and how these relate to paramedic stress.
- Identify and describe the defence mechanisms and management techniques commonly used to deal with stress.
- Describe the components of critical incident stress management (CISM).
- Provide examples of situations in which CISM would likely be beneficial to paramedics.

- Given a scenario involving a stressful situation, formulate a strategy to help cope with the stress.
- Describe the stages of the grieving process (Kübler-Ross).
- Describe the needs of the paramedic when dealing with death and dying.
- Describe the unique challenges for paramedics in dealing with the needs of children and other special populations related to their understanding or experience of death and dying.
- Discuss the importance of universal precautions and body substance isolation practices.
- Describe the steps to take for personal protection from airborne and bloodborne pathogens.
- Given a scenario in which equipment and supplies have been exposed to body substances, plan for the proper cleaning, disinfection, and disposal of the items.
- Explain what is meant by an exposure and describe principles for management.

Affective

- Advocate the benefits of working toward the goal of total personal wellness.
- Serve as a role model for other ambulance service providers in regard to a total-wellness lifestyle.
- Value the need to assess his/her own lifestyle.
- Challenge him/herself to each wellness concept in his/her role as a paramedic.
- Defend the need to treat each patient as an individual, with respect and dignity.
- Assess his/her own prejudices related to the various aspects of cultural diversity.
- Improve personal physical well-being through achieving and maintaining proper body weight, regular exercise, and proper nutrition.
- Promote and practise stress management techniques.
- Defend the need to respect the emotional needs of dying patients and their families.
- Advocate and practice the use of personal safety precautions in all scene situations.
- Advocate and serve as a role model for other ambulance service providers relative to body substance isolation practices.

Psychomotor

- Demonstrate safe methods for lifting and moving patients in emergency and non-emergency situations.
- Demonstrate the proper procedures to take for personal protection from disease.

Introduction

Clive Owens is a long-serving paramedic who has been in the ambulance service for more than 25 years. Clive has arthritis in his knees and hips, and his back is chronically stiff and sore. He avoids most kinds of exercise because everything he has tried hurts.

When Clive attended his first emergency call, few people thought about paramedic wellness. The slogan of the times was "the patient always comes first". Every week, Clive was given five shifts that were so busy the crews did not have time to cook. Clive and most of his colleagues resorted to takeaway food while they were on duty, often putting off eating until their last late-night call when they were ravenous. They ate large portions and gulped down large soft drinks and great volumes of coffee to get them through their busy nights.

Ambulance trolleys typically had to be lifted into and out of ambulances, with or without patients. Two people managed that job by themselves, because there were no first responders. The only way a provider could load or unload one of those beds was by lifting from the side. To avoid straining his or her back, a provider would try to stand very close to the trolley, spreading his or her thighs widely and lifting with the hands between the knees, about 46 cm apart. The whole procedure put a lot of stress on the lifter's knees and hips.

Between calls, most crews sat and waited—or slept, bracing themselves for repeated wake-up calls. Many smoked more than a packet of cigarettes a day. Providers were generally young (usually in their early 20s) with no plans to stay in medical health care. Like most people their age, they gave little thought to the long-term consequences of their on-duty lifestyle. But many of them developed life-altering injuries.

Even an expert in human occupational health care could not have devised a more torturous test of the human mind or body. Thirty years ago no research project tracked the injuries or the impact of sleep loss and bad eating and exercise habits on ambulance crews. The research about the impact of stress on all health care providers has grown in the past 30 years, culminating in a better understanding of (and hopefully the prevention of) the damage to the physical and mental health of the dedicated professionals on either side of the accident and emergency department door.

Paramedics need to know how to ensure their own well-being and to share what they have learned with other professionals and the public.

Components of Well-Being

Wellness is a baseline state of adjustment to the rigours of life that makes us happy and pain-free most of the time, often brings

You are the Paramedic Part 1

You are fresh out of training school. Your supervisor has paired you with an experienced paramedic, who is knowledgeable but somewhat bad tempered. You and your partner have had a long day. Just as you sit down to eat dinner, you are dispatched to a nonemergency transport from a local nursing care home. As you get up from the table, your partner lets out a big sigh and mumbles something under his breath.

When you arrive, you are greeted by one of the care centre's registered nurses. She tells you this patient is being transported for evaluation by his doctor and, as she begins to tell you about the patient's recent history of illness, your partner says, "That's OK. We've got it. Do you have the guy's notes?" She quickly hands you the patient's medical file, and you enter the room to find a morbidly obese 55-year-old man. You estimate his weight to be about 20 stones. You take an initial set of vital signs.

As your partner is getting the stretcher ready, you ask him if it would be a good idea to call for additional help. He tells you, "No, let's just get this over with".

Initial Assessment	Recording Time: 0 Minutes
Appearance	Eyes open, no apparent distress
Level of consciousness	Alert and oriented
Airway	Open
Breathing	Adequate rate and tidal volume
Circulation	Radial pulse present
Vital Signs	
Skin	Warm, pink, and dry
Pulse	90 beats/min, regular and strong
Blood pressure	160/94 mm Hg
Respirations	22 breaths/min
S_PO_2	94% on 2 l/min nasal cannula

1. What is your main concern at the moment?
2. What concerns do you have, if any, regarding your partner's behaviour?
3. Does your partner's attitude have any effect on patient care?

us joy, and generally produces interactions with others that are mutually supportive and fulfilling Figure 2-1 ▸ . Wellness has at least three dimensions: the physical, the mental, and the emotional. Many people believe that a fourth dimension, the spiritual, is also essential.

Physical Well-Being

Health care providers have known for years that they are less likely to get hurt if they show up in shape for the work. Your muscle strength, the flexibility of your joints, your cardiac endurance, your emotional equilibrium, your posture (both sitting and standing), your state of hydration, the quality of the foods you eat, and even the amount of sleep you get affect your quality of life. And each of these factors directly impacts the likelihood that you will get through a shift without injury and be able to deal with the mental stress inherent in the job. Let's take a closer look at these factors.

Nutrition

Supervisors and shift planners understand a lot more about scheduling for good nutrition and hydration today than they did 30 years ago. Even food and drink containers have improved. Researchers learned a lot about the consequences of poor nutrition—cardiac illness, type 2 diabetes, obesity, and possibly even Alzheimer's disease. But many ambulance service providers still work long shifts, sometimes without scheduled meal breaks. The ambulance service system is clearly challenged.

Many years ago, nutritional education in schools suggested eating foods from the four main food groups (fruits and vegetables, meats, grains, and dairy products) in carefully prescribed amounts. Research has shown that one size does not fit all, and people must adjust their diets to meet their individual energy needs.

The British government's document *Balance of Good Health* is a model of how to eat healthily and is based on the 8 guidelines for a healthy diet. It shows the types and proportions of different foods that should be eaten over a period of time. The *Balance of Good Health* applies to all healthy individuals over five years of age, but does not apply to individuals with special dietary requirements. The 8 guidelines for a healthy diet include:

1. Enjoy your food
2. Eat a variety of different foods
3. Eat the right amount to be a healthy weight
4. Eat plenty of foods rich in starch and fibre
5. Eat plenty of fruit and vegetables (five portions a day)
6. Don't eat too many foods that contain a lot of fat
7. Don't have sugary foods and drinks too often
8. If you drink alcohol, drink sensibly; do not binge.

You should choose a variety of foods from each of these four food groups every day:

- Bread, other cereals and potatoes
- Fruit and vegetables
- Milk and dairy foods
- Meat, fish, and alternatives

Foods in the fifth group, i.e. foods containing fat and foods containing sugar, can be eaten sparingly as part of a healthy balanced diet, but should not be eaten instead of foods from the other food groups, or too often or in large amounts. Having a variety of foods in the diet is important for health—it is not necessary to follow the model at every meal, but rather over a day or two Figure 2-2 ▾ .

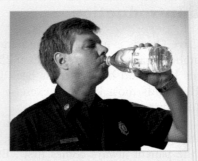

Figure 2-1 Because of the special demands of their job, paramedics must be continually focused on staying both physically and emotionally healthy.

So, what is the best way for a paramedic to sustain energy? Perhaps the best answer to nutrition is to plan your meals before you report for duty. You can keep yourself better hydrated by carrying bottled water instead of buying soft drinks, and minimising your intake of caffeine. You can stay better nourished and more alert by carrying numerous small snacks (like raisins, nuts, and fruits) you can eat slowly. Taking these steps will also save you lots of money. This is better than speed-eating big, expensive, high-fat, high-salt meals.

Weight Control

Emergency work demands active people who can quickly and accurately assess, access, observe, cope with, and control chaotic situations. Staying fit is a necessity in public service. Patterns of living you develop in your youth are hard to modify in later life—and impose lasting effects on your overall health.

It is generally accepted that in order to lose weight we should reduce calorie intake, increase physical activity, and make wiser food choices. We should discourage crash-dieting and instead recommend "eating fewer calories while increasing physical activity [as] the keys to controlling body weight".

Gradual weight reduction, like an exercise programme, requires you to plan your meals and your breaks. Rather than taking coffee breaks, some paramedics take breaks by walking or doing other forms of aerobic activity. These ambulance service providers often split a meal between two people when they eat in a restaurant, and they are hearty eaters of salad, vegetables, and fresh-caught grilled fish. You too can do this, with some planning. If you have to eat out, you could order oatmeal or cold cereal for breakfast, a salad (with lowfat dressing) and soup for lunch, and roast turkey for dinner.

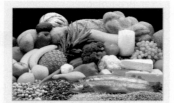

Figure 2-2 Having a variety of foods in the diet is important for health.

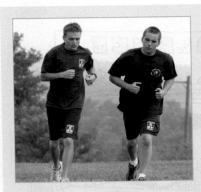

Figure 2-3 Regular exercise—apart from the work you do on calls—should be part of your daily or weekly routine.

Exercise

Regular vigorous exercise is closely linked to your body weight, nutritional status, and hydration, and has been shown to improve your sleep, sex life, mental capacity, ability to cope with stress, and overall long-term health. The best exercise programme for you depends on your personal preferences. It should be something you enjoy and should be targeted at maintaining, or improving, three areas: your cardiovascular endurance, your flexibility, and your physical strength. More specifically, it should involve enough moderate to vigorous daily physical activity to keep you from gaining weight.

It is recommended that adults engage in at least 30 minutes of moderate to vigorous physical activity most days of the week to help build optimal cardiovascular endurance. Working in a busy station, you probably feel that you get that workout on every call. Back at the station, it is very tempting to prop your feet up and vegetate until the next call. But to stay in good physical condition, you need to find a healthy balance between full-out physical activity (when you are "running hot") and no activity at all Figure 2-3 ▲ .

You should know your target heart rate and attempt to reach this goal every time you exercise. To find your target heart rate, calculate the following:

1. Measure your resting heart rate.
2. Subtract your age from 220. This total is your estimated maximum heart rate.
3. Subtract your resting heart rate from your maximum heart rate. Multiply that figure by 0.7.
4. Add this figure to your resting heart rate.

For example, a 40-year-old man has a resting heart rate of 70 beats/min. Calculations would be as follows:

1. **Resting heart rate.**
   70 beats/min
2. **Maximum heart rate.**
   220 − 40 = 180 beats/min
3. **Maximum heart rate minus resting heart rate multiplied by 0.7.**
   180 − 70 = 110 × 0.7 = 77
4. **Target heart rate.**
   77 + 70 = 147 beats/min

At the Scene

Being a paramedic is physically and mentally demanding. Following simple guidelines for nutrition, exercise, and mental health will greatly enhance and prolong your career. Recruiting others you work with to join a health maintenance plan that includes these elements will foster teamwork as well as help maintain a balance between your career and your health.

Smoking

If you don't already, *please* don't start! If you do, *please* stop! Not only does this habit fly in the face of everything the ambulance service is about, it also produces many of the most terrible cardiovascular and pulmonary disasters that paramedics confront during the span of their careers. In addition, it sets an awful example for the public—especially to people who have breathing disorders such as asthma. And it makes us look and smell (*Yes, smell!*) like anything but professional caregivers.

Are you a smoker who is trying to quit? Several strategies can help you. First, try to cultivate a relationship with a mentor who was once truly addicted to smoking but who has successfully quit. Use that person as a support, and draw on his or her advice and encouragement. There are also programmes that attack a smoker's psychological dependency. These programmes may include instructions and audiotapes, and provide ongoing support.

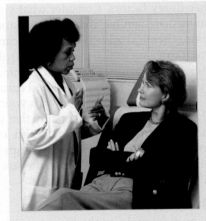

Figure 2-4 Both traditional and alternative health care providers offer a variety of ways to help smokers deal with nicotine addiction.

Talk to your general practitioner (GP). Your doctor should be familiar with many useful techniques Figure 2-4 ▲ . All of these solutions are cheaper than cigarettes and their attendant health risks.

Circadian Rhythms and Shift Work

The ambulance service imposes schedules on paramedics that conflict with the body's circadian rhythms, or natural timing system. These rhythms are controlled by special areas of the brain, called the suprachiasmatic nuclei, which govern our "internal clocks". Ignoring our circadian rhythms can cause some of us to experience consistent difficulty with sleep, higher thought functions, physical coordination, and even with social functions. You can have trouble focusing during some parts of the day or night (so that you simply cannot function as a paramedic) if you don't know what your natural rhythms are, try hard to understand them, and determine a schedule that is best for you. Research on circadian rhythms is only beginning to appear in medical journals, suggesting that some day we might be able to alter our internal clock.

Some tips for dealing with shift work:

- Avoid caffeine.
- Eat healthy meals and try to eat at the same times every day.
- Keep a regular sleep schedule.

The most important point for all paramedics is: don't overlook the need for rest, whatever your rhythms Figure 2-5 ▶. Many ambulance service providers depend on overtime as part of their normal income. But a paramedic who has been awake and working for 18 hours straight is only human, and needs rest. You cannot continue to operate an emergency vehicle or administer medications without necessary sleep.

Periodic Health Risk Assessments

Besides sleep, diet, exercise, hydration, and all the other things that make up a healthy lifestyle, you need to be aware of your hereditary factors. Consider what you might know about your immediate family's and your ancestors' health. Alzheimer's disease, chemical addiction, cancer, cardiac illness, hypertension, migraine, mental illness, and stroke all feature prominent hereditary factors. The most common of all inherited health risk factors are heart disease and cancer.

Share this information with your GP. Your GP is bound by the same oath of confidentiality that you are. Work with him or her to set up a schedule for health assessments, building them into your routine physical checkups. Your GP should be your ally in screening for these diseases and in assessing your lifestyle as well as your heredity.

Body Mechanics

A professional weight lifter typically performs a 30-minute warm-up routine before he or she lifts his or her personal maximum weight. Obviously, that's not an option in any emergency service. But there are a number of habits you can develop that are sure to reduce your exposure to damage from lifting your maximum weight. They include the following:

- Minimise the number of total body-lifts you have to perform. When patients need to be lifted, they need to be lifted. But remember that you risk an injury every time you do it. A patient with an arm laceration can stand for a moment while someone rolls the trolley behind him or her

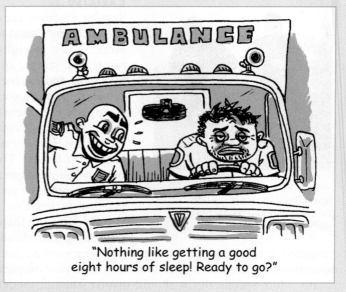

"Nothing like getting a good eight hours of sleep! Ready to go?"

Figure 2-5

and then helps the patient sit down. You can also cut your total number of lifts from ground level by having the ambulance trolley ready in a hands-height position—never fully lowered. That way, you need bend down only once—to lift the patient on a long board or accessory stretcher (scoop/basket). Then, stand where you are and ask a bystander to roll the trolley underneath the long board or accessory stretcher. (Don't forget, whenever you walk, you are balancing on only one foot at a time.)

- Coordinate every lift in advance. Make sure that every member of the team knows what you expect him or her to do. It is equally important to make sure the patient knows it as well. The last thing you want is for him or her to panic in midlift and grab someone around the neck, throwing everyone off balance.
- Minimise the total amount of weight you have to lift. If you have access to a second person who can help lift and load at the foot end of the trolley, why not ask for his or her help? Additionally, ask your service to fit tail lifts on the rear of the ambulance.
- Never lift with your back, not ever. Anyone who has spent a few years in the ambulance service has made this mistake at least a few times, citing the pressure of the moment. That pressure can finish your career, unless you're lucky.

You are the Paramedic Part 2

As you pull the patient across to the trolley, you feel a slight twinge in your lower back. You hope it's nothing, and prepare to lift your end of the stretcher. As you lift, although you are using proper lifting techniques, you feel a sharp pain in the area of your lumbar spine. You are fairly certain you've just hurt yourself. You tell your partner, who replies, "OK. Well, let's just get this guy to his appointment, and then we'll call the shift supervisor". Reservedly, you agree, but you must still load the patient in the ambulance.

4. Is this the best course of action?

5. What is the best way to handle this situation?

6. What factors could affect your decisions?

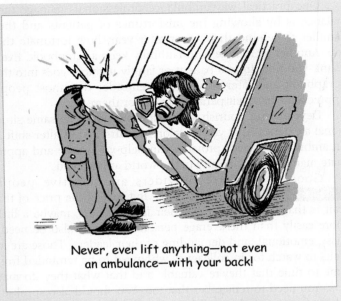

Never, ever lift anything—not even an ambulance—with your back!

Figure 2-6

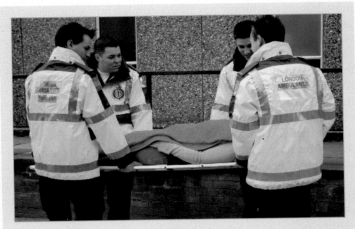

Figure 2-7 Never hesitate to ask for help from your colleagues, or to provide it when you are asked.

You cannot trust luck. The human back is a great weight bearer, but it's a terrible lifter. To protect your back, follow these precautions **Figure 2-6 ▲** :

- Always keep your back in a straight, vertical position and lift without twisting.
- When lifting, spread your legs about shoulder-width apart and place your feet so that your centre of gravity is properly balanced.
- Hold your back upright as you bring your upper body down by bending your legs at the knees.
- Lift by raising your upper body and arms and by straightening your legs until you are standing.
- Always lift with your legs, not with your back!

- Don't carry what you can put on wheels. Get the ambulance, and the trolley, as close to the patient as you can. Use a carry chair if you have to. (Tip: If you have access to a wheelchair, and the stairs are not too narrow, remember that a wheelchair makes a better carrying chair than a carry chair!)
- Ask for help any time, without embarrassment or hesitation—and offer it liberally to others. Anytime you need to move a patient who cannot or should not walk, consider the possibility of asking an extra person to help you **Figure 2-7 ▶** . That's not laziness. It's good sense, and it almost always enhances your body mechanics.

Mental Well-Being

The ambulance service can be a challenging and demanding profession because paramedics are no less vulnerable to diseases and injuries than their patients. Paramedics, like the

loved ones of their patients, can be frazzled by the stress of addressing the immediate and inflexible needs of others.

Mild stress can be a good thing, because it can enhance your mental acuity. But overwhelming stress can push us into fight-or-flight syndrome, a physiological response to a profound stressor, featuring increased sympathetic tone and resulting in dilation of the pupils, increased heart rate, dilation of the bronchi, mobilisation of glucose, shunting of blood away from the gastrointestinal tract and cerebrum, and increased blood flow to the skeletal muscles. It helps you deal with the situation right now, but can lead to crushing physical and mental strain if you do not learn appropriate coping skills.

Let's say you need to get away from a dangerous situation. Your body quickly modifies its performance to enable you to run from the scene. It borrows blood from your gastrointestinal tract and cerebrum, and shunts the blood to your skeletal muscles, your adrenal glands, your lungs, and your brain (your cerebellum and medulla). Your pupils dilate, enhancing your night vision. You become a running machine—at least for a short time. But you do that at the expense of your higher mental faculties. Your speech becomes clumsy. With those big pupils, you forfeit your depth perception and visual acuity. Your skeletal muscles perform well but, for the time being, you don't feel most kinds of pain such as muscle strain. You lose your fine motor control, so you might have trouble performing actions that require manual dexterity. You might experience a case of the jitters. And all of that would occur in less than 20 seconds. Your body is preparing you for trouble. You need coping strategies for behaviour that would be most effective in dealing with the situation.

A paramedic needs to be a great observer and a sharp thinker with a two-fisted grip on his or her emotions. Is there a way to control your reactions? It can be difficult, because some events are simply overwhelming. But there are some immediate and long-term techniques that you can use. Remember, the most important thing you can do in modeling your behaviour is to plan for it. Try any or all of these techniques long before you feel yourself melting down in the field.

You can look and act the part of a professional; take pride in what you do. Caring for people is an ancient pursuit, perhaps the oldest in history. Remind yourself that the world is full of caregivers who do what they do without support, rewards, or recognition from anyone—much less payment. Accept that you are a caregiver with a trust from the public you serve. You have a responsibility to that public in the same way as any other health care professional.

And remember, the ambulance service is a lot bigger than your job, but your life is more important than the ambulance service. Keep your lifelong perspective as broad as possible by cultivating relationships with people who are not part of the ambulance service.

Emotional Well-Being

Any professional caregiver needs to have a natural interest in and liking for people. The key to remaining happy in the lifelong practice of critical care medicine is making a deliberate effort to create a healthy balance between life at work and life away. Although many practitioners become very involved in the ambulance service and very dedicated to it, the ambulance service should never be a paramedic's whole life.

The ambulance service does satisfy some of its practitioners' deeply felt needs—especially the need for self-esteem. But, as a popular saying goes, "Don't love something that can't love you back". In fact, many ambulance service practitioners will say that the more energy you pour into the ambulance service, the more energy it will require to deal with the stress of its importance to you. Why? Because, as another popular saying goes, "Nobody gets out of here alive". Patients can die, regardless of how good their paramedics, nurses, or trauma surgeons are. And you need to recognise that patient death is not your fault, unless you allow your skills, education, or professionalism to decay.

One practical way ambulance professionals manage their balance is by allowing the misfortunes of patients and their families to remind them, year after year, how fortunate they are. Another technique is to faithfully keep a scrapbook. Every thank-you note from a patient or family member goes into that scrapbook and later serves as a reminder that most people appreciate what their paramedics do for them.

Develop and nourish your realisation that the same situational awareness that you develop in yourself shift after shift as an ambulance service provider can help you to see and appreciate many kinds of beauty in the world around you.

Good health care providers are sensitive people **Figure 2-8 ▶**. They have to be. But part of the price of that trait is that they tend to get their feelings hurt, maybe a little more easily than the average person. They can also be needy, fussy, emotional, and demanding of their leaders. Those are all traits to watch for in colleagues who need to be reminded from time to time that they're valuable and that what they do matters. You need to remember that too. You should also speak up when you notice that colleagues are not taking care of themselves. You may feel uncomfortable about broaching the subject, but letting them know that you are worried about them can make a difference.

Spiritual Well-Being

Human spirituality is an unseen dimension of human experience. Some people address it with formal religion, but those who do not may still recognise the existence of supernatural power and even of one or more divine entities. Few experienced emergency medical workers deny the possibility of a plane of life beyond our understanding. This possibility may have been reinforced from witnessing the effectiveness of the portable defibrillator, which seems to interrupt the death process, giving ambulance service providers credible and consistent stories from patients.

Medical care supports the dignity and value of life, and the sacredness of individuals. It is essential for you to respect the beliefs of others—those you work with, and patients and their

You are the Paramedic Part 3

Because you are on probation, you are afraid to contradict your partner. You assist him in loading the patient into the ambulance, and you are now in great pain. It is all you can do to focus on caring for your patient. He is stable and in a position of comfort. You wish the same statement held true for you.

Vital Signs	Recording Time: 15 Minutes
Skin	Warm, pink, and dry
Pulse	90 beats/min, regular and strong
Blood pressure	162/94 mm Hg
Respirations	22 breaths/min
S_PO_2	95% on 2 l/min nasal cannula

7. What decisions could you have made to prevent this situation?
8. Has patient care been affected?

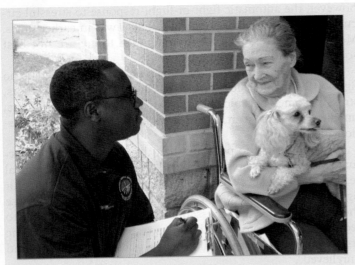

Figure 2-8 One thing that draws people to work as a paramedic is the pleasure of interacting closely with people.

families—to whom those beliefs can be all-important. Your respect for patients' beliefs will also help you in managing effective patient care. Many ambulance service providers describe a rich sense of their own spirituality that keeps their lives in good perspective.

Stress

All of us have experienced the effects of stress at one time or another. In fact, virtually every human activity involves some degree of stress—sometimes pleasant, sometimes unpleasant, sometimes mild, sometimes intense. And virtually all living creatures are equipped with some sort of inborn stress reaction that enables them to deal effectively with their environment. Hans Selye, considered the "father of stress theory", has defined biological stress as the "nonspecific response of the body to any demand made upon it".

So, stress is a reaction of the body to any agent or situation (stressor) that requires the individual to adapt. Adaptation of one sort or another is necessary all the time, for growth, for development, or just for meeting the demands of everyday life. By itself, then, stress is neither a good thing nor a bad thing, nor should all stress be avoided. After all, self-

Documentation and Communication

People from certain cultures and some older patients may believe that showing emotion is a sign of weakness. They may not show the emotions you may readily see in other people in the same situations. Do not assume because they don't indicate stress in the usual ways that they are not distressed. Try to read their body language and hear what they are saying. Also make sure they understand you.

preservation, one of the most basic requirements of life, would be impossible without a stress-alarm mechanism. Think about that dangerous situation we talked about earlier. That mechanism also serves you in other ways, for example, motivating you to study for examinations!

It is important to distinguish between injurious and noninjurious stress responses. Selye, for that reason, has classified stress into two categories: eustress (positive stress), the kind of stress that motivates an individual to achieve; and distress (negative or injurious stress), the stress that a person finds overwhelming and debilitating Figure 2-9 ▲. In the rest of this chapter, when we speak about stress, we shall in fact be talking about distress, the negative kind of stress.

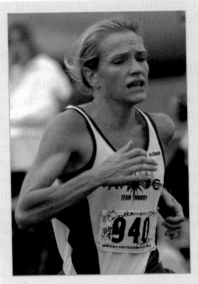

Figure 2-9 Some types of stress, called eustress, are positive and help push us to greater achievements.

What Triggers Stress

The stress response often begins with events that are perceived as threatening or demanding, but the specific events that trigger the reaction vary enormously from individual to individual. One person may go into a cold sweat even at the *thought* of air travel, while another de-stresses among the clouds piloting an aircraft. Learned attitudes strongly affect the situations people find stressful.

The following factors trigger stress in the vast majority of people:
- Loss of a loved one (death of a spouse or family member or going through a divorce) or of a valued possession
- Personal injury or illness
- Major life event (starting or finishing school, marriage, pregnancy, or having children leave home)
- Job-related stress (conflicts with others, excessive responsibility, the possibility of losing your job, or changing a job)

To deal effectively with stress, each of us needs to make a personal appraisal of the stress triggers in his or her life and take action to minimise their effects.

The Physiology of Acute Stress

One of the fundamental models for stress evolved from studies of how humans and other animals responded to threats. It was observed that when a person or a laboratory animal was confronted with a situation that he or she perceived as threatening, a standard series of physiological reactions was triggered, whatever the threat (this is why Selye referred to stress as a nonspecific response).

Typically, these physiological reactions prepare the animal for fight-or-flight syndrome by activating the sympathetic nervous system. The sympathetic nervous system is the part of the autonomic, or involuntary, nervous system that prepares the body to deal with an emergency. We will discuss the sympathetic nervous system more fully in Chapter 22.

Generally, the first stage of the stress response is an alarm reaction, which occurs within a fraction of a second after being confronted with a strong stimulus—for instance, a sudden loud noise. The alarm reaction begins with a quick alert response, in which you immediately stop whatever you are doing and focus on the source of the stimulus Figure 2-10.

Anyone who has ever startled a grazing deer remembers how the deer exhibited an alert response: it stopped grazing, looked toward the sound that had startled it, and stood absolutely still. Along with the alert response, there is sudden stimulation of the sympathetic nervous system, producing constricted blood vessels, increased heart rate, dilated pupils, erect hair follicles, increased perspiration, and a variety of other physiological effects. Indeed, we often describe our reactions to a stressful experience in terms of the sympathetic nervous system: "My heart was pounding in my chest". "I broke out in a cold sweat". These are all part of the body's fight-or-flight response to a perceived threat.

For most animals, the fight-or-flight response is a very useful and adaptive mechanism, mobilising them either to defend themselves (fight) or to run away (flight) in the face of possible danger. Taking either of these steps dissipates the stress, and the animal then goes through a stage of relaxation ("I breathed a sigh of relief when it was over".) and finally returns to its original internal balance. In the modern world,

however, the automatic fight-or-flight response to stressful circumstances is probably not as useful as it was in earlier times. Most of the stressors that humans face today are not best solved by fighting or running away.

When a loved one dies or when you lose a job, there is no fight-or-flight outlet for the stress. Under such circumstances, stress becomes chronic, placing our bodies in a continuous, unrelieved state of alert, possibly leading eventually to exhaustion and ill health.

It is important to point out that the stress response is normal. Many people misunderstand the normal physiological reactions to stressors and interpret the body's preparations for fight or flight as signs of disease, which only serves to increase the level of anxiety. It is essential for paramedics to learn to recognise the symptoms of the stress response, because chronic stress can exact a high toll when it goes unrecognised and unrelieved.

Coping With Your Own Stress

Some early warning signs of your own stress include heart palpitations, rapid breathing, chest tightness, and sweating. Learn to feel yourself entering your fight-or-flight mode. You may notice rapid breathing and breathlessness, unnecessary shouting, and use of swear words that you would not normally use. You may also feel yourself perspiring despite the weather. It is important to the care of your patients that you try keeping calm to help control the fight-or-flight mechanism in emergencies. Take appropriate action. Initial management techniques include the following steps:

1. **Controlled breathing.** On emergency calls, controlled breathing or taking deep breaths in through the nose and out through the mouth may be the least obvious way to control your anxiety.

2. **Reframing.** Reframing is using your head to look at the situation from a different viewpoint. Instead of thinking "I can't do this", reframe your thoughts to "I trust my training, I can do this".

3. **Progressive relaxation.** After the call, you may find yourself still stressed. Progressive relaxation is a strategy in which you tighten and then relax specific muscle groups to initiate muscle relaxation throughout the body.

Other coping strategies include focusing on the immediate situation while on duty. Off duty, remind yourself (even aloud, although not within the hearing of a patient or his or her loved ones), "I will do my very best, but what I can do to help may not be enough" Figure 2-11.

Coffee is not your friend in avoiding stress reactions. Avoid excessive amounts of stimulants such as caffeine. Faithfully get enough rest, and avoid alcohol during the 12 hours before a duty day. Exercise vigorously and regularly, especially during the hours preceding a shift. Find plenty of things to laugh and joke about, and find compatible partners at work.

A sense of scepticism is valuable to a paramedic, but don't let yourself become cynical and judgemental. Don't spend too long in environments where people don't care about the ambu-

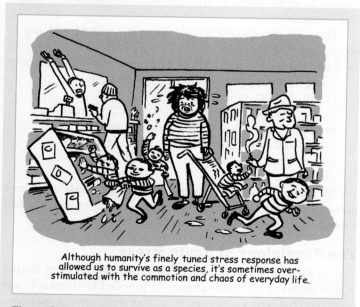

Although humanity's finely tuned stress response has allowed us to survive as a species, it's sometimes over-stimulated with the commotion and chaos of everyday life.

Figure 2-10

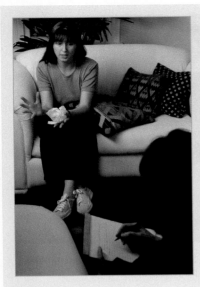

Figure 2-11 Consulting with a professional counsellor or therapist can be an important part of dealing with stress and maintaining your emotional well-being.

lance service and avoid prolonged or frequent assignments with cynical people. Study routinely, and keep your Continuing Professional Development Portfolio up-to-date. The social element of continuing education is invaluable in managing stress.

How People React to Stressful Situations

Anyone—the patient, the family, bystanders, or health care professionals—who confronts critical illness or injury responds in some way to the stresses of each emergency.

At the Scene

Learn to look for signs of stress in your colleagues and patients. Early discovery can often prevent the situation from worsening.

Responses of Patients to Illness and Injury

Patients' responses to emergencies are determined by their personal methods of adapting to stress. It will help you as a paramedic to recognise certain common patterns of coping. If the emergency is a medical illness, most people first become aware of some painful or unpleasant sensations and perhaps a decrease in energy and strength as well. The common response to that awareness is anxiety. Some people exhibit their anxiety by denying it; others become irritable or angry. Once the patient accepts that he or she is ill or injured, any of several common reactions may occur:

- **Fear.** Patients in these situations have realistic fears, such as fear of pain, disability, or death (or fear of their economic knock-on effects).
- **Anxiety.** Patients can also experience diffuse anxiety, often stemming from a feeling of helplessness. People who find themselves transformed into patients experience a loss of control. They must place themselves in the hands of a stranger whom they must depend on completely and whose competence they cannot really evaluate. People whose self-esteem depends on being active, independent, and aggressive are particularly vulnerable to anxiety when they become ill or injured.
- **Depression.** Depression is a natural response to loss. The patient with a critical illness or injury has lost some

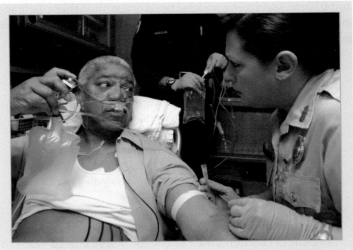

Figure 2-12 The sudden loss of control a patient feels when being treated during an emergency can lead to surprising and sometimes extreme reactions.

bodily function as well as some control. The patient who has had a stroke, for example, may have lost the ability to move an arm or leg on one side of the body and even the ability to speak. It is only natural to feel low and depressed in such circumstances.

- **Anger.** Anger is one of the most difficult problems for many caregivers to deal with. Suppose a paramedic arrives at the scene of a collision and starts tending immediately to the patient, but the patient becomes hostile and abusive Figure 2-12 ▲ . The paramedic's natural tendency, under the circumstances, is to think, "Here I am trying to save this guy's life, and he's venting his anger and being difficult. Well, he can just go and get stuffed". It is crucial, therefore, to understand that often people respond to discomfort or limitation of function by becoming resentful and suspicious of those around them. A patient who feels angry may vent anger on the rescuer by becoming impatient and irritable or excessively demanding, simply because the rescuer is the most convenient target. A *professional* caregiver realises in these circumstances that the patient's anger stems from fear and discomfort, and is not really directed at the paramedic.
- **Confusion.** Confusion is especially common among older patients, in whom illness or injury may precipitate disorientation. Such confusion is furthered by the presence of unfamiliar people and equipment, which may seem overwhelming. When a patient appears confused, therefore, it is very important to explain carefully at the outset who you are and what your mission is; thereafter, you should keep up a running commentary on what you are doing to help orient the patient to your role.

In addition to experiencing the reactions just described, most people who have a sudden illness or injury will mobilise one or more psychologic <u>defence mechanisms</u>. Patients and ambulance service providers usually employ these defence mechanisms automatically and subconsciously as a way of relieving personal stress. Here are some examples:

- **Denial.** Many patients tend to ignore or diminish the seriousness of their medical emergencies, because of the anxiety they cause. Denial is often evident in a tendency to dismiss all symptoms with words such as *only* or *a little* (for example, the middle-aged man with chest pain who says, "I'm fine, I'm fine. It's only a little indigestion".). When a patient tries to minimise his or her symptoms in that way, it may be necessary to find a reliable informant among the patient's family or friends so you can obtain more details. Treat for the worst.

- **Regression.** Regression is a return to an earlier age level of behaviour or emotional adjustment. Regression is often evident in children under stress; for instance, a 10-year-old may suddenly start wetting the bed at night after a stressful experience. Adults too can revert to more childish behaviours under stress. Indeed, when people are injured or become ill, their roles as patients *force* them into a state of dependency, very much like children.

- **Projection.** Projection is attributing your own (sometimes unacceptable) feelings, motives, desires, or behaviour to others. Patients who express vehement indignation or anger at the behaviour of others can unconsciously be denying their own "bad" behaviour by attributing it to other people.

- **Displacement.** Displacement occurs when someone redirects an emotion from the original cause of the emotion (like a cardiac problem) to a more immediate substitute (like a paramedic). Displacement is often the operative mechanism when patients express anger at the paramedic. In reality, patients are angry at someone else—themselves, a family member, fate, God—but they unconsciously redirect their anger toward the stranger who comes to provide medical care. A professional caregiver recognises that, and accepts it without complaint.

As noted, most of the psychological stress responses are not under your patients' conscious control. Injured patients who respond with anger toward the paramedic often have no perspective on their unpleasant behaviour. The reaction is automatic for the stressed patient.

Just as patients have their own ways of reacting to stress, you have subconscious expectations of how the patient *should* behave when stressed. You might expect a child to cry or to reach out to someone for comfort. But do you allow or tolerate that same reaction in adults?

Often, reactions to illness or injury are rooted in the patient's culture. We live in a multicultural society. Some cultures may openly exhibit their anxieties in what might be termed inappropriate behaviour in another culture. You will not be able to manage patient care well if you do not respect the culture of your patient.

For example, many patients may react to a situation in what you may think of as quite an emotional way. They may

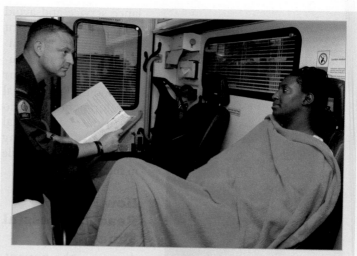

Figure 2-13 Always maintain an open and non-judgemental attitude when dealing with all patients.

take comfort in having many family members around them for support. This can be quite overwhelming if you come from a cultural background where people are often rather stoic.

Many northern Europeans place great emphasis on making eye contact, having a firm handshake, and respecting personal space. Some patients may not make eye contact with you because, in their culture, lowered eyes show deference to your authority and uniform. Many people are not comfortable with physical contact (even with their own health care provider) until they have developed a rapport. Obtain permission, if possible, before any hands-on encounters. It is difficult to learn about another culture in an emergency situation, but we need to recognise cultural differences. Learn the cultural differences of the populations you serve, realising that the reactions you see are only different, not wrong or abnormal   **Figure 2-13 ▲** .

Responses of Family, Friends, and Bystanders
Bystanders and family members can exhibit many of the responses that patients exhibit. Family members can be anxious, panicky, or—especially if they are struggling with guilt—angry. Suppose you are called to a 4-year-old child who has been struck by a car. The parents of the child are at the scene. Consciously or unconsciously, they feel guilty for what has happened; they may believe, deep down, that if they had kept a closer eye on the child, he or she would not have run out into the street. But, using the mechanisms of projection and displacement, the parents express their guilty feelings as aggression and/or anger toward the rescuers.

They may demand instant action or put pressure on you to move immediately to the hospital. Especially galling may be their implications that you are not competent to handle the situation ("Hurry up and get her to the hospital so that she can be seen by a *doctor!*"). The paramedic needs to recognise that the patient's family and friends have concerns too and that their behaviour, however irritating, arises from distress.

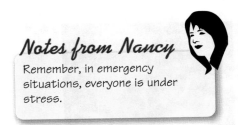

Step back emotionally from the situation for a moment. Keep your cool. Whether dealing with the behaviour of the patient or of those around him or her, the paramedic must constantly remain aware of the distress that lies behind the behaviour. When you are called to an emergency, it will not normally be a picnic. You are entering a situation in which *everyone is under stress,* and you cannot guarantee that people are going to behave appropriately. People who are ordinarily calm and polite in everyday life may not be calm and polite in an emergency. But if *you* can stay calm and polite, no matter what is going on around you, you can improve the behaviour of everyone else at the scene, including yourself.

Special Considerations

When children are seriously ill or injured, family members and other people at the scene may become frantic. You need to remain calm and confident in your skills, as this may be all that is needed to provide reassurance to everyone at the scene. Remind yourself (and, if you can, the anxious people around you) that scientific studies indicate that paramedic care and stabilisation will improve the patient's chances of a positive outcome.

Responses in Multiple-Casualty Incidents

In a situation involving multiple casualties, for example a train derailment, building collapse, or natural disaster (such as a flood), both victims and bystanders may react by becoming dazed, disorganised, or overwhelmed. The American Psychiatric Association has identified five categories of reactions in such circumstances. In general, people with these reactions should be removed from the scene.

- **Anxiety.** The normal reactions to such incidents are signs of extreme anxiety, including sweating, trembling, weakness, nausea, and sometimes vomiting. People experiencing this response can recover fully within a few minutes and provide useful assistance if properly directed. Ambulance service personnel are not immune to this type of reaction. If you see one of your crew looking a little shaky, the best remedy is to give him or her a specific task ("Get this IV started".).

- **Blind panic.** A more worrisome reaction is blind panic, in which the individual's judgement seems to disappear entirely. Blind panic is particularly dangerous because it is "catchy", and it may precipitate mass panic among others present. For this reason, a panicky bystander needs to be separated quickly from others and, if at all possible, placed under the supervision of a calmer person.

- **Depression.** This can be seen in individuals who sit or stand in a numbed, dazed state. The depressed bystander needs to be brought back to reality and removed from the scene.

- **Overreaction.** People who overreact tend to talk compulsively, joke inappropriately, become overly active, and race from one task to another without accomplishing anything useful. The person who is overreacting needs to be removed from the area where casualties are being treated.

- **Conversion hysteria.** Some patients subconsciously convert anxiety into a bodily dysfunction. They may be unable to see or hear or may become paralysed in an extremity.

We shall go into more detail on how to cope with bystanders in Chapter 48 where we discuss mass-casualty incidents.

Responses of the Paramedic

Health care professionals are not immune to the stresses of emergency situations, and it is to be expected that those dealing with the critically ill and injured will experience a multitude of feelings, not all of them pleasant. The paramedic may feel angry at the demands of the family or the patient, anxious in the face of life-threatening injuries, defensive at any suggestion that he or she is not competent to handle the situation, sad in response to the death of a patient, or any number of these sensations at the same time. These feelings are all perfectly natural, but it is preferable to keep them to yourself during an emergency. An attitude of outward calm and confidence on your part will do much to relieve the anxieties of others at the scene—and that too is part of the paramedic's therapeutic role.

One reaction that is common among health care professionals is a feeling of irritation at the patient who does not appear to be particularly ill. That reaction is especially prevalent among emergency personnel, who are psychologically geared to deal with life-threatening and catastrophic cases and who therefore tend to regard an apparently minor complaint as a burdensome annoyance. Try hard to remember that people define their own emergencies. Also, consider the possibility that people who call 999 with seemingly minor complaints are not calling for something minor at all—like the woman who called 999 because she couldn't get to sleep. Her problem was that it was her first night back home after the funeral of her husband. She was scared to death of her first night alone and she had no one else to call. Anyone who has ever been truly alone knows what an emergency that can be. These victims are not abusing us. They are precisely the ones we're here for.

At the Scene

Do not assume that seemingly non-emergency complaints are not a sign of something wrong. Tunnel vision can cause many mistakes in patient assessments and ultimately in their outcomes.

Burnout

What's this? We've scarcely started the paramedic course, and already we're talking about burnout! Why should we start worrying now about something that may (or may not) happen 10 years down the line?

We need to consider burnout now—at the earliest stage of paramedic training—because now is the time to start developing attitudes and habits that will help prevent burnout, whether 1 year or 20 years down the line.

The dictionary defines <u>burnout</u> as the exhaustion of physical or emotional strength. Burnout is, in fact, a consequence of chronic, unrelieved stress. The paramedic's job, by its very nature, is full of potential stresses. There are the obvious stresses imposed by having to deal, day after day, with mutilating trauma or catastrophic illness. There are, as well, more subtle stresses associated with interpersonal relations, pay, prestige, fringe benefits, and other issues. These complaints and stresses are, no doubt, legitimate. But burnout does not occur solely because of stress. Burnout develops because of the way a person *reacts* to stress.

One person's eustress may be another's distress **Figure 2-14 ▶**. The reason is that distress is a *learned* reaction, based on the way an individual perceives and interprets the world around him or her. In other words, distress is nearly always the result of what a person *believes*. Some beliefs are more likely than others to produce stress. Here are some beliefs that are common among ambulance service personnel:

- I have to be perfect all the time.
- My safety depends on being able to anticipate every possible danger.
- I am totally responsible for what happens to patients; if they die, it is wholly my fault.
- If there's something I don't know, people will think less of me.
- A good paramedic never makes mistakes.

These perfectionist beliefs are very likely to produce stress. They are also false beliefs. Prevention and relief of stress among ambulance service personnel begin with the recognition that such beliefs are unrealistic and invalid.

Like many of the conditions we will study in this textbook, burnout is also a sort of illness. And like any other illness, it has signs and symptoms. Learn to look for the symptoms of burnout in yourself and in your colleagues. These symptoms are warning signals, telling you to stop and reexamine your beliefs and your ways of responding to stress. Symptoms of impending burnout include:

- Chronic fatigue and irritability
- Cynical, negative attitudes
- Lack of desire to report to work
- Emotional instability (crying easily, flying off the handle without provocation, laughing inappropriately)
- Changes in sleep patterns (insomnia or sleeping more than usual), and waking without feeling refreshed
- Feelings of being overwhelmed or being helpless or hopeless
- Loss of interest in hobbies

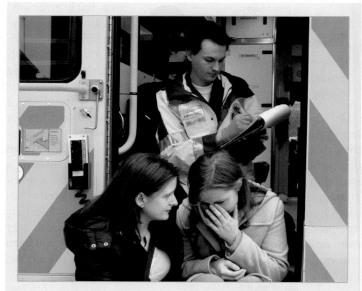

Figure 2-14 Dealing with stress as a paramedic requires the ability to emotionally distance yourself from the situation, and accept the limits of what you personally can do. Draw upon the help of others.

- Decreased ability to concentrate
- Declining health—having lots of colds, stomach upsets, and muscle aches and pains (especially headaches or backaches)
- Constant tightness in your muscles
- Overeating, smoking, or abusing drugs and alcohol

It is preferable, of course, not to wait until symptoms of burnout develop. There are paramedics who have been in the field for 20 years and show no signs whatsoever of burnout, who still report to work every day with the same enthusiasm they did at the start. What is their secret? In general, the paramedics who do not suffer burnout are those who have learned to respect and value *themselves*. That is not as easy as it sounds. The type of person who chooses to become a paramedic is usually altruistic—someone who puts the needs of others ahead of his or her own needs. In theory, that is very laudable. But in fact, no one can give their best to others for very long if they ignore their own personal needs.

Practically speaking, what does it mean to respect and value yourself? How can you translate that attitude into concrete action? Some of the steps you can take to protect yourself from burnout are summarised in **Table 2-1 ▶**.

■ Coping With Death and Dying

We all deal with death (remember the quote, "Nobody gets out of here alive"?). What do you say to people who know they're dying? What do you say to a bereaved parent or spouse? How do you deal with your own feelings when a patient has died while under your care? These are all questions we need to be able to answer for ourselves eventually, and it can take a lifetime to sort them out.

TABLE 2-1	Nancy's Guidelines for Preventing Burnout

1. **Paramedic heal thyself!** Take care of your own health.
   - Get enough rest.
   - Eat a balanced diet.
   - Get regular physical exercise—at least 30 minutes of aerobic activity (walking, running, or swimming) three to four times a week.
   - Don't abuse your body. Smoking, overindulgence in alcohol, taking recreational drugs, or self-prescribing any other drugs are all forms of self-abuse.
2. Give yourself some "me" time every day. Some of the most stress-resistant paramedics are those who have learned the techniques of reflective practice and can thereby escape now and then to a quiet place within themselves. Try different methods of relaxation and see which one works best for you.
3. Learn how to relax (Figure 2-15 ▾).
   - Take time for hobbies.
   - Engage in social activities with people not involved in the ambulance service.
   - Try to leave your job behind when your shift is over.
4. Do not make unreasonable demands on yourself.
   - Forget the idea that you have to be perfect. No one is perfect. If you do the best job you can, that is good enough.
   - You don't have to be right all the time. Accept the fact that now and then you will make a mistake—and that the world will not come to an end on account of it.
5. Do not make unreasonable demands on others.
6. Stay in touch with your feelings.
   - Find someone you can talk to. Share the situational stress.
   - Cry when you need to. There's no shame in being sad sometimes.
7. Learn techniques for shedding stress while on duty. Don't let stress accumulate.
8. Debrief after tough calls.

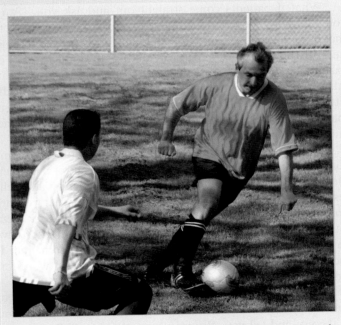

Figure 2-15 One of the best ways of dealing with the stress of working as a paramedic is to invest in relationships and activities outside of work that are meaningful to you.

Death in the Western hemisphere is generally regarded as a very traumatic experience, something to be feared and postponed as long as possible. It's not that way everywhere in the world. It may help you to know that many seasoned paramedics reveal in candid discussion that they are not afraid to die. Think about it. The average person's only experience with death has been the death of a loved one. It was a rare event. Chances are it was surprising, it was frightening, and it was painful for the survivor.

As a paramedic, you will be there when a lot of people are born and you will be there when a lot of them die. Every one of these encounters is an honour—a most private moment in someone's life, to which you and a small number of your colleagues are invited. Why an honour? Because, in many cultures, these moments are a holy time. And because you are meeting someone for the very first time in his or her life—or seeing him or her alive for the very last time. Many of the latter group will exhibit great dignity with their dying, and perhaps show you how to die well someday.

You don't need to experience great frustration because you tried to resuscitate someone and he or she died anyway. For you to resuscitate someone, everything has to go just right. As a paramedic, you will have the opportunity to help a great many people, but you will not be involved in many successful resuscitations, even in the course of a long career. Accept your profession as a calling, and be fulfilled by it. Keep a good grip on your ego, and you will find that "losing" someone will rarely be an issue for you.

What follows here are some general guidelines and techniques for dealing with the dying, their families, and your own stress.

Stages of the Grieving Process

In her classic study, *On Death and Dying*, Elisabeth Kübler-Ross defined five stages through which grieving people—usually the dying, but sometimes their survivors—often proceed (Figure 2-16 ▾). Each of these stages in some way helps

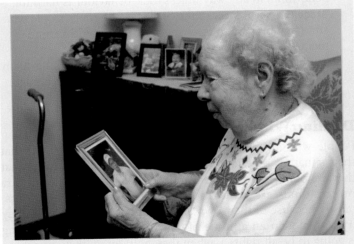

Figure 2-16 People usually go through a lengthy process of grieving before fully accepting the death of a loved one.

the dying or their family members adapt to their own reality. It helps to be aware of these stages, and to consider the behaviour of dying patients or their families in the context of the grieving process.

- **Stage 1: Denial.** We have already mentioned denial as a mechanism by which people attempt to ignore a problem or pretend it does not exist. Denial is a way of buffering bad news until we can mobilise the resources to deal with that news more effectively.

- **Stage 2: Anger.** When people can no longer deny the reality of a situation, anger over the loss replaces denial. They may ask, "Why me?" and displace their anger randomly to those around them. As we mentioned earlier, such anger may be very difficult for health care personnel to deal with, and it is necessary again and again to remind yourself, "This patient (or this family member) is not really angry at me. She is angry at the hand life has just dealt her".

- **Stage 3: Bargaining.** When anger does not change the painful reality of a situation, people may resort to bargaining, that is, trying to make some sort of deal in hopes of postponing the inevitable ("If I can just live long enough to see my daughter's wedding, then I'll die in peace".).

- **Stage 4: Depression.** When bargaining fails to change the reality of a loss and people must come to terms with dying, there is suddenly an enormous sense of loss. They may become very quiet. Other people may make the mistake of trying to "cheer them up" at this point. But the people who have experienced the loss typically do not *want* to be cheered up. They want permission to express their sorrow—in words, in tears, or in what Kübler-Ross calls "the silence that goes beyond words". Acknowledge their loss and sadness, and if they act like they want to cry, offer some tissues or a towel and encourage them to "let it out". If they seem to want a hug, offer it. If they seem to just want to be quiet by themselves, do what you can to accommodate that as well. But try hard not to steer their behaviours in any way unless their behaviour is harmful.

- **Stage 5: Acceptance.** In the final stage of grief, people who are dying prepare to disengage from the world around them. They shed their fears and most of their other feelings as well and begin to loosen the ties that bind them to the living. When the dying enter this acceptance stage, it is often the family that is in need of the most help.

Dealing With the Dying Patient

People who are dying generally know, at the very least, that their situation is serious; they may, in fact, be well aware that they are dying and may want to talk about it. Many health care professionals are reluctant to discuss death with patients, mostly because of their own anxiety about the subject. So they try to maintain an attitude of cheery reassurance ("Everything is going to be all right".), when they both know that everything will *not* be all right. The message patients get is that the subject of dying is taboo and that they'd better keep their feelings

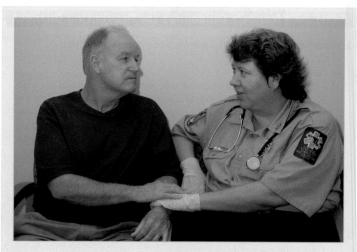

Figure 2-17 Be aware that each patient will have different ways of dealing with his or her immediate situation. Some may be relieved to talk openly about how they feel, while others may have a greater sense of privacy or stoicism.

about dying to themselves. In fact, perhaps the most important thing you can do for dying patients is to let them know that it's OK to talk about it. There are many ways of doing so. You don't need to come right out and ask, "Do you want to talk about dying?" It's enough to say, "If there's anything worrying you, I'd be glad to listen".

Having made the offer to listen, be prepared to do so. Let patients talk as much as they wish Figure 2-17 ▲. Make some physical contact. Hold their hand, put a hand on their shoulder, or make some other unmistakable gesture of empathy.

What if patients come straight out and ask you, "Am I going to die?" There is no simple answer as to how to reply to that question, but the answer should acknowledge the seriousness of their condition without taking away all hope. For example, you might say, "You seem to have had a severe heart attack. We're going to give you the best care available, but the situation *is* serious". For patients who know they are dying, it may be a great relief to have someone else acknowledge the fact and thereby give them permission to talk about it.

Dying patients also need to feel that they still have some control over their life. When people lose all control over their life, they may lose a large measure of their dignity and self-respect. As much as possible, explain to them what you are doing and allow them to participate in the treatment. Ask them if there is anyone they would like you to contact or if they have any special instructions they want conveyed to someone. If they *do* ask you to convey a message, *write it down* word-for-word as they state it to you.

Experience tells us that people who know they're going to die usually don't *ask* you if they are going to die. They look you in the eye and *tell* you, "I think I'm going to die". People who ask tend to be fairly stable, but that doesn't mean they're not scared to death. If they appear to be doing OK, let them know that, and tell them not to be afraid, that you've "got them".

Dealing With a Grieving Family

Suppose you are called to the scene where a child has been run over by a lorry. You can see at a glance that the child has significant head injury and is beyond resuscitation. Two police officers are restraining the child's mother, who is crying hysterically.

The fact that there is nothing you can do for the child does *not* mean that the call is over. There is another "patient" at the scene—the child's mother—and the call is not over until you have done all you can for her Figure 2-18 ▾ .

What kinds of things *can* you do for a grieving family? How can you help them begin the process of dealing with their loss? Here are a few guidelines:

- Do *not* try to hide the body of the deceased from the family, even if the body has been badly mutilated. (*Do* conceal it from the general public, however.) People who are prevented from seeing the body of a loved one may later have enormous difficulty working through their grief, for they may not be able to get beyond their denial.
- For similar reasons, do not use euphemisms for death, such as "expired" or "passed away". The family needs to hear the word "dead".
- Do not be in a hurry to clear away all your resuscitation equipment. Let the family see the equipment before you start tidying up and packing away your gear, so that they will know that everything possible was done to try to save the patient.
- Give the family some time with the body, especially when the victim is a child. If the death occurred in a public place—as in the hypothetical road traffic collision described—move the body into the ambulance and let the family be alone for a short while. Give them a chance to say goodbye in their own way. Offer them the opportunity to travel with you to hospital.

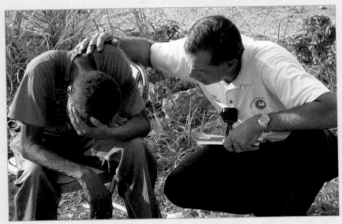

Figure 2-18 While on the scene, one of your responsibilities is to help family members through the initial period after the death of a loved one.

- Try to arrange for further support; neighbours and friends are often happy to assist.
- Accept the family's right to experience a variety of feelings—guilt, shock, denial, or anger. And when family members do respond with anger, remind yourself yet again, "They aren't really angry at *me*, just the situation".

Dealing With a Grieving Child

You need to be particularly sensitive to the emotional needs of children and how they differ depending on their age group. Children up to 3 years of age will be aware that something has happened and people are sad. Family members should be advised to try to maintain the child's routine. They should also watch for irritability and monitor the child's eating and sleeping patterns. Children 3 to 6 years of age believe that death is temporary and may continually ask when the person will return. Family members should be informed that the child may feel responsible for the death and may worry that everyone else they love may also die. The family should emphasise to the child that he or she was not responsible for the death and also that it's OK to cry when you are sad.

Children 6 to 9 years of age may mask their feelings in an effort to not look babyish. Family members should discuss the normal feelings of grieving with the child. Also, they should not hesitate to cry in front of the child. This will convey to the child that crying is a helpful and acceptable behaviour after the loss of a loved one.

Children 9 to 12 years of age may want to know details surrounding the incident. Family members should encourage the sharing of feelings and memories to facilitate the grieving process.

After the Call Is Over

Some kinds of calls can be real shockers, like the London bombings or the World Trade Center attack. In those cases, everyone involved in the call is likely to experience some strong feelings. If these feelings stay bottled up, there may be all sorts of problems later. Every ambulance service, therefore, needs to develop routine procedures for debriefing after any call that involved the death of a patient. All those who participated in the call need a chance to sit down together, in an atmosphere of confidentiality, and air their feelings about what happened.

By definition, a critical incident is one that overwhelms the ability of an ambulance service worker or an ambulance service system to cope with the experience, either at the scene or later. In some areas, it has become standard practice for ambulance services to deploy specially trained staff to assist emergency personnel who have been involved in particularly traumatic calls or other painful incidents. The sorts of incidents that are apt to require debriefing include:

- Serious injury or death of a fellow worker whilst at work
- Suicide of a fellow worker
- Multiple-casualty incidents, such as an airliner crash or rail accident

- Serious injury or death of a child
- Intense media attention to an incident

It is impossible to predict how any given person will react to a particular incident. A call that may be very disturbing to one paramedic may not bother his or her partner at all. People should be offered opportunities to debrief but debriefings should never be forced upon them.

Controversies

There are definitely two sides of the fence on the effectiveness of critical incident stress debriefing (CISD). Psychology professionals and ambulance service professionals alike have debated this issue for some time now. Take part in a debriefing whenever you can. Be open-minded about the experience and then draw your own conclusion as to which side of the fence you are on.

Post Traumatic Stress Disorder

Most calls should not disrupt your normal life functions. But, depending on a number of variables, some especially traumatic calls can preoccupy even well-adjusted providers for weeks or even months afterward. This is called post traumatic stress disorder (PTSD). Most paramedics never experience it, but it's what debriefings were developed to prevent. Let your superiors know if you experience one or more of the following signs of PTSD:

- You have trouble getting an incident out of your thoughts.
- You keep having flashbacks of an incident.
- You have nightmares or other sleep disturbances after an incident.
- Your appetite is not the same after an incident.
- After an incident, you laugh or cry for no good reason.
- You find yourself withdrawing from colleagues and family members after an incident.

The purpose of a debriefing is to accelerate the normal recovery process and to help ambulance service personnel realise that they are normal people having normal reactions to *ab*normal events Figure 2-19 ▶ . As mentioned, ambulance services have management teams to provide support after a traumatic call—and sometimes even during the incident itself. The intervention may take the form of a brief (usually about 30 minutes) defusing session right after the call, in which all who were involved in the incident are offered an opportunity to express their feelings about what happened. As the name implies, a defusing session is intended to remove the explosive potential from a situation and thereby prevent more serious psychological consequences later on.

A formal debriefing is usually coordinated by one or more professional counsellors 24 to 72 hours after an incident, when it becomes clear that the incident has had a serious impact and is causing persistent symptoms among the crew. A debriefing usually takes about 3 hours, and is conducted away from the workplace and in a confidential atmosphere so participants can feel free to say what's on their minds.

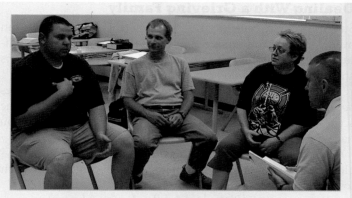

Figure 2-19 A debriefing with colleagues after an especially traumatic or difficult call can help everyone voice their feelings.

Emergency Vehicle Operations

An emergency vehicle is a four-sided billboard that communicates to the public all the time, whether we realise it or not. It communicates our respect for—or lack of respect for—the safety of others. It communicates our courtesy—or complete lack of it. And it communicates our concern for the comfort and safety of that patient and caregiver—or our complete lack of it.

A paramedic's first job is to come home safe to loved ones. There are plenty of paramedics (some whose careers span 20 or 30 years) who have never been involved in an ambulance collision, and not by good luck. They understand that safety is deliberate. They understand that operating an ambulance is a public trust. And they never forget that driving an ambulance is potentially dangerous.

Here are some proven safety tips you can use in your daily driving:

1. Think of your warning equipment as tools you can use to *ask for* (never demand) the right of way.
2. Always allow for the incompetence of other drivers.
3. Come to a full and complete rolling stop when you encounter a red traffic light. Proceed only after you have given other drivers time and cause to anticipate your intentions.
4. Expect some drivers to panic Figure 2-20 ▶ . If that happens, turn off your siren, and give them time to move out of your way.
5. Remember, other drivers may not immediately hear your siren when you are travelling at motorway speed or if they have the stereo on loud. Stay far enough behind other drivers so they can see your lights in their rear-view mirrors. Anticipate that, when they notice you, their first instinct will be to slam on their brakes.
6. As frustrating as it may be, control your emotions when it appears that a driver is refusing to give way. Avoid reacting to the situation, which will cause you to lose your cool and potentially worsen it.

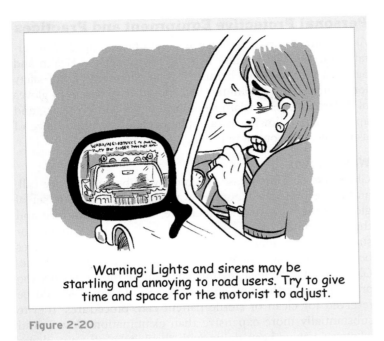

Warning: Lights and sirens may be startling and annoying to road users. Try to give time and space for the motorist to adjust.

Figure 2-20

Besides the general use of lights and the siren, some additional aspects of operating an emergency vehicle deserve special mention.

Using Escorts

When you find yourself responding in tandem with an escort vehicle, remember that the average driver is not likely to understand that one vehicle is escorting another. Most drivers have not had a course in emergency driving. Typically, drivers on the road hear one siren and, especially in their rear-view mirrors, will see only the first vehicle in a convoy. Deliberately using an escort is not only a bit pompous, but also dangerous. Do yourself a favour. Minimise the number of times you use any warning equipment and the number of vehicles on a given response. You'll live longer, and so will the public.

Adverse Environmental Conditions

Most of us have enough trouble keeping ourselves visible and trying to predict other drivers' behaviour on clear, sunny days. Add a little bad weather, fog, heavy rain and spray, or slippery tarmac from black ice and the average driver can be overwhelmed. Try to be as careful, alert, and predictable for other drivers as you can under the circumstances. When you lose

Documentation and Communication

When considering transporting a patient with lights and siren on, ask yourself, "Can I justify the potential risk to my safety, my patient's safety, and the safety of others to save a few minutes?" Make sure you can legitimately justify why you transported in this way and document the need to do so.

even the slightest visibility, be super observant and expect the worst decision-making from your fellow travellers. In fact, don't even trust yourself under these conditions. Remember to drive slowly and especially careful in adverse weather conditions.

Parking at Emergency Scenes

Many of us were taught years ago that when we park in traffic, we should shield ourselves with our equipment and aim the front wheels into traffic. That works fine if you're in law enforcement and you need the illumination from your headlamps anyway. But it does you no good at all if you're going to end up loading an ambulance, because ambulances load from the rear. Protect your back; park in the best position for loading, preferably at the front of the accident scene **Figure 2-21 ▾** .

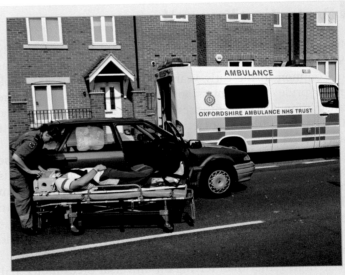

Figure 2-21 Place your vehicle beyond the accident to allow a safe working area and easy egress.

You are the Paramedic Part 4

Your partner drives to the ambulance entrance of the hospital. It takes every ounce of your concentration to aid your partner in unloading the patient. You tell yourself that you can finish the call but, as you and your partner lower the stretcher to the height of the hospital bed, you are unable to hold up your end. It drops to the floor, and the patient drops with it. Although he appears to be uninjured, the patient screams loudly and immediately threatens to sue you. Your partner now seems to be injured, and the hospital staff members appear to be horrified at what has just transpired.

9. What parts of this situation were preventable?

10. Beyond the physical injuries, what other damage has occurred?

There is an exception, and that's if the ambulance happens to be the first vehicle on the scene. Just remember: it may need to be moved later on. (Chapter 46 provides a more detailed discussion of this situation.)

Due Regard for the Safety of Others

Anyone who operates an emergency vehicle needs to have profound respect for the pain ambulance service drivers can inflict on the public by driving too close and too fast, or by insisting on the right-of-way.

People who have abused this privilege tell us that they can't describe the horror they felt on the morning after causing a fatality (especially the death of a colleague). These events are always horrible, and they can usually be traced to something that took no more than a couple of seconds to occur. There is no "undo" button in ambulance service driving, and no amount of shock or grief can ever give us those seconds back.

While speed is sometimes perceived as the essence of ambulance service, rest secure in this advice: knowledge is the essence of professional ambulance service. As you become a paramedic, you will have the most training and the most experience of any ambulance service worker. Be professional.

▌Protecting Yourself

Much has changed in the ambulance service since the early 1990s. The use of personal protective equipment (PPE) was not common in the early years. Surgeons in the 1800s took similar pride in their messy operating aprons, but they were transmitting infectious diseases by the score. Paramedics in the 2000s take pride in not endangering themselves or their patients.

Thanks to the research and reporting done by disease control bodies (dcb), we are now more aware that biohazards are an integral part of our profession and can have long-term effects on the health care worker if certain precautions are not adhered to. The dcb developed a set of <u>universal precautions</u> for health care workers to use in treating patients. The ambulance service follows <u>body substance isolation (BSI)</u> precautions rather than relying on universal precautions. BSI differs from universal precautions in that it is designed to approach all body fluids as being potentially infectious. In observing universal precautions, you assume that only blood and certain body fluids pose a risk for transmission of hepatitis B and human immunodeficiency virus (HIV).

Use the personal tools that are at your disposal that are designed not only to protect you from your sick patients but to protect them from you! In addition to these tools, consider adopting a practice that doesn't necessarily involve tools, but has proven its worth over the years. Wash your hands and wash them properly!

Personal Protective Equipment and Practices

At a minimum, each ambulance should be equipped with certain PPE, not just because it is the law under the Health and Safety at Work Act, but because it is an important part of safety for yourself. At a minimum, you should have access to gloves of difference sizes, facial protection (masks and eyewear), and aprons. The following paragraphs explain the importance of using infection control practices.

Wear Gloves

Gloves are absolutely essential on any ambulance service call, and some patient encounters warrant more than one set of gloves, depending on the procedure, the patient's history, and the environment (Figure 2-22 ▾). Anytime you intubate or start an IV, consider following that with a new set of gloves before loading the patient and jumping aboard that ambulance. Gloves are a good idea anytime you sanitise the ambulance too or even handle the mop and bucket. Sterile gloves should be reserved for clean or sterile patient care procedures; they're substantially more expensive than examination gloves. And whatever you've been doing with them, take off your gloves before you drive.

Wash Your Hands

Wash your hands, routinely and often. Long before it was common practice for ambulance personnel (or any clinical workers) to wear gloves during nonsterile procedures, we learned to wash our hands—sometimes more than 30 times a day, depending on our caseloads. Turn that into a habit. Habits are reliable, even when we're stressed.

Use Lotion

To replenish the natural oils you wash off your skin, and to keep the skin on your hands from cracking, use hand lotion several times a day both on and off duty. For you lads, it's not

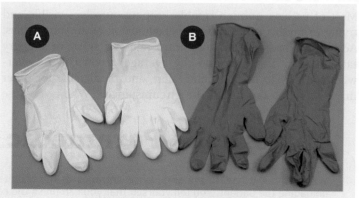

Figure 2-22 Two commonly used types of gloves are **A.** latex and **B.** nitrile.

At the Scene

Get used to washing your hands before and after using the bathroom, before ingesting anything by mouth, before getting into your personal car, and before and after any physical contact between you and a patient or a medical instrument.

Any advanced medical text on infection control starts with "wash your hands" and ends with it, too.

When you do wash your hands, wash them vigorously with antibacterial soap for at least 30 seconds before rinsing with clean water. If you don't have access to soap and water, carry waterless hand cleaner wipes in your ambulance and use them instead. Isopropyl alcohol, the active ingredient they contain, is a very effective bactericide.

Whatever else you do, wash your hands.

just for sissies; it's good sense. Your skin is a very effective barrier to pathogens, as long as it hasn't been breached by the drying effects of frequent washing. And the job of a professional caregiver warrants frequent washing.

Use Eye Protection

Many experienced paramedics make it their standard practice to wear antisplash eyewear throughout certain patient contacts. It's an absolute necessity during suctioning or intubation procedures. In fact, during intubation, it may be a good idea to use a face shield instead.

Consider Wearing a Mask

Have a cold? Wear a mask—not only to protect your patients and your colleagues from you, but to protect you from additional infections while you are in a weakened state. Have an infection? Stay home.

Protect Your Body

Masks and gowns are appropriate whenever you deal with a patient who is extremely messy or bloody **Figure 2-23** . A bin bag can be used as a two-armed glove to slide a patient from a couch or bed onto a trolley bed if the patient is covered with faeces, urine, or blood. Once the patient has been moved, the crew can simply turn the bag inside-out, squeeze the air out of it, tie a knot in its open end, and place it in a clinical waste bag.

Incontinence pads should be laid out on a surface when the patient is leaking any type of fluid or has skin lesions.

Clean Your Ambulance and Equipment

Sanitise the surfaces in the back of the ambulance frequently, but especially the trolley, the seat, the hand rails, the floor and floor brackets, and the interior and exterior areas around

the door handles. These surfaces should be cleaned daily and after every call. The same is true for the door handles inside (and outside) the cab, the steering wheel and gear stick, the handbrake, and anything else that you or your colleagues may have handled while wearing contaminated gloves. Clean the trolley mounts at least once a week to get rid of any unseen dirt that tends to accumulate there. Disinfect the phones and microphones as a matter of routine which you are bound to handle while wearing contaminated gloves.

Disinfect or replace your pen often. Typically, you handle it several times during every call, with your gloves on. Then, you handle it after the call, after you've washed your hands. Likewise, disinfect your stethoscope with alcohol after every call.

Decontamination of equipment and supplies that have been exposed to body substances requires a different cleansing routine than just soap and water. First, any piece of equipment that is intended for single use should be discarded in an appropriate clinical waste bag. Second, use a commercial disinfecting agent on any piece of equipment that has had direct contact with the patient's skin. Bleach diluted in water (1:10) can also be used as a disinfecting agent. Disinfection kills many of the microorganisms on the surface of your equipment.

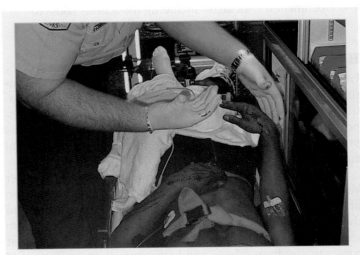

Figure 2-23 Paramedics always need to protect themselves from contact with any type of body fluids.

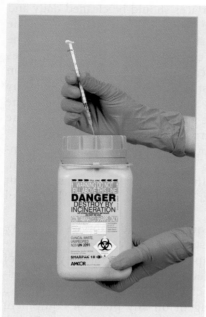

Figure 2-24 Any needles or blades must be disposed of in special bins.

Properly Dispose of Sharps

Disposal bins (large for the ambulance and small for carry-in gear) for sharps, such as needles and blades, are essential to protect crews against needlesticks or cuts **Figure 2-24 ◄**.

Consider Wearing Body Armour

Body armour can be bulky, expensive, and uncomfortable. It's not nearly as protective against bullets as are self-protective avoidance strategies. But it can protect the wearer from many kinds of chest and abdominal trauma from knives.

Management of an Exposure

In the event that you have been exposed to a patient's blood or body fluids, follow your local ambulance service guidelines. Generally, any ambulance service provider who has been exposed should do the following:

- Wash the affected area immediately with soap and water.
- Comply with all reporting requirements.
- Get a medical evaluation.
- Obtain proper immunisation boosters.
- Document the incident, including the actions taken to reduce chances of infection.

Hostile Situations

Until very recently, ambulance service providers were routinely thrust without assistance into situations involving hostile patients who needed to be restrained, treated, and transported against their will. There is a no more dangerous prospect than confronting someone like that without special equipment and plenty of help.

But ambulance service providers are also exposed to other kinds of hostile situations. If the element of hostility is known or can be anticipated in advance, ambulance service crews and their first responders should never be allowed to arrive on scene first. Discipline yourself to scrutinise all information that comes to you from others, and keep yourself on "yellow alert" any time you are on duty. Specifically, beware any call dis-

patched as a fight, stabbing, shooting, domestic disturbance, "collapse", or "abandoned call". Every one of these calls is suspicious and warrants an initial response by police **Figure 2-25 ▼**. In addition, you should have the prerogative to ask for a police response to any call that your intuition says is violent. Whether or not you ask for police backup may depend on your knowledge of the response area and your analysis of the information you receive from your communications centre.

Do not be afraid of being less than a good caregiver if you ask for police to go in first. You will not be able to treat your patient if you are hurt.

You are likely to find your intuition a reliable tool that warrants your trust; and it will become more and more sensitive as you gain experience and additional training.

Once you are in contact with a hostile patient, try hard to listen a lot more than you talk. Avoid arguing. Concentrate on de-escalating his or her emotions, because people who are upset don't listen well and they don't reason well either. (Remember fight-or-flight?) Many hostile patients who started out willing to go to the hospital became unwilling because a crew member couldn't resist a "witty" comment.

Remember that whenever you are on someone else's turf, they have a clear advantage. You can expect them to know everything about their environment while you know nothing (including locations of weapons). Volatile patients in their home environment are much more dangerous there than anywhere else—especially in poor lighting.

Finally, some situations get out of hand due to the paramedic's inability to communicate effectively and build a rapport. Show empathy and understanding on the scene, and you will develop the trust of your patients. Knowledge of diverse

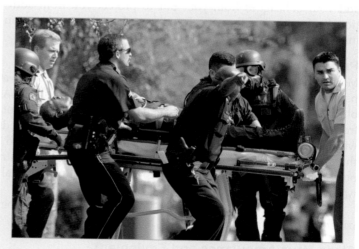

Figure 2-25 Do not hesitate to call for the police if anyone's safety is in question.

cultures plays a major role in effective communication. "Know your audience" is not just a catch phrase for entertainers. The more you know about the people you serve, the more likely you will know their customs and expectations. You must also be diligent in your pursuit of treating all patients with respect and dignity. Put your personal prejudices aside every time you step on the scene.

Traffic Scenes

The most dangerous kinds of calls you will run are the everyday ones, because you naturally get comfortable with them. But regardless of where you are, vehicles move at high speeds, may carry hazardous substances, and may crash into one another in locations that are both dangerous for you and sure to attract spectators. It is important to stay aware of your surroundings, even the familiar ones that you see day in and day out.

Like any scene, your approach to traffic scenes always begins with your familiarity with the response area and your awareness of what the system's other public servants have been doing for the past few hours (because we know you've been paying attention to their frequencies!). This is critical information, because it lets you know your best routing and who might be available to help you with traffic control, air support, hazardous materials, terrain issues, and potential destinations.

Traffic may be only one of the many hazards at the scene of a road traffic collision **Figure 2-26**. The undercarriage of our vehicles are quite hot, especially after travelling 5 to 10 minutes to get to a scene. Parking a hot, running vehicle on the side of the road in dry grass is just inviting a grass fire. Watch where you park, and the type of material you park over, very carefully. If you arrive at a scene in the early morning hours, before the sun starts heating up, and park over a liquid spill long enough, it may trigger combustion of the liquid. Sometimes we create our own hazards by carelessly throwing equipment and its packaging all around us at the scene. Not only can people trip over them but we often lose pieces because they get kicked under the vehicles.

Remember that your primary concern at any scene is safety; safety for yourself as well as for those around you. Identify as many hazards as you can before even leaving your vehicle.

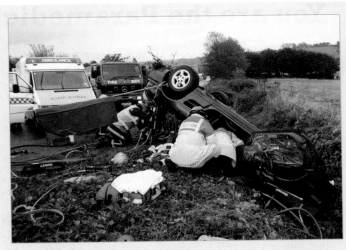

Figure 2-26 At a busy accident scene, it is important to place your vehicle in a safe, visible location, and to minimise the risk of any additional accidents.

Reviewing the scene before leaving your ambulance goes a long way toward identifying hazards such as fire, unstable vehicles or buildings, unruly crowds, or hazardous materials.

Begin making physical observations well before you arrive on the scene. Watch the traffic, pay attention to the wind direction, look for smoke, and begin planning for evolving darkness and for weather-related issues. As you get closer, note the kinds of vehicles and obstacles involved. Make an educated guess about what may have happened. If someone is not yet handling traffic, decide how to control the flow of traffic initially.

How big an incident do you have, both in size and scope? Are you dealing with commercial carriers of industrial products? What resources will you need immediately? What is the topography? Where will fluids drain naturally? Remember that if you do not have a fire on the scene now, it could start quickly as some kinds of fuel begin leaking on hot metal exhaust systems or as a result of electrical arcing.

Where do you eventually want to park? What will your working space be? These are all important considerations, and they will be covered in more detail in Section 7. For now, concentrate more on seeing and protecting the whole scene and not so much on what's wrong with individual patients.

You are the Paramedic Summary

1. What is your main concern at the moment?

Your main concern should be the safety of yourself, your partner, and, finally, your patient. Lifting patients of this size should be performed by an adequate number of responders (no less than four). Your patient is stable, so there is no need for immediate action.

2. What concerns do you have, if any, regarding your partner's behaviour?

It's possible that your partner is having a bad day, is generally disagreeable, or is suffering from burnout. Because you do not know him well yet, it is hard to determine definitively. Employee assistance programmes exist to help responders when they are overwhelmed and in need of help.

3. Does your partner's attitude have any effect on patient care?

He dropped the ball on obtaining essential information regarding this patient's medical history and, most likely, his attitude has affected his patient care on other calls. People suffering from burnout can be more likely to cut corners, make mistakes, and experience problems with colleagues, other medical professionals, and patients. Depending on their condition, these responders may also have difficulty in their personal lives as well.

4. Is this the best course of action?

The best course of action was your first reaction, to call for additional resources. This is appropriate whenever you feel that the number of ambulances, supplies, equipment, or personnel that you have on the scene is inadequate.

5. What is the best way to handle this situation?

Although you might experience grumbling and resistance from your partner, you should tell him that you feel it is unsafe for you and your partner to lift this patient without additional personnel. If you stress the issue of safety, he will likely cooperate with your suggestion.

6. What factors could affect your decisions?

When you are newly recruited, no matter how supportive the service is that you work for, you will be under pressure to perform well. Most services have a probationary period for new members during which you can be fired. Obviously, this is a source of stress. No matter how much you are concerned about your employee evaluation, you must, however, put safety first.

7. What decisions could you have made to prevent this situation?

You could have called for additional resources despite the complaints of your partner. You could have requested aid from other employees within the nursing home. Certified nursing assistants are familiar with appropriate lifting techniques, and with some communication, could aid you in safely moving and lifting the patient. Some departments forbid any nondepartmental personnel from engaging in activities such as this, so always follow local standard operating guidelines.

8. Has patient care been affected?

Obviously, you must obtain information regarding this patient's medical history and reason for transport. To do otherwise could place the patient at risk. Because the patient's condition was stable, patient care was not jeopardised a great deal. However, if the patient's condition changed rapidly and you were not able to care for the patient because of your own pain, patient care could very well have been compromised.

9. What parts of this situation were preventable?

This situation was entirely avoidable. Don't hesitate to protect yourself. In the end, it was your responsibility to speak up regardless of whether or not it would create an uncomfortable situation with your partner.

10. Beyond the physical injuries, what other damage has occurred?

Because you chose to be agreeable rather than use your common sense and instincts, you not only hurt yourself but also your partner and possibly the patient. Beyond the physical injuries and their associated costs (treatment, rehabilitation, and lost work hours and the resultant overtime), you have damaged the image of your department. This last type of injury is very difficult to fix. The patient will remember what happened, and may choose to sue you, your partner, the department, the city, and the hospital. Depending on what transpires, word of this story could travel to outside parties, including local or national newspapers and/or websites.

Prep Kit

■ Ready for Review

■ Paramedics need to know how to ensure their own well-being.

■ Wellness has at least three dimensions: physical, mental, and emotional. It is important to keep all three dimensions healthy and balanced.

■ Nutrition plays a key role in maintaining day-to-day energy and maintaining a healthy body for life.

■ Practise proper lifting techniques to protect your body and lengthen your career.
  - Minimise the number of total body-lifts you have to perform.
  - Coordinate every lift in advance.
  - Minimise the total amount of weight you have to lift.
  - Never lift with your back.
  - Don't carry what you can put on wheels.
  - Ask for help anytime, without embarrassment or hesitation, and offer it liberally to others.

■ Learn how to control stress effectively so that it does not affect your wellness. Take appropriate action. Initial management techniques include:
  - Controlled breathing
  - Reframing
  - Progressive relaxation

■ A patient's reaction to stress may include fear, anxiety, depression, anger, confusion, denial, regression, projection, and displacement. Most of these reactions are not under the patient's conscious control. Remember, in emergency situations, everyone is under stress.

■ Health care professionals are not immune to the stresses of emergency situations and experience a multitude of feelings, not all of them pleasant. These feelings are normal, but it is better to keep them to yourself during an emergency.

■ Burnout is a consequence of chronic, unrelieved stress. Perfectionist beliefs are likely to produce stress.

■ As a paramedic, you will be present when a lot of people are born and you will be there when a lot of people die. Every one of these encounters is an honour.

■ The patient who is dying may be aware of that fact, and may want to talk about it. One of the most important things you can do for a dying patient is to let him or her know that it is OK to talk about it. Be prepared to listen and provide empathy.

■ Debriefings are provided to emergency personnel who have been involved in traumatic calls or other painful incidents.

■ An emergency vehicle is an instrument that can either earn its crew a living or kill them. It deserves respect and it warrants understanding.

■ Protect yourself by washing your hands; using hand lotion; wearing gloves, eye protection, and a mask and gown (when necessary); cleaning your ambulance and equipment; and properly disposing of sharps.

■ Decontamination of equipment and supplies that have been potentially exposed to body substances require a different cleansing routine than just soap and water; sterilisation may be required.

■ Keep yourself on "yellow alert" while you are on duty. Do not be afraid to ask for the police to enter a scene first. You will not be able to treat a patient if you or your partner is hurt.

■ The most dangerous calls are your everyday ones because you become comfortable with them and let down your guard.

■ Your primary concern at any scene is safety—safety for yourself as well as those around you.

■ Vital Vocabulary

alarm reaction The body's first, "startle" response to a stressor.

alert response The first reaction in the alarm reaction, in which you immediately stop whatever you are doing and focus on the source of the stimulus.

blind panic A fear reaction in which a person's judgement seems to disappear entirely; it is particularly dangerous because it may precipitate mass panic among others.

body substance isolation (BSI) An infection control concept and practice that assumes that all body fluids are potentially infectious.

burnout The exhaustion of physical or emotional strength.

conversion hysteria A reaction in which a person subconsciously transforms his or her anxiety into a bodily dysfunction; the person may be unable to see or hear or may become partially paralysed.

critical incident An event that overwhelms the ability to cope with the experience, either at the scene or later.

defence mechanisms Psychological ways to relieve stress; they are usually automatic or subconscious. Defence mechanisms include denial, regression, projection, and displacement.

denial An early response to a serious medical emergency, in which the severity of the emergency is diminished or minimised. Denial is the first coping mechanism for people who believe they are going to die.

displacement Redirection of an emotion from yourself to another person.

distress A type of stress that a person finds overwhelming and debilitating.

eustress A type of stress that motivates an individual to achieve.

fight-or-flight syndrome A physiological response to a profound stressor that helps one deal with the situation at hand; features increased sympathetic tone and resulting in dilation of the pupils, increased heart rate, dilation of the bronchi, mobilisation of glucose, shunting of blood away from the gastrointestinal tract and cerebrum, and increased blood flow to the skeletal muscles.

post traumatic stress disorder (PTSD) A delayed stress reaction before an incident, often the result of one or more unresolved issues concerning the incident.

projection Blaming unacceptable feelings, motives, or desires on others.

regression A return to more childish behaviour while under stress.

stress A nonspecific response of the body to any demand made upon it.

stressor Any agent or situation that causes stress.

universal precautions Protective measures that have traditionally been developed by disease control bodies (dcb) for use in dealing with objects, blood, body fluids, or other potential exposure risks of communicable disease.

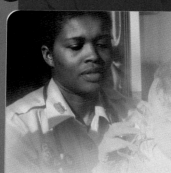

Assessment in Action

On duty, paramedics are expected to be able to perform all the functions of their job. This includes lifting, handling stress, prioritising patient care, assessing the situation quickly and accurately, keeping themselves and their crew safe, controlling chaotic situations, and dealing with grieving family members. In order to do all of these things, paramedics must take care of themselves outside of the job. They need to keep physically fit, know safe lifting techniques, maintain flexibility, eat properly, and much more, as suggested in this book. The following questions pertain to taking care of yourself in order to perform your job at the highest level you can.

1. **Wellness has how many defined dimensions?**
   A. Two—physical and mental
   B. Three—physical, mental, emotional
   C. Three—physical, mental, and spiritual
   D. Four—physical, mental, emotional, and spiritual

2. **Which of these is NOT recommended for ambulance service providers to help themselves stay fit and prepared for their job duties?**
   A. Carrying bottled water instead of buying soft drinks during shifts
   B. Making sure to take vitamins daily
   C. Eating several small, nutritious snacks
   D. Minimising intake of caffeine

3. **During any given shift you go on approximately seven calls that involve moving quickly, lifting patients, and other related movement. Does this meet the criteria for "regular vigorous exercise"?**
   A. Yes. It gets your heart rate up and exercises various muscles several times during shifts.
   B. No. Regular vigorous exercise means approximately 30 minutes of cardiovascular exercise involving various muscle groups four to five times a week.

4. **What is the suggested exercise programme for ambulance service providers?**
   A. Muscle size improvement, cardiovascular endurance, and lifting capabilities
   B. Cardiovascular endurance, flexibility, and physical strength
   C. Flexibility, increasing amounts of weight able to be lifted, and cardiovascular endurance
   D. Physical strength, cardiovascular strength, and concentration on developing muscles most frequently injured in the ambulance service

5. **True or false? Fight-or-flight syndrome can always help in the ambulance service by giving you the energy boost you need to handle a crisis situation.**
   A. True
   B. False

6. **True or false? There is good stress (eustress) and bad stress (distress).**
   A. True
   B. False

7. **Which one of the following is NOT a reaction identified as occurring in multiple-casualty incidents?**
   A. Overreaction—talking or joking inappropriately or racing from one task to another without accomplishing anything
   B. Blind panic—person's judgement seems to disappear entirely
   C. Coping—finding small ways to cope with a situation
   D. Conversion hysteria—patient or bystander subconsciously converts own anxiety into a bodily dysfunction

8. **A patient with serious internal injuries asks you point blank, "Am I going to die?" What would be the best response to this question?**
   A. Be honest, and say that the outlook is not good.
   B. Reassure her that things will be fine.
   C. Be honest but reserved. Assure her that you and all other medical personnel will do your very best to take care of her, but that the situation is serious.
   D. Avoid the question by explaining each procedure you perform on the way to the hospital.

9. **Which of the following is NOT a suggested guideline for helping a grieving family cope with their loved one's death?**
   A. Do not try to hide the body of their loved one from them; give them time alone with the body if requested.
   B. Do not be in a hurry to clear away all resuscitation equipment that was used. Let them see everything possible was done to save their loved one.
   C. Use softer words to present the information, such as "he passed away" or "he's expired".
   D. Accept any feelings the family may go through in your presence, including anger directed toward you.

Challenging Questions

10. If you cannot easily stay up late at night, be alert during the night, or get up early, can you still successfully work in the ambulance service?

11. List some activities and approaches that will help you keep a positive perspective while working in a stressful field.

12. A common reaction among ambulance service providers is irritation at being called to help a patient who does not seem particularly ill. When you receive this kind of call, what should you consider?

■ Points to Ponder

You are called to the home of a frequent caller for the general complaint of "not feeling well". This person usually calls when she is depressed and lonely, and does not usually have any medical conditions that you can treat. Sometimes, after talking, she says she feels better and refuses transport. Your partner is familiar with her as well. Because of past situations, your partner says you should take your time getting to the scene, neither of you should waste a pair of gloves going in because she is never ill or injured, and the two of you should get through the call as quickly as possible so that you can respond to those who actually need help.

Should you listen to your partner? Should you wear gloves?

Issues: Treating Each Patient, Serving as a Role Model for Scene Safety, Empathy, Working With Other Providers.

3 Illness and Injury Prevention

Objectives

Cognitive

- Describe the incidence, morbidity, and mortality of unintentional and alleged unintentional events.
- Identify the human, environmental, and socio-economic impact of unintentional and alleged unintentional events.
- Identify health hazards and potential crime areas within the community.
- Identify local municipal and community resources available for physical, socio-economic crises.
- List the general and specific environmental parameters that should be inspected to assess a patient's need for preventative information and direction.
- Identify the role of the ambulance service in local municipal and community prevention programmes.
- Identify the local prevention programmes that promote safety for all age populations.
- Identify patient situations where the paramedic can intervene in a preventative manner.
- Document primary and secondary injury prevention data.

Affective

- Value and defend tenets of prevention in terms of personal safety and wellness.
- Value and defend tenets of prevention for patients and communities being served.
- Value the contribution of effective documentation as one justification for funding of prevention programmes.
- Value personal commitment to success of prevention programmes.

Psychomotor

- Demonstrate the use of protective equipment appropriate to the environment and scene.

Table 3-1	Childhood Motor Vehicle Occupant Injuries Using the Haddon Matrix		
	Host (Human)	**Agent (Car Seat/Vehicle)**	**Environment**
Pre-event	• Wear seatbelt and use car seat at all times. • Make sure babysitter, day care, and extended family members use car seat. • Drive defensively. • Reduce driving during high-risk times, such as rush hour, holiday weekends, or high-speed long distance travel.	• Maintain up-to-date recall information on car seats. • Manufacture easy-to-use car seats. • Provide 3-point seatbelts in rear seating positions. • Regulate good maintenance and safety features of vehicle.	• Enforce seatbelt and car seat laws. • Encourage safer roads with lower speeds and central reservations. • Encourage low-cost car seat programmes. • Conduct media and education campaigns about seatbelts, car seats, driving under the influence of alcohol, and enforcement.
Event	• Driver maintains control of vehicle. • Driver is belted. • Child is restrained.	• Seatbelts and correctly fitted car seats restrain and protect. • Vehicle design provides accident protection.	• Breakaway signs and light poles are in place. • Crash barriers and central reservations are in place.
Post-event	• Bystanders are trained in first response. • Ambulance service personnel are expertly trained in treating paediatric injuries as well as car seat and seatbelt extrications.	• Ambulances are outfitted with up-to-date supplies and equipment designed for children.	• Roadside call boxes are in place. • 999 and emergency medical dispatch systems are in place. • Adequate road shoulders for emergency use are in place. • There is quality ambulance service response and transport. • A hospital equipped to deal with major trauma is nearby.

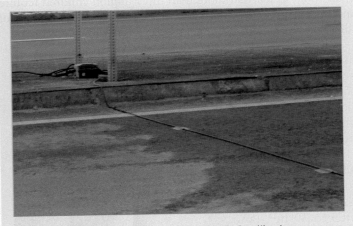

Figure 3-7 One type of surveillance that is familiar to anyone who drives is the use of technology that can tally the number of cars using a particular roadway.

will give you and your community a good feeling to address a problem that will have the maximum impact on the community's well-being.

Recognising Injury Patterns in Your Community

To be effective in prevention, you need to understand the patterns of injuries that occur in your community and learn the

Documentation and Communication

Good documentation on prehospital care reports allows for more consistencies in data gathering, surveillance, and predictions of injury trends.

characteristics of its population and environment and the types of risks that are present. Your ambulance service or public health department will have the most data about injury statistics and is a good starting place to gather information. Many trusts have this information on the Internet. There are a wide variety of other resources readily available online, including detailed information about specific problems, case studies, and expert assistance.

Intentional Injuries

Intentional injuries include suicides and suicide attempts, murders, nonfatal batterings, violent assaults on women (including rapes and domestic abuse), and child and elder abuse.

Ambulance service providers are frequently called to treat the victims of assault. In England and Wales, 2002–03, there were 1,045 murders and 140,000 reported cases of deliberate self harm, including 3,499 cases of suicide. Alarmingly, the use of firearms resulted in 572 serious injuries **Figure 3-8 ▶**. Certain factors emerge as numerically connected with intentional

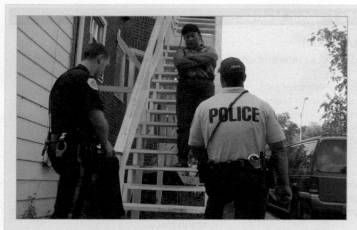

Figure 3-8 Intentional injuries include all cases of domestic and child abuse. As citizens and medical professionals, we are obliged to report all incidents of abuse or potentially abusive situations.

Table 3-2	Top Seven Causes of Deaths from Unintentional Injuries in 2004

1. Transport accidents
2. Falls
3. Accidental exposure to unspecified factor
4. Accidental drowning and submersion
5. Other causes
6. Exposure to smoke, fire, and flames
7. Accidental poisoning by and exposure to noxious substances

Source: Adapted from Health Protection in the 21st Century—10 Injuries (2004).

At the Scene

Remember, you are also a member of "the public" so practice a safe lifestyle on and off the job. Wear seatbelts, safety helmets, and observe safety laws in everything you do.

violence: being male, access to firearms, alcohol abuse, history of childhood abuse, mental illness, and poverty. These are all risk factors—characteristics that increase the chances of disease or injury.

It is often overwhelming to consider solutions when the challenges are linked to deeply rooted social ills. How can ambulance service personnel prevent intentional violence when it is clear that the scope of the problem is a wide one?

One way ambulance service providers have played important supporting roles in programmes that seek to reduce suicide, domestic violence, and child abuse is by carefully reporting data and noting risk factors while on the scene. Also, ambulance service providers can be taught to identify injuries and risk factors associated with domestic violence or child abuse, and report them to the proper authorities.

Remember, you are about to become a paramedic. What you do, your expectations of yourself, and your role will filter down to the other members of your crew. Being a conscientious observer will set an example.

Unintentional Injuries

Unintentional injuries have no premeditation; we often call them accidents. **Table 3-2 ▶** shows the top seven causes of deaths from unintentional injuries in 2004. Transport accidents account for the most unintentional deaths (28%), followed by falls (27%), accidental exposure to unspecified factor (26%), accidental drowning and submersion (9%), other causes (5%), exposure to smoke, fire and flames (3%) and accidental poisoning by and exposure to noxious substances (2%).

Unintentional Injuries in Children

Many prevention programmes have been strongly linked to children, for good reason. Each year 20% to 25% of *all* children sustain an injury sufficiently severe to require medical attention, missing school, and/or require bed rest. Their devel-

oping bodies, including a larger head in proportion to the body, thinner skin, and a smaller airway, put them at higher risk of injury and of being more seriously affected by the injury than adults. Each year more than three million children require medical treatment; in the UK children account for 25–30% of all A&E department attendances. **Figure 3-9 ▾** .

Grants, partners, and commercial sponsors support car seat inspections or donations of bike helmets for children because communities recognise that children are at risk. An additional reason to focus on children's issues is the "pass-along effect". Other family members benefit from the message too, such as when a four-year-old insists that Daddy put his seatbelt on too.

Health promotion initatives such as the SAFEKIDS campaign, coordinated by the Child Accident Prevention Trust with sponsorship from Johnson & Johnson, aim to promote child safety while cycling, rollerblading, skateboarding, etc. The SAFEKIDS scheme emphasises the

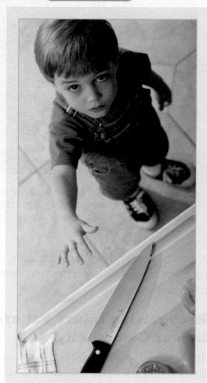

Figure 3-9 Children are at higher risk of sustaining serious injuries from an accident. Parents should always be aware of the potential dangers in reach of a child.

use of protective equipment, such as helmets and pads; SAFEKIDS also aims to encourage any activities that provide positive health benefits in children.

Risk Factors for Children

Children at greatest risk of injury are of lower socio-economic status. The patterns of injury will differ from community to community, but just as the poorest children statistically are at risk of contracting a physiological disease, they are also at risk of injury.

The American CDC reports that home injuries of children occur most frequently where there is/are:

- Water, such as in the kitchen or bathroom.
- Intense heat, such as in the kitchen or a patio barbecue.
- Toxic agents, such as in the kitchen, bathroom, garage, or in a hand bag.
- High potential "energy", such as in stairwells or loaded guns not returned to locked cabinets.

Many community members have a common belief that schools have become more violent and that intentional injuries are an increasing threat to students. However, *unintentional* injuries—accidents—still represent a much greater threat to health.

School injuries occur most frequently during sports activities, industrial arts classes, and on playgrounds. Each year in the UK approximately 40,000 children sustain injuries while playing on playgrounds.

With the wide variety of injuries affecting children, how do we prioritise prevention efforts? Experts in public health suggest focusing on injuries that have high mortality (death) rates or hospitalisation rates, that have a high long-term disability rate, or that have effective countermeasures. The highest priorities are assigned to those types of injuries that are common, severe, and readily preventable.

Community Organising

Those in the ambulance service who have created successful prevention programmes give the following advice as you build your team and create an implementation plan:

- Identify a lead person to coordinate the effort.
- Build as broad a base of support as possible.
- Create a realistic time line for any project, keeping in mind that most must be ongoing to be effective.
- Gather data and facts that pinpoint who is being injured where, with what, and how frequently.

- Choose goals and objectives that are SMART—Simple, Measurable, Accurate, Reportable, and Trackable; build consensus in the community on the need for action.
- Make sure you understand the religious, ethnic, cultural, and language challenges that you may face in implementing an intervention in your community.
- Don't reinvent the wheel—seek out others who have had success with similar interventions or who have expertise in public health.
- Anticipate opposition and expect some losses; turf battles are common but not inevitable.
- As you lobby to legislators, be brief in phone calls, visits, and testimony.
- Set up your programme so that you can measure results and make changes as needed.
- Establish self-sustaining funding sources.
- Keep a sense of humour and persist—change doesn't happen overnight.

At the Scene

For your first project, start small with realistic goals.

The Five Steps to Developing a Prevention Programme

This step-by-step approach to establishing an injury prevention programme has been advocated in the United States by the EMS for Children (EMSC), an American organisation that provides millions of US dollars in funding to injury prevention and research programmes. EMSC emphasises the need to establish goals and objectives carefully, with measurable outcomes. (This method can be applied other age groups and problems.)

1. Conduct a Community Assessment

Bring individuals and groups together to assess what is already being accomplished in your region and to establish what resources (expertise, time, money) are potentially available. Make sure to invite people who represent the community at large, in all its diversity, including survivors of injuries and their families Figure 3-10 ▸ . Potential partners include:

- Out-of-hospital care groups (private and public ground and air ambulance services, fire fighter unions, volunteer services, rescue services, lifeguards)
- Police services

You are the Paramedic Part 3

You have enlisted the help of many different organisations who are now as determined as you are to minimise the recurrence of crashes in this stretch of road. They aid you in performing assessments of the area and making plans to prevent crashes.

4. What groups are potential partners to enlist in a prevention programme in this situation?

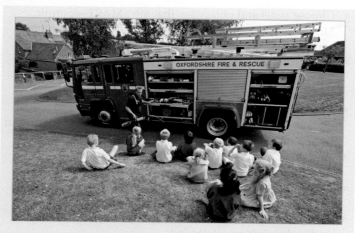

Figure 3-10 An example of an injury prevention programme is training to avoid injury in the event of a fire in the home.

- School groups (parent-teacher associations, student clubs, school governing bodies, staff)
- The media (management, editorial board members, staff reporters)
- Public health officials and health care providers (groups representing emergency doctors and nurses, paediatricians, managed care organisations, hospitals, clinics)
- Members of the business community (including those related to insurance, cars, sports, home improvements, safety equipment, local chambers of commerce)
- Religious organisations, civic groups, and service clubs (such as the Boy Scouts and Girl Guides)
- Sports-related organisations (such as kid's football and rugby clubs or YMCAs)
- Local chapters of nonprofit groups (such as SAFEKIDS Coalitions, British Red Cross, Alzheimer's Society)
- Local and national celebrities, community leaders, and elected officials
- Research groups (such as those at university departments, independent foundations, community colleges)

2. Define the Injury Problem

On the basis of the community assessment and the data you've been able to gather, define the problem in specific quantifiable terms. For example, you should be able to answer the following questions for your community:

- What are the most frequent causes of fatal and nonfatal childhood injuries?
- What populations (by age, location, and other characteristics) are at highest risk of these injuries? When and where are they occurring?
- Using the Haddon matrix, what other factors are associated with these causes?
- What, if anything, is already being done to prevent these injuries?

- Is there an effective intervention available? What resources do you have in order to develop, implement, and evaluate different interventions?

3. Set Goals and Objectives

Goals Make this a broad, general statement about the long-term changes the prevention initiatives are designed to make. (For example, a goal can be to decrease preventable injuries to children on the community's roadways.)

Objectives Make these specific, time-limited, and quantifiable. There are two types: process objectives (1,000 child safety seats will be distributed to low income families within the next 18 months) and outcome (impact) objectives (the bicycle safety programme will increase the rate of helmet use by children younger than 18 years from 30% to 50% within the next 18 months).

4. Plan and Test Interventions

Interventions are the actions you take to accomplish your goals and objectives. Using the 4 Es of prevention and the Haddon matrix, mind-map options. Consider the resources you have available to commit, and make sure you have thoroughly reviewed what others have already done. You may find communities have had success with similar interventions in similar populations. In that case, you can reliably duplicate their efforts as a process objective. (For example, other groups have shown that bike helmets reduce head injuries; you then need only to demonstrate increased usage of helmets in your targeted population.) Experienced prevention specialists also suggest that you be keenly aware of timing and cultural considerations as you plan your intervention. Getting a sample group together and testing the intervention before actually rolling out the entire programme usually helps to improve your chances of success.

5. Implement and Evaluate Interventions

To be credible, your intervention needs to be established so that the results can be measured quantitatively; that is, a formal evaluation will definitively tell you whether you met your goals and objectives. One American out-of-hospital service knew from previous surveys that the seatbelt usage rate in their community was well below the national average. They established an objective of improving seatbelt usage in their community by 50%. Working with the department of public health in their county, they enacted a series of prevention programmes. To measure the effectiveness of different interventions, they put volunteers at selected junctions around the city. They counted physically, with a clicker, every belted and nonbelted motorist who stopped in front of them. This is extremely important so that your experience can be shared with others. You want to spend your time and resources on efforts you can *show* make a difference. There is a science to planning, implementing, and evaluating an intervention. Seek out others who have knowledge and experience in this facet of injury prevention; it will make for a better programme.

Finally, be aware that many if not most interventions demand ongoing attention to be effective. In one American state, EMS providers who had initial success in reducing drownings in

Assessment in Action

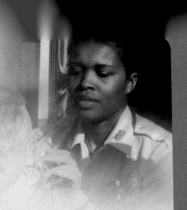

Each year, more than 10,000 people die as a direct result of trauma in the UK, and over half a million will sustain injuries severe enough to require hospital admission. There are several things, besides treating injuries, that the paramedic can do to cut down on the number of injuries sustained each year. There is also information about injuries that is important for all paramedics to know. The following questions concern the information that is important to know, and what things paramedics and other health care professionals can do to cut down on the number of injuries sustained each year.

1. **Paramedics are responsible for many duties. However, what is the number one priority of paramedics in their community?**
   A. To be ready to stop and help, whether off duty or on duty.
   B. To be prepared to respond and treat injuries that will inevitably occur in their community.
   C. To make sure their skills are always up-to-date.
   D. To make sure they are good role models in their community.

2. **Injuries are defined by the National Center for Injury Prevention and Control as:**
   A. intentional or unintentional.
   B. resulting from exposure to thermal, mechanical, electrical, or chemical energy.
   C. resulting from the absence of essentials such as heat or oxygen.
   D. all of the above.

3. **One way to measure the cost of injuries to society and the full impact of injury and disease is by using the concept of years of potential life lost. This means:**
   A. assume a productive life until age 65 years for all people, then deduct the year of age at death.
   B. estimate how long that person would have lived given his or her socio-economic background and genetic makeup, then subtract that number from his or her age at death.
   C. factor in all the patient's health issues at the time of death and estimate how long he or she may have lived based on that information.
   D. compare the cost to society of injuries versus other diseases.

4. **The most successful interventions need to combine education with three other factors. What are they?**
   A. Enforcement, persuasion, modelling of safe behaviour
   B. Legislation, litigation, regulation
   C. Regulatory change, behavioural feedback, economic incentives
   D. Enforcement, engineering/environment, economic incentives

5. **The public health model identifies three influences that cause a health problem. What are they?**
   A. Disease, heredity, lifestyle
   B. Host, agent, environment
   C. Accidents, murders, suicides
   D. Noneducation, bad lifestyle choices, not using safety measures such as seatbelts

6. **A doctor developed a method to help find ways to prevent people from being killed on highways. He identified several principles of injury prevention and summarised them in a matrix. The host, agent, and environment are seen as factors that interact over time to cause injury. The factors correspond to three phases of the event: pre-event, event, post-event. The matrix discusses nine separate components that contribute to injury. This matrix encourages creative thinking in understanding injury causes and potential interventions. Who was this person, and what is the matrix called?**
   A. William Haddon, Jr, MD; the Haddon matrix
   B. Paul Maxwell; the Maxwell matrix
   C. Ricardo Martinez, MD; the Martinez matrix
   D. Frank Holden; the Holden matrix

7. **Passive interventions in preventing injuries are things such as:**
   A. making seatbelt use a law and adding crash barriers to the sides of hazardous roads.
   B. putting safety caps on medicine bottles and putting air bags in cars.
   C. offering monetary discounts for safe driving records.
   D. offering educational classes such as CPR and safe babysitting classes often.

Challenging Questions

8. **You are given the statistics for accidental falls in your town, and asked to develop a plan that may reduce the number of falls, given your experience as a paramedic. List some ideas to help reduce the number of falls in your area in the year ahead?**

9. **What could you and other health care professionals do to decrease the number of people in your area who contract diseases such as measles, tuberculosis (TB), hepatitis, and influenza?**

Objectives

Cognitive

- Differentiate between legal and ethical responsibilities.
- Describe the structure of the legal system in the United Kingdom.
- Differentiate between civil and criminal law as it pertains to ambulance personnel.
- Identify and explain the importance of laws pertinent to ambulance personnel.
- Differentiate between certification, registration and regulation as they apply to ambulance personnel including paramedics.
- List the specific problems or conditions that ambulance personnel may encounter while providing care and that they are required to report.
- Define the following terms:
  - Advance directives
  - Assault
  - Battery
  - Breach of duty
  - Confidentiality
  - Consent
  - Defamation
  - Do not attempt resuscitation (DNAR) orders
  - Duty of care
  - False imprisonment
  - Immunity
  - Liability
  - Libel
  - Minor
  - Negligence
  - Nuisance
  - Proximate cause
  - Scope of practice
  - Slander
  - Standard of care
  - Tort/delict
  - Trespass
  - Vicarious liability
- Differentiate between the scope of practice and the standard of care for clinical practice.
- Discuss the concept of medical direction, including remote access medical direction and on scene medical support, and its relationship to the standard of care of ambulance personnel.
- Describe the four elements that must be present in order to prove negligence.
- Critically review scenarios in which patients are injured while ambulance personnel are providing care, to determine whether negligence has occurred.
- Using case presentations, identify patient care behaviours that may protect ambulance personnel from claims of negligence.
- Explain the concept of liability as it applies to ambulance personnel.
- Discuss the legal concept of immunity as it applies to ambulance personnel.

- Explain the importance and necessity of patient confidentiality and the standards for maintaining patient confidentiality that apply to ambulance personnel.
- Differentiate between expressed, informed, and implied consent.
- Describe the process used to obtain consent when caring for conscious and unconscious patients.
- Identify the steps to take where patients refuse care.
- Critically review patient management and communication techniques that may prove useful when dealing with refusal of care situations.
- Describe the concept of duty of care as it relates to clinical practice.
- Identify the legal issues involved in decisions not to transport patients, and decisions to reduce the level of care being provided during transport.
- Describe how hospitals are selected to receive patients based on patient need and hospital capability and capacity, and the role of ambulance personnel in such selection.
- Differentiate between assault and battery and describe how to avoid each.
- Describe the conditions under which the use of force, including restraint, is acceptable.
- Explain the purpose of advance directives in relation to patient care and how ambulance personnel should care for patients who are covered by advance directives.
- Discuss the responsibilities of ambulance personnel in relation to resuscitation efforts for patients who are potential organ donors.
- Describe the actions that ambulance personnel should take to preserve evidence at scenes of crime or incident scenes.
- Describe the importance of providing accurate documentation in relation to incidents and care delivered.
- Describe the characteristics of patient records required to make them effective legal documents.
- Using case presentations prepare concise and effective patient records.
- Describe the components of effective clinical records, and their importance as legal documents.

Affective

- Critically assess personal attitudes towards patient care and the importance of demonstrating respect for the rights and feelings of patients.
- Critically assess personal commitment to protecting patient confidentiality.
- Explain the importance of obtaining consent for adult patients and those who are minors.
- Critically assess personal beliefs regarding withholding treatment or stopping patient care episodes.
- Critically assess the role of advance directives and personal attitudes towards them.

Psychomotor

None

Introduction

All medical providers who provide care must do so in accordance with the laws of the land and ensure that respect for individual choice, privacy, and dignity are maintained. On joining the profession, paramedics are also governed by legal and professional rules that affect how they must treat patients. Ethical responsibilities, which underpin the clinical care of patients and the decision-making process, differ from legal obligations in a number of ways. Ethics are principles, both personal and societal, that are involved in providing justification for actions taken and relate to the degree of rightness or wrongness involved Figure 4-1 ▶ . A key difference between law and ethics is that laws involve sanctions for violation that are enforceable by the courts whereas ethics impose no such sanctions. Registrant bodies may, however, consider the appropriateness and ethical basis of behaviour when considering allegations of poor practice while laws define obligations and protect the rights and welfare of citizens. Ambulance personnel responding to emergencies work within a framework comprising various laws that are laid down by the government through statutes.

Paramedics may find themselves called to court to provide evidence of their involvement in patient care situations and to relay their clinical findings in cases under investigation, or to testify regarding their role in litigation claims involving complaints or claims of alleged negligence Figure 4-2 ▶ . It is here that the importance of accurate, complete, and contemporaneous clinical records is most evident, and should never be underestimated.

It is essential, therefore, that ambulance personnel have an understanding of the law as it applies to emergency care. Failing to perform their role within the confines of the law can result in civil liability, rendering ambulance personnel including paramedics and their employing bodies potentially liable for claims of alleged negligence or misconduct, or criminal liability in the

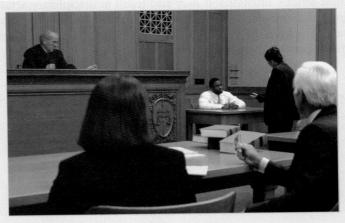

Figure 4-1 Laws are enforceable rules that all citizens are obliged to follow.

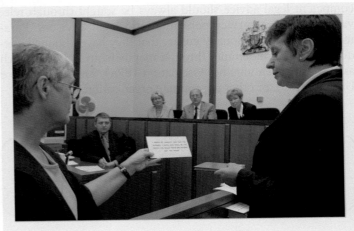

Figure 4-2 Paramedics may be called to court.

You are the Paramedic Part 1

You are dispatched to 28 Wilfred Street to a 63-year-old man who has taken an overdose of his co-codomal medication with five pints of bitter. As your arrive on scene, you are greeted by the neighbours of the patient who had called 999 after he turned up at their doorstep and admitted taking the overdose. You are invited into the living room and find Roland, your patient, reclining on the sofa. He appears sleepy and on seeing you states that he does not want to go to hospital, but be left to die.

Initial Assessment	Recording Time 0 Minutes
Appearance	Lying on sofa, smoking a cigarette. Speaks to you and his neighbours, but slurs his words and looks groggy
Level of consciousness	A (Alert to person, place, and day)
Airway	Open
Breathing	Adequate rate and tidal volume
Circulation	Radial pulse present

1. What are your immediate medical concerns?
2. How might these conflict with the legal, ethical, and professional issues?

most serious situations. It may also result in disciplinary action from the ambulance service and the imposition of a range of sanctions from the Health Professions Council (HPC), the paramedic profession's regulatory body.

At the Scene

The best legal protection is to undertake a careful, detailed patient assessment and appropriate medical care, followed by complete and accurate documentation as soon as possible after the event. The patient should be either taken to definative care, or if transport is declined, left with a competent adult and advice given on how to re-call the ambulance service if the situation changes.

This chapter will focus on the more important legal concepts affecting ambulance personnel, and will provide a framework to develop understanding of their legal responsibilities. This is not, however, a definitive legal reference guide, and competent legal advice should always be sought through relevant ambulance service personnel and legal advisors. Paramedics should additionally ensure that they have obtained adequate personal indemnity through membership of bodies such as the British Paramedic Association (BPA), Medical Defence Union (MDU), or other appropriate organisation.

At the Scene

Many ambulance services have web sites with information on laws that affect paramedics. It is a good idea to review the laws of the country in which you are working.

The Legal System in the United Kingdom

The United Kingdom (UK) comprises Scotland, England, Wales, and Northern Ireland. Its legal system consists of three branches each of which has clearly defined functions and each of which is vested in distinct bodies: the executive, legislative, and judiciary.

The executive generally refers to the Prime Minister and his/her chosen government ministers. The executive is responsible for formulating and executing policies, and for implementing legislation.

The legislative branch refers to Parliament which comprises the Crown, the House of Lords, and the House of Commons, each of which is assigned different tasks. The House of Commons represents the views and grievances of all sections of society, scrutinises the executive and legitimises government actions. The House of Lords provides a forum for debate on matters of public interest, revises Bills from the House of Commons, initiates Bills, considers delegated legislation, scrutinises the executive, and serves as the Supreme Court of Appeal. The Crown retains some powers, invariably those of national interest, most of which are exercised by the executive in the name of the Crown, or are exercised by the Crown under the advice of the executive.

Although laws governing the UK are made in Parliament, some of these powers have been devolved to the constituent countries themselves through Acts of Parliament thus enabling decision and policy-making at a more local level. However, some centrally administered matters, particularly those vital to national interests, remain with the State and the Crown, and cannot be devolved.

The third branch, the judiciary, which comprises the court system, is responsible for interpreting and enforcing laws, and for resolving disputes based upon the interpretation of laws. Several levels exist within the court system including magistrate's court, crown court, high court, and appellate court, and the coroner's court which is of particular interest to paramedics.

Matters concerning health are typically addressed by the Department of Health, with a degree of devolved responsibility to national bodies.

Types of Law

Two kinds of law govern ambulance service practice: civil law under which patients can claim for injuries caused by alleged negligence or substandard care, and criminal law in which prosecutions may be brought for alleged criminal offences such as gross negligence, manslaughter, or instances involving a breach of the law. Negligence or malpractice claims are tried under civil law, while instances involving the misuse of drugs may be tried under criminal law.

A substantial part of civil law is concerned with establishing liability, or responsibility. Where people experience injuries and seek redress for them, the judicial process must determine who was responsible. This may arise where for example, patients or their survivors are dissatisfied with the clinical care that was received. They may believe that inadequate or substandard care led or contributed to a poor outcome, and that the actions of the ambulance personnel were in some way responsible. People have a constitutional right to take legal action against doctors, nurses, paramedics, ambulance personnel or other involved parties. However, the parties bringing the claim must prove that the clinical providers in question caused harm by failing to provide care that met accepted standards of practice. Poor outcomes alone do not prove negligence; rather all components of negligence must be satisfied for actions to be successful.

Legal action of this sort is known as a civil claim, ie, an action instituted by private individuals or corporations (the claimants) against other private individuals or corporations (the defendants). The wrongful act that gives rise to a civil claim is referred to as a tort in England, Wales, and Northern Ireland, and as a delict in Scotland. The primary objective of a civil claim is typically some form of financial compensation,

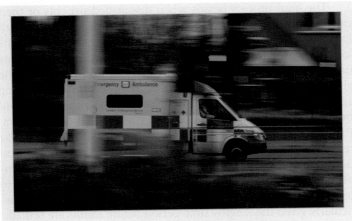

Figure 4-3 The majority of civil claims against ambulance personnel arise from emergency vehicle collisions.

At the Scene

The distinction between civil and criminal law is reflected in the court structure and lies in the actions or consequences that may follow proceedings. Breach of the criminal law may be followed by prosecution in the criminal courts, whereas liability in civil law is actionable in the civil courts and may or may not constitute a crime.

usually <u>damages</u>, for the injury the claimant sustained, although explanations or apologies often suffice, with assurances given of practice changes to prevent future recurrences. In addition to seeking compensation for physical injury, claimants may also claim for psychiatric injury or harm caused through pain, suffering, and loss of amenity. To succeed in civil claims, claimants must satisfy the legal burden of proof, ie, on a balance of probabilities, whereas the burden of proof in criminal cases is somewhat higher and requires claimants to prove their case beyond a reasonable doubt.

A number of claims against ambulance personnel results from emergency vehicle collisions. The importance of safe driving and its relation to personal health and well-being should, therefore, not be underestimated nor should it be forgotten that safe driving is the key to preventing such claims. Road traffic collisions (RTCs) are all too common and, each year, cause serious harm to patients, bystanders, and ambulance personnel, as well as resulting in expensive property damage **Figure 4-3 ▲** .

Other types of claims against ambulance personnel are also prevalent with numerous instances arising each year. Many relate to dispatch and transport issues involving delayed response, cases of non-conveyance where patients are not transported and their condition subsequently deteriorates; or involve the quality of clinical care provided by ambulance personnel while on scene or on route to definitive care.

Sometimes the same alleged wrongful or harmful acts that gave rise to civil claims may also result in <u>criminal prosecutions</u>. This may arise in response to actions where the defendants are believed to have violated criminal laws. The criminal laws most likely to apply in prehospital care situations include assault, battery, and false imprisonment. These typically arise in response to complaints about the behaviour of paramedics, for example involving the improper use of restraints, not obtaining consent before touching patients or making physical contact with them, or transporting patients against their will **Figure 4-4 ▶** .

In cases of assault, battery, and false imprisonment, there may also be grounds for civil actions, although claims of this nature against ambulance personnel are rare. It is important to note that <u>assault</u> is said to occur when one person instills the fear or threat of immediate bodily harm or breach of bodily security in another, and does not require this threat to be carried out, ie, it does not require any physical contact or touching. <u>Battery</u>, on the other hand, occurs when the defendant actually touches another person or interferes with his or her bodily integrity, without first obtaining consent. Virtually all clinical actions and interventions carry the risk of constituting either assault or battery, for most involve a real or perceived risk of violating patients' bodily integrity. Communicating clearly and effectively, ensuring patient understanding, and obtaining informed consent are, therefore, essential for all actions taken.

This also applies to situations involving <u>false imprisonment</u> which occur when people are intentionally and unjustifiably detained against their will. In prehospital care, charges of false imprisonment may arise where ambulance personnel transport patients to hospital or other facilities without their consent, or use restraints inappropriately or improperly. Where

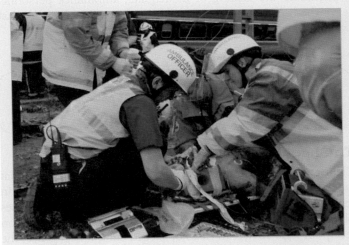

Figure 4-4 Most criminal cases focus on the behaviour of ambulance personnel during calls. The best deterrent to prevent legal action in such cases is to ensure that all actions taken are in the best interests of patients, to ensure that patients' needs remain your first priority, and to document all actions and interventions accurately as soon as possible after the event.

restraints are considered necessary, it may be advisable to seek the assistance of the police to ensure safe handling of the situation. As previously stated, it is essential to obtain informed consent for all actions taken; where this proves to be impossible it is not only good practice but also advisable from a professional perspective to ensure that a second ambulance provider or emergency team member acts as a witness.

Ambulance personnel may also find themselves charged with defamation, which is the intentional making of a false statement through written or verbal communication that injures the good name or reputation of another person. Libel refers to situations involving *written* false statements, or statements that are made in other permanent forms such as email or fax. When completing clinical records it is important to ensure that only clinically relevant information is included, and that terms that may be considered insulting or offensive are omitted, such as "the patient appears to be drunk". Whatever subjective or personal views may be held, the clinical record is a legal document that may later be relied upon in court, and should be treated as such.

Slander refers to the *verbal* making of false statements that injure another person's good name or reputation. As with libel, terms that could be considered offensive to the patient should be avoided when communicating information to emergency department personnel or other clinical colleagues.

How Laws Affect Ambulance Personnel

In recent years the public has become aware of the increasing capabilities of ambulance personnel. Where ambulance responses are perceived as delayed or the efforts of its personnel considered incompetent, the public will often file claims seeking compensation for injuries that they believe were caused by inadequate or substandard care or treatment. Where explanations are lacking or inadequate, ambulance personnel leave themselves open to criticism and possible reprisal, that could ultimately find its way into the courtroom.

At the Scene

Courteous, honest, and professional behaviour and actions will prevent most patients from complaining or proceeding with a filed claim.

The Legal Process: Anatomy of a Claim

Claims typically arise as a consequence of adverse outcomes that are either real or perceived as such by patients or their carers. In many cases, realisation of claims or potential claims only takes place months or years after the events in question, often upon receipt of legal advice. In cases of alleged clinical negligence, the limitation period ie, the time limit within which claims can be brought, is three years although this may be extended in certain circumstances. These include cases involving people who are incapable by reason of mental disorder (for as long as they remain under such a disability), and children, who have a three-year period from their 18th birthday in which to bring claims based on events that arose during their age of minority.

The legal process begins when dissatisfied patients or their carers seek advice from solicitors who in turn file claims with local courts on their behalf. These contain the allegations lodged against the ambulance personnel in question, but may not contain specific details. All named parties involved in the allegation are required to respond, although in cases involving ambulance personnel it is likely that the ambulance service will be named as the defendant and not individual pracitioners. Paramedics or other involved personnel will, however, be required to provide statements relating to the events in question. Accurate and comprehensive documentation that is completed as soon as possible after the original event will prove to be invaluable in defending claims, and to recalling events particularly given the lengthy time period before claims are settled.

Responses, or answers to complaints will be filed by the solicitor representing the ambulance service. A discovery period then follows, during which time solicitors on both sides seek to learn as much about the case as possible. Written documents including the patient's clinical records are exchanged outlining questions that must be answered by the parties under oath, and depositions or statements taken under oath. Many cases are settled out of court through mediation proceedings, thus avoiding the expense and stress associated with trials and arduous court proceedings, and the inevitable pressures and difficulties associated with protecting personal and professional reputations.

Ambulance personnel who find themselves on the receiving end of such claims must ensure that they remain in close contact with their clinical supervisors and managers, not only to provide additional information that may be required but also to ensure that they remain supported throughout the process. Given that paramedics are recognised as professionals in their own right, they would be well advised to obtain personal professional indemnity through organisations such as the British Paramedic Association or the Medical Defence Union.

At the Scene

Many cases are settled either inside or outside of the courtroom, a significant proportion of which are based on absent or inadequate documentation. This may prevent a complete defence, rather than signifying negligence on the part of practitioners.

Legal Accountability of Paramedics

Accountability refers to the extent to which individuals can be held to account for their actions, and encompasses legal, professional, moral, and ethical arenas. Although there is some overlap with responsibility, the concepts differ in that responsibility refers to liability to be called to account whereas accountability refers to being answerable or accountable for actions, omissions or decisions taken. Of particular concern to ambulance personnel and paramedics are legal and professional accountability, and their awareness and knowledge of the limits to their practice that are imposed on them by the law, particularly given increased public knowledge of complaints, litigation procedures, and access to legal representation.

All ambulance personnel are directly accountable to their employer, the ambulance service, and to their clinical director in relation to clinical standards and procedures. As professionals in their own right, paramedics have an extra line of accountability, with the addition of their professional and/or governing body. As such, paramedics are held accountable for their actions; however the service itself will be held accountable for ensuring the provision of adequate training, education, and supervision of its staff and for failing to take action in response to poor performance or incompetence. Such actions may include restriction of clinical activities or the practitioner's scope until competence has been achieved and remedial training or recertification is undertaken.

The Health Professions Council (HPC) regulates paramedic practice and is responsible for laying down clinical and professional standards. All clinical interventions and decisions taken must be based on doing what is best for patients, and acting in their best interests. Paramedics and other ambulance personnel, who have this principle as their goal and who ensure that they follow established national clinical guidelines, are likely to be able to defend their actions and thus be well protected against allegations of negligence or misconduct.

All paramedics are required to act in accordance with their professional and clinical standards and to perform to the level of the *reasonable* paramedic; similar rulings apply to other ambulance personnel with ambulance technicians judged with reference to the standard of a *reasonable* ambulance technician and so on.

At the Scene

Where it is considered necessary to deviate from guidelines, advice must first be sought from medical or clinical directors of the relevant ambulance service. This must be documented in the patient's clinical record or the patient report form (PRF).

Scope of Practice

Only those activities for which ambulance personnel have been trained and deemed competent and which are authorised by their employer, and regulatory body in the case of paramedics, can be said to be within their *scope of practice*.

The Standards of Proficiency that underpin the paramedic scope of practice are issued by the Health Professions Council, while the detailed clinical content of their application can be found in national clinical guidelines and associated training manuals. Ambulance technicians do not have an associated scope of practice document as they are not professionals in their own right. They are, however, required to follow national protocols and guidelines which govern their practice. Where paramedics carry out procedures or otherwise practise beyond their scope

You are the Paramedic Part 2

You and your colleague attempt to persuade the patient to come with you to hospital. Despite adopting various techniques, including explaining the consequences of leaving his current condition untreated, Roland still refuses to come with you or let you perform any observations. He threatens to hit you if you don't "get out of my face" and leave. On hearing this, your colleague moves into the hall and calls for police backup.

Vital Signs	Recording Time: 15 Minutes after Arrival
Level of consciousness	Glasgow Coma Scale score of 15
Skin	Appears normal
Pulse	Unable to assess
Blood pressure	Unable to measure
Respirations	12 breaths/min
Oxygen saturation	Unable to measure

3. If you left scene now, would you be in breach of your duty of care?

4. Could the patient's threat be seen as assault?

of practice or level of competence, they are considered as acting outwith their clinical scope or sphere of responsibility, and as such are liable to sanctions from both their employing ambulance service and possibly their regulatory body.

Data Protection Act 1998

Those who care for patients are given information that would not be disclosed to them in any other circumstances. This information is required to ensure that a clinical diagnosis can be reached and a treatment plan formulated, and to ensure that patients receive the required treatment. In order to reveal this information, patients must know that it will be held secure and will not be disclosed to third parties, exceptions being only those situations where disclosure is required by law or by virtue of being in the patient's best interests, the latter being restricted to those who are closely involved in the patient's care.

This duty of confidentiality is supplemented by statutes such as the Data Protection Act 1998 which enable the law to protect the privacy rights of individuals in respect of their personal data, such data referring to any information relating to identified or identifiable persons. The law regulates the processing of such data by reference to principles that, among other things, ensure that data is only processed so far as it is fair and lawful to do so and only so far as it is necessary for the purposes for which it was obtained. From the ambulance service perspective, it is thus unacceptable for prehospital reports or other clinical data to be left in public areas or to be otherwise accessible to those who have no need to know the information contained therein for the reasons stated above. It is also unacceptable to discuss or share patient-sensitive or patient-identifiable information in public fora without that patient's consent.

In health care organisations such as those involving ambulance service personnel, these principles are often encapsulated within the auspices of clinical governance. A senior executive of ambulance trusts is also typically assigned the role of Caldicott Guardian, with ultimate responsibility for ensuring that all patient identifiable information is dealt with appropriately.

The Freedom of Information Act 2000

The Freedom of Information Act 2000 which gives patients a right of access to information held by public authorities, such as ambulance services and other National Health Service (NHS) bodies, came into force in 2005. Requests for access to personal data are, however, inappropriate under this Act and should instead be brought under the Data Protection Act 1998. Requests for access to material containing information that would identify other individuals would also be refused where disclosure would breach data protection principles or the common law duty of confidence. Exceptions that would restrict access to such information include information provided in confidence and legal professional privilege.

Emergency Vehicle Laws

Statutes define those vehicles that may be determined emergency vehicles and outline the rules that should be followed and adhered to when driving such vehicles and when being approached by them. It is essential to remember that these statutes still require emergency vehicles to be operated in a safe and prudent manner, and do not offer exemptions from offences of reckless, dangerous or careless driving, or from driving without reasonable consideration for other road users. Laws governing emergency vehicle operation do not authorise speeding or ignoring red lights, or driving vehicles in an unsafe manner.

Vehicles being used for emergency ambulance purposes may treat red light signals as "give way" signs where observance of the red lights is likely to hinder their use and purpose. They may also ignore keep left and keep right signs, but only in a manner or at times not likely to cause danger to anyone. Similarly, statutory speed limits do not apply to emergency vehicles where observance of those limits would hinder their emergency purpose. The prohibition on sounding audible warning instruments while stationary or in built up areas between the hours of 23:00 and 07:00 is also lifted when emergency vehicles are being used for relevant purposes, and where it is necessary or desirable to do so to indicate to other road users the urgency of the purpose or to warn other road users of the presence of the vehicle on the road.

In the event of road traffic collisions involving the ambulance service, ambulance personnel may find themselves to have been at fault and thus the subject of civil actions, or even criminal prosecution in particularly serious situations. Ambulance personnel must, therefore, ensure vigilance to the rules of road safety and courtesy and must not ignore these obligations in their haste to reach their destination.

Immunity

Generally speaking, members of the community who stop to volunteer their services at the scene of incidents or emergencies will be immune from liability in the event of possible claims. As laypersons with no duty of care to the victim(s), they would incur no liability for omissions to act, but having stopped to help they would be expected to do the best that they could to help, and would be considered as acting instinctively due to their moral or social conscience. The situation regarding off-duty ambulance personnel is, however, somewhat different.

In these situations, ambulance personnel are not under a legal duty of care to the victim(s) as they are not operating in the course of their employment. Having stopped to help, however, the standard of care that would be expected of them would be the same as that which would have been expected had they been on duty, albeit within the confines of medical equipment available to them at that time. Although under no legal obligation to stop to help, they may feel under a moral obligation (beyond that felt by an ordinary layperson) to assist given their level of knowledge and skill. Having embarked upon this course of action, they have accepted a duty of care, a duty that they are obligated to perform until further professional help arrives. Should paramedics be faced with untoward events resulting from their intervention (ie, a "Good Samaritan" act), they may be covered by personal indemnity that they have taken out with the British Paramedic Association (BPA) Medical Defence Union (MDU) or similar organisation.

Other Kinds of Immunity
Crown Immunity and Crown Indemnity

An abiding principle of English law is that the Queen (or King) cannot be sued because "the Queen can do no wrong". In the past, public authorities such as NHS bodies were considered to be acting in the name of the Queen (ie, the Crown), and were thus protected from liability for civil actions arising from alleged clinical negligence. This legal principle of Crown immunity was, however, changed to Crown indemnity in 1991 when NHS Trusts were formed, meaning that the NHS as a public service now has legal responsibility for such situations, no longer rendering them immune from prosecution.

To protect themselves from liability and exposure to possible legal claims and potentially large financial settlements, the majority of ambulance service Trusts and other NHS bodies now subscribe to the Clinical Negligence Scheme for Trusts (CNST). Established in 1966 the CNST administers a voluntary scheme where compensation is met from a pooling system, payment into which is dependent on an assessment of the risk presented by that particular trust. The scheme has established standards for the management of risks and claims, some of which have a substantial impact on promoting good practice and go some way to mitigating the failure of the common law to set standards. Liabilities prior to April 1995 are covered by the Existing Liabilities Scheme (ELS) which is centrally funded. Those arising since April 1st 1995 are overseen by the NHS Litigation Authority (NHSLA), a special health authority set up to supervise the CNST in handling claims. The NHSLA uses an approved list of solicitors to handle litigation thus enabling expertise in defending clinical negligence claims to be focused in a small number of relatively experienced firms.

▌Negligence and Protection Against Negligence Claims

Unless there is some type of immunity, nothing can protect ambulance personnel from liability for negligence. For negligence to have occurred, the following elements must be satisfied:

- Ambulance technicians and paramedics owe a duty of care to the patient.
- There has been a breach of that duty of care. This may arise when the person accused of negligence has failed to act in accordance with the standard expected of another reasonable person with similar training and expertise in the same circumstances. Such breaches of duty may apply to actions and omissions to act.
- The patient suffered harm, loss or injury that was directly caused by the breach of duty, or the breach materially contributed to the harm, ie, the breach was the proximate cause (the first event in a chain of events) that caused the claimant's injury.

Ambulance personnel are likely to be protected from liability provided that they perform according to the standards expected of them and adhere to national guidelines and directives. Although these standards are not enshrined in law and thus are not legally binding, they may be introduced as evidence in litigation and may affect the outcome of a claim. Failure to adhere to these standards is likely to be heavily scrutinised and may result in sanctions or reprisals.

In addition to duty of care, breach of care and causation of harm, another significant component in establishing negligence is that of foreseeability. This concept implies that the injury, harm or loss could have been predicted, or known in advance, and therefore could have been avoided had the proper precautions been taken. For example, it is foreseeable that giving an incorrect dose or concentration of a drug may result in harm to patients, just as it is foreseeable that ignoring a red light while en route to a call may result in a road traffic collision.

Duty

A prerequisite to a successful legal claim is that the person or institution claimed against owed a legal duty of care to the injured person, ie, a duty that must be recognised by the law as giving rise to liability. The relationship between ambulance personnel and patients is one that creates such a duty, and is usually clearly established with little or no difficulty or controversy. The overriding duty of ambulance personnel is to do no harm to their patients (*primum non nocere*) and to avoid further harm. Thereafter, their prevailing duty is to act in their patients' best interests and to provide the best quality of care possible.

The first element of negligence that must be proven for claims to be successful is that of duty. Curzon's *Dictionary of Law* defines duty as "*an act that is due by legal or moral obligation*". It goes on to define duty of care in terms of the dictum laid down by Lord Atkin in the case of <u>*Donoghue v Stevenson*</u> [1932], where he states that you must take reasonable care to avoid acts or omissions that you can reasonably foresee would be likely to injure your neighbour, your neighbour in law being persons who are so closely and directly affected by your act that you ought reasonably to have them in your thoughts as being so affected when performing the acts or omissions in question.

In addition to this legal duty of care, paramedics and other ambulance personnel have a professional duty to ensure that they remain clinically updated and familiar with all procedures and guidelines. This extends to ensuring their attendance at continuing education programmes including clinical skills refresher updates and recertification courses, and in the case of paramedics, to ensure that their registration with the HPC and the ongoing continual professional development (CPD) remains current and valid. Emotional and psychological well-being are also key attributes of effective prehospital care providers as well as physical health, all of which are the responsibility of individual practitioners and their crewmates. Ensuring the provision and maintenance of safe and functional equipment at the start of each shift is also vital to effective clinical care, and the practitioner's duty in this regard should not be underestimated. Lastly, the duty to respect each patient's right to privacy and dignity, in addition to their basic human rights as defined in the Human Rights Act 1998, should always be remembered as well as their right to refuse treatment or otherwise limit the level of care provided to them.

Breach of Duty

Anyone who engages the help of professionals to perform a particular role or function expects this to be carried out properly, the legal standard to be met being that of the ordinary skilled person exercising and professing to have that particular skill. This is particularly relevant to the second element of negligence that must be proven for claims to be successful, ie, that the practitioner breached his or her duty of care and failed to perform to the required standard. This standard of care is the standard that would be expected of the competent post holder, ie, a reasonable practitioner of the same level when faced with the same or similar situation.

After the claim has been prepared, the testimony of independent expert witnesses will be sought and presented to assist the court, and a decision taken regarding whether the practitioner's care reached the required standard of reasonableness, ie, whether it satisfied the "Bolam test", named after the case in which it was applied (*Bolam v Friern Hospital Management Committee* [1957]. In medical cases this standard of reasonableness is met if it is one that is accepted as proper by a responsible body of medical opinion. The existence of a common practice in a profession, however, does not automatically mean that negligence cannot be established. Indeed, in cases subsequent to *Bolam*, most notably that of *Bolitho v City and Hackney Health Authority* [1997], the courts sought confirmation that the body of medical opinion in question withstood the test of logical analysis ie, that it had a logical basis and endured rigorous scrutiny. The courts also need to be satisfied that, in forming their opinions, the experts directed their minds to assessing comparative risks and benefits, and reached a defensible conclusion on the matter. For example, the courts are unlikely to accept an expert's opinion that it was reasonable to withhold thrombolytic therapy from a patient presenting with an acute myocardial infarction, who had no contraindications to treatment, on the basis of weak or flimsy evidence.

Causation

Curzon's *Dictionary of Law* defines causation as the relationship between cause and effect, and proximate cause as the immediate, rather than the remote, cause that should be considered. In cases where the legal duty of care has been established and the practitioner breached his or her duty, the claim will fail unless the claimant can link the events and show that the breach caused, or materially contributed to, the loss or harm suffered. In many cases this will not cause a problem such as those situations involving surgery performed on the wrong limb. However, where patients seek to establish loss or harm as a consequence of alleged clinical negligence, this may prove to be more problematic. This is particularly the case where more than one possible cause exists. Here claimants must prove on a balance of probabilities that it was the breach that led to the loss or harm in question, ie, that it was more likely than not (greater than 50% likelihood) that the breach caused the harm.

Thus causation may be seen as the natural and continuous sequence of events, unbroken by any intervening cause, that produces injury and without which the result would not have occurred. Simply stated, the claimant must prove that the practitioner's improper action, or failure to act, caused his or her injury. For example, failure of ambulance personnel to secure a patient safely on a long board may be found to be the proximate cause of severing of the spinal cord. Proving that an action or failure to act proximately caused an injury is often the most difficult part of a claim. It is also the element of the claim on which defence solicitors spend most of their time. For example, in the case of practitioners who treat the victim of a road traffic collision who later suffers a spinal cord injury, but who drop the stretcher while caring for him or her, the patient may try to show that the injury resulted from the dropped stretcher and not from the incident itself. In such instances, careful documentation of assessments and clinical findings throughout the entire patient care episode will prove to be invaluable to the defence.

Harm

The final element that must be proven in negligence claims is that claimants were harmed or suffered a loss. Although physical injury is commonly part of clinical negligence claims, patients also may claim damages for pain, suffering, emotional distress, loss of income, loss of enjoyment of life and loss of future earning capacity. To be successful they will have to demonstrate that the practitioner's actions or omissions proximately caused each of these kinds of damage.

Typically the injured parties set out to investigate the possibility of obtaining compensation. Cases may arise, however, where their perception of their loss is greater than the actual loss. In circumstances such as these which may, for example, arise following a delayed diagnosis, assuming that the outcome would have been the same, then compensation is likely to be awarded for the pain, suffering, and perhaps psychiatric consequences that occurred between the date at which the diagnosis should have been made and the time that it was actually made. If no loss has been suffered, the claim will fail and no compensation will be awarded. The aim of the law in such situations is to return the patient as far as possible to the position that she or he would have been in had negligence not occurred; compensation is the means by which this is achieved.

Continuity of Care and Patient Handover

Having responded to an emergency call, it is imperative that ambulance personnel communicate with health care professionals, transfer the patient's care to them and relay details of the patient's journey in a timely and appropriate way. It is the responsibility of ambulance personnel to remain with patients until the transfer of care has been completed. This includes leaving a copy of the patient's clinical record with relevant staff in the receiving hospital, including details of prehospital clinical findings, physiological observations, medications administered, and procedures performed. If the patient declines transport, it is good practice to leave a copy of the patient report form at the house for subsequent health professionals to view if called back to the patient.

Advance Directives

Advance directives are written documents that express the wants, needs, and desires of patients with regard to their future medical care. They state the medical care that patients wish or do not wish to receive when they are unable to independently express their wishes, and the care and treatment that they are consenting to. Living wills, do not attempt resuscitation (DNAR) orders, organ donation cards, and other related documents are all types of advance directives.

In order for these to be binding, advance directives must be made by individuals with the necessary capacity, be applicable to the circumstances that arise, be understood by the patient who has fully appreciated the significance and consequences of the refusal of such treatment, and must be made without duress. Where advance directives have been made fulfilling these criteria, they are binding upon all health care pro-

fessionals and any contravention of the refusal of treatment is likely to constitute an assault. There is no legal requirement for advance directives to be written; however, it is clearly much easier to establish the patient's wishes if they are both written and communicated to all involved in the patient's care as soon as possible after they have been devised. Legal advice should always be sought where there is uncertainty over an advance refusal of treatment. Where ambulance personnel are faced with such advance directives, patients should be transported to hospital and all relevant information relayed to the clinician responsible for the patient's care as well as to emergency team members.

Do not attempt resuscitation (DNAR) orders are a specific type of advance directive that states those life-sustaining emergency procedures that should be performed on patients in situations when their hearts have stopped working or where respirations have ceased. They are required to be updated at regular intervals. The ethics of advance directives and issues surrounding organ procurement will be discussed in Chapter 5.

▋ Certification, Registration, and Regulation

Certification generally refers to evidence of completion of a certain level of training, such as a certificate of completion of basic training awarded upon satisfactory completion of specified hours of training and examination. It addresses minimum competency levels and indicates the level to which practitioners will practise. Registration, on the other hand, is the process by which professionals are authorised to practise at a defined level by a governing body, with their names, details, and individual registration number being retained on a centrally administered database. Given that paramedics are the only ambulance personnel who are recognised as professionals in their own right, it is only paramedics to whom registration

You are the Paramedic Part 3

You continue to try and persuade Roland to go to hospital, but he adamantly refuses. He is becoming increasingly groggy and falls asleep frequently, requiring a raised voice or gentle shake to rouse him.

Vital Signs	Recording Time: 30 Minutes after Arrival
Level of consciousness	GCS score of 13
Skin	Appears normal
Pulse	Unable to assess
Blood pressure	Unable to measure
Respirations	10 to 12 breaths/min
Oxygen saturation	Unable to measure

5. How does patient consent affect your management of Roland?

6. Consent has to be valid or informed, what does this mean?

applies. Regulation refers to the process by which professions ensure that standards are established and maintained, monitor their members to ensure that they are fit to practise and account for their actions and omissions, and monitor defined standards of education, training, behaviour, and competence.

Ambulance Personnel–Patient Relationships

Confidentiality

Ambulance personnel have a duty of confidentiality to patients in relation to the private information disclosed to them by virtue of their privileged relationship. In addition to this legal duty, health care professionals have a similar duty imposed by their regulatory bodies and through their contracts of employment. Release of this privileged information may be permitted where patients give their consent to such disclosure. To give their consent, patients must have the necessary capacity and be aware of the circumstances and purpose of the release. Breach of this duty of confidentiality represents a major breach of trust as well as a violation of legal, professional, and ethical codes of practice and conduct. Exceptions to this arise in a number of situations where disclosure of information is required by the law. These include notifiable diseases, certain road traffic offences, prevention of terrorism, and in response to a court order.

Caution must be exercised regarding the choice of location where patients are spoken to. Every effort should be made not to confer in front of bystanders, whether at the scene of an incident or in hospital corridors.

Consent and Refusal of Treatment

The concepts of consent and refusal of treatment provide the backbone of health care law. Any touching of a patient's body without his or her consent may give rise to charges of assault and battery. Thus to enable emergency medical care to be given, consent must first be obtained. The concept of consent is predicated on patients who have reached the age of legal majority, ie, 18 years and over, and who possess the capacity to make clinical decisions having been able to retain and assimilate information and assess the risks, benefits and consequences of the options presented to them. Adult patients who have this capacity are entitled to refuse all or part of the emergency medical care offered to them. This does not apply to minors; however, as they are not considered in law to be able to make a binding refusal of treatment.

For consent to exist three components are necessary, namely patients must have the necessary capacity to consent to treatment, they must have been given sufficient information, and they must have been under no duress or undue influence in reaching their decision. Consent may be obtained in a number of ways that ambulance personnel must be familiar with, the most notable of these being implied consent and informed consent.

Informed consent must be obtained from every competent adult patient who has decision-making capacity and consists of two elements. Firstly, patients must be told about the proposed actions or interventions, and have the opportunity to ask questions, have issues clarified and have the risks explained. A number of factors could distract them from giving matters their full attention thereby preventing their understanding such as pain, injury, hypoglycaemia, hypoxia, confusion, anxiety and fear. It is imperative, therefore, that ambulance personnel limit these distractions and their impact as far as possible, for example by giving pain relief, and that they carry out consultations and procedures in appropriate environments such as in the ambulance or in the patient's home, having taken all necessary measures to limit external influences. Secondly, patients must give their permission to be touched in the manner proposed, and must do so free from duress. This permission may be given verbally, ie, expressed consent, or may be implied by actions such as rolling up a sleeve to enable blood pressure to be taken.

In unconscious patients, or adults who are too ill or injured to consent to emergency lifesaving treatment, their consent to treatment is implied. In these circumstances, clinicians including ambulance personnel assume that this implied consent would reflect the patients' wishes, particularly given the severity of their condition. Such treatment is often administered under the doctrine of necessity which reflects the life-saving nature of their actions and the degree of urgency involved. The two requirements for necessity to apply are that it is impossible to communicate with the patient and the action taken must be what a reasonable person would have done in the circumstances.

Minors present particular issues for ambulance personnel to deal with. The position for patients who are aged below 18 years, ie, minors, is different to that of adults. For the purposes of consenting to treatment as opposed to refusing it, minors aged 16 and 17 are treated as adults. Children who are below the age of maturity, ie, 18 years, and who are not "Gillick competent" as defined in the Children Act 1989, ie, who have not reached the level of sufficient age and understanding, are deemed by law to be incapable of giving their consent to treatment. Where, however, children have sufficient intelligence and understanding to enable them to understand fully what is proposed and the likely consequences, then they are said to have capacity and may consent to treatment. Whether or not children have capacity will be determined as a matter of fact in each case. The situation regarding refusal of treatment is, however, somewhat different for in these situations parental consent must be obtained. Under the current law parental consent may be given by anyone with parental responsibility. Married parents and all mothers have this automatically. Unmarried fathers do not have this responsibility and must either apply for this or enter into an agreement with the child's mother. Those who have responsibility for the physical care of children are permitted to do what is reasonable in all the circumstances of the case for the purpose of safeguarding or promoting the child's welfare.

Adults aged over 18 years who have capacity may refuse treatment for any reason, whether rational or irrational, or for no reason at all. Where such patients have capacity the law is clear: the refusal must be accepted. However, patients must have been given a complete explanation of the consequences of the decision, including the risks of death or serious injury. Failure to do this would mean that the patient's decision was not informed as it was not based on all the relevant information. Any refusal of treatment should be documented in full, including details of the consultation and explanations given, the fact that the patient had capacity and his or her reasons for reaching their decision. Where possible, this should be witnessed by another health care professional and signed.

Where patients refuse treatment and ambulance personnel are concerned regarding their clinical condition or safety, senior medical advice should be sought immediately. In these circumstances, patients should not be left unattended but should be observed and monitored as far as possible. In some circumstances, particularly those involving mental health emergencies, patients may require to be detained against their will under the Mental Health Act 1983 and transported to hospital where this is considered to be in their best interests. In many cases management of these situations may require police assistance.

Refusal of treatment by those aged under 18 years is not recognised in law. In theory, the ability to give consent lies with those with parental responsibility, however in situations involving more mature minors it may become more difficult to administer treatment and the situation may become more complicated. Where difficulties arise, senior medical advice and legal counsel should be sought.

Communication

The role of ambulance personnel in managing such situations is crucial. In many cases involving adults refusing treatment, calm, reassuring and supportive explanations that are provided in terms and language that patients understand can make all the difference between consent to treatment or refusal. Those refusing treatment often do so based on fear, misunderstanding and lack of knowledge, which can sometimes be projected as aggression or hostility. By eliciting the source of the patient's refusal to treatment and acting as his or her advocate, the patient's perspective can be more clearly understood often resulting in the formulation of a clinical action plan that is acceptable to all. Where treatment continues to be refused despite these efforts, measures should be taken to ensure that patients remain supervised by competent and reliable professionals, appropriate follow-up has been arranged, and actions to be taken should a patient have a change of mind and wish clinical intervention.

Throughout this consultation ambulance personnel must be convinced of the absence of altered mental status or unstable vital signs that could interfere with decision-making capacity **Figure 4-5**. Criteria for determining mental competence should always be checked including:

- orientation to time, place, and person
- appropriate responses to questions
- lack of significant mental impairment from alcohol, drugs, head injury, or other organic illness
- confirmation from family members, where possible, that patients are behaving normally

- confirmation that patients understand the nature of their condition and the risks of not being transferred to hospital
- vital signs, oxygen saturation levels, and blood glucose levels are all within normal limits

Use of Force: Violent and Aggressive Patients and the Use of Restraints

Patients with acute mental health problems may be detained against their will under the Mental Health Act 1983 when they are considered to be at risk of harming themselves or others, and may be transferred to hospital for clinical assessment and treatment. In some instances police assistance may be required to accompany such patients, particularly where the risk of violence or aggression is evident.

Today's society is associated with increasing levels of violence from which ambulance personnel are not immune. The reality of prehospital care is such that they are likely to encounter actual or potential violence from patients or others, and may be called upon to defend themselves against these forces. Under the law, the only force that ambulance personnel, or indeed other individuals, may use to defend themselves is that which is proportionate to the force used against them. In any situations involving actual or potential violence that suggest a threat to the safety of ambulance personnel, police assistance must be sought immediately and entry to the potentially dangerous or unsecured situation avoided until the arrival of police officers.

Transport

Patients should be transported to the hospital of their choice where possible and practicable. However, when making decisions about the preferred hospitals or receiving facilities, the capability of each hospital to meet the individual patient's needs must be borne in mind, particularly when specialist

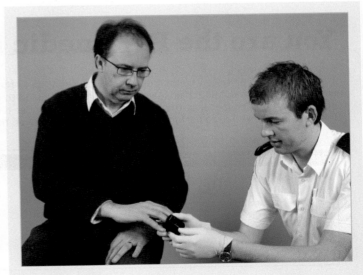

Figure 4-5 Remember that a patient's decision-making ability can be affected by the intake of alcohol or drugs, and by abnormal blood glucose or oxygen saturation levels.

facilities such as trauma teams, neurological assessment, burns expertise and cardiac units are required.

Decisions made by ambulance personnel not to transport patients to hospital at all, known as non-conveyance, may be associated with controversy and may become the subject of complaints, particularly where patients later deteriorate and their conditions give cause for concern. Where non-conveyance has been decided upon, ambulance personnel must ensure that they document all actions taken including the patient's response, and all follow-up arrangements made. Senior medical advice should be sought where concern exists or where further clinical support is required.

Incident Sites and Scenes of Crime

When involved in situations involving death or potential crime scenes, ambulance personnel must exercise extreme caution to ensure that they do not disturb or destroy potential evidence. Where road traffic collisions are involved, only debris that obstructs access to patients should be moved. Similarly, where fatalities are involved, the bodies should remain in situ until death is pronounced and authorisation given to remove the deceased person to hospital or to the mortuary. Where dead bodies obstruct access to live patients, particularly where critical illnesses or injuries are concerned, these may be removed, taking all precautions necessary to preserve the incident site.

Where the incident has occurred indoors, touching of objects should be limited to only that which is essential, to avoid interfering with evidence such as fingerprints. Statements made by potential witnesses to the event should be documented carefully and contact details obtained. The number of emergency personnel who enter the scene should also be limited as each person who enters may further contaminate what may later turn out to be a crime scene.

In cases involving sexual assault or rape, all evidence must be preserved including that retained on victims, such as fibres or hair. This should be preserved as far as possible. Ambulance personnel should refrain from wrapping patients in blankets or similar garments, and should ensure that victims do not change their clothing or bathe until forensic medical examinations have been completed.

Where scenes involve death, ambulance personnel must remain with the body until police support arrives to preserve any potential chain of evidence, and to protect the scene from contamination by bystanders, family members, or other emergency personnel.

At the Scene

Be aware that at crime scenes the perpetrator may still be at or near the scene and could be a factor in deciding when, where, and how you care for your patient.

Documentation

Importance of Documentation

Even the most skilled and conscientious health care professional may at some point during their career have to attend court as a witness or defendant in a civil or criminal action. The best protection for ambulance personnel in court is a *thorough and accurate clinical record* outlining details of the patient's prehospital care journey Figure 4-6 ▶ . Effective clinical records should contain the following elements which characterise the principles of good record-keeping:

- **Date and times.** Document when the call was received, scene arrival, departure from the scene, and the time of arrival at hospital.

You are the Paramedic Part 4

The police finally arrive on scene. You explain the situation to them. The neighbours have had enough of Roland by this point and ask him to leave. Once outside, you again try to persuade Roland to come with you. The police officer tells Roland that he either goes to hospital in the ambulance, or they will take him to A&E under the Mental Health Act. Roland grudgingly agrees to travel with you to hospital and allows you to perform a vital signs check. However, he will not let you administer any drugs.

Reassessment	Recording Time: 60 Minutes
Level of consciousness	GCS score 14/15
Skin	Warm and pink
Pulse	54 beats/min, regular
Blood pressure	134/76 mm Hg
Respirations	12 breaths/min
SpO$_2$	96%, on air

7. Could calling the police be considered a breach of confidentiality?
8. Does the Mental Health Act allow the police to force Roland to go to hospital?

Figure 4-6 A. Professional documentation. **B.** Unprofessional documentation.

- **History.** Include details of information elicited from patients and bystanders, and their contact details. Where appropriate it may be prudent to document statements in quotation marks.
- **Observations.** Details of the scene, particularly where they provide information relating to the mechanism of injury.
- **Physical examination.** A detailed description of physical assessments and clinical findings should be noted including all pertinent negatives, for example, any part of the body you examine and find to be normal.
- **Treatment.** Details of clinical interventions and actions taken should be documented including the dose, route and strength of medicines given, and details of invasive procedures such as intravenous access.
- **Changes.** All changes in the patient's status throughout their prehospital period should be accurately documented including actions taken in response to these.

All clinical records are legal documents and should be completed as soon as possible after the event, as memory recall and accuracy and reliability of information is known to deteriorate with time. All records should be clear, concise, contemporaneous and legible, and must be completed in ink, preferably black ink. They must also include the signature of the author and his or her printed name at the end of the document. From a legal perspective it is important to remember that if something is not documented, this suggests that it was not done and provides no evidence to the contrary.

The quality of clinical records and record keeping should never be underestimated. When later produced in court, incomplete and illegible records suggest that the care of the patient may also have been unprofessional, sloppy and incomplete. All relevant events influencing the patient's care should be included, and should be documented factually and concisely.

The Ambulance Report Is Part of the Medical Record

A copy of the patient clinical record (also known as the patient report form) should remain at the accident and emergency department with the hospital and should be handed to the clinician assuming responsibility for the patient's care **Figure 4-7 ▾**. This will aid understanding of the mechanism of injury or original event, ensure continuity of the patient's care and enable any trends in his or her clinical condition to be detected. This document will become part of the patient's permanent medical record. Where photographs have been taken to provide information relating to incident scenes or mechanisms of injury, these should be treated in a similar manner.

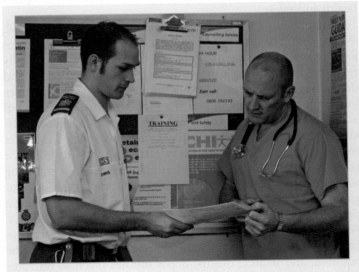

Figure 4-7 To ensure competent and continuous care for each patient, each patient's clinical record should be handed over to appropriate medical personnel at the hospital.

Retention of Medical Records

Statute dictates that clinical records should be retained for a minimum period of eight years after the last treatment episode. Obstetric records should be kept for 25 years, and children's records until their 25th birthday or their 26th birthday if treatment ended when they were 17. The retention period is extended in relation to patients suffering from mental health problems; here, records are kept for 20 years from the date when no further treatment was considered necessary. Where patients die, it is recommended that the notes are kept for eight years from the date of death. Ambulance personnel should *never* make personal copies of patient records due to the confidential nature of the information involved.

▌Reportable Cases

The Health and Safety at Work Act 1974 came into force to impose a statutory duty on employers to ensure the health, safety and welfare at work of all its employees, so far as is reasonably practicable. It is enforceable through the criminal and civil courts, and requires employers to lay down safe systems of work, ensure that their employees have the necessary skill, instruction and supervision, and to ensure that they are provided with safe premises and equipment with which to work. It also imposes a duty on all employees to take responsibility for their health and safety. Examples include the safe disposal of equipment, maintenance of a safe environment, and responsibility for performing regular risk assessments. Under the Act employers also have a duty of care to non-employees to ensure their health and safety, this duty extending to patients, visitors and the general public. Health and safety regulations came into force on January 1st 1993 as a result of European Directives relating to the provision and use of equipment, manual handling, personal protective equipment and general workplace health and safety.

Submitted by the Health and Safety at Work Act, RIDDOR, the Reporting of Injuries, Diseases and Dangerous Occurrences Regulations 1995 came into force on 1st April 1996, and legally requires the reporting of work-related accidents, diseases and dangerous occurrences. The Act applies to all work activities but not to all incidents and involves the immediate reporting of accidents connected with work where employees or self-employed people working on the premises are killed or suffer major injury, or where members of the public are killed or taken to hospital. The information obtained enables enforcing authorities to identify where and how risks arise and to investigate serious accidents. It also enables them to give advice on preventive action to reduce injury, ill health and accidental loss. For the most part reportable accidents, dangerous occurrences or cases of disease are comparatively rare events which must be reported, and include deaths; major injuries (such as fractures other than to fingers, thumbs or toes); amputations; dislocations of the shoulder, hip, knee or spine; temporary or perma-

nent loss of sight; chemical or hot metal burns to the eye or penetrating injuries of the eye; injuries resulting from electric shock or electrical burn; injuries requiring admission to hospital for more than 24 hours; acute illnesses requiring medical treatment; or loss of consciousness arising from absorption of any substance by inhalation, ingestion, or through the skin; and accidents resulting in three or more days off work.

Ambulance personnel are also required to report all cases of suspected child abuse. As such they must be familiar with child protection reporting mechanisms and the identity, location and contact details of the child protection leads for their region. Warning signs that may alert ambulance personnel to possible physical, emotional, psychological or sexual child abuse should be identified and immediate action taken to ensure the child's safety. In many instances this will involve transporting the child to hospital for assessment by paediatric specialists, often accompanied by parents or carers. In many prehospital care situations it may not be possible to determine whether children have already been identified as being at risk and placed on the child protection register. It should also be remembered that not all at-risk children have been entered onto the child protection register, and a high index of suspicion and awareness should be employed at all times.

A high index of suspicion and heightened awareness should also be maintained regarding potential abuse or neglect of those in the vulnerable groups such as the elderly. In many instances the presenting complaint may be symptomatic of more serious underlying problems including physical, emotional, psychological, social, sexual, or financial abuse. As with children, immediate steps should be taken to ensure their safety and welfare and referrals made to the relevant social services or other protection agencies to investigate matters further.

Special Considerations

Elder abuse is as prevalent as child abuse in our society. Heightened awareness of this should be maintained and any suspicious signs or symptoms reported to the appropriate authorities.

Coroner's Inquests

As an agent of the court the coroner is required to hold inquests into deaths where there is reasonable cause to suspect that the death was violent or unnatural, of sudden and unknown cause, or where it occurred in prison or police custody or elsewhere where an Act of Parliament requires an inquest to be held.

Every death must be registered with the Registrar of Births, Marriages and Deaths within five days. Any doctor who has attended the deceased during his last illness must complete a death certificate which states the cause of death. Cases which fall under the coroner's jurisdiction should be reported to the coroner's officer, and the relatives told that the death cannot be registered until the coroner has completed his investigation. Those cases which *must* be reported to the coroner include those where:

- The deceased was not attended by a doctor during his last illness
- A completed death certificate has not been obtained
- The deceased was not seen by the doctor completing the death certificate either after death or within 14 days before death
- The cause of death is unknown
- The death was unnatural or caused by violence, neglect, abortion, or in suspicious circumstances
- The death occurred during or within 24 hours of surgery or before recovery from the effects of an anaesthetic
- The cause of death was due to an industrial disease or industrial poisoning.

Notification of an inquest is usually given by the coroner's officer, who has responsibility for conducting investigations on behalf of the coroner. This may or may not involve a post mortem being carried out. Upon completion of these investigations, an inquest will be held if the coroner believes that the death was violent, unnatural, unexplained, sudden, or occurred in custody. The inquest itself takes the form of an inquiry by the coroner, who seeks to determine the facts surrounding the death in order to answer the questions that must be addressed. It is not an adversarial process. Here, there are no parties, no claimant or defendant, and no case is presented. Ambulance personnel may, however, be called upon to give evidence to the coroner regarding the death, having first submitted a written statement of events. Those who find themselves in this situation are advised to seek senior medical support and possibly legal advice. Legal advice may also be recommended in particularly complex or sensitive cases.

You are the Paramedic Summary

1. What are your immediate medical concerns?

The patient has consumed an unknown quantity of an opiate drug, which when combined with alcohol can depress his level of consciousness and respiratory rate. Therefore Roland's airway and respiratory sufficiency are at risk and he requires careful monitoring and transport to hospital. Even if you were to administer naloxone, the half life of codeine is far longer and will put Roland at risk once the naloxone wears off.

2. How might these conflict with the legal, ethical, and professional issues?

All patients have a basic right to decide what happens to them. All health care providers must respect the wishes of the patient, even if that goes against our own desires to preserve and promote life. At the same time, we have a duty of care to our patients and a professional registration to protect, which can make the management of patients who refuse assistance difficult.

3. If you left scene now, would you be in breach of your duty of care?

You have a responsibility as a health care professional to treat and care for patients with an appropriate degree of skill and care. Since the patient has threatened you, it is necessary to perform a risk assessment to determine whether you are in danger, in which case it might be acceptable to withdraw from the patient. In this case, given the current condition of the patient, it is unlikely he could follow through with his threat if you keep out of arms reach. It is important to realise that you must make a genuine and concerted effort in persuading the patient to consent to treatment, thus avoiding potential claims of negligence.

4. Could the patient's threat be seen as assault?

Yes, remember that the patient only has to threaten you with immediate bodily harm, ie, there does not have to be any physical contact.

5. How does patient consent affect your management of Roland?

Before you can touch, treat or care for a patient, you need their permission, or consent. Failure to obtain this could lead to charges of battery or assault. Although it is often frustrating with patient's who refuse your help, it is important that you always consider the patient's best interest above your own.

6. Consent has to be valid and informed, what does this mean?

Roland needs to be able to understand and retain the relevant information relating to his current medical condition, not feel under any pressure to accept or refuse treatment and have sufficient information provided by you regarding what you propose to do, have the opportunity to ask questions, have issues clarified and be able to ask questions. He must also be able to assimilate information and make reasoned decisions based upon all information and options available to him. In this case, it could be argued that the influence of alcohol and opiate drugs have diminished Roland's capacity to consent, but at the present time it would be inappropriate to administer treatment without his consent. Should he become unconscious, then consent could be implied and administered under a doctrine of necessity.

7. Could calling the police be considered a breach of confidentiality?

Breaching the patient's confidentiality is a major breach of trust as well as violation of legal, professional and ethical codes of practice. If the patient consents to the disclosure, then this is acceptable and there are a number of situations where breaches are required by law. The police have a right of access to a patient's personal information such as their name and address in relation to any crime, but health information can only be disclosed if they are investigating a serious crime (for example a rape or an act of terrorism). The actual offence does not necessarily have to have been committed either; they also have the right to the information when trying to prevent a serious crime being committed to. In this case, it would not be appropriate for you to make health information available to the police, but it is quite likely that the patient or his neighbours would do so.

8. What part of the Mental Health Act allows the police to force Roland to go to hospital?

Section 136 of the Mental Health Act (Place of Safety Order–public) allows the Police to remove (forceably if necessary) a person who appears to be suffering from a mental disorder in a public place and remove them to a place of safety to be assessed by a doctor or relevant health care professional and a social worker. Two definitions are important to understand here; mental disorder and place of safety. The Mental Health Act defines a mental disorder as a mental illness, arrested or incomplete development of mind, psychopathic disorder, and any other disorder or disability of mind. It could be argued that this patient could be suffering from a mental disorder which warrants further investigation. A place of safety is usually either a police station or a hospital. Locations are generally agreed at a local level and in advance.

Prep Kit

Ready for Review

- Ambulance personnel operate in an environment that exposes them to legal liability. Failing to perform their role and failure to deliver care to the required standard could expose them to civil and/or criminal liability.
- Three branches of government, the executive, judiciary, and legislative branches form the framework within which the law works.
- There are two types of law: civil and criminal.
  - Civil cases result in financial compensation.
  - Criminal cases result in some form of punishment.
- Ambulance personnel are vulnerable to allegations of assault and battery. Assault is said to occur when the fear of bodily harm is instilled in another. Battery occurs when one person unlawfully touches another without his or her consent.
- False imprisonment can occur when ambulance personnel restrain patients against their will. Accurate, detailed, and comprehensive documentation can help protect against this allegation.
- Defamation, slander, and libel present risks to ambulance personnel when they make statements, whether verbal, written or in some other permanent form, which injure a person's reputation. Care should be taken to document objectively all clinical findings and the concerns that ambulance personnel may have.
- Claims follow a general process that involves the lodging of a complaint, a response or answer by the defendant, a discovery period, settlement discussions, and trial process.
- Ambulance personnel are subject to multiple jurisdictions including the law of the land, professional regulations, national guidelines and local policy.
- Ambulance personnel must ensure that all actions are aimed at doing what is in the best interests of their patients and doing them no further harm.
- Paramedics must ensure that they act within their scope of professional practice at all times. All other ambulance personnel must ensure that they act in accordance with guidelines and protocols.
- The Data Protection Act 1998 and Freedom of Information Act 2000 govern the management of patient identifiable information and access to information by professionals and the public alike.
- Emergency vehicles must always be operated in a safe and courteous manner in order to protect the public from further injury. There is no excuse for reckless or careless driving or for driving without due care or attention.
- Ambulance personnel may provide care when they are off duty. However, they must remember that in so doing they are not covered by their employer and must take out some form of personal insurance to protect themselves in such situations. This particularly applies to paramedics who should obtain individual membership of organisations such as the British Paramedic Association or the Medical Defence Union.
- Ambulance personnel are no longer protected from liability by Crown immunity. Where complaints suggesting allegations of negligence are made, such personnel may be covered vicariously by their employers through vicarious liability if it can be shown that they were acting within the scope of their employment at the time the alleged negligence occurred.
- Negligence can only be said to occur when four elements are present:
  - Duty of care. The ambulance service provider must have owed a duty to care to the patient.
  - Breach of duty of care. This duty of care was breached in some way, for example by acting in a way that could not be said to be reasonable by the standard of the ordinary ambulance person skilled in that particular art.
  - Causation. This breach of duty caused or materially contributed to the claimant's injury.
  - Harm, injury or loss resulted as a consequence of the above.
- Patients have the right to determine their own care. Ambulance personnel must understand their responsibilities when faced with advance directives issued by patients.
- Do not attempt resuscitation (DNAR) orders are a specific type of advance directives that generally define those lifesaving procedures that patients are consenting to. This does not represent a signal to avoid caring for patients or to avoid administering other forms of treatment.
- Ambulance personnel must respect the fact that all adult patients with capacity have the right to consent to treatment and to refuse it.
- Patients must be provided with all relevant information regarding any proposed examination, treatment or intervention to enable them to make an informed decision regarding giving their consent.
- When faced with unconscious patients or those incapacitated by virtue of injury or illness from whom it is not possible to obtain consent, ambulance personnel may administer that life-saving treatment that would be considered reasonable in the circumstances under the doctrine of necessity.
- For the purposes of consenting to treatment minors aged 16 and 17 are treated as adults. Where children aged less than 16 are deemed to have sufficient understanding and intelligence to enable them to fully comprehend the treatment proposed, ie, they have capacity, and they are permitted to consent to treatment. This is referred to as "Gillick competence".
- Minors aged under 18 years are not permitted to refuse treatment. In these circumstances consultation must be made with those who have parental responsibility for them. Where those with parental responsibility refuse treatment that clinicians deem to be in the best interests of patients, a court order may be sought to determine the way forward.
- A detailed and comprehensive clinical record must be made of all calls attended by ambulance crews. This documentation should include demographic information, the date and time of events, the history of events including mechanism of injury, details of the physical examination, treatment given including medications administered and vital signs, noting any changes in the patient's condition and response to interventions.
- Accurate, detailed and comprehensive clinical records that are completed as soon as possible after the event will prove invaluable in defending claims of alleged negligence.
- Violence is prevalent in today's society. Ambulance personnel must be vigilant to ensure their safety and that of their team members. Joint guidelines and protocols must be devised by ambulance, police and other emergency services for the management of such situations.
- Ambulance personnel have a key role to play in preserving evidence at incident sites or scenes of crime. Effective communication between ambulance, police and other emergency services is essential to managing such situations, and to ensuring a collaborative approach in investigations. Concise and accurate documentation may prove invaluable in these instances.

www.Paramedic.EMSzone.com/UK/

Prep Kit

Vital Vocabulary

advance directives Written documents that set out in advance patients' wishes regarding those types of medical treatment the authors of the directives do or do not wish to receive in specific circumstances, should they be incapable of expressing their wishes and giving or refusing their consent.

assault A crime and a tort resulting from an act by which any person directly, negligently, or possibly recklessly, causes another to fear immediate bodily harm or invasion of bodily security.

battery A crime and a tort (or delict) involving unwanted touching or the infliction of unlawful violence by the defendant against the claimant. This includes even the slightest force, and need not result in actual harm.

causation The relationship between cause and effect.

civil claim An action instituted by a private individual or corporation against another private individual or corporation. Formerly known as a civil action.

consent Compliance with or deliberate approval of a course of action. It is not legally binding if obtained by coercion, fraud, undue influence or duress.

criminal prosecution An action instituted by the state against a private individual for violation of the criminal law.

damages The court's estimated compensation in financial terms for detriment or injury sustained by the claimant.

defamation The publishing of statements which lower the level of esteem in which individuals are held by right-thinking members of society, or damage their reputation.

defendant A person against whom a claim is made.

delict Term used in Scots law. (*tort* is the equivalent term in English law) Obligation of a person to compensate another who has suffered loss as a result of the wrongful actions of that person.

doctrine of necessity Doctrine under which necessary and urgent life-saving treatment may be administered to patients in their best interests in the absence of their ability to give consent.

do not attempt resuscitation (DNAR) orders A type of advance directive that states those life-sustaining emergency procedures to which patients have consented should their heart fail or respirations cease.

duty An act that is due by legal or moral obligation.

duty of care A duty of care is said to exist where one's actions are reasonably likely to cause harm to another person.

ethics A set of values in society that differentiates right from wrong.

expressed consent A type of consent where patients indicate through their words that they are permitting another to do something such as provide care.

false imprisonment The direct, intentional (or negligent) infliction of some bodily restraint involving complete deprivation of liberty, for any period of time, which is neither expressly nor impliedly authorised by law.

implied consent A type of consent where patients indicate through their actions or behaviour that they are permitting another to do something such as provide care.

informed consent A patient's agreement to something, eg treatment after being informed of the nature of the disease, the risks and benefits of the proposed treatment, alternative treatments, or the choice of no treatment at all.

liability Legal obligation or duty.

libel The publication in permanent form, such as writing or email, of a statement which injures another's good name or reputation, or exposes them to hatred, ridicule or contempt.

minors People under the age of 18 years.

negligence Failure to perform to the ordinary objective standard of conduct expected of a reasonable person performing that skill or art. This may be due to actions or omissions. For negligence to be proven there must have been a duty of care owed, breach of this duty and resultant harm that was either caused by, or materially contributed to by, the breach.

Parliament Comprises the Crown, the House of Lords, and the House of Commons, each of which is assigned different tasks.

proximate cause The immediate cause that should be considered, rather than a remote cause.

scope of practice The limits to practice that are imposed by the regulatory or professional body.

slander Spoken words or gestures that amount to defamation ie, that injure another's good name or reputation.

standard Measure to which others conform or by which the accuracy or quality of others is judged.

standard of care The standard of care that would be expected from a reasonable person with similar training in the same or similar circumstances.

tort A wrongful act that gives rise to a civil claim.

▇▇ Points to Ponder

You and your colleague are dispatched to a dying patient who has an advance directive dated 1 month ago; this is signed by the patient and her general practitioner. The advance directive states that the patient requests that no resuscitative measures be taken. The only care requested is that which is required to ensure that she remains comfortable and pain-free.

A hospice volunteer is on scene and requests that you transport the patient to hospital. The patient's daughter, who holds power of attorney for her, is also on scene. She was unaware that the volunteer phoned the emergency services and refuses to allow her mother to be transported to hospital. The other family members are very upset and become angry telling you that the patient wanted to die in the bed her husband died in 40 years ago. They ask you to leave.

Did the volunteer have the right to call the emergency services without first speaking to the family and in particular to the patient's daughter who holds medical power of attorney for her? Does the daughter have the right to refuse her mother being transported to hospital? How do you and your partner resolve these issues?

Issues: Defending the Patient's Right to Die With Dignity, Defending the Value of Advance Directives.

Assessment in Action

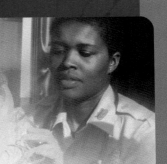

You are called to a scene in which a man with altered mental status is bleeding heavily from an open wound on his forehead. His neighbours called 999 after seeing him having difficulty walking in his garden and attempting to mow the lawn whilst it is raining heavily. When you arrive, the man is angry that you have been called and insists that he is well. He cannot recall how he sustained the injury to his head. He is incoherent and seems confused. He refuses your help, does not allow you to examine him, and refuses to answer any questions. He declines your offer to transport him to hospital for further assessment. What would be the appropriate response to the following questions?

1. **What is the difference between *assault* and *battery*?**
   A. Assault is harmful physical contact; battery is severe injury.
   B. Assault relates to verbal or other threats that instill fear in someone; battery is actually touching someone without their consent.
   C. Assault relates to verbal threats actually carried out; battery is physically harming someone without any kind of warning to that person.
   D. Assault is any form of physical contact only; battery is verbal and psychological harm.

2. **Which of the following is *the most important* principle underpinning paramedic practice?**
   A. Always acting in the patient's best interests
   B. Always seeking senior medical advice prior to advanced clinical interventions
   C. Always ensuring that patients are treated without discrimination
   D. Always obtaining details of past medical history, medications taken, and allergies prior to attending the scenes of incidents

3. **Which of the following situations does NOT apply to information obtained in relation to the patient in the given scenario?**
   A. Information may be relayed to clinicians and emergency team members who may be directly involved in the patient's care at a later stage.
   B. Information may be divulged to all police officers who attend the scene including those involved in restraining the patient.
   C. Information obtained by virtue of the privileged relationship between ambulance personnel and their patients must be dealt with in a confidential manner.
   D. Ambulance personnel must ensure that patient-identifiable information is not released to unauthorised parties and that clinical records are not left unsupervised or are otherwise made accessible to unauthorised parties.

4. **The man in the scenario tells you that one of the reasons he is refusing transport is fear of being taken to the local hospital as his wife died there 6 months ago. Which of the following statements is true?**
   A. Patients must always be taken to the nearest receiving facility irrespective of the nature of their illness or injury.
   B. No further assessment is required at this stage. It would be reasonable to leave this patient at home with instructions to call you if he changes his mind regarding transport to hospital.
   C. Patients may be permitted to exercise a degree of choice in relation to the receiving hospital to which they may be taken as long as this is in their best interests and does not adversely affect their clinical management.
   D. This patient may be taken to hospital despite refusing your help and intervention.

5. **There are certain elements that must be present for an allegation of negligence to be successful. They are:**
   A. duty of care, breach of duty of care, and harm caused that was directly attributable to the breach of duty.
   B. duty, breach of duty, and lack of informed consent.
   C. breach of duty, harm, and lack of informed consent.
   D. duty of care, breach of duty of care, and harm caused that was not directly attributable to the breach of duty.

6. **With regard to the patient's entitlement to refuse care, please answer true or false to the following.**
   A. The patient is not orientated to place, time, or person.
   B. You are concerned that the patient does not understand his condition or the need for medical attention.
   C. You believe that the patient has ingested a significant quantity of alcohol which has contributed to his injuries.
   D. The patient has sustained an obvious head injury and is not answering questions appropriately.

7. **What is the paramedic's *best* protection in court, irrespective of the charge or case against him or her?**
   A. A good attitude and proper maintenance of skills
   B. His or her reputation—professionally and personally
   C. A thorough and accurate medical record on all patients treated
   D. An exceptional memory of all calls and patients treated

Challenging Questions

You and your colleague have responded to a road traffic collision. There was only one person injured and her injuries were minor. You have transported her to the local accident and emergency (A&E) department, which is extremely busy. You know that your ambulance station is understaffed, that the weather is hazardous, and understand that you will soon be called to another incident. While in the A&E department you engage the attention of a nurse and tell her about your patient and her condition/injuries. The nurse tells you that she will see to her as soon as possible but that she is currently attending to another patient with serious injuries. You leave a copy of the patient clinical record at the nurses' station and leave the patient on the trolley so that you can respond to your next call.

8. **What actions have you performed for which you could later be the subject of litigation?**

You are called to a scene of domestic violence. The man who attacked his wife has been taken into custody by the local police who are still on scene. The man has injuries that you know require sutures. He is refusing clinical care. The officers tell you that you can treat him and transport him to hospital (in their presence) based on the concept of involuntary consent.

9. **Why is this reasoning unacceptable?**

5 Ethical Issues

Objectives

Cognitive

- Define ethics.
- Distinguish between ethical and moral decisions.
- Identify the premise that should underlie the paramedic's ethical decisions in out-of hospital care.
- Analyse the relationship between the law and ethics in the ambulance service.
- Compare and contrast the criteria that may be used in allocating scarce ambulance service resources.
- Identify the issues surrounding the use of advance directives in making a prehospital resuscitation decision.
- Describe the criteria necessary to honour an advance directive in your service.

Affective

- Value the patient's autonomy in the decision-making process.
- Defend the following ethical positions:
  - The paramedic is accountable to the patient.
  - The paramedic is accountable to the medical director.
  - The paramedic is accountable to the ambulance service.
  - The paramedic is accountable for fulfilling the standard of care.

- Given a scenario, defend or challenge a paramedic's actions concerning a patient who is treated against his/her wishes.
- Given a scenario, defend a paramedic's actions in a situation where a doctor orders therapy the paramedic feels to be detrimental to the patient's best interests.

Psychomotor

None

Medical Ethics

Ethics is the philosophy of right and wrong, of moral duties, and of ideal professional behaviour. Morality is a code of conduct that can be defined by society, religion, or a person, affecting character, conduct, and conscience.

Paramedics need to be ethical in their practice and be aware of their own moral standards in their daily work. Do not assume that your patients share your moral standards. Your moral standards may conflict with your patients' wishes or your patients' best interests, and it is important that you put your patients' interests before your own Figure 5-1 ▼.

Often, however, the word *ethics* becomes blurred with the word *morals*. Morality is what *you* think about an issue and ethics are the foundations for the actions you take.

Medical ethics or more accurately health care ethics is a discipline within ethics that discusses and debates the health care of human beings, your patients. Your understanding of health care ethics must be formed as a part of, and consistent with, the general codes of the health care professional Figure 5-2 ▼. Throughout the ages, there have been many published codes of ethics for health professionals. The Oath of Geneva, drafted by the World Medical Association in 1948, provides a good example; it is the oath taken by many medical students on completion of their studies, at the time of being admitted to the medical profession:

"I solemnly pledge myself to consecrate my life to the service of humanity; I will give to my teachers the respect and gratitude which is their due; I will practice my profession with conscience and dignity; the health of my patient will be my first consideration; I will respect the secrets which are confided in me; I will maintain by all the means in my power the honour and noble traditions of the medical profession; my colleagues will be my brothers; I will not permit considerations of religion, nationality, race, party politics, or social standing to intervene between my duty and my patient; I will maintain the utmost respect for human life from the time of conception; even under threat, I will not make use of my medical knowledge contrary to the laws of humanity. I make these promises solemnly, freely and upon my honour".

Very similar principles underlie the more detailed *Standards of conduct, performance, and ethics*, which was issued by

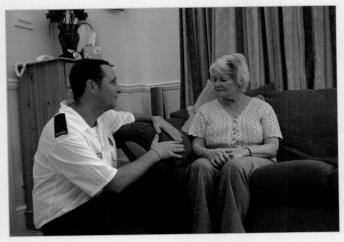

Figure 5-1 As a paramedic serving a diverse public, you will frequently work with people who have cultural backgrounds that are different from your own. Work to set aside your own personal beliefs when making decisions on the patient's behalf.

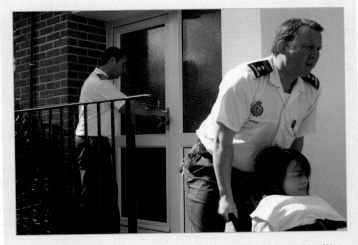

Figure 5-2 When people call 999, they trust you not only with providing proper medical care, but also with using sound ethical judgement—including the safeguarding of their personal possessions.

You are the Paramedic Part 1

You are dispatched to 75a High Street for a 50 year-old-man with an unknown medical problem. En route to the scene, ambulance control informs you that "CPR is in progress". Your estimated time of arrival to the scene is approximately 15 minutes, but you feel confident this patient has a good chance for survival because your ambulance service has a tiered-response system.

In a brief radio report, technicians on-scene advise you that this was a witnessed cardiac arrest. The patient complained of chest pain just prior to collapse, and CPR was started immediately by a family member. No other information is provided. When you ask if the patient has been defibrillated, no one replies. You find this odd, and wonder if something is wrong.

1. Are career and volunteer staffing held to the same standards of patient care?
2. If sensitive information needs to be relayed regarding patient care, what other communication options should the technicians have available?

the Health Professions Council in 2003 and is still in effect today. As a health professional, you must protect the health and well-being of people who use or need your services in every circumstance.

This means that you must always keep high standards of conduct. You must always:

1. act in the best interests of your patients, clients, and users;
2. respect the confidentiality of your patients, clients, and users;
3. maintain high standards of personal conduct; and,
4. provide any important information about conduct, competence, or health.

Also, you must always keep high standards of performance. You must always:

5. keep your professional knowledge and skills up to date;
6. act within the limits of your knowledge, skills, and experience and, if necessary, refer on to another professional;
7. maintain proper and effective communications with patients, clients, users, carers, and professionals;
8. effectively supervise tasks you have asked others to carry out for you;
9. get informed consent to give treatment (except in an emergency);
10. keep accurate patient, client, and user records;
11. deal fairly and safely with the risks of infection; and,
12. limit your work or stop practising if your performance or judgement is affected by your health.

Finally, you must always keep high standards of ethics. You must always:

13. carry out your duties in a professional and ethical way;
14. behave with integrity and honesty;
15. follow our guidelines for how you advertise your services; and,
16. make sure that your behaviour does not damage your profession's reputation.

These standards, and others like them, are simply an amplification of a very basic concept: concern for the welfare of others. All of the various codes of right and wrong must ultimately arise from that concern, and it is a safe generalisation that *if you place the welfare of the patient ahead of all other considerations, you will rarely if ever commit an unethical act in medical care* **Figure 5-3 ▶**. It would be impossible to enumerate here all the ethical dilemmas with which you may at one time or another be faced in your work as a paramedic. However, if each time you are confronted with a dilemma of right and wrong you ask yourself, "What is in the best interest of the *patient?*" you will be on a firm footing.

To expand this even more, the following principles will help you to deal with a situation where a moral maze may occur:

- *Beneficence* relates to you, the paramedic, acting in the best interests of the patient. Everything you do, or don't do, should be intended to benefit the patient.
- *Nonmaleficence* supports beneficence; your actions should not cause any harm or suffering to any patient. The doctrine of "first do no harm" is applicable here.

You are the Paramedic Part 2

When you arrive, you learn that the AED could not be used because the battery failed. The staff on-scene were relief technicians, and no one had been able that weekend to check the equipment because they had all been at other ambulance stations. They ask you not to tell anyone, and promise it will never happen again.

You don't have time to become involved in a detailed discussion, but gather information pertinent to caring for your patient. As you proceed to hospital, the patient's wife identifies herself, tells you that she is an RN and asks if she can ride with you to hospital. En route to the accident and emergency department, she asks you why the AED failed to operate.

Initial Assessment	Recording Time: 15 Minutes
Level of consciousness	Unresponsive
Airway	Patent
Breathing	Bag-valve-mask ventilations
Circulation	Carotid pulse detected with compressions
Vital Signs	
Skin	Cool, mottled with blue mucosa
Blood pressure	None
SpO_2	Unable to obtain
ECG	Asystole in three leads (I, II, and III)
Pupils	Fixed and dilated

3. Is it ever appropriate to conceal information regarding patient care?
4. How should you answer the wife's question?
5. How and when should you address her concerns?

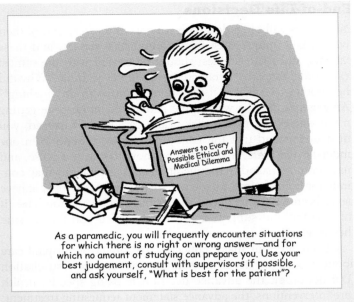

As a paramedic, you will frequently encounter situations for which there is no right or wrong answer—and for which no amount of studying can prepare you. Use your best judgement, consult with supervisors if possible, and ask yourself, "What is best for the patient"?

Figure 5-3

Controversies

Some religious beliefs influence a patient's decision about being treated and may be different from what you think is best for a patient. Patients sometimes refuse standard life-saving therapies and treatments based on their religious convictions.

- *Justice* is a principle where your decisions are fair and just, not only to your patient, but the wider community. You need to consider whether any action you take may prejudice the availability or standard of care to others and ultimately, are your actions in the best interests to all?
- *Dignity* is exactly what it says it is; all patients have the right to be assessed and treated in a dignified way, just as does the person who is undertaking the assessment and treatment. The patient should not be lied to and the truth about their condition is paramount.

Patient's Rights: Autonomy

As you learned in the previous chapter, patients have the right to direct their own care and to decide how they want their end of life medical care provided to them. This right, known as patient autonomy, has come to the forefront of health care ethics.

As medical technology has made the line between life and death more imprecise, a number of high-profile cases have brought the issue of patient autonomy to the forefront of the health care ethics debate in the past 20 years.

Under the Mental Capacity Act 2005, a person who has mental capacity may make an advance directive refusing life-sustaining treatment in the event that they become mentally incapacitated. In your role as a paramedic, you must ensure that when dealing with advance directives, they were made by a person who has capacity at the time, must be clear about the treatment being refused, and must specify in writing if the refusal is intended to apply to life-sustaining treatment.

In England and Wales, the Mental Capacity Act 2005 allows a patient with mental capacity to appoint a proxy decision-maker (who need not be a relative) to make decisions about care and treatment should the patient lose decision-making capacity. This is called a lasting power of attorney. If the patient wishes the attorney to have the power to refuse life-sustaining treatment, this must be specified in writing in the document granting the power. If a person loses capacity and has not taken out a lasting power of attorney, the Court of Protection may appoint a deputy to make health care decisions. The deputy does not have a power to refuse life-sustaining treatment.

In Scotland, the legal position on advance directives is the same as in England and Wales. The Adults with Incapacity (Scotland) Act allows people over 16 to appoint a proxy decision-maker who has the legal power to give consent to medical treatment when the patient loses capacity. Unless to do so is unreasonable or impracticable, the proxy must be consulted about treatment decisions. Proxy decision-makers cannot demand treatment that is judged to be against the patient's interests. The Act also requires doctors to take account, so far as is reasonable and practicable, of the views of the patient's nearest relative and his or her primary carer.

It is good practice to involve people close to the patient in decisions. If the patient is mentally capable, their consent should be sought before friends or relatives are involved and capable patients should be asked whom they would like to be involved in their decision-making should they become mentally incapacitated. Refusal by a mentally capable person to allow information about their treatment to be divulged to specified relatives should be respected. If the wishes of a mentally incapacitated patient regarding treatment are not known, those providing care have a duty to act in the person's best interests. In determining best interests, paramedics and other health care professionals must, where practicable and appropriate, consider the views of anyone named by the person to be consulted, any carer of the person interested in his or her welfare, anyone who exercises a lasting power of attorney granted by the person (England and Wales) or who is a treatment proxy (Scotland), or any deputy appointed by the Court of Protection.

Patients' decisions may not be accepted by other members of the public or other members of the patient's family, but it is important for the paramedic to remember that each of us has the right to make decisions about our own medical care. Patients may well make decisions, such as refusals of treatment, that the paramedic does not agree with, but the paramedic must respect that patient's wishes, assuming the patient has decision-making capacity. Ethics has become the subject of many paramedic discussions because paramedics find themselves in the unique position of being accountable to more systems than the average health care provider in trying to respect the wishes of the patient

Figure 5-4 ▾ . The ambulance service you work for and your community's standard of care could compete with the wishes of the patient. These competing interests can create an ethical conflict that you will want to resolve. How? Communicate, communicate, communicate. Occasionally, a doctor will give an order that the paramedic feels is detrimental to the patient's best interests. It is important for the paramedic to discuss why they feel that way with the doctor immediately. Remember, you are often in a better position to see what is going on with the patient, and a big part of your job is to communicate fully with the doctor. A paramedic should never perform a procedure or administer a medication that he or she believes will be deliberately detrimental to the patient. If a doctor, for example, mistakenly asks you to perform a procedure in which you are not trained, it is important for you to ask the doctor to repeat the order. However, if the dispute is not resolved, you need to be a patient advocate and act in the patient's best interest. If the doctor is insistent, there are several ways to handle the problem: (1) Tell the doctor that your standing orders are never to perform this procedure; can he or she suggest another alternative? (2) Tell the doctor that you can only perform the procedure if your medical director approves. None of these are even half as good as having a good, trusting relationship between you as a paramedic and the staff of the accident and emergency department. Communicate!

A situation that is much more common is the necessity of treating patients against their wishes. As a paramedic, you have a duty to take such steps as are reasonable in the circumstances to assess the patient's capacity   Figure 5-5 ▸ . If you form the reasonable belief that the person lacks mental capacity to make the decision, you have a duty to give treatment which you reasonably believe to be in the patient's best interests. In making that decision, you have a duty to take into account the patient's wishes and feelings expressed while competent.

End-of-Life Decisions

Paramedics will often deal with patients at the very end of their lives. It is a unique trust in the ambulance service, and these patients, and their families, should be treated with the utmost respect and empathy. Paramedics should never think: "Why did they bother to call 999 if they don't want us to do anything"? (An example, by the way, of the paramedic moral code getting in the way of the paramedic's health care ethics.) Instead, you must understand that the family of a dying patient, even one under hospice care, may not know how to check a pulse, and may not understand that difficult, agonal respirations may continue for hours before a patient actually dies. Many people have never been with someone at the moment of death. You have. If information and support is what they called you for, be sure they receive it—it is part of your job.

There are four major concepts that direct prehospital care about end-of-life decisions: the do not attempt resuscitation (DNAR) order; the advance decision refusing specific health care interventions; the advance statement requesting treatment; and the lasting power of attorney (England and Wales) or treatment proxy (Scotland).

DNAR Orders

During the last decade, DNAR orders were finally recognised in the prehospital setting. The ambulance service has now joined the medical community in recognising that patients have the same rights to direct their care, and to refuse care, outside the hospital that they do inside the hospital. Many trusts now have protocol specific to the ambulance service, and most trusts have laws that govern the process of dying and what rights patients have to direct that process.

Although the technicalities may vary from service to service, ambulance service DNAR orders are written orders designed to tell ambulance service technicians and paramedics when resuscitation is or is not appropriate. Trusts have their

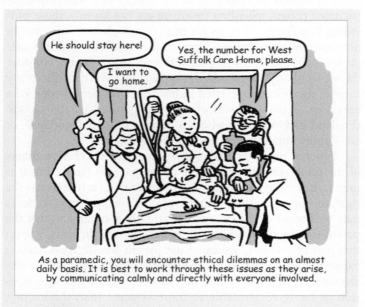

As a paramedic, you will encounter ethical dilemmas on an almost daily basis. It is best to work through these issues as they arise, by communicating calmly and directly with everyone involved.

Figure 5-4

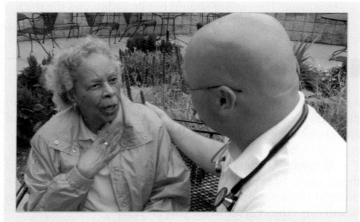

Figure 5-5 Remember that the decision to accept medical treatment is a difficult one. Give the patient time to think and to consider what feels right. Often, this is the first time the patient has had to face the reality of his or her medical condition.

own procedure for how to recognise a valid DNAR order. Some United Kingdom (UK) ambulance trusts rely on a written doctor order (which might not be available at the time to the ambulance service clinician), while others may require the patient to wear a bracelet or necklace. In some cases, such jewellery indicates that the patient has consented to the release of stored information, such as the patient's DNAR status, to medical personnel Figure 5-6 ▶ . In some trusts, DNAR orders expire within a specified time frame, and must be renewed in order to remain valid, while others may have no expiration date. You should be familiar with the documents used in your trust, and what you are expected to do if the documents are not available.

You, the paramedic, should avoid imposing your own moral code on a patient whose value system may be very different from your own. Paramedics will be called to assist with dying patients with varied cultural beliefs and should be prepared to respect a patient's wishes even if the patient's lifestyle or religious beliefs differ greatly from the paramedic's.

Paramedics are likely to encounter confusing scenarios when the DNAR paperwork may not be immediately available. It is permissible to begin resuscitation efforts, and then to discontinue them if and when the paperwork is confirmed. In other situations, the paperwork may be present, but family members may disagree with the DNAR order and insist that you begin resuscitation. In these situations, avoid any hostile encounters while carrying out the patient's wishes to the best of your ability. Contact control in confusing situations involving resuscitation questions.

Advance Decisions, Advance Statements, and Lasting Power of Attorney

The term living will has no legal significance in the UK, but is an umbrella term covering different types of arrangements made by a patient while they are still capable to enable their wishes to be respected when they lose mental capacity to make decisions for themselves. There are three types of arrangements which may be made: the advance decision refusing specified medical treatments, the advance statement requesting a specified intervention, and the lasting power of attorney or treatment proxy whereby a person is appointed to make decisions after the patient loses mental capacity. In each case, the precondition which activates the arrangements is the patient losing decision-making capacity.

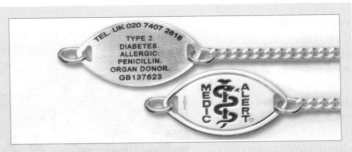

Figure 5-6 Medical ID bracelets can provide access to vital information about a patient, including important medical conditions and possible DNAR orders. In the case of MedicAlert®, the ambulance service provider can obtain stored patient information from the MedicAlert Foundation.

Advance decisions refuse specified medical treatments. Under the Mental Capacity Act 2005, a person who has mental capacity may make an advance decision refusing life-sustaining treatment in the event that they become mentally incapacitated. To be binding on health care professionals, an advance decision must be made by a person who has capacity at the time, must be clear about the treatment being refused, and specify in writing if the refusal is intended to apply to life-sustaining treatment. Advance decisions may be made in oral form, but if they are to refuse life-sustaining treatment, they must be in writing.

An advance directive requesting treatment is known as an advance statement. Unlike an advance decision refusing treatment, an advance statement cannot bind a clinician to provide treatment which is futile, or which is contrary to that clinician's assessment of the patient's best interests. However, such a statement must be considered by anyone making a decision about what is in the patient's best interests.

At the Scene

Do not be confused: A living will is not the same as a DNAR order. The living will allows for decisions to be made regarding DNAR orders if a patient becomes incapacitated or unable to make his or her own decisions.

You are the Paramedic Part 3

After you arrive at hospital your patient is pronounced dead. At this point, there is no way for you to know whether the patient could have been saved with the prompt use of the AED. You contact your supervisor, notify him of this issue and contact medical control to report the incident to her. You then carefully document all of the pertinent patient care information in the patient record form.

6. Beyond the documentation required to complete the patient record form, what else should you document and how?

7. Why is it important to completely and concisely document a call, especially a call such as this one?

8. What is the purpose of continuous quality improvement?

In England and Wales, the Mental Capacity Act 2005 allows a patient with mental capacity to appoint a proxy decision-maker (who need not be a relative) to make decisions about care and treatment should the patient lose decision-making capacity. This is called a lasting power of attorney. If the patient wishes the attorney to have the power to refuse life-sustaining treatment, this must be specified in writing in the document granting the power. If a person loses capacity and has not taken out a lasting power of attorney, the Court of Protection may appoint a deputy to make health care decisions. The deputy does not have a power to refuse life-sustaining treatment.

In Scotland, the legal position on advance decisions and advance statements is the same as in England and Wales. The Adults with Incapacity (Scotland) Act allows people over 16 to appoint a proxy decision-maker who has the legal power to give consent to medical treatment when the patient loses capacity. Unless to do so is unreasonable or impracticable, the proxy must be consulted about treatment decisions. Proxy decision-makers cannot demand treatment that is judged to be against the patient's interests. The Act also requires doctors to take account, so far as is reasonable and practicable, of the views of the patient's nearest relative and his or her primary carer.

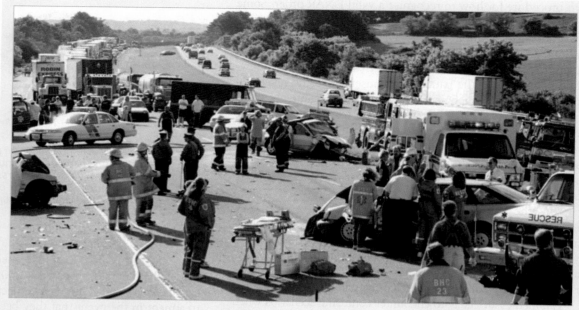

Figure 5-7 Although our instincts are always to try to sustain life at whatever cost, sometimes it is clear that resuscitation efforts will be futile, and should be withheld per local protocols.

▌Withholding or Withdrawing Resuscitation

Modern health care ethical guidelines rely on the use of common sense and reasonable judgement in deciding when to stop CPR and resuscitation efforts, as well as when it is appropriate for paramedics to decline to initiate them at all. Numerous medical studies have shown that resuscitation of medical as well as trauma patients is sometimes futile at the onset or may become futile at some point. Futile resuscitation efforts—interventions that studies have shown do not benefit patients—are not medically or ethically indicated (Figure 5-7 ▲).

Paramedics, especially those working in rural situations, will need to carefully consider the time it will take for a patient to reach definitive care at the hospital.

You are the Paramedic Part 4

An internal investigation was initiated by medical control to determine the appropriate course of action regarding this call. You learn that evidence normally gathered by the AED, including an audio recording of the event, as well as a cardiac strip, are now missing. Without these pieces to the puzzle, the investigation comes to a halt.

You receive a call from one of the technicians, and he tells you that he witnessed one of the other technicians destroying the evidence. Even more unnerving, he tells you this has happened before. He is a fairly new technician and is afraid that he will be let go if anyone learns that he called you.

9. What should you do?

10. Can ambulance service trusts be sued? Can ambulance service clinicians be sued?

4. **Medical control gives you an order to give one of the patients 2 mg of morphine for pain. The patient says he is not in that much pain, and although he is not allergic to opioids, he doesn't like the effect they have on him. Should you follow the medical director's order?**
   A. Give medical control the information the patient has shared with you, and ask that he reconsider his order.
   B. Tell the patient that medical control is your boss, and what he says has to be done.
   C. Tell medical control you will administer the morphine, but don't actually administer it to the patient.
   D. Tell the patient that he may not be in much pain yet, but he will, and medical control knows best.

5. **On an off-duty Friday night, some friends call and ask you to a party. You don't have a designated driver, and you can't stay out too late because you have a shift in the morning. What do you do?**
   A. Go out and have a good time; life is short. You can drive slowly on the way home and be very careful because it's not too far from your house.
   B. If you go, don't drink. You have a reputation to uphold.
   C. Go, but drink very little, so you're only driving under the influence a little, not a lot.
   D. Just make sure you're completely sober before hitting the road home.

6. **The older woman in the second vehicle tells you she has a terminal illness. When she begins having chest pains, she requests that you do nothing to save her if she should go into cardiac arrest. She does not have her DNAR orders with her, however. She is relatively calm, and seems to be of sound mind in making her decision. She does not even want the ECG put on her. What do you do?**
   A. Comply with her wishes if she is competent to make the decision.

   B. You cannot comply with her request unless she has her DNAR order with her.
   C. Tell her that you must hook up the ECG machine and treat her until she is at hospital, where she and a doctor can decide what is best.
   D. Call medical control, explain the situation, and ask for advice.

Challenging Questions

You are called to the scene of a two-car accident involving several teenage girls. They all claim to be injured only slightly. One of the members of your team jokingly says that in any trauma, the rule is to "strip them" and check them thoroughly. You know they should have a complete physical examination—many patients don't feel other injuries until the adrenaline of the situation has worn off. However, you also know that at least one person on your team is hinting at taking advantage of the situation.

7. **Do you give the patients a thorough examination, while also giving your colleague(s) a cheap thrill?**

8. **Do you point out to your colleague(s) that what they are doing is unethical and unprofessional, and has no place in the field of prehospital care?**

9. **Do you report what you saw and heard to your line manager after the incident is taken care of?**

Points to Ponder

The more time you spend with your new colleague, the more you think he may have a substance abuse problem that is getting worse. He is having trouble remembering things and making quick decisions on the job. You see him taking pills often, but nothing you recognise. When you question him even subtly, he gets defensive and angry. His actions may cause a mistake, or put someone in danger. You like him, and he's a good colleague when he isn't affected by whatever he is taking, and you don't want to get him in trouble.

What do you do?

Issues: Working With Other Providers, Accountability to the Ambulance Service System and the Patient, Maintaining and Encouraging the Standard of Care.

www.Paramedic.EMSzone.com/UK/

6 Pathophysiology

This chapter on pathophysiology has been adapted from *Paramedic: Pathophysiology* (Bob Elling, Mikel A. Rothenberg, MD, and Kirsten M. Elling, 2006, Jones and Bartlett Publishers). It is dedicated to the late Dr Rothenberg, who, like Dr Caroline, spent his life helping health care providers understand the complexity of the human body in crisis and injury.

Objectives

Cognitive

- Discuss cellular adaptation.
- Describe cellular injury and cellular death.
- Describe the factors that precipitate disease in the human body.
- Describe the cellular environment.
- Discuss analysing disease risk.
- Describe environmental risk factors.
- Discuss combined effects and interaction among risk factors.
- Describe ageing as a risk factor for disease.
- Discuss family diseases and associated risk factors.
- Discuss hypoperfusion.
- Define cardiogenic, hypovolaemic, neurogenic, anaphylactic, and septic shock.
- Describe multiple organ dysfunction syndrome.
- Define the characteristics of the immune response.
- Discuss induction of the immune system.
- Discuss fetal and neonatal immune function.
- Discuss ageing and the immune function in the elderly.
- Describe the inflammation response.
- Discuss the role of mast cells as part of the inflammation response.
- Describe the plasma protein system.
- Discuss the cellular components of inflammation.
- Describe the systemic manifestations of the inflammation response.
- Describe the resolution and repair from inflammation.
- Discuss the effect of ageing on the mechanisms of self-defence.
- Discuss hypersensitivity.
- Describe deficiencies in immunity and inflammation.
- Describe homeostasis as a dynamic steady state.
- List types of tissue.
- Describe the systemic manifestations that result from cellular injury.
- Describe neuroendocrine regulation.
- Discuss the inter-relationships between stress, coping, and illness.
- Identify the characteristics of the inflammatory process.
- Identify the difference between cellular and humoral immunity.
- Identify alterations in immunological response.
- Describe the function of coagulation factors, platelets, and blood vessels necessary for normal coagulation.
- Identify blood groups.
- Describe how acquired factor deficiencies may occur.
- Define fibrinolysis.

Affective

- Advocate the need to understand and apply the knowledge of pathophysiology to patient assessment and treatment.

Psychomotor

None

Introduction

The human body is made up of cells, tissues, and organs, which function in a constantly changing microenvironment. The study of living organisms with regard to their origin, growth, structure, behaviour, and reproduction is known as biology. Pathophysiology refers to the study (*logos*) of the functioning of the organism (*physiology*) in the presence of suffering/disease (*pathos*). When the normal condition or functioning of the cellular systems breaks down in response to stressors, and the systems can no longer maintain homeostasis, disease may result. Determining the aetiology (cause) of this disease process often helps the paramedic identify an informed approach to both evaluation and initial treatment of the patient.

To understand how disease may alter cellular function, it is first necessary to understand normal cellular structure and function. This chapter begins by reviewing the structure and function of the cellular system and environment. Following that review is a discussion of how alterations of the environment and normal homeostasis may result in the state of disease. Next, the impact of genetics on the development of disease states, the role of immunity and self-defence mechanisms in protecting the organism from disease, the states of inflammation and shock, and the role of stress on the development of disease are described and discussed in detail.

Review of the Basic Cellular Systems

Cells

The cell is the basic self-sustaining unit of the human body. As cells grow and mature, they become specialised (eg, kidney cells) through the process of differentiation. Groups of cells form tissues, various types of tissues make up organs, and groups of organs constitute organ systems.

Nearly all cells of higher organisms, except mature red blood cells and platelets, have three main components: the cell membrane, the cytoplasm containing the internal components or organelles, and a nucleus.

The cell membrane consists of fat and protein. It surrounds the cell and protects the internal components within the cytoplasm.

At the Scene

Chemically, fatty compounds—like those in the cell membrane—are neutral (uncharged), whereas electrolytes (sodium and potassium) are water-based (charged). Fats are soluble in oil but not in water. Thus, for a charged molecule to enter through a cell membrane, it has to travel through a special pathway. These transport channels—the so-called ion channels—consist of protein-lined pores that are specifically sized for each substance (calcium and potassium). Local anaesthetics (eg, lignocaine) and antiarrhythmic drugs (eg, amiodarone) exert their effects by blocking ion channels.

The organelles, which are found within the cell's cytoplasm (fluid), operate in a cooperative and organised fashion to maintain the life of the cell. They include the following components Figure 6-1 ▶ :

Ribosomes contain RNA and protein. They interact with RNA from other parts of the cell, joining amino acid chains together to form proteins. When ribosomes attach to endoplasmic reticulum, they create rough endoplasmic reticulum.

You are the Paramedic Part 1

You are complaining to your colleague about how taking a pathophysiology review course has nothing at all to do with being a paramedic when you are called to a local dialysis centre for an unknown medical emergency. You are met by a health care assistant who takes you to a 67-year-old woman who appears to be in moderate distress. The nurse caring for the patient states that 30 minutes into dialysis, the patient's blood pressure dropped to 86/44 and she became short of breath. They immediately stopped therapy and called 999. This occurred approximately 15 minutes prior to your arrival. The nurse further mentions that the patient has a fever of 38.8°C. When questioned, the patient tells you that she missed her last two dialysis sessions because she was not feeling well. She admits to having malaise and a fever for 3 days. She further complains of pain in her right forearm at the site of the dialysis shunt and slight shortness of breath. The patient denies experiencing chest pain, nausea, vomiting, abdominal pain, or dizziness.

Initial Assessment	Recording Time: 0 Minutes
Appearance	Awake and anxious
Level of consciousness	A (Alert to person, place, and day)
Airway	Open
Breathing	Slightly elevated rate with accessory muscle use noted
Circulation	Weak radial pulses with pale, warm, moist skin

1. What are some of the potential complications that can occur from missing dialysis?
2. Does renal disease affect other organ systems?

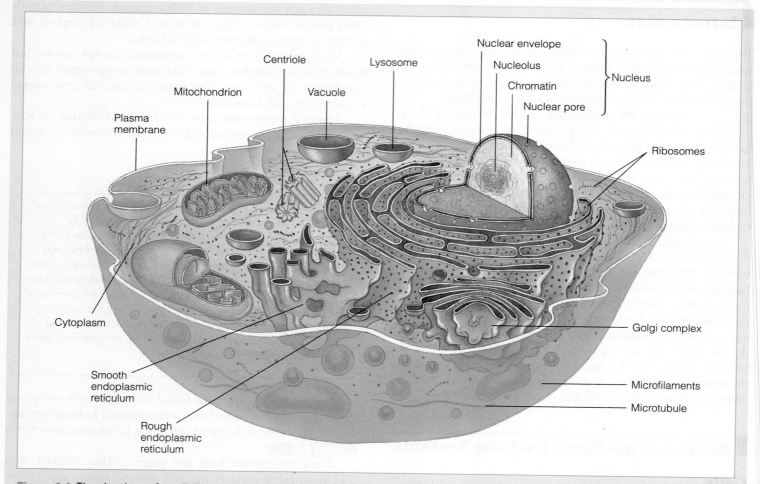

Figure 6-1 The structure of a cell. The cell is divided into nuclear and cytoplasmic compartments. The cytoplasm is packed with organelles, the structures in which the cell carries out many functions.

The *endoplasmic reticulum* is a network of tubules, vesicles, and sacs. Rough endoplasmic reticulum is involved in building proteins. Smooth endoplasmic reticulum is involved in building lipids (fats), such as those found in the cell membranes and those found in carbohydrates.

The *Golgi complex* is located near the nucleus of the cell. It is involved in the synthesis and packaging of various carbohydrates (sugar) and complex protein molecules such as enzymes.

Lysosomes are membrane-bound vesicles that contain digestive enzymes. These enzymes function as an intracellular digestive system, breaking down bacteria and organic debris that have been taken into the cell.

Similar to lysosomes, *peroxisomes* are found in high concentrations in the liver and neutralise toxins such as alcohol.

Mitochondria are small, rod-like organelles that function as the metabolic centre of the cell. They produce adenosine triphosphate (ATP), which is the major energy source for the body.

The nucleus contains the genetic material, called chromatin, and the nucleoli, which are rounded, dense structures

that contain ribonucleic acid (RNA). The RNA is responsible for controlling the cellular activities. The nucleus is surrounded by a membrane called the nuclear envelope; the nucleus itself is embedded in the cytoplasm.

Tissues

Tissues are composed of groups of similar cells that work together for a common function. There are four types of tissues: epithelial, connective, muscle, and nerve tissue.

Epithelium covers the external surfaces of the body. Epithelial tissue also lines hollow organs within the body, such as the intestines, blood vessels, and bronchial tubes. In addition to providing a protective barrier, epithelial tissues play roles in the absorption of nutrients in the intestines and the secretion of various body substances. For example, the sweat glands in the dermis layer of the skin—specifically, the stratified squamous epithelial cells—produce a solution containing urea and salt. In contrast, the simple columnar epithelium lines the small intestine and absorbs nutrients from the foods we eat. The epithelial cells that line the inside of blood vessels are called endothelial cells; they regulate the flow of blood through the vessel as well as clotting of the blood (coagulation).

Connective tissue binds the other types of tissue together. The extracellular matrix is a nonliving substance consisting of protein fibres, nonfibrous protein, and fluid that separates connective tissue cells from one another. Collagen is the major protein within the extracellular matrix. At least 12 types of collagen exist, with types I, II, and III being the most abundant. Alterations in collagen structure resulting from abnormal genes or abnormal processing of collagen proteins result in numerous diseases (eg, scurvy). Bone and cartilage are subtypes of connective tissue. Adipose tissue is a special type of connective tissue that contains large amounts of lipids (fat).

Muscle tissue is characterised by its ability to contract. It is enclosed by fascia, which is the layer of fibrous connective tissue that separates individual muscles. Muscles overlie the framework of the skeleton and are classified in terms of both their structure and their function. Structurally, muscle tissue is either striated (ie, microscopic bands or striations can be seen) or nonstriated (also called smooth). Functionally, muscle is either voluntary (consciously controlled) or involuntary (not normally under conscious control).

The three types of muscle are skeletal muscle (striated voluntary), cardiac muscle (striated involuntary), and smooth muscle (nonstriated involuntary). Most of the muscles used voluntarily in day-to-day activities are skeletal muscles. The heart consists of cardiac muscle and has the ability to both contract and generate impulses. Smooth muscle lines most glands, digestive organs, lower airways, and vessels. When a person's brain senses the need to respond to an environmental stimulus by vasoconstriction, the vessels in the periphery react. For example, the smooth muscle in the bronchioles may vasoconstrict during an asthma attack, leading to wheezing and difficulty moving air out of the lungs. Smooth muscle is also responsible for constriction and dilation of the pupil of the eye when it is exposed to changes in light levels.

Nerve tissue is characterised by its ability to transmit nerve impulses. The central nervous system (CNS) consists of the brain and the spinal cord. Peripheral nerves extend from the brain and spinal cord, exiting from between the vertebrae to various parts of the body.

Neurons are the main conducting cells of nerve tissue, and the cell body of the neuron is the site of most cellular functions. Dendrites receive electrical impulses from the axons of other nerve cells and conduct them toward the cell body, whereas axons typically conduct electrical impulses away from the cell body. Each neuron has only one axon, but it may have several dendrites. Nerve cells are separated by a gap called the synapse. Electrical impulses travel down the nerve and trigger the release of neurotransmitters, which carry the impulse from axon to dendrite.

Homeostasis

Adaptive responses to various stimuli allow the cells and tissues to respond and function in stressful environments, in a constant effort to preserve a degree of stability or equilibrium.

This adaptation process is known as homeostasis (from the Greek words for "same" and "steady"); it is also called the *dynamic steady state*.

Homeostasis is maintained in the body because normal regulatory systems are counterbalanced by counter-regulatory systems. Thus, for every cell, tissue, or organ that performs one function, there is always at least one component that performs the opposing function. For example, the autonomic nervous system consists of the sympathetic and parasympathetic components, which act to speed up or slow down the activity of target organs. Other homeostatic mechanisms include the body's control of its internal temperature despite fluctuations in the external temperature, the regulation of pH and acid–base balance in the body, and the balance of water or hydration in the cells and body of the organism.

Regulatory systems communicate within the body mainly at the cellular level. Cells communicate electrochemically through a process called cell signalling, in which they release molecules (such as hormones) that bind to proteins called receptors, located on the surface of the receiving cells. This signalling triggers chemical reactions in the receiving cells that lead to a biological action. When the action is completed, the opposing system "turns off" the action through a process called feedback inhibition or negative feedback `Figure 6-2 ▶`.

The thermostat mechanism in a house is a good example of a feedback mechanism. In the middle of the winter, heat is constantly being lost through the house's windows, doors, and any poorly insulated areas. The thermostat detects this decrease in temperature and signals the boiler to produce heat to rewarm the house. Once the temperature rises to a certain point, the thermostat gives negative feedback to the boiler, causing it to shut down to prevent overheating. This feedback process keeps the house temperature within a selected range `Figure 6-3 ▶`. Similarly, the body is constantly generating heat through its cellular processes. Five primary mechanisms help the body eliminate excess temperature or heat: convection, conduction, radiation, evaporation, and respiration. In short, the body's thermostat works to balance the generation of heat with the processes of heat elimination.

The human body maintains homeostasis by balancing what it takes in with what it puts out. For example, the body takes in chemicals and electrolytes, food, and water. It utilises the nutrients, proteins, sugars, and oxygen and then eliminates the unnecessary chemicals and byproducts through respiration (carbon dioxide), urine and sweat (excess liquids), and faeces (solid waste). `Figure 6-4 ▶` illustrates this normal balance.

When normal cell signalling is interrupted, disease occurs. The normal counterbalances within the body are rendered ineffective, such that normal regulatory systems begin to operate autonomously. The system stops providing critical negative feedback; instead, it gives unopposed positive feedback.

Excessive output can rapidly upset homeostasis (eg, severe diarrhoea kills millions of children each year in some countries, and severe perspiration can cause excessive water loss and dehydration). Likewise, changes in input can alter homeostasis

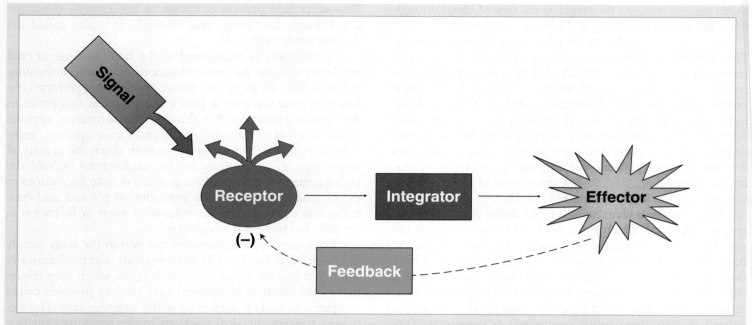

Figure 6-2 Most cellular communication includes a component of negative feedback in which the product of a reaction feeds back information about its own "assembly line", thereby stopping its own production.

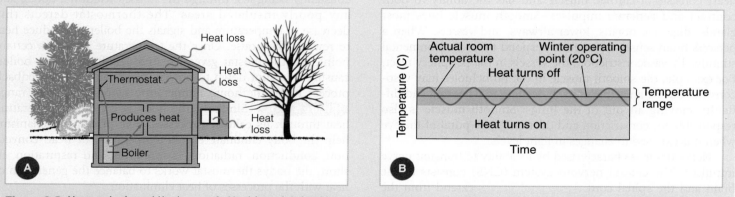

Figure 6-3 Homeostasis and the house. **A.** Heat is maintained in a house by a boiler, which compensates for heat loss. The thermostat monitors the internal temperature and switches the boiler on and off in response to temperature changes. **B.** A hypothetical temperature graph showing temperature fluctuation around the set point.

(eg, going without water for 3 or more days can be life-threatening, and excess salt intake can cause hypertension) **Figure 6-5** ▶.

The degree of fluid imbalance required to alter homeostasis and result in illness depends on the individual's size, age, and underlying medical conditions. In healthy adults, loss of more than 30% of total body fluid is required, but a loss of only 10% to 15% of total body fluid in a small child could easily result in symptoms. For this reason, fluid therapy is part of the basics of resuscitation.

Ligands

Ligands are molecules that are either produced by the body (endogenous) or given as a drug (exogenous), and that bind any receptor, anywhere, leading to any reaction. In addition to medications, common ligands include hormones, neurotransmitters, and electrolytes.

Hormones are substances that are formed in very small amounts in one specialised organ or group of cells and then carried to another organ or group of cells in the same organism to perform regulatory functions. Endocrine hormones (eg,

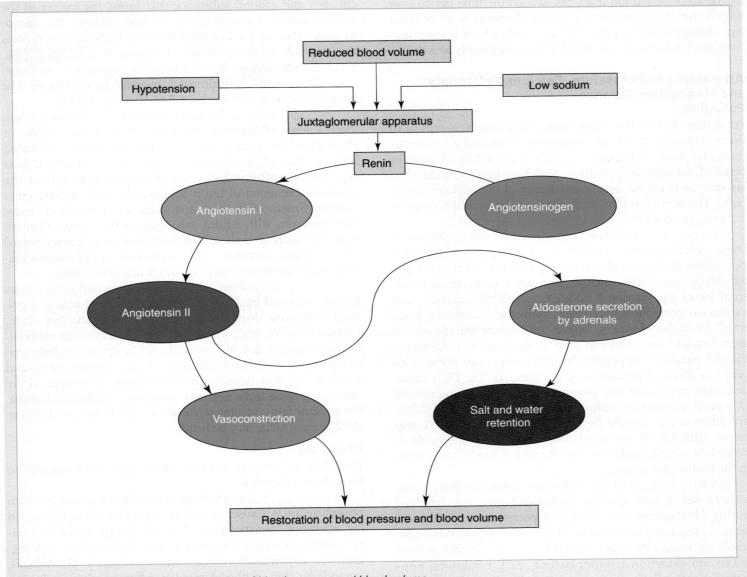

Figure 6-8 Role of the kidneys in regulation of blood pressure and blood volume.

water movement across the cell membrane. When cells are placed in an isotonic solution (ie, one with the same osmolarity as intracellular fluid—280 mOsm/kg), they neither shrink nor swell. When cells are placed in a hypertonic solution, water is pulled out of the cells and they shrink. When cells are placed in a hypotonic solution, they swell.

An isotonic fluid deficit is a decrease in extracellular fluid with proportionate losses of sodium and water. An isotonic fluid excess is a proportionate increase in both sodium and water in the extracellular fluid compartment; common causes include kidney, heart, and liver failure. Manifestations of these problems depend on the serum sodium level. When dehydration exists, orthostatic hypotension and decreased urine output (oliguria) are common. Hyperthermia, delirium, and coma may be seen with very high sodium levels (> 160 mmol/l).

A hypertonic fluid deficit is caused by excess body water loss without a proportionate sodium loss (a relative water loss exists). The result is hypernatraemia, which is clinically defined as a serum sodium level greater than 148 mmol/l and a serum osmolarity greater than 295 mOsm/kg. A hypotonic fluid deficit is caused by excessive sodium loss with less water loss (a relative water excess exists). This results in hyponatraemia, which is characterised by a serum sodium level less than 135 mmol/l and a serum osmolarity less than 280 mOsm/kg.

Causes of hypernatraemia and hyponatraemia may include excess sweating from hot environmental conditions or exercise as well as gastrointestinal losses through vomiting, diarrhoea, inappropriate intravenous fluids, or diuretics. Some patients have nausea and headaches, and others go on to develop convulsions and coma. Clinical findings typically depend not only on the absolute sodium level, but also on the time period over which the abnormality developed. Patients who become hyponatraemic over a period of days tend to have fewer symptoms than individuals who develop the abnormality acutely.

Alterations in Potassium, Calcium, Phosphate, and Magnesium Balance

Potassium

Potassium (K$^+$), as the major intracellular cation, is critical to many functions of the cell. Potassium is necessary for neuromuscular control, regulation of the three types of muscles (skeletal, smooth, and cardiac), acid–base balance, intracellular enzyme reactions, and maintenance of intracellular osmolarity. The normal serum level of potassium is in the range of 3.5 to 5.0 mmol/l.

Hypokalaemia is defined as a decreased serum potassium level. Common causes include decreased potassium intake, potassium shifts into the cells (eg, insulin, alkalosis, beta-adrenergic stimulation such as with adrenaline), renal potassium losses (eg, increased aldosterone activity, diuretics), and extrarenal potassium losses (eg, vomiting, diarrhoea, laxatives). Muscular weakness, fatigue, and muscle cramps are the most frequent complaints in mild to moderate hypokalaemia. Flaccid paralysis, hyporeflexia, and tetany may occur with very low levels of potassium (< 2.5 mmol/l). The ECG shows decreased amplitude and broadening of T waves, prominent U waves, premature ventricular contractions and other arrhythmias (eg, torsade de pointes), and depressed ST segments. Although acute hypokalaemia can be treated with IV potassium supplementation, this therapy is rarely undertaken in the prehospital setting.

Hyperkalaemia is an elevated serum potassium level. Common causes include spurious causes (repeated fist-clenching during phlebotomy, with release of potassium from forearm muscles; specimen drawn from an arm with a potassium infusion), decreased excretion (renal failure, drugs that inhibit potassium excretion [spironolactone, ACE inhibitors, non-steroidal anti-inflammatory drugs (NSAIDs)]), shifts of potassium from within the cell (eg, burns, metabolic acidosis, insulin deficiency), and excessive intake of potassium. The elevated potassium level interferes with normal neuromuscular function, leading to muscle weakness and, rarely, flaccid paralysis. ECG changes occur in fewer than half of patients with a serum potassium level greater than 6.5 mmol/l and include peaked T waves, widening of the QRS complex, and arrhythmias (eg, ventricular tachycardia).

Hyperkalaemia can be life-threatening due to its cardiac manifestations; therefore, urgent transfer to definitive care is essential. Calcium administered intravenously immediately antagonises cardiac conduction abnormalities. Bicarbonate, insulin, and salbutamol shift potassium into the cells during a 15- to 30-minute period.

Calcium

The majority (98%) of the body's calcium is found in the bone and teeth. This element provides strength and stability for the collagen and ground substance that forms the matrix of the skeletal system. Calcium enters the body through the gastrointestinal tract and is absorbed from the intestine in a process that depends on the presence of vitamin D Figure 6-9. Vitamin D is largely obtained through exposure to sunlight, stored in the bone, and ultimately excreted by the kidney. The normal serum calcium level is 8.5 to 10.5 mg/100 ml.

Hypocalcaemia is defined as a decreased serum calcium level. Causes of hypocalcaemia include decreased intake or absorption (eg, malabsorption, vitamin D deficit), increased loss (eg, alcoholism, diuretic therapy), and endocrine disease (eg, hypoparathyroidism, sepsis). Symptoms reflect the increased excitation of the neuromuscular and cardiovascular systems. Spasm of skeletal muscle causes cramps and tetany. Laryngospasm with stridor can obstruct the airway. Convulsions can occur as well as abnormal sensations (paraesthesias) of the lips and extremities. Prolongation of the QT interval predisposes to the development of ventricular arrhythmias.

Hypercalcaemia is an increased serum calcium level. Causes include increased intake or absorption (eg, excess antacid ingestion), endocrine disorders (eg, primary hyperparathyroidism, adrenal insufficiency), neoplasms (eg, cancers), and miscellaneous causes (eg, diuretics, sarcoidosis). Symptoms include constipation and frequent urination (polyuria). Stupor, coma, and renal failure may develop in severe cases. Treatment of the underlying cause is the mainstay of dealing with hypercalcaemia. On an acute basis, volume replacement with boluses of 0.45% or 0.9% normal saline may be helpful.

Phosphate

Phosphate is primarily an intracellular anion and is essential to many body functions.

Hypophosphataemia is characterised by a decrease in serum phosphate levels. Causes include decreased supply or absorption (eg, starvation, malabsorption, blocked absorption [aluminum-containing antacids]), excessive loss of phosphate ion (eg, diuretics, hyperparathyroidism, hyperthyroidism, alcoholism), intracellular shift of phosphorus (eg, administration of glucose, anabolic steroids, oral contraceptives, respiratory alkalosis, salicylate poisoning), electrolyte abnormalities (eg, hypercalcaemia, hypomagnesaemia, metabolic acidosis), and abnormal losses followed by inadequate repletion (eg, diabetic ketoacidosis, chronic alcoholism). Symptoms include muscle weakness, decreased deep tendon reflexes, mental obtundation, and confusion. Weakness is common. Acute, severe hypophosphataemia can lead to acute haemolytic anaemia and increased susceptibility to infection. Muscle death (rhabdomyolysis) may also occur. Treatment involves oral replenishment in mild to moderate cases. Severe cases and symptomatic patients require IV phosphate replacement.

Hyperphosphataemia is defined as an increased serum phosphate level. Causes include massive loading of phosphate into the extracellular fluid (eg, excess vitamin D, laxatives or enemas containing phosphate, IV phosphate supplements, chemotherapy, metabolic acidosis) and decreased excretion into the urine (eg, renal failure, hypoparathyroidism, excessive growth hormone [acromegaly]). Symptoms vary widely, but

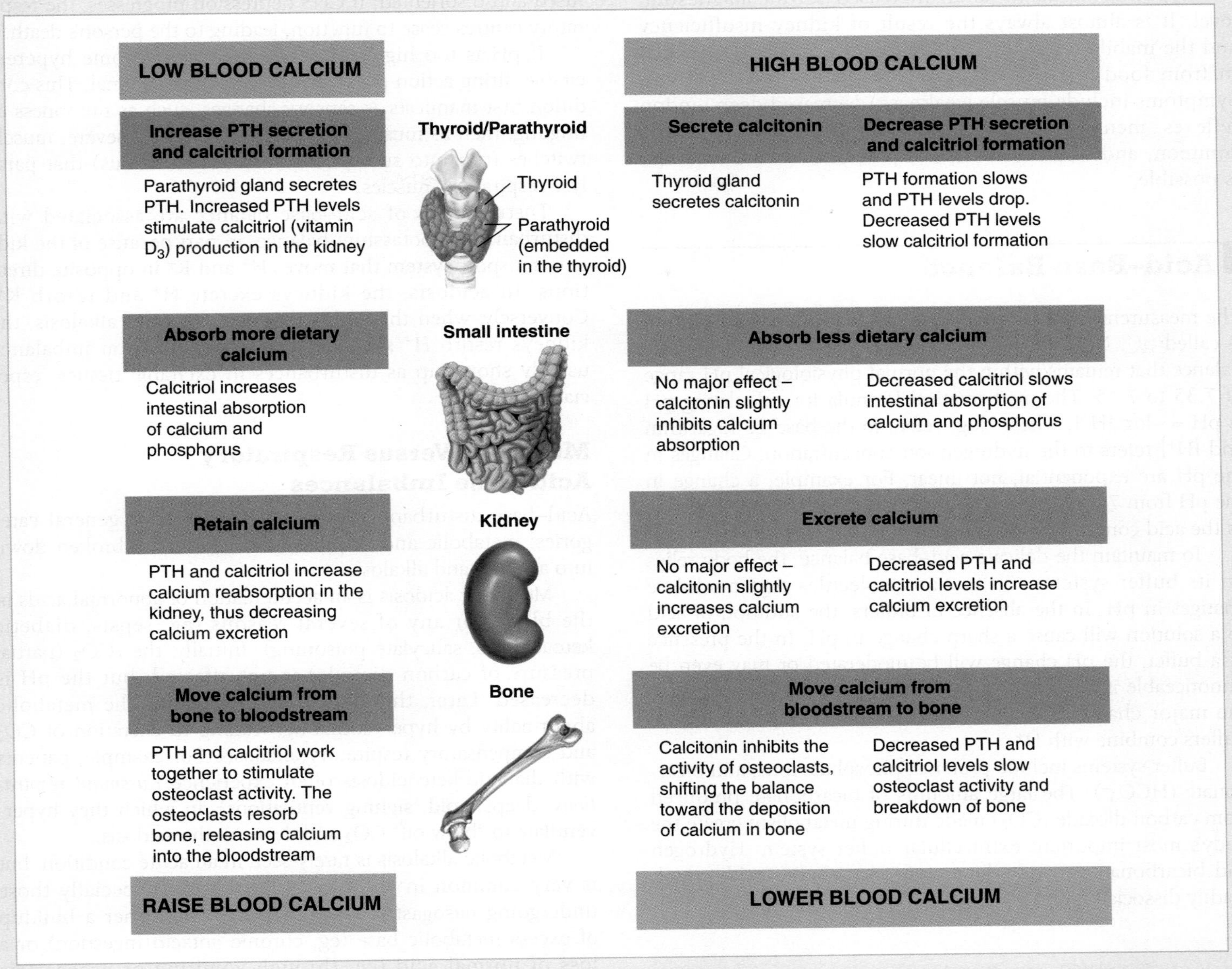

LOW BLOOD CALCIUM

Increase PTH secretion and calcitriol formation

Parathyroid gland secretes PTH. Increased PTH levels stimulate calcitriol (vitamin D_3) production in the kidney

Thyroid/Parathyroid

Thyroid

Parathyroid (embedded in the thyroid)

Absorb more dietary calcium

Calcitriol increases intestinal absorption of calcium and phosphorus

Small intestine

Retain calcium

PTH and calcitriol increase calcium reabsorption in the kidney, thus decreasing calcium excretion

Kidney

Move calcium from bone to bloodstream

PTH and calcitriol work together to stimulate osteoclast activity. The osteoclasts resorb bone, releasing calcium into the bloodstream

Bone

RAISE BLOOD CALCIUM

HIGH BLOOD CALCIUM

Secrete calcitonin

Thyroid gland secretes calcitonin

Decrease PTH secretion and calcitriol formation

PTH formation slows and PTH levels drop. Decreased PTH levels slow calcitriol formation

Absorb less dietary calcium

No major effect – calcitonin slightly inhibits calcium absorption

Decreased calcitriol slows intestinal absorption of calcium and phosphorus

Excrete calcium

No major effect – calcitonin slightly increases calcium excretion

Decreased PTH and calcitriol levels increase calcium excretion

Move calcium from bloodstream to bone

Calcitonin inhibits the activity of osteoclasts, shifting the balance toward the deposition of calcium in bone

Decreased PTH and calcitriol levels slow osteoclast activity and breakdown of bone

LOWER BLOOD CALCIUM

Figure 6-9 Regulation of blood calcium levels. Calcitonin has only a weak effect on calcium ion concentration. It is fast-acting, but any decrease in calcium ion concentration triggers the release of parathyroid hormone (PTH), which almost completely overrides the calcitonin effect. In prolonged calcium excess or deficiency, the parathyroid mechanism is the most powerful hormonal mechanism for maintaining normal blood calcium levels.

may include tremor, paraesthesia, hyporeflexia, confusion, convulsions, muscle weakness, stupor, coma, hypotension, heart failure, and prolonged QT interval. Treatment of the underlying cause and of any accompanying hypocalcaemia is the most common therapeutic approach. Saline boluses (forced diuresis) are often helpful.

Magnesium

Magnesium is the second most abundant intracellular cation, after potassium. About 50% of the body's magnesium is stored in the bones, 49% in the body cells, and the remaining 1% in the extracellular fluid. Normal serum levels are 1.5 to 2.0 mmol/l.

Hypomagnesaemia is defined as a decreased serum magnesium level. Causes include diminished absorption or intake (eg, malabsorption, chronic diarrhoea, laxative abuse, malnutrition), increased renal loss (eg, diuretics, hyperaldosteronism, hypercalcaemia, volume expansion), and miscellaneous causes (eg, diabetes, respiratory alkalosis, pregnancy). Common symptoms are weakness, muscle cramps, and tremor. Patients develop marked neuromuscular and central nervous system hyperirritability with tremors and jerking. There may be hypertension, tachycardia, and ventricular arrhythmias. In some patients, confusion and disorientation are prominent features. Treatment consists of IV fluids containing magnesium.

Hypermagnesaemia is an increased serum magnesium level. It is almost always the result of kidney insufficiency and the inability to excrete the amount of magnesium taken in from food or drugs, especially antacids and laxatives. Symptoms include muscle weakness, decreased deep tendon reflexes, mental obtundation, and confusion. Weakness is common, and respiratory muscle paralysis or cardiac arrest is possible.

Acid–Base Balance

The measurement of hydrogen ion concentration of a solution is called pH. Normal body functions depend on an acid–base balance that remains within the normal physiological pH range of 7.35 to 7.45. The mathematical formula for calculating pH is $pH = -\log [H^+]$, where "log" refers to the base-10 logarithm and $[H^+]$ refers to the hydrogen ion concentration. Changes in the pH are exponential, not linear. For example, a change in the pH from 7.40 to 7.20 results in a 10^2 (ie, 100-fold) change in the acid concentration.

To maintain the delicate acid–base balance, the body relies on its buffer systems. Buffers are molecules that modulate changes in pH. In the absence of buffers, the addition of acid to a solution will cause a sharp change in pH. In the presence of a buffer, the pH change will be moderated or may even be unnoticeable in the same situation. Because acid production is the major challenge to pH homeostasis, most physiological buffers combine with H^+.

Buffer systems include proteins, phosphate ions, and bicarbonate (HCO_3^-). The large amounts of bicarbonate produced from carbon dioxide (CO_2) made during metabolism create the body's most important extracellular buffer system. Hydrogen and bicarbonate ions combine to form carbonic acid, which readily dissociates into water and carbon dioxide:

$$H + HCO_3 \Leftrightarrow H_2CO_3 \Leftrightarrow H_2O + CO_2$$

In the bicarbonate buffer system, excess acid (H^+) combines with bicarbonate (HCO_3), forming H_2CO_3. This compound rapidly dissociates into water and CO_2, which is then exhaled. Because the acid is eliminated as water and CO_2, the total pH does not change significantly. A similar process occurs with the production of metabolic base (bicarbonate).

Acidosis Versus Alkalosis

When the buffering capacity of the body is exceeded, acid–base imbalances occur. A blood pH greater than 7.45 is called alkalosis; a blood pH less than 7.35 is called acidosis.

If the pH is too low (acidosis), neurons become less excitable and CNS depression results. Patients become con-fused and disoriented. If CNS depression progresses, the respiratory centres cease to function, leading to the person's death.

If pH is too high (alkalosis), neurons become hyperexcitable, firing action potentials at the slightest signal. This condition first manifests as sensory changes, such as numbness or tingling, then as muscle twitches. If alkalosis is severe, muscle twitches turn into sustained contractions (tetanus) that paralyse respiratory muscles.

Disturbances of acid–base balance are associated with disturbances in potassium balance, in part because of the kidney transport system that moves H^+ and K^+ in opposite directions. In acidosis, the kidneys excrete H^+ and resorb K^+. Conversely, when the body goes into a state of alkalosis, the kidneys resorb H^+ and excrete K^+. A potassium imbalance usually shows up as disturbances in excitable tissues, especially the heart.

Metabolic Versus Respiratory Acid–Base Imbalances

Acid–base disturbances are classified into two general categories: metabolic and respiratory. Each is then broken down into acidosis and alkalosis.

Metabolic acidosis is an accumulation of abnormal acids in the blood for any of several reasons (eg, sepsis, diabetic ketoacidosis, salicylate poisoning). Initially, the pCO_2 (partial pressure of carbon dioxide) is not affected, but the pH is decreased. Later, the body compensates for the metabolic abnormality by hyperventilating, leading to excretion of CO_2 and compensatory respiratory alkalosis. For example, patients with diabetic ketoacidosis often experience *Kussmaul respirations* (deep, rapid, sighing ventilations), in which they hyperventilate to "blow off" CO_2 and decrease the acidosis.

Metabolic alkalosis is rarely seen in an acute condition, but is very common in chronically ill patients, especially those undergoing nasogastric suction. It involves either a buildup of excess metabolic base (eg, chronic antacid ingestion) or a loss of normal acid (eg, through vomiting or nasogastric suctioning). The pH is high and the pCO_2 unchanged initially. On a chronic basis, the body compensates by slowing ventilation and increasing the pCO_2, thereby creating a compensatory respiratory acidosis.

At the Scene

Respiratory compensation for metabolic problems (acidosis or alkalosis) occurs rapidly and is relatively predictable. Metabolic compensation for respiratory problems (acidosis or alkalosis), if it occurs at all, takes hours to days. Compensation returns the pH toward normal. Acutely, compensation is never complete. Chronic compensation, as in chronic obstructive pulmonary disease (COPD), often results in a completely normal pH.

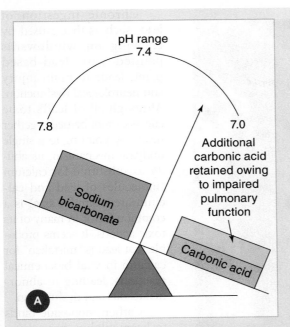
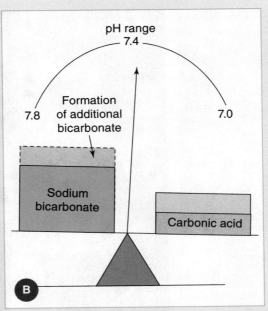

Figure 6-10 **A.** Derangement of acid-base balance in respiratory acidosis. **B.** Compensation by formation of additional bicarbonate.

Respiratory acidosis occurs when CO_2 retention leads to increased pCO_2 levels. It also occurs in situations of hypoventilation (eg, heroin overdose) or intrinsic lung diseases (eg, asthma or COPD) Figure 6-10 ▲.

Excessive "blowing off" of CO_2 with a resulting decrease in the pCO_2 causes respiratory alkalosis. Although often called hyperventilation, many potentially serious diseases (eg, pulmonary embolism, acute myocardial infarction, severe infection, diabetic ketoacidosis) may be responsible for increased ventilatory levels.

Cell Injury

Cellular injury may result from various causes, such as hypoxia (lack of oxygen), ischaemia (hypoxia due to lack of blood supply), chemical injury, infectious injury, immunological (hypersensitivity) injury, physical damage (mechanical injury), and inflammatory injury. The manifestations of cell injury and death depend on how many and which types of cells are damaged.

Manifestations of cellular injury occur at both the microscopic (structural) and the functional levels. Common microscopic abnormalities (eg, those observed in the cardiac cell undergoing necrosis from hypoxaemia for an extended period of time) include cell swelling, rupture of cell membranes or nuclear membranes, and breakdown of nuclear material (chromosomes) Figure 6-11 ▶. This damage often results in a change in cell shape and function. Functional changes may include an inability to use oxygen appropriately, development of intracellular acidosis, accumulation of toxic waste products,

and an inability to metabolise nutrients.

Damage and functional changes in individual cells often have an impact on the entire organism. In some cases, only minor systemic abnormalities are noted, such as fever. At other times, entire organ systems fail and the patient's situation becomes critical (eg, kidney failure). Because all body systems are connected in some manner, dysfunction in one system inevitably affects other systems. When the homeostatic balance in the body is upset, the "scales" can shift in an unfavourable direction.

Cell injury may, up to a point, be repaired with proper treatment. Irreversible injury occurs once cells have passed the "point of no return", after which no treatment will help. Cell death is followed by necrosis, a process in which the cell breaks down. The cell membrane becomes abnormally permeable, leading to an influx of electrolytes and fluids. The cell and its organelles swell. Lysosomes also release enzymes that destroy intracellular components. These processes occur both during and after actual cell death.

Hypoxic Injury

Hypoxic injury is a common—and often deadly—cause of cellular injury. It may result from decreased amounts of oxygen in the air or loss of haemoglobin function (eg, carbon monoxide poisoning), a decreased number of red blood cells (eg, bleeding), disease of the respiratory or cardiovascular system (eg, COPD), or loss of cytochromes (mitochondrial proteins that convert oxygen to ATP, like that seen in cyanide poisoning).

Although hypoxia by itself has deleterious effects on cells, the damage does not stop there. Cells that are hypoxic for more than a few seconds produce mediators (substances) that may damage other local or distant body locations. The result is a positive feedback cycle in which mediators lead to more cell damage, which leads to more hypoxia, which leads to further mediator production, and so forth.

The earliest and most dangerous mediators produced by cells in response to hypoxia are free radicals. These molecules are missing one electron in their outer shell. The presence of an odd, unpaired electron results in chemical instability Figure 6-12 ▶. Free radicals randomly attack cells and membranes in an attempt to "steal back" the missing electron. The result is widespread and potentially deadly tissue damage.

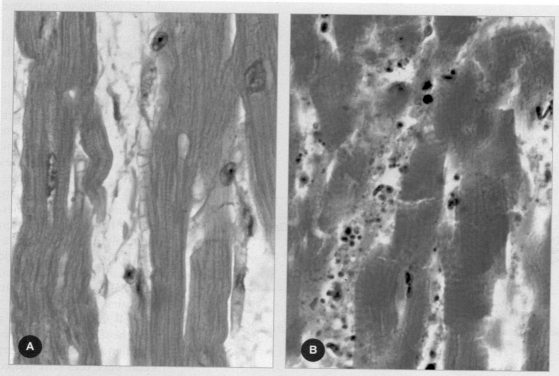

Figure 6-11 Comparison of cardiac muscle fibres. **A.** With necrotic fibres. **B.** Note fragmentation of fibres, loss of nuclear staining, and fragmented bits of nuclear debris. When the cell is injured it swells, resulting in nuclear membrane rupture and breakdown of the nuclear material (original magnification, ×400).

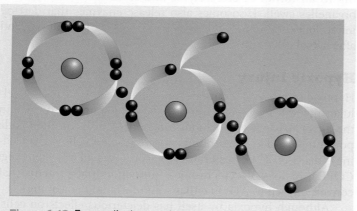

Figure 6-12 Free radicals are missing one electron in their outside orbit. This molecular structure results in chemical instability. Each black dot represents an electron in the outer shell.

Chemical Injury

A variety of chemicals may injure and ultimately destroy cells, including poisons, lead, carbon monoxide, ethanol, and pharmacological agents. Common poisons include cyanide and pesticides. Cyanide induces cell hypoxia by blocking oxidative phosphorylation in the mitochondria and preventing the metabolism of oxygen. Pesticides block an enzyme, acetylcholinesterase, thereby preventing proper transmission of nerve impulses.

Chronic ingestion of lead, such as that caused by chewing on windowsills painted with lead-based paint, leads to brain injury and neurological dysfunction. Although all of lead's toxic effects cannot be tied together neatly by pointing to a single unifying mechanism, its ability to substitute for calcium (molecules of lead and calcium are a similar size) is a common factor in many of its toxic actions. It seems probable that lead is "mistaken" for calcium in vital biochemical reactions, leading to abnormal results and dysfunction.

Carbon monoxide binds to haemoglobin, preventing adequate oxygenation of the tissues. Low levels cause nausea, vomiting, and headache. Higher levels result in death.

In lower doses, ethanol causes the well-known effects of inebriation. Higher doses result in severe CNS depression, hypoventilation, and cardiovascular collapse.

Some pharmacological agents produce toxic products when they are metabolised in the body, especially in "overdose conditions". Paracetamol in doses of more than 140 mg/kg in an adult, results in acute overdose, causing the accumulation of toxic intermediates that poison the liver and may lead to death.

Infectious Injury

Infectious injury to cells occurs as a result of an invasion of either bacteria or viruses. Bacteria may cause injury either by direct action on cells or by the production of toxins. Viruses often initiate an inflammatory response that leads to cell damage and patient symptoms.

Virulence measures the disease-causing ability of a microorganism. The pathogenicity of any particular microorganism is a function of its ability to reproduce and cause disease within the human body. In particular, the growth and survival of bacteria in the body depend on the effectiveness of the body's own defence mechanisms and the bacteria's ability to resist those mechanisms. A depressed immune system is less able to fight off microorganisms that the body perceives as harmful; populations with weaker immune systems may include newborn infants, elderly patients, people with diabetes, and people with cancer or other chronic diseases.

Bacteria

Many bacteria possess a capsule that protects them from ingestion and destruction by phagocytes—cells (eg, white blood cells) that engulf and consume foreign material such as microorganisms and cellular debris Figure 6-13 ▾ . Not all bacteria are encapsulated, however. *Mycobacterium tuberculosis*, for example, lacks a capsule, yet stubbornly resists destruction; it can be transported by phagocytes throughout the body. Gram-positive bacteria are distinguished by very thick cell walls composed of many layers of peptidoglycan (amino acids and sugar); conversely, the cell walls of gram-negative bacteria consist largely of lipids. The pathogenic qualities of gram-negative bacteria, which include the microorganism that causes bubonic plague, make them especially problematic for humans.

Bacteria also produce exotoxins or endotoxins—substances such as enzymes or toxins—that can injure or destroy cells. Staphylococci, streptococci, and *Clostridium tetani*, for example, secrete exotoxins into the medium surrounding the cell. Endotoxins are lipopolysaccharides that are part of the cell walls of gram-negative bacteria. When large amounts of endotoxins are present in the body, a person may develop septic shock.

When cells are injured, circulating white blood cells are attracted to the site of injury. White blood cells release endogenous pyrogens, which then cause a fever to develop. Indeed, the body's most common reaction to the presence of bacteria is inflammation. Some bacteria have the ability to produce hypersensitivity reactions. The proliferation of microorganisms in the blood is called bacteraemia or sepsis.

Viruses

Viruses are intracellular parasites that take over the metabolic processes of the host cell and then use the cell to help them replicate. A virus consists of a nucleic acid core of either RNA or DNA. Surrounding the viral core is a layer of protein known as the capsid, which protects the virus from phagocytosis. Some viruses have an additional protective coat known as the envelope.

The replication of a virus occurs inside the host cell because viruses do not contain any of their own organelles. Viral infection of a host cell leads to a decreased synthesis of macromolecules that are vital to the host cell. Unlike bacteria, however, viruses do not produce exotoxins or endotoxins.

There may be a symbiotic relationship between a virus and normal cells that results in a persistent unapparent infection. Viruses have been known to evoke a strong immune response and can rapidly produce an irreversible, lethal injury in highly susceptible cells, as is the case with acquired immunodeficiency syndrome (AIDS).

Immunological and Inflammatory Injury

Inflammation is a protective response that can occur even without bacterial invasion. Infection is characterised by an invasion of microorganisms that causes cell or tissue injury, which leads to the inflammatory response. The immune system protects the body by providing defences to attack and remove foreign organisms such as bacteria or viruses.

Cellular membranes may be injured when they come in direct contact with the cellular and chemical components of the immune or inflammatory process, such as phagocytes (neutrophils and macrophages), histamine, antibodies, and lymphokines. In such a case, potassium leaks out of the damaged cell and water flows inward, causing the cell to swell. The nuclear envelope, organelle membranes, and cell membrane may all rupture, leading to cell death. The degree of swelling and chance of membrane rupture depend on the severity of the immune and inflammatory responses.

Other Injurious Factors

Genetic factors that may damage cells include chromosomal disorders, premature development of atherosclerosis, and obesity (in some cases). There are two ways an abnormal gene may develop in an individual: by mutation of the gene during meiosis, which affects the newly formed fetus, or by heredity. In trisomy 21 (Down's syndrome), the child is born with an extra chromosome, usually number 21.

Good nutrition is required to maintain good health and assist the cells in fighting off disease. Nutritional disorders that can injure cells and the organism as a whole include obesity, malnutrition, vitamin excess or deficiency, and mineral excess or deficiency. These conditions can lead to alterations in physical growth, mental and intellectual impairment, and even death in some circumstances.

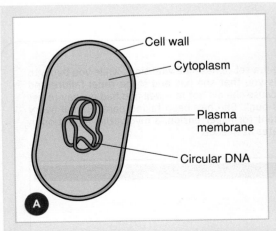
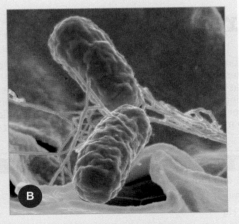

Figure 6-13 General structure of a bacterium. **A.** Bacteria come in many shapes and sizes, but all have a circular strand of DNA, cytoplasm, and a plasma membrane. A cell wall surrounds the membrane in many bacteria. **B.** An electron micrograph of salmonella bacteria. Many bacteria have a capsule that protects them from ingestion and destruction by phagocytes.

Physical agents, such as heat, cold, and radiation, may also cause cell injury—for example, burns, frostbite, radiation sickness, and tumours. The degree of cell injury that results is determined by both the strength of the agent and the length of exposure.

Apoptosis

Apoptosis is normal cell death. It is unique in that it is genetically programmed into the cell as a part of normal development, organogenesis, immune function, and tissue growth. It plays a normal role in ageing, early development, menses, lactating breast tissue, thymus involution, and red blood cell turnover.

During apoptosis, cells exhibit characteristic nuclear changes, and they typically die in well-defined clusters rather than in a random fashion. The molecular mechanism underlying apoptosis involves the activation of genes that code for proteins known as caspases. These proteins are essentially cellular "cyanide"—in essence, their production leads to cell suicide. Unlike in the case of cell death from disease processes, proteins and DNA undergo controlled degradation that allows their remnants to be taken up and reused by neighbouring cells. In this way, apoptosis allows the body to eliminate a cell but still "recycle" many of its components. Pathologically, areas that have undergone apoptotic death do not show any evidence of inflammation. In contrast, an inflammatory response is typically observed when cells undergo necrosis from hypoxia or cellular toxins.

Apoptosis can be activated prematurely by pathological factors such as cell injury. This sort of premature stimulation results in early cell death, which occurs in some forms of heart failure. Another example of pathological apoptosis is the death of hepatocytes (liver cells) in patients with viral hepatitis. The dying cells form

lumps of chromatin known as Councilman's bodies. Factors that inhibit the normal course of apoptosis result in unwanted cellular proliferation, as in cancer and rheumatoid arthritis (uncontrolled synovial tissue proliferation). **Figure 6-14 ▾** illustrates the process by which cancerous cells develop from normal cells.

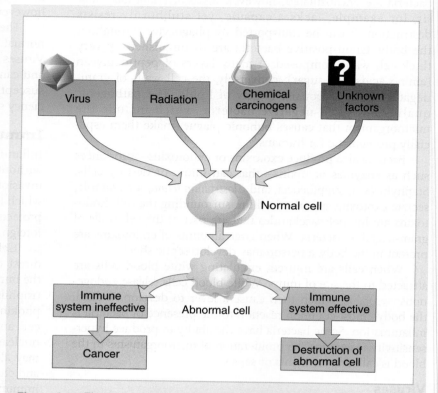

Figure 6-14 The onset of cancer. Viruses and other factors induce a normal cell to become abnormal. When the immune system is working effectively, it destroys the abnormal cells, so no cancer develops. When abnormal cells evade the immune system, they form a tumour and then may become a spreading cancer.

You are the Paramedic Part 2

You ask your colleague to place the patient on oxygen via a nonrebreathing mask and get a set of baseline vital signs while you begin to question her regarding her current illness and past medical history. The patient tells you that she has end-stage renal failure and requires dialysis every other day. She was unable to make it to her last appointment because she did not feel well and had no way to get there. She did not call her doctor, stating that she thought she could "shake off this bug". She had been taking paracetamol every 4 hours for the fever and the pain in her forearm. Her past medical history is significant for hypertension, a myocardial infarction in 2003, and congestive heart failure. Daily medications include captopril, aspirin, and nitrates as needed.

Vital Signs	Recording Time: 5 Minutes
Skin	Pale, warm, and moist
Pulse	140 beats/min, regular; weak radial
Blood pressure	86/50 mm Hg
Respirations	28 breaths/min, accessory muscle use, rales auscultated half way up the back bilaterally
SpO_2	93% on nonrebreathing mask at 15 l/min of supplemental oxygen

3. What should you monitor your patient for?

4. Which interventions should you consider at this point, if any?

Abnormal Cell Death

If the injury leading to cell degeneration is of sufficient intensity and duration, irreversible cell injury will lead to cell death. Necrosis is the result of the morphological changes that occur following cell death in living tissues. It may be either simple necrosis (coagulation) or derived necrosis.

Simple necrosis refers to areas of necrosis where the gross and microscopic tissue and some of the cells are recognisable. It may be caused by acute ischaemia, acute toxicity (eg, from heavy metals), or direct physical injury (eg, from caustic chemicals and burns).

Derived necrosis includes caseation necrosis, dry gangrene, fat necrosis, and liquefaction necrosis. Caseation necrosis is manifested by the loss of all features of the tissue and cells, so that they come to resemble cheese when viewed through a microscope. Dry gangrene results from invasion and putrefaction of necrotic tissue, after the blood supply is compromised to the tissue and the tissue undergoes coagulation necrosis. Fat necrosis results from the destruction of fat cells, usually by enzymes (ie, pancreatic proteases and lipases). Liquefaction necrosis results from coagulation necrosis followed by liquefaction necrosis of tissues and invasion by putrefying bacteria that grow rapidly in a warm moist environment; the bacteria then produce lytic enzymes and gas.

▌Genetics and Family Disease

Factors Causing Disease

Genetic, environmental, age-related, and sex-associated factors can all cause disease. Genetic factors are present at birth and are passed on through a person's genes to future generations. Environmental factors include microorganisms, immunological and toxic exposures, personal habits and lifestyle, exposures to chemicals, the physical environment, and the psychosocial environment.

Age- and sex-associated factors interact with a combination of genetic and environmental factors, lifestyle, and anatomic or hormonal differences. The risk of a particular disease often depends on the patient's age. For example, newborns are at greater risk of certain diseases because their immune systems are not fully developed (see Chapter 41). Teenagers are at high risk of other diseases due to trauma, drugs, and alcohol. The older we become, the greater the risk of cancer, heart disease, stroke, and Alzheimer's disease (see Chapter 42). Some diseases are more prevalent in men, such as lung cancer, gout, and Parkinson's disease. Women are more likely to have osteoporosis, rheumatoid arthritis, and breast cancer.

Some uncontrollable factors (eg, genetics) influence a disease process, but many other factors can be controlled. For example, behaviours such as smoking, drinking alcohol, poor nutrition (eg, excessive fat, salt, and sugar intake; insufficient intake of protein, fruits, vegetables, and fibre), lack of exercise, and stress can all be modified.

Analysing Disease Risk

Analysing disease risk involves consideration of disease rates and disease risk factors (both causal and noncausal). All studies of a disease should consider the incidence, prevalence, and mortality of the disease. The incidence is the frequency of disease occurrence (eg, one in four patients has this disease). The prevalence is the number of cases in a particular population over time (eg, last year, more than 100,000 patients had this disease). The mortality is the number of deaths from a disease in a given population (eg, 1 in 50 affected individuals in the United Kingdom with this disease will die).

Risk factors, age, and sex differences often interact. For example, suppose a person has a genetic tendency toward coronary artery disease; the risk of myocardial infarction or sudden death is higher in this individual even if he or she exercises regularly and has no other risk factors. A person who smokes heavily but has no other risk factors may have a similarly elevated risk.

Common Family Diseases and Associated Risk Factors

The terms *genetic risk* and *family tendency* are often used interchangeably. A true genetic risk is one that is passed through generations by inheritance of a gene. In contrast, with a family tendency, diseases may "cluster" in family groups despite lack of evidence for heritable gene-associated abnormalities.

Table 6-2 ▶ lists some of the traits and diseases carried on human chromosomes. Autosomal recessive is a pattern of inheritance that involves genes located on autosomes (any chromosome other than sex chromosomes). A person needs to inherit two copies of a particular form of such a gene to show that trait. A parent who carries the gene for an autosomal recessive trait but does not display the trait has a 25% chance of passing the inherited condition to his or her child if the other parent is also a carrier for the trait. If both parents actually have the inherited condition, then all of their children will have the condition. Haemochromatosis, which causes people to accumulate too much iron in their bodies, shows an autosomal recessive pattern of inheritance—a person must inherit a copy of the haemochromatosis gene from each parent to develop the disease.

In autosomal dominant inheritance, a person needs to inherit only one copy of a particular form of a gene to show that trait; it does not matter which form of the gene is inherited from the other parent. A parent has at least a 50% chance of passing on an autosomal dominant inherited condition to his or her child. Family adenomatous polyposis, which places people at extremely high risk of developing colon cancer, shows an autosomal dominant pattern of inheritance.

Immunological Disorders

Immunological diseases are caused by either hyperactivity or hypoactivity of the immune system. Most immunological diseases that exhibit family tendencies involve an overactive immune system—for example, allergies, asthma, and rheumatic fever. Often there is significant overlap between causative factors, including the patient's environment. **Table 6-3 ▾** lists common respiratory diseases that may be caused by environmental pollutants, viruses, or bacteria.

Allergies are acquired following initial exposure to a stimulant, known as an allergen. Repeated exposures cause the immune system to react to the allergen **Figure 6-15 ▸** . Although the clinical presentation varies, it usually includes swelling and itching, runny nose, coughing, sneezing, wheezing, and nasal congestion. A person who has an allergic tendency is said to be atopic. Environmental conditions may also increase a person's susceptibility toward an allergic reaction.

Asthma is a chronic inflammatory condition resulting in intermittent wheezing and excess mucus production. Nearly 60% of attacks are precipitated by viral infections. Allergies account for another 20% of asthma attacks, with stress and emotions causing the remainder. In addition to the family component, chromosomal differences in certain individuals may enhance their susceptibility to asthma.

Rheumatic fever is an inflammatory disease that occurs primarily in children. This disease results from a delayed reaction to an untreated streptococcal infection of the upper respiratory tract (eg, strep throat). Symptoms, which appear several weeks after the acute infection, may include fever, abdominal pain, vomiting, arthritis, palpitations, and chest pain. Recurrent episodes of rheumatic fever may cause permanent myocardial damage, especially to the cardiac valves. A family history of acute rheumatic fever may predispose an individual to the disease.

Cancer

Cancer includes a large number of malignant growths (neoplasms). The prognosis often depends on the extent of its spread (metastasis) and the effectiveness of treatment.

Table 6-2 | Traits and Diseases Carried on Human Chromosomes

Autosomal recessive	
Albinism	Lack of pigment in eyes, skin, and hair
Cystic fibrosis	Pancreatic failure, mucus buildup in lungs
Sickle cell anaemia	Abnormal haemoglobin leading to sickle-shaped red blood cells that obstruct vital capillaries
Tay-Sachs disease	Improper metabolism of gangliosides in nerve cells, resulting in early death
Phenylketonuria	Accumulation of phenylalanine in blood; results in mental impairment
Attached earlobe	Earlobe attached to skin of the neck
Hyperextendable thumb	Thumb bends past 45° angle
Autosomal dominant	
Achondroplasia	Dwarfism resulting from a defect in epiphyseal plates of forming long bones
Marfan's syndrome	Defect manifest in connective tissue, resulting in excessive growth and aortic rupture
Widow's peak	Hairline coming to a point on forehead
Huntington's disease	Progressive deterioration of the nervous system beginning in late 20s or early 30s; results in mental deterioration and early death
Brachydactyly	Disfiguration of hands, shortened fingers
Freckles	Permanent aggregations of melanin in the skin

Table 6-3 | Common Respiratory Diseases

Disease	Symptoms	Cause	Treatment
Emphysema	Breakdown of alveoli; shortness of breath	Smoking and air pollution	Administer oxygen to relieve symptoms; quit smoking; avoid polluted air. No known cure.
Chronic bronchitis	Coughing, shortness of breath	Smoking and air pollution	Quit smoking; move out of polluted area; if possible, move to warmer, drier climate.
Acute bronchitis	Inflammation of the bronchi; yellowy mucus coughed up; shortness of breath	Many viruses and bacteria	If bacterial, take antibiotics, cough medicine; use vapouriser.
Sinusitis	Inflammation of the sinuses; mucus discharge; blockage of nasal passageways; headache	Many viruses and bacteria	If bacterial, take antibiotics and decongestant tablets; use vapouriser.
Laryngitis	Inflammation of larynx and vocal cords; sore throat; hoarseness; mucus buildup and cough	Many viruses and bacteria	If bacterial, take antibiotics, cough medicine; avoid irritants, such as smoke; avoid talking.
Pneumonia	Inflammation of the lungs ranging from mild to severe; cough and fever; shortness of breath at rest; chills; sweating; chest pains; blood in mucus	Bacteria, viruses, or inhalation of irritating gases	Consult doctor immediately; go to bed; take antibiotics, cough medicine; stay warm.
Asthma	Constriction of bronchioles; mucus buildup in bronchioles; periodic wheezing; difficulty breathing	Allergy to pollen, some foods, food additives; dandruff from dogs and cats; exercise	Use inhalants to open passageways; avoid irritants.

Table 6-4	Signs and Symptoms in the Phases of Hypoperfusion
Compensated	**Decompensated**
■ Agitation, anxiety, restlessness ■ Sense of impending doom ■ Weak, rapid (thready) pulse ■ Clammy (cool, moist) skin ■ Pallor with cyanotic lips ■ Shortness of breath ■ Nausea, vomiting ■ Delayed capillary refill in infants and children ■ Thirst ■ Normal blood pressure	■ Altered mental status (verbal to unresponsive) ■ Hypotension ■ Laboured or irregular breathing ■ Thready or absent peripheral pulses ■ Ashen, mottled, or cyanotic skin ■ Dilated pupils ■ Diminished urine output (oliguria) ■ Impending cardiac arrest

vasoconstriction (increased systemic vascular resistance). In addition, the RAAS is activated and antidiuretic hormone is released from the pituitary gland. Together these actions trigger salt and water retention as well as peripheral vasoconstriction, thereby increasing blood pressure and cardiac output. Depending on the severity of the insult, variable amounts of fluid will shift from the interstitial tissues into the vascular compartment. The spleen also releases some red blood cells that are normally sequestered there, to augment the oxygen-carrying capacity of the blood. The overall response of the initial compensatory mechanisms is to increase the preload (venous return), stroke volume, and heart rate. The result is usually an increase in cardiac output and myocardial oxygen demand.

As hypoperfusion persists, the myocardial oxygen demand continues to increase. Eventually, the above-normal compensatory mechanisms can no longer keep up with the demand. Myocardial function worsens, with decreased cardiac output and ejection fraction. Tissue perfusion decreases, leading to impaired cell metabolism. Often, the blood pressure decreases, especially in progressive hypoperfusion. Fluid may leak from the blood vessels, causing systemic and pulmonary oedema. At this point, other signs of hypoperfusion may be present, such as dusky skin, oliguria, and impaired mental status.

Types of Shock

Shock is an abnormal state associated with inadequate oxygen and nutrient delivery to the metabolic apparatus of the cell, resulting in impairment of cell metabolism and inadequate perfusion of vital organs (see Chapter 18). Once a certain level of tissue hypoperfusion is reached, cell damage proceeds in a similar manner regardless of the type of initial insult. Impairment of cellular metabolism prevents the body from properly using oxygen and glucose at the cellular level. Cells revert to anaerobic metabolism, which causes increased lactic acid production and metabolic acidosis, decreased oxygen affinity for haemo-

globin, decreased ATP production, changes in cellular electrolytes, cellular oedema, and release of lysosomal enzymes. Glucose impairment leads to elevated blood glucose levels due to release of catecholamines and cortisol. In addition, fat breakdown (lipolysis) with ketone formation may occur.

Shock can occur due to inadequacy of the central circulation (eg, the heart and the great vessels) or of the peripheral circulation (the remaining vessels, including the microscopic circulation [eg, arterioles, venules, and capillaries, as illustrated in Figure 6-21 ▸]). From a mechanistic approach, two types of shock are distinguished: central and peripheral. Central shock consists of cardiogenic shock and obstructive shock. Peripheral shock includes hypovolaemic shock and distributive shock.

Cardiogenic shock occurs when the heart cannot circulate enough blood to maintain adequate peripheral oxygen delivery. In the case of ischaemic heart disease, this requires loss of 40% or more of functioning myocardium. The most common cause of cardiogenic shock is myocardial infarction, either as a single event or by cumulative damage. Other forms of cardiac dysfunction may also result in cardiogenic shock (ie, large ventricular septal defect or haemodynamic significant arrhythmias) (see Chapter 27).

Obstructive shock occurs when blood flow becomes blocked in the heart or great vessels. In pericardial tamponade Figure 6-22 ▸, diastolic filling of the right ventricle is impaired due to significant amounts of fluid in the pericardial sac surrounding the heart, leading to a decrease in the cardiac output. Aortic dissection leads to a false lumen (aortic opening), with loss of normal blood flow Figure 6-23 ▸. A left atrial tumour may obstruct flow between the atrium and ventricle and decrease cardiac output. Obstruction of either the superior or inferior vena cava (vena cava syndrome) decreases cardiac output by decreasing venous return. A large pulmonary embolus or a tension pneumothorax may prevent adequate blood flow to the lungs, resulting in inadequate venous return to the left side of the heart.

In hypovolaemic shock, the circulating blood volume is unable to deliver adequate oxygen and nutrients to the body. Two types of hypovolaemic shock—exogenous and endogenous—are possible, depending on where the fluid loss occurs. The most common type of exogenous hypovolaemic shock is external bleeding (eg, from an open wound); it may also result from loss of plasma volume caused by diarrhoea or vomiting. Endogenous hypovolaemic shock occurs when the fluid loss is contained within the body.

Distributive shock occurs when there is widespread dilation of the resistance vessels (small arterioles), the capacitance vessels (small venules), or both. The circulating blood

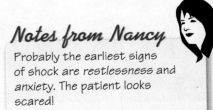

Notes from Nancy

Probably the earliest signs of shock are restlessness and anxiety. The patient looks scared!

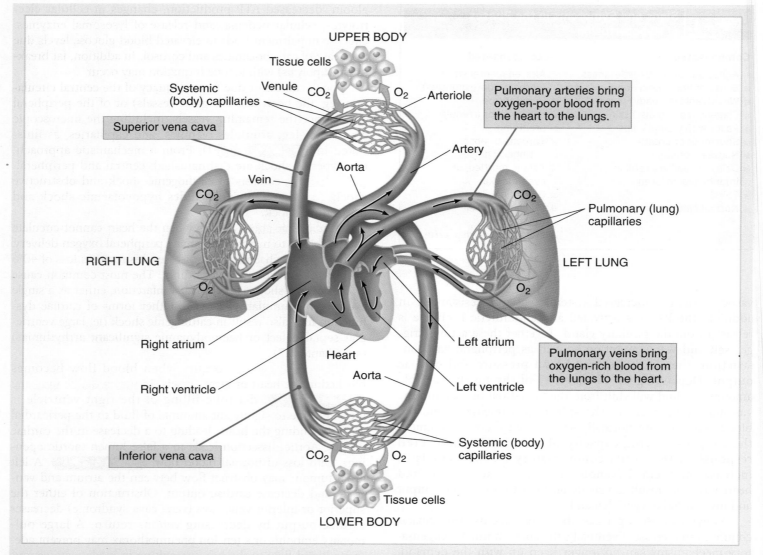

UPPER BODY

Tissue cells

Systemic (body) capillaries

Venule CO_2 O_2 Arteriole

Superior vena cava

Aorta

Vein

Artery

CO_2 CO_2

RIGHT LUNG   **LEFT LUNG**

O_2 O_2

Right atrium

Heart   Left atrium

Aorta

Right ventricle

Left ventricle

Inferior vena cava

CO_2 O_2 Systemic (body) capillaries

Tissue cells

LOWER BODY

Pulmonary arteries bring oxygen-poor blood from the heart to the lungs.

Pulmonary (lung) capillaries

Pulmonary veins bring oxygen-rich blood from the lungs to the heart.

Figure 6-21 The circulatory system includes the heart, arteries, veins, and interconnecting capillaries. The capillaries—the smallest vessels—connect with venules and arterioles. At the centre of the system, and providing its driving force, is the heart.

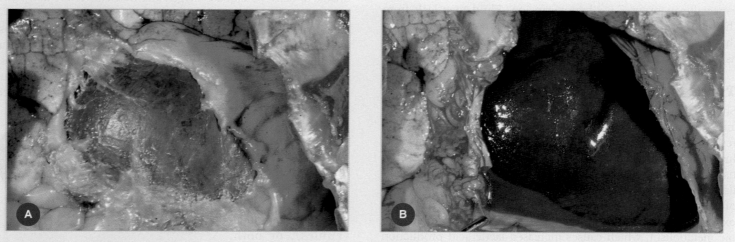

Figure 6-22 Cardiac tamponade secondary to myocardial rupture. **A.** Distended pericardial sac. **B.** Pericardial sac opened, showing clotted blood surrounding the heart, which compressed the heart and prevented filling of the right ventricle in diastole.

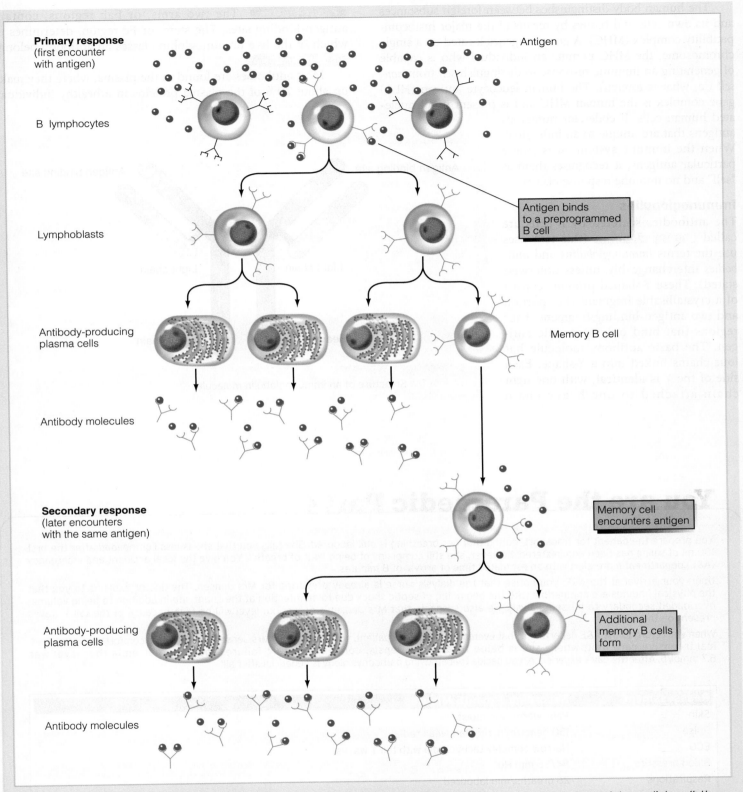

Figure 6-29 B-cell activation. Immunocompetent B cells are stimulated by the presence of an antigen, producing an intermediate cell, the lymphoblast. The lymphoblasts divide, producing plasma cells and some memory B cells. Memory B cells respond to subsequent antigen encroachment, yielding a rapid secondary response.

The human body distinguishes between foreign substances and its own cells and tissues by means of the major histocompatibility complex (MHC). A group of genes located on a single chromosome, the MHC permits an individual who is capable of generating an immune response to distinguish *self* from *non-self* (ie, what is foreign). The human leucocyte antigen (HLA) gene complex is the human MHC and is present in all nucleated human cells. It codes for numerous antigens that are unique to an individual. When the immune system "sees" these particular antigens, it recognises them as "self" and no immune response occurs.

Immunoglobulins

The antibodies secreted by B cells are called immunoglobulins (this text uses use the terms *immunoglobulins* and *antibodies* interchangeably, unless otherwise stated). These Y-shaped proteins consist of a crystallisable fragment (Fc) portion and two antigen-binding fragment (Fab) regions that bind only a specific antigen. The basic antibody molecule has four chains linked into a Y-shape. Each side of the Y is identical, with one light chain attached to one heavy chain **Figure 6-30 ▾** . The two arms, or Fab regions, contain antigen-binding sites. The stem, or Fc region, determines to which of the five immunoglobin classes an antibody belongs **Figure 6-31 ▸** .

Most antibodies are found in the plasma, where they make up about 20% of the plasma proteins in a healthy individual.

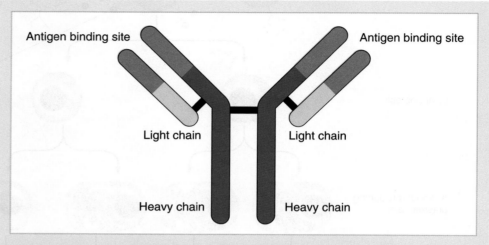

Figure 6-30 Structure of an immunoglobulin molecule.

You are the Paramedic Part 4

You prepare the patient for transport, noting that her breathing is still laboured. She tells you that she is less lightheaded after the first 100 ml of saline has been administered; however, she still complains of being "out of breath". You give the local accident and emergency (A&E) department a pre-alert with an estimated time of arrival of 8 minutes.

Upon your arrival at the A&E, you notice that the dialysis nurse is already preparing for Mrs Jensen. The doctor explains to you that the physical findings are compatible with the beginning of septic shock due to an infection at the shunt site in addition to being volume-overloaded secondary to missed dialysis. He also suspects that Mrs Jensen's potassium level will be high because of the tall T waves present on the ECG.

When you return to the A&E department that evening with another patient, you check up on Mrs Jensen. She's resting comfortably in the medical intensive care unit, where she is being treated for sepsis, congestive heart failure, and hyperkalaemia (her level was 6.7 mmol/l). After the day's experience, you decide that studying pathophysiology is beneficial after all!

Reassessment	Recording Time: 15 Minutes
Skin	Pale, warm, and moist
Pulse	150 beats/min, regular; weak radial
ECG	Narrow complex tachycardia with tall T waves
Blood pressure	84/56 mm Hg
Respirations	26 breaths/min laboured
SpO_2	93% on nonrebreathing mask at 15 l/min of supplemental oxygen
Pupils	Equal and reactive to light

7. How did the inflammatory process manifest itself in this patient?

8. What are other signs and symptoms of hyperkalaemia?

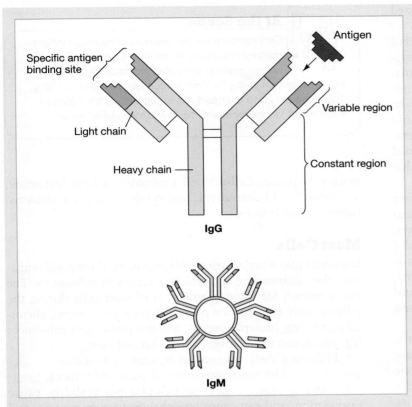

Figure 6-31 General structure of an antibody.

Antibodies make antigens more visible to the immune system in three ways:

- Antibodies act as opsonins. In opsoninisation, an antibody coats an antigen to facilitate its recognition by immune cells. Antibodies are not toxic by themselves, but they label antigens so that other immune cells will attack them.
- Antibodies cause antigens to clump for easier phagocytosis (precipitation, also known as agglutination).
- Antibodies bind to and inactivate some toxins produced by bacteria. Macrophages can then ingest and destroy the inactivated toxins.

Antibodies are divided into five general classes of immunoglobulins ◆ **Table 6-6** ▶. Fetal immunity is a passive acquired immunity that is derived primarily from maternal IgG and IgM antibodies. Following delivery, these antibodies persist until the neonate's own B cells take over. A substantial number of antibodies are also transferred through breast milk, which is one of many reasons why experts favour breastfeeding.

Cell-Mediated Immune Response

In cell-mediated immunity, T-cell lymphocytes recognise antigens and contribute to the immune response in two major ways: (1) by secreting cytokines that attract other cells or (2) by becoming cytotoxic and killing infected or abnormal cells. There are four subgroups of T cells:

- *Killer T cells* (also called cytotoxic T cells) destroy the antigen. Cytotoxic T cells help rid the body of cells that

have been infected by viruses as well as cells that have been transformed by cancer. They are also responsible for the rejection of tissue and organ grafts.

- *Helper T cells* activate many immune cells, including B cells and other T cells (also called T4 or CD4+ cells).
- *Suppressor T cells* (also called T8 or CD8+ cells) suppress the activity of other lymphocytes so they do not destroy normal tissue.
- *Memory T cells* remember the reaction for the next time it is needed.

During the cell-mediated response, macrophages ingest pathogens. When a macrophage digests a pathogen, it releases small particles of antigen. This antigen pushes its way to the macrophage surface, where it is recognised by specific T cells. Other T cells, such as helper T cells and killer T cells, bind to the antigen and macrophage, destroying the invader.

Cellular Interactions in the Immune Response

There are remarkable similarities in how the body responds to different kinds of immune challenges. Although the details depend on the particular challenge, the basic pattern is the same—the innate response starts first and is then reinforced by the more specific acquired response. These two pathways are interconnected.

Consider what happens when bacteria enter the body. If the bacteria are not encapsulated, macrophages begin to ingest them immediately. If the bacteria are encapsulated, antibodies

Table 6-6	General Classes of Immunoglobulins
IgG	The most common immunoglobulin. Accounts for 75% of the antibodies in the blood. Found in lymph, synovial fluid, peritoneal fluid, cerebrospinal fluid, and breast milk. IgG is the only immunoglobulin that crosses the placenta, giving infants immunity in the first few months of life.
IgA	Accounts for 15% of the antibodies in the blood. Also found in tears, saliva, respiratory tract secretions, and the stomach. IgA combines with a protein in the mucosa and defends body surfaces against invading microorganisms.
IgM	Accounts for 5% to 10% of the antibodies in the blood and is the dominant antibody in ABO (blood type) incompatibilities. IgM is the initial antibody formed in most infections.
IgE	Accounts for less than 1% of the antibodies in the blood and is associated with allergic reactions. When mast cell receptors combine with IgE and antigen, the mast cells degranulate and release chemical mediators such as histamine.
IgD	Accounts for less than 1% of the antibodies in the blood. The physiological role of IgD is unclear.

(opsonins) must coat the capsule before they can be ingested by phagocytes.

Components of the cell wall then activate the complement system. Some components of the activated complement system, termed chemotaxins, attract leucocytes from the circulation to help fight the infection. The complement cascade ends with the formation of a set of proteins called the membrane attack complex (MAC). These molecules insert themselves into the bacterial membrane, weakening those areas in the membrane. Ions and water enter the cell through the weakened areas, leading to lysis of the bacterium (a chemical process that does not involve immune cells).

If antibodies to the bacteria are already in the body, they will help the innate response by acting as opsonins and neutralising bacterial toxins. Although it often takes several days, memory B cells attracted to the infection site will be activated if they encounter an antigen they recognise. If the infection is new to the body (preexisting antibodies are not present), B cells will be activated. Combined with helper T cells and cytokine release, antibodies are produced and memory B and T cells are formed.

T-cell and B-cell function is deficient in older patients. Depressed lymphocyte function is accompanied by a decrease in macrophage activity. Therefore, older people are more prone to experience infections and recover slowly. In addition, older people have increased levels of autoantibodies (antibodies directed against the patient), which partly explains why older people are prone to autoimmune disease.

Acute and Chronic Inflammation

Inflammation is a dynamic process that, once initiated, triggers a complex cascade of events involving both local and systemic events. The two most common causes of inflammation are infection (eg, bacterial or viral) and injury.

The acute inflammatory response involves both vascular and cellular components. After transient arteriolar constriction, the arterioles dilate, allowing an influx of blood under increased pressure. This active hyperaemia (increased intravascular pressure) causes the blood vessel to expand; as in a balloon that is being inflated, the vessel walls become thinner. The higher pressure combined with increased vessel wall permeability causes fluid to leak into the interstitial spaces (oedema). When enough fluid has escaped into the surrounding area and the intravascular pressure has been released, the vessel wall contracts and the outflow slows, leading to stasis of blood in the capillaries.

A variety of blood cells participate in tissue inflammatory reactions: white blood cells (leucocytes), platelets, mast cells, and plasma cells (B lymphocytes that create antibodies). Specific cell types include neutrophils, monocytes, lymphocytes, eosinophils, basophils, and activated platelets. Chemical mediators, primarily produced by the mast cells, account for the vascular and cellular events that occur during the acute inflam-

matory response. Cell-derived mediators include histamine, arachidonic acid derivatives, and cytokines (eg, interleukins, tumour necrosis factor).

Mast Cells

Mast cells play a major role in inflammation. During inflammation, they degranulate and release a variety of substances. The major stimuli for the degranulation of mast cells during the inflammatory response are physical injury (eg, trauma), chemical agents (eg, bacterial toxins), and immunological substances (eg, interaction of an antigen and an IgE antibody).

Following their degranulation, mast cells release vasoactive amines. The most important of these substances, histamine and serotonin, increase vascular permeability, cause vasodilation, and can cause bronchoconstriction, nausea, and vomiting. Because histamine is a preformed vasodepressor amine that is stored in mast cells, it can be released quickly, so its actions are seen early in the inflammatory response. Mast cells also synthesise chemotactic factors that attract neutrophils (neutrophil chemotactic factor) and eosinophils (eosinophilic chemotactic factor).

Mast cells also synthesise leucotrienes. Leucotrienes—also known as slow-reacting substances of anaphylaxis (SRS-A)—are a family of biologically active compounds derived from arachidonic acid. The clinically important leucotrienes participate in host defence reactions and pathophysiological conditions that paramedics commonly see in the prehospital environment, such as immediate hypersensitivity and inflammation. Leucotrienes have potent actions on many parts of the body, including the cardiovascular, pulmonary, immune, and central nervous systems, and the gastrointestinal tract.

Leucotrienes are primarily endogenous mediators of inflammation. They contribute to the signs and symptoms seen in acute inflammatory responses, including responses resulting from the interaction of allergens with IgE antibodies on mast cells. Certain leucotrienes are bronchoconstrictors, stimulate airway mucus secretion, and are very potent at increasing the permeability of postcapillary venules (including those in the bronchial circulation), thereby causing plasma protein exudation (oozing out of the tissue) and oedema. Certain leucotrienes may also promote eosinophil migration into the airways of animals and asthmatic patients, and they may also increase bronchial hyperresponsiveness through their action on sensory nerves.

Finally, mast cells synthesise prostaglandins. These substances, which are derived from arachidonic acid, comprise a group of about 20 lipids that are modified fatty acids attached to a five-member ring. Prostaglandins are found in many vertebrate tissues, where they act as messengers involved in reproduction, the inflammatory response to infection, and pain. Aspirin and other NSAIDs inhibit prostaglandin synthesis, leading to reduced inflammation and pain.

Plasma Protein Systems

The plasma-derived mediators that modulate the inflammatory process are called plasma protein systems. They include the complement system, the coagulation (clotting) system, and the kinin system. The interaction of these systems is vital to a normal inflammatory response. Each system consists of a cascade of biochemical reactions such that as one compound is produced, it catalyses the formation of the next compound—much like knocking over a line of dominoes.

Complement System

The complement system is a group of plasma proteins that attract white blood cells to sites of inflammation, activate white blood cells, and directly destroy cells. The central compound in this complement cascade is called C3. C3 is produced by one of the two "complement pathways": the classic pathway or the alternate pathway. The classic pathway starts when an antigen–antibody complex binds to a complement component (C1); activation of this pathway is dependent on the presence of antibodies. The alternate pathway can be triggered by bacterial toxins and does not need antibodies to be activated.

Regardless of which pathway is taken, the main products are the same: C3b, anaphylatoxins, and the MAC. C3b coats bacteria, making it easier for macrophages to engulf them. Anaphylatoxins (C3a, C4a, and C5a) stimulate smooth-muscle contraction and increase vascular permeability by stimulating the release of histamine from mast cells and platelets. The MAC is a set of complement proteins (C5b, C6, C7, C8, and C9) that bind to form a hollow tube, much like a short straw, that can puncture into the plasma membrane of a cell. In this way, transmembrane channels are formed that allow ions, water, and other small molecules to pass through, resulting in loss of cellular osmolarity and death of the cell.

Coagulation System

The coagulation system plays a vital role in the formation of blood clots in the body and facilitates repairs to the vascular tree. Inflammation triggers the coagulation cascade, initiating a complex series of reactions that result in the formation of fibrin. Fibrin is the protein that polymerises (bonds) to form the fibrous component of a blood clot. The various coagulation factors are counterbalanced by a variety of inhibitors, so that the coagulation is restricted to one area. Simultaneously, the fibrinolysis cascade is activated to dissolve the fibrin and create fibrin split products (ie, fragments of the dissolving clot).

Kinin System

The kinin system leads to the formation of the vasoactive protein bradykinin from kallikrein. Kallikrein is an enzyme that is normally found in blood plasma, urine, and body tissue in an inactive state. When it becomes activated, it can dilate blood vessels, influence blood pressure, modulate salt and water excretion by the kidneys, and influence cardiac remodelling after acute myocardial infarction. Bradykinin increases vascular permeability, dilates blood vessels, contracts smooth muscle, and causes pain when injected into the skin.

The kinin system is spurred into action by the activation of Hageman factor (coagulation factor XII). (**Table 6-7 ▶** lists the various coagulation factors.) In addition to its role in the kinin system, Hageman factor participates in the clotting, fibrinolytic, and complement cascades. Its activators include bacterial lipopolysaccharides and endotoxin. Activated factor XII triggers the intrinsic clotting cascade, which occurs when blood is exposed to collagen or other substances. For example, when a blood vessel is cut, the skin cells are damaged and the blood comes in contact with collagen. The extrinsic clotting cascade is activated by substances released from injured cells when tissue damage occurs.

Cellular Components of Inflammation

The goal of the cellular component of acute inflammatory response is for inflammatory cells—namely, polymorphonuclear neutrophils (PMNs)—to arrive at the sites within tissue where they are needed. This process involves two major stages: an intravascular phase and an extravascular phase. During the intravascular phase, leucocytes move to the sides of blood vessels and attach to the endothelial cells. During the extravascular phase, leucocytes travel to the site of inflammation and kill organisms. The cellular event sequence is as follows:

1. **Margination.** Loss of fluid from the blood vessels into the inflamed or infected tissue causes the blood left in the vessels to have increased viscosity, which slows the flow of blood and produces stasis. PMNs, which usually travel toward the centre of the vessel, settle toward the sides of the vessel as the blood flow slows down. As stasis develops, leucocytes also move (marginate) toward the sides of blood vessels, where they bump into the endothelial cells and bind to them. Stress can lead to demargination of some white blood cells, which stimulates the bone marrow to produce more white blood cells, which in turn increases the white blood cell count.

2. **Activation.** Mediators of inflammation trigger the appearance of selectins and integrins on the surfaces of endothelial cells and PMNs, respectively.

3. **Adhesion.** PMNs attach to endothelial cells, as mediated by selectins and integrins.

4. **Transmigration (diapedesis).** The PMNs permeate through the vessel wall, moving into the interstitial space.

5. **Chemotaxis.** PMNs move toward the site of inflammation in response to chemotactic factors that are released by

Table 6-7	Coagulation Factors	
Factor Number	**Name**	**Functions**
I	Fibrinogen	Protein synthesised in liver; converted into fibrin in stage 3
II	Prothrombin	Protein synthesised in liver (requires vitamin K); converted into thrombin in stage 2
III	Tissue thromboplastin	Released from damaged tissue; required in extrinsic stage 1
IV	Calcium ions	Required throughout entire clotting sequence
V	Proaccelerin (labile factor)	Protein synthesised in liver; required to form prothrombin activator in both intrinsic and extrinsic stage 1
VII	Serum prothrombin conversion accelerator (stable factor, proconvertin)	Protein synthesised in liver (requires vitamin K); functions in extrinsic stage 1
VIII	Antihaemophilic factor (antihaemophilic globulin)	Protein synthesised in liver; required for intrinsic stage 1
IX	Plasma thromboplastin component	Protein synthesised in liver (requires vitamin K); required for intrinsic stage 1
X	Stuart factor (Stuart-Prower factor)	Protein synthesised in liver (requires vitamin K); required to form prothrombin activator in both intrinsic and extrinsic stage 1
XI	Plasma thromboplastin antecedent	Protein synthesised in liver; required for intrinsic stage 1
XII	Hageman factor	Protein required for intrinsic stage 1
XIII	Fibrin-stabilising factor	Protein required to stabilise the fibrin strands in stage 3

bacteria or formed from activated complement, chemokines, or arachidonic acid derivatives (eg, leucotrienes) in response to cell injury. Figure 6-32 ▶ illustrates the inflammatory response.

Cellular Products of Inflammation

Cytokines are products of cells that affect the function of other cells. Monocytes release monokines, and lymphocytes release lymphokines.

Interleukins include IL-1 (interleukin-1) and IL-2 (interleukin-2), which attract white blood cells to the sites of injury and bacterial invasion. Interferon is a protein produced by cells when they are invaded by viruses. This cytokine is released into the bloodstream or intercellular fluid to induce healthy cells to manufacture an enzyme that counters the infection.

Lymphokines stimulate leucocytes. Macrophage-activating factor stimulates macrophages to help engulf and destroy foreign substances. Migration inhibitory factor keeps white blood cells at the site of infection or injury until they can perform their designated task.

Injury Resolution and Repair

Normal wound healing involves four steps—repair of damaged tissue, removal of inflammatory debris, restoration of tissues to a normal state, and regeneration of cells. Healing after tissue injury or loss caused by inflammation depends on the type of cells that make up the affected organ. Labile cells divide continuously, so organs derived from these cells (eg, skin or intestinal mucosa) heal completely. Stable cells are replaced by

regeneration from remaining cells, which are stimulated to enter mitosis. These cells are found in the liver and kidney. Permanent cells, such as nerve cells and cardiac myocytes, cannot be replaced; scar tissue is laid down instead.

Wounds may heal by either primary or secondary intention. Healing by primary intention occurs in clean wounds with opposed margins (eg, a clean surgical wound). First, blood fills the defect and coagulates, forming a scab, which is a mesh-like structure composed of fibrin and fibronectin. If the inflammatory process was severe, tissue may be destroyed and require repair. Next, macrophages remove cellular debris and secrete growth factors. These growth factors stimulate angiogenesis and growth of fibroblasts, leading to the formation of granulation tissue. The epithelium then regenerates, covering the surface defect. Deposition of collagen results in fibrous union. By the end of the first week, 10% of the preoperative strength is regained. Scar maturation occurs as collagen cross-linking takes place. By the end of 3 months, 80% of the normal tensile strength of the tissue has been restored.

Healing by secondary intention occurs in large gaping or infected wounds. Wounds that heal by secondary intention have a more pronounced and prolonged inflammatory phase, causing the neutrophils to persist for days. They also have more abundant granulation tissue. Wound contraction is mediated by myofibroblasts, which help to draw the margins of the wound closer to each other as time passes.

Factors that can lead to dysfunctional wound healing may be either local or systemic. Local factors include infection (when the body's healing efforts are diverted to fight off the cause of the infection); an inadequate blood supply (as in diabetes) that produces tissue hypoxia, which slows wound

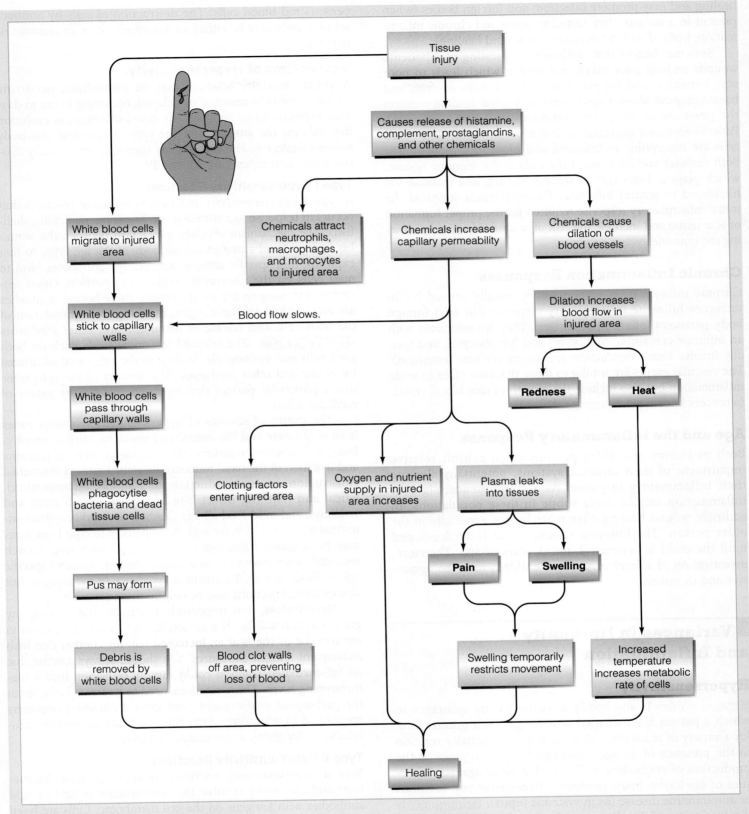

Figure 6-32 The inflammatory response.

healing and may promote infection; and foreign bodies (when present in a wound, they stimulate acute and chronic inflammation, both of which interfere with wound healing).

Systemic factors that influence the healing of a patient's wounds include poor nutritional intake, which leads to poor scar formation and suppression of the immune system, and haematological abnormalities (proper wound healing requires the presence of adequate numbers of white blood cells). Patients who have impaired bone marrow stores of white blood cells are susceptible to infection and often heal more slowly. Both diabetes and AIDS affect the cells of the immune system, which plays a direct role in wound healing, and increase the likelihood of wound infection. Corticosteroids suppress the initial inflammatory response required for the proper formation of scar tissue and increase the risk of wound infection by slowing the immune system response.

Chronic Inflammation Responses

Chronic inflammation responses are usually caused by an unsuccessful acute inflammatory response due to a foreign body, persistent infection, or antigen. They are associated with an infiltrate containing monocytes and lymphocytes, and usually involve tissue destruction and repair (or scar formation). The vascular events are similar to those that take place in acute inflammation but also include the growth of new blood vessels (a process known as angiogenesis).

Age and the Inflammatory Response

Both newborns and older persons often exhibit relative impairment of their immune systems, potentially slowing their inflammatory response. As a consequence, signs of inflammation may be more subtle in these populations. In addition, wound healing often takes longer, especially in the older person. The immune system is not fully developed until the child is between 2 and 3 years of age. Therefore, investigation of a fever in younger children must be aggressive and thorough.

▌Variances in Immunity and Inflammation

Hypersensitivity

Hypersensitivity is any bodily response to any substance to which a patient has increased sensitivity. It is a generic term for a variety of reactions. Allergy is a hypersensitivity reaction to the presence of an agent (allergen). Autoimmunity is the production of antibodies or T cells that work against the tissues of one's own body, producing hypersensitivity reactions or autoimmune disease (as in systemic lupus). Isoimmunity is the formation of T cells or antibodies directed against the antigens on another person's cells (typically after the transplantation of an organ or tissues). A blood transfusion reaction is an example of an isoimmune reaction to another

person's red blood cells. The destruction of cells by antibodies or T cells may be either an autoimmune or an isoimmune reaction.

Mechanisms of Hypersensitivity

A hypersensitivity reaction may be immediate, occurring within seconds to minutes, or delayed, occurring hours to days after exposure to an antigen. The speed of symptom evolution depends on the antigen and the type of response the body mounts against it. Hypersensitivity reactions are typically classified into four types: I, II, III, and IV.

Type I Hypersensitivity Reactions

A type I hypersensitivity reaction is an acute reaction that occurs in response to a stimulus (eg, bee sting, penicillin, shellfish). The mechanism involves interaction between the stimulus (antigen) and a preformed antibody of the IgE type. At first exposure to a specific antigen, specific IgE antibodies bind to mast cells via the nonspecific region (Fc) portion. Upon secondary exposure to the same antigen, these bound antibodies are cross-linked by the antigen, resulting in degranulation of the mast cell, and release of histamine and other mediators **Figure 6-33 ▶**). The released histamine feeds back on both mast cells and eosinophils, leading to the release of additional histamine and other mediators. The severity of the symptoms that a particular patient develops depends on the extent of mediator release.

The degree of severity of hypersensitivity reactions varies from very severe and life-threatening reactions, such as anaphylaxis, to less severe reactions, such as allergic rhinitis (oedema and irritation of the nasal mucosa), bronchial asthma (bronchial constriction, mucus production, and airway inflammation), wheal and flare (ie, insect bite leading to vasodilation and swelling), and mild food allergy (leading to diarrhoea, gastrointestinal distress, and vomiting). A propensity to type I reactions may be diagnosed through skin tests (eg, patch test, scratch test) and other laboratory procedures (measurement of specific IgE antibody levels). Treatment is avoidance of the antigen, but desensitising injections may be helpful in severe cases.

Nevertheless, it is impossible to predict how severe any given reaction will be. If a person has had a severe reaction in the past, he or she is at an increased risk for another one with subsequent antigen exposures. You should always assume that an IgE-mediated reaction could rapidly transition into a life-threatening event. These reactions need to be treated quickly in the prehospital environment, and most prehospital providers are trained to administer adrenaline by using an EpiPen auto-injector or by giving a subcutaneous injection.

Type II Hypersensitivity Reactions

Type II hypersensitivity reactions are cytotoxic (cell destructive) and classically involve the combination of IgG or IgM antibodies with antigens on the cell membrane. Cells are lysed (destroyed), either by complement fixation or by other antibodies. This process also destroys many of the body's healthy cells. Histamine release from mast cells is not involved, and IgG-mediated allergic responses occur within a few hours of

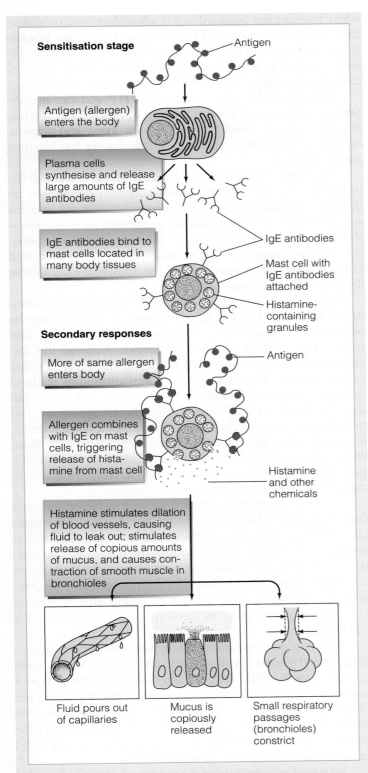

Sensitisation stage

Antigen

Antigen (allergen) enters the body

Plasma cells synthesise and release large amounts of IgE antibodies

IgE antibodies bind to mast cells located in many body tissues

IgE antibodies

Mast cell with IgE antibodies attached

Histamine-containing granules

Secondary responses

More of same allergen enters body

Antigen

Allergen combines with IgE on mast cells, triggering release of hista-mine from mast cell

Histamine and other chemicals

Histamine stimulates dilation of blood vessels, causing fluid to leak out; stimulates release of copious amounts of mucus, and causes con-traction of smooth muscle in bronchioles

Fluid pours out of capillaries

Mucus is copiously released

Small respiratory passages (bronchioles) constrict

Figure 6-33 Type I allergic reaction. The antigen stimulates the production of massive amounts of IgE, a type of antibody produced by plasma cells; the IgE, in turn, attaches to mast cells. This is a sensitisation stage. When the antigen enters again, it binds to the IgE antibodies on the mast cells, triggering a massive release of histamine and other chemicals. Histamine causes blood vessels to dilate and become leaky, and it promotes increased production of mucus in the respiratory tract. Mast cell degranulation may also cause bronchospasm in some people.

antigen exposure. Examples of IgG-mediated responses include transfusion reactions and newborn haemolytic disease.

Type III Hypersensitivity Reactions

Type III hypersensitivity responses involve primarily IgG antibodies that form immune complexes with antigen to recruit phagocytic cells, such as neutrophils, to a site where they can release inflammatory cytokines. Since histamine release from mast cells is not involved, IgG-mediated allergic responses occur within a few hours of antigen exposure. Reactions may be systemic or localised.

The systemic form is called <u>serum sickness</u> and results from a large, single exposure to an antigen, such as horse antibody serum. Antigen–antibody complexes formed in the bloodstream are then deposited in sites around the body, most notably in the kidney, with resultant inflammatory reactions (eg, serum sickness from penicillin). Signs and symptoms of serum sickness may include fever, malaise, rashes, joint aches, lymphademopathy, and splenomegaly.

The localised form of type III response is called an <u>Arthus reaction</u>. Arthus reactions consist of a circumscribed area of vascular inflammation (<u>vasculitis</u>). An example of an Arthus reaction is farmer's lung (a hypersensitivity pneumonitis), which is a local hypersensitivity reaction in the lung to moulds that grow on hay.

Type IV Hypersensitivity Reactions

Type IV allergic responses, also known as cell-mediated hypersensitivity, are primarily mediated by soluble molecules that are released by specifically activated T cells. These reactions are classified into two subtypes: delayed hypersensitivity and cell-mediated cytotoxicity.

Delayed hypersensitivity involves lymphocytes and macrophages. T cells respond to an antigen and activate CD4 (a helper T cell) lymphocytes. These lymphocytes release mediators that are designed to destroy the foreign substance. Examples include contact hypersensitivity to poison ivy, or the local induration due to mononuclear cell infiltrates from a PPD (tuberculin) skin test.

Cell-mediated cytotoxicity involves only sensitised T cells (CD8 lymphocytes or <u>T killer cells</u>). These cells kill the antigen-bearing target cells rather than activating the CD4 lymphocyte to do so. Examples include the body's response to viral infections, tumour immune surveillance, and the mechanism by which transplant rejection occurs.

Targets of Hypersensitivity

The immune system targets different molecules, depending on the type of hypersensitivity reaction. In allergic reactions, the target is an antigen or allergen. Allergens are substances that cause a hypersensitivity reaction, such as those listed in **Table 6-8 ▶**.

In autoimmune reactions, the target is a person's own tissues. For reasons that are unclear, normal tolerance of "self" tissues breaks down and the immune system treats the body's own tissues as foreign.

Graves' disease is an autoimmune disease caused by thyroid-stimulating or thyroid-growth immunoglobulins.

Table 6-8	Allergens That Can Cause Hypersensitivity Reactions	
Type	**Examples**	
Inhalants	Pollen, dust, smoke, fungi, plastic, odours	
Foods	Eggs, milk, wheat, chocolate, strawberries	
Drugs	Aspirin, antibiotics, serums, codeine	
Infectious agents	Bacteria, viruses, fungi, animal parasites	
Contactants	Animals, plants, metals, chemicals	
Physical agents	Light, pressure, radiation, heat, and cold	

These antibodies activate receptors for thyroid-stimulating hormone, causing increased activity by the thyroid gland. In addition to hyperthyroidism, Graves' disease is associated with characteristic eye changes—lid retraction, stare, and exophthalmus (protrusion of the eyes)—and skin changes (pretibial myxoedema—localised oedematous skin in the pretibial area).

Type 1 diabetes mellitus is also considered an autoimmune disease. Although the exact insult is unknown (but is suspected to be a viral infection), some agent stimulates the body to produce autoantibodies against beta cells in the pancreas that produce insulin. The result is a deficiency of insulin, and diabetes.

Rheumatoid arthritis is a chronic systemic disease that affects the entire body. One of the most common forms of arthritis, it is characterised by inflammation of the synovium (the connective tissue membrane lining the joint) with resulting pain, stiffness, warmth, redness, and swelling. Inflammatory cells release enzymes that cause damage to bone and cartilage. The involved joint can lose its shape and alignment, resulting in pain and loss of movement. Rheumatoid arthritis is associated with the formation of rheumatoid factor—that is, IgM antibodies to tissue IgG. In the joints, the synovial membrane is thickened due to infiltration of inflammatory cells (lymphocytes).

Myasthenia gravis is an acquired autoimmune disease that is characterised by autoimmune attack on the nerve–muscle junction. The circulating autoantibodies cause abnormal muscle fatigability and typically involve the smallest motor units first, such as the extraocular muscles. This produces ptosis (droopy eyelid) and diplopia (double vision). Other muscles may be involved, causing problems with swallowing (dysphagia). Characteristically, repeated contraction of the affected muscles makes the symptoms worse. Two thirds of patients with myasthenia gravis have thymic abnormalities, with the most common being thymic hyperplasia. A minority of patients have a tumour of the thymus, called a thymoma.

Immune thrombocytopenia purpura (ITP) is a blood disorder in which the patient forms antibodies to blood platelets that cause their destruction. Thrombocytopenia describes a decrease in blood platelets; purpura are purplish areas of the skin and mucous membranes (such as the lining of the mouth)

where bleeding has occurred as a result of decreased or ineffective platelets. Some cases of ITP are caused by drugs, whereas others are associated with infection, pregnancy, or immune disorders such as systemic lupus erythematosus. About half of all cases are classified as "idiopathic" (ie, the cause is unknown).

Bleeding is the main symptom of ITP and can include bruising and tiny red dots on the skin or mucous membranes. In some instances, bleeding from the nose, gums, and digestive or urinary tracts may occur. Rarely, the patient has bleeding within the brain.

Treatment of idiopathic ITP is based on the severity of the symptoms and the patient's platelet count. In some cases, no therapy is needed. In most cases, drugs that alter the immune system's attack on the platelets are prescribed, such as corticosteroids (eg, prednisolone) and IV infusions of immunoglobulin. Another treatment that usually results in an increased number of platelets is removal of the spleen, the organ that destroys antibody-coated platelets.

Systemic lupus erythematosus (SLE) is a chronic autoimmune disease with many manifestations. In this disease, the body's own immune system is directed against the body's own tissues. The aetiology of SLE is not known. Although this disease is more common in young women, it can occur in either sex at any age. The production of autoantibodies leads to immune complex formation. These immune complexes can then be deposited in glomeruli, skin, lungs, synovium, and mesothelium, among other places. Symptoms include arthritis, a red rash over the nose and cheeks, fatigue, weakness, fever, and photosensitivity. Glomerulonephritis (kidney disease), pericarditis, anaemia, and neuritis may develop. In addition, many SLE patients develop renal complications.

Rh factor is an antigen that is present in the erythrocytes (red blood cells) of about 85% of the population. Erythrocytes contain antigens on their surface, which are proteins recognised by the immune system. Within the plasma are antibodies, which are proteins that react with antigens. Individuals are classified as having one of four blood types based on the presence or absence of these specific antigens. This process of classification is referred to as blood typing, or determining the ABO blood group.

Type A blood contains erythrocytes with type A surface antigens and plasma containing type B antibodies; type B blood contains type B surface antigens and plasma containing type A antibodies. Type AB blood contains both types of antigens but the plasma contains no ABO antibodies. Type O contains neither A nor B antigens but contains both A and B plasma antibodies. A person's blood type determines which type of blood he or she may receive in a blood transfusion.

Rh blood groups involve a complex of antigens first discovered in rhesus monkeys. The presence of any of the 18 separate Rh antigens makes an individual's blood Rh positive. If an individual with Rh negative blood were to be exposed to Rh positive blood, antibodies to the antigens could be produced.

Persons who have the factor are designated Rh-positive; those who lack the factor are termed Rh-negative. Blood for transfusions must be classified in terms of its Rh factor, as well as the ABO blood group, to prevent possible incompatibility reactions. If an Rh-negative person receives Rh-positive blood, for example, haemolysis and anaemia can result. A similar reaction can occur if an Rh-negative mother exposes her Rh-positive fetus to antibodies to the factor.

Immune and Inflammation Deficiencies

Immunodeficiency is an abnormal condition in which some part of the body's immune system is inadequate, and consequently resistance to infectious disease is decreased. It may be congenital or acquired.

Congenital Immunodeficiencies

Patients with severe combined immunodeficiency disease have defects that involve lymphoid stem cells. As a consequence, both T cells (cellular immunity) and B cells (humoral immunity) are affected. Patients are at risk for infection with all types of organisms (eg, bacteria, mycobacteria, fungi, viruses, parasites). There are two forms of this disease, both of which are inherited.

X-linked agammaglobulinaemia is one of the most common forms of primary immunodeficiency. This disease, which affects male infants, is caused by a defect in the differentiation of pre-B cells into B cells. The result is markedly decreased levels of all immunoglobulins and of mature B lymphocytes. T lymphocytes, however, function normally. Patients develop recurrent pyrogenic infections, but have no problems with fungal and viral infections because their cell-mediated immunity is unaffected. These infections first emerge in affected infants at about 6 months of age when maternal immunoglobulin levels have decreased.

Isolated deficiency of IgA is probably the most common form of immunodeficiency. This disease results from a block in the terminal differentiation of B lymphocytes. Most patients are asymptomatic, but some may develop chronic sinus infections. Patients also have an increased incidence of autoimmune disease.

Acquired Immunodeficiencies

Any nutritional deficiency can hamper normal immune function and the inflammatory response. Nutritional deficiencies may depress bone marrow function and diminish white blood cell development **Figure 6-34 ▶**. A lack of protein in the diet, for example, decreases the liver's ability to manufacture inflammatory mediators and plasma proteins.

The stress of trauma can also cause immunodeficiency. Other contributors to this condition may include hypoperfusion or shock, mediator production, damage to vital organs, and the decreased nutrition occurring during trauma states.

Iatrogenic (treatment-induced) immunodeficiency is most frequently caused by drugs. Corticosteroids, whether taken orally or inhaled, suppress the immune system. Often, this results in therapeutic benefit to the patient. In a small number of patients, however, the resulting immunosuppression leads to other diseases (eg, tuberculosis). Usually doctors are very careful about the prescribed duration of this therapy because of its

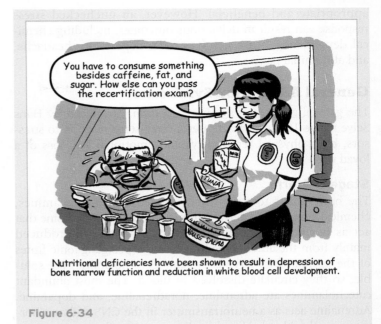

Nutritional deficiencies have been shown to result in depression of bone marrow function and reduction in white blood cell development.

Figure 6-34

potential for adverse effects. In addition, idiosyncratic reactions to antibiotics may result in bone marrow suppression, as is the case with chemotherapeutic drugs for cancer. Many cases of bone marrow suppression in cancer are direct and predictable side effects of chemotherapy, and not true idiosyncratic, "out of the blue" reactions.

Physical or mental stress has been shown to decrease white blood cell and lymphocyte function. It may also lead to decreased production of various antibodies.

AIDS is an immunodeficiency disease that is caused by the RNA retrovirus HIV (human immunodeficiency virus). HIV binds to the CD4 surface protein of helper T cells, infects these cells, and kills them. Their destruction causes decreased humoral and cell-mediated reactions.

Treatment of Immunodeficiencies

Replacement therapy is available for some types of immunodeficiencies (eg, common variable immunodeficiency). Intravenous gamma globulin has been used in the therapy of a number of immunological disorders of the nervous system, especially myasthenia gravis and inflammatory neuropathies, with considerable success. Bone marrow transplantation may restore immune competence in persons with acquired causes of immunodeficiency, such as following chemotherapy for cancer. In the future, gene therapy may be useful for treatment of both congenital and acquired causes of immunodeficiency.

Stress and Disease

Stress is the medical term for a wide range of strong external stimuli, both physiological and psychological, that can cause a physiological response. Usually, the response to stress is appropriate and beneficial. However, an unchecked stress response can result in deleterious outcomes, including chemical dependency, heart attack, stroke, depression, headache, and abdominal pain.

General Adaptation Syndrome

The general adaptation syndrome, a term introduced by Hans Selye in the 1920s, characterises a three-stage reaction to stressors, both physical (eg, injury) and emotional (eg, loss of a loved one).

Stage 1: Alarm

The body reacts to stress first by releasing catecholamines, chemical compounds derived from the amino acid tyrosine that act as hormones or neurotransmitters. They are produced mainly from the adrenal medulla and the postganglionic fibres of the sympathetic nervous system. Catecholamines are soluble, so they circulate dissolved in blood. The most abundant catecholamines are adrenaline, noradrenaline, and dopamine. Adrenaline acts as a neurotransmitter in the CNS and as a hormone in the blood. Noradrenaline is primarily a neurotransmitter of the peripheral sympathetic nervous system but is also present in the blood (mostly through "spillover" from the synapses of the sympathetic system).

Normally, the "fight-or-flight" response that occurs in the alarm reaction prepares the body to deal with stress, but it can also weaken the immune system, leading to infection.

Stage 2: Resistance

Stage 2, the resistance stage, is the body's way of adapting to stressors. It does so primarily by stimulating the adrenal gland to secrete two types of corticosteroid hormones that increase the blood glucose level and maintain blood pressure: glucocorticoids and mineralocorticoids. The most significant glucocorticoid in the body is cortisol, which controls carbohydrate, fat, and protein metabolism. Cortisol also has potent anti-inflammatory actions. Mineralocorticoids (predominantly aldosterone) control electrolyte and water levels in the body, mainly by promoting sodium retention by the kidney.

Continuation of stress and accompanying corticosteroid release eventually leads to fatigue, lapses in concentration, irritability, and lethargy.

Stage 3: Exhaustion

After a long period of stress, the person enters the exhaustion stage. The adrenal glands become depleted, leading to decreased blood glucose levels. The result is decreased stress tolerance, progressive mental and physical exhaustion, illness, and collapse. At this point, the body's immune system is compromised, significantly reducing a person's ability to resist disease. Heart attack, high blood pressure, or severe infection may result.

Effects of Chronic Stress

The hypothalamic-pituitary-adrenal axis (HPA axis) is a major part of the neuroendocrine system that controls reactions to stress. The HPA axis triggers a set of interactions among the glands, hormones, and parts of the midbrain that mediate the general adaptation syndrome. Continued stress, however, leads to loss of these normal control mechanisms. As a result, the adrenals continue to produce cortisol, which exhausts the stress mechanism and leads to fatigue and depression. Cortisol also interferes with serotonin activity, furthering the depressive effect.

Consistently high cortisol levels lead to suppression of the immune system through increased production of interleukin-6, an immune system messenger. Not surprisingly, then, research indicates that stress and depression have a negative effect on the immune system. Reduced immunity renders the body more susceptible to everything from colds and flu to cancer. For example, the incidence of serious illness, including cancer, is significantly higher among people who have suffered the death of a spouse in the previous year. Although severe, prolonged stress does not cause death directly, it does cause the body to lose its ability to fight disease in its effort to manage the stress. Stress also causes the body to release fat and cholesterol into the bloodstream, which in turn leads to clogging of the arteries and may eventually result in heart attack or stroke.

Many people start drinking alcohol to excess to combat their stress. Other manifestations of chronic stress include depression, headaches, insomnia, ulcers, and asthma. Fortunately, this immune suppression process can be corrected with psychotherapy, medication, or any number of other positive influences that restore hope and a feeling of self-esteem. The ability of human beings to recover from adversity is remarkable.

You are the Paramedic Summary

1. What are some of the potential complications that can occur from missing dialysis?

Patients who have end-stage renal failure depend on dialysis to take on the workload of the kidneys, such as being a filter for toxins and maintaining proper fluid balance and electrolyte balance. An interruption in these vital functions can lead to the development of problems such as congestive heart failure, myocardial infarction, pulmonary oedema, arrhythmias, electrolyte imbalances, and medication toxicity.

2. Does renal disease affect other organ systems?

Yes, all organ systems are affected by renal failure. Patients can develop problems similar to those experienced by patients with diabetes or hypertension. For example, patients with renal disease often develop problems with peripheral neuropathy, gastrointestinal disturbances, and anaemia.

3. What should you monitor your patient for?

The patient is presenting with a number of issues, any of which could potentially lead to problems. First and foremost, she is hypotensive and in respiratory distress. You need to keep a watchful eye on her blood pressure and respiratory status, being prepared to intubate if necessary. The tall T waves on the ECG are characteristic of hyperkalaemia. The heart does not behave in an environment in which the potassium is out of line. Check the monitor frequently for the development of ventricular arrhythmias such as premature ventricular contractions, ventricular tachycardia, and ventricular fibrillation.

4. Which interventions should you consider at this point, if any?

At this point, Mrs. Jensen is receiving high-flow supplemental oxygen. The patient definitely requires cardiac monitoring and intravenous access for possible fluid and medication administration.

5. Is the patient going into shock? If so, what type?

Yes, the patient is going into shock, but which type can be a little tricky. We know from her clinical presentation that septic shock is a possibility due to the signs of infection at the shunt site. With a history of a past myocardial infarction and congestive heart failure, cardiogenic shock cannot be ruled out as a possible cause.

6. Why is a fluid bolus appropriate in this setting?

Hypotension is a common side effect of dialysis that can result from the change in fluid and/or electrolyte distribution. Most patients will respond favourably to a small fluid bolus (200 to 250 ml) returning fluid back to the blood vessels. This small amount of fluid should not have a negative effect in the respiratory status of your patient.

7. How did the inflammatory process manifest itself in this patient?

The inflammatory process manifested itself in both local and systemic effects. Local effects include the development of redness, swelling, tenderness, and heat at the shunt site. Systemic involvement of the inflammatory process is seen in the presence of fever.

8. What are other signs and symptoms of hyperkalaemia?

Patients who have hyperkalaemia may also present with irritability, abdominal distention, nausea, diarrhoea, oliguria, weakness, or paralysis. Good history taking will help you clue into this serious electrolyte imbalance and initiate therapy!

Prep Kit

Ready for Review

- All cells except red blood cells and platelets have three main components: a nucleus, cytoplasm, and a cell membrane.
- There are four major tissue types: epithelial tissue; connective tissue, muscle tissue, and nervous tissue.
- When cells are exposed to adverse conditions, they go through a process of adaptation (which can be temporary or permanent) to protect themselves from injury. Examples of adaptations include atrophy, hypertrophy, hyperplasia, dysplasia, and metaplasia.
- The cellular environment refers to the distribution of cells, molecules, and fluids throughout the body. It changes with ageing, exercise, pregnancy, medications, disease, and injury. Body fluids contain water, sodium, chloride, potassium, calcium, phosphorus, and magnesium.
- pH is a measurement of hydrogen ion concentration. Normal body functions depend on an acid-base balance that remains within the normal physiological pH range of 7.35 to 7.45.
- Cellular injury results from causes such as chemical exposure, infectious agents, immunological responses, inflammatory responses, prolonged periods of hypoxia, genetic factors, nutritional imbalances, and physical agents.
- Age- and sex-associated factors interact with a combination of genetic and environmental factors, lifestyle, and anatomic or hormonal differences to cause disease.
- Analysing disease risk involves consideration of disease rates (incidence, prevalence, mortality) and disease risk factors (causal and noncausal). These risk factors, age, and sex differences interact to influence an individual's level of risk.
- A true genetic risk is passed through generations on a gene. In contrast, a family tendency may "cluster" in family groups despite lack of evidence for heritable gene-associated abnormalities. In autosomal dominant inheritance, a person needs to inherit only one copy of a particular form of a gene to show that trait. In autosomal recessive inheritance, the person must inherit two copies of a particular form of a gene to show the trait.
- Immunological diseases occur because of hyperactivity or hypoactivity of the immune system. Allergies are acquired following initial exposure to a stimulant, known as an allergen. Repeated exposures cause a reaction by the immune system to the allergen.
- Perfusion is the delivery of oxygen and nutrients to cells, organs, and tissues through the circulatory system. Hypoperfusion occurs when the level of tissue perfusion falls below normal.
- Shock is an abnormal state associated with inadequate oxygen and nutrient delivery to the metabolic apparatus of the cell, resulting in an impairment of cell metabolism.
- Multiple organ dysfunction syndrome (MODS) is a progressive condition usually characterised by combined failure of several organs, such as the lungs, liver, and kidney, along with some clotting mechanisms. It occurs after severe illness or injury.
- The immune system includes all of the structures and processes that mount a defence against foreign substances and disease-causing agents. The body has three lines of defence: anatomic barriers, the inflammatory response, and the immune system.
- The immune system has two anatomic components: the lymphoid tissues of the body and the cells that are responsible for the immune response.
- The primary cells of the immune system are the white blood cells, or leucocytes.
- There are two general types of immune response: native and acquired.
- Immunity may be either humoral or cell-mediated.
- The antibodies secreted by B cells are called immunoglobulins. Antibodies make antigens more visible to the immune system in three ways: by acting as opsonins, by making antigens clump, and by inactivating bacterial toxins.

- The inflammatory response is a reaction of the tissues of the body, triggered by cellular injury, to irritation or injury that is characterised by pain, swelling, redness, and heat.
- The two most common causes of inflammation are infection and physical agents.
- Cytokines are products of cells that affect the functioning of other cells; they include interleukins, lymphokines, and interferon.
- Chronic inflammatory responses are usually caused by an unsuccessful acute inflammatory response after the invasion of a foreign body, persistent infection, or antigen.
- Normal wound healing involves four steps: repair of damaged tissue, removal of inflammatory debris, restoration of tissues to a normal state, and regeneration of cells.
- Wounds may heal by either primary or secondary intention.
- Hypersensitivity is an increased bodily response to any substance to which the person is abnormally sensitive. A hypersensitivity reaction may be immediate, occurring within seconds to minutes, or delayed, occurring hours to days after exposure to the antigen.
- Immunodeficiency may be congenital or acquired.
- Stress does not cause death directly, but it can permit diseases that ultimately lead to the patient's death to flourish.
- The general adaptation syndrome describes the body's short-term and long-term reactions to stress.

Vital Vocabulary

acidosis A blood pH of less than 7.35.

acquired immunity A highly specific, inducible, discriminatory, and permanent method by which literally armies of cells respond to an immune stimulant.

activation Mediators of inflammation trigger the appearance of molecules known as selectins and integrins on the surfaces of endothelial cells and PMNs, respectively.

active hyperaemia The dilation of arterioles after transient arteriolar constriction, which allows influx of blood under increased pressure.

adhesion The attachment of PMNs to endothelial cells, mediated by selectins and integrins.

adipose tissue A connective tissue containing large amounts of lipids.

aetiology The cause of a disease process.

alkalosis A blood pH greater than 7.45.

allergen Any substance that causes a hypersensitivity reaction.

allergy Hypersensitivity reaction to the presence of an agent (allergen) that is intrinsically harmless.

anaphylactic shock A severe hypersensitivity reaction that involves bronchoconstriction and cardiovascular collapse.

angiogenesis The growth of new blood vessels.

antibodies Proteins secreted by certain immune cells that bind antigens to make them more visible to the immune system.

antigen A foreign substance recognised by the immune system.

apoptosis Normal, genetically programmed cell death.

Arthus reaction A localised reaction involving vascular inflammation in response to an IgG-mediated allergic response.

asthma A chronic inflammatory lower airway condition resulting in intermittent wheezing and excess mucus production.

atopic The medical term for having an allergic tendency.

atrophy A decrease in cell size due to a loss of subcellular components.

autoantibodies Antibodies directed against the patient.

autocrine hormone A hormone that acts on the cell that has secreted it.

autoimmunity The production of antibodies or T cells that work against the tissues of a person's own body, producing autoimmune disease or a hypersensitivity reaction.

autosomal dominant A pattern of inheritance that involves genes that are located on autosomes or the nonsex chromosomes. You only need to inherit a single copy of a particular form of a gene to show the trait.

autosomal recessive A pattern of inheritance that involves genes located on autosomes or the nonsex chromosomes. You must inherit two copies of a particular form of a gene to show the trait.

axon Part of the neuron that conducts the impulses away from the cell body.

basophils Approximately 1% of the leucocytes, they are essential to nonspecific immune response to inflammation due to their role in releasing histamine and other chemicals that dilate blood vessels.

bone marrow Specialised tissue found within bone.

buffers Molecules that modulate changes in pH to keep it in the physiological range.

capillary refill time A test done on the fingers or toes by briefly squeezing the toe or finger, then evaluating the time it takes for the pink colour to return.

cardiogenic shock A condition caused by loss of 40% or more of the functioning myocardium; the heart is no longer able to circulate sufficient blood to maintain adequate oxygen delivery.

cell-mediated immunity Immune process by which T-cell lymphocytes recognise antigens and then secrete cytokines (specifically lymphokines) that attract other cells or stimulate the production of cytotoxic cells that kill the infected cells.

cell signalling The process by which cells communicate with one another.

central shock A term that describes shock secondary to central pump failure, it includes both cardiogenic shock and obstructive shock.

chemotaxins Components of the activated complement system that attract leucocytes from the circulation to help fight infections.

chemotaxis The movement of additional white blood cells to an area of inflammation in response to the release of chemical mediators, such as neutrophils, injured tissue, and monocytes.

coagulation system The system that forms blood clots in the body and facilitates repairs to the vascular tree.

complement system A group of plasma proteins whose function is to do one of three things: attract leucocytes to sites of inflammation, activate leucocytes, and directly destroy cells.

connective tissue Tissue that serves to bind various tissue types together.

cytokines Products of cells that affect the function of other cells.

dendrites Part of the neuron that receives impulses from the axon and contains vesicles for the release of neurotransmitters.

distributive shock Occurs when there is widespread dilation of the resistance vessels (small arterioles), the capacitance vessels (small venules), or both.

dysplasia An alteration in the size, shape, and organisation of cells.

endocrine hormones Hormones that are carried to their target or cell group in the bloodstream.

endothelial cells Specific types of epithelial cells that serve the function of lining the blood vessels.

eosinophils Cells that make up approximately 1% to 3% of leucocytes, which play a major role in allergic reactions and bronchoconstriction in an asthma attack.

epithelium Type of tissue that covers all external surfaces of the body.

exocrine hormones Hormones that are secreted through ducts into an organ or onto epithelial surfaces.

feedback inhibition Negative feedback resulting in the decrease of an action in the body.

fibrin A whitish, filamentous protein formed by the action of thrombin on fibrinogen. Fibrin is the protein that polymerises (bonds) to form the fibrous component of a blood clot.

fibrinolysis cascade The breakdown of fibrin in blood clots, and the prevention of the polymerisation of fibrin into new clots.

free radicals Molecules that are missing one electron in their outer shell.

general adaptation syndrome A three-stage description of the body's short-term and long-term reactions to stress.

gut-associated lymphoid tissue (GALT) The lymphoid tissue that lies under the inner lining of the oesophagus and intestines.

hapten A substance that normally does not stimulate an immune response but can be combined with an antigen and at a later point initiate an antibody response.

haemochromatosis An inherited disease in which the body absorbs more iron than it needs and stores it in the liver, kidneys, and pancreas.

haemolytic anaemia A disease characterised by increased destruction of the red blood cells. It can occur from an Rh factor reaction, exposure to chemicals, or a disorder of the immune system.

haemophilia An inherited sex-linked disorder characterised by excessive bleeding.

helper T cell A type of T lymphocyte that is involved in both cell-mediated and antibody-mediated immune responses. It secretes cytokines that stimulate the B cells and other T cells.

histamine A vasoactive amine that increases vascular permeability and causes vasodilation.

homeostasis is a term derived from the Greek words for "same" and "steady". All organisms constantly adjust their physiological processes in an effort to maintain an internal balance.

hormones Proteins formed in specialised organs or glands and carried to another organ or group of cells in the same organism. Hormones regulate many body functions, including metabolism, growth, and temperature.

humoral immunity The immunity that utilises antibodies made by B-cell lymphocytes.

hypercalcaemia A condition in which calcium levels are elevated.

hypercholesterolaemia An elevated blood cholesterol level.

hyperkalaemia An elevated blood serum potassium level.

hypermagnesaemia An increased serum magnesium level.

hypernatraemia A blood serum sodium level greater than 148 mmol/l and a serum osmolarity greater than 295 mOsm/kg.

hyperphosphataemia An elevated blood serum phosphate level.

hyperplasia An increase in the actual number of cells in an organ or tissue, usually resulting in an increase in size of the organ or tissue.

hypersensitivity A generic term for bodily responses to a substance to which a patient is abnormally sensitive.

hypertonic solution A solution with an osmolarity greater than intracellular fluid.

hypertrophy An increase in the size of the cells due to synthesis of more subcellular components, leading to an increase in tissue and organ size.

hypocalcaemia A decreased serum calcium level.

hypokalaemia A decreased blood serum potassium.

hypomagnesaemia A decreased serum magnesium level.

hyponatraemia A blood serum sodium level that is below 135 mmol/l and a serum osmolarity that is less than 280 mOsm/kg.

hypoperfusion A condition that occurs when the level of tissue perfusion decreases below that needed to maintain normal cellular functions.

hypophosphataemia A decreased blood serum phosphate level.

hypothalamic-pituitary-adrenal (HPA) axis A major part of the neuroendocrine system that controls reactions to stress. It is the mechanism for a set of interactions among glands, hormones, and parts of the midbrain that mediate the general adaptation syndrome.

hypotonic solution A solution with an osmolarity lower than intracellular fluid.

hypovolaemic shock A condition that occurs when the circulating blood volume is inadequate to deliver adequate oxygen and nutrients to the body.

immune response The body's defence reaction to any substance that is recognised as foreign.

immune system The body system that includes all of the structures and processes designed to mount a defence against foreign substances and disease-causing agents.

immunodeficiency An abnormal condition in which some part of the body's immune system is inadequate, and consequently resistance to infectious disease is decreased.

immunogen An antigen that activates immune cells to generate an immune response against itself.

immunoglobulins Antibodies secreted by the B cells.

incidence The frequency with which a disease occurs.

inflammatory response A reaction by tissues of the body to irritation or injury, characterised by pain, swelling, redness, and heat.

interferon Protein produced by cells in response to viral invasion. Interferon is released into the bloodstream or intercellular fluid to induce healthy cells to manufacture an enzyme that counters the infection.

interleukins Chemical substances that attract white blood cells to the sites of injury and bacterial invasion.

isoimmunity Formation of antibodies or T cells that are directed against antigens or another person's cells.

isotonic solution A solution with the same osmolarity as intracellular fluid (280 mOsm/l).

kinin system A general term for a group of polypeptides that mediate inflammatory responses by stimulating visceral smooth muscle and relaxing vascular smooth muscle to produce vasodilation.

leucocytes The white blood cells responsible for fighting off infection.

leucotrienes Arachidonic acid metabolites that function as chemical mediators of inflammation. Also known as slow-reacting substances of anaphylaxis (SRS-A).

ligand Any molecule that binds a receptor leading to a reaction.

lymph A thin, watery fluid that bathes the tissues of the body.

lymphatic system A network of capillaries, vessels, ducts, nodes, and organs that helps to maintain the fluid environment of the body by producing lymph and transporting it through the body.

lymphocytes The white blood cells responsible for a large part of the body's immune protection.

lymphokines Cytokines released by lymphocytes, including many of the interleukins, gamma interferon, tumour necrosis factor beta, and chemokines.

macrophages Cells that developed from the monocytes that provide the body's first line of defence in the inflammatory process.

margination Loss of fluid from the blood vessels into the tissue, causing the blood left in the vessels to have an increased viscosity, which in turn slows the flow of blood and produces stasis.

mast cells The cells that resemble basophils but do not circulate in the blood. Mast cells play a role in allergic reactions, immunity, and wound healing.

membrane attack complex (MAC) Molecules that insert themselves into the bacterial membrane, leading to weakened areas in the membrane.

metaplasia A reversible, cellular adaptation in which one adult cell type is replaced by another adult cell type.

mitochondria The metabolic centre or powerhouse of the cell. They are small and rod-shaped organelles.

monocytes Mononuclear phagocytic white blood cells derived from myeloid stem cells. They circulate in the bloodstream for about 24 hours and then move into tissues to mature into macrophages.

mortality The number of deaths from a disease in a given population.

mucosal-associated lymphoid tissue (MALT) The lymphoid tissue associated with the skin and the respiratory, urinary, and reproductive traits as well as the tonsils.

multiple organ dysfunction syndrome (MODS) A progressive condition usually characterised by combined failure of several organs, such as the lungs, liver, and kidney, along with some clotting mechanisms, which occurs after severe illness or injury.

native immunity A nonspecific cellular and humoral response that operates as the body's first line of defence against pathogens.

negative feedback The concept that once the desired effect of a process has been achieved, further action is inhibited until it is needed again; also called feedback inhibition.

neurogenic shock This condition usually results from spinal cord injury. The effect is loss of normal sympathetic nervous system tone and vasodilation.

neurotransmitters Proteins that transmit signals between cells of the nervous system.

neutrophils Cells that make up approximately 55% to 70% of leucocytes responsible in large part for the body's protection against infection. They are readily attracted by foreign antigens and destroy them by phagocytosis.

nucleus A cellular organelle that contains the genetic information. The nucleus controls the function and structure of a cell.

obstructive shock This occurs when there is a block to blood flow in the heart or great vessels.

oliguria Decreased urine output.

opsoninisation Occurs when an antibody coats an antigen to facilitate its recognition by immune cells.

organelles Internal cellular structures that carry out specific functions for the cell.

osmosis The movement of water down its concentration gradient across a membrane.

paracrine hormones Hormones that diffuse through intracellular spaces to their target.

pathophysiology The study of how normal physiological processes are affected by disease.

perfusion The delivery of oxygen and nutrients to the cells, organs, and tissues of the body. Also involves the removal of waste.

pericardial tamponade Impairment of diastolic filling of the right ventricle due to significant amounts of fluid in the pericardial sac surrounding the heart, leading to a decrease in cardiac output.

peripheral nerves All of the nerves of the body extending from the brain and spinal cord.

peripheral shock A term that describes shock secondary to peripheral circulatory abnormalities—includes both hypovolaemic shock and distributive shock.

pH The measure of acidity or alkalinity of a solution.

phagocyte A kind of cell that engulfs and consumes foreign material such as microorganisms and debris.

phagocytosis Process in which a cell eats or engulfs a foreign substance to destroy it.

polymorphonuclear neutrophils (PMNs) A type of white blood cell formed by bone marrow tissue that possesses a nucleus consisting of several parts or lobes connected by fine strands; a variety of leucocyte.

polyuria Frequent and plentiful urination.

prevalence The number of cases of a disease in a specific population over time.

prostaglandins A group of lipids that act as chemical messengers.

pyrogens Chemicals or proteins that travel to the brain and affect the hypothalamus, and stimulate a rise in the body's core temperature.

renin-angiotensin-aldosterone system (RAAS) A complex feedback mechanism responsible for the kidney's regulation of sodium in the body.

Rh factor An antigen present in the erythrocytes (red blood cells) of about 85% of people.

ribonucleic acid (RNA) Nucleic acid associated with controlling cellular activities.

septic shock This occurs as a result of widespread infection, usually bacterial. Untreated, the result is multiple organ dysfunction syndrome (MODS) and often death.

serotonin A vasoactive amine that increases vascular permeability to cause vasodilation.

serum sickness A condition in which antigen antibody complexes formed in the bloodstream deposit in sites around the body, most notably in the kidney, with resultant inflammatory reactions.

slow-reacting substances of anaphylaxis (SRS-A) Biologically active compounds derived from arachidonic acid called leucotrienes.

T killer cells Cells released during a type IV allergic reaction that kill antigen-bearing target cells.

tonicity Tension exerted on a cell due to water movement across the cell membrane.

transmigration (diapedesis) The PMNs permeate through the vessel wall, moving into the interstitial space.

urticaria Multiple small, raised areas on the skin that may be one of the warning signs of impending anaphylaxis. Also known as hives.

vasculitis An inflammation of the blood vessels.

vasoactive amines Substances such as histamine and serotonin that increase vascular permeability.

virulence A measure of the disease-causing ability of a microorganism.

■ Points to Ponder

You have a new partner for the day and you respond to a "difficulty breathing" call. Once there, your patient advises that he has an "autoimmune disease". Your partner leans over to you and says quietly, "Oh no, this guy has AIDS and we're going to get it".

How are you going to explain this patient's medical condition to your partner without doing so in front of your patient?

Issues: Bloodborne Pathogens, Autoimmune Diseases, Universal Precautions.

Assessment in Action

You have responded to a 40-year-old male patient who crashed on his motorcycle. The patient is wearing a helmet and is conscious but agitated and restless. You notice a large amount of blood on the ground around the patient's lower body. As you complete your assessment, you find the patient has an unstable pelvis and an open femur fracture. Your initial vital signs are blood pressure, 136/70 mm Hg; pulse, 100 beats/min; and respiration, 16 breaths/min. You know your patient has lost a considerable amount of blood and are concerned the patient may start exhibiting signs of shock.

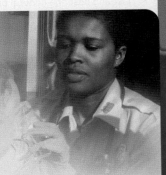

1. **What are the two types of shock?**
   A. Arterial and venous
   B. Central and peripheral
   C. Hypovolaemic and systemic
   D. Peripheral and distributive

2. **What type of shock involves fluid loss?**
   A. Anaphylactic
   B. Cardiogenic
   C. Hypovolaemic
   D. Septic

3. **What are the two types of hypovolaemic shock and which one is exhibited by this patient?**
   A. Exogenous and endogenious
   B. Aerobic and anaerobic
   C. Kallikrein and kinin
   D. Angiotensin and aldosterone

4. **Based on your assessment of this patient, his agitation, anxiety, and restlessness may be a sign of:**
   A. decompensated shock.
   B. compensated shock.
   C. neurogenic shock.
   D. distributive shock.

5. **Which adult blood pressure reading would represent decompensated shock?**
   A. The systolic blood pressure is greater than 5% for the age range
   B. The systolic blood pressure is less than 5% for the age range
   C. The diastolic blood pressure is greater than 5% for the age range
   D. The diastolic blood pressure is less than 5% for the age range

6. **A normal capillary refill time should be:**
   A. more than 4 seconds.
   B. 3 to 4 seconds.
   C. greater than 2 seconds.
   D. less than 2 seconds.

Challenging Question

7. **What is your main priority—stabilising the patient or transporting the patient?**

Pharmacology

Objectives

Cognitive

- Describe historical trends in pharmacology.
- Differentiate between the chemical, generic (nonproprietary), and trade (proprietary) names of a drug.
- List the four main sources of drug products.
- Describe how drugs are classified.
- List the authoritative sources for drug information.
- List legislative acts controlling drug use and abuse in the United Kingdom.
- Differentiate among Schedule I, II, III, IV, and V substances.
- List examples of substances in each schedule.
- Discuss standardisation of drugs.
- Discuss special considerations in drug treatment with regard to pregnant, paediatric, and older patients.
- Discuss the paramedic's responsibilities and scope of management pertinent to the administration of medications.
- Review the specific anatomy and physiology pertinent to pharmacology with additional attention to autonomic pharmacology.
- List and describe general properties of drugs.
- List and describe liquid and solid drug forms.
- List and differentiate routes of drug administration.
- Differentiate between enteral and parenteral routes of drug administration.
- Describe mechanisms of drug action.
- List and differentiate the phases of drug activity, including the pharmaceutical, pharmacokinetic, and pharmacodynamic phases.

- Describe the process called pharmacokinetics, pharmacodynamics, including theories of drug action, drug-response relationship, factors altering drug responses, predictable drug responses, iatrogenic drug responses, and unpredictable adverse drug responses.
- Differentiate among drug interactions.
- Discuss considerations for storing and securing medications.
- List the component of a drug profile by classification.
- List and describe drugs that the paramedic may administer.
- Integrate pathophysiological principles of pharmacology with patient assessment.
- Synthesise patient history information and assessment findings to form an initial impression.
- Synthesise an initial impression to implement a pharmacological management plan.
- Assess the pathophysiology of a patient's condition by identifying classifications of drugs.

Affective

- Serve as a model for obtaining a history by identifying classifications of drugs.
- Support the administration of drugs by a paramedic to effect positive therapeutic effects.
- Advocate drug education through identification of drug classifications.

Psychomotor

None

1914–1918 war. A series of Dangerous Drugs Acts brought the various international agreements into force in the UK. In 1961, the Single Convention on Narcotic Drugs replaced all the earlier international agreements. This was the basis of the Dangerous Drugs Act of 1965 in the UK.

The misuse of amphetamines and other psychotropic drugs widened the problems of abuse. As problems of drug abuse continued to increase, the law was extended by the Misuse of Drugs Act of 1971. In the UK today, the Medicines Act of 1968 and the Poisons Act of 1972, together with the Misuse of Drugs Act of 1971, regulate the use of all medicines and poisons:

- The Medicines Act of 1968 controls the manufacture and distribution of medicines.
- The Poisons Act of 1972 regulates the sale of non-medicinal poisons.
- The Misuse of Drugs of Act 1971 deals with the abuse of drugs.

The Medicines Act of 1968

There are three classes of product under the Medicines Act of 1968. These are:

1. **General-sales-list medicines (GSL):** those which can be sold to the public without the supervision of a pharmacist.
2. **Pharmacy medicines (P):** these may only be sold under the supervision of a pharmacist.
3. **Prescription-only medicines (POM):** medicinal products that may be sold or supplied by retail in accordance with a prescription given by an appropriate practitioner. There are some exemptions from POM status and these include all preparations of insulin. No one may administer a POM except to himself, unless he is a practitioner or acting in accordance with the directions of a practitioner. There is a list of medicines for use by parenteral administration that is exempt from this restriction when administered to save a life in an emergency. This list includes adrenaline, atropine, and glucagon.

The Misuse of Drugs Act of 1971

The Misuse of Drugs Act came into operation on 1 July, 1973. It controls the export, import, production, supply, and possession of dangerous or otherwise harmful drugs and consolidates and extends earlier legislation. The Advisory Committee on the Misuse of Drugs was established on 1 February, 1972 and advises ministers. The drugs subject to control are termed *controlled drugs*.

- Part I (Class A), eg, diamorphine, cocaine, lysergide (LSD), methadone
- Part II (Class B), eg, oral amphetamines, barbiturates, codeine
- Part III (Class C), eg, buprenorphine, diazepam, anabolic steroids, cannabis

The use of controlled drugs in medicine is permitted by the Misuse of Drugs Regulations of 1985. The drugs controlled are

classified into five schedules in descending order of control. The most stringent controls apply to those drugs in Schedule 1.

- **Schedule 1.** These drugs may not be used for medicinal purposes and their possession is limited to involvement in research and other special cases. Examples are coca leaf, lysergide, and raw opium.
- **Schedule 2.** These drugs have a very high abuse potential including opiates (such as heroin, morphine, and methadone) and major stimulants (such as the amphetamines). Requirements for safe custody and control over destruction apply to these drugs and the keeping of records must be observed.
- **Schedule 3.** These drugs include a number of minor stimulant drugs and barbiturates that may lead to low or moderate physical dependence or high psychological dependence. Buprenorphine, pentazocine, and temazepam are in this class.
- **Schedule 4.** This schedule contains benzodiazepines, such as diazepam. Anabolic steroids and androgenic steroids are also in this class. Records do not have to be kept by retailers and there are no safe custody requirements.
- **Schedule 5.** These are preparations of controlled drugs that have only minimal risk of abuse. Examples are medicinal opium containing not more than 0.2% morphine and preparations containing no more than 0.1% cocaine.

At the Scene

It is important for you to become familiar with "street" names of these commonly used and abused drugs. Most users will not tell you they took methylenedioxymethamphetamine; you are more likely to hear terms like ecstasy, XTC, E, disco biscuits, or Adams. Research or look up these common street terms.

Legal Issues

This chapter gives a broad overview of pharmacology, and therefore the legal aspects of how staff obtain their rights to both carry and administer drugs will not be covered in any depth. In the UK, the law that pertains to the carrying and administration of drugs within the ambulance service arena is to be found in the Prescription Only Medicines (Human Use) Order of 1997 (as amended). This is most commonly referred to as the "POMs Order". Within the POMs Order, it is Schedule 5, Part III that gives paramedics registered with the Health Professions Council (HPC) the legal right to administer the range of drugs detailed therein. Emergency Medical Technicians have the right to administer those drugs that are detailed in Article 7 of the POMs Order. Both of these parts of the POMs Order give a legal exemption from Section 58(2) of the Medicines Act of 1968, which essentially states that no-one, other than a registered medical practitioner, can administer prescription-only medicines.

Morphine is a Class A controlled drug under Schedule 2 of the Misuse of Drugs Act of 1985. It is therefore subject to full controlled drug requirements relating to administration, safe custody, and the requirement to keep and register records. HPC registered paramedics gain their ability to carry and administer morphine sulphate by virtue of a group authority issued under The Misuse of Drugs Regulations of 2001.

The Joint Royal Colleges Ambulance Liaison Committee National Clinical Guidelines gives details of those drugs that are available for administration by ambulance clinicians within the legal framework detailed above. Other prescription-only medicines may be available to registered health care staff working in the public sector under a device known as a Patient Group Direction (PGD). PGDs are written instructions for the supply or administration of medicines to groups of patients who may not be individually identified before presentation for treatment. The main piece of legislation that applies here is the Prescription Only Medicines (Human Use) Amendment Order of 2003.

It is strongly recommended that all practitioners familiarise themselves with the law that pertains to their area of practice. If you have any doubts, first and foremost consult your employer. The best organisations to consult additionally are:

- The Medicines and Healthcare products Regulatory Agency
- The National Prescribing Centre
- The Department of Health
- The Joint Royal Colleges Ambulance Liaison Committee
- The Health Professions Council

Manufacturing-Related Regulations

Legislation also focuses on guaranteeing standardisation of doses. Standardisation assures patients that when they take a medication with a stated amount of the active ingredient, they will, in fact, receive that amount of the drug. Clearly, no one would want to be prescribed a certain dose of a drug and find that the actual medication contained twice (or half) the amount of active ingredient stated on the drug's label.

The Drug-Approval Process

New drugs are constantly being developed. The commercialisation process, however, takes years—the average time for a drug to be developed, tested, and approved is about 9 years. In some cases, manufacturers spend most of those 9 years developing a drug only to find out that the drug does not work as envisioned or is too dangerous for human consumption.

All new drugs must go through animal studies and clinical trials in humans before they are approved for distribution.

Animal Studies

Animal studies are designed to identify tissues and organs sensitive to the drug's actions and to determine its pharmacodynamic and pharmacokinetic properties. Testing in at least two animal species is required by law. After successful completion of animal studies, a new drug under investigation may enter clinical trials in humans.

Clinical Trials

Clinical trials proceed in four phases:

- **Phase I.** The new drug is tested in healthy volunteers to compare human data with those in animals, to determine safe doses of the drug, and to assess its safety.
- **Phase II.** These trials are performed in homogenous populations of patients (50 to 300 patients). In double-blind studies, one group receives the drug and the other group receives a placebo. These studies are designed to evaluate the drug's efficacy and safety and to establish which form is the most effective dose.
- **Phase III.** In these clinical trials, the drug is made available to a larger group of patients (several thousand). These studies, which usually last several years, evaluate the drug's efficacy and monitor the nature and incidence of side effects.
- **Phase IV.** After successful completion of Phase III clinical trials, the drug company can apply to the MHRA for approval to market the drug. Phase IV trials compare the new drug with others on the market and examine the drug's long-term efficacy and cost-effectiveness.

Special Considerations in Drug Therapy

Pregnant Patients

Administration of any medication to a pregnant woman poses two pharmacological challenges: Pregnancy causes several physiological changes that affect the way drugs are handled by the body, and it has the potential to harm the fetus directly. For this reason, you must be familiar with how a particular medication might affect the fetus before you consider giving it to a pregnant patient. In the prehospital environment, you must be able quickly to evaluate the risks versus the benefits of the drug's administration. Does the potential benefit to the mother outweigh the risk to the fetus? If the drug is the only option for saving the mother's life, then that consideration would be paramount.

To see how the twin concerns of mother and fetus play into your decision to administer a particular medication, let's examine information from the British National Formulary (BNF) about amiodarone:

- **Drug information:** Amiodarone is used in the treatment of arrhythmias, particularly when other drugs are ineffective or contraindicated.
- **Pregnancy:** Use in the second and third trimesters carries the risk of neonatal goiter; use only if no alternative.
- **Breastfeeding:** Avoid; present in milk in significant amounts; theoretical risk from release of iodine.

Note: At present, paramedics only administer amiodarone for refractory ventricular fibrillation. This is one of the times when saving the life of the mother is more important than any possible side effects on the fetus. As a result, pregnancy is not a contraindication to the administration of amiodarone in a cardiac arrest.

Paediatric Patients

Medications have very different effects in adults from those they have in children—whether the paediatric patient is a newborn, a neonate, an infant, or a toddler. In particular, infants do not achieve the same level of hepatic (liver) function as adults until they reach about 6 months of age; as a consequence, babies have a sharply reduced metabolic capacity. Similarly, the products of metabolism in children can vary from those seen in adults, which may sometimes result in unexpected responses. At the same time, children can metabolise some medications much more quickly than adults do, so they may require relatively higher doses or more frequent administration of some medications. The incomplete development of the gastrointestinal tract in young infants slows absorption of oral medications and delays elimination, so the same medication would be more potent in an infant than in an adult.

Elderly Patients

The changes in pharmacokinetics in elderly patients are comparable to those observed in young children. In elderly people, hepatic functions and gastrointestinal activity slow, which in turn delays absorption and elimination. In addition, elderly patients are often taking several medications; these concomitant therapies may interact and modify one another's effects. Furthermore, because they may have a large number of medications to be taken and alterations in their normal mental status, elderly patients may unintentionally overdose on a particular drug or forget to take it.

Special Considerations

Paediatric and elderly patients often have slower absorption and elimination times, necessitating modification of the doses administered. Pregnant patients are limited in the medications they can take because of risk to the fetus.

The Scope of Management

Safe and Effective Drug Administration

The wrong drug or the wrong dose of the right drug can kill a patient as effectively as a lethal weapon. For this reason, you must be intimately familiar with the pharmacological agents used in the prehospital environment—their indications and contraindications, their side effects, and their dangers. Nowhere in prehospital care can ignorance or carelessness on the part of paramedics do so much harm as in the administration of drugs. As a paramedic, you will be responsible for ensuring that administration of medications in the prehospital environment is safe, therapeutic, and effective.

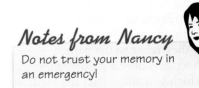

Notes from Nancy
Do not trust your memory in an emergency!

You are the Paramedic Part 2

You ask your colleague to place the patient on oxygen via nonrebreathing mask at 15 l/min and obtain a set of vital signs while you begin to question the patient further about his current illness and past medical history. The patient's son explains that his father was discharged from the hospital last week for problems associated with his heart. He hands you an index card that contains his father's medical history and list of medications. You note that the patient has a history of atrial fibrillation, congestive heart failure, and stable angina. Daily medications include digoxin, 0.125 mg every morning; warfarin, 3 mg every morning; furosemide, 60 mg with breakfast and 60 mg at bedtime; diltiazem, 60 mg three times daily; and glyceryl trinitrate as required for chest pain. As you are looking over the list, the son pulls you over to side of the room and quietly expresses his concern about his father's medication compliance, as he has noticed that his father can be forgetful and may be taking his medication more often than it is prescribed.

Vital Signs	Recording Time: 5 Minutes
Skin	Pale, cool, and moist
Pulse	45 beats/min, irregular; weak radial
Blood pressure	72/50 mm Hg
Respirations	24 breaths/min, rales auscultated at bases
SpO₂	96% on nonrebreathing mask at 15 l/min of supplemental oxygen

3. What type of drug is diltiazem and how does it work?

At the Scene

The ever-growing variety of medications available makes it impossible for you to know everything about each drug. Do not hesitate to contact your local hospital or consult a reference guide when faced with a medication you are not intimately familiar with.

Legal, Moral, and Ethical Responsibilities

When administering medications to a patient, you are legally responsible for the appropriate use and documentation of that therapy. Even if another paramedic prepares the medication and hands a syringe to you to administer, you are still the person responsible. Always have a clear understanding of which medication you are administering and why you are administering it.

Put yourself in the shoes of your patient. How much confidence would you have in the person providing your care if he or she did not have a complete understanding of each drug, when to use it, and how it works? In addition to the obvious legal responsibility, we have a moral and ethical responsibility to ensure that we administer drugs safely.

The following guidelines will help you fulfil your responsibilities.

- Make certain you understand the precautions and contraindications associated with each medication. In addition, consider the precautions and contraindications as they relate to the patient.
- Practise proper administration techniques. The manner in which you administer the medication will have a direct effect on how the drug works and may prevent complications such as infection.
- Know the side effects associated with the particular medication, and understand how to observe for, and document, side effects experienced by your patient. Being familiar with the medication's classification will assist you in understanding its side effects.
- Understand the pharmacokinetics and pharmacodynamics of the medications.

As health care has evolved in the prehospital setting, the list of medications administered by paramedics has expanded in tandem. Keeping abreast of all the information is a challenge that you will face throughout your entire career. Do not hesitate to use references to refresh your memory. Having appropriate material readily available will prove beneficial, especially when you need to make important decisions.

Notes from Nancy

There are, in fact, tens of thousands of possible drug interactions, particularly in a society like ours, in which people take a lot of pills. The books on drug interactions are often the size of the London telephone directory, and no human brain could be expected to absorb all that information.

Try to obtain concise yet thorough information about the patient's medication use. It is essential to get an accurate list of the patient's current prescribed medications because this list may reveal clues about the patient's medical history. It is also necessary for deciding appropriate drug therapy so that you may avoid potentially dangerous drug interactions. Determine what, if any, GSL medications the patient may have taken. Find out whether the patient is taking any recreational drugs, vitamins, herbal remedies, or homeopathy. All of these substances can have significant interactions with the medications used in emergency settings—and they may even be the culprit causing the patient's current condition.

Finally, remember that the patient has the right to refuse treatment. Be sure to inform your patient fully about the care that you are giving, including any medications that may be administered and the potential effects and side effects that he or she may experience.

▌Pharmacology and the Nervous System

Medications administered as part of the care provided in the prehospital setting exert their effects largely by acting on the nervous system. For this reason, it is critical that you understand the functioning of the nervous system as it relates to pharmacology.

Anatomically, the nervous system is made up of the central nervous system (CNS; the brain and spinal cord) and various types of peripheral nerves. The two major types of peripheral nerves are the afferent nerves (Latin: *ad,* "to" + *ferre,* "to carry"), which carry sensory impulses from all parts of the body to the brain, and the efferent nerves (Latin: *e,* "from" + *ferre,* "to carry"), which carry messages from the brain to the muscles and all other organs of the body.

Functionally, the nervous system is divided into two primary components (Figure 7-3 ▶): the CNS and the peripheral nervous system (PNS).

Central Nervous System

The CNS functions as the control centre for all other nervous system functions. One can easily think of the CNS like the CPU (central processing unit) in a home computer. The CPU in a computer carries out all calculations, coordinating a wide array of incoming and outgoing information from the many cables and connections of the computer. The CNS receives input from many receptors throughout the body, interprets the stimulus received via these sensory neurons, and makes decisions and directs actions to be carried out at target sites and organs throughout the body. These messages are then sent back out to the body via motor neurons or effectors, which carry out the desired action in various muscles and glands throughout the body. Computers work in a similar manner—the CPU interprets data from the keyboard, mouse, disk drives, and so forth and makes decisions and produces output actions such as printing. The whole system is connected by cables that function like the efferent and afferent nerves, sending and receiving information back and forth between the various components.

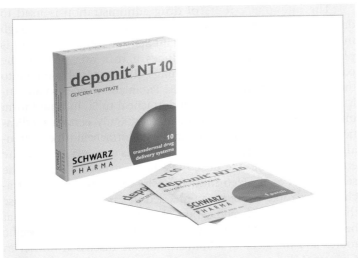

Figure 7-7 GTN patch.

- **Capsule.** A cylindrical gelatin container enclosing a dose of medication, for example, some antibiotics, such as amoxicillin
- **Tablet.** A powdered drug that has been moulded or compressed into a small disc, such as aspirin and glyceryl trinitrate (GTN) tablets
- **Suppository.** A drug mixed in a firm base that melts at body temperature and is shaped to fit the rectum; may be used for local action (for example, glycerin suppositories to promote evacuation of the rectum) or for systemic effect (for example, diazepam suppositories to treat convulsion disorders and status epilepticus in children). Diazepam is also available as a rectal solution given from a rectal tube.
- **Ointment.** A semisolid preparation for external application to the body, usually containing a medicinal substance, for example, neomycin ointment, a topical antibiotic
- **Patch.** A medication impregnated into a membrane or adhesive that is applied onto the surface of the skin, for example, GTN patch (Figure 7-7 ▲)

Gaseous Drug Forms

Medications may also come in the form of a vapour. Gaseous medications are primarily used in general anaesthesia. To create the gas, a medication in liquid form is placed into a machine that promotes vaporisation. The vapours are inhaled by the patient to induce anaesthesia. An example of a medication administered as a vapour is sevoflurane.

Overview of the Routes of Drug Administration

Rates of Drug Absorption

How you choose to administer a drug—that is, the mode of administration—affects the rate at which the body absorbs the drug and, ultimately, the onset of its therapeutic effects.

The action of a drug, especially the speed with which it works, is also influenced by the way it enters the body—that is, the route of administration. Obviously, drugs injected directly into the circulation, such as IV or intraosseous (IO) injections, enter the bloodstream the most rapidly. Nearly as fast is the absorption across the respiratory mucosa when drugs are breathed in from an inhaler. Other mucosal surfaces, such as those found in the rectum, provide for rapid absorption as well, albeit at an unpredictable rate. Intramuscular (IM) injection is slower because the drug must be picked up from the muscles by the circulating blood; the same is true of subcutaneous (SC) injections, which are absorbed more slowly than IM injections. Near the slowest end of the scale are drugs administered orally (PO). The slowest absorption of all is across intact skin. (Table 7-2 ▼) summarises the rates of absorption. Note that the route of administration that is appropriate for one drug may be unsuitable for another drug, so for any given drug it is essential to know the routes by which it may be given.

Local or Systemic Effects

Drugs may produce their effects locally, systemically, or both. Local effects result from the direct application of a drug to a tissue—for example, when you apply a lotion to the skin to relieve itching. Systemic effects occur after the drug is absorbed by any route and distributed by the bloodstream; they almost invariably involve more than one organ, although the response of one or another organ may predominate.

The action of a drug is rarely a completely fixed property of the medication. Instead, the effect of any given drug typically varies depending on the patient, the dose, the route by which the drug is given, and the drug's metabolic rate.

Table 7-2	Rates of Absorption by Different Routes
Route of Administration	**Time Until Drug Takes Effect***
Topical	Hours to days
Oral (PO)	30–90 min
Rectal (PR)	5–30 min (unpredictable)
SC injection	15–30 min
IM injection	10–20 min
Sublingual tablet	3–5 min
Sublingual injection	3 min
Inhalation	3 min
Endotracheal (ET)	Unknown; unpredictable
IO	60 s
IV	30–60 s
Intracardiac (IC)	15 s
*In a healthy person with normal perfusion.	

Routes of Drug Administration

The routes of administration are classified into three categories based on how the medication is absorbed and distributed: percutaneous, enteral, and parenteral. Medications given via the percutaneous routes are applied to and absorbed through the skin or mucous membranes. Enteral medications are administered and absorbed somewhere along the gastrointestinal tract, usually orally. Any route of administration that does not cause the drug to be absorbed through the skin, mucous membranes, or gastrointestinal tract is considered parenteral. The actual route of administration you select in the prehospital environment is dependent on the medication and the intended effect.

Percutaneous Routes

Percutaneous routes of medication administration are those for any medication that is absorbed through the skin or through a mucous membrane. Drugs may be applied topically—that is, on the surface of the body. Ordinarily, the intact skin is an effective barrier to absorption of drugs, but some drugs have been specially prepared to cross the barrier at a very slow rate, so the route is useful for sustained release of drugs for a long period. Thus, some patients take GTN in the form of a patch pasted onto the skin. Oestrogens (female hormones) are also sometimes given in the form of a patch.

Administration via the transdermal route is generally performed by placing medication directly onto the patient's skin. It is also easily controlled by simply removing and wiping the medication from the skin, which causes the effect to subside quickly. Although the rate of absorption is consistent, steady, and predictable, it can be affected by the thickness of the skin and the presence of scar tissue at the site of administration. It can also be affected by the amount of peripheral circulation. Conditions that decrease peripheral circulation, such as hypothermia and hypotension, will lead to a slower rate of absorption. In a febrile patient, the rate of absorption would be much quicker than anticipated.

At the Scene

Make absolutely certain you use gloves when administering any medication, particularly topical drugs. If the medication can be absorbed into the patient's skin, it can be absorbed into yours as well.

Administering medications through mucous membranes is becoming increasingly popular in the prehospital setting. This route allows for the medication to be absorbed at a moderate to rapid rate. Sublingual (SL) administration refers to giving a medication—GTN, for example—under the tongue. Drugs given sublingually are usually rapidly absorbed, with effects becoming apparent within a few minutes. The buccal route (between the cheeks and gums) may be used to give glucose gel to hypoglycaemic patients with diabetes.

The pulmonary route of drug administration is used to deliver medications directly to the pulmonary system through inhalation or injection. In the inhalation route, the drug is placed in a nebuliser that reduces it to a mist, which the patient then breathes in. In the lungs, the drug is absorbed into the bronchioles and alveolar sacs. Paramedics can also administer medications through an endotracheal tube, in liquid form into the bronchioles and alveolar sacs. Only certain medications are suitable to be given via the endotracheal tube. Adrenaline is an example. If medications are given via the endotracheal route, the dose must be increased to achieve the same effects as if given intravenously. Currently, the endotracheal tube route is not recommended in cardiac arrest because the effectiveness of medication absorption is questionable at best. The IV and IO routes are preferred in these cases. Specific routes and the steps of administration are discussed further in Chapter 8.

Enteral Routes

Medications that are given via one of the enteral routes are absorbed somewhere along the gastrointestinal tract. Most patients take their daily medications at home by the oral route (per os, or PO) because that route is painless, convenient, and economical. Drugs taken by mouth are absorbed at an unpredictable but generally slow rate from the stomach and intestines—usually somewhere between 30 and 90 minutes. Because absorption is slow and unpredictable, drugs are rarely given by the oral route in emergency situations. The one exception is aspirin for patients suspected of having acute coronary syndrome (ACS); its administration requires an adequate level of consciousness to prevent aspiration, however.

Drugs may be administered rectally for their local effect; they may also be given rectally because they are irritating if given orally or because the patient cannot take an oral medication (for example, if vomiting). In the prehospital setting, the rectal route can be considered if quick IV access is impractical. The extreme vascularity of the rectum promotes rapid but sometimes unpredictable absorption. Medications administered rectally (per rectum, or PR) generally do not pass through the liver and, therefore, are not subjected to hepatic alterations.

Parenteral Routes

Parenteral routes include those in which medications are administered via any route other than the alimentary canal (digestive tract), skin, and mucous membranes. They are generally administered via syringes and needles. In most cases, parenteral routes allow for the fastest absorption rate.

The IV route is the most rapidly effective—but also the most dangerous route of administration. Drugs given intravenously go directly into the bloodstream and to the target organs, without any appreciable delay in absorption. Thus, IV injection enables you to deliver a known quantity of drug over a known period; that is, it allows the most accurate control of dosage. It is a dangerous route, however, precisely because the entire dose of the drug is delivered in one blast, so a toxic reaction is much more likely. Absorption of an IV drug into the tissues usually takes about 30 to 60 seconds. The absorption rate will be slowed in heart failure (because of the longer circulation time). In cardiac arrest with CPR in progress, an IV drug will take 3 to 4 times longer than usual to reach its target organ because the cardiac output is only one third of the normal rate. As a consequence, it will take at least 1 or 2 minutes after giving an emergency drug during CPR to ensure that the drug has circulated adequately. Always prepare to administer a medication in cardiac arrest by drawing it up ahead of time. Administer drugs during compression cycles to enhance distribution whenever possible, and never interrupt compressions to administer a medication during cardiac arrest. In general, IV drugs should be given *slowly*, unless you receive contrary orders. In the prehospital environment, it is unacceptable to administer a medication by direct venepuncture because this technique may result in infiltration of the drug. Infiltration is the escape of fluid into the surrounding tissue, which causes a localised area of oedema, and is discussed in more detail in Chapter 8.

The intraosseous (IO) route is becoming increasingly popular in the prehospital setting. This route has long been used for paediatric patients, but with the advent of convenient devices for adult use, it is quickly becoming standard when quick IV access is not practical. Any medication that can be given intravenously can be given intraosseously. The rate of absorption and time of onset have been shown to be identical if not better because the medicine enters a noncollapsible channel with rapid flow into the central circulation.

Drugs given by the intramuscular (IM) route take longer to act than those given intravenously because they must first be absorbed from the muscle into the bloodstream. By the same token, IM medications have a longer duration of action than IV drugs because they are absorbed gradually during a period of minutes to hours. Obviously, absorption of medications given by the IM or SC route depends on adequate blood flow to muscles and peripheral tissues, which is not the case in shock or cardiac arrest. Therefore, IM injections should be given only to patients with adequate perfusion.

An IM injection usually involves volumes of about 1 to 5 ml and is usually given into the deltoid muscle of the upper arm or the antero-lateral aspect of the thigh (the preferred site for prehospital applications). (The technique for IM injection is described later in this chapter.) Should dyspnoea, dizziness, itching, oedema, urticaria, wheezing, or any other sign of an allergic reaction develop following an IM (or SC) injection in the arm, you should manage the patient as described in Chapter 30.

At the Scene

Do not give IM or SC injections to patients with impaired peripheral perfusion.

With the subcutaneous (SC) route, a small amount (usually less than 2 ml) of drug is injected into the fat or connective tissue beneath the skin. Medications administered by this route are absorbed more slowly and over a more prolonged period than when they are given intravenously; the peak drug effect usually occurs within about 30 minutes. These injections are usually given under the skin of the upper outer arm, anterior thigh, or abdomen.

You are the Paramedic Part 3

You perform a physical examination on the patient whilst your colleague prepares an IV-giving set. You document the following findings: positive JVD; crackles auscultated at the bases; slight swelling around the ankles; and a slow, irregular, weak pulse. You ask the patient to describe his vision problems. He explains that for the past 2 days his sight has been blurry and objects have had a yellow-green circle around them. He jokingly tells you that this blurriness interferes with him being able to complete the morning crossword puzzle and watch the soaps in the evenings.

Before leaving for hospital you perform a 12-lead ECG, which shows atrial fibrillation at a rate in the 40s with frequent PVCs. Recalling the information on cardiac medication from a recent in-service training session you know that both digoxin and diltiazem can lower the heart rate. You also know that the patient is symptomatic from the low heart rate and PVCs. Unsure of how to proceed with treatment, you decide to contact the A&E consultant for guidance.

Reassessment	Recording Time: 10 Minutes
Skin	Pale, cool, and moist
Pulse	42 beats/min, irregular; weak radial
ECG	Atrial fibrillation with a slow ventricular response and frequent PVCs
Blood pressure	78/44 mm Hg
Respirations	24 breaths/min, slight increase work of breathing
SpO₂	96% on nonrebreathing mask at 15 l/min of supplemental oxygen
Pupils	Equal and reactive to light

4. Does the patient present with signs and symptoms of possible drug toxicity? If so, which medications are in question?

5. What treatment will increase the patient's blood pressure?

Pharmacokinetics

Every medication has varying effects on the body. Pharmacokinetics is the study of the movement of a drug through the body, with particular emphasis on the time required for absorption, duration of action, distribution in the body, and method of excretion.

Absorption

Absorption of medications refers to the transfer of a medication from its site of administration to the general circulation and thus to specific target organs and tissues. The ultimate goal is for the medication to reach a therapeutic concentration in the bloodstream. Achieving this therapeutic concentration depends partially on the rate and extent to which the drug is absorbed. The rate and extent are, in turn, dependent on the ability of the medication to cross the cell membrane.

Mechanisms of Medication Absorption

A medication may cross the cell's membrane by one of two mechanisms: active transport or passive diffusion (discussed in Chapter 8). In active transport, specialised proteins that span the membrane of a cell facilitate the movement of the medication inside target tissues and cells. This energy-dependent process uses a carrier-mediated mechanism to assist the medication into the cell and can move the drug across the concentration gradient (from an area of lower concentration to an area of higher concentration). In contrast, passive diffusion of a medication does not use energy or carrier-mediated mechanisms. Instead, medications move from an area of high concentration to an area of low concentration. Lipid-soluble medications move easily across most cell membranes, as do water-soluble drugs via aqueous channels.

Blood Flow and Medication Absorption

A properly functioning circulatory system greatly enhances the rate of medication absorption. If the body area to which a medication is applied (for example, transdermal route) or injected (for example, IM route) has a good vascular system and a rich blood supply, the rate of absorption is enhanced. In contrast, areas of the body with poor blood supply or particular routes of administration (for example, SC route) may be associated with a delay in the rate of absorption. As mentioned earlier, medications administered via the IV route are immediately passed throughout the circulatory system, absorbed, and delivered to target tissues and organs. In patients in profound states of shock or circulatory compromise, absorption may be delayed with any of the administration methods.

Surface Areas and Medication Absorption

All medications must pass through nontarget cells to reach their intended receptor target; these nontarget cells may include the skin, mucosa, and intestinal tissue. The larger the surface area that is available to the medication as a "launching pad", the greater the amount of absorption and the more quickly the medication can reach its target and take effect.

Another factor affecting the absorption rate is the nature of the cells that the medication is trying to pass through. Single layers of cells, like the tissue of the intestines, readily transport medications. In contrast, multilayer tissues, like the skin, require more time for absorption.

Medication Concentration and Absorption

The concentration of the medication administered affects its absorption as well. Pharmaceutical manufacturers use this fact to their advantage—for example, by altering a medication's coating to tweak the ultimate rate of absorption. Medications that are administered in high doses are generally absorbed more quickly than medications that are administered at lower doses.

When medications are administered to a patient, they eventually become distributed throughout the entire body. Thus, the higher the concentration in the body, the greater the absorption. For this reason, giving very high concentrations or doses to speed absorption is not a good idea. Once a medication is administered, it will continue to circulate in the body and affect its target receptors until the drug is eliminated. Typically, when continued doses are required, two approaches to administration are used. First a loading dose— a large dose of the same concentration that temporarily exceeds the body's ability to eliminate the medication—is given to quickly reach a therapeutic level. It is followed by a maintenance dose—a smaller dose administered over time and intended to maintain a therapeutic level of the medication at the receptor site. Loading doses are typically based on the volume of distribution, which takes into account the patient's weight; maintenance doses are selected based on the body's ability to eliminate the medication.

Environmental pH and Medication Absorption

Most medications are weak acids or weak bases. Once in solution, they become ionised (electrically charged). Most medications reach a state of equilibrium between their ionised and nonionised forms, facilitating their absorption. The pH of a medication affects its ability to ionise. Medications that are weak acids are able to ionise much better in an alkaline environment, whereas medications that are weak bases are able to ionise more completely in an acidic environment.

Medications administered by any route inevitably undergo side reactions—that is, reactions with nontarget cells and tissues—before they reach their intended destination. A critical consideration for the effectiveness of any drug is how much of it is still active by the time it reaches its target organ. This property, called the drug's bioavailability, must be taken into account when selecting the dose to ensure that enough medication is being absorbed at the target organ to achieve the desired effect.

Distribution

Medication distribution is the process by which a medication moves throughout the body. Blood is the primary distribution vehicle. Factors that change the way blood flows through the body will change the way medications are transported to the target tissue. If the patient's overall cardiac output is diminished, the medication will not move as quickly. Along the same lines, if blood is not moving efficiently to a particular part of the body, the distribution may be slowed. For example, if the patient is cold, the blood is shunted away from the skin and peripheral extremities. In such a case, an antibiotic intended to fight an infection in the foot will not arrive at that area as quickly as intended.

The only way a medication molecule can actually be used by the body is if it is not bound with anything else—that is, it must be "free drug". Because of this, the extent to which the medication binds with nontarget cells affects its intensity and duration of action. Not all of the medication molecules are floating around the blood at the same time. Medications have a tendency to collect in certain areas of the body that act as storage sites. Typically, drugs will become bound to fat, muscle tissue, and bone, thereby limiting the amount of medication that is free in the bloodstream. In particular, lipid-soluble medications have a high affinity for adipose (fat) tissue. As a consequence, low blood flow may allow for their extended retention in the adipose tissue. Some medications have an unusual affinity for bone tissue. Molecules of these drugs will accumulate after the drug is absorbed onto the bone crystal surface.

In contrast, while roaming around the body in the bloodstream, the medication may become bound to plasma proteins. Such a drug-protein complex cannot be used by the body, so its formation lowers the therapeutic concentration of the drug. The amount of free drug is always proportional to the amount of bound drug. Thus, as the free drug is used and eliminated, the drug-protein complexes break down and release more free drug to replace what has been used.

In particular, molecules of a medication may become bound to the plasma protein known as albumin. Albumin, which is too large to diffuse out of the bloodstream, essentially kidnaps drug molecules, making them ineffective. Albumin is not in endless supply, however. Furthermore, other medications may be competing to bind to the same albumin. As such, the amount of free drug is influenced by the amount of available albumin. Some conditions may cause a decrease in the albumin levels, particularly those that involve decreased liver functions. Even if the albumin levels are normal, the amount of affinity for albumin that one medication has compared with another can affect free-drug levels (think of it like magnets and a metal screw for the albumin, with one magnet being stronger than the other).

Other aspects of the body may also prevent medication molecules from being distributed to certain tissue. The blood-brain barrier allows only lipid-soluble medications to enter the brain and cerebrospinal fluid. In a pregnant patient, the placental barrier consists of membrane layers separating blood vessels of the mother and the fetus. Much like the blood-brain barrier, the placental barrier does not permit most non–lipid-soluble medications to pass to the fetus. This is not an impregnable barrier, however; some non–lipid-soluble medications can cross the placental barrier, so you must understand which medications can be given to a pregnant patient and in which situations.

Biotransformation

The manner in which the body metabolises medications is referred to as biotransformation. It occurs in one of two ways: by transforming the medication into a metabolite or by making the medication more water soluble. Only medication molecules that are in a free-drug form are able to be biotransformed. Drug manufacturers use this fact to their advantage when creating medications, known as prodrugs, that become active only *after* they undergo biotransformation. Most of the biotransformation takes place in the liver. The endoplasmic reticulum of hepatocytes contains the enzymes primarily responsible for biotransformation.

The biotransformation of a medication directly affects the route chosen to deliver a medication. All blood that comes from the gastrointestinal tract must pass through the liver before moving on to the rest of the body. This gives the liver the opportunity to partially or completely inactivate drugs long before they reach the intended target tissue, a scenario known as the first-pass effect. Because of the first-pass effect, some medications can be given only parenterally. For example, insulin must always be given subcutaneously—never orally. The liver would completely inactivate insulin if it were to undergo the first-pass effect, making it useless. Even medications that are not completely inactivated by the first-pass effect sometimes require a higher dose when given orally to ensure that enough of the drug survives to have a therapeutic effect.

Liver enzymes can act on a drug in two ways, or phases. In phase 1, the enzymes may oxidise the drug or bind it with oxygen molecules. The enzymes may also hydrolyze the medication, decomposing it by a reaction with water. In either case, the medication becomes more soluble with water. In phase 2, the medication molecules combine with a chemical found in the body; this interaction is known as a conjugation reaction. Phase 1 and phase 2 allow the drug to move to the next stage, excretion.

Excretion

In excretion, the body eliminates the remnants of the drug, which could be toxic or inactive metabolites. (Remember that the liver may have inactivated at least some of the drug through biotransformation.) Excretion occurs primarily through the kidneys via three mechanisms:

- **Glomerular filtration.** A passive process in which blood flows through the glomeruli of the kidneys. These structures are bundles of capillaries within a capsule. A differential in pressure forces wastes away from the blood into the capsule where it is transported for excretion via the urine.
- **Tubular secretion.** An active transport process in which medications are bound to specific transporters aiding in their elimination.
- **Partial reabsorption.** This occurs when some amount of the drug is reabsorbed after being filtered.

The same factors that affect absorption can also affect excretion, particularly the environmental pH—in this case, the pH of the urine. In this case, if the medication is acidic in an alkaline urine, the medication will move more readily into the urine for excretion. Conversely, an alkaline medication in an acidic urine environment will also readily move to the urine. The closer the pH, the slower the medication will be excreted.

Pharmacodynamics

Pharmacodynamics is the way in which a medication produces the response we intended, also known as the mechanism of action. It also encompasses the factors that may alter the intended response and any side effects or unexpected effects.

Theories of Drug Action

Medications cause their action on the body by four mechanisms:

- They may bind to a receptor site.
- They may change the physical properties of cells— typically, by changing the osmotic balance.
- They may chemically combine with other chemicals (such as with the goal of turning the substance into a nonproblematic chemical).
- They may alter a normal metabolic pathway (such as by interrupting the normal growth process of cells).

Medications that bind to a receptor site are the most prevalent, particularly in the prehospital setting. Receptor sites are specialised proteins on a cell that receive chemical mediator messages to stimulate a particular response. For example, when ACh attaches to receptor sites in the heart, it causes the heart rate to slow. Cellular responses can be wide ranging depending on the chemical mediator and the cells being stimulated. A medication molecule will have one of two effects when it attaches to a receptor site: It may stimulate the receptor site to cause the response it normally does (agonist), or it may block the receptor site from being stimulated by other chemical mediators and inhibit the normal response (antagonist). Some medications can also act as agonist-antagonists, or partial agonists, by performing both roles. In any event, the medication molecule must compete with the naturally occurring chemical mediator. To win this battle, the medication molecule must have a higher affinity for the receptor than the chemical mediator does. In addition, more than one medication may compete for the same receptor.

Once the medication is bound to the receptor site, it initiates a chemical change that produces the expected effect. In some cases, this chemical change *is* the intended effect. In other cases, the initial chemical change releases a second compound (known as a second messenger) that actually causes the intended effect. Cyclic adenosine monophosphate (cAMP) is the most common second-messenger chemical related to pharmacology. Once cAMP enters the cell, it triggers the release of other enzymes, which then carry out their own functions.

The number of available receptors is inconsistent and can be affected by the actual number of sites present, the number already occupied by another chemical mediator, and the number occupied by another medication. As medication molecules bind to the receptor sites, the number of receptors decreases, a process known as down-regulation. However, some medications can actually increase the number of available receptor sites, a process known as up-regulation.

Drug-Response Relationship

Once the medication finds the target tissue, it needs to accumulate to a sufficient concentration to produce its desired effect. The drug-response relationship correlates the amount of medication given and the response it causes. Most of this information comes from the plasma-level profiles, which describe the length of onset, duration, and termination of action. They also allow pharmacologists to determine the minimum level of medications to be effective and how much it would take to become toxic to the patient. When administering a medication, we need to know how long it will take for the concentration of the medication at the target tissue to reach the minimum effective level—that is, the onset of action. We also need to know how long the medication can be expected to remain above that minimum level to provide the intended action—that is, the duration of action. The termination of action is the amount of time after the concentration level falls below the minimum level to the time it is eliminated from the body. All of these factors affect the therapeutic index—the ratio of a drug's lethal dose for 50% of the population (LD_{50}) to its effective dose for 50% of the population (ED_{50}). In other words, the therapeutic index gives an indication of a medication's margin of safety. The plasma profile also provides information about the medication's biological half-life—that is, the time it takes the body to eliminate half of the drug.

Factors Affecting Drug Responses

A chief variable affecting the action of a drug is patient characteristics. Patients differ from one another in several ways with respect to how they react to medications:

- **Age.** Patients of different ages may have very different responses to the same drug. Older people, for example, tend to be much more sensitive to the effects of drugs and often require smaller doses than younger patients. It is not, however, solely a matter of dose. Some drugs actually have different effects altogether in different age groups. Barbiturates, for example, act as sedatives in most adults, but in older patients, they may produce excitement or agitation.
- **Weight.** Many drugs are formulated for an average adult, usually considered to be a 70-kg person. Clearly, however, the ultimate concentration in the body of a given dose of a drug will be quite different if the same drug is taken by a 48-kg person and a 136-kg person. To correct for differences in weight between patients, when specifying drug doses for prehospital care, we usually give the dose in milligrams of the drug per kilogram of the patient's body weight (mg/kg).

Depression is a common disorder for which many treatments are available. In particular, it is often treated with selective serotonin reuptake inhibitors (SSRIs) and monoamine oxidase inhibitors (MAOIs), which block the metabolism of monoamines in the brain. Tricyclic antidepressants (TCAs) are also used as antidepressants. The TCAs have powerful inhibitory effects:

- They block the neurotransmitters noradrenaline and serotonin from being reabsorbed in the brain.
- They block ACh from reaching its receptors, which may lead to tachycardia.
- They block alpha-1 receptors, which may produce postural hypotension.

Drugs for Specific CNS and PNS Dysfunctions

The central nervous system (CNS) agents are a class of drugs that produce physiological and psychological effects through a variety of mechanisms. These agents can be divided into two groups: specific agents, which bring about an identifiable mechanism with unique receptors for the agent, and nonspecific agents, which produce effects on different cells through a variety of mechanisms. The nonspecific agents are generally classified by the focus of action or specific therapeutic use, for example, anti-obesity agents.

Another common group of CNS agents is stimulants, which exert their action by excitation of the CNS. Some of the specific drugs included in this group are caffeine, cocaine, and various amphetamines. All of these drugs are used to enhance alertness and reduce drowsiness and fatigue. However, high doses of these agents can cause increased nervousness, irritability, tremors, and headache. Some people may also experience withdrawal symptoms when they stop taking stimulants.

In other cases, patients may be prescribed CNS depressants. These agents are used to slow brain activity. They may be prescribed to treat anxiety, muscle tension, pain, insomnia, stress, panic attacks, and, in some cases, convulsions. Some other CNS depressants are used as anaesthetics. Examples of CNS depressants include lorazepam (Ativan), and diazepam (Valium).

Drugs Affecting the Parasympathetic Nervous System

Stimulation of the parasympathetic nervous system produces myriad effects. For example, it causes the pupils to constrict and produces bronchoconstriction. It has cardiac effects, too—it causes the heart to slow and reduces its contractile force. In the digestive system, increased activity of the parasympathetic nervous system stimulates secretions from digestive glands and enhances the activity of the smooth muscles found along the digestive tract.

Cholinergic Medications

All preganglionic and postganglionic parasympathetic nerves use ACh as the neurotransmitter. Acetylcholine, which has a short life span, is deactivated by AChE. Two types of ACh receptors, collectively known as cholinergic receptors, are found in the parasympathetic system: nicotinic receptors and muscarinic receptors. The nicotinic receptors are found in all autonomic ganglia and at the neuromuscular junctions. The muscarinic receptors, which are widespread throughout the body, enable the parasympathetic nervous system to respond to stimulation. Cholinergic medications (also known as parasympathomimetics) stimulate the cholinergic receptors. Anticholinergic medications (also known as parasympatholytics) block the cholinergic receptors.

Cholinergic medications may act directly or indirectly on cholinergic receptors. A drug that has direct action binds with these receptors, thereby blocking ACh from exerting its effects. A drug that has indirect action interacts with AChE, thereby allowing ACh to avoid deactivation. If excessive cholinergics are present, the patient may exhibit the SLUDGE phenomena: increased Salivation/sweating, Lacrimation, Urination, Defecation/drooling/diarrhoea, Gastric upset/cramps, and Emesis. Patients exposed to certain fertilisers, insecticides, VX (a nerve agent), and sarin gas exhibit SLUDGE symptoms because all of these substances have cholinergic properties. Weapons of mass destruction are covered in Chapter 48.

Anticholinergic Medications

Anticholinergic medications work in opposition to the parasympathetic nervous system by blocking the muscarinic and nicotinic receptors:

- **Muscarinic cholinergic antagonists** block ACh exclusively at the muscarinic receptors. Atropine, for example, is a muscarinic cholinergic antagonist; it decreases secretions, increases heart rate, dilates the pupils, and decreases gastrointestinal system activity.
- **Nicotinic cholinergic antagonists** block ACh exclusively at the nicotinic receptors. This inhibition effectively disables the ANS, so it is virtually never used.

Neuromuscular blocking agents affect the parasympathetic nervous system by inducing paralysis. Two classes of paralytics are used to induce paralysis in the prehospital setting: depolarising neuromuscular blocking agents and nondepolarising neuromuscular blocking agents. All neuromuscular blocking agents bind to the parasympathetic neurotransmitter receptor site for ACh at the neuromuscular junction. Depolarising medications stimulate depolarisation of the muscle cells, which manifests as fasciculations (muscle twitches). The medication then produces continuous stimulation of the muscle cell, which does not allow it to return to its resting (repolarised) state. In contrast, nondepolarising agents bind in a competitive but nonstimulatory manner to part of the ACh receptor. As a result, these drugs do not cause fasciculations. The lack of fasciculations, coupled with the availability of reversal agents, might suggest that nondepolarising neuromuscular blocking agents would be preferred over depolarising agents. In reality, nondepolarising agents tend to have a long onset and duration of action, which significantly reduces their desirability in prehospital care.

Suxamethonium is a depolarising neuromuscular blocking agent that is the paralytic of choice for prehospital airway management. Despite its promotion of depolarisation, it is favoured because of its rapid onset of action (less than 45 seconds) and its short duration of action (4 to 5 minutes).

Some newer versions of nondepolarising neuromuscular blocking agents offer shorter onset times relative to suxamethonium, but little progress has been made in shortening their duration of action. The extended duration of action is a problem because if an endotracheal intubation attempt is unsuccessful, the patient is left without spontaneous respiration for more than 30 minutes. Vecuronium is a newer nondepolarising neuromuscular blocker that produces paralysis in as little as 30 seconds but has an intermediate duration of action of approximately 30 minutes.

Rocuronium works similarly to vecuronium. It also has a fairly rapid onset of 45 seconds, but its duration of action can be as long as 45 minutes. Rocuronium may be substituted for succinylcholine if the extended recovery time is acceptable, such as following successful endotracheal intubation.

Pancuronium is another neuromuscular blocking agent that may be used in the prehospital setting. It is important to keep in mind that acceptable conditions for endotracheal intubation generally take 90 to 120 seconds after administration of the drug, and ventilation and oxygenation must be ensured during the interval. In addition, the paralysis can last anywhere from 45 to 90 minutes. Some consider this unfavourable in situations calling for paralysing the patient for airway management, which are time critical situations. The 90-plus-second onset time, especially compared with other shorter acting paralytics, does not make this drug the best choice. Furthermore, the duration of 45 to 90 minutes means that if the intubation attempt were unsuccessful, we would have a completely paralysed patient for upwards of an hour without appropriate means of ventilation.

Drugs Affecting the Sympathetic Nervous System

Medications may be given to a patient in an effort to stimulate the sympathetic nervous system (sympathomimetics) or inhibit the sympathetic nervous system (sympatholytics). These medications can be selective or nonselective in terms of the receptors they affect.

Sympathomimetics stimulate the adrenal medulla so that it releases noradrenaline and adrenaline, the major neurotransmitters in the sympathetic nervous system. Noradrenaline and adrenaline, in turn, stimulate one of two types of sympathetic receptors: dopaminergic receptors and adrenergic receptors.

Stimulation of dopaminergic receptors produces dilation of the renal, coronary, and cerebral arteries. As yet, no medications have been marketed that specifically target these receptors.

Four types of adrenergic receptors are distinguished, based on their effects when stimulated:

- **Alpha-1 receptors.** Produce peripheral vasoconstriction, are associated with mild bronchoconstriction, and releases energy stores from the liver

- **Alpha-2 receptors.** Inhibits noradrenaline and ACh release, promotes platelet aggregation, contracts vascular smooth muscle, and inhibits insulin release
- **Beta-1 receptors.** Increase the heart rate, cause cardiac muscle to contract, produce automaticity, and trigger cardiac electrical conduction
- **Beta-2 receptors.** Stimulate vasodilation and bronchodilation

A medication that agonises (stimulates) the alpha-1 receptors increases blood pressure by increasing cardiac preload and afterload. When these receptors are antagonised (suppressed), the blood pressure is lowered by preventing vasoconstriction. This tends to cause feedback responses as the body attempts to compensate for the decreased blood pressure. Most notably, the heart rate increases and the body attempts to increase blood volume by reabsorbing sodium and water in the kidneys.

In the prehospital setting, we often agonise the beta-1 receptors in an attempt to treat cardiac arrest and hypotension. Stimulation of these receptors increases myocardial contractility (also known as inotropic). In contrast, antagonising the beta-1 receptors lowers the blood pressure by limiting the myocardial contractility and the heart rate (chronotropic). It also decreases impulse generation in the heart and slows the conduction at the atrioventricular node, thereby treating tachycardia.

Stimulation of the beta-2 receptors allows us to treat asthma and other diseases that cause excessive narrowing of the bronchioles. Keep in mind that when using beta-2 agonists, the patient may exhibit some beta-1 effects as well. Beta-2 antagonism serves no clinical purpose; there are no circumstances in which we want to reduce the amount of air getting to the lungs via bronchoconstriction.

Skeletal Muscle Relaxants

Overstimulation of the nicotinic cholinergic transmission process can cause skeletal muscle spasms, which are very uncomfortable at best and painful at worst. Three types of skeletal muscle relaxants may provide relief: central acting, direct acting, and neuromuscular blocking. Central-acting medications work by producing CNS depression in the brain. Direct-acting medications target the muscles themselves to produce relaxation. Neuromuscular blockers produce complete paralysis.

Drugs Affecting the Cardiovascular System

The walls of the heart are composed of many interconnected cells. These cells are specialised to serve particular functions: Some conduct electrical impulses; others cause the heart to contract. Medications targeting the cardiovascular system are classified according to their effects on these specialised cells.

Medications that affect the heart rate are said to have a chronotropic effect. Inotropic effects are changes in the force of contraction. When a drug alters the velocity of the conduction of electricity through the heart, it is said to have a dromotropic effect. All three types of effects can be positive or negative. In other words, if there is a positive chronotropic effect, the heart rate has increased. If there is a negative inotropic effect, the heart is not squeezing as forcefully.

Cardiac glycosides are a class of medications that are derived from plants. These drugs block certain ionic pumps in the heart cells' membranes, which indirectly increases calcium concentrations. Digoxin, for example, may have positive inotropic effects or a combination of modest negative chronotropic and more dramatic negative dromotropic effects. Cardiac glycosides in general have a small therapeutic index (margin of safety), however, and are associated with numerous side effects.

Anti-arrhythmic medications have long been used in the prehospital setting to treat and prevent cardiac rhythm disorders. These medications can have direct and indirect effects on cardiac tissue. Anti-arrythmics are further classified into four groups according to their fundamental mode of action on the heart:

- **Sodium channel blockers** slow the conduction through the heart; in other words, they have a negative dromotropic effect.
- **Beta blockers** reduce the adrenergic stimulation of the beta receptors.
- **Potassium channel blockers** increase the heart's contractility (positive inotropic effect) and work against the reentry of blocked impulses.
- **Calcium channel blockers** block the inflow of calcium into the cardiac cells, thereby decreasing the force of contraction and automaticity. They may also decrease the conduction velocity (negative dromotropic effect).

Anti-hypertensive Medications

As many as 16 million people in the UK have hypertension or prehypertension. Medications administered to treat hypertension, known as anti-hypertensives, have the following treatment goals: keep blood pressure within normal limits, maintain or improve blood flow, and reduce the stress placed on the heart. Because these drugs are often administered for many years (even on a lifelong basis), the agent selected for a particular patient should not produce tolerance or have unbearable side effects.

Diuretic medications cause the kidneys to remove excess amounts of salt and water in the body. By lowering the total fluid volume, they reduce the level of stress placed on the cardiovascular system. In particular, they lower the preload on the heart and decrease the stroke volume. Thiazides, a type of diuretic medication often given with other anti-hypertensive medications, control the sodium and water quantities excreted by the kidneys and have some vasodilatory action. Loop diuretics lower the concentration of sodium and calcium ions in the body; unfortunately, their use may also lead to excessively low levels of potassium.

Vasodilator medications act on the smooth muscles of the arterioles and veins. This property explains why GTN, a vasodilator, is so beneficial in treating myocardial ischaemia. Unfortunately, the dilation of these vessels prompts a response from the sympathetic nervous system. As a consequence, when vasodilators are used to lower blood pressure, the patient must also take medications that inhibit the sympathetic nervous system.

Sympathetic blocking agents include beta blockers and adrenergic inhibitors. Beta blockers compete with adrenaline to bind with available receptor sites, thereby diminishing the effects of beta stimulation. The exact mechanism of action of adrenergic inhibitors has not been clearly elucidated but, like beta blockers, these medications decrease cardiac output and diminish the production of renin. Renin is one component of the renin-angiotensin-aldosterone system, which partially controls blood pressure.

Angiotensin-converting enzyme (ACE) inhibitors also target the renin-angiotensin-aldosterone system. ACE inhibitors suppress the conversion of angiotensin I to angiotensin II.

In contrast, angiotensin II receptor antagonists block angiotensin II from binding to its receptor sites. These drugs have been used to treat congestive heart failure and vascular diseases.

Calcium channel blockers have anti-arrhythmic and anti-hypertensive properties. By causing the dilation of coronary arteries, they enable more oxygen to reach the heart via coronary artery dilation. In addition, they prevent the contraction of smooth vascular muscle, which reduces resistance in the peripheral vascular system.

Anti-coagulants, Fibrinolytics, and Blood Components

Platelets play an important role in haemostasis and the repair of damaged blood vessels. This function is critical because defects in blood vessels can cause blood flow to slow, sometimes enough to result in the formation of a blood clot (also known as a thrombus). Abnormal thrombi may cause a life-threatening crisis such as ACS or stroke. A variety of medications are used to prevent or minimise the detrimental effects of thrombi.

Anti-platelet agents interfere with the aggregation, or collection, of platelets. They do not break down aggregated platelets but simply prevent further buildup of these blood cells. Aspirin has significant anti-platelet properties and has proved important in the prehospital setting thanks to its ability to minimise the damage to the myocardium in ACS.

Anti-coagulant drugs, as their name suggests, work against coagulation, thereby preventing thrombi from forming. Some patients can be prescribed anti-coagulants on a long-term basis as a preventive measure, thereby avoiding the formation of thrombi associated with surgeries and certain cardiovascular conditions. You need to be aware of anti-coagulant use, particularly when patients are involved in some sort of traumatic injury. Just as anti-coagulants prevent blood coagulation in the vascular system, they can also prevent the lifesaving coagulation needed to prevent blood loss.

Once a blood clot has formed, a fibrinolytic agent may be administered to dissolve the thrombus and prevent it from breaking off and entering the bloodstream, where it might do further damage. Fibrinolytic agents actually promote the digestion of fibrin. These drugs have shown to reduce mortality when administered by paramedics for acute myocardial infarction, although percutaneous coronary intervention (PCI) is now the treatment of choice. However, not all hospitals are able to offer this in the time frame required and you should follow local guidelines when choosing between treatments.

Anti-hyperlipidaemic Medications

Research has shown that treating raised cholesterol levels can reduce the incidence of coronary heart disease. Several types of medications are available to control cholesterol levels. HMG (3-hydroxy-3-methylglutaryl) coenzyme A reductase inhibitors—commonly referred to as statins—are especially popular choices. These medications disrupt the cholesterol production pathway in the body.

Mucokinetic and Bronchodilator Drugs

Serious respiratory emergencies often arise from severe narrowing of any portion of the respiratory tract. The respiratory tract is lined by smooth muscle fibres that influence the diameter of the airway. Control of the smooth muscles is maintained by the ANS. The parasympathetic nervous system stimulates the airway to constrict, whereas the sympathetic nervous system causes the airway diameter to dilate. Sympathetic stimulation is a result of adrenaline stimulation of the beta-2 receptors.

Many respiratory emergency treatments attempt to expand the respiratory tract by using sympathomimetic medications. These medications are classified according to their effects on the receptors. Some medications are nonselective: They affect alpha, beta-1, and beta-2 receptors alike. Stimulation of alpha receptors reduces vasoconstriction, which in turn reduces mucosal oedema. Stimulation of beta-1 receptors increases the patient's heart rate and the force of myocardial contraction. Most beneficial to patients with respiratory issues, stimulation of the beta-2 receptors produces bronchodilation and vasodilation.

Complications arise when patients with respiratory emergencies eventually experience decreased amounts of oxygen to the vital organs, including the heart. As nonselective sympathomimetics begin exerting their effects, the increased heart rate and greater force of contraction lead to a higher demand for oxygen—but, of course, oxygen is already in short supply in a respiratory emergency. For this reason, it is preferable to treat respiratory emergencies with medications specific to beta-2 receptors. Such drugs produce smaller increases in heart rate and force of contraction and, thereby, dramatically decreases the body's rate of oxygen consumption.

A second-line treatment in a respiratory emergency is the class of drugs known as xanthines. These drugs relieve airway constriction by relaxing the smooth muscles of the bronchioles and stimulating cardiac muscles to work harder, thereby increasing blood flow. They also stimulate the CNS—in fact, one notable xanthine is the well-known CNS stimulant, caffeine.

Other respiratory medications suppress the inflammatory response that typically causes acute distress for patients with restrictive airway diseases. In the acute care setting, steroids.

Oxygen and Miscellaneous Respiratory Drugs

Oxygen is the most commonly used medication in the prehospital setting. And it is, in fact, a medication—which means it has appropriate and inappropriate uses and some side effects. Supplementary oxygen therapy is covered in depth in Chapter 11.

Patients may be taking a range of medications to treat respiratory problems, depending on their symptoms. Especially during the cold and influenza seasons, use of GSL decongestant medications is common. Try to find out what medications your patient is taking, and know the effects that these drugs may have on other medications and the signs and symptoms they can produce. Although each decongestant varies slightly in terms of its mechanism of action, all such medications seek to reduce tissue oedema, facilitate drainage, and maintain the patency of the sinuses.

Unfortunately, the fact that these and other medications are readily available sometimes leads to their illicit use. People looking for a high have been known to overdose on decongestants—particularly dextromethorphan, and pseudoephedrine.

Drugs Affecting the Gastrointestinal System

Several classes of medications that target the gastrointestinal system are available; the exact choice of drug depends on the specific complaint. Patients experiencing nausea and vomiting may be treated in the prehospital setting with antiemetic medications such as metoclopramide. **Table 7-3 ▶** lists other gastrointestinal agents.

Eye Medications

Ophthalmic (eye) medications are virtually always administered in the form of drops directly to the eye. The exact treatment depends on the patient's particular condition but often includes anti-infective agents and drugs intended to reduce swelling (such as NSAIDs and steroids). Ophthalmic administration of medications in the prehospital setting is generally limited to anaesthetic purposes to relieve isolated irritation or to ease flushing of the eye.

Patients may be prescribed anti-glaucoma drugs that are used to treat glaucoma, an eye disease characterised by abnormally high intraocular fluid pressure, damaged optic disc, hardening of the eyeball, and partial to complete loss of vision. Common examples include dorzolamide, pilocarpine, and timolol (a beta-adrenergic antagonist). All of these agents are prepared as eye drops or ointments. Other agents include mydriatic and cycloplegic agents. Mydriatic agents are used to dilate the pupils, and cycloplegics are used in the treatment and evaluation of eye problems and include tropicamide, cyclopentolate, and topical atropine. Several medications used by paramedics are cautioned in the presence of glaucoma, so having an idea of which medications the patient may be taking for this condition will assist you in making appropriate decisions about your patient's care.

Ear Medications

In the same way as ophthalmic medications, medications affecting the ear (otic) are generally administered in the form of drops directly to the ear. The exception occurs in the rare case of a significant infection of the ear, which may require systemic anti-microbial medications. Most otic medications have anti-infective and anti-inflammatory effects. Prehospital administration of otic medications is not indicated.

Table 7-3	Gastrointestinal Agents
Agent(s)	Action
Antacids	Neutralise stomach acid, used to relieve acid indigestion, upset stomach, "sour stomach", and heartburn; typically are GSL preparations, for example, milk of magnesia
Anti-flatulents	Prevent or are used to treat excessive gas in the intestinal tract.
Digestants	Used to aid in or stimulate the digestive process.
Anti-emetics	Prevent or arrest vomiting, examples include prochlorperazine metoclopramide, and ondansetron
Cannabinoids	Provide relief to people whose chemotherapy drug causes *minimal* nausea and vomiting; believed to work in an area of the brain thought to be partly responsible for causing nausea and vomiting; mild drowsiness, dizziness, and euphoria are common side effects
Cytoprotective agents	Predominantly used to treat peptic ulcer disease; provide protection to the lining of the stomach and the duodenum to allow ulcers to heal
H_2-receptor antagonists	Reduce acid production in the stomach; act by blocking acid-producing cells in the stomach, examples include ranitidine and omeprazole
Laxatives	Stimulate loosening, relaxation, or evacuation of the bowels; sometimes abused by patients with eating disorders and can lead to profound dehydration if taken improperly; often used for in-hospital management of ACS patients to avoid vagal stimulation during bowel movements
Anti-diarrhoeals	Used to prevent or treat diarrhoea and frequently found as GSL preparations

Drugs Affecting the Pituitary Gland

Although not used in the prehospital setting, medications are available to treat pituitary disorders. These drugs may be administered to shrink or eradicate pituitary tumours. They can also block the pituitary gland from making too much hormone.

Drugs Affecting the Parathyroid and Thyroid Glands

Thyroid disorders are a fairly common finding in patients treated by paramedics. Medications either suppress the activity of the thyroid (used in hyperthyroidism) or replace missing thyroid hormones (used in hypothyroidism). Levothyroxine is a popular medication used to replace the hormones missing in hypothyroidism.

Drugs Affecting the Adrenal Cortex

Most of the treatment for disorders of the adrenal cortex involves the use of corticosteroids. Corticosteroids have anti-inflammatory properties and can have profound metabolic effects.

Drugs Affecting the Pancreas

A variety of medications are available to affect the pancreas. Still others may not act on the pancreas directly, but rather alter the way insulin (produced by the pancreas) is utilised by the body.

To affect the pancreas directly, sulphonylureas increase insulin secretion from the pancreatic beta cells. This medication is effective only if patients have residual beta cell function. Insulin sensitivity is increased by thiazolidinediones and biguanides, which are oral hypoglycaemic agents.

Drugs for Labour and Delivery

The use of medications for women in labour is generally limited to situations in which the delivery is abnormal or complicated, which is relatively rare. Of course, if the labour were normal, you probably would not be there. The medications administered in this situation have one of two effects: precipitating labour or inhibiting labour. Oxytocin is a naturally occurring hormone that has multiple reproductive functions. Boosting the levels of oxytocin increases the force and frequency of contractions. This drug is also used to reduce postpartum haemorrhage.

If labour begins before the baby is fully developed or if the labour is causing danger to the mother or baby, medications with tocolytic properties can be used. Tocolytic medications suppress the force and frequency of uterine contractions. Ritodrine, a selective beta-2 adrenergic stimulant, is used to inhibit or prevent pre-term labour. Salbutamol, from a metered-dose inhaler, is also used to promote uterine relaxation in awake patients. Magnesium sulphate also relaxes the smooth muscles, including those located in the uterus.

Drugs Affecting the Reproductive System
Medications and the Male Reproductive System

With the exception of antibiotics and antivirals for specific infections, a majority of the medications prescribed to affect the male reproductive system are intended to treat erectile dysfunction. Although you will not need to be involved in the treatment of erectile dysfunction, you need to be aware of whether the patient is being treated because of the complications that can arise in prehospital care. Phosphodiesterase inhibitors—for example, sildenafil (Viagra), is commonly prescribed to relax the smooth muscles of the corpora cavernosa and induce vasodilation. Using other vasodilatory medications, particularly GTN, within 24 to 48 hours of having taken a phosphodiesterase inhibitor can have serious implications for the patient's blood pressure. Always ask patients if they have used erectile dysfunction medications before administering GTN to avoid profound hypotension

Figure 7-8 ▶.

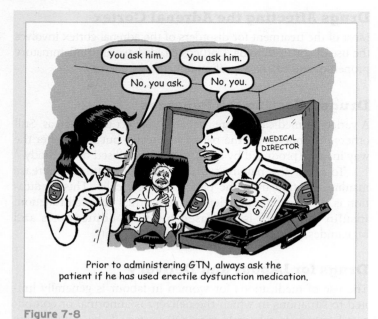

Prior to administering GTN, always ask the patient if he has used erectile dysfunction medication.

Figure 7-8

Medications and the Female Reproductive System

Female reproductive medications perform a variety of functions, from contraception to promoting conception. Most of the medications carry out their functions by altering the reproductive hormones. Contraceptive medications contain synthetic hormones that trick the body into believing the ovary has already released an ovum, which in turn prevents an ovum from being released for fertilisation. Antibiotics and anti-fungal medications may be used for specific conditions. Involvement of paramedics in administering medications affecting the female reproductive system is not indicated.

Anti-neoplastic Drugs

Anti-neoplastic medications are designed to combat cancer. Most chemotherapy medications are anti-neoplastic drugs that work by targeting the DNA within the cancerous cells. As yet, these medications do not have the ability to single out cancerous cells, so their systemic side effects are typically significant. As paramedics, we are called to care for cancer patients from time to time; an understanding of their condition and treatments will assist you in treating them effectively.

Drugs Used in Infectious Diseases and Inflammation

Drugs Used to Treat HIV Infection

The MHRA has approved a number of drugs for treating HIV infection. The first group of drugs used to treat HIV infection, called nucleoside reverse transcriptase inhibitors, interrupts the virus during an early stage of replication (that is, when the virus is making copies of itself). These drugs may slow the spread of HIV in the body and delay the acquisition of opportunistic infections. This class of drugs is also referred to as nucleoside analogues.

A second class of drugs for treating HIV infection, called protease inhibitors, interrupts the virus during replication at a later step in its life cycle.

Another class of drugs are fusion inhibitors, such as enfuvirtide, that prevent the HIV-1 virus from entering immune cells by blocking the merger of the virus with the cell membranes. This drug is designed for use in combination with other anti-HIV treatment. It reduces the level of HIV infection in the blood and may be active against HIV that has become resistant to current antiviral treatment schedules.

You are the Paramedic Part 4

You monitor the patient's vital signs closely. Upon safe transfer of the patient at the hospital the doctor explains that the patient is probably experiencing the effects of digitalis and calcium channel blocker toxicity.

Reassessment	Recording Time: 15 Minutes
Skin	Pink, warm, and dry
Pulse	74 beats/min, irregular; strong radial
ECG	Atrial fibrillation
Blood pressure	118/84 mm Hg
Respirations	22 breaths/min
SpO2	98% on nonrebreathing mask at 15 l/min of supplemental oxygen
Pupils	Equal and reactive to light

6. What does it mean when a medication has a low therapeutic index?

7. What occurs when one drug potentiates a second drug?

Antibiotics

Antibiotic medications are actually a subclassification of anti-microbial medications. Antibiotics are themselves classified into several categories based on their composition and the types of bacteria they target. Not all antibiotics affect all types of infections. Antibiotics generally work by killing the bacteria (bactericidal) or by preventing multiplication of the bacteria and thereby allowing the body's immune system to overcome the infectious invaders. Many patients are allergic to certain antibiotics.

Anti-fungal, Antiviral, and Anti-parasitic Medications

Treating fungal infections in humans, particularly systemic infections, can be much more difficult than treating bacterial or viral infections. The basic cellular structure is nearly identical between humans and fungi. Because anti-microbial medications target a specific structure within the infective organism, it is a challenge to identify a medication that will not harm human cells as well. One difference between human and fungal cells is that fungal cells use ergosterol instead of cholesterol as part of the cellular wall. Polyene medications cause the fungal cells' contents to leak out, causing them to die. Two other classes of anti-fungal medications, the imidazoles and the triazoles, work by inhibiting certain enzymes, thereby blocking fungal cell wall synthesis.

Antiviral medications work by a variety of mechanisms. Some antiviral medications inhibit the replication of RNA and DNA in the virus. Others inhibit the penetration and uncoating of the virus in the host cell. Still others can act as prodrugs, boosting the effectiveness of other antiviral medications given concurrently.

Anti-parasitic medications target parasites (organisms that live in or on the living tissue of a host organism at the expense of that host). **Table 7-4 ▸** lists types of anti-fungal, antiviral, and anti-parasitic agents.

Nonsteroidal Anti-inflammatory Drugs

The NSAIDs are designed to reduce pain, inflammation, and fever. They work by inhibiting Cyclo-oxygenase (COX) enzymes, which produce the chemical prostaglandin; prostaglandin, in turn, promotes pain, inflammation, and fever. There are two COX enzymes, known as COX-1 and COX-2. Some NSAIDs can be nonselective or semiselective in targeting only the COX-2 enzymes. It has been shown that COX-2 medications are associated with a lower incidence of bleeding and ulcers, but may result in an increased risk of myocardial infarction in certain at-risk patients.

Aspirin differs slightly from other NSAIDs in that it targets the COX-1 enzymes to reduce platelet aggregation, which provides great benefit in patients who are suspected of having a myocardial infarction. This selectivity also explains why you cannot substitute another NSAID such as ibuprofen, which targets COX-2 to a much greater extent, for aspirin in this situation.

Uricosuric Drugs

Uric acid is found in the blood and is excreted by the kidneys. If uric acid levels are too high, this chemical can be deposited in the form of solid crystals in the joints—a condition known as gout. Uricosuric medications are designed to lower the uric acid levels in the blood by increasing its excretion by the kidneys into the urine.

Serums, Vaccines, and Other Immunising Agents

Serums, vaccines, and other immunising agents all fall into the immunobiological medications category. Immunisations can consist of antigens (vaccines, toxoids) or antibodies (immune globulins, antitoxins). A toxoid is a modified bacterial toxin that has been made nontoxic but retains the ability to stimulate the formation of antibodies. A vaccine, a suspension of whole (live or inactivated) or fractionated bacteria or viruses that have been made nonpathogenic, is given to induce an immune response and prevent disease.

Drugs Affecting the Immunological System

Patients who undergo organ transplantation or have an autoimmune disease are often prescribed immunosuppressant medications. Immunosuppressants are intended to inhibit the body's ability to attack the "foreign" organ or, in the case of autoimmune diseases, the medications inhibit the body's attack on itself. These drugs are generally derived from fungi or bacteria and tend to have a complicated mechanism of action. Put succinctly, they inhibit lymphocytes and T cells from carrying out their immune functions.

Table 7-4	Anti-fungal, Antiviral, and Anti-parasitic Agents
Agent(s)	**Action**
Anti-malarial	Any drug used to prevent or treat malaria: chloroquine, an anti-malarial drug used to treat malaria and amoebic dysentery; mefloquine hydrochloride (Larium), an anti-malarial drug effective in cases that do not respond to chloroquine and said to produce harmful neuropsychiatric effects in some people; primaquine, a bitter alkaloid extracted from cinchona bark
Antituberculous	A group of medications used in the treatment of tuberculosis, including isoniazid, rifampicin, pyrazinamide, and ethambutol
Amoebicides	Medications used to treat amoebas in the body
Anthelmintics	Medications used to treat parasitic intestinal worms
Leprostatic	A group of medications used in the treatment and management of leprosy

Dermatological Drugs

A wide variety of afflictions can affect a patient's skin, from infections to cancer. The specific medication used will be determined by the condition itself. Although several systemic medications can be used to treat dermatologic disorders, a majority of the drugs used will be applied topically. In addition, medications used to affect other areas of the body can be given through the skin (that is, transdermally). GTN for patients with chest pain and fentanyl for pain management, for example, are commonly encountered medications that are administered transdermally.

Vitamins and Minerals

Vitamins and minerals are necessary substances that allow for normal metabolism, growth and development, and cellular function. Patients may be taking vitamin and mineral supplements to replace deficient items or as a preventive measure. Vitamins affect a wide variety of functions, but one particular we focus on in the prehospital setting is thiamine (vitamin B_1). Thiamine aids in converting carbohydrates into energy. People with alcoholism, among others, have a propensity to be deficient in this vitamin. It is sometimes appropriate to give thiamine intravenously to patients with risk factors for thiamine deficiency before administering glucose in an attempt to facilitate effective metabolism.

Fluids and Electrolytes

Several types of IV fluids may be administered to patients. Crystalloid solutions are typically used in the prehospital setting and can be isotonic, hypotonic, or hypertonic. Isotonic solutions provide a stable medium for the administration of medication and provide effective fluid and electrolyte replacement. Hypertonic solutions help provide nutrition. Hypotonic solutions are beneficial in dehydration situations but not in hypovolaemic cases. IV fluids are discussed in detail in Chapter 8.

Antidotes and Overdoses

The management of overdose reflects the agent that the patient has consumed. Antidotes can function antagonistically by blocking receptor sites that would otherwise be stimulated by the agent. They can transform the agent into an inert, non-hazardous form to facilitate excretion. Alternatively, they may bind to the agent to prohibit its absorption into the bloodstream. Overdoses and their antidotes are discussed in depth in Chapter 33.

◼ Tying It All Together

As you review the various classifications of medications on the preceding pages, you will probably ask yourself why you need to know all of these because you don't administer them in the prehospital setting. And that is a very good question.

The answer is that there is a tremendous amount of information that can be obtained about your patient's current condition and medical history based on the medications taken. Having an understanding of which types of medications have specific functions allows you to assess your patient's condition(s) more effectively. If your patient is unresponsive and you find a spilled bottle of GTN tablets, what will you suspect? Knowing what GTN is used for and the effects it has on the body allows you to significantly narrow down the possible conditions your patient might have.

In addition to the assessment of the current condition, you can also gather significant information about the patient's medical history. Again, a general understanding of the uses and effects of different medications provides the clues you need to obtain a large portion of the patient's medical history even when the patient is unable to answer. Furthermore, it is common for patients to forget about a medical condition or not consider it a medical *problem.* For example, a patient may tell you that you he does not have high blood pressure, but when you review his prescription medications, you find labetalol. Because you know that labetalol is often used to treat hypertension, you question him again. He may respond this way: "I don't have high blood pressure because that medication lowers it". This proves to be very useful information that you might have missed had you not understood the classifications of medications.

In addition, a patient's medications may alter the clinical presentation of some conditions. As you probably already know, a patient who is in hypovolaemic shock will have an increased pulse rate followed by a decrease in blood pressure. What do you think you will see in a patient with hypovolaemic shock but who is taking a prescription medication intended to block beta adrenergic receptors?

Once you have an idea of the condition the patient has and know the medical history, you can begin to develop your pharmacological treatment plan. Understanding the classifications of medications has a role in this situation as well. You need to develop a treatment plan that will treat the patient's condition while considering the negative effects and interactions with the patient's other medications.

You are the Paramedic Summary

1. What are some potential differential diagnoses?

Your patient presents with a combination of symptoms: palpitations, mild shortness of breath and visual disturbances. Looking at this trio of symptoms, cardiac problems such as a silent MI, high blood pressure, and abnormal heart rate or rhythm are good possibilities. The mention that he has a history of "heart problems" also helps to tip the scale in this direction.

2. What types of medications might your patient be taking?

There are a variety of different types of medications that he could be taking for heart problems—including a diuretic, a beta blocker, a calcium channel blocker, or an ACE inhibitor.

3. What type of drug is diltiazem and how does it work?

Diltiazem is a calcium channel blocker. This drug lowers blood pressure by decreasing peripheral vascular resistance. It helps decrease the work load of the heart by diminishing myocardial and smooth muscle contraction. Calcium channel blockers are also effective in the management of fast cardiac rhythm disturbances because of their ability to decrease the conduction of electrical impulses through the heart.

4. Does the patient present with signs and symptoms of possible drug toxicity? If so, which medications are in question?

Yes, drug toxicity, specifically digoxin and diltiazem, is a possibility. When taken in excess, either medication can cause a significant drop in a patient's haemodynamic status, which explains the problems with the heart rate and blood pressure, but what about the vision disturbances? One of the other side effects of digoxin toxicity is visual disturbances, including the presence of a yellow-green halo around objects and blurred vision.

5. What treatment will increase the patient's blood pressure?

The best treatment is to reverse the effects of the calcium channel blocker, diltiazem. Calcium salts may be used for this purpose if digoxin toxicity is not also present.

6. What does it mean when a medication has a low therapeutic index?

The therapeutic index measures the safety of the drug. It is calculated by dividing the lethal dose 50 (LD_{50}) by the effective dose 50 (ED_{50}). The closer the answer is to 1, the more harmful the drug is. Since the therapeutic index for digoxin is close to one, the amount of medication between a normal dose and a toxic dose is very small, making it easy for toxic levels to develop. Because of this, patients who take digoxin frequently have their blood levels checked to make sure that they are within the therapeutic range.

7. What occurs when one drug potentiates a second drug?

When potentiation occurs, the effect of one drug increases the effect of another. In your patient, the administration of diltiazem increased the amount of digoxin in the blood, leading to the increased effects of digoxin and an increased chance of toxicity.

Prep Kit

■ Ready for Review

- In the prehospital setting, the goal of emergency pharmacology is to use medications to reverse, prevent, or control various diseases and illnesses, chronic and acute.
- Medications must always be delivered according to the *six rights:* the Right patient, the Right dose, the Right route, the Right time, the Right medication, and Right documentation on your PCR.
- A medication is a drug that has been approved by the government agency that regulates pharmaceuticals for the purpose of curing or reducing the symptoms of an illness or medical condition or to assist in the diagnosis, treatment, or prevention of a disease. A drug may also be given in an attempt to alter the disease process.
- The manufacture of pharmaceuticals in the UK and most other countries is subject to a variety of laws and regulations that aim to prohibit manufacturers from making false claims about their drugs' benefits and advising patients to administer the drugs incorrectly.
- Drugs are derived from four principal sources: animal, vegetable, mineral, and synthetic compounds.
- Special considerations exist when administering medications to pregnant women, children, and older people.
- Paramedics are legally responsible for the appropriate use of medications and documentation of medication therapy. Always have a clear understanding of which medication you are administering and why you are administering it.
- Medications administered as part of the care provided in the prehospital setting exert their effects largely by acting on the nervous system.
- The peripheral nervous system is separated into two divisions: the somatic nervous system and the ANS. The ANS is particularly vulnerable to the administration of prehospital medications. It is considered to be "automatic" or involuntary because we cannot control its functioning or force functions under its control to happen or not happen. The sympathetic nervous system, which gives the fight-or-flight response, is the dominant system during periods of stress and activity. The parasympathetic nervous system is the dominant system during periods of rest and relaxation.
- Neurotransmission is the process of chemical signalling between cells.
- Receptors are unique molecular structures or sites on the surface or interior of a cell that bind with substances such as hormones, drugs, and neurotransmitters. Receptors are highly specialised and, in most cases, respond only to a particular substance, much like a lock and key.
- Normal neurotransmission can be altered by using drugs that mimic or inhibit neurotransmission. Some medications inhibit the release of neurotransmitters, and others work by blocking the receptor sites along the neural pathway.
- Drugs adjust or influence the body's existing functions by interacting with various cells and tissues in the body, and they typically work through several mechanisms of action rather than relying on a single action. In most cases, medications may bind to a receptor site and trigger a stimulus; in some cases, they change the chemical properties of cells and tissues. They may also combine with other chemicals within cells or organ systems to aid in elimination or bind to receptors to alter the normal metabolic functions of cells and tissues.
- Drugs are available in a wide array of forms, including liquids, solids, and vapours. In the prehospital environment, you use only a limited subset of drug forms.
- The mode of administration affects the rate at which the body absorbs the drug, and the route of administration affects the speed with which a drug works.
- Local effects result from the direct application of a drug to a tissue. Systemic effects occur after the drug is absorbed by any route and distributed by the bloodstream.
- The routes of administration are classified into three categories based on how the medication is absorbed and distributed: percutaneous (applied to and absorbed through the skin), enteral (absorbed somewhere along the gastrointestinal tract), and parenteral (any route of administration that does not cause the drug to be absorbed through the skin, mucous membranes, or gastrointestinal tract).
- Every medication has varying effects on the body. The study of the metabolism and action of medications within the body is called pharmacokinetics, which focuses particularly on the time required for absorption, duration of action, distribution in the body, and method of excretion.
- A medication's ability to reach a therapeutic concentration in the bloodstream depends partially on the rate and extent to which the drug is absorbed. Rate and extent are dependent on the ability of the medication to cross the cell membrane, which occurs by active transport or passive diffusion.
- Blood is the primary distribution vehicle for medications. Factors that change the way blood flows through the body will change the way medications are transported to the target tissue.
- Biotransformation, or the way in which the body metabolises medications, occurs by transforming the medication into a metabolite or by making the medication more water-soluble.
- Excretion occurs primarily through the kidneys via glomerular filtration, tubular secretion, and partial reabsorption.
- Medications cause their action on the body by binding to a receptor site, changing the physical properties of cells, chemically combining with other chemicals, or altering a normal metabolic pathway.
- The drug-response relationship correlates to the amount of medication given and the response it causes.
- Factors affecting how patients react to medications include age, weight, sex, environment, time of administration, condition of the patient (overall state of health), genetic factors, and psychological factors.
- Every medication has some side effects that are known and anticipated, although occasionally unanticipated adverse reactions (iatrogenic responses) are seen.
- Extremes of temperature, exposure to direct sunlight, or excessive humidity may decrease the potency of some medications or degrade the actual molecular components and make the medication inactive.
- Understanding drug profiles will help you select the most appropriate medication for your patients.
- Classifications of drugs are based on the effect the drugs will have on a particular part of the body or on a specific condition.

■ Vital Vocabulary

absorption The process by which a medication's molecules are moved from the site of entry or administration into the body and into systemic circulation.

adrenal medulla The inner portion of the adrenal glands that synthesises, stores, and eventually releases adrenaline and noradrenaline.

adrenergic Pertaining to nerves that release the neurotransmitter noradrenaline (such as adrenergic nerves, adrenergic response). The term also pertains to the receptors acted on by noradrenaline, that is, the adrenergic receptors.

afferent nerves The nerves that carry sensory impulses from all parts of the body to the brain.

affinity The force attraction between medications and receptors causing them to bind together.

agonist A substance that mimics the actions of a specific neurotransmitter or hormone by binding to the specific receptor of the naturally occurring substance.

anaesthetic A type of medication intended to induce a loss of sensation to touch or pain.

analgesia The absence of the sensation of pain.

analgesics A classification for medications that relieve pain, or induce analgesia.

angiotensin converting enzyme (ACE) inhibitors Medications that suppress the conversion of angiotensin I to angiotensin II.

angiotensin II receptor antagonists Medications that are similar to ACE inhibitors but work by selectively blocking angiotensin II at their receptor sites.

antagonist A molecule that blocks the ability of a given chemical to bind to its receptor, preventing a biological response.

anti-arrhythmic medications The medications used to treat and prevent cardiac rhythm disorders.

antibiotic medications The medications that fight bacterial infection by killing the bacteria or by preventing multiplication of the bacteria to allow the body's immune system to overcome them.

anticholinergic Of or pertaining to the blocking of acetylcholine receptors, resulting in inhibition of transmission of parasympathetic nerve impulses.

anti-coagulant drugs The medications used to prevent intravascular thrombosis by preventing blood coagulation in the vascular system.

anti-hypertensives The medications used to control blood pressure.

anti-neoplastic medications The medications designed to combat cancer.

anti-platelet agents The medications that interfere with the collection of platelets.

autonomic nervous system (ANS) The component of the peripheral nervous system that sends sensory impulses from internal structures (such as blood vessels, the heart, and organs of the chest, abdomen, and pelvis) through afferent autonomic nerves to the brain.

barbiturates Any medications of a group of barbituric acid derivatives that act as central nervous system depressants and are used as sedatives or hypnotics.

benzodiazepines Any medications of a group of psychotropic agents used as anti-anxiety, muscle relaxants, sedatives, or hypnotics.

bioavailability The amount of a medication that is still active once it reaches its target tissue.

biological half-life The time it takes the body to eliminate half of the drug.

biotransformation A process by which a medication is chemically converted to a different compound or metabolite.

buccal route A medication route in which medication is administered between the cheeks and gums.

calcium channel blockers The medications that suppress arrhythmias, provide more oxygen to the heart via coronary artery dilation, and reduce peripheral vascular resistance.

capsule A cylindrical gelatin container enclosing a dose of medication.

cardiac glycosides A classification of medications that naturally occur in plant substances and that block certain ionic pumps in the heart cells' membranes, which indirectly increases calcium concentrations; an example is digoxin.

chemical name A description of the drug's chemical composition and molecular structure.

cholinergic Fibres in the parasympathetic nervous system that release a chemical called acetylcholine.

chronotropic Affecting the rate of rhythmic movements, such as the heartbeat. A positive chronotropic effect would result in increasing the heart rate.

CNS stimulants Any medications or agents that increase brain activity.

contraindications In health care, conditions or factors that increase the risk involved in using a particular drug, carrying out a medical procedure, or engaging in a particular activity.

cross-tolerance A form of drug tolerance in which patients who take a particular medication for an extended period can build up a tolerance to other medications in the same class.

cumulative effect An effect that occurs when several successive doses of a medication are administered or when absorption of a medication occurs faster than excretion or metabolism.

depolarising neuromuscular blocking agents Medications designed to keep muscles in a contracted state.

distribution The movement and transportation of a medication throughout the bloodstream to tissues and cells of the body and, ultimately, to its target receptor.

diuretic medications The medications designed to promote elimination of excess salt and water by the kidneys.

dopaminergic receptors The receptors believed to cause dilation of the renal, coronary, and cerebral arteries.

dromotropic Relating to or influencing the conductivity of nerve fibres or cardiac muscle fibres.

drugs Any chemical compounds that may be used on humans to help in diagnosis, treatment, cure, mitigation, or prevention of disease or other abnormal conditions.

duration of action How long the medication concentration can be expected to remain above the minimum level needed to provide the intended action.

efferent nerves The nerves that carry messages from the brain to the muscles and all other organs of the body.

elixir A syrup with alcohol and flavouring added.

emulsion A preparation of one liquid (usually an oil) distributed in small globules in another liquid (usually water).

enteral routes The medication administration routes in which medications are absorbed somewhere along the gastrointestinal tract.

excretion The elimination of toxic or inactive metabolites from the body. This is primarily done by the kidneys, intestines, lungs, and assorted glands.

extract A concentrated preparation of a drug made by putting the drug into solution (in alcohol or water) and evaporating off the excess solvent to a prescribed standard.

fibrinolytic agents The only medications available to dissolve blood clots after they have already formed; the drugs promote the digestion of fibrin.

fluid extract A concentrated form of a drug prepared by dissolving the crude drug in the fluid in which it is most readily soluble.

ganglia Groupings of nerve cell bodies located in the peripheral nervous system.

generic drug A medication that is not patented.

generic name A general name for a drug that is not manufacturer-specific; usually the name given to the drug by the company that first manufactures it.

iatrogenic response An adverse condition inadvertently induced by the treatment given.

idiosyncrasy An abnormal (and usually unexplained) reaction by a person to a medication, to which most other people do not react.

immunobiological medications The medications that include serums, vaccines, and other immunising agents.

immunosuppressant medications The medications intended to inhibit the body's ability to attack the "foreign" organ or, in the case of autoimmune diseases, the medications that inhibit the body's attack on itself.

indications The reasons or conditions for which the medication is given.

inotropic affecting the contractility of muscle tissue, especially cardiac muscle.

interference A direct biochemical interaction between two drugs.

intramuscular (IM) route A method of delivering a medication into the muscle of the body. This is accomplished by placing a needle into a muscle space and injecting the medication into the tissue.

www.Paramedic.EMISzone.com/UK/

intraosseous (IO) route A method of delivering a medication into the marrow cavity of a bone. This is accomplished by placing a rigid needle into the marrow cavity and flushing a medication into the space.

liniments Liquid preparations of drugs for external use, usually to relieve some discomfort (such as pain, itching) or to protect the skin.

local anaesthesia A type of anaesthesia that causes a loss of sensation to touch or pain at a specific isolated spot on the body where a procedure is to take place.

local effects The effects that result from the direct application of a drug to a tissue, for example when lotions are applied to the skin to relieve itching.

loop diuretics Medications that inhibit the reabsorption of sodium and calcium ions and that can cause an excessive loss of potassium.

mechanism of action The way in which a medication produces the intended response.

medication A licensed drug taken to cure or reduce symptoms of an illness or medical condition or as an aid in the diagnosis, treatment, or prevention of a disease or other abnormal condition.

milk In the context of pharmacology, an aqueous suspension of an insoluble drug.

muscarinic cholinergic antagonists Medications that block acetylcholine exclusively at the muscarinic receptors; an example is atropine.

neuromuscular blocking agents Medications that affect the parasympathetic nervous system by inducing paralysis.

neurotransmission The process of chemical signalling between cells.

nicotinic cholinergic antagonists Medications that block the acetylcholine only at nicotinic receptors.

nonbarbiturate hypnotics Medications designed to sedate without the side effects of a barbiturate.

nondepolarising neuromuscular blocking agents Medications designed to cause temporary paralysis by binding in a competitive but nonstimulatory manner to part of the ACh receptor. Do not cause fasciculations.

nonopioid analgesics Medications designed to relieve pain without the side effects of opioids.

nonspecific agents Medications that produce effects on different cells through a variety of mechanisms. Generally classified by the focus of action or specific therapeutic use.

nonsteroidal anti-inflammatory drugs (NSAIDs) Medications with analgesic and fever reducing properties.

ointment A semisolid preparation for external application to the body, usually containing a medicinal substance.

onset of action The time needed for the concentration of the medication at the target tissue to reach the minimum effective level.

opioid agonist-antagonists Medications designed to relieve pain without the side effects of opioids.

opioid agonists Chemicals that are similar to or derived from the opium plant.

opioid antagonists A classification of medications that reverses the effects of opioid drugs.

para-aminophenol derivatives Medications designed to reduce fevers and relieve pain.

parenteral routes Medication routes in which medications are administered via any route other than the alimentary canal (digestive tract), skin, or mucous membranes.

patch A solid medication impregnated into a membrane or adhesive that is applied to the surface of the skin.

percutaneous routes The medication routes of any medication absorbed through the skin or a mucous membrane.

peripheral nervous system (PNS) Consists of all nervous tissue outside of the brain and spinal cord and is subdivided into two divisions, the *somatic* and *autonomic* nervous systems.

pharmacodynamics The branch of pharmacology that studies reactions between medications and living structures, including the processes of body responses to pharmacological, biochemical, physiological, and therapeutic effects.

pharmacokinetics The study of the metabolism and action of medications with particular emphasis on the time required for absorption, duration of action, distribution in the body, and method of excretion.

pharmacology The branch of medicine dealing with the actions of drugs in the body—therapeutic and toxic effects—and development and testing of new drugs and new uses of existing ones.

pill A drug shaped into a ball or oval to be swallowed; often coated to disguise an unpleasant taste.

potentiation In health care, the effect of increasing the potency or effectiveness of a drug or other treatment; may occur by administering two medications concurrently, and one increases the effect of the other.

powder A drug that has been ground into pulverised form.

pulmonary route A medication route in which medication is administered directly to the pulmonary system through inhalation or injection.

regional anaesthesia A type of anaesthesia that focuses on a particular portion of the body, such as the legs or the arms.

sedation An effect in which the patient experiences decreased anxiety and inhibition.

side effects Reactions that can manifest as signs or symptoms that are not desired but are expected based on how the medication works.

skeletal muscle relaxants Medications that provide relief of skeletal muscle spasms.

sodium channel blockers Anti-arrhythmic medications that slow conduction through the heart.

solution A liquid containing one or more chemical substances entirely dissolved, usually in water.

specific agents Medications that bring about an identifiable mechanism with unique receptors for the agent.

spirits A preparation of a volatile substance dissolved in alcohol.

stimulants An agent that increases the level of body activity.

subcutaneous (SC) route A medication route in which injections are given beneath the skin into the fat or connective tissue immediately underlying it.

sublingual (SL) A medication route in which medication is administered under the tongue.

summation effect The process whereby multiple medications can produce a response that the individual medications alone do not produce.

suppository A drug mixed in a firm base that melts at body temperature and is shaped to fit the rectum.

suspension A preparation of a finely divided drug intended to be (or already) incorporated in a suitable liquid.

sympathetic blocking agent An anti-hypertensive medication that decreases cardiac output and renin secretions.

sympathomimetics The medications administered to stimulate the sympathetic nervous system.

synergism An interaction of two or more medications that results in an effect that is greater than the sum of their effects if taken independently.

syrup A drug suspended in sugar and water to improve its taste.

systemic anaesthesia A type of anaesthesia often done through the inhalation of volatile vapourised liquids and predominantly reserved for operating theatre use; also called general anaesthesia.

systemic effects The effects that occur after the drug is absorbed by any route and distributed by the bloodstream; almost invariably involve more than one organ.

tablet A powdered drug that has been moulded or compressed into a small disc.

tachyphylaxis A condition in which the patient rapidly becomes tolerant to a medication.

termination of action The amount of time after the medication's concentration falls below the minimum effective level until it is eliminated from the body.

therapeutic The desired or intended action of a medication.

therapeutic index The ratio of a drug's lethal dose for 50% (LD_{50}) of the population to its effective dose for 50% (ED_{50}) of the population; a medication's margin of safety.

thiazides A type of diuretic medication that specifically controls the sodium and water quantities excreted by the kidneys.

tincture A dilute alcoholic extract of a drug.

tolerance A physiological response that requires a patient to take an increased medication dose to produce the same effect that formerly was produced by the lower dose.

toxoid A modified bacterial toxin that has been made nontoxic but retains the ability to stimulate the formation of antibodies.

trade name The brand name registered to a specific manufacturer or owner; also called proprietary name.

transdermal route A medication route generally performed by placing medication directly onto the patient's skin.

uricosuric medications The medications designed to lower the uric acid level in the blood by increasing the excretion by the kidneys into the urine.

vaccine A suspension of whole (live or inactivated) or fractionated bacteria or viruses that have been made nonpathogenic; given to induce an immune response and prevent disease.

vapour A gaseous medication form primarily used in operating room anaesthesia.

vasodilator medications The medications that work on the smooth muscles of the arterioles and/or the veins.

xanthines A classification of medications that affect the respiratory smooth muscle and that relax bronchiole smooth muscles, stimulate cardiac muscle, and stimulate the central nervous system.

Assessment in Action

You and your colleague have responded to a call for chest pain. The patient is a 68-year-old man who describes the pain as being a 20 on a 0-to-10 scale with 10 being the worst pain ever. As your colleague connects the patient to the monitor, you start gathering your patient's history. The patient has had a previous cardiac event and has been prescribed a "beta blocker".

1. **What is the primary action of a beta blocker?**
   A. It reduces the adrenergic stimulation of the beta receptors in the heart.
   B. It increases the adrenergic stimulation of the beta receptors in the heart.
   C. It reduces the cholinergic stimulation of the beta receptors in the heart.
   D. It increases the cholinergic stimulation of the beta receptors in the heart.

2. **You decided to give your patient aspirin once you determine that he is not allergic to it. Aspirin is a(n):**
   A. calcium channel blocker.
   B. sympathomimetic.
   C. anti-platelet agent.
   D. anti-hypertensive.

3. **Your patient has not taken any of his own GTN, so you decide to give him a dose of yours. How are you going to deliver the medication?**
   A. IV push
   B. Sublingual
   C. Intramuscular
   D. Subcutaneous

4. **How long should it take for the GTN to take effect through this route of administration?**
   A. 15 to 20 minutes
   B. 10 to 15 minutes
   C. 5 to 10 minutes
   D. Less than 5 minutes

5. **Your patient is still having substantial chest pain after the GTN, and you decide that he will benefit greatly from analgesia. Which medication is an analgesic?**
   A. Morphine
   B. Narcan
   C. Oxygen
   D. Salbutamol

6. **What is a specific cardiac action of the analgesic mentioned in question 5 that should benefit this patient?**
   A. It has a chronotropic action that slows the heart rate.
   B. It decreases the workload on the heart.
   C. It increases the workload on the heart.
   D. It decreases ectopic beats.

Challenging Question

7. **If this patient had taken three doses of his own GTN, would you still give him three doses of yours?**

Points to Ponder

You are called to assist a neighbouring ambulance service with a cardiac arrest. On scene, you find that a paramedic has already secured the airway and inserted an IV line. You introduce yourself and your colleague and assume responsibility for administering the medications. You ask your colleague to hand you some adrenaline. Your colleague pulls the unfamiliar drug box over and starts rummaging through looking for a particular colour of label, which he cannot find. All of the medications are unboxed and stored in elastic loops in a soft-sided pack. You look back at your colleague to see what the hold-up is and you see the medication pack.

Are all medication boxes standardised by the colour of the box? Who has the responsibility to select the correct medication?

Issues: Working With Other Responders, Properly Administering Medication.

Objectives

Cognitive

- Review the specific anatomy and physiology pertinent to medication administration.
- Review mathematical principles.
- Review mathematical equivalents.
- Discuss formulas as a basis for performing drug calculations.
- Discuss applying basic principles of mathematics to the calculation of problems associated with medication dosages.
- Describe the indications, equipment needed, technique used, precautions, and general principles of peripheral venous or external jugular cannulation.
- Describe the indications, equipment needed, technique used, precautions, and general principles of intraosseous needle placement and infusion.
- Discuss legal aspects affecting medication administration.
- Discuss the "six rights" of drug administration and correlate these with the principles of medication administration.
- Discuss medical asepsis and the differences between clean and sterile techniques.
- Describe use of antiseptics and disinfectants.
- Describe the use of universal precautions when administering a medication.
- Differentiate among the different dosage forms of oral medications.
- Describe the equipment needed and general principles of administering oral medications.
- Describe the indications, equipment needed, techniques used, precautions, and general principles of administering medications by the inhalation route.
- Describe the indications, equipment needed, techniques used, precautions, and general principles of administering medications by the gastric tube.
- Describe the indications, equipment needed, techniques used, precautions, and general principles of rectal medication administration.
- Differentiate among the different parenteral routes of medication administration.
- Describe the equipment needed, techniques used, complications, and general principles for the preparation and administration of parenteral medications.

- Differentiate among the different percutaneous routes of medication administration.
- Describe the purpose, equipment needed, techniques used, complications, and general principles for obtaining a blood sample.
- Describe disposal of contaminated items and sharps.
- Synthesise a pharmacological management plan including medication administration.
- Integrate pathophysiological principles of medication administration with patient management.

Affective

- Comply with paramedic standards of medication administration.
- Comply with universal precautions.
- Defend a pharmacological management plan for medication administration.
- Serve as a model for medical asepsis.
- Serve as a model for advocacy while performing medication administration.
- Serve as a model for disposing contaminated items and sharps.

Psychomotor

- Use universal precautions and medical asepsis during medication administration procedures.
- Demonstrate cannulation of peripheral or external jugular veins.
- Demonstrate intraosseous needle placement and infusion.
- Demonstrate aseptic technique during medication administration.
- Demonstrate administration of oral medications.
- Demonstrate administration of medications by the inhalation route.
- Demonstrate administration of medications by the gastric tube.
- Demonstrate rectal administration of medications.
- Demonstrate preparation and administration of parenteral medications.
- Demonstrate preparation and techniques for obtaining a blood sample.
- Perfect disposal of contaminated items and sharps.

Introduction

Vascular access is often needed in emergency medicine for patients in haemodynamically unstable condition and in need of intravenous (IV) fluids, various medications, or both. A number of techniques are used to gain vascular access in the prehospital setting, including cannulation of a peripheral extremity vein, external jugular vein cannulation, and intraosseous infusion. In critically ill or injured patients, survival often depends on your ability to obtain vascular access quickly and effectively. Because these procedures are invasive, you must be proficient, yet cautious. Significant harm to the patient can result from improper technique and/or insufficient knowledge of the medication(s) being administered.

This chapter begins with an overview of fluids and electrolytes—balanced and imbalanced—and the processes of osmosis and diffusion. Next, it discusses the various types of IV solutions used in the prehospital setting and the techniques of IV therapy and intraosseous infusion. Finally, it describes the mathematical principles used in pharmacology, calculating medication doses (bolus and maintenance infusion), and the various routes for administering medications.

Fluids and Electrolytes

The human body is composed mostly of water, which provides the environment in which the chemical reactions necessary to life take place. Water also serves as a transport medium for nutrients, hormones, and waste materials. The total body water (TBW) constitutes 60% of the weight of an adult man and is distributed among the following compartments (Figure 8-1 ▶):

- Intracellular fluid (ICF) is the water contained inside the cells; it normally accounts for 45% of body weight.
- Extracellular fluid (ECF), the water outside the cells, accounts for 15% of body weight and is further divided into two types of fluids:
  - Interstitial fluid, the water bathing the cells, accounts for about 10.5% of body weight. The interstitial fluid also includes special fluid collections, such as cerebrospinal fluid and intraocular fluid.
  - Intravascular fluid (plasma), the water within the blood vessels, carries red blood cells, white blood cells, and vital nutrients. Intravascular fluid normally accounts for about 4.5% of body weight.

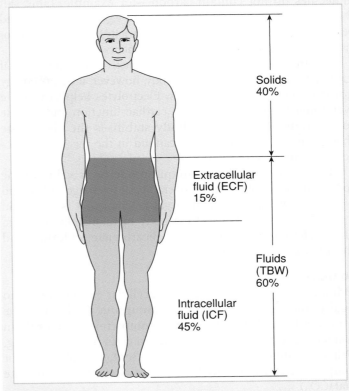

Figure 8-1 Distribution of water throughout the body.

The fluids in the body are composed of dissolved elements and water, a combination known as a solution. A solution is a mixture of two things:

- Solvent. The fluid that does the dissolving, or the solution that contains the dissolved components
- Solute. The dissolved particles contained in the solvent

Water in the body serves as the universal solvent, dissolving a variety of solutes. These solutes can be classified as electrolytes or nonelectrolytes.

Electrolytes

Atoms carry charges—some positive, some negative. Two or more atoms that bond together form a molecule. When atoms bond together, they share and disperse their charges throughout the molecule. Organic molecules contain carbon atoms—for example, table sugar ($C_6H_{12}O_6$). By contrast, inorganic

You are the Paramedic Part 1

You are dispatched to the home of a 70-year-old woman who has diabetes. A neighbour found her lying on a sofa in her living room. The neighbour tells you she tried to wake up the patient, but was unable to do so. The patient appears to be unconscious; she is pale and noticeably perspiring. She is breathing, but her respirations are rapid and shallow.

1. Is this a medical patient or a trauma patient?
2. What are your initial priorities of care?

molecules do not contain carbon—for example, table salt (NaCl). Inorganic molecules give rise to electrolytes (so called because of their ability to conduct electricity) when they dissociate in water into their charged components.

Electrolytes, also called ions, are reactive and dangerous if left to circulate in the body. The body, however, uses the energy stored in these charged particles. Electrolytes help to regulate everything from water levels to cardiac function and muscle contractions. Water in the body stabilises the electrolyte charges so that the electrolytes can aid in the metabolic functions that are necessary for life.

Each electrolyte has a unique property or value to the body. If the electrolyte has an overall *positive* charge, it is called a cation; if it has an overall *negative* charge, it is called an anion. The major cations of the body include sodium, potassium, calcium, and magnesium. Bicarbonate, chloride, and phosphorous are the major anions.

Sodium

Sodium (Na^+) is the principal extracellular cation needed to regulate the distribution of water throughout the body in the intravascular and interstitial fluid compartments. Its role in maintaining adequate cellular perfusion gives rise to the saying, "Where sodium goes, water follows". Sodium is also a major component of the circulating buffer, sodium bicarbonate ($NaHCO_3$).

Potassium

About 98% of all the body's potassium (K^+) is found inside the cells of the body, making it the principal intracellular cation. Potassium plays a major role in neuromuscular function and in the conversion of glucose into glycogen. Cellular potassium levels are regulated by insulin. The sodium-potassium (Na^+-K^+) pump is helped by the presence of insulin and adrenaline. Low potassium levels—hypokalaemia—in the serum (blood plasma) can lead to decreased skeletal muscle function, gastrointestinal disturbances, and alterations in cardiac function. High potassium levels in the serum—hyperkalaemia—can lead to hyperstimulation of neural cell transmission, resulting in cardiac arrest.

Calcium

Calcium (Ca^{++}) is the principal cation needed for bone growth. It also plays an important part in the functioning of heart muscle, nerves, and cell membranes and is necessary for proper blood clotting.

Low serum calcium levels—hypocalcaemia—can lead to overstimulation of nerve cells. Signs and symptoms of hypocalcaemia include skeletal muscle cramps, abdominal cramps, carpopedal spasms, hypotension, and vasoconstriction.

High serum calcium levels—hypercalcaemia—can lead to decreased stimulation of nerve cells. Signs and symptoms of hypercalcaemia include skeletal muscle weakness, lethargy, ataxia, vasodilation, and hot, flushed skin.

Magnesium

Magnesium (Mg^{++}) has an important role as a coenzyme in the metabolism of proteins and carbohydrates. In addition, it acts in a manner similar to calcium in controlling neuromuscular irritability.

Bicarbonate

Bicarbonate (HCO_3^-) levels are the determining factor between acidosis and alkalosis in the body. Bicarbonate is the primary buffer used in all circulating body fluids.

Chloride

Chloride (Cl^-) primarily regulates the pH of the stomach. It also regulates extracellular fluid levels.

Phosphorous

Phosphorous (P) is an important component in adenosine triphosphate (ATP), the body's powerful energy source.

Nonelectrolytes

The body also contains solutes that have no electrical charge. These nonelectrolytes include glucose and urea. The normal concentration of glucose in the blood, for example, is 70 to 110 milligrams (mg) per 100 millilitres (ml).

▌Fluid and Electrolyte Movement

Water and electrolytes move among the body's fluid compartments according to some basic chemical and biological tenets. One governing principle is that unequal concentrations on different sides of a cell membrane will move to balance themselves equally on both sides of the membrane. Balance across a cell membrane has two components:

- Balance of compounds (for example, water and electrolytes) on either side of the cell membrane
- Balance of charges [the positive ($^+$) or negative ($^-$) charges carried on the atoms] on either side of the cell membrane

When concentrations of charges or compounds are greater on one side of the cell membrane than on the other side, a gradient is created. The natural tendency for materials is to flow from an area of higher concentration to one of lower concentration, establishing a concentration gradient. Gradients are categorised according to the type of material that flows down them: Chemical compounds flow down chemical gradients;

electrical currents flow down electrical gradients. The process of flowing down a gradient depends on whether the cell membrane will allow the material to pass through it. Certain compounds can travel freely across the cell membrane (a kinetically favourable situation that requires little energy), whereas others require active transport across the membrane because of the size of the compound or because of an incompatible charge.

Diffusion

When compounds or charges concentrated on one side of a cell membrane move across it to an area of lower concentration, the process is called diffusion. To visualise this situation, imagine that too many people show up for a theatre performance. The management decides to open another seating area to accommodate the crowd. Patrons (charges or compounds) are concentrated in a small area (the cell) outside the door (the cell membrane) leading to the new seating area. When the theatre manager opens the door, patrons can move through it (selective cell membrane permeability) from the congested area (down a concentration gradient). The patrons spread themselves out evenly (diffuse) throughout the total area, with some choosing to stay behind in the original seating area as others move into the new area, until all have an equal amount of room.

Filtration

Filtration, another type of diffusion, is commonly used by the kidneys to clean blood. Water carries dissolved compounds across the cell membranes of the tubules of the kidney. The tubule membrane traps these dissolved compounds but lets the water pass through in much the same way that a coffee filter traps the grounds as water passes through it. This cleans the blood of wastes and removes the trapped compounds from cir-culation so they can be flushed out of the body. The anti-diuretic hormone (ADH) prevents the loss of water from the kidneys by causing its reabsorption into the tubules.

Active Transport

Often, the cell must maintain an imbalance of compounds across its membrane to achieve some metabolic purpose. For example, in the sodium-potassium pump, the cell uses sodium outside the cell and potassium inside the cell for depolarisation. To maintain this imbalance, the cell must use energy in the form of ATP and actively transport compounds across its membrane. Even though active transport demands a high-energy expenditure, its benefits outweigh the initial use of ATP. Pumping sodium out of the cell and potassium into the cell has the added benefit of moving glucose into the cell at the same time.

Osmosis

As noted earlier, fluid compartments in the body are separated from one another by membranes, such as the cell membranes and the membranes lining blood vessels. The concentration of fluid in those compartments—that is, the number of solute particles—is chiefly influenced by the process called osmosis. If two solutions are separated by a semipermeable membrane (eg, a cell wall), water will flow across the membrane *from* the solution of *lower* solute concentration *to* the solution of *higher* solute concentration. The net effect is to equalise the solute concentrations on both sides of the membrane.

The effects of osmotic pressure on a cell constitute the tonicity of the solution Figure 8-2 ▶ . Tonicity reflects the concentration of sodium in a solution and the movement of water in relation to the sodium levels inside and outside the cell.

You are the Paramedic Part 2

Your general impression of the patient and her environment reveals no signs of injury. After carefully moving the patient to the floor, you perform an initial assessment. Your partner opens the primary response bag in preparation for treatment.

Initial Assessment	Recording Time: 0 Minutes
Level of consciousness	U (Unresponsive)
Airway	Patent; airway is clear of secretions
Breathing	Respirations, rapid and shallow
Circulation	Radial pulses, rapid and weak; skin, pale and perspiring; no obvious gross bleeding

3. What is the most appropriate initial airway management for this patient?

4. Does this patient require immediate medication therapy?

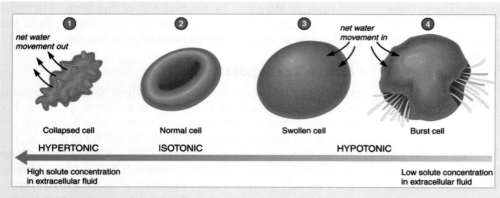

Figure 8-2 Tonicity.

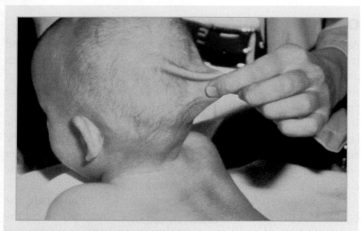

Figure 8-3 Dehydration.

Abnormal States of Fluid and Electrolyte Balance

The healthy body maintains a delicate balance between intake and output of fluids and electrolytes, ensuring that the internal environment remains fairly constant. The internal environment's resistance to change is called homeostasis. The ill or injured body, however, may be unable to maintain homeostasis, and excesses or deficits of fluids and electrolytes may occur. You need to know when IV fluids are indicated, what kinds of fluids are required in different situations, and when IV fluids can be dangerous. Although national clinical guidelines and local service procedures largely guide the use of IV fluids in the prehospital environment, you must still use your own judgement when administering IV fluids in order to function independently.

A healthy person loses approximately 2 to 2.5 litres of fluid daily through urine output and through the lungs (exhalation) and skin. These losses are replaced by intake of fluids and by nutrients that are partially converted to water in their metabolism. In illness, abnormal states of hydration may occur in which intake and output are no longer in balance.

Dehydration

Dehydration is defined as inadequate total systemic fluid volume Figure 8-3 ◄ . It is usually a chronic condition of elderly or very young people and may take days to manifest. As fluid is lost from the vascular compartment, the body reacts by shifting interstitial fluid into the vascular area; fluid also shifts from the intracellular to the extracellular compartments. As a consequence, a total systemic fluid deficit occurs.

Signs and symptoms of dehydration include decreased urine output, decreased level of consciousness, postural hypotension, tachypnoea, dry mucous membranes, tachycardia, poor skin turgor, and flushed, dry skin. Causes of dehydration include diarrhoea, vomiting, gastrointestinal drainage, haemorrhage, and insufficient fluid or food intake.

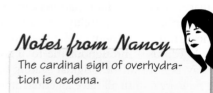

Notes from Nancy

The cardinal sign of overhydration is oedema.

Overhydration

When the body's total systemic fluid volume increases, overhydration occurs. Fluid fills the vascular compartment, filters into the interstitial compartment, and is forced from the engorged interstitial compartment into the intracellular compartment. This fluid backup can lead to death Figure 8-4 ▶ .

Signs and symptoms of overhydration include shortness of breath, puffy eyelids, oedema, polyuria, moist crackles (rales), and acute weight gain. Causes of overhydration include unmonitored IVs, kidney failure, and prolonged hypoventilation.

▌IV Fluid Composition

The use of IV fluids can significantly alter the patient's condition and facilitate patient treatment. Each bag of IV solution must be sterile and safe; therefore, each bag of IV solution is individually sterilised Figure 8-5 ▶ . The compounds and ions dissolved in the solutions are identical to the ones found in the body.

Sodium is used as the benchmark to calculate a solution's tonicity. The concentration of sodium in the cells of the body is approximately 0.9%. Altering the concentration of sodium in the IV solution, therefore, can move the water into or out of any fluid compartment in the body.

Types of IV Solutions

There are two basic types of IV solutions, crystalloid and colloid, of which crystalloids can be isotonic, hypotonic, or hypertonic. IV fluids use combinations of these solutions to create the desired effects inside the body.

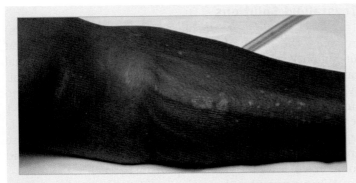

Figure 8-4 In an overhydrated patient, fluid backup occurs.

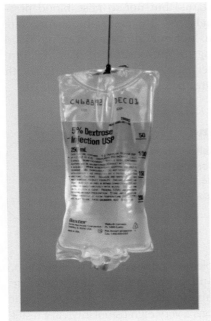

Figure 8-5 Each bag of IV solution must be sterile and safe.

Fluid movement across a cell membrane resulting from hypertonic, isotonic, and hypotonic solutions is illustrated in **Figure 8-6 ▾**. IV fluids introduced into the circulatory system can affect the tonicity of the extracellular fluid, resulting in dire consequences unless care is used.

Isotonic Solutions

Isotonic solutions such as normal saline (0.9% sodium chloride) have almost the same osmolarity (concentration of sodium) as serum and other body fluids. As a consequence, isotonic solutions expand the contents of the intravascular compartment without shifting fluid to or from other compartments, or changing cell shape—an important consideration when dealing with hypotensive or hypovolaemic patients. When administering isotonic solutions, you must be careful to avoid fluid overloading. Patients with hypertension and congestive heart failure are at greatest risk of this problem. The extra fluid increases preload, which in turn increases the workload of the heart, creating fluid backup in the lungs.

Lactated Ringer's (LR) (Hartmann's solution) solution is generally used in the prehospital setting for patients who have lost large amounts of blood. It contains lactate, which is metabolised in the liver to form bicarbonate—the key buffer that combats the intracellular acidosis associated with severe blood loss. LR solution should not be given to patients with liver problems because they cannot metabolise the lactate.

Glucose 10% in water is a unique type of isotonic solution. As long as it remains in the bag, it is considered an isotonic solution. Once it is administered, however, the glucose is quickly metabolised, and the solution becomes hypotonic.

Hypotonic Solutions

A hypotonic solution has an osmolarity less than that of serum. When this fluid is placed in the vascular compartment, it begins diluting the serum. Soon the serum osmolarity is less than that of the interstitial fluid; water is pulled from the vascular compartment into the interstitial fluid compartment, causing cells to swell and possibly burst from the increased intracellular osmotic pressure.

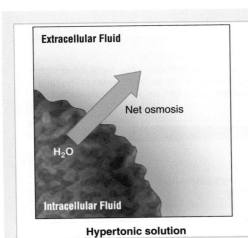
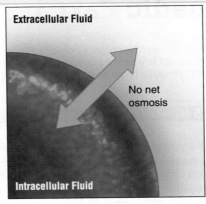
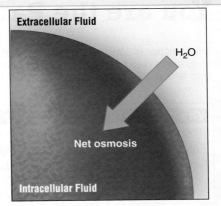

Figure 8-6 Fluid movement with hypertonic, isotonic, and hypotonic solutions.

Hypotonic solutions hydrate the cells while depleting the vascular compartment. They may be needed for a patient who is receiving dialysis when diuretic therapy dehydrates the cells. They may also be used for hyperglycaemic conditions such as diabetic ketoacidosis, in which high serum glucose levels draw fluid out of the cells and into the vascular and interstitial compartments.

Hypotonic solutions can cause a sudden fluid shift from the intravascular space to the cells, leading to cardiovascular collapse and increased intracranial pressure from shifting fluid into the brain cells. For example, giving glucose 10% for an extended period can increase intracranial pressure. This makes hypotonic solutions dangerous for patients with stroke or any head trauma. Administering these solutions to patients with burns, trauma, malnutrition, or liver disease is also hazardous because these patients are at risk for developing third spacing, an abnormal fluid shift into the interstitial compartment.

Hypertonic Solutions

A hypertonic solution has an osmolarity higher than that of serum, meaning that the solution has more ionic concentration than serum and pulls fluid and electrolytes from the intracellular and interstitial compartments into the intravascular compartment. The danger is that the cells may collapse from the increased extracellular osmotic pressure. Hypertonic solutions shift body fluids into the vascular spaces and help stabilise blood pressure, increase urine output, and reduce oedema. These fluids are rarely, if ever, used in the prehospital setting.

Often the term "hypertonic" is used to refer to solutions that contain high concentrations of proteins. These proteins have the same effect on fluid as sodium. Careful monitoring is needed to guard against fluid overloading when using hypertonic fluids, especially with patients with impaired heart or kidney function. Also, hypertonic solutions should not be given to patients with diabetic ketoacidosis or others at risk of cellular dehydration.

Crystalloid Solutions

Crystalloid solutions are dissolved crystals (eg, salts or sugars) in water. The ability of these fluids to cross membranes and alter fluid levels makes them the best choice for prehospital care of injured patients who need body fluid replacement. When you use an isotonic crystalloid for fluid replacement to support blood pressure after blood loss, remember the 3-to-1 replacement rule: *3 ml of isotonic crystalloid solution is needed to replace 1 ml of patient blood.* This amount is needed because approximately two thirds of the infused isotonic crystalloid solution will leave the vascular spaces in about 1 hour.

When you replace lost volume, it is imperative to remember that crystalloid solutions cannot carry oxygen. Boluses of 20 ml/kg should be given to maintain perfusion (ie, radial pulses, adequate mental status) but not to raise blood pressure to the patient's normal level. Increasing blood pressure too much with IV solutions not only dilutes remaining blood volume, thereby decreasing the proportion of haemoglobin, but also may increase internal bleeding by interfering with haemostasis—the body's internal blood-clotting mechanism.

At the Scene

Isotonic crystalloid solutions—normal saline and LR—replace lost volume but do not carry oxygen. Replace lost volume to maintain perfusion, but recognise the need for rapid transport.

Colloid Solutions

Colloid solutions contain molecules (usually proteins) that are too large to pass out of the capillary membranes and, therefore, remain in the vascular compartment. These very large protein molecules give colloid solutions a very high osmolarity. As a result, they draw fluid from the interstitial and intracellular compartments into the vascular compartments. Colloid solutions work very well in reducing oedema (eg, in pulmonary or cerebral

You are the Paramedic Part 3

Your partner is appropriately managing the patient's airway. The patient remains unconscious and unresponsive. Your rapid head-to-toe assessment reveals no gross injury or bleeding. The patient is wearing a medical ID bracelet that identifies her as having diabetes. The neighbour tells you that she was talking to the patient approximately 1 hour earlier and she was fine. Baseline vital signs reveal the following:

Vital Signs	Recording Time: 5 Minutes
Blood pressure	100/60 mm Hg
Pulse	120 beats/min, weak and regular
Respirations	30 breaths/min and shallow (baseline); your partner is assisting ventilation with a bag-valve-mask device connected to 15 l/min of supplemental oxygen via a reservoir
SpO_2	99% (with assisted ventilation and 15 l/min of oxygen)

5. Given the patient's history, what additional assessment should you perform?

6. When starting an IV for this patient, what solution should you use?

oedema) while expanding the vascular compartment. They could cause dramatic fluid shifts and place the patient in considerable danger if they are not administered in a controlled setting. For this reason, colloids are rarely used in the prehospital setting. Examples of colloids are albumin, dextran, hetastarch (Hespan), haemaccel, and gelofusine.

Oxygen-Carrying Solutions

Obviously, the best fluid to replace lost blood is whole blood. Unlike the crystalloid and colloid solutions, whole blood contains haemoglobin, which carries oxygen to the body's cells. On occasion (eg, aeromedical transports, major incidents), O-negative blood—a universally compatible blood type—may be used outside a hospital setting. However, because of the refrigeration requirements and other storage issues, general use of whole blood is impractical in the prehospital setting.

Synthetic blood substitutes, which do have the ability to carry oxygen, are being researched and, in some places, field-tested. They show great potential for improving the way you treat patients who have lost large amounts of blood. Not only would these synthetic blood substitutes expand circulating volume, but they also would carry and deliver oxygen to the part of the body that needs it the most—the cell.

▌ IV Techniques and Administration

Intravenous means "within a vein". Intravenous (IV) therapy involves cannulation of a vein with a cannula to access the patient's vascular system. It is one of the most frequent invasive techniques you will perform as a paramedic. Peripheral vein cannulation involves cannulating veins of the periphery—that is, veins that can be seen and/or palpated (eg, veins of the hand, arm, or lower extremity and the external jugular vein).

The most important point to remember about IV therapy is to keep the IV equipment sterile. Forethought and attention to detail will help prevent mental and procedural errors while starting the IV. One way to ensure proper technique is to develop a routine to follow as you assemble the appropriate equipment.

Assembling Your Equipment

To avoid delays and IV site contamination, gather and prepare all your equipment before you attempt to start an IV. In some cases, the patient's condition may make full preparation difficult, so working as a team becomes critical. The members of your own crew, by anticipating your needs, often make the assembly of IV equipment possible.

Choosing an IV Solution

When choosing the most appropriate IV solution, you must identify the needs of your patient. Ask yourself these questions:

- Is the patient's condition critical?
- Is the patient's condition stable?
- Does the patient need fluid replacement?
- Will the patient need medications?

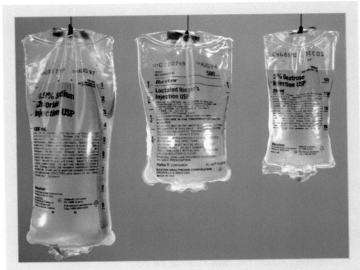

Figure 8-7 IV solution bags come in different fluid volumes.

In the prehospital setting, the choice of IV solution is usually limited to two isotonic crystalloids, normal saline and LR solution. Glucose 10% is often reserved for administering medication because the presence of dextrose has the potential to alter fluid and electrolyte levels in the body.

Each IV solution bag is wrapped in a protective sterile plastic bag and is guaranteed to remain sterile until the posted expiry date. Once the protective wrap is torn and removed, however, the IV solution must be used within 24 hours. The bottom of each IV bag has two ports: an injection port for medication and an access port for connecting the administration set. A removable blue pigtail protects the sterile access port. Once this pigtail is removed, the bag must be used immediately or discarded.

IV solution bags come in different fluid volumes **Figure 8-7 ▲**. Volumes commonly used in hospitals are 1,000 ml, 500 ml, 250 ml, 100 ml, and 50 ml; the more common prehospital volumes are 1,000 ml and 500 ml. The smaller volumes (250 ml and 100 ml) typically contain glucose 10% or saline and are used for mixing and administering maintenance medication infusions.

Choosing an Administration Set

An administration set moves fluid from the IV bag into the patient's vascular system. IV administration sets are sterile as long as they remain in their protective packaging. Each set has a piercing spike protected by a plastic cover. Once this spike is exposed and the seal surrounding the cap is broken, the set must be used immediately or discarded.

On most drip sets, a number on the package indicates the number of drops it takes for a millilitre of fluid to pass through the orifice and into the drip chamber **Figure 8-8 ▶**. Administration sets come in two primary sizes: microdrip and macrodrip. Microdrip sets allow 60 gtt (drops) per millilitre

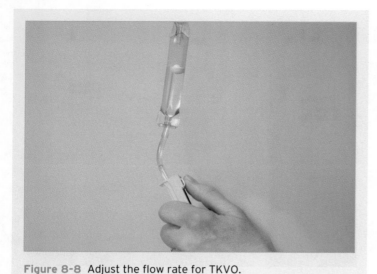

Figure 8-8 Adjust the flow rate for TKVO.

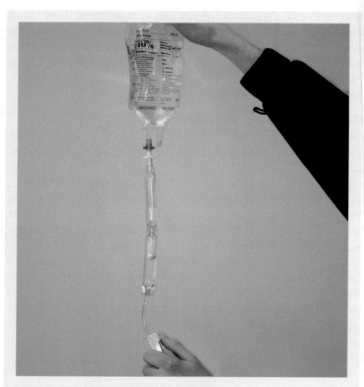

Figure 8-9 An adult fluid administration set.

(ml) through the needlelike orifice inside the drip chamber. They are ideal for medication administration or paediatric fluid delivery because it is easy to control their fluid flow. Macrodrip sets allow 10 or 15 gtt/ml through a large opening between the piercing spike and the drip chamber. They are best used for rapid fluid replacement.

Preparing an Administration Set
After choosing the IV administration set and the IV solution bag, verify the expiry date of the solution and check for solution clarity. Prepare to spike the bag with the administration set. The steps for this procedure are shown here and illustrated in **Skill Drill 8-1 ▶**:

1. Remove the rubber pigtail found on the end of the IV bag by pulling on it. The bag is still sealed and will not leak until the piercing spike punctures this port. Remove the protective cover from the piercing spike. (Remember, this spike is sterile!) **Step 1**.
2. Close the roller clamp, if it is still open. Slide the spike into the IV bag port until you see fluid enter the drip chamber **Step 2**.
3. Squeeze the drip chamber, to fill it halfway. Open the roller clamp, allowing the solution to run freely through the drip chamber and into the tubing, to prime the line and expel all the air **Step 3**.
4. Twist the protective cover on the opposite end of the IV tubing to allow air to escape. Do not remove this cover yet, because the cover keeps the tubing end sterile until it is needed. Let the fluid flow until air bubbles are removed from the line before turning the roller clamp wheel to stop the flow **Step 4**.

5. Go back and check the drip chamber; it should be only half-filled. The drip chamber is often more than half filled. The fluid level must be visible to calculate drip rates. If the fluid level is too low, squeeze the chamber until it fills; if the chamber is too full, invert the bag and the chamber and squeeze the chamber to empty the fluid back into the bag **Step 5**. Hang the bag in an appropriate location with the end of the IV tubing easily accessible.

Other Administration Sets
Blood tubing is a macrodrip administration set that is designed to facilitate rapid fluid replacement by manual infusion of IV fluids or blood products. The central drip chamber has a special filter designed to filter the blood during transfusions.

Fluid control for paediatric patients and certain older patients is very important. A microdrip set called a burette allows you to fill a 100- or 200-ml calibrated drip chamber with a specific amount of fluid and administer only that amount to avoid inadvertent fluid overload **Figure 8-9 ▲**. These are commonly used in paediatric patients. A proximal roller clamp enables you to shut off the burette drip chamber from the IV bag. If the patient needs additional fluids, simply open the proximal roller clamp and fill the burette with more fluid.

Skill Drill 8-1: Spiking the Bag

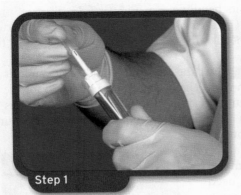

Step 1

Pull on the rubber pigtail on the end of the IV bag to remove it. Remove the protective cover from the piercing spike.

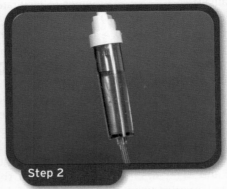

Step 2

Slide the spike into the IV bag until you see fluid enter the drip chamber.

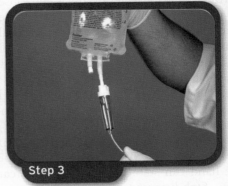

Step 3

Allow the solution to run freely through the drip chamber and into the tubing to prime the line and flush the air out of the tubing.

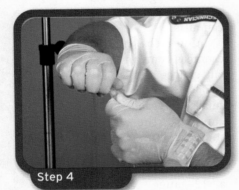

Step 4

Twist the protective cover of the opposite end of the IV tubing to allow air to escape. Do not remove this cover yet. Let the fluid flow until air bubbles are removed from the line before turning the roller clamp wheel to stop the flow.

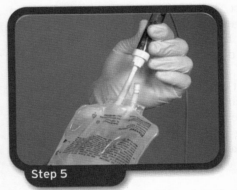

Step 5

Check the drip chamber; it should be only half-filled. If the fluid level is too low, squeeze the chamber until it fills; if the chamber is too full, invert the bag and the chamber and squeeze the chamber to empty the fluid back into the bag. Hang the bag in an appropriate location, above the height of the cannulation site.

Choosing an IV Site

It is important to select the most appropriate vein for IV cannula insertion. Avoid areas of the vein that contain valves because a cannula will not pass through these areas easily and the needle may cause damage. Valves can be recognised as small bumps located in the vein. Use the following criteria to select a vein:

- Locate the vein section with the straightest appearance
  Figure 8-10 ▶ .
- Choose a vein that has a firm, round appearance or is springy when palpated.
- Avoid areas where the vein crosses over joints.
- Avoid oedematous extremities and any extremity with a dialysis fistula or on the side a mastectomy was done.

If IV therapy is being given for a life-threatening illness or injury, this choice is often limited to the areas that remain open during hypoperfusion. Otherwise, limit IV access to the more distal areas of the extremities: *Start distally, work proximally.* If the most distal site ruptures or infiltrates, you can

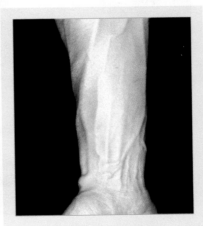

Figure 8-10 Look for veins that are relatively straight and spring back when palpated.

move up the extremity to the next appropriate site. Because failed cannulation brings the possibility of leakage into the surrounding tissues, any fluid introduced immediately below an open wound has the potential to enter the tissue and cause damage.

Large protruding arm veins can be deceiving in terms of their ease of cannulation. Often these bulging veins can roll from side to side during a cannulation attempt, causing you to miss the vein. A remedy is to apply manual traction to the vein to lock it into position. Traction techniques differ depending on the location chosen for cannulation. Hold hand veins in place by pulling the skin over the vein taut with the thumb of your free hand as you flex the patient's hand [**Figure 8-11 ▾**]. Stabilise wrist veins by flexing the wrist and pulling the skin taut over the vein. Applying lateral traction to the vein with your free hand can stabilise veins in the forearm and antecubital areas. Stabilising and cannulating the external jugular vein requires a different approach (discussed later in this chapter).

The patient's opinion should also be considered when selecting an IV site because he or she may know an IV location that has worked in the past. Avoid attempts to insert an IV in an extremity if it shows signs of trauma, injury, or infection; if it has an arteriovenous shunt for renal dialysis; or if it is on the same side a mastectomy was done. Also, pay careful attention to areas of the vein that have track marks; they are usually a sign of sclerosis caused by frequent cannulation or puncture of the vein, for example from IV drug abuse.

Some protocols allow IV cannulation of leg veins. Use caution when cannulating veins in these areas because they can place the patient at greater risk of venous thrombosis and subsequent pulmonary embolism.

Choosing an IV Cannula

Cannula selection should reflect the purpose of the IV, the age of the patient, and the location for the IV. The most common types used in the prehospital setting are over-the-needle cannulas and butterfly cannulas. An over-the-needle cannula

[**Figure 8-12 ▾**] is a Teflon cannula inserted *over* a hollow needle (eg, Angiocath, Jelco, Venflon, Accuvance). A butterfly cannula is a hollow, stainless steel needle with two plastic wings to facilitate its handling [**Figure 8-13 ▾**]. Through-the-needle cannulas (Intracaths) are plastic cannulas inserted *through* a hollow needle; these cannulas are rarely used in the prehospital setting.

[**Table 8-1 ▸**] lists the advantages and disadvantages of over-the-needle cannulas. These cannulas are preferred for use in the prehospital setting for infusing IV fluids or medications in adults and children. They are more readily secured, are less cumbersome than the butterfly cannula, and allow for greater patient movement without the need to immobilise the entire limb.

[**Table 8-2 ▸**] lists the advantages and disadvantages of butterfly cannulas.

Over-the-needle cannulas come in different gauges and lengths [**Figure 8-14 ▸**]. The smaller the gauge of the cannula, the larger the diameter. Thus a 14-gauge cannula is of larger diameter than a 22-gauge cannula; 14 gauge is the largest, 27 gauge is the smallest. The larger the diameter, the more fluid that can be delivered through it.

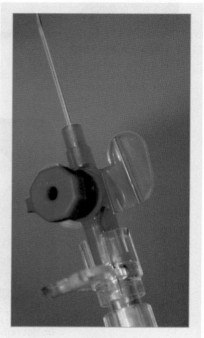
Figure 8-12 Over-the-needle cannula.

Select the largest-diameter cannula that will fit the vein you have chosen or that will be the most appropriate and comfortable for the patient. An 18- or 20-gauge cannula is usually a good size for adults who do not need fluid replacement. Metacarpal veins

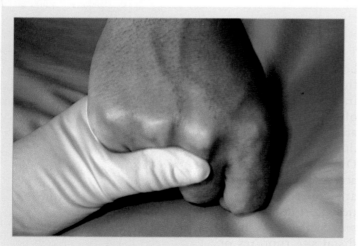
Figure 8-11 Hold hand veins in place by pulling the skin over the vein taut with the thumb of your free hand as you flex the patient's hand.

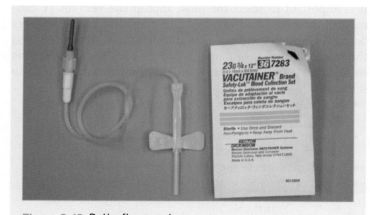
Figure 8-13 Butterfly cannula.

At the Scene

As a general rule, you should start distally and work your way up the patient's extremity when starting an IV. For patients who need rapid fluid replacement, are in cardiac arrest, or are otherwise haemodynamically unstable, however, you should use the antecubital fossa. Unlike other extremity veins (eg, hand, forearm), this vein is usually visible and easier to palpate. A neck vein or an adult IO are other options.

Special Considerations

If you are using an over-the-needle cannula to start an IV in a paediatric patient, choose among the 20-, 22-, 24-, or 26-gauge cannulas, depending on the child's age. Butterfly cannulas can be placed in the same locations as over-the-needle cannulas and in visible scalp veins in paediatric patients. Scalp veins are best used in young infants.

Table 8-1	Advantages and Disadvantages of Over-the-Needle Cannulas	
Advantages	**Disadvantages**	
■ Less likely to puncture the vein than a butterfly cannula	■ Risk of sticking the paramedic with contaminated needle as it is withdrawn	
■ More comfortable once in position	■ More difficult to insert than other devices	
■ Radiopaque for easy identification during X-ray	■ Possibility of cannula shear	

Table 8-2	Advantages and Disadvantages of Butterfly Cannulas	
Advantages	**Disadvantages**	
■ Easiest venepuncture device to insert	■ May easily cause infiltration	
■ Useful for scalp veins in infants and in small, difficult veins in older patients for obtaining blood samples	■ Possible blood cell damage when drawing blood through the butterfly cannula	
■ Small, short needles	■ Small-gauge needles limit fluid flow	

of the hand can usually accommodate 18- or 20-gauge cannulas. A 14- or 16-gauge cannula should be used when the patient requires fluid replacement (eg, for hypovolaemic shock). You should be able to insert a 14- or 16-gauge cannula into an antecubital fossa or external jugular vein in the average adult.

In recent years, an attempt has been made to create over-the-needle cannulas that minimise the risk of a needlestick—when a paramedic or technician punctures his or her skin with the same cannula that was used to cannulate the vein of a patient. For example, some of these newer cannulas offer automatic needle retraction after insertion, usually accomplished with a locking slide mechanism or a spring-loaded slide mechanism.

Inserting the IV Cannula

Each paramedic has a unique technique to insert an IV, and you should observe many different techniques to determine what works best for you. Two considerations, however, apply to *any* technique: (1) Keep the bevelled side of the cannula up when inserting the needle in a vein Figure 8-15 ▼ , and (2) maintain adequate traction on the vein during cannulation.

Apply a tourniquet above the site you have chosen for the insertion to allow blood to fill the veins. This creates additional vascular pressure to engorge the veins with blood below the band. It should be snug enough to diminish venous flow significantly but should not hamper arterial flow. The tourniquet should be left in place only long enough to complete the IV insertion, obtain blood samples (if needed), and

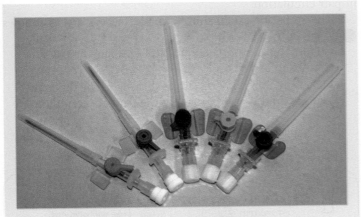

Figure 8-14 Note the difference in the lengths and diameters of over-the-needle cannulas.

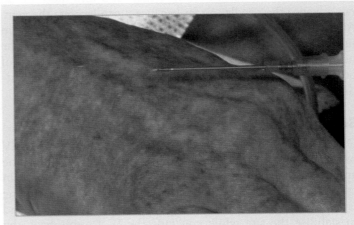

Figure 8-15 Keep the bevelled side of the cannula up when inserting the needle into a vein.

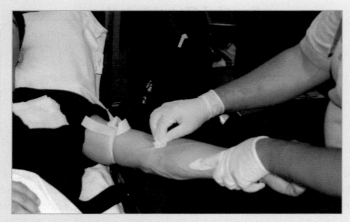

Figure 8-16 When cleansing the site for IV cannulation, use the first alcohol pad or iodine swab to clean in a circular motion from the inside out, then use the second to wipe straight down the centre of the vein.

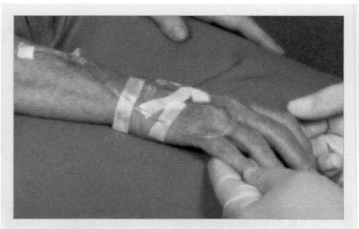

Figure 8-17 Tape the area so that the cannula and tubing are securely anchored.

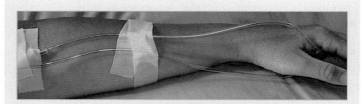

Figure 8-18 Loosely wrap the IV line around the patient's thumb and secure it to the forearm.

attach the line. *Do not leave the tourniquet in place while you assemble IV equipment.*

Tourniquets can be difficult to manage, especially if you are wearing gloves. You should develop a technique that will allow you to release the tourniquet with a small tug on one end. Items that can be used as tourniquets include a blood pressure cuff.

Once you have selected an insertion site, prep it with an alcohol swab   Figure 8-16 ▲ . Apply gentle downward or lateral traction on the vein with your free hand while holding the cannula, bevel side up, in your dominant hand. Take care as you apply traction to avoid collapsing the vein. Begin by establishing an insertion angle of about 45°. Advance the cannula through the skin until the vein is pierced (you should see a flash of blood in the cannula flash chamber); then immediately drop the angle down to about 15° and advance the cannula a few more centimetres to ensure the cannula sheath is in the vein. Slide the sheath off the needle and into the vein; do not advance the needle too far because it can lacerate the vein. After the cannula is fully advanced, apply pressure to the vein just proximal to the end of the indwelling cannula, remove the needle, and dispose of it in a sharps bin, or in the case of other style cannulas, trigger the shielding device before putting it in a sharps bin.

Securing the Line

Once the cannula is in position and the contents of the IV bag are flowing properly, you must secure the IV. Tape the area so that the cannula and tubing are securely anchored in case of a sudden pull on the line   Figure 8-17 ▶ . Tear the tape before you start the IV, because you will need one hand to stabilise the site while you tape the IV. Double back the tubing to create a loop that will act as a shock absorber if the line is pulled accidentally. Cover the insertion site with an

At the Scene

Iodine helps to make veins more visible in dark-skinned people. As with any patient, make sure the patient is not allergic to iodine.

adhesive IV dressing such as opsite, tegaderm, or veccafix. Avoid circumferential taping around any extremity, as it may impair circulation.

The steps for establishing vascular access are as follows   Skill Drill 8-2 ▶ :

1. Choose the appropriate fluid, and examine the bag for clarity and expiry date.

   Make sure that no particles are floating in the fluid and that the fluid is appropriate for the patient's condition.

At the Scene

To further stabilise the IV line, loosely wrap it around the patient's thumb and secure it to the forearm   Figure 8-18 ▲ . This will prevent disruption of the IV if the line is pulled.

2. Choose the appropriate drip set, and attach it to the fluid. A macrodrip set (eg, 10 gtt/ml) should be used for a patient who needs volume replacement; a microdrip set (eg, 60 gtt/ml) should be used for a patient who needs a medication route.

3. Fill the drip chamber by squeezing it (Step 1).

4. Flush or "prime" the tubing to remove any air bubbles by opening the roller clamp (Step 2). Make sure no errant bubbles are floating in the tubing.

5. Prepare the tape before venepuncture, or have a commercial device available (Step 3).

6. Apply gloves before making contact with the patient. Palpate a suitable vein (Step 4). Veins should be "springy" when palpated. Stay away from areas that are hard when palpated.

7. Apply the tourniquet above the intended IV site (Step 5). It should be placed approximately 15 to 25 cm above the intended site.

8. Clean the area using aseptic technique. Use an alcohol pad to wipe straight down the centre (Step 6).

9. Choose the appropriately sized cannula, twist the cannula to break the seal. Do not advance the cannula upward, as this may cause the needle to shear the cannula. Examine the cannula and discard it if you discover any imperfections (Step 7). Occasionally you will find "burrs" on the edge of the cannula.

10. Insert the cannula at an angle of approximately 45° with the bevel up while applying proximal traction with the other hand (Step 8). This traction will stabilise the vein and help to keep it from "rolling" as you work.

11. Observe for "flashback" as blood enters the cannula (Step 9). The clear chamber at the top of the cannula should fill with blood when the cannula enters the vein. If you note only a drop or two, you should gently advance the cannula further into the vein. Safety cannulas have a low flashback due to the extra mechanism.

12. Occlude the cannula to prevent blood leaking while removing the stylet (Step 10). Place the thumb of the hand not holding the cannula over the end of the cannula that is currently situated inside the vein to prevent blood running out when you remove the needle. With practice, you will be able to feel the cannula.

13. Immediately dispose of all sharps in the proper container (Step 11).

14. Attach the prepared IV line (Step 12).

15. Remove the tourniquet (Step 13).

16. Open the IV line to ensure fluid is flowing and the IV is patent. Observe for any swelling or infiltration around the IV site (Step 14). If the fluid does not flow, check whether the tourniquet has been released. If infiltration is noted, immediately stop the infusion and remove the cannula while holding pressure over the site to prevent bleeding.

17. Secure the cannula with tape or a commercial device (Step 15).

18. Secure IV tubing and adjust the flow rate while monitoring the patient (Step 16).

Documentation and Communication

To document an IV, you need to include four things:
- The gauge of the needle
- The site (for example, left forearm, left external jugular)
- The type of fluid you are administering
- The rate at which the fluid is running

For example, you may write: 16G cannula in the left ante-cubital fossa, flushed with 10 ml normal saline. Commenced infusion of normal saline at 14:45 at 120 ml per hour.

At the Scene

Helpful IV Hints
- Allow the arm to hang off the stretcher.
- Pat or rub the area.
- If you meet resistance from a valve, elevate the extremity.
- After two misses, let your colleague try (Figure 8-19 ▶).
- Try sticking without a tourniquet if the IV keeps infiltrating.
- Never pull the cannula back over the needle.
- The more IVs you perform, the more proficient you will become.

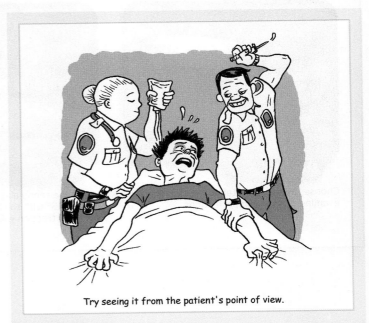

Try seeing it from the patient's point of view.

Figure 8-19

Skill Drill 8-2: Obtaining Vascular Access

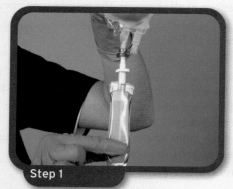

Step 1

Fill the drip chamber by squeezing it.

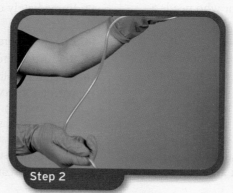

Step 2

Flush or "prime" the tubing to remove any air bubbles by opening the roller clamp.

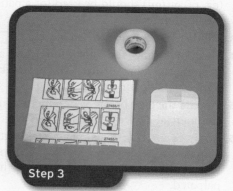

Step 3

Prepare the tape before venepuncture, or have a commercial device available.

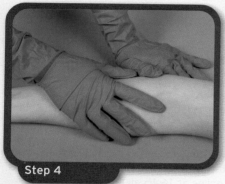

Step 4

Apply gloves before making contact with the patient. Palpate a suitable vein.

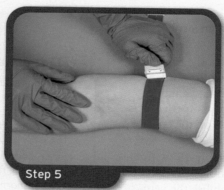

Step 5

Apply the tourniquet above the intended IV site.

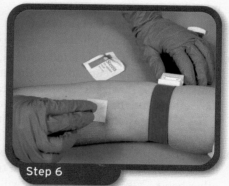

Step 6

Clean the area using aseptic technique. Use the alcohol pad to wipe straight down the centre.

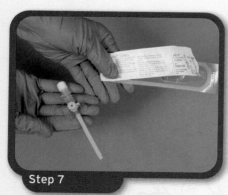

Step 7

Choose the appropriately sized cannula, and examine it for any imperfections.

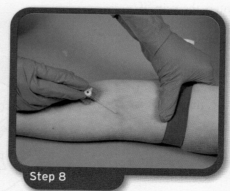

Step 8

Insert the cannula at an angle of approximately 45° with the bevel up while applying proximal traction with the other hand.

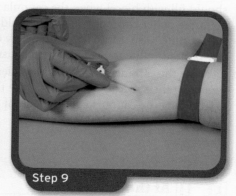

Step 9

Observe for "flashback" as blood enters the cannula.

Skill Drill 8-2: Obtaining Vascular Access (*continued*)

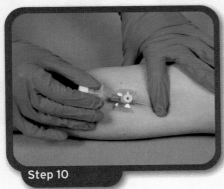

Step 10

Occlude the cannula to prevent blood leaking while removing the stylet.

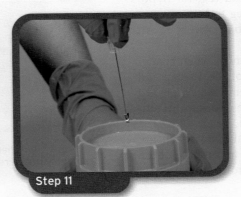

Step 11

Immediately dispose of all sharps in the proper container.

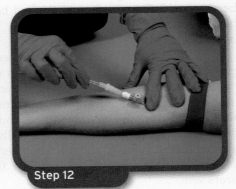

Step 12

Attach the prepared IV line.

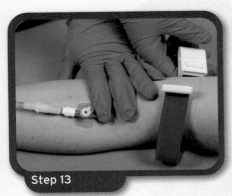

Step 13

Remove the tourniquet.

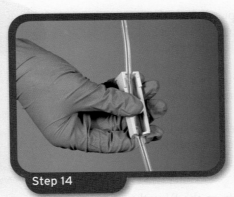

Step 14

Open the IV line to ensure fluid is flowing and the IV is patent. Observe for swelling or infiltration around the IV site.

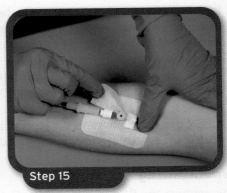

Step 15

Secure the cannula with tape or a commercial device.

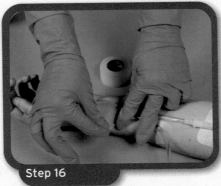

Step 16

Secure the IV tubing and adjust the flow rate while monitoring the patient.

Changing an IV Bag

You may have to change the IV bag for some patients, particularly those who require larger volumes of IV fluid (eg, for hypovolaemic shock). Do not allow an IV fluid bag to become *completely* depleted of fluid. Change the bag when about 25 ml of fluid is left.

There are two important points to remember when changing an IV bag. First, like the initial setup of the IV bag and administration set (see Skill Drill 8-1), replacing the IV bag is a sterile process. If the equipment becomes contaminated, replace it and use new equipment. Second, never allow the administration set to become depleted of fluid; always ensure that some fluid remains in the drip chamber and tubing of the set. This simple action will prevent air from entering the patient's vein.

The steps for changing an IV fluid bag are as follows:

1. Stop the flow of fluid from the depleting bag by closing the roller clamp.
2. Prepare the new IV bag by removing the pigtail from the piercing spike port. Inspect the new bag of IV fluid for clarity and discolouration and to ensure that the expiry date has not passed.
3. Remove the piercing spike from the depleted bag and insert it into the port on the new bag. *Do not touch the piercing spike of the administration set.*
4. Ensure that the drip chamber is appropriately filled, and then open the roller clamp and adjust the fluid rate accordingly.

Discontinuing the IV Line

To discontinue the IV line, shut off the flow from the IV with the roller clamp. Gently peel the tape back toward the IV site. As you get closer to the site and the cannula, stabilise the cannula while you loosen the remaining tape holding the cannula in place. Do not remove the IV tubing from the hub of the cannula. Fold a 10 cm × 10 cm piece of gauze and place it over the site, holding it down while you pull back on the hub of the cannula. Gently pull the cannula and the IV line from the patient's vein while applying pressure to control bleeding Figure 8-20 ▶ .

External Jugular Vein Cannulation

The external jugular (EJ) vein Figure 8-21 ▶ runs downward and obliquely backward behind the angle of the jaw until it pierces the deep fascia of the neck just above the middle of the clavicle. It ends in the subclavian vein, where valves retard backflow of blood. The EJ vein is fairly large and usually easy to cannulate; however, because the vein lies so near the surface of the skin, it rolls if the vein is not appropriately anchored during cannulation. It is also very near other vessels (such as the carotid artery) that may be damaged during cannulation.

You should exhaust all other means of cannulating a peripheral vein (eg, in the arm or hand) before attempting cannulation of the EJ vein. Although it is a "peripheral" vein, more

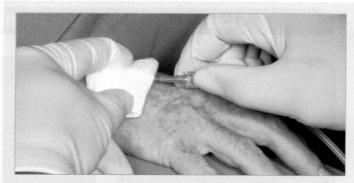

Figure 8-20 When removing a cannula and IV line, pull gently and apply pressure to control bleeding.

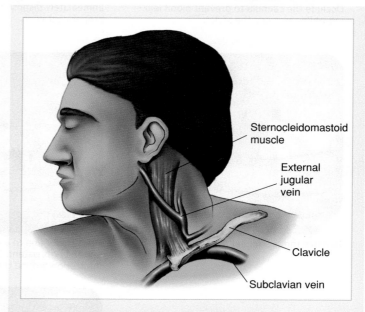

Figure 8-21 Anatomy of the external jugular vein.

risks are associated with cannulation of this vein—namely, inadvertent puncture of the carotid artery, a *rapidly* expanding haematoma if infiltration occurs, and air embolism.

Follow these steps to cannulate the external jugular vein:

1. Place the patient in a supine, head-down position to fill the jugular vein. Turn the patient's head to the side opposite the intended venepuncture site. ***Always** feel carefully for a pulse before cannulating an external jugular vein. It is imperative not to pierce the carotid artery.*
2. Appropriately cleanse the venepuncture site.
3. Occlude the jugular vein with your finger, distal to the cannula insertion site, to facilitate backflow of blood; this will allow the vein to become more visible.
4. Align the cannula in the direction of the vein, with the point aimed toward the shoulder on the side of the venepuncture Figure 8-22 ▶ .

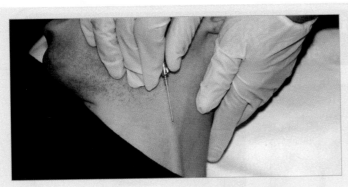

Figure 8-22 The external jugular vein requires a specific insertion site midway between the angle of the jaw and the midclavicular line with the cannula pointed toward the shoulder on the same side as the venepuncture.

5. Make the puncture midway between the angle of the jaw and the midclavicular line. Stabilise the vein by placing a finger lightly on top of it just above the clavicle.

6. Proceed as described for cannulation of a peripheral vein. *Do not let air enter the cannula once it is in the vein.*

7. Tape the line securely but do *not* put circumferential dressings around the neck.

Factors Affecting IV Flow Rates

Several factors can influence the flow rate of an IV. For example, if the IV bag is not hung high enough, the flow pressure will not be sufficient. Perform the following checks after completing IV administration and whenever a flow problem occurs:

- *Check the IV fluid.* Thick, viscous fluids such as blood products and colloid solutions infuse slowly and may be diluted to help speed delivery. Cold fluids run more slowly than warm fluids. If possible, warm IV fluids before administering them in a cold environment, according to your guidelines.
- *Check the administration set.* Macrodrips are used for rapid fluid delivery; microdrips deliver a more controlled flow.
- *Check the height of the IV bag.* The IV bag must be hung high enough to overcome gravity. Hang it about 1 m above IV site.
- *Check the type of cannula used.* The larger the diameter of the cannula (the smaller the number—for example a 14-gauge is of larger diameter than a 20-gauge), the more fluid can be delivered.
- *Check the tourniquet.* Do not leave the tourniquet on the patient's arm after completing the IV. (A common mistake with new paramedics.)

Potential Complications of IV Therapy

Problems associated with IVs can be categorised as local or systemic reactions. Local reactions include problems such as infiltration and thrombophlebitis. Systemic complications include allergic reactions and circulatory overload.

Local IV Site Reactions

Most local reactions require you to discontinue the IV and re-establish the IV in the opposite extremity. Examples of local reactions include infiltration; thrombophlebitis; occlusion; vein irritation; haematoma; nerve, tendon, or ligament damage; and arterial puncture.

Infiltration

Infiltration is the escape of fluid into the surrounding tissue, which causes a localised area of oedema. Causes of infiltration include the following problems:

- The IV passes completely through the vein and out the other side.
- The patient moves excessively.
- The tape used to secure the IV becomes loose or dislodged.
- The cannula is inserted at too shallow an angle and enters only the fascia surrounding the vein (this problem is more common with IVs in larger veins, such as those in the upper arm and neck).

Signs and symptoms of infiltration include oedema at the cannula site, continued IV flow after occlusion of the vein above the insertion site, and patient complaints of tightness and pain around the IV site.

If infiltration occurs, discontinue the IV and re-establish it in the opposite extremity or in a more proximal location on the same extremity. Apply direct pressure over the swollen area to reduce further swelling or bleeding into the tissue. Avoid wrapping tape completely around the extremity, as it could restrict the circulation distally.

Thrombophlebitis

Infection and thrombophlebitis (inflammation of the vein) may occur in association with venous cannulation; both conditions are most frequently caused by lapses in aseptic technique. Thrombophlebitis is commonly encountered in patients who abuse drugs as well as in patients who are receiving long-term IV therapy in a hospital or hospice setting or with vein-irritating solutions (eg, glucose solutions, which have a very low pH, or hypertonic solutions of any sort). It can also be produced by mechanical factors, such as excessive motion of the IV needle or cannula after it has been placed.

Thrombophlebitis is usually manifested by pain and tenderness along the vein and redness and oedema at the venepuncture site. These signs generally do not appear until after several hours of IV therapy, so you are unlikely to see a case of thrombophlebitis in the prehospital setting unless you are doing an interhospital transport of a patient with an established IV. In such a case, stop the infusion and discontinue the IV at that site. Warm compresses applied to the site may provide some relief.

It is far better to prevent thrombophlebitis or infection than to treat it afterward. To prevent thrombophlebitis, take the following measures:

- Use a povidone-iodine preparation to scrub and disinfect the skin over the venepuncture site; then do a final wipe with an alcohol swab. Make certain the site is dry before initiating the venepuncture.

- Always wear gloves when doing a venepuncture.
- After inserting the cannula, cover the puncture site with a sterile dressing.
- Anchor the cannula and tubing securely to prevent motion of the cannula within the vein.

Occlusion

Occlusion is the physical blockage of a vein or cannula. If the flow rate is not sufficient to keep fluid moving out of the cannula tip such that blood enters the cannula, a clot may form and occlude the flow. The first sign of an occlusion is a decreasing drip rate or the presence of blood in the IV tubing. With a positional IV site, fluid flows at different rates depending on the position of the cannula within the vein; these differences can produce occlusions. Positional IVs may be necessary because of proximity to a valve or because of patient movement that allows the line to become physically blocked, such as resting on the line or crossing arms. Occlusion may also develop if the IV bag is almost empty and the patient's blood pressure overcomes the flow, causing fluid backup in the line.

If occlusion occurs, follow the steps shown in **Skill Drill 8-3 ▸** to determine whether the IV should be re-established:

1. Select and assemble a sterile 10-ml syringe and large-gauge needle or a blunt-ended drawing up needle **Step 1** .
2. Draw up a 10 ml ampoule of either saline 0.9% or water for injections (depending on local policy). Expel any remaining air from the syringe **Step 2** .
3. Open the drug administration port on the top of the IV cannula and swab with an alcohol wipe (dependent on the type of cannula used). Attach the 10-ml syringe containing the flush, ensuring a snug fit **Step 3** .
4. Do not adjust the roller clamp, instead fold the tubing backwards and clip this into the rear of the roller clamp assembly. This will clamp off the line. As a secondary measure, kink the tubing with your hand, closer to the IV cannula site.

5. Apply gentle pressure to the syringe plunger to flush the line, disrupting the occlusion and re-establishing the flow. Once flushed, un-pinch and unclamp the line, to allow the IV to run freely.
6. If the flow is re-established, ensure that the line is free and that the rate has not altered from that previously set.
7. If the occlusion does not dislodge, discontinue the IV and re-establish in the opposite extremity or at a proximal location in the same extremity **Step 4** .

Skill Drill 8-3: Determining Whether an IV Is Viable

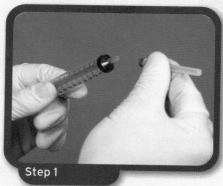

Step 1

Select and assemble a sterile 10-ml syringe and large-gauge needle or a blunt-ended drawing up needle.

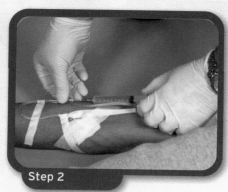

Step 2

Draw up a 10-ml ampoule of either saline 0.9% or water for injections, (depending on local policy). Expel any remaining air from the syringe.

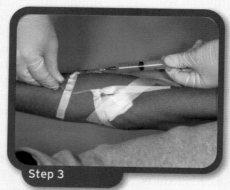

Step 3

Open the drug administration port on the top of the IV cannula and swab with an alcohol wipe. Attach the 10 ml syringe containing the flush, ensuring a snug fit.

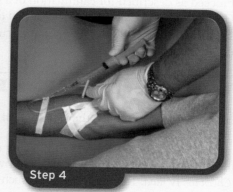

Step 4

Do not adjust the roller clamp; instead fold the tubing backwards and clip this into the rear of the roller clamp assembly. This will clamp off the line. As a secondary measure, kink the tubing with your hand, closer to the IV cannula site. Apply gentle pressure to the syringe plunger to flush the line, disrupting the occlusion and re-establishing the flow. Once flushed, un-pinch and unclamp the line, to allow the IV to run freely.

If the occlusion does not dislodge, discontinue the IV and re-establish in the opposite extremity or at a proximal location in the same extremity.

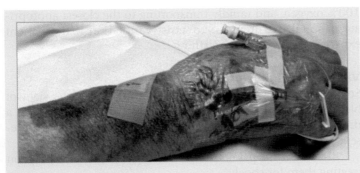

Figure 8-23 Haematomas can be caused by the improper removal of a cannula, resulting in pooling of blood around the IV site, leading to tenderness and pain.

Vein Irritation

Occasionally, a patient will experience vein irritation from the IV fluid. Patients who have this problem often complain immediately that the solution is bothering them (ie, tingling, stinging, itching, and burning). In such cases, observe the patient closely in case an allergic reaction to the fluid develops.

Vein irritation is usually caused by a too-rapid infusion rate. If redness develops at the IV site—a sign suggesting thrombophlebitis—discontinue the IV and save the equipment for later analysis. Re-establish the IV in the other extremity with new equipment in case the old equipment contained unseen contaminants.

Haematoma

A haematoma is an accumulation of blood in the tissues surrounding an IV site, often resulting from vein perforation or improper cannula removal. Blood can be seen rapidly pooling around the IV site, leading to tenderness and pain Figure 8-23 ▲ . Patients with a history of vascular diseases (including diabetes) and patients taking certain medications (eg, corticosteroids or a blood thinner like Warfarin) can have a predisposition to vein rupture or to haematoma development with IV insertion.

If a haematoma develops while you are attempting to insert a cannula, stop and apply direct pressure to help minimise bleeding. If a haematoma develops after a successful cannula insertion, evaluate the IV flow and the haematoma. If the haematoma appears to be controlled and the flow is not affected, monitor the IV site and leave the line in place. If the haematoma develops as a result of discontinuing the IV, apply direct pressure with a 10 cm × 10 cm gauze pad to the site.

Nerve, Tendon, or Ligament Damage

Incorrect identification of anatomical structures around the IV site can lead to perforation of tendons, ligaments, and nerves. Selecting an IV site located near joints increases the risk for perforation of these structures. When this type of injury occurs, patients will experience sudden and severe shooting pain. Numbness or tingling in the extremity after the incident is common. Immediately remove the cannula and select another IV site.

Arterial Puncture

You may accidentally puncture the wrong blood vessel if the vein selected for cannulation lies near an artery. *The risk of arterial puncture is especially high when cannulating an external jugular vein—be careful!* If you insert a cannula into an artery by mistake, bright red blood will spurt back through the cannula. The blood's colour and its flow characteristics will alert you to your error. *Immediately withdraw the cannula, and apply direct pressure over the puncture site for at least 5 minutes or until bleeding stops.*

To avoid cannulating an artery, always check for a pulse in any vessel you intend to cannulate. Under normal circumstances, veins are near the skin surface and arteries lie much deeper. On occasion, an anatomical anomaly occurs and the vessels become transpositioned, resulting in an artery being very superficial.

Systemic Complications

Systemic complications can evolve from reactions or complications associated with IV insertion. They usually involve other body systems and can be life-threatening. If the IV line is established and patent in such a patient, do not remove it because it may be needed for treatment. Potential systemic complications include allergic reactions, pyrogenic reactions, circulatory overload, air embolus, vasovagal reactions, and cannula shear.

Allergic Reactions

Often, allergic reactions associated with IV therapy are minor. However, anaphylaxis—a potentially life-threatening condition— is possible and must be treated aggressively. Allergic reactions can result from a person's unexpected sensitivity to an IV fluid or medication. Such sensitivity could be unknown to the patient, so you must maintain vigilance with any IV for a possible allergic reaction.

The patient presentation depends on the extent of the reaction. Common signs and symptoms of an allergic reaction include itching (pruritus), shortness of breath, oedema of the face and hands, urticaria (hives), bronchospasm, and wheezing.

If an allergic reaction occurs, discontinue the IV and remove the solution. Leave the cannula in place as an emergency medication route. Maintain an open airway. Monitor the patient's ABCs and vital signs. Keep the solution or medication for evaluation by the hospital (Chapter 30 covers allergic reactions and anaphylaxis in more detail).

Pyrogenic Reactions

Pyrogens are foreign proteins capable of producing fever. Their presence in the infusion solution or administration set may induce a pyrogenic reaction, which is characterised by an abrupt rise in temperature (as high as 41.1°C) with severe chills, backache, headache, weakness, nausea, and vomiting. Occasionally vascular collapse occurs, with all the signs and symptoms of shock. The reaction usually begins within 30 minutes after the IV infusion has been started.

If you observe *any* signs of such a reaction—for example, if the patient complains of a headache or backache after you have started running fluids—*stop the infusion immediately!* Start a new IV in the other arm with a *fresh infusion solution,* and then remove the first IV. If the patient is showing signs of shock, treat as any other case of shock.

Pyrogenic reactions can be largely avoided by inspecting the IV bag carefully before use. If the bag has any leaks or if the fluid looks cloudy or discoloured, select another bag.

Circulatory Overload

Healthy adults can handle as much as 2 to 3 extra litres of fluid without compromise. Problems occur, however, when the patient has cardiac, pulmonary, or renal dysfunction; these types of dysfunction do not tolerate any additional demands from increased circulatory volume. The most common cause of circulatory overload in the prehospital setting is failure to readjust the drip rate after flushing an IV line immediately after insertion. Always monitor the IV to ensure the proper drip rate. If available, consider using a burette administration set for patients who are at risk for circulatory overload.

Signs and symptoms of circulatory overload include dyspnoea, jugular vein distention, and hypertension. Crackles (rales) are often heard when evaluating breath sounds. Acute peripheral oedema can also be an indication of circulatory overload.

To treat a patient with circulatory overload, slow the IV rate to keep the vein open and raise the patient's head to ease respiratory distress. Administer high-flow oxygen, and monitor vital signs and breathing adequacy. Certain drugs can be given to reduce the circulatory volume.

> **Special Considerations**
>
> It is easy to overload older patients who need large amounts of IV fluids. Administer small boluses of fluid (200 to 300 ml), and check breath sounds before and after each bolus to ensure that the lungs remain "dry".

Air Embolus

Healthy adults can tolerate as much as 200 ml of air introduced into the circulatory system. For patients who are already ill or injured, however, *any* air introduced into the IV line can present a problem. Properly flushing an IV line will help eliminate the likelihood of air embolus. Although IV bags are designed to collapse as they empty to help prevent this problem, this collapse does not always occur. Be sure to replace IV bags with full ones when down to 25 ml.

If your patient begins developing respiratory distress with unequal breath sounds, consider the possibility of an air embolus. Other associated signs and symptoms include cyanosis (even in the presence of high-flow oxygen), signs and symptoms of shock, loss of consciousness, and respiratory arrest.

Treat a patient with a suspected air embolus by placing the patient on his or her left side with the head down to trap any air inside the right atrium or right ventricle, administering

100% oxygen, and rapidly transporting to the closest appropriate hospital. Be prepared to assist ventilation if the patient experiences inadequate breathing.

Vasovagal Reactions

Some patients have anxiety concerning needles or the sight of blood. Such anxiety may cause vasculature dilation, leading to a drop in blood pressure and patient collapse. Patients can present with anxiety, diaphoresis, nausea, and syncopal episodes.

Treatment for patients with vasovagal reactions centres on treating them for shock:

1. Place patient in shock position.
2. Apply high-flow oxygen, at 15 l/min.
3. Monitor vital signs.
4. Establish an IV in case fluid resuscitation is needed.

Cannula Shear

Cannula shear occurs when part of the cannula is pinched against the needle, and the needle slices through the cannula, creating a free-floating segment. The cannula segment can then travel through the circulatory system and possibly end up in the pulmonary circulation, causing a pulmonary embolus. Treatment involves surgical removal of the sheared tip. If you suspect a cannula shear, place the patient in a left lateral recumbent position with his or her legs down and head up to try to keep the cannula remnant out of the pulmonary circulation.

Cannula hubs are radiopaque (ie, they appear white in an X-ray) to aid in diagnosing this type of problem. Never rethread a cannula. Dispose of the used one and select a new cannula.

Patients who have experienced cannula shear with pulmonary artery occlusion present with sudden dyspnoea, shortness of breath, and possibly diminished breath sounds. Their symptoms mimic the presentation of an air embolus and can be treated the same way. Such patients need continued IV access, and you must try to obtain an IV site in the right arm or leg.

> *Notes from Nancy*
>
> Once a cannula has been advanced over a needle, never, never, never pull it back!

Whenever your patients experience complications at the scene, remember to document these complications accurately.

Obtaining Blood Samples

Blood samples are sometimes taken in the prehospital setting. This is an area of practice that is generally agreed locally, between ambulance service providers and the hospitals within their region. If local policy includes obtaining blood samples, this should be done at the same time as starting the IV. If you have difficulty drawing blood, however, stop and finish the IV.

To obtain blood samples, you will need a cylindrical device that can either be used in conjunction with a needle, or which can be attached to the end of a cannula, this is known as a Vacutainer. The blood sample tubes are inserted into the Vacutainer, after it has been attached to an already sited cannula, or after the Vacutainer and needle have entered a vein. This is the safest recommended method for obtaining samples, as it forms a relatively needleless system.

In the absence of a Vacutainer, a conventional syringe and needle assembly can be used. This however, is not a recommended practice, particularly in the prehospital setting, as it involves recurrent tube punctures with a "live" needle and is extremely hazardous.

To obtain blood samples using a Vacutainer, connected to an established IV cannula, follow these steps:

1. Ensure that the tourniquet is still applied, or reapply it at this stage, to promote venous filling. Ensure you adopt universal precautions.

2. Following the recommended order of draw (explained later), insert each blood tube in turn, allowing it to fill to the line Figure 8-24 ▶ .

3. Once the desired amount of blood has been obtained, remove the tourniquet and apply pressure over the cannula site. Disconnect the Vacutainer and attach either IV fluids or a stopper to the open cannula port.

4. Discard the Vacutainer in a sharps bin.

5. Label each tube with the patient's details to prevent the risk of mixing up samples with those from another patient. Do it immediately.

The types of blood sample tubes available will vary depending on local laboratory systems, so it is important that you familiarise yourself with locally agreed systems and equipment. Each tube top is colour coded. Generally, the red- or pink-topped tube contains no additives and is used to obtain samples for typing and cross-matching of blood products. The blue-topped tube contains additives facilitating clotting screens. The green- or yellow-topped tubes contain additives facilitating evaluation of urea and electrolytes and other biochemistry tests, and purple-topped tubes contain additives facilitating examination of a patient's full blood count and some other haematology tests. Get to know the systems used in your area of work. The order of draw refers to the order in which the samples are obtained. This is important, due to the potential cross-contamination of samples with differing additives. The order of draw will be decided locally, dependant upon the tube system used, so it is important that you ensure familiarity with local systems and guidelines. Generally, samples are drawn in the following order: tubes with no additives, followed by coagulation samples and finally, tubes with any other additives.

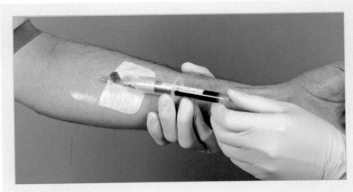

Figure 8-24 Obtaining blood samples with a Vacutainer.

Once the sample tubes have been filled, gently turn them back and forth several times to mix the additives and blood evenly. The exception to this is the tube for transfusion blood typing and crossmatch, which is intended to separate the serum from other blood components. Avoid shaking this tube after the blood has clotted, because the motion may destroy the sample.

For blood samples to be viable for testing, they must be at least three quarters full or to the line. Follow local guidelines relating to this.

Intraosseous Infusion

Intraosseous means "within the bone". Intraosseous (IO) infusion is a technique of administering fluids, blood and blood products, and medications into the intraosseous space of a long bone, usually the proximal tibia.

Long bones consist of a shaft (diaphysis), the ends (epiphyses), and the growth plate (epiphyseal plate) Figure 8-25 ▶ .

The intraosseous (IO) space collectively comprises the spongy cancellous bone of the epiphyses and the medullary cavity of the diaphysis. Its vasculature drains into the central circulation by a network of venous sinuses and canals.

When a patient is in shock, cardiac arrest, or an otherwise haemodynamically compromised condition, peripheral veins often collapse, making IV access extremely difficult, if not impossible. However, the IO space remains patent, unless the patient has suffered trauma to its bony structure (eg, a fracture). For this reason, the IO space is commonly referred to as a "noncollapsible vein". It quickly absorbs IV fluids and medications and rapidly gets them to the central circulation—as rapidly as is possible with the IV route. Anything that can be given via the IV route—crystalloids, medications, and blood and blood products—can be given via the IO route.

IO infusion is indicated when you are unable to obtain IV access in a critically ill or injured patient (eg, in profound shock, cardiac arrest, or status epilepticus). Historically, IO

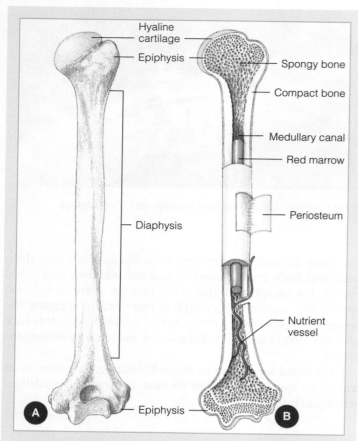

Figure 8-25 The components of a long bone. **A.** The humerus. Note the long shaft and dilated ends. **B.** Longitudinal section of the humerus showing compact bone, cancellous (spongy) bone, and marrow.

infusion was reserved for children younger than 6 years when IV access could not be obtained within 3 attempts or 90 seconds. Although this still holds true, IO infusion is also advocated as an alternative means of establishing vascular access in critically ill or injured adults. This practice is, however, governed by local ambulance service provider policy.

Equipment for IO Infusion

Several products are used for placing an IO needle into the IO space: manually inserted IO needles, the F.A.S.T.1, the EZ-IO, and the Bone Injection Gun (BIG). Use of these devices requires specialised training and thorough familiarity with each device's features, functionality, and clinical application. If your ambulance service uses any of these devices, follow local guidelines regarding their application.

Manually inserted IO needles (eg, Jamshedi needle, Cook cannula) were the original devices used for establishing IO access in children and are still widely used in the prehospital setting. They consist of a solid boring needle (trocar) inserted through a sharpened hollow needle (Figure 8-26 ▶). The IO

needle is pushed into the bone with a screwing, twisting action. Once the needle pops through the bone, the solid needle is removed, leaving the hollow steel needle in place. The IV tubing is attached to this cannula.

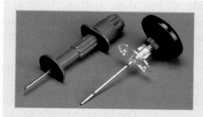

Figure 8-26 Manually inserted IO needles.

Because manually inserted IO needles are long, rest at a 90° angle to the bone, and are easily dislodged, they require full and careful stabilisation. Stabilisation is critical for these lines to maintain adequate flow. Stabilise the IO needle in the same manner that you would any impaled object, rolls of tape work well.

The F.A.S.T.1 (First Access for Shock and Trauma) was the first IO device approved for use in adults; *it is not used in children.* Four design elements allow for this device's IO placement in the sternum: an infusion tube and subcutaneous portal, an introducer, a target/strain relief patch, and a protective dome (Figure 8-27 ▾). The company that developed the F.A.S.T.1 chose sternum placement based on the ease of locating the manubrium and the easier penetration than other bones.

The EZ-IO features a hand-held battery-powered driver, to which a special IO needle is attached (Figure 8-28 ▶). This device is used to insert an IO needle into the proximal tibia of adults and children when IV access is difficult or impossible to obtain. The battery-powered driver of the EZ-IO is universal, but different sizes of needles are available for adults and children.

The Bone Injection Gun (BIG) is a spring-loaded device that is used to insert an IO needle into the proximal tibia of adult and paediatric patients. It comes in an adult size (Figure 8-29 ▶) and a paediatric size (Figure 8-30 ▶), though both versions offer the same operational features.

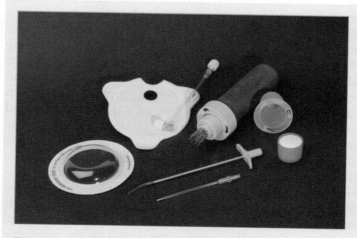

Figure 8-27 F.A.S.T.1 sternal IO device.

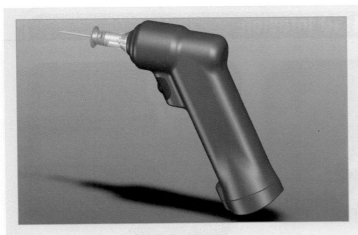

Figure 8-28 EZ-IO.

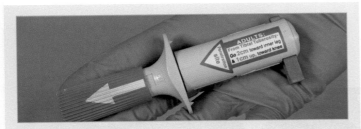

Figure 8-29 Adult BIG.

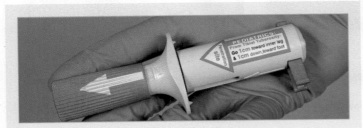

Figure 8-30 Paediatric BIG.

Performing IO Infusion

The technique for performing IO infusion requires proper anatomical landmark identification. The flat bone of the proximal tibia—the most commonly used site—is located medial to the tibial tuberosity, the bony protuberance just below the knee.

Follow these steps to perform IO infusion using a manually inserted IO needle **Skill Drill 8-4 ▶**.

1. Check the selected IV fluid for proper fluid, clarity, and expiry date. Look for discolouration and for particles floating in the fluid. If found, discard the bag and choose another bag of fluid.

2. Select the appropriate equipment, including an IO needle, syringe, saline, and extension set **Step 1**. A three-way

tap may also be used to facilitate easier fluid administration.

3. Select the proper administration set. Connect the administration set to the bag.

   Prepare the administration set. Fill the drip chamber and flush the tubing. Make sure all air bubbles are removed from the tubing.

4. Prepare the syringe and extension tubing.

5. Cut or tear the tape. This can be done at any time before IO puncture.

6. Adopt universal precautions **Step 2**. *This must be done before IO puncture.*

7. Identify the proper anatomical site for IO puncture **Step 3**. When using the BIG in an adult, go 2 cm from the tibial tuberosity toward the inner leg, and then 1 cm up toward the knee. When using the EZ-IO, go down 2 cm from the patella to the tibial tuberosity, then 1 cm toward the inner leg. It is important to avoid penetrating the epiphyseal (growth) plate in children. When using the BIG in a child, go 1 to 2 cm from the tibial tuberosity toward the inner leg, and then 1 cm down toward the foot.

8. Cleanse the site appropriately. Follow aseptic technique by cleansing in a circular manner from the inside out.

9. Perform the IO puncture, by first stabilising the tibia, then placing a folded towel or bag of fluid under the knee, and finally holding in a manner to keep your fingers away from the site of puncture.

10. Insert the needle at a 90° angle to the leg. Advance the needle with a twisting motion until a "pop" is felt **Step 4**. Unscrew the cap, and remove the stylet from the needle **Step 5**.

11. Attach the syringe and extension set to the IO needle. Pull back on the syringe to aspirate blood and particles of bone marrow to ensure proper placement.

12. Slowly inject saline to ensure proper placement of the needle. Watch for extravasation, and stop the infusion immediately if it is noted. It is possible to fracture the bone during insertion of the IO. If this happens, you should remove the IO and switch to the other leg.

13. Connect the administration set and adjust the flow rate as appropriate **Step 6**. Fluid does not flow as rapidly through an IO cannula as through an IV line; therefore, crystalloid boluses should be given with a syringe in children and a pressure infuser device in adults.

14. Secure the needle with tape, and support it with a bulky dressing. Stabilise in place in the same manner that an impaled object is stabilised. Use bulky dressings around the cannula, and tape securely in place. Be careful not to tape around the entire circumference of the leg, as this could impair circulation and potentially result in compartment syndrome **Step 7**.

15. Dispose of the needle in the proper container.

Skill Drill 8-4: IO Infusion

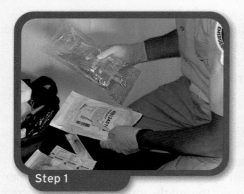

Step 1

Check selected IV fluid for proper fluid, clarity, and expiry date.
Select the appropriate equipment, including an IO needle, syringe, saline, and extension tubing.
Select the proper administration set. Connect the administration set to the bag. Prepare the administration set, syringe, and extension tubing.

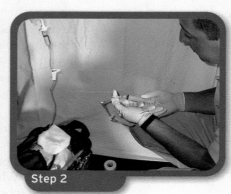

Step 2

Take universal precautions.

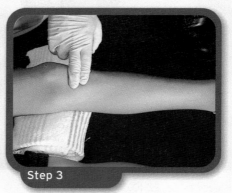

Step 3

Identify the proper anatomical site for IO puncture.

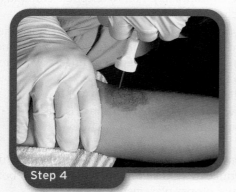

Step 4

Cleanse the site appropriately.
Stabilise the tibia, and insert the needle at a 90° angle, advancing it with a twisting motion until a "pop" is felt.

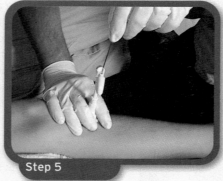

Step 5

Unscrew the cap, and remove the stylet from the needle.

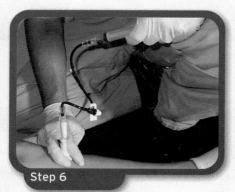

Step 6

Attach the syringe and extension set to the IO needle.
Pull pack on the syringe to aspirate blood and particles of bone marrow to ensure proper placement.
Slowly inject saline to ensure proper placement of the needle.
Watch for extravasation, and stop the infusion immediately if it is noted.
Connect the administration set, and adjust the flow rate as appropriate.

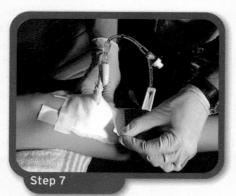

Step 7

Secure the needle with tape, and support it with bulky dressing.

Potential Complications of IO Infusion

If proper technique is used (ie, proper anatomical landmark identification, aseptic technique), IO infusion is associated with a relatively low complication rate. The same potential complications associated with IV therapy—thrombophlebitis, local irritation, allergic reaction, circulatory overload, and air embolism—can occur with IO infusion, as well as several others unique to this method of infusion.

Extravasation occurs when the IO needle does not rest in the IO space, but rather rests outside the bone (because the bone was missed completely or is fractured). In such a case, IV fluid will collect in the soft tissues. The risk of extravasation can be reduced significantly by using the proper insertion technique: *Insert the IO needle at a 90° angle to the bone.* Extravasation should be suspected if the infusion does not run freely or if the site—especially the posterior aspect of the leg—rapidly becomes oedematous. If this occurs, discontinue the infusion immediately and reattempt insertion in the opposite leg. Undetected extravasation could result in compartment syndrome.

Osteomyelitis is inflammation of the bone and muscle caused by an infection. According to several studies, osteomyelitis occurs in fewer than 0.6% of IO insertions.

Failure to identify the proper anatomical landmark can damage the growth plate, potentially resulting in long-term bone growth abnormalities in children.

If your insertion technique is too forceful, or if you use an IO needle that is too large for the patient's age or size, fractures can occur.

Through-and-through insertion occurs when the IO needle passes through *both* sides of the bone. To avoid this, stop inserting the needle when you feel a pop. If you feel a "pop, pop", it is probable you have passed the needle through both sides of the bone. Remove the needle and attempt insertion on the opposite extremity with a new needle.

A pulmonary embolism (PE) can occur if particles of bone, fat, or marrow find their way into the systemic circulation and lodge in a pulmonary artery. Suspect a PE if the patient experiences acute shortness of breath, pleuritic chest pain, and cyanosis.

Contraindications to IO Infusion

Cannulation of a peripheral vein remains the preferred route for administering IV fluids and medications. If a functional IV line is available—in a paediatric patient or an adult—IO cannulation is *not* indicated. Other contraindications to IO cannulation and infusion include fracture of the bone intended for IO cannulation, osteoporosis, osteogenesis imperfecta (a congenital disease resulting in fragile bones), and bilateral knee replacements (obviously more relevant in adults).

At the Scene

With the exception of the F.A.S.T.1 sternal IO device, all IO devices—manual, spring-loaded, and battery-powered—are primarily used to insert an IO needle into the IO space of the proximal tibia. However, other anatomical locations, such as the distal tibia and distal femur, may also be acceptable locations for IO needle insertion.

Calculating Fluid Infusion Rates

Once the IV or IO cannula is in place, you need to adjust the flow rate according to the patient's clinical condition. To do so, you must know the following information:

- The volume to be infused
- The period over which it is to be infused
- The properties of the administration set you are using—that is, how many drops per millilitre (gtt/ml) it delivers

Documentation and Communication

When you start an IV for the purpose of administering a medication, you should set the flow rate just slow enough to keep the vein patent. This slow flow rate can be documented using the acronym TKVO, which stands for To Keep Vein Open.

By knowing in advance the volume to be infused, the period over which it will be infused, and the properties of the administration set, you can easily calculate the flow rate:

$$\text{gtt/min} = \frac{\text{volume to be infused} \times \text{gtt/ml of administration set}}{\text{total time of infusion } in \text{ minutes}}$$

For example, suppose an infusion of 1 l (1,000 ml) of normal saline is to be infused in 4 hours, and the macrodrip administration set provides 10 gtt/ml:

Total volume to be infused = 1,000 ml
gtt/ml of the administration set = 10
Time of infusion (in minutes) = 240

$$\text{gtt/min} = \frac{1,000 \text{ ml} \times 10 \text{ gtt/ml}}{240 \text{ minutes}} = \text{approximately 42 gtt/min}$$

At the Scene

If a specific number of millilitres to be administered per hour (ml/h), a quick and easy way to calculate the number of drops per minute (gtt/min) is to divide the number of millilitres per hour:

- By 6, if using a macrodrip that provides 10 gtt/ml
- By 4, if using a macrodrip that provides 15 gtt/ml
- By 1, if using a microdrip set that provides 60 gtt/ml

Medication Administration

Before administering any medication to a patient, you must have a thorough understanding of how the medication will affect the human body—negatively and positively. This includes familiarity with the medication's mechanism of action, indications, contraindications, side effects, routes of administration, paediatric and adult doses, and antidotes (if available) for adverse reactions (see Chapter 7).

The first rule of medicine is *primum non nocere,* "The first thing (is) to do no harm". For example, administering the drug atropine to a patient with asymptomatic bradycardia could result in undesirable tachycardia and potential haemodynamic compromise. As a result, you have caused harm to the patient who otherwise did not need the drug. It is, therefore, paramount to ensure that a particular drug is clearly indicated to treat the patient's condition.

You must also have an understanding of basic maths for pharmacology to calculate the appropriate medication dose. This section begins with a review of basic mathematical principles as they apply to pharmacology and concludes with the various methods of medication administration.

Drug doses and flow rate calculations are often sources of confusion for many prehospital personnel, yet they are skills you will need to utilise frequently in the prehospital environment and during your initial training while practising at skill stations. As a paramedic, you must learn to calculate medication doses quickly and accurately, to maximise the chance for a positive patient outcome. Disastrous results, including death, may be the outcome if you administer an inappropriate drug or dose, give it by the wrong route, or give the medication too rapidly or too slowly.

Mathematical Principles Used in Pharmacology

The Metric System

The metric system is a decimal system based on multiples of ten (**Figure 8-31 ▾**). In this system, the basic unit of length is the metre (m), the basic unit of volume is the litre (l), and the basic unit of weight is the gram (g). Prefixes indicate the fraction of the base being used. Commonly used prefixes, from smallest to largest, include *micro-* (0.000001), *milli-* (0.001), *centi-* (0.01), and *kilo-* (1,000).

Drugs are supplied in a variety of weights and volumes, and you will be required to convert those weights to volume to administer the appropriate dose of a medication to your patient. (**Table 8-3 ▸**) lists the symbols of weight and volume, with their respective abbreviations, that are used in the metric system. (**Table 8-4 ▸**) lists the metric units of weight and volume and their equivalents.

Weight and Volume Conversion

To administer the appropriate dose of a medication to a patient, you must be able to convert larger units of weight to smaller ones (for example, g to mg) and larger units of volume to smaller ones (for example, l to ml). Conversely, you must be able to convert smaller units of weight to larger ones (for example, mg to g) and smaller units of volume to larger ones (for example, ml to l).

Drugs are packaged in different units of weight and volume. However, the weight (for example, µg, mg, g) and volume (for example, ml) of the drug to be administered usually comprise only a fraction of the total amount of its packaged form. For example, you may order 50 mg of a drug for a patient, but the drug is packaged in grams. Therefore, you must be able to convert grams to milligrams and then determine how much volume is required to achieve the desired dose.

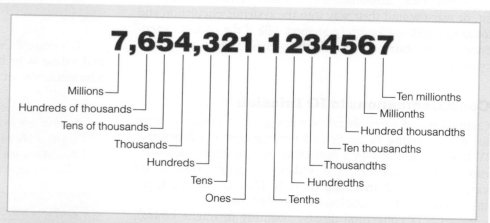

Figure 8-31 Decimal scale.

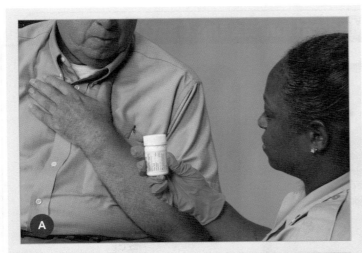

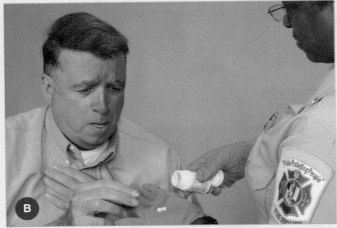

Figure 8-35 Administering an oral medication. **A.** Check the medication and its expiry date. **B.** Have the patient take the medication. Provide a glass or cup of water if necessary.

1. Take universal precautions.
2. Confirm proper gastric tube placement. Attach a 60-ml cone-tipped syringe to the gastric tube and slowly inject air as you or your partner auscultates over the epigastrium (Step 1).

    To further confirm proper placement, withdraw on the plunger of the syringe and observe for the return of gastric contents in the tube. Leave the gastric tube open to air.
3. Draw up 30 to 60 ml of normal saline into the syringe, and irrigate the gastric tube (Step 2). If you meet resistance, ensure that the tube is not kinked.
4. Draw up the appropriate amount of medication, and slowly inject it into the gastric tube (Step 3).
5. Inject 30 to 60 ml of normal saline into the gastric tube following administration of the medication (Step 4). This will ensure that the tube is flushed and that the patient has received the entire dose of the medication.
6. Clamp off the proximal end of the gastric tube (Step 5). Do not attach the gastric tube to suction because this will result in removal of the medication from the stomach.

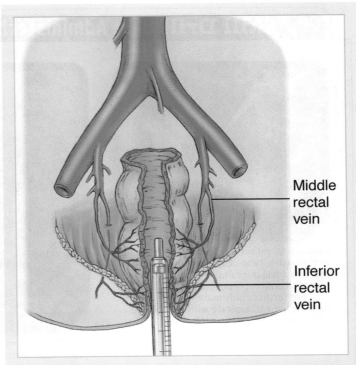

Figure 8-36 The rectal mucosa is highly vascular. It rapidly and predictably absorbs medications.

Monitor the patient for adverse reactions. Repeat the medication dose if indicated.

Rectal Medication Administration

Certain drugs may be administered rectally if you are unable to establish IV or IO access. In the prehospital environment, diazepam (Valium) can be administered rectally in paediatric patients because IV access can be challenging enough under normal circumstances, and even more so when the child is having a seizure. Because the rectal mucosa is highly vascular, medication absorption is rapid and predictable (**Figure 8-36** ▲). Certain antiemetic medications are available in suppository form (eg, promethazine [Phenergan]), and under certain circumstances, you might be asked to administer them. A suppository is a drug mixed in a firm base that melts at body temperature and is shaped to fit the rectum.

Follow these steps to administer a drug via the rectal route:

1. Take universal precautions.
2. Determine the need for the medication based on patient presentation.
3. Obtain a focused history and physical examination, including any drug allergies.
4. Follow clinical guidelines or contact medical control for advice.
5. Determine the appropriate dose, and check that the medication is the right medication, there is no cloudiness or discolouration, and the expiry date has not passed.

Skill Drill 8-5: Administering Medication via the Gastric Tube

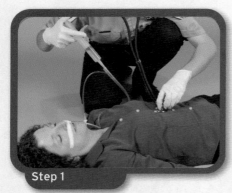

Step 1

Attach a 60-ml syringe to the proximal end of the gastric tube, and slowly inject air into the tube while auscultating over the epigastrium to confirm proper placement.

For further confirmation of correct tube placement, aspirate with the syringe and observe for gastric contents.

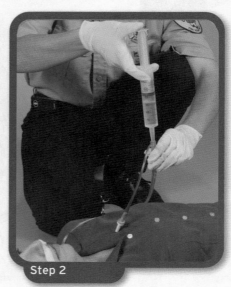

Step 2

Inject 30 to 60 ml of normal saline into the gastric tube to irrigate the tube.

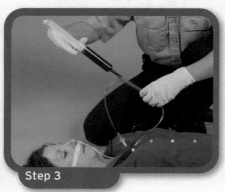

Step 3

Inject the appropriate amount of medication into the gastric tube.

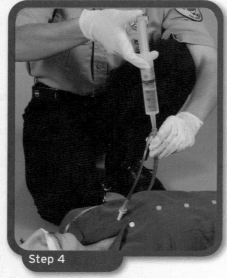

Step 4

Flush the gastric tube with 30 to 60 ml of normal saline to ensure dispersal of the drug into the stomach.

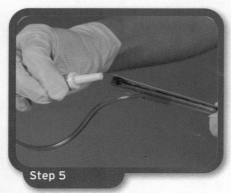

Step 5

Clamp off the proximal end of the gastric tube; do not reattach the tube to suction.

Monitor the patient for adverse reactions, and repeat the medication dose if indicated.

6. When inserting a suppository, use a water-soluble gel for lubrication. Insert the suppository into the rectum approximately 2 to 3 cm while instructing the patient to relax and not to bear down.

7. For medications in liquid form, some modifications are needed. You may use a nasopharyngeal airway or a small endotracheal tube as your delivery device.
   - Lubricate the end of the nasal airway or endotracheal tube with a water-soluble gel, and gently insert it approximately 2 to 3 cm into the rectum (Figure 8-37 ▶).
   - Instruct the patient to relax and not to bear down.
   - With a *needleless* syringe, gently push the medication through the tube.
   - Once the medication has been delivered, remove and dispose of the tube or syringe in an appropriate container.

8. Monitor the patient's condition, and document the medication given, route, time of administration, and response of the patient.

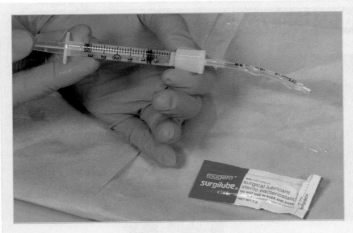

Figure 8-37 Syringe attached to an endotracheal tube.

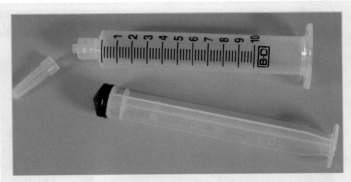

Figure 8-38 A syringe consists of a plunger, body or barrel, flange, and tip.

At the Scene

Diazepam (Valium) is available in a specially designed container, which is marketed under the name Stesolid. The distal end of the container is tapered, which facilitates insertion into the rectum. This feature eliminates the need for syringes or other methods of injecting the medication into the rectum.

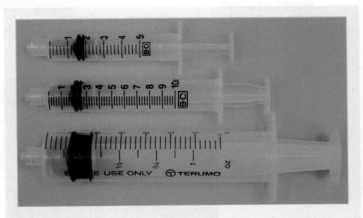

Figure 8-39 Syringes come in a variety of sizes. Some come with needles already attached, others without needles attached.

Parenteral Medication Administration

The parenteral route refers to any route other than the gastrointestinal tract. Parenteral routes for medication administration include the subcutaneous, intramuscular, intravenous, intraosseous, and percutaneous routes. Compared with enterally administered medications (eg, oral, gastric tube), parenterally administered medications are absorbed into the central circulation more quickly and at a more predictable rate, thus achieving their therapeutic effects faster. Of the parenteral drug routes, IV administration is the route most commonly used in the prehospital setting and generally is the quickest route for getting medication into the central circulation.

Syringes and Needles

A variety of needles and syringes are used for administering parenteral medications. The needles and syringes are usually packaged separately. Syringes consist of a plunger, body or barrel, flange, and tip 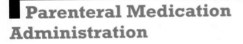. Most syringes are marked with 10 calibrations per millilitre on one side of the barrel, where each small line represents 0.1 ml; the other side of the barrel is marked in minims. Syringes vary from 1 ml to 60 ml. Syringe selection is based on the volume of medication that you will administer Figure 8-39 ▸ .

Hypodermic needle lengths vary from 16 mm to 29 mm for standard injections. As with IV cannulas, the gauge of the needle refers to the diameter: The smaller the number, the larger the diameter. Common needle gauges range from 18 to 26. The needle gauge used depends on the route of parenteral medication administration. Smaller-gauge needles, for example, are used for subcutaneous injections, whereas larger-gauge needles are used for intramuscular and IV injections.

The proximal end of the needle, or hub, attaches to the standard fitting on the syringe. The distal end of the needle is bevelled.

Packaging of Parenteral Medications
Ampoules

Ampoules are breakable sterile glass containers that are designed to carry a single dose of medication Figure 8-40 ▸ . They may contain as little as 1 ml or as much as 10 ml, depending on the medication.

When drawing a medication from an ampoule, follow the steps in Skill Drill 8-6 ▸ .

1. Check the medication to be sure that the expiry date has not passed and that it is the correct drug and concentration.

Skill Drill 8-6: Drawing Medication From an Ampoule

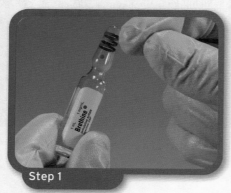

Step 1

Gently tap the stem of the ampoule to shake medication into the base.

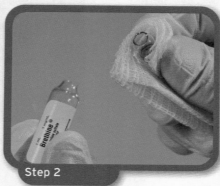

Step 2

Grip the neck of the ampoule using a 10 cm × 10 cm gauze pad, and snap the neck off.

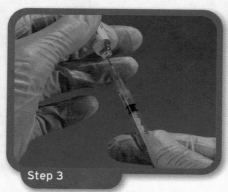

Step 3

Without touching the outer sides of the ampoule, insert the needle into the medication in the ampoule, and draw the solution into the syringe.

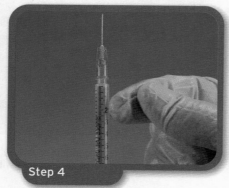

Step 4

Holding the syringe with the needle pointing up, gently tap the barrel to loosen air trapped inside.

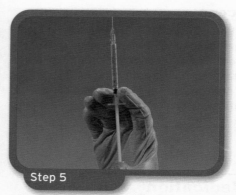

Step 5

Gently press on the plunger to dispel any air bubbles, and recap the needle using the one-handed method, if necessary.

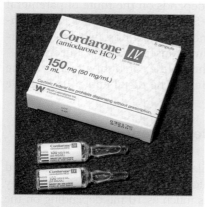

Figure 8-40 Ampoules.

2. Shake the medication into the base of the ampoule. If some of the drug is stuck in the neck, gently thump or tap the stem (Step 1).

3. Using a 10 cm × 10 cm gauze pad or an alcohol prep, grip the neck of the ampoule and snap it off. Drop the stem in the sharps bin (Step 2).

4. Insert the needle into the ampoule without touching the outer sides of the ampoule. Draw the solution into the syringe, and dispose of the ampoule in the sharps bin (Step 3).

5. Hold the syringe with the needle pointing up, and gently tap the barrel to loosen air trapped inside and cause it to rise (Step 4). Press gently on the plunger to dispel any air bubbles (Step 5).

6. Recap the needle using the one-handed method, if necessary.

Vials

Vials are small glass or plastic bottles with a rubber-stopper top; they may contain single or multiple doses of a medication (Figure 8-41 ▶). When using a vial of medication, you must first determine how much of the drug you will need and how many doses are in the vial.

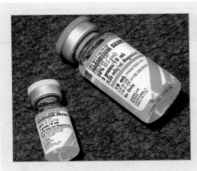

Figure 8-41 Vials (single-dose and multidose).

For a single-dose vial, you will draw up the entire amount in the vial. For multiple-dose vials, you should draw up only the amount needed. Remember that once you remove the cover from a vial, it is no longer sterile. If you need a second dose, clean the top of the vial with alcohol before withdrawing the medication.

Some medications that are stored in vials may need to be reconstituted, such as methylprednisolone sodium succinate (Solu-Cortef) and glucagon. Glucagon is stored in two vials, one with the powdered form of the drug and the other with sterile water. Drug reconstitution involves injecting the sterile water (or provided diluent) from one vial into the vial that contains the powder, thereby making a solution for injection. To reconstitute the contents of two vials, draw the fluid out of the first vial and inject it into the vial that contains the powder. Shake the vial vigorously to mix the medication before drawing out the contents for administration.

Solu-Cortef is stored in a single vial divided into two compartments by a rubber stopper. To reconstitute a drug that is contained in a dual vial, squeeze the two vials together, which releases the centre stopper and allows the contents to mix. Shake vigorously to mix the contents before drawing out the medication.

When drawing medication from a vial, follow the steps in **Skill Drill 8-7 ▸** .

1. Check the medication to be sure that the expiry date has not passed and that it is the correct drug and concentration (**Step 1**).
2. Remove the sterile cover, or clean the top with alcohol if the vial was previously opened.
3. Determine the amount of medication that you will need, and draw that amount of air into the syringe (**Step 2**). Allow a little extra room to expel some air while removing air bubbles.
4. Invert the vial, and insert the needle through the rubber stopper into the medication. Expel the air in the syringe into the vial and then withdraw the amount of medication needed (**Step 3**).
5. Once you have the correct amount of medication in the syringe, withdraw the needle from the vial and expel any excess air in the syringe and needle (**Step 4**).
6. Recap the needle using the one-handed method (**Step 5**).
7. Before administering medication to a patient, use a new needle if the first needle drew medication through a rubber bung.

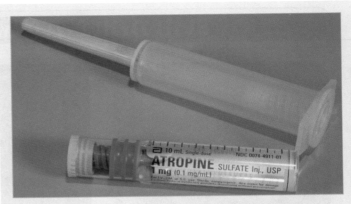

Figure 8-42 Two-part prefilled syringes are separated into a glass drug cartridge and a syringe (for example, Minijet).

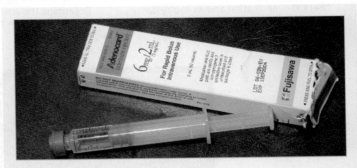

Figure 8-43 Preassembled prefilled syringe.

Prefilled Syringes

Prefilled syringes are packaged in tamper-proof boxes. Two types of prefilled syringes exist: those that are separated into a glass drug cartridge and a syringe, **Figure 8-42 ▴** , and preassembled prefilled syringe **Figure 8-43 ▴** . These syringes are designed for ease of use. After all, it is much easier and quicker to use a prefilled syringe when you are treating a patient in cardiac arrest than it is to draw up each individual dose.

To assemble the two-part prefilled syringe, pop the yellow caps off of the syringe and the drug cartridge, insert the drug cartridge into the barrel of the syringe, and screw them together. Remove the needle cover, and expel air in the manner previously described. Follow the steps for the route the medication is to be given.

Subcutaneous Medication Administration

Subcutaneous (SC) injections are given into the loose connective tissue between the dermis and the muscle layer **Figure 8-44 ▸** . Volumes of a drug administered subcutaneously are usually 1 ml or less. The injection is performed using a 24- to 26-gauge needle. Common sites for SC injections—in both adults and

Skill Drill 8-7: Drawing Medication From a Vial

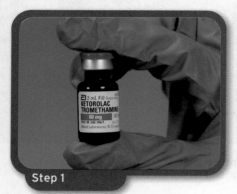

Step 1

Check the medication and its expiry date.

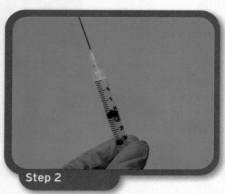

Step 2

Determine the amount of medication needed, and draw that amount of air into the syringe.

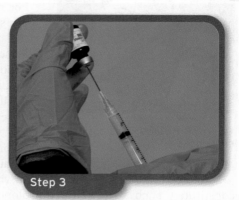

Step 3

Invert the vial, and insert the needle through the rubber stopper. Expel the air in the syringe into the vial, and then withdraw the amount of medication needed.

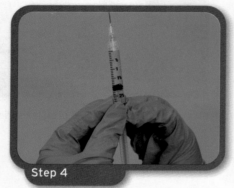

Step 4

Withdraw the needle, and expel any air in the syringe.

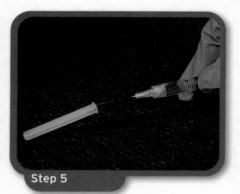

Step 5

Recap the needle using the one-handed method.

At the Scene

Whenever you use a needle to draw up medication from an ampoule or vial, hold the syringe against your palm with the needle pointing up and draw the ampoule or vial down onto the needle using the thumb and forefinger of the palm the syringe is braced against to avoid sticking yourself. This especially applies if you are in a moving ambulance. Time this on straight stretches of roads or at traffic lights.

children—include the upper arms, anterior thighs, and the abdomen **Figure 8-45 ▶**. Patients who take insulin injections usually vary the sites owing to the multiple (usually daily) injections they require.

Follow the steps in **Skill Drill 8-8 ▶** to administer a medication via the subcutaneous route:

1. Take universal precautions.
2. Determine the need for the medication based on patient presentation.
3. Obtain a focused history and physical examination, including any drug allergies and vital signs.
4. Check the medication to ensure that it is the correct one, that it is not cloudy or discoloured, and that the expiry date has not passed, and determine the appropriate amount and concentration for the correct dose **Step 1**.
5. Advise the patient of potential discomfort while explaining the procedure.

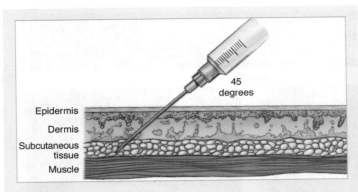

Figure 8-44 A subcutaneous injection is below the dermis and above the muscle.

6. Assemble and check equipment needed: alcohol preps and an appropriate sized syringe with a 24- to 26-gauge needle. Draw up the correct dose of medication (Step 2).

7. Cleanse the area for the administration (usually the upper arm or thigh) using aseptic technique (Step 3).

8. *Pinch the skin* surrounding the area, advise the patient of a stick, and insert the needle at a *45° angle*. Note: Before administering medication to a patient, use a new needle if the first needle drew medication through a rubber bung.

9. Pull back on the plunger to aspirate for blood. The presence of blood in the syringe indicates you may have entered a blood vessel. In such a case, remove the needle, and hold pressure over the site. Discard the syringe and needle in the sharps bin. Prepare a new syringe and needle, and select another site.

10. If there is no blood in the syringe, inject the medication and remove the needle. Immediately dispose of the needle and syringe in the sharps bin (Step 4).

11. To disperse the medication through the tissue, rub the area in a circular motion with your gloved hand.

12. Store any unused medication properly.

13. Monitor the patient's condition, and document the medication given, route, administration time, and response of the patient (Step 5).

Intramuscular Medication Administration

Intramuscular (IM) injections are given by penetrating a needle through the dermis and subcutaneous tissue and into the muscle layer (Figure 8-46 ▾). This technique allows administration of a larger volume of medication (up to 5 ml) than the subcutaneous route. Because there is also the potential for damage to nerves due to the depth of the injection, it is important to choose the appropriate site. Common

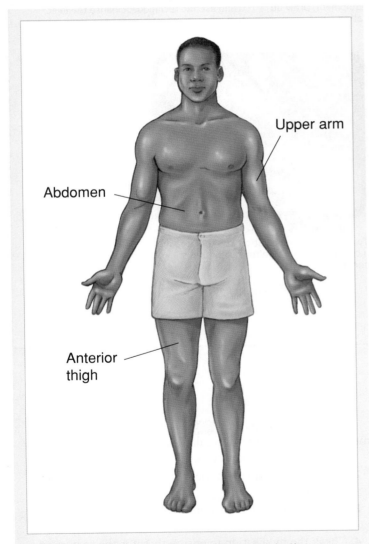

Figure 8-45 Common sites for subcutaneous injections.

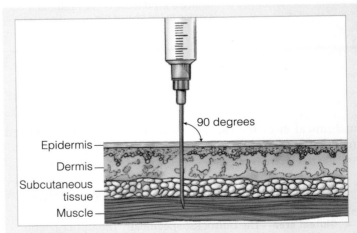

Figure 8-46 An intramuscular injection is below the dermis and subcutaneous layer and into the muscle.

Skill Drill 8-8: Administering Medication via the Subcutaneous Route

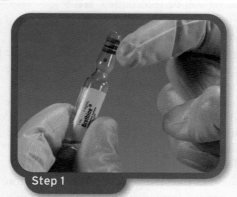

Step 1

Check the medication to ensure that it is the correct one, that it is not discoloured, and that the expiry date has not passed.

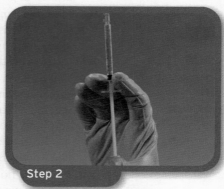

Step 2

Assemble and check the equipment. Draw up the correct dose of medication.

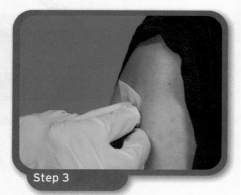

Step 3

Using aseptic technique, cleanse the injection area.

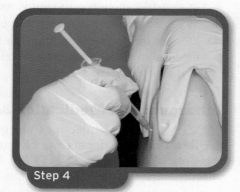

Step 4

Pinch the skin surrounding the area, and insert the needle at a 45° angle. Pull back on the plunger to aspirate for blood. If there is no blood, inject the medication, remove the needle, and hold pressure over the area. Immediately dispose of the needle and syringe in the sharps bin.

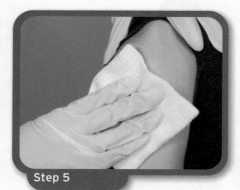

Step 5

To disperse the medication, rub the area in a circular motion. Monitor the patient's condition.

anatomical sites for IM injections for adults and children include the following:

- **Vastus lateralis muscle**—the large muscle on the lateral side of the thigh.
- **Rectus femoris muscle**—the large muscle on the anterior side of the thigh.
- **Gluteal area**—the buttocks, specifically the upper lateral aspect of either side.
- **Deltoid muscle**—the muscle of the upper arm that covers the prominence of the shoulder. The site for injection is approximately 3 to 5 cm below the acromion process on the lateral side (Figure 8-47 ▶).

Follow the steps in (Skill Drill 8-9 ▶) to administer a medication via the intramuscular route:

1. Take universal precautions.
2. Determine the need for the medication based on patient presentation.
3. Obtain a focused history and physical examination, including any drug allergies and vital signs.
4. Check the medication to ensure that it is the correct one, that it is not cloudy or discoloured, and that the expiry date has not passed, and determine the appropriate amount and concentration for the correct dose (Step 1).

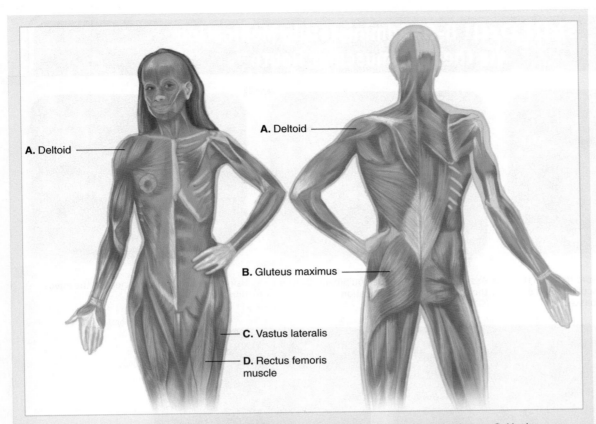

A. Deltoid

A. Deltoid

B. Gluteus maximus

C. Vastus lateralis

D. Rectus femoris muscle

Figure 8-47 Common sites for intramuscular injections. **A.** Deltoid muscle. **B.** Gluteal area. **C.** Vastus lateralis muscle. **D.** Rectus femoris muscle.

10. If there is no blood in the syringe, inject the medication and remove the needle. Immediately dispose of the needle and syringe in the sharps bin (Step 4).

11. To disperse the medication through the tissue, rub the area in a circular motion with your gloved hand (Step 5).

12. Store any unused medication properly.

13. Monitor the patient's condition, and document the medication given, route, administration time, and response of the patient.

IV Bolus Medication Administration

The IV route places the drug directly into the circulatory system. It is the fastest route of medication administration because it bypasses most barriers to drug absorption. As a result, *there is no room for error with IV administration.* (See "Potential Complications of IV Therapy" earlier in this chapter for details on what can go wrong.) Drugs are administered by direct injection with a syringe into an established peripheral IV. The syringe simply screws into the injection port of the IV cannula.

A bolus is a single dose, usually given by the IV route. When given in one mass, it may consist of a small or large quantity of a drug and can be given rapidly or slowly, depending on the drug. Some medications, such as lignocaine and amiodarone, require an initial bolus and then may require a continuous IV infusion to maintain a therapeutic level of the drug.

Follow the steps in (Skill Drill 8-10 ▶) when administering a medication via the IV bolus route:

1. Take universal precautions.

2. Determine the need for the medication based on patient presentation.

3. Obtain a focused history and physical examination, including any drug allergies and vital signs.

4. Check the medication to ensure that it is the correct one, that it is not cloudy or discoloured, and that the expiry date has not passed, and determine the appropriate amount and concentration for the correct dose.

At the Scene

Effective absorption of medications administered by the subcutaneous and intramuscular routes requires adequate peripheral perfusion. This is clearly not the case in patients in profound shock or cardiac arrest. Therefore, subcutaneous and intramuscular injections should not be given to patients with inadequate perfusion.

5. Advise the patient of potential discomfort while explaining the procedure. Don't say "it won't hurt".

6. Assemble and check equipment needed: alcohol preps and an appropriate sized syringe with a 21-gauge needle. Draw up the correct dose of medication (Step 2).

7. Cleanse the area for administration (usually the upper arm or the hip) using aseptic technique (Step 3).

8. *Stretch the skin* over the cleansed area, advise the patient of a pricking sensation, and insert the needle at a *90° angle.* Note: Before administering medication to a patient, use a new needle if the first needle drew medication through a rubber bung.

9. Pull back on the plunger to aspirate for blood. The presence of blood in the syringe indicates you may have entered a blood vessel. In such a case, remove the needle, and hold pressure over the site. Discard the syringe and needle in the sharps bin. Prepare a new syringe and needle, and select another site.

Skill Drill 8-9: Administering Medication via the Intramuscular Route

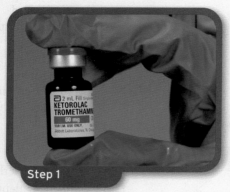

Step 1

Check the medication to ensure that it is the correct one, that it is not discoloured, and that its expiry date has not passed.

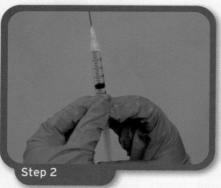

Step 2

Assemble and check the equipment. Draw up the correct dose of medication.

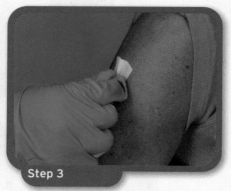

Step 3

Using aseptic technique, cleanse the injection area.

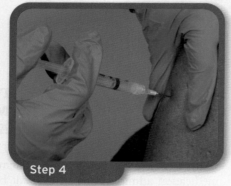

Step 4

Stretch the skin over the area, and insert the needle at a 90° angle. Pull back on the plunger to aspirate for blood. If there is no blood, inject the medication and remove the needle. Immediately dispose of the needle and syringe in the sharps bin.

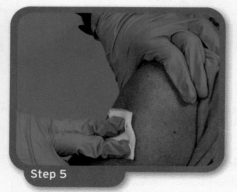

Step 5

To disperse the medication, rub the area in a circular motion. Monitor the patient's condition.

5. Explain the procedure to the patient and the need for the medication.

6. Assemble needed equipment, and draw up medication. Expel any air in the syringe. Draw up 20 ml of normal saline to use as a flush for the medication.

7. Remove the protective cap if using the needleless system.

8. Administer the correct dose of the medication at the appropriate rate. Some medications must be administered very quickly, while others must be pushed slowly to prevent adverse effects (Step 1). Note: Before administering medication to a patient, use a new needle if the first needle drew medication through a rubber bung.

9. Remove the syringe, ensuring that you close the injection port cover. Dispose of syringe in sharps bin.

10. Unclamp the IV line to flush the medication into the vein. Allow it to run briefly wide open.

11. Readjust the IV flow rate to the original setting (Step 2).

12. Properly store and label any unused medication.

13. Monitor the patient's condition, and document the medication given, route, time of administration, and response of the patient.

Adding Medication to an IV Bag

Certain medications are added to the IV solution itself to be administered as a maintenance infusion—for example,

Skill Drill 8-10: Administering Medication via the Intravenous Bolus Route

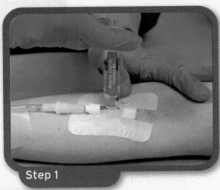

Step 1

Assemble and check the equipment. Remove the protective cap if using the needleless system. Administer the correct dose at the appropriate rate.

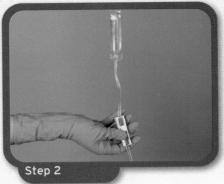

Step 2

Unclamp the IV line to flush the medication into the vein, allowing it to run briefly wide open. Readjust the IV flow rate to the original setting, and monitor the patient's condition.

dopamine, lignocaine, and adrenaline. All of these medications require careful titration to achieve the desired effect.

The steps for adding medication to an IV bag are as follows:

1. Check the fluid in the IV bag for clarity or discolouration, and ensure that the expiry date has not passed.
2. Check the *drug name* on the ampoule, vial, or prefilled syringe. Check the *concentration of the drug* it contains (for example, mcg/ml or mg/ml).
3. *Calculate the volume* of the drug to be added to the IV bag. Draw up that amount in a syringe (if a prefilled syringe is used, note the proportion of the volume of the syringe required).
4. Cleanse the medication injection port on the IV bag with an alcohol swab.
5. Inject the desired volume of medication into the IV bag by puncturing the rubber stopper on the medication injection port **Figure 8-48 ▶** .
6. Withdraw the needle, and dispose of the needle and syringe in the sharps bin. Agitate the IV bag gently to ensure that the added drug is well mixed in the solution.

You are the Paramedic Part 5

After administering 50 ml of glucose 10%, the patient's level of consciousness rapidly improves. She pushes the bag-valve-mask away from her face but will tolerate a nonrebreathing mask. She is obviously confused about what happened, but consents to ambulance transport to hospital. You explain to her what has happened to her, and reassess her. Your colleague retrieves the stretcher from the ambulance.

Reassessment	Recording Time: 12 Minutes
Level of consciousness	A (Alert to person, place, and day)
Airway and breathing	Airway remains patent; respirations, 18 breaths/min with adequate depth
Blood pressure	112/70 mm Hg
Pulse	88 beats/min, strong and regular
SpO_2	99% (with 100% oxygen) on 15 l/min
Blood glucose	8 mmol/l

10. Does this patient require an additional dose of glucose 10%?
11. Does this patient require an IV bolus of normal saline?

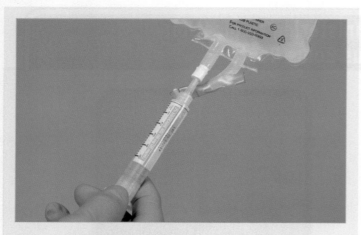

Figure 8-48 Adding medication to an IV bag.

At the Scene

Medications that are used for maintenance infusions (for example, lignocaine and dopamine) are commonly premixed and prepackaged, which eliminates the need to calculate and draw up the appropriate amount of medication to add to the bag. However, you must still be aware of the concentration (for example, µg/ml or mg/ml) of drug in the premixed solution and the appropriate maintenance infusion rate.

7. *Label the IV bag* with the name of the medication added, the amount added, the concentration of medication in the IV bag (for example, µg/ml or mg/ml), the date and time, and your name.
8. Attach the IV administration set, and prepare the IV bag as discussed earlier in this chapter.

Electromechanical Infusion Pumps

When administering a medication maintenance infusion, you should use an electromechanical infusion pump, if available. The infusion pump can also be used to deliver IV fluid maintenance infusions in children and elderly patients to minimise the risk of a "runaway IV" and subsequent circulatory overload.

Most infusion pumps allow you to set the parametres of medication administration—drug concentration and volume to be infused—and will then calculate the appropriate infusion rate. This feature allows for precise medication dosing, minimising the risk of delivering too little or too much medication.

Electromechanical infusion pumps deliver fluids or medications via positive pressure. Although medications delivered in this manner can result in infiltration of a vein, most infusion pumps are equipped with an alarm that indicates a change in the flow pressure. Other common safety features include alarms that alert you to the presence of occlusion (eg, air in the tubing) or depletion of the medication. Some infusion pumps are designed to accommodate the IV tubing to regulate the flow of IV fluids or medications **Figure 8-49 ▸**, whereas others are designed to accommodate a needleless syringe **Figure 8-50 ▸**.

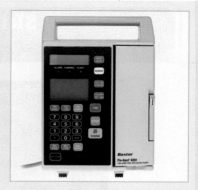

Figure 8-49 Infusion pump that accommodates IV tubing.

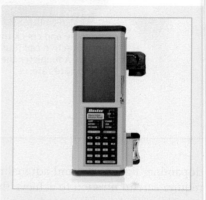

Figure 8-50 Syringe-type infusion pump.

IO Medication Administration

The IO route is used for critically ill or injured children and adults when IV access is difficult or impossible to obtain. Any fluid or medication that may be given through an IV line—bolus or maintenance infusion—can be given by the IO route. Shock, status epilepticus, and cardiac arrest are but a few of the reasons for establishing IO access. Unlike with an IV line, fluid does not flow well into the bone because of resistance; therefore, it is necessary to use a large syringe to infuse the fluid. A <u>pressure infuser device</u>—a sleeve placed around the IV bag and inflated to force fluid from the IV bag—should be used when infusing fluids in adults.

Complications of using the IO route are similar to those of the IV route. Along with the complications discussed earlier in this chapter, there is also the potential for compartment syndrome if fluid leaks outside the bone and into the osteofascial compartment.

Follow the steps in **Skill Drill 8-11 ▸** to administer a medication via the IO route:

Skill Drill 8-11: Administering Medication via the IO Route

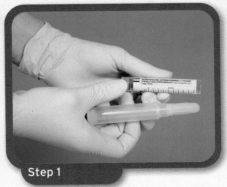

Step 1

Check the medication to ensure that it is the correct one, that it is not discoloured, and that the expiry date has not passed.
Assemble the equipment, and draw up the medication.

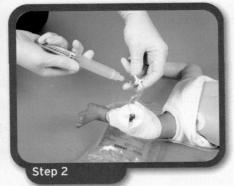

Step 2

Close the 3-way tap.

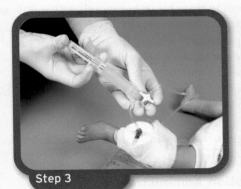

Step 3

Attach the drug to the 3-way tap.

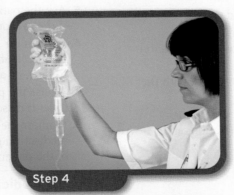

Step 4

Use the 3-way tap to flush with a 20 ml bolus of normal saline.

1. Take universal precautions.
2. Determine the need for the medication based on patient presentation.
3. Obtain a focused history and physical examination, including any drug allergies and vital signs.
4. Check the medication to ensure that it is the correct one, that it is not cloudy or discoloured, and that the expiry date has not passed, and determine the appropriate amount and concentration for the correct dose.

5. Explain the procedure to the patient and/or parent and the need for the medication.
6. Assemble needed equipment, and draw up the medication (Step 1).
7. Close the 3-way tap (Step 2).
8. Attach the drug to the 3-way tap (Step 3).
9. Use the 3-way tap to flush with a 20 ml bolus of normal saline (Step 4).

Percutaneous Medication Administration

With <u>percutaneous</u> routes of administration, medications are applied to and absorbed through the skin and mucous membranes. Because percutaneously administered medications bypass the gastrointestinal tract, their absorption is more predictable. Percutaneous routes of medication administration include the transdermal, sublingual, buccal, ocular, aural, and nasal routes.

Transdermal Medication Administration

<u>Transdermal</u> medications are applied topically—that is, on the surface of the body. Ordinarily, intact skin is an effective barrier to absorption of drugs. However, some drugs have been specially prepared to cross that barrier at a very slow steady rate, so the transdermal route is useful for the sustained release of certain medications.

Glyceryl trinitrate (GTN), oestrogen, nicotine, and analgesic patches, for example, are applied to the skin and release medications over a specified period. Creams, lotions, and pastes (eg, GTN paste, corticosteroid cream) are also transdermally administered medications.

Factors that can increase the speed of transdermal absorption include administration of too much of the medication (ie, inadvertent or intentional overdose) and thin or nonintact skin. Decreased speed of transdermal absorption can be caused by factors such as thick skin, scar tissue in the area to which the medication is applied, and peripheral vascular disease. The skin temperature and subsequent peripheral circulation will also effect absorption rate.

Other than assisting a patient with his or her transdermal medication, there is rarely a need to use this route of administration in the prehospital setting. Should a situation arise that requires you to administer a transdermal medication patch or paste, follow these steps:

1. Take universal precautions.
2. Determine the need for the medication based on patient presentation.
3. Obtain a focused history and physical examination, including any drug allergies and vital signs.
4. Check the medication patch or cream to ensure that it is the correct one and that the expiry date has not passed, and determine the appropriate amount for the correct dose.
5. Explain the procedure to the patient and the need for the medication.
6. Clean and dry the area of the skin where the medication will be applied.
7. Apply the medication to the area in accordance with the manufacturer's specifications.
8. Monitor the patient's condition, and document the medication given, route, time of administration, and response of the patient.

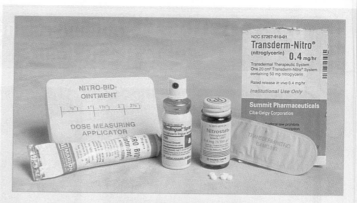

Figure 8-51 GTN is often given sublingually as a spray or a tablet. It is also available as a transdermal patch or paste and can be administered as an IV drip.

3. Obtain a focused history and physical examination, including any drug allergies and vital signs.
4. Check the medication to ensure that it is the correct one and that its expiry date has not passed, and determine the appropriate amount for the correct dose.
5. Ask the patient to rinse his or her mouth with a little water if the mucous membranes are dry Step 1 .
6. Explain the procedure, and ask the patient to lift his or her tongue. Place the tablet or spray the dose under the tongue, or ask the patient to do so.
7. Advise the patient not to chew or swallow the tablet, but to let it dissolve slowly.
8. Monitor the patient's condition, and document the medication given, route, administration time, and response of the patient Step 2 .

Buccal Medication Administration

The buccal region, which is also highly vascular, lies in between the cheek and gums. Most medications administered via the buccal route are in the form of tablets. Unlike the sublingual route, you will occasionally administer medications via the buccal route in the prehospital setting.

To administer a medication via the buccal route, follow these steps:

1. Take universal precautions.
2. Determine the need for the medication based on patient presentation.
3. Obtain a focused history and physical examination, including any drug allergies and vital signs.
4. Check the medication to ensure that it is the correct one and that its expiry date has not passed, and determine the appropriate amount for the correct dose.
5. Explain the procedure to the patient and the need for the medication.
6. Place the medication in between the patient's cheek and gum, or ask the patient to do so.
7. Advise the patient not to chew or swallow the tablet, but to let it dissolve slowly.

At the Scene

During assessment of your patient, look for transdermal medication patches, especially narcotic and GTN patches, which can result in hypotension. If the patient is already in a haemodynamically unstable condition, narcotics and GTN may complicate the clinical picture.

Sublingual Medication Administration

The sublingual (under the tongue) region is highly vascular, so medications given via the sublingual route are rapidly absorbed. Sublingually administered medications, relative to enterally administered medications, get into the circulation much faster. GTN—spray or tablet—is a drug that is most commonly administered via the sublingual route Figure 8-51 ▶ .

To administer a sublingual medication, follow these steps Skill Drill 8-12 ▶ .

1. Take universal precautions.
2. Determine the need for the medication based on patient presentation.

Skill Drill 8-12: Administering Medication via the Sublingual Route

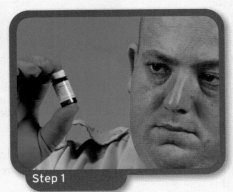

Step 1

Check the medication for drug type and its expiry date, and determine the appropriate amount for the correct dose.

Have the patient rinse his or her mouth with a little water if the mucous membranes are dry.

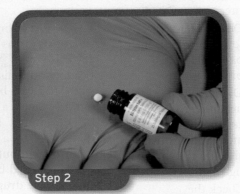

Step 2

Explain the procedure to the patient, and ask the patient to lift his or her tongue. Place the tablet or spray the dose underneath the tongue, or have the patient do so.

Advise the patient not to chew or swallow the tablet, but to let it dissolve slowly.

Monitor the patient, and document the medication given, the route, administration time, and the response of the patient.

At the Scene

Wear gloves when administering GTN. Otherwise, the medication can be absorbed through your own skin.

8. Monitor the patient's condition, and document the medication given, route, administration time, and response of the patient.

Ocular Medication Administration

Drops or ointments are commonly administered via the <u>ocular</u> route. Ocular medications are typically administered for pain relief, allergies, drying of the eyes, or infections. Other than assisting a patient with his or her ocular medication or irrigating a patient's eyes following a toxic exposure, none of the medications used in the prehospital setting are administered via the ocular route.

If a patient asks you to assist him or her with ocular medication administration, follow these steps:

1. Take universal precautions.
2. Confirm that the medication is prescribed to the patient.
3. Place the patient in a supine position, or have the patient place his or her head back and look up.
4. *Without touching the eyeball,* expose the conjunctiva by gently pulling down on the lower eyelid.

5. Administer the required amount of medication on the conjunctival sac by using an eye dropper. Do not apply the medication directly onto the eyeball.
6. Advise the patient to close his or her eyes for 1 to 2 minutes.
7. Document the medication name, dose, and administration time.

Aural Medication Administration

Certain medications—mainly antibiotics, analgesics, and ear-wax removal preparations—are administered via the mucous membranes of the <u>aural</u> (ear) canal. As with ocular medications, the aural route is rarely, if ever, used in the prehospital setting.

If you are asked by the patient to assist in administering his or her aural medication, follow these steps:

1. Take universal precautions.
2. Confirm that the medication is prescribed to the patient.
3. Place the patient on his or her side with the affected ear facing up.
4. Expose the ear canal by pulling the ear up and back (adults) or down and back (infants and children).
5. Administer the medication in the appropriate dose with a medicine dropper.
6. Document the medication name, dose, and administration time.

Intranasal Medication Administration

<u>Intranasal</u> (within the nose) medications include nasal spray for congestion or solutions to moisten the nasal mucosa. In recent years, this route of medication administration has become increasingly more popular in the prehospital setting outside of the UK. Intranasally administered medications are rapidly absorbed, providing a more rapid onset of action than IM injections. Administration of emergency medications via the intranasal route is performed with a <u>mucosal atomiser device (MAD)</u> **Figure 8-52 ▶**. The MAD attaches to a syringe and allows you to spray (atomise) select medications into the nasal mucosa.

Owing to the molecular structure of drugs, only a few emergency medications can be given intranasally, including naloxone and midazolam.

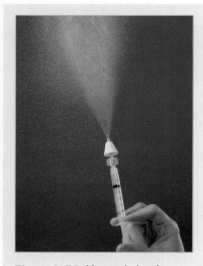

Figure 8-52 Mucosal atomiser device (MAD).

To administer a drug via the intranasal route, follow these steps:

1. Take universal precautions.
2. Determine the need for the medication based on patient presentation.
3. Obtain a focused history and physical examination, including any drug allergies and vital signs.
4. Check the medication to ensure that it is the correct one, that it is not cloudy or discoloured, and that the expiry date has not passed.
5. Draw up the appropriate dose of medication in the syringe.
6. Attach the mucosal atomiser device to the syringe.
7. Explain the procedure to the patient (or to a relative if the patient is unconscious) and the need for the medication.
8. Spray *half* of the medication dose into each nostril.
9. Dispose of the atomiser device and syringe in the appropriate container.
10. Monitor the patient's condition, and document the medication given, route, time of administration, and response of the patient.

Medications Administered by the Inhalation Route

Nebuliser and Metered-Dose Inhaler

Many medications used in the treatment of respiratory emergencies are administered via the inhalation route. The most common inhaled medication is oxygen. Beta-2 agonist bronchodilators (eg, salbutamol) are often administered in the prehospital setting for patients experiencing respiratory distress caused by certain obstructive airway diseases, such as asthma, bronchitis, and emphysema. Other medications, such as ipratropium bromide—an anticholinergic bronchodilator—are also administered via the inhalation route. Check your drug reference guide or the package insert for the indications, contraindications, and precautions

before giving any of these medications.

A patient with a history of respiratory problems will usually have a metered-dose inhaler (MDI) to use on a regular basis or as needed Figure 8-53 ▶ . Medications administered by the MDI can be delivered through a mouthpiece held by the patient or by a mask—

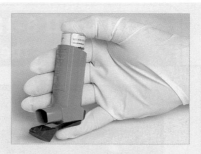

Figure 8-53 Some medications are inhaled into the lungs with an MDI so that they can be absorbed quickly into the bloodstream.

with or without a spacer device. Increasingly, spacer devices are being used by many patients as the patients tend to receive more of the drug this way Figure 8-54 ▼ .

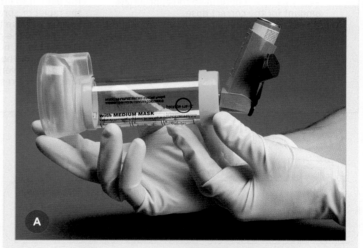

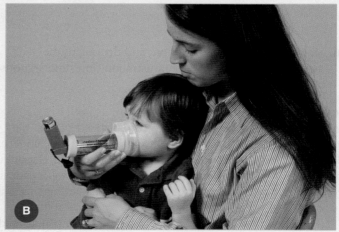

Figure 8-54 A. In children, an MDI and spacer can be used with or without a mask. **B.** Children as young as 6 months can use a mask and spacer device.

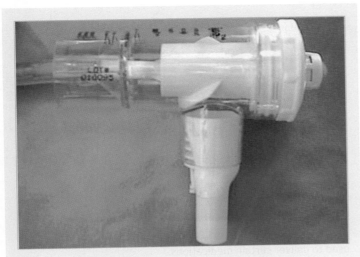

Figure 8-55 A small-volume nebuliser is used to deliver medications via aerosolised mist.

6. Set the flowmeter at 6–8 l/min to produce a steady mist (Step 3).

7. Instruct the patient on the proper way to breathe. Have the patient breathe as deeply as possible and hold his or her breath for 3 to 5 seconds before exhaling. Continue to coach the patient as needed.

8. Monitor the patient's condition, and document the medication given, route, time of administration, and response of the patient to the medication (Step 4).

9. Cardiac monitoring is essential when administering a beta agonist. If cardiac dysrhythmias are noted, stop the administration of the medication, administer high-flow oxygen.

Some patients with respiratory emergencies may be breathing inadequately (ie, inadequate tidal volume, fast or slow respiratory rate) and will not be able to effectively inhale beta-agonist medications into the lungs via a nebuliser or an MDI.

For more severe problems, liquid bronchodilators may be aerosolised in a nebuliser for inhalation. Small-volume nebulisers are the most commonly used method of administration of inhaled medications in the prehospital setting (Figure 8-55 ▲). Oxygen or a compressed air source is connected to the nebuliser to produce the aerosolised mist.

Follow the steps in Skill Drill 8-13 ▶ to administer a medication via small-volume nebuliser:

1. Take universal precautions.

2. Determine the need for an inhaled bronchodilator based on patient presentation.

3. Obtain a focused history and physical examination, including any drug allergies and vital signs.

4. Check the medication and its expiry date. Make sure that you have the right medication and that it is not cloudy or discoloured (Step 1).

5. Add medication to the chamber (Step 2).

Skill Drill 8-13: Administering a Medication via Small-Volume Nebuliser

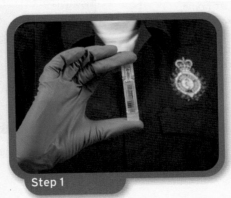

Step 1
Check the medication and the expiry date.

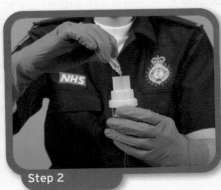

Step 2
Add medication to the chamber.

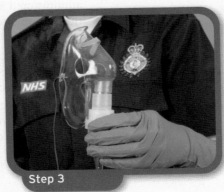

Step 3
Set the flowmeter at 6 l/min.

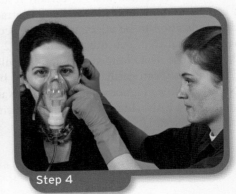

Step 4
Instruct the patient to breathe as deeply as possible and hold his or her breath for 3 to 5 seconds before exhaling. Monitor the patient for effects.

In these cases, ventilation should be assisted with a bag-valve-mask. A T-piece nebuliser with catheter mount assembly attached to it, should be connected between the bag-valve and the mask. This same T piece assembly can also be connected to a laryngeal mask or endotracheal tube if a definitive airway adjunct has been used Figure 8-56 ▸.

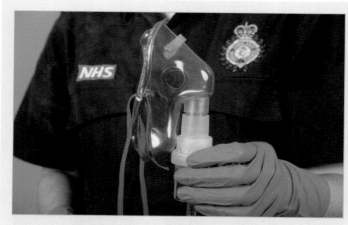

Figure 8-56 A nebuliser connected to an oxygen mask can be used to deliver certain medications.

Controversies

In the past, nebulisers were considered the preferred method of delivering beta-agonist medications for the treatment of asthma attacks. Recent studies, however, have shown that MDIs—especially when used with spacing devices—are at least as effective as nebulisers and have several distinct advantages:

- MDIs are *more convenient* than nebulisers. They do not require any setup time or a source of compressed gas.
- MDIs are *more reliable* than nebulisers. With a nebuliser, one cannot be certain that the patient is getting the full dose of the drug. MDIs deliver a more consistent amount of drug aerosol.
- Because most people with asthma use MDIs at home, using the MDI in an emergency provides an excellent opportunity to educate the patient in proper use of the device. Studies have shown that more than half of patients using MDIs at home employ an incorrect and ineffective technique. Showing a patient the correct technique and demonstrating its effectiveness can improve the outcome of subsequent asthma attacks.

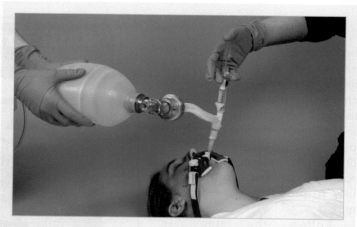

Figure 8-57 Administering medication via the ET tube.

Endotracheal Medication Administration

If IV or IO access is unavailable, certain resuscitative medications can be administered down the endotracheal (ET) tube. For the medication to be adequately dispersed throughout the tracheobronchial tree, you must administer 2 to 2.5 times the standard IV dose. *Only* four medications should be given down the ET tube; they can easily be remembered by the mnemonic ALAN: Adrenaline, Lignocaine, Atropine, Naloxone. Another mnemonic is LEAN (Lignocaine, Epinephrine [adrenaline], Atropine, Naloxone).

To administer medications via the ET tube, follow these steps:

1. Draw up the appropriate dose of the medication to be administered as your partner ventilates the patient. Dilute the appropriate dose of the medication in 10 ml of normal saline.
2. Disconnect the bag-valve-mask device from the ET tube, and rapidly instill the medication down the ET tube or use the drug port of the ET catheter mount Figure 8-57 ▴.
3. Immediately reconnect the bag-valve-mask device to the ET tube, and ventilate the patient briskly to facilitate passage of the drug down the trachea and into the lungs.

Controversies

Although current practice calls for administering certain resuscitative medications via the ET tube, recent studies have suggested that this route of medication administration may not be particularly effective. Follow local guidelines, or contact medical control as needed regarding endotracheal drug administration. The 2005 European Resuscitation Council guidelines provide greater detail on this topic.

Rates of Medication Absorption

The speed at which a drug is absorbed is directly related to the route by which it is given. Obviously, drugs injected directly into the bloodstream (ie, as IV or IO injections) gain access to the central circulation the fastest. Oral medications take longer to achieve their therapeutic effects, because they must be absorbed through the gastrointestinal tract first. Table 8-6 ▶ summarises the various medication routes and their rates of absorption.

Table 8-6	Medication Routes and Rates of Absorption
Route of Administration	**Onset of Action***
Intraosseous	30–60 s
Intravenous	30–60 s
Endotracheal	2–3 min†
Inhalation	2–3 min
Sublingual	3–5 min
Intramuscular injection	10–20 min
Subcutaneous injection	15–30 min
Rectal	5–30 min
Oral	30–90 min
Topical	Minutes to hours

*In a healthy person with adequate perfusion.

†Recent data suggest that ET drug administration may be less effective than previously thought, especially in poor perfusion states.

You are the Paramedic Summary

1. Is this a medical patient or a trauma patient?

You have not obtained enough information to be able to establish whether this is a medical patient or a trauma patient. Your index of suspicion should increase for the potential for trauma in this case, especially because no one witnessed the events preceding the patient's condition. Further assessment of the patient and her surroundings is required. If there is *any* potential for trauma, then treat her accordingly (ie, spinal immobilisation). Paramedics should not be too hasty to "label" a patient as being a medical or trauma patient; this requires a careful assessment. Some patients have *both* medical and traumatic elements to their condition.

2. What are your initial priorities of care?

Immediate care for this patient involves carefully moving her to the floor (with spinal precautions if trauma is suspected) and performing an initial assessment. This is the most important aspect of initial patient care. You *must* be able to *rapidly identify and correct* immediate threats to life. This patient is unresponsive; clearly, her condition requires immediate treatment.

3. What is the most appropriate initial airway management for this patient?

The patient is unconscious and unresponsive, so you must immediately ensure that her airway is open and clear of secretions. Furthermore, her respirations are rapid and shallow (reduced tidal volume). Initial airway management should include inserting an oral or nasal airway adjunct and assisting ventilation with bag-valve-mask ventilation and 100% oxygen. Rapid, shallow respirations will result in decreased minute volume. If this is not *immediately* treated, significant hypoxia and acidosis will develop.

4. Does this patient require immediate medication therapy?

Other than 100% oxygen, which you have already administered, further assessment is required before determining whether medication therapy is indicated. Although the patient's history of diabetes and clinical presentation are highly suggestive of hypoglycaemia, they are not conclusive. In some patients who have diabetes, it may be difficult to differentiate between hypoglycaemia and hyperglycaemia, especially if the patient is unconscious.

5. Given the patient's history, what additional assessment should you perform?

Obviously, you should test the blood glucose level of any unconscious patient—with or without a history of diabetes. This is especially true if you observe signs suggesting hypoglycaemia. Adequate glucose to the brain is just as critical as oxygen; without it, permanent brain damage or death can occur. Because hypoglycaemia is an easily correctable condition, rapid blood glucose testing should be performed and, if necessary, treated immediately.

6. When starting an IV for this patient, what solution should you use?

An isotonic crystalloid (usually normal saline) is the fluid of choice for the vast majority of patients that you will treat in the prehospital setting. A glucose 10% solution (or any glucose-containing solution) should not be used in patients with diabetes. Glucose 10% is a more appropriate choice when mixing a medication to deliver in a maintenance infusion. Patients with diabetic ketoacidosis, for example, are typically dehydrated from the osmotic diuresis caused by excess blood glucose levels. Isotonic crystalloids, because they remain in the vascular space for longer periods, are needed for rehydration and maintenance of adequate perfusion.

7. What does the % in glucose 10% mean?

In terms of medication concentration, percent refers to the number of grams present in 100 ml (1 dl) of volume. Therefore, glucose 10% contains a concentration of 10 g (10,000 mg) in 100 ml of volume. Since glucose 10% is dispensed in a 500 ml volume, there are 50 g of medication in the container.

8. What is the concentration of glucose you have on hand?

The concentration on hand represents the total amount of weight (mcg, mg, or g) present in 1 ml. Glucose 10% represents 10 g of glucose in 100 ml volume; however, because glucose 10% is contained in 500 ml you have 50 g available. To determine the concentration on hand, divide the total number of milligrams (50 g = 50,000 mg) by the total volume (500 ml); 50,000 mg ÷ 500 ml = 100 mg/ml.

9. What are the "six rights" of medication administration?

Before administering any medication, you must review the six rights to ensure that safe and effective patient care is given: (1) right patient, (2) right drug, (3) right dose, (4) right route, (5) right time, and (6) right documentation. You can cause further harm to the patient if a drug—even if it's the right drug—is given at the wrong time, by an inappropriate route, or in the wrong dose.

10. Does this patient require an additional dose of glucose 10%?

Based on a reading of 8 mmol/l and the patient's obvious clinical improvement, additional doses of glucose 10% are not indicated. However, the question remains as to why her blood glucose level dropped initially. Ask further questions to explore this issue, such as when she last ate, what she ate (if she ate), if she took her insulin and how much, and if she has any other medical problems. During transport, continue to monitor the patient's level of consciousness and reassess her blood glucose level as needed.

11. Does this patient require an IV bolus of normal saline?

The IV line can remain at a TKVO rate; there is no need for fluid boluses. At present, the patient's vital signs indicate haemodynamic stability. Her heart rate, which was 120 beats/min initially, was likely due to a sympathetic nervous system discharge in response to hypoglycaemia, not hypovolaemia. Following administration of the glucose 10%, the patient's heart rate promptly recovered. No mechanism for volume loss has been identified (eg, vomiting, diarrhoea).

Prep Kit

■ Ready for Review

- The cellular environment contains charged ions, called electrolytes, that are used by the cell for different purposes. These electrolytes include sodium, potassium, calcium, bicarbonate, chloride, and phosphorous. Their electrical charges must remain in balance on either side of the cell membrane.
- There must be a balance of compounds on either side of the cell membrane. If an imbalance occurs, the cell can move chemicals or charges across its membrane by various methods, including osmosis, diffusion, active transport, and filtration.
- Understanding the workings of the intracellular and extracellular chemicals and charges will provide you with a better foundation for understanding why different types of IV solutions are administered for different conditions.
- Techniques for gaining vascular access include cannulation of a peripheral extremity vein, cannulation of the external jugular vein, and cannulation of the IO space. Although the ultimate goal of vascular access is to be able to administer fluids and medications, each of these techniques requires a different approach and must be practised frequently for initial and ongoing proficiency.
- Several different IV administration sets exist, and you must know which one is most appropriate for a given patient condition. Microdrip sets (60 gtt/ml) are commonly used for medication infusions. Macrodrip sets (10 or 15 gtt/ml) are used when the patient requires IV fluid boluses to treat dehydration, hypovolaemic shock, and other states of haemodynamic instability.
- You must consider two factors when choosing an IV cannula: gauge and length. The larger the gauge (the smaller the number), and the shorter the length, the more fluid that can be infused through it. Over-the-needle cannulas are the most commonly used IV cannulas in the prehospital setting.
- Cannulation of a peripheral extremity vein is the preferred initial means of establishing vascular access. If it is unsuccessful and the patient is critically ill or injured, proceed with IO cannulation without delay. External jugular vein cannulation is usually attempted only after all other techniques of gaining vascular access have failed.
- IO cannulation and infusion are no longer reserved for children only; they can also be used to establish emergency vascular access in adults. The IO space, which acts like a sponge, quickly absorbs fluids and medications and rapidly transports them to the central circulation.
- Although peripheral veins often collapse when a patient is in shock or cardiac arrest, the IO space tends to remain patent. Thus IO cannulation and infusion—in children and adults—may be lifesaving measures if peripheral venous access is not possible. Any fluid or medication that can be administered via the IV route can be administered via the IO route and can travel to the central circulation just as rapidly.
- You must be thoroughly familiar with the equipment you are using when performing IO cannulation. Follow local guidelines and attend in-service training regarding the specific equipment used for IO cannulation in your ambulance service.
- Use aseptic technique when performing any invasive procedure to minimise the risk of patient contamination. Always use universal precautions when performing an invasive procedure to maximise your own safety.
- Along with the dispensing of medications comes the responsibility to be thoroughly familiar with each medication carried on your ambulance. Carry a pocket guide or other reference to look up unfamiliar drugs or to confirm the doses and routes of drugs that you are familiar with. Remember: *First do no harm.*
- Good maths skills and a thorough understanding of the metric system are imperative to providing the right dose of a drug to your patient. The six rights of medication are right patient, right drug, right dose, right route, right time, and right documentation. Administering the wrong drug, using the wrong route, or giving the wrong dose can have disastrous effects.
- All equipment used in the administration of medications must be kept sterile to prevent contamination of the patient. Use proper universal precautions to protect yourself. Needleless systems have made older needle systems increasingly obsolete, as the former systems decrease the incidence of needlesticks.
- As a paramedic, you must be familiar with the various routes of medication administration, including the proper use of equipment and proper anatomical locations for administration via each route.
- Enteral medication administration includes the administration of all drugs that may be given through any portion of the gastrointestinal tract. The parenteral route includes any method of drug administration that does not pass through the gastrointestinal tract.
- The IV and IO routes are the fastest routes of medication administration; the oral and transdermal (topical) routes are the slowest.
- When in doubt, always follow local guidelines or contact medical control as needed for advice when administering a medication. *Never make a critical decision in haste or without consulting a doctor!*

■ Vital Vocabulary

access port A sealed hub on an administration set designed for sterile access to the IV fluid.

acidosis A pathological condition resulting from the accumulation of acids in the body.

administration set Tubing that connects to the IV bag access port and the cannula to deliver IV fluid.

alkalosis A pathological condition resulting from the accumulation of bases in the body.

ampoules Small glass containers that are sealed and the contents sterilised.

anion An ion that contains an overall negative charge.

antecubital The anterior aspect of the elbow.

antidiuretic hormone (ADH) A hormone produced by the pituitary gland that signals the kidneys to prevent excretion of water.

antiseptics Chemicals used to cleanse an area before performing an invasive procedure, such as starting an IV; not toxic to living tissues; examples include isopropyl alcohol and iodine.

aseptic technique A method of cleansing used to prevent contamination of a site when performing an invasive procedure, such as starting an IV.

ataxia A staggered walk or gait.

aural Pertaining to the ear.

blood tubing A special type of macrodrip administration set designed to facilitate rapid fluid replacement by manual infusion of IV bags or IV-blood replacement.

bolus A term used to describe "in one mass"; in medication administration, a single dose given by the IV or IO route; may be a small or large quantity of the drug.

Bone Injection Gun (B.I.G.) A spring-loaded device that is used for inserting an IO needle into the proximal tibia in adult and paediatric patients.

buccal Between the cheek and gums.

burette A special type of microdrip set that features a 100- or 200-ml calibrated drip chamber; used for fluid regulation in patients prone to circulatory overload, such as paediatric and elderly patients; also called a Buretrol.

butterfly cannula A rigid, hollow, venous cannulation device identified by its plastic "wings" that act as anchoring points for securing the cannula.

cannula shear Occurs when a needle is reinserted into the cannula, and it slices through the cannula, creating a free-floating segment.

cannulation The insertion of a cannula, such as into a vein to allow for fluid flow.

carpopedal spasms Hand or foot spasms; usually the result of hyperventilation or hypocalcaemia.

cation An ion that contains an overall positive charge.

clinical guidelines A broad outline of best practice relating to specific aspects of care.

colloid solutions Solutions that contain molecules (usually proteins) that are too large to pass out of the capillary membranes and, therefore, remain in the vascular compartment.

concentration The total weight of a drug contained in a specific volume of liquid.

concentration gradient The natural tendency for substances to flow from an area of higher concentration to an area of lower concentration, within or outside the cell.

crystalloid solutions Solutions of dissolved crystals (for example, salts or sugars) in water; contain compounds that quickly dissociate in solution.

dehydration Depletion of the body's systemic fluid volume.

depolarisation The rapid movement of electrolytes across a cell membrane that changes the cell's overall charge. This rapid shifting of electrolytes and cellular charges is the main catalyst for muscle contractions and neural transmissions.

desired dose The amount of drug that you decide the patient requires.

diaphysis The shaft of a long bone.

diffusion A process in which molecules move from an area of higher concentration to an area of lower concentration.

diluent A solution (usually water or normal saline) used for diluting a medication.

disinfectants Chemicals used on nonliving objects to kill organisms; toxic to living tissues; examples include Virex, Cidex, and Microcide.

drip chamber The area of the administration set where fluid accumulates so that the tubing remains filled with fluid.

drug reconstitution Injecting sterile water or saline from one vial into another vial containing a powdered form of the drug.

electrolytes Charged atoms or compounds that result from the loss or gain of an electron. These are ions that the body uses to perform certain critical metabolic functions.

enteral route A route of medication administration that involves the medication passing through a portion of the gastrointestinal tract.

epiphyseal plate The growth plate of a bone; a major site of bone development during childhood.

epiphyses The ends of a long bone.

external jugular (EJ) vein Large neck vein that is lateral to the carotid artery.

extracellular fluid (ECF) The water outside the cells; accounts for 15% of body weight.

EZ-IO A hand-held, battery-powered driver to which a special IO needle is attached; used for insertion of the IO needle into the proximal tibia of children and adults.

fascia The fibrous connective tissue that covers arteries, veins, tendons, and ligaments.

F.A.S.T.1 A sternal IO device used in adults; stands for First Access for Shock and Trauma.

flash chamber The area of an IV cannula that fills with blood to help indicate when a vein is cannulated.

gastric tubes Tubes that are occasionally inserted in patients in the prehospital setting to decompress the stomach; can also be used to administer certain enteral medications.

gauge The internal diameter of an IV cannula or needle.

glucose 10% An intravenous solution made up of glucose 10% in water.

gtt A unit of measure that indicates drops.

haematoma An accumulation of blood in the tissues beneath the skin; a potential complication of IV therapy.

haemostasis The body's natural blood-clotting mechanism.

homeostasis The balance of all body systems of the body; also known as homeostatic balance.

hyercalcaemia A high serum calcium level.

hyperkalaemia A high serum potassium level.

hypertonic solution A solution that has a greater concentration of sodium than does the cell; the increased osmotic pressure can draw water out of the cell and cause it to collapse.

hypocalcaemia A low serum calcium level.

hypokalaemia A low serum potassium level.

hypotonic solution A solution that has a lower concentration of sodium than does the cell; the increased osmotic pressure lets water flow into the cell, causing it to swell and possibly burst.

infiltration The escape of fluid into the surrounding tissue; the result of vein perforation during IV cannulation.

inhalation Breathing into the lungs; a medication delivery route.

interstitial fluid The water bathing the cells; accounts for about 10.5% of body weight; includes special fluid collections, such as cerebrospinal fluid and intraocular fluid.

intracellular fluid (ICF) The water contained inside the cells; normally accounts for 45% of body weight.

intramuscular (IM) Into a muscle; a medication delivery route.

intranasal Within the nose.

intraosseous Within the bone.

intraosseous (IO) infusion A technique of administering fluids, blood and blood products, and medications into the intraosseous space of a long bone, usually the proximal tibia.

intraosseous (IO) space The spongy cancellous bone of the epiphyses and the medullary cavity of the diaphysis, collectively.

intravascular fluid Plasma; the water within the blood vessels, which carries red blood cells, white blood cells, and vital nutrients; normally accounts for about 4.5% of body weight.

intravenous Within a vein.

intravenous (IV) therapy Cannulation of a vein with an IV cannula to access the patient's vascular system.

ionic concentration The amount of charged particles found in a particular area.

ions Charged atoms or compounds that results from the loss or gain of an electron.

isotonic crystalloids Intravenous solutions that do not cause a fluid shift into or out of the cell; examples include normal saline and lactated Ringer's solutions.

isotonic solution A solution that has the same concentration of sodium as does the cell. In this case, water does not shift, and no change in cell shape occurs.

lactated Ringer's (LR) solution A sterile isotonic crystalloid IV solution of specified amounts of calcium chloride, potassium chloride, sodium chloride, and sodium lactate in water. Also called Hartmann's solution.

local reactions Reactions that occur in a localised area; a potential complication of IV therapy.

macrodrip sets Administration sets named for the large orifice between the piercing spike and the drip chamber; allow for rapid fluid flow into the vascular system; allow 10 or 15 gtt/ml, depending on the manufacturer.

medical asepsis A term applied to the practice of preventing contamination of the patient by using aseptic technique.

metabolic Pertaining to the breakdown of ingested foodstuffs into smaller and smaller molecules and atoms that are used as energy sources for cellular function.

metered-dose inhaler (MDI) A pressurised canister that delivers a specific dose of a medication; commonly used for beta-agonist bronchodilators.

metric system A decimal system based on tens for the measurement of length, weight, and volume.

microdrip sets Administration sets named for the small needlelike orifice between the piercing spike and the drip chamber; allow for carefully controlled fluid flow and are ideally suited for medication administration; allow for 60 gtt/ml.

mucosal atomiser device (MAD) A device that attaches to the end of a syringe that is used to spray (atomise) certain medications via the intranasal route.

nebuliser A device for producing a fine spray or mist that is used to deliver inhaled medications.

needlestick The puncturing of an emergency care provider's skin with a needle or cannula that was used on a patient.

nonelectrolytes Solutes that have no electrical charge; include glucose and urea; measured in milligrams (mg).

normal saline A solution of 0.9% sodium chloride; an isotonic crystalloid.

occlusion Blockage, usually of a tubular structure such as a blood vessel or IV cannula.

ocular Pertaining to the eye.

online medical control Type of medical control in which the paramedic is in direct contact with a doctor, usually via two-way radio or telephone.

osmolarity The ability to influence the movement of water across a semipermeable membrane.

osmosis The movement of water across a semipermeable membrane (for example, the cell wall) from an area of lower to higher concentration of solute molecules.

osteogenesis imperfecta A congenital bone disease that results in fragile bones.

osteomyelitis Inflammation of the bone and muscle caused by infection.

overhydration An increase in the body's systemic fluid volume.

over-the-needle cannula A Teflon (plastic) cannula inserted over a hollow needle.

parenteral route A route of medication administration that involves any route other than the gastrointestinal tract.

percutaneous Through the skin or mucous membrane.

peripheral vein cannulation Cannulating veins of the periphery, that is, those that can be seen and/or palpated. Examples of peripheral veins include those of the hand, arm, and lower extremity and the external jugular vein.

piercing spike The hard, sharpened plastic spike on the end of the administration set designed to pierce the sterile membrane of the IV bag.

postural hypotension Symptomatic drop in blood pressure related to the patient's body position; detected by measuring pulse and blood pressure while the patient is lying supine, sitting up, and standing. An increase in pulse rate and a decrease in blood pressure in any one of these positions is considered a positive sign for this condition.

prefilled syringes Medication syringes that are prepackaged and prepared with a specific concentration.

pressure infuser device A sleeve that is placed around the IV bag and inflated to force fluid to flow from the IV bag and into the tubing.

pulmonary embolism A blood clot or foreign matter trapped within the pulmonary circulation.

pyrogenic reaction A reaction characterised by an abrupt temperature elevation (as high as 41°C) with severe chills, backache, headache, weakness, nausea, and vomiting; a potential complication of IV or IO therapy.

radiopaque Feature of an IV cannula (or any other object) that allows it to appear on an X-ray.

sharps Any contaminated item that can cause injury; includes IV needles and cannulas, broken ampoules or vials, or anything else that can penetrate or lacerate the skin.

sodium-potassium (Na^+-K^+) pump The mechanism by which the cell brings in two potassium (K^+) ions and releases three sodium (Na^+) ions.

solute The dissolved particles contained in the solvent.

solution Combination of dissolved elements (solutes) and water (solvent).

solvent The fluid that does the dissolving, or the solution that contains the dissolved components.

sterile The destruction of all living organisms; achieved by using heat, gas, or chemicals.

subcutaneous (SC) Into the tissue between the skin and muscle; a medication delivery route.

sublingual Under the tongue; a medication delivery route.

syncopal episodes Fainting; brief losses of consciousness caused by transiently inadequate blood flow to the brain.

systemic complications Reactions that affect systems of the body.

third spacing The shifting of fluid into the tissues, creating oedema.

thrombophlebitis Inflammation of a vein.

through-the-needle cannulas Plastic cannulas inserted through a hollow needle; referred to as Intracaths.

tonicity The osmotic pressure of a solution, based on the relationship between sodium and water inside and outside the cell, that takes advantage of their chemical and osmotic properties to move water to areas of higher sodium concentration.

total body water (TBW) Total amount of water in the human body; accounts for approximately 60% of the weight of an average man; divided into various compartments.

track marks The visible scars from repeated cannulation of a vein; commonly associated with illicit drug use.

transdermal Across the skin; a medication delivery route.

tubules Sections of the kidney where the filtration of wastes, electrolytes, and water is controlled.

Vacutainer A cylindrical device that attaches to an 18- or 20-gauge sampling needle; accommodates self-sealing blood tubes when obtaining blood samples.

venous thrombosis The development of a stationary blood clot in the venous circulation.

vials Small glass or plastic bottles that contain medication; may contain single or multiple doses.

Assessment in Action

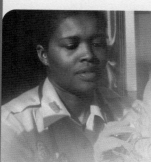

You and your colleague are dispatched to a block of flats because of a possible overdose. Police officers are already present and inform you that the scene is secure and safe. When you enter the flat, you find the patient, a 30-year-old man, unconscious in the sofa. With the assistance of the police, you and your colleague quickly move the patient to the floor and perform an initial assessment. The patient has reduced respirations and a slow, weak radial pulse. There is no gross bleeding or evidence of trauma.

1. **How will you treat this patient initially?**
   A. Apply oxygen via nonrebreathing mask.
   B. Suction his oropharynx for 15 seconds.
   C. Provide bag-valve-mask ventilation and 100% oxygen.
   D. Manually open his airway and insert an airway adjunct.

2. **Your partner assesses the patient's respirations and notes that they are slow and shallow. What should you direct him to do?**
   A. Apply a nonrebreathing mask set at 15 l/min.
   B. Provide bag-valve-mask ventilation and 100% oxygen at 15 l/min.
   C. Assess the patient's oxygen saturation with a pulse oximeter.
   D. Help you prepare to perform immediate endotracheal intubation.

3. **Following additional assessment of the patient, you suspect a narcotic overdose. While your partner continues to manage the patient's airway, you prepare to establish vascular access. Which of the following statements regarding vascular access is MOST correct?**
   A. You should immediately insert an IO cannula into the patient's proximal tibia.
   B. External jugular vein cannulation is preferred when patients are deeply unconscious.
   C. Glucose 10% in water is the fluid of choice for patients who may require volume expansion.
   D. The antecubital fossa is the preferred vein to use when starting an IV on a critically ill or injured patient.

4. **Which of the following IV cannulas will allow you to deliver the greatest amount of volume in the *shortest* period?**
   A. 14-gauge
   B. 16-gauge
   C. 18-gauge
   D. 20-gauge

5. **Vascular access has been obtained. Your guidelines call for the administration of naloxone (Narcan) in a dose of 400 mcg. You have a pre-filled syringe of naloxone containing 1 mg in 5 ml. How many millilitres of naloxone will you administer to achieve the desired dose of 400 mcg?**
   A. 1 ml
   B. 2 ml
   C. 3 ml
   D. 4 ml

6. **Compared with medications administered via the enteral route, parenteral medications:**
   A. must be instilled through a gastric tube.
   B. can be delivered only by the IV route.
   C. do not pass through the gastrointestinal tract.
   D. reach the central circulation at a much slower rate.

7. **Which of the following medication routes has the *slowest* rate of absorption?**
   A. Intravenous
   B. Transdermal
   C. Subcutaneous
   D. Intramuscular

8. **Shortly after administering naloxone to your patient, the IV line infiltrates. You obtain a blood glucose reading of 2 mmol/l and must administer glucagon via the IM route. However, glucagon must be reconstituted before being administered. What does drug reconstitution involve?**

   A. Administration of the drug during a period of at least 5 seconds

   B. Delivering the medication in the form of a maintenance infusion

   C. Diluting the drug with at least 5 ml of normal saline or sterile water

   D. Adding diluent to the powdered form of the drug to make a solution

Challenging Questions

A 54-year-old male is found unconscious in his home by a close friend. The patient is unresponsive, breathing slowly and shallowly, and is bradycardic. As your colleague begins ventilation assistance with a bag-valve-mask device and 100% oxygen, you find a bottle of hydrocodone—a potent narcotic analgesic—on an adjacent table. The prescription was filled 2 days earlier and is now empty. According to the friend, the patient recently had bilateral knee replacements, and was prescribed the medication for pain relief. He further states that the patient has "emotional problems". Recognising that the patient will require naloxone, you attempt to establish a peripheral IV line, but are unsuccessful after several attempts. Your partner reports that she is not having difficulty with bag-valve-mask ventilation.

9. **Should you intubate this patient?**

10. **What alternate medication routes are available to administer the Narcan?**

Points to Ponder

You and your colleague are treating a 35-year-old man with a headache. The patient is conscious and alert and denies chest pain or shortness of breath. His blood pressure is 130/84 mm Hg, heart rate is 44 beats/min and regular, and respirations are 16 breaths/min and unlabored. Further assessment reveals that the patient's skin is pink, warm, and dry, and his lungs are clear to auscultation bilaterally. The cardiac monitor reveals sinus bradycardia at 40 beats/min.

An IV line is established and set at a to keep vein open (TKVO) rate. As you are obtaining the patient's medical history, your paramedic partner administers 1 mg of atropine sulphate to the patient. Following administration of the atropine, the patient experiences tachycardia at a rate of 130 beats/min and becomes anxious and nauseous. However, his symptoms have resolved by the time you arrive at hospital.

Analyze this situation and explain what happened.

Issues: Recognising a Patient in Stable Versus Unstable Condition, Understanding the Need to Verify the "Six Rights" of Medication Administration, Documenting and Reporting a Medication Error.

9

Human Development

Objectives

Cognitive

- Compare the physiological and psychosocial characteristics of an infant with those of an early adult.
- Compare the physiological and psychosocial characteristics of a toddler with those of an early adult.
- Compare the physiological and psychosocial characteristics of a pre-school child with those of an early adult.
- Compare the physiological and psychosocial characteristics of a school-aged child with those of an early adult.
- Compare the physiological and psychosocial characteristics of an adolescent with those of an early adult.
- Summarise the physiological and psychosocial characteristics of an early adult.

- Compare the physiological and psychosocial characteristics of a middle aged adult with those of an early adult.
- Compare the physiological and psychosocial characteristics of a person in late adulthood with those of an early adult.

Affective

- Value the uniqueness of infants, toddlers, pre-school, school aged, adolescent, early adulthood, middle aged, and late adulthood physiological and psychosocial characteristics.

Psychomotor

None

Another type of attachment, referred to as <u>anxious avoidant attachment</u>, is observed in infants who are repeatedly rejected. These children develop an isolated lifestyle where they do not have to depend on the support and care of others.

<u>Trust and mistrust</u> refers to a stage of development from birth to about 18 months of age. Most infants desire that their world be planned, organised, and routine. When their caregivers and parents provide this environment for them, the infant gains trust in those individuals. The opposite also holds true (**Figure 9-5 ▸**).

Toddlers and Preschoolers

Physical Changes

In <u>toddlers</u> (ages 1 to 3 years (**Figure 9-6 ▸**) and <u>preschoolers</u> (ages 3 to 5 years (**Figure 9-7 ▸**)), the heart rate and respiratory rate are slower than the corresponding vital signs in infants, whereas the systolic blood pressure is higher (approximately 100 mm Hg). At the same time, weight gain should level off.

At the Scene

When dealing with patients who are very young, try to keep their routine the same by keeping family and familiar items nearby.

A toddler's cardiovascular system isn't dramatically different from that of an adult. A toddler's lungs continue to develop more bronchioles and alveoli. Although toddlers and preschoolers have more lung tissue, they do not have well-developed lung musculature. This anomaly prevents them from sustaining deep or rapid respirations for an extended period of time.

The loss of passive immunity in the immune system is possibly the most obvious development at this stage of human life. "Colds" often develop that may manifest as gastrointestinal distress or upper respiratory tract infections. As toddlers spend

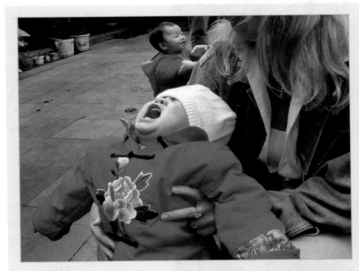

Figure 9-5 If an infant perceives that his or her parents or caregivers will not provide an organised, routine environment, the infant can develop behavioural problems.

You are the Paramedic Part 2

You apply supplemental high-flow oxygen to your patient, place her in a position of comfort, and begin your focused assessment and history. Your assessment reveals right-sided lower abdominal pain rated as 9 on a 10-point scale, with radiation to the back and groin. You continue to ask your patient questions about her history. Her father provides answers about her prior knee surgery a few years ago, and the fact that she takes salbutamol and beclometasone inhalers for her allergies and asthma.

When you ask the patient about her last menstrual period, you discover that she is taking extended-cycle birth control pills for regulation of her menstrual cycle and that her last period was a little less than 2 months ago. Per her medication schedule, her next menstrual period is due in about a month and a half. When you ask the patient whether there is any chance she may be pregnant, she adamantly denies the possibility, and her father is insulted that you would ask such a question.

Assessment	Recording Time: 10 Minutes
Skin	Pale, warm, and moist
Pulse	118 beats/min
Blood pressure	130/88 mm Hg
Respirations	24 breaths/min
SpO₂	100% on 15 l/min nonrebreathing mask on supplemental oxygen

4. What are your differential diagnoses now?
5. What is your next step in treatment of this patient?

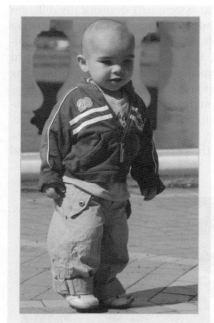

Figure 9-6 A toddler.

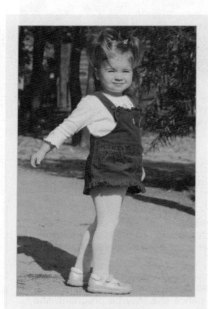

Figure 9-7 A preschooler.

more time around play-mates and classmates, they acquire their own immunity as the body is exposed to various viruses and germs.

Neuromuscular growth also makes considerable progress at this age. Toddlers and preschoolers spend a great deal of time finding out exactly how to use their expansive nervous system and the muscles it controls by walking, running, jumping, and playing catch Figure 9-8 ▶ . This stage also includes the continued development of the renal system and of elimination patterns (ie, toilet training).

Other developments that occur during this time frame include the emergence of "baby" teeth. Teething (ie, "breaking teeth" through the gums) can be painful and accompanied by pyrexia. In addition, parents and toddlers are enthralled with sensory development—for example, tickling.

Psychosocial Changes

This period of development is often exciting for parents. The toddler or preschooler is learning to speak and express himself or herself, thereby taking a major step toward independence. By the age of 3 or 4 years,

most children can use and understand full sentences. As they progress through this stage of their life, they will go from using language to communicate what they want, to using language creatively and playfully.

This is also the time when toddlers begin to interact with other playmates and start to play games. Playing games teaches control, following of rules, and even competitiveness. A lot of learning and development takes place by the child watching his or her peers during group outings, such as "school visits" with other children. Of course, behaviour observed on television and computers can also be learned, which is why some parents limit their children's viewing choices or the amount of time they devote to these activities. During this phase of development, children also learn to recognise sexual differences by observing their role models.

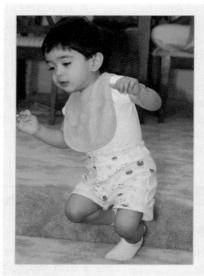

Figure 9-8 Toddlers learn to walk, one of the major milestones in life.

School-Age Children

Physical Changes

From ages 5 to 12 years, a school-age child's vital signs and body gradually approach those observed in adulthood Figure 9-9 ▶ . Obvious physical traits and body function changes become apparent as most children grow about 2 kg and 6 cm each year. Their permanent teeth also come in during this period.

Psychosocial Changes

Children are engaged in a lot of psychosocial growing up during the school years. Parents as a whole do not devote as much time to their children during this

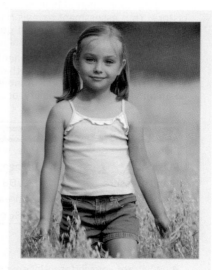

Figure 9-9 A school-age child.

At the Scene

With toddlers and preschoolers, you might try to "break the ice" by giving them a teddy bear and explaining what you are going to do by showing them on the teddy bear. Such children may be able to understand by show-and-tell more clearly than using only a verbal description.

phase. Nevertheless, it is at this critical time in human development that children learn various types of reasoning. In preconventional reasoning, children act almost purely to avoid discipline and to get what they want. In conventional reasoning, they look for approval from their peers and society. In postconventional reasoning, children make decisions guided by their conscience.

During this stage, children begin to develop their self-concept and self-esteem. Self-concept is our perception of ourselves; self-esteem is how we feel about ourselves and how we "fit in" with our peers.

Adolescents (Teenagers)

Physical Changes

The vital signs of adolescents (ages 12 to 18 years Figure 9-10 ▼) begin to level off within the adult ranges, with

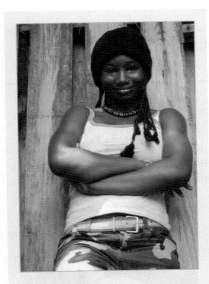

Figure 9-10 An adolescent.

a systolic blood pressure generally between 90 and 110 mm Hg, a pulse rate between 60 and 100 beats/min, and respirations in the range of 12 to 16 breaths/min. Adolescence is also the time of life when humans experience a growth spurt (ie, an increase in muscle and bone growth) and blood changes. As a whole, boys experience this stage of development later in life than girls do. When this period of growth has finished, however, boys are generally taller and stronger than girls.

One of the more subtle changes during this phase of life is the maturation of the human reproductive system. Secondary sexual development begins, along with enlargement of the external sex organs. Pubic hair and axillary hair begin to appear. Voices start to change in range and depth. In females, the breasts and thighs increase in size as adipose tissue is deposited there. Menstruation begins during this time; menarche is starting to occur at increasingly younger ages, however, so it is not uncommon to begin menstruation prior to becoming a teenager. Another key development in female teenagers is the release of follicle-stimulating hormone and luteinising hormone, both of which increase oestrogen and progesterone production. In contrast, the hormone gonadotrophin is secreted in males and results in the production of testosterone. Acne can occur due to hormonal changes.

Psychosocial Changes

Adolescents and their families often deal with conflict as teenagers try to gain control of their lives from their parents. Privacy becomes an issue among adolescents, their siblings, and their parents. Adolescents may struggle to create their own identity—to define who they are Figure 9-11 ▼ . They may also show greater interest in sexual relations. Many adolescents

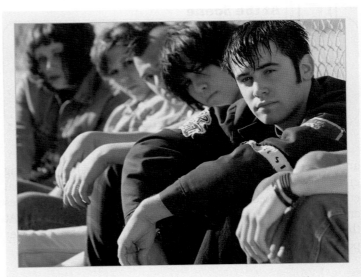

Figure 9-11 Adolescents want to fit in and may struggle to create an identity.

You are the Paramedic Part 3

You and your partner load your frightened patient into the back of your ambulance, whilst her father returns to the house for his wallet and keys. In a professional manner, you tactfully repeat your prior questions regarding her sexual activity and the possibility of pregnancy, acknowledging her previous answers may have been for the benefit of her father and reminding her that it is important to her health that you know the truth. She confides in you that she is sexually active and that she missed taking a couple of her birth control pills in the past few months. She says, "I'm freaking out. I think I'm pregnant and my dad's going to kill me"! You try to calm the patient and continue to provide care, including the initiation of an IV line. At hospital, you give your report to the accident and emergency department nurse and your partner shows the patient's father to the waiting area.

6. What is your primary differential diagnosis now?

7. Did this diagnosis alter your care?

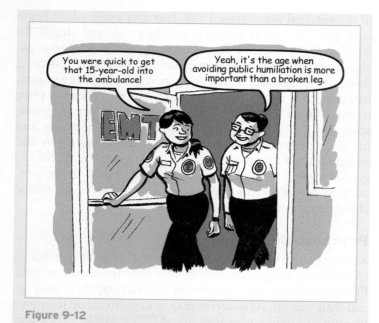

Figure 9-12

At the Scene

When you interview adolescents in the presence of their family, they may not tell you the complete truth so as to protect their privacy or image. It is best to ask these patients certain questions in total privacy, where they feel they can answer without constraint.

are fixated on their public image and are terrified of being embarrassed Figure 9-12 ▲. At this age, a code of personal ethics is developed, based partly on parents' ethics and values and partly on the influence of the teenager's environment. At this tumultuous time, teenagers are at a higher risk than other populations for suicide and depression.

Early Adults

Physical Changes

Early adults range in age from 19 to 40 years Figure 9-13 ▶. Their vital signs do not vary greatly from those seen throughout adulthood. Ideally, the human heart rate will stay around 70 beats/min, the respiratory rate will stay in the range of 12 to 20 breaths/min, and the systolic blood pressure will be approximately 120/80 mm Hg.

From age 19 years to just a little after 25 years, the human body should be functioning at its optimal level. After this point, the discs in the spine begin to settle, and height can sometimes be affected, causing a "shrinking". Fatty tissue increases, which leads to weight gain. Muscle strength

decreases, and the reflexes slow. For all these reasons, accidents are common causes of death in this age group.

Psychosocial Changes

Three words best describe a human's world during this stage of life: work, family, stress. During this period, humans strive to create a place for themselves in the world, and many do everything they can to "settle down". Along with this natural tendency to settle comes love and childbirth. Despite all of this stress and change, this age group enjoys one of the more stable periods of life.

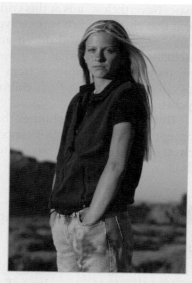

Figure 9-13 An early adult.

Middle Adults

Physical Changes

Middle adults are ages 41 to 60 years Figure 9-14 ▾ . This group is vulnerable to vision and hearing loss. Cardiovascular health also becomes an issue in many of these individuals, as does the greater incidence of cancer. In women, menopause—the cessation of menstruation—begins in the late 40s or early 50s.

Psychosocial Changes

Middle adults tend to focus on achieving their life's goals, as they realise that they are approaching the halfway point in human life expectancy. At this point, many parents must cope with becoming a married couple

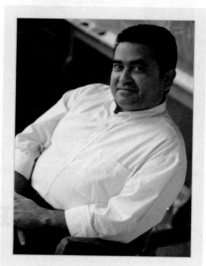

Figure 9-14 A middle adult.

again and reprioritise their lives as their children leave the home, creating "empty nest" syndrome. Finances may become a worrying issue, as people look forward to retirement and experience small crisis moments. The term *mid-life crisis* describes a person who makes a dramatic gesture in a bid to reclaim his or

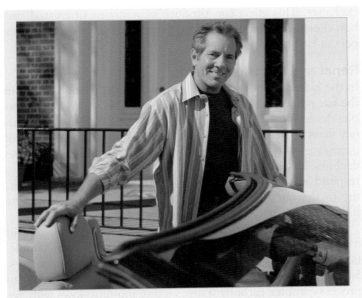

Figure 9-15 The classic example of the mid-life crisis is the middle-aged man who buys a fancy, expensive sports car!

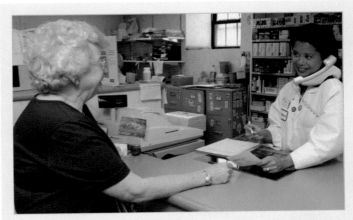

Figure 9-17 Older people are often on multiple medications to help them stay active.

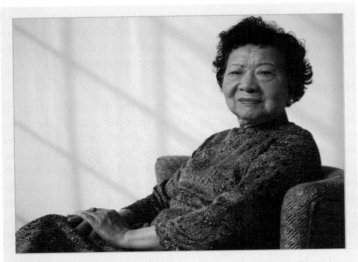

Figure 9-16 A late adult.

her youth. The classic example is the 45-year-old father of three who buys a bright red, two-seat convertible sports car Figure 9-15 ▲ .

▌Late Adults

Physical Changes

Late adults include those ages 61 and older Figure 9-16 ▲ . Life expectancy is constantly changing. When the first edition of this text was printed in 1979, life expectancy was about 73 years. It is approximately 77 years at this time, with maximum life expectancy estimated at 120 years.

Later in life, the vital signs depend on the patient's overall health, medical conditions, and medications taken. Today's late adults are staying active longer than their ancestors. Thanks to medical advances, they are often able to overcome numerous medical problems, but may need multiple medications to do so Figure 9-17 ▲ .

Cardiovascular System

Cardiac function declines with age consequent to anatomic and physiological changes that are largely related to atherosclerosis. In this disorder, which is most likely to affect coronary vessels, cholesterol and calcium build up inside the walls of blood vessels, forming plaque. The accumulation of plaque eventually leads to partial or complete blockage of blood flow. Atherosclerosis can also contribute to development of an aneurysm, or weakening and bulging of the blood vessel wall; an aneurysm may potentially rupture if it is subjected to high stretching forces. More than 60% of people older than age 65 have atherosclerotic disease.

Other age-related changes typically include a decrease in heart rate, a decline in cardiac output (the amount of blood circulated each minute), and the inability to elevate cardiac output to match the demands of the body. The vascular system also becomes stiff. For example, the pressure of systole increases with age. The left ventricle must then work harder, so it becomes thicker, losing its elasticity in this process. The thickening and stiffening of this muscle hinders filling in the ventricle, thereby decreasing cardiac output. Similar stiffening occurs in the heart valves, which may impede normal blood flow into and out of the heart. As the blood passes through these stiffened valves, a heart murmur may be heard, even in the absence of disease. Decreases in elastin and collagen in blood vessel walls, in turn, reduce the elasticity of the peripheral vessels by as much as 70%. Compensation for blood pressure changes will be hampered because these vessels are less able to distend and contract.

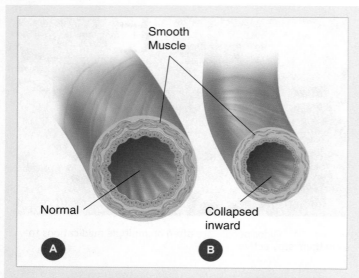

Smooth Muscle

Normal

Collapsed inward

A

B

Figure 9-18 **A.** Healthy muscle in a younger patient's airway helps maintain the open airway during the pressures of inhalation. **B.** Muscle weakening with age can lead to airway collapse that may produce wheezing.

Respiratory System

In late adults, the size of the airway increases and the surface area of the alveoli decreases. The natural elasticity of the lungs also decreases, forcing them to use their intercostal muscles more to breathe. In addition, the chest becomes more rigid because of calcification of the ribs to the sternum, which adds to the difficulty breathing.

The loss of the mechanisms that protect the upper airway can include a decreased ability to clear secretions as well as decreased cough and gag reflexes. The cilia that line the airways diminish with age, while the innervation of the structures in the airway provides increasingly less sensation. Without the ability to maintain the upper airway, aspiration and obstruction become more likely.

When a younger patient inhales, the airway maintains its shape, allowing air to enter. As the smooth muscles of the lower airway weaken with age, strong inhalation can make the walls of the airway collapse inward and cause inspiratory wheezing (Figure 9-18 ▲). The collapsing airways result in low flow rates, because less air can move through the smaller airways, and air trapping, because air does not completely exit the alveoli (incomplete expiration).

By the age of 75 years, the vital capacity (the volume of air moved during the deepest inspiration and expiration) may amount to only 50% of the vital capacity noted in young adulthood. Factors contributing to this decline include loss of respiratory muscle mass, increased stiffness of the thoracic cage, and decreased surface area available for the exchange of air.

Physiologically, vital capacity decreases and residual volume (the amount of air left in the lungs after expiration of the maximum possible amount of air) increases with age. As a consequence, stagnant air remains in the alveoli and hampers gas exchange. This effect can produce hypercarbia (increased carbon dioxide in the bloodstream) and acidosis, even when the person is at rest.

Renal and Gastric Systems

In the kidneys, both structural and functional changes occur in the late adult. The filtration function of these organs, for example, declines by 50% between the ages of 20 and 90 years. Kidney mass decreases by 20% over the same span. The number of nephrons—the basic filtering units in the kidneys—also declines between the ages of 30 and 80 years. Ageing kidneys respond less efficiently to haemodynamic stress (ie, stress relating to the circulation of blood) and to fluid and electrolyte imbalances.

Changes in gastric and intestinal function may inhibit nutritional intake and utilisation in older adults. For example, tastebud sensitivity to salty and sweet sensations decreases. Saliva secretion decreases, which reduces the body's ability to process complex carbohydrates. Gastric motility slows with age because of the loss of intestinal tract neurons, which can lead older adults to feel constipated or not hungry. Likewise, gastric acid secretion diminishes. Blood flow in the mesenteries (membranes that connect organs to the abdominal wall) may drop by as much as 50%, decreasing the ability of the intestines to extract nutrients from digested food. Gallstones become increasingly common with age, and anal sphincter changes reduce elasticity and can produce faecal incontinence.

Nervous System

Nervous system changes can result in the most debilitating of age-related ailments. In the central nervous system, the brain weight may shrink 10% to 20% by age 80 years. A selective loss of 5% to 50% of neurons occurs, and the surviving neurons shrink in size. The frontal lobe may lose as much as 20% of its synapses (the junctions between neurons) over the course of a person's life. Motor and sensory neural networks become slower and less responsive. The metabolic rate in the older brain does not change, however, and oxygen consumption remains constant throughout life.

The brain, which is surrounded by the meninges, takes up almost all of the space in the skull. Cerebrospinal fluid protects the brain inside these membranes. Unfortunately, age-related shrinkage creates a void between the brain and the outermost layer of the meninges, which provides room for the brain to move when stressed. This shrinkage also stretches the bridging veins that return blood from inside the brain to the dura mater. If trauma moves the brain forcibly, the bridging veins can tear and bleed (Figure 9-19 ▶). Bleeding can empty into this void, resulting in a subdural haematoma, which may go unnoticed for some time. Increased intracranial pressure is required for signs of head trauma to be present; the intracranial pressure will not rise—and, therefore, its signs will not be present—until the void has been filled and pressurised. (For more information, see Chapter 21.)

Functioning of the peripheral nervous system also slows with age. Sensation becomes diminished and misinterpreted.

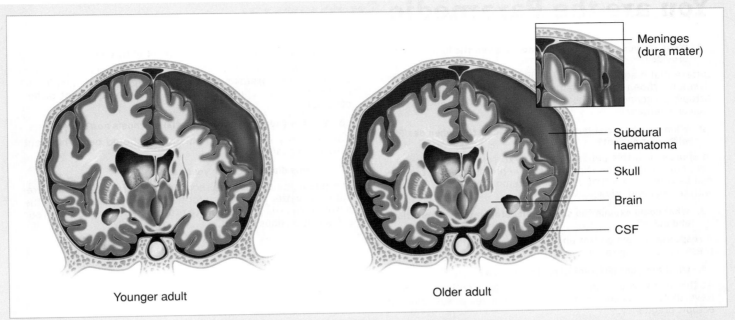

Figure 9-19 Brain atrophy with age can make tearing of the bridging veins more likely with trauma. It may also create a space into which bleeding can occur without producing immediate signs of increased intracranial pressure.

The resulting slowdown in reflexes may contribute to the incidence of trauma. Nerve endings deteriorate, and the ability of the skin to sense the surroundings becomes hindered. Hot, cold, sharp, and wet items can all create dangerous situations because the body cannot sense them quickly enough.

Sensory Changes

Pupillary reaction and ocular movements become more restricted with age. The pupils are generally smaller in older patients, and the opacity of the eye's lens diminishes visual acuity and makes the pupils sluggish when responding to light. Visual distortions are also common in older people. Thickening of the lens makes it harder for the eye to focus, especially at close range. Peripheral fields of vision become narrower, and a greater sensitivity to glare constricts the visual field.

Hearing loss is about four times more common than loss of vision in late adults. Changes in several hearing-related structures may lead to a loss of high-frequency hearing, or even deafness.

Psychosocial Changes

Paramedics should treasure their opportunities to spend time with and communicate with late adults. Many of them have amazing stories and experiences to share with us, yet we often take them for granted. Our elderly share with us a great amount of wisdom, and we need to remind them of their self-worth. Indeed, until about 5 years before death, most late-stage adults retain high brain function. In the 5 years preceding death, however, mental function is presumed to decline, a theory referred to as the terminal drop hypothesis.

As the elderly population continues to grow, we have the responsibility to seek out unique ways to accommodate their

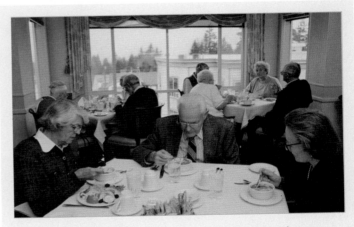

Figure 9-20 Many older adults live in sheltered housing communities.

needs during their last 20 to 40 years of life. While many older adults refuse to give up the independence of having their own home, the number of sheltered housing communities is growing across the nation. These facilities allow older adults to live in warden controlled communities with people in their own age group, while enjoying the privacy of their own accommodation Figure 9-20 ▲ . Unfortunately, these facilities can be expensive.

Most people need to deal with financial issues throughout their lives. Few things in life produce more worry and stress than money problems. Late adults, in particular, may constantly worry about rising costs of health care and are often forced to make decisions such as whether to pay for groceries or their medication.

You are the Paramedic Summary

1. What are your differential diagnoses given the information provided?

Differential diagnoses should include, but are not limited to, dysmenorrhoea (period pains), gastroenteritis, appendicitis, ectopic pregnancy, hernia, urinary tract infection, and psychological emergency.

2. What psychosocial factors need consideration when dealing with your patient?

In approaching this patient, you need to remember that she is very much capable of being a woman in physical terms, but may still be a teenage girl at a social and emotional level. Treat her with respect and privacy.

3. What could explain the slightly elevated patient respirations and pulse?

A response to pain and/or anxiety can increase the pulse, blood pressure, and respirations.

4. What are your differential diagnoses now?

At this point, you cannot rule out any differential diagnosis. Nevertheless, you should maintain a high index of suspicion for ectopic pregnancy.

5. What is your next step in treatment of this patient?

The paramedic should initiate IV access and should draw blood samples if local protocol allows while keeping the patient in the best position for comfort and repeated reassessment of her condition.

6. What is your primary differential diagnosis now?

Your primary diagnosis at this point should be to rule out ectopic pregnancy.

7. Did this diagnosis alter your care?

The possibility of ectopic pregnancy shouldn't alter your care, but it will better prepare you for transition of patient care at the hospital. You will also be able to provide better comfort for your extremely anxious patient.

Prep Kit

■ Ready for Review

- While each developmental stage is marked by different changes and characteristics, infants (1 month to 1 year) develop at a startling rate.
- The vital signs of toddlers (aged 1 to 3 years) and preschoolers (aged 3 to 5 years) differ somewhat from those of an infant.
- From ages 5 to 12 years, the school-age child's vital signs and body gradually approach those observed in adulthood.
- The vital signs of adolescents (aged 12 to 18 years) begin to level off within the adult ranges.
- Early adults are those who are age 19 to 40 years.
- Middle adults are those who are age 41 to 60 years.
- Late adults are those who are age 61 years and older.
- Vital signs do not vary greatly through adulthood.

■ Vital Vocabulary

adolescents Individuals who are 12 to 18 years of age.

aneurysm A swelling or enlargement of part of a blood vessel, resulting from weakening of the vessel wall.

anxious avoidant attachment A bond between an infant and his or her parent or caregiver in which the infant is repeatedly rejected and develops an isolated lifestyle that does not depend upon the support and care of others.

atherosclerosis A disorder in which cholesterol and calcium build up inside the walls of the blood vessels, forming plaque, which eventually leads to partial or complete blockage of blood flow.

barotrauma Injury resulting from pressure disequilibrium across body surfaces, for example from too much pressure in the lungs.

bonding The formation of a close, personal relationship.

conventional reasoning A type of reasoning in which a child looks for approval from peers and society.

ductus arteriosus A duct that is present before birth that connects the pulmonary artery to the aorta in order to move unoxygenated blood back to the placenta.

ductus venosus A duct that is present before birth that connects the placenta to the heart in order to move oxygenated blood to the foetus.

early adults Individuals who are 19 to 40 years of age.

fontanelles Areas where the infant's skull has not fused together; usually disappear at approximately 18 months of age.

foramen ovale An opening in the septum of the heart before birth, and which closes after birth.

growth plates Structures located on either end of an infant's bone, which aid in lengthening bones as the child grows.

hypercarbia Increased carbon dioxide levels in the bloodstream.

infants Individuals who are from 1 month to 1 year of age.

late adults Individuals who are 61 years old or older.

life expectancy The average amount of years a person can be expected to live.

mesenteries The membranes that connect organs to the abdominal wall.

middle adults Individuals who are 41 to 60 years of age.

moro reflex An infant reflex in which, when an infant is caught off guard, the infant opens his or her arms wide, spreads the fingers, and seems to grab at things.

nephrons The basic filtering units in the kidneys.

palmar grasp An infant reflex that occurs when something is placed in the infant's palm; the infant grasps the object.

postconventional reasoning A type of reasoning in which a child bases decisions upon his or her conscience.

preconventional reasoning A type of reasoning in which a child acts almost purely to avoid discipline to get what he or she wants.

preschoolers Individuals who are 3 to 5 years of age.

rooting reflex An infant reflex that occurs when something touches an infant's cheek, and the infant instinctively turns his head toward the touch.

school age A person who is 5 to 12 years of age.

secure attachment A bond between an infant and his or her parent or caregiver, in which the infant understands that his parents or caregivers will be responsive to his needs and take care of him when he needs help.

sucking reflex An infant reflex in which the infant starts sucking when his or her lips are stroked.

terminal drop hypothesis The theory that a person's mental function declines in the last 5 years of life.

toddlers Individuals who are 1 to 3 years of age.

trust and mistrust A phrase that refers to a stage of development from birth to approximately 18 months of age, during which infants gain trust of their parents or caregivers if their world is planned, organised, and routine.

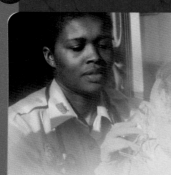

Assessment in Action

Your ambulance has arrived on the scene of an accident in which a people carrier has gone into the back of another vehicle at a fairly low speed. The people carrier's airbag did not deploy. Inside the people carrier you have four patients. The driver of the vehicle is a 38-year-old woman who was wearing a seatbelt. In the passenger seat is a 70-year-old woman who was also wearing a seatbelt. In the back seat are an infant who is restrained in a car seat and a toddler who has freed himself from his car booster seat.

1. **Which of your patients will be most prone to having airway occlusion problems?**
   A. Infant
   B. Adolescent
   C. Early adult
   D. Late adult

2. **When you assess the infant's vital signs, what should a normal respiratory rate be?**
   A. 12 to 20 breaths/min
   B. 18 to 24 breaths/min
   C. 30 to 60 breaths/min
   D. 26 to 40 breaths/min

3. **When you assess the infant's respiratory rate, you notice that the infant's chest is not moving but his abdomen is moving with his respirations. Is this a normal finding?**
   A. No, there is obviously an injury to the infant's chest.
   B. No, loosen the car seat straps and see if that makes a difference.
   C. No, remove the infant from the car seat immediately.
   D. Yes, infants are normally "abdominal breathers".

4. **The toddler in the vehicle is withdrawing from your attempts at a hands-on assessment. How will you continue to assess this toddler?**
   A. Reason with him.
   B. Explain what you want to do.
   C. Show the child what you are going to do using a prop.
   D. Let a family member continue the assessment.

5. **When doing your assessment on the 70-year-old patient, you attempt to check the pulse, motor function, and sensation on her lower extremities. The pulse is very hard to locate, and sensation appears to be nonexistent. You see no signs of trauma to the patient's lower extremities. To what source can you attribute this loss of sensation?**
   A. Peripheral nerve function slows with ageing.
   B. You must be missing a traumatic injury.
   C. There is no change to nerve function but there is with circulation.
   D. The patient is cold and does not adjust well.

6. **The female patient in the driver's seat is approximately 38 years old. What would you expect her normal vital signs to be if she had not been involved in this accident?**
   A. P = 70, R = 30, BP = 180/90
   B. P = 70, R = 16, BP = 120/80
   C. P = 100, R = 30, BP = 180/90
   D. P = 100, R = 16, BP = 120/80

Challenging Question

You have notified dispatch that you will need a second ambulance to respond to this location due to the number of patients. All of the patients appear to have non-time-critical injuries, which allows you to choose which patients will travel together.

7. **How will you use your knowledge of human development to make this decision?**

Points to Ponder

You are about to transport a toddler to hospital for a minor laceration that will need a few stitches. The toddler will not lie down on the stretcher and fights your attempts to calm him down. The mother of the child is willing to ride with you to hospital.

Where will you have her ride—in full view of the toddler or in one of the seats in the saloon where the toddler cannot see her?

Issues: Physical and Psychological Changes in Human Development, Stranger Anxiety.

10 Communication Skills

Objectives

Cognitive

- Define communication.
- Identify internal and external factors that affect a patient/bystander interview conducted by a paramedic.
- Restate the strategies for developing patient rapport.
- Provide examples of open-ended and closed or direct questions.
- Discuss common errors made by paramedics when interviewing patients.
- Identify the nonverbal skills that are used in patient interviewing.
- Restate the strategies to obtain information from the patient.
- Summarise the methods to assess mental status based on interview techniques.
- Discuss the strategies for interviewing a patient who is not motivated to talk.
- Differentiate the strategies a paramedic uses when interviewing a patient who is hostile compared to one who is cooperative.
- Summarise developmental considerations of various age groups that influence patient interviewing.
- Restate unique interviewing techniques necessary to employ with patients who have special needs.
- Discuss interviewing considerations used by paramedics in cross-cultural communications.

Affective

- Serve as a model for an effective communication process.
- Advocate the importance of external factors of communication.
- Promote proper responses to patient communication.
- Exhibit professional nonverbal behaviours.
- Advocate development of proper patient rapport.
- Value strategies to obtain patient information.
- Exhibit professional behaviours in communicating with patients in special situations.
- Exhibit professional behaviours in communication with patients from different cultures.

Psychomotor

None

Introduction

The scenario with the Browns in *You are the Paramedic Part 1* illustrates the importance of something we all need to remember throughout our careers. However well-intentioned we may be, some of us see people not as people but as their medical problems. That's a shallow approach to prehospital emergency medicine. It always begins with something else that's hard to teach, and which most of us never hear much about. The following pages are intended to guide you through the art and skills of communicating with people on the worst days of their lives.

People are not just medical puzzles for you to solve, and they're certainly not just nuisances or interruptions. They're the reason paramedics exist. And they deserve your best efforts at service.

Being a good paramedic requires a major talent for multitasking. When you're kneeling in front of Mr Brown, who is sitting there on his sofa and denying his symptoms, you should also be aware that Mrs Brown, seated right there next to him, is scared to death that she could lose him. More than that, you have to *feel* something for both of them. These are abilities you would not expect to find, and probably wouldn't need, in most other jobs. These abilities are the gifts of carers.

Internal Factors for Effective Communication

You need to be able to *naturally like people* (which is difficult for some people). You don't have to like them all, and you don't have to like them every day. But liking them has to be real for you, and it has to come easily. Why? Because when they defaecate in your ambulance, vomit on your shoes, or bleed all over your clean uniform, you have to be able to toler-

ate that without so much as a syllable of protest. These events are all part of a paramedic's job.

This chapter is based on the presumption that you like people, you care about them, and you honestly want to serve them. You'd better. Because if you don't, they will pick up your true feelings and poor attitude in the blink of an eye—and so will their families. And if you don't like people, you're pretty much guaranteed to hate doing what paramedics do every day: serving people, in their own time and on their own terms. As a paramedic you may see people looking their worst. They may smell like urine, vomit, digested blood, stale perspiration, faeces, or worse. But that's how real people really are, especially when they're sick. If you go into the prehospital environment expecting anything else, the mistake will be all yours and your patients will pay for it in the marginal care they may get from you. And you'll pay for it by having a really short career.

More than half of the calls you will attend as a paramedic will take you into people's homes, day and night and in the most private moments of their lives. Try to see every invitation into the home of someone else as a personal honour in a time and place where no one else would be welcome Figure 10-1 ▶ . You will be there when a lot of people are born, and you will be there when a lot of people die. In many cultures, people believe that God is present in times like these. Whether you subscribe to that belief or not, try hard to sense the privilege of being invited. It can make your career a lasting and fulfilling experience, instead of a source of drudgery.

External Factors for Effective Communication

A paramedic who looks the part of a professional inspires a lot more confidence in patients, in family members, and in the public than one who pays no attention to his or her appearance

You are the Paramedic Part 1

Mary and Bill Brown have been married for 44 years. Their four children have all moved away, and the two of them share a quiet rural home. Late one evening while watching TV, Mary notices that one side of her husband's face appears flaccid. When she asks him if he is all right, he says he's fine, but his words are slurred and difficult to understand. She waits only a few more minutes before announcing that she is going to call for help, and she dials 999 despite his protests. The paramedics who arrive a few minutes later are obviously tired from a busy shift.

Initial Assessment	Recording Time: 0 Minutes
Appearance	Flaccid and weak muscles on left side of patient's face
Level of consciousness	Alert (orientated to person, place, and day)
Airway	Open
Breathing	Normal rate; adequate depth
Circulation	Radial pulse present

1. What communication difficulties do you immediately anticipate in this scenario?

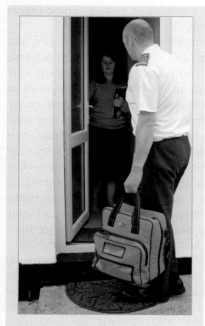

Figure 10-1 Think of it as an honour to be asked into a patient's home. Be respectful, and always be kind.

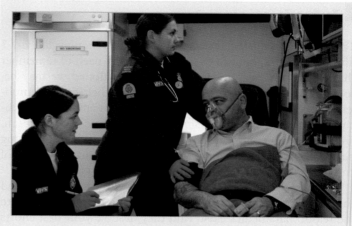

Figure 10-2 One way to comfort patients is to look as though you can help them, to look in charge. Be sure that your uniform is clean and that your shoes are clean, in good shape, and polished.

Figure 10-2 ▶ . You've heard this in other chapters but listen to this advice once again: polish your leather shoes and iron your shirt before you show up for work. Learn the principles of professional etiquette, and make sure your over-all behaviour inspires respect in people you don't know. That's more than being nice; it's what a professional does.

If you want people to tell you about their problems, convince them you want to hear what they have to say. Com-munication is the act of transmitting information to another person—and, for paramedics, it can be verbal or through body language. Give patients your undivided attention; don't treat them like nuisances. There's nothing worse than talking about someone in his or her presence, as though he or she is an inanimate object—or worse, as though the person doesn't even exist. And it's unforgivable to ask someone a question you're just going to repeat later because you didn't pay attention to the answer the first time. Write it down. When it's time to communicate, *communicate*. That means listen, don't just talk. Listening is part of communicating too, because it transmits information as well.

An excellent way to convince someone that you're really listening to him or her is a technique called "active listening". Almost all professional interviewers use it routinely. Active listening is repeating the key parts of a patient's responses to

At the Scene

Patients will pick up on how you treat or are treated by other ambulance staff at the scene. If you are treated with respect, and if you treat the other ambulance staff with respect, the patient will see this and have more confidence in you as well.

You are the Paramedic Part 2

Mary gets the impression from the paramedics' demeanour that they would prefer to be somewhere else. Twice she asks them what they think is happening to Bill, but they don't reply. Instead, they focused on giving oxygen, starting an IV, attaching electrodes, and performing various other skills and assessments. They don't talk to the patient except to ask questions, and they don't seem to appreciate or address the fact that Mary is terrified.

Vital Signs	Recording Time: 3 Minutes
Skin	Pale and cool; perspiring
Pulse	88 beats/min, irregular
Blood pressure	184/94 mm Hg
Respirations	18 breaths/min
SpO_2	97% on 15 l/min via nonrebreathing mask

2. Describe what the phrase "total patient care" means to you.

questions. Especially when you're taking notes at the same time, it helps you to convince patients that you really want to hear what they're saying. Active listening also helps confirm the information patients are providing. This ensures there is no misunderstanding between you and your patients.

Some specific expressions that are helpful are:

- When patients thank you, say, "You're very welcome"! (not "No problem". "No problem" implies, "That's OK; you aren't too much of a nuisance". It's definitely not as nice as saying, "You're welcome".)
- When patients apologise to you because they're incontinent or vomiting or because you have to carry them down a flight of stairs, tell them something like, "It's OK; you don't need to be sorry. This is what we do, *and we're here because we want to be"*.

If you like serving people, these kinds of expressions will feel natural to you, and no doubt you will find your colleagues imitating you after only a short time.

Try hard not to shout. Some scenes are very noisy. But even so, when you shout, so does everyone else. And when people are shouting, they tend to get excited. If you're answering a call in a noisy place such as a bar, ask the barstaff to help by turning off the music, turning up the lights, and keeping an eye on the other patrons. (In this type of situation, get your patient out of there as soon as you can.) Move the patient to your "office"—the back of the ambulance. If fire fighters must use a compressor or run a noisy generator on the scene, shut it off as soon as you can to cut down on the noise level. Meanwhile, try to talk close to your patient's ears in a calm voice. It lets him or her know that you have your emotions under control, which helps him or her stay calm as well. Try managing your history-taking all at one time. Taking the patient's medical and health history helps you stay organised and encourages people to take your questions seriously.

If you want reliable answers to personal questions, try to manage your scene so you can ask these kinds of questions quietly and in private. Even if you do earn a patient's trust, there are things people just don't want to talk about in front of others. Don't forget to ask a few patient centred questions— questions that don't fall under the category of routine medical history but that, time after time, will net you information that's critical to a presumptive diagnosis. Some patient centred questions are listed and explained later in this chapter.

Some scenes are easy to manage. But paramedics very often work in bizarre, noisy, difficult, and sometimes dangerous environments that are challenging at best Figure 10-3 ▶ . Under these circumstances, communicating with patients (and their family members) is especially critical to the skills of assessment and the art of bringing about calm (and therefore healing).

▍Developing Rapport

When you find yourself standing at someone's bedside in the middle of the night, if you really don't want to be there, if you

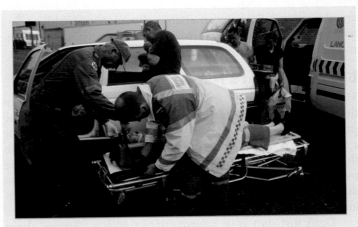

Special Considerations

Do not assume that all elderly patients are hard of hearing. You will be put in your place if you begin by talking loudly or too slowly to an older patient only to be told by the patient, "I'm not deaf".

Figure 10-3 Even in the most chaotic conditions, try to create a safe zone for your patient. Shut out everything else as best as you can, and focus on helping this one person.

really don't care how he or she feels, and if you just want to get back to the station, he or she will get the message, *whether you intended to give it or not.* Nothing you pretend, say, or do will fool your patient. If you really *do* want to be there, you really *do* care, your patient will get that message too.

People in crisis are highly perceptive, and there is no greater crisis than being scared to death that you're about to lose someone you love more than anyone in the whole world. Your most essential challenge as a therapeutic communicator is to convey calm, unmistakable, genuine concern for someone you've never met. People in crisis do much better if someone like you can help them to relieve their fear.

Watch Your Inflection

Your voice is just as important in communication as your words. You know what someone's voice sounds like when he or she is really concerned for you. Think about how the voice of someone who cares for you sounds when you are hurt or upset. Use that calm and steady tone of reassurance to reinforce your interest in and concern for the patient.

Respond to the Patient

There is probably nothing as insulting to a patient as asking or telling a paramedic something and receiving no response at all. Regardless of what the patient says, acknowledge what he or she said. If you are not comfortable responding, simply nod or restate what the patient said, without providing a definitive answer right away. If you later figure out how you can give more information, you may tell the patient at that point.

Tell People Who You Are

Once you break that initial ice with someone, tell him or her who you are. That's just common courtesy, but it is often overlooked by medical professionals. Tell them something more too. Tell them you're a paramedic. Remember, they're about to entrust their privacy and their medical well-being to someone they didn't know a moment ago. They deserve to know what you know (and what you don't). By introducing yourself, you are also saying, "You are in charge of your own health care. I will be your advocate, and ensure that we maintain good communications at all times".

Use the Patient's Name

Most of us use the same few words to greet our patients, both in the prehospital environment and in the hospital: "Hi. What's the problem"? That's OK for an amateur, but it doesn't say much for a professional. Why? Because people's names are important to them and to their families. Your name is the first thing you receive after birth, and it's the only thing you keep when you die (think about every gravestone you've ever seen). As a paramedic, use the importance of a person's name like a tool.

Don't just start your patient contact with a question about the medical problem. Introduce yourself, and then ask patients their name. That simple practice tells them their discomfort is important, but it also opens a window through which you can quickly assess a lot. Think about that for a few moments.

When you address patients with an expression like, "Hi. My name is Lee Jones and I'm a paramedic. What's your name"? what do they have to be able to do in order to answer appropriately? They have to go through a very specific sequence of physical and mental processes, which amounts to a mini-mental status examination. Consider the following:

- They have to hear your words.
- They have to locate the source of your voice and meet your gaze.
- They have to process the meaning of your words (in your common language).
- They have to formulate a meaningful, accurate response from memory.
- They have to put their response into coherent speech.
- They have to be able to do all of that within about 1 second.

During that second, if you're close enough to see the size of their pupils, you can assess their mental state and the function of at least six pairs of cranial nerves. That's a fair amount of assessment.

In addition, you've communicated something very important to the patient and his or her family just by asking that question—your respect. Part of your respectful behaviour is to introduce yourself with your name and your profession. Finally, using the names of people is good for us and for our colleagues. It reminds us that we're not just dealing with damaged bodies and broken hearts day after day. Instead, we're dealing with *people*.

You are the Paramedic Part 3

As the paramedics assess Mr Brown, his wife hears them casually discussing the likelihood of stroke. This is her worst nightmare as their GP had warned Bill about the risks of his high blood pressure and high cholesterol. After repeated attempts to communicate with the paramedics have failed, she becomes so frustrated that she screams, "Why do you keep ignoring me"?

Reassessment	Recording Time: 7 Minutes
Level of consciousness	Alert (orientated to person, place, and day)
Skin	Pale and cool; perspiring
Pulse	88 beats/min, irregular
Blood pressure	184/98 mm Hg
Respirations	18 breaths/min
SpO_2	96% on 15 l/min via nonrebreathing mask
ECG	Atrial fibrillation

3. Although the paramedics in this scenario are attending to the patient's medical needs, could the wife have a valid complaint regarding their caregiving?
4. How can your introductions (or lack of) and general demeanour affect your ability to communicate with your patients as well as with their friends and family members?

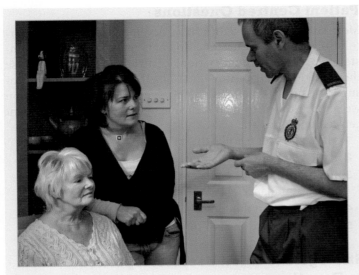

Figure 10-4 As soon as possible, you or your partner should explain to the patient's family members what is happening and what they can do. This information can help them deal with their fear and worry.

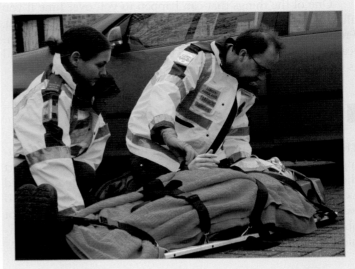

Figure 10-5 Show your patient the same respect you'd want others to show your father or brother or your mother or sister. Protect modesty with a blanket or towel.

Anticipate and Deal With Fear

Usually, after a few weeks of ambulance calls, you will be impressed with the fact that most patients are scared to death of the situation. If the patient isn't afraid, consider that one or more of his or her loved ones may be absolutely terrified 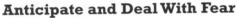. Reassurance may be one of the most important treatments you can provide.

How do you control fear? First, by your own sense of competence and professional calm. Second, by honestly caring about someone (a fact that, like kindness, patients and family members alike can easily detect). Third, by giving people information. When someone wakes up in the middle of the night with a dull, crushing chest pain, that person doesn't want to be treated like a child or someone who cannot understand what is happening. Tell your patients what you think is happening. Show patients what their ECG reveals, tell them their blood pressure, explain how you're planning to help them, and let them know how they're doing.

Respect the Importance of Pain Relief

When someone tells you he or she is in pain, let that person know you grasp and appreciate the situation, and then do something about it. One of the most grievous offences by carers (in and out of hospitals) is ignoring pain. People deserve to have their pain relieved as completely as possible, then and there—with a medical consultation if necessary. Don't make them wait. You wouldn't want your loved ones to wait for pain relief. A patient should never have to be patient about any pain you can alleviate, whether in the prehospital environment or in the hospital.

Respect and Protect People's Modesty

Modesty matters—no matter how acute the medical condition. It's especially important to the very old, adolescents, and sometimes, the very young. If the patient is not personally sensitive to modesty (because of an impaired mental state, for example), family members most certainly are Figure 10-5 ▲.

Help, Don't Judge

As a paramedic, you will need to know a person's medical history in order to help him or her. For example, you will need to use naloxone to treat an opiate addict. Sadly, drug and alcohol addicts support their addictions by lying. Few addicts will admit to drinking more than two pints, let alone to taking an opiate. Here's where your own moral code has to take a backseat to professional ethics. Try to avoid judging patients because the causes of addiction can be very complex. We can't pretend to know why people make the choices they make; we, as health care providers, see only the results of these choices.

When you ask someone an uncomplicated question in plain, simple English, and he or she responds with an unnecessarily complicated or inappropriate response, one of the things you should probably consider is the possibility that the patient is lying. Of course, that's not always true. Patients may also be mentally impaired (by chemicals, hypoxia, psychiatric disorders, or other causes of disorganised thinking). But lying does happen often enough, so you should anticipate it.

One of the things that can happen to you over time if you allow yourself to judge people is that you can become cynical. Professional scepticism is a useful tool; it facilitates sound, clinical decision-making. But cynicism is scepticism gone wild and is unproductive to you and your patients.

Conducting the Interview

The reason we question people is to find out how they're feeling, what happened that may have made them sick or hurt them, and what their lives have been like. But to quote the old expression about computers: "Rubbish in, rubbish out". If we're not careful about what questions we ask, we may not obtain the information we need. The following three techniques can make your questioning more productive.

Open-Ended Questions

When you need to know how someone feels, first try asking a question that makes the patient do the thinking. This is an open-ended question—a question that does not have a yes or no answer, and which does not give the patient specific options to choose from. For instance, if you ask patients to describe their own chest pain, don't suggest qualities like sharpness, dullness, or pressure. Instead, let them think of a word that describes how the pain feels; their own words will probably more accurately describe what they are feeling. Some examples of open-ended questions are:

- How have you been feeling lately?
- Do you have an idea of what is causing this?
- Do you have any other concerns about your health?
- Is there anything else you would like to discuss?

Closed-Ended Questions

Sometimes (for example, when you're trying to find out about a patient's medical history) you need answers to specific questions. In these cases, try a direct, or closed-ended question. In fact, it's a good idea to develop a standard set of questions concerning medical history that you ask almost all patients. Avoid talking down to them (that's insulting), but avoid using medical terms. Instead, try using words that people without medical training can understand. Your standard questions may include the following:

- Have you ever had any heart problems?
- Any lung problems?
- Any high or low blood pressure?
- Diabetes?
- Convulsions?
- Fainting spells?
- Any previous head injury?
- Do you have both of your lungs and kidneys?

If the patient is female and of childbearing age (generally, 12 to 50 years old), be sure to ask about her history of pregnancies, deliveries, miscarriages, and abortions, when her last menstrual period was and if it was normal, and if she has had any gynaecological surgery.

Patient Centred Questions

Most seasoned paramedics have developed their own repertoire of additional questions for patients in specific circumstances. We call them patient centred questions because they're like icebergs—tiny questions that can reveal huge subsurface issues. Sometimes these issues are the hidden reason we've been called to help someone. Some examples of patient centred questions are:

1. Have you ever felt like this before?
2. Have you been upset about anything lately?
3. Are you afraid of someone? (Save this one for the privacy of the ambulance.)
4. Have you been thinking about hurting yourself?
5. What happened the last time you felt this way?

Strategies to Elicit Useful Responses to Questions

To get the right answers, it's not always enough just to ask the right questions. Why? Because when people are in crisis, some of them are terrible communicators. It can be almost impossible to think and organise your thoughts when you are scared. Fortunately, good interviewers also have the following tools to use to get answers.

Facilitate the Response

If patients hesitate to answer questions completely, encourage them to provide you with more information. One useful expression is simply, "Please say more". Another is, "Please feel free to tell me about that".

Be Quiet

If you sense that patients are trying to put something into words but are having trouble expressing themselves, try this famous tip "Never miss a good opportunity to shut up". Be patient. Don't say anything at all for a few seconds. Let them talk.

Documentation and Communication

If you must stop patients from talking to get an urgent task done, explain to them why they need to be quiet and that they will be able to talk to you when you finish your task.

Clarify the Response

If you don't understand what patients have told you, ask them to explain what they mean. This communicates that you are listening and taking their comments seriously. It may also help you understand what they are trying to tell you.

Redirect the Response

Sometimes patients will mention something in passing or will avoid answering a specific question. You can politely redirect their attention to that question (several times, if necessary) until you get them to answer it.

Interpret the Response

If you've tried clarification and you're still not sure what patients are trying to tell you, sometimes it helps to say what you think they've said and invite them to correct you.

Simplify and Summarise the Response

Some patients have a hard time speaking plainly, no matter how hard they try. It can be difficult to communicate with people who have psychiatric problems, who fabricate their diseases, and who are afraid or upset. If patients give you a confusing or disorganised response, try putting their comments into simpler terms and see if they agree with your synopsis. It can help them focus their thoughts and help you as an interviewer.

Common Interviewing Errors

None of us are perfect, and all of us have made errors in the course of questioning patients. Learn to improve your interviewing skills by observing what other paramedics have done:

Assume Nothing!

Most mistakes carers make have happened as the result of assuming things. Assuming that a patient is faking unconsciousness or convulsions, assuming that a companion is a spouse, assuming that a fight victim is a member of a gang, or assuming that a patient is inebriated are very common mistakes. Try hard to become a careful observer and to keep your mind open to a wide range of possibilities. Remember that when we assume, sometimes it makes an "ass" out of "u" and "me".

Giving Medical Advice

Patients and their families often ask their paramedics for medical advice, in much the same way as they would consult a doctor. That's an honour because it conveys their trust. Patients may even ask you to comment on a decision by their GP. Don't fall for that one (however well-intentioned the question may be). Instead, suggest they obtain their medical advice from a doctor.

Providing False Hope

Try not to over encourage patients or their family members if a patient is very ill. You can't possibly see in advance what's going to happen to someone. But remember that the question, "Am I going to die"? is very different from the statement, "I think I'm going to die". Lots of patients whose status seems very stable will ask you if they're going to die. A good answer to that one is, "One day—but you look ok at the moment". Another option is "I don't know, but I hope not". Invite their family members to give them a kiss before taking them to the emergency department. It may be their last opportunity, and they will treasure that memory forever.

If the patient or a family member asks you if the patient is going to die, and the patient is not in stable condition, you could say, "We think he (or she) is very sick, but we're doing everything we possibly can to help".

Assuming Excessive Authority

Just as we're not qualified to judge people, it's important to remember that we're not police officers either. Adopting the no-nonsense demeanour of a police officer can frighten your patient, and make your job of caring for that patient nearly impossible. (How do *you* feel when you are pulled over by a police officer, just for having a faulty brake light?)

Sidestepping the Truth

Patients deserve to know what their blood pressure is, and what their ECG reveals about them. Their blood sugar (blood glucose) level isn't a secret you need to keep from them. When patients ask you what you think is wrong, remember that you

You are the Paramedic Part 4

Upon seeing his wife distraught, Mr Brown becomes upset as well. He tries to explain that she has recently had a heart attack, but his words are garbled and the paramedics are unable to understand him, in spite of his best efforts, so his message goes undelivered.

Reassessment	Recording Time: 10 Minutes
Level of consciousness	Alert (orientated to person, place, and day)
Skin	Pale, cool, and moist
Pulse	98 beats/min, irregular
Blood pressure	190/104 mm Hg
Respirations	18 breaths/min
SpO2	96% on 15 l/min via nonrebreathing mask
ECG	Atrial fibrillation
Blood glucose	4.0 mmol/l

5. How has this crew's lack of people skills affected this call?
6. Can this situation be mended?

are serving them. Remind them that you don't have definitive answers and that you're not a doctor, but tell them what you think may be going on. Be honest and sincere about what you're telling them, but never harsh.

Distancing Yourself From Patients as People

Another Western medical technique for maintaining the relationship between supposedly all-powerful doctors and impotent patients is professional distancing—that is, avoiding contact with patients as people. This can take the form of using lots of big, complicated medical words you hope they won't understand, and answering patients' questions with half-truths. No matter who uses these techniques, do not adopt them as your own. They will not serve your own or your patients' well-being in the long run.

Nonverbal Skills

People in crisis are still people, and you can use many of the same methods that other professional interviewers use to get them to tell you things. Following are a few of those skills or tools.

Eye Contact

Direct eye contact is something you avoid with animals; they perceive it as a sign of aggression. But people expect brief, frequent, direct eye contact, especially when they need reassurance. "Seeing eye-to-eye" with people generally communicates honesty and concern and is considered a baseline necessity of sincere communication of any kind **Figure 10-6 ▸** . Think about that when you consider interviewing a patient with your mirrored sunglasses on.

You won't always have time to fully interview some patients, especially if they're very sick. But try to remember that when a patient's status is subacute, your busy hands may correlate to you engaging in less (or no) eye contact. If the patient needs someone to talk to, take the time to listen when you can.

Touch

Some people don't like to be touched at all; to others, it's a valuable assurance that someone cares about them. You should try gently touching patients on a neutral part of the body, such as a shoulder or arm, especially when you're trying to reassure them or mitigate their fear **Figure 10-7 ▸** . But watch how they react. If they pull away from you, chances are that touch in this instance won't be a valuable strategy. If they react positively (for instance, by leaning toward you or seeming to relax), than touch as a form of reassurance will work with them.

Gentleness

Being gentle is actually a quality of touch (mentioned above). You can use it even with a patient who prefers not to be touched. Gentleness can be the easy way you place the head of your stethoscope against the patient's chest or the way you apply a blood pressure cuff or blanket.

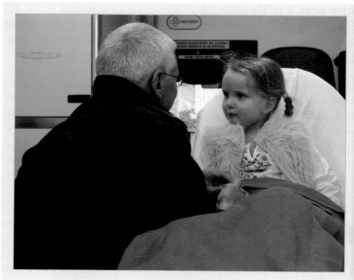

Figure 10-6 Whenever possible, put yourself at eye level with your patient. This is especially important when you're treating a child.

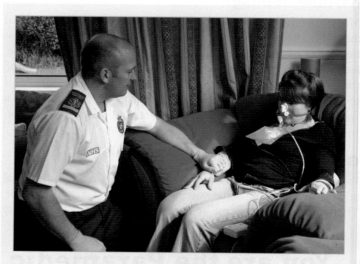

Figure 10-7 A gentle touch on the hand, arm, or shoulder can comfort someone who is sick or hurt and very scared.

Posture

When you're dealing with patients who are terrified, don't stand in front of them with your arms folded across your chest. That conveys confrontation, not concern. Instead, try to position yourself at the same level as (or below the level of) their eyes. Sit or kneel at an angle that would not encroach on their personal space. For instance, lots of paramedics squat on the floor or ground in front of people who are seated in a car or on a bus seat. Some choose to sit on the paramedic box.

Demeanour

A pleasant demeanour comes easily to people who like people. To others, it doesn't come at all; and it's one of the reasons we emphasised liking people earlier in this chapter. It's absolutely necessary when you're dealing with people in crisis, because

At the Scene

Avoid whispering, laughing, or sniggering with your partner or other responders in front of or within hearing distance of the patient. It is unprofessional. Even if it is not about them, they will feel as if it is.

they need to see you as someone who is safe to be with, who does not pose a threat, and who honestly cares. With that comes the belief that you are going to handle the crisis.

Therapeutic Smile

Anyone who has dealt with even a few scared people can tell you that a smile can greatly help relieve stress. Think back to a time when you were troubled by something and someone's smile told you that everything was going to be OK. Your ability to smile can be just as valuable when you're dealing with people in crisis.

Assessing Mental Status

Excellent communication is vital in assessing how alert and orientated your patients are. There are many useful techniques for assessing mental status, and most of them are simple and based on plain old common sense. We have already discussed the most versatile first step ever invented: asking a patient for his or her name. Beyond that, consider the patient's ability to express himself or herself in the following ways.

Appropriate Humour

The highest form of mental function is the spontaneous expression of appropriate humour. To generate that degree of mental status, a person has to possess a high degree of cognitive function and an intact memory. People who aren't thinking clearly don't have the neuronal function to invest in spontaneous humour.

Timing of Responses to Questions

Assess how long it takes a patient to respond appropriately to your questions. A patient who is thinking clearly should be able to answer simple questions that make sense within 1 second.

Memory (Person, Place, Day, and Event)

Patients should be able to tell you quickly and accurately who they are and who you are, where they are, what day of the week it is, and what happened that necessitated you being called. Incorrect responses to any of these constitute a memory dysfunction and possibly decreased blood flow to the brain.

Ability to Obey Simple Commands

Any disruption in a patient's ability to comply with requests in the preceding steps may indicate a brain dysfunction in the cerebrum or possibly the cerebellum. The dysfunction may be acute and could even be pre-existing.

Special Interview Situations

There are situations in paramedic practice that may require special communication techniques. Some of these may include uncommunicative patients, hostile patients, very old or very young patients, and patients with special needs. Stereotyping any of these groups of patients, however, will only work against effective communication. A good paramedic is never judgemental

You are the Paramedic Part 5

The paramedics attempt to calm Mrs Brown and apologise to her. She is now crying uncontrollably, and says she's experiencing chest pain and shortness of breath. She sits down next to her husband and self-administers a GTN tablet under her tongue. An IV of normal saline has been established to keep vein open.

Reassessment	Recording Time: 15 Minutes
Level of consciousness	Alert (orientated to person, place, and day)
Skin	Pale and cool; perspiring
Pulse	118 beats/min, irregular
Blood pressure	188/102 mm Hg
Respirations	18 breaths/min
SpO$_2$	98% on 15 l/min via nonrebreathing mask
ECG	Atrial fibrillation

7. What would be the best course of action in this situation?
8. What are the different forms of communication and how do they impact patient care?

about his or her patients. No one calls you to judge them or their circumstances; they call for your medical care! But you can and should try the following techniques when you find yourself *not* communicating well with some patients.

People Who Are Not Wanting to Talk

There's nothing wrong with a little quiet; in fact, people who talk too much can be fairly irritating. When patients refuse to talk and you're not seeing signs of decreased mental status, there's no need to force the issue. Instead, make lots of eye contact, express your concern in every way possible, explain everything you are doing, invite them repeatedly to answer questions, and let them know it's all right if they don't wish to talk. This strategy of accepting them as they are can be very effective at breaking down barriers.

People Who Are Hostile

You are guaranteed to receive some unpleasant insults from people who are in crisis, and the insults will probably happen quite frequently. It's especially predictable when you're dealing with people who are chemically impaired. Discipline yourself never to respond in kind. Nothing escalates a situation faster than trading insults. Very often, when it involves a patient or bystanders, there are plenty of witnesses. It makes no sense and it can be very dangerous, especially when you're on their turf (about which you know nothing and they know everything). Remember, you're a helper. Remember, just as you can't fix everybody medically, you can't fix everybody emotionally either. Consider the possibility that you may not be able to defuse someone's anger. If the situation gets out of control, you should request police assistance.

At the Scene

Learn to look for aggressive body language that signals increased anger and a possible attack such as clenched fists, intense staring directed at you, and breathing heavily through clenched teeth.

People Who Are Very Old or Very Young

Try not to presume that older people are any harder to communicate with than anyone else just because they're older. Their illnesses may tend to be more complex than the illnesses of younger people because they may have more than one disease or disorder and they may be taking more kinds of medicines concurrently. You may note individual differences among the older population related to hearing, eyesight, mental status, and mobility; you need to adapt to them. The fact remains, older people are individuals and their differences are individual. See Chapter 42 for more information on communicating with older people.

Children can be difficult patients because they pose communication challenges, even to the best paramedic. They tend

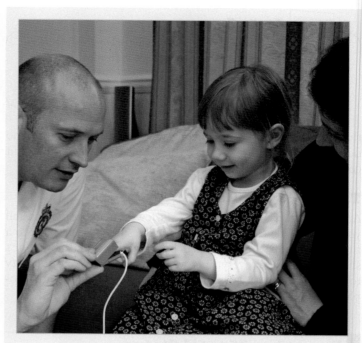

Figure 10-8 When you're examining a very young child, involve the parents. Have the father hold the child on his lap, or ask the mother to keep the toddler occupied while you work.

to protest pain vigorously, they may be afraid of strangers (like you). With a little practice, we can become comfortable treating them too.

Equipment (such as stethoscopes or needles) is not as important early in our contact with children as are friendly eye contact, smiles, and calm, subdued explanations, geared to match each child's age. Discipline yourself to minimise your movements, lower your voice, and touch as gently as you can. Try placing yourself at or below the child's eye level, for instance by sitting on the floor and placing the child on the cot or on a parent's lap Figure 10-8 ▲ . If possible, involve a parent in the hands-on care of a conscious small child (for instance, by holding an extremity while you insert a cannula). This is much less helpful when treating older children but is more important with infants and toddlers.

When parents are not available, toys are very useful for bridging the emotional gap between paramedics and some children. Some crews stock their ambulances with teddy bears for toddlers. Short of those, you can make a serviceable chicken out of an examination glove by inflating the glove and marking its eyes with a felt marker Figure 10-9 ▶ . You are more likely to connect with the child if you do this right in front of the child rather than if you ask someone else to do it.

Adolescents (from around the age of 12) may not want their parents present at all during questioning or examination. In fact, an adult who insists on monitoring your conversation with an adolescent should raise questions in your mind. Don't refuse the prerogative of a parent, but be sure you communi-

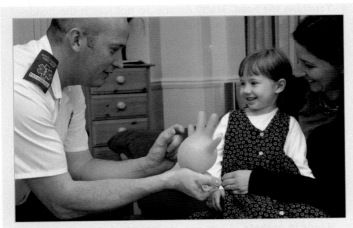

Figure 10-9 An examination-glove chicken can put a youngster at ease.

cate the situation to the accident and emergency department doctor, and document it accurately. Generally, it's a good idea to deal with adolescents as adults. You gain better cooperation from them by offering them options and honouring their choices. (Hint: Never offer an option you know you can't honour.) Make special efforts to protect the modesty of adolescents in particular. They are, for the most part, obsessed with their image and what others think of them.

People Who Live With Special Challenges

It would be a mistake to overlook the needs of people who have speech, hearing, sight, or other kinds of communication disorders. Many carers enroll in sign-language or lip-reading classes to facilitate communication with these patients.

When you encounter a patient who has trouble communicating, remember that family members or primary carers who know these patients well can facilitate your efforts. Just as importantly, they can also help you to alleviate fear.

Many carers find that touch and eye contact are helpful bridging mechanisms when dealing with these patients. For example, a light touch on a patient's shoulder can convey kindness, while a firm grasp can express reassurance. Some patients respond well to brief, one-armed hugging. In still other situations, you can grasp a patient's face between your hands and use your eyes to convey concern or to calm him or her down.

Documentation and Communication

Many hospitals and ambulance communication centres have interpreter capabilities (language line) and are a good resource for communicating with patients who speak a language that is different from yours. Know what resources are available for patients who use sign language as a means of communication as well.

Cross-Cultural Communication

To effectively communicate to save lives, you must strive to understand the differences inherent in all peoples, then you can adjust your efforts to accommodate and overcome cultural barriers. The most common barriers to communication include the barriers of race, ethnicity, age, gender, language, education, religion, geography, and even economic status. The combination of all these groups can be defined as "culture". No matter who we are, or where we come from, or how open-minded we think ourselves to be, we *all* have some level of prejudice we must be conscious of. You cannot treat your patients effectively if you use your own culture as your only reference—it is much like imposing your own morality on patients. While understanding other cultures is not necessarily an ethical issue, it still is best not to have preconceived ideas about how you should communicate when you care for a patient.

Cultural sensitivity and cultural diversity have become important buzzwords in business today. There are literally thousands of classes and seminars on how to deal with cultural differences of both employees and business contacts. What do all these classes and seminars actually teach? In a word, "respect".

Sounds simple enough in theory, but in practice? Many people fall short of giving even basic respect in everyday interactions, let alone in a health care environment. In the United Kingdom, emphasis falls on getting the job done, and many people seem to be too hurried and busy, and too self-absorbed, to be really concerned about how we are viewed. We can offend with the abruptness of our behaviour. In other cultures, appearance and manners mean everything and lack of respect is unforgivable.

While the social practices, mannerisms, etiquette, and idiosyncrasies of all cultures are too numerous to list in one book, let alone in a chapter, it is highly important that you be open to educating yourself. It is the responsibility of the individual paramedic to research what cultural groups, ethnic groups, or religious groups are prevalent in his or her area of practice and learn how to deal with each culture accordingly. You may not get everything right when you encounter a representative from one of these groups, but your efforts at communicating will translate the idea of respect and that makes all the difference in the world.

Manners

Manners are also important. British culture has come to a place where many young people no longer have even a rudimentary understanding of the concept of good manners. Pop culture has destroyed many concepts of appropriateness in dress and behaviour. Take for instance, the ubiquitous baseball cap. Not too long ago, it was considered rude for a man to wear a hat indoors, when a woman walked by, or even in a pub or cafe. While wearing a baseball cap has become accepted practice in some places, many people are offended if they see a hat worn indoors. However, in other cultures, covering your head by wearing a hat at all times is considered a demonstration of your faithfulness to God. It is important for the paramedic to know the difference.

Additionally, many of the polite forms of address have fallen by the wayside. Patients have been referred to as "dude", "mate", "man", and even "guv". Responses to patient's questions have included "naw", "yep", "yeah", and "uh-huh". This is slang, it is lazy, and it is not professional. Get used to saying "Yes sir", "No madam", "Thank you", and "Please". You would be amazed at how far such niceties go in instilling confidence and establishing a professional relationship with your patient.

"Would you . . .", "Could you . . .", and "May I . . .". are equally important. Most people like to give permission before being touched. Lack of address and assumption of permission is particularly demeaning to an older person in a nursing home. You are nonverbally communicating, "You are not important enough or mentally competent enough to be asked for permission".

Hand Gestures

Another British usage that may be looked upon with disfavour is our use of hand gestures. The thumbs-up sign that Britons use to indicate "everything is OK" or "ready to go" is actually the equivalent of an extended middle finger in many Arabic and some Latin countries.

The OK sign, made with thumb and index finger circled, and the other three fingers extended, is standard British for "everything's alright". In Latin countries, it is a reference to a circular orifice located posteriorly. It also has this meaning in Germany, Italy, and Russia. In France, the gesture means zero and can be used to indicate something is worthless. In other cultures, it represents the evil eye. In Japan, it indicates that money is needed, or that coins are preferred.

The extended middle finger is probably the rudest gesture in the British gesture catalogue. In Japan, the middle digit is used as the index finger and has the same significance as pointing. Please remember this fact when providing care to a Japanese family; they are not being rude when you ask to be shown where it hurts.

Body Language

Body language and gestures are common the world over, but an innocent gesture in one country may be a serious insult in another. Perhaps the most cross-cultural gesture, and the easiest to remember, is the simple smile. A smile is readily received by almost every culture on earth and has the tendency to convey good will and acceptance.

Every culture in the world has its own peculiarities and social and religious practices that are unique. The list below is by no means all-inclusive, but illustrates some of the differences you may see when providing cross-cultural care:

- **Bowing.** Shows rank and status in Japan. The deeper the bow, the more respect is communicated.

- **Touching the head.** Many Asians do not touch the head. The head is considered the most sacred part of the body and is the residence of the soul. Touching the head may put the soul in jeopardy.
- **Touching with the left hand.** Islamic and Hindu cultures avoid touching with the left hand, as traditionally this hand was used for unclean functions. It is considered rude and offensive to offer the left hand in greeting.
- **Feet.** Showing the bottom of the feet is considered offensive in Muslim nations, as well as most of Thailand. To point the soles of your shoes or the soles of your feet at someone is to say "you are beneath my feet" or "you are worth less than dirt".
- **Slouching.** Considered rude in Japan.
- **Hands in pockets.** A gesture of disrespect in Turkey.
- **Sitting with legs crossed.** Disrespectful in Turkey and Ghana.
- **Hands on hips.** Sign of hostility in Mexico and Argentina.
- **Eye contact.** Avoid direct eye contact to show respect in most Asian, African, Latin American, and Caribbean cultures (Somalian and Brazilian cultures are exceptions). Prolonged eye contact is acceptable in Arab, Somalian, and Brazilian cultures; in these cultures, it is believed prolonged eye contact communicates honesty and interest in the recipient.
- **Nodding.** Indian and Arabic people may signal agreement by moving the head from side-to-side (the Western "no" gesture). They may indicate no by tipping the head back, and clicking the tongue against the roof of the mouth.

Communication in Difficult Circumstances

Sometimes the paramedic has the difficult role in the setting of a patient's death. After death is declared, comfort the patient's family. Offering sensitive support to the family helps the surviving family members. This can be challenging because the paramedic may be struggling with personal emotional responses related to the loss of a patient.

Talking to the family can be difficult. There are techniques that may improve the quality of these interactions:

- **Use the patient's name.** This acknowledges the patient as an individual rather than "the patient".
- **Try to find a quiet area to talk to the patient's family.** Often the scene can become noisy with activity. Finding an area where the family can concentrate on your conversation will help to keep your message clear.
- **Use concrete terms.** The use of euphemisms to soften the news can make it harder for the family to understand what has happened.

You are the Paramedic Summary

Your ability to communicate compassion, care, and understanding can be just as important as your ability to start IVs and perform other advanced life-support skills. If you rebel against acquiring the emotional intelligence that will help you communicate effectively, you are likely to experience a bumpy road as an ambulance service provider. Possessing a high emotional intelligence quotient will positively affect your relationships with subordinates, peers, and superiors, as well as with your patients. Possessing an understanding of the human side of the ambulance service is essential to becoming an outstanding ambulance service provider.

1. What communication difficulties do you immediately anticipate in this scenario?

Patients experiencing a stroke can have difficulties understanding and communicating language. You should immediately be concerned with communication when you suspect your patient is experiencing a stroke. As you can imagine, it would be very frustrating and frightening to understand speech but be unable to respond (or vice versa). If normal methods of communication fail, think outside the box to effectively communicate with your patient.

2. Describe what the phrase "total patient care" means to you.

Total patient care involves caring for all of the patient's needs, including his or her physical, mental, and emotional needs. To ignore any of these is not caring for the entire patient and is therefore considered incomplete care. To ignore a patient's pain, for instance, is not only poor patient care but can also be considered grounds for a lawsuit if you have the ability to medicate or otherwise ease the patient's pain and fail to do so.

3. Although the paramedics in this scenario are attending to the patient's medical needs, could the wife have a valid complaint regarding their caregiving?

Yes! Although the paramedics are tired, they should not ignore questions from the wife, nor should they treat the patient as though he is a manikin. It's important to remember that ambulance service personnel exist to care for life-threatening conditions. Your care needs to include an education and communication component. If you choose not to work on your people skills or to learn the qualities needed for emotional intelligence, you are likely to experience difficulties in communicating and caring for your patients.

4. How can your introductions (or lack thereof) and general demeanour affect your ability to communicate with your patients as well as with their friends and family members?

Failing to establish a connection with your patients is likely to cause problems with your patients right from the start. You need to quickly establish a bond of trust between yourself and your patient. It can be difficult if you are tired, hungry, or otherwise having a bad day, but failing to do so will translate these feelings to your patients who may respond negatively to them.

5. How has this crew's lack of people skills affected this call?

Their failure to address the softer aspects of patient care really made this call more difficult than it needed to be. Total patient care should also encompass the needs of family members or other loved ones. Failure to address their questions or concerns can directly and negatively affect patient care and, in some instances, can exacerbate a patient's medical condition. If you don't have time to address every issue, at the very least, you should acknowledge questions and explain that you will address their questions after you have finished with the task at hand.

6. Can this situation be mended?

It is very difficult to undo a situation such as this one. One bad PR move can cost an ambulance or fire service and its personnel in many ways. It is very important to keep and maintain the public's trust, and one incident can destroy years of good relations between members of the public and an ambulance service.

7. What would be the best course of action in this situation?

Calling an additional crew to diffuse the situation (as well as to transport Mrs Brown to the hospital for her chest pain) would be the best course of action. Consider the possibilities of what would happen if her condition suddenly worsened (for example, if she had an acute myocardial infarction and had a cardiac arrest). Obviously, offering a sincere apology is ideal, although it may not be enough in this situation. Requesting an additional crew to interject new faces may be required to calm both patients as well as to provide the required medical care they both need.

8. What are the different forms of communication and how do they impact patient care?

Much of how we communicate as people is done without the use of words. Body language is very powerful and can send a very different message than what is being communicated through words. Be mindful of your facial expressions, stance, and tone of voice as these will communicate your true intention or message beyond your words. Sometimes it's not what you say but how you say it that has the biggest impact on what is communicated between you and your patient.

Prep Kit

▇ Ready for Review

- People are not just medical puzzles for us to solve; they are the reason we as paramedics exist.
- Most of the people you will meet during responses will be in crisis, and having the worst days of their lives.
- At least half of the calls you will attend as a paramedic will take you into people's homes, day and night, and in the most private moments of their lives. Try to see every invitation into the home of someone else as a personal honour in a time and place where no one else would be welcome.
- If you want people to tell you about their problems, convince them you want to hear what they have to say. Give them your undivided attention.
- Active listening is repeating the key parts of a patient's responses to questions. It helps confirm the information the patient is providing. This assures there is no misunderstanding.
- Your most essential challenge as a therapeutic communicator is to convey calm, unmistakable, genuine concern for someone you've never met.
- When you first meet your patients, introduce yourself and ask them for their name. By doing so, you communicate your respect for them.
- Even if you're not convinced that patients are in real trouble, consider the possibility that they're scared to death.
- When patients tell you they're in pain, let them know you grasp and appreciate their situation, and then do something about it.
- Modesty matters, no matter how acute the medical condition. If the patient is not personally sensitive to it, family members most certainly are.
- When you need to know how patients feel, try asking open-ended questions—questions that do not have a yes or no answer, and which do not give them specific options to choose from.
- When you're trying to find out about facts (for example, a medical history), use the closed-ended, or direct, question.
- If you sense that patients are trying to put something into words, but are having trouble, be patient. Don't say anything at all for a few seconds. Let them talk.
- Never assume. Try hard to become a careful observer and to keep your mind open to a wide range of possibilities.
- Nonverbal communication can be as powerful as words.
- Direct eye contact generally communicates honesty and concern.
- Posture is important. Try to position your eyes at the same level or below the level of the patient's eyes.

- A smile can greatly help relieve a stressful situation. Your ability to smile can be valuable when you're dealing with people in crisis.
- The highest form of mental function is the spontaneous expression of appropriate humour.
- Assess how long it takes for a patient to respond appropriately to your questions. Patients who are thinking clearly should be able to answer simple questions within 1 second.
- Patients should be able to tell you accurately who they are and who you are, where they are, what time of day it is, and what happened that necessitated your being called.
- When you ask patients to perform a simple task, they should be able to do the task correctly within about 1 second.
- When a patient refuses to talk and you're not seeing signs of decreased mental status, there's no need to force the issue. Instead, make lots of eye contact, express your concern in every way possible, explain everything you are doing, invite them repeatedly to answer questions, and let them know it's all right if they don't wish to talk.
- Try not to presume that older people are any harder to communicate with than anyone else, just because they're older.
- Children can pose treatment and communication challenges even to the best of us. Minimise your movements, lower your voice, and touch them as gently as you can—possibly without gloves at first. Try keeping your eye level at or below the child's, by sitting on the floor and placing the child on the cot or on a parent's lap.
- When you encounter a patient who has trouble communicating, remember that family members or primary carers who know these patients well can facilitate your efforts. Just as importantly, they can also help you alleviate fear.
- Dealing with people of cultures different from your own can be challenging. It's always considered a mark of your respect if you make an effort to learn about their language and culture.

▇ Vital Vocabulary

closed-ended question A question that is specific and focused, either demanding a yes or no answer, or an answer chosen from specific options.

communication The transmission of information to another person—whether it be verbal or through body language.

open-ended question A question that does not have a yes or no answer, and which does not give the patient specific options to choose from.

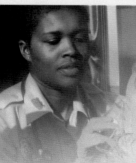

Assessment in Action

You get a call to the home of an elderly couple. The man has been sick with a cough and fever and is now vomiting. His wife is extremely concerned. She is also lonely and happy for the chance to talk to anyone at all. When you arrive, she takes her time telling you how his illness started, how he is doing now, and then starts talking about how long they've been married, their children, and so on. In this situation, how would you answer the following questions?

1. **The act of communicating involves:**
   A. talking as much as listening.
   B. listening as much as talking.
   C. listening only.
   D. talking only.

2. **If the man or woman in this scenario were hard of hearing, how would you handle it?**
   A. Scream at him or her at the top of your voice.
   B. Get closer to him or her, but try not to be exceptionally loud.
   C. Tell him or her to turn up his or her hearing aid.
   D. Do whatever it takes to get the information you need, including talking loudly or writing notes.

3. **If the woman in this scenario were a person who calls paramedics for every ache and pain and, as much as you like people, she drives you crazy, how would you react?**
   A. Let your impatience show, hoping she will get to the point of the visit so you can do your job.
   B. Ignore her and concentrate on talking to her ill husband since he is the patient.
   C. Be patient and redirect her when she gets off track, without letting your impatience show.
   D. Listen to her whole story, picking out what's needed, and thinking about what job you'd like to switch to when you're done with that shift.

4. **Just in case your patient has chest pain or cardiac issues, you need to ask if he's taking any erectile dysfunction medication. Since this couple is elderly, how would you go about this?**
   A. Explain that you need to know some personal information in case of any cardiac issues, and explain the possible interaction with GTN or other cardiac medications.
   B. Ask her directly, making a joke out of it to make her more comfortable.
   C. Ask him instead, elbowing him jokingly and referring to "keeping her happy".
   D. Ask them both very professionally, and see who answers.

5. **With this older couple, would you call them by their first names or use their last names with Mr and Mrs?**
   A. Call them whatever you want, you are in charge and they are the patients.
   B. Call them by their first name to let them know you remember who they are and are on a very personal level with them.
   C. Call them pet names like "honey" and "darling".
   D. Call them by their last names preceded by Mr and Mrs unless they say otherwise.

6. **What if the woman in this scenario were so scared for her husband that she was having trouble staying calm and answering questions?**
   A. Tell her to calm down and that she's doing him no good acting like that.
   B. Keep your voice calm and even. Get close enough to him so that you can do some assessments while you try to calm her down with your own calm demeanour.
   C. Have your partner take her out of the room so she isn't a distraction, and try to get the information that you need from her husband.
   D. Let your partner try to talk to her about her family while you try to talk with the patient.

7. **After examining the man in this scenario, you have no idea what may be wrong with him, or if taking him to the hospital will make any difference. His wife asks you what you think. What is your best option?**
   A. Tell her the truth; you have no idea, he's just sick.
   B. Talk in big medical terms she won't understand, and get busy transporting him so she can't ask for clarification.
   C. Tell her that she must face that they're both getting old and they will be more and more ill as time goes on, she should just get used to it.
   D. Tell her that you have some ideas, but it's best to let the doctor check him out. He'll be taken care of by you and the hospital staff.

Challenging Questions

8. **An older woman fell in the shower and hurt her hip badly. You are told she has a history of osteoporosis. When you arrive, she is still lying in the bathtub with a towel covering her; her family didn't want to move her. You can see and sense that she is very modest and doesn't want that towel moved so that you can assess her injury. What is the best way to handle this situation?**

9. **You have been called to the home of a 14-year-old girl who has severe cramps and heavy vaginal bleeding. You need to ask her about her sexual activity, and if there is any chance that she may be pregnant. Her parents are standing right there. What should you do?**

■ Points to Ponder

You are called to the scene of a road traffic collision in which the driver of one car has significant leg injuries. He is conscious and alert, and is also deaf.

How would you best communicate with this patient?

Issues: Communicating With Patients in Special Situations, Alternative Strategies for Communication.

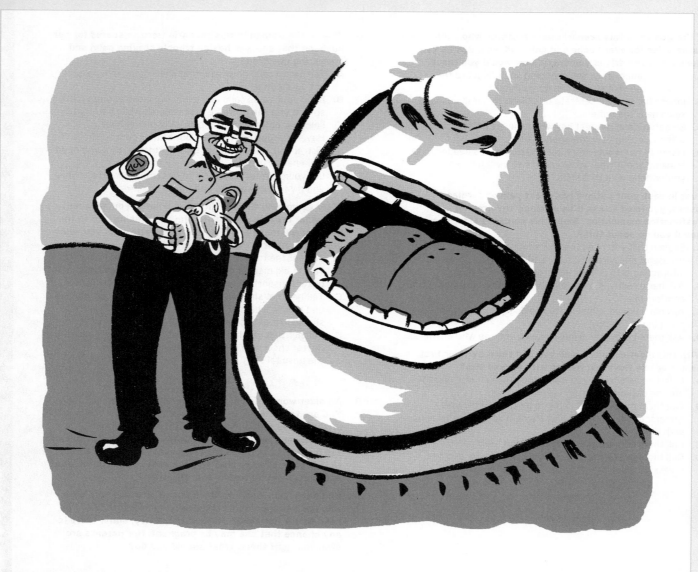

> My five rules of airway management are pretty simple. 1. Blue is bad. 2. Oxygen is good. 3. Air should go in and out. 4. Noisy breathing is obstructed breathing. 5. Bare the chest!"
>
> —Ronald D. Stewart, OC, MD, FRCPC, DSc

Airway

Section Editor: Bob Fellows

2

Section

11 Airway Management and Ventilation

Objectives

Cognitive

- Explain the primary objective of airway maintenance.
- Identify commonly neglected prehospital skills related to airway.
- Identify the anatomy of the upper and lower airway.
- Describe the functions of the upper and lower airway.
- Explain the differences between adult and paediatric airway anatomy.
- Define gag reflex.
- Explain the relationship between pulmonary circulation and respiration.
- List the concentration of gases that comprise atmospheric air.
- Describe the measurement of oxygen in the blood.
- Describe the measurement of carbon dioxide in the blood.
- Describe peak expiratory flow.
- List factors that cause decreased oxygen concentrations in the blood.
- List the factors that increase and decrease carbon dioxide production in the body.
- Define atelectasis.
- Define and differentiate between hypoxia and hypoxaemia.
- Describe the voluntary and involuntary regulation of respiration.
- Describe the modified forms of respiration.
- Define normal respiratory rates and tidal volumes for the adult, child, and infant.
- List the factors that affect respiratory rate and depth.
- Explain the risk of infection to ambulance service clinicians associated with ventilation.
- Define pulsus paradoxus.
- Define and explain the implications of partial airway obstruction with good and poor air exchange.
- Define complete airway obstruction.
- Describe causes of upper airway obstruction.
- Describe causes of respiratory distress.
- Describe manual airway manoeuvres.
- Describe the Sellick (cricoid pressure) manoeuvre.
- Describe complete airway obstruction manoeuvres.
- Explain the purpose of suctioning the upper airway.
- Identify types of suction equipment.
- Describe the indications for suctioning the upper airway.
- Identify types of suction catheters, including hard or rigid catheters and soft catheters.
- Identify techniques of suctioning the upper airway.
- Identify special considerations of suctioning the upper airway.
- Describe the indications, contraindications, advantages, disadvantages, complications, equipment and technique of tracheobronchial suctioning in the intubated patient.
- Describe the use of an oropharyngeal and nasopharyngeal airway.
- Identify special considerations of tracheobronchial suctioning in the intubated patient.
- Define gastric distension.
- Describe the indications, contraindications, advantages, disadvantages, complications, equipment and technique for inserting a nasogastric tube and orogastric tube.
- Identify special considerations of gastric decompression.
- Describe the indications, contraindications, advantages, disadvantages, complications, and technique for inserting an oropharyngeal and nasopharyngeal airway.
- Describe the indications, contraindications, advantages, disadvantages, complications, and technique for ventilating a patient by:
  - Mouth-to-mouth
  - Mouth-to-nose
  - Mouth-to-mask
  - One person bag-valve-mask
  - Two person bag-valve-mask
  - Three person bag-valve-mask
  - Flow-restricted, oxygen-powered ventilation device
- Explain the advantage of the two person method when ventilating with the bag-valve-mask.
- Compare the ventilation techniques used for an adult patient to those used for paediatric patients.
- Describe indications, contraindications, advantages, disadvantages, complications, and technique for ventilating a patient with an automatic transport ventilator (ATV).
- Explain safety considerations of oxygen storage and delivery.
- Identify types of oxygen cylinders and pressure regulators (including a high-pressure regulator and a therapy regulator).
- List the steps for delivering oxygen from a cylinder and regulator.
- Describe the use, advantages and disadvantages of an oxygen humidifier.
- Describe the indications, contraindications, advantages, disadvantages, complications, litre flow range, and concentration of delivered oxygen for supplemental oxygen delivery devices.
- Define, identify and describe a tracheostomy, stoma, and tracheostomy tube.
- Define, identify, and describe a laryngectomy.
- Define how to ventilate with a patient with a stoma, including mouth-to-stoma and bag-valve-mask-to-stoma ventilation.
- Describe the special considerations in airway management and ventilation for patients with facial injuries.
- Describe the special considerations in airway management and ventilation for the paediatric patient.
- Differentiate endotracheal intubation from other methods of advanced airway management.
- Describe the indications, contraindications, advantages, disadvantages and complications of endotracheal intubation.
- Describe laryngoscopy for the removal of a foreign body airway obstruction.
- Describe the indications, contraindications, advantages, disadvantages, complications, equipment, and technique for direct laryngoscopy.
- Describe visual landmarks for direct laryngoscopy.
- Describe use of cricoid pressure during intubation.
- Describe the indications, contraindications, advantages, disadvantages, complications and equipment for rapid sequence intubation with neuromuscular blockade.
- Identify neuromuscular blocking drugs and other agents used in rapid sequence intubation.

- Describe the indications, contraindications, advantages, disadvantages, complications and equipment for sedation during intubation.
- Identify sedative agents used in airway management.
- Describe the indications, contraindications, advantages, disadvantages and complications for performing an open cricothyroidotomy.
- Describe the equipment and technique for performing an open cricothyroidotomy.
- Describe the indications, contraindications, advantages, disadvantages, complications, equipment and technique for translaryngeal cannula ventilation (needle cricothyroidotomy).
- Describe methods of assessment for confirming correct placement of an endotracheal tube.
- Describe methods for securing an endotracheal tube.
- Describe the indications, contraindications, advantages, disadvantages, complications, equipment and technique for extubation.
- Describe methods of endotracheal intubation in the paediatric patient.

Affective

- Defend the need to oxygenate and ventilate a patient.
- Defend the necessity of establishing and/or maintaining patency of a patient's airway.
- Comply with universal precautions to protect against infectious and communicable diseases.

Psychomotor

- Perform universal precautions during basic airway management, advanced airway management, and ventilation.
- Perform pulse oximetry.
- Perform end-tidal CO_2 detection.
- Perform peak expiratory flow testing.
- Perform manual airway manoeuvres, including:
  - Opening the mouth
  - Head tilt–chin lift manoeuvre
  - Jaw-thrust manoeuvre
- Perform manual airway manoeuvres for paediatric patients, including:
  - Opening the mouth
  - Head tilt–chin lift manoeuvre
  - Jaw-thrust manoeuvre

- Perform the Sellick manoeuvre (cricoid pressure).
- Perform complete airway obstruction manoeuvres, including:
  - Heimlich manoeuvre (abdominal thrust)
  - Finger sweep
  - Chest thrusts
  - Removal with Magill forceps
- Demonstrate suctioning the upper airway by selecting a suction device, catheter, and technique.
- Perform tracheobronchial suctioning in the intubated patient by selecting a suction device, catheter, and technique.
- Demonstrate insertion of an oropharyngeal airway.
- Demonstrate insertion of a nasopharyngeal airway.
- Demonstrate ventilating a patient by the following techniques:
  - Mouth-to-mask ventilation
  - One person bag-valve-mask
  - Two person bag-valve-mask
  - Three person bag-valve-mask
  - Flow-restricted, oxygen-powered ventilation device
  - Automatic transport ventilator
  - Mouth-to-stoma
  - Bag-valve-mask-to-stoma ventilation
- Ventilate a paediatric patient using the one and two person techniques.
- Perform ventilation with a bag-valve-mask with a nebuliser.
- Perform oxygen delivery from a cylinder and regulator with an oxygen delivery device.
- Perform oxygen delivery with an oxygen humidifier.
- Deliver supplemental oxygen to a breathing patient using the following devices: nasal cannula, simple face mask, partial rebreather mask, nonrebreather mask, and Venturi mask.
- Perform stoma suctioning.
- Perform retrieval of foreign bodies from the upper airway.
- Perform assessment to confirm correct placement of the endotracheal tube.
- Intubate the trachea by the following methods:
  - Orotracheal intubation
  - Open cricothyroidotomy
- Adequately secure an endotracheal tube.
- Perform endotracheal intubation in the paediatric patient.
- Perform transtracheal cannula ventilation (needle cricothyroidotomy).
- Perform extubation.
- Perform replacement of a tracheostomy tube through a stoma.

Maintaining a Patent Airway: A Critical Concern

Establishing and maintaining a patent (open) airway and ensuring effective oxygenation and ventilation are vital aspects of effective patient care. Attempting to stabilise a patient whose airway is compromised is futile. No airway, no patient—it's that simple! The human body needs a constant supply of oxygen to carry out the physiological processes necessary to sustain life; the airway is where it all begins. Few situations will cause such acute deterioration and death more rapidly than airway and ventilation compromise. Therefore, the patient's airway must remain patent at all times.

The function of the respiratory system is quite simple. It brings in oxygen and eliminates carbon dioxide (the primary waste product of oxygen metabolism). If this process is interrupted, vital organs of the body will not function properly. For example, the brain can survive for only 6 minutes or so without oxygen before permanent brain damage is virtually assured.

Failure to manage the airway or inappropriate management of the airway is a major cause of preventable death in the prehospital setting. Unfortunately, basic techniques to secure a patent airway are commonly neglected or performed improperly in the rush to proceed to advanced interventions. Poor technique (eg, improper bag-valve-mask seal, improper airway positioning) and failure to reassess the patient's condition merely serve to increase mortality and morbidity.

Paramedics must understand the importance of early detection of airway problems, rapid and effective intervention, and continual reassessment of a patient with airway or breathing compromise.

This chapter examines the airway in detail, beginning with a review of the anatomy and physiology of the respiratory system. It follows a "basic-to-advanced" approach, just as airway management should be performed in the prehospital environment. The chapter describes the various techniques of opening and maintaining a patent airway, recognising and treating airway obstructions, assessing a patient's ventilation status, administering supplemental oxygen, and providing ventilatory assistance. Advanced techniques, including advanced airway devices and procedures, are then discussed in detail. Remember to operate only within your scope of practice until trained and authorised to move to the next level of practice.

Anatomy of the Upper Airway

The upper airway consists of all anatomical airway structures above the level of the vocal cords. Its major functions are to warm, filter, and humidify air as it enters the body through the nose and mouth. The first portion of the upper airway, the pharynx (throat), is a muscular tube that extends from the nose and mouth to the level of the oesophagus and trachea. The pharynx is composed of the nasopharynx, oropharynx, and laryngopharynx (also called the hypopharynx). The laryngopharynx is the lowest portion of the pharynx; it opens into the larynx anteriorly and the oesophagus posteriorly **Figure 11-1 ▼**.

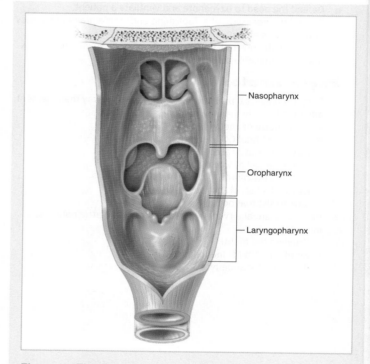

— Nasopharynx

— Oropharynx

— Laryngopharynx

Figure 11-1 The pharynx.

You are the Paramedic Part 1

You are dispatched to a corner shop for a 50-year-old man with difficulty breathing. You and your colleague reach the scene in approximately 5 minutes. Upon arrival, you find the patient sitting on a bench in front of the shop. He is conscious, alert, and in mild respiratory distress. He tells you, in complete sentences, that he suddenly began having trouble breathing while inside the shop.

1. Is this patient's airway open?
2. How will you proceed with your assessment of this patient?

Nasopharynx

On inhalation, air normally enters the body through the nose and passes into the nasopharynx, which is formed by the union of the facial bones.

The entire nasal cavity is lined with a ciliated mucous membrane that keeps contaminants such as dust and other small particles out of the respiratory tract. In illness, the body produces additional mucus to trap potentially infectious agents. This mucous membrane is extremely delicate and has a rich blood supply. Any trauma to the nasal passages, such as improper or overly aggressive placement of airway devices, may result in profuse bleeding from the posterior nasal cavity. Bleeding from this area cannot be controlled by direct pressure. Extrinsic factors (eg, cocaine use) can also damage the delicate nasal passages or the septum, which separates the two nares.

Three bony shelves, called turbinates, protrude from the lateral walls of the nasal cavity and extend into the nasal passageway, parallel to the nasal floor. The turbinates serve to increase the surface area of the nasal mucosa, thereby improving the processes of warming, filtering, and humidification of inhaled air.

The nasopharynx is divided into two passages by the nasal septum, a rigid partition composed of bone and cartilage. Normally, the nasal septum is in the midline of the nose. In some people the septum may be deviated to one side or the other—a condition that becomes important when contemplating insertion of a nasopharyngeal airway.

The sinuses are cavities formed by the cranial bones. Fractures of these bones may cause cerebrospinal fluid (CSF) to leak from the nose (cerebrospinal rhinorrhoea) or the ears (cerebrospinal otorrhoea). The sinuses prevent contaminants from entering the respiratory tract and act as tributaries for fluid to and from the eustachian tubes and tear ducts.

Oropharynx

The oropharynx forms the posterior portion of the oral cavity, which is bordered superiorly by the hard and soft palates, laterally by the cheeks, and inferiorly by the tongue Figure 11-2 ▾. The 32 adult teeth are embedded in the gums in such a manner that significant force is required to dislodge them. However, trauma of lesser severity may result in fracture or avulsion of the teeth, potentially obstructing the upper airway or causing aspiration of tooth fragments into the lungs.

The tongue is a large muscle attached to the mandible and the hyoid bone—a small, horseshoe-shaped bone to which the jaw, epiglottis, and thyroid cartilage attach as well. From an airway perspective, the most important anatomical consideration regarding the tongue is its tendency to fall back and occlude the posterior pharynx when the mandible relaxes. In fact, the tongue is the most common cause of anatomical upper airway obstruction, especially in patients with a decreased level of consciousness.

The palate forms the roof of the mouth and separates the oropharynx and nasopharynx. Its anterior portion, which is

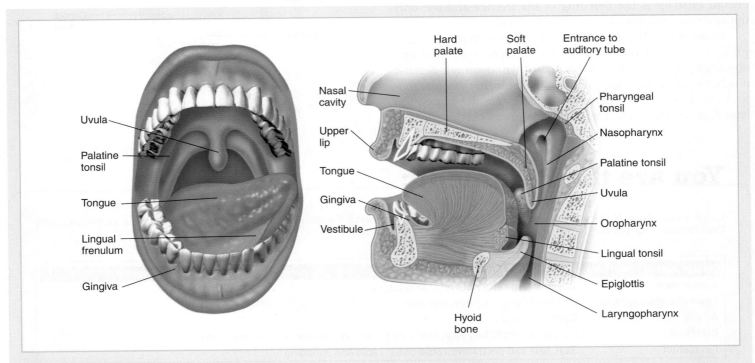

Figure 11-2 The oral cavity.

formed by the maxilla and palatine bones, is called the hard palate. The soft palate is posterior to the hard palate.

The adenoids, which are located on the posterior nasopharyngeal wall, are lymphatic tissues that filter bacteria. The tonsils, which are also made of lymphatic tissue, are located in posterior pharynx; they help to trap bacteria. The adenoids and tonsils often become swollen and infected. Severe swelling of the tonsils can potentially cause obstruction of the upper airway.

The uvula, a soft-tissue structure that resembles a punch bag, is located in the posterior aspect of the oral cavity, at the base of the tongue.

The superior border of the glottic opening is the epiglottis. This leaf-shaped cartilaginous flap prevents food and liquid from entering the larynx during swallowing.

The vallecula is an anatomical space, or "pocket", located between the base of the tongue and the epiglottis. It is an important landmark for endotracheal intubation.

Larynx

The larynx is a complex structure formed by many independent cartilaginous structures **Figure 11-3 ▸** . It marks where the upper airway ends and the lower airway begins.

The thyroid cartilage is a shield-shaped structure formed by two plates that join in a "V" shape anteriorly to form the laryngeal prominence known as the Adam's apple. The thyroid cartilage is suspended in place by the thyroid ligament and is directly anterior to the glottic opening.

The cricoid cartilage, or cricoid ring, lies inferiorly to the thyroid cartilage; it forms the lowest portion of the larynx. The cricoid cartilage is the first ring of the trachea and the only upper airway structure that is circumferential.

Between the thyroid and cricoid cartilages is the cricothyroid membrane, which is a site for emergency surgical and nonsurgical access to the airway (cricothyroidotomy). Because it is bordered laterally and inferiorly by the highly vascular thyroid gland, ambulance personnel must locate the anatomical landmarks carefully when accessing the airway via this site.

The glottis, also called the glottic opening, is the space in between the vocal cords and the narrowest portion of the adult's airway **Figure 11-4 ▸** . Airway patency in this area is heavily dependent on adequate muscle tone. The lateral borders of the glottis are the vocal cords. At rest, these white bands of tough tissue are partially separated (ie, the glottis is partially open). During forceful inhalation, the vocal cords open widely to provide minimum resistance to air flow.

The arytenoid cartilages are pyramid-like cartilaginous structures that form the posterior attachment of the vocal cords; they are valuable guides for endotracheal intubation. As the arytenoid cartilages pivot, the vocal cords open and close, which regulates the passage of air through the larynx and controls the production of sound; hence, the larynx is sometimes called the "voice box".

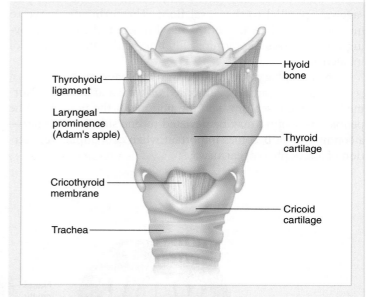

Figure 11-3 The larynx.

You are the Paramedic Part 2

Closer examination of the patient reveals that he has mild use of accessory muscle and intercostal recession. As your colleague opens the response bag, you perform an initial assessment and note the following:

Initial Assessment	Recording Time: 0 Minutes
Appearance	Obvious respiratory distress; anxious; pale
Level of consciousness	A (Alert to person, place, and day)
Airway	Open and clear
Breathing	Increased respiratory rate, laboured breathing with adequate tidal volume
Circulation	Skin, pale and perspiring; radial pulse, rapid and bounding

3. What immediate management is indicated for this patient?

4. What questions would be pertinent to ask this patient?

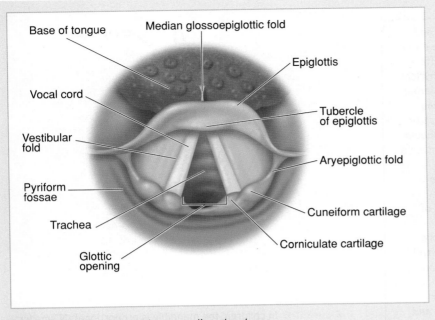

Figure 11-4 The glottis and surrounding structures.

The <u>pyriform fossae</u> are two pockets of tissue on the lateral borders of the larynx. Airway devices are occasionally inadvertently inserted into these pockets, resulting in a tenting of the skin under the jaw.

When the airway is stimulated (eg, during aspiration of foreign material or a water submersion incident), defensive reflexes cause a <u>laryngospasm</u>—spasmodic closure of the vocal cords, which seals off the airway. This reflex normally lasts a few seconds. Persistent laryngospasm can threaten the airway by preventing ventilation altogether.

■ Anatomy of the Lower Airway

The function of the lower airway is to exchange oxygen and carbon dioxide. Externally, it extends from the fourth cervical vertebra to the xiphoid process. Internally, it spans the glottis to the pulmonary capillary membrane.

The <u>trachea</u>, or windpipe, is the conduit for air entry into the lungs. This tubular structure is approximately 10 to 12 cm in length and consists of a series of C-shaped cartilaginous rings. The trachea begins immediately below the cricoid cartilage and descends anteriorly down the midline of the neck and chest to the level of the fifth or sixth thoracic vertebra. It divides into the right and left mainstem bronchi at the

level of the <u>carina</u>. These bronchi are lined with mucus-producing cells and beta-2 receptors that, when stimulated, result in bronchodilation.

The right bronchus is somewhat shorter and straighter than the left bronchus. Thus an endotracheal tube that is inserted too far will often come to lie in the right mainstem bronchus.

All of the blood vessels and the bronchi enter each lung at the <u>hilum</u>. The lungs consist of the entire mass of tissue that includes the smaller bronchi, bronchioles, and alveoli **Figure 11-5 ▼**.

The right lung has three lobes and the left lung has two lobes, which are covered with a thin, slippery outer lining called the <u>visceral pleura</u>. The <u>parietal pleura</u> lines the inside of the thoracic cavity. A small amount of fluid is found between the pleurae, which decreases friction during breathing.

Upon entering the lungs, each bronchus divides into increasingly smaller bronchi, which in turn subdivide into <u>bronchioles</u>. The bronchioles, which are made of smooth muscle, dilate or constrict in response to various stimuli. The smaller bronchioles branch into alveolar ducts that end at the alveolar sacs.

The balloon-like clusters of single-layer air sacs known as <u>alveoli</u> are the functional site for the exchange of oxygen and carbon dioxide. This exchange occurs by simple diffusion between the alveoli and the pulmonary capillaries.

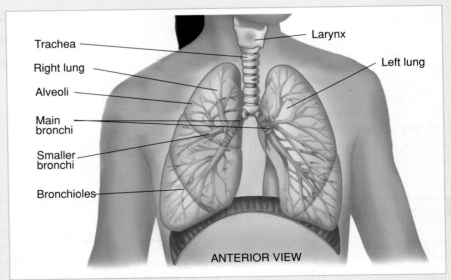

Figure 11-5 The trachea and the lungs (lower airway structures).

Special Considerations

Although the manoeuvres, techniques, and indications for airway management are essentially the same in children as they are in adults, several anatomical differences in the child make mastery of these techniques critical.

Infants and small children have a proportionately larger occiput, which causes the head to flex when the child lies supine; this position itself can cause an airway obstruction. When positioning the airway of an infant or child, you should place a folded towel under his or her shoulders to maintain a neutral position of the head.

Compared to adults, children have a proportionately smaller mandible and a proportionately larger tongue **Figure 11-6 ▶**. Both factors increase the incidence of airway obstruction in children.

The child's epiglottis is horse-shoe shaped and more floppy than an adult's. As a consequence, it must be lifted out of the way to visualise the vocal cords for intubation **Figure 11-7 ▶**.

In general, the infant's and child's airway is smaller and narrower at all levels. The larynx lies more superior and anterior than in an adult—an important consideration when visualising the vocal cords for intubation. The larynx is also funnel-shaped due to the narrow, underdeveloped cricoid cartilage. In children younger than 10 years, the narrowest portion of the airway is at the cricoid ring. Further narrowing of the child's inherently narrow airway, such as that caused by soft-tissue swelling or foreign body aspiration, can result in a major decrease in airway resistance and breathing inadequacy.

Children do not have well-developed chest musculature, and their ribs and cartilage are softer and more pliable than an adult's. As a result, the thoracic cavity cannot optimally contribute to lung expansion. Children rely heavily on their diaphragm for breathing, which moves their abdomen in and out. For this reason, infants and children are commonly referred to as "belly breathers".

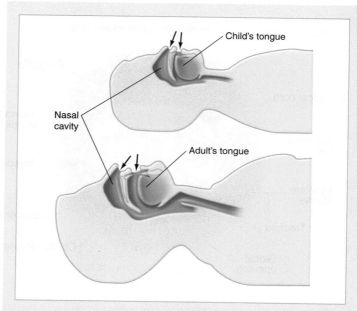

Figure 11-6 In children, the mandible is proportionately smaller and the tongue is proportionately larger than in an adult.

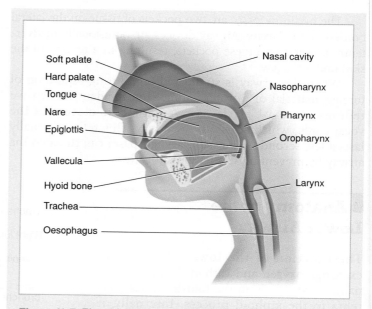

Figure 11-7 The child's epiglottis and surrounding structures.

The alveoli are lined with a proteinaceous substance called surfactant, which decreases surface tension on the alveolar walls and keeps them expanded. If the amount of pulmonary surfactant is decreased or the alveoli are not inflated, they will collapse—a condition called atelectasis.

■ Lung and Respiratory Volumes

The total lung capacity in the average adult male is approximately 6 litres, but only a fraction of this capacity is used during normal breathing. While a small amount of gas exchange occurs in the alveolar ducts and terminal bronchioles, most of the gas exchange occurs in the alveoli.

Tidal volume (V_T), a measure of the depth of breathing, is the volume of air that is inhaled or exhaled during a single respiratory cycle. Normal tidal volume is 5 to 7 ml/kg. Inspiratory reserve volume is the amount of air that can be inhaled in addition to the normal tidal volume; it is normally about 3,000 ml.

In the adult, about 30% of the normal tidal volume remains in the upper airway passages; this so-called dead space volume

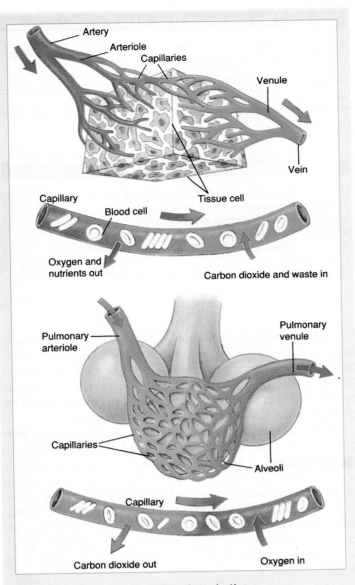

Figure 11-10 Internal and external respiration.

may also result in decreased blood-oxygen levels. These conditions decrease the surface area of the alveoli either by damaging the alveoli or by leading to an accumulation of fluid in the lungs. Nonfunctional alveoli inhibit the diffusion of oxygen and carbon dioxide. As a result, blood entering the lungs from the right side of the heart will bypass the alveoli and will return to the left side of the heart in an unoxygenated state, a condition called intrapulmonary shunting.

Causes of Abnormal Carbon Dioxide Concentrations in the Blood

The pCO_2 in the arterial blood represents a balance between the CO_2 produced in metabolism and the CO_2 eliminated during ventilation. The amount of CO_2 produced normally remains relatively constant. As the metabolic rate goes up (eg, fever), however, more CO_2 is produced. As the metabolic rate falls (eg, hypothermia), the production of CO_2 declines. The type of metabolism also influences CO_2 production, with any metabolic process that results in the formation of acids increasing the amount of CO_2 in the blood. For example, excess lactic acid in the blood (caused by anaerobic metabolism) or excess ketoacids in the blood (caused by fat metabolism due to absent cellular glucose) will increase the circulating levels of CO_2.

If CO_2 production exceeds the body's ability to eliminate it by ventilation, the level of pCO_2 rises to produce hypoventilation. Theoretically, hypoventilation can occur in two ways: CO_2 production can exceed the body's ability to eliminate it, or CO_2 elimination can be depressed to the extent that it no longer keeps up with normal metabolism.

At the other extreme is hyperventilation, which occurs when CO_2 elimination exceeds CO_2 production. For example, patients experiencing an anxiety attack tend to breathe very deep and very fast (eg, minute volume is increased), so they eliminate CO_2 at a rate faster than their body produces it. The level of CO_2 in their blood then falls below normal and they experience symptoms such as dizziness and numbness/tingling in the face and extremities.

You are the Paramedic Part 4

As you continue with your focused history and physical examination of the patient, you note that his level of consciousness has diminished and that cyanosis is developing around his mouth. You perform an immediate reassessment.

Reassessment	Recording Time: 5 Minutes
Level of consciousness	V (Responsive to verbal stimuli); confused
Respirations	32 breaths/min, shallow
Pulse	130 beats/min, weak and regular
Skin	Pale and perspiring, developing peripheral cyanosis
Blood pressure	130/78 mm Hg
SpO_2	82% while breathing oxygen via nonrebreathing mask on 15 l/min

7. How should you adjust your treatment for this patient? Why?

Table 11-2	Carbon Dioxide Balance	
	Hypoventilation	**Hyperventilation**
Minute volume	↓	↑
CO_2 elimination	↓	↑
pCO_2	↑ (hypercarbia)	↓ (hypocarbia)

Table 11-3	Normal Respiration Rate Ranges
Adults	12 to 20 breaths/min
Children	15 to 30 breaths/min
Infants	25 to 50 breaths/min
Note: Ranges presented in other courses or texts may vary.	

Given a steady rate of CO_2 production and CO_2 elimination, pCO_2 is directly proportional to minute volume (Table 11-2 ▲). Decrease the minute volume, and you decrease CO_2 elimination, so CO_2 builds up in the blood (hypercarbia). Increase the minute volume, and you increase carbon dioxide elimination, so the level of CO_2 in the blood falls (hypocarbia).

The Measurement of Gases

Dalton's law of partial pressure states that the total pressure of a gas is the sum of the partial pressure of the components of that gas, or the pressure exerted by a specific atmospheric gas. The major components of air are nitrogen (78.62%); oxygen (20.84%); CO_2 (0.04%); and water vapour (0.50%).

◼ Airway Evaluation

The importance of carefully assessing a patient's airway and ventilatory status cannot be overemphasised. In the field, you will encounter patients with a variety of airway problems— some of these problems are easily corrected, others require aggressive management. *The care you provide to a patient with an airway or breathing problem is only as good as the assessment you perform.*

Essential Parameters

If you can hear a patient breathing, there is usually a problem. Breathing at rest should appear effortless, not laboured. Normally, an adult at rest should have a respiratory rate between 12 and 20 breaths/min (Table 11-3 ▶). The respirations should be of adequate depth (tidal volume) and follow a regular pattern of inhalation and exhalation.

Patients experiencing respiratory distress often attempt to compensate with preferential positioning, such as an upright tripod position (elbows out), or a semi-recumbent (semi-sitting) position. Obviously, patients with respiratory distress will avoid a supine position.

Recognition of Airway Problems

A patient who is conscious, alert, and able to speak to you in complete sentences has no immediate airway or breathing problems. Nonetheless, you must still closely monitor a patient's airway and breathing status and be prepared to intervene should

Table 11-4	Signs of Inadequate Breathing

- Slow (< 12 breaths/min) or fast (> 20 breaths/min) respirations
- Shallow breathing (reduced tidal volume)
- Adventitious (abnormal) breath sounds
- Altered mental status
- Cyanosis (blue or purple skin; indicates low blood oxygen saturation)

his or her condition deteriorate. Changes in respiratory rate, depth, and regularity may be subtle. If these subtleties are overlooked, and the appropriate care is not provided, the patient's outcome may be less than desirable. In case of inadequate breathing, it is critical to intervene immediately with some form of positive-pressure ventilation and high flow oxygen.

The adult patient with an abnormal respiratory rate must be evaluated for other signs of inadequate ventilation (Table 11-4 ▲). Causes of inadequate ventilation include severe infection (sepsis), trauma, brain stem insult, a noxious or oxygen-poor atmosphere, and renal failure, to name a few. In addition to inadequate ventilation, causes of respiratory distress may include upper and/or lower airway obstructions, impairment of the respiratory muscles (eg, spinal cord injury), or impairment of the nervous system (eg, head injury, drug overdose).

Dyspnoea is defined as any difficulty in respiratory rate, regularity, or effort. It may result from hypoxaemia, a decrease in arterial oxygen levels. If left untreated, hypoxaemia will progress to hypoxia, a lack of oxygen to the body's cells and tissues. Untreated hypoxia will lead to anoxia, an absence of oxygen that results in cellular and tissue death.

If a patient's airway is not patent, or if breathing is absent or inadequate, all therapies that you may attempt will prove futile. Proper airway management involves opening the airway, clearing the airway, assessing breathing, and providing the appropriate intervention(s)—in that order.

Evaluation of the airway includes the techniques of look, listen, and feel. Visual techniques should be used at first sight of the patient. The following questions must be answered when assessing the patient with respiratory distress:

- How is the patient positioned?
  - Is he or she in a tripod position?

– Is the patient experiencing <u>orthopnoea</u> (positional dyspnoea)?

■ Is rise and fall of the chest adequate (eg, adequate tidal volume)?

■ Is the patient gasping for air (air hunger)?

■ What is the skin colour?

■ Is there flaring of the nostrils?

■ Is the patient breathing through pursed lips?

■ Do you note any <u>recession</u> (skin pulling in between and around the ribs during inhalation):

 – Intercostal?

 – At the suprasternal notch?

 – At the supraclavicular fossa?

 – Subcostal?

■ Is the patient using <u>accessory muscles</u> to breathe? (Accessory muscles, which are not normally used during normal breathing, include the sternocleidomastoid muscles in the neck.)

■ Is the patient's chest wall moving symmetrically? (<u>Asymmetric chest wall movement</u>, when one side of the chest moves less than the other, indicates that airflow into one lung is decreased.)

Listen for air movement at the patient's nose and mouth. Is the patient taking a series of quick breaths, followed by a prolonged exhalation phase? If so, this is a sign of inadequate ventilation.

Auscultate breath sounds with a stethoscope. Breath sounds should be clear and equal on both sides of the chest (bilateral), anteriorly and posteriorly. Compare each apex (top) of the lung to the opposite apex and each base (bottom) of the lung to the opposite base **Figure 11-11 ▼** .

If you are ventilating the patient with a bag-valve-mask device, note any resistance or change in ventilatory compliance. Increased compliance (decreased resistance) means that air can be forced into the lungs with relative ease; decreased compliance (increased resistance) suggests an upper or lower airway obstruction.

Assess for <u>pulsus paradoxus</u> (paradoxical pulse), which occurs when the systolic blood pressure drops more than 10 mm Hg during inhalation. A change in pulse quality, or even the disappearance of a pulse during inhalation, may also be detected. Pulsus paradoxus is typically seen in patients with decompensating COPD, severe pericardial tamponade, or other conditions that increase intrathoracic pressure (eg, tension pneumothorax, severe asthma attack).

A history of the patient's present illness is a vital part of your assessment of the patient with respiratory distress. You should ask questions to determine the evolution of the current problem:

■ Was the onset of the problem sudden or gradual over time?

 – Some people may perceive respiratory distress that occurred 2 days prior as arising gradually, when, in fact, the onset was sudden; the patient may have simply waited 2 days before calling for help.

■ Is there any known cause or "trigger" of the event?

 – Asthma is commonly exacerbated by stress or cold weather. A foreign body airway obstruction is commonly preceded by a sudden onset of difficulty in breathing during a meal or, in children, while playing with small toys or other objects.

■ What is the duration (is it constant or recurrent)?

■ Does anything alleviate or exacerbate the problem?

■ Are there any other associated symptoms, such as a productive cough, chest pain or pressure, or fever?

■ Were any interventions attempted prior to ambulance arrival?

■ Has the patient been evaluated by a doctor or admitted to the hospital for this condition in the past?

 – Determine specifically whether the patient was hospitalised or merely seen in the accident and emergency (A&E) department and then released. If the patient was hospitalised, ask whether the patient was admitted to an intensive care unit (ICU) or a regular, unmonitored ward. A condition that warranted an ICU admission is clinically significant.

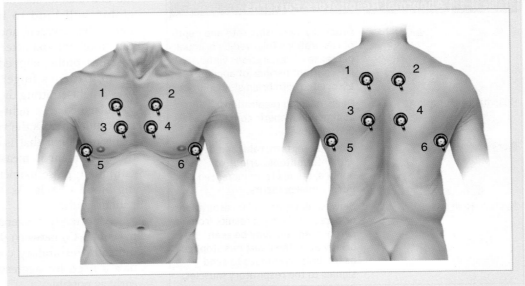

Figure 11-11 Auscultation of breath sounds (1 to 6).

- Is the patient currently taking any medications?
  - Don't simply ask which medications were taken today. Instead, determine the *overall* compliance by asking whether the patient has been taking the medications as prescribed. Verify this information by looking at the prescription date on the medication bottle(s), reading the prescription directions, and counting the pills remaining in the bottle (if you have sufficient time).
  - Ask whether the patient has had any changes to a current prescription, such as a new medication or changes in the prescribing directions of an existing medication.
- Does the patient have any risk factors that could cause or exacerbate his or her condition, such as alcohol or illicit drug use, cigarette smoking, or a poor diet?

Evaluate the patient for any modified forms of respiration. Protective reflexes of the airway include coughing, sneezing, and gagging. Coughing is a forceful exhalation produced with a greater than normal volume of breath. The patient whose cough mechanism is suppressed—whether by drugs, pain, trauma, or by any other cause—is at serious risk of aspirating foreign material.

Gagging is a forceful muscular contraction of the pharyngeal muscles and the glottis. This reaction is automatic when something touches an area deep in the oral cavity. The gag reflex helps protect the lower airway from aspiration, or entry of fluids or solids into the trachea, bronchi, and lungs.

Patients with serious injuries or illness may present with changes in their respiratory pattern. **Table 11-5 ▾** shows various abnormal respiratory patterns and their causes.

Table 11-5	Abnormal Respiratory Patterns
Cheyne-Stokes respirations	Gradually increasing rate and depth of respirations followed by gradual decrease of respirations with intermittent periods of apnoea; associated with brain stem injury.
Kussmaul respirations	Deep, gasping respirations; common in diabetic coma (ketoacidosis).
Biot respirations	Irregular pattern, rate, and depth with intermittent periods of apnoea; results from increased intracranial pressure.
Agonal respirations	Slow, shallow, irregular respirations or occasional gasps; results from cerebral anoxia; may be seen briefly after the heart has stopped as the brain continues to send signals to the respiratory muscles.

At the Scene

A critical question to ask the patient with respiratory distress is if he or she has ever been intubated for the same problem. A condition serious enough to warrant intubation requires urgent attention to prevent a repeated occurrence. Also, determine whether other interventions (eg, defibrillation, transcutaneous pacing) were required to treat the same problem in the past. This information will increase your index of suspicion and prepare you for a potential rapid deterioration in the patient's condition. Use layperson's language when talking to the patient.

Diagnostic Testing

Several methods and devices are used to quantify oxygenation and ventilation. Pulse oximetry is a simple, rapid, safe, and noninvasive method of measuring—minute by minute—how well a person's haemoglobin is saturated with oxygen.

A pulse oximeter **Figure 11-12 ▸** measures the percentage of haemoglobin in the arterial blood that is saturated. Under normal circumstances, haemoglobin is saturated with oxygen. When carbon monoxide is available, haemoglobin will bind to it rather than oxygen, and can "fool" the oximeter. A sensor probe, clipped to the patient's finger,

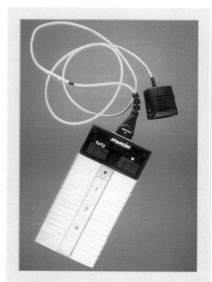

Figure 11-12 A pulse oximeter.

uses a light-emitting diode (LED) to transmit light through the vascular bed to a light-sensing detector. The amount of light transmitted across the vascular bed depends on the proportion of haemoglobin that is saturated with oxygen. To ensure that the instrument is measuring arterial and not venous oxygen saturation, pulse oximeters are designed to assess only pulsating blood vessels. As a consequence, they also measure the patient's pulse.

A normally oxygenated, normally perfused person should have an SpO_2 between 95% and 99%. Any reading below 95% indicates respiratory compromise; a reading below 90% signals a need for aggressive oxygen therapy, act upon this as early as possible.

Situations in which pulse oximeters may be useful in pre-hospital emergency care include the following:

- **Monitoring the oxygenation of a patient during an intubation attempt or during suctioning.** The low-saturation alarm on the pulse oximeter can signal that the paramedic should abort the intubation attempt and ventilate the patient.
- **Identifying deterioration in a trauma victim.** In the patient with multiple trauma, the signs of a developing tension pneumothorax, for instance, may not be evident until the problem is quite advanced. A declining SpO_2 level can alert the paramedic that something bad is happening and prompt a search for the cause of the problem.
- **Identifying deterioration in the cardiac patient.** Pulse oximetry may enable early identification of patients who are experiencing congestive heart failure in the wake of an acute myocardial infarction.
- **Identifying high-risk patients with respiratory problems.** For example, pulse oximetry may identify patients with asthma who are having serious attacks or patients with emphysema who are in severe decompensation.
- **Assessing vascular status in orthopaedic trauma.** Pulse oximetry is routine practice in assessing a fractured extremity to evaluate the pulse distal to the fracture. Loss of a pulse means that the limb is in jeopardy and may require urgent action at the scene if transport time is long. A pulse oximeter clipped to a finger or toe on a broken limb might provide critical information about the ongoing circulation to the limb.

The usefulness of a pulse oximeter depends on its ability to provide accurate information. A pulse oximeter that gives a reading of 99% when the patient is actually severely hypoxaemic will not be much help to anyone. Be aware of circumstances that might produce erroneous readings:

- **Bright ambient light** may enter the spectrophotometer of the pulse oximeter and create an incorrect reading. Protect the sensor clip by covering it with a towel or blanket.
- **Patient motion** can confuse the pulse oximeter, as it may mistake motion for arterial pulsation and read the oxygen saturation from a vein rather than an artery.
- **Poor perfusion** makes it difficult for the oximeter to sense a pulse and therefore to generate a reading. Poor perfusion occurs in conditions such as shock, cardiac arrest, and exposure to cold.

- **Nail varnish** will prevent the sensor from working properly.
- **Venous pulsations** may occur in some patients with right-sided heart failure. If a vein is pulsating, the oximeter may regard it as an artery and measure venous oxygen saturation.
- **Abnormal haemoglobin** may produce a falsely high SpO_2. Carboxyhaemoglobin, for example, is formed by the attachment of CO to the haemoglobin molecule. Because the pulse oximeter cannot distinguish between oxyhaemoglobin (haemoglobin that is occupied by oxygen) and carboxyhaemoglobin, it may give a high SpO_2 reading for a patient who is severely hypoxaemic from CO poisoning. The results of pulse oximetry should therefore be interpreted cautiously in victims of smoke inhalation or other circumstances likely to have produced CO poisoning.

When in Doubt, Look at the Patient!

Always weigh the information provided by pulse oximetry (or any other device) against clinical observations. If the patient is turning blue and struggling to breathe, you may ignore the pulse oximeter reading that says the patient is adequately oxygenated.

The steps for performing pulse oximetry are listed here and shown in **Skill Drill 11-1 ▾**.

Skill Drill 11-1: Performing Pulse Oximetry

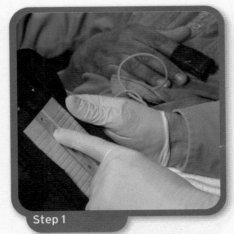

Step 1

Clean the patient's finger tip and nail bed and place his or her finger in the pulse oximeter probe. Turn on the pulse oximeter and note the SpO_2 display.

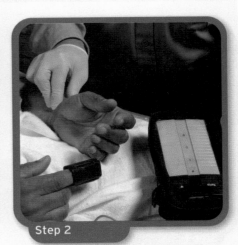

Step 2

Palpate the radial pulse to ensure that it correlates with the display on the pulse oximeter.

1. Clean the patient's finger and remove nail varnish as needed. Dark, shiny, or metallic flake nail varnish are particularly problematic. Place the index or middle finger into the pulse oximeter probe. Turn on the pulse oximeter and note the S_PO_2 reading (**Step 1**).

2. Palpate the radial pulse to ensure that it correlates with the display on the pulse oximeter (**Step 2**).

In patients with certain reactive airway diseases (eg, asthma), bronchoconstriction can be evaluated by measuring the peak rate of a forceful exhalation with a peak expiratory flow monitor. An increasing peak expiratory flow suggests that the patient is responding to treatment (eg, inhaled bronchodilators). A decreasing peak expiratory flow may be an early indication that the patient's condition is deteriorating.

Peak expiratory flow varies based on sex, height, and age. Normal adults have a peak expiratory flow rate of 350 to 750 ml.

The steps for performing peak expiratory flow measurement are listed here and shown in (**Skill Drill 11-2** ▾).

1. Place the patient in a seated position with the legs dangling. Assemble the peak flowmeter and make sure that it is reset to zero (**Step 1**).

2. Ask the patient to take a deep breath, place the mouthpiece in his or her mouth, and ask the patient to exhale as forcefully as possible. Make sure no air leaks around the device or comes from the patient's nose (**Step 2**).

3. Perform the test three times, and take the average of the three readings (**Step 3**).

Airway Management

Clearly, a patient who is conscious and talking, screaming, or crying has an open airway. In a patient with an altered LOC, however, the airway is often not patent and manual manoeuvres will be required to open it. In addition, artificial airway adjuncts may be needed to assist in maintaining the airway.

Positioning the Patient

If patients are found unconscious and in a prone position, however, you must position them properly so that you can open the airway, assess respirations, and provide ventilation or CPR if needed.

To move a patient to a supine position, log roll the individual as a unit. Once the patient is in a supine position, open the airway and assess breathing status. The recovery position, which involves placing the patient in a right lateral recumbent position, should be used in all nontrauma patients with a decreased LOC who are able to maintain their own airway spontaneously and are breathing adequately (**Figure 11-13** ▸). This also ensures they face into the centre of the ambulance during subsequent transport.

Skill Drill 11-2: Peak Expiratory Flow Measurement

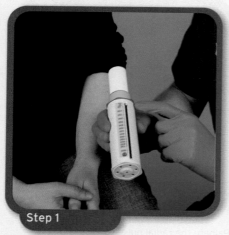

Step 1

Assemble the peak flowmeter and make sure it is reset to zero.

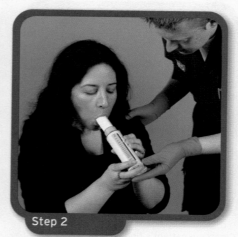

Step 2

Ask the patient to take a deep breath, place the mouthpiece in his or her mouth, and ask the patient to exhale as forcefully as possible. Make sure no air leaks around the device or comes from the patient's nose.

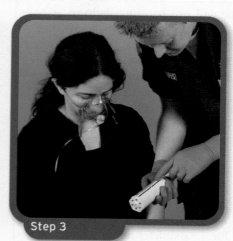

Step 3

Perform the test three times, and take the average of the three readings.

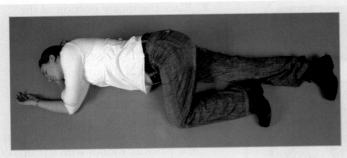

Figure 11-13 The recovery position.

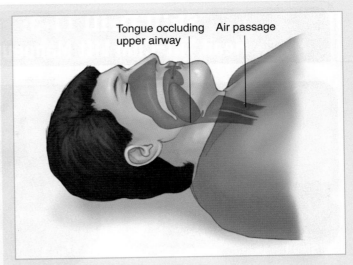

Figure 11-14 When the tongue falls back and occludes the posterior pharynx, it may obstruct the airway.

Manual Airway Manoeuvres

In the unresponsive patient, the most common cause of airway obstruction is the patient's tongue (Figure 11-14 ▸). To correct this problem, manually manoeuvre the patient's head to propel the tongue forward and open the airway. Techniques used to accomplish this include the head tilt–chin lift manoeuvre and the jaw-thrust manoeuvre (with or without head tilt).

Head Tilt–Chin Lift Manoeuvre

Opening the airway to relieve an obstruction can often be done quickly and easily by simply tilting the patient's head back and lifting the chin, known as the head tilt–chin lift manoeuvre. Occasionally, this simple manoeuvre is all that is required for the patient to resume breathing. Following are some considerations when using the head tilt–chin lift manoeuvre:

- **Indications.** An unresponsive patient, no mechanism for cervical spine injury, or a patient who is unable to protect his or her own airway.
- **Contraindications.** A responsive patient or a possible cervical spine injury.
- **Advantages.** No equipment is required, and the technique is simple, safe, and noninvasive.
- **Disadvantages.** It is thought to be hazardous to patients with spinal injury and does not protect from aspiration. Perform the head tilt–chin lift manoeuvre in the following manner (Skill Drill 11-3 ▸).

1. With the patient in a supine position, position yourself beside the patient's head (Step 1).
2. Place one hand on the patient's forehead, and apply firm backward pressure with your palm to tilt the patient's head back (Step 2). This extension of the neck will propel the tongue forward, away from the posterior pharynx and clear the airway.
3. Place the tips of your fingers of your other hand under the lower jaw near the bony part of the chin (Step 3). Do not compress the soft tissue under the chin, as this may block the airway.
4. Lift the chin upward, bringing the entire lower jaw with it, helping to tilt the head back (Step 4). Do not use your thumb to lift the chin. Lift so that the teeth are nearly brought

together, but avoid closing the mouth completely. Continue to hold the forehead to maintain backward tilt of the head.

Jaw-Thrust Manoeuvre

If you suspect that the patient has experienced a cervical spine injury, open his or her airway with the jaw-thrust manoeuvre. In this technique, you open the airway by placing your fingers behind the angle of the jaw and lifting the jaw forward. The jaw is displaced forward at the mandibular angle. You can easily seal a mask around the patient's nose and mouth while performing this manoeuvre. Following are some considerations when using the jaw-thrust manoeuvre:

- **Indications.** An unresponsive patient, possible cervical spine injury, or a patient who is unable to protect his or her own airway.
- **Contraindications.** A responsive patient with resistance to opening the mouth. The jaw-thrust manoeuvre may be needed in the responsive patient who has sustained a jaw fracture to keep the tongue away from the back of the throat.
- **Advantages.** May be used in patients with cervical spine injury, may use with cervical collar in place, and does not require special equipment.
- **Disadvantages.** Cannot maintain if patient becomes responsive or combative, difficult to maintain for an extended period of time, very difficult to use in conjunction with bag-valve-mask ventilation, thumb must remain in place to maintain jaw displacement, requires second ambulance person for bag-valve-mask ventilation, and does not protect against aspiration. Perform the jaw-thrust manoeuvre in the following manner (Skill Drill 11-4 ▸).

1. Position yourself at the top of the supine patient's head (Step 1).

Skill Drill 11-3:
Head Tilt-Chin Lift Manoeuvre

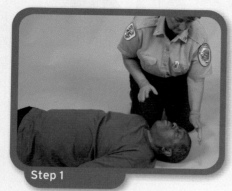

Step 1

Position yourself at the side of the supine patient.

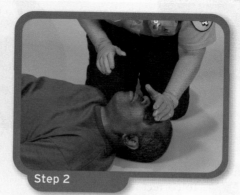

Step 2

Place your hand closest to the patient's head on the forehead.

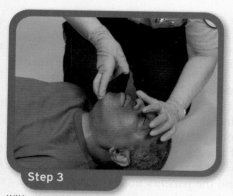

Step 3

With your other hand, place two fingers on the bony part of the patient's chin.

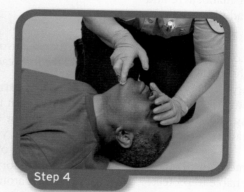

Step 4

Simultaneously apply backward and downward pressure to the patient's forehead and lift the jaw straight up. Do not depress the soft tissue below the chin.

2. Place the meaty portion of the base of your thumbs on the zygomatic arches and hook the tips of your index fingers under the angle of the mandible, in the indent below each ear (**Step 2**).
3. While holding the patient's head in a neutral inline position, displace the jaw upward and open the patient's mouth with the tips of your thumbs (**Step 3**).

If you are unable to open the airway with the jaw-thrust manoeuvre, you should carefully perform the head tilt–chin lift manoeuvre.

Jaw-Thrust Manoeuvre With Head Tilt

The jaw-thrust manoeuvre with head tilt is similar to the head tilt–chin lift manoeuvre, with a few exceptions. Following are some considerations when using the jaw-thrust manoeuvre with head tilt:

- **Indications.** An unresponsive patient or a patient unable to protect his or her own airway.
- **Contraindications.** A responsive patient or a patient with a possible cervical spine injury.
- **Advantages.** It is noninvasive and does not require special equipment.
- **Disadvantages.** It is difficult to maintain, requires a second rescuer for bag-valve-mask ventilation, and does not protect against aspiration.

You are the Paramedic Part 5

You are now assisting the patient's breathing with a bag-valve-mask device and oxygen at 25 l/min, attached to the reservoir bag. You call control and ask for an additional crew to respond for assistance. Your colleague quickly reassesses the patient and notes the following:

Reassessment	Recording Time: 8 Minutes
Level of consciousness	P (Responsive to painful stimuli)
Respirations	36 breaths/min, shallow and gurgling; you are assisting ventilations with a bag-valve-mask device and oxygen at 25 l/min
Pulse	150 beats/min, regular and weak
Skin	Pale and perspiring extremities and trunk; facial cyanosis
Blood pressure	118/70 mm Hg
S_PO_2	86% while being ventilated with a bag-valve-mask device and oxygen on 25 l/min

8. Why is your patient's condition not improving with assisted ventilation?

9. What must you do to correct the situation?

Skill Drill 11-4: Jaw-Thrust Manoeuvre

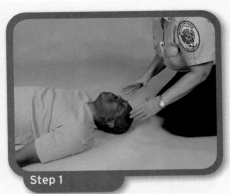

Step 1

Position yourself at the top of the patient's head.

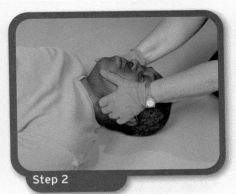

Step 2

Place the meaty portion of the base of your thumbs on the zygomatic arches, and hook the tips of your index fingers under the angle of the mandible, in the indent below each ear.

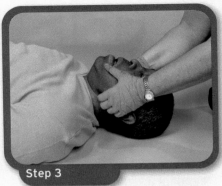

Step 3

While holding the patient's head still, displace the jaw upward and open the patient's mouth with your thumb tips.

Skill Drill 11-5: Jaw-Thrust Manoeuvre With Head Tilt

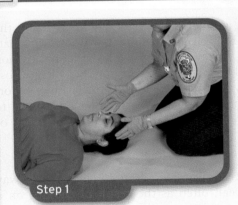

Step 1

Position yourself at the top of the patient's head.

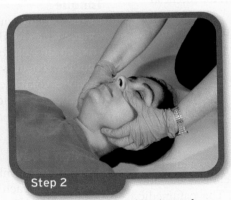

Step 2

Place the meaty portion of the base of your thumbs on the zygomatic arches, and hook the tips of your index fingers under the angle of the mandible, in the indent below each ear.

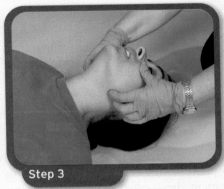

Step 3

Displace the jaw upward and tilt the head back.

Perform the jaw-thrust manoeuvre with head tilt in the following manner **Skill Drill 11-5 ▲**.

1. Position yourself at the top of the patient's head **Step 1**.
2. Place the meaty portion of the base of your thumbs on the zygomatic arches, and hook the tips of your index fingers under the angle of the mandible, in the middle indent below the patient's ear **Step 2**.

3. Displace the jaw upward and tilt the head back **Step 3**.

Tongue-Jaw Lift Manoeuvre

The tongue-jaw lift manoeuvre is used more commonly to open a patient's airway for the purpose of suctioning or inserting an oropharyngeal airway. It cannot be used to ventilate a patient, because it will not allow for an adequate mask seal on

Skill Drill 11-6: Tongue-Jaw Lift Manoeuvre

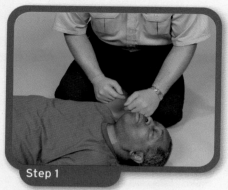

Step 1

Position yourself at the patient's side.

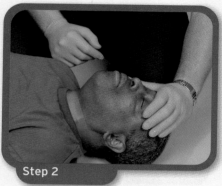

Step 2

Place the hand closest to the patient's head on the forehead.

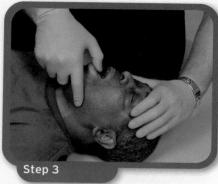

Step 3

With your other hand, reach into the patient's mouth and hook your first knuckle under the incisors or gum line. While holding the patient's head and maintaining the hand on the forehead, lift the jaw straight up.

the patient's face. Perform the tongue-jaw lift in the following manner **Skill Drill 11-6** ▲ .

1. Position yourself at the side of the patient **Step 1** .
2. Place the hand closest to the patient's head on the forehead **Step 2** .
3. With the other hand, reach into the patient's mouth and hook your first knuckle under the incisors or gum line. While holding the patient's head and maintaining the hand on the forehead, lift the jaw straight up **Step 3** .

▌ Airway Obstructions

The airway connects the body to the life-giving oxygen in the atmosphere. If it becomes obstructed, this lifeline is cut and the patient dies—often within a few minutes. The paramedic must recognise the signs of an obstructed airway and immediately take corrective action.

Causes of Airway Obstruction

In an adult, sudden foreign body airway obstruction usually occurs during a meal. In children, it typically occurs while eating or playing with small toys. An otherwise healthy child who presents with a sudden onset of difficulty breathing—especially in the absence of fever—should be suspected of having a foreign body airway obstruction. A multitude of other conditions can cause an airway obstruction, including the tongue, laryngeal oedema, laryngeal spasm (laryngospasm), trauma, and aspiration.

When the airway is obstructed secondary to an infectious process or a severe allergic reaction, repeated attempts to clear the airway as if it were obstructed by a foreign body will be unsuccessful and potentially harmful. These patients require specific management (discussed in Chapter 26) and prompt transport to the nearest A&E deparment.

Tongue

In the patient with an altered LOC, the jaw relaxes and the tongue tends to fall back against the posterior wall of the pharynx, closing off the airway. A patient with partial obstruction from the tongue will have snoring respirations; a patient whose airway is completely obstructed will have no respirations. Fortunately, obstruction of the airway by the tongue is simple to correct using a manual manoeuvre (eg, head tilt–chin lift, or jaw-thrust).

Foreign Body

A significant number of people die from foreign body airway obstructions each year, often as the result of choking on a piece of food. The typical victim is middle-aged or older and wears dentures. He or she has usually had a few alcoholic drinks, which depresses protective reflexes and adversely affects a person's judgement regarding how large a piece of food can be prudently placed in the mouth. Additionally, patients with conditions that decrease their airway reflexes (eg, stroke) are at an increased risk for a foreign body airway obstruction. A foreign body may cause a mild or severe airway obstruction, depending on the size of the object and its location in the airway.

Signs may include choking, gagging, stridor, dyspnoea, aphonia (inability to speak), and dysphonia (difficulty speaking). Treatment for the patient depends on whether he or she is effectively moving air. Techniques for foreign body airway obstruction removal will be discussed later in this chapter.

Laryngeal Spasm and Oedema

A laryngeal spasm (laryngospasm) results in spasmodic closure of the vocal cords, completely occluding the airway. It is often caused by trauma during an overly aggressive intubation attempt or immediately upon extubation, especially when the patient has an altered LOC.

Laryngeal oedema causes the glottic opening to become extremely narrow or totally closed. Conditions that commonly cause this problem include epiglottitis, anaphylaxis, or inhalation injury (eg, burns to the upper airway).

Airway obstructions caused by laryngeal spasm or oedema may be relieved by aggressive ventilation to force air past the narrowed airway or a forceful upward pull of the jaw in an attempt to reposition the airway. The patient should be transported to the hospital for evaluation.

Fractured Larynx

Airway patency depends on good muscle tone to keep the trachea open. Fracture of the larynx increases airway resistance by decreasing airway size secondary to decreased muscle tone, laryngeal oedema, and ventilatory effort. An advanced airway may be required to maintain an open airway.

Aspiration

Aspiration of blood or other fluid significantly increases mortality. In addition to potentially obstructing the airway, aspiration destroys delicate bronchiolar tissue, introduces pathogens into the lungs, and decreases the patient's ability to ventilate (or be ventilated).

Suction should be readily available for any patient who is unable to maintain his or her own airway. Patients requiring emergency care should always be assumed to have a full stomach.

Recognition of an Airway Obstruction

A foreign body lodged in the upper airway can cause a mild (partial) or severe (complete) airway obstruction. A rapid but careful assessment is required to determine the seriousness of the obstruction, as the differences in managing mild versus severe cases are significant.

A patient with a mild airway obstruction is conscious and able to exchange air, but may show varying degrees of respiratory distress. The patient will usually have noisy respirations and may be coughing. The patient may wheeze between coughs but does not become cyanotic. *Patients with a mild airway obstruction should be encouraged to give a forceful cough, as this is the most effective means of dislodging the obstruction.* Attempts to manually remove the object could force it farther down into the airway and cause a severe obstruction.

A patient with a severe airway obstruction typically experiences a sudden inability to breathe, talk, or cough—classically during a meal. The patient may grasp at his or her throat, begin to turn cyanotic, and make frantic, exaggerated attempts to breathe Figure 11-15 ▶ . Patients with a severe airway obstruction have a weak, ineffective, or absent cough and are in marked respiratory distress; weak inspiratory stridor and cyanosis are often present.

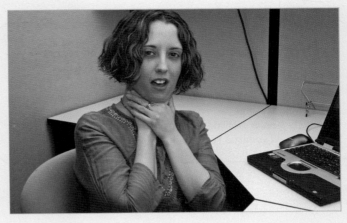

Figure 11-15 The universal sign of choking.

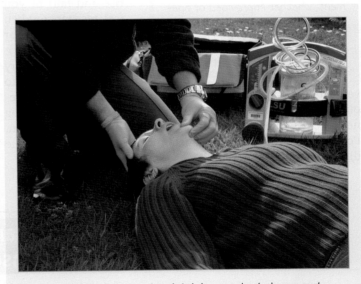

Figure 11-16 Securing and maintaining a patent airway and ensuring adequate ventilation are among the most important steps in caring for an unconscious patient.

Emergency Medical Care for Foreign Body Airway Obstruction

If the patient with a suspected airway obstruction is conscious, ask, "Are you choking?" If the patient nods "yes", begin treatment immediately. If the obstruction is not promptly cleared, the amount of oxygen in the blood will decrease dramatically, resulting in severe hypoxia, unconsciousness, and death.

Open and maintain the airway with the appropriate manual manoeuvre, assess for breathing, and provide artificial ventilation if necessary Figure 11-16 ▲ .

At the Scene

Causes of Airway Obstruction

- Relaxation of the tongue in an unresponsive patient
- Foreign objects—food, small toys, dentures
- Blood clots, broken teeth, or damaged oral tissue following trauma
- Airway tissue swelling—infection, allergic reaction
- Aspirated vomitus (stomach contents)

Special Considerations

According to current clinical guidelines, a child is defined as a patient from 1 year of age to the onset of puberty.

Notes from Nancy

Blind insertion of any instrument, whether improvised or specially designed, into a patient's pharynx is extremely dangerous. Don't do it!

If, after opening the airway, you are unable to ventilate the patient (no chest rise and fall) or you feel resistance when ventilating (poor lung compliance), reopen the airway and again attempt to ventilate the patient. Lung compliance is the ability of the alveoli to expand when air is drawn into the lungs, either during negative-pressure ventilation or positive-pressure ventilation. Poor lung compliance is characterised by increased resistance during ventilation attempts.

If large pieces of vomitus, mucus, loose dentures, or blood clots can be seen in the upper airway, sweep them forward and out of the mouth with your gloved index finger. *Blind finger sweeps of the mouth—regardless of the patient's age—are not recommended and may cause further harm.* After the patient's airway is open, insert your gloved index finger down along the inside of the patient's cheek and into his or her throat at the base of the tongue, then try to hook the foreign body to dislodge it and manoeuvre it into the mouth. Take care not to force the foreign body deeper into the airway. Do *not* blindly insert any object other than your finger into the patient's mouth to remove a foreign body, as an instrument jammed into the throat can damage the delicate structures of the pharynx and compound the obstruction with haemorrhage. Suctioning should be used to clear the airway of secretions as needed.

The steps for managing a severe airway obstruction in a conscious adult or child are listed here and shown in **Skill Drill 11-7 ▾** .

1. Determine whether the patient is choking by asking, "Are you choking"? If the patient nods "yes", then your help is needed (**Step 1**).

Skill Drill 11-7: Managing Severe Airway Obstruction in a Conscious Adult or Child

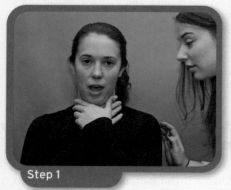

Step 1

Determine whether the patient is choking by asking, "Are you choking"? If the patient nods "yes", then your help is needed.

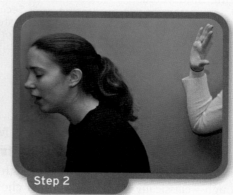

Step 2

Provide five back slaps between the shoulder blades. Check after each slap to see whether the obstruction has been relieved.

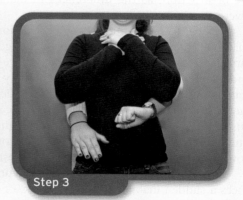

Step 3

If the airway remains obstructed, perform five abdominal thrusts. If the obstruction still is not relieved, continue to alternate between back slaps and abdominal thrusts until the airway is clear or the patient is unconscious.

Skill Drill 11-8: Managing Severe Airway Obstruction in an Unconscious Adult or Child

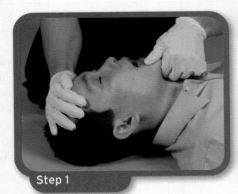

Step 1

Open the airway and look in the mouth. If you see the object, carefully remove it from the patient's mouth.

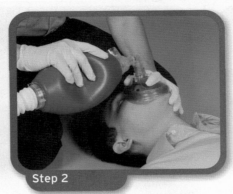

Step 2

Attempt two ventilations. If unsuccessful, reopen the airway and again attempt ventilation.

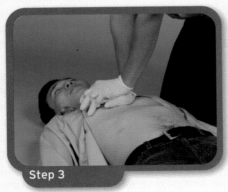

Step 3

Perform 30 chest compressions.

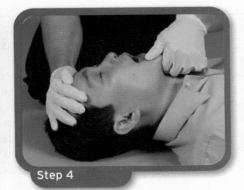

Step 4

Open the airway and look in the mouth. If you see the object, carefully remove it from the patient's mouth. Repeat steps 2 through 4 until successful.

2. Provide five back slaps between the shoulder blades with the heel of one hand. Check after each slap to see whether the obstruction has been relieved (Step 2).

3. If the airway remains obstructed, perform five abdominal thrusts; if the obstruction is still not relieved, continue to alternate five back slaps with five abdominal thrusts until the airway is clear or patient is unconscious (Step 3).

The steps for managing a severe airway obstruction in an unconscious adult or child are listed here and shown in Skill Drill 11-8 ▲ .

1. Open the airway with the head tilt–chin lift manoeuvre and look in the patient's mouth (Step 1). If you see the object, carefully remove it from the patient's mouth.

2. Attempt two ventilations (Step 2). If unsuccessful, reopen the airway and again attempt ventilation.

3. Perform 30 chest compressions (Step 3).

4. Open the airway with the head tilt–chin lift manoeuvre and look in the patient's mouth (Step 4). If you see the object, carefully remove it from the patient's mouth. Repeat steps 2 through 4 until successful.

The steps for managing a severe airway obstruction in a conscious infant are listed here and shown in Skill Drill 11-9 ▶ .

1. Perform five back slaps (Step 1).

2. Perform five chest thrusts (Step 2). Repeat steps 1 and 2 until the object is expelled or the infant becomes unresponsive.

The steps for managing a severe airway obstruction in an unconscious infant are listed here and shown in Skill Drill 11-10 ▶ .

1. Open the infant's airway with slight extension of the neck and look in the mouth (Step 1). If you see the object, carefully remove it from the infant's mouth.

2. Attempt to ventilate (Step 2). If unsuccessful, reopen the airway and again attempt ventilation.

3. Perform 30 chest compressions (Step 3).

4. Open the infant's airway with slight extension of the neck and look in the mouth (Step 4). If you see the object, carefully remove it from the infant's mouth. Repeat steps 2 through 4 until successful.

Abdominal thrusts (Heimlich manoeuvre) are the most effective method of dislodging and forcing an object out of the airway. It aims to create an artificial cough by forcing residual air out of the victim's lungs, thereby expelling the object. You should perform abdominal thrusts on a conscious child (but not infants) or adult with a severe airway obstruction until the obstructing object is expelled or until

Skill Drill 11-9: Managing Severe Airway Obstruction in a Conscious Infant

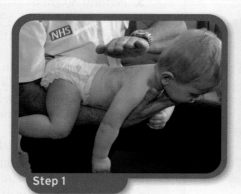

Step 1

Perform five back slaps.

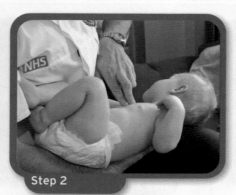

Step 2

Perform five chest thrusts. Repeat steps 1 and 2 until the object is expelled or the infant becomes unresponsive.

fully remove it from the upper airway with your Magill forceps, a special type of curved forceps **Figure 11-17 ▲** . The steps for removal of an upper airway obstruction with Magill forceps are listed here and shown in **Skill Drill 11-11 ▶** .

1. With the patient's head in the sniffing position, open the patient's mouth and insert the laryngoscope blade **Step 1** .
2. Visualise the obstruction, and grasp the object with the Magill forceps **Step 2** .
3. Remove the object with the Magill forceps **Step 3** .
4. Attempt to ventilate the patient **Step 4** .

At the Scene

A patient with a severe upper airway obstruction has very little time before severe hypoxia develops. If several attempts to relieve the obstruction with conventional BLS methods fail, you should proceed with direct laryngoscopy without delay. As you are performing BLS manoeuvres, your partner should be preparing the correct size endotracheal tube, laryngoscope blade, and handle.

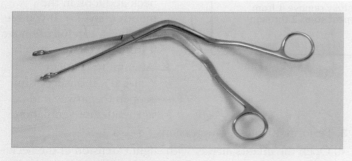

Figure 11-17 Magill forceps.

the patient becomes unresponsive. If the conscious patient with a severe airway obstruction is in the advanced stages of pregnancy or is morbidly obese, perform chest thrusts instead of abdominal thrusts.

If you are unable to relieve a severe airway obstruction in an unconscious patient with the basic techniques previously discussed, you should proceed with direct laryngoscopy (visualisation of the airway with a laryngoscope) for the removal of the foreign body in unresponsive patients. Insert the laryngoscope blade into the patient's mouth. If you see the foreign body, care-

▌Suctioning

When the patient's mouth or throat becomes filled with vomitus, blood, or secretions, a suction apparatus enables you to remove the liquid material quickly and efficiently, thereby allowing you to ventilate the patient. Ventilating a patient with secretions in his or her mouth will force material into the lungs, resulting in an upper airway obstruction or aspiration. Therefore, clearing the patient's airway with suction, if needed, is your next priority after opening the patient's airway. *If you hear gurgling, the patient needs suctioning! Noisy airways are not good.*

Suctioning Equipment

Ambulances should carry both an ambulance mains/battery power suction unit and a portable suction unit, which is often taken into the call with the primary response bag **Figure 11-18 ▶** . Regardless of your location—in the patient's residence, the middle of a field, or in the back of the ambulance—you must have quick access to suction. It is essential for resuscitation.

Mechanical or vacuum-powered suction units should be capable of generating a vacuum of 300 mm Hg within 4 seconds of clamping off the tubing. The amount of suction should be adjustable for use in children and intubated patients. Check the vacuum on the mechanical suction unit at the beginning of every shift by turning on the device, clamping (or kinking) the tubing, and making sure the pressure gauge registers 300 mm Hg. Ensure that all battery-charged units have fully charged batteries. **Table 11-6 ▶** lists the advantages and disadvantages of the most common types of suction devices.

In addition to the suctioning unit, the following supplies should be readily accessible at the patient's head:

- Wide-bore, thick-walled, nonkinking tubing

Skill Drill 11-10: Managing Severe Airway Obstruction in an Unconscious Infant

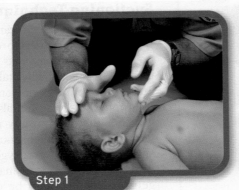

Step 1

Open the infant's airway and look in the mouth. If you see the object, carefully remove it from the infant's mouth.

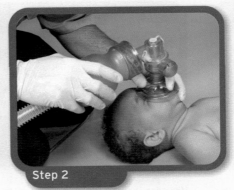

Step 2

Attempt to ventilate. If unsuccessful, reopen the airway and again attempt ventilation.

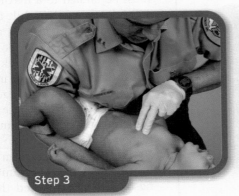

Step 3

Perform chest compressions.

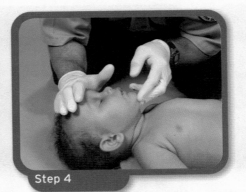

Step 4

Open the infant's airway and look in the mouth. If you see the object, carefully remove it from the infant's mouth. Repeat steps 2 through 4 until successful.

- Soft and rigid suction catheters of different gauges and lengths
- A nonbreakable, disposable collection bottle

A Yankeur catheter is a good option for suctioning the pharynx in adults. These plastic-tip catheters have a large diameter and are rigid, so they do not collapse. Rigid catheters are capable of suctioning large volumes of fluid rapidly. Tips with a curved contour allow for easy, rapid placement in the pharynx **Figure 11-19 ▶**.

Soft plastic, nonrigid catheters can be placed in the oropharynx or nasopharynx or down an endotracheal (ET) tube. They come in various sizes and have a smaller diameter than hard-tip catheters. Soft catheters are used to suction the nose and liquid secretions in the back of the mouth and in situations in which you cannot use a rigid catheter, such as for a patient with a stoma **Figure 11-20 ▶**. For example, a rigid catheter could break a tooth in a patient with clenched teeth, whereas a flexible catheter may be worked along the cheeks without causing injury. The use of suction tubing without the attached catheter

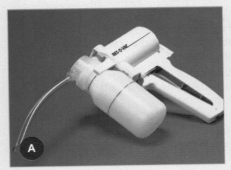

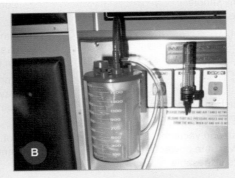

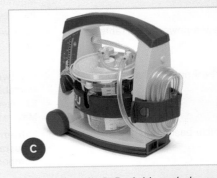

Figure 11-18 Suctioning equipment is essential for resuscitation. **A.** Hand-operated device. **B.** Fixed ambulance unit. **C.** Portable ambulance suction unit.

Skill Drill 11-11: Removal of an Upper Airway Obstruction With Magill Forceps

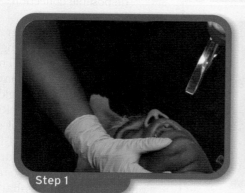

Step 1

With the patient's head in the sniffing position, open the patient's mouth and insert the laryngoscope blade.

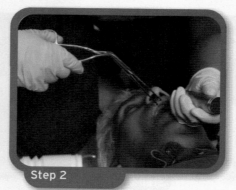

Step 2

Visualise the obstruction, and grasp the object with the Magill forceps.

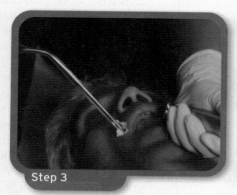

Step 3

Remove the object with the Magill forceps.

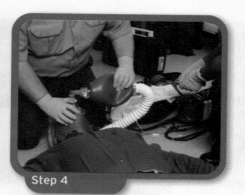

Step 4

Attempt to ventilate the patient.

facilitates suctioning of large debris in the oropharynx and allows access to the back of the pharynx in a patient with clenched teeth.

Suctioning Techniques

Mortality increases significantly if a patient aspirates; therefore, suctioning the upper airway is critical to avoid this potentially fatal event. Suctioning removes not only liquids from the airway, but also oxygen. For that reason, any patient who is to be suctioned should ideally be adequately preoxygenated first; this will provide a small oxygen reserve that can be drawn upon while you are suctioning. Even so, each suctioning attempt must be limited to a maximum of 15 seconds in the adult (less in infants and children). Try actually counting from 1 to 15. Be careful not to stimulate the back of the throat of a young child or infant as the vagal stimulus can cause the heart rate to drop. After the patient has been suctioned, continue ventilation and oxygenation.

Soft-tip catheters must be lubricated when suctioning the nasopharynx and used through an ET tube. The catheter is inserted, and suction is applied during extraction of the catheter

Table 11-6	Suction Devices		
Suction Device	**Advantages**		**Disadvantages**
Hand powered	• Lightweight • Portable • Mechanically simple • Inexpensive		• Limited or reduced total volume • Manually powered • Components not always disposable
Oxygen-powered portable	• Lightweight • Small		• Limited suction power • Uses a lot of oxygen at the scene for limited suctioning power
Battery-operated portable	• Lightweight • Portable • Excellent suction power • May resolve most problems with the device		• More complicated mechanics • May lose battery integrity over time • Some fluid contact
Vehicle-based unit	• Extremely strong vacuum • Adjustable vacuum power • Components disposable		• Not portable • Cannot use in the prehospital environment

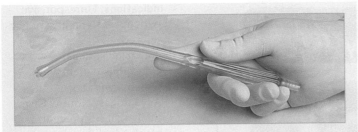

Figure 11-19 Yankeur catheters are a good choice for suctioning the oropharynx because they have wide-diameter tips and are rigid.

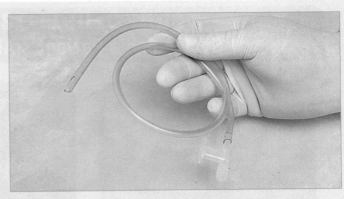

Figure 11-20 Soft-tip catheters are used in situations in which rigid catheters cannot be used, such as when a patient has a stoma or if the patient's teeth are clenched.

Notes from Nancy

Carry your paramedic kit which includes intubation kit whenever you respond to a call in a restaurant.

to clear the airway. After the patient has been suctioned, reevaluate the patency of his or her airway, and continue to ventilate and oxygenate as needed.

Before inserting any suction catheter into a patient, make sure you measure for the proper size, going from the corner of the mouth to the earlobe.

The steps for suctioning a patient in a non-emergency are listed here and shown in **Skill Drill 11-12 ▶**.

1. Turn on the assembled suction unit **Step 1**.
2. Measure the catheter from the corner of the mouth to the earlobe.
3. Before applying suction, open the patient's mouth by using the crossfinger technique or tongue-jaw lift, and insert the tip of the catheter to the predetermined depth. Do not suction while inserting the catheter.
4. Apply suction in a circular motion as you withdraw the catheter. Do not suction an adult for more than 10 seconds **Step 2**.

At the Scene

Suctioning Time Limits

Adult	15 seconds
Child	10 seconds
Infant	5 seconds

Airway Adjuncts

The first step in the initial management of an unconscious patient is to open the airway, initially by manual methods (eg, head tilt–chin lift, jaw-thrust). If the patient has an altered LOC, an artificial airway may then be needed to help maintain an open air passage. Even after an airway adjunct has been inserted, the appropriate manual position of the head must be maintained.

You are the Paramedic Part 6

The patient's airway has been cleared appropriately and bag-valve-mask ventilation with oxygen is continued. The second ambulance crew arrives and two colleagues assist you in loading the patient into your ambulance, where you attach a cardiac monitor, cannulate, and perform a reassessment. The closest appropriate hospital is approximately 40 miles away.

Reassessment	Recording Time: 11 Minutes
Level of consciousness	V (Responsive to verbal stimuli)
Respirations	28 breaths/min, shallow (baseline); you are assisting ventilation with a bag-valve-mask device and oxygen connected to a reservoir bag
Pulse	120 beats/min, regular and weak
Skin	Remains pale and perspiring; facial cyanosis is improving
Blood pressure	114/72 mm Hg
S_PO_2	95% while receiving assisted ventilations with a bag-valve-mask device and supplemental oxygen

10. What is your most appropriate action at this point?

Skill Drill 11-12: Suctioning a Patient's Airway

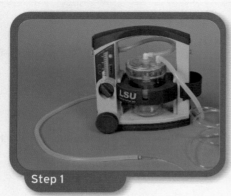

Step 1
Make sure the suctioning unit is properly assembled, and turn on the suction unit.

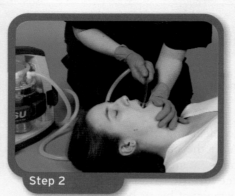

Step 2
Measure the catheter from the corner of the mouth to the earlobe. Open the patient's mouth, and insert the catheter to the predetermined depth without suctioning. Apply suction in a circular motion as you withdraw the catheter. Do not suction an adult for more than 15 seconds.

- **Indications.** Unresponsive patients with an absent gag reflex.
- **Contraindications.** Conscious patients and patients with a gag reflex.
- **Advantages.** Noninvasive, easily placed, prevents blockage of the glottis by the tongue.
- **Disadvantages.** Does not prevent aspiration.
- **Complications.** Unexpected gag may cause vomiting, pharyngeal or dental trauma with poor technique.

If the oropharyngeal airway is improperly sized or is inserted incorrectly, it could actually push the tongue back into the pharynx, creating an airway obstruction. Rough insertion of the airway can injure the hard palate, resulting in oropharyngeal bleeding and creating a risk of vomiting or aspiration. Prior to inserting an oropharyngeal airway, suction the oropharynx as needed to ensure that the mouth is clear of blood or other fluids. The steps for inserting an oropharyngeal airway are listed here and shown in **Skill Drill 11-13 ▲**.

1. To select the proper size, measure the vertical distance from the angle of the jaw to the centre of the patient's incisors **Step 1**.
2. Open the patient's mouth with the crossfinger technique or tongue-jaw lift. Hold the airway upside down with your other hand. Insert the airway with the tip facing the roof of the mouth **Step 2**.

At the Scene

Wear a face mask and protective glasses whenever you are managing a patient's airway. Body fluids can become aerosolised, and the mucous membranes of the paramedic's mouth, nose, and eyes can easily come in contact with these contaminants.

Oropharyngeal Airway

The oropharyngeal airway is a curved, hard plastic device that fits over the back of the tongue with the tip in the posterior pharynx **Figure 11-21 ▶**. It is designed to hold the tongue away from the posterior pharyngeal wall, and its use makes it much easier to ventilate patients with a bag-valve-mask device. The oropharyngeal airway can also serve as an effective bite-block, preventing an intubated patient from chomping down on the ET tube.

An oropharyngeal airway should be inserted promptly in unresponsive patients—breathing or not—who have no gag reflex. Because its distal end sits in the back of the throat, this device will stimulate gagging and retching in a conscious or semiconscious patient. For that reason, the oropharyngeal airway should be used only in unconscious, unresponsive patients without a gag reflex. *If the patient gags during insertion of the oropharyngeal airway, remove the device immediately and be prepared to suction the oropharynx.* Following are some considerations when using an oropharyngeal airway:

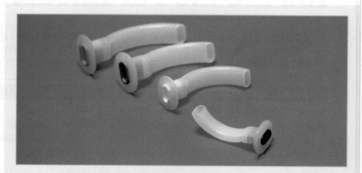

Figure 11-21 An oropharyngeal airway is used for unconscious patients who have no gag reflex. It helps to keep the tongue from blocking the airway.

Skill Drill 11-13: Inserting an Oropharyngeal Airway

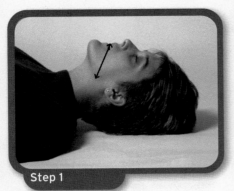

Step 1

Determine the size of the airway by measuring the vertical distance from the angle of the jaw to the patient's incisors.

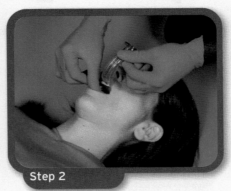

Step 2

Open the patient's mouth with the crossfinger technique or tongue-jaw lift. Hold the airway upside down with your other hand. Insert the airway with the tip facing the roof of the mouth and slide it in until it touches the roof of the mouth.

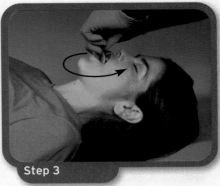

Step 3

Rotate the airway 180°, flipping it over the tongue. Insert the airway until the flange rests on the patient's lips. In this position, the airway will hold the tongue away from the posterior pharynx.

3. Rotate the airway 180°, flipping it over the tongue. When inserted properly, the airway will rest in the mouth, with the curvature of the airway following the contour of the teeth. The flange should rest against the lips, with the distal end in the posterior pharynx Step 3.

At the Scene

An easy way to insert an oropharyngeal airway is to use the "hard palate, soft palate, rotate" technique. As the airway is gliding across the hard palate, you should feel a slight bump as the airway reaches the soft palate. Because the soft palate is just above the curvature of the tongue, you should rotate the airway 180° as soon as you feel the bump; this will allow the airway to catch the base of the tongue and propel it forward.

If you encounter difficulty while inserting the oropharyngeal airway, try this alternative technique Skill Drill 11-14.

1. Use a wooden or plastic tongue blade to depress the tongue, ensuring that the tongue remains forward Step 1.
2. Insert the oropharyngeal airway sideways from the corner of the mouth, until the flange reaches the lips Step 2.
3. Rotate the oropharyngeal airway 90°, removing the tongue blade as you exert gentle backward pressure on the oropharyngeal airway, until the flange rests securely in place against the lips Step 3.

Special Considerations

In children, using a tongue blade to hold the tongue down while inserting an oropharyngeal airway is the preferred method. Because the airways of children are less developed than those of adults, rotating the oropharyngeal airway in the posterior pharynx may cause damage.

Nasopharyngeal Airway

The nasopharyngeal airway is a soft, plastic tube that is inserted through the nose into the posterior pharynx behind the tongue, thereby allowing passage of air from the nose to the lower airway. The nasopharyngeal airway is much better tolerated than an oropharyngeal airway in patients who have an intact gag reflex yet an altered LOC Figure 11-22. Do not use this device when is the patient has experienced trauma to the nose or you have reason to suspect a possible skull fracture (eg, CSF leakage from the nose). Inserting the airway in such cases may cause it to enter the brain through the hole caused by the fracture.

The nasopharyngeal airway must be inserted gently to avoid precipitating epistaxis (nosebleed). Lubricate the nasopharyngeal airway generously with a water-soluble jelly, and slide it gently, tip downward, into one nostril. *Do not try to force it.* If you meet resistance, try to pass the airway down the

Skill Drill 11-14: Inserting an Oropharyngeal Airway With a 90° Rotation

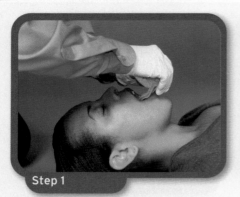

Step 1

Depress the tongue with a tongue blade so the tongue remains forward.

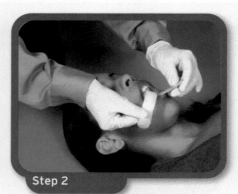

Step 2

Insert the oropharyngeal airway sideways from the corner of the mouth, until the flange reaches the lips.

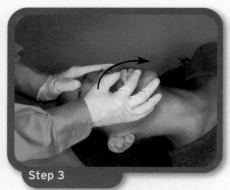

Step 3

Rotate the oropharyngeal airway 90°, and remove the tongue blade as you exert gentle backward pressure on the oropharyngeal airway until the flange rests securely in place against the lips.

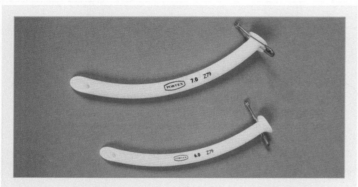

Figure 11-22 An nasopharyngeal airway is better tolerated by patients who have an intact gag reflex.

other nostril. Following are considerations when using a nasopharyngeal airway:

- **Indications.** Unresponsive patients, patients with an altered mental status who have an intact gag reflex.
- **Contraindications.** Patient intolerance, presence of facial fracture, skull fracture, Battle's sign, or nasal polyps.
- **Advantages.** Can be suctioned through, provides a patent airway, can be tolerated by awake patients, can be safely placed "blindly", does not require the mouth to be open.
- **Disadvantages.** Poor technique may result in severe bleeding (resulting epistaxis may be extremely difficult to control), does not protect from aspiration.

The steps for inserting a nasopharyngeal airway are listed here and shown in **Skill Drill 11-15** .

1. Before inserting the airway, make sure you have selected the proper size. Measure the distance from the tip of the nostril to the tragus of the ear. In almost all individuals, one nostril is larger than the other. The diameter should be roughly equal to the patient's little finger.

At the Scene

Oxygen is one of the most powerful drugs for saving lives that you will carry in your ambulance. Don't be afraid to use it and don't let it run out!

2. After lubricating the nasopharyngeal airway with a water-soluble gel, place the airway in the larger nostril (usually the right nostril), with the curvature of the device following the curve of the floor of the nose and the bevel facing the septum (**Step 1**).

3. Place the bevel toward the septum and insert it gently along the nasopharyngeal floor, parallel to the mouth. *Do not force the airway* (**Step 2**).

4. When completely inserted, the flange should rest against the nostril. The distal end of the airway will open into the posterior pharynx (**Step 3**).

If the nasopharyngeal airway is too long, it may obstruct the patient's airway. If the patient becomes intolerant of the nasopharyngeal airway, gently remove it from the nasopharyngeal passage. Although the nasopharyngeal airway is not as likely to cause vomiting as the oropharyngeal airway, you should still have suction readily available.

■ Supplemental Oxygen Therapy

Supplemental oxygen should be administered to any patient with potential hypoxia, regardless of his or her clinical appearance. In some conditions, a part of the patient's body does not receive enough oxygen, *even though the oxygen supply to the body as a whole is entirely adequate.* For example, when a patient experiences an acute myocardial infarction (heart attack), a portion of the myocardium is hypoxic, *even though the rest of the*

Skill Drill 11-15:
Inserting a Nasopharyngeal Airway

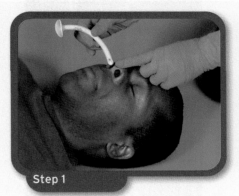

Step 1

Determine the size of the airway by measuring the distance from the tip of the nose to the tragus of the ear. Coat the tip with a water-soluble lubricant.

Insert the lubricated airway into the larger nostril, with the curvature following the floor of the nose and the bevel facing the septum.

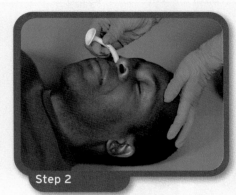

Step 2

Gently advance the airway. If using the left nostril, insert the nasopharyngeal airway until it meets with resistance, then rotate the airway 180° into position. *This rotation is not required if you are using the right nostril.*

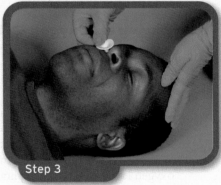

Step 3

Continue until the flange rests against the nostril. If you feel any resistance or obstruction, remove the airway and insert it into the other nostril.

Oxygen delivery is measured in terms of litres per minute (l/min). As a precaution against running out at an inconvenient moment, you should replace an oxygen cylinder with a full one when the pressure falls to 200 psi or below. That level is called the safe residual pressure, indicating that it is *unsafe* to continue using the oxygen cylinder (traditionally, ambulance crews replace tanks at 1/4 full). On the basis of the pressure in the oxygen cylinder and the flow rate of oxygen delivery, you can calculate how long the supply of oxygen in the cylinder will last—that is, the tank life **Table 11-7 ▶** .

Oxygen Regulators and Flowmeters

The pressure of gas in a full oxygen cylinder is approximately 2,000 psi. Clearly, this is far too much pressure to deliver directly into a patient's airway. Instead, gas flow from an oxygen cylinder to the patient is controlled by a therapy regulator, which attaches to the stem of the oxygen cylinder and reduces the high pressure of gas to a safe range (about 50 psi). CD cylinders come ready prepared with an inbuilt regulator.

Flowmeters, which are usually permanently attached to the therapy regulator, allow the oxygen delivered to the patient

body is well oxygenated. Increasing the available oxygen supply also enhances the body's compensatory mechanisms during shock and other distressed states.

The oxygen-delivery method must be appropriate for the patient's ventilatory status and should be reassessed frequently and adjusted accordingly based on the patient's clinical condition and breathing adequacy. When a patient needs oxygen, the paramedic's first priority is to provide that oxygen quickly.

Oxygen Sources

Pure (100%) oxygen is stored in steel (old style), aluminum, or carbon wrap cylinders, whose colour is conventionally black with white shoulders **Figure 11-23 ▶** .

Oxygen cylinders are available in various sizes. You will most often use the CD-(portable) or the F-sized (vehicle-based) cylinder. These contain 425 litres and 1,360 litres respectively.

At the Scene

It should be routine procedure at the beginning of every shift to open the main cylinder valve on the ambulance's oxygen supply and check the pressure remaining in the cylinder or cylinders. Check the pressure gauges on all portable cylinders after every call in which oxygen is used. It is very unprofessional—not to mention negligent—to arrive at the scene of a gasping patient, only to discover that your oxygen cylinder is empty. Replace oxygen cylinders when their pressure reaches or falls below 200 psi. Always carry at least one backup cylinder in the ambulance—you may not have a chance to return to your station for a full cylinder after that cardiac arrest call. Scenes involving entrapment may require additional oxygen to be brought to the scene by a supplementary crew.

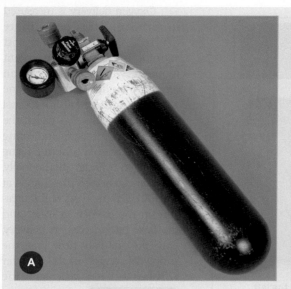
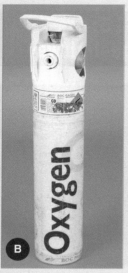

Figure 11-23 Oxygen cylinders. **A.** Old style. **B.** New style.

Table 11-7	Oxygen Cylinders: Duration of Flow
Formula	

Formula

$$\frac{\text{Tank pressure in psi} - 200\ \text{psi}}{\text{(the safe residual pressure)} \times \text{cylinder constant}}{\text{Flow rate in l/min}} = \text{Duration of flow in minutes}$$

Cylinder Constant

D = 0.16	G = 2.41
E = 0.28	H = 3.14
M = 1.56	K = 3.14

Calculation

Determine the life of a D cylinder that has a pressure of 2,000 psi and a flow rate of 15 l/min.

$$\frac{(2{,}000\ [\text{psi}] - 200\ [\text{safe residual pressure}] \times 0.16\ [\text{cylinder constant}])}{15} = \frac{288}{15\ (\text{l/min})} = 19.2\ (19)\ \text{min}$$

Note: psi indicates pounds per square inch.

to be adjusted within a range of 1 to 25 l/min. The two types of flowmeters most commonly used are the pressure-compensated flowmeter and the Bourdon-gauge flowmeter.

A <u>pressure-compensated flowmeter</u> incorporates a float ball within a tapered calibrated tube; this float rises or falls based on the gas flow in the tube. The gas flow is controlled by a needle valve located downstream from the float ball. Because this type of flowmeter is affected by gravity, it must remain in an upright position to obtain an accurate flow reading **Figure 11-24 ▸**.

By contrast, the <u>Bourdon-gauge flowmeter</u> is not affected by gravity and can be placed in any position. This pressure gauge is calibrated to record the flow rate **Figure 11-25 ▸**. The major disadvantage of this type of flowmeter is that it does not compensate for backpressure. As a result, it will usually record a higher flow rate when there is any obstruction to gas flow downstream.

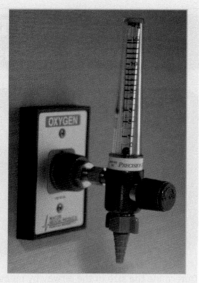

Figure 11-24 Pressure-compensated flowmeters contain a float ball that rises or falls based on the gas flow in the tube. It must remain in an upright position for an accurate flow reading.

Preparing an Oxygen Cylinder for Use

Prior to administering supplemental oxygen to your patient, you must prepare the oxygen cylinder and therapy regulator. To place an oxygen cylinder into service, follow these steps **Skill Drill 11-16 ▸**.

1. Inspect the cylinder and its markings. Remove the plastic seal covering the valve stem opening. Inspect the opening to ensure that it is free of dirt or other debris (**Step 1**). With the tank facing away from yourself and others, use an oxygen key to "crack" the cylinder—opening and closing the valve to ensure that dirt particles and other contaminants do not enter the oxygen flow.

2. Attach the regulator/flowmeter to the valve stem, ensuring that the pin-index system is correctly aligned. A Bodock seal is placed around the oxygen port to optimise the airtight seal between the collar of the regulator and the valve stem (**Step 2**).

3. Place the regulator collar over the cylinder valve, with the oxygen port and pin-indexing pins on the side of the valve stem that has two holes. Align the

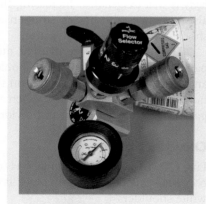

Figure 11-25 The flowmeter is not affected by gravity and can be placed in any position.

Skill Drill 11-16: Placing an Oxygen Cylinder Into Service

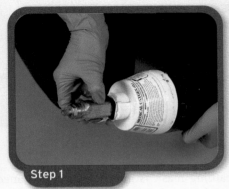

Step 1

Remove plastic shrinkwrap and red seal on a full cylinder.

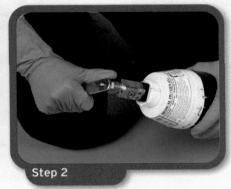

Step 2

Using an oxygen key, turn the valve anti-clockwise to "crack" the cylinder. Attach the regulator/flowmeter to the valve stem and make sure that the Bodock seal is in place.

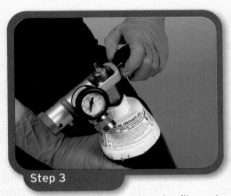

Step 3

Align the regulator so that the pins fit snugly into the correct two-pin indexing holes on the yoke and hand-tighten the regulator.

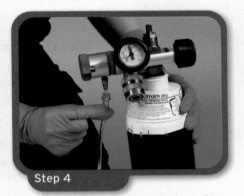

Step 4

Attach the oxygen connective tubing to the flowmeter.

Safety Considerations

Any cylinder containing compressed gas under high pressure has the potential, under the right conditions (actually, the *wrong* conditions!), to assume the properties of a rocket. Furthermore, oxygen presents the additional hazard of fire, because it supports the combustion process. For these reasons, safety precautions are necessary when you are handling oxygen cylinders:

- Keep combustible materials, such as oil or grease, away from contact with the cylinder itself, the regulators, fittings, valves, or tubing.
- Do not permit smoking in any area where oxygen cylinders are in use or on standby.
- Store oxygen cylinders in a cool, well-ventilated area. Do not subject the cylinders to temperatures above 50°C.
- Use an oxygen cylinder only with a safe, properly fitting regulator valve. Regulator valves for one gas should never be modified for use with another gas.
- Close all valves when the cylinder is not in use, even if the tank is empty.
- Secure cylinders so that they will not topple over. In transit, keep them in a proper carrier or rack, or strap them onto the stretcher with the patient.
- When working with an oxygen cylinder, always position yourself to its side. Never place any part of your body over the cylinder valve! A loosely fitting regulator can be blown off the cylinder with sufficient force to demolish any object in its path.

regulator so that the oxygen port and the pins fit into the correct holes on the valve stem; align the screw bolt on the opposite side with the dimpled depression. Tighten the screw bolt until the regulator is firmly attached to the cylinder. At this point, you should not see any space between the sides of the valve stem and the interior walls of the collar (Step 3).

4. With the regulator firmly attached, open the cylinder and read the pressure level on the regulator gauge. Follow your local protocols regarding minimum cylinder pressures, or minimum gauge readings.

5. A second gauge or a selector dial on the flowmeter indicates the oxygen flow rate. Attach the oxygen connective tubing to the "Christmas tree" spigot on the flowmeter and select the oxygen flow rate that is appropriate for your patient's clinical condition (Step 4).

Supplemental Oxygen-Delivery Devices

The most common oxygen-delivery devices that you will use in the prehospital setting are the nonrebreathing mask, aerosolised oxygen driven nebuliser masks, nasal cannula, and bag-valve-mask device. However, your ambulance service may encounter other oxygen-delivery devices, such as the medium

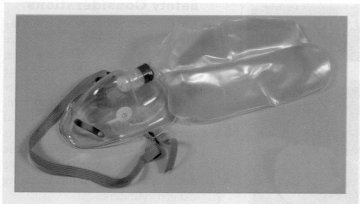

Figure 11-26 Nonrebreathing mask.

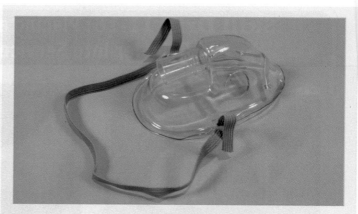

Figure 11-28 A medium concentration face mask.

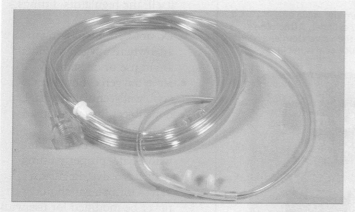

Figure 11-27 Nasal cannula.

concentration face mask, partial rebreathing mask, nasal cannulas, Kneck breather, and Venturi mask.

Nonrebreathing Mask

The nonrebreathing mask is the preferred device for delivering supplemental oxygen to spontaneously breathing patients in the prehospital setting. With a good mask-to-face seal and a flow rate of 15 l/min, it is capable of delivering around 90% inspired oxygen.

The nonrebreathing mask is a combination mask and reservoir bag system. Oxygen fills a reservoir bag that is attached to the mask by a one-way valve. This permits the patient to inhale from the reservoir bag but not to exhale back into it. The only gas that can enter the reservoir, therefore, is pure oxygen piped in from the oxygen cylinder. Exhaled gas escapes through one-way flapper valves located on the side of the mask Figure 11-26 ▲ .

Prior to administering oxygen to a patient with a nonrebreathing mask, you must ensure that the reservoir bag is completely filled. The oxygen flow rate is adjusted from 12 to 15 l/min to prevent collapse of the bag during inhalation. Use a paediatric nonrebreathing mask, which has a smaller reservoir bag, for infants and small children; they inhale smaller volumes of air.

The nonrebreathing mask is indicated for spontaneously breathing patients who require high-flow oxygen concentrations (eg, shock, hypoxia from any cause) and have adequate tidal volume (ie, good chest rise). A patient with reduced tidal volume (shallow breathing) will benefit very little, if any, from the nonrebreathing mask.

Nasal Cannula

The nasal cannula delivers oxygen via two small prongs that fit into the patient's nostrils Figure 11-27 ◄ . With an oxygen flow rate of 1 to 6 l/min, the nasal cannula can deliver an oxygen concentration of 24% to 44% depending on the manufacturer. Higher flow rates will merely irritate the nasal mucosa without increasing the delivered oxygen concentration.

The nasal cannula provides low to moderate oxygen enrichment and is most beneficial to patients who require long-term oxygen therapy (eg, for COPD). In the prehospital setting, the nasal cannula is primarily used when patients who need oxygen cannot tolerate a nonrebreathing mask.

Medium Concentration Face Mask

A medium concentration face mask is a full mask enclosure with open side ports. Room air is drawn in through the side ports on inhalation, diluting the concentration of inspired oxygen Figure 11-28 ▲ . Exhaled air is vented through holes on each side of the mask. The simple face mask will deliver around 40% oxygen at 10 l/min. If there is a leak around the face, however, the

At the Scene

Oxygen-Delivery Devices

Device	Flow Rate	Oxygen Delivered
Nasal cannula	1–6 l/min	24%–44%
Nonrebreathing mask	15 l/min	> 90%
Bag-valve-mask device with reservoir	15 l/min – flush	> 85%

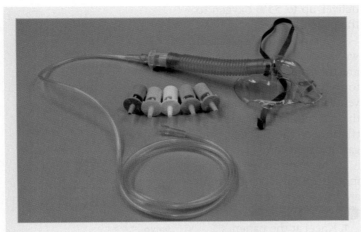

Figure 11-29 Venturi mask with various spigots.

amount of inspired oxygen decreases. The simple face mask can deliver oxygen concentrations slightly higher than those delivered by the nasal cannula. These devices are used less frequently but are still common in some services.

Venturi Mask

The Venturi mask draws room air into the mask along with the oxygen flow, allowing for the administration of highly specific oxygen concentrations Figure 11-29 ▲ . Depending on the adapter used, the Venturi mask can deliver a variety of percentages of oxygen to the patient, typically, 24%, 28%, 35%, 40%, 50%, or 60% oxygen. Venturi masks are especially useful in the hospital management of patients with COPD and other chronic respiratory diseases. They offer less advantage in prehospital care, except in the long-range transport of such patients. They are more expensive but are still popular in some areas.

Nebuliser

A nebuliser is used primarily to deliver aerosolised salbutamol. Oxygen enters an aerosol chamber that contains the fluid poured in from the opened nebule, appropriate for the age and size of the patient. The pressurised oxygen in this chamber aerosolises the fluid, and the mist assists the inhalation of the drug deep into the lungs. Some nebulisers are operated on air and not pure oxygen.

▌ Assisted and Artificial Ventilation

A patient who is not breathing needs artificial ventilation with a bag-valve-mask that is attached to free flow supplemental oxygen. The same is true of patients who are breathing inadequately, such as those with fast or slow respirations, reduced tidal volume, or an irregular pattern of respirations. These patients need ventilation assistance to improve oxygenation and facilitate CO_2 elimination from the body.

Inadequate negative-pressure ventilation is treated with some form of positive-pressure ventilation, which involves forcing air into the patient's lungs. The techniques used differ only in the

At the Scene

Airway management and ventilation procedures often expose you to blood, vomitus, and oropharyngeal secretions. While blood is the most potentially infectious body fluid, you should exercise great caution to avoid contact with all body fluids. Wear gloves for all airway and ventilation procedures and when handling airway equipment that has been contaminated with body fluids. To mitigate the risk of splashing or droplets of body fluid coming in contact with your mouth, nose, and eyes, wear a mask and protective eyewear or a face shield, especially when placing an advanced airway. In cases of significant blood splashing, such as in trauma, you should also wear a protective apron, if possible.

At the Scene

A nebuliser with saline or sterile water placed in the medication chamber may be used in place of humidified oxygen. Simply attach an oxygen mask to the aerosol chamber and set the flowmeter at 7 l/min.

power source used to generate the pressures and the airflows required for inflating a patient's lungs Table 11-8 ▼ .

Mouth-to-Mouth and Mouth-to-Nose Ventilation

Consider the following scenario: You are relaxing by the side of a local swimming pool when you see a teenager being pulled out of the water, apparently unconscious. You run over to him and tilt his head back to open his airway; then you look, listen, and feel for breathing and determine that he is apnoeic. What should you do next? Because you don't ordinarily bring resuscitation equipment to the pool, you will have to initiate positive-pressure ventilations with the only equipment immediately available to you—your own mouth and lungs.

Mouth-to-mouth is the most basic form of ventilation. Mouth-to-nose simply involves ventilating through the nose, rather than through the mouth.

The disadvantages of mouth-to-mouth or nose ventilation include psychological barriers secondary to sanitary and communicable disease issues. There is a potential for exposure to blood and other body fluids through direct contact with the patient's mouth or nose. Although mouth-to-mouth or mouth-to-nose ventilation requires no special equipment, allows you

Table 11-8	Methods of Positive-Pressure Ventilation

- Mouth-to-mask
- Two-person bag-valve-mask device
- Flow-restricted, oxygen-powered ventilation device
- One-person bag-valve-mask device

Note: The methods are listed in order of preference, because research has demonstrated that personnel who ventilate patients infrequently have great difficulty maintaining an adequate seal between the mask and the patient's face.

to deliver excellent tidal volume, and provides 16% oxygen to the patient (adequate to sustain life), other methods of providing positive-pressure ventilation are safer for the rescuer.

There are also some potential complications associated with mouth-to-mouth or mouth-to-nose ventilation. Hyperventilation of the patient's lungs may occur, especially if the patient is small and the rescuer is overzealous. Hyperventilation of the rescuer is another potential complication. Rapid, deep breathing, especially for prolonged periods of time, decreases carbon dioxide levels in the blood and, in severe cases, could cause the rescuer to lose consciousness. Gastric distension may also occur, increasing the risk of vomiting and aspiration; this clearly would be detrimental to the patient but would also expose the rescuer to the patient's vomitus.

To avoid putting yourself in a position where mouth-to-mouth or mouth-to-nose ventilation is the only option, ensure that you have access to a pocket mask or carry a face shield on your key ring—or anything with a barrier device—regardless of where you are.

Mouth-to-Mask Ventilation

Mouth-to-mask ventilation employs the same readily available power source as mouth-to-mouth or mouth-to-nose (the rescuer's lungs), but eliminates direct contact with the patient's mouth or nose. Use of a one-way valve over the mask's mouthpiece virtually eliminates any possibility of contact with the patient's secretions and diverts the patient's exhaled air away from the rescuer's mouth **Figure 11-30 ▶** .

Because you are able to use both hands to hold the mask to the patient's face, it is easier to maintain an effective seal and deliver excellent tidal volume. If the pocket face mask is not equipped with an oxygen inlet valve, then you will deliver 16% oxygen to the patient. When its inlet valve is connected to an oxygen source at a flow rate of 15 l/min, the pocket mask can

deliver up to 55% oxygen to the patient.

Complications associated with using a pocket face mask are the same as for mouth-to-mouth or mouth-to-nose ventilation—hyperinflation of the patient's lungs, hyperventilation of the rescuer, and gastric distension.

The steps for performing mouth-to-mask ventilations are listed here and shown in **Skill Drill 11-17 ▾** .

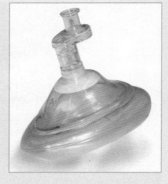

Figure 11-30 Pocket mask with a disposable one-way valve.

1. Kneel at the patient's head. Open the airway with the appropriate manual manoeuvre. Connect the one-way valve to the face mask. Place the mask over the patient's face, ensuring that the top is over the bridge of the nose and the bottom is in the groove between the lower lip and chin. Grasp the patient's lower jaw with the first three fingers on each hand. Place your thumbs on the dome of the mask. Make an airtight seal by applying firm pressure between the thumbs and the fingers. Maintain an upward and forward pull on the lower jaw with your fingers to keep the airway open **Step 1** .
2. Take a breath and exhale through the open port of the one-way valve. Breathe into the mask for 1 second, observing visible chest rise **Step 2** .
3. Remove your mouth, and watch for the patient's chest to fall during passive exhalation **Step 3** .

Ventilation effectiveness is best determined by watching the patient's chest rise and fall and feeling for resistance of the patient's

---

Skill Drill 11-17: Mouth-to-Mask Ventilation

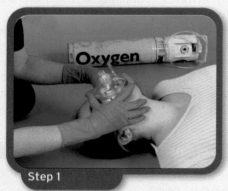

Step 1
Once the patient's head is properly positioned, place the mask on the patient's face. Seal the mask to the face using both hands.

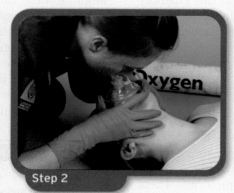

Step 2
Exhale into the open port of the one-way valve for 1 second as you watch for visible chest rise.

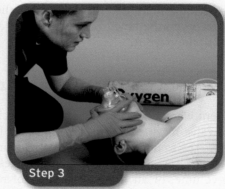

Step 3
Watch for the patient's chest to fall during exhalation.

Table 11-9	Ventilation Rates

Adult*

- Apnoeic with a pulse: 10 to 12 breaths/min
  - With *or* without an advanced airway in place (eg, ET tube, LMA)
- Apnoeic and pulseless: 8 to 10 breaths/min
  - After an advanced airway has been inserted

Infant and Child*

- Apnoeic with a pulse: 12 to 20 breaths/min
  - With *or* without an advanced airway in place (eg, ET tube, LMA)
- Apnoeic and pulseless: 8 to 10 breaths/min
  - After an advanced airway has been inserted

*Avoid hyperventilating *any* patient; hyperventilated lungs may "squeeze" the heart, thus impeding venous return and subsequent cardiac output. Hyperventilation also increases the risk of regurgitation and aspiration.

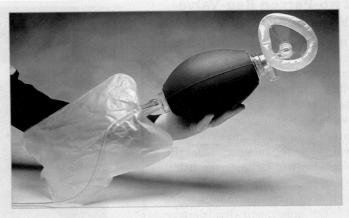

Figure 11-31 A disposable bag-valve-mask device.

lungs as they expand. You should also hear and feel air escape as the patient exhales. Make sure that you provide the correct number of breaths per minute for the patient's age Table 11-9 ▲ .

One-Person Bag-Valve-Mask Ventilation

The bag-valve-mask device is the most common device used to ventilate patients in the field Figure 11-31 ▶ . With an oxygen flow rate of at least 15 l/min and a reservoir attached, the bag-valve-mask device can deliver around 85% oxygen to the patient. Bag-valve-mask ventilations are indicated for apnoeic patients and for patients who are breathing inadequately, as long as they can tolerate the device. This technique provides an excellent barrier from blood and other body fluids and allows the paramedic to ventilate the patient for extended periods of time without fatigue.

A major challenge (and disadvantage) is maintaining an effective mask-to-face seal. The single person operating a bag-valve-mask device must be able to perform three tasks with only two hands: keeping the airway properly positioned, maintaining a mask seal, and squeezing the bag. Complications associated with the one-person bag-valve-mask ventilation technique are typically related to inadequate tidal volume delivery, which usually occurs secondary to poor technique, inadequate mask-to-face seal, or gastric distension.

The steps for performing the one-person bag-valve-mask ventilation technique are listed here and shown in Skill Drill 11-18 ▼ .

1. Choose the proper mask size to seat the mask from the bridge of the nose to the chin Step 1 .
2. Position the mask on the patient's face and ensure an adequate seal Step 2 .
3. Open the patient's airway and hold the mask in place with one hand. Squeeze the bag completely over 1 second with the other hand and watch for visible chest rise. Allow the bag to reinflate slowly and completely Step 3 .

Skill Drill 11-18: One-Person Bag-Valve-Mask Ventilation

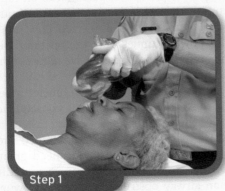

Step 1

Choose the proper mask size to seat the mask from the bridge of the nose to the chin.

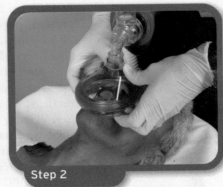

Step 2

Position the mask on the patient's face and ensure an adequate seal.

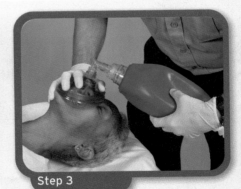

Step 3

Open the patient's airway and hold the mask in place with one hand as you squeeze the bag with the other hand. Allow the bag to reinflate slowly and completely.

Two-Person Bag-Valve-Mask Ventilation

In contrast to the one-person technique, two-person bag-valve-mask ventilation is a much more efficient means of providing artificial or assisted ventilations. With two rescuers, one can maintain an adequate mask-to-face seal, while the other squeezes the bag. This will facilitate the delivery of excellent tidal volume and high oxygen concentrations.

The only major disadvantage of the two-person bag-valve-mask technique is that it requires additional personnel, who are not always present on every call. Complications include hyperinflation of the patient's lungs and gastric distension. For these reasons, the patient must be constantly monitored for adequate chest rise and ventilation compliance.

The steps for performing the two-person bag-valve-mask ventilation technique are listed here and are shown in (**Skill Drill 11-19** ▲).

1. The first paramedic or technician maintains a mask seal by the most appropriate method (**Step 1**).
2. The second paramedic squeezes the bag completely with both hands over 1 second, observing for visible chest rise (**Step 2**).

Flow-Restricted, Oxygen-Powered Ventilation Device

A third potential source for artificial ventilation is the <u>flow-restricted, oxygen-powered ventilation device (FROPVD)</u>, also referred to as a manually triggered ventilator or demand valve (**Figure 11-32** ▼). The FROPVD can be used to ventilate apnoeic

Skill Drill 11-19: Two-Person Bag-Valve-Mask Ventilation

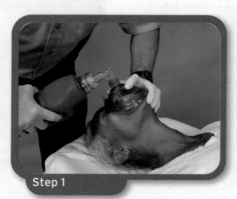

Step 1
The first paramedic maintains the mask seal by the most appropriate method.

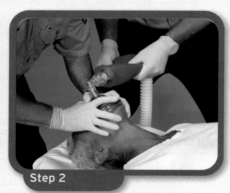

Step 2
The second paramedic squeezes the bag completely over 1 second to provide visible chest rise.

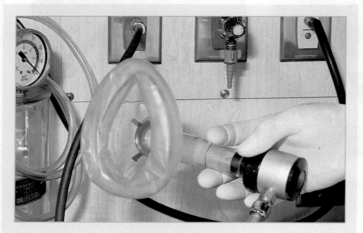

Figure 11-32 Flow-restricted, oxygen-powered ventilation device.

patients or to administer supplemental oxygen to spontaneously breathing patients. Its plastic housing includes a 15/22-mm adapter designed to fit onto standard ventilation masks as well as advanced airways (eg, ET tube, LMA).

The FROPVD has a demand valve that is triggered by the negative pressure generated during inhalation. This valve automatically delivers pure oxygen as the spontaneously breathing patient begins to inhale and stops the flow of gas at the end of inhalation. Generally, patients find it most comfortable if they hold the mask to their face themselves. The FROPVD delivers only the volume needed by the patient during inhalation, rather than wasting oxygen by providing a constant flow. Because the FROPVD makes an airtight seal with the patient's face, the patient inhales almost 100% oxygen.

For ventilation of apnoeic patients, a pushbutton on top of the FROPVD can control the release of oxygen. When the button is depressed, pure oxygen streams out at a fixed flow rate of around 40 l/min. This flow continues until the operator takes his or her finger off the button or the pop-off valve releases when the device reaches the preset pressure limit.

The valve opening pressure at the cardiac sphincter (opening into the stomach) is also about the same. As a consequence, the FROPVD may reduce (but not eliminate) gastric distension, compared with bag-valve-mask ventilation. This limited pressure is a disadvantage for certain patients who need greater pressure to overcome increased airway resistance, including those with COPD or an airway obstruction. Therefore, whenever you are ventilating patients with a FROPVD, ensure that they are receiving enough volume by observing the chest for adequate rise.

Unlike a bag-valve-mask device or pocket mask, the FROPVD requires an oxygen source to function—a potential disadvantage. In addition, the operator cannot feel whether the patient is being adequately ventilated with this device. Changes in compliance can be an important early indication of an impending problem. You must closely monitor the patient being ventilated mechanically and remain vigilant for changes in his or her condition.

The steps for ventilating an apnoeic patient with the FROPVD are listed here and shown in **Skill Drill 11-20 ▸**.

1. Choose the proper mask size to seat the mask from the bridge of the nose to the chin **Step 1**.

2. Open the patient's airway and hold the mask in place with a "C" grip, maintaining an adequate mask-to-face seal **Step 2**.

3. Press the ventilation button until you see visible chest rise **Step 3**.

4. Allow the patient to exhale passively **Step 4**.

The steps for administering supplemental oxygen to a spontaneously breathing patient with the FROPVD are listed here and shown in **Skill Drill 11-21 ▸**.

1. Prepare your equipment by attaching the appropriate-sized mask to the FROPVD and ensuring that it is connected to an oxygen source.

2. Whenever possible, have the patient hold the mask to his or her own face to maintain a good seal **Step 1**.

Skill Drill 11-20: Flow-Restricted, Oxygen-Powered Ventilation for Apnoeic Patients

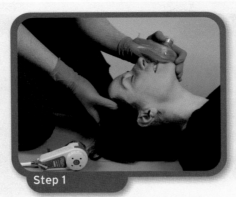

Step 1

Choose the proper mask size to seat the mask from the bridge of the nose to the chin.

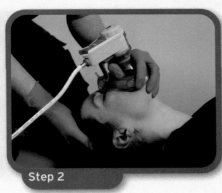

Step 2

Open the patient's airway and hold the mask with a "C" grip.

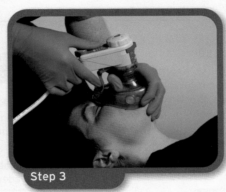

Step 3

Press the ventilation button until you achieve visible chest rise.

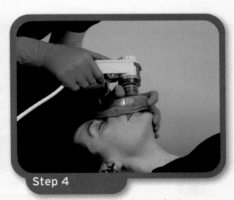

Step 4

Allow the patient to exhale passively.

3. When the patient inhales, the negative pressure created will trigger the valve within the FROPVD and deliver pure oxygen **Step 2**.

Automatic Transport Ventilators

Although the FROPVD delivers a constant flow rate that subsequently controls the upper airway pressure, the paramedic's hands are still needed to maintain a mask seal and ventilate the patient. Additionally, variations in the rate and duration of ventilation are possible with the FROPVD. The automatic transport ventilator (ATV) solves these problems.

The ATV is essentially a FROPVD attached to a control box that allows the variables of ventilation—tidal volume and respiratory rate—to be set. Therefore, one can control the patient's minute volume with considerable accuracy **Figure 11-33 ▸**. The ATV is indicated when patients need extended periods of ventilation, such as those in cardiopulmonary arrest after the patient has been intubated.

At the Scene

Indications That Artificial Ventilation Is Adequate*

- Adequate and equal chest rise and fall with ventilation
- Ventilations are delivered at the appropriate rate:
  - 10 to 12 breaths/min for adults
  - 12 to 20 breaths/min for infants and children
- Heart rate returns to a normal range

Indications That Artificial Ventilation Is Inadequate

- Minimal or no chest rise and fall
- Ventilations delivered too fast or too slow for patient's age
- Heart rate does not return to a normal range

*In patients who are apnoeic with a pulse (ie, not in cardiac arrest).

Skill Drill 11-21: Flow-Restricted, Oxygen-Powered Ventilation Device for Conscious, Spontaneously Breathing Patients

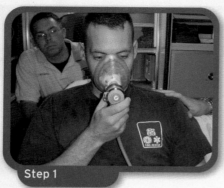

Step 1

Prepare your equipment. Whenever possible, get the patient to hold the mask to his or her own face to maintain a good seal.

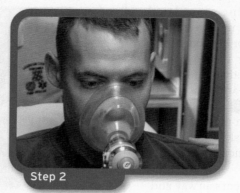

Step 2

When the patient inhales, the negative pressure created will trigger the valve within the FROPVD and deliver pure oxygen.

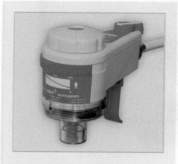

Figure 11-33 Automatic transport ventilator.

In all cases, the respiratory rate on the ATV should be set on the lowest child setting so that the device does not actually overinflate a child's lungs when used in the field. Settings vary from device to device; read the instructions.

Table 11-10 ▶ describes the steps for ventilating a patient with an ATV.

Table 11-10	Ventilating a Patient With an Automatic Transport Ventilator

1. Preferably attach the ATV to the wall-mounted oxygen source.
2. Set the tidal volume and ventilatory rate on the ATV as appropriate for the patient's age and clinical condition.
3. Connect the ATV to the 15/22-mm fitting on the ET tube.
4. Auscultate the patient's breath sounds and observe for chest rise to ensure adequate ventilation.

Special Considerations

Artificial Ventilation of the Paediatric Patient

The flat nasal bridge of the paediatric patient makes achieving an effective mask-to-face seal more difficult in children than in adults. Furthermore, compressing the mask against the face to improve mask seal may result in obstruction.

A paediatric bag-valve-mask device with a minimum tidal volume of 450 ml should be used for full-term neonates and infants. In children (1 year of age to the onset of puberty), consider the size of the child when determining bag size. An adult bag with a 1,500-ml volume may be used, but a paediatric bag-valve-mask is preferred. Children older than 12 to 14 years of age require the adult-sized bag-valve-mask for adequate ventilation. Choose a size to ensure a proper mask fit. The mask should reach from the bridge of the nose to the cleft of the chin. A length-based resuscitation tape may also be used to determine the most appropriate-sized bag-valve-mask device for paediatric patients who weigh up to 34 kg.

When you are ventilating a paediatric patient, ensure that there is a proper mask seal by using the EC-grip technique **Figure 11-34 ▶** . Place the mask over the mouth and nose, avoiding compression of the eyes. With one hand, place your thumb on the mask at the apex (over the nose) and your index finger on the mask at the chin to form a "C". With gentle pressure, push down on the mask to establish an adequate seal. Maintain the airway by lifting the bony prominence of the chin with your remaining fingers, forming an "E". Avoid placing pressure on the soft area under the chin, as this may cause an airway obstruction.

During ventilation, look for adequate chest rise. Listen for bilateral lung sounds at the third intercostal space on the midaxillary line. Also assess the patient for improvement in skin colour and heart rate.

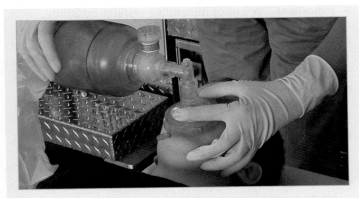

Figure 11-34 The EC-grip technique will facilitate proper hand placement to maintain a good mask-to-face seal.

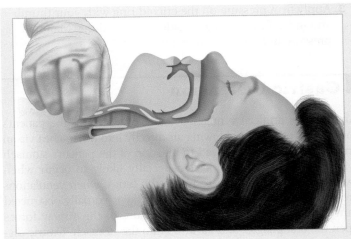

Figure 11-35 Cricoid pressure, or the Sellick manoeuvre.

Cricoid Pressure (Sellick Manoeuvre)

When ventilating any patient who is not intubated, you must be alert for gastric distension. This problem can be partially prevented or alleviated by using the Sellick manoeuvre, also called cricoid pressure. When performed properly, this non-invasive procedure can also help prevent passive regurgitation with aspiration during positive-pressure ventilation.

When you apply posterior pressure to the cricoid cartilage, the oesophagus is partially occluded between the cricoid ring and the cervical vertebrae, providing more air delivery into the lungs and less air delivery into the stomach Figure 11-35 ▶ . Cricoid pressure is indicated only in unconscious patients who cannot protect their own airway and are at imminent risk for vomiting (or if vomiting is occurring). This technique can also be used during endotracheal intubation to move the larynx posteriorly and facilitate an adequate view of the vocal cords.

Disadvantages of this technique include extreme or a large quantity of emesis if pressure is removed; therefore, cricoid pressure should be maintained until the patient is intubated. In addition, the procedure requires two clinicians. If a cervical spine injury is present, cricoid pressure may cause further injury, so this technique is contraindicated in these patients. Potential complications associated with cricoid pressure include trauma to the larynx if excessive force is used, oesophageal rupture from unrelieved high gastric pressures, and obstruction of the trachea when the technique is used in small children.

The steps for performing cricoid pressure are listed here and shown in Skill Drill 11-22 ▾ .

1. Visualise the cricoid cartilage Step 1 .
2. Palpate the cricoid cartilage to confirm its location—inferior to the thyroid cartilage Step 2 .

Skill Drill 11-22: Cricoid Pressure (Sellick Manoeuvre)

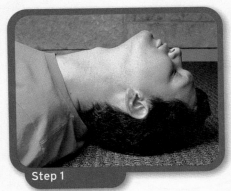

Step 1
Visualise the cricoid cartilage.

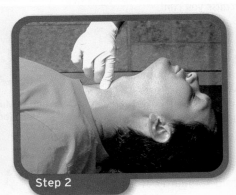

Step 2
Palpate to confirm its location.

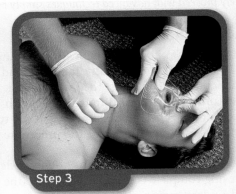

Step 3
Apply firm pressure with your thumb and index finger on either side of the midline.

3. Apply firm pressure on the cricoid ring with your thumb and index finger on either side of the midline. Maintain pressure until the patient is intubated (Step 3).

Gastric Distension

Any form of artificial ventilation that blows air into the patient's mouth—as opposed to blowing air directly into the trachea via an endotracheal tube—may lead to inflation of the patient's stomach with air. Gastric distension is especially likely to occur when excessive pressure is used to inflate the lungs, when ventilations are performed too fast, or when the airway is partially obstructed during ventilation attempts. The pressure in the airway forces open the oesophagus, and air flows into the stomach. Gastric distension occurs most frequently in children but is common in adults as well.

A distended stomach is harmful to the patient for at least two reasons. First, it promotes regurgitation of stomach contents, and vomitus creeping up the back of the throat rapidly finds its way into the patient's lungs (aspiration). Second, a distended stomach pushes the diaphragm upward into the chest, reducing the amount of space in which the lungs can expand.

Signs of gastric distension include an increase in the diameter of the stomach, an increasingly distended abdomen, and increased resistance to bag-valve-mask ventilations. If these signs are noted, you should reassess and reposition the airway as needed, apply cricoid pressure, and observe the chest for adequate rise and fall as you continue ventilating. In addition, limit ventilation times to 1 second or the time needed to produce adequate chest rise.

Advanced Airway Management

One of the most common mistakes in the situation of respiratory or cardiac arrest is to proceed with advanced airway management too early, forsaking the basic techniques of establishing and maintaining a patent airway in a patient who is already hypoxaemic. *Never abandon the basics of airway management and immediately proceed with advanced techniques simply because you can!*

Endotracheal Intubation

Endotracheal intubation is defined as passing an endotracheal (ET) tube through the glottic opening and sealing the tube with a cuff inflated against the tracheal wall. When the tube is passed into the trachea through the mouth, the procedure is called endootracheal intubation. When the tube is passed into the trachea through the nose, the procedure is called nasotracheal intubation.

Intubation of the trachea is the *most* definitive means of achieving complete control of the airway (the gold standard). A solid understanding of the basics of this technique is needed when making urgent decisions about when to intubate a patient. Following are considerations when performing endotracheal intubation:

- **Indications.** Present or impending respiratory failure, apnoea, inability of the patient to protect own airway.
- **Contraindications.** None in emergency situations. However with inexperienced personnel, other advanced airways may be easier, such as an LMA.
- **Advantages.** Provides a secure airway, protects against aspiration, provides an alternate route to IV/IO for certain medications (as a last resort).
- **Disadvantages.** Requires special equipment, bypasses physiological functions of the upper airway (warming, filtering, humidifying).
- **Complications.** Bleeding, hypoxia, laryngeal swelling, laryngospasm, vocal cord damage, mucosal necrosis, barotrauma.

The basic structure of an endotracheal (ET) tube (Figure 11-36 ▾) includes the proximal end, the tube itself, the cuff and pilot balloon, and the distal tip. The proximal end is equipped with a standard 15/22-mm adapter that allows it to be attached to any ventilation device. It also includes an inflation port with a pilot balloon; the distal cuff is inflated with a syringe attached to the inflation port, which has a one-way valve. The pilot balloon indicates whether the distal cuff is inflated or deflated once the tube has been inserted into the mouth.

Markings along the length of the tube provide a measurement of its depth in centimetres. The distal end of the tube has a beveled tip to facilitate insertion and an opening on the side called Murphy's eye, which enables ventilation to occur even if the tip becomes occluded by blood, mucus, or the tracheal wall.

At the Scene

Perform ventilations with a bag-valve-mask device and pure oxygen for *a few minutes* prior to attempting intubation. The patient needs an oxygen reserve to tolerate the period of time without ventilation that will occur during insertion of an advanced airway. You also need the time to check your equipment properly, ideally before the shift commences, so that you are very familiar with the location of each item when on scene.

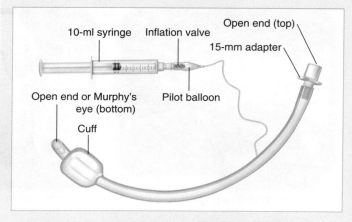

10-ml syringe   Inflation valve   Open end (top)

15-mm adapter

Open end or Murphy's eye (bottom)   Pilot balloon

Cuff

Figure 11-36 Endotracheal tube.

Endotracheal tubes range in size from 2.5 to 11.0 mm inside diameter, and their length ranges from 12 to 32 cm Figure 11-37 ▶ . Sizes ranging from 6.0 to 11.0 mm are equipped with a distal cuff that, when inflated, makes an airtight seal with the tracheal wall. A tube that is too small for the patient will lead to an increased resistance to airflow and difficulty in ventilating. A tube that is too large can be difficult to insert and may cause trauma. Normally, an adult female will require a 7.0- to 8.0-mm tube, while an adult male will require a 8.0- to 9.0-mm tube.

ET tubes ranging from 2.5 to 6.5 mm are used in paediatric patients. In children the funnel-shaped cricoid ring (the narrowest portion of the paediatric airway) forms an anatomical seal with the ET tube, eliminating the need for a distal cuff in most cases. There are limited situations where a cuffed paediatric tube may be used in the prehospital setting. The proximal end of the tube still has a 15/22-mm adapter for use with standard ventilation devices, and the distal end has a bevelled tip with distal end markings. However, because it lacks a balloon cuff, there is no pilot balloon.

A number of anatomical clues can help determine the proper size of ET tube for adults and children. The internal diameter of the nostril is a good approximation of the diameter of the glottic opening. The diameter of the little finger or the size of the thumbnail is also a good approximation of airway size. In children, the formula of (age ÷ 4) + 4 will give the internal diameter relatively accurately. Because all attempts to predict the tube size required for a given patient are estimates, however, you should always have *three* ET tubes ready: one tube of the size you *think* will be appropriate, one a size larger, and one a size smaller.

The laryngoscope and blade are required to perform orotracheal intubation by direct laryngoscopy—a procedure in which the vocal cords are directly visualised for safe and effective placement of the ET tube. The laryngoscope consists of a handle and interchangeable blades Figure 11-38 ▶ . The handle contains the power source for the light on the laryngoscope blade. Most laryngoscopes run on batteries, but a few are rechargeable. The handle has a bar designed to connect with a notch on the blade Figure 11-39 ▶ . When the blade is moved into the perpendicular position, the bright light shines near the tip of the blade.

The two most common types of laryngoscope blades are the straight (Miller) blade and the curved (Macintosh) blade. The straight laryngoscope blade is designed so that its tip will extend beneath the epiglottis and lift it up Figure 11-40 ◀ —a particularly useful fea-

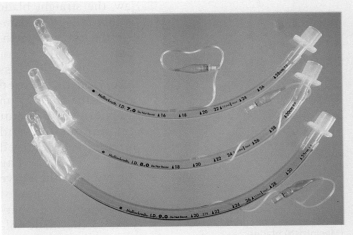

Figure 11-37 Endotracheal tubes are available in a variety of sizes, both cuffed and uncuffed.

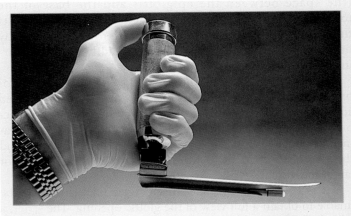

Figure 11-38 A laryngoscope with blade (Miller) attached.

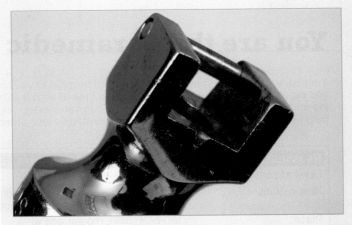

Figure 11-39 The laryngoscope's handle has a bar designed to connect with a notch on the blade.

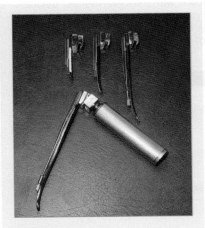

Figure 11-40 A straight (Miller) blade.

ture in infants and small children, who often have a long, floppy epiglottis that is difficult to elevate out of the way with a curved blade. In the adult, use of a straight blade requires great care; if used improperly and levered across the upper

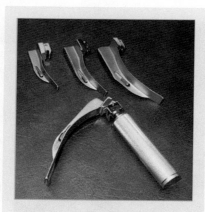

Figure 11-41 A laryngoscope and an assortment of curved (Macintosh) blades.

jaw, the straight blade is more likely to damage the patient's teeth. The curved laryngoscope blade is less likely to be levered against the teeth by an inexperienced doctor or paramedic and is usually preferred **Figure 11-41** . The direction of the curve conforms to that of the tongue and pharynx, so the blade follows the outline of the pharynx with relative ease. The tip of the curved blade is placed in the vallecula (the space between the epiglottis and the base of the tongue) rather than beneath the epiglottis; it indirectly lifts the epiglottis to expose the vocal cords. You should ideally have *both* curved and straight blades readily available during an orotracheal intubation attempt.

Blade sizes range from 0 to 4. Sizes 0, 1, and 2 are appropriate for infants and children, whereas 3 and 4 are considered adult sizes. For paediatric patients, blade sizes are often recommended based on the child's age or height. Most paramedics choose the blade for adults based on experience and the size of the patient (3 for average-sized adults and 4 for larger individuals).

It is common, especially in emergency situations, to be unable to obtain a full view of the glottic opening. The stylet, a semirigid wire that can be inserted into the ET tube to mould and maintain the shape of the tube, enables you to guide the tip of the tube over the arytenoid cartilage, even if you cannot see the entire glottic opening. This device should be lubricated with a water-soluble gel to facilitate its removal, and its end should be bent to form a gentle "hockey stick" curve. The end of the stylet should rest at least 1 cm back from the end of the ET tube; if the stylet protrudes beyond the end of the tube, it may damage the vocal cords and surrounding structures. Bend the other end of the stylet over the proximal tube connector, so that the stylet cannot slip farther into the tube.

Magill forceps have two uses in the emergency setting. First, they are used to remove airway obstructions under direct visualisation, as discussed earlier in this chapter. Second, they are used to guide the tip of the ET tube through the glottic opening if you are unable to get the proper angle with simple manipulation of the tube or stylet.

Endotracheal Intubation by Direct Laryngoscopy

Orotracheal intubation by direct laryngoscopy involves inserting an ET tube through the mouth and into the trachea while visualising the glottic opening with a laryngoscope; it is by far the most common method of performing endotracheal intubation in the emergency setting. Following are some considerations when performing orotracheal intubation by direct laryngoscopy:

- **Indications.** Apnoea, hypoxia, poor respiratory effort, suppression or absence of a gag reflex.
- **Contraindications.** Caution in an unsuppressed gag reflex.
- **Advantages.** Direct visualisation of anatomy and tube placement, ideal method for confirming placement, may be performed in breathing or apnoeic patients.

You are the Paramedic Part 7

Your colleague begins immediate transport to hospital as you continue to assist the patient's ventilations with a bag-valve-mask device and supplemental oxygen. With an estimated time of arrival at hospital of 20 minutes, you find that you are having difficulty maintaining an adequate mask-to-face seal with the bag-valve-mask device; the patient looks worse. You ask one of the additional crew members to assist you maintaining the patient's airway. Reassessment of the patient reveals the following:

Reassessment	Recording Time: 16 Minutes
Level of consciousness	U (Unresponsive)
Respirations	30 breaths/min and shallow (baseline); you are having difficulty maintaining an adequate mask-to-face seal with the bag-valve-mask device
Pulse	160 beats/min, regular and weak
Skin	Severe facial cyanosis
Blood pressure	98/58 mm Hg
S_PO_2	83% while receiving assisted ventilations with a bag-valve-mask device and oxygen at 15 l/min

11. What are the signs of inadequate artificial ventilation?

12. What management is required to prevent further deterioration of this patient's condition?

- **Disadvantages.** Requires special equipment.
- **Complications.** Dental trauma, laryngeal trauma, misplacement (right main stem bronchus, oesophagus).

Universal Precautions

Intubation may expose you to blood or other body fluids, so take proper precautions when performing this procedure. In addition to gloves, wear a face mask that will protect you if the patient vomits or coughs during intubation.

Preoxygenation

Adequate preoxygenation with a bag-valve-mask device and oxygen is a critical step prior to intubating a patient. You should mildly hyperoxygenate (approximately 24 breaths/min) the apnoeic or hypoventilating patient for 2 to 3 minutes. During the intubation attempt, the patient will undergo a period of forced apnoea when he or she will not be ventilated. The goal of preoxygenation is to prevent hypoxia from occurring during this time.

The consequences of even brief periods of hypoxia can be disastrous. Do not rely solely on pulse oximetry to quantify a patient's oxygenation status; it can produce falsely high readings, even if the patient is severely hypoxic. Although some sequelae of hypoxia are dramatic and occur immediately, most are subtle and occur gradually. Clearly, some of the poor neurological outcomes following aggressive airway management result from intubation-induced hypoxia.

At the Scene

Ideally, the patient should have an SpO_2 of 100% (or as close to it as possible) prior to the intubation attempt. If you are unable to obtain an SpO_2 reading, however, you should moderately hyperoxygenate (24 breaths/min) the patient for at least 2 minutes before attempting to intubate. If you are attempting to preoxygenate the patient, and the SpO_2 continues to drop despite your best efforts at manual airway management and ventilation, it is best to proceed with intubation without delay.

Positioning the Patient

Successful laryngoscopy will be extremely difficult—if not impossible—to perform without proper positioning of the patient's head. The airway has three axes: the mouth, the pharynx, and the larynx. When the head is in a neutral position, these axes are at acute angles, facilitating entry of food into the oesophagus rather than into the trachea Figure 11-42A ▶. Although this positioning is advantageous to the conscious, spontaneously breathing patient, the angles of these axes make laryngoscopy difficult.

To facilitate visualisation of the airway, the three axes must be aligned to the greatest extent possible. This is most effec-

tively achieved by placing the patient in the "sniffing the morning air" position (the position of the head when intentionally sniffing). The position involves approximately a 20° extension of the atlanto-occipital joint and a 30° flexion of the neck at C6 and C7 for patients with short necks and/or no chins, increasing the angle even further will help improve visualisation. The Sellick manoeuvre further improves the ability to see the vocal cords Figure 11-42B ▾.

At the Scene

If the patient has experienced a possible neck injury, his or her head must be placed in a neutral in-line position. Do not use the sniffing position or extend the patient's head in any way. Intubation of the trauma patient is most effectively performed by two paramedics.

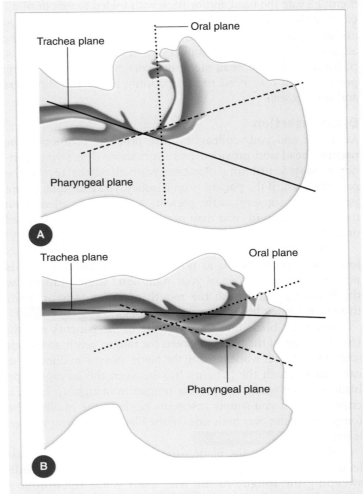

Figure 11-42 Three axes of the airway: oral plane, pharyngeal, and tracheal. **A.** Neutral position. **B.** Sniffing the morning air position.

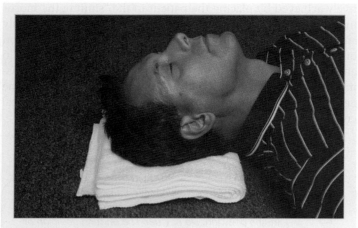

Figure 11-43 Head elevation is best achieved with folded towels positioned under the head and/or neck.

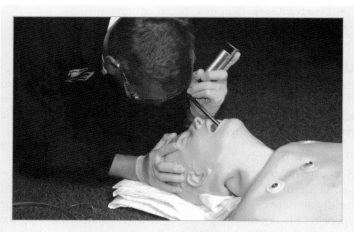

Figure 11-44 If the patient is on the floor or ground, you may need to kneel and lean forward or lie on the floor to get into the proper position.

In most supine patients, the sniffing position can be achieved by extending the head and elevating the occiput 2.5 to 5 cm. Elevate the head and/or neck with folded towels until the ear is at the level of the sternum (**Figure 11-43 ▲**). When you are using towels or blankets, their thickness can easily be adjusted by changing the number of folds. With obese patients, padding under the head alone may not result in the sniffing position; you may need to add padding under the shoulders and neck as well.

Blade Insertion

After you and your colleagues have properly positioned the patient's head and provided preoxygenation, direct your partner to stop ventilating. Position yourself at the top of the patient's head. If the patient is on a trolley, you can squat to put your head at the level of the patient's head. If the patient is on the floor or ground, you may need to kneel and lean forward or lie down to get into the proper position (**Figure 11-44 ▶**).

Grasp the laryngoscope with your left hand and hold it as low down on the handle as possible. If the patient's mouth is not open, place the side of your right-hand thumb just below the bottom lip and push the mouth open, or "scissor" your thumb and index finger between the molars (**Figure 11-45 ▶**).

Insert the blade into the *right* side of the patient's mouth. Use the flange of the blade to sweep the tongue gently to the left side of the mouth while moving the blade into the midline. Take care not to catch the patient's lips between the laryngoscope blade and the teeth. Moving the tongue from right to left is a critical step. If you simply insert the blade in the midline, the tongue will hang over both sides of the blade and all you will see is the tongue (**Figure 11-46 ▶**).

Slowly advance the blade—the curved blade into the vallecula or the straight blade beneath the epiglottis—while sweeping the tongue to the left. Exert *gentle* traction at a 45° angle to the floor as you lift the patient's jaw. *Do not "lever" back on the laryngoscope;* this will cause you to use the patient's upper teeth as a fulcrum, resulting in breaking and potential aspiration of teeth (**Figure 11-47 ▶**). Keeping your back and

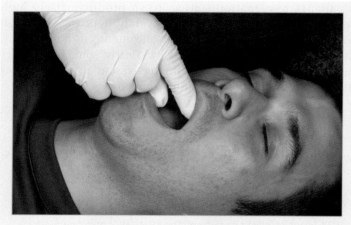

Figure 11-45 Place the side of your right-hand thumb just below the bottom lip and push the mouth open, or scissor your thumb and index finger between the molars.

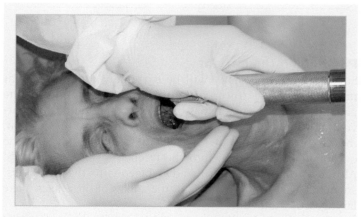

Figure 11-46 The tongue is a sticky, amorphous structure that can be a major hindrance to visualising the airway. Proper use of the laryngoscope is critical to controlling the tongue.

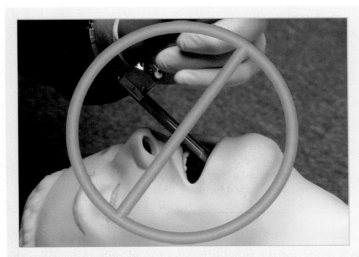

Figure 11-47 Levering against the upper teeth with the laryngoscope can result in breaking and potential aspiration of the teeth. Don't do it!

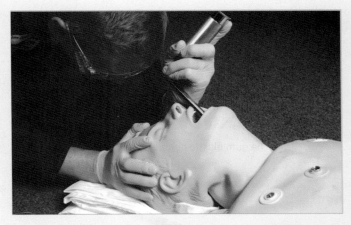

Figure 11-48 Keep your back and your left arm straight as you pull upward. This allows you to use the strength of your shoulders to lift the patient's jaw.

your left arm straight as you pull upward allows you to use the strength of your shoulders to lift the patient's jaw and decreases the likelihood of levering the laryngoscope blade against the patient's teeth Figure 11-48 ▸. The correct motion is similar to holding a wine glass and offering a toast.

Visualisation of the Glottic Opening

Continue lifting the laryngoscope as you look down the blade. You should see some familiar anatomic landmarks—the epiglottis or the arytenoid cartilage. Identifying these structures enables to you make small adjustments in the position of the blade to aid in visualisation of the glottic opening.

With the curved blade, walk the blade down the tongue because you know that the vallecula and the epiglottis lie at the base of the tongue. With the straight blade, insert the blade straight back until the tip touches the posterior pharyngeal wall.

As you continue to work the tip of the blade into position (lifting the epiglottis with the straight blade or the vallecula with the curved blade), the glottic opening should come into full view. The vocal cords are the white fibrous bands that lie vertically within the glottic opening; they should be slightly open Figure 11-49 ▸.

If you are having difficulty seeing the glottic opening, consider cricoid pressure with the help of a colleague.

The gum elastic bougie, also called the Eschmann stylet, is a flexible device that is approximately 3 mm in diameter and 60 cm long Figure 11-50 ▸. It can make intubation possible in some difficult situations, especially when your view of the glottic opening is limited. The bougie is rigid enough that it can be easily directed through the glottic opening, yet flexible enough that it does not cause damage to the tracheal walls.

The bougie is inserted through the glottic opening under direct laryngoscopy. The angle at its distal tip facilitates entry into the glottic opening and enables you to "feel" the ridges of the tracheal wall Figure 11-51 ▸. Once the bougie is placed

At the Scene

Improving Your Laryngoscopic View: The Sellick Manoeuvre and the BURP Manoeuvre

When the angle of the pharynx and the larynx is particularly acute, it is often difficult to see the entire glottic opening. You can do two things to increase the percentage of the glottic opening that you can see: the Sellick manoeuvre or the BURP manoeuvre. The Sellick manoeuvre, which reduces the incidence of gastric distension during positive-pressure ventilation, also moves the larynx more posteriorly. If applied by an assistant during direct laryngoscopy, it reduces the acuity of the angle between the pharynx and larynx and can improve your laryngoscopic view.

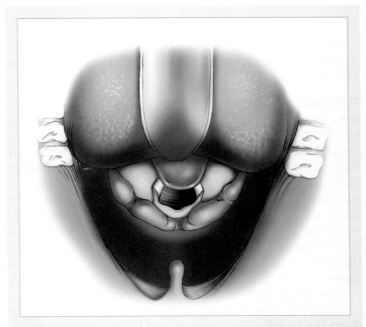

Figure 11-49 Laryngoscopic view of the vocal cords (white fibrous bands).

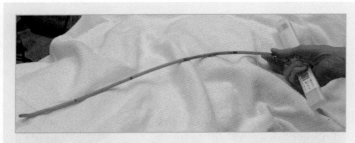
Figure 11-50 The gum elastic bougie device.

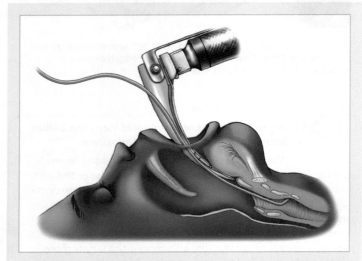
Figure 11-51 The angle at the distal tip of the gum elastic bougie facilitates entry into the glottic opening and enables you to feel the ridges of the tracheal wall.

deeply into the trachea, it becomes a guide for the ET tube. Simply slide the tube over the bougie and into the trachea. Remove the bougie, ventilate, and confirm proper ET tube placement.

Tube Insertion

Once you have visualised the glottic opening, pick up the endotracheal tube in your right hand. Under direct vision, insert the tube from the right corner of the patient's mouth through the vocal cords. Continue to insert the tube until the proximal end of the cuff is 1 to 2 cm past the vocal cords. *You must see the tip of the ET tube pass through the vocal cords. If you cannot see the vocal cords, do not insert the tube!* The only way to be certain that the tube has passed through the vocal cords is to *see* it pass through the vocal cords. If you take your eye off the tip of the tube (and the vocal cords), even for a second, you significantly increase the likelihood of allowing the tube to slip into the oesophagus.

A major mistake of beginners is to try to pass the tube down the barrel of the laryngoscope blade—especially when using a straight blade. The laryngoscope blade is not designed

At the Scene

An intubation attempt should not take more than 30 seconds. If you are unable to intubate the patient within 30 seconds, abort the attempt and reoxygenate the patient for at least 30 seconds to 1 minute with 100% oxygen before attempting intubation again.

Multiple intubation attempts, provided that you perform appropriate oxygenation and ventilation in between attempts, will generally not harm your patient; however, a prolonged individual attempt will. During CPR, compressions should not be stopped for more than 10 seconds.

as a guide for the tube; it is a tool used only to visualise the glottic opening. Placing the tube down the barrel of the blade will obscure your view of the glottic opening **Figure 11-52 ▾**.

Ventilation

After you have seen the cuff of the ET tube pass roughly 1 to 2 cm beyond the vocal cords, gently slide out the blade, hold the tube securely in place with your right hand, and remove the stylet from the tube. Inflate the distal cuff with 5 to 10 ml of air and then detach the syringe from the inflation port. If the syringe is not removed immediately following inflation of the distal cuff, air from the cuff may leak back into the syringe, resulting in a loss of an adequate seal between the cuff and the tracheal wall. Avoid inflating the distal cuff with excess pressure as this may cause tissue necrosis of the tracheal wall.

Instruct your colleague to attach the bag-valve-mask device to the ET tube and continue ventilation. As the first ventilations are delivered, look at the patient's chest to ensure that it rises with each ventilation. At the same time, listen with a

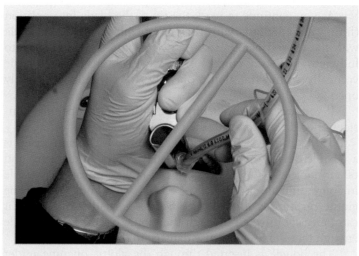
Figure 11-52 Placing a tube down the barrel of the blade obscures your view of the glottic opening.

Skill Drill 11-25: Securing an Endotracheal Tube With a Commercial Device

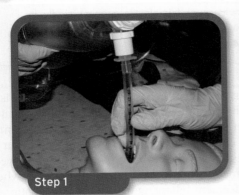

Step 1

Note the centimetre marking on the tube at the level of the patient's teeth.

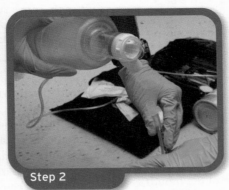

Step 2

Remove the bag-valve-mask device from the ET tube.

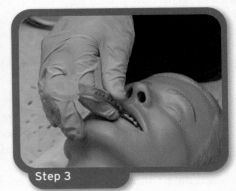

Step 3

Position the ET tube in the centre of the patient's mouth.

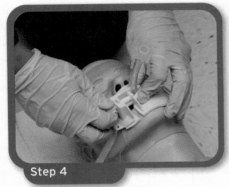

Step 4

Place the commercial device over the ET tube. Tighten the screw and fasten the strap around the nape of the neck to secure.

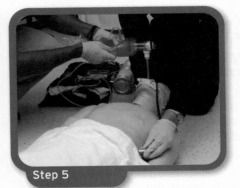

Step 5

Reattach the bag-valve-mask device, and auscultate again over the apexes and bases of the lungs and over the epigastrium.

You are the Paramedic Part 8

After definitively securing the patient's airway, you attach an automatic transport ventilator (ATV) and continue transport. En route, you note marked improvement in his condition. Your reassessment reveals the following:

Reassessment	Recording Time: 22 Minutes
Level of consciousness	P (Responsive to painful stimuli); improving, patient is becoming resistant to the ET tube
Respirations	Ventilated with an ATV and pure oxygen at a rate of 12 breaths/min
Pulse	118 beats/min, regular and stronger
Skin	Cyanosis is dissipating; skin is cool and dry
Blood pressure	118/70 mm Hg
SpO$_2$	97% while being ventilated with an ATV

13. Should you extubate this patient? Why or why not?

The steps for orotracheal intubation by direct laryngoscopy are summarised here and shown in **Skill Drill 11-26 ▶**.

1. Use universal precautions (gloves and face shield) **Step 1**.
2. Preoxygenate the patient for 2 to 3 minutes with a bag-valve-mask device and oxygen **Step 2**.
3. Assemble and prepare your equipment which has been checked pre-shift **Step 3**.
4. Place the patient's head in the "sniffing the morning air" position **Step 4**.
5. Insert the blade into the right side of the patient's mouth, and displace the tongue to the left **Step 5**.
6. Gently lift the long axis of the laryngoscope handle until you can visualise the glottic opening and the vocal cords **Step 6**.
7. Insert the ET tube through the right corner of the mouth, and visualise its entry between the vocal cords **Step 7**.
8. Remove the laryngoscope from the patient's mouth **Step 8**.
9. Remove the stylet (if used) from the ET tube **Step 9**.
10. Inflate the distal cuff of the ET tube with 5 to 10 ml of air, and detach the syringe from the inflation port **Step 10**.
11. Attach an end-tidal carbon dioxide detector to the ET tube **Step 11**.
12. Attach the bag-valve-mask device, ventilate, and auscultate over the apexes and bases of both lungs and over the epigastrium. Check the $ETCO_2$ reading **Step 12**.
13. Secure the ET tube with tape or a professional device **Step 13**.
14. Place an oropharyngeal airway in the patient's mouth if using tape **Step 14**.
15. Print off the $ETCO_2$ reading.

Nasotracheal Intubation

Nasotracheal intubation is the insertion of a tube into the trachea through the nose. When performed, it is usually performed without directly visualising the vocal cords—hence the term "blind" nasotracheal intubation. It is not a practice used regularly in the prehospital setting in the UK.

Documentation and Communication

On the patient clinical record, document the means of assessing placement of the ET tube, such as breath sounds, visualisation, and capnography or capnometry prints from the monitor. The depth of the tube, as noted by the centimetre marking at the patient's teeth, should also be documented. Additionally, indicate when correct placement was confirmed: at the time the ET tube was placed, when the patient was moved into the ambulance, and upon arrival at hospital.

At the Scene

Keep a laryngoscope and Magill forceps within easy reach in case the patient becomes apnoeic during the procedure or you are unable to thread the tip of the tube through the glottic opening blindly. In these cases, you will need to complete the procedure under direct laryngoscopy.

On the downside, because nasotracheal intubation is a blind technique, the paramedic cannot use one of the major tube confirmation methods—visualising the tube passing through the vocal cords. Confirming proper tube position is important, regardless of which intubation method is employed; however, the paramedic should be even more diligent when confirming tube placement following nasotracheal intubation.

Digital Intubation

Intubation can be performed without the use of a laryngoscope. Digital intubation (also referred to as "blind" or "tactile" intubation) involves directly palpating the glottic structures and elevating the epiglottis with your middle finger while guiding the ET tube into the trachea by feel. This rarely used technique should not be attempted without adequate training.

At the Scene

Always check your intubation equipment at the beginning of each shift to ensure that it is fully functional. Failure to do so increases the risk of equipment breakdown when it is needed the most. Digital intubation, although an extreme emergency technique, is clearly the least desirable option. Having functional equipment when you need it will avoid the need to stick your fingers down the patient's throat to place the ET tube.

Successful placement of the ET tube via digital intubation depends on frequency of practice, experience, manual dexterity, and the size and length of the paramedic's fingers. Paramedics with short fingers or fingers that are large in diameter will have greater difficulty performing digital intubation.

Transillumination Techniques for Intubation

Transillumination intubation, like digital intubation, is rarely considered a first-line technique to definitively secure the airway, but it may prove valuable in some situations. The tissue that overlies the trachea is relatively thin. Therefore, a bright light source placed inside the trachea emits a bright, well-circumscribed light that is visible on the outside of the trachea and the external soft tissue that overlies it.

Skill Drill 11-26: Intubation of the Trachea Using Direct Laryngoscopy

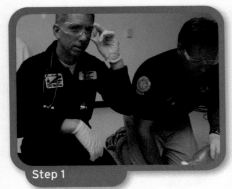

Step 1

Use universal precautions (gloves and face shield).

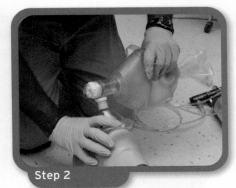

Step 2

Preoxygenate the patient for 2 to 3 minutes with a bag-valve-mask device and oxygen.

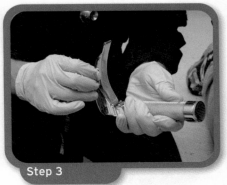

Step 3

Assemble and prepare your equipment.

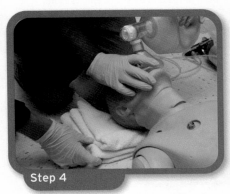

Step 4

Place the patient's head in the "sniffing the morning air" position.

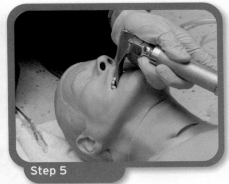

Step 5

Insert the blade into the right side of the patient's mouth, and displace the tongue to the left.

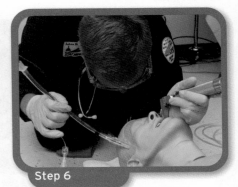

Step 6

Gently lift the long axis of the laryngoscope handle until you can visualise the glottic opening and the vocal cords.

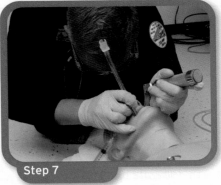

Step 7

Insert the ET tube through the right corner of the mouth, and visualise its entry between the vocal cords.

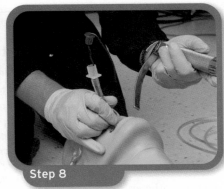

Step 8

Remove the laryngoscope from the patient's mouth.

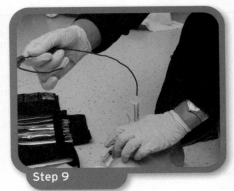

Step 9

Remove the stylet (if used) from the ET tube.

Skill Drill 11-26: Intubation of the Trachea Using Direct Laryngoscopy (*continued*)

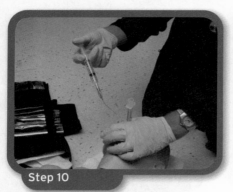

Step 10

Inflate the distal cuff of the ET tube with 5 to 10 ml of air, and detach the syringe from the inflation port.

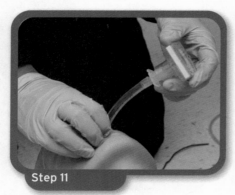

Step 11

Attach an end-tidal carbon dioxide detector to the ET tube.

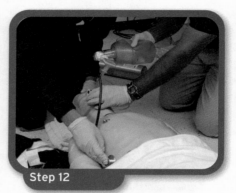

Step 12

Attach the bag-valve-mask device, ventilate, and auscultate over the apexes and bases of both lungs and over the epigastrium.

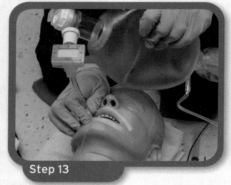

Step 13

Secure the ET tube with tape or professional device.

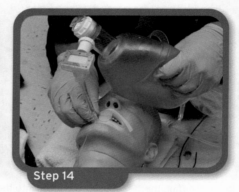

Step 14

Place an oropharyngeal airway in the patient's mouth if not using a professional securing device.

A number of devices can be used to intubate the trachea with the transillumination technique. You should be familiar with your specific equipment and consult the product documentation for instructions in its use. In this section, the term "lighted stylet" will be used generically to describe any malleable stylet with a bright light source at its distal end that can be used to guide intubation.

Tracheobronchial Suctioning

Tracheobronchial suctioning involves passing a suction catheter into the ET tube to remove pulmonary secretions. The first rule to remember about performing tracheobronchial suctioning is this: Don't do it if you don't have to! This kind of suctioning requires strict attention to sterile technique, which is nearly impossible to maintain when you're in a ditch by the side of the road. Suctioning the trachea can also cause cardiac arrhythmia; cardiac arrest has been reported during tracheobronchial suctioning. For these reasons, you should avoid suctioning through an ET tube *unless secretions are so massive that they interfere with ventilation.* If tracheobronchial suctioning must be performed, use a

At the Scene

Endotracheal Intubation: Points to Remember

- Never attempt endotracheal intubation before the patient has been adequately preoxygenated.
- Assemble and check all your equipment before you begin.
- Position is everything! Ensure that the patient's head is in the proper position to align the airway axes.
- Don't rush! Work with *deliberate* speed.
- Get it right the first time. The second attempt is likely to be more difficult. Remember that a patent BLS airway is acceptable until a more experienced provider has time to pass an advanced airway.
- Confirm that the ET tube is in the right place. Take *nothing* for granted.
- Secure the ET tube appropriately. Otherwise, you'll soon be trying to put it back in again.
- Even when the tube is properly secured, stabilise it with your hand as you ventilate the patient.

sterile technique (if possible), and monitor the patient's cardiac rhythm and oxygen saturation during the procedure.

Preoxygenation of the patient is essential prior to performing tracheobronchial suctioning. Prelubricate a soft-tip catheter and hyperoxygenate the patient for at least 2 to 3 minutes. It may be necessary to inject 3 to 5 ml of sterile water down the ET tube to loosen thick pulmonary secretions.

Gently insert the suction catheter down the ET tube until resistance is felt. Apply suction as the catheter is extracted, taking care not to exceed 15 seconds in the adult patient. After tracheobronchial suctioning is complete, reattach the bag-valve-mask device, continue ventilations, and reassess the patient.

The steps for performing tracheobronchial suctioning are listed here and shown in (Skill Drill 11-27 ▶).

1. Check, prepare, and assemble your equipment (Step 1).
2. Lubricate the suction catheter (Step 2).
3. Preoxygenate the patient (Step 3).
4. Detach the bag-valve-mask device and inject 3 to 5 ml of sterile water down the ET tube, **if** the secretions are very thick (Step 4).
5. Gently insert the catheter into the ET tube until resistance is felt (Step 5).
6. Occlude the catheter finger port and withdraw the catheter. Monitor the patient's cardiac rhythm and oxygen saturation during the procedure (Step 6).
7. Reattach the bag-valve-mask device and resume ventilation and oxygenation. Check the ETCO$_2$ print-out (Step 7).

Prehospital Extubation

Extubation is the process of removing the tube from an intubated patient. Patients are rarely extubated in the prehospital setting. Generally, the only reason to consider performing extubation in the prehospital environment is if the patient is *unreasonably* intolerant of the ET tube (eg, extremely combative, gagging, or retching).

The most obvious risk associated with extubation is overestimation of the patient's ability to protect his or her own airway. Additionally, when extubation is performed on conscious patients, there is a high risk of laryngospasm, and most patients experience some degree of upper airway swelling because of the trauma of having the tube in the trachea. These two facts, along with the ever-present potential for vomiting, make successful reintubation challenging, if not impossible. If you are not *absolutely* sure that you can reintubate the patient, do not remove the tube! Prehospital extubation is absolutely contraindicated if there is *any* risk of recurrent respiratory failure or if you are uncertain that the patient can maintain his or her own airway spontaneously.

If prehospital extubation is indicated, you must first hyperoxygenate the patient. Discuss the procedure with the patient, and explain what you plan to do. Assemble and have available all equipment to suction, ventilate, and reintubate, if necessary. After confirming that the patient remains responsive enough to protect his or her own airway, suction the oropharynx to remove any secretions or debris that may threaten the airway once the tube has been removed. Deflate the distal cuff on the ET tube as the patient begins to exhale so that any accumulated secretions proximal to the cuff are not aspirated into the lungs. On the next exhalation, *remove the tube in one steady motion,* following the curvature of the airway. Consider placing a towel or sick bowl in front of the patient's mouth in case vomiting occurs.

The steps for performing extubation are listed here and shown in (Skill Drill 11-28 ▶).

1. Hyperoxygenate the patient (Step 1).
2. Ensure that ventilation and suction equipment are immediately available (Step 2).
3. Confirm patient responsiveness (Step 3).
4. Lean the patient on his or her side.
5. Suction the oropharynx with a rigid catheter (Step 4).
6. Deflate the distal cuff of the ET tube (Step 5).
7. Remove the ET tube as the patient coughs or begins to exhale (Step 6).

You are the Paramedic Part 9

The patient is now calm and compliant with the ET tube and mechanical ventilations, but you note a decrease in his oxygen saturation and an increase in his heart rate. You immediately reassess breath sounds and epigastric sounds and determine that the ET tube is still correctly placed; the ETCO$_2$ detector confirms this.

Reassessment	Recording Time: 27 Minutes
Level of consciousness	Unresponsive
Respirations	Ventilated with an ATV and pure oxygen at a rate of 12 breaths/min; gurgling is heard in the ET tube
Pulse	130 beats/min, strong and regular
Skin	Pink and moist
Blood pressure	122/74 mm Hg
SpO$_2$	90% while being ventilated with an ATV and the use of oxygen

14. What is most likely to have caused this patient's increased heart rate and decreased SpO$_2$?
15. How will you remedy the situation?

Skill Drill 11-27: Performing Tracheobronchial Suctioning

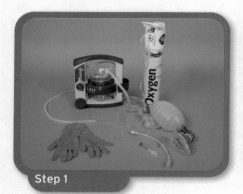

Step 1

Check, prepare, and assemble your equipment.

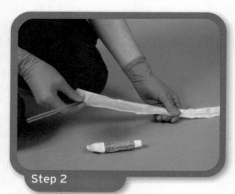

Step 2

Lubricate the suction catheter.

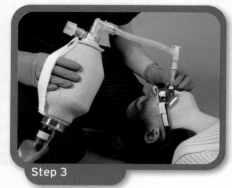

Step 3

Preoxygenate the patient.

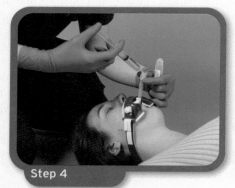

Step 4

Detach the bag-valve-mask device and inject 3 to 5 ml of sterile water down the ET tube, if the secretions are very thick.

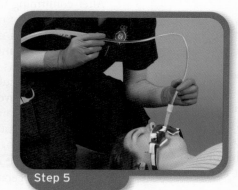

Step 5

Gently insert the catheter into the ET tube until resistance is felt.

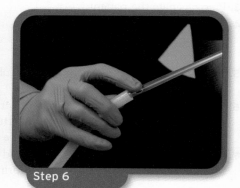

Step 6

Occlude the catheter finger port and withdraw the catheter. Monitor the patient's cardiac rhythm and oxygen saturation during the procedure.

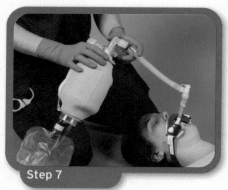

Step 7

Reattach the bag-valve-mask device and resume ventilation and oxygenation. Check the ETCO$_2$ print-out.

Chapter 11 Airway Management and Ventilation

Skill Drill 11-28: Performing Extubation

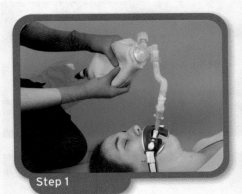

Step 1

Hyperoxygenate the patient.

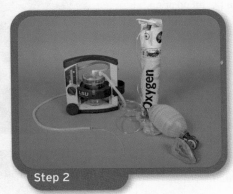

Step 2

Ensure that ventilation and suction equipment are immediately available.

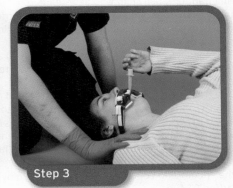

Step 3

Confirm patient responsiveness.

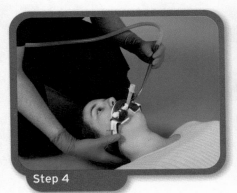

Step 4

Suction the oropharynx with a rigid catheter.

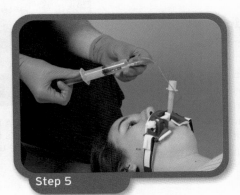

Step 5

Deflate the distal cuff of the ET tube.

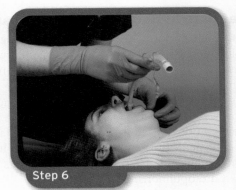

Step 6

Remove the ET tube as the patient coughs or begins to exhale.

Table 11-11	Differences in the Paediatric Airway

- Infants have a larger, rounder occiput, which causes the head of an infant or small child who lies supine to be in a flexed position.
- In children, the tongue is proportionately larger and the mandible is proportionately smaller—differences that increase children's propensity for airway obstruction.
- The epiglottis in a child is horse-shoe shaped and floppy, so it must be lifted, or positioned, out of the way to visualise the vocal cords.
- The trachea in a child is smaller, shorter, and narrower than an adult's, and it is positioned more anteriorly and superiorly.
- The narrowest portion of the child's airway is the cricoid ring, which is below the vocal cords (subglottic), and the anatomy below the vocal cords is funnel-shaped. This makes a cuff less necessary for occluding the trachea; the developing cartilage of the cricoid ring could potentially be injured by inflation of a cuffed ET tube.

Paediatric Endotracheal Intubation

Although endotracheal intubation has been considered the gold standard for definitive prehospital airway management in adults, recent studies suggest that effective bag-valve-mask ventilations in the paediatric patient can be as effective as intubation for ambulance services that have short transport times. However, if bag-valve-mask ventilations are not producing adequate ventilation and oxygenation, the infant or child should be intubated. Indications for endotracheal intubation in paediatric patients are the same as those in adults:

- Cardiopulmonary arrest
- Respiratory failure/arrest
- Traumatic brain injury
- Unresponsiveness
- Inability to maintain a patent airway
- Need for prolonged ventilation
- Need for endotracheal administration of resuscitative medications (if no IV or IO)

Certain anatomical differences between children and adults Table 11-11 ▲ play a key role in performing a successful intubation, as proper airway positioning is critical.

Laryngoscope and Blades

Although any laryngoscope handle can be used to intubate a child, most paramedics prefer the thinner paediatric handles. Straight blades facilitate lifting of the floppy epiglottis. If a curved blade is used, the tip of the blade is positioned in the vallecula to lift the jaw and epiglottis to visualise the vocal cords.

The blade should extend from the child's mouth to the tragus of the ear. Acceptable means of measuring this length include use of a length-based resuscitation tape measure or using the following general guidelines:

- Premature newborn: size 0 straight blade
- Full-term newborn to 1 year of age: size 1 straight blade
- 2 years of age to adolescent: size 2 straight blade

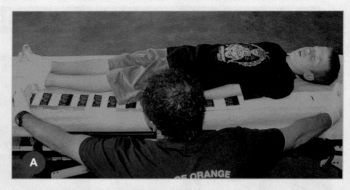
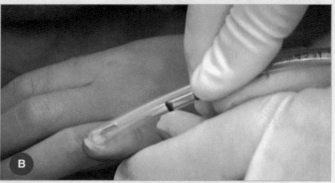

Figure 11-57 **A.** A length-based resuscitation tape can help estimate a child's ET tube size. **B.** The width of the child's small fingernail can be used to estimate ET tube size.

- Adolescent and older: size 3 straight or curved blade
- Have a spare blade of a different size

Endotracheal Tubes

ET tube size can be selected by using a length-based resuscitation tape measure Figure 11-57A ▲ . For children older than 1 year of age, the following formula can be used:

- (Age [in years] ÷ 4) + 4 =
  - A 4-year-old child would need a 5.0-mm tube (4 [age in years] ÷ 4 + 4) = 5.0

Certain anatomical clues, such as the nares or the width of the child's small fingernail Figure 11-57B ▲ can be used to estimate tube size, or you can follow general guidelines based on the child's age.

Uncuffed ET tubes should be used in the prehospital environment until the child is 8 to 10 years of age. A cuff at the cricoid ring is unnecessary to obtain a seal in children in this age range. Furthermore, a cuff can cause ischaemia and damage the tracheal mucosa at the level of the cricoid ring. When selecting the appropriate size ET tube, you should have a tube one size smaller as well as one size larger than expected for situations in which there is variability in the child's upper airway diameter.

The appropriate depth of insertion of the ET tube is 2 to 3 cm beyond the vocal cords. After the tube has been inserted, the depth at the corner of the child's mouth should be recorded and monitored. For uncuffed tubes, a black band—the vocal cord guide—often encircles the tube at its distal end. When you see this band at the level of the vocal cords, stop. Cuffed tubes should be inserted until the cuff is just below the level of the vocal cords.

Paediatric Stylet

The use of a stylet, for the most part, is a matter of personal preference when intubating the paediatric patient. If a stylet is used, insert it into the ET tube, stopping at least 1 cm from the end of the tube. Paediatric stylets will fit into tubes of size 3.0 to 6.0 mm, whereas the adult stylets are used for tubes of size 6.0 mm and larger. After inserting the stylet into the ET tube, bend the tube into a gentle upward curve. In some cases, bending the tube into the shape of a hockey stick is beneficial.

Preoxygenation

Adequate preoxygenation with a bag-valve-mask device and high flow oxygen for at least 30 seconds prior to attempting intubation cannot be overemphasised—respiratory failure or arrest is the most common cause of cardiac arrest in the paediatric population. While preoxygenating the child, you must also ensure that the child's head is in the proper position; this is the neutral position for patients with suspected trauma or the sniffing position otherwise. If needed, insert an airway adjunct; in conjunction with proper manual positioning of the head, it will maintain airway patency and facilitate effective ventilation.

Additional Preparation

Stimulation of the parasympathetic nervous system with resultant bradycardia can occur during intubation in children; therefore, you should apply a cardiac monitor, if available. A pulse oximeter should be used throughout the intubation attempt to monitor the child's heart rate and oxygen saturation. In addition, suction should be readily available to clear oral secretions from the child's airway.

Intubation Technique

With the child's head in a sniffing position, open his or her mouth by applying thumb pressure on the chin. Some children may require use of the crossfinger technique: use your thumb and index finger or thumb and middle finger to push the upper and lower teeth apart. If an oropharyngeal airway has been inserted, remove it. If needed, suction the child's mouth and pharynx to remove any secretions.

Hold the laryngoscope handle in your left hand, using your thumb, index finger, and middle finger to hold the handle (the "trigger finger" position). Insert the laryngoscope blade in the right side of the child's mouth, sweeping the tongue to the left side and keeping it under the blade.

Advance the blade straight along the tongue, while applying gentle traction upward along the axis of the laryngoscope handle at a 45° angle. *Never use the teeth or gums as a fulcrum for the blade.* A child's teeth could easily be loosened or cracked during a traumatic intubation attempt.

When the blade passes the epiglottis, gently lift the epiglottis if you are using a straight blade. If you are using a curved blade, place the tip of the blade in the vallecula, and lift the jaw, tongue, and blade gently at a 45° angle.

Identify the vocal cords and other normal anatomical landmarks. If they are not visible, ask your partner to apply gentle cricoid pressure. Additional gentle suctioning may be needed to facilitate your view of the vocal cords.

Hold the ET tube in your right hand, and insert the tube from the right-side corner of the child's mouth. Do not pass the tube through the channel of the laryngoscope blade, as you will lose sight of the vocal cords. Guide the tube through the vocal cords, and advance the tube until the glottic/vocal cord mark (black band) is positioned just beyond the vocal cords (approximately 2 to 3 cm). Record the depth of the tube as measured at the right-side corner of the child's mouth, and remove the laryngoscope blade.

Carefully remove the stylet if one was used, while holding the tube securely in place. Next, recheck the tube depth to ensure that it did not become displaced during removal of the stylet. If you are using a cuffed ET tube, inflate the cuff until the pilot balloon is full. Suction the tracheal tube if fluid is present. Attach the tube to a bag-valve-mask device with oxygen.

Confirm proper ET tube placement by using one or more techniques. Observe the patient for bilateral chest rise during ventilation. Auscultate the lungs bilaterally at the midaxillary line at the third intercostal space, listening for two breaths in each location. If breath sounds are decreased on the left side, the tube may be positioned too deep and aimed toward or in the right mainstem bronchus. To correct this problem, listen to the left side of the chest while ventilating and *carefully* withdrawing the tube, until breath sounds are equal on both sides of the chest. Re-record the depth of the tube.

Breath sounds travel easily in a child because of a child's small chest size. Auscultate over the epigastrium to ensure that no bubbling or gurgling sounds are present. These sounds indicate oesophageal intubation, mandating immediate removal of the tube, suctioning as needed, and ventilation with a bag-valve-mask device and oxygen prior to reattempting intubation.

Additional clinical methods to confirm proper ET tube placement include improvement in the child's skin colour, pulse rate, and oxygen saturation, as well as use of an $ETCO_2$ detector or oesophageal detector device. When using these devices in children, remember two important points: (1) The adult colourimetric $ETCO_2$ detector cannot be used in children weighing less than 15 kg; and (2) the oesophageal bulb or syringe cannot be used in children weighing less than 20 kg.

After you confirm proper tube placement, hold the ET tube firmly in place and secure it with tape or a commercially available device. Although several methods for securing an ET tube exist, no single method is foolproof. Ideally one person should always hold the tube in place while another properly secures it.

It is important to reconfirm tube placement not only after securing the tube but also following any patient movement (eg, onto the stretcher or into the ambulance), because tubes can easily become dislodged. To do so, auscultate for bilateral breath sounds and epigastric sounds. Once tube position has been confirmed, resume ventilations with oxygen at the appropriate rate.

If you realise the tube is too large or you cannot identify the vocal cords and glottic landmarks, abort the intubation attempt and ventilate the child with the bag-valve-mask device and oxygen. Modify your equipment selection accordingly, and start the procedure from the beginning. If intubation cannot be accomplished after two attempts, discontinue attempts, and resume bag-valve-mask ventilation for the remainder of the transport.

The steps for performing paediatric endotracheal intubation are listed here and shown in **Skill Drill 11-29 ▶**.

1. Take universal precautions (gloves and mask) (Step 1).
2. Check, prepare, and assemble your equipment (Step 2).
3. Manually open the child's airway and insert an adjunct if needed (Step 3).

4. Preoxygenate the child with a bag-valve-mask device attached to oxygen for at least 30 seconds (Step 4).
5. Insert the laryngoscope in the right side of the mouth and sweep the tongue to the left. Lift the tongue with firm, gentle pressure. Avoid using the teeth or gums as a fulcrum (Step 5).
6. Identify the vocal cords. If the cords are not yet visible, instruct your partner to apply cricoid pressure (Step 6).
7. Introduce the ET tube in the right corner of the child's mouth.
8. Pass the ET tube through the vocal cords to approximately 2 to 3 cm below the vocal cords. Inflate the cuff if a cuffed tube is used (Step 7).
9. Attach an ETCO$_2$ detector.
10. Attach the bag-valve-mask device, and auscultate for equal breath sounds over each lateral chest wall high in the axillae. Ensure absence of breath sounds over the epigastrium (Step 8).
11. Secure the ET tube, noting the placement of the distance marker at the child's teeth or gums and reconfirm tube placement (Step 9).

If an intubated child's condition acutely deteriorates, you must take immediate action to identify and correct the underlying problem. The DOPE mnemonic (Displacement, Obstruction, Pneumothorax, and Equipment failure) can be used to recall the common causes of acute deterioration in the intubated child **Table 11-12 ▼**.

Table 11-12	Troubleshooting Acute Deterioration With the DOPE Mnemonic in the Intubated Child
Displacement	■ Reauscultate breath sounds and over the epigastrium ■ If breath sounds are stronger on the right, slowly withdraw the tube until they are equal bilaterally ■ If breath sounds are absent and you hear epigastric gurgling, immediately remove the ET tube, suction as needed, and ventilate with a bag-valve-mask device and using oxygen
Obstruction	■ If thick pulmonary secretions are interfering with your ability to effectively ventilate the intubated child, perform tracheobronchial suctioning ■ Consider tube obstruction if ventilation compliance is decreased (eg, it is hard to squeeze the bag)
Pneumothorax	■ Suspect a pneumothorax if breath sounds are stronger on the *left* and decreased or absent on the right; such findings are not consistent with right mainstem intubation ■ Ventilation compliance may also be decreased in a child with a pneumothorax ■ Prepare to perform needle decompression
Equipment failure	■ Ensure that you are delivering pure oxygen ■ Check the reservoir bag on the bag-valve-mask device for tears, ensure that the device is attached to an oxygen source, and check the bag itself for tears ■ Replace defective or damaged equipment as soon as possible

Skill Drill 11-29: Performing Paediatric Endotracheal Intubation

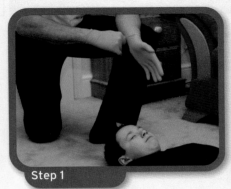

Step 1

Take universal precautions (gloves and mask shield).

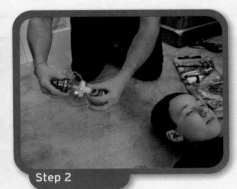

Step 2

Check, prepare, and assemble your equipment.

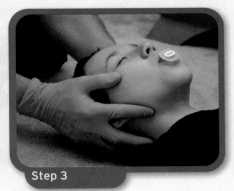

Step 3

Manually open the child's airway and insert an adjunct if needed.

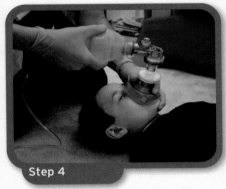

Step 4

Preoxygenate the child with a bag-valve-mask device and 100% oxygen for at least 30 seconds.

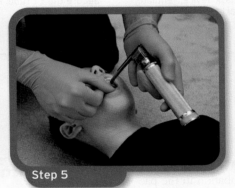

Step 5

Insert the laryngoscope in the right side of the mouth and sweep the tongue to the left. Lift the tongue with firm, gentle pressure. Avoid using the teeth or gums as a fulcrum.

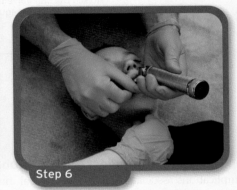

Step 6

Identify the vocal cords. If the cords are not yet visible, instruct your partner to apply cricoid pressure.

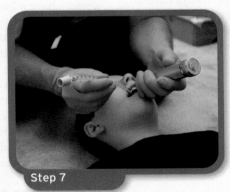

Step 7

Introduce the ET tube in the right corner of the child's mouth. Pass the ET tube through the vocal cords to approximately 2 to 3 cm below the vocal cords. Inflate the cuff if a cuffed tube is used.

Skill Drill 11-29: Performing Paediatric Endotracheal Intubation

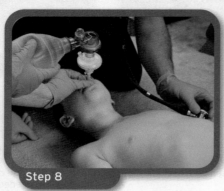

Step 8

Attach the bag-valve-mask device, ventilate, and auscultate for equal breath sounds.

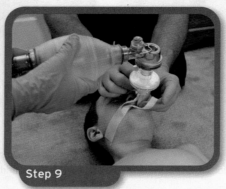

Step 9

Secure the ET tube. Reconfirm tube placement.

Complications of Endotracheal Intubation

Complications associated with endotracheal intubation in the paediatric patient are essentially the same as those for adult patients:

- **Unrecognised oesophageal intubation.** *Frequently* monitor the position of the tube, especially after *any* major patient move.
- **Induction of vomiting and possible aspiration.** *Always* have a suctioning device immediately available and working.
- **Hypoxia resulting from prolonged intubation attempts.** Limit any paediatric intubation attempt to *20 seconds*. Monitor the child's cardiac rhythm and oxygen saturation during intubation.
- **Damage to teeth, soft tissues, and intraoral structures.** Technique, technique, technique!

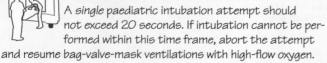

At the Scene

A single paediatric intubation attempt should not exceed 20 seconds. If intubation cannot be performed within this time frame, abort the attempt and resume bag-valve-mask ventilations with high-flow oxygen.

Multilumen Airways

The Combitube and the pharyngeotracheal lumen airway (PtL) have been shown to provide good airway management and ventilation in patients over 150 cm tall Figure 11-58 ▶ . Both devices have a long tube that is blindly inserted into the airway. This tube can be used for either oesophageal obturation or endotracheal intubation; as a result, ventilation is possible regardless of whether the tube is placed into the oesophagus or the trachea. The presence of an oropharyngeal balloon also eliminates the need for a mask seal.

These devices have two lumens, each with a 15/22-mm ventilation adapter. The proper port for ventilation depends on where the tube is positioned during insertion. Both types of multilumen airways have a proximal cuff, which is inflated in the oropharynx to eliminate the need for a face mask.

Indications and Contraindications

Multilumen airways are indicated only for use in deeply unresponsive, apnoeic patients without a gag reflex. If the patient regains consciousness, the device must be removed.

These devices are contraindicated in paediatric patients, and they should be used only for patients between 150 and 215 cm tall.

At the Scene

Hypersensitivity to sedative medications is the primary contraindication to the use of these drugs. Obtain an accurate medical history prior to giving any drug to any patient.

easier and safer to perform. If used improperly, however, it can cause further harm.

The complications associated with sedation in airway management are related primarily to undersedation or oversedation. Undersedation can result in poor patient cooperation, the complications of gagging (eg, trauma, tachycardia, hypertension, vomiting, or aspiration), and incomplete amnesia of the event. Oversedation can result in uncontrolled general anaesthesia, loss of protective airway reflexes, respiratory depression, complete airway collapse, and hypotension.

The level of sedation desired dictates the amount of the medication administered. The patient's response to sedatives is dose dependent. The paramedic should follow local guidelines or should contact medical advice via control for further guidance.

At the Scene

Combativeness, aggressiveness, and belligerence should be considered signs of cerebral hypoxia until proven otherwise. You must be firm and direct, but still treat your patients with respect and empathy. Keep in mind that they are fighting for their lives, not with you.

Neuromuscular Blockade in Emergency Intubation

Cerebral hypoxia can make an ordinarily docile person combative, aggressive, belligerent, and uncooperative. This can make for a very difficult and potentially dangerous situation—both for the patient and for the paramedics. The patient with cerebral hypoxia must be treated with aggressive oxygenation and ventilation, but his or her combativeness often makes this a difficult, if not impossible, task to perform. Clenching of the patient's teeth due to spasm of the jaw muscles (trismus) and vocal cords spasm (laryngospasm) can also hamper your efforts to obtain a definitive airway.

Neuromuscular Blocking Agents

Although sedatives alone can be used to facilitate intubation, the incidence of complications and side effects is unacceptably high. It is much more effective to administer a drug specifically designed to induce paralysis. Paralytic drugs affect every skeletal muscle in the body, including the diaphragm and the inter-

costal muscles. Within about a minute of receiving an IV dose of a paralytic, a patient will become *totally* paralysed. That is, the patient will stop breathing; his or her jaw muscles will go slack, and the base of the tongue will flop back against the posterior pharynx and obstruct the airway. Put bluntly, paralytics convert a breathing patient with a marginal airway into an apnoeic patient with no airway. Before you bring about such a change, you must be *absolutely* sure that you can place an ET tube into the patient's trachea within the next 30 seconds. Once a patient is paralysed, you are completely responsible for that patient's breathing and well-being. Fortunately, paralytic agents do not affect cardiac or smooth muscle.

A paralysed patient will *appear* to be asleep or unconscious, but is not! Paralytic agents, unlike sedatives, have no effect on level of consciousness. The patient is fully aware and can hear, feel, and think.

Pharmacology of Neuromuscular Blocking Agents

To understand how medications induce paralysis, recall how skeletal muscles contract. All skeletal (striated) muscles are voluntary and require input from the somatic nervous system to initiate contraction. As an impulse to contract reaches the terminal end of a motor nerve, acetylcholine (ACh) is released into the synaptic cleft (the junction between the nerve cell and the muscle cell). This neurotransmitter diffuses across the short distance of the synaptic cleft and binds to receptor sites on the motor end plate. Acetylcholine occupying the receptor sites triggers changes in electrical properties of the muscle fibre, a process called depolarisation. When enough motor end plates have been depolarised, a threshold is reached and the muscle fibre contracts. Depolarisation lasts for only a few milliseconds because of the presence of acetylcholinesterase, an enzyme that quickly removes acetylcholine from the synaptic cleft and from the receptors on the motor end plate.

Paralytic medications all function at the neuromuscular junction and relax the muscle by impeding the action of acetylcholine. Collectively, all paralytics are referred to as

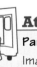

At the Scene

Paralysis Versus Sedation

Imagine what it must be like to be completely paralysed. You can't blink, talk, move, and, most importantly, breathe! You are completely dependent upon others to keep you alive. Paralytic agents to do not induce sedation or amnesia. If you administer only a paralytic agent, the patient will be fully conscious and remember the entire event. Therefore, unless contraindicated, you must sedate a patient who is paralysed. **Paralysis without sedation is a form of patient abuse!**

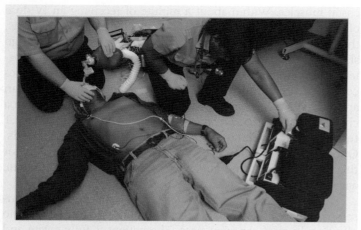

Figure 11-63 Preoxygenate the patient prior to performing rapid-sequence intubation.

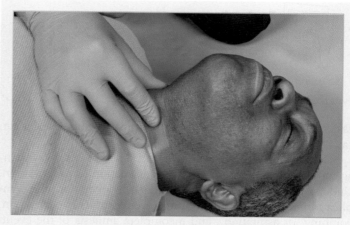

Figure 11-64 A second paramedic should apply posterior cricoid pressure to reduce the risk of regurgitation.

neuromuscular blocking agents. They are classified into two categories: depolarising and nondepolarising agents.

Rapid-Sequence Intubation

Rapid-sequence intubation (RSI) represents a culmination and integration of all of your airway, problem-solving, and decision-making skills into one procedure. It includes the safe, smooth, and rapid induction of sedation and paralysis followed immediately by intubation. Although RSI has been successfully performed in the operating theatre for years, its use in the prehospital setting is relatively new. It is generally used for conscious or combative patients who need to be intubated but who are unable or unwilling to cooperate.

Preparation of the Patient and Equipment

The experience of being intubated is frightening for patients, so you must explain what you are going to do and reassure the patient that he or she will be asleep during the procedure and will not feel or remember anything. Place the patient on a cardiac monitor and pulse oximeter. Check, prepare, and assemble your equipment and ensure that it is in good working order. In particular, have suction *immediately* available.

Preoxygenation

Adequately preoxygenate the patient with oxygen to ensure that positive-pressure ventilation will not be necessary until the patient has been successfully intubated Figure 11-63 ▲ . If the patient is not ventilating adequately, you will need to assist ventilations during the procedure itself.

Premedication

Stimulation of the glottis associated with intubation can cause arrhythmia and a substantial increase in intracranial pressure (ICP)—a particularly problematic issue for patients with closed head injuries or other conditions associated with increased ICP. If you are performing RSI on a patient with closed head trauma, administer lignocaine to decrease the risk of arrhythmias and the spike in ICP associated with stimulation of the upper airway.

 You should administer a defasciculating dose (typically 10% of a normal dose) of a nondepolarising paralytic, if time

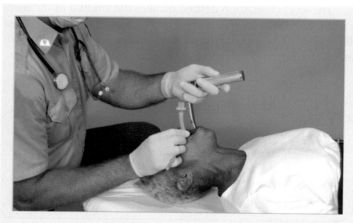

Figure 11-65 Intubate the trachea.

permits. Atropine sulphate should also be administered to decrease the incidence of bradycardia associated with the administration of suxamethonium.

Sedation and Paralysis

As long as the patient is haemodynamically stable (systolic BP > 90 mm Hg), administer a sedative agent to induce sedation and amnesia. Immediately thereafter, administer suxamethonium. Paralysis will begin in 30 seconds and will be complete within 2 minutes.

Posterior Cricoid Pressure

Immediately after the patient is sedated and paralysed, get an assistant to apply posterior cricoid pressure Figure 11-64 ▲ . As long as the patient's oxygen saturation is maintained, do not provide positive-pressure ventilation, as this will significantly increase the risk of regurgitation and aspiration.

Intubation

Intubate the trachea as carefully as possible Figure 11-65 ▲ . If you cannot accomplish the intubation within 30 seconds, stop and ventilate the patient for up to 1 minute with a bag-valve-mask device and the use of oxygen before trying again. *If you must ventilate the patient with a bag-valve-mask, do so slowly*

(1 second per breath [enough to produce visible chest rise]) while maintaining cricoid pressure to minimise the risk of regurgitation. If the patient is inadequately paralysed, you may give a second dose of suxamethonium.

Once the tube is in the trachea, inflate the cuff, remove the stylet, verify correct position of the ET tube, and release cricoid pressure. Secure the tube in place as normal and continue ventilations at the appropriate rate.

Maintenance of Paralysis and Sedation

When you are *absolutely* sure that you have successfully intubated the trachea, administer a nondepolarising blocker to maintain long-term paralysis. Continue to administer a sedative if the patient's blood pressure is adequate. Monitor the patient's heart rate and blood pressure to ensure that sedation is not wearing off.

While the general steps of RSI are the same for all patients, some modification is necessary for unstable patients. If the patient's oxygen saturation drops at any point, you have no choice except to ventilate (just do it slowly). If the patient is haemodynamically unstable, you must judge whether sedation is appropriate or whether the risk of profound hypotension is too great to sedate the patient prior to inducing paralysis. **Table 11-13 ▸** lists sample protocols for RSI in haemodynamically stable and unstable patients.

■ Surgical and Nonsurgical Airways

In most cases, the paramedic is able to secure a patent airway with relative ease using either basic (bag-valve-mask device with oropharyngeal airway) or advanced (endotracheal intubation) methods. In some situations, however, the patient's condition or other factors preclude the use of conventional airway techniques, and a more aggressive and invasive approach should be considered to secure the airway and maximise survival.

Two methods of securing a patent airway can be used when conventional techniques and methods fail: the open (surgical) cricothyroidotomy and translaryngeal cannula ventilation (nonsurgical, or needle cricothyroidotomy). To per-

Table 11-13	Sample Protocols for Rapid-Sequence Intubation

For haemodynamically stable patients
1. Prepare patient and equipment.
2. Preoxygenate with oxygen for at least 2 to 3 minutes.
3. Consider a defasciculating dose of nondepolarising paralytic, lignocaine, or atropine.
4. Sedate.
5. Administer suxamethonium.
6. Apply cricoid pressure.
7. Intubate, verify tube placement, and release cricoid pressure.
8. Administer a nondepolarising paralytic and maintain adequate sedation.

For haemodynamically unstable patients
1. Prepare patient and equipment.
2. Preoxygenate and ventilate as necessary.
3. Consider sedation.
4. Administer suxamethonium.
5. Apply cricoid pressure.
6. Intubate, verify tube placement, and release cricoid pressure.
7. Administer a nondepolarising paralytic.

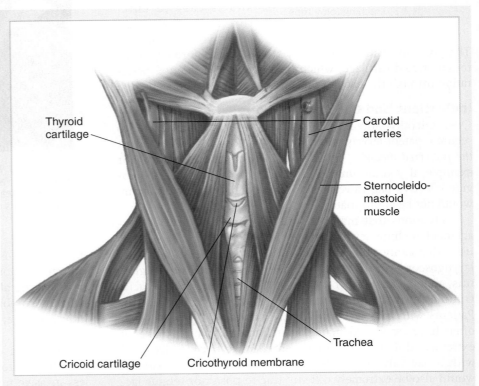

Figure 11-66 Anatomy of the anterior part of the neck.

form these procedures, you must be familiar with the key anatomical landmarks that lie in the anterior aspect of the neck **Figure 11-66 ▲**.

In addition, you must be familiar with the important blood vessels in this area. The superior cricothyroid vessels run at a transverse angle across the upper third of the cricothyroid membrane. The external jugular veins run vertically and are located lateral to the cricothyroid membrane. If the cricothyroid membrane is incised vertically when performing a cricothyroidotomy, the jugular veins can be avoided altogether.

When performing cricothyroidotomy, you should expect to encounter some minor bleeding from the subcutaneous and small skin vessels as you incise the cricothyroid membrane. This bleeding should be easily controlled with light pressure after the tube has been inserted into the trachea.

Open Cricothyroidotomy

Open cricothyroidotomy (surgical cricothyroidotomy) involves incising the cricothyroid membrane with a scalpel and inserting an endotracheal or tracheostomy tube Figure 11-67 ▼ directly into the subglottic area (below the vocal cords) of the trachea. The cricothyroid membrane is the

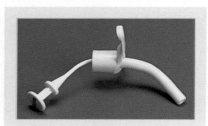

Figure 11-67 Tracheostomy tube.

ideal site for making a surgical opening into the trachea because no important structures lie between the skin and the airway. The airway at this level lies relatively close to the skin and is easy to enter through the thin cricothyroid membrane. The posterior wall of the airway at this level is formed by the tough cricoid cartilage, which helps prevent accidental perforation through the back of the airway into the oesophagus.

Indications and Contraindications

Open cricothyroidotomy is indicated when you are unable to secure a patent airway with more conventional means. *It is not the preferred means of initially securing a patient's airway.* For example, if you are unable to intubate a patient but can provide effective bag-valve-mask ventilations, cricothyroidotomy would not be appropriate.

Situations that may preclude conventional airway management include severe foreign body upper airway obstructions that cannot be extracted with Magill forceps and direct laryngoscopy, airway obstructions from swelling (eg, epiglottitis, anaphylaxis, upper airway burns), massive maxillofacial trauma, and the inability to open the patient's mouth. Patients with massive maxillofacial trauma Figure 11-68 ▶ often have associated mandibular fractures, which makes it extremely difficult to maintain an effective mask-to-face seal with a bag-valve-mask device. Intubation in these patients would also be extremely difficult due to posterior tongue lacerations with profuse bleeding. In such cases, frequent suctioning to prevent aspiration would delay intubation and increase patient hypoxia.

Patients with head injuries and trismus (clenched teeth) may require cricothyroidotomy, especially if you do not have the resources or protocols to perform RSI. Furthermore, head

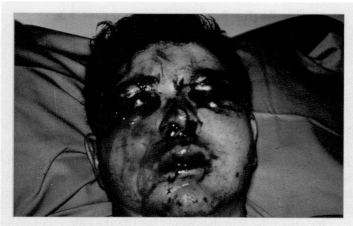

Figure 11-68 Patients with massive maxillofacial trauma often have mandibular fractures or profuse oral bleeding, both of which can make bag-valve-mask ventilations or intubation extremely difficult, if not impossible, to perform.

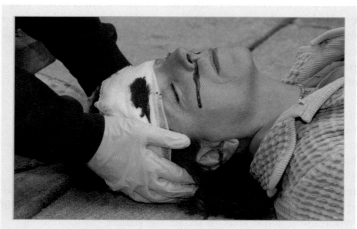

Figure 11-69 Endotracheal intubation may not be possible in patients with a head injury and trismus. Nasotracheal intubation is contraindicated in patients with head injury and fluid drainage from the ears or nose.

injury, which is commonly accompanied by facial trauma, is a contraindication for nasotracheal intubation or placement of a nasopharyngeal airway, especially if fluid is draining from the patient's ears or nose Figure 11-69 ▲ . If this fluid is CSF, it indicates either a basilar skull fracture or a fracture of the cribriform plate.

As noted earlier, the main contraindication for open cricothyroidotomy is the ability to secure a patent airway by less invasive means. Other contraindications include inability to identify the correct anatomical landmarks (cricothyroid membrane), crushing injuries to the larynx and tracheal transection, underlying anatomic abnormalities (eg, trauma, tumours, or subglottic stenosis), and age younger than 8 years. The larynx of a small child is generally unable to support a tube large enough to produce effective ventilation without causing damage to the larynx; you would be safer performing a needle cricothyroidotomy (discussed later in this chapter) in young children.

In situations where cricothyroidotomy is contraindicated, the paramedic must rapidly transport the patient to the closest A&E department, where an emergency tracheostomy can be performed.

Advantages and Disadvantages

Open cricothyroidotomy can be performed quickly, is technically easier than performing a tracheostomy, and can be performed without manipulating the cervical spine. The latter characteristic is especially advantageous because many cricothyrotomies involve patients with massive facial trauma.

Disadvantages of cricothyroidotomy include difficulty in performing the procedure in children (younger than 8 years) and in patients with short, muscular, or fat necks. In contrast to needle cricothyroidotomy, an open cricothyroidotomy is more difficult to perform; however, inserting a large-bore tube (eg, an ET tube or tracheostomy tube) enables you to achieve greater tidal volume, which facilitates more effective oxygenation and ventilation.

Complications

You should expect some minor bleeding when performing an open cricothyroidotomy. More severe bleeding is usually the result of inadvertent laceration of the external jugular vein. Incising the cricothyroid membrane vertically, instead of horizontally, will minimise this potential complication. It will also minimise the risk of damaging the highly vascular thyroid gland. After the incision has been made, *gently* inserting the tube will minimise the risk of perforating the oesophagus or damaging the laryngeal nerves.

An open cricothyroidotomy must be performed quickly. Taking too long to complete a cricothyroidotomy will result in unnecessary hypoxia to the patient, which may result in cardiac arrhythmias, permanent brain injury, or cardiac arrest.

> ### At the Scene
>
> Frequent practice on a special cricothyroido-tomy manikin, will maximise your ability to perform cricothyroidotomy quickly. In general, skills that are not frequently performed in the field should be routinely practised to maintain proficiency and competence within your scope of practice.

Tube misplacement should be suspected when subcutaneous emphysema is encountered after performing a cricothyroidotomy. Subcutaneous emphysema occurs when air infiltrates the subcutaneous (fatty) layers of the skin, and is characterised by a "crackling" sensation when palpated.

Any invasive procedure performed in the prehospital setting carries the risk of infection to the patient. Therefore, you

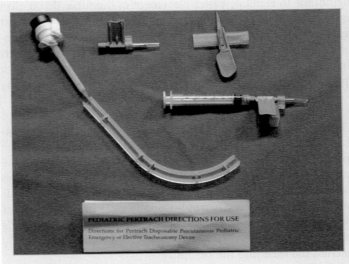

Figure 11-70 Cricothyroidotomy kit.

should make all attempts to maintain aseptic technique when performing an open cricothyroidotomy.

Equipment

Commercially manufactured cricothyroidotomy kits are available **Figure 11-70 ▲** . If such a kit is not available, however, you must prepare the following equipment and supplies:

- Bag-valve-mask device attached to oxygen
- Commercial device (or tape) for securing the tube
- Curved haemostatic forceps
- ETCO$_2$ equiment
- Iodine or equivalent
- New scalpel blade on a new handle
- Sterile gauze pads for minor bleeding control
- Stethoscope
- Suction apparatus and appropriate catheters
- Tape
- Tracheotomy tube (6.0 mm minimum)

Technique for Performing Open Cricothyroidotomy

Once you determine that an open cricothyroidotomy is needed, you must proceed rapidly, yet cautiously. Identify the cricothyroid membrane by palpating for the V notch of the thyroid cartilage, which feels like a high, sharp bump. Stabilise the larynx between your thumb and middle fingers while you palpate with your index finger. When you have located the V notch, slide your index finger down into the depression between the thyroid and cricoid cartilage; that is the cricothyroid membrane.

While you are locating and preparing the site, your partner should be preparing your equipment as well as ensuring that the cardiac monitor and pulse oximeter are attached to the patient.

Maintain aseptic technique as you cleanse the area with iodine or equivalent; avoid touching the area once cleansed. While stabilising the larynx with one hand, make a 1- to 2-cm vertical incision over the cricothyroid membrane. Some advocate making an additional 1-cm incision horizontally across the membrane to facilitate easier placement of the tube. If you elect to do so, remember that the thyroid gland and external jugular veins are lateral to the area and can be damaged if the horizontal incision is too long. Once the incision has been made, insert the curved haemostatic forceps into the opening and spread it apart. Your partner should be readily available to control any bleeding that might occur.

With the trachea exposed, gently insert a 6.0-mm cuffed ET tube or a 6.0 tracheostomy tube and direct it into the trachea. Once the tube is in place, inflate the distal cuff with the appropriate volume of air—typically 5 to 10 ml. Attach the bag-valve-mask device to the standard 15/22-mm adapter on the tube and ventilate the patient while your partner auscultates to ensure the presence of bilaterally clear breath sounds as well as the absence of epigastric sounds. If epigastric sounds are heard, it is likely you have perforated and inadvertently inserted the tube into the oesophagus.

Additional confirmation of correct tube placement can be accomplished by attaching an ETCO₂ detector in between the tube and bag-valve-mask device. After confirming proper tube placement, ensure that any minor bleeding has been controlled, properly secure the tube, and continue to ventilate the patient at the appropriate rate.

The steps for performing an open cricothyroidotomy are listed here and shown in Skill Drill 11-31 ▼ .

1. Take universal precautions (gloves and goggles) Step 1 .
2. Check, assemble, and prepare the equipment Step 2 .
3. With the patient's head in a neutral position, palpate for and locate the cricothyroid membrane Step 3 .
4. Cleanse the area with an iodine-containing solution Step 4 .
5. Stabilise the larynx and make a 1- to 2-cm vertical incision over the cricothyroid membrane Step 5 .
6. Puncture the cricothyroid membrane and make a horizontal cut 1 cm in each direction from the midline Step 6 .
7. Spread the incision apart with curved haemostatic forceps Step 7 .
8. Insert the tube into the trachea Step 8 .
9. Inflate the distal cuff of the tube Step 9 .

Skill Drill 11-31: Performing an Open Cricothyroidotomy

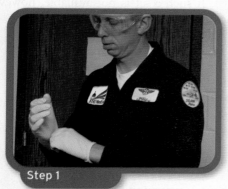

Step 1

Take universal precautions (gloves and goggles).

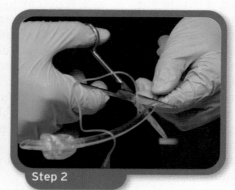

Step 2

Check, assemble, and prepare the equipment.

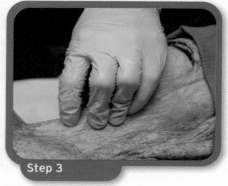

Step 3

With the patient's head in a neutral position, palpate for and locate the cricothyroid membrane.

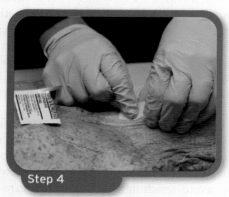

Step 4

Cleanse the area with an iodine-containing solution.

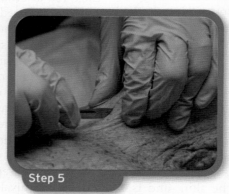

Step 5

Stabilise the larynx and make a 1- to 2-cm vertical incision over the cricothyroid membrane.

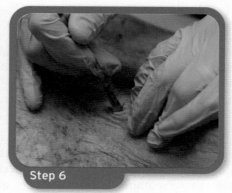

Step 6

Puncture the cricothyroid membrane and make a horizontal cut 1 cm in each direction from the midline.

Skill Drill 11-32: Performing Needle Cricothyroidotomy and Translaryngeal Cannula Ventilation (*continued*)

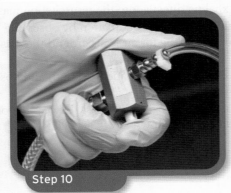

Step 10

Open the release valve on the jet ventilator and adjust the pressure accordingly to provide adequate chest rise.

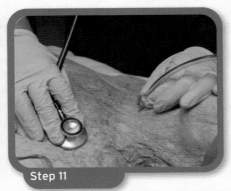

Step 11

Auscultate the apexes and bases of both lungs and over the epigastrium to confirm correct cannula placement.

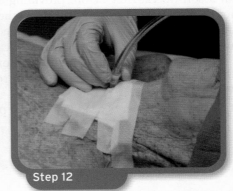

Step 12

Secure the cannula with a 10 × 10 cm gauze pad and tape. Continue ventilations while reassessing for adequate ventilations and potential complications.

Skill Drill 11-33: Suctioning of a Stoma

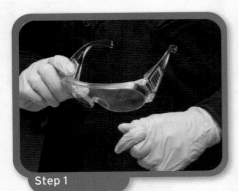

Step 1

Take universal precautions (gloves and face shield).

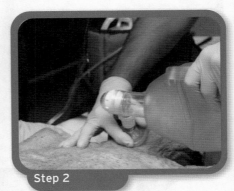

Step 2

Preoxygenate the patient with a bag-valve-mask device and oxygen.

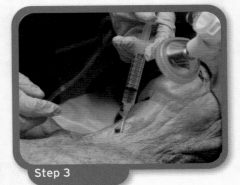

Step 3

Inject 3 ml of saline through the stoma and into the trachea.

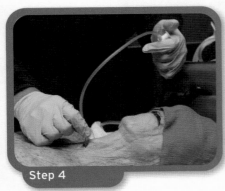

Step 4

Instruct the patient to exhale, and insert the catheter (without providing suction) until resistance is felt (no more than 12 cm).

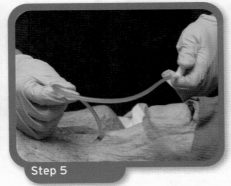

Step 5

Suction while withdrawing the catheter as you instruct the patient to cough or exhale.

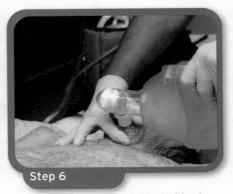

Step 6

Resume oxygenating the patient with a bag-valve-mask device and oxygen.

be needed to perform bag-valve-mask device-to-stoma ventilations: one to seal the nose and mouth and the other to squeeze the bag-valve-mask device. If you are unable to ventilate a patient who has a stoma, try suctioning the stoma and mouth with a soft-tip catheter before providing artificial ventilation through the nose and mouth. If you seal the stoma during ventilation, the ability to artificially ventilate the patient in this way may be improved, or it may help to clear any obstructions.

The steps for performing mouth-to-stoma ventilation with a resuscitation mask are listed here and shown in **Skill Drill 11-34 ▾**.

1. Position the patient's head in a neutral position with the shoulders slightly elevated (**Step 1**).

2. Locate and expose the stoma site (**Step 2**).
3. Place the resuscitation mask (paediatric mask preferred) over the stoma, and ensure an adequate seal (**Step 3**).
4. Maintain the patient's neutral head position, and ventilate the patient by exhaling directly into the resuscitation mask.
5. Assess the patient for adequate ventilation by observing his or her chest rise and feeling for air leaks around the mask (**Step 4**)
6. If air leakage is evident, seal the patient's mouth and nose and ventilate (**Step 5**).

The steps for performing bag-valve-mask device-to-stoma ventilation are listed here and shown in **Skill Drill 11-35 ▸**.

Skill Drill 11-34: Mouth-to-Stoma Ventilation (Using a Resuscitation Mask)

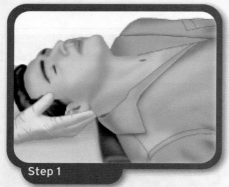

Step 1

Position the patient's head in a neutral position with the shoulders slightly elevated.

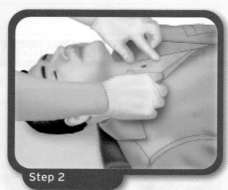

Step 2

Locate and expose the stoma site.

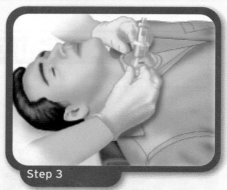

Step 3

Place the resuscitation mask (paediatric mask preferred) over the stoma, and ensure an adequate seal.

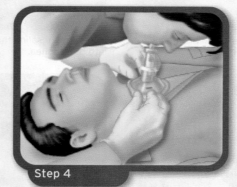

Step 4

Maintain the patient's neutral head position, and ventilate the patient by exhaling directly into the resuscitation mask.

Assess the patient for adequate ventilation by observing his or her chest rise and feeling for air leaks around the mask.

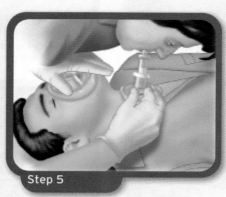

Step 5

If air leakage is evident, seal the patient's mouth and nose and ventilate.

Prep Kit

Ready for Review

- The upper airway consists of all structures above the vocal cords—the larynx, oropharynx, nasopharynx, and tongue. Its functions include warming, filtering, and humidification of inhaled air.

- The lower airway consists of all structures below the vocal cords—the trachea, mainstem bronchi, bronchioles, pulmonary capillaries, and alveoli. Pulmonary gas exchange takes place at the alveolar level in the lungs.

- The diaphragm is the major muscle of breathing; it is innervated by the phrenic nerves. The intercostal muscles, the muscles between the ribs, are innervated by the intercostal nerves. Accessory muscles, which are used during times of respiratory distress, include the sternocleidomastoid muscles of the neck.

- The primary breathing stimulus in a healthy patient is based on increasing arterial carbon dioxide levels. The hypoxic drive—a backup system for breathing—is based on decreasing arterial oxygen levels.

- Ventilation is the movement of air into and out of the lungs. Negative-pressure ventilation is the drawing of air into the lungs due to changes in intrathoracic pressure. Positive-pressure ventilation is the forcing of air into the lungs and is provided via bag-valve-mask device, pocket mask, or mechanical ventilation device to patients who are not breathing (apnoeic) or are breathing inadequately.

- Manual airway manoeuvres include the head tilt–chin lift, jaw-thrust (with and without head tilt), and the tongue-jaw lift.

- Regardless of the patient's condition, his or her airway must remain patent at all times. Clearing the airway means removing obstructing material; maintaining the airway means keeping it open, manually or with adjunctive devices.

- Airway obstruction can be caused by choking on food (or, in children, on toys), epiglottitis, inhalation injuries, airway trauma with swelling, and anaphylaxis. It is critical to differentiate between a mild (partial) airway obstruction and a severe (complete) airway obstruction.

- Chest compressions, ventilations, and airway inspection should be performed to relieve an obstructed airway in an unconscious patient.

- Back slaps and chest thrusts are performed to relieve a severe airway obstruction in conscious infants. Chest compressions are performed in unconscious infants with a severe airway obstruction.

- Patients with a mild airway obstruction should be closely monitored and transported. Encourage the patient who is coughing forcefully to continue coughing, as it is the most effective way of clearing the airway.

- If conventional methods of airway obstruction removal fail, perform direct laryngoscopy and attempt to retrieve the object with Magill forceps.

- Basic airway adjuncts include the oropharyngeal airway and the nasopharyngeal airway. The oropharyngeal airway keeps the tongue off of the posterior pharynx; it is used only in unresponsive patients without a gag reflex. The nasopharyngeal airway is better tolerated in patients with altered mental status who have an intact gag reflex.

- Oropharyngeal suctioning may be required after opening a patient's airway. Rigid catheters are preferred when suctioning the pharynx. Soft-tip catheters are used to suction secretions from the nose, and can be passed down the endotracheal tube to suction pulmonary secretions.

- Oropharyngeal suction should be limited to 15 seconds in the adult, 10 seconds in the child, and 5 seconds in the infant.

- The recovery position involves placing the patient in a left lateral recumbent position. It is the preferred position to maintain the airway of unconscious patients without traumatic injuries, who are breathing adequately.

- Adequate breathing features a respiratory rate between 12 and 20 breaths/min, adequate depth (tidal volume), a regular pattern of inhalation and exhalation, symmetrical chest rise, and bilaterally clear and equal breath sounds.

- Inadequate breathing features a rate that is too slow (< 12 breaths/min) or too fast (> 20 breaths/min), a shallow depth of breathing (reduced tidal volume), an irregular pattern of inhalation and exhalation, asymmetrical chest movement, adventitious airway sounds, cyanosis, and an altered mental status.

- The nonrebreathing mask is the preferred device for delivering oxygen to patients who are breathing adequately in the prehospital setting; it can deliver up to 98% oxygen when the flow rate is set at 15 l/min. The nasal cannula should be used if the patient cannot tolerate the nonrebreathing mask; it can deliver oxygen concentrations of 24% to 44% when the flowmeter is set at 1 to 6 l/min. Other types of oxygen delivery devices include the simple medium concentration mask, partial rebreathing mask, and Venturi mask.

- The pulse oximeter measures the percentage of blood that is saturated with oxygen (SpO_2). This type of measurement depends on adequate perfusion to the capillary beds and can be inaccurate when the patient is cold, is in shock, or has been exposed to carbon monoxide.

- Peak expiratory flow is a fairly reliable assessment of the severity of a patient's bronchoconstriction. It is also used to gauge the effectiveness of treatment, such as an inhaled beta-2 agonists.

- Patients with inadequate breathing require some form of positive-pressure ventilation; patients with adequate breathing who are suspected of being hypoxaemic require supplemental oxygen via nonrebreathing mask. Never withhold oxygen from any patient suspected of being hypoxaemic.

- Unrecognised inadequate breathing will lead to hypoxia, a dangerous condition in which the body's cells and tissues do not receive adequate oxygen.

- The methods of providing artificial ventilation—in order of preference—include the mouth-to-mask technique; the two-person bag-valve-mask technique; the flow-restricted, oxygen-powered ventilation device (FROPVD); and the one-person bag-valve-mask technique. Use extreme caution with the FROPVD and never use this device in children and those with cervical spine or thoracic injuries.

- Combined with your own exhaled breath, mouth-to-mask ventilation with supplemental oxygen attached will deliver approximately 55% oxygen to the patient. A bag-valve-mask device with supplemental oxygen, a reservoir, and an adequate mask-to-face seal can deliver < 95% oxygen.

- Ventilating too forcefully or too fast can cause gastric distension, which can cause regurgitation and aspiration. Delivering ventilations over 1 second and the use of posterior cricoid pressure (Sellick manoeuvre) will reduce the incidence of gastric distension and the associated risk of regurgitation/aspiration.

- Unresponsive patients or patients who cannot maintain their own airway should be considered candidates for endotracheal intubation, the insertion of an endotracheal (ET) tube into the trachea.

www.Paramedic.EMSzone.com/UK/

- Tracheobronchial suctioning is indicated if the condition of the intubated patient deteriorates due to pulmonary secretions in the ET tube.
- Extubation should not be performed in the prehospital setting unless the patient is unreasonably intolerant of the tube. It is generally best to sedate the intubated patient who is becoming intolerant of the ET tube.
- Alternative airway devices, which may be used if endotracheal intubation is not possible or is unsuccessful, include the laryngeal mask airway (LMA).
- Paediatric endotracheal intubation involves a similar technique as for adult patients, but with smaller equipment.
- Patients with a tracheal stoma or tracheostomy tube may require ventilation, suctioning, or tube replacement. Ventilation through a tracheostomy tube involves attaching the bag-valve-mask device to the 15/22-mm adapter on the tube; ventilation of the patient with a stoma and no tracheostomy tube can be performed with a pocket mask or bag-valve-mask device. Use paediatric-size masks when ventilating a patient through his or her stoma.
- Open (surgical) cricothyroidotomy involves incising the cricothyroid membrane, inserting a tracheostomy tube or ET tube into the trachea, and ventilating the patient with a bag-valve-mask device. Needle cricothyroidotomy involves inserting a 14 gauge over-the-needle cannula through the cricothyroid membrane and ventilating the patient with a high-pressure jet ventilation device.
- Rapid-sequence intubation (RSI) involves using pharmacological agents to sedate and paralyse the patient to facilitate placement of an ET tube. It should be considered when a conscious or combative patient requires intubation but cannot tolerate laryngoscopy.
- Drugs used for RSI include sedatives, such as diazepam and midazolam, and neuromuscular blocking agents (paralytics) to induce complete paralysis. The latter agents are classified into depolarising paralytics (eg, suxamethonium) and nondepolarising paralytics (eg, vecuronium, pancuronium).
- Check for loose dental appliances in a patient before providing artificial ventilation. Loose dental appliances should be removed to prevent them from obstructing the airway; tight-fitting dental appliances should be left in place during artificial ventilation.
- Dental appliances should be removed before intubating a patient. Removing them after the patient has been intubated may result in inadvertent extubation.
- Patients with massive maxillofacial trauma are at high risk for airway compromise due to oral bleeding. Assist ventilations and provide oral suctioning as needed.

■■ Vital Vocabulary

accessory muscles Muscles not normally used during normal breathing; includes the sternocleidomastoid muscles of the neck.

acetylcholine (ACh) Chemical neurotransmitter of the parasympathetic nervous system.

adenoids Lymphatic tissues located on the posterior nasopharyngeal wall that filter bacteria.

alveolar volume Volume of inhaled air that reaches the alveoli and participates in gas exchange; equal to tidal volume minus dead space volume and is approximately 350 ml in the average adult.

alveoli Balloon-like clusters of single-layer air sacs that are the functional site for the exchange of oxygen and carbon dioxide in the lungs.

anatomic dead space Includes the trachea and larger bronchi. The air remaining in these areas is the result of residual gas in the upper airway at the end of inhalation.

anoxia An absence of oxygen.

aphonia Inability to speak.

arytenoid cartilages Pyramid-like cartilaginous structures that form the posterior attachment of the vocal cords.

aspiration Entry of fluids or solids into the trachea, bronchi, and lungs.

asymmetric chest wall movement When one side of the chest moves less than the other; indicates decreased airflow into one lung.

atelectasis Collapsing of the alveoli.

atlanto-occipital joint Joint formed at the articulation of the atlas of the vertebral column and the occipital bone of the skull.

automatic transport ventilator (ATV) Portable mechanical ventilator attached to a control box that allows the variables of ventilation (eg, rate, tidal volume) to be set.

bag-valve-mask device Manual ventilation device that consists of a bag, mask, one-way valves, reservoir, and oxygen inlet; capable of delivering up to 95% oxygen.

barotrauma Trauma resulting from excessive pressure.

Bourdon-gauge flowmeter An oxygen flowmeter that is commonly used because it is not affected by gravity and can be placed in any position.

bronchioles Subdivision of the smaller bronchi in the lungs; made of smooth muscle and dilate or constrict in response to various stimuli.

capnographer Device that attaches in between the endotracheal tube and bag-valve-mask device; contains colorimetric paper, which should turn yellow during exhalation, indicating proper tube placement.

capnometer Device that attaches in the same way as a capnographer, but provides a light-emitting diode (LED) readout of the patient's exhaled carbon dioxide.

carboxyhaemoglobin Abnormal haemoglobin that is formed by the attachment of carbon monoxide to the haemoglobin molecule.

carina Point at which the trachea bifurcates into the left and right mainstem bronchi.

cerebrospinal otorrhoea Cerebrospinal fluid drainage from the ears.

cerebrospinal rhinorrhoea Cerebrospinal fluid drainage from the nose.

chemoreceptors Monitor the levels of O_2, CO_2, and the pH of the CSF and then provide feedback to the respiratory centres to modify the rate and depth of breathing based on the body's needs at any given time.

Combitube Multilumen airway device that consists of a single tube with two lumens, two balloons, and two ventilation ports; an alternative device if endotracheal intubation or an LMA is not possible or has failed.

cricoid cartilage Forms the lowest portion of the larynx; also referred to as the cricoid ring; the first ring of the trachea and is the only upper airway structure that forms a complete ring.

cricoid pressure The application of posterior pressure to the cricoid cartilage to reduce the risk of regurgitation during positive-pressure ventilation; also called the Sellick manoeuvre.

cricothyroid membrane A thin, superficial membrane located between the thyroid and cricoid cartilages that is relatively avascular and contains few nerves; the site for emergency surgical and nonsurgical access to the airway.

curved laryngoscope blade Also called the Macintosh blade; designed to fit into the vallecula, indirectly lifting the epiglottis and exposing the vocal cords.

dead space Any portion of the airway that does not contain air and cannot participate in gas exchange.

defasciculating dose A drug dose to limit or stop the involuntary twitching and jerking of nerve ends and muscles.

diaphragm The major muscle of breathing. It is the anatomical point of separation between the thoracic cavity and the abdominal cavity.

diffusion Movement of a gas from an area of higher concentration to an area of lower concentration.

digital intubation Method of intubation that involves directly palpating the glottic structures and elevating the epiglottis with your middle finger while guiding the ET tube into the trachea by feel.

direct laryngoscopy Visualisation of the airway with a laryngoscope.

dysphonia Difficulty speaking.

dyspnoea Any difficulty in respiratory rate, regularity, or effort.

endotracheal (ET) tube Tube that is inserted into the trachea; equipped with a distal cuff, proximal inflation port, a 15/22-mm adapter, and cm markings on the side.

end-tidal carbon dioxide (ETCO$_2$) detectors Device that detects the presence of carbon dioxide in exhaled air.

epiglottis Leaf-shaped cartilaginous structure that closes over the trachea during swallowing.

exhalation Passive movement of air out of the lungs; also called expiration.

expiration Passive movement of air out of the lungs; also called exhalation.

expiratory reserve volume The amount of air that you can exhale following a normal exhalation; average volume is about 1,200 ml.

external respiration The exchange of gases between the lungs and the blood cells in the pulmonary capillaries; also called pulmonary respiration.

extubation The process of removing the tube from an intubated patient.

face mask A full mask enclosure with open side ports. Room air is drawn in through the side ports on inhalation, diluting the concentration of inspired oxygen. Exhaled air is vented through holes on each side of the mask. The face mask will deliver between 40% and 60% oxygen at 10 l/min.

flow-restricted, oxygen-powered ventilation device (FROPVD) Also referred to as a manually triggered ventilator or demand valve. Can be used to ventilate apnoeic or to administer supplemental oxygen to spontaneously breathing patients.

fraction of inspired oxygen (FiO$_2$) The percentage of oxygen in inhaled air.

functional reserve capacity The amount of air that can be forced from the lungs in a single exhalation.

gag reflex Automatic reaction when something touches an area deep in the oral cavity; helps protect the lower airway from aspiration.

gastric distension Inflation of the patient's stomach with air.

glottis The space in between the vocal cords that is the narrowest portion of the adult's airway; also called the glottic opening.

gum elastic bougie Also called the Eschmann stylet; a flexible device that is inserted in between the glottis under direct laryngoscopy. The ET tube is then threaded over the device, facilitating its entry into the trachea.

haemoglobin An iron-containing protein within red blood cells that has the ability to combine with oxygen.

head tilt-chin lift manoeuvre Manual airway manoeuvre that involves tilting the head back while lifting up on the chin; used to open the airway of a semiconscious or unconscious nontrauma patient.

Heimlich manoeuvre Abdominal thrusts performed to relieve a foreign body airway obstruction.

Hering-Breuer reflex A protective mechanism that terminates inhalation, thus preventing overexpansion of the lungs.

hilum Point of entry of all of the blood vessels and the bronchi into each lung.

hyoid bone A small, horseshoe-shaped bone to which the jaw, tongue, epiglottis, and thyroid cartilage attach.

hypercarbia Increased CO$_2$ content in arterial blood.

hyperventilation Occurs when CO$_2$ elimination exceeds CO$_2$ production.

hypocarbia Decreased CO$_2$ content in arterial blood.

hypoventilation Occurs when CO$_2$ production exceeds the body's ability to eliminate it by ventilation.

hypoxaemia A decrease in arterial oxygen levels.

hypoxia A lack of oxygen to the body's cells and tissues.

hypoxic drive Secondary control of breathing that stimulates breathing based on decreased pO_2 levels.

inspiration The active process of moving air into the lungs; also called inhalation.

inspiratory reserve volume The amount of air that can be inhaled after a normal inhalation; the amount of air that can be inhaled in addition to the normal tidal volume.

intercostal nerves Nerves that innervate the external intercostal muscles, the muscles between the ribs.

internal respiration The exchange of gases between the blood cells and the tissues; also called cellular respiration.

intrapulmonary shunting Bypassing of oxygen-poor blood past nonfunctional alveoli.

jaw-thrust manoeuvre Manual airway manoeuvre that involves stabilising the patient's head and thrusting the jaw forward; the preferred method of opening the airway of a semiconscious or unconscious trauma patient.

jaw-thrust manoeuvre with head tilt Manual airway manoeuvre that involves thrusting the jaw forward while tilting back on the head.

laryngeal mask airway (LMA) Device that surrounds the opening of the larynx with a silicone cuff positioned in the hypopharynx; an alternative device to bag-valve-mask ventilation.

laryngectomy A surgical procedure in which the larynx is removed.

laryngospasm Spasmodic closure of the vocal cords.

larynx A complex structure formed by many independent cartilaginous structures that all work together; where the upper airway ends and the lower airway begins.

lung compliance The ability of the alveoli to expand when air is drawn into the lungs, either during negative-pressure ventilation or positive-pressure ventilation.

Magill forceps A special type of forcep that is curved, thus allowing the paramedic to manoeuvre it in the airway.

minute volume The amount of air that moves in and out of the respiratory tract per minute.

Murphy's eye An opening on the side of an endotracheal tube at its distal tip that enables ventilation to occur even if the tip becomes occluded by blood, mucus, or the tracheal wall.

nasal cannula Delivers oxygen via two small prongs that fit into the patient's nostrils. With an oxygen flow rate of 1 to 6 l/min, the nasal cannula can deliver an oxygen concentration of 24% to 44%.

nasal septum A rigid partition composed of bone and cartilage; divides the nasopharynx into two passages.

nasopharyngeal airway A soft rubber tube that is inserted through the nose into the posterior pharynx behind the tongue, thereby allowing passage of air from the nose to the lower airway.

nasopharynx The nasal cavity; formed by the union of the facial bones.

nasotracheal intubation Insertion of an endotracheal tube into the trachea through the nose.

nebuliser Device used primarily to deliver aerosolised medications. Oxygen enters an aerosol chamber that contains 3 to 5 ml of fluid. The pressurised oxygen in this chamber aerosolises the medication for inhalation.

needle cricothyroidotomy Insertion of a 14- to 16-gauge over-the-needle IV catheter (angiocath) through the cricothyroid membrane and into the trachea.

negative-pressure ventilation Drawing of air into the lungs; airflow from a region of higher pressure (outside the body) to a region of lower pressure (the lungs); occurs during normal (unassisted breathing).

nonrebreathing mask A combination mask and reservoir bag system. Oxygen fills a reservoir bag that is attached to the mask by a one-way valve. This permits the patient to inhale from the reservoir bag but not to exhale back into it. With a good mask-to-face seal and a flow rate of 15 l/min, it is capable of delivering up to 90% inspired oxygen.

oesophageal detector device (EDD) Bulb or syringe that is attached to the proximal end of the ET tube; a device used to confirm proper ET tube placement.

open cricothyroidotomy Also referred to as a surgical cricothyroidotomy; an emergent procedure that involves incising the cricothyroid membrane with a scalpel and inserting an endotracheal or tracheostomy tube directly into the subglottic area of the trachea.

oropharyngeal airway A hard plastic device that is curved in such a way that it fits over the back of the tongue with the tip in the posterior pharynx.

orthopnoea Positional dyspnoea.

oxyhaemoglobin Haemoglobin that is occupied by oxygen.

palate Forms the roof of the mouth and separates the oropharynx and nasopharynx.

parietal pleura Thin membrane that lines the chest cavity.

partial laryngectomy Surgical removal of a portion of the larynx.

patent Open.

peak expiratory flow An approximation of the extent of bronchoconstriction; used to determine whether patients are improving with therapy (eg, inhaled bronchodilators).

pharyngeotracheal lumen airway (PtL) Multilumen airway device that consists of two tubes and two cuffs; an alternative device if endotracheal intubation is not possible or has failed.

pharynx Throat.

phrenic nerves Nerves that innervate the diaphragm.

physiological dead space Additional dead space created by intrapulmonary obstructions or atelectasis.

pneumotaxic centre Area of the brain stem that has an inhibitory influence on inspiration.

positive-pressure ventilation Forcing of air into the lungs.

pressure-compensated flowmeter An oxygen flowmeter that incorporates a float ball within a tapered calibrated tube. The float rises or falls according to the gas flow within the tube. Because this type of flowmeter is affected by gravity, it must remain in an upright position to obtain an accurate flow reading.

primary respiratory drive Normal stimulus to breathe; based on fluctuations in $_PCO_2$ and pH of the CSF.

pulse oximeter Device that measures oxygen saturation.

pulsus paradoxus A drop in the systolic BP of 10 mm Hg or more; commonly seen in patients with pericardial tamponade or severe asthma.

pyriform fossae Two pockets of tissue on the lateral borders of the larynx.

rapid-sequence intubation (RSI) A specific set of procedures, combined in rapid succession, to induce sedation and paralysis and intubate a patient quickly.

recession Skin pulling in between and around the ribs during inhalation.

recovery position Left-lateral recumbent position; used in all semiconscious and unconscious nontrauma patients, who are able to maintain their own airway spontaneously and are breathing adequately.

residual volume The air that remains in the lungs after maximal expiration.

respiration The exchange of gases between a living organism and its environment.

safe residual pressure A term that implies that it is unsafe to continue using an oxygen cylinder with a pressure of less than 200 psi.

sedation Reduction of a patient's anxiety, induction of amnesia, and suppression of the gag reflex.

Sellick manoeuvre The application of posterior pressure to the cricoid cartilage to minimise the risk of regurgitation during positive-pressure ventilation; also referred to as cricoid pressure.

sinuses Cavities formed by the cranial bones that trap contaminants from entering the respiratory tract and act as tributaries for fluid to and from the eustachian tubes and tear ducts.

stenosis Narrowing.

stoma The resultant orifice of a tracheostomy that connects the trachea to the outside air; located in the midline of the anterior neck.

straight laryngoscope blade Also called the Miller blade; designed to lift the epiglottis and expose the vocal cords.

surfactant A proteinaceous substance that lines the alveoli; decreases alveolar surface tension and keeps the alveoli expanded.

therapy regulator Attaches to the stem of the oxygen cylinder, and reduces the high pressure of gas to a safe range (about 50 psi).

thyroid cartilage The main supporting cartilage of the larynx; a shield-shaped structure formed by two plates that join in a "V" shape anteriorly to form the laryngeal prominence known as the Adam's apple.

tidal volume A measure of the depth of breathing; the volume of air that is inhaled or exhaled during a single respiratory cycle.

tongue-jaw lift manoeuvre A manual manoeuvre that involves grasping the tongue and jaw and lifting; commonly used to suction the airway and to place certain airway devices.

tonsils Lymphatic tissues that are located in the posterior pharynx; they help to trap bacteria.

total laryngectomy Surgical removal of the entire larynx.

total lung capacity The total volume of air that the lungs can hold; approximately 6 l in the average adult male.

trachea The conduit for all entry into the lungs; a tubular structure that is approximately 10 to 12 cm in length and is composed of a series of C-shaped cartilaginous rings; also called the windpipe.

tracheobronchial suctioning Passing a suction catheter into the endotracheal tube to remove pulmonary secretions.

tracheostomy Surgical opening into the trachea.

tracheostomy tube Plastic tube placed within the tracheostomy site (stoma).

translaryngeal cannula ventilation Used in conjunction with needle cricothyroidotomy to ventilate a patient; requires a high-pressure jet ventilator.

upper airway Consists of all anatomical airway structures above the level of the vocal cords.

uvula A soft-tissue structure that resembles a punch bag; located in the posterior aspect of the oral cavity, at the base of the tongue.

vallecula An anatomical space, or "pocket", located between the base of the tongue and the epiglottis; an important anatomic landmark for endotracheal intubation.

ventilation The process of moving air into and out of the lungs.

Venturi mask A mask that has a number of interchangeable adapters that draws room air into the mask along with the oxygen flow; allows for the administration of highly specific oxygen concentrations.

visceral pleura Thin membrane that lines the lungs.

vocal cords White bands of tough tissue that are the lateral borders of the glottis.

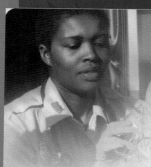

Assessment in Action

You are dispatched to a house for an "unconscious male". You arrive at the scene 6 minutes after being dispatched and are met at the door of the residence by a frantic woman.

Your initial assessment reveals that the man is unresponsive. His respirations are slow and shallow, and his pulse is rapid and weak. Further assessment reveals facial cyanosis and vomitus around his mouth. The patient's wife tells you that she thinks her husband has had a stroke. You and your partner begin immediate treatment.

1. **Vomitus that has been aspirated into the lungs will:**
   A. cause a rapid, fatal infection.
   B. impair pulmonary diffusion.
   C. increase ventilation compliance.
   D. require deep tracheal suctioning.

2. **The goal of providing assisted ventilation to a hypoventilating patient is to:**
   A. minimise hypocarbia.
   B. reduce gastric distension.
   C. improve cardiac output.
   D. maintain minute volume.

3. **Signs of adequate ventilation in the adult include:**
   A. pink mucous membranes.
   B. a prolonged exhalation phase.
   C. a shallow depth of breathing.
   D. respirations of 30 breaths/min.

4. **Positive-pressure ventilation is defined as:**
   A. forcing air into the lungs.
   B. drawing air into the lungs.
   C. deep spontaneous breathing.
   D. a reduction in tidal volume.

5. **Which of the following oxygen delivery devices is MOST appropriate for a patient with suspected hypoxaemia and adequate tidal volume?**
   A. Nasal cannula
   B. Simple face mask
   C. Nonrebreathing mask
   D. bag-valve-mask device with reservoir

6. **Negative-pressure ventilation occurs when:**
   A. the diaphragm relaxes and ascends.
   B. pressure within the thoracic cavity decreases.
   C. air is blown into the lungs with a bag-valve-mask device.
   D. a patient is ventilated with a demand valve.

7. **The volume of air moved into and out of the lungs per breath is called:**
   A. tidal volume.
   B. stroke volume.
   C. minute volume.
   D. alveolar volume.

8. **The primary respiratory drive in a healthy individual is based on:**
   A. decreasing pO_2 levels.
   B. the pH of venous blood.
   C. progressive hypocarbia.
   D. increasing pCO_2 levels.

9. **In contrast to hypoxia, hypoxaemia is defined as:**
   A. a complete lack of oxygen to the brain.
   B. a deficiency of oxygen in the arterial blood.
   C. decreased oxygen to the body's tissues and cells.
   D. an insufficient supply of oxygen to the myocardium.

10. **What is the MOST commonly encountered problem when ventilating a patient with the one-person bag-valve-mask technique?**
    A. Inability to squeeze the bag
    B. Forgetting to attach the reservoir
    C. Difficulty maintaining a mask seal
    D. Not manually positioning the head

11. **The phrenic nerves innervate the:**
    A. diaphragm.
    B. intercostal muscles.
    C. accessory muscles.
    D. pons and medulla.

12. **Physiological dead space would increase with:**
    A. atelectatic alveoli.
    B. increased tidal volume.
    C. reduced minute volume.
    D. gastric distension.

13. **Alveolar surface tension would increase with:**
    A. positive-pressure ventilation.
    B. inadvertent oesophageal intubation.
    C. increased ventilatory compliance.
    D. a deficiency of pulmonary surfactant.

14. **What is the usual anatomical dead space volume in the average adult male?**
    A. 70 ml
    B. 150 ml
    C. 200 ml
    D. 350 ml

15. **The exchange of gases between a living organism and its environment is called:**
    A. ventilation.
    B. respiration.
    C. expiration.
    D. inhalation.

16. **If performed properly, the Sellick manoeuvre will minimise the risk of:**
    A. shallow breathing.
    B. excessive tidal volume.
    C. gastric distension.
    D. tracheal intubation.

17. **The volume of air that remains in the lungs after maximal expiration is called:**
    A. residual volume.
    B. expiratory reserve volume.
    C. inspiratory reserve volume.
    D. functional reserve capacity.

18. **A patient who has an altered mental status and has shallow respirations should be treated initially with:**
    A. immediate endotracheal intubation.
    B. a nonrebreathing mask at 15 l/min.
    C. insertion of a laryngeal mask airway.
    D. some form of positive-pressure ventilation.

19. **Which of the following MOST accurately describes pulsus paradoxus?**
    A. An increase in the heart rate during inhalation
    B. A decrease in systolic BP during inhalation
    C. An increase in diastolic BP during exhalation
    D. A decrease in the heart rate during exhalation

20. **Which of the following respiratory patterns is characterised by occasional, irregular, shallow breaths?**
    A. Biot breathing
    B. Agonal breathing
    C. Cheyne-Stokes breathing
    D. Kussmaul breathing

21. **Immediately after inserting an endotracheal tube through the vocal cords, the paramedic should:**
    A. begin ventilations.
    B. attach an ETCO$_2$ detector.
    C. inflate the distal cuff.
    D. auscultate for breath sounds.

22. **To properly align the three airway axes prior to endotracheal intubation, the patient's head should be placed in what position?**
    A. Sniffing
    B. Flexed
    C. Extended
    D. Neutral

23. **Multilumen airway devices are not intended to be used in patients who:**
    A. are deeply unconscious.
    B. weigh more than 75 kg.
    C. have an oesophageal disease.
    D. are in cardiopulmonary arrest.

24. **Following a needle cricothyroidotomy, ventilations are MOST effectively performed with which of the following devices?**
    A. bag-valve-mask device and oxygen
    B. Flow-restricted oxygen-powered device
    C. ET tube adapter and a 10-ml syringe
    D. High-pressure jet ventilation device

25. **Medications used during rapid-sequence intubation (RSI) include which of the following?**
    A. Adrenaline
    B. Suxamethonium
    C. Amiodarone
    D. Furosemide

Points to Ponder

Your colleague is attempting to perform endotracheal intubation on a middle-aged unconscious, apnoeic man. The patient is attached to a cardiac monitor, which is displaying a normal sinus rhythm, and a pulse oximeter, which is reading 98%. Approximately 15 seconds into the intubation attempt, you note that the patient's heart rate has dropped approximately 30 beats/min and the pulse oximeter now reads 82%. You immediately advise your colleague of the change in the patient's condition, to which he replies, "I still have 15 seconds left". He continues with the intubation attempt, which is successful.

As you are in the process of securing the ET tube in place, the patient experiences cardiac arrest. Despite aggressive management and prompt transport to hospital, the patient dies.

Why did this patient experience cardiac arrest? What could have been done to prevent it?

Issues: Knowing When to Abort an Intubation Attempt, Understanding the Importance of Adequate Oxygenation and Ventilation, Working Effectively as a Team.

www.Paramedic.EMSzone.com/UK/

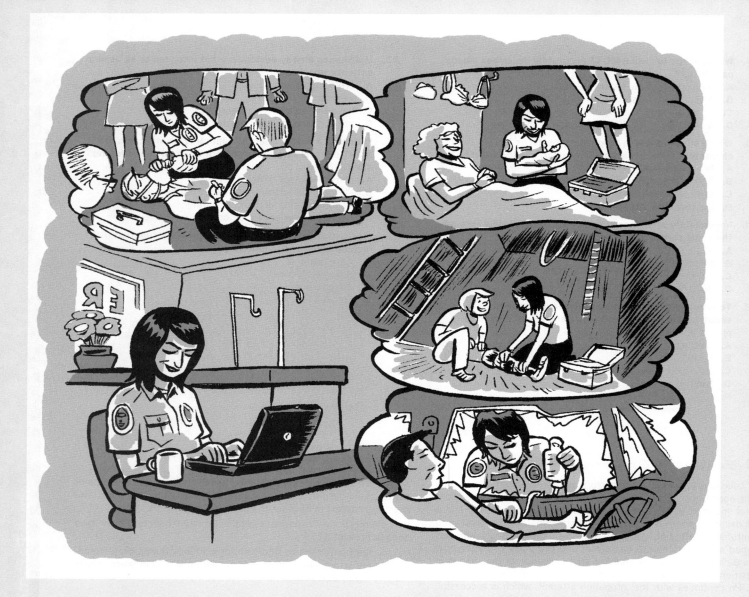

"

I learned the special stresses and constraints of rendering care outside the controlled conditions of a hospital: CPR in a crowded restaurant, childbirth in the lingerie section of a department store, splinting at the bottom of an elevator shaft, intravenous infusions inside a wrecked automobile".

—Nancy L. Caroline, MD

Patient Assessment

Section Editor: Richard Pilbery

Section 3

Objectives

Cognitive

- Describe the techniques of history taking.
- Discuss the importance of using open ended questions.
- Describe the use of facilitation, reflection, clarification, empathetic responses, confrontation, and interpretation.
- Differentiate between facilitation, reflection, clarification, sympathetic responses, confrontation, and interpretation.
- Describe the structure and purpose of a health history.
- Describe how to obtain a comprehensive health history.
- List the components of a comprehensive history of an adult patient.

Affective

- Demonstrate the importance of empathy when obtaining a health history.
- Demonstrate the importance of confidentiality when obtaining a health history.

Psychomotor

None

Introduction

Most practising technicians, paramedics, nurses, and doctors quickly learn that patient assessment is one of the most important parts of their job. Assessment combines a number steps—assessing the scene, getting your patient's <u>chief complaint</u>, taking care of life-threatening problems, taking your patient's medical history, and doing a physical examination. One of the most unique things about your patient assessment skills is that *there is no limit to how good they can be*. With a positive attitude and a commitment to excellence, you will have the opportunity to continue to polish and improve these critical skills throughout your career as a paramedic.

Paramedics often work with dangerously ill or injured patients without the input of specialised resources, like clinical laboratories and X-ray departments Figure 12-1 ▶ . However, you can be confident in a good initial diagnosis if you learn excellent history-taking skills. Many doctors say that hospital tests more often than not confirm a diagnosis the doctor arrived at *by taking a patient history.*

To the patient, the entire assessment process should appear to be a seamless process. To the provider, more often than not, it is a blend of questions and answers with a physical examination. What varies from patient to patient is the number and types of questions that must be asked and to what extent the patient should be examined before an initial diagnosis is reached. Never forget that the entire patient assessment process should be organised and systematic, but, at the same time, be reasonably flexible.

Aside from performing the initial assessment, which focuses on the identification and correction of any life threats to the patient, virtually all of the remaining history-gathering and physical examination components come with a lot of latitude as to when each is sequenced into the patient assessment

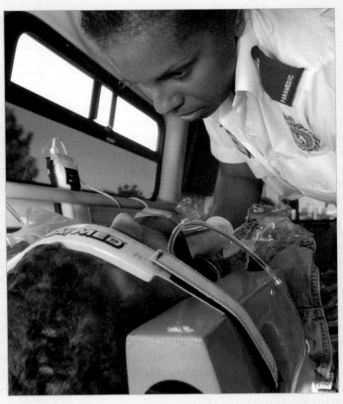

Figure 12-1 As a paramedic, you will work with dangerously ill or injured patients.

process. In other words, you can do the majority of your assessment and examination in the order that is in the best interest of patient care, *once the initial assessment and correction of life threats is completed.*

You are the Paramedic Part 1

You are dispatched to 11 Broomhall Road for a 65-year-old man who has "passed out". En route to the scene, dispatch informs you that your patient is now conscious and alert and reportedly was stung by a bee.

As you arrive on the scene, someone waves for you from the garden of the residence. As you approach, you see a man seated at a picnic table surrounded by an obviously concerned group of people. There are a few large bowls of food placed in the middle of the table, and several insects are flying around them. You introduce yourself to the group, and they introduce you to your patient, Lawrence Smith. Your patient's adult daughter tells you that they were all eating dinner when the patient was stung by a bee. He is complaining of itching at the sting site and dizziness.

Initial Assessment	Recording Time: 0 Minutes
Appearance	Eyes open, talking with family members
Level of consciousness	A (Alert to person, place, and day)
Airway	Patent
Breathing	Adequate rate and tidal volume
Circulation	Radial pulse present

1. What are your immediate concerns?
2. At this point, what would you want to know about his medical history?

At the Scene

For peak efficiency, communicate your patient assessment findings with your partner(s) and share with them the patient care plan.

Most ambulance teams are made up of two people working in tandem to quickly identify and address the patient's needs. The ambulance team may be composed of two paramedics, or, it may be a split team, with one paramedic and a technician. In either case, with the limited physical resources of a two-person team, working in the dynamic, often unstable out-of-hospital environment, providing quality patient care can be quite a challenge.

A key part of making your practice of prehospital care successful is for you to develop and cultivate your own style of assessment and an overall strategy for evaluating and providing care for the patients you will encounter in the unique and varied circumstances in the out-of-hospital setting. You will have to work within the parameters of the published standards of care in your system, adding your own personal touches, for example, what gear you take in on a given call or whether you like to kneel or sit while you interview the patient.

Always remember that your overall job as a paramedic is to quickly identify your patient's problem(s), set your care priorities, develop a patient care plan, and quickly and efficiently execute the patient care plan.

At the Scene

In prehospital emergency care, the priorities of evaluation and treatment are based on the degree of threat to the patient's life.

Sick Versus Not Sick

The most important assessment skill for a paramedic to acquire, and one that comes only from lots of experience, is quickly determining whether the patient is *sick* or *not sick*. This quick visual assessment is based on the chief complaint, respirations, pulse, mental status, and skin signs and colour. For trauma patients, the mechanism of injury and obvious trauma should be factored in as well. These items together reflect the overall performance of the respiratory, cardiovascular, and neurological systems and can quickly provide you with a sound medical basis for determining whether a patient is in stable or unstable condition. Abnormalities in any of these areas could indicate a life-threatening condition.

If the patient is sick, the next step is to determine "how sick". On one end of the sick scale is a patient with a miserable sinus infection. Is the patient sick? Yes. Is this a life-threatening event? Probably not. On the other end of the scale is a patient who is a dusky grey, struggling to answer your questions, and so short of breath that only one- or two-word bursts are possible. Is the patient sick? Yes. Is this a life-threatening event? Unlike the previous scenario, the answer is yes.

Documentation and Communication

The key to getting a good patient history is to develop rapport with your patient—even though you spend only a short time with him or her.

Every time you assess a patient, you have to *qualify* whether your patient is sick or not sick, and then you must *quantify* how sick the patient is. Once this has been accomplished, you are in a position to decide what, if any, care needs to be provided at the scene versus in the ambulance, en route to the hospital.

Making Your Initial Diagnosis

More often than not, you will make your initial diagnosis on scene based on the *patient history* and the *chief complaint*. Your ability to obtain quality information from patients with differing educational, cultural, and ethnic backgrounds; patients with various levels of cognitive ability; and patients impaired by alcohol or drugs is no small challenge. In addition, you still have to ask the right questions to get the information needed to make the best decisions for your patient.

For the most part, being good at patient assessment is a lot like being a good detective. As you interview your patient, you will sift through the information you obtain, and throughout that process, you will continuously glean clues **Figure 12-2 ▾** . On the basis of clues, you will ask more questions to seek information relevant to the patient's chief complaint. You may pursue one line of questioning about current medications that yields nothing important, yet the next line of questioning about medical history is a goldmine.

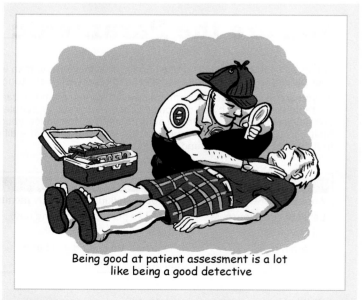

Being good at patient assessment is a lot like being a good detective

Figure 12-2

Controversies

There is much controversy about paramedics making a "diagnosis" at the scene. However, an "initial diagnosis" must be made to understand which treatment guideline to use.

Just as the veteran detective methodically collects and analyses clues to ultimately "solve the case", so must you use a similar process to best meet your patient's needs.

In time, every paramedic develops his or her own *style* of patient assessment. As you work at developing this most important job skill, it is critical that you to think of patient assessment as a "fluid" process. The overall assessment process must be organised and systematic but still flexible enough to allow you to maximise your information gathering. As the patient interview unfolds, you need be able to change the sequence of your questioning as the situation or patient's condition dictates. You must know when to expand your questioning to elicit more information and when to focus your questioning to ascertain the most relevant facts.

Medical Versus Trauma

Last, keep in mind that there are two basic categories of patient problems: medical and trauma. For patients with medical problems, identifying their chief complaint and sifting carefully through their medical history will allow you to provide the quality care the patients need.

Unlike medical emergencies, trauma calls are generally the result of unexpected events. When trauma is the primary culprit, the patient's medical history often has little or no impact on your care plan. Because of that, trauma cases require a modified approach to assessment. That will be covered in more detail in Chapter 13.

That said, it is important to never forget that medical events can cause trauma; for example, a person with diabetes takes insulin, forgets to eat breakfast, the blood glucose level drops, and, as a result, the person falls down the steps. By comparison, traumatic events can produce medical problems; for example, a person with asthma wrecks a new car and the stress of the event results in an asthma attack. Keep your mind open to the varied patient care scenarios you may encounter in your practice so you are mentally ready to respond to your patient's needs.

Evaluation of the Emergency Scene

Regardless of when and where you respond to an emergency call, the *very first* step, *before patient care is initiated*, is to *take a look around* and evaluate the overall safety and stability of the emergency scene for any risks to you or any other member of the emergency services, the patient, and any friends, family, and bystanders Figure 12-3 ▶ .

If you do not take a few moments to evaluate the scene and address safety issues, you may find that you and/or your partner have joined the list of casualties. An injured paramedic simply adds to the list of injured and subtracts from the list of rescue resources, making more work for the rest of the rescue team.

Notes from Nancy

Dead heroes can't save lives. Injured heroes are a nuisance. So check the scene for hazards before you lunge in.

Content of the Patient History

Patient Information

There are a number of components that collectively make up the patient history. On most incidents, the two most important pieces of patient history information that you need to obtain are the patient's name and the chief complaint. After that, you can obtain the rest of the patient history in whatever order is most conducive to good patient care and most convenient.

Your first step in approaching your patient is to introduce yourself and to explain that you are a paramedic. Then you can ask your patient his or her name and why he or she asked for your help (the chief complaint). Along with the patient's *name*, you need to ask about the *date, time, location,* and *events* surrounding the current situation. This is important information and gives you the chance to quickly determine if the patient is orientated to person, place, time, and events. Your ambulance service may require you to collect some additional identifying data such as age, sex, address, and occupation. You will also

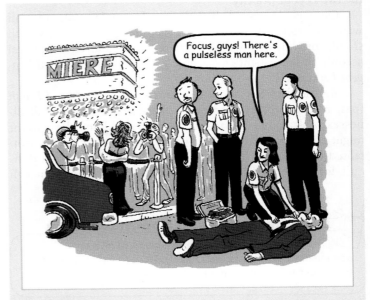

Figure 12-3

want to know who called 999; did the patient place the call for help, or was it a friend, family member, or bystander who placed the call?

If first responders are already on the scene, find out the information they have already obtained and the results of any care they provided. This information saves time by avoiding your having to ask the same questions again, which in turn, keeps the patient from getting frustrated.

Learning About the Present Illness

Once the meet-and-greet phase is over, start gathering information. Again, take a moment to make sure the patient is as comfortable as possible before you start—warm or cool enough, privacy ensured—and that you have gained the patient's confidence and trust.

The history of the present illness starts with one of the most open-ended of all medical questions: "What's going on today that made you call 999"? An open-ended question cannot be answered with a "yes" or "no". This or a similar question gets the ball rolling. More often than not, the answer you get involves some problem(s) with the person being in pain or discomfort. If your patient's behaviour is inappropriate, consider the possibility that it might be a psychiatric emergency.

Sometimes patients will have multiple complaints. Let's say a 64-year-old man tells you, "I'm really weak, and it feels like there are butterflies in my chest". You will need to figure out whether these symptoms are related. If you believe that they are related, to provide appropriate care, you need to identify the *origin of the problem*. In this case, you may want to ask, "Have you had this problem before"?

On the other hand, let's say your patient is complaining of "being dizzy and having pain in her left ankle". You can ask a couple of questions and may determine, for example, that the two complaints are not related. You must then decide which of the two is your priority.

Once you've established the chief complaint(s), you will want to flesh out the history of the present illness, which should provide you with a clear sequence and chronological account of the patient's signs and symptoms, that is, *what happened* and *when*.

You need to ask about the patient's *general state of health* (past medical history) and any serious childhood or adult illnesses. Ask about any mental health problems the patient might be having and whether he or she has ever been hospitalised for a mental health problem. Although it is often difficult for patients and families to admit to mental health

Documentation and Communication

The history of present illness should always be documented clearly and accurately. This is often the most important information, medically and legally.

problems, if you are matter-of-fact and dignified in asking the question, you can get a "straight" answer.

You will also need to ask about any accidents or injuries the patient had within the last month or so and about any operations or hospitalisations within the last 6 months or so.

One of the more challenging aspects of the history-taking process is that of pulling together the patient's *current health status,* because it is made up of many unrelated pieces of information. However, it often ties together some of the past medical history with the history of the current event, so it has definite value to the assessment process. The simple fact of the matter is, you don't need to obtain each and every piece of information on the following list for every patient. It takes time and practice and a certain amount of common sense for you to know the right questions to ask each patient.

Questions that will be most helpful in getting a useful history include the following:

- What prescription medicines are you currently taking? How much and how often? (Patients can and do confuse when and how to take their medications—and if your patient has, you could be witnessing a drug reaction. Also, as you gain paramedic experience, your familiarity with the drugs will give you an idea of the patient's illness. Medications will also give you a clue about mental health problems or dementia without your needlessly antagonising a reluctant patient.)
- Do you take any over-the-counter medication like aspirin, herbs, or vitamins?
- Are you allergic to any medicines or other substances?
- Do you smoke? How much? Do you drink alcohol? How much and how often?
- Have you been smoking or taking drugs other than cigarettes? Assure your patient of confidentiality.
- What did you have to eat yesterday and today?
- Ask about screening tests that are appropriate. For example, for difficulty breathing ask: "Have you had a chest X-ray lately"?
- Are your immunisations up-to-date? How about a flu jab or pneumococcal vaccine? Ask about children's immunisations, too.
- Have you been getting a good night's sleep? Look for maladaptive sleep patterns.
- Do you like to exercise? How much?
- What kinds of chemical cleaners do you have in your house? Do you have any strong chemicals where you work? You might need to probe for environmental hazards.
- Does the family use seatbelts and car seats for the children? Do you have baby gates? Are medicines locked away (if it seems necessary)?
- Do you have a history of any specific diseases in your family?
- Where do you live? What do you like to do at home? Is there anyone in your life that you might be afraid of? You might need to assess a difficult home situation.

- How do you spend your time during the day?
- Do you have anything in your religion that would prevent me from administering treatment?
- Are you an optimistic person? You might feel it important to get your patient's overall outlook on life.

Special Considerations

In some cases, a patient's religious beliefs may be relevant, for example if the beliefs pertain directly to medical care. If your patient indicates that such beliefs are important, this information should be passed along to accident and emergency (A&E) department staff.

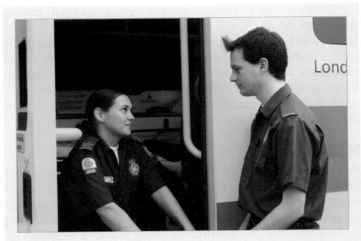

Figure 12-4 Your appearance should be professional and your demeanour positive and friendly.

You have to decide which of the listed items you want to explore and which you do not. For a really sick patient with immediate life threats, you may have no time to explore any of them. For a patient in stable condition who appears to be in no apparent distress, you may have time and decide to explore all relevant topics.

Last, you'll want to do a quick check on the body systems. A great way to gain insight is to ask, "Has your doctor ever told you that you have a heart, lung, or brain problem"? After that, you can ask about things like bowel movements, and so on, which tend to be non–life threatening.

Techniques for History Taking

Setting the Stage for Quality Patient Care

Every time you care for a patient, you must first establish a professional relationship. In most cases, this is a *short-term* relationship, less than 2 hours' duration, until you hand-over the patient to the A&E staff.

Your Demeanour and Appearance

Although time is short, you will want to have a positive patient outcome in the care you provide and the communication you establish with all involved. When you first meet your patient, your appearance should be that of a clean, neat, health care provider. You should have good personal hygiene and grooming and attire that is professional, clean, and pressed **Figure 12-4** ▶. If you look professional, your patient will be likely to develop a good first impression of you.

Along with your appearance, there is the matter of your demeanour. On every call, your attitude is always on display. If you are unhappy, a look of unhappiness is almost certainly on your face. Your facial expression and body language can send powerful messages. If you have come to believe that calls to 999 need to meet *your* expectations, *you are wrong*. If patients

think a problem is serious enough to merit a call to 999, you have an obligation to treat patients and their complaints accordingly—professionally and to the best of your ability.

Be sure to introduce yourself and your partner to the patient.

Try to interview the patient in a private setting. Don't hesitate to ask any nonessential personnel to leave the room or to at least step back because you will frequently find yourself asking your patients personal or intimate questions. Most people do not want to admit some bad habits (for example, cigarettes) that have a negative impact on their health. But you need to know. If the setting makes the patient uncomfortable, the patient may choose to not answer your questions or to answer inaccurately. Working to ensure the patient's privacy, confidentiality, and comfort level goes a long way toward establishing positive patient rapport and encourages more honest, open communication.

Confidentiality

As discussed in Chapter 4, it is your duty to maintain confidentiality of the patient's information. You need to be familiar with the relevant laws that govern the disclosure of patient information. Also, showing the patient that you respect the confidentiality of his or her medical information helps build rapport and contributes to total patient care.

How to Address the Patient

After introducing yourself, ask the patient his or her name and how he or she would like to be addressed. Err on the side of formality, using Mr., Miss, Mrs., or Ms. There is a world of difference in Mr. John Markham (formal), John (more casual), or Johnnie (really casual). Your patient will say, "Call me John" if that is what he prefers. Calling patients by the name of their choosing is professional, but assuming formality will help establish more rapport than being too familiar.

Avoid "catch-all names" or "pet names" like pal, buddy, sport, love, friend, honey, sweetie, poppet, and darling. You can bog down the process of obtaining a history by demeaning the patient and treating the patient unprofessionally. Using casual nicknames also can be problematic when there are cultural differences. Some terms have negative connotation in some cultures. You need to be familiar with the cultural groups in your area and with issues that could lead to misunderstanding.

Note Taking

As you get ready to start the assessment process, let the patient know that you are going to be asking a number of questions and that while he or she is answering, you or your partner will be taking notes. This lets patients know they aren't being ignored and that the information being provided is important enough to write down   Figure 12-5 ▶ .

Too often, ambulance clinicians read off a list of questions to patients to fill in all the blanks on the patient clinical record. With this approach comes the problem of making little to no eye contact with the patient. Don't bury your nose in the clipboard! If possible, position yourself at the eye level of your patient.

Reviewing the Medical History and Information Reliability

Frequently, you will obtain information not just from your patient but also from other sources. It is important that you document the source of this information in your record. Family members are commonly involved at emergency scenes, as are friends. Police personnel and bystanders also can be valuable sources of information.

A large number of the patient contacts in day-to-day calls are routine patient transfers from sheltered or warden controlled housing to the hospital and back. Take a few moments to review the transfer paperwork. You need to know the medical history of the patient so you are prepared to provide care should your planned routine transfer suddenly deteriorate.

Keep in mind the importance of evaluating your sources of information for reliability. Although the medical records in the doctor's letter should be assumed to be reasonably accurate, it may be a locum writing the referral who has never met the patient before. When all is said and done, you are responsible for patient care decisions, so make sure you work with information that is as accurate as possible.

> **Notes from Nancy**
> Never assume that it is impossible to talk to a patient until you have tried.

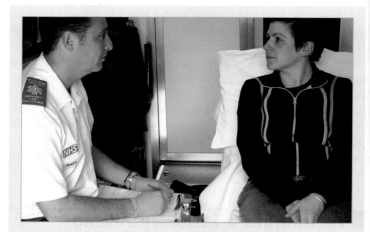

Figure 12-5 You may want to take notes during the patient history.

You are the Paramedic Part 2

After moving the bowls of food out of the immediate area and asking the other members of the family to give you and your patient some privacy, you notice localised swelling and redness at the sting site and a venom sac embedded in his skin. You scrape the stinger away with a tongue depressor, obtain vital signs, give the patient high-flow supplemental oxygen, and insert an 18-gauge cannula in the right antecubital vein to give normal saline to keep the vein open. The patient denies having shortness of breath and any history of severe allergic reactions. He also denies carrying or using an EpiPen or having taken any antihistamines before your arrival. When you ask about his medical history, he says he has occasional chest pain with exertion and that his only medication is GTN. He has no allergies to medication. He tells you that currently he has no chest pain.

Vital Signs	Recording Time: 3 Minutes
Skin	Localised redness and swelling at the sting site and hives on the abdomen
Pulse	98 beats/min, regular
Blood pressure	108/58 mm Hg
Respirations	24 breaths/min
S$_P$O$_2$	100% with oxygen at 12 to 15 l/min via nonrebreathing mask

3. What medication(s) would you administer to this patient?

4. What other assessment tools would you like to use?

Communication Techniques

Encourage Dialogue

On the basis of the questions asked and answers received, you will make patient care decisions. A number of approaches and conversation techniques can help to improve the volume and quality of information you obtain during the patient interview.

Facilitation

A dictionary definition of facilitation is to "make easy or easier". Facilitation in communication means using techniques that permit your patient to feel open to giving you some of the most delicate information he or she can share. Patients of all ages are hesitant to share private or embarrassing information. Your job is to make your patients feel so secure with you that they will give you the information you need.

The most important thing you can do to facilitate the information exchange is pay attention. Good eye contact is essential. It's hard to believe that someone who never makes eye contact is really listening. Use phrases that encourage the patient to share more information such as, "That's helpful", "Anything else you can think of"? or "Please go on". Nodding your head and using an appropriately placed, "Okay", every now and then lets the patient know you are getting the message.

Documentation and Communication

Do not put ideas into the patient's head, such as, "Is the pain in your chest a dull ache that is behind your sternum and radiates into your jaw"?

Another helpful facilitation technique is repeating key information from the patient's answers.

Patient: *"I've been feeling very odd since I got up, and my chest really aches. It never felt like this before".*
Paramedic: *"Your chest aches"?*
Patient: *"Really badly. I've never had an ache like this before".*
Paramedic: *"You've had chest pain before"?*
Patient: *"Yes, I've been seeing my GP pretty regularly for 5 years now. Before I used to get a kind of squeezing feeling in my chest, I'd take GTN, and it would go away. Well, this is nothing like that! I took two GTN as soon as it started, and that must be about an hour and a half ago, and nothing has changed".*

In this case, with just two short questions, you greatly expanded what you knew about the patient. You now know that the patient:

- Has a history of heart disease.
- Has been seeing their GP for 5 years.
- Is having pain today that is different from and more serious than pain in the past.
- Is having pain today that is the worst it has ever been.

- Has taken GTN for symptom relief in the past.
- Took two GTN doses today that failed to relieve the symptoms.

Reflection

Reflection is the *repetition* of a word or phrase that a patient has used to encourage more detail.

Your patient might say: *"I couldn't catch my breath".*
You could respond: *"You couldn't catch your breath, Mrs. Brown"?*
Your patient might elaborate: *"I don't know. I recall my heart just all of a sudden seemed to start beating really fast, and then I got scared, and all of a sudden I was breathing really fast but not getting enough air".*

Reflection is a powerful tool for getting a good patient history for two reasons: (1) Reflection usually does not break the flow or your patient's thoughts. It helps you both stay focused. (2) The information you will obtain is not biased by "leading" the patient. You are using the words the patient used, not your own description, which is very important in good histories.

Clarification

Clarification is the technique of asking your patients for more information when some aspect of the history is vague or unclear to you Figure 12-6 ▾ . The clearer you are about your patient's condition, the more helpful and appropriate your care will be. On the other hand, if you are unsure about your patient's problem, the more likely your care is based on guesswork and happenstance.

Paramedic: *"What's going on today, Mrs. Hendrickson"?*
Patient: *"Oh I don't know. I'm just . . . well I'm just not feeling like myself".*
Paramedic: *"I'm sorry. Could you try to be a little more specific? If you could do that, it will help me figure out what's going on with you today".*
Patient: *"I'm always full of energy first thing in the morning, but I'm so weak right now that I couldn't even take Princess out to do her business".*

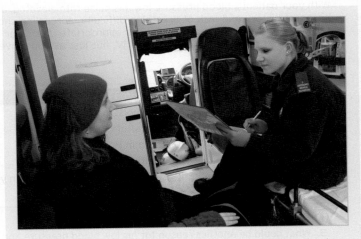

Figure 12-6 Use clarification to gain more information about the patient's chief complaint.

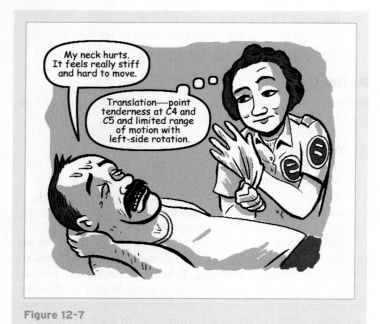

My neck hurts. It feels really stiff and hard to move.

Translation—point tenderness at C4 and C5 and limited range of motion with left-side rotation.

Figure 12-7

With this example, having identified the chief complaint as "weakness" is medically clearer than the complaint of "not feeling like myself".

Clarification is one of the more frequently used interview techniques in emergency situations. By the nature of your job, you may want to speak and listen to the language of medicine, but the average layperson has a limited medical vocabulary. Patients will generally use nonmedical terms to answer your assessment questions **Figure 12-7 ◂**. You will need to clarify what they mean.

Empathetic Response

Empathy is often described as one step further than sympathy; empathy is a psychological gift that allows you to feel what your patient is feeling—putting yourself into his or her shoes. At times, you will hear sad and tragic information from your patients. Do not hesitate to communicate your feelings and address the emotional impact of what has been said **Figure 12-8 ▸**.

Paramedic: *"What is the reason you called for help today, Mr. King"?*
Patient: *"I've just been horribly depressed".*
Paramedic: *"And why is that, Mr. King"?*
Patient: *"My wife and two kids were hit and killed by a drunk driver 6 months ago, and I just can't get over it".*
Paramedic: *"I am so sorry to hear that, Mr. King. That seems so wrong to me".*

Mr. King, the man who has lost his entire family, might not have an overt medical problem, but certainly you should consider the possibility that he might be so depressed that some kind of mental health referral is needed.

Documentation and Communication

Layman's Lingo	Paramedic Lingo
My sugars	I'm a diabetic
Passed out	Had a syncopal episode
Has the fits	History of convulsions
Water tablets	Diuretics (eg Furosemide)

You are the Paramedic Part 3

With your patient's blood pressure low, his pulse rate elevated, and the presence of hives, you consider adrenaline administration. With his heart history and lack of breathing difficulty, adrenaline should be administered with caution. You decide that the intramuscular route of 500 micrograms of 1:1,000 is appropriate, and your partner begins preparing the equipment and site. You also choose to administer chlorphenamine (Piriton) IV, but just as you move your patient to the trolley, you see a small, open pill bottle lying on his chair.

Reassessment	Recording Time: 5 Minutes
Skin	Slightly moist, pale, and warm
Pulse	100 beats/min, regular
Blood pressure	108/58 mm Hg
Respirations	24 breaths/min
SpO_2	100% with oxygen at 12 to 15 l/min via nonrebreathing mask
ECG	Sinus rhythm with no ectopy

5. What could be another reason for his low blood pressure and elevated pulse rate?
6. What should you immediately ask your patient?
7. Should you consider rethinking your diagnosis and treatment plans now?

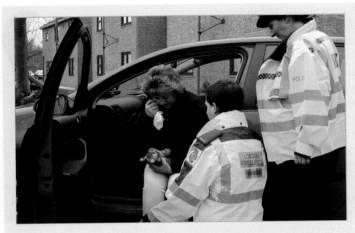

Figure 12-8 Be empathetic when the patient conveys sad or tragic information.

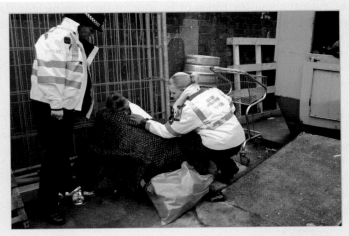

Figure 12-9 Use a nonjudgemental approach when confronting a patient.

Paramedics, unlike most other health care providers, see people when the illness or trauma just occurred. Your patients are uniquely vulnerable and uniquely demanding. Try your best to develop empathy for your patients.

Remember that in earlier chapters we discussed being active in your community to keep yourself aware of other sources of help for your patients. Empathy can help you set your patient on a path to healing—no matter what the diagnosis.

Confrontation

Confrontation is making your patients aware that you perceive something that is not consistent with their behaviour, the actual scene, or the information the patient is giving you. Nevertheless, avoiding confrontations with your patients is a good practice. If you must confront a patient, for example about using illegal drugs or alcohol, a professional approach can help you get medically appropriate information. Sometimes patients want a chance to deal with their problems. The key is to remain professional and nonjudgemental Figure 12-9 ▶.

Patient: *"My life just sucks. I don't why I even go on living"*.
Paramedic: *"Are you considering suicide"*?
Patient: *"I'm thinking that might just be the best thing"*.
Paramedic: *"Have you made plans on how you are going to do it"*?
Patient: *"I don't know, I haven't given it that much thought"*.

This patient's response clearly points toward possible suicide. Use a direct approach and ask the patient about whether he is contemplating suicide and if so, if he has a plan. This information helps you assess how distressed the patient is so that you can decide how to best ensure safe transport of the patient.

Interpretation

If your patient refuses to give you information, you need to deduce what could be causing the distress and then ask the patient if you are right. (In the preceding situation, the para-

medic, who spoke with a clearly distressed patient used interpretation about whether the patient was suicidal.)

The skill of interpretation demands that paramedics use their best diplomatic skills. One of the best phrases with which to begin a deduction is the ever-reliable, "So, if I understand you correctly . . ".

Asking About Feelings

Asking about feelings is one of the most difficult roles of a paramedic. But as part of a good health history, you will need to ask if a patient is tired, depressed, or any number of feelings that are most easily dealt with by denial. (You will even need to ask these questions of a colleague if you see the symptoms.)

Try to keep possible unpleasant sights, sounds, and smells from your patient who is feeling badly. You can also validate feelings. "This is a tough situation". That's empathy in action. Do your best to attend to psychological needs at the scene. It is a tough job, but these needs profoundly affect physical health.

Be effective. Do not ask, "Are you okay"? This is the most tempting of all questions (and it *can* be answered with a yes or no!). Instead, ask for facts first, then follow up. Even with someone you know quite well, you need to establish rapport to ask a question about how he or she is feeling. Most of us would deny that we are exhausted, frazzled, scared, or depressed. Your patients met you only a few minutes ago. Establish that you are a caring health professional during a series of "safe" questions about physical health.

Getting More Information

You've got a lot of information from your patient, but in many cases, you need to refine your thinking to come up with a valid diagnosis. Let's say you were exploring a particular symptom such as "abdominal pain" with your patient. (As you will soon learn, abdominal pain can suggest a startlingly large number of diagnoses.) Some possible questions you might ask the patient about the *region* or location of the pain include the following:

- Where exactly does it hurt?
- Does it hurt in one particular spot or in a general area?
- Can you point to where it hurts with one finger?
- Does the pain stay right there, or does it move or radiate anywhere else?
- If your pain does move or radiate, where does it go?

Questions you may ask about the *quality* of the abdominal pain include the following:

- What type of pain is it: a sharp pain or more of a dull ache?
- Does the pain come and go, or is it constant?
- If you wanted me to feel the same feeling that you do, what would you do to me to make me feel that way?

At the Scene

Letting patients describe their pain in their own words will be very helpful for your assessment.

Questions you may ask about the *severity* of the abdominal pain include the following:

- In your opinion, how bad is this pain?
- Is it more of an uncomfortable feeling or a feeling of hurt?
- Would you say the pain is similar to or worse than with previous episodes?
- On a scale of 1 to 10, with 10 being the *worst* pain you've ever felt and 1 being very minor, how would you rate your pain?

The questions in these lists are not exhaustive or all-inclusive. Add and modify questions to the patient interview as you need to. Subtract questions if time is of the essence. Use open-ended questions whenever you can (**Figure 12-10 ▾**). Pin your patient down

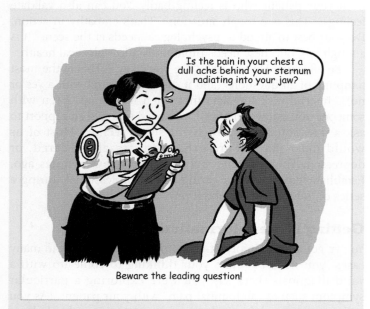

Is the pain in your chest a dull ache behind your sternum radiating into your jaw?

Beware the leading question!

Figure 12-10

with a closed question if that's what the situation requires.

Try to be *orderly* and *systematic* in your information gathering and assessment, while at the same time *flexible* in your approach. Being flexible in an emergency is a lot harder than it sounds, but it is attainable with practice—lots and lots of practice.

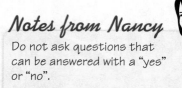

Notes from Nancy

Do not ask questions that can be answered with a "yes" or "no".

You could probably use some help in remembering what to cover. The mnemonic OPQRST offers an easy-to-remember approach to analysing a patient's chief complaint that is simple and effective.

- **Onset.** When did you start to feel pain?
- **Provocation.** What do you think brought on your pain?
  - Did the pain start all of a sudden or come on over a period of time?
  - Does anything make the pain go away or feel better or feel worse?
- **Quality.** How would you describe this type of pain (is it sharp, dull, etc.)?
- **Region/Radiation/Referral.**
  - Can you point to the place where it hurts with one finger?
  - Does the pain stay there, or does it go somewhere else?
- **Severity.** On a scale of 1 to 10, with 1 being insignificant and 10 the worst pain you've ever felt, how would you score this?
- **Time.** How long have you felt this way?

Documentation and Communication

Documenting pain severity ratings is important. Also note how distressed the patient appears: mild, moderate, or severe.

Clinical Reasoning

The results of your questions should expand your thinking about problems and other body systems that are associated with the symptoms your patient has mentioned. In Chapter 15, you will learn the details of critical thinking. Critical thinking consists of (1) concept formation, (2) data interpretation, (3) application of principles (guidelines or algorithms), (4) reflection in action (being willing to change course as you interpret your patient's condition), and (5) reflection on action (doing honest and thorough debriefs to benefit learning).

Being able to think and perform well under pressure is a big part of being able to be a good paramedic. In many ways, critical thinking and decision making are just two more skills you will need to work on, not just while you are a student, but for the rest of your career as a practicing paramedic.

One of the most important elements of the interview process is for you to be a *great listener,* and a big part of being a great listener is also being a *patient listener.* For a number of reasons, patients can be slow to respond. Maybe they didn't hear your question. Maybe they didn't understand you. Maybe they are afraid to answer. There are many possible explanations. Ask, then wait, and give your patients time to gather their thoughts so they can answer you.

Communicate with your patients by using terminology matched to their knowledge and understanding. For example, a patient who is an A&E nurse or a retired surgeon will understand medical terminology. On the other hand, a patient who speaks little English needs simple and focused communication.

Throughout the assessment process, look for nonverbal communication, such as changes in facial expression, heavy sighs, or aggressive gestures (finger pointing), any of which can impact your information processing.

Direct Questions

To complete the history, direct questions could be required. Patients might not be giving you easy-to-digest facts about themselves, and if you need a date, time, or other specific information, you should ask for it.

Getting a History on Sensitive Topics

As a paramedic, you will be privileged to care for people who depend on you during some of the worst moments of their lives. You represent hope and comfort no matter how difficult, even horrific, your patient's situation might be.

Some sensitive factors like drug and alcohol abuse can stand in the way of your best efforts for the health of your patients. Here are some ways that can help you be the paramedic you want to be, no matter how sensitive the situation.

Alcohol and Drug Abuse

People who regularly abuse drugs or alcohol become adept at hiding the signs and symptoms from their friends, family, and workplace associates and denying there is a problem. Such denial can go on for years, and the signs and symptoms can be hidden even from people closest to the patient.

If asked how much alcohol or drug has been consumed, the amount is often understated. Some experienced paramedics say the standard answer to the question about how many drinks is "two", when the behaviour indicates many more. Slightly *fewer* than half of all motor vehicle crashes involve alcohol. Just *more* than half of all motor vehicle crashes that result in fatalities involve alcohol **Figure 12-11 ▶**.

It is probable that an alcohol-impaired patient will give an unreliable history. Do not assume that all that you are told is completely accurate. Keep in mind that alcohol can mask any number of signs and symptoms. When a patient who experienced a significant traumatic event denies neck or back pain, if

you smell what you believe to be an alcoholic beverage on the patient's breath or behaviour raises your suspicion of alcohol or drug use, take precautions to restrict spinal motion.

Alcohol is a legal drug. If your patient is using other substances to "get high", using them is likely to be illegal. The fear of punishment for illegal use of drugs might lead patients to deny their use. Let your patient know that you are a medical person and anything that he or she tells you will be kept in confidence. Do your best to win your patient's trust because you need the information to provide proper treatment.

Keep your best professional attitude as you work with patients you suspect of using drugs or alcohol. Paramedics should never judge their patients by appearances or behaviour. An unkempt homeless person might be in desperate need of assessment for head trauma, not alcoholism. A city executive might have hit his head during a crash, but drinking alcohol might be the cause of the accident.

Physical Abuse and Domestic Violence

As a paramedic, you are required to report a case if you have reason to suspect physical abuse or domestic violence. Although it is inappropriate for you to accuse someone of abuse at the scene, never hesitate to call for the police if you have reason to believe that abuse has occurred. They will help stabilise the scene and provide another set of professional eyes.

A number of clues may lead you to suspect domestic violence. Injuries inconsistent with the information you are being given are common, as are multiple injuries in various stages of healing. Unspoken messages can be given by the family's behaviour. Maybe it's the cowering posture of the woman at the kitchen table as her husband or partner towers over her and answers your questions for her. If the injured family member does not give you the information but waits for someone else to speak up, that's a clue that the injured family member is being repressed. You can suggest that the partner who is doing all the talking go to the ambulance to

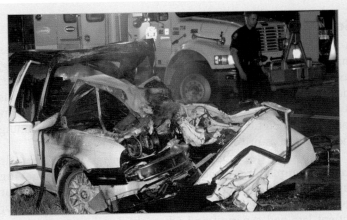

Figure 12-11 Many crashes involve alcohol. In these cases, the patient history may not be reliable.

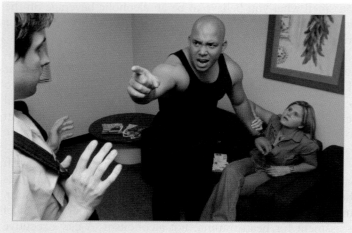

Figure 12-12 Do not handle potentially violent calls alone. Summon the police.

At the Scene

If you find yourself suddenly in a potentially dangerous position and your partners are not aware of it, use a predetermined code word to alert them. One inconspicuous code is to use the trade name of something in your ambulance—"could you get the Ferno cot"? Your partners should know that it means there is danger and that they should summon the police.

help with the trolley. The moment the door shuts, you may receive valuable information, such as, "My partner is beating me and I'm scared to death. You've got to get me out of here before he kills me or one of the kids". *Immediately* request the police if this or if anything close to this happens.

Emergency scenes involving domestic violence are some of the most dangerous for ambulance clinicians and police alike Figure 12-12 ▲). Don't even think of handling them without the police on hand.

Sexual History

A number of factors may influence a patient about being less than forthcoming about sexual history. Religious upbringing, cultural or societal mores, and exotic or bizarre sexual tastes may inhibit a patient from sharing sexual history because this is truly one of the most private and personal aspects of a person's life. When the topic is someone's sexual history, obtaining the history in as private a setting as possible is essential.

Keep your questions focused and on task. For a female patient complaining of acute abdominal pain, foul smelling vaginal discharge, pain on urination, genital lesions, or similar complaints, you will need to know such things as when your patient last had a period and when she last had sexual intercourse. You will also need to find out if there is vaginal bleeding, whether she has had multiple sexual partners, the

Special Considerations

Some younger teens may be confused when asked about sexual issues. Be direct and avoid using questions like, "Are you sexually active"? because they may think active means often.

characteristics of the vaginal discharge, and whether she uses a birth control method.

Male patients with complaints of pain on urination, discharge from the penis, genital lesions, and so forth, need to be asked about their most recent sexual encounter, whether they use condoms, the characteristics of their discharge and lesions, and so forth.

You may need to ask female and male patients if they have ever been tested for HIV, AIDS, or hepatitis. Do not interject any opinions or biases about sexual choices or behaviour. Their choices aren't your choices, just as your choices are not theirs. Every patient you care for deserves to be treated with compassion and respect.

Special Assessment Challenges

Simply put, it is impossible to address every scenario you may encounter in your work as a paramedic, but there are a number of special assessment challenges that occur often enough to be worth talking about.

Silence

When you are on a mission to obtain your patient's history in a timely manner, a period of silence on the part of your patient can make you uneasy. Don't let it. Your patient may be simply trying to gather his or her thoughts, trying to recall possibly distant details relative to the questions(s) you just asked, or trying to decide if he or she trusts you enough to answer your question(s) truthfully or at all. In any case, be patient.

Keep your antennae extended for nonverbal signs of distress. Pain, psychological distress, or fear often register in body movements and facial expression.

As you work in the prehospital setting while you are a student, you will learn how to read the many nonverbal cues that patients give. The paramedics you work with will help, as will working with experienced carers in the A&E department and the hospital. Although paramedics work outside the hospital, you will still find help in learning to read nonverbal cues from everyone you work with.

Another pair of essential skills you can learn from these seasoned veterans are how to time your questions and how to be patient. Learn to ask questions and then *wait*. What seems like an eternity to you is but 1 or 2 seconds to your patients, as they think, retrieve facts, or assess your trustworthiness.

Over Talkative Patients

On the other side of the coin are overly talkative patients. Some people learn to talk endlessly as a way of socialising, but you must consider possible clinical reasons for the chattiness. Recovering from a fight-or-flight situation, consuming a triple espresso 15 minutes ago, or an illegal drug—cocaine, crack, or methamphetamine—might be the reason. Whatever the cause, the first requirement of dealing with a talkative patient is to keep your patience (again). Try giving the patient free reign for the first few minutes. You might not be able to get as comprehensive a history as you would like with such a patient, given the limits on your time.

After a few minutes, try interrupting your patient to ask for clarification of a piece of information. This gives you an opportunity to quickly summarise what you have just heard.

One thing is certain: you are better off with too much information than with too little or no information.

Patients With Multiple Symptoms

Although your calls would be much simpler if your patients had only a single complaint, that is not reality. Sometimes you will be presented with "linked" complaints such as, "It feels like my heart is just fluttering, and I'm really dizzy". In this case, both symptoms can be tied to the patient having a high pulse rate.

Then again, especially with the older population, it is entirely possible and, in many cases, entirely likely that you are dealing with multiple causes. A patient with diabetes who is having a cardiac crisis may easily forget that he or she has taken insulin and takes it again. One of the classic musts is to *always check the blood glucose level* on patients with an altered mental state, whether they have a history of diabetes or not.

You need to learn to prioritise your patient's complaints. Only when that is accomplished can you develop an appropriate care plan as you decide which of your patient's problems you need to address and in which order you need to address them.

Notes from Nancy

If you don't ask, you won't find out.

No matter how sure you are about your initial diagnosis, *always* remain open to the possibility that something else is going on with your patient.

Anxious Patients

Believe it or not, you are the cause of many of your patients being overly anxious. No matter much the public loves to watch emergencies on TV, it is frightening to see an ambulance, fire appliance, or police car pull up and stop in front of the house. You should expect your patient to initially be somewhat anxious, but he or she should start to calm down shortly after your arrival. If not, it's time to open your mind up to other

At the Scene

A common cause of anxiety is hypoxia, or lack of oxygen in the blood. The patient may be sweaty and restless and become agitated very easily. Hypoxia is often misinterpreted as panic.

possibilities. High anxiety is a sign of physiological shock beginning to set in. You will need to be ready to treat immediately. Or your patient could be hiding something, such as physical abuse or the use of illegal drugs.

Whatever the case, be sensitive to verbal and nonverbal clues, always keeping in mind that any information you fail to obtain could be the information you need to treat your patient.

Reassurance

When communicating with patients, you should be poised and confident, with a positive demeanour. With that positive demeanour also comes the temptation to reassure your patients, sometimes inappropriately. Be cautious about what you tell your patients so that you don't make promises you can't deliver.

For example, it can be tempting to reassure a metal worker who caught his wedding ring on a piece of metal that a couple of stitches should make him good as new. However, many circumferential finger cuts can result in an amputation. Imagine how much distress you will cause your patient when he arrives at the hospital and the news is not so cheery.

In addition, if your reassurance is inappropriate, your patient could choose not to share quite as much information as he or she might have under other circumstances, leaving you with less information rather than more.

Anger and Hostility

Frequently you will find yourself the target of patients' and family members' frustrations, which may manifest as anger or outright hostility. Anger and hostility at unfairness and harsh realities are normal. Remember, don't take these situations personally—take them professionally.

The most important skill that you can use is not to get angry yourself. When you are in control of your own anger, you can work to calm the situation. Be attentive to changes in body language, such as threatening gestures or an escalating volume of the conversation or, worse yet, having a heated dialogue melt down into an outright yelling match. When people are angry or hostile, the worst thing you can do is get angry yourself.

As with any call, establishing a safe and secure scene is your first order of business. If you cannot calm the patient or family members, it's time to consider possibly calling for the police. If the patient or a family member is hostile, you might need to tell the person directly that if he or she continues to shout, you will not feel safe enough to do your assessment and

Special Considerations

Many patients are older than the paramedics taking care of them. They can feel threatened by strange "youngsters" telling them what is best for them. Listen to them. They often do know what is best for themselves.

will need to call the police. However, if the patient and/or the family members are already angry, telling them that the police are on the way is not going to make them any happier. In worst case scenarios, you may have to withdraw to the safety of your ambulance to wait for the police to arrive.

If the hostile person suddenly leaves the room, especially in the middle of the conversation, you or your colleague should follow the person, while working to calm him or her and defuse the situation. What you are also doing is making certain that the person doesn't go into the kitchen, get a knife, and come back and stab you, your partner, and maybe even the spouse.

Intoxication

When your patient is intoxicated, whether from alcohol or drugs, taking a good medical history becomes very difficult. Intoxication may mask symptoms, such as pain. With intoxication also comes a decrease in patience; while the patient is trying to explain to things to you, his or her hostility or anger can escalate faster than if he or she were not intoxicated. A common scenario for this type of situation occurs at minor RTC, where the intoxicated person wants to get back in the car and continue on his or her way after having run into a bollard or lamp post. The person's behaviour can become explosive. Your ability to be patient and diplomatic with your communication is paramount.

As frustrating as dealing with intoxicated people can be, do your best to remain objective and nonjudgmental. Remember, one of the keys to being a good paramedic is that *you have to like people,* but that in no way means that you *have to like what people do.*

Crying

Sometimes people cry because they are happy or sad. Although these are certainly common reasons for crying, other possibilities exist.

When the unexpected strikes, it can overwhelm people emotionally. Patients and their family members, along with their friends and neighbours, can suddenly find themselves under extreme levels of stress as a result of the emergency situation at hand. Just as some people react with anger and hostility to a stressful situation, others cry.

Once again, patience goes a long way. You can't expect the crying to immediately stop by yelling, "Stop crying"! Be patient.

Fortunately, the presence of an ambulance arriving on the scene often exerts a calming effect. During the course of your career, you will be surprised at how often you hear someone say, usually the very moment you walk in the door, something like, "Thank goodness, the paramedics are here"! Collectively, your calm demeanour and patient approach; appropriate touch, such as a hand on the shoulder; and a quiet, "I'm in control now", tone of voice will help get the crying to stop and allow you to move on to other matters.

Depression

Depression is a common reason for seeking medical attention. If a patient seems sad, hopeless, restless, and irritable; has sleep or eating disruptions; says that he or she feels his or her energy is low; or has pain for which you cannot find a source, consider that your patient might be depressed.

You are the Paramedic Part 4

Your patient admits to taking his GTN after being stung. He tells you that his doctor told him to "take it when he feels bad". So he did.

Reassessment	Recording Time: 10 Minutes
Skin	Localised redness and swelling at the sting site and hives on the abdomen
Pulse	96 beats/min, regular
Blood pressure	108/58 mm Hg
Respirations	24 breaths/min
SpO_2	100% with oxygen at 12 to 15 l/min via nonrebreathing mask
ECG	Sinus rhythm; no ectopy

8. What could have happened if you had continued to treat according to your original diagnosis?

9. What is your updated assessment and treatment plan?

10. What is important to remember when talking with the average person about medications and medical history?

5. **You must ask the patient what medication he is taking. This is important because medications can suggest past and present illnesses. To best determine medications that are being taken, you should:**
   A. review his pharmacy receipts.
   B. call his doctor.
   C. consult his relatives.
   D. ask him what medications, including prescription, over-the-counter, and herbal supplements he is taking.

6. **The posture of the patient's wife stiffens, and she begins to look angry. She starts yelling at you and your partner, telling you to hurry up and do something. You should:**
   A. have your partner take her aside and calmly explain what you are doing.
   B. call for back up at the first opportunity.
   C. have police stand by during the history taking.
   D. ignore her.

7. **You smell beer on the patient's breath. You wonder if he might be intoxicated. Problems encountered with intoxicated patients include which of the following?**
   A. Intoxicated patients may not understand what you are trying to say, making effective communications difficult or impossible.
   B. Intoxication may mask symptoms, making treatment decisions difficult.
   C. Intoxicated patients can present potentially violent situations.
   D. All of the above.

8. **You are dispatched to an unknown injury. You and your partner arrive on scene and hear loud noises and yelling from inside the residence. You then hear the sound of glass breaking. What should you do?**

9. **You arrive on scene at the home of a patient with hearing difficulty. What can you do to better enable effective communications?**

▄▄ Points to Ponder

You respond to a medical call involving a 46-year-old man. On arrival you recognise the patient as a teacher at the local school. You ask why you were called today and the patient tells you that he has been experiencing serious anxiety. You inquire about medical history, and your patient tells you that he checked himself into a psychiatric hospital during the summer break to get treatment for paranoia.

After shift, you are eating dinner at a popular restaurant with your partner and two other paramedics from your service. They ask if anything interesting happened today. You begin to tell them about the teacher, and your eyes meet those of your partner. You realise that this is not appropriate.

Why is this not appropriate, and what should you do now?

Issues: Confidentiality, History Taking.

13 Physical Examination

Objectives

Cognitive

- Define the terms inspection, palpation, percussion, auscultation.
- Describe the techniques of inspection, palpation, percussion, and auscultation.
- Describe the evaluation of mental status.
- Evaluate the importance of a general survey.
- Describe the examination of skin, hair, and nails.
- Differentiate normal and abnormal findings of the assessment of the skin.
- Distinguish the importance of abnormal findings of the assessment of the skin.
- Describe the examination of the head and neck.
- Differentiate normal and abnormal findings of the scalp examination.
- Describe the normal and abnormal assessment findings of the skull.
- Describe the assessment of visual acuity.
- Explain the rationale for the use of an ophthalmoscope.
- Describe the examination of the eyes.
- Distinguish between normal and abnormal assessment findings of the eyes.
- Explain the rationale for the use of an otoscope.
- Describe the examination of the ears.
- Differentiate normal and abnormal assessment findings of the ears.
- Describe the examination of the nose.
- Differentiate normal and abnormal assessment findings of the nose.
- Describe the examination of the mouth and pharynx.
- Differentiate normal and abnormal assessment findings of the mouth and pharynx.
- Describe the examination of the neck.
- Differentiate normal and abnormal assessment findings of the neck.
- Describe the survey of the thorax and respiration.
- Describe the examination of the posterior chest.
- Describe percussion of the chest.
- Differentiate the percussion notes and their characteristics.
- Differentiate the characteristics of breath sounds.
- Describe the examination of the anterior chest.
- Differentiate normal and abnormal assessment findings of the chest examination.
- Describe special examination techniques related to the assessment of the chest.
- Describe the examination of the arterial pulse including rate, rhythm, and amplitude.
- Distinguish normal and abnormal findings of arterial pulse.
- Describe the assessment of jugular venous pressure and pulsations.
- Distinguish normal and abnormal examination findings of jugular venous pressure and pulsations.
- Describe the examination of the heart and blood vessels.
- Differentiate normal and abnormal assessment findings of the heart and blood vessels.
- Describe the auscultation of the heart.
- Differentiate the characteristics of normal and abnormal findings associated with the auscultation of the heart.
- Describe special examination techniques of the cardiovascular examination.
- Describe the examination of the abdomen.
- Differentiate normal and abnormal assessment findings of the abdomen.
- Describe auscultation of the abdomen.
- Distinguish normal and abnormal findings of the auscultation of the abdomen.
- Describe the examination of the female genitalia.
- Differentiate normal and abnormal assessment findings of the female genitalia.
- Describe the examination of the male genitalia.
- Differentiate normal and abnormal findings of the male genitalia.
- Describe the examination of the anus and rectum.
- Distinguish between normal and abnormal findings of the anus and rectum.
- Describe the examination of the peripheral vascular system.
- Differentiate normal and abnormal findings of the peripheral vascular system.
- Describe the examination of the musculoskeletal system.
- Differentiate normal and abnormal findings of the musculoskeletal system.
- Describe the examination of the nervous system.
- Differentiate normal and abnormal findings of the nervous system.
- Describe the assessment of the cranial nerves.
- Differentiate normal and abnormal findings of the cranial nerves.
- Describe the general guidelines of recording examination information.
- Discuss the considerations for examination of an infant or child.

Affective

- Demonstrate a caring attitude when performing physical examination skills.
- Discuss the importance of a professional appearance and demeanour when performing physical examination skills.
- Appreciate the limitations of conducting a physical examination in the prehospital environment.

Psychomotor

- Demonstrate the examination of skin, hair, and nails.
- Demonstrate the examination of the head and neck.
- Demonstrate the examination of the eyes.
- Demonstrate the examination of the ears.
- Demonstrate the assessment of visual acuity.
- Demonstrate the examination of the nose.
- Demonstrate the examination of the mouth and pharynx.
- Demonstrate the examination of the neck.
- Demonstrate the examination of the thorax and ventilation.
- Demonstrate the examination of the posterior chest.
- Demonstrate auscultation of the chest.
- Demonstrate percussion of the chest.

- Demonstrate the examination of the anterior chest.
- Demonstrate special examination techniques related to the assessment of the chest.
- Demonstrate the examination of the arterial pulse including location, rate, rhythm, and amplitude.
- Demonstrate the assessment of jugular venous pressure and pulsations.
- Demonstrate the examination of the heart and blood vessels.
- Demonstrate special examination techniques of the cardiovascular examination.
- Demonstrate the examination of the abdomen.
- Demonstrate auscultation of the abdomen.
- Demonstrate the external visual examination of the female genitalia.
- Demonstrate the examination of the male genitalia.
- Demonstrate the examination of the peripheral vascular system.
- Demonstrate the examination of the musculoskeletal system.
- Demonstrate the examination of the nervous system.

Introduction

Physical examination is the process by which quantifiable, objective (based on fact or observable) information is obtained from a patient about his or her overall state of health. This information is compared with subjective (perceived by the patient) and historical information that is obtained from the patient. Armed with these two types of information, you can make a comprehensive assessment of the patient. While performing an assessment, you may see the patient's condition as a clinical manifestation; however, a caring and empathetic approach will yield better results and a more accurate evaluation. Likewise, a professional appearance and demeanour will instill trust and confidence in the abilities of the ambulance clinician.

The physical examination consists of two elements—obtaining vital signs that measure overall body function, and performing a head-to-toe survey that evaluates the workings of specific body organ systems. This survey is done in a sequential manner, ensuring that every aspect of the body's function is evaluated. Of course, the conditions in the prehospital setting may determine precisely how the physical examination is performed. Sometimes, the physical examination may be condensed. For example, for a patient with a significant mechanism of injury (MOI), it may only be appropriate to perform a rapid trauma assessment before transporting the patient.

The overall patient assessment is intended to determine whether a problem exists, so that actions can be taken to manage that problem. Before you can appreciate abnormalities on examination, you must understand the wide variety of normal presentations. This is something that can be learned only through direct hands-on experience and interaction with patients. Thus every patient encounter represents an opportunity for you to gain experience about the normal and abnormal human state of health.

Examination Techniques

The techniques of inspection, palpation, percussion, and auscultation allow you to obtain physical information and to understand the normal (versus abnormal) functions of a patient's body. Inspection involves looking at the patient, either in general or at a specific area (ie, a patient's overall appearance from the doorway versus looking specifically at the chest wall for abnormalities/deformities) **Figure 13-1 ▾**. Palpation is physical touching for the purpose of obtaining information—for example, tenderness (elicited pain), deformity, crepitus, mass effect, pulse quality, and abnormal organ enlargement **Figure 13-2 ▸**.

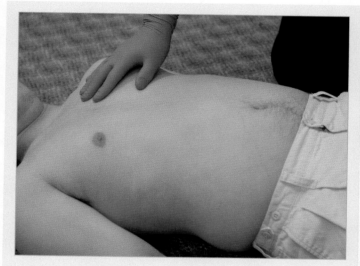

Figure 13-1 Inspection.

You are the Paramedic Part 1

You and your colleague brave the harsh winter winds as you leave the protective warmth of the accident and emergency (A&E) department and go quickly to your ambulance. It is one of the coldest days of the year and, unfortunately, one of the busiest. Just as you manage to get the ambulance heated, you and your partner are dispatched to a GP surgery for a patient complaining of shortness of breath. When you arrive, you are immediately taken to an examination room where you find a 75-year-old man in acute respiratory distress.

Initial Assessment	Recording Time: 0 Minutes
Appearance	Patient is leaning forward in tripod position
Level of consciousness	A (Alert to person, place, and day)
Airway	Patent
Breathing	Rapid and shallow, visible recession and audible wheezes, pursed lip breathing
Circulation	Strong radial pulses; pale, warm skin with cyanotic lips and nail beds

1. What is your general impression of the patient? Is he sick or not sick?
2. What do you think is the most valuable assessment tool at your disposal?

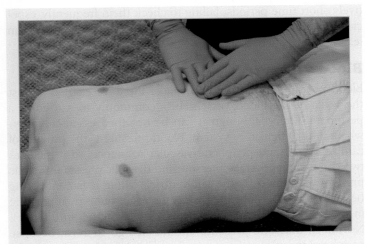

Figure 13-2 Palpation.

Percussion is a skill that requires a lot of practice to perfect. Follow the steps in Skill Drill 13-1 ▾:

1. Place your nondominant hand lightly against the surface to be examined Step 1.
2. Hyperextend the middle finger and apply firm pressure to the surface to be percussed Step 2.
3. Directly strike the middle phalanx of the middle finger with one or two fingertips of the other hand Step 3.
4. Apply the same force over each area of the body for an accurate comparison of the sounds produced by percussion.

Auscultation involves listening with a stethoscope Figure 13-3 ▸. The body generates a variety of high- and low-frequency sounds—both normal and abnormal—that can be detected via auscultation. Bowel sounds can be assessed via auscultation, as can lung sounds. Recognising the presence and differences in auscultated sounds requires practice.

At the Scene

When done properly, palpation should never cause harm. Deep palpation requires practice and knowing when to stop; it is generally outside the scope of practice of most paramedics.

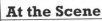Percussion entails gently striking the surface of the body, typically where it overlies various body cavities. This technique allows the paramedic to detect changes in the densities of the underlying structures. For example, percussion of a normal lung will yield medium to loud, low-pitched, resonant sounds. Percussion sounds over muscle and bone should be soft, high-pitched, and flat. Percussion sounds over hollow organs such as the intestines are often described as loud, high-pitched, and tympanic (like a drum).

Vital Signs

Vital signs consist of a measurement of pulse rate, rhythm, and quality; respiratory rate, rhythm, and quality; blood pressure; temperature; and pulse oximetry. Other than overall patient

At the Scene

There are important differences between the bell and diaphragm of the stethoscope. The bell is cup-shaped and is used to listen for deep and low-pitched sounds (heart murmurs). It is placed very lightly on the skin, just enough to make a seal. The diaphragm is flat-shaped and is used to listen for high-pitched sounds (breath, bowel, and normal heart sounds); it is placed firmly on the skin.

Skill Drill 13-1: Percussion

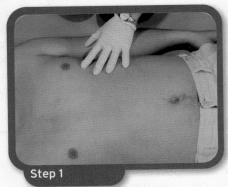

Step 1

Place your hand lightly against the surface to be examined.

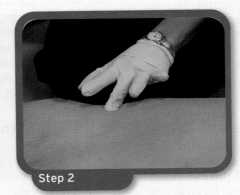

Step 2

Hyperextend the middle finger and apply firm pressure.

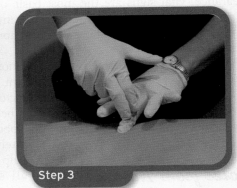

Step 3

Strike the middle phalanx of the middle finger with one or two fingertips of the other hand.

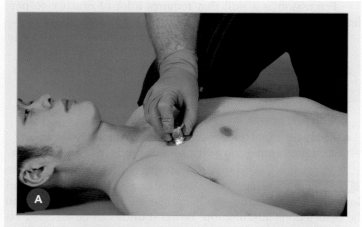

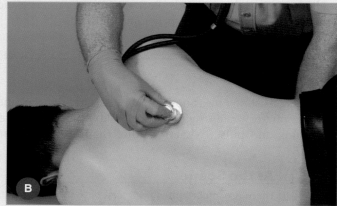

Figure 13-3 Auscultation of the (**A**) anterior chest and the (**B**) posterior chest.

At the Scene

Be aware that the patient's age, underlying physical and mental conditions, and current medications can affect the patient's vital signs. Like any other assessment tool, consider the vital signs but devote your attention to the patient.

appearance, vital signs are the most basic objective data for determining patient status. Their measurement requires the paramedic to use the techniques of inspection, palpation, and auscultation.

Vital signs are aptly named; strict attention should be paid to the assessment of these critically important parameters. Normal limits can vary depending on several factors, including age and medication use, and vital signs should be interpreted with those factors in mind. Vital signs should be obtained both accurately and serially to help determine overall stability of the patient. Because vital signs can change dramatically over rela-

Notes from Nancy
Measure vital signs frequently.

tively short time periods, failing to check them frequently, especially in the context of a significantly ill or injured patient, can lead to poor patient care.

Blood Pressure

Blood pressure is the measurement of the force exerted against the walls of the blood vessels. It is commonly measured in a peripheral artery, although it can be obtained essentially anywhere in the circulatory system. Blood pressure is the product of cardiac output and peripheral vascular resistance, so it includes two components: systolic pressure and diastolic pressure. Systolic pressure is created by the left ventricle while it is contracting (ie, in systole). Diastolic pressure is the result of residual pressure in the system while the left ventricle is relaxing (ie, in diastole). Normally, diastolic pressure should not go to zero, because peripheral vascular resistance in the arteriolar side of the circulatory system should continually provide for a diastolic pressure. The coronary arteries receive blood flow by this mechanism, so lower diastolic pressure means less myocardial perfusion.

At the Scene

Many patients exhibit an increase in blood pressure due to anxiety and the stress of an acute injury or illness. Look at your patient, as well as at trends in vital signs, before concluding that the blood pressure is truly abnormal.

Blood pressure must be measured using a cuff that is appropriate to the patient's size and habitus (physique or body build). Too small or tight a cuff will yield an artificially high pressure; too large or loose a cuff will give inappropriately low results. If blood pressure is not measured with an automatic blood pressure monitor, it should ideally be auscultated. If this is not possible, you can palpate the systolic blood pressure, although this will only provide an estimate.

Pulse

Pulse measurements should assess the presence, location, quality, rate, and rhythm of the pulses. To palpate the pulse, gently compress an artery against a bony prominence, which allows you to feel the pressure wave generated by the heart's contraction. Pulses can be obtained at several points in the body, including the radial, brachial, femoral, and carotid arteries Figure 13-4 ▶ . When formally counting the pulse rate, time the pulses for a minimum of 15 seconds and then multiply by 4 to obtain the rate per

At the Scene

Whenever possible, avoid taking a blood pressure on a painful/injured extremity, an arm with an arteriovenous shunt or fistula, or on a post-mastectomy side. This can cause pain and/or result in inaccurate readings.

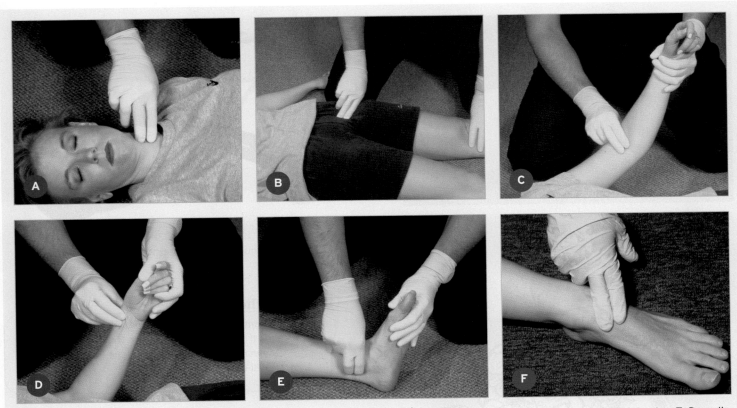

Figure 13-4 Common pulse points. **A.** Carotid pulse. **B.** Femoral pulse. **C.** Brachial pulse. **D.** Radial pulse. **E.** Posterior tibial pulse. **F.** Dorsalis pedis pulse.

Special Considerations

Palpating the carotid pulse in an infant may present a problem. Because an infant's neck is often very short and fat, and its pulse is often quite fast, you may have a hard time finding the pulse. Therefore, in infants younger than 1 year, you should palpate the brachial artery to assess the pulse.

minute. Palpating a pulse is a basic way to evaluate perfusion and cardiac output. Ambulance clinicians should compare proximal and distal pulses during patient evaluations.

Although it is appropriate to check for the presence of a central pulse in an unresponsive patient, the actual pulse rate should be counted in the most peripheral location that can be palpated, to aid with rapid estimation of the blood pressure. In the responsive patient, you may want to determine respiratory rate while you appear to be checking the pulse; this may decrease patients' tendency to inadvertently alter their breathing pattern or rate when they become aware of being evaluated.

Respiration

The respiratory rate is typically measured by inspection of the patient's chest, but respiratory movements can also be assessed by visualising portions of the abdominal wall, neck, face, and overall accessory muscle use. Although the absolute respiratory rate is important, the quality of the respiratory effort should be evaluated as well. In particular, you should learn to recognise pathological respiratory patterns or rhythms (eg, tachypnoea, Kussmaul, and Cheyne-Stokes). Similarly, you should recognise breathing difficulties when patients exhibit tripod positioning, accessory muscle use, or recession. This information is especially helpful in the assessment of paediatric patients. Respiratory rate should be measured for the full minute to gauge the exact rate.

Temperature

Many methods can be used to evaluate body temperature. If you use a tympanic device for obtaining a patient's body temperature, however, be aware of extrinsic factors that may increase or decrease the temperature reading.

At the Scene

The accuracy of tympanic membrane temperatures has been called into question by some research, especially in patients with severe infections. If your patient looks sick, feels warm, and the tympanic membrane temperature is "normal", consider using a different type of thermometer.

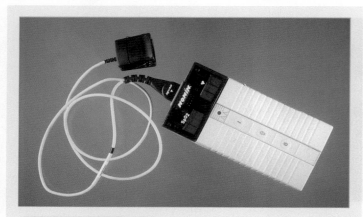

Figure 13-5 Pulse oximeter.

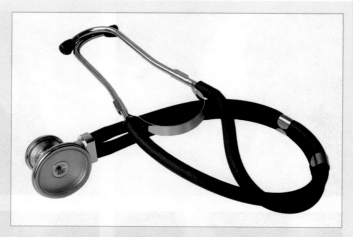

Figure 13-7 Sprague Rappaport stethoscope.

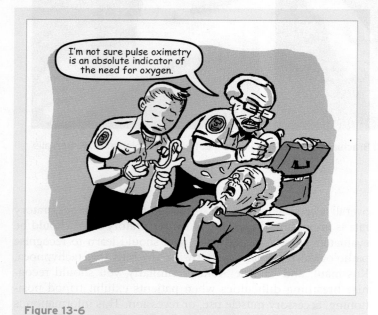

"I'm not sure pulse oximetry is an absolute indicator of the need for oxygen."

Figure 13-6

Pulse Oximetry

Measuring arterial oxygen saturation by <u>pulse oximetry</u> has earned a place in emergency health care as part of regular vital signs monitoring Figure 13-5 ▲ . Although pulse oximetry is a valuable tool, it should never be used as an absolute indicator of the need for oxygen therapies. Pulse oximetry measures the percentage of haemoglobin saturation and can provide inaccurate information in certain situations. Ambulance clinicians need to understand potential complications with pulse oximetry in order to process appropriately the information it provides Figure 13-6 ▲ . Inaccurate readings may be obtained for a variety of reasons—a hypotensive or cold patient, carbon monoxide poisoning, abnormal haemoglobin (ie, sickle-cell disease), vascular dyes, patient motion, incorrect placement, or even a dirty sensor.

At the Scene

Remember to look at your patient, not the "number". If the patient looks sick, and the pulse oximetry reading is "normal", then the patient is still sick.

Equipment Used in the Physical Examination

Equipment that can be used to perform the physical examination includes a stethoscope, blood pressure cuff (sphygmomanometer), <u>ophthalmoscope</u>, <u>otoscope</u>, scissors, a reliable light source, gloves, and a sheet or blanket.

Stethoscopes Figure 13-7 ▲ are available in two forms: acoustic and electronic. Today's acoustic stethoscope, which is the most commonly seen in the prehospital setting, consists of two earpieces attached to an air-filled tube that connects to a chest piece. The chest piece has two sides—a diaphragm (plastic disc) and a bell (hollow cup)—that can be placed against the patient to sense sounds. The diaphragm is vibrated by the sounds of the body, which are then transmitted up to the stethoscope's earpieces; thus the diaphragm side is used to pick up higher-frequency sounds. The bell, which usually transmits lower-frequency sounds, senses the sounds directly off the skin of the patient.

The acoustic stethoscope doesn't amplify sounds; rather, it simply blocks out ambient noises, allowing the paramedic to hear and appreciate the sounds of the body. In contrast, the electronic stethoscope converts the acoustic sound waves into an electronic signal that is then amplified.

The sphygmomanometer, or blood pressure cuff, is used in the measurement of the patient's blood pressure Figure 13-8 ▶ . This device consists of an inflatable cuff, which occludes blood flow, and a manometer (pressure meter),

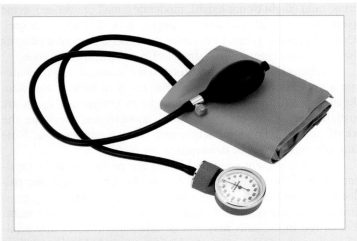

Figure 13-8 Sphygmomanometer.

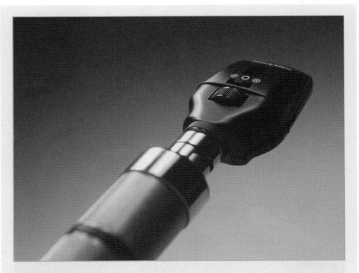

Figure 13-9 Ophthalmoscope.

which is used to determine the pressure in the artery at various points in the physical examination. These two components are connected via tubing. In manual cuffs, a separate tube connects to an inflation bulb.

Many sizes of blood pressure cuffs are available, and using the appropriate size for the patient is essential to obtain an accurate reading. The cuff should be one half to two thirds the size of the upper arm. The blood pressure measurement is separated into systolic and diastolic pressures and is reported in millimetres of mercury (mm Hg).

The ophthalmoscope allows the clinician to look into a patient's eyes and view the retina and aqueous fluid. This tool consists of a concave mirror and a battery-powered light, which

is usually contained in the device's handle   **Figure 13-9 ▲** . The clinician looks through a monocular eyepiece that is usually equipped with a rotating disc of lenses; selection of a lens allows for adjustment of the depth and magnification. Use of the ophthalmoscope is usually reserved for hospital and GP surgery examination, because effective evaluation requires dilation of the patient's pupils with medication.

The otoscope is used to evaluate the ears of a patient. This instrument consists of a head and a handle. The head contains an electric light source and a low-power magnifying lens. The front of the headpiece has an attachment for a disposable plastic

You are the Paramedic Part 2

Your colleague starts to obtain the patient's vital signs and you begin your patient assessment. The GP tells you that the patient made an emergency appointment this morning for increasing shortness of breath that began last night around 22:00. He presented in severe respiratory distress with increased work of breathing and audible wheezes. He was nebulised with 5 mg of salbutamol 20 minutes prior to the ambulance service being called. Your examination reveals that the patient is still experiencing severe respiratory distress. He has a barrel-shaped chest with marked intercostal and supraclavicular recession, pursed lipped breathing, audible inspiratory and expiratory wheezes, and can only speak in one- or two-word sentences. You also observe cyanosis around his mouth and nail beds with clubbing of the fingers. The GP provides you with the patient's medical history, which is significant for a 60-year smoking habit, emphysema, and hypertension. He is prescribed 2.5 mg of salbutamol/normal saline via nebuliser four times a day, two puffs of budesonide inhaler twice a day, 200 mg of metoprolol once a day, and home oxygen at 3 l/min. He has an allergy to iodine and penicillin.

Vital Signs	Recording Time: 5 Minutes
Skin	Pale, warm, with cyanotic lips and nail beds
Pulse	130 beats/min, regular; strong radial
Blood pressure	168/82 mm Hg
Respirations	40 breaths/min, laboured, audible wheezes
SpO_2	80% with a Venturi mask administering 28% O_2

3. Which signs and symptoms are acute? Which are chronic?

4. Which interventions should you consider at this point?

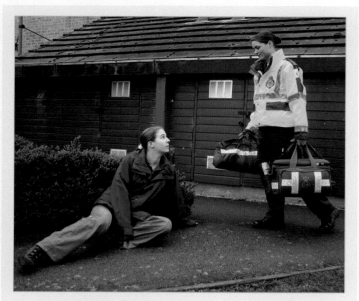

Figure 13-10 Get a general impression of the overall situation as you approach the patient.

earpiece (speculum). The clinician inserts the speculum into the ear and looks through a lens on the rear of the headpiece. Some otoscopes include a sliding rear window that allows for the insertion of an additional instrument (eg, to remove ear wax). Most have an insertion point for a bulb that is used to push air into the ear canal, allowing the clinician to visualise the movement of the tympanic membrane. The batteries are located in the handle unless it is a wall-mounted unit, such as those found in a GP surgery.

The General Survey

The general survey begins as you approach the scene, simultaneously assessing the situation and the patient's overall presentation   Figure 13-10 ▲ . A quick look at the environment in which the patient is found and the general appearance of the patient provides a substantial amount of information before you ask the first question. An important skill that many paramedics develop is a sense as to when a patient is seriously ill, based primarily on his or her initial appearance. The expression "sick or not sick?" sums up this approach.

Look for signs of significant distress such as mental status changes, anxiousness, laboured breathing, difficulty speaking, diaphoresis, obvious pain, obvious deformity, and guarding of a painful area. It is not uncommon for individuals experiencing substantial and incapacitating pain to show little external sign, so use your history to help you.

Other aspects that may be readily apparent and worth noting during the general survey include dress, hygiene, expression, overall size, posture, untoward odours, and overall state of health. When characterising the overall state of the patient, be sure to use appropriate terms to describe degree of distress: no apparent dis-

tress, mild (slight or not harsh), moderate (small or average), acute (very great or bad), and severe (dangerous or difficult to endure). Other acceptable terms to describe the general state of a patient's health include chronically ill, frail, feeble, robust, and vigorous.

Perhaps the quickest and most reliable initial way to evaluate a patient's overall degree of distress is to look at the skin. Relatively subtle but serious changes in overall perfusion are usually seen early on in the skin's appearance. Evaluate the skin's colour, relative moisture, and relative temperature. Note any obvious lesions or deformities.

Pallor is present when red blood cell perfusion to the capillary beds of the skin is poor. You may also be able to detect pallor by looking at the patient's lips or eye conjunctiva. Cyanosis indicates a relative lack of oxygen perfusion, although the number of red blood cells may still be adequate to carry any available oxygen. Cyanosis correlates extremely well with low arterial oxygen saturation. It can be visualised generally in the skin, but more specifically in the fingernail beds, face, and lips.

Ecchymosis is localised bruising or blood collection within or under the skin. Evaluate large ecchymoses for the possibility of serious underlying soft-tissue, bony, or organ injury. Serious wounds to the head, neck, and torso should also be noted, as well as any evidence of a potential haemorrhage.

The Physical Examination

The physical examination of a patient in the prehospital setting is the most important skill a health care provider can master. This ability is first developed as a technician and should be refined as an advanced practitioner. Starting intravenous access, administering medications, and performing endotracheal intubation are simply mechanical skills that require only practice to achieve proficiency. The skills of patient assessment and interpreting the findings of a physical examination, by comparison, truly separate the accomplished paramedic from the technician. The physical examination consists of a comprehensive review of systems to determine the nature and extent of the patient's illness or injury.

Mental Status
Evaluation of a patient's mental status involves assessing cognitive function (ie, ability to use reasoning or perception). At a minimum, evaluate the patient's degree of alertness. This assessment is accomplished by using the AO × 4 method, which means the patient is alert and orientated to person, place, time, and events leading up to this particular moment. The AVPU scale is a rapid method of assessing the patient's level of consciousness using one of the following four designations:

A *Alert* (orientated to person, place, and day)
V Responds to *Verbal* stimuli
P Responds to *Painful* stimuli
U *Unresponsive*

When classifying the response to stimuli, grade the patient according to the best response you can elicit. For example, a patient passed out on the street who moans in response to a loud shout from the paramedic would score a V on the AVPU scale. Response to tactile stimuli (eg, pinching the earlobe, applying supraorbital pressure) would earn a P. No response to verbal or tactile stimuli would be classified as U.

Skin, Hair, and Nails
Skin

The skin, which is the largest organ system in the body, serves three major functions: It regulates the temperature of the body, transmits information from the environment to the brain, and protects the body in the environment.

The skin is the major organ governing the body's thermoregulation. In a cold environment, constriction of the blood vessels shunts blood away from the skin to decrease the amount of heat radiated from the body surface (observed as pale skin). When the outside environment is hot, the vessels in the skin dilate, the skin becomes flushed or red, and heat radiates from the body surface. Also, in a hot environment, sweat is secreted to the skin surface from the sweat glands. Energy, in the form of body heat, is lost during the evaporation process, which causes body temperature to fall.

Information from the environment is carried to the brain through a rich supply of sensory nerves that originate in the skin. Nerve endings that lie in the skin are adapted to perceive and transmit information about heat, cold, external pressure, pain, and the position of the body in space. In this way, the skin recognises changes in the environment. It also reacts to pressure, pain, and pleasurable stimuli.

The skin is composed of two layers: the epidermis and the dermis Figure 13-11 ▶ . The epidermis, or outermost layer, is the body's first line of defence. It serves as the principal barrier against water, dust, microorganisms, and mechanical stress.

Underlying the epidermis is the dermis—a tough, highly elastic layer of connective tissues. This complex material is composed chiefly of collagen fibres, elastic fibres, and a mucopolysaccharide gel. Numerous fibroblasts (cells that secrete collagen, elastin, and ground substance) are found within the dermis as well.

The dermis is subdivided into the papillary dermis and a reticular layer. The vasculature inside the papillary dermis serves two functions—it provides nutrients to the epidermis, and aids in thermoregulation. Dilation of these vessels increases blood flow to the skin, allowing heat to dissipate. Conversely, blood vessel constriction results in retention of heat. The reticular layer consists of dense, irregular connective tissue, which provides both strength and elasticity. With age, the skin undergoes significant changes, including loss of the collagen connective tissues and diminished capillary supply.

Examination of the skin involves both inspection and palpation. Pay careful attention to the skin colour, moisture, temperature, texture, turgor, and any significant lesions. Look for evidence of diminished perfusion, evaluate for pallor and cyanosis, and be wary of diaphoresis. Reddened or pink skin can be seen in a variety of normal states, but it is also evident in states of relative vasodilatation (flushing). Flushed skin is usually apparent in patients with fever, and it may be seen in patients experiencing an allergic process. Reddened skin should also be considered in the context of superficial burns.

Examining the skin for changes in perfusion is usually best accomplished in areas where the epidermis is thinnest, such as the fingernails, lips, and conjunctivae. It is sometimes useful to examine the palms and soles as well. Pale skin is a relatively common finding in the seriously ill patient and may indicate severe vasoconstriction, as seen in profound anaemia, acute cardiovascular events, other shock-like states, and hypothermia. Local areas of blanched, cool, white skin are typical of

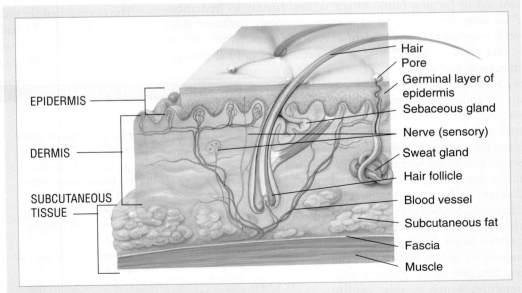

Figure 13-11 The skin is composed of a tough external layer (the epidermis) and a vascular inner layer (the dermis).

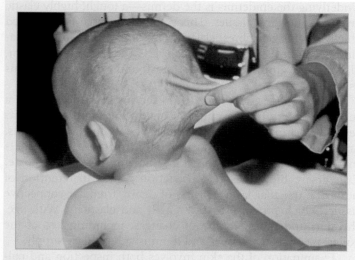

Figure 13-12 Tenting is evident with extreme dehydration.

Special Considerations

When assessing skin turgor in an older patient, use the skin of the upper chest. This is a much more reliable indicator than the extremities.

frostbite. Although cyanotic skin is commonly seen in states of oxygen desaturation, it can also be a function of hypothermia, especially in very young patients. Mottling is a typical finding in states of severe protracted hypoperfusion and shock and is readily evident in paediatric patients.

It takes practice to gauge patients' relative perfusion and hydration status accurately. Becoming familiar with the abnormal findings of the skin and mucous membranes is an excellent aid in judging both. Turgor relates directly to hydration. Poor skin turgidity is an expression of poorly hydrated skin, with associated tenting evident in extreme cases, particularly in young children (Figure 13-12 ▲). Because of normal changes in elastin and connective tissues with advanced age, skin turgor is an insignificant indicator in older patients, as is skin that is abnormally dry to the touch. Paying attention to skin temperature can sometimes prove useful when trying to determine the aetiologies of different problems (eg, respiratory distress). Sometimes making a clinical distinction between congestive heart failure with pulmonary oedema versus pneumonia is a function of the patient's temperature, which may be readily apparent from tactile examination of the skin.

At the Scene

When inspecting the skin, always be alert for signs of possible abuse or maltreatment. Multiple bruises at different stages of healing or even pressure sores may raise concerns about possible physical abuse and should be reported.

Skin lesions may sometimes be the only external evidence of a serious internal injury. Take note of any large areas of bruising, palpable crepitus (palpable fractures), and open wounds. Devastating internal injuries can result from wounds whose only external signs are relatively benign-appearing penetrations. Be aware of any body areas that are hidden by clothing or by devices such as a longboard and head immobiliser. Always visually inspect and manually palpate the patient's back and expose body parts. Likewise, evaluation for rashes is usually best accomplished by discreetly examining areas of skin otherwise hidden by clothing.

Hair

Examination of the hair is done by inspection and palpation. In this survey, note the quantity, distribution, and texture of the hair. Recent changes in the growth or loss of hair can indicate an underlying endocrine disorder, such as diabetes, or may result from treatment modalities for disease processes (eg, chemotherapy or radiation treatment of cancer). Although the recent loss of hair may be related to a disease process, the thinning and loss of hair can also be a normal finding in the older patient.

Nails

The examination of the fingernails and toenails can reveal many subtle findings (Table 13-1 ▼). The colour, shape, texture, and presence or absence of lesions should all be assessed. The normal nail should be firm and smooth on palpation. Normal changes to the nails with ageing include the development of striations and a change in colour (yellowish tint) related to the reduction in body calcium.

Table 13-1	Abnormal Findings in the Nails	
Condition	**Findings**	**Possible Cause**
Beau's lines	Transverse depressions in the nail inhibiting growth	Systemic illness, severe infection, or nail injury
Clubbing	The angle between the nail and the nail base approaches or exceeds 180°	Flattening and enlargement of the fingertips is associated with chronic respiratory disease
Psoriasis	Pitting, discolouration, and subungual thickening of the nail	
Splinter haemorrhages	Red or brown linear streaks in the nail bed	Bacterial endocarditis or trichinosis
Terry's nails	Transverse white bands that cover the nail except for the distal tip	Cirrhosis (liver)

Head, Ears, Eyes, Nose, and Throat

The head, ears, eyes, nose, and throat (HEENT) examination consists of a comprehensive evaluation of the head and related structures. It is crucial because the head contains the brain, numerous important sensory organs, and all of the upper airway anatomy. The eyes are a nervous system structure that involves both motor pathways (lids, extraocular muscles, pupillary constrictors, corneal blink reflex) and sensory pathways. The ears provide for both hearing and balance control. The nose is a sensory organ involved with the senses of smell and taste; it also plays an important role in assisting with breathing. The throat consists of the mouth and posterior pharynx, and all the structures intrinsic to them. This complicated organ simultaneously coordinates many motor and sensory functions, while also coordinating the initial activities of both the respiratory and digestive systems.

Head

The head is divided into two parts: the cranium and the face. The cranium, or skull, contains the brain. The brain connects to the spinal cord through the foramen magnum, a large opening at the base of the skull. The most posterior portion of the cranium is the occiput. On each side of the cranium, the lateral portions are called the temples or temporal regions. Between the temporal regions and the occiput lie the parietal regions. The forehead is called the frontal region. Just anterior to the ear, in the temporal region, you can feel the pulse of the superficial temporal artery. A layer of muscle fascia covers the skull. The thick skin covering the cranium, which usually bears hair, is called the scalp.

Within the skull lie the meninges, three distinct layers of tissue that suspend the brain and the spinal cord within the skull and the spinal canal. The dura mater is the tough, fibrous, outer layer that resembles leather. It forms a sac that contains the central nervous system (CNS), with small openings through which the peripheral nerves exit. The inner two layers of the meninges, called the arachnoid and the pia mater, are much thinner than the dura mater. They contain the blood vessels that nourish the brain and spinal cord. Cerebrospinal fluid (CSF) is produced in a chamber inside the brain, called the third ventricle. CSF fills the space between the meninges and acts as a shock absorber.

When you are examining the head, you should inspect it visually and feel it. This step is important in the management of potential trauma patients and with patients who have altered mental status or are unresponsive. If you find evidence of external bleeding, attempt to separate the hair manually and irrigate the clot; this should allow you to identify the source of bleeding.

Special Considerations

Always inspect the fontanelle in infants.
Bulging = Increased intracranial pressure in a quiet child
Sunken = Dehydration

Evaluate the skull for any deformity, step-off, or tenderness. Observe the general shape and contour of the skull.

In children younger than 18 months, routinely palpate the anterior fontanelle (the "soft spot"). Prior to its normal physiological closure, it can serve as an excellent relative indicator of hydration and intracranial pressure. The fontanelle is usually characterised as open and flat (the normal state), bulging (common while crying, pathological when observed in a quiet child), and sunken (in severe dehydration).

When you are evaluating the face, observe the colour and moisture of the skin, as well as expression, symmetry, and contour of the face itself. Also pay attention to any swelling or apparent areas of injury, and note any signs of respiratory distress. Use the mnemonic DCAP-BTLS—Deformities, Contusions, Abrasions, Punctures/penetrations, Burns, Tenderness, Lacerations, and Swelling—to assist you during the physical examination. Follow the steps in **Skill Drill 13-2** to assess the head:

1. Visually inspect the head, looking for any obvious DCAP-BTLS **Step 1**.
2. Palpate the top and back of the head to locate any subtle abnormalities **Step 2**. Use a systematic approach, going from front to back, to ensure that nothing is missed.
3. Part the hair in several places to examine the condition of the scalp. Identify any lesions under the hair **Step 3**.
4. Note any pain during the process (this examination should not cause the patient any pain).
5. Palpate the structure of the face noting any DCAP-BTLS. Pay attention to the condition of the skin, hair distribution, and shape of the face **Step 4**.

At the Scene

Protecting fragile CNS structures from further damage is vital to the patient's prospects for living a normal life. Lean toward caution and overprotection in assessing and treating possible brain and spinal cord injuries.

Eyes

The eyes are a tremendously complex sensory organ **Figure 13-13**. They process light stimuli for the brain, so that the brain is able to decode light impulses presenting to the eyes and form a visual image. The eyes are a critical link to the CNS, and as such they allow the examiner to more precisely assess the functions of the CNS.

Each eye consists of an anterior chamber and a posterior chamber, which are always assessed in a standardised fashion (ie, from "front to back"). The outer aspects of the eye are checked first, with deeper structures subsequently evaluated. General issues to ask about include any pain or redness, loss of vision, diplopia (double vision), photophobia, blurring, discharge, and corrective contact lens use.

After addressing these general questions, assess for visual acuity (VA)—that is, the ability or inability to see, and how

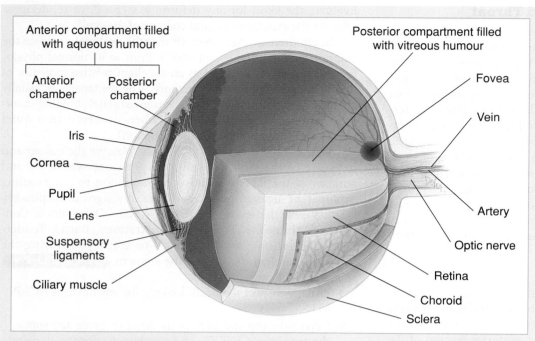

Anterior compartment filled with aqueous humour

Anterior chamber

Posterior chamber

Iris

Cornea

Pupil

Lens

Suspensory ligaments

Ciliary muscle

Posterior compartment filled with vitreous humour

Fovea

Vein

Artery

Optic nerve

Retina

Choroid

Sclera

Figure 13-13 The structure of the eye.

Skill Drill 13-2: Assessing the Head

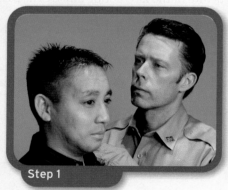

Step 1

Visually inspect the head, looking for any obvious DCAP-BTLS.

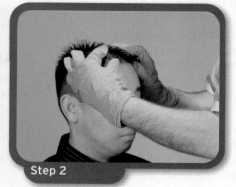

Step 2

Palpate the top and back of the head to locate any subtle abnormalities.

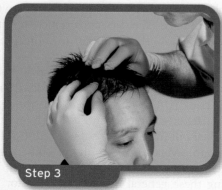

Step 3

Part the hair in several places to examine the condition of the scalp.

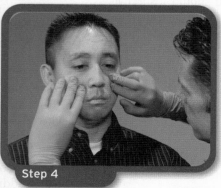

Step 4

Palpate the structure of the face, noting any DCAP-BTLS.

well the patient can see. Check VA by examining each eye in isolation. If prescription corrective lenses are normally worn, check VA with the correction in place. The standard device for checking VA is the Snellen ("E") chart Figure 13-14 ▶, although it is not an appropriate tool in the prehospital setting. More appropriate tools in this environment include simple tests such as light/dark discrimination and finger counting. Finger counting should be done from a noted distance, typically 2 m, 1 m, and 30 cm. Reporting on VA must include the distance from which finger counting was measured.

The pupil is a circular opening in the centre of the pigmented iris of the eye. The diameter and reactivity of the patient's pupil to light reflect the status of the brain's perfusion, oxygenation, and condition. The pupils are normally round and of approximately equal size; they serve as optical diaphragms, adjusting their size depending on the available light. In normal room light, the pupils appear to be midsized. With less light, they dilate to allow more light to enter the eye, making it possible to see even in dim light. With high light levels or when a bright light is suddenly introduced, the pupils instantly constrict, allowing less light to enter and protecting the sensitive receptors in the inner eye from damage. When a brighter light is introduced into one eye (or higher levels of light enter one eye only), both pupils should constrict equally to the appropriate size for the pupil receiving the most light.

In the absence of any light, the pupils will become fully relaxed and dilated. When light is introduced, each eye sends sensory signals to the brain, indicating the level of light received. Pupil size is regulated

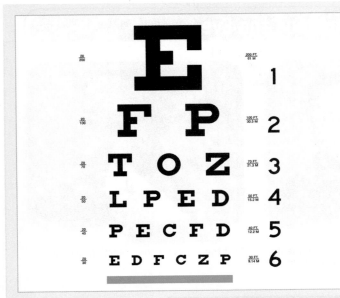

Figure 13-14 Due to its size and complexity, the Snellen chart is not a good prehospital tool.

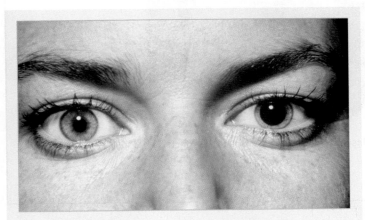

Figure 13-15 Asymmetric pupils may be normal or may signify a severe brain injury.

by a series of continuous motor commands that the brain automatically sends through the oculomotor nerves (third cranial nerve) to each eye. Normally, pupil size changes instantly to any change in light level.

When assessing the pupils, check for size (in millimetres), shape, and symmetry. Also check for a reaction to light shined on them, performing this assessment in as darkened an environment as possible. Asymmetric pupils (anisocoria, which can be found in 20% of the population) may indicate significant ocular or neurological pathology, but must be correlated with the patient's overall presentation Figure 13-15 ▲ . Topical applications of certain medicines and substances can also provoke pupillary changes.

Muscles are responsible for physically moving the eyes from side to side and up and down, which allows for seamless binocular vision. When asked to follow a finger moved in a "Z" or "H" pattern, the eyes should move smoothly and symmetrically with the finger. Visual field examination assesses the

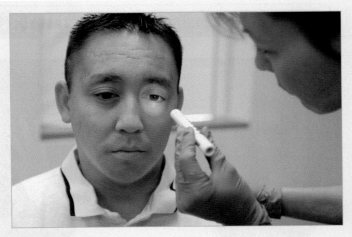

Figure 13-16 Pen light examination of the eye.

retina's (and therefore the optic nerve's) ability to perceive light. This is done by checking the patient's peripheral vision, examining each eye in isolation.

Following the general eye examination, a more precise pen light examination is typically undertaken Figure 13-16 ▲ . Check the lids, lashes, and tear ducts. Look for foreign bodies, evidence of wounds and trauma, and discharge. Turn up the lids to look for foreign bodies, and inspect the conjunctivae and sclera. The sclera ought to be white, not jaundiced or injected (red). Painless subconjunctival haemorrhage is a common but benign presentation. The conjunctivae ought to be pink—not cyanotic, pale, or overly reddened. The cornea and lens will be difficult to examine without additional assessment tools—although in a trauma situation, you should note whether the globe is patent. Next, examine the anterior chamber and iris for clarity, noting any cloudiness or bleeding. Finally, examine the posterior chamber and retina; however, this examination is more useful after chemical dilation of the pupil and appropriate use of an ophthalmoscope. Follow the steps in Skill Drill 13-3 ▶ and Skill Drill 13-4 ▶ :

1. Examine the exterior portion of the eye. Look for any obvious trauma or deformity Step 1 .
2. Ask the patient about any pain, altered vision (eg, blurred or double vision), discharge, or sensitivity to light.
3. Measure visual acuity by having the patient count the number of fingers you are holding up at varying distances (usually 2 m, 1 m, and 30 cm away from the patient). Perform this examination on each eye independently of the other Step 2 .
4. Examine the pupils for size, shape, and symmetry. They should be equal.
5. Test the pupils for their reaction to light. Both pupils should constrict when exposed to light, and they should be equal in their response Step 3 .
6. Test for cranial nerve function by asking the patient to follow your fingers in a "Z" or "H" pattern. Note any abnormal movement of the eyes Step 4 .
7. Inspect the eyelids, lashes, and tear ducts for evidence of trauma, foreign bodies, or discharge Step 5 .

Skill Drill 13-3: Examining the Eye

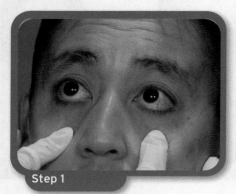

Step 1

Examine the exterior portion of the eye.

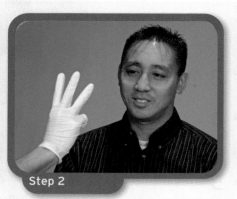

Step 2

Measure visual acuity by having the patient count the number of fingers you are holding up at varying distances.

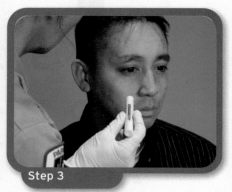

Step 3

Test the pupils for their reaction to light.

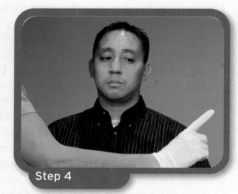

Step 4

Test for cranial nerve function by asking the patient to follow your fingers in a "Z" or "H" pattern.

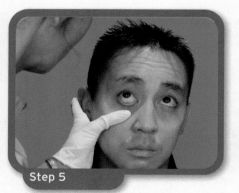

Step 5

Inspect the eyelids, lashes, and tear ducts.

At the Scene

Eye movement is not parallel. Failure to follow in a certain direction indicates weakness of an extraocular muscle or dysfunction of a cranial nerve innervating it.

At the Scene

Cataracts appear as opaque black areas against the red reflex.

1. Darken the environment as much as possible.
2. Ask the patient to look straight ahead and focus on a distant object (Step 1).
3. Set the light on the ophthalmoscope to a setting no brighter than necessary and the lens to 0 unless another setting works better for your eyes.
4. Use your right hand and eye to examine the patient's right eye; use your left hand and eye to examine the patient's left eye (Step 2).
5. Place the scope to your eye and look into the patient's pupil from 25 to 50 cm away at a 45° angle to the eye. You should see the retina as a "red reflex" or a bright orange glow (Step 3).
6. Slowly move toward the patient to appreciate the structures of the fundus. Adjust the lens as needed to improve the focus. Locate a blood vessel and follow it back to the disc. Use this blood vessel as a point of reference.
7. Inspect for the size, colour, and clarity of the disc. Note the integrity of the blood vessels and any lesions present on the retina. Move nasally to observe the macula (yellow spot near the centre of the retina) (Step 4).
8. Repeat the process with the other eye.

Skill Drill 13-4: Eye Examination With an Ophthalmoscope

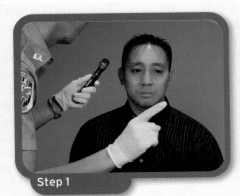

Step 1

Ask the patient to look straight ahead and focus on a distant object.

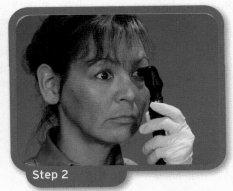

Step 2

Use your right hand and eye to examine the patient's right eye; use your left hand and eye to examine the patient's left eye.

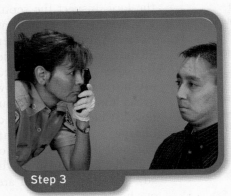

Step 3

Place the scope to your eye and look into the patient's pupil from 25 to 50 cm away at a 45° angle to the eye.

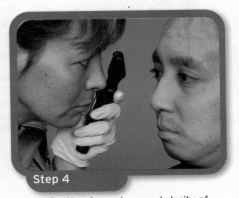

Step 4

Inspect for the size, colour, and clarity of the disc.

At the Scene

Use of the ophthalmoscope requires frequent practice. It is not routinely used in prehospital care.

Ears

The ear is a sensory organ that is chiefly involved with hearing and sound perception but is also intimately involved with balance control. The ear consists of an outer portion, a middle portion, and an inner portion Figure 13-17 ▶.

The external ear consists of the pinna, or auricle (the part lying outside of the head), and the external auditory canal, which leads in toward the tympanic membrane, or eardrum.

The middle ear contains three small bones, the malleus, incus, and stapes (hammer, anvil, and stirrup), that move in response to sound waves hitting the tympanic membrane. This mechanism controls how we hear and differentiate sounds. The middle ear is connected to the nasal cavity by the Eustachian tube, or internal auditory canal. This connection permits equalisation of pressure in the middle ear when external atmospheric pressure changes.

The inner ear consists of bony chambers filled with fluid. As the head moves, so does the fluid. In response, fine nerve endings within the fluid send impulses to the brain, indicating the position of the head and the rate of change of position.

Assessing the ears essentially involves checking for new aberrations in hearing perception plus inspecting and palpating for wounds, swelling, or drainage (pus, blood, CSF). Often the mastoid process of the skull, which is palpated immediately posterior to the auricle, is assessed for discolouration and tenderness (Battle's sign). Abnormalities of the external canal and tympanic membrane are visualised by use of an otoscope. Follow the steps in Skill Drill 13-5 ▶ :

1. Select an appropriately sized speculum. Dim the lights as much as possible.
2. Ensure that the ear is free of foreign bodies.
3. Place your hand firmly against the patient's head and gently grasp the patient's auricle. Move the ear to best visualise the canal, usually upward and back in the adult patient Step 1 .
4. Instruct the patient not to move during the examination to avoid damaging the ear.
5. Turn on the otoscope and insert the speculum into the ear Step 2 . Insertion toward the patient's nose usually provides the best view. Don't insert the speculum deeply into the canal.

At the Scene

When looking for a foreign body, don't advance an otoscope tip blindly; you may accidentally push the foreign body in further.

6. Inspect the canal for any lesions or discharge. A small amount of cerumen (ear wax) is normal (Step 3).

7. Visualise the tympanic membrane (eardrum), and inspect it for integrity and colour. It should be translucent or a pearly grey colour. Note any signs of inflammation, including swelling or discolouration (pink or redness in the canal or tympanic membrane).

Nose

The nose is a sensory organ involved with smell and taste; it is also part of the respiratory system. In assessing injuries involving the nose, it helps to picture the inside of the nose itself **Figure 13-18 ▶**. The nasal cavity is divided into two sections or chambers by the nasal septum, which is made of cartilage. Each nasal chamber contains three layers of bone (the turbinates) that are covered with a moist lining. Both chambers have superior, middle, and inferior turbinates. During nasal breathing, the air moves through the nasal chambers and is humidified as it passes over the turbinates.

When checking the nose, assess it both anteriorly and inferiorly. Look for evidence of asymmetry, deformity, wounds, foreign bodies, discharge or bleeding, and tenderness. Note any evidence of respiratory distress, such as flaring of the nostrils. Inspect the exterior of the nose, looking for colour changes, symmetry, and structural abnormalities. The nose should be firm and the nares clear of obstruction. Examine the column of the nose; it should be midline with the face. Inspect the septum for any deviation from midline. The nares should be symmetrical. Slight deviation or asymmetry of the nares, septum, and column are normal findings; however, gross abnormalities should be noted. Note any drainage or discharge. Small amounts of mucosal discharge are normal, but large amounts of mucus and any blood or CSF fluid are serious findings.

Throat

Assessment of the throat should include an evaluation of the

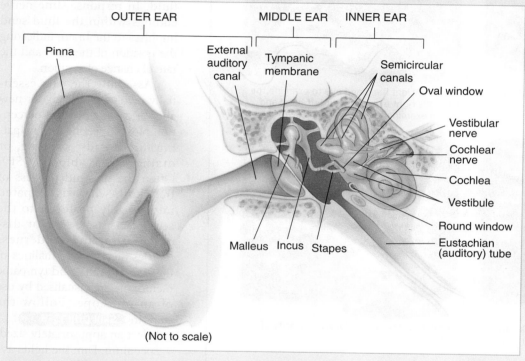

Figure 13-17 The structure of the outer, middle, and inner ear.

Skill Drill 13-5: Examining the Ear With an Otoscope

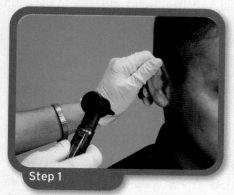

Step 1

Place your hand firmly against the patient's head and gently grasp the patient's auricle.

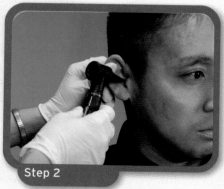

Step 2

Turn on the otoscope and insert the speculum into the ear.

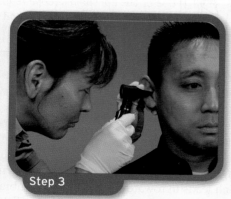

Step 3

Inspect the canal for any lesions or discharge.

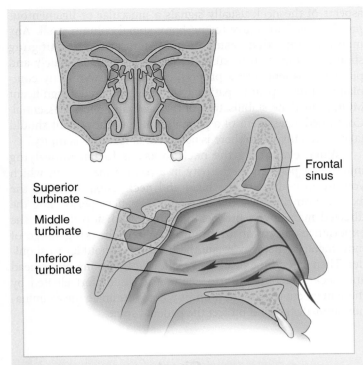

Figure 13-18 The nose has two chambers, divided by the septum. Each chamber is composed of layers of bone called turbinates. Above the nose are the frontal sinuses. On either side of the nose are the orbits of the eyes.

Frontal sinus

Superior turbinate

Middle turbinate

Inferior turbinate

At the Scene

Frank blood or clear, watery drainage (CSF) from the ears or nose following trauma suggests a basilar skull fracture.

mouth, the pharynx, and sometimes the neck. The throat is a conduit for both respiration and digestion, and it is in close proximity to numerous vital neurovascular structures.

As part of the assessment of overall hydration status, pay close attention to the lips, teeth, oral mucosa, and tongue. In patients who present with markedly altered mental status, you'll need to rapidly determine upper airway status; prompt assessment of the throat and upper airway structures is mandatory. Depending on the situation, assess for the presence of a foreign body or aspiration in either the throat or lower airway structures. Situations requiring removal of foreign bodies, secretions, or blood can manifest in many types of emergency cases. Always be prepared to assist with clearing the pharynx using manual techniques and suction.

The examination of the mouth begins with the lips, which should be pink and free of oedema or surface irregularities. Confirm that the mouth is symmetrical. The gums should be pink, with no lesions or oedema. Inspect the airway to ensure that it is free of obstructions. Visualise the tongue, noting its colour, size, and moisture. The tongue should be located at midline, without swelling, and moist. Examine the oropharynx, identifying any discolouration or pustules that might indicate an infection. Note

any unusual odours on the breath, as they can indicate certain illnesses. Inspect the uvula for oedema and redness.

The neck is an extraordinarily muscular region, through which many vital structures pass. External anatomy includes the jaw, cricothyroid membrane, external jugular veins, thyroid cartilage, suprasternal notch, and cervical spinous processes. When assessing the neck, take the time to look for any abnormalities, including those related to symmetry, masses, and venous distension. In order to measure the jugular venous pulse, the patient needs to be positioned reclining at 45°. This is not appropriate if you suspect a spinal injury! Make sure that the neck muscles are relaxed and look across the neck from the side of the patient. Estimate the height of the venous pulsation from the sternal angle. Usually, it is just visible above the clavicle. Any higher, and it is considered to be raised. Palpate the carotid pulses and note relative strength of impulse. Look for any pulsating or expanding mass near the carotid pulse point. Palpate the suprasternal notch in an effort to identify any tracheal deviation. Have the patient open and close the jaws while you palpate over the temporomandibular joint during your examination of the jaw. To examine the neck, follow the steps in Skill Drill 13-6 ▸ :

1. If trauma is suspected, take precautions to protect the cervical spine (Step 1).
2. Assess for the usage of accessory muscles during respiration.
3. Palpate the neck to find any structural abnormalities or subcutaneous air, and to ensure the trachea is midline. Begin at the suprasternal notch and work your way toward the head (Step 2). Be careful about applying pressure to the area of the carotid arteries, as it may stimulate a vagal response.
4. Assess the lymph nodes and note any swelling, which may indicate infection (Step 3).
5. Assess the jugular veins for distension; it may indicate a problem with blood returning to the heart (Step 4).

Cervical Spine

The cervical spine is the pathway by which the spinal cord makes its way out of the brain and into the torso, enabling the spinal nerves to branch out and innervate the rest of the body Figure 13-19 ▸ . It is also the point at which the head connects to the body. The spine is supported by a large mass of muscle, as well as multiple tendinous and ligamentous supports. Cervical injury can present in a variety of ways, and the assessment for such injury must be conducted in a careful manner.

Evaluate the patient first for the MOI and then for the presence of pain. Does the patient have an altered mental status, or did a loss of consciousness occur at the time of the event? Is there a significant MOI, or do multiple or serious distracting injuries make assessment of the cervical spine difficult? Is the patient under the influence of any intoxicating substances? Being able to confidently answer all of those questions will allow you to decide which patients may (or may not) require further treatment of a potential cervical spine injury.

When examining the cervical spine, inspect and palpate it, looking for evidence of tenderness and deformity. Midline posterior tenderness involving the bony spinous processes should always raise concerns. Palpable discomfort over the lateral

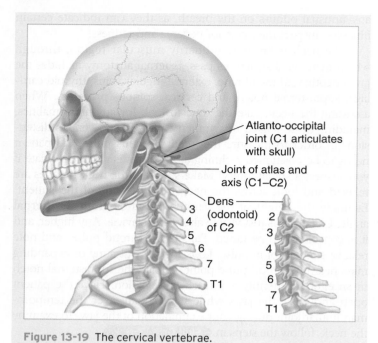

Figure 13-19 The cervical vertebrae.

Labels in figure:
- Atlanto-occipital joint (C1 articulates with skull)
- Joint of atlas and axis (C1–C2)
- Dens (odontoid) of C2
- 3 4 5 6 7 T1
- 2 3 4 5 6 7 T1

aspects of the neck usually signals a muscular or ligamentous problem, not an injury to the bony spinal column itself. Any manipulations that result in pain, tenderness, or tingling should prompt you to stop the examination *immediately* and place the patient into a properly sized collar. With any complaints of neck pain in patients who have suffered a significant MOI, immediate stabilisation of the head and neck is essential. Continued assessment of a patient's range of movement should take place only when there is *no* potential for serious injury.

When examining the neck to assess for an underlying injury, first perform the activity in a passive manner, in which you are in control of the head and neck. Next, conduct the examination actively—that is, with the patient performing the directed manoeuvres but being cautioned to stop if he or she experiences any pain or tingling. When checking range of movement, first slowly rotate the head from shoulder to shoulder. Then extend the head back, followed by flexing of the head and neck, touching chin to chest. Any discomfort elicited by these manoeuvres should prompt you to terminate the examination immediately and protect the patient's spine.

Skill Drill 13-6: Examining the Neck

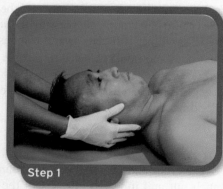

Step 1

If trauma is suspected, take precautions to protect the cervical spine.

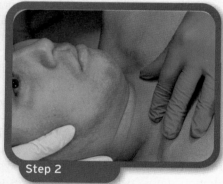

Step 2

Palpate the neck to find any structural abnormalities or subcutaneous air, and to ensure the trachea is midline. Begin at the suprasternal notch and work your way toward the head.

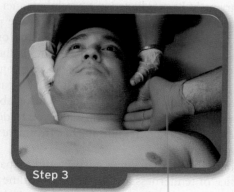

Step 3

Assess the lymph nodes.

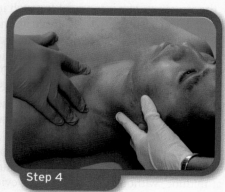

Step 4

Assess the jugular veins for distension.

Chest

The chest (or thorax) consists of the superior aspect of the torso, from the base of the neck to the diaphragm as delineated by the costal arch **Figure 13-20 ▶**. The chest wall is divided into anterior and posterior portions—literally, the patient's front and back. The back of the chest extends down the patient's back, to the level of the diaphragm posteriorly, which tends to move up and down with breathing. The chest contains many vital structures, including the lungs and mediastinal elements (heart, great vessels). The chest wall serves as a protective covering for the internal components. It consists of numerous musculoskeletal, vascular, nervous, connective, and lining structures.

Typically, the chest examination proceeds in three phases. The chest wall is checked, a pulmonary evaluation is conducted, and finally the cardiovascular assessment is performed. The chest must be inspected to assess for deformities in wall patency as well as to look for external clues of respiratory distress. Expose the chest and then begin its assessment, using the techniques of inspection, palpation, percussion, and auscultation. The examination of the posterior

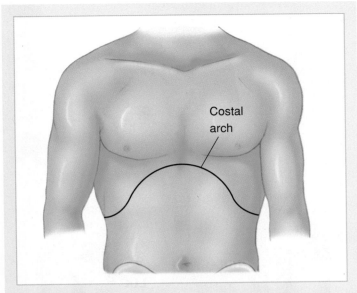

Figure 13-20 The chest (thorax) consists of the superior aspect of the torso, from the base of the neck to the diaphragm as delineated by the costal arch.

Compare the two sides of the chest for symmetry. Observe the chest wall for respiratory effort, and document the respiratory rate, depth, and rhythm. Listen to the patient's breathing, and note the general shape of the chest wall. Pay close attention to any signs of abnormal breathing movements (paradox, accessory muscle use, impaired or diminished breathing movement) and recession (suprasternal, sternal, intercostal, and subcostal). The presence of recession is an important indicator of pulmonary issues, especially in children. Note any chest deformities, such as barrel chest (chronic obstructive pulmonary disease [COPD]), flail segments/subcutaneous air (trauma), kyphoscoliosis of the spine (compression fractures, COPD), significant bruising, and any suspicious wounds.

When palpating the chest wall, note any tenderness or crepitus. Be sure to palpate areas that were initially noted to be abnormal on inspection. Palpation will also enable you to better appreciate respiratory symmetry and expansion. Although often impractical in the prehospital environment, percussion of the chest wall can allow for enhanced evaluation of the underlying chest cavity by distinguishing either dullness or hyperresonance versus normal resonance.

Auscultate the breath sounds **Figure 13-21 ▸**. The lungs consist of five discrete lobes: The right side contains the right upper, right middle, and right lower lobes; the left side contains

chest is the same as the examination of the anterior chest. Follow the steps in **Skill Drill 13-7 ▸**:

1. Ensure the patient's privacy as best you can.
2. Inspect the chest for any obvious DCAP-BTLS **Step 1**.
3. If you find any open wounds, dress them appropriately.
4. Note the shape of the patient's chest—it can give you clues to many underlying medical conditions (eg, emphysema or bronchitis) **Step 2**.
5. Look for any surgical scars that may be a result of pacemaker implantation or a midline scar (a "zipper") that indicates previous cardiothoracic surgery. Palpation of the chest may also reveal air under the skin (ie, subcutaneous emphysema).
6. Use percussion to detect any abnormalities **Step 3**.
7. Auscultate the lung fields, noting any abnormal lung sounds **Step 4**.
8. Auscultate for heart sounds.
9. Repeat the appropriate portions of the examination for the posterior aspect of the thorax.

Skill Drill 13-7: Examining the Chest

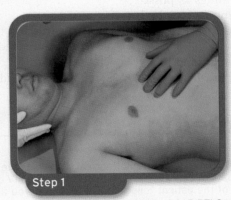

Step 1
Inspect the chest for any obvious DCAP-BTLS.

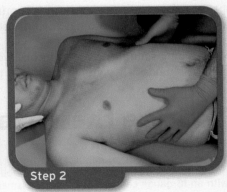

Step 2
Note the shape of the chest.

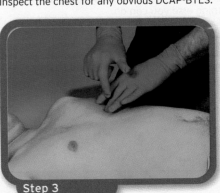

Step 3
Percuss the chest to detect any abnormalities.

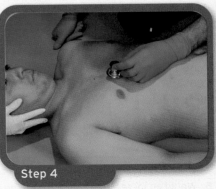

Step 4
Auscultate the lung fields, noting any abnormal lung sounds.

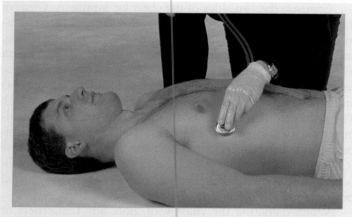

Figure 13-21 Auscultate the breath sounds on both sides of the chest.

At the Scene

Lungs are hyperinflated with chronic emphysema, resulting in hyperresonance where you would expect cardiac dullness.

the left upper and left lower lobes (Figure 13-22 ▸). During your examination, listen over each lobe, both anteriorly and posteriorly. Have the patient take as deep a breath as he or she can via an open mouth to facilitate your auscultatory assessment. Listen to as many portions of the lungs as possible, preferably avoiding any bony prominences, attached medical equipment, or clothing. Always use the best stethoscope available.

Normal lung sounds include bronchial, vesicular, and bronchovesicular sounds. They are a function of the particular pul-

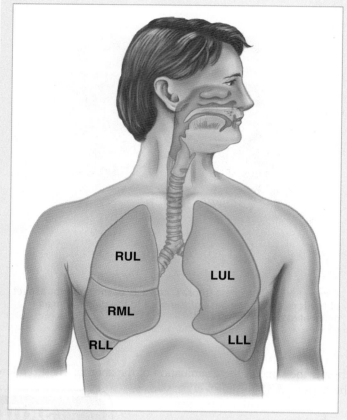

Figure 13-22 The five lobes of the lungs.

monary structure that air is passing through. Pathological or adventitious (added) breath sounds include wheezes, <u>rales</u> (or crackles), and <u>rhonchi</u> (or low wheezes). They are indications of lung tissue consolidation, atelectasis, oedema, mucus collection,

You are the Paramedic Part 3

You administer another nebuliser treatment with 5 mg of salbutamol/normal saline via face mask on 15 l/min as you prepare him to be moved to the ambulance. Once you have your patient safely in the back you establish an IV of normal saline in his right antecubital vein with an 18-gauge cannula. Upon reassessment of the patient following the nebuliser, you find that he still has audible inspiratory and expiratory wheezes and increased work of breathing evidenced by intercostal and supraclavicular recession. The patient states that he does not feel any relief and asks if there is anything else you can do.

Reassessment	Recording Time: 12 Minutes
Skin	Pale, warm, and dry with cyanotic nail beds and lips
Pulse	138 beats/min, regular, strong distal pulses
ECG	Sinus tachycardia
Blood pressure	164/82 mm Hg
Respirations	38 breaths/min, laboured
SpO_2	78% on a nebuliser at 15 l/min
Pupils	Equal and reactive to light

5. Would an increased work of breathing be present upon reassessment of the patient if your treatment was effective?

6. How should your patient management progress?

At the Scene

Percussion of the chest produces hyperresonance when the thorax is full of air and hyporesonance, or dullness, when it's full of blood.

and haemorrhage. <u>Stridor</u> is an abnormal respiratory sound of the upper airway that is often apparent on general examination, but can also be auscultated in more subtle presentations. <u>Rubs</u> can be heard emanating from either the lungs or the heart. A rub is produced by a partial loss of intrapleural integrity, when an abnormal collection of fluid has accumulated between a portion of the visceral and parietal pleura, resulting in "pleuritic" pain and a perceived rub on auscultation.

One of the most important—and perhaps most often overlooked—aspects of pulmonary assessment is appreciating when breath sounds are diminished or absent. You can't be aware of this phenomenon without first developing an appreciation of the wide spectrum of normal presentations that exist. Before going out into the prehospital environment, you should spend many hours listening to normal breath sounds, in order to develop an understanding of what constitutes the many variations of normal breathing. After that, you'll spend time listening to patients with respiratory difficulty, preferably alongside an experienced paramedic practitioner who can point out the significant variations in the presenting abnormalities.

Decreased breath sounds can be localised to a portion of one lung, or they can encompass the entire chest. When hypoventilation is suspected, you must take immediate action. Decreased breath sounds typically signal a lack of respiratory excursion or decreased tidal volume. Numerous problems can cause decreased breath sounds, including pneumothorax, haemothorax, pleural effusion, pulmonary oedema, atelectasis, consolidation, exacerbated COPD, status asthmaticus, opiate intoxication, pneumonia, bronchitis, and altered mental status.

At the Scene

Normal breathing should be quiet and not grossly evident to you. If you can see or hear the patient breathe, there's a problem.

Cardiovascular System

The cardiovascular system circulates blood throughout the body, an activity that maintains perfusion of the body's tissues (Figure 13-23 ▶). The cardiovascular system comprises a pump (the heart), a set of pipes (the blood vessels), and a liquid transported within those pipes (blood).

Blood consists of plasma, red blood cells, white blood cells, and platelets. Plasma is essentially a mild saline solution, but it also contains blood-clotting factors and particles that play important roles in the body's immune response.

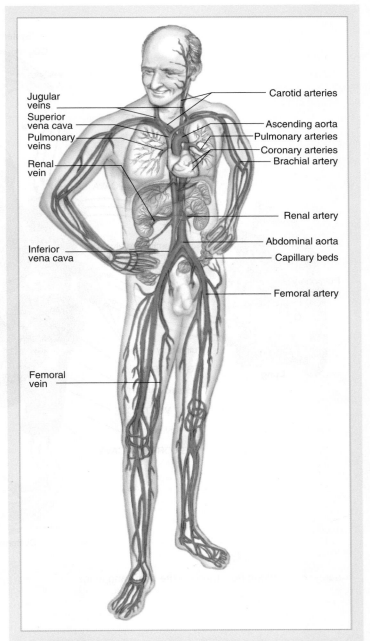

Figure 13-23 The cardiovascular system.

The complex arrangement of connected tubes in the circulatory system includes the arteries, arterioles, capillaries, venules, and veins. This system is entirely closed, with capillaries connecting the arterioles and the venules.

Blood flows through two circuits in this system: the systemic circulation in the body and the pulmonary circulation in the lungs. The systemic circulation carries oxygen-rich blood from the left ventricle through the body and back to the right atrium. As this blood passes through the tissues and organs, it gives up oxygen and nutrients and absorbs cellular wastes and carbon dioxide. The cellular wastes are, in turn, eliminated as the blood flows through the liver and the kidneys. The

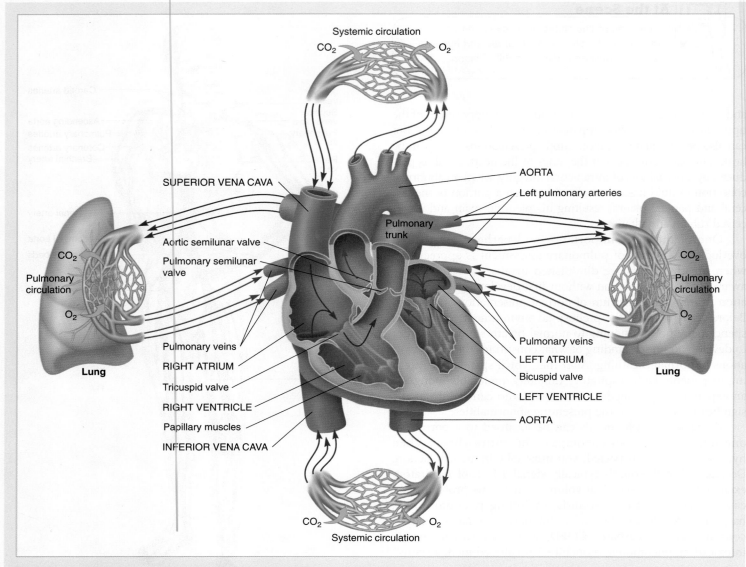

Figure 13-24 Blood flow through the heart and lungs.

pulmonary circulation carries oxygen-poor blood from the right ventricle through the lungs and back into the left atrium.

The cardiac cycle involves the events of cardiac relaxation (diastole), filling, and contraction (systole). These mechanical events are coordinated electrically with the heart's pacing and conduction system. The heart consists of four chambers: two atria (upper chambers) and two ventricles (lower chambers). Each side of the heart contains one atrium and one ventricle. The interatrial septum (membrane) separates the two atria; a thicker wall, the interventricular septum, separates the right and left ventricles. Each atrium receives blood that is returned to the heart from other parts of the body; each ventricle pumps blood out of the heart. The upper and lower portions of the heart are separated by the atrioventricular valves, which prevent backward flow of blood. The semilunar valves, which are

located between the ventricles and the arteries into which they pump blood, serve a similar function Figure 13-24 ▲.

Blood enters the right atrium via the superior and inferior vena cavae and the coronary sinus, which consists of veins that collect blood returning from the walls of the heart. Blood from four pulmonary veins enters the left atrium. Between the right and left atria is the fossa ovalis, a depression that represents the former location of the foramen ovale, an opening between the two atria that is present in the foetus.

The cardiac cycle coordinates the movement of blood between the chambers of the heart. The atria always relax and contract together, as do the ventricles. While the atria are contracting (and filling the ventricles), the ventricles are relaxing. Conversely, when the ventricles are contracting, the atria are relaxing, being filled by either the vena cava or the pulmonary veins.

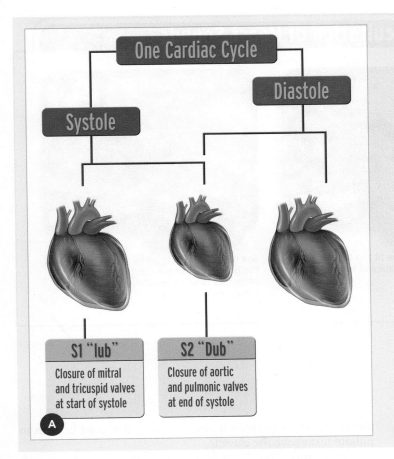

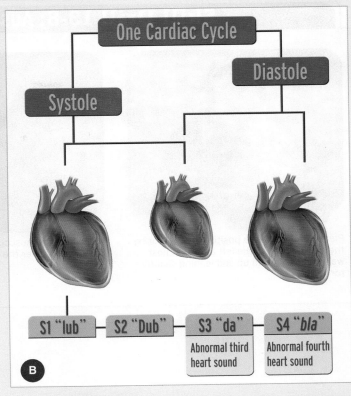

Figure 13-25 Heart sounds. **A.** The normal S_1 and S_2 heart sounds. **B.** The abnormal S_3 and S_4 heart sounds.

The contraction and relaxation of the heart, combined with the flow of blood, generates characteristic heart sounds during auscultation with a stethoscope. The normal pattern sounds much like this: "lub-DUB lub-DUB, lub-DUB . . ." The "lub" is referred to as the first heart sound or S_1, and the "DUB" (emphasised because it is often louder) as the second heart sound or S_2. Pathological heart sounds include S_3 and S_4 **Figure 13-25 ▲**. The S_3 or third heart sound is a soft, low-pitched heart sound that occurs about one third of the way through diastole. Although S_3 is sometimes present in healthy young people and during pregnancy, it most commonly is associated with abnormally increased filling pressures in the atria secondary to moderate to severe heart failure. The resulting rhythm is classically described as a gallop. S_4 is a moderately pitched sound that occurs immediately before the normal S_1 sound; it's always abnormal. The S_4 sound represents either decreased stretching (compliance) of the left ventricle or increased pressure in the atria.

Heart sounds can be appreciated by listening to the chest wall in the parasternal areas superiorly and inferiorly as well as in the region superior to the left nipple. Follow the steps in **Skill Drill 13-8 ▶**:

1. Place the patient in one of these positions, to bring the heart closer to the left anterior chest wall:
   - Sitting up and leaning slightly forward **Step 1**
   - Supine
   - Recovery position
2. Place your stethoscope at the fifth intercostal space over the apex of the heart **Step 2**.
3. To appreciate the S_1 sound, ask the patient to breathe normally and hold the breath on expiration.
4. To appreciate the S_2 sound, ask the patient to breathe normally and hold the breath on inhalation **Step 3**.
5. Auscultate the area above the left nipple to listen for S_3 and S_4 heart sounds.

Korotkoff sounds are detected while listening to a patient's blood pressure. A bruit is an abnormal "whoosh"-like sound that indicates turbulent blood flow moving through a narrowed artery (most significant in the carotid arteries). A murmur is an abnormal whoosh-like sound heard over the heart that indicates turbulent blood flow around a cardiac valve. Murmurs are graded as a range of intensity from 1 (softest) to 6 (loudest). Many people have normal, physiological murmurs. In some patients, they can represent a degree of pathology, depending on the nature of the underlying problem and the specific anatomy

At the Scene

The S_3 sound is associated with heart failure and is always abnormal in patients over 35 years of age, except in the case of pregnancy.

Skill Drill 13-8: Auscultation of Heart Sounds

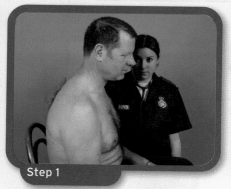

Step 1

Place the patient in a position that will bring the heart closer to the left anterior chest wall, such as sitting up and leaning slightly forward.

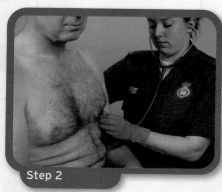

Step 2

Place your stethoscope at the fifth intercostal space over the apex of the heart.

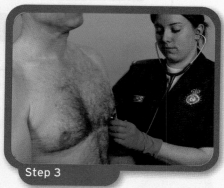

Step 3

Ask the patient to breathe normally and hold the breath on exhalation. Then ask the patient to breathe normally and hold the breath on inhalation.

of the valve involved. To fully appreciate the nature and quality of normal heart sounds and murmurs, you must practise your listening skills thoroughly, using a good quality stethoscope.

Arterial pulses are a physical expression of systolic blood pressure. They are caused when contraction of the left ventricle and ejection of blood into the systemic circulation generate a pressure wave, which then travels throughout the arterial system. Arterial pulses are palpable wherever an artery crosses a bony prominence.

Venous pressure tends to be very low. In fact, in the normal setting, the pressure in the vena cava just before blood is received into the right atrium is close to zero. Veins are relatively nonmuscular, thin-walled vessels that have no effect on systemic vascular resistance and do not assist in promoting systemic blood pressure. Blood flows through the venous system and returns to the heart in part because it is propelled from behind in a continuous fashion, draining the capillary network. Most venous return of blood is a function of the respiratory cycle, generated by negative intrathoracic pressure that is developed at inspiration during normal breathing.

You can estimate the capacity of the venous system by observing a patient's jugular venous pressure, also known as jugular venous distension (JVD). In right-sided heart failure, blood tends not to be readily accepted into the right atrium. Venous capacitance increases in an effort to compensate for this failure, which in turn results in elevated pressures and corresponding JVD. This can be most readily observed by evaluating the anterolateral aspects of the neck. Position the patient reclining at 45°. Measure the vertical height of the JVD from the sternal angle in centimetres. Normally, it should be seen to pulsate just above the clavicle.

In situations involving hypotension, there may be no evidence of JVD, even while the patient is supine. Hypotensive patients with JVD must be carefully assessed as to the nature of their condition, however. Depending on the clinical situation, patients with JVD may be experiencing cardiogenic shock or have a ruptured cardiac valve. In the setting of chest trauma, neck vein distension and hypotension may symbolise a tension pneumothorax or pericardial tamponade.

The ability of the circulatory system to constrict and dilate can diminish markedly as a person ages. Although this limitation may vary considerably from patient to patient, an older patient's ability to compensate for cardiovascular insults may be profoundly curtailed by age-related changes, especially arterial atherosclerosis and diabetes. In addition, many medications that older individuals use for routine management of problems such as high blood pressure can negatively affect the body's ability to handle sudden changes in the demand for blood supply. By contrast, children and young adults have an enhanced ability to vasoconstrict and increase the pulse rate to compensate for a vascular insult; this compensation mechanism can fool paramedics into believing that young patients are "less sick" than they actually are.

When you are examining the cardiovascular system, pay attention to arterial pulses, noting their location, rate, rhythm, and quality. Obtain an accurate blood pressure, and repeat this measurement periodically to assess the patient's haemodynamic stability. Examine the jugular veins for distension. While inspecting and palpating the chest, listen for heart sounds. Feel the chest wall to locate the point of maximum impulse (PMI), and then listen over the areas where the cardiac valves are. The aortic valve is found near the second intercostal space, to the right of the sternum. The pulmonic valve lies near the second intercostal space, to the left of the sternum. The tricuspid valve is auscultated over the lower left sternal border. The mitral valve can be appreciated over the cardiac apex, lateral to the lower left sternal border near the midclavicular line. Note the intensity of the heart sounds, and listen for S_1, S_2, and any extra sounds and murmurs.

Abdomen

Because of the large number of organs within the abdomen, the location of organs and their related medical complaints are most easily described by dividing the abdomen into imaginary quadrants. The umbilicus (navel) serves as the central reference point. The diaphragm, the large dome-shaped muscle used for respiration, is at the top of the abdominal cavity, and the pelvis is at the bottom. The quadrants are divided by a set of imaginary perpendicular lines intersecting at the umbilicus **Figure 13-26 ▾**.

The abdomen contains almost all of the organs of digestion, the organs of the urogenital system, and significant neurovascular structures. The abdominal wall is a relatively thick muscular organ that overlies the peritoneum. The peritoneum is itself a well-defined layer of fascia made up of the parietal and visceral peritoneum. Abdominal organs are often characterised as being either intraperitoneal or extraperitoneal, depending on where they reside in relation to this layer. Intraperitoneal organs include the stomach, proximal duodenum of the small intestine, pancreas, jejunum, ileum, appendix, caecum, transverse colon, sigmoid colon, proximal rectum, liver, gallbladder, spleen, omentum, and female internal genitalia. Extraperitoneal organs include the mid- and distal duodenum, abdominal aorta, mid- and lower rectum, kidneys, pancreatic tail, adrenal glands, ureters, renal blood vessels, gonadal blood vessels, ascending colon, descending colon, and urinary bladder.

The abdominal organs can be topographically organised and sequentially assessed by viewing the overlying abdominal wall in a subdivided fashion. This is typically done in quadrants—left upper quadrant (LUQ), right upper quadrant (RUQ), left lower quadrant (LLQ), right lower quadrant (RLQ)—or ninths: right hypochondrial, RH; epigastric, E; left hypochondrial, LH; right lumbar, RL; umbilical, U; left lumbar, LL; right iliac, RI; hypogastric, H; left iliac, LI **Figure 13-27 ▾**.

Abdominal pain and associated concerns are common complaints, but their cause is often difficult to identify. Obtaining any appropriate history relevant to the situation is critical to help determine the nature of the problem. Historical information should include the location, quality, and severity of the discomfort; time of onset and duration of symptoms; significant activities at onset of distress; any aggravating or alleviating factors; and any associated symptoms, including nausea, vomiting, febrile symptoms, or changes in dietary, bowel, or bladder habits.

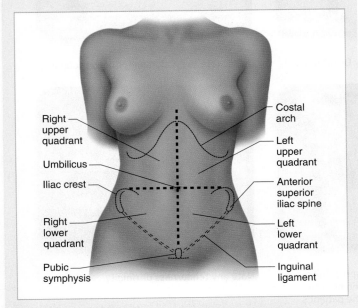

Figure 13-26 The abdomen is divided into four quadrants by imaginary vertical and horizontal lines.

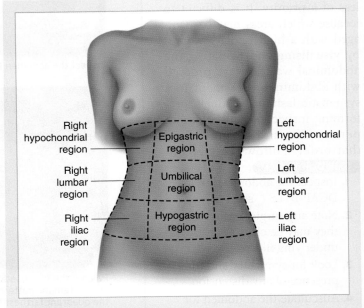

Figure 13-27 The abdomen can also be divided into nine regions.

At the Scene

Assess the abdomen for the following:
- Tenderness
- Rigidity
- Swelling
- Guarding
- Distension

When you are examining a patient's abdomen, generally it is best to make the patient as comfortable as possible. Sometimes this requires giving some pain medication first, as the patient may be more cooperative and better able to focus with less discomfort. To assess the abdomen, the patient must be in a supine position. To examine and palpate/percuss over the posterior aspects of the abdomen, however, you should either sit the patient up or log roll him or her at some point.

Prior to palpating the abdomen, ask the patient to point to the area of greatest discomfort. Avoid touching that area until last. Work slowly and avoid quick movements. When appropriate, speak with the patient about the nature of the illness while palpating the abdomen. Once an area of tenderness has been localised, attempt to visualise which structures may underlie it and think about what might potentially be causing the problem. In situations of penetrating trauma, this step is less of a priority: It is difficult to localise which areas may be damaged with a high-velocity wound by visualising and palpating the abdominal wall. Always proceed with abdominal assessment in a systematic fashion, routinely performing inspection, auscultation, percussion, and palpation, in that order. Follow the steps in **Skill Drill 13-9 ▸** :

1. Inspect the abdomen for any DCAP-BTLS (**Step 1**).
2. Note any surgical scars, as they may be clues to an underlying illness.
3. Look for symmetry and the presence of any distension.
4. Auscultate the abdomen for bowel sounds (**Step 2**).
5. Perform percussion.

6. Palpate the four quadrants of the abdomen in a systematic pattern, beginning with the quadrant farthest from the patient's complaint of pain (**Step 3**).
7. Note any tenderness or rigidity, and pay special attention to the patient's expressions as they may yield valuable information (**Step 4**).

When you are inspecting the abdomen, look at the skin as well as the contour and overall appearance of the abdominal wall. Identify any scars, wounds, striae, dilated veins, bruises, rashes, and discolourations. Note any generalised distension or localised masses.

At the Scene

When palpating the abdomen, always begin on the side opposite the site of pain.

Skill Drill 13-9: Examining the Abdomen

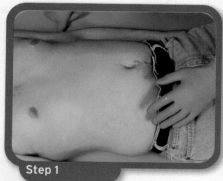

Step 1

Inspect the abdomen for any DCAP-BTLS.

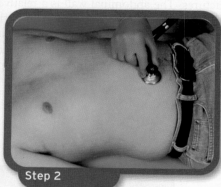

Step 2

Auscultate the abdomen for bowel sounds.

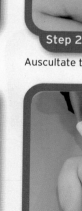

Step 3

Palpate the four quadrants of the abdomen in a systematic pattern, beginning with the quadrant farthest from the patient's complaint of pain.

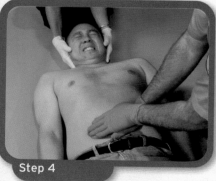

Step 4

Note any tenderness or rigidity.

At the Scene

Restlessness and constant repositioning occur with colicky pain of gastroenteritis or bowel obstruction. Absolute stillness, resisting any movement, is demonstrated with the pain of peritonitis. Knees flexed, facial grimacing, and rapid/uneven respirations also indicate signs of pain.

The abdomen can be described as flat, rounded, protuberant (bulging out), scaphoid (where the anterior wall is hollowed), or pulsatile. Any abdominal distension needs to be distinguished from obesity. An obese abdomen tends to be more protuberant than distended, and is typically exceptionally pliable. A patient with intra-abdominal pathology who also happens to have significant obesity will present a challenge in this regard.

Some patients may have ascites, a collection of fluid within the peritoneal cavity. Ascites is consistent with an underlying oedema, but instead of affecting the interstitial tissues of the legs, it involves the abdomen. The patient's abdomen may appear markedly distended, and a visible or palpable fluid wave may be evident during examination, with shifting dullness noted to percussion. Ascites is most typically seen in patients who suffer from liver disease, but it can also be appreciated with underlying malignancy and, to a certain extent, with renal and cardiac insufficiency.

Auscultation of the abdomen is commonly performed as part of the routine abdominal examination, although it may have limited utility in the prehospital setting. To hear bowel sounds, the setting must be fairly optimal and you should take enough time to ensure an adequate assessment. Differentiating normal from abnormal can sometimes be challenging, so you should practise this skill on as many healthy individuals as you can.

When you are assessing bowel sounds, make note of their presence or absence. Sometimes the abnormality is characterised by hyperactivity or hypoactivity, rather than a total lack of sounds. Bowel sounds can also be described as increased, decreased, or absent. In the case of hyperactive sounds, note their frequency and character. With an obstruction, the sounds are often referred to as high-pitched and tinkling.

Palpation yields perhaps the most significant diagnostic information during the abdominal examination—that is, tenderness (elicited pain). You may then be able to correlate historical information related to the patient's current illness or

At the Scene

High-pitched, rushing, or tinkling sounds can signal bowel obstruction. Hypoactive or absent sounds follow recent abdominal surgery or are a sign of inflammation of the peritoneum.

situation and the findings from the examination, and determine what is wrong.

A patient who contracts his or her abdominal muscles shows the sign called guarding. Guarding can be either a voluntary or involuntary act, and is typically encountered when the patient has peritoneal irritation. Such irritation may arise when an organ underlying the peritoneum becomes inflamed, or when a hollow organ ruptures and empties its contents into the peritoneal cavity. In trauma cases, however, solid-organ bleeding does not always result in peritoneal irritation and guarding. Large-volume bleeding with peritoneal distension will result in this phenomenon. Marked peritoneal irritation and guarding is referred to as abdominal rigidity. This clinically important feature often results in urgent surgical evaluation and intervention. Guarding and rigidity are often encountered in trauma patients, but may also be seen in cases of appendicitis, cholecystitis, hollow-organ perforation, pancreatitis, and diverticulitis.

At the Scene

Pain upon release of pressure confirms rebound tenderness, which is a reliable sign of peritoneal inflammation such as with appendicitis.

Patients with more generalised guarded tenderness to palpation may have a more visceral problem. Although this may represent an early manifestation of a serious condition, it can also be associated with various degrees of bowel obstruction, renal colic, biliary colic, or urinary tract infection. Often the pain is less localised on palpation, and is deep-seated and poorly described by the patient. Cases of colic typically involve a problem with peristalsis, the wave-like contraction motion of a hollow tubular structure (eg, small and large intestine, common bile duct, or ureter). A stone may obstruct the tube, for example, or an adhesion or hernia may prevent proper intestinal peristalsis. Some patients will describe the pain as "wave-like", or waxing and waning in nature. Other lower abdominal sources of pain and tenderness include genitourinary processes.

Vascular sources can cause significant abdominal pain, most notably aortic aneurysm. Occasionally a markedly dilated aorta can be seen pulsating in the upper midline abdomen. Palpation will enable the provider to estimate its diameter. A ruptured aortic aneurysm also tends to be tender to palpation, and care should be taken to minimise manipulation of an aneurysm once it is suspected. The aorta is a retroperitoneal structure, however, so a lack of obvious findings while assessing the anterior abdomen does not rule out this diagnosis in an otherwise proper clinical setting. Other notable palpable abdominal wall masses include hernia, a localised weakening of the abdominal wall musculature. Hernias are usually acquired, for example by lifting heavy loads, but can be congenital. They can result in strangulation of the underlying intestine.

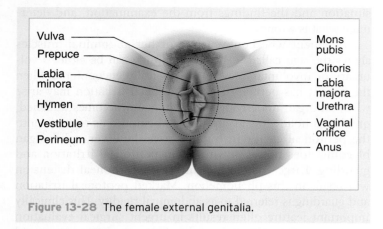

Figure 13-28 The female external genitalia.

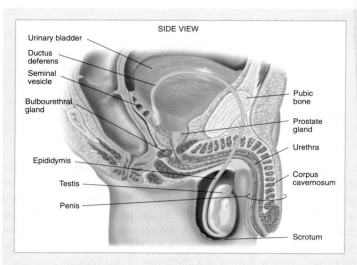

Figure 13-29 The male genitalia.

Female Genitalia

The female genitalia consist of the ovaries, fallopian tubes, uterus, vagina, and external genitalia Figure 13-28 ▲. The ovaries lie in the lowermost abdomen, in the inguinal regions, just superior to the inguinal creases. During a woman's reproductive years, the ovaries produce specialised hormones and ova. Hormonal regulation results in the maturation and release of an ovum roughly once a month as part of the menstrual cycle during that time.

After its release by the ovary, the ovum enters the fallopian tube and travels to the uterus. In the nonpregnant state, the uterus is a small structure, which is not palpable on external examination. This hollow, very muscular organ opens via the cervix into the vagina. Its inner lining thickens in response to hormonal stimulation, corresponding with the ripening and release of an ovum from the ovary.

The uterus receives sperm via the vagina and cervix. Pregnancy can result if sperm and ova successfully combine and become implanted in the lining of the uterine wall. If such fertilisation does not occur, the uterine lining will slough and pass from the body with the menstrual flow.

In general, assessment of female genitalia is performed in a very limited and discreet fashion. Always keep the patient appropriately draped during the course of the examination. Male paramedics should be assisted by a female. Reasons to examine the genitalia include concern over life-threatening haemorrhage or imminent delivery in childbirth.

While assessing the abdomen, palpate both the bilateral inguinal regions and the hypogastric region. If the decision is made to examine the genitalia specifically, limit the examination to inspection only. Pain and tenderness in the fallopian tubes and ovaries can be elicited during patient assessment. Clinically significant causes of this pain include ectopic pregnancy, complications of third-trimester pregnancy, and nonpregnant ovarian problems or pelvic infections. In the trauma patient where pelvic fracture is a concern, genital bleeding is a possibility, albeit an unlikely one. In the case of injury involving intentional trauma, significant bleeding is possible; if you must intervene in this kind of situation, be sure to preserve any garments, blankets, etc. and give them to the police as soon as possible. In general, make note of the amount and quality of any bleeding, as well as any inflammation, discharge, swelling, or lesions of the genitalia.

Male Genitalia

The male reproductive system consists of the testes, reproductive ducts, prostate, penis, and urethra Figure 13-29 ▲. The testes are analogous to the ovaries, in that they are the principal organs of reproduction and are responsible for manufacturing sperm. The testes, which lie outside the torso in a sac called the scrotum, produce hormones, seminal fluid (semen), and reproductive cells (sperm). The sperm and seminal fluid are transported from the testes to the lower abdomen, where they are stored in the seminal vesicles.

During sexual intercourse, sperm and semen are ejaculated through the urethra. During its passage through the urethra, the prostate gland adds fluids to the semen. The urethra passes through the penis, which is a highly vascular structure. Reflexive arteriolar dilation within the penis results in penile engorgement and subsequent erection.

When you are examining male genitalia, make certain that your partner is present and perform the examination in a very limited and discreet fashion. In the prehospital setting, situations requiring assessment of the male genitalia are limited. Female practitioners should ideally be assisted by a male colleague. Always assess the entire abdomen and note any pertinent findings, as occasionally lower abdominal problems are referred from the genitalia. Situations of testicular torsion or inguinal hernia sometimes present with a complaint of lower abdominal pain but minimal abdominal tenderness. In the case of a trauma patient, assess for the possibility of significant genital bleeding and injury, or underlying fracture. Note any inflammation, discharge, swelling, or lesions.

Anus

The anus—the distal orifice of the alimentary canal—is often evaluated at the same time as the genitalia. It is examined in only a very limited number of circumstances, and is always done with the patient appropriately draped and your colleague present. Examination usually occurs with the patient lying in a laterally recumbent position, and involves inspection only. Examine the sacrococcygeal and perineal areas, noting obvious bleeding, trauma, lumps, ulcers, inflammation, rash, and abrasions.

Musculoskeletal System

The extremities consist of both soft tissues and bones. Joints are areas where bone ends abut each other and form a kind of hinge, creating a jointed appendage. Joints are filled with shock-absorbing linings and fluid (synovium), and are held together by ligaments. They allow the body to perform mechanical work. Indeed, the mechanical process of motion becomes possible when the joints are flexed and extended by skeletal (or striated) muscles that traverse the joints. Skeletal muscles are anchored to bone via tendons, with each muscle being named according to its location and function.

The principal joints of the upper extremities include the shoulder (acromioclavicular and glenohumeral joints), elbow (olecranon), and wrist (radiocarpal). The principal joints of the lower extremities include the hip (acetabulum), knee (patellar), and ankle (tibiotalar).

As joints age, they become more vulnerable to repetitive motion stress and trauma, and they lose much of their articular abilities due to inflammation and breakdown of the synovium. Disruption of the bones, joints, and soft tissues can take a variety of forms, and discomfort or disability may be a manifestation of an acute problem, a chronic problem, or a combination of the two.

Common types of musculoskeletal and soft-tissue injuries include fractures, sprains, strains, dislocations, contusions, haematomas, and open wounds. Fractures may be characterised in a number of ways. For example, an open fracture is essentially a fracture with direct communication to the exterior surface of the body, or simply an open wound in close proximity to the site of a presumed fracture.

Although fractures always involve a pathological process, it is important to distinguish a pathological fracture from a physiological fracture. A physiological fracture occurs when abnormal forces are applied to normal bone structures, producing a fracture. A pathological fracture occurs when normal forces are applied to abnormal bone structures, producing a fracture. Physiological fractures occur in the setting of high-force injury. Pathological fractures often occur in settings of decreased bone density, such as osteoporosis or occult malignancy.

At the Scene

Point tenderness is the most reliable indicator of an underlying closed fracture.

When you are examining the skeleton and joints, pay attention to both their structure and their function. Consider how the joint and associated extremity look and how well they work. Does the extremity look normal, and does it move easily? In particular, note any limitation in range of movement, pain with range of movement, or bony crepitus. When assessing the joints and extremities, look for evidence of inflammation or injury, such as swelling, tenderness, increased heat, redness, bruising, or decreased function. Also evaluate the joint or extremity for obvious deformity, diminished strength, atrophy, or asymmetry from one side to the other. The examination of the musculoskeletal system should not cause the patient any pain; if any occurs, it should be considered an abnormal finding. Follow the steps in **Skill Drill 13-10 ▶**:

1. Beginning with upper extremities, inspect the skin overlying the muscles, bones, and joints for soft-tissue damage **Step 1**.
2. Note any deformities or abnormal structure.
3. Check for adequate distal pulse, movement, and sensation in each extremity **Step 2**.
4. Inspect and palpate the hands and the wrists, noting any DCAP-BTLS.
5. Ask the patient to flex and extend the joints of the fingers, hands, and wrist, noting any abnormalities in the range of movement. If the patient experiences any discomfort, stop that portion of the examination immediately **Step 3**.
6. Inspect and palpate the elbows, noting any abnormalities. Ask the patient to flex and extend the elbow to determine the range of movement.
7. Ask the patient to turn the hand from the palm-down position to the palm-up position and back again, noting any pain or abnormalities **Step 4**.
8. Inspect and palpate the shoulders. Ask the patient to shrug the shoulders and raise and extend both arms **Step 5**.
9. Inspect the skin overlying the lower extremities.
10. Beginning with the feet, inspect and palpate the bony structures, noting any abnormalities **Step 6**.
11. Ask the patient to point and bend the toes to establish the range of movement **Step 7**.
12. Ask the patient to rotate the ankle, checking for pain or restricted range of movement **Step 8**.
13. Inspect and palpate the knee joints and patella. Ask the patient to bend and straighten both to establish the range of movement **Step 9**.
14. Check for structural integrity of the pelvis by applying gentle pressure to the iliac crests and pushing in and then down **Step 10**.
15. Ask the patient to lift both legs by bending at the hip and then turning the legs inward and outward. Note any abnormalities **Step 11**.

Often the diagnosis of a problem involving the shoulders and related structures can be made simply by noting the patient's posture at the time of first contact with paramedics **Figure 13-30 ▶**. For example, a glenohumeral joint

Skill Drill 13-10: Examining the Musculoskeletal System

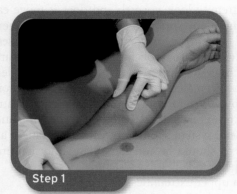

Step 1

Inspect the skin overlying the muscles, bones, and joints for soft-tissue damage.

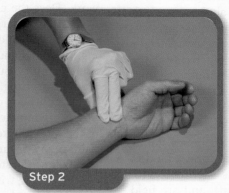

Step 2

Check for adequate distal pulse, motor, and sensation to each extremity.

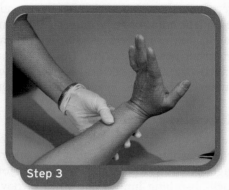

Step 3

Ask the patient to flex and extend the joints of the fingers, hands, and wrist to establish range of movement.

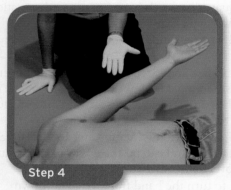

Step 4

Ask the patient to turn the hand from the palm-down position to the palm-up position and back again.

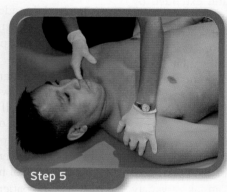

Step 5

Inspect and palpate the shoulders.

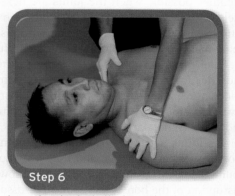

Step 6

Inspect and palpate the bony structures.

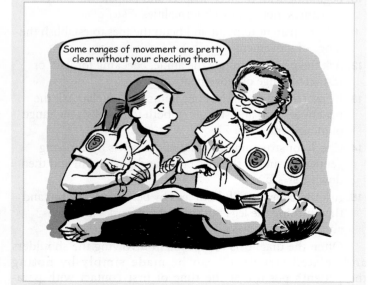

Some ranges of movement are pretty clear without your checking them.

Figure 13-30

dislocation may be manifested as the loss of normal contour of the shoulder, with abnormal squaring of the lateral aspect of the shoulder and the humeral head visible and/or palpable in the soft tissues of the chest wall, in the subacromial region **Figure 13-31 ▶**.

When you are palpating the proximal upper extremity and shoulder, be sure to assess the sternoclavicular joint, acromioclavicular joint, subacromial area, and bicipital groove (origin of the biceps, just distal to the anterior aspect of the humeral head). Note any tenderness, swelling, crepitus, deformity, rotation, or bruising in these areas.

When possible, check the patient's range of movement by asking the patient to raise the arms to the vertical position, above the head. Next, ask the patient to demonstrate external rotation

At the Scene

When you are assessing a patient with a possible shoulder dislocation, position yourself behind the patient and compare the shoulders. The dislocated side is usually lower than the uninjured side.

Skill Drill 13-10: Examining the Musculoskeletal System (*continued*)

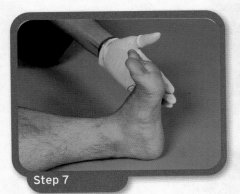

Step 7

Ask the patient to point and bend the toes to establish range of movement.

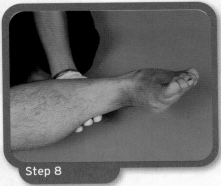

Step 8

Ask the patient to rotate the ankle, checking for pain or restricted range of movement.

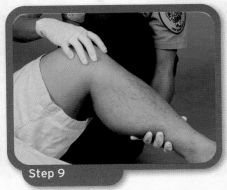

Step 9

Inspect and palpate the knee joints and patella. Ask the patient to bend and straighten both to establish range of movement.

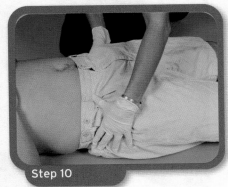

Step 10

Check for structural integrity of the pelvis by applying gentle pressure to the iliac crests and pushing in and then down.

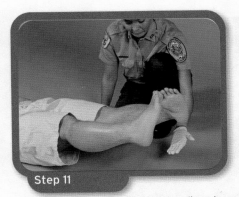

Step 11

Ask the patient to lift both legs, bending at the hip and then turning the legs inward and outward.

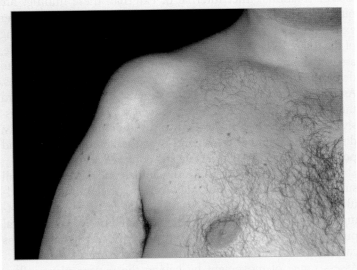

Figure 13-31 Abnormal squaring of the shoulder.

and abduction by placing both hands behind the neck with the elbows out to the sides. Finally, perform internal rotation by having the patient place both hands behind the lower back.

Evaluation of the elbows should start with an overall inspection for gross deformity or abnormal rotation. Palpate the elbow between the epicondyles and olecranon, and palpate the epicondyles and olecranon themselves (**Figure 13-32 ▶**). Note any tenderness, crepitus, swelling, or thickening. Range-of-movement testing should be performed last, as suspicion of significant pathology or fracture of the elbow mandates appropriate immobilisation as soon as possible. When examining the elbows, flex and extend them both passively and actively. Then have the patient supinate and pronate the forearms while the elbows are flexed at the patient's sides.

When you are checking the hands and wrists, inspect them for any abnormalities, including swelling, redness, contusions, wounds, nodules, deformities, or atrophy. Palpate the hands, feeling the medial and lateral aspects of each interphalangeal joint on each finger (**Figure 13-33 ▶**). Squeeze the hands, compressing the metacarpophalangeal joints. Palpate the carpal

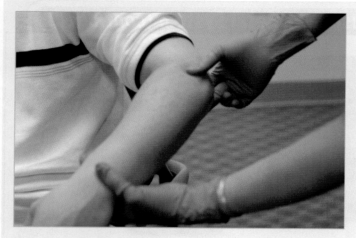
Figure 13-32 Palpate the elbow.

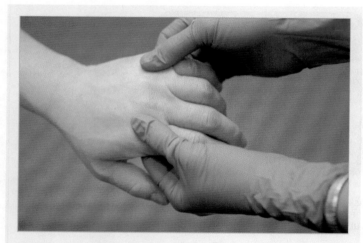
Figure 13-33 Palpate the fingers.

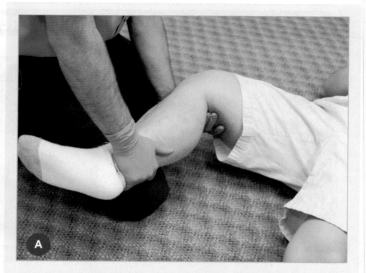

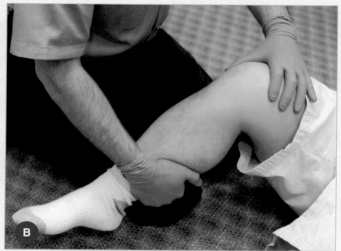
Figure 13-34 Examination of the lower extremities. **A.** Hip. **B.** Knee.

At the Scene

Heberden's and Bouchard's nodules are hard and not tender to the touch, and occur with osteoarthritis.

bones of the wrists, noting any areas of swelling, tenderness, or bogginess (soft and unstable). Perform range-of-movement evaluations by asking the patient to make fists with both hands, then extend and spread the fingers, then flex and extend the wrists, and finally move the hands laterally and medially with the palms facing down. Check capillary refill, symmetry of radial pulses, and overall limb temperature at this point.

A rapid appreciation of injury or disability involving the lower extremities can be made by evaluating the patient's ability to walk. Of course, this may not be a practical first approach to assessment in many prehospital cases.

Examination of the knees and hips begins with inspection of overall alignment and deformity of the lower extremities **Figure 13-34** . Identify any lower extremity shortening

and/or rotation, either internal or external; these findings are often evident with an injury to the proximal aspects of the lower extremity. Look for evidence of thickening, swelling, or bruising of the thigh. Note any crepitus or palpable tenderness. If possible, assess the range of movement of the knees and hips in an effort to determine the presence of underlying injury to those structures. Ask the patient to bend each knee and raise the bent knee toward the chest. Assess for rotation and abduction of the hips, both passively and actively. Palpate each hip individually—specifically, distal to the inguinal crease and over the anterior, lateral, and posterior aspects. Finally, palpate and compress the pelvis.

When you are examining the ankles and feet, observe all surfaces. Note any wounds, deformities, discolourations, nodules, or swelling. Palpate all aspects of the feet and ankles, noting tenderness, bogginess, swelling, or crepitus. Measure distal pulses over the dorsalis pedis and posterior tibialis, and assess capillary refill and overall limb temperature at this point. Assess range of movement by having the patient plantar flex, dorsiflex, and invert and evert the ankles and feet. Be sure to

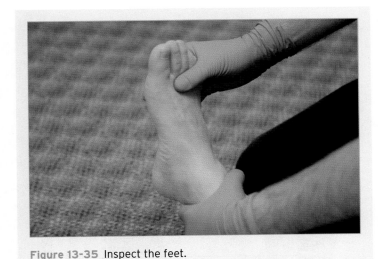

Figure 13-35 Inspect the feet.

check the forefoot and toes by inspection, palpation, and range-of-movement testing Figure 13-35 ▲ .

Peripheral Vascular System

The peripheral vascular system comprises all aspects of the circulatory system, except for the heart, the great vessels immediately involved with the mediastinum, and the coronary circulation. Thus it includes all of the body's arteries, veins, arterioles, venules, capillaries, lymphatic system, and the respective fluids that fill these structures.

The lymphatic system is an intricate network of nodes and ducts of various sizes that are dispersed throughout the body Figure 13-36 ▶ . The ducts contain a fat-rich fluid known as lymph, which transports materials from the lymph tissue into the central venous circulation via the thoracic ducts. Lymph nodes are larger accumulations of lymphatic tissue, and smaller amounts of lymph are distributed in tissue throughout the body. All lymphatic tissue contains large numbers of immunologically active cells; thus the lymphatics manage a key function in the body's immune system.

Perfusion occurs in the peripheral circulation via the network of capillary beds. Blood cells and plasma in close proximity to tissue offload substances required by the cells for proper metabolic functioning, and simultaneously pick up metabolic wastes for transport out of the tissues, ultimately for elimination from the body. Impaired functioning of the peripheral vascular system means that the capillary beds can't provide sufficient blood for adequate tissue and organ perfusion—this is a significant source of morbidity and mortality. Diseases of the peripheral vascular system are often seen in patients who smoke and/or have other underlying medical conditions, such as diabetes, hypertension, dyslipidaemia, and obesity. These disease processes typically target and cause malfunctioning of the smaller-diameter vessels of the peripheral vascular system, resulting in disease states of the tissues and organs that depend on those vessels for proper functioning. With age and the occurrence of these various disease processes, the vasculature becomes less able to rapidly manage changes in perfusion requirements, so it can itself become a source of illness.

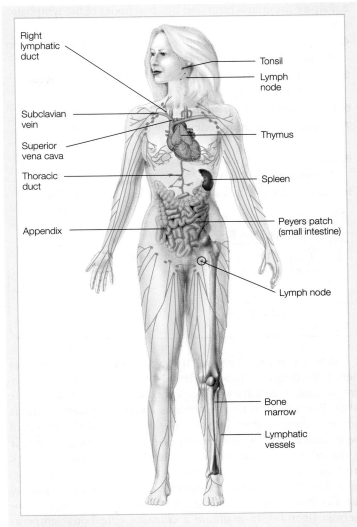

Figure 13-36 Lymphatic system.

When you are assessing the peripheral vascular system, pay attention to both the upper and lower extremities. Look for signs indicative of either acute or chronic vascular problems. A wide range of disorders can affect the peripheral vascular system—from chronic venous stasis and lymphoedema to intermittent claudication (cramp-like pain in the lower legs due to poor circulation) and acute arterial occlusion. Peripheral vascular disease can manifest in many forms, depending on the point in the vasculature where the abnormality is located. Carotid artery disease can manifest as a stroke, for example, while arterial embolisation involving the mesenteric vessels can result in bowel ischaemia and necrosis. In the extremities, involvement of the peripheral vasculature can result in limb ischaemia. Follow the steps in Skill Drill 13-11 ▶ :

1. While examining the upper extremities, note any abnormalities in the radial pulse, skin colour, or condition Step 1 .

2. If abnormalities are noted in the distal pulse, work your way proximally, checking these pulse points and noting your findings Step 2 .

3. Palpate the epitrochlear and brachial nodes of the lymphatic system, noting any swelling or tenderness (Step 3).

4. Examine the lower extremities, noting any abnormalities in the size and symmetry of the legs (Step 4).

5. Inspect the skin colour and condition, noting any abnormal venous patterns or enlargement (Step 5).

6. Check distal pulses, noting any abnormalities (Step 6).

7. Palpate the inguinal nodes for swelling or tenderness (Step 7).

8. Evaluate the temperature of each leg relative to the rest of the body and to each other.

9. Evaluate for pitting oedema in the legs and feet (Step 8).

At the Scene

Pitting oedema 4-point scale:
+1 = 0–0.75 cm
+2 = 0.75–1.25 cm
+3 = 1.25–2 cm
+4 ≥ 2 cm

When you are checking the upper extremities, inspect them from fingertips to shoulders. Note the extremity's relative size, and evaluate it for symmetry by comparing one side to the other. Pay attention to any obvious swelling, unusual venous patterns, the colour and texture of the skin, and the colour of the nail beds. Palpate the radial pulses, and compare each side to the other. In situations of unilaterally absent pulses, check proximally over the brachial pulse sites. When you are evaluating a limb for ischaemia, consider the five Ps of acute arterial insufficiency: Pain, Pallor, singular Paraesthesia/paresis, Poikilothermia (inability to maintain a constant core body temperature independent of ambient temperature), and Pulselessness. The loss of a palpable pulse is probably the worst indicator of such a problem, as it is considered a late finding. If indicated, palpate the epitrochlear and axillary lymph nodes, noting their size, tenderness, overlying redness, and mobility.

Proper evaluation of the vascular status of the lower extremities requires the patient to be lying down and draped appropriately. Remove the patient's socks, stockings, and shoes before proceeding with the examination. Inspect the lower extremities from the groin and buttocks to the feet. Always examine the lower extremities by comparing the right side to the left. Look at the size and symmetry of the legs, noting any localised versus generalised swelling. Pay attention to any remarkable superficial venous patterns or venous enlargement. Observe the skin pigmentation, as well as the skin colour and texture. Rubor, bruising, or pallor may all be encountered in patients who are suffering from significant vascular insufficiency. Also note the presence of any rashes, scars, and ulcers, and determine whether they are shallow or deep.

Palpate pulses in the lower extremities to assess the arterial circulation. In particular, palpate pulses over the dorsalis pedis, the posterior tibialis, and the femoral regions. The popliteal pulse can also occasionally be appreciated. Note the tempera-

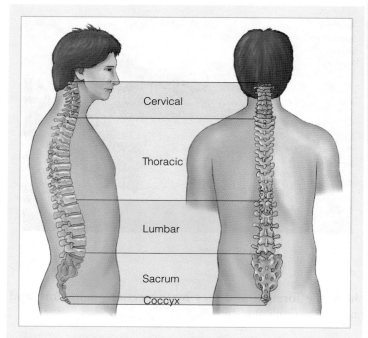

Figure 13-37 The five sections of the spinal column.

At the Scene

Bilateral, dependent, pitting oedema occurs with systemic conditions such as heart failure and hepatic cirrhosis. Unilateral oedema occurs with local conditions such as occlusion of a deep vein.

ture of the feet and legs, and attempt to palpate oedema in the legs. To do so, press your thumb over the dorsum of the foot and anteriorly over the tibias, holding the thumb with firm, gentle pressure for at least 5 seconds. If indicated, palpate the superficial inguinal lymph nodes, noting their size, tenderness, any overlying redness, and mobility.

Spine

The spine represents the core of the axillary skeleton. It consists of 33 individual vertebrae, the lower nine of which are fused (Figure 13-37). The vertebrae are irregularly shaped bones that articulate with each other in a complex fashion. The spine provides anchoring points for the skull, shoulders, ribs, and pelvis. It also protects the spinal cord and provides the passageway through which spinal nerves travel to and from the peripheral nervous system.

When you are assessing the spine, begin by inspecting the back from both the posterior and lateral aspects. The spine features several curves, representing the cervical, thoracic, and lumbar regions. Lordosis refers to the inward curve of the lumbar spine just above the buttocks. An exaggerated form of lordosis results in swayback. Kyphosis refers to the outward curve of the thoracic spine. It is frequently exaggerated in older people due to degenerative joint disease, osteoporosis,

Skill Drill 13-11: Examining the Peripheral Vascular System

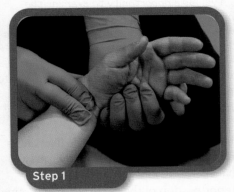

Step 1

Note any abnormalities in the radial pulse, skin colour, or condition.

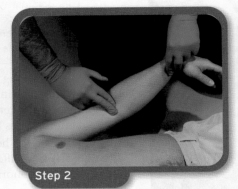

Step 2

If abnormalities are noted in the distal pulse, work your way proximally, checking these pulse points and noting your findings.

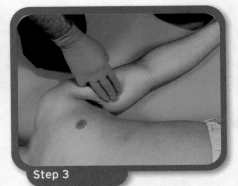

Step 3

Palpate the epitrochlear and brachial nodes of the lymphatic system, noting any swelling or tenderness.

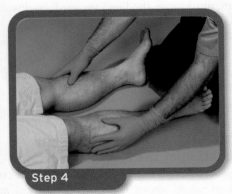

Step 4

Examine the lower extremities, noting any abnormalities in the size and symmetry of the legs.

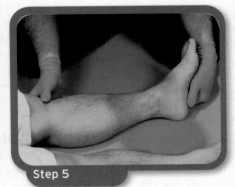

Step 5

Inspect the skin colour and condition, noting any abnormal venous patterns or enlargement.

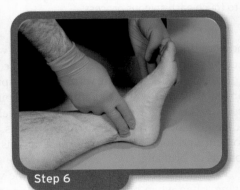

Step 6

Check distal pulses.

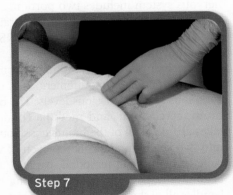

Step 7

Palpate the inguinal nodes for swelling or tenderness.

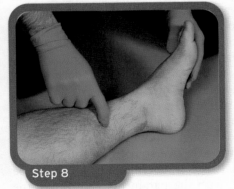

Step 8

Evaluate for pitting oedema in the legs and feet.

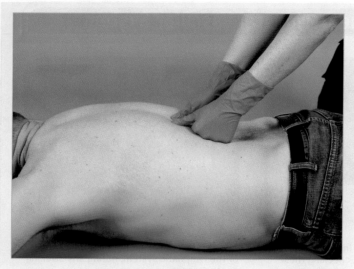

Figure 13-38 When you are palpating the spine, use the thumb to touch each spinous process.

and vertebral compression fractures. At its worst, kyphosis can become a source of restrictive lung disease, a form of COPD. Scoliosis is a sideways curvature of the spine, and is always abnormal. When you are examining the spine, look for differences in the height of the shoulders as well as differences in the heights of the iliac crests of the pelvis. Be sure to take a moment and look at the entire back at this point, noting any wounds or bruising.

Palpation of the spine is typically done while the patient is supine, often when he or she has been log rolled onto one side to facilitate access to the back and placement of a spinal immobilisation device. When you are palpating the spine, use the thumb to touch each spinous process Figure 13-38 ▲ . This allows you to identify any tenderness, step-off, or crepitus. Identification of an abnormality should prompt you to institute proper splinting and protective measures.

While you are examining the spine, it's also appropriate to check the rest of the back for any other significant findings on palpation. Tap over the costovertebral angles, and palpate the scapulae, paraspinal areas, and base of the neck. Also check the buttocks.

Finally, perform a range-of-movement evaluation. Although this evaluation may be of limited utility in the prehospital setting, in areas that practise selective spinal immobilisation, it may prove quite helpful. Range of movement should always be checked passively first, with the paramedic controlling the range. It is then done actively, with the patient controlling the range. If at any time during the examination you elicit pain in the spine or tingling in the extremities, stop that phase of assessment immediately and immobilise the spine. Examination of the cervical spine should require rather limited movements. In contrast, examining the remainder of the spine may include somewhat exaggerated motions, including flexion and extension, with the patient front- and back-bending. Lateral bending can also be appreciated, as can leftward and rightward rotation. Pay attention to the smoothness and symmetry of the patient's

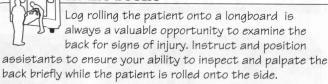

At the Scene

Log rolling the patient onto a longboard is always a valuable opportunity to examine the back for signs of injury. Instruct and position assistants to ensure your ability to inspect and palpate the back briefly while the patient is rolled onto the side.

movements, along with the actual degree of movement elicited. Follow the steps in Skill Drill 13-12 ▶ :

1. Inspect the cervical, thoracic, and lumbar curves for any abnormalities Step 1 .
2. Evaluate the heights of the shoulders and the iliac crests Step 2 . Differences from one side to the other may indicate abnormal curvature of the spine.
3. Palpate the posterior portion of the cervical spine, noting any point tenderness or structural abnormalities Step 3 .
4. In the nontrauma patient, and in the absence of reported pain, ask the patient to move the head forward, backward, and from side to side Step 4 .
5. Move down the spine, palpating each vertebra with the thumbs to note any tenderness or instability Step 5 .
6. In the absence of pain or trauma, ask the patient to bend at the waist in each direction to establish the range of movement Step 6 .

Nervous System
Structure and Function of the Nervous System

The nervous system is the body's master control system. It constantly receives information about the body's internal and external environments, and it continuously readjusts the body's systems in response to changes in those environments. The nervous system includes two portions: the central nervous system (CNS), which consists of the brain and spinal cord, and the peripheral nervous system (PNS), which includes the remaining motor and sensory nerves.

The brain is an extraordinarily complex structure, with an enormous perfusion requirement. It is constantly active at both conscious and unconscious levels. The brain comprises the cerebrum, cerebellum, and medulla (brain stem). The cerebrum takes charge of all of the brain's conscious processes; it is divided into two cerebral hemispheres; each of which contains four discrete lobes (frontal, temporal, parietal, and occipital). The cerebellum is responsible for coordinating balance. The brain stem handles all of the unconscious deeper processes.

With the exception of the cranial nerves, all nerves are ultimately channelled to the brain via the spinal cord. The spinal cord plays the role of a large conduit, passing information back and forth along itself. The peripheral nerves that emanate from the spinal cord, which are known as spinal nerves, have both motor and sensory pathways. Motor nerves control some aspect of motion or movement, whereas sensory nerves receive external signals and send them to the brain for processing and motor response. Motor tracts run from the spinal cord to the body outwardly; sensory nerves run from the body to the cord inwardly.

Skill Drill 13-12: Examining the Spine

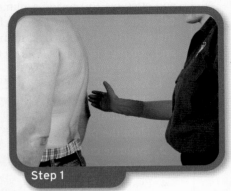

Step 1

Inspect the cervical, thoracic, and lumbar curves for any abnormalities.

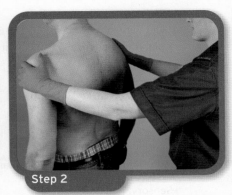

Step 2

Evaluate the heights of the shoulders and the iliac crests.

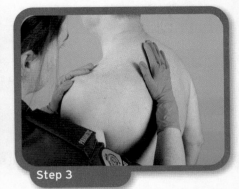

Step 3

Palpate the posterior portion of the cervical spine, noting any point tenderness or structural abnormalities.

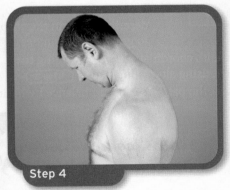

Step 4

In the nontrauma patient, and in the absence of reported pain, ask the patient to move the head forward, backward, and from side to side.

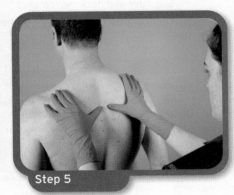

Step 5

Palpate each vertebra with the thumbs.

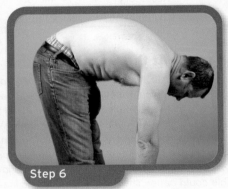

Step 6

In the absence of pain or trauma, ask the patient to bend at the waist in each direction to establish the range of movement.

Cranial nerves are not mediated by the spinal cord but rather go directly to and from the brain, originating at the medulla. They innervate the face, head, and parts of the neck, with the exception of the vagus nerve, which runs down the neck and into the chest and abdomen. There are 12 cranial nerves in total. They play roles in a wide variety of motor and sensory functions **Table 13-2** that involve both the voluntary and autonomic nervous systems (discussed later in this section).

The peripheral nerves are covered with a sheet-like material called myelin. Myelin promotes rapid transmission of impulses along the nerve. In the newborn, several of the major motor pathways (or long tracts) are not fully myelinated. Over time, however, myelin is completely deposited and the motor pathways become fully functional. Conversely, with advancing age and the occurrence of various disease states, neurological functions can deteriorate. This failure may take the form of a cognitive problem (eg, dementia), or it may lead to a physical

disability (eg, the problems seen with Parkinsonism and cerebrovascular disease).

In addition to the central/peripheral distinctions, the nervous system may be divided into involuntary (autonomic) and voluntary portions, with the autonomic nervous system being further subdivided into the sympathetic and parasympathetic systems. Reflexes are involuntary motor responses to specific sensory stimuli, such as a tap on the knee or stroking the eyelash. The location of what is stimulated determines which muscle will contract to produce a reflexive response. Spinal reflexes occur when sensory input comes from receptors in the muscles, joints, and skin. The motor response to this stimulation occurs entirely within the spinal cord; no brain processing is required. Other reflexes include the deep tendon reflexes and the superficial and brain stem reflexes. Primitive reflexes—including the Babinski, grasping, and sucking signs—are normal findings in infants. In older people, once the long motor pathways of the PNS have become fully

Table 13-2	Cranial Nerves		
Number	**Name**	**Motor vs Sensory**	**Functions**
I	Olfactory	Sensory	Smell
II	Optic	Sensory	Light perception and vision
III	Oculomotor	Motor	Pupil constriction, eye movements
IV	Trochlear	Motor	Eye movements
V	Trigeminal	Motor and sensory	Motor: chewing Sensory: face, sinuses, teeth
VI	Abducens	Motor	Eye movements
VII	Facial	Motor	Facial movements
VIII	Vestibulocochlear	Sensory	Hearing, balance perception
IX	Glossopharyngeal	Motor and sensory	Motor: throat and swallowing, gland secretion Sensory: tongue, throat, ear
X	Vagus	Motor and sensory	Heart, lungs, palate, pharynx, larynx, trachea, bronchi, GI tract, external ear
XI	Accessory	Motor	Shoulder and neck movements
XII	Hypoglossal	Motor	Tongue, throat, and neck movements

At the Scene

A Babinski test may be used to check for neurological function in an unresponsive patient. This is accomplished by stimulating the sole of the foot by rubbing with your thumb or running a pen or other pointed object along the sole of the foot. In a normal reaction, the big toe will flex. However, do NOT perform a Babinski test on a patient who has injuries to the lower extremities. This could cause the patient to pull the leg back, causing pain.

myelinated, the primitive reflexes represent abnormal findings, typical of injury or disconnection between the cerebral cortex and the brain stem.

The Neurological Examination

When you are performing a neurological examination, you need to focus on several key concepts (Skill Drill 13-12). At a bare minimum, the neurological examination should determine the patient's baseline mental status (AVPU), cranial nerve function (pupils, eyes, smile, speech, swallow, shoulder shrug), distal motor function (ability to move), and distal sensory function (ability to feel). It may also test the deep tendon reflexes if necessary.

First, assess the patient's overall mental status. Is the patient awake? If so, is the patient alert, and to what degree? If a change in level of consciousness has occurred, what kind of stimulus does it take to get a response, and to what degree does the patient's mental status improve? In the case of an altered mental status, do you observe any unusual postures? Is there any alteration in physical status (eg, is the ability to move successfully and symmetrically preserved)?

The Glasgow Coma Scale was designed as a tool to assist in better assessing subjects with significant alterations in mental status; it was originally intended for use in the trauma setting. It

simultaneously scores several parameters, including eye opening, verbal acuity, and motor activity, and attempts to provide a numerical score as a rapid means of defining severity of brain dysfunction and potential prognosis. Follow the steps in **Skill Drill 13-13**:

1. Assess the patient's mental status by using the AVPU mnemonic.
2. Note the patient's posture.
3. Evaluate cranial nerve function **Step 1**.
4. Evaluate the patient's neuromuscular status by checking muscle strength against resistance **Step 2**. Use the grading system described later in the chapter to grade all extremities.
5. Evaluate the patient's coordination by performing the finger-to-nose test using alternating hands **Step 3**.
6. If appropriate, test the patient's gait and balance by having the patient walk heel-to-toe or perform the heel-to-shin stance **Step 4**.
7. Perform the pronator drift test by asking the patient to close his or her eyes and hold both arms out in front of the body **Step 5**. There should be no difference in movement on either side.
8. Evaluate the patient's sensory function by checking his or her responses to both gross and light touch.
9. If appropriate, check for deep tendon reflexes.

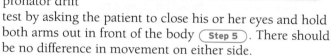

Notes from Nancy

Restlessness is a danger signal!

After assessment of the patient's overall mental status, you should begin the comprehensive neurological examination. Of course, such an examination is not needed in every case. Its details may vary greatly, depending on the nature of the patient's problem. Also, many portions of the neurological examination may have been completed earlier, during other aspects of the patient assessment. Keep track of these initial findings so that you can report them, they are not needlessly repeated, and any subsequent changes in status can be noted. Are left- and right-sided motor and sensory findings symmetrical? If not, how do they differ? Does the presenting problem appear to be more of a CNS or a PNS malfunction?

When testing the cranial nerves, a number of simple manoeuvres can be employed to determine the presence and degree of disability **Table 13-3**. With practice, the entire cranial nerve examination can be performed in less than 3 minutes.

Adequate evaluation of the motor system involves assessment of several distinct areas. Although motor activity may

Skill Drill 13-13: Examining the Nervous System

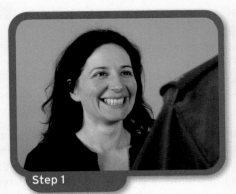

Step 1

Evaluate cranial nerve function.

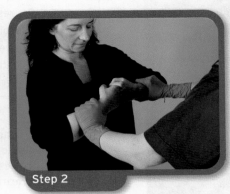

Step 2

Evaluate the patient's neuromuscular status by checking muscle strength against resistance.

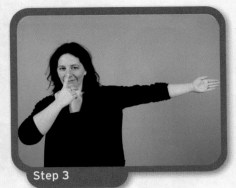

Step 3

Evaluate the patient's coordination by performing the finger-to-nose test using alternating hands.

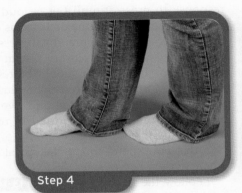

Step 4

If appropriate, test the patient's gait and balance by having the patient walk heel-to-toe or perform the heel-to-shin stance.

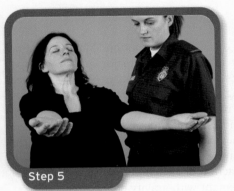

Step 5

Perform the pronator drift test by asking the patient to close his or her eyes and hold both arms out in front of the body.

Cranial Nerve	Test
Table 13-3	**Tests for Disability in Cranial Nerves**
I	Check smell
II	Check visual acuity and fields
III	Check pupil size, shape, symmetry, response to light, eye movements
IV	Check eye movements
V	Check jaw clench; touch both sides of face at forehead, cheeks, and jaw
VI	Check eye movements
VII	Check facial symmetry; look for abnormal movements; raise eyebrows, grin broadly, frown, shut eyes tightly, puff out cheeks; note any asymmetry
VIII	Check hearing and balance
IX, X	Check pharyngeal sensation, palate movements, and gag reflex
XI	Check shoulder shrug; turn head from left to right and back
XII	Check swallowing

represent the localised workings of the musculoskeletal system, the nervous system has an overriding influence on motor activity. Observe the patient's initial posture and body position **Figure 13-39 ▸** as well as the body position both at rest and with movement, if appropriate. Watch for any apparent involuntary movements, and document their quality, rate, rhythm, and amplitude. Try to determine whether these involuntary movements are related to the patient's posture or activity, and think about whether their presentation

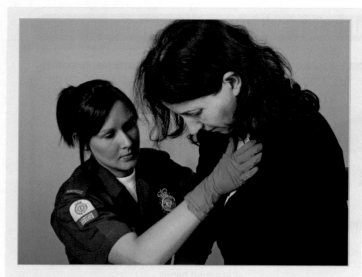

Figure 13-39 Note the patient's posture and body position.

Table 13-4	Scoring of Deep Tendon Reflexes
Grade	Deep Tendon Reflex Response
0	No response
1+	Sluggish
2+	Active (expected response)
3+	Slightly hyperactive
4+	Hyperactive

includes a component of fatigue or emotion. Make a general assessment of the bulk of the patient's major muscle groups. Compare these muscles' sizes and contours. Note associated muscle tone by checking for resistance to passive movement.

Probably the single most important part of the motor examination is the evaluation of overall muscle strength. To perform this assessment, get the patient to move actively against the examiner's resistance. Strength is graded on a scale of 1 to 5:

1: No muscle contraction or twitch detectable

2: Only active movement with gravity eliminated

3: Active movement against gravity obtained

4: Active movement against some resistance or with fatigue evident

5: Active movement against full resistance without evident fatigue

Strength is expressed as a ratio—for example, "strength is 4 over 5 (4/5) in the bilateral upper and lower extremities"; 5/5 is a state of normal muscle tone. When checking strength, and depending on the location of the muscle groups involved, be prepared to test for flexion, extension, grip, abduction, adduction, and opposition.

Checking coordination is an important part of the neurological examination because it tests a variety of nervous system functions, especially those involving cerebellar functioning. Coordination is assessed by evaluating a patient's ability to perform rapid alternating movements, point-to-point movements (including finger-to-nose and heel-to-shin testing), stance, and gait. Gait and stance should be evaluated only in those subjects whose status allows them to be safely placed in a standing position. Note any upper extremity tremors, flaps, or pronator drift at this point as well.

Just as evaluation of motor function tests the workings of the nervous system from the brain outward to the body, testing sensory function checks the workings of the nervous system from the body inward to the brain. In general, sensory

processes are tested bilaterally, looking for changes in symmetry from one side to the other, as well as comparing proximal to distal processes. When performing the initial assessment on a patient appearing in extremis, a sensory examination is typically the first evaluation done. Initial "shake and shout" manoeuvres represent an attempt to find evidence of preserved higher cerebral functioning. Typically these tests look for any response to gross stimuli (eg, a loud shout in the face) or implementation of more noxious forms of stimuli (eg, pinching the earlobe, applying supraorbital pressure). As part of a general examination of the sensory system, minimal perception of gross versus light touch should be tested (no equipment is required). More involved sensory evaluation involves checking sharp versus dull perception and two-point discrimination. Sensation is commonly reported in relation to dermatomal location on the body's surface. Dermatomes are distinct areas of skin that correspond to specific spinal or cranial nerve levels where sensory nerves enter the CNS.

Follow the steps in Skill Drill 13-14 ▶ to evaluate deep tendon reflexes. Scoring of deep tendon reflexes is covered in Table 13-4 ▲ .

1. Place the patient in the sitting position Step 1 .

2. Flex the patient's arm to 45° at the elbow. Locate the biceps tendon in the antecubital fossa. Place your thumb over the tendon, with your fingers behind the elbow. Strike your thumb with the reflex hammer, noting the flexion of the elbow Step 2 .

3. With the patient's arm remaining at a 45° angle, rest the patient's forearm on your arm with the hand slightly pronated. Strike the patient's brachioradial tendon proximal to the wrist, noting the flexion of the elbow Step 3 .

4. Flex the patient's arm at the elbow 90° and rest his or her hand against the body. Locate and strike the triceps tendon, noting contraction of the triceps or extension of the elbow Step 4 .

5. Flex the patient's knee to 90°, allowing the leg to dangle. Support the upper leg with your hand, and strike the patellar tendon just below the patella. Note the contraction of the quadriceps and the extension of the lower leg Step 5 .

6. With the patient's leg in the same position, hold the heel of the patient's foot in your hand. Strike the Achilles tendon, noting the plantar flexion of the foot Step 6 .

Skill Drill 13-14: Evaluation of Deep Tendon Reflexes

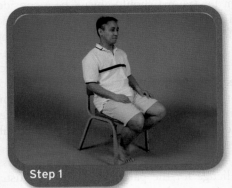

Step 1

Place the patient in the sitting position.

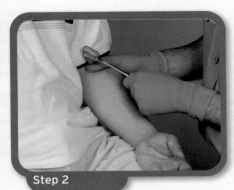

Step 2

Flex the patient's arm to 45° at the elbow. Locate the biceps tendon in the antecubital fossa. Place your thumb over the tendon, with your fingers behind the elbow. Strike your thumb with the reflex hammer, noting the flexion of the elbow.

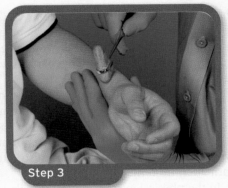

Step 3

With the patient's arm remaining at a 45° angle, rest the patient's forearm on your arm with the hand slightly pronated. Strike the patient's brachioradialis tendon proximal to the wrist, noting the flexion of the elbow.

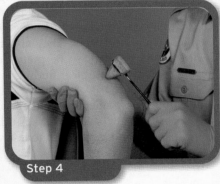

Step 4

Flex the patient's arm at the elbow 90° and rest his or her hand against the body. Locate and strike the triceps tendon, noting contraction of the triceps or extension of the elbow.

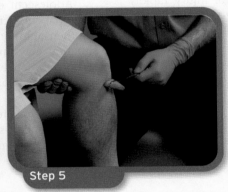

Step 5

Flex the patient's knee to 90°, allowing the leg to dangle. Support the upper leg with your hand, and strike the patellar tendon just below the patella.

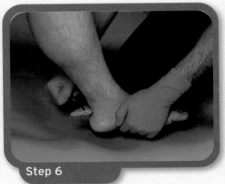

Step 6

With the patient's leg in the same position, hold the heel of the patient's foot in your hand. Strike the Achilles tendon.

Results of the Neurological Examination

Abnormal findings on the neurological examination can take a wide variety of forms. The most common of these are mental status changes that can represent any number of acute and chronic processes, many of which have a nonneurological origin. Changes in mental status often represent changes in perfusion or are encountered as a subtle indicator of early sepsis (which is very common in the older population).

Distinguishing between delirium and dementia, when dealing with a patient with abnormal mental status, is also important. Delirium is more consistent with an acute sudden change in mental status, secondary to some significant underlying aberration. Dementia is representative of a gradual and pervasive deterioration of cognitive cortical functions, typically secondary to the slow progression of some disease state.

Commonly encountered motor abnormalities include facial and extremity strength asymmetry along with difficulty in speaking (dysphasia). These signs are very typical of cerebrovascular disease. Other commonly encountered abnormalities include ataxia, dystonia, convulsions, vertigo, visual changes, tinnitus, and tremor. In the setting of trauma, global changes in mental status are more indicative of intracranial mass lesions, whereas decreased extremity motor function may present with proximal versus distal asymmetry and objective paraesthesia (tingling or sensory changes), which is more consistent with a spinal lesion.

Physical Examination of Infants and Children

When caring for infants and children, you'll need to alter your approach to patient assessment in general. Because a young child might not be able to speak, your assessment of his or her condition must be based in large part on what you can see and hear yourself.

Examining a child requires understanding that you may have to deal with several sources of information. Families may be helpful in providing vital information about the injury or illness. If possible, and if the patient is of an adequate age and developmental status, you should also attempt to elicit some information from the patient.

In the physical examination, the goals of assessment in children are the same as those for adult patients. If possible, obtain the permission of the parent or guardian before conducting an examination. Explain to the child that you're going to check him or her because you're a paramedic, and that you're here to help. In a situation of acute life-threatening illness or injury, rapidly conduct the initial assessment and manage life-threatening conditions as with an adult patient.

When time permits, consider certain age-related strategies for attempting to facilitate the examination. Overall, children tend to do better being examined from toe to head, as opposed to the reverse method commonly used with adults. This strategy tends to gain trust and decreases the child's fear. Infants generally appear not to be particularly distressed by being manipulated by adults, so the basic approach to assessment is reasonable with

them. Pay close attention to vital signs and physical findings, as the ability to obtain a helpful history is limited.

Children are prone to dehydration and infection (eg, sepsis), and assessment for trauma should always be a consideration as well. Children from 1 to 3 years of age can be challenging to work with, and as a rule will strenuously object to being touched or manipulated by a stranger. The toe-to-head approach is a good strategy in this age group. Decide which aspects of the examination must be performed, set some reasonable ground rules for the examination, and then examine the patient accordingly. Practise ways to hold young patients safely and adequately, to facilitate the assessment. If possible, have family members assist with this task.

Children from 4 to 5 years of age are typically much less of a management challenge for the paramedic. They are usually cooperative and helpful with the examination, and the standard head-to-toe approach can usually be employed. School-age children tend to be cooperative as well, and should be actively engaged in the examination process. Be sure to take the time to explain what you're doing while you're examining them.

Adolescent evaluation can be a bit more demanding, as these patients tend to have feelings more directed at preserving their autonomy, and can be concerned about how a given situation may involve either parents or peers. They also tend to be very concerned with bodily integrity, so be prepared to reassure them that things are okay if a physical finding is not worrying.

When you are dealing with the assessment of children, some general principles apply. No matter how stressful or disturbing the situation, remain calm, patient, and gentle. Be honest with

You are the Paramedic Part 4

Your patient's oxygen saturations have risen slightly, but are still insufficient. You are just preparing another 5 mg of salbutamol when the patient grabs you by the arm and whispers that he can't keep breathing any longer and loses consciousness. You ask your partner to pull over so that you can intubate. Using a size 3 Macintosh blade you are able to visualise the vocal cords and insert an 8.0 mm endotracheal tube. Endotracheal tube placement is further confirmed with bilateral breath sounds, equal and symmetric, chest rise, and a positive end-tidal CO_2 waveform. After confirming tube placement you secure the tube and ventilate the patient.

You arrive at hospital approximately 12 minutes later. The patient is immediately placed on a hospital ventilator. Three hours later he is admitted to the medical intensive care unit with an exacerbation of his emphysema. He is treated successfully with antibiotics and aggressive respiratory therapy and is discharged home 8 days later.

Reassessment	Recording Time: 25 Minutes
Skin	Pale, warm, and dry, with cyanotic lips and nail beds
Pulse	120 beats/min, regular, with strong distal pulses
ECG	Sinus tachycardia
Blood pressure	150/88 mm Hg
Respirations	12 breaths/min on bag-valve-mask ventilation
S_PO_2	86% on bag-valve-mask ventilation at 100% supplemental oxygen
Pupils	Equal and reactive to light

7. Why is it important to reassess your patient after each treatment intervention?

children; if something is likely to hurt, say so—but without much else in the way of fanfare. If at all possible, attempt to keep children and parents together. It is normal for children to harbour fears over separation; in the setting of acute illness or injury, these anxieties will only be worsened. Remember that paediatric patients presenting in the prehospital setting are often victims of trauma. Be sure to appropriately assess for injury, and treat appropriately. Don't neglect a child's pain.

Recording Examination Findings

Medical information may be presented in both oral and written forms. Recording of information should always be done in as orderly and concise a fashion as possible, without omitting important information. The obtained information may then be practically and accurately relayed to the receiving medical staff. In addition, documentation ensures that an accurate historical accounting of the patient's problems prior to entering the hospital will legally exist in the formal medical record. You must use the patient clinical record forms that are issued by your ambulance service.

A physical examination requires a physical interaction between the patient and the care provider, and it can be successfully performed on a patient who can't communicate. When you are recording examination findings, note objective signs, pertinent negatives, and other similar relevant information. Objective information is commonly recorded in a standard format, in the same order as used for the verbal or written report.

At the Scene

Remember the legal and ethical components to the physical examination:

1. Respect the patient's autonomy in decision making.
2. Be accountable to the patient.
3. Respect the patient's confidentiality and privacy.
4. Obtain consent.
5. Recognise assault.
6. Understand and respect advance directives.
7. Document facts accurately and nonjudgementally.

Limits of the Physical Examination

The ability to competently perform a physical examination is one of the most valuable skills a paramedic can possess. This examination can, for example, uncover information that the patient is unable or unwilling to share. An accomplished practitioner will use this skill in conjunction with the patient interview and other diagnostic tools to form an impression and formulate a treatment plan.

Nevertheless, despite the emphasis placed on a comprehensive physical examination, it has limitations. Even the most experienced doctor understands that not everything can be discovered in the examination. In the prehospital setting, it is important to remember that evaluation by a fully trained doctor and laboratory and radiographic studies may be needed for a definitive diagnosis.

You are the Paramedic Summary

1. What is your general impression of the patient? Is he sick or not sick?

You see an older man in a tripod position in obvious respiratory distress. His breathing is rapid and shallow. He has recession and audible wheezes, and cyanosis is present not only in the fingertips but in the lips as well. Your general impression should be "I have a sick patient here"!

2. What do you think is the most valuable assessment tool at your disposal?

Cardiac monitor? No, try again. Blood pressure cuff? Nah! Pulse oximeter? Keep trying! Stethoscope? Good guess, but not quite. You are the most valuable assessment tool that you have! Think about it. You are able to gather information and form the general impression of a patient without using any equipment, right? If the patient is talking to you upon arrival, he or she has a patent airway. Checking a radial pulse will not only tell you the pulse rate, but the quality of pulse and skin temperature as well. You can visualise skin colour, check for symmetric chest rise, recession, and work of breathing. Abnormal breath sounds such as wheezes, stridor, and rhonchi may be severe enough to be heard without a stethoscope. Don't forget about smell. The nose knows when odours such as ketones, alcohol, and cyanide are present. All of this information can be obtained without the use of any equipment.

3. Which signs and symptoms are acute? Which are chronic?

The chronic signs and symptoms of COPD are clubbing of the fingers, cyanotic nail beds, barrel-shaped chest, and pursed-lipped breathing. Acute signs and symptoms include abnormal breath sounds. A decreased oxygen saturation, shallow breathing, and rapid respiratory rate may be both acute and chronic. This is where you need to ask the patient what is normal for him and move forward from there. For example, your patient's normal oxygen saturation may be 84%, which is definitely decreased; therefore, an oxygen saturation level of 70% indicates an acute condition requiring your attention.

4. Which interventions should you consider at this point?

The focus of treatment needs to be decreasing your patient's work of breathing. Supplemental oxygen can be applied via a nonrebreathing mask. (Yes, it is safe to do this provided you keep reassessing your patient to make sure he doesn't become apnoeic or develop altered mental status!) Pharmacological treatment is achieved by the administration of a bronchodilator such as salbutamol and ipratropium. Bronchodilators will help by relaxing the muscles surrounding the bronchioles, allowing air to flow more freely into and out of the lungs.

5. Would an increased work of breathing be present upon reassessment of the patient if your treatment was effective?

This is a tough question. It may take a while for the patient's work of breathing to return to what is normal for him. Don't get discouraged if after the first treatment he is still experiencing increased work of breathing. Remember to also reassess breath sounds, pulse rate, and pulse oximetry and be sure to document your findings.

6. How should your patient management progress?

Listen to your patient; he knows his condition better than you! He is telling you that the breathing treatment is not working. Administering additional nebuliser treatments with salbutamol is appropriate.

7. Why is it important to reassess your patient after each treatment intervention?

Imagine being put in the middle of an unfamiliar country without a map, compass, or means of communication. How would you find your way out? Without reassessing your patient, how would you get the information necessary to guide further treatment? In your patient, it would be important to note respiratory rate and effort, changes in breath sounds, an improvement in his ability to speak, mental status, pulse rate, and pulse oximetry. Are the breathing treatments working or do you need to consider adding other medications? Can the patient maintain his own airway or do you need to control it via bag-valve-mask ventilation or endotracheal intubation? Remember, your patient can provide you with the clues you need as long as you look for them.

Prep Kit

Ready for Review

- Physical examination is the process by which quantifiable, objective information is obtained from a patient about his or her overall state of health.
- The physical examination consists of two elements: obtaining vital signs that measure overall body function, and performing a head-to-toe survey that evaluates the workings of specific body organ systems. This survey is done in a sequential manner, ensuring that every aspect of the body's function is evaluated.
- The techniques of inspection, palpation, percussion, and auscultation allow you to use your physical senses to obtain physical information and to understand the normal (versus abnormal) functions of a patient's body.
- Vital signs consist of a measurement of blood pressure; pulse rate, rhythm, and quality; respiratory rate, rhythm, and quality; temperature; and pulse oximetry. Other than overall patient appearance, vital signs are the most basic objective data for determining patient status.
- The general survey begins as you approach the scene, simultaneously assessing the overall situation and the patient's appearance. Review the environment in which the patient is found and the general state of the patient's health.
- The physical examination consists of a comprehensive review of systems to determine the nature and extent of the patient's illness or injury.
- Evaluate the patient's mental status using the AVPU scale.
- When you are examining the head, you should both feel it and inspect it visually. This step is important in the management of potential trauma patients and with patients who have altered mental status or are unresponsive.
- When you are evaluating the face, observe the colour and moisture of the skin, as well as expression, symmetry, and contour of the face itself. Pay attention to any swelling or apparent areas of injury, and note any signs of respiratory distress. Use the mnemonic DCAP-BTLS.
- When you are assessing the pupils, check for size (in millimetres), shape, and symmetry. Also check for a reaction to light shined on them.
- Cervical injury can present in a variety of ways, and the assessment for such injury must be conducted in a careful manner. Evaluate the patient first for the MOI and then for the presence of pain.
- Any manipulations of the spine that result in pain, tenderness, or tingling should prompt you to stop the examination *immediately* and place the patient into a properly sized collar. With any complaints of neck pain in patients who have suffered a significant MOI, immediate stabilisation of the head and neck is essential.
- Typically, the chest examination proceeds in three phases: the chest wall is checked, a pulmonary evaluation is conducted, and finally the cardiovascular assessment is performed. Inspect the chest to assess for deformities in wall patency and to look for external clues of respiratory distress.
- Heart sounds can be best heard at the fifth intercostal space over the apex of the heart.
- Because of the large number of organs within the abdomen, the location of organs and their related medical complaints are most easily described by dividing the abdomen into imaginary quadrants.
- When you are inspecting the abdomen, look at the skin as well as the contour and overall appearance of the abdominal wall. Identify any scars, wounds, striae, dilated veins, bruises, rashes, and discolourations. Note any generalised distension or localised masses.
- When you are examining the skeleton and joints, pay attention to both their structure and their function. Consider how the joint and associated extremities look and how well they work.
- When you are assessing the joints and extremities, look for evidence of inflammation or injury, such as swelling, tenderness, increased heat, redness, bruising, or decreased function. Also evaluate the joint or extremity for obvious deformity, diminished strength, atrophy, or asymmetry from one side to the other.
- The examination of the musculoskeletal system should not cause the patient any pain; if any occurs, it should be considered an abnormal finding.
- Palpation of the spine is typically done while the patient is supine, often when he or she has been log rolled onto one side to facilitate access to the back and placement of a spinal immobilisation device.
- When you are palpating the spine, use the thumb to touch each spinous process. Identification of an abnormality should prompt you to institute proper splinting and protective measures.
- The neurological examination should determine the patient's baseline mental status (AVPU), cranial nerve function (pupils, eyes, smile, speech, swallow, shoulder shrug), distal motor function (ability to move), and distal sensory function (ability to feel). It may also test the deep tendon reflexes if necessary.
- You need to alter your approach to patient assessment when dealing with infants and children. Because a young child might not be able to speak, your assessment of his or her condition must be based in large part on what you can see and hear yourself. Family members or carers may also be able to provide useful information.
- Medical information may be presented in both verbal and written forms. Recorded information should be orderly, concise, and complete.

Vital Vocabulary

ascites Abnormal accumulation of fluid in the peritoneal cavity.

auscultation The method of listening to sounds within the body with a stethoscope.

bruit An abnormal "whoosh"-like sound of turbulent blood flow moving through a narrowed artery.

crepitus Crackling, grating, or grinding that is often felt or heard when two ends of bone rub together.

cyanosis A bluish-grey skin colour that is caused by reduced levels of oxygen in the blood.

delirium Change in mental status that is marked by the inability to focus, think logically, and maintain attention.

dementia The slow onset of progressive disorientation, shortened attention span, and loss of cognitive function.

dermatomes Distinct areas of skin that correspond to specific spinal or cranial nerve levels where sensory nerves enter the CNS.

dysphasia The impairment of language that affects the production or understanding of speech and the ability to read or write.

ecchymosis Localised bruising or blood collection within or under the skin.

foramen magnum A large opening at the base of the skull.

Glasgow Coma Scale Scoring system used to determine level of consciousness.

guarding Tensing of the abdominal wall muscles to minimise movement of inflamed organs within the abdomen.

hernia Protrusion of any organ through an opening into a body cavity where it does not belong.

inspection Looking at the patient, either in general or at a specific area (ie, a patient's overall appearance from the doorway, versus looking specifically at the chest wall for abnormalities/deformities).

Korotkoff sounds Sounds related to blood pressure that are heard by stethoscope.

kyphosis Outward curve of the thoracic spine, giving a stooped appearance.

lordosis Inward curve of the lumbar spine just above the buttocks. An exaggerated form of lordosis results in the condition known as swayback.

mottling A blotchy pattern on the skin; a typical finding in states of severe protracted hypoperfusion and shock.

murmur An abnormal "whoosh"-like sound heard over the heart that indicates turbulent blood flow around a cardiac valve.

occiput The most posterior portion of the cranium.

ophthalmoscope An instrument used to look into a patient's eyes and view the retina and aqueous fluid; consists of a concave mirror and a battery-powered light that is usually contained in the handle.

otoscope An instrument for examing the ear drum.

pallor Paleness.

palpation Physical touching for the purpose of obtaining information.

paraesthesia Tingling or sensory change.

pathological fracture A fracture that occurs when normal forces are applied to abnormal bone structures.

percussion Gently striking the surface of the body, typically overlying various body cavities to detect changes in the densities of the underlying structures.

perfusion The circulation of blood within an organ or tissue in adequate amounts to meet the cells' needs.

physical examination The process by which quantifiable, objective information is obtained from a patient about his or her overall state of health.

physiological fracture A fracture that occurs when abnormal forces are applied to normal bone structures.

primitive reflexes Reflex reactions such as Babinski, grasping, and sucking signs normally found in very young patients.

pulse oximetry An assessment tool that measures oxygen saturation of haemoglobin in the capillary beds.

rales Rattling, bubbling, or crackling lung sounds.

reflexes Involuntary motor responses to specific sensory stimuli, such as a tap on the knee or stroking the eyelash.

rhonchi Lung sounds that resemble snoring.

rubor Redness; one of the classic signs of inflammation.

rubs Lung sound produced by a partial loss of intrapleural integrity, when an abnormal collection of fluid has accumulated between a portion of the visceral and parietal pleura, resulting in "pleuritic" pain and a perceived rub on auscultation.

scoliosis Sideways curvature of the spine.

stridor A harsh, high-pitched, crowing inspiratory sound, such as the sound often heard in acute laryngeal obstruction.

tenting A condition in which the skin slowly retracts after being pinched and pulled away slightly from the body; a sign of dehydration.

turgor Loss of elasticity in the skin.

vasoconstriction Narrowing of a blood vessel, such as with hypoperfusion or cold extremities.

vasodilatation Widening of a blood vessel.

visual acuity (VA) The ability or inability to see, and how well one can see.

Assessment in Action

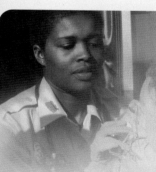

You're dispatched to the home of a 24-year-old woman who is complaining of abdominal pain. On your arrival, she is bent over, grasping her abdominal wall, and tells you the pain is very intense. Her vital signs are within normal limits. You begin to ask questions and perform your physical examination.

1. _____ is a rapid method of assessing the patient's level of consciousness.
   A. APU
   B. C&O×3
   C. AVPU
   D. AO×4

2. Inspection involves:
   A. looking at the patient, either in general or at a specific area.
   B. the physical touching for the purpose of obtaining information.
   C. gently striking the surface of the body, typically overlying various body cavities.
   D. listening with a stethoscope.

3. Measuring _____ require(s) the paramedic to utilise the techniques of auscultation, palpation, and inspection.
   A. blood pressure
   B. pulse rate
   C. heart rate
   D. vital signs

4. Blood pressure must be measured with a cuff that's appropriate to the patient's size. If you use a blood pressure cuff that is too small or tight you will yield a(an):
   A. artificially low blood pressure.
   B. artificially normal blood pressure.
   C. artificially high blood pressure.
   D. normal pressure.

5. Because of the large number of organs within the abdomen, the _____ serves as a central reference point.
   A. lower rib cage
   B. pelvic girdle
   C. xyphoid process
   D. umbilicus

6. The above patient is complaining of pain near her gallbladder. This would be located in the:
   A. RUQ.
   B. LUQ.
   C. RLQ.
   D. LLQ.

7. When a patient is contracting his or her abdominal muscles, this is called:
   A. rigidity.
   B. guarding.
   C. soft.
   D. not tender.

Challenging Question

8. Are there any special considerations you should take based on your patient's gender?

▇ Points to Ponder

You are dispatched to the home of a 65-year-old woman who is complaining of a feeling of general malaise that began about 4 days ago. When you arrive on scene, the patient appears to be in no distress. You introduce yourself and begin your physical examination. The patient denies having any chest pain, shortness of breath, nausea, or vomiting. Her vital signs are as follows: respiratory rate, 18 breaths/min; pulse oximetry reading, 99% on room air; blood pressure, 110/70 mm Hg; and pulse rate, 75 beats/min with a normal sinus rhythm on the monitor. The patient states that she "hasn't felt right" for a few days and she called now because she had no way to get to the doctor.

Where should you begin your examination?

Issues: Understanding the Importance of a Complete Physical Examination, Understanding the Need for a Caring Attitude When Performing a Physical Examination, Understanding the Importance of a Professional Appearance and Demeanour When Performing a Physical Examination.

14 Patient Assessment

Objectives

Cognitive

- Recognise hazards/potential hazards.
- Describe common hazards found at the scene of a trauma and a medical patient.
- Determine hazards found at the scene of a medical or trauma patient.
- Differentiate safe from unsafe scenes.
- Describe methods to making an unsafe scene safe.
- Discuss common mechanisms of injury/nature of illness.
- Predict patterns of injury based on mechanism of injury.
- Discuss the reason for identifying the total number of patients at the scene.
- Organise the management of a scene following assessment.
- Explain the reasons for identifying the need for additional help or assistance.
- Summarise the reasons for forming a general impression of the patient.
- Discuss methods of assessing mental status.
- Categorise levels of consciousness in the adult, infant, and child.
- Differentiate between assessing the altered mental status in the adult, child, and infant patient.
- Discuss methods of assessing the airway in the adult, child, and infant patient.
- State reasons for management of the cervical spine once the patient has been determined to be a trauma patient.
- Analyse a scene to determine whether spinal precautions are required.
- Describe methods used for assessing if a patient is breathing.
- Differentiate between a patient with adequate and inadequate minute ventilation.
- Distinguish between methods of assessing breathing in the adult, child, and infant patient.
- Compare the methods of providing airway care to the adult, child, and infant patient.
- Describe the methods used to locate and assess a pulse.
- Differentiate between locating and assessing a pulse in an adult, child, and infant patient.
- Discuss the need for assessing the patient for external bleeding.
- Describe normal and abnormal findings when assessing skin colour.
- Describe normal and abnormal findings when assessing skin temperature and condition.
- Explain the reason for prioritising a patient for care and transport.
- Identify time critical patients.
- Describe the evaluation of a patient's perfusion status based on findings in the initial assessment.
- Describe orthostatic vital signs and evaluate their usefulness in assessing a patient in shock.
- Apply the techniques of physical examination to the medical patient.
- Differentiate between the assessment that is performed for a patient who is unresponsive or has an altered mental status and other medical patients requiring assessment.
- Discuss the reasons for reconsidering the mechanism of injury.
- State the reasons for performing a rapid trauma assessment.
- Recite examples and explain why patients should receive a rapid trauma assessment.
- Apply the techniques of physical examination to the trauma patient.
- Describe the areas included in the rapid trauma assessment and discuss what should be evaluated.
- Identify cases where the rapid assessment may be altered in order to improve patient care.
- Discuss the reason for performing a focused history and physical examination.
- Describe when and why a detailed physical examination is necessary.
- Discuss the components of the detailed physical examination in relation to the techniques of examination.
- State the areas of the body that are evaluated during the detailed physical examination.
- Explain what additional care should be provided while performing the detailed physical examination.
- Distinguish between the detailed physical examination that is performed on a trauma patient and that of the medical patient.
- Differentiate patients requiring a detailed physical examination from those who do not.
- Discuss the reasons for repeating the initial assessment as part of the on-going assessment.
- Describe the components of the on-going assessment.
- Describe trending of assessment components.
- Discuss medical identification devices/systems.

Affective

- Explain the rationale for crew members to evaluate scene safety prior to entering.
- Serve as a role model for others by explaining how patient situations affect your evaluation of mechanism of injury or illness.
- Explain the importance of forming a general impression of the patient.
- Explain the value of performing an initial assessment.
- Demonstrate a caring attitude when performing an initial assessment.
- Attend to the feelings that patients with medical conditions might be experiencing.
- Value the need for maintaining a professional caring attitude when performing a focused history and physical examination.
- Explain the rationale for the feelings that these patients might be experiencing.
- Demonstrate a caring attitude when performing a detailed physical examination.
- Explain the value of performing an on-going assessment.

- Recognise and respect the feelings that patients might experience during assessment.
- Explain the value of trending assessment components to other health professionals who assume care of the patient.

Psychomotor

- Observe various scenarios and identify potential hazards.
- Demonstrate the scene assessment.
- Demonstrate the techniques for assessing mental status.
- Demonstrate the techniques for assessing the airway.
- Demonstrate the techniques for assessing if the patient is breathing.
- Demonstrate the techniques for assessing if the patient has a pulse.
- Demonstrate the techniques for assessing the patient for external bleeding.
- Demonstrate the techniques for assessing the patient's skin colour, temperature, and condition.
- Demonstrate the ability to prioritise patients.
- Using the techniques of examination, demonstrate the assessment of a medical patient.

- Demonstrate the patient care skills that should be used to assist with a patient who is responsive with no known history.
- Demonstrate the patient care skills that should be used to assist with a patient who is unresponsive or has an altered mental status.
- Perform a rapid medical assessment.
- Perform a focused history and physical examination of the medical patient.
- Using the techniques of physical examination, demonstrate the assessment of a trauma patient.
- Demonstrate the rapid trauma assessment used to assess a patient based on mechanism of injury.
- Perform a focused history and physical examination on a non-critically injured patient.
- Perform a focused history and physical examination on a patient with life-threatening injuries.
- Perform a detailed physical examination.
- Demonstrate the skills involved in performing the on-going assessment.

Patient Assessment

Scene Assessment

Body Substance Isolation
Scene Safety
Consider Mechanism of Injury/Nature of Illness
Determine the Number of Patients
Consider Additional Resources
Consider C-Spine Immobilisation

Initial Assessment

Approach and Form a General Impression
Assess Mental Status
Assess the Airway
Assess Breathing
Assess Circulation
Identify Priority Patients and Make Transport Decisions

Trauma Patients

Focused History and Physical Examination

Reconsider Mechanism of Injury

Significant Mechanism of Injury	No Significant Mechanism of Injury
Rapid Trauma Assessment	Focused Trauma Assessment Based on Chief Complaint
Baseline Vital Signs	Baseline Vital Signs
SAMPLE History	SAMPLE History
Re-evaluate Transport Decision	Re-evaluate Transport Decision

Detailed Physical Examination

Perform the Detailed Physical Examination
Re-assess Vital Signs

Medical Patients

Focused History and Physical Examination

Evaluate Responsiveness

Responsive	Unresponsive
History of Illness	Rapid Medical Assessment
SAMPLE History	Baseline Vital Signs
Focused Medical Assessment Based on Chief Complaint	SAMPLE History
Baseline Vital Signs	Re-evaluate Transport Decision
Re-evaluate Transport Decision	

On-going Assessment

Repeat the Initial Assessment
Re-assess and Record Vital Signs
Repeat the Focused Assessment
Check Interventions

Introduction

Patient assessment is the platform on which quality prehospital care is built and the single most important skill you bring to bear on patient care. Patient assessment is a complex skill made up of two primary components: information gathering and physical examination. In the first component, called history-taking, you try to determine the nature of the patient's problems by asking questions, listening to and analysing answers, and observing the way the patient presents and the setting in which he or she is found. In the second component, called physical assessment, you perform a hands-on evaluation of the patient to further explore the chief complaint(s) and to detect injuries or signs of illness.

This chapter describes the skill of patient assessment, focusing primarily on the *what* aspects of patient assessment (that is, what needs to done as part of an organised, systematic assessment). Chapters 12 and 13 presented the *how* aspects of the patient assessment in more detail. Now you will learn how to pull everything together. Please note that paediatric assessment is covered in detail in Chapter 41: *Paediatrics*.

The information gleaned during the patient assessment process helps you make key patient care decisions. The first and most important question during the initial assessment is always "Does my patient have any life-threatening conditions"? If life threats are present, you must quickly decide how to address them. Patient findings obtained early in the assessment process often dictate whether the patient needs to be transported by ground or by air ambulance and to which hospital. For these reasons, your patient assessment skills are the single most important tools in your toolbox. While *some* of your patients may need spinal immobilisation and *others* may need a respiratory treatment, *all of your patients* need excellent patient assessment.

The fundamental components of your job are to identify problems (the chief complaint, or why someone called 999), set priorities (rank the problems from most to least serious), develop a care plan (address the problems), and execute the plan (provide care for the patient). As you gain prehospital experience and attend more incidents, however, the breadth and depth of your knowledge base should increase and you should see a corresponding increase in your assessment skills. Patient assessment is a skill that you should hone *throughout your entire paramedic career.*

The Elements of Patient Assessment

Several elements make up the skill of patient assessment, with each being used in some way to gather information. The primary source of information during your assessment is usually the patient, but you will also gather information from sources such as the patient's family and friends or eyewitnesses to the emergency event. That information is then added to information gathered from the emergency scene itself, along with the data you obtain from your diagnostic tools and tests (such as cardiac monitor, glucometer, and pulse oximeter).

Care in the prehospital setting is very similar to the process used in solving a "whodunit" murder mystery. In this case, however, you are the detective, and the mystery is finding out what is wrong with your patient and what you can do about it. To solve the mystery, you gather "clues" about your patient's problem, sift through the clues, and analyse the data. Missed clues resulting from a weak, disorganised, or incomplete patient assessment may prevent you from solving the mystery, which in the real world of patient care equates with your patient getting less than optimal care.

You are the Paramedic Part 1

You are sent to a motorbike rally track for a collapsed male. Upon arrival, you find a 17-year-old male lying on the ground, unconscious. His friends report that Mike suddenly collapsed from standing and was not riding his bike at the time of the incident. They also state that Mike had no complaints just before the event and seemed to be "just fine".

In your initial assessment, the patient responds only to deep, painful stimuli, and you find no obvious signs of trauma. Mike's friends aren't sure if he has any medical conditions, and they can't provide any further information.

Initial Assessment	Recording Time: 0 Minutes
Appearance	Wearing full protective gear; supine
Level of consciousness	P (Responsive to painful stimuli)
Airway	Patent
Breathing	Slightly fast but adequate
Circulation	Strong, full radial pulse

1. What is the best method of airway assessment and management for a patient who is wearing a helmet?
2. Although his friends deny the occurrence of any trauma, should you immobilise this patient?

Scene Assessment

Patient Assessment

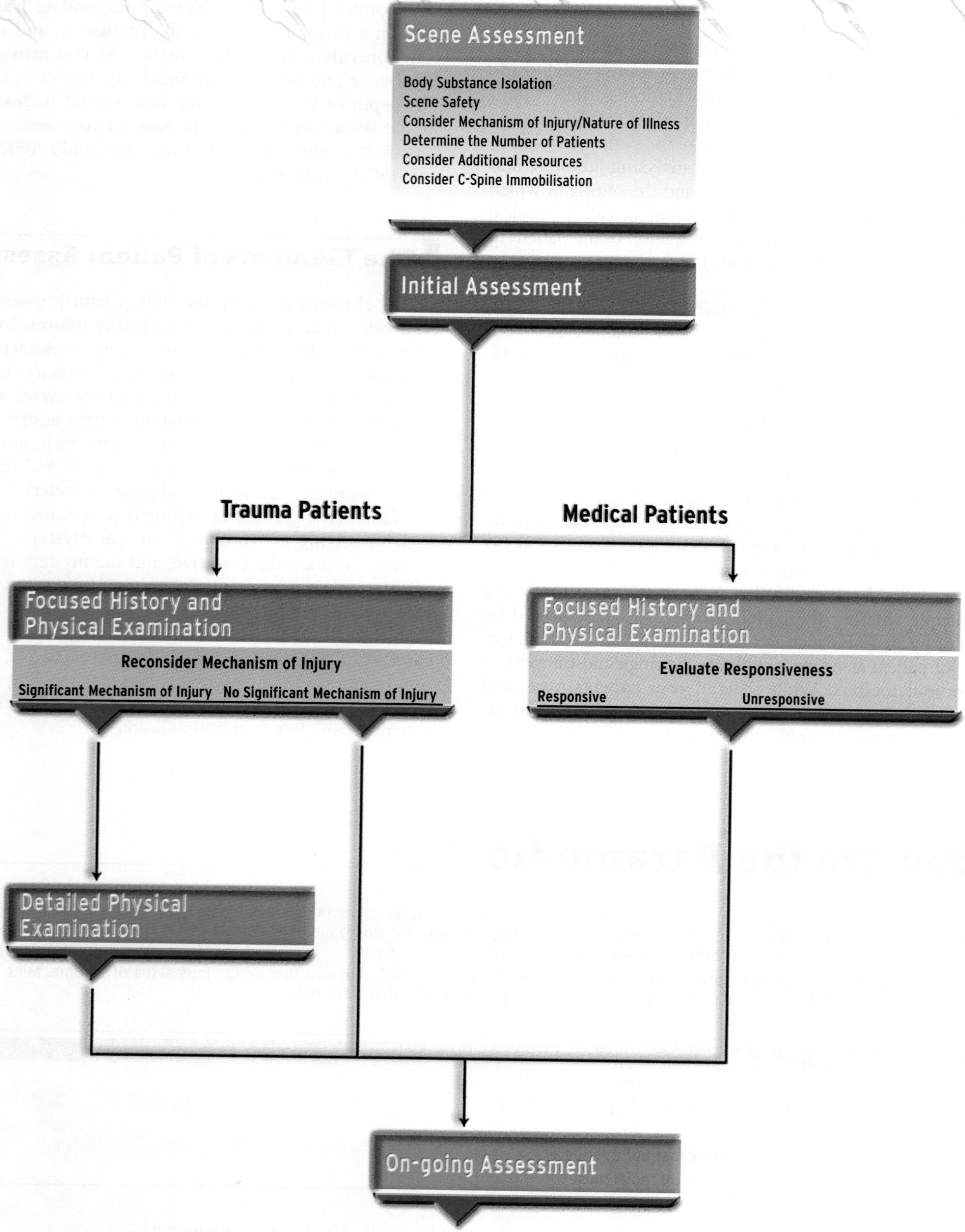

Scene Assessment

Body Substance Isolation
Scene Safety
Consider Mechanism of Injury/Nature of Illness
Determine the Number of Patients
Consider Additional Resources
Consider C-Spine Immobilisation

Initial Assessment

Trauma Patients

Medical Patients

Focused History and Physical Examination

Reconsider Mechanism of Injury

Significant Mechanism of Injury   No Significant Mechanism of Injury

Focused History and Physical Examination

Evaluate Responsiveness

Responsive   Unresponsive

Detailed Physical Examination

On-going Assessment

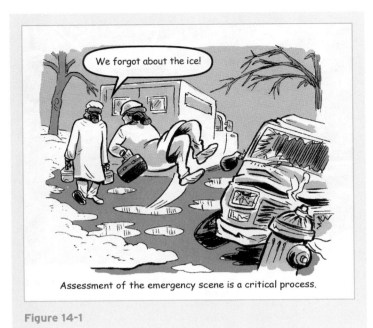

We forgot about the ice!

Assessment of the emergency scene is a critical process.

Figure 14-1

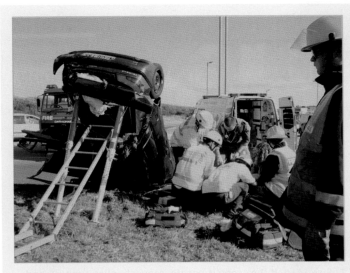

Figure 14-2 Accident scenes have many risks to you, your colleagues, and the patient.

Scene Assessment and Evaluation

Body Substance Isolation and Universal Precautions

The first step of the patient assessment process is the scene assessment. Your first and foremost concern on any call is ensuring your own safety and the safety of your colleagues 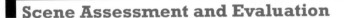 Figure 14-1 ▲. You are of no value to the patient if you get injured and can't provide care. Suppose you get an infectious disease because you neglected to follow universal precautions and body substance isolation (BSI) procedures; you may then miss time from work because you are sick. In the worst-case scenario, you might contract a career-ending or life-threatening disease, all because you chose to ignore a simple but important set of rules—the rules of BSI and universal precautions.

You should wear properly sized gloves on every call. If blood or other fluids could potentially splash or spray, wear eye protection. When inhaled particles are a risk factor, wear a properly sized and fitted mask. Always take the steps necessary to protect yourself on calls. When in doubt about the nature of the threat, it's always better to err on the side of caution and protect yourself too much rather than too little. Infection control is covered in depth in Chapters 2 and 36.

Scene Safety

In the assessment and evaluation of the emergency scene, the main focus is to ensure the safety and well-being of the team. Ask yourself, "Is it safe for me and my colleague to enter this scene and to approach the patient"? To answer that question, you need to use a "wide-angle lens" thought process when you

assess and evaluate the scene. Some of the issues you might encounter in particular scenes are described next.

Crash and rescue scenes often include multiple risks, such as unstable vehicles, moving traffic, jagged metal and broken glass, fire or explosion hazards, fallen power lines, and, possibly, hazardous materials Figure 14-2 ▲.

Toxic substances are found at many scenes. From the lawn and garden chemicals found in almost every home to the countless chemicals used in industry and manufacturing, you should always be alert for the presence of toxic substances. You should also be wary of working in toxic environments (that is, the atmosphere itself). Smoke is the by-product of incomplete combustion and can contain many toxins, pathogens, and carcinogens. In these cases, having proper body and respiratory protection is a must before entering the scene and initiating patient care Figure 14-3 ▶.

Don't just think of crime scenes in the past tense because there is always the possibility that more violence may occur. Under ideal circumstances, when sent to a potential crime scene, the police should enter and secure the scene first. All too frequently, however, paramedics arrive first and unknowingly enter a crime scene. For example, ambulance control

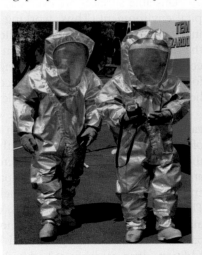

Figure 14-3 Scenes involving toxic substances may require specially trained rescuers with extra protective equipment.

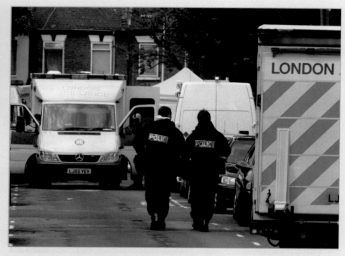

Figure 14-4 If the scene is unsafe, request police support, and wait in your vehicle at a safe distance.

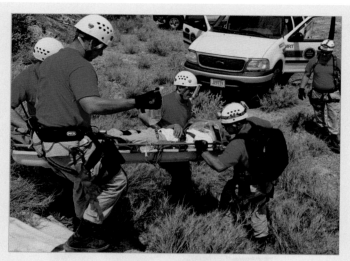

Figure 14-5 At times you may need a team to carry patients out of areas with unstable terrain.

might receive a call for a collapsed patient; on arrival, the paramedics might discover that the patient has been stabbed three times in the chest. The police should be requested immediately in such cases because it is nearly impossible for you and your partner to control the scene and care for the patient at the same time (**Figure 14-4 ▲**)—and because the assailant could return.

When faced with a currently unstable scene or a scene that begins deteriorating (for example, people become progressively louder or more unruly or make aggressive gestures or threats), consider retreating to the ambulance until the scene is secured and deemed safe. If you believe that you can pull it off safely, remove the patient from the scene with you, but making such an attempt is clearly a judgement call on your part.

Unstable surfaces are everyday occurrences in the prehospital environment. Thus, working on unstable surfaces is an inevitable part of prehospital medicine (**Figure 14-5 ▶**). Take the time to make all of your patient lifts and moves as safe and controlled as possible. Just making a mental commitment to focus on this aspect of your practice will go a long way toward helping prevent a fall and a possible injury.

Behavioural emergencies are common and challenging calls, and they always present with the possibility of some sort of violent outbreak occurring. With the continued increase in the manufacture and abuse of recreational drugs, paramedics are seeing a growing number of patients who are on the tail end of multiple sleepless days fuelled by recreational drugs. These people are often paranoid, emotionally unstable, and may be armed, making them far more a threat than an average patient with a non–drug-induced behavioural emergency. In addition, drug users are at high risk of experiencing excited or

agitated delirium, such that they may present in a blind rage and be almost uncontrollable. Never hesitate to call for police assistance when managing any patient who has the potential for becoming violent.

While protecting the team is clearly a priority, so is protecting the patient and bystanders. Establishing a perimeter around an emergency scene may prevent bystanders from entering a dangerous scene and potentially becoming patients themselves. If the police and fire service are already on scene, then this may have already been done. However, you will need to liaise closely with both services to maintain scene safety and determine resource priorities. Environmental issues can also influence scene safety and the patient care process. The longer a patient is exposed to wind and rain, the more likely it is that hypothermia will become a factor. When the environment is unfriendly, perform the initial assessment, address life threats, and get the patient into the controlled environment of the ambulance as quickly as possible.

Mechanism of Injury/Nature of Illness

Most calls to 999 will be for a medical emergency or some form of trauma. A generic-sounding call such as a "sick person" in no way guarantees that a sick, hypoglycaemic patient didn't also fall and injure himself as a result of a low blood glucose level. Or, a trauma patient may have crashed her car when she passed out because of an abnormal heart rhythm. Prudent paramedics keep their minds open to multiple possibilities when trying to figure out just what's going on with patients. The mechanism of injury (MOI) is the way in which traumatic injuries occur—the forces that act on the body to cause damage. Assessing and evaluating the MOI can help you predict the likelihood of certain injuries having occurred and estimate their severity. (The patterns of injuries sustained in traumatic events are discussed in detail in Chapter 17.)

On purely medical calls, you should quickly determine from the patient (or family, friends, or bystanders) why ambulance services were requested. The nature of illness (NOI) is the general type of illness a patient is experiencing.

At this point, if there is more than one patient or the patient is obese, you can call for additional resources. If multiple patients are present and have similar symptoms or complaints, you might consider carbon monoxide poisoning (or contact with some other noxious agent), a possible terrorist attack, or food poisoning as prime candidates. Irrespective of the cause of the problem, the presence of multiple patients means that they must be triaged to determine which additional resources you need and how you will allocate the resources.

Likewise, when you have multiple patients at a trauma scene, you must triage all patients. Once you have identified the total number of patients and estimated the severity of their injuries, you should request any additional resources—for example, fire and rescue, police, or specialised teams—needed to support the efforts of those already on the scene.

The process of scene assessment is completed in a very short time. Once you have digested the ambulance control information, evaluated the overall scene and safety, determined the MOI or NOI, and summoned additional help, you are ready to manage patient care. By contrast, if you can manage the situation without further assistance, you assess the need for spinal immobilisation and continue with patient care. Based on the scene assessment and MOI, paramedics must ensure that spinal immobilisation takes place on reaching the patient. Indications for spinal immobilisation will be covered further in Chapter 22.

At the Scene

Assessing the safety of a scene before entering may be the single most important way in which paramedics can attend to their own well-being. Subtle signs of danger not immediately recognised and neutralised—or avoided—at this point can become more threatening without being noticed once you shift your attention to patient assessment and care. Initial scene assessment often allows you to distinguish between a manageably safe scene and one that could spin dangerously out of control without further warning.

The Initial Assessment

The initial assessment is the most time-intensive portion of the assessment process because it focuses on the identification and management of life-threatening problems. In the first 60 to 90 seconds, as you look at, talk with, and touch your patient, you should be able to identify threats to the ABCs. More often than not, you will form the general impression of your patient based almost solely on the initial presentation and chief complaint.

Each of us, without even trying or being conscious of doing so, makes dozens of observations about the appearance

You are the Paramedic Part 2

As you secure the patient's airway, your colleague applies a pulse oximeter and obtains vital signs. High-flow supplemental oxygen is applied, venous access is established, and the patient is prepared for transport.

Vital Signs	Recording Time: 5 Minutes
Level of consciousness	P (Responsive to painful stimuli) with a Glasgow Coma Scale score of 9
Skin	Pink, warm, and moist
Pulse	70 beats/min, regular
Blood pressure	104/68 mm Hg
Respirations	24 breaths/min
S_PO_2	100% while breathing room air

3. Because this patient is a minor, what are some important considerations for treatment and transport?

4. Of all your differential diagnoses, which ones should be considered a diagnosis of exclusion?

Initial Assessment

Patient Assessment

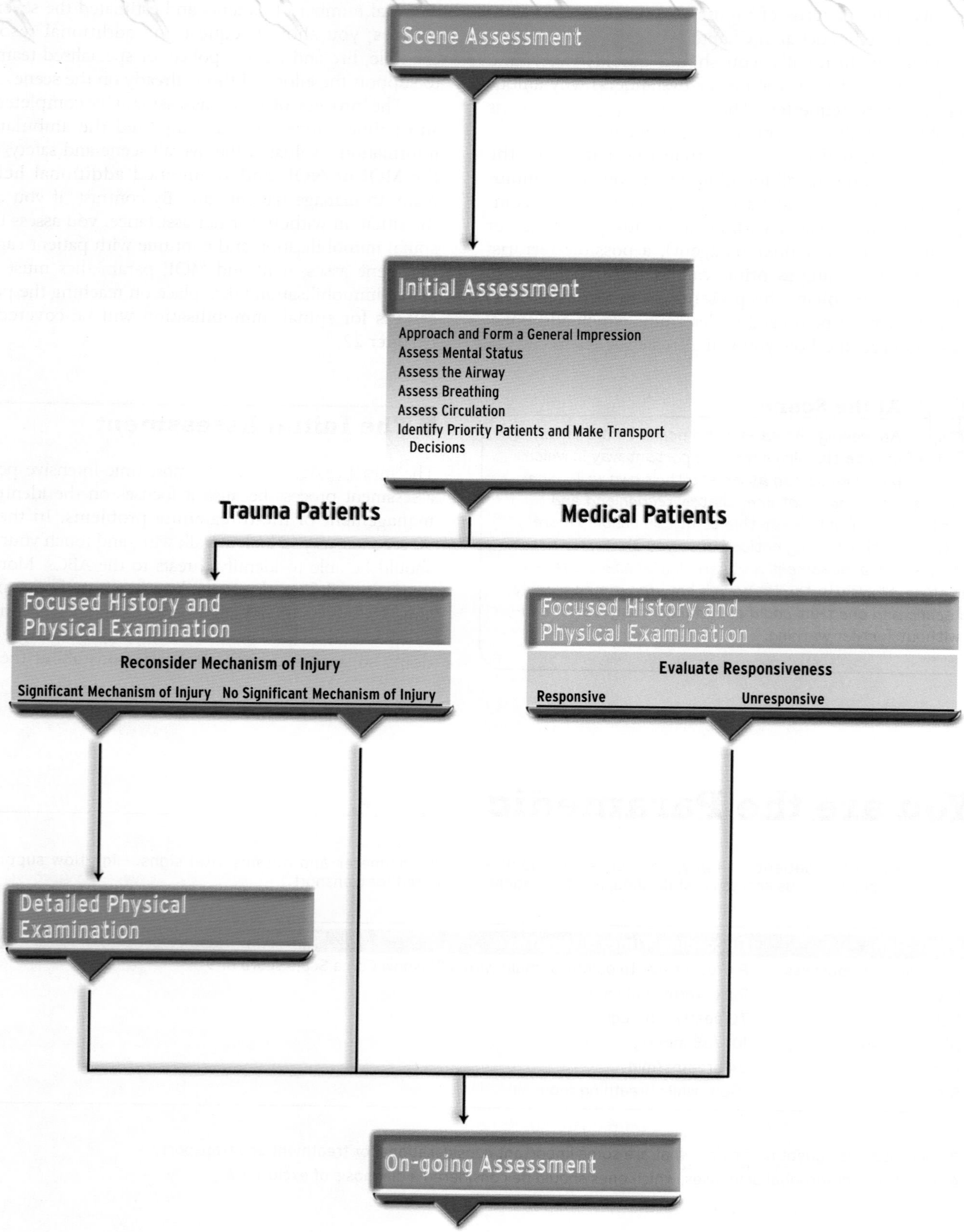

Scene Assessment

Initial Assessment

Approach and Form a General Impression
Assess Mental Status
Assess the Airway
Assess Breathing
Assess Circulation
Identify Priority Patients and Make Transport
   Decisions

Trauma Patients   **Medical Patients**

Focused History and Physical Examination

Reconsider Mechanism of Injury

Significant Mechanism of Injury   No Significant Mechanism of Injury

Focused History and Physical Examination

Evaluate Responsiveness

Responsive   Unresponsive

Detailed Physical Examination

On-going Assessment

of another person during the first few seconds of an encounter—for example, whether the other person is sitting or standing, overweight or thin, smiling or frowning, dressed neatly or sloppily. In assessing a patient, we must make similar observations, but in a much more conscious, objective, and systematic manner, looking for specific clues to give us an immediate sense of the seriousness of the situation. A complaint of "I just can't catch my breath" that comes to you in one- or two-word bursts clearly points to a very sick patient. A patient complaining of "chest pain" after being stabbed in the chest is an even more obvious example of a priority.

You are trying to answer two questions: Is my patient sick? If so, how sick is he or she? In the case of trauma, the questions take a slightly different form: Is my patient hurt? If so, how badly hurt is the patient?

Whether it is medical or trauma, the first question is a qualification and the second is a quantification. "Is my patient sick"? has a yes or no answer, whereas "How sick is my patient"? attempts to rate the event's severity. With time and experience, you should be able to answer both questions in that 60- to 90-second window, forming your general impression.

Once these questions are answered, you can move forward with determining your priorities of care, developing a care plan, and putting the care plan into action. If the primary problem seems to be a traumatic injury, identify and evaluate the MOI. If the primary problem seems to be medical, identify the NOI. As you mentally move through this process, keep in mind that an injured patient might have a medical component to his or her problem, just as a patient with a medical emergency might have a trauma component to his or her problem.

You will also need to identify the age and sex of your patient because each can change how your patient presents. For example, an older woman having a heart attack may have an atypical presentation (no chest pain) compared with the more traditional presentation seen with an older man with the same condition. Likewise, a teenage girl will often be more emotionally mature than a boy of the same age, changing how each answers your questions and reacts to the emergency itself.

The information gleaned from the initial assessment is crucial to the overall outcome for your patient. Treat life threats as you find them, but also decide what additional care is needed, what needs to be done on scene versus en route, when to initiate transport, and which hospital is most appropriate given your patient's needs.

Assess the Patient's Mental Status and Neurological Function

The patient's mental status is often one of the prime indicators of how sick the patient really is. Changes in the state of consciousness may provide the first clue to an alteration in the patient's condition, so establish a baseline as soon as you encounter the patient. At the same time as you are assessing mental status, if trauma is involved, you need to decide whether you will implement spinal immobilisation procedures.

The quickest and simplest way to assess the patient's mental status or level of consciousness (LOC) is to use the AVPU process:

A *Alert* to person, place, and day
V Responsive to *Verbal* stimuli
P Responsive to *Pain*
U *Unresponsive*

You can further assess mental status by considering whether the patient is alert and orientated (A + O) in four areas: person, place, day, and the event itself. Assessing whether the patient can recall his or her name and the day tests long-term memory, whereas assessing whether the patient knows where he or she is and what happened tests short-term memory.

The most reliable and consistent method of assessing mental status and neurological function is the Glasgow Coma Scale (GCS), which assigns a point value (score) for eye opening, verbal response, and motor response; these values are totalled for a total score **Table 14-1 ▶**. While it may take slightly longer to perform than the AVPU, the GCS provides much greater insight into the patient's overall neurological function.

Let's work through a scenario. You encounter an older man who tracks you with his eyes as you enter his room. As you speak with the man, you note that his verbal response is disorientated, even though he follows your commands. His GCS values would be 4, 4, and 6, for a total score of 14. By comparison, if the patient opened his eyes only to pain, moaned as the only verbal response, and withdrew to pain, he would be assigned GCS values of 2, 2, and 4, for a total score of 8. Clearly, a child or infant will respond differently from an adult. A modified assessment should be used for these patients. This is addressed in Chapter 41.

Documentation and Communication

Be aware of how your body language and physical presence might affect a frightened patient. Standing over and looking down on a patient can be intimidating. In such a case, try to get even with the patient's eye level so that you present a more "equal" impression of communication.

At the Scene

Regardless of the method you use to evaluate mental status, avoid using phrases such as "semiconscious", "lethargic", and "sluggish". These terms are too vague to be useful from a clinical perspective.

Table 14-1 | Glasgow Coma Scale

Eye Opening		Best Verbal Response		Best Motor Response	
Spontaneous	4	Orientated and converses	5	Obeys commands	6
To voice	3	Confused conversation	4	Localises pain	5
To pain	2	Speaking but nonsensical	3	Withdraws to pain	4
No response	1	Moans or makes unintelligible sounds	2	Decorticate flexion	3
		No response	1	Decerebrate extension	2
				No response	1

Scores:
14–15: Mild dysfunction
9–13: Moderate dysfunction
3–8: Severe dysfunction (The lowest possible score is 3.)

Assess the Patient's Airway Status

Assessment of the patient's airway status focuses on two questions: Is the airway open and patent? Is it likely to remain so? For air to be drawn into the lungs, the airway has to be properly positioned and not obstructed (open from an anatomical perspective). If you hear sonorous respirations (snoring), think "position problem"—the sounds you are hearing are probably from the tongue partially obstructing the airway. If you hear gurgling or bubbling sounds, think "suction"—there are likely to be fluids such as blood, mucus, or vomit in the mouth or posterior pharynx.

When approaching airway management, think from the simple to the complex. The easiest problem to solve is one of position. Its resolution requires no equipment and can be done quickly. The possibility of a spine injury (or lack thereof) drives the decision of which technique to use to open the airway (head tilt–chin lift or jaw-thrust manoeuvre). In the case of obstruction, such as by food, procedures to clear the obstruction that require no equipment can be done quickly.

Assessment of a patient's airway is completed in the same way regardless of the patient's age. In responsive patients of any age, talking or crying will give clues about the adequacy of the airway. For all unconscious patients, you must establish responsiveness and look, listen, and feel for breathing. If breathing is ineffective or absent, you must open the airway with a head tilt–chin lift (in nontrauma patients) or jaw thrust (in trauma patients).

When performing the head tilt–chin lift manoeuvre, remember the anatomical differences in the various age groups and make sure that you do not create an airway obstruction with an improper position of the head. Infants and young children do not have the developed tracheal rings that provide support, which means the trachea is easily collapsed or occluded when the head position changes.

Suctioning takes longer (because of the need to set up and use the equipment) and is a more complicated procedure than positioning. If you suction the patient for too long, you create a new problem: hypoxia.

If a mechanical means is required to keep the airway open and patent, you must choose an airway adjunct. If you opt to place an oropharyngeal or nasopharyngeal airway, you must retrieve the equipment, choose the right size for the specific patient, and then place the airway.

If you determine that the patient cannot maintain his or her airway and you cannot maintain it by any other means, you need to use a more invasive technique, such as endotracheal intubation. This invasive procedure involves several pieces of equipment: a laryngoscope handle, a laryngoscope blade, a properly sized endotracheal tube, a syringe, a stylet, an oropharyngeal aiway, a bag-valve-mask device, and a method to secure the tube once it is placed. Obviously, gathering the equipment, preparing the patient, and performing the intubation procedure is more time-intensive than previously mentioned interventions.

Other advanced airway management options include use of a multilumen airway, laryngeal mask airway, or surgical airway (discussed in Chapter 11).

Assess the Patient's Breathing

The assessment of breathing focuses on two questions: First, is the patient breathing? If not, then you have to breathe for the patient. Second, if the patient is breathing, is breathing adequate?

Recall from Chapter 11 that the respiratory rate multiplied by the tidal volume inspired with each breath equals the minute volume. For example, a patient breathing slowly and deeply at 10 breaths/min and 500 ml/breath has a minute volume of 5,000 ml. By comparison, a patient breathing faster and shallower at a rate of 24 breaths/min and 200 ml/breath would have a minute volume of 4,800 ml. On a per-minute basis, the volumes of the two patients are virtually identical, even though the second patient is breathing more than twice as fast as the first patient. Always keep in mind that the amount of air actually moved in and out of the lungs each minute is the best measure of breathing adequacy. Besides the assessment of tidal volume, note the patient's breathing rate, effort of breathing (accessory muscle use), breath sounds, skin colour, and LOC or mental status as part of the breathing assessment.

The techniques used to assess a patient's breathing status are not new: Look, listen, and feel. Look for chest rise and fall, noting symmetry of the chest wall and depth of respirations. Listen for breath sounds by using your sense of hearing or by auscultation with a stethoscope. Note adventitious lung sounds, and treat the patient accordingly. Finally, feel for air movement by placing your cheek or the palm of your hand near the patient's mouth.

Assess the Patient's Circulation

Assessing the pulse gives a rapid check of the patient's cardiovascular status and provides information about the rate, strength, and regularity of the heartbeat. In adults and children, the pulse is best palpated over the radial (responsive) and carotid or femoral (unresponsive) artery by using the tips of your index and middle fingers. In responsive or unresponsive infants, palpate the pulse over the brachial artery. First measure the pulse rate by counting the number of beats during 15 seconds; then multiply by 4. If the pulse is irregular or slow, it is best to count for a full minute.

As you count the pulse rate, note the force of the pulse. A normal pulse feels "full", as if a strong wave has passed beneath your fingertips. When there is severe vasoconstriction or in the case of hypotension with a fast pulse, the pulse may feel weak or "thready". By comparison, a patient who is hypertensive will produce a pulse that is more forceful than usual—a "bounding" pulse.

Finally, note the rhythm of the pulse. A normal rhythm is regular, like the ticking of a clock. If some beats come early or late or are skipped, the pulse is irregular. Although many cardiac arrhythmias are not life threatening, in the case of heart blocks, an irregular pulse can indicate a serious condition. As such, consider all patients with an irregular pulse at risk until proven otherwise.

Report your findings by describing the rate, force, and rhythm of the pulse. For example, state that "The patient's pulse was 72, full, and regular", or "The pulse was 138, thready, and regular".

As part of this phase of the initial assessment, assess the patient's skin for colour, temperature, and moisture. Collectively, these criteria provide insight into the patient's overall perfusion. Use the back of your hand to assess the warmth and moisture of the patient's skin because it tends be more sensitive than your palm **Figure 14-6 ▶** .

The colour of the skin **Table 14-2 ▶** , especially in light-skinned patients, reflects the status of the circulation immediately underlying the skin, including the oxygen saturation of the blood. In people with darker skin, changes may not be readily evident in the skin but may be assessed by examining the mucous membranes (such as the lips or conjunctivae). When the blood vessels supplying the skin are fully dilated, the skin becomes warm and pink. When the blood vessels supplying the skin constrict or the cardiac output drops, the skin

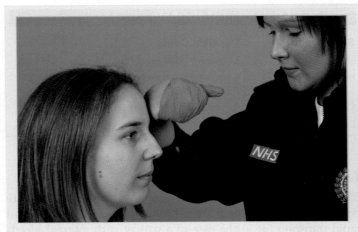

Figure 14-6 Assessing the skin condition. Use the back of the hand to assess the temperature and moisture of the skin.

Table 14-2	Inspection of the Skin
Skin Colour	**Possible Cause**
Red	Fever Hypertension Allergic reactions Carbon monoxide poisoning
White (pallor)	Excessive blood loss Fright
Blue (cyanosis)	Hypoxaemia
Mottled	Cardiovascular embarrassment (as in shock)

becomes pale or mottled and cool. If the patient does not get enough oxygen, as in the case of an opiate overdose where the patient is breathing four times per minute, the blood will desaturate as the oxygen level drops; the skin will turn a dusky grey or blue (cyanosis). Pallor occurs if arterial blood flow ceases to part of the body, as in the case of a blood clot or massive bleeding. Hypothermia will also result in pallor as the body shunts blood to the core and away from the extremities.

Skin temperature rises as peripheral blood vessels dilate; it falls as blood vessels constrict. Fever and high environmental temperatures usually stimulate vasodilation, whereas shock elicits vasoconstriction. Normal skin is moderately warm and dry. The dryness or moisture of the skin is largely determined by the sympathetic nervous system. Stimulation of the sympathetic nervous system, as in shock or any other severe stress, causes sweating. Depression of the sympathetic nervous system, as in an injury to the thoracic or lumbar spine, can cause the skin in the affected area to become abnormally dry and cool **Table 14-3 ▶** .

Initial Assessment

Table 14-3	Palpation of the Skin
Skin Condition	**Possible Cause**
Hot, dry	Excessive body heat (heat stroke)
Hot, wet	Reaction to increased internal or external temperature
Cool, dry	Exposure to cold
Cool, wet	Shock

Identify Priority Patients

Early in the assessment process, you need to identify priority patients who will benefit from limited time at the scene and rapid transport, as in the case of a patient with internal bleeding from trauma. Such a patient needs to see a surgeon who will sew up the holes and replace the lost blood, neither of which can be accomplished in the prehospital setting.

When you have a priority patient, you need to expedite transport, doing only what is absolutely necessary at the scene and handling everything else en route, including the appropriate focused history and physical examination. Determining a priority patient requires that you think through a variety of possibilities:

- **Poor general impression.** The patient is in obvious distress and does not "look well".
- **Unresponsive patients.** Unresponsiveness is never a good sign and typically points to a patient in serious or critical condition.
- **Responsive but does not or cannot follow commands.** Altered mental state is another bad sign; the question you need to answer is "How bad"?

- **Difficulty breathing.** Breathing problems are one of the most common chief complaints in prehospital care. Patients who have difficulty breathing are in trouble; those who are "working to breathe" are in serious trouble.
- **Hypoperfusion or shock.** Without question, hypoperfusion or shock is an obvious sign of a high-risk patient. Weak or absent peripheral pulse, sustained tachycardia, and pale, cool, wet skin all point to serious consequences.
- **Complicated childbirth.** Anything that presents from the birth canal other than the newborn's head represents a situation not likely to be managed in the prehospital setting.
- **Chest pain with a systolic blood pressure less than 90 mm Hg.** Especially in the context of tachycardia, this sign indicates cardiac compromise and a high-risk patient in an unstable condition.
- **Uncontrolled bleeding.** Whether internal or external, such bleeding is a serious life threat.
- **Severe pain anywhere.** Any person with severe pain, especially enough to wake the person up in the middle of the night, should be considered a priority patient.
- **Multiple injuries.** While a patient may have multiple minor injuries that by themselves aren't serious, several small problems can add up to one big problem.

Don't forget to pre-alert the hospital if you have identified a priority patient. It is not much good to rapidly transport a patient only to have to wait while a team is assembled at hospital. Guidance for when to pre-alert a hospital about your arrival varies between services (and hospitals), so follow your local pre-alert policy.

You are the Paramedic Part 3

The patient's mother is contacted at work. She reports that, other than mild scoliosis identified 2 years previously, Mike's past medical history is unremarkable. When asked, she denies Mike having any recent history of significant trauma and drug use beyond "sneaking a few beers with friends".

Re-assessment	Recording Time: 15 Minutes
Level of consciousness	P (Responsive to painful stimuli) with a Glasgow Coma Scale score of 9
Skin	Pink, warm, and moist
Pulse	72 beats/min, regular
Blood pressure	106 mm Hg by palpation
Respirations	24 breaths/min with adequate depth
SpO_2	100% on room air
Temperature	37.2°C
Pupils	3 mm/PEARRL
Blood glucose	5.8 mmol/l

5. Does this patient need high-flow supplemental oxygen? Why or why not?

6. Should this patient be intubated? Why or why not?

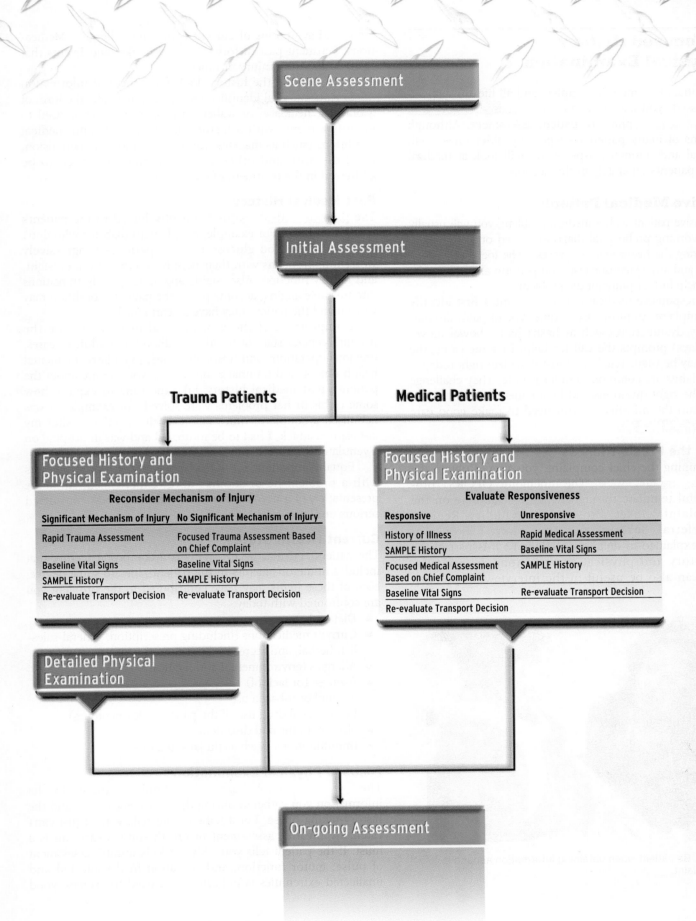

The Focused History and Physical Examination

Once the initial assessment is complete and all life threats have been addressed, you can move into the focused history and physical examination phase of patient assessment. Although the problems of many patients—especially older ones—will have medical and traumatic aspects, we will look at medical and trauma patients separately in this section.

Responsive Medical Patients

For a responsive patient with a medical problem, you will usually form your working prehospital diagnosis based on information gathered during the history-taking process. The focused physical examination and any diagnostic tests you perform after taking the history will help further pinpoint the problem.

With a responsive medical patient, you must first identify the chief complaint. In most cases, some type of pain, discomfort, or body dysfunction (such as hasn't had a bowel movement in 4 days) prompts the call for help. In some cases, the complaint may be vague (such as "I just don't feel right today"). Vague complaints are common in older people. They challenge you to ask the right questions and be a patient listener as you work to obtain the information you need to make good care decisions Figure 14-7 ▾ .

History of the Present Illness

After determining the chief complaint, you should obtain the history of the present illness. The mnemonic OPQRST provides a helpful template through which to elaborate on the chief complaint: Onset, Provocation, Quality, Region/radiation/referral, Severity, and Timeframe. (The use of OPQRST is explained in detail in Chapter 12.) As part of the focused history and physical examination, the SAMPLE mnemonic can also be useful in the interviewing process:

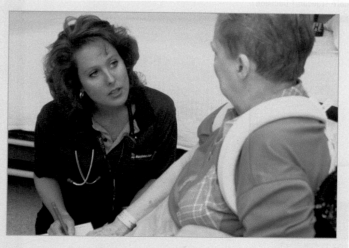

Figure 14-7 Be patient when obtaining information about a vague complaint.

Signs and symptoms of current complaint; Allergies; Medications; Medications; Pertinent past history; Last oral intake; and Events that led to the current injury or illness.

While taking the history, look for a medical information tag or card. Medical identification devices may take the form of a bracelet, necklace, or wallet card. Such a device is used to identify patients with a history of allergies, certain medical conditions (such as diabetes, cardiac conditions, hypertension, renal disease), and other conditions that may need to be addressed in the treatment of the patient.

Past Medical History

The past medical history is frequently linked to the patient's current problem. For example, people with diabetes who don't manage their blood glucose levels experience progressively worsening problems with their peripheral circulation, eyesight, and kidney function. Also, stable angina frequently transitions into unstable angina; at some point, the patient's condition may worsen and the patient may have a heart attack.

Components of the past medical history include the patient's general state of health, childhood and adult diseases, previous operations and hospitalisations, psychiatric or mental health illness, and traumatic injuries. As you inquire about the patient's past medical history, take the time to explore how some of his or her problems were solved (for example, "I was nebulised a couple of times before I felt better" or "After my last asthma attack, I had to be intubated and was in hospital on a ventilator for a week").

Equally important is the case in which the patient presents with a problem he or she has never experienced. An acute presentation of a new problem or condition is best considered serious until proven otherwise.

Current Health Status

The patient's current health status is a composite picture that includes numerous factors in the patient's life. To some degree, each of these items may have contributed to the problem you are confronted with today:

- Dietary habits
- Current medications (including prescription, general-sales-list, herbal, and recreational drugs)
- Allergies (environmental and medication)
- Exercise (or lack of)
- Alcohol or tobacco use
- Recreational drug use (if the patient is forthcoming)
- Sleep patterns and disorders
- Immunisations (such as flu jabs, tetanus)

Focused Physical Examination

The focused physical examination should be driven by the information you gathered during the initial assessment and the history-taking phase. For a patient who tells you, "I just can't catch my breath", assessment of breath sounds early on is a must. If the patient tells you, "My leg feels numb", assessment of pulse, motor function, and sensation in the affected and unaffected extremities is indicated. You need to exercise good judgement to make the best use of your time. Don't waste time palpating a patient's abdomen or auscultating heart sounds if the person complains of a stiff neck.

The most common complaints from a responsive medical patient will involve the head, heart, lungs, or abdomen, individually or in combination.

For patients with a "head" problem (confusion, headache, altered mental state), you should assess and palpate the head looking for signs of trauma. Check for facial asymmetry, such as facial droop or other signs of a suspected stroke. Dilated or constricted pupils may point to recreational drug use, whereas red conjunctiva may suggest drug or alcohol use. Elevated blood pressure often accompanies a headache, possibly secondary to hypertension.

For a suspected heart problem, assess the pulse for regularity and examine the skin for signs of hypoperfusion (pallor, cool, wet) or oxygen desaturation (cyanosis). Listen to breath sounds—many cardiac problems are associated with respiratory problems (such as crackles secondary to pulmonary oedema). Obtain baseline vital signs. Serious hypotension with sustained or progressive tachycardia is common in cardiogenic shock; stay alert for this condition because its mortality rate is more than 80%. Check for jugular venous distension because it can indicate heart failure or pneumothorax. Examine the extremities for signs of peripheral oedema that may result from right-sided heart failure.

For patients with respiratory complaints, assess breath sounds early and often. Possible findings or problems include the following:

- Lung fields with absent breath sounds: pneumothorax
- Silent breath sounds: status asthmaticus
- Lung fields with areas of consolidation: pneumonia
- Wheezing (localised or diffuse): asthma or bronchoconstriction
- Crackles (wet lung sounds): pulmonary oedema, heart failure, toxic inhalation, submersion

For any patient with a respiratory complaint, be alert for the appearance of accessory muscle use or recession, both of which are signs of increased work of breathing. Also, keep an eye out for the signs of ventilatory fatigue, such as decreased mental state or a tired, worn-out appearance that often precedes ventilatory failure and respiratory or cardiac arrest. Watch for the appearance of jugular venous distension with respiratory patients because it may point to pneumothorax or heart failure.

One of the most challenging complaints in the prehospital setting is that of abdominal pain because it can result from multiple causes and often presents with little or no external signs. Three basic mechanisms produce abdominal pain:

- *Visceral pain* results when hollow organs are obstructed, thereby stretching the smooth muscle wall, which in turn produces cramping and more diffuse, widespread pain.
- *Inflammation* or irritation of the somatic pain fibres located in the skin, the abdominal wall, and the musculature may produce sharp, localised pain, as in the case of pelvic inflammatory disease or appendicitis. If gastric contents,

blood, or urine enters the peritoneum, it will also produce somatic pain, albeit usually much less localised and more diffuse.

- *Referred pain* has its origin in a particular organ but is described by the patient as pain in a different location. Examples include scapular pain from cholecystitis, back pain from pancreatitis, and inner thigh pain from renal colic.

Inspection and palpation of the abdomen can provide valuable information, although it is often general. Tightness or guarding can result from internal bleeding, an inflamed organ, and many other causes. With upper left quadrant pain, possible sources include a ruptured spleen from a sickle cell crisis and glandular fever. Patients with lower left abdominal pain, especially if they have a history of constipation, nausea, vomiting, and fever, should be suspected of having diverticulitis. With lower right abdominal pain, appendicitis is a likely culprit. Generalised abdominal pain in women of childbearing age can be the result of an ectopic pregnancy, a ruptured ovarian cyst, or some other obstetric or gynaecological problem.

During the focused physical examination, along with history taking, obtain a full set of vital signs, including blood pressure, pulse and respiratory rates, and the patient's temperature. Use other diagnostic tools as indicated.

Baseline vital signs are an integral part of any focused history and physical examination. Clues provided will help you determine the seriousness of the patient's condition and the function of internal organs. Remember that shock, whether medical or trauma-related, is seen in different stages. Changes in a patient's blood pressure may be the last piece of evidence providers see when shock changes from one level to the next. Keep in mind that blood pressure must be sufficient to maintain adequate end-organ perfusion.

Test for postural hypotension by measuring the blood pressure (and heart rate, if possible) of your patient in a lying or sitting position and then on standing. A drop in blood pressure of more than 20 mm Hg systolic or 10 mm Hg diastolic is considered significant.

Normally, baroreceptors in the body sense changes in the blood pressure and volume and stipulate a catecholamine and rennin-aldosterone response. This, in turn, causes peripheral vasoconstriction, increased heart rate, and fluid retention, which puts more blood into core circulation and increases volume.

In patients with significant postural hypotension, this physiological process does not work as it should. There are three main reasons why this occurs:

- Inadequate blood volume to maintain sufficient blood flow to the brain on standing. This has a wide variety of causes including vomiting, diarrhoea, haemorrhage, and overuse of diuretics.
- Medication such as beta blockers interfering with the body's response to the release of catecholamines, such as adrenaline and noradrenaline.
- Diseases of the nerve fibres (neuropathy) responsible for making blood vessels constrict.

Focused History and Physical Examination

At the Scene

Many technological devices are available to paramedics to aid in patient assessment. Just remember that you are assessing a patient—not a machine. Take the time to explain what your tools are and why you are using them. This simple action may help lessen patient anxiety.

Don't forget to document the blood pressure and the rate and regularity of the pulse. If the patient is monitored, then include the rhythm strip and note any other symptoms. If fluid replacement is given, repeat the test if possible.

An Unresponsive Medical Patient

With an unresponsive medical patient, you start at a disadvantage in your assessment because your most reliable source of information—the patient—can't answer your questions. Owing to this serious limitation, assessment of an unresponsive medical patient looks much like a trauma assessment. You must rely on a thorough head-to-toe physical examination plus the normal diagnostic tools (pulse oximetry, cardiac monitor, and glucometer) to acquire the information needed to care for your patient. If family or friends are present, they may be able to provide information about the chief complaint, history of the present illness, past medical history, and possibly current health status. Nevertheless, the information they offer is almost never as good as that provided directly by the patient.

After completing the initial assessment, and assuming you have ruled out trauma, position unresponsive medical patients in the recovery position to facilitate drainage of vomit, blood, or other fluids and to help prevent aspiration. If trauma is a factor, position the patient in neutral alignment, place a properly sized and fitted rigid cervical collar, and implement spinal immobilisation procedures as per local guidelines.

Perform a thorough assessment of the head, neck, chest, abdomen, pelvis, posterior body, and extremities, looking for signs of illness such as rash or urticaria, fever, unusual or excessive bruising, pulmonary or peripheral oedema, and irregular pulse. Follow up your examination with at least two sets of vital signs—one taken now and another taken a few minutes after you've started your initial interventions (such as supplemental oxygen and IV therapy). The first set establishes a baseline (baseline vital signs); the second and additional sets (serial vital signs) provide comparative data to help you evaluate whether the patient's condition is improving, stable, or worsening. If time allows, additional sets of vital signs add further data, allowing you to map trends (such as a progressively increasing pulse rate). Make sure the vital signs include a blood pressure, pulse and respiratory rates, and the patient's temperature. A recheck of breath sounds is always a prudent choice as well.

Unconscious, unresponsive medical patients should always be considered in an unstable condition and at high risk, so rapid transport to the appropriate hospital is indicated. Throughout transport, perform on-going assessment, which includes rechecking the ABCs and re-assessing anything associated with the patient's chief complaint.

Trauma Patients
Focused History and Physical Examination

Trauma patients may be classified into two major groups: patients with an isolated injury and patients with multi-system trauma. The biggest difference from an assessment perspective is that an isolated injury allows you to immediately focus on the main problem. In contrast, with multi-system trauma, you must first find all (or as many as you can reasonably find) of the various problems (for example, a haematoma on the forehead, a fractured arm, and neck and lower back pain). Then you need to prioritise the injuries by severity and the order in which you plan to address them. During the assessment, you must continually think about how each injury or condition relates to the others. For example, the mortality rate for a patient with a serious traumatic brain injury who has just a single episode of hypotension doubles. In such a case, not recognising and addressing the hypotension and the lack of adequate perfusion pressure has a huge impact—in some cases, a fatal impact.

Another important consideration is the "high visibility factor" of many injuries, which sometimes creates a visual distraction. A compound fracture of the lower leg and ankle, with the foot twisted sideways and jammed under the brake pedal in a car, is not a pretty sight—but it is not a life-threatening injury. Because of the visual distraction, you might focus on the grossly deformed ankle and miss the early signs and symptoms of shock caused by the internal injuries and bleeding that you can't see.

Notes from Nancy

The salvage of lives takes precedence over the salvage of limbs.

As you move into the focused history and physical examination of a trauma patient, quickly revisit all of the information from your initial assessment, including reconsidering the mechanism of injury. Collectively, these data may help you identify patients who need to be priority transports to hospital.

A number of mechanisms have the potential to produce life-threatening injuries **Figure 14-8 ▶** :

- Ejection from *any* vehicle (car, motorcycle, or all-terrain vehicle)
- Death of another patient in the same passenger compartment
- Falls from more than 6 m (or three times the patient's height)
- Vehicle rollover (unrestrained occupant)

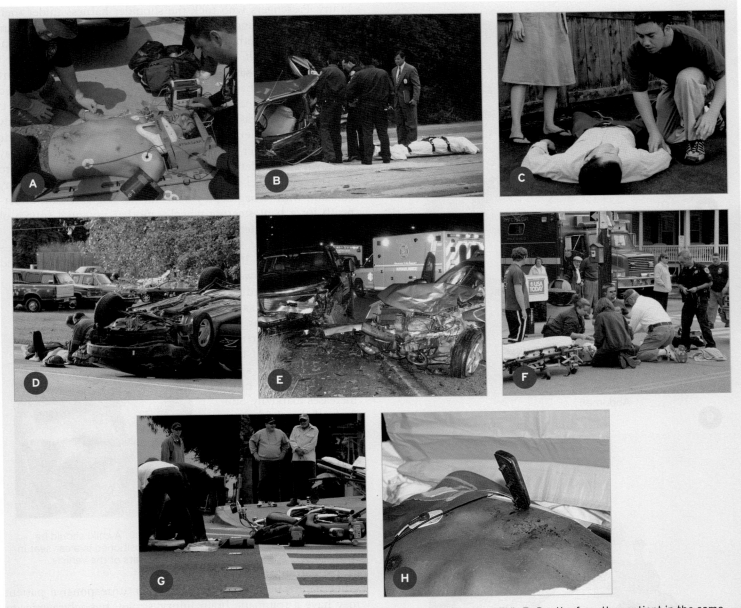

Figure 14-8 Significant mechanisms of injury. **A.** Ejection from *any* vehicle (car, motorcycle, ATV). **B.** Death of another patient in the same passenger compartment. **C.** Falls from more than 6 m. **D.** Vehicle rollover. **E.** High-speed road traffic collision. **F.** Vehicle-pedestrian collision. **G.** Motorcycle crashes. **H.** Penetrating wounds to the head, chest, or abdomen.

- High-speed road traffic collision
- Vehicle-pedestrian collision
- Motorcycle crash
- Penetrating wounds to the head, chest, or abdomen

If the patient is an infant or a child, mechanisms of injury that would indicate a high-priority patient include falls from more than 3 m (or twice the child's height), a bicycle collision, or being struck by a vehicle **Figure 14-9 ▶**.

In many cases, multiple mechanisms of injury have come into play—for example, a T-bone collision that leaves the patient with a crushed upper arm and pelvic girdle and also penetrating trauma from the piece of door trim impaled in his chest. A patient with any of the previously mentioned mechanisms should immediately raise your index of suspicion. Two or more mechanisms of injury markedly increase the chance of a patient sustaining a serious or fatal injury.

Several other mechanisms of injury are also worth considering. Seatbelts, even when properly positioned, can cause injuries as the car and its occupants decelerate in a crash. Check the clavicles where the shoulder strap crosses. The clavicles are

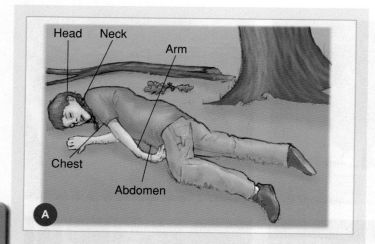

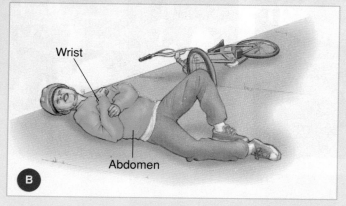

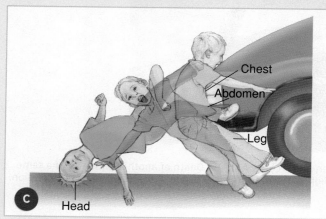

Figure 14-9 Significant mechanisms of injury for an infant or child. **A.** Falls from more than 3 m. **B.** Bicycle collision. **C.** Pedestrian–vehicle collision.

small bones, and the subclavian vein and arteries run directly underneath them. In shorter patients, the shoulder strap can ride up across the neck, increasing the risk of soft-tissue and cervical spine injury. Examine the area where the lap belt crosses the pelvic girdle. If the belt is not across the iliac crest but has ridden up over the lower abdomen, the patient has an increased risk of organ damage and thoracic or lumbar spine

injury. Passengers who tuck the shoulder harness under their arms for comfort and are then involved in rollover collisions are at high risk of death from liver injuries caused by the improperly positioned belt.

Airbags have saved countless lives, but many people don't realise that an airbag is a secondary restraint system, designed to work with seatbelts to reduce injuries. When the seatbelt is not used and a crash occurs, the airbag deploys, momentarily catching the patient. As the airbag deflates, it releases the driver or passenger, who continues moving forward and may go down-and-under (into the dashboard) or up-and-over (into the steering wheel and/or windscreen). When attending any collision with airbag deployment, lift the bag and look underneath for a bent steering wheel—another potential source of life-threatening internal injuries.

Child safety seats have also saved countless lives Figure 14-10 ▶ . If they are improperly installed or positioned in the vehicle, however, they can be rendered useless as a safety device. If the car seat comes loose during a crash, the risk of face, head, neck, and spine trauma to the child increases markedly. Similarly, if the child is too large or too small for the seat, the seat will not provide the intended level of protection.

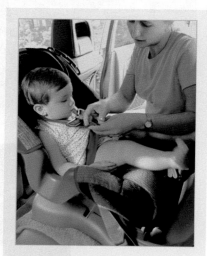

Figure 14-10 A child should be properly positioned in a car seat in the rear seats of the vehicle.

Any trauma patient who is unresponsive or has altered mental state should be considered a high-risk, priority patient and requires immediate transport. An unconscious, unresponsive patient may have a traumatic brain injury, stroke, hypoglycaemia, or alcohol or drug intoxication. All are bad—even potentially lethal—events, with some (such as traumatic brain injury) being devastating injuries.

Rapid Trauma Assessment

The rapid trauma assessment is a specialised tool that is typically sandwiched between the initial assessment and the focused physical examination of a trauma patient. This assessment is usually performed on patients with any significant mechanism of injury. As with any aspect of patient assessment involving inspection, always stay alert for any medical alert bracelets or devices and take note of any scars indicating that the patient has had open heart surgery or had a pacemaker or automated internal cardioverter-defibrillator implanted in the chest wall.

The rapid trauma assessment is usually performed after the initial assessment and all life threats to airway, breathing, and circulation have been identified and addressed. If the patient is responsive, identify the chief complaint(s) and symptoms, and then use this information to guide and direct your assessment. Give the patient who has been involved in any kind of significant traumatic event a quick once-over from head-to-toe by performing a rapid trauma assessment. Keep in mind that the most visible injury you may be looking at (the scalp laceration) or the most painful injury the patient complains about (the fractured and dislocated ankle) may not be nearly as serious as the most lethal injury the patient has (the ruptured spleen). A splenic injury, for example, is less visible and less painful than the other two injuries.

Before you begin the rapid trauma assessment, make sure that the patient's cervical spine is manually immobilised in the neutral position. Quickly re-assess the patient's current mental status, comparing it with the baseline you established when you first encountered the patient. Last, revisit your transport decision. If you decide the patient needs immediate transport, you should perform the rapid trauma assessment while the patient is being immobilised and prepared for transport, so that the moment you get the patient loaded, you can head to the hospital.

The model of rapid trauma assessment discussed here is organised and systematic. While it isn't the only way to perform such a assessment, it's a good way to do one. **Skill Drill 14-1 ▶** shows the steps of the rapid trauma assessment, which are also described in the following paragraphs. As you evaluate each region, use the mnemonic, DCAP-BTLS:

1. Start the rapid trauma assessment at the patient's head, inspecting and palpating the skull for any asymmetry (such as depressions) or bleeding (Step 1).
2. Palpate down the posterior cervical spine, feeling for and looking for any signs of trauma (Step 2). Be alert for a

facial grimace or moan that may indicate tenderness on the cervical spine.

3. Quickly look in and behind the patient's ears for blood, cerebrospinal fluid (CSF), or bruising (all signs of a possible skull fracture or traumatic brain injury) (Step 3). Move your head to look; *don't turn the patient's head.*
4. Check the pupils, and quickly palpate the orbits, doing both sides in unison. Feel from the nose out to the lateral edge, including upper and lower ridges (Step 4).
5. Inspect the nose for bleeding and other signs of trauma (Step 5).
6. Assess the mouth for blood or other fluids that may need suctioning (Step 6). Ask a responsive patient to run the tongue around the inside of the teeth to feel whether anything seems to be broken or displaced. If the patient is unresponsive, open the mouth and look for injury or a need for suctioning.
7. Assess the neck for subcutaneous emphysema (a sign of air leaking from the chest), or tracheal shift (a very late sign of a pneumothorax) (Step 7). Note whether a medical identification tag is present.
8. On completing your inspection of the head and neck, examine your gloves for signs of bleeding, and apply a properly sized rigid cervical collar (Step 8).
9. Inspect and palpate the chest. Place your thumbs in the suprasternal notch and follow both clavicles out to the shoulder girdle, keeping the clavicles (commonly fractured bones) between your thumb and finger. This technique allows you to feel most of the entire length of the bone while maintaining continuous contact (Step 9). At the same time, inspect the chest for symmetrical rise and fall

You are the Paramedic Part 4

You continue to provide supplemental high-flow oxygen at a rate of 15 l/min. The patient's oxygen saturations rise to 100% and his ECG shows a sinus rhythm.

Upon arrival at hospital, the patient is transferred to the care of the accident and emergency (A&E) department staff with no change in his status. Blood is drawn, and all laboratory values are unremarkable, including the drug screen, which comes back negative. However, the patient remains unconscious for approximately 2 hours.

Re-assessment	Recording Time: 20 Minutes
Level of consciousness	Glasgow Coma Scale score of 9
Skin	Pink, warm, and moist
Pulse	72 beats/min, regular
Blood pressure	106 by palpation
Respirations	24 breaths/min with adequate depth
SpO2	100% on supplemental oxygen
Pupils	3 mm (PEARRL)

7. If no initial diagnosis is possible, what should your patient care goals be?
8. Under normal circumstances, when an abrupt loss of consciousness occurs, which four primary probabilities should you consider as part of your differential diagnosis?

and for any signs of recessions or other excessive "work of breathing".

10. Gently place your palm on the sternum; press down and then side-to-side to check stability as you assess for a flail chest or fractured sternum (Step 10).

11. Barrel-hoop the rib cage under the armpits and then at the costal margin to assess for fractured ribs (commonly broken bones) or a flail chest (Step 11). Be firm but gentle. Fractured ribs are painful enough without undue pressure being placed on them. If you find large bruised areas, make special mental note: You may be looking at a flail segment but one that does not show the classic paradoxical ("seesaw") movement because the body is still "splinting" the segment with muscle spasm.

12. If you log roll the patient to move him or her to a longboard, examine and palpate the thoracic and lumbar spine for deformity, dislocation, and tenderness as you also look for puncture wounds or other signs of trauma (Step 12).

13. Inspect and palpate all four quadrants of the abdomen, being alert for rigidity, guarding, bruising, and tenderness (Step 13). While you are palpating the abdomen, be alert for a grimace or moan from the patient, which indicates that you touched something that caused pain or discomfort. Given the number of organs in and adjacent to the abdomen, one or more is likely to be injured in any significant traumatic event. Be quick but thorough with your assessment of the abdomen.

14. Move to the pelvic girdle, and gently but firmly assess flexion and compression by pressing down and then inward on the iliac crest, feeling for any sign (instability or pain) that the pelvic girdle is damaged (Step 14).

15. Gently palpate over the bladder (Step 15). If the groin area is wet or bloody or if the patient complains of pain in the area, quickly examine the groin and the genitalia.

16. Inspect and palpate both lower extremities from hip to ankle, looking for signs of bleeding or swelling (Step 16). Note whether one extremity is shorter than the other or if either or both are rotated abnormally (signs of fracture or dislocation).

17. After you have inspected and palpated both legs, simultaneously assess pedal pulses (Step 17), noting whether they feel similar. A difference in pulse quality (one weaker than the other) points to a potentially serious vascular disruption. Bilateral loss of motor function suggests a spinal cord injury, whereas unilateral loss of function is likely to be musculoskeletal in origin, except in the case of a suspected stroke. In a responsive patient, check motor function and sensation of the extremities as well (distal pulse, motor function, and sensation).

18. Check your gloves for blood (Step 18).

19. Inspect and palpate the arms, and assess the pulse, motor function, and sensation (Step 19) just as you did with the legs. Check for a medical identification tag.

20. Check your gloves for blood (Step 20).

21. Assess the back. You can slide your hands under the retroperitoneal area to palpate the bottom of the thoracic spine and some of the lumbar spine. Unless you log roll the patient, however, you won't be able to inspect and palpate the entire back. Inspect and palpate the back to whatever extent you can (Step 21).

22. One last time, check your gloves for blood (Step 22).

When you complete the rapid trauma assessment, obtain a set of baseline vital signs. If you have the resources, have another provider take the vital signs while you do your rapid trauma assessment; it is efficient, saves time, and is a good practice.

Also, mentally piece together all that you now know about your patient, including the chief complaint, the history of the present event, the medical history, and any information about the patient's current health status. Combine that knowledge with the other information and insights you have gained from your various assessments, along with the information obtained from your diagnostics, and you should have more than enough information to make good clinical choices for your patient.

The rapid trauma assessment will help you find any life threats you may have missed in the initial assessment, but it needs to be done quickly. While it generally follows the pattern of a detailed physical examination, the rapid trauma assessment is much, much quicker. A detailed physical examination can take 15 minutes or more; with practise, you can perform a rapid trauma assessment in 2 or 3 minutes. *But you must understand that it takes lots and lots of practise* (Figure 14-11 ▾).

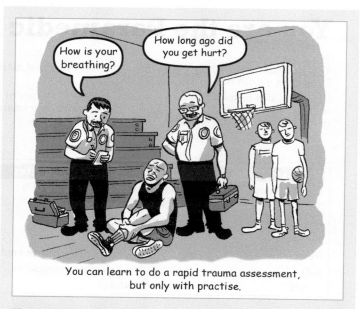

You can learn to do a rapid trauma assessment, but only with practise.

Figure 14-11

Skill Drill 14-1: The Rapid Trauma Assessment

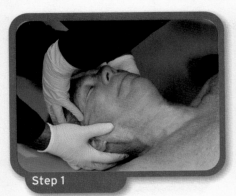

Step 1

Inspect and palpate the skull.

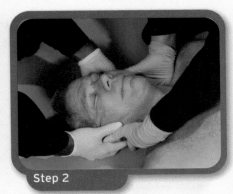

Step 2

Palpate down the posterior cervical spine.

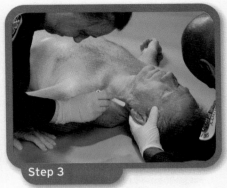

Step 3

Look in and behind the patient's ears.

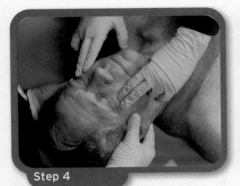

Step 4

Check the pupils, and quickly palpate the orbits.

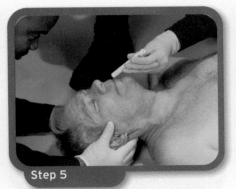

Step 5

Inspect the nose.

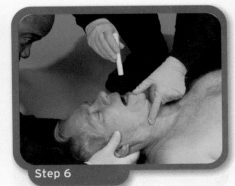

Step 6

Assess the mouth.

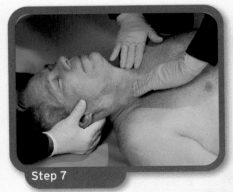

Step 7

Assess the neck.

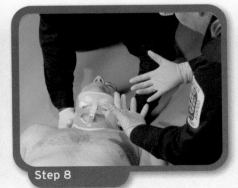

Step 8

Check your gloves for any signs of bleeding. Apply a properly sized rigid cervical collar.

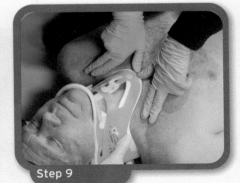

Step 9

Inspect and palpate the chest.

Focused History and Physical Examination

Skill Drill 14-1: The Rapid Trauma Assessment (*continued*)

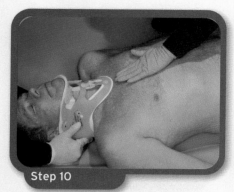

Step 10

Assess for a flail chest or fractured sternum.

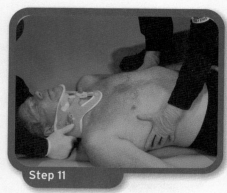

Step 11

Assess for fractured ribs or a flail chest.

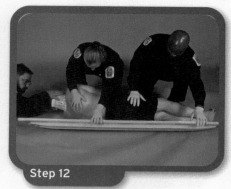

Step 12

If you log roll the patient to a longboard, examine and palpate the thoracic and lumbar spine.

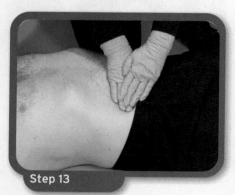

Step 13

Inspect and palpate all four quadrants of the abdomen.

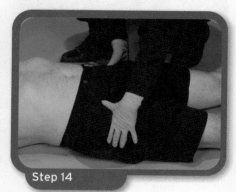

Step 14

Assess the pelvic girdle.

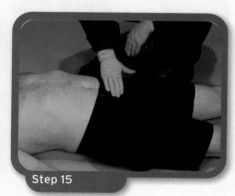

Step 15

Palpate over the bladder.

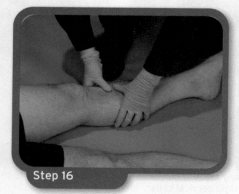

Step 16

Inspect and palpate both lower extremities from hip to ankle.

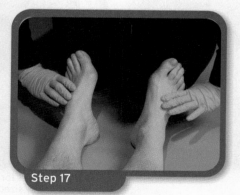

Step 17

Simultaneously assess pedal pulses.

You are the Paramedic Part 5

As the neurosurgeon begins evaluation of the patient, he shakes the patient's big toe and speaks to him. To his surprise, Mike says, "I'm fine, thank you"! On re-assessment of his mental status, the patient receives a GCS score of 15 and shows no neurological deficits. A comprehensive assessment by the neurosurgeon includes a computed tomography scan and magnetic resonance imaging, both with negative results.

The patient was discharged home the following day, and cleared for motorbike riding 1 week later. No final determination for the transient loss of consciousness was identified.

Skill Drill 14-1: The Rapid Trauma Assessment (*continued*)

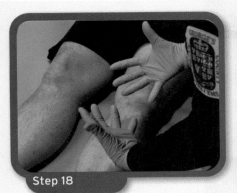

Step 18

Check your gloves for blood.

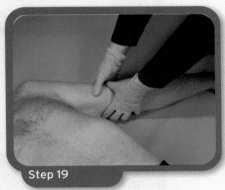

Step 19

Inspect and palpate the arms, and assess pulse, motor function, and sensation.

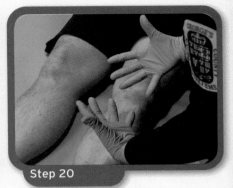

Step 20

Check your gloves for blood.

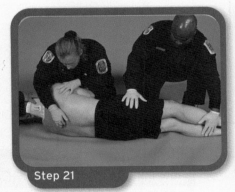

Step 21

Inspect and palpate the back.

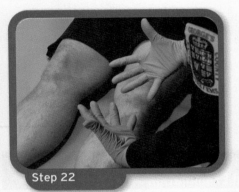

Step 22

Check your gloves for blood.

At the Scene

It may be difficult to assess the stability of a large patient's chest for paradoxical motion. Try fanning out the fingers of both of your hands as wide as possible; then assess the up-and-down motion of the patient's breathing. This will give you a better assessment of equality and movement of the chest with respiration.

Patients With Minor Injuries or No Significant Mechanism of Injury

Most trauma calls involve patients with a single, isolated injury or, on occasion, several minor injuries. In almost all of these cases, the lack of serious or critical injuries is consistent with the lack of a significant mechanism of injury: A collision on the football pitch results in a sprained ankle; a skater crashes and ends up with a Colles fracture; a loose piece of metal spins off a lathe in the machine shop, lacerating the machinist's forearm. Patients should not show any signs of systemic involvement (hypotension). If they do, there is more going on than an isolated injury. You need to continue with your assessment with the goal of finding the more serious problem.

Detailed Physical Examination

Patient Assessment

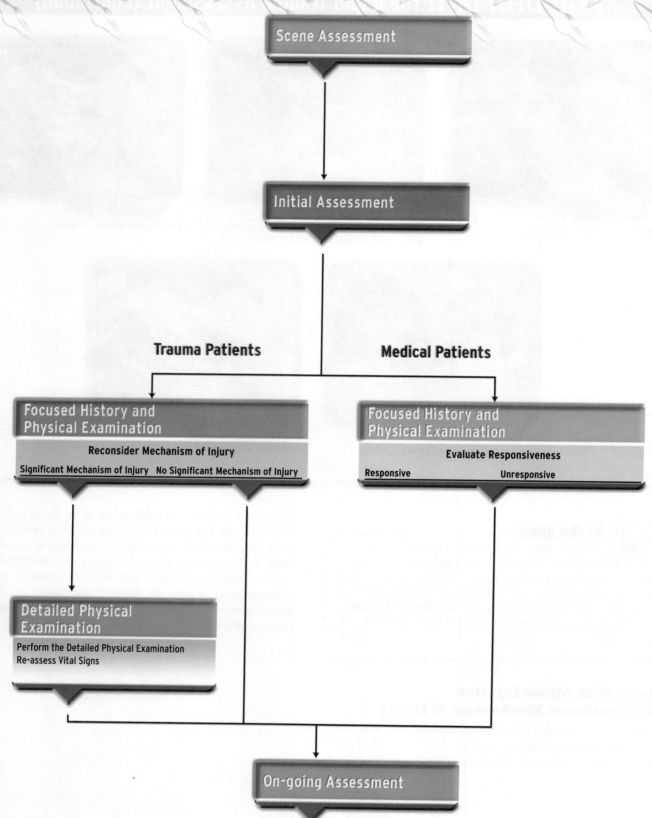

Scene Assessment

Initial Assessment

Trauma Patients

Medical Patients

Focused History and Physical Examination

Reconsider Mechanism of Injury

Significant Mechanism of Injury   No Significant Mechanism of Injury

Focused History and Physical Examination

Evaluate Responsiveness

Responsive   Unresponsive

Detailed Physical Examination

Perform the Detailed Physical Examination
Re-assess Vital Signs

On-going Assessment

The Detailed Physical Examination

The <u>detailed physical examination</u> is another specialised form of patient assessment. In many cases, you won't need to do this assessment (such as for a finger laceration) or won't have time (such as when you have a patient in serious or critical condition). The detailed physical examination can take 15 minutes or more to gather comprehensive history and perform a thorough physical examination (such as checking range of movement [ROM]).

In the majority of cases when you perform a detailed physical examination, it will be done on a trauma patient en route when you have extended transport time (usually more than 15 minutes). Frequently, you will find yourself modifying the examination based on the patient's chief complaint. Use this tool as you see fit—or not at all, if you don't think it will provide meaningful information.

The detailed physical examination can be stressful and produce anxiety in patients because you are asking them to divulge personal information to a paramedic they have known for 10 minutes, and they would normally share such information only with their general practitioner, whom they may have known for 10 years. Be respectful of patients' privacy, and maintain your most professional demeanour as you perform a detailed physical examination.

As you prepare to perform this examination, you will want to review the patient data gathered when you identified the chief complaint and performed the initial assessment. Add in the history of the present injury, the medical history, and the current health status. Keeping this information in mind will help keep you focused and on task as you delve into your patient's problem(s).

A detailed physical examination seeks to define complaints or problems that were not identified in the focused history and physical examination. During this process, paramedics reevaluate any treatment that is under way, based on new information gathered. New treatments are also started to deal with problems found during the detailed physical examination. In addition, paramedics reevaluate the patient's vital signs and assess trends in any changes.

Begin your detailed physical examination by evaluating the patient's mental status:

- Is the patient's appearance and behaviour appropriate?
- How is the patient's posture and general motor behaviour?
- Evaluate the patient's speech and language by listening to what the patient says and how he or she says it.
- Pay attention to the patient's thought process and perceptions.
- Assess the insights the patient does or does not have, along with the judgements the patient makes. (The patient is really sick but doesn't want to go to hospital today ". . . but maybe tomorrow".)
- Assess memory and attention in the remote and the recent domains. For example, ask about memorable past birthdays, then about the events of the day.
- Evaluate new learning ability. For example, give the patient a simple phrase to remember (such as "You can't teach an old dog new tricks" or "Jack and Jill went up the hill") and explain that you plan to ask the patient about the phrase in a little while. Wait 5 minutes and do just that.

After you complete the mental status examination, begin the general survey of the patient. Assess the patient's LOC and compare it with baseline data. Has the LOC changed? If so, how? What is the skin colour? Are there any visible lesions? Look carefully at the patient's facial expression. Does the patient show obvious signs of anxiety or distress, or does the patient look pale and lethargic as if he or she might be in end-stage shock? Assess the patient's apparent state of health and ask yourself that all-important question: "Sick or not sick"? (In the case of trauma, this question becomes "Hurt or not hurt"?)

Other considerations covered in the detailed physical examination include the following:

- The patient's height and weight (Are they proportional to the patient's build?)
- Dress, grooming, and personal hygiene
- General posture, gait, and motor activity
- Unusual breath or body odours
- Skin colour, temperature, moisture, and turgor

Head and Face

Start your hands-on assessment at the patient's head. Inspect and feel the entire cranium for signs of deformity or asymmetry, being careful not to palpate any depressions, as you might push bone fragments into the cranial vault or the brain **Figure 14-12 ▼** . Note any warm, wet areas; they usually represent blood, CSF, or a combination of the two.

Carefully inspect and palpate the upper and lower orbits, starting at the nose and working toward the lateral edge. Assess the eyes for shape and symmetry, and check the pupils for size and reactivity (fixed, dilated, sluggish). Evaluate whether the eyes move in harmony (conjugate gaze) and whether they can track in all fields (up, down, left, right, across). Note periorbital bruising (raccoon's eyes).

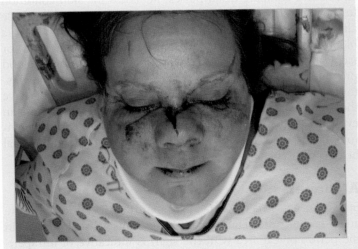

Figure 14-12 Do not palpate any depressions in the skin; you could push bone fragments into the cranial vault or brain.

Inspect and palpate the nose for structural integrity, and look inside for signs of trauma and fluids that may need suctioning. If there is drainage, determine whether it is bloody or clear (in which case, it could be mucus or CSF). Inspect and palpate the maxilla and the mandible, assessing the integrity and symmetry of both structures. Open the mouth, and look for signs of trauma (such as cracked or missing teeth, missing crowns). Check the bite for fit. Be alert for any unusual odours on the patient's breath (such as alcohol or ketones). Check the posterior pharynx for fluids that may need to be suctioned.

Check in, around, and behind the ears for fluids or bruising (Battle's sign). Look carefully into the ear canal, and examine the structure of the ear for signs of trauma. Inspect the anterior part of the neck, assessing for swelling, and other signs of trauma. Assess for midline placement of the trachea.

Chest and Lungs

Before starting the physical examination of the chest, look at the overall symmetry, then assess for equal rise and fall, and finally look for recession, accessory muscle use, and other signs of increased work of breathing. Remember—flail segments may not have paradoxical movement early on due to the splinting effect of muscle spasms. When you re-assess lung sounds later, look for signs of flail segments that may just be presenting.

Inspect and palpate the clavicles from the suprasternal notch out to the shoulder girdles. Assess the ROM of the acromioclavicular joint. Confirm that the sternum is structurally intact. By using the flat surface of your palms, barrel-hoop the rib cage, feeling for asymmetry, deformities, and unstable segments, and evaluate the overall integrity of the chest wall. If the environment is quiet enough, percuss the chest for hyper resonance (pneumothorax, asthma, chronic obstructive pulmonary disease) and hyporesonance (haemothorax). Finally, assess breath sounds in a minimum of six fields.

Cardiovascular System

Check and compare distal pulses. Re-assess the skin condition for pallor and perspiration (signs of sympathetic discharge). Be alert for patients with sustained bradycardia (which lowers blood pressure and may decrease the patient's mental state) or tachycardia (increases cardiac workload and may lower blood pressure). Run a 3-lead ECG for all patients with a cardiac history. If the patient has a significant heart history and you have the time, acquire a 12-lead ECG. It would be tragic to miss an evolving MI due to hypotension caused by trauma. If the environment is quiet enough, consider auscultating for abnormal heart sounds.

Abdomen

Start your assessment of the abdomen by inspecting the entire area for signs of swelling or bruising. Bluish discolouration in the periumbilical area (Cullen's sign) is indicative of intraperitoneal haemorrhage, with two of the more common causes

being ruptured ectopic pregnancy and acute pancreatitis. Look for a rash or other signs of an allergic reaction. Take note of scars from previous trauma or surgeries.

Palpate each quadrant gently but firmly, and recognise that the patient may respond in many ways. A moan, a guarding posture or withdrawing, or a facial grimace all send the same message: You have touched something or somewhere that causes pain or discomfort. That information is worth pursuing with your assessment. Consider any signs or symptoms of abdominal injury as serious and indicative of a high-priority patient in unstable condition.

Rebound tenderness checks are rarely done in the prehospital setting primarily because they can be painful for the patient as you slowly push down and then rapidly release sections of the abdomen. A positive sign (the patient cries out or withdraws) indicates peritoneal irritation.

Genitalia

Unless the patient complains of pain or discomfort or of feeling that he or she is bleeding, there is no reason to examine the genitalia. If you note wetness or bleeding during your examination, you should examine the genitalia because these vascular organs can bleed extensively when injured. Take note of priapism in male patients; a prolonged erection is usually the result of a spinal cord injury or the use of drugs such as sildenafil (Viagra).

In cases of sexual assault or rape, handle all clothing per local guidelines and bag it with any other evidence (not in biodegradable bags). Sexual assault and rape have huge psychological impacts. Be as supportive, caring, and nonjudgemental as possible throughout your care for the patient. It is almost always helpful to have a member of the team who is the same sex as the patient involved in care. If that is not possible, however, do not delay care of the patient because of it.

Anus and Rectum

Unless the patient has a history or indication of trauma to the anus or rectum, there is generally no reason to examine this area. With a positive history or signs or symptoms of trauma, examine the area to assess the need for bleeding control or another intervention (such as treatment for shock, care of eviscerated parts).

Peripheral Vascular System

Moving from the upper extremities to the lower limbs, inspect the extremities for asymmetry and any skin signs, such as bruising, pallor, mottling, or other signs of trauma. Check skin temperature and moisture. When you assess pulses in the extremities, do both sides simultaneously so that you can compare pulse strength, rate, and regularity from side to side. A significant variation in pulse strength in one extremity, especially when associated with pallor or cyanosis, points to vascular compromise.

Musculoskeletal System

Start your assessment of the musculoskeletal system by performing a global inspection of the patient. Do all extremities appear to be properly positioned and functioning normally? If the patient is standing or seated, assess his or her posture for signs of scoliosis or the telltale lean of a suspected stroke. Look for redness or inflammation at the joints (signs of arthritis). Stay alert for red, swollen areas on the extremities, especially those that are warm to the touch (signs of a clot or thrombus).

Check the ROM. First, ask patients to move the extremities by themselves; significantly decreased ROM in this setting may be attributed to joint-related problems. Next, get patients to work their extremities through a normal ROM, only this time with you providing resistance against their movements. Decreased or diminished ROM under these circumstances usually points to muscular weakness or atrophy or possibly problems with innervation. Assess for equality of grips.

Nervous System

The check of the nervous system is one of the most time-consuming elements of the detailed physical examination, mainly because it involves five separate mini-assessments: mental status, motor response, cranial nerve function, reflexes, and sensory response.

The mental status examination essentially repeats the examination done in the rapid trauma assessment. Think of it as checking "mental vital signs". Assess the patient's LOC, and compare it with your baseline and any other LOC checks during other parts of your assessment. A handy mnemonic to guide you through the mental status examination is the mnemonic COASTMAP:

- **Consciousness.** Along with LOC, note the patient's ability to pay attention and concentrate. Is the patient easily distracted?
- **Orientation.** Ask about the year, season, month, day, and date. Have the patient identify the present location—that is, county, town, and specific location. Can the patient recall and describe the event(s) currently going on?
- **Activity.** Does the patient appear anxious or restless? Is he or she sitting very still, scarcely moving at all? Is he or she making any strange or repetitive motions (possibly because of drug use)?
- **Speech.** Note the rate, volume, articulation, and intonation of the patient's speech. Does it sound pressured? Does the speech have a flat, monotone delivery consistent with depression? Is the speech garbled or slurred? Garbled or slurred speech may have many causes, including alcohol or drug impairment, stroke, and head injury.
- **Thought.** Listen to the patient's story. What's on his or her mind? Is the patient making sense? Is there anything unusual about his or her reasoning? Is the patient expressing apparently false ideas (delusions)? Are voices telling the patient what to do or think (psychotic)? Does the patient report that people are "out to get me" (paranoia)?
- **Memory.** You can usually form an impression of the patient's memory by listening to his or her reconstruction of events. A more precise assessment requires asking a few questions. Ask the patient if you may test his or her memory. If the patient assents, slowly say the names of three unrelated subjects (such as apple, bicycle, sewing machine). Now ask the patient to repeat those words; that will test registration. A few minutes later, ask the patient if he or she can remember the three words you named before; that tests retention and memory.
- **Affect.** The patient's affect (mood) may be most apparent in his or her body language. The patient sitting with shoulders drooping and head bent, for example, conveys depression. Note whether the affect—the expression of inner feelings—seems appropriate to the situation.
- **Perception.** Detecting disorders of perception may be difficult because patients are often hesitant to answer questions about hallucinations. Sometimes it is helpful to ask the patient, "Do you ever hear things that other people can't hear"?

It is also helpful to assess the following:

- **Cranial nerves.** Quickly assess the cranial nerves, as described in Chapter 13.
- **Motor system.** Take an overall look at how the patient moves. Are his or her movements smooth or jerky? Note unusual or repetitive movements. Check for muscle strength by assessing bilateral grips.
- **Reflexes.** By using a reflex hammer, evaluate the patient's deep tendon reflexes in the knees and elbows for diminished or heightened responses. Additional reflex checks are probably not warranted in the prehospital environment.
- **Sensory system.** By using the appropriate tools, test the patient for pain (dull versus sharp), sensation, position, and vibration. Compare distal sensation and proximal sensation and one side with the other as you assess the dermatomes.

After completing this assessment, make certain that all assessment findings have been accurately recorded, take one more set of vital signs, and recheck breath sounds.

On-going Assessment

Patient Assessment

```
Scene Assessment
        │
        ▼
Initial Assessment
        │
```

Trauma Patients   **Medical Patients**

```
┌──────────────────────────────┐   ┌──────────────────────────────┐
│ Focused History and          │   │ Focused History and          │
│ Physical Examination         │   │ Physical Examination         │
├──────────────────────────────┤   ├──────────────────────────────┤
│ Reconsider Mechanism of Injury│  │ Evaluate Responsiveness      │
│ Significant Mechanism of Injury  No Significant Mechanism of Injury │  Responsive          Unresponsive │
└──────────────────────────────┘   └──────────────────────────────┘
        │              │                    │
        ▼              │                    │
┌──────────────────┐   │                    │
│ Detailed Physical │  │                    │
│ Examination       │  │                    │
└──────────────────┘   │                    │
        │              │                    │
        └──────────────┴────────┬───────────┘
                                ▼
                    ┌──────────────────────────┐
                    │ On-going Assessment      │
                    ├──────────────────────────┤
                    │ Repeat the Initial Assessment │
                    │ Re-assess and Record Vital Signs │
                    │ Repeat the Focused Assessment │
                    │ Check Interventions      │
                    └──────────────────────────┘
```

The On-going Assessment

After the initial assessment, the on-going assessment is the single most important assessment process you will perform. It represents a continuous, yet cyclical, process that you perform throughout transport, right up to the time you turn patient care over to the A&E department staff. For patients in a stable condition, you should do an on-going assessment every 15 minutes or so. For patients in an unstable condition, you need to make a concerted effort to repeat the on-going assessment every 5 minutes.

Re-assessment of Mental Status and the ABCs

The on-going assessment combines repetition of the initial assessment, re-assessment of vital signs and breath sounds, and repetition of the focused assessment. During the on-going assessment, you continue to evaluate and re-evaluate the patient's status and any treatments already administered. Trends in the patient's current condition may give clues about the effectiveness of treatments: Have they improved the patient's condition? Are identified problems better or worse? This information indicates which changes have occurred and which critical conditions have been addressed and corrected.

First, compare the patient's LOC with your baseline assessment. Is the LOC changing? If so, how?

Second, review the patient's airway. Is it patent? Swelling, bleeding, or just a change of position can obstruct the airway in the blink of an eye, so make certain that the airway is properly positioned and dry. Always be prepared to suction, and don't delay if you hear gurgling in the upper airway. It's far better to prevent aspiration than to treat it later. If the airway needs to be secured, *do it immediately,* and intubate the patient. Once intubation is accomplished, recheck lung sounds and perform pulse oximetry and capnography periodically to confirm that the tube is properly placed.

Third, re-assess breathing. Is the patient breathing adequately? If not, figure out why and fix the problem. For hypoventilation, assist breathing with oxygen and a bag-valve-mask device. Correct hypoxia with high-concentration oxygen therapy. For patients with diminished or absent breath sounds, jugular venous distension, and progressive dyspnoea (signs of pneumothorax), decompress the chest.

Stay alert for signs that the patient is experiencing ventilatory fatigue (for example, decreasing pulse oximetry reading, looks increasingly tired). Be especially alert for this possibility in children because it a classic sign that precedes disaster for the patient. Patients of any age who are going into ventilatory fatigue need to have their airway managed for them.

Finally, re-assess the patient's circulation. Assess overall skin colour as an initial measure of cardiovascular function and haemodynamic status. With pale, cool, wet skin, think shock; with cyanosis, think oxygen desaturation; with mottling, think end-stage shock.

Make certain that all bleeding is controlled. If you find blood-soaked dressings, add more fresh dressings to the stack and rebandage in place. Re-assess the blood pressure, watching closely for signs that the patient is beginning to decompensate.

Re-assess the pulse, including its rate, strength, and regularity. Progressive tachycardia may indicate that the patient is still bleeding, is hypoxic, or is developing cardiogenic shock. In contrast, sustained or progressively worsening bradycardia may reflect rising intracranial pressure (from trauma or a stroke) or end-stage shock.

Re-assessment of Patient Care and Transport Priorities

After repeating the initial assessment as part of your on-going assessment, think about your present care plan. Have you addressed all life threats? Based on what you now know, do you need to revise your priority list? If so, make the change and get on with patient care. In contrast, if your plan is working well and you've addressed most or all of the patient's complaints, there is no need to revise the care plan.

While you are re-evaluating your patient care priorities, you should re-assess the transport plan as well. Should routine transport be stepped up to priority? Is the patient's condition worsening to the point that you need to consider diverting to a closer hospital? Do you need to set up a rendezvous with an air ambulance and fly the patient to hospital? If your patient's condition has improved and stabilised, you should step down from priority and transport the patient as a routine case.

Get another complete set of vital signs, and compare them with the expected outcomes from your therapies. For example, if you administered a 250-ml bolus of normal saline to a patient with gastrointestinal bleeding, you usually would expect a rise in blood pressure and a decrease in pulse rate. With any priority patient, you should have, at a minimum, three sets of vital signs—and that would be if you had a short transport. With most priority patients, you will have four or five sets of vital signs. Thus, you can look for trends or patterns such as a slowing pulse, rising blood pressure, and erratic respiratory patterns that represent the Cushing's triad, a grave sign for patients with head trauma. Alternatively, narrowed pulse pressure, muffled heart tones, and jugular venous distension are associated with cardiac tamponade (Beck's triad), usually secondary to penetrating chest trauma.

The last element of the on-going assessment is to revisit the patient's complaints (from the focused history), along with your interventions. Have any complaints improved or resolved? Has the 9 over 10 chest pain improved with the GTN you administered? Did the second salbutamol treatment ease the patient's breathing? Which situations remain unresolved? Situations that are worsening are especially concerning because they could mean an unseen problem or ineffective interventions. If you have not reached the receiving hospital, get ready to do the on-going assessment again—that's why it's called the on-going assessment.

You are the Paramedic Summary

1. What is the best method of airway assessment and management for a patient who is wearing a motorbike helmet?

Even with a flip-up-front motorbike helmet, optimum airway and cervical management can only occur once you have removed the helmet, so this needs to be a priority, especially with full-face helmets. With the helmet removed, it is possible to manage the airway and keep the spine in a neutral position should the patient require spinal immobilisation (spinal immobilisation is covered in Chapter 22).

2. Although the bystanders deny any trauma, should you immobilise this patient?

There is no evidence to suggest that this patient requires spinal precautions. When in doubt, err on the side of caution and immobilise the patient. This will be a decision for you to make in accordance with your local guidelines.

3. Because this patient is a minor, what are some important considerations for treatment and transport?

In such cases every effort should be made to contact an adult with parental responsibility for the child. If the parents are unavailable, this patient would be treated and transported without consent, but acting in the patient's best interest.

4. Of all your differential diagnoses, which ones should be considered a diagnosis of exclusion?

Although at some point during the course of your career you will likely encounter patients who exaggerate signs or falsify symptoms (including feigning unconsciousness), this should be the last thing you suspect, even in patients who have a history of malingering. Consider this possibility only after you've carefully reviewed all other potential causes. Doing otherwise is likely to cause a misdiagnosis and/or delay of essential care and prompt transport.

5. Does this patient need high-flow supplemental oxygen? Why or why not?

It is appropriate to apply high-flow oxygen because the patient is unconscious and can benefit from supplemental oxygen therapy. Be ever mindful of what you're doing and why, especially when administering drugs, including oxygen. Note that pulse oximetry is not always accurate, even when it provides a reading. Patients with carbon monoxide poisoning may have an acceptable or even a 100% oximetry reading. Patients who have cold hands or who wear nail varnish may initially have a lower pulse oximetry reading but, in fact, be better oxygenated than their carbon monoxide-poisoned counterparts.

6. Should this patient be intubated? Why or why not?

This patient is adequately ventilating but his airway is at risk because he is unconscious. Using a simple airway adjunct such as an oropharyngeal airway and placing the patient in the recovery position may be all that is required for this patient. If he is immobilised on a longboard, then care needs to be taken that suction is available and more advanced airway management techniques need to be considered such as endotracheal intubation. In this particular scenario, intubation may not be successful since some airway reflexes will probably be present. If this is the case, then the patient would require sedation, which is not within the scope of practice of most paramedics.

7. If no initial diagnosis is possible, what should your patient care goals be?

As a paramedic, your goals are to assess and treat any life-threatening conditions, monitor ABCs, provide supportive measures, and continue to search for underlying causes of the patient's signs and symptoms.

8. Under normal circumstances, when an abrupt loss of consciousness occurs, which four primary probabilities should you consider as part of your differential diagnosis?

Any sudden change in mentation should make you question the presence of underlying illnesses or injuries related to the neurovascular system as well as hypoglycaemia, drug toxicity, and cardiac arrhythmias.

Prep Kit

■ Ready for Review

- Patient assessment is the platform on which quality prehospital care is built and the single most important skill you bring.
- Patient assessment is a complex skill made up of two primary components: information gathering and physical examination.
- Several elements make up the skill of patient assessment, with each being used in some way to gather information.
- The first step of the patient assessment process is the scene assessment because your first and foremost concern on any call is ensuring your own safety and the safety of your colleagues.
- During the initial assessment, in the first 60 to 90 seconds, as you look at, talk with, and touch your patient, you should be able to identify threats to the ABCs.
- Once the initial assessment is complete and all life threats have been addressed, you can move into the focused history and physical examination phase of patient assessment.
- The detailed physical examination can take 15 minutes or more for a comprehensive history and a thorough physical examination (such as checking ROM).
- After the initial assessment, the on-going assessment is the single most important assessment process you will perform.

■ Vital Vocabulary

alert and orientated (A + O) A decision made when assessing mental status by looking at whether the patient is orientated to four elements: person, place, time, and the event itself. Each element provides information about different aspects of the patient's memory.

AVPU A method of assessing mental status by determining whether a patient is awake and Alert, responsive to Verbal stimuli or Pain, or Unresponsive; used principally in the initial assessment.

Beck's triad The combination of a narrowed pulse pressure, muffled heart sounds, and jugular venous distension associated with cardiac tamponade; usually resulting from penetrating chest trauma.

current health status A composite picture of a number of factors in a patient's life, such as dietary habits, current medications, allergies, exercise, alcohol or tobacco use, recreational drug use, sleep patterns and disorders, and immunisations.

Cushing's triad The combination of a slowing pulse, rising blood pressure, and erratic respiratory patterns; a grave sign for patients with head trauma.

detailed physical examination The part of the assessment process in which a detailed area-by-area examination is performed on patients whose problems cannot be readily identified or when more specific information is needed about problems identified in the focused history and physical examination.

focused history and physical examination The part of the assessment process in which the patient's major complaints or any problems that are immediately evident are further and more specifically evaluated.

focused physical examination The examination done on a responsive medical patient, driven by the information gathered during the initial assessment and the history-taking phase.

general impression The overall initial impression that determines the priority for patient care; based on the patient's surroundings, the mechanism of injury, signs and symptoms, and the chief complaint.

Glasgow Coma Scale (GCS) An evaluation tool used to determine level of consciousness, which evaluates and assigns point values (scores) for eye opening, verbal response, and motor response, which are then totalled; effective in helping predict patient outcomes.

history of the present illness Information about the chief complaint, obtained using the OPQRST mnemonic.

initial assessment The part of the assessment process that helps you identify immediately or potentially life-threatening conditions so that you can initiate lifesaving care.

mechanism of injury (MOI) The way in which traumatic injuries occur; the forces that act on the body to cause damage.

nature of illness (NOI) The general type of illness a patient is experiencing.

on-going assessment The part of the assessment process in which problems are reevaluated and responses to treatment are assessed.

past medical history Information obtained during the patient history, such as the patient's general state of health, childhood and adult diseases, surgeries and hospitalisations, psychiatric and mental illnesses, or traumatic injuries, which may relate to the patient's current problem.

rapid trauma assessment A unique and specialised assessment performed between the initial assessment and the focused physical examination of a trauma patient, usually on patients with a significant mechanism of injury, assessing specific parts of the entire body.

scene assessment A quick assessment of the scene and its surroundings made to provide information about scene safety and the mechanism of injury or nature of illness, before you enter and begin patient care.

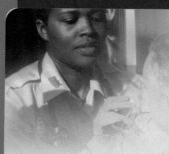

Assessment in Action

You have been dispatched to a road traffic collision in which a small car has struck a pole. Ambulance control has advised you that there appears to be one patient in the vehicle. As you arrive on the scene, you notice that the pole is leaning at a 45° angle toward the car, and the wires are hanging low over the vehicle but not touching it. Without leaving the ambulance, you see a person sitting in the driver's seat who appears to be leaning over the steering wheel but is not moving. You are not sure, but you believe you see the top of a child's car seat in the rear of the car. No traffic or crowd control has been started, and you do not see the electricity board on the scene.

1. **What is the first step in your patient assessment?**
   A. Assess the patient's chief complaint.
   B. Perform a detailed physical examination to determine the extent of the condition.
   C. Perform a scene assessment.
   D. Assess AVPU.

2. **What is the first and foremost concern during your scene assessment?**
   A. The patient's level of consciousness
   B. The patient's breathing
   C. The safety of you and the rest of your colleagues
   D. The safety of the patient and their family members

3. **What best describes the term mechanism of injury?**
   A. The forces that act on the body to cause damage
   B. The internal forces of the human body
   C. The way an accident happened
   D. The external circumstances that caused an accident to happen

4. **How long should your initial assessment take?**
   A. 10 to 20 seconds
   B. 30 to 40 seconds
   C. 60 to 90 seconds
   D. More than 90 seconds

5. **A rapid trauma assessment be should performed on any trauma patient with a:**
   A. fracture.
   B. significant MOI.
   C. significant medical history.
   D. significant NOI.

6. **When should a detailed physical examination be done?**
   A. For every patient encounter
   B. When you have time on scene to complete it
   C. While you are transporting the patient to hospital
   D. During the scene assessment

Challenging Questions

You arrive at a building site where a worker fell approximately 6 m from a ladder and landed on his left side. Your initial assessment does not reveal threats to the ABCs. The patient, who is conscious and alert, complains of pain to the left side of his body; he denies having chest pain and shortness of breath and states that he did not lose consciousness. Other than some minor abrasions to the patient's left arm and lateral thigh, the remainder of your examination is unremarkable. Your partner reports the following vital signs: blood pressure, 126/76 mm Hg; pulse rate, 86 beats/min and regular; and respirations, 14 breaths/min and unlaboured.

7. **Does this patient require transport to hospital?**

8. **Could you defend a pre-alert call and emergency transport for this patient?**

■ Points to Ponder

You and your colleague have been sent to a patient complaining of "chest pain". When ambulance control provides an update, they state that the patient is a 70-year-old woman who started having chest pain about 2 hours ago. The patient has a cardiac history, but the extent of the history is unclear because of a language barrier. Ambulance control also states that there is an 8-year-old child with the patient.

Upon arrival, you find the patient sitting upright in a chair. She is leaning slightly forward, with her arms folded across her chest. You introduce yourself and ask her for information about her chief complaint. She looks up at you and says, "No English", in a heavy accent that you do not recognise. You have already formed your initial impression of the patient and have determined that she is in considerable distress.

How do you proceed with your physical assessment given that this patient does not speak English and you do not speak her native language? Would you consider using the 8-year-old as an interpreter? How will you address a time delay in your assessment progression?

Issues: Assessing People of Differing Cultures, Communications Barriers, Time Delay During Assessment.

15

Critical Thinking and Clinical Decision Making

Objectives

Cognitive

- Compare the factors influencing medical care in the prehospital environment to other medical settings.
- Differentiate between critical life-threatening, potentially life-threatening, and non–life-threatening patient presentations.
- Evaluate the benefits and shortfalls of protocols/guidelines, standing orders and patient care pathways.
- Define the components, stages and sequences of the critical thinking process for paramedics.
- Apply the fundamental elements of critical thinking for paramedics.
- Describe the effects of the "fight or flight" response and the positive and negative effects on a paramedic's decision making.

- Summarise the "six Rs" of putting it all together: Read the scene, Read the patient, React, Reevaluate, Revise the management plan, Review performance.

Affective

- Defend the position that clinical decision making is the cornerstone of effective paramedic practice.
- Practise facilitating behaviours when thinking under pressure.

Psychomotor

None

The hormonal response has an impact on you both positively and negatively. On the positive side, you may have enhanced visual and auditory acuity as well as improved reflexes and muscle strength. On the negative side, you may have impaired critical thinking skills and diminished concentration and assessment abilities. One way to counter these negative effects is to improve your mental conditioning. Practise your skills until you can do them almost instinctively and can perform them on command, almost flawlessly, in the skills lab setting. Once you reach that level, you can draw on these skills in a real-life setting, allowing you to better focus on patient assessment or other decision-making areas.

Facilitate better thinking under pressure by memorising the following mental checklist for all calls:

1. Take a moment to *scan the situation.*
2. Take another moment to *stop and think.*
3. *Make decisions and act* on behalf of the patient.
4. *Stay calm,* and maintain clear, concise *mental control.*
5. Plan to regularly and continually *reevaluate the patient.*

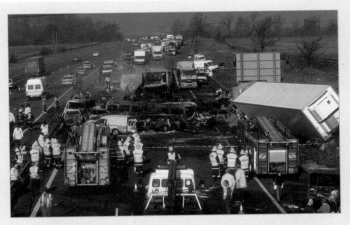

Figure 15-10 Although you need to focus on treating patients as soon as possible, always take a moment to register important information about the scene. What has happened that will help you assess each patient's condition?

Taking It to the Streets

Having now looked at the science side of critical thinking, let us move on to the practical side. When you are out on a call, critical thinking can be summed up with the *Six Rs.*

1. Read the Scene

The emergency scene is a relative goldmine of information readily available to you, if you are wise enough to mine it. Equally important to consider is that this information is *only* available at the scene and becomes unavailable once you initiate transport to the hospital. Some of the primary elements involved in reading the scene are: evaluating the overall safety of the situation, the environmental conditions, the immediate surroundings, access and exit issues, and finally evaluating the mechanism of injury Figure 15-10 . In particular, when you are looking at the mechanism of injury, take time to evaluate all aspects. For example, with a car crash look at the length of the skid marks or note whether there are none, what the vehicle struck, how much intrusion there is into the passenger compartment, and whether seat belts were worn. In another example, the case of a fall, you would look for the height of a fall, how the patient landed, and what the patient landed on.

Other issues when you "read the scene" include assessing the environment in which the patient was found. Was it hot, cold, wet? Also, are there eyewitnesses or friends or family to provide additional information?

2. Read the Patient

Probably one of the greatest skills you can develop is learning to read a patient quickly. As you approach the patient, does the patient see you and track you with his or her eyes? Offer the patient your hand to shake, and introduce yourself and ask why 999 was called. If the patient takes your hand and answers you appropriately, you have just determined that the patient has a Glasgow Coma Scale score of 15 (spontaneous eye opening, follows commands, appropriate verbal response). Other components of effectively reading a patient include:

- **Observe** the patient. What's the patient's LOC and level of comfort or discomfort? Skin colour? Position? Work of breathing? Any obvious deformity or asymmetry? Figure 15-11 ▶
- **Talk** to the patient. Determine the chief complaint. Is this a new problem or the worsening of a pre-existing condition? Obtain the medical history and the history of the present problem.
- **Touch** the patient. What's the skin temperature and moisture level like? Assess the pulse rate for regularity and strength.
- **Auscultate** lungs sounds. Confirm the adequacy or inadequacy of respirations and reassess the patency of the airway.
- **Identify** life threats. Correct any life threats relative to airway, breathing, and circulation in the order you find them.

Notes from Nancy

If you do not take a few moments to survey the scene . . . you are very likely to become one of the casualties yourself. And a paramedic who is injured because he or she rocketed out of the ambulance without taking a good look around, will be of no benefit to the patient(s). Indeed, an injured paramedic just increases the number of victims that the remaining rescue personnel have to care for, and that will very likely detract from the care given to the other patients. The moral is: Dead heroes can't save lives. Injured heroes are a nuisance, so check the scene for hazards before you lunge in.

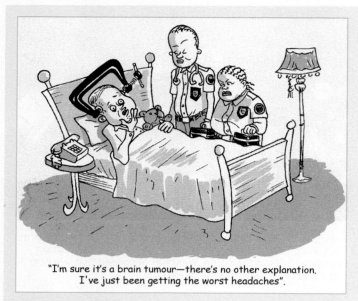

"I'm sure it's a brain tumour—there's no other explanation.
I've just been getting the worst headaches".

Figure 15-11

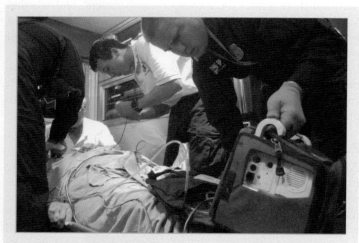

Figure 15-12 The more accurate your patient readings, the more reliable your diagnosis will be. Take the time to collect two sets of baseline vital signs on every patient.

■ **Obtain** complete and accurate vital signs (Figure 15-12 ▲). For every patient, even for transfer patients, a baseline set of vital signs is a must. For patients with serious problems, two sets of vital signs provide comparative data. With critical patients, three or more sets of vital signs allow you to assess trends and to reassess whether the patient's condition is stabilising, getting better, or getting worse. If your patient's condition is getting worse, multiple sets of vital signs provide some indication of how fast the patient's condition is deteriorating.

3. React

You must begin patient care by addressing life threats in the order you find them. Next, consider the worst-case scenario that

Controversies

Ambulance services have for many years treated patients with prophylactic treatments even when there is no evidence to support the need. Should every trauma patient be immobilised on a longboard? Should every unconscious person be given Narcan?

could be causing your patient's symptoms, and either rule it out or rule it in. After that, your primary focus should be to determine the most common and statistically probable cause for the patient's current condition. By addressing the worst-case scenario, you can try to avoid any serious complications in patient care and then can take the time to look for less lethal problems.

If, at the end of your assessment, you haven't been able to develop a working diagnosis, it is acceptable to provide care based on the presenting signs and symptoms. If your patient is having difficulty breathing, you administer high-flow oxygen and place the patient in a position of comfort. For symptoms of shock, you elevate the feet, provide a cover for warmth, administer high-flow oxygen, and establish a large-bore IV line while you continue to try to search for the cause of the condition. When you put the limited physical and technical resources of the prehospital environment up against the number of possible diagnoses a patient might have, you will find that you will regularly be treating patients who cannot be diagnosed until they reach the hospital. In some cases, the diagnosis may elude the doctor as well, so this is nothing to be ashamed of or worried about. It is simply a reality of medicine and has to be dealt with in a professional fashion.

4. Reevaluate

As patient care is continuing, another key element of good care is to make certain that you follow up on any interventions. See whether the splint you applied has eased the pain in your patient's injured leg. If you are treating frequent PVCs (premature ventricular contractions) with an antidysrhythmic medication, check the monitor to see whether the contractions have resolved. On challenging calls, once paramedics get into the treatment mode, they can fall into the trap of focusing on *doing things,* forgetting to monitor whether the *things they are doing* are actually improving the patient's situation.

As you reassess your patient, take the time to add any information you may have gathered from the detailed or focused physical examination and add it to the information you found in the initial assessment. Say you find that your patient has no breath sounds in the upper right lobes secondary to a fractured rib that caused a small pneumothorax. By itself, the small pneumothorax is not an immediate life threat to a relatively healthy individual. But let's say the patient also has bilateral fractured femurs, significant blood loss, and a minor head injury. Under those circumstances, a small pneumothorax may complicate matters far more than if it were the only condition. When you encounter patients, especially trauma patients, with multiple pathophysiologies, it is up to you to add them up as

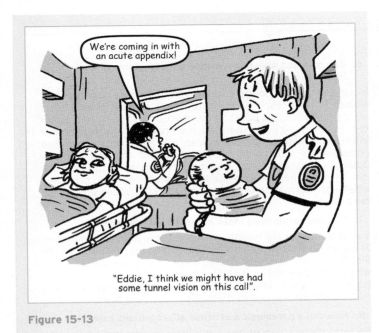

"Eddie, I think we might have had some tunnel vision on this call".

Figure 15-13

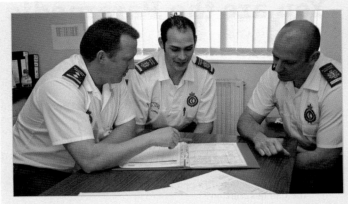

Figure 15-14 You will learn something new with every patient encounter. One of the best ways to review your performance—and to learn—is to talk it over with peers.

you develop your care plan to make sure nothing is overlooked that can be addressed in the prehospital environment.

5. Revise the Plan

As you continue to care for your patient, you may get indications that what you once thought was a head injury is a problem secondary to glue sniffing: two very different causes. The thinking paramedic, no matter how sure he or she is of the working diagnosis, always keeps part of the thought process open to other possibilities Figure 15-13 ▲ . As other information becomes available as the call unfolds, you should always be prepared to change directions as necessary. By remaining mentally "light on your feet", you position yourself to be receptive to changing presentations or circumstances, which in turn helps you avoid tunnel vision.

6. Review Your Performance

Again, once a call is over, you as a provider have the opportunity to look back and reexamine your work Figure 15-14 ▶ . Whether this review is in the formal setting of a continuous

quality improvement (CQI) meeting or just back at the station reviewing the call with your partner, taking the time to critically look at your work allows you real growth opportunities. This is particularly true when you have made a mistake. While success is satisfying and certainly feels good, there is little growth opportunity to be had. However, when you make a mistake, take the time to analyse the call so that you can avoid repeating your behaviour and making the same mistake. Mistakes will only change if you want to find out what they were, and why they recurred. Excellence in prehospital care is the gradual result of you as a provider constantly striving to improve your practice, which requires that you *always* have an attitude that is open to life-long learning.

Being a thinking paramedic will happen only if you choose to work on your critical thinking skills throughout your career. As you continue to improve the way you think and make decisions, your patient care will improve as well. Your reward will be excellence in your practice—the ultimate job satisfaction.

You are the Paramedic Summary

1. When do you begin patient assessment?

Most people consider patient assessment to begin as early as being activated on a call. Good ambulance providers know their primary service areas, and can use this information to add further understanding to information that dispatchers provide regarding their patients. As a good paramedic, your antennae would go up if you are dispatched to a local orchard for difficulty breathing. Could your patient be suffering from anaphylaxis related to a bee sting or a respiratory emergency related to the inhalation of a pesticide?

2. What are the benefits and the risks of diagnosing based on the call description?

Ambulance control are adept at gathering and distilling information from 999 callers. They not only gather information, but also calm callers, provide instructions, and send appropriate resources to a caller's location. Despite control's best efforts, the information gained from callers may or may not be accurate. Oftentimes, this information gives you a good list of possible causes related to a patient's chief complaint, but it is very important to refrain from making a diagnosis. Information provided should be used to see the big picture, where you can begin to determine whether other resources are likely to be necessary and discuss en route to the scene what role you and the other provider will play. The bottom line—generate a list of possible causes, but be flexible!

3. What are pertinent negatives?

Pertinent negatives are findings you would expect to see in a medical condition, but do not. If a paramedic suspects an infection, you would ask questions about the recent history of a productive cough, fever, or chills—all indicators of infection. If your patient denies having any of these signs and symptoms, you are faced with a pertinent negative—it is possible that your patient does not have an infection.

4. What information is missing from the above assessment?

Temperature can yield a wealth of information, particularly in this case. The presence or lack of fever can aid you in narrowing down your list of possible causes. All of your assessment tools aid you in narrowing your list of differential diagnoses.

5. How can a patient's opinion affect treatment and transport decisions?

Patients sometimes self-diagnose, although they are not trained to see what you can. Don't let a patient talk you into a different diagnosis. Of course, you will consider your patient's feelings and opinions but only in conjunction with your physical findings. Patients' feelings and opinions are important, but you make the final determination about treatment based on your training.

6. Can men and women have different symptoms of acute illness?

More and more is learned about the differences of men and women in their response to acute illness. In most classic heart attack scenarios, the patient experiences chest pain. This symptom is not required to question the presence of a myocardial infarction. Postmenopausal women may have only associated complaints of a sudden onset of generalised weakness, fatigue, dizziness, or shortness of breath. Obtaining an adequate medical history to include all possible risk factors can also provide a wealth of information to aid you in narrowing your list of possible causes.

7. Do good paramedics make mistakes like this one?

Yes. Because we are human, we are capable of making mistakes in our work. Mistakes are not welcomed and may result in loss of life. This is why we must assess and reassess our patients and why we must strive to maintain our skills and improve our knowledge. The key is to learn from mistakes (both your mistakes and mistakes by others) and to try to avoid repeating them.

8. How can a paramedic's attitude affect patient care?

Because we are human, we can allow our personal feelings to affect patient care. This is not always a bad thing, but our personal attitudes should never have a negative impact on patient care. Being tired, hungry, or otherwise distracted is not your patient's concern. Your patient's needs come first, and second only to the safety of yourself and your crew.

9. What was done right in this call?

You erred on the side of the patient. Although you failed to gather adequate data about your patient's condition, you encouraged her to seek evaluation by a doctor. Being genuinely concerned for the patient's well-being will oftentimes prevent poor patient care or outcomes. You also provided oxygen, established an IV, and placed her on the cardiac monitor. Your assessment and care, albeit incomplete, did have a positive effect. When reviewing calls, it is important to note what you do right as well as what you can improve on.

10. How could this mistake have been avoided?

For all calls, you should have a list of possible causes. Always be suspicious for serious, life-threatening conditions. Rule out the worst possible scenario. Don't make assumptions or be complacent or lazy. Every patient deserves a thorough assessment regardless of time of day or if your needs are or aren't being met at the time. It is also important to continue to read the latest in medical research. Medicine is an evolving field, and each year more is learned about the human body and its response to various treatments.

Prep Kit

Ready for Review

- The first cornerstone of your practice as a paramedic is having the ability to *gather, evaluate,* and *synthesise* information.
- Once you have gathered information, you must assess and evaluate this information as to its validity and the impact it will have on the patient care plan you are developing.
- Once you have evaluated the information you obtained from the scene, the patient, or any bystanders and determined what information is valid, then you need to process—or *synthesise*—that information.
- The second cornerstone of your practice is the *development and implementation of patient care plans.*
- Your care plan is nearly always defined by the patient care guidelines and local operating procedures in the ambulance service you work for.
- The third cornerstone is *judgement and making independent decisions.*
- The fourth and final cornerstone of your practice is your ability to *think and work under pressure.*
- The first stage of the thought process in prehospital care is gathering information—things you see, hear, smell, or feel. This is *concept formation.*
- The second stage of the critical thinking process is data interpretation—evaluating the information you have gathered.
- The last stage in the critical thinking process occurs after the call is over and is commonly associated with debriefing. Look back at the total call and reflect on how you processed the signs and symptoms and reached the decisions that you did.

- The *six Rs* can be used to summarise what must be done on a call:
  - –Read the scene
  - –Read the patient
  - –React
  - –Reevaluate
  - –Revise the plan
  - –Review your performance
- Excellence in prehospital care results from a constant striving to improve your practice, which requires that you ALWAYS have an attitude that is open to learning.

Vital Vocabulary

concept formation Pattern of understanding based on initially obtained information.

cookbook medicine Treatment based on a guideline without adequate knowledge of the patient being treated.

data interpretation The process of formulating a conclusion based on comparing the patient's condition with information from your training, education, and past experiences.

medical ambiguity Uncertainty regarding the specific cause of the patient's condition.

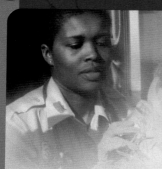

Assessment in Action

You are called to a scene where a 16-year-old male has had a convulsion, is vomiting, and isn't making much sense to his family. By the time you get there, he is making a little more sense, and is no longer actively vomiting. The family tells you he came home from a party, began vomiting almost immediately, and had a mild convulsion that lasted about a minute. He has not answered any of their questions, and they have no idea what he may have eaten or taken at the party.

1. **You introduce yourself to the family and the patient, and ask him how he is feeling. He doesn't answer. You tell him you'd really like to help him feel better, and need for him to answer your questions and be honest. You can see that his pupils are very dilated, he is sweating, and his face is very pale. He doesn't want to answer any of your questions, but does shake his head "no" when you ask if he drank or took any kind of drugs at the party. What do you do?**
   A. Continue with your evaluation as you normally would, in front of his family, despite his denial of having drunk alcohol or taken any drugs.
   B. Tell him you know he's lying based on what his body is telling you, and be confrontational until he tells you what he drank or took.
   C. Try to embarrass him in front of his family so he will tell you the truth.
   D. Continue your evaluation as normal, until you can get him in a private setting so that he may be more inclined to be honest because he is not in front of his family.

2. **In the back of your ambulance, the patient still denies having taken or drank anything. The symptoms he is experiencing tell you otherwise. What do you do?**
   A. Try to scare him by telling him that he will get much worse, and could even die, if he is not honest so you can treat him appropriately.
   B. Call the receiving hospital, give them all known information, and ask what you should do.
   C. Treat him based on what you *think* he may have taken, without confirmation from the patient himself.
   D. Take him to the hospital and let the doctor deal with him.

3. **In the back of the ambulance, the patient admits to drinking some cider at the party. He says he is not on any medications, has no known allergies, has never had any type of convulsion previously, and has never taken drugs. His pupils are still dilated, he is still somewhat confused, he is sweating and pale, and he is developing stomach cramps. He begins vomiting again, but does not smell like cider at all. He seems to be getting worse. He does not want to go to hospital, and begs you not to tell his parents about the cider. What do you do?**
   A. Tell his parents you believe he may have a stomach virus, keeping his secret for him. After all, you were a teenager once too and have had your share of partying days.
   B. Tell his parents the truth—that you believe he has taken some kind of drug and that he needs to be taken to the accident and emergency department for treatment, asking their permission to take him against his will for treatment.
   C. Honour the patient's request to deny treatment, tell him what risks he is facing, and that you will be happy to return and take him to the accident and emergency department if he changes his mind.
   D. Tell his parents nothing except that you are taking him to hospital for evaluation and that he cannot refuse treatment because he has an altered mental status.

4. **While in the ambulance, your partner suggests the possibility that the patient, based on his symptoms, is experiencing some kind of blood glucose issue. What do you do?**
   A. Consider this possibility and check the patient's blood glucose level.
   B. Tell your partner that you are the paramedic, and you've already made up your mind about what is wrong with the patient, and that is that.
   C. Call the receiving hospital and ask if you should even consider any possibility of blood glucose issues.
   D. Tell your partner when he has the experience and knowledge that you have, he can make the decision.

5. **The patient's family is impatiently waiting outside your ambulance. His mother begins knocking on the door, then banging on it, insisting she know exactly what is being said and done to her son. She begins yelling and swearing that you are not doing your job right, she doesn't trust you, and she no longer wants you to treat her son. What do you do?**
   A. Send your partner out to calm her down, explaining that you are evaluating her son and doing what is best for him.
   B. Ignore her and continue to evaluate and treat her son.
   C. Explain to her how sick her son is, and that he must be treated based on his altered mental status, with or without her consent.
   D. Let her into the ambulance, apologise, explain what you are doing, what you believe is wrong, what you think will happen if he is not treated at all, and ask that she give her consent.

6. **If the young man mentioned in the above scenario had a rapidly deteriorating mental status (confusion that got worse and worse in a short amount of time) and other signs such as his breathing rate also deteriorated, how would this affect your evaluation and treatment?**
   A. It would not affect it; you would evaluate and treat him as you would in other questions listed above.
   B. You would panic, tell his parents the outlook was not good, and take him to the accident and emergency department as quickly as possible.
   C. You would tell his parents that their son's condition was his own fault for drinking alcohol while under age or taking drugs, and he should have known better.
   D. You would consider it an ALS call, and treat all symptoms as they occurred on your way to the accident and emergency department.

7. **What if the patient in the scenario became combative, stubborn, and mean, and insisted that you give him opiate pain medication before you do anything else? What if he would not allow you to examine or otherwise treat him unless you did this first? You know he needs to go to hospital, and that he has more problems than just the pain he is dealing with. What would you do?**

   A. Give him the pain medication to make him more cooperative, and to make your assessment, diagnosis, and treatment easier.

   B. Bribe him—tell him if he's cooperative for the evaluation and treatment, you will give him what he wants (even if you have no intention of doing so).

   C. Tell him that you have to follow guidelines, which do not allow you to administer pain medication without a full examination.

   D. Tell him that if he does not cooperate and let you do your job, you will tell his parents that you believe he has taken drugs, and may even get the police involved.

Challenging Questions

You are called to the home of an older man whose neighbours saw him walking around his house and garden late in the evening in his underwear, seeming confused. When you arrive, he does not answer his open front door. You walk in, calling his name, and take note of some small insulin syringes lying on the kitchen counter. You find him standing in the garden, looking confused. When you introduce yourself and question him, he says he has no idea why he's in the garden and had no idea he wasn't dressed. You note that he is also wearing a medical identification bracelet, but it does not have a condition listed on it. He asks you at least four times who you are, and why you're there. You ask him how he's feeling; he says he's fine. You ask him about his medical history, asking specifically if he is diabetic. He tells you he is not. But you know from neighbours that he lives alone. He is extremely confused and irrational.

8. **Do you listen to your patient's answers and put faith into them, assuming he knows what he is talking about, and try to assess and diagnose him based on that information? Or do you take into account his behaviour and what you have seen (insulin syringes, medical identification bracelet), heard, and observed?**

9. **If the patient in this scenario were naked and began saying inappropriate things to your young female partner, how would you (and your partner) handle it?**

■ Points to Ponder

You are sent to a "two-vehicle crash that occurred at a slow speed; minor or no injuries reported by bystander".

How should you prioritise this call?

Issues: Preparation, Priorities, Response Time to Scene.

16 Documentation and Communications

Objectives

Cognitive

- Identify the importance of communications when providing prehospital care.
- Identify the role of verbal, written, and electronic communications in the provision of prehospital care.
- Describe the phases of communications necessary to complete a typical ambulance service event.
- Identify the importance of proper terminology when communicating during an ambulance service event.
- Identify the importance of proper verbal communications during an ambulance service event.
- List factors that impede effective verbal communications.
- List factors which enhance verbal communications.
- Identify the importance of proper written communications during an ambulance service event.
- List factors which impede effective written communications.
- List factors which enhance written communications.
- Recognise the legal status of written communications related to an ambulance service event.
- State the importance of data collection during an ambulance service event.
- Identify technology used to collect and exchange patient and/or scene information electronically.
- Recognise the legal status of patient medical information exchanged electronically.
- Identify the components of the local ambulance service communications system and describe their function and use.
- Identify and differentiate among the following communications systems:
  - Simplex
  - Multiplex
  - Duplex
  - Trunked
  - Digital communications
  - Mobile telephone
  - Facsimile
  - Computer
- Describe how an emergency medical dispatcher functions as an integral part of the emergency medical team.
- List appropriate information to be gathered by the emergency medical dispatcher.
- Identify the role of emergency medical dispatch in a typical ambulance service event.
- Identify the importance of pre-arrival instructions in a typical ambulance service event.
- Describe the purpose of verbal communication of patient information to the hospital.
- Organise a list of patient assessment information in the correct order for electronic transmission to medical direction according to the format used locally.
- Identify the general principles regarding the importance of ambulance service documentation and ways in which documents are used.

- Identify and use medical terminology correctly.
- Recite appropriate and accurate medical abbreviations and acronyms.
- Record all pertinent administrative information.
- Analyse the documentation for accuracy and completeness, including spelling.
- Identify and eliminate extraneous or nonprofessional information.
- Describe the differences between subjective and objective elements of documentation.
- Evaluate a finished document for errors and omissions.
- Evaluate a finished document for proper use and spelling of abbreviations and acronyms.
- Evaluate the confidential nature of a patient clinical record.
- Describe the potential consequences of illegible, incomplete, or inaccurate documentation.
- Describe the special considerations concerning patient refusal of transport.
- Record pertinent information using a consistent narrative format.
- Explain how to properly record direct patient or bystander comments.
- Describe the special considerations concerning major incident documentation.
- Apply the principles of documentation to computer charting, as access to this technology becomes available.
- Identify and record the pertinent, reportable clinical data of each patient interaction.
- Note and record "pertinent negative" clinical findings.
- Correct errors and omissions, using proper procedures as defined under local guidelines.
- Revise documents, when necessary, using locally approved procedures.
- Assume responsibility for self-assessment of all documentation.
- Demonstrate proper completion of an ambulance service event record used locally.

Affective

- Show appreciation for proper terminology when describing a patient or patient condition.
- Advocate among peers the relevance and importance of properly completed documentation.
- Resolve the common negative attitudes toward the task of documentation.

Psychomotor

- Demonstrate the ability to use the local dispatch communications system.
- Demonstrate the ability to use a radio.
- Demonstrate the ability to use the biotelemetry equipment used locally.

Introduction

In ambulance service communication, relaying information from one person to another becomes extremely urgent in the short time that you will have to care for a patient. That information needs to move rapidly, efficiently, and effectively. As a paramedic, you must be able to effectively communicate verbally and in writing with many other people.

You need to know what constitutes an ambulance service communications system, who needs to be able to talk with whom, what technical resources are available to you to make those conversations possible, and what you can do to make communications as efficient as possible. You also need to understand the crucial role of the emergency medical dispatcher (EMD) in facilitating all phases of ambulance service communications. You need to know how to organise patient information into a brief, orderly verbal report that can be transmitted by radio or by telephone.

Written communication in the form of reports or documentation is as vital to your patient care as following clinical guidelines. Learning to write effectively and accurately with only the absolutely necessary subjective information is an important paramedic skill. Subjective information includes the symptoms patients describe—the degree of pain, for example. Objective information includes the measurable signs that you observe and record, such as blood pressure. You must record subjective *and* objective information and the details of patient care for every call in a written or computer-based report, and in some cases, both. This report needs to be complete, accurate, and legible because it can provide the basis of defence in legal proceedings and is of vital importance to your trust for many other reasons as well, including facilitation of quality care and continuity. Your written report should "paint a picture" of the entire call that is clear and accurate to the reader.

Phases of Communication

Communication during an emergency call has several phases that are essential to appropriate patient care and transportation. You will be exchanging information with many people, including the patient, bystanders with valuable information, the patient's family, the receiving hospital staff, your ambulance control, police officers, and other members of the ambulance service team. One paramount responsibility in an emergency is communication with your colleague. Staying in constant touch will keep each of you on top of your responsibilities and working effectively as a team while caring for your patient.

Each phase of the communication process requires using terminology understood by the people you are communicating with. Patients might need you to explain their medical condition in terms they know and understand. When you relay information to the receiving hospital, you can use the medical terminology you have learned to make your radio report clear. The old saying, "When in Rome, do as the Romans do", applies in the ambulance service. Using medical terminology and avoiding slang terms shows your professionalism and respect for everyone you work with.

Although you might not think of yourself as a "number-crunching" scholar, collecting information and data is essential to prehospital care. You can help gather the data, analyse it, and determine what changes are necessary by writing clear, accurate, and easy-to-read reports. Although data collection

You are the Paramedic Part 1

It is a beautiful summer day when you and your partner receive a call to a person who has fallen off their bike outside 52 Lanyon Road. On arrival, you are greeted by a member of the public who tells you that during his usual afternoon walk he found a woman lying next to the road. He said he was worried she had been hit by a car or was otherwise injured, so he didn't move her and immediately called 999.

You find a 45-year-old woman lying on the ground and unresponsive. Her bike is lying on top of her, and she is wearing a helmet, bike shorts, and a T-shirt.

Initial Assessment	Recording Time: 0 Minutes
Appearance	Pale, obviously perspiring
Level of consciousness	U (Unresponsive)
Airway	Open; secretions present
Breathing	Noisy breathing present
Circulation	Rapid radial pulse present

1. Why did the call taker supply very little information for this call?
2. What immediate challenges do you foresee regarding this call?
3. How does the initial information you're given from EMDs, family, bystanders, or other responders impact your decisions regarding patient care?

may seem time-consuming, ensure that the information you record and report to your ambulance service is accurate for data collection and reporting purposes. Even in cases of major incidents (MIs), collecting data is especially essential for determining patient care totals, severity of injuries, outcomes, and mass care procedures.

Who Needs to Communicate With Whom?

For the ambulance service system to work, a number of people have to be able to contact a number of other people. Let's follow an emergency call from its inception to its conclusion to see who needs to reach whom.

The first stage of the ambulance service response is notification, that is, someone has to tell the ambulance service that an emergency exists. Usually notification is carried out by telephone or mobile phone, and the person requesting help communicates with the call taker. A universal emergency telephone number—999 in the United Kingdom—and the availability of telephones and mobile phones in most places has greatly helped notification.

The next step is dispatch, communicating from the emergency communications centre with the responding paramedic team. The person who directs that crew to the scene of the emergency is called the emergency medical dispatcher (EMD) **Figure 16-1 ▾** . Dispatch may be accomplished by telephone, pager, fax, or two-way radio that may include push-to-talk technology. Push-to-talk devices can include mobile phones or walkie-talkies known as half-duplex devices. These allow the voice to be transmitted when a button is pushed and allow the listener to hear if the button is released. Most telecommunications equipment today uses digital technology rather than direct or analogue transmission and radio tubes. Digital technology offers many advantages in terms of speed, privacy, programmability, and the global positioning system, or GPS. Many communication centres use computer-aided dispatch systems, automated computer systems that process the information received and assist EMDs with multiple functions and tasks.

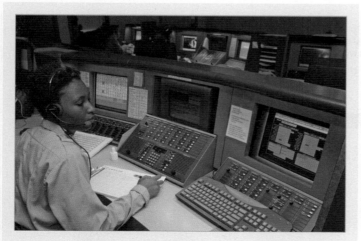

Figure 16-1 The emergency medical dispatcher is aware of the location of all resources and dispatches the nearest ambulance to an incident.

Your EMD may update you en route with further information, such as the patient's current condition or relevant scene information. For example, if the patient has been assaulted with a weapon, you will need to ensure that the scene is safe and perhaps even wait for police attendance before approaching the patient's location.

Once on scene, it may be necessary to contact the EMD for additional resources, such as ambulances or fire service and police attendance. When preparing to leave, consider whether you need to alert the receiving hospital. If you do, make sure that you have the relevant patient information ready beforehand. The mnemonic ASHICE is commonly used to organise this information:

- **Age**—the patient's age
- **Sex**—male or female
- **History**—briefly what happened
- **Injuries/Illness**—that are currently affecting the patient.
- **Condition**—the patient's vital signs such as blood pressure, heart rate, respiratory rate, oxygen saturation and GCS. Also include any treatment such as drugs you have administered.
- **Estimated time of arrival** at the receiving hospital.

This needs to be concise but contain enough information to enable the receiving hospital to prepare for your arrival.

▌Components of an Ambulance Service Communications System

Even though the digital revolution has improved communications, most ambulance service communications systems today still use radios, so you need to learn about what radio signals are and what equipment is available for sending and receiving radio signals.

Radio Communications and Telemetry

Radio transmits signals by electromagnetic waves. Remember, energy can be emitted in the form of waves or particles. When energy is emitted in the form of waves, the energy can be characterised by the length of the waves it produces. Energy of a relatively long wavelength produces audible sound; energy of shorter wavelength is in the infrared light spectrum. Between sound and infrared light are the wavelengths for radio transmission. Radio wavelengths are used for tuning by adjusting your radio to the proper frequency—how frequently the wave recurs in a given time (usually 1 second). Short wavelengths are repeated more often—with higher frequency—than longer wavelengths. Radio frequencies are designated by their cycles per second, or hertz (Hz) (named after the man who first described the propagation of electromagnetic waves). The following abbreviations are commonly used:

- hertz (Hz)—cycles per second
- kilohertz (kHz)—1,000 cycles per second
- megahertz (MHz)—1 million cycles per second
- gigahertz (GHz)—1 billion cycles per second

Radio waves are confined to the part of the electromagnetic frequency spectrum extending from 3 kHz to about 3,000 GHz. A normal voice channel requires a minimum of 3 kHz. Frequency bands are portions of the radio frequency spectrum assigned for specific uses. The most commonly used bands for medical communications are the very high frequency (VHF) band and the ultrahigh frequency (UHF) band. The VHF band extends from roughly 30 to 175 MHz and has been arbitrarily divided into a low band (30 to 50 MHz) and a high band (150 to 175 MHz). The low-band frequencies may have ranges up to 3,200 kilometres, but are unpredictable because changes in ionospheric conditions may cause "skip interference", with patchy losses in communication. The high-band frequencies are almost wholly free of skip interference, but at a price—a much shorter transmission range. The most commonly used of the VHF high-band frequencies for emergency medical purposes are in the 150 to 160 MHz range. The UHF band extends from 300 to 3,000 MHz, with most medical communications occurring around 450 to 470 MHz. At these frequencies, communications are entirely free of skip interference and have minimal noise (signal distortion). The UHF band has better penetration in dense metropolitan areas, and UHF reception is usually quite adequate inside buildings. The UHF band, however, has a shorter range than the VHF band, and energy at UHF is more readily absorbed by rain and environmental objects, such as trees and undergrowth.

Radios that operate at 800 MHz are common in ambulance service systems. This frequency offers excellent penetration of buildings and has minimal interference and reduced channel noise. Because of this, it works quite well in urban areas; 800 MHz also allows for trunking, in which multiple agencies or systems can share frequencies. An 800-MHz radio can also be linked to a computer system to transmit voiceless communications. The use of trunked systems has allowed the EMD to reprogramme the radios so that agencies that do not routinely talk to each other can easily do so at the scene of an MI, a rescue, a hazardous materials incident, or other special operations.

Biotelemetry

Biotelemetry (usually called simply telemetry) is the capability of measuring vital life signs and transmitting them to a distant terminal. Biotelemetry started out with ECGs but often is used for other measurements. Telemetry is even used to send the pulse and respiratory rate of astronauts from space to a receiving station on earth.

The term *biotelemetry* in emergency medical care is usually shortened to *telemetry*. Most often, telemetry is a short way of saying you are transmitting an ECG signal from your patient to a distant receiving station. The standard ECG is composed of low-frequency signals (100 Hz or less), which would be filtered out by a voice communications system. To make sure voice communication doesn't filter the ECG out, the ECG signal must be encoded if it is to be sent over the same radio channels used to transmit voice. The ECG signal is encoded by using a reference audio tone, for example at 1,000 Hz,

which is made to vary with the voltage generated by the electric events in the heart. The reference tone, or calibration, of a varying 1,000-Hz tone is used to modulate the frequency of the transmitter to ensure that all signals are being transmitted. When the ECG signal is received at the distant terminal at the receiving hospital, it is amplified and decoded to produce a voltage that is an exact replica of the original. That voltage is then converted to the graphic plot seen on the oscilloscope or printout.

ECG telemetry over UHF frequencies is confined to one lead of a 12-lead ECG, so it can be used to interpret cardiac rhythms. For a more complete diagnosis of an ECG, such as in the case of examining the ECG of a patient with suspected acute coronary syndrome, one must examine all 12 leads of the ECG. Some ambulance services use facsimile technology to allow transmission of ECGs, including 12-lead ECGs, to receiving hospitals before the arrival of the ambulance at the hospital.

Distortion of the ECG signal by extraneous spikes and waves is known as noise and may arise from a variety of sources:

- Muscle tremor
- Loose ECG electrodes
- Sources of 60-cycle alternating current (AC), such as transformers, power lines, and electric equipment
- Attenuation (reduction) of transmitter power, caused by weak batteries or transmission beyond the range of the transmitter

In the past several years, as paramedics have become more and more skilled in dysrhythmia recognition, the trend has been to make less and less use of ECG telemetry; rather, most systems rely solely on the paramedic's assessment of the patient's cardiac rhythm and rarely require confirmation of the assessment by a doctor. Just as ECG telemetry seemed headed for the fate of the horse-drawn ambulance, however, two developments occurred to bring about a reassessment of prehospital ECG telemetry. First, conclusive research on the use of fibrinolytic agents indicated that the earlier the agents were given during an acute myocardial infarction, the better the chances of myocardial reperfusion. Second, mobile telephone and facsimile technology made it possible to transmit a 12-lead ECG from a moving ambulance to a hospital and, therefore, to diagnose myocardial infarction before the patient reaches the hospital. At the least, such early diagnosis enables the hospital to gear up for administration of fibrinolytic therapy immediately as the patient arrives; and in some ambulance service systems, the fibrinolytics are actually administered in the prehospital setting. Because technology can facilitate assessment and treatment in the prehospital setting, it is probable that telemetry in one form or another will remain a part of emergency care for some time. Information other than ECGs may also be transmitted to the receiving hospital before the patient arrives. Because advances in technology are occurring rapidly, ambulance service systems must keep up with the technology that will allow better methods for communication of patient information.

Mobile Telephones

Mobile telephones are becoming more common in ambulance service communications systems. These telephones are simply low-power portable radios that communicate through a series of interconnected repeater stations called "cells". Cells are linked by a sophisticated computer system and connected to the telephone network. Mobile telephones are also popular with other public safety agencies, particularly as more cell sites are constructed in rural areas.

Mobile phones have advantages that radio does not: (1) The public is encouraged to make use of the free service for 999 or other emergency numbers. (2) Mobile phone technology incorporates GPS to let emergency responders know where the patient is.

The public is often able to call 999 or other emergency numbers on a mobile telephone free of charge. However, this easy access may result in overloading and jamming of mobile systems in MCI and disaster situations, and you should have a backup communications plan in your service to circumvent these overloads.

Modes of Radio Operation

Assigned radio frequencies may be used in a variety of systems. In a simplex system, portable units can transmit only in one mode (voice or telemetry) or receive (voice) at any given time. A simplex system requires only a single radio frequency. A network that uses two different frequencies at the same time, to permit simultaneous transmission and reception (like a tele-phone), is referred to as duplex. Another alternative is to combine, or multiplex, two or more signals—such as the paramedic's voice and the patient's ECG—for simultaneous transmission on one frequency.

Building Blocks of a Communications System

Although ambulance service communications systems vary considerably, most systems serving moderate to large populations are constructed of the following components.

Base Stations

The base station is a collection of radio equipment consisting, at minimum, of a transmitter, receiver, and aerial. The base station serves as a dispatch and coordination area and ideally should be in contact with all other elements of the system. Base stations generally use relatively high power output (45 to 275 W).

The base station must be equipped with an aerial mast sited in suitable terrain, preferably on a hill or high building, close to the base. The aerial system has a vital part in transmission and reception efficiency.

Mobile Transmitter/Receivers (Transceivers)

A mobile transmitter/receiver, or mobile transceiver, is a two-way radio mounted in a vehicle. Mobile transmitter/receivers come in a variety of power ranges, and the power output largely determines the distance over which the signal can be effectively transmitted. A transmitter in the 7.5 W range, for example, will transmit for distances of 10 to 12 miles over slightly hilly terrain. Transmission distances are greater over water or flat terrain

You are the Paramedic Part 2

You see that additional assistance will be required to extricate the patient from under her bike, and you request it. Another crew is dispatched from a nearby ambulance station. You and your partner err on the side of caution and initiate spinal precautions. Your partner controls the patient's cervical spine while you manage the airway.

The crew are soon on scene and extricate the patient and place her on the longboard. You next insert an intravenous (IV) line and perform a blood glucose check. No trauma is noted beyond a few minor abrasions to her right arm, shoulder, and leg.

Vital Signs	Recording Time: 5 Minutes
Level of consciousness	Unresponsive, with a Glasgow Coma Scale score of 5
Skin	Pale, cool, and perspiring
Pulse	128 beats/min, strong and regular
Blood pressure	132/86 mm Hg
Respirations	22 breaths/min
SpO_2	92% ambient air

4. How did this call change from dispatch to arrival?
5. Given her level of consciousness, what concerns do you have regarding her airway?
6. What are your top priorities at the moment?

and reduced in mountainous areas or where there are many tall buildings. Mobile transmitters with higher outputs have proportionally greater transmission ranges. Today, the typical mobile transmitter operates at between 20 and 50 W.

Portable Transmitter/Receivers

Portable, hand-held radios are useful when paramedics must work at a distance from their vehicle but need to stay in communication with the base or with one another (Figure 16-2 ▾).

Repeaters

A repeater is a miniature base station used to extend the transmitting and receiving range of a telemetry or voice communications system (Figure 16-3 ▸). Repeaters may be stationary in one location (fixed repeaters) or carried in emergency vehicles (mobile repeaters). A repeater picks up a weak signal and retransmits it at a higher power on another frequency, so it extends the range of low-power portables and allows more members of the system to hear one another.

Remote Consoles

A remote console, usually located in the accident and emergency (A&E) department, is a terminal that receives transmissions of telemetry and voice from the field and transmits messages back, usually through the base station. Remote consoles are connected to the base station by dedicated telephone lines, microwave, or radio. They contain an amplifier and speaker for incoming voice reception, a decoder for translating the telemetry signal into an oscilloscope tracing or printout, and a microphone for voice transmission.

Backup Communications Systems

In addition to radio communications, most systems use landline (telephone) backup to link various fixed components of the system, such as hospitals, public safety services, and poison control. Telephones may also be patched into radio transmissions through the base station, enabling, for example, communication between paramedics using radios in the field and the A&E staff. Finally, as mentioned earlier, mobile telephones are becoming an increasingly important part of ambulance service communications, overcoming many of the problems of overcrowded ambulance service radio frequencies. Mobile phones are cheaper than radios and generally give a much clearer signal. Furthermore, they enable a paramedic in the field to communicate with anyone who has a telephone—the patient's family GP, an injured child's parent, an expert in another part of the country who can advise on a hazardous materials situation. The possibilities are as varied as the listings in the telephone directory.

Communicating by Radio

The effectiveness of an ambulance service communications network depends on the technical hardware and on the people who use it. Communicating effectively by radio under emergency conditions requires skill and experience. Some paramedics "freeze" at the microphone, whereas others find themselves acting out their latent ambitions as disc jockeys with unlimited streams of patter. Neither behaviour is appropriate or useful. Effective radio communication in the ambulance service requires knowledge of the rules that govern the communications and an understanding of conventions for transmitting medical information by radio. It is not complicated if you bear in mind that the purpose of talking on the radio is to transmit pertinent information. Keep communications simple, brief, and direct.

You should practice effective communications skills and be familiar with all of the various methods of communication that will be required through your radio. As part of your job, you

Notes from Nancy
The purpose of talking on the radio is to transmit pertinent information.

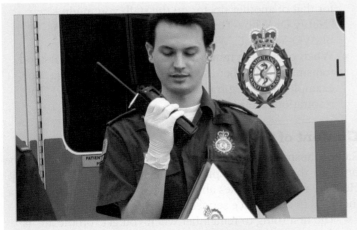
Figure 16-2 A portable radio is essential if you need to communicate with the EMD when you are away from the ambulance.

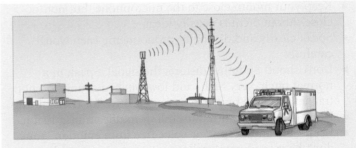
Figure 16-3 A message is sent from the control centre by a landline to the transmitter. The radio carrier wave is picked up by the repeater for rebroadcast to outlying units. Return radio traffic is picked up by the repeater and rebroadcast to the control centre.

will need to demonstrate how to communicate effectively with your EMD for the call, from call receipt to call end. In addition, you must be able to effectively communicate with the receiving hospital and deliver a precise and direct radio report in an organised and systematic manner.

Clarity of Transmission

The basic model of communication, whether by radio, intercom, telephone, or face-to-face involves a *sender,* a clear message, a *receiver,* and a *feedback loop* to ensure that the exact message that was sent is received and interpreted properly by the receiver. The purpose of communications equipment is to permit communication. That sounds obvious, yet it is often forgotten. Simply blurting something into a microphone is not communicating. For communication to occur, someone at the other end of the radio has to be able to hear and understand what you say. The first principle of communicating by radio is clarity.

A number of guidelines can help you improve the clarity of transmissions:

- Before you begin to transmit, listen to make sure the channel is clear. If another radio transmission is in progress, wait until the parties have finished transmitting before you try to get on the air. Cutting in on someone else's transmission will only ensure that neither of you will be adequately heard.
- Once the channel is quiet, press the transmit key for at least 1 second before you start speaking to ensure that the beginning of your message is not lost.
- Start your transmission with the identifying information: give the number or the name of the unit being called first, then your own identification (for example, "Control, this is BRAVO YANKEE 1, over"). That way, the unit being called is alerted immediately and will be listening when you give your own identification, so they can reply at once, "Go ahead, BRAVO YANKEE 1". If you do say, for example, "BRAVO YANKEE 1 calling control", the recipients might listen only when you've mentioned their identification and, therefore, will miss your identification. "St. Wilfred's Hospital. What vehicle is calling"? That extra transmission is a waste of time.
- Keep your mouth close to the microphone, but not too close. About 5 cm is usually ideal.
- Speak clearly and distinctly, pronouncing each word carefully.
- Don't shout! Shouting distorts the signal. Speak in a normal pitch; very high- and low-pitched sounds do not transmit well. Whispering is not effective for transmitting.
- Don't talk with your mouth full. It muffles transmission.
- Keep calm and keep your voice free from emotion. You don't have to imitate a talking computer; a normal conversational tone is fine. Just keep your voice and mind free of panic, anger, excitement, and other feelings that can distort your transmission and your judgement.

	Table 16-1		International Phonetic Alphabet		
A	Alpha	**J**	Juliet	**S**	Sierra
B	Bravo	**K**	Kilo	**T**	Tango
C	Charlie	**L**	Lima	**U**	Uniform
D	Delta	**M**	Mike	**V**	Victor
E	Echo	**N**	November	**W**	Whisky
F	Foxtrot	**O**	Oscar	**X**	X-ray
G	Golf	**P**	Papa	**Y**	Yankee
H	Hotel	**Q**	Quebec	**Z**	Zulu (or Zebra)
I	India	**R**	Romeo		

- Keep your transmissions brief. Air time is precious, and emergency medical frequencies are not the place for long philosophical dialogues. Try having your radio reports taped at some point to critique your own transmissions and perfect your style.

Notes from Nancy
Anyone may be listening!

- If you have a long message to transmit, break up the message into 30-second segments, checking at the end of each segment to determine whether it was received and understood.
- Don't waste air time with unnecessary phrases, such as "be advised". Also bear in mind that courtesy is taken for granted; there is no need to use air time for social graces such as "please", "thank you", and "how nice to hear your voice".
- When speaking a word or name that might be misunderstood, spell it out, using the international phonetic alphabet Table 16-1 ▲ or a similar system. Suppose, for example, you are asking the EMD to notify the patient's family doctor whose name might be mistaken for that of another doctor on the staff; you might say, "Notify Dr Wilby. That's Dr WHISKY-INDIA-LIMA-BRAVO-YANKEE, Wilby".
- When presenting numbers that might be misunderstood, transmit the number as a whole, then digit by digit. For example, if the respirations are 16, you would say, "The respirations are sixteen, that is, one-six".

Content of Transmissions

Radio transmissions for emergency medical services should be brief, to the point, and professional in tone Figure 16-4 ▶. Here are some guidelines about what should and should not be included in ambulance service radio communications:

- The first thing to remember when you get "on the air" is that your words are, quite literally, in the air, floating around for anyone to hear. Remember, anyone may be listening Figure 16-5 ▶.

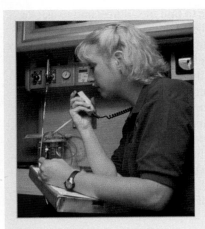

Figure 16-4 The patient report should be given in an objective, accurate, professional manner.

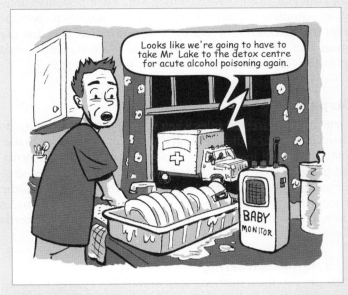

Figure 16-5

The medical staff at the local A&E department, a patient signing in at the front desk of another A&E department, a 12-year-old radio buff playing with his scanner at home . . . any of them may be listening with great attention to your transmission. Therefore, it is essential to protect the privacy of the patient at all times. Do not use the patient's name on the air, and do not transmit personal information about the patient. Certain types of cases, such as rape or psychiatric problems, confidential communicable disease history (such as HIV status), are best identified on the air by an established code or given in face-to-face communications when you arrive in the A&E.

Don't assume that your mobile telephone offers you protected conversations. There are scanners on the market that can tune into the local mobile frequencies. So don't say anything on the radio or the mobile phone that you don't want everyone in town to hear.

- Be impersonal. Use "we", not "I", to refer to yourself, and use proper names and titles ("Dr York", not "Billy") to refer to others when necessary.
- Don't try to be a comedian or a critic. There is no place for unprofessional behaviour, sarcasm, or other poor conduct on emergency medical radio frequencies.
- Don't use profane language on the air. Aside from the reflection on your professional character, you may face disciplinary action.
- Use professional language, but don't show off. Once again, remember that the object of the exercise is to communicate information, not to stun your listener into awe and admiration. Using proper medical terminology is advisable when done correctly.
- Avoid using words that are difficult to hear. The word "yes", for example, is easily lost in transmission; use "affirmative" instead. Similarly, use "negative" instead of "no".
- Use standard formats agreed on by your ambulance service for transmission of information. The patient's history, for example, should always be presented in the same order. When the listeners know what they are listening for, they are less likely to miss parts of the transmission.
- When you finish transmitting, obtain confirmation that the transmission was received. When you receive instructions by radio from the EMD, echo the order back to make certain you have understood it correctly.
- Question any orders you did not hear clearly or did not understand.

- Use ambulance service frequencies only for emergency medical communications.

Codes

Some ambulance services still use radio codes; most do not. Codes were used for several reasons:

- To maintain security of communication
- To keep air time as brief as possible
- To diminish the likelihood of misunderstanding or noise
- To prevent the patient, family, and bystanders from understanding what is being said

The last-mentioned reason is particularly important when the information you need to convey to the EMD or doctor could alarm the patient. Suppose that you want to tell the doctor that your patient is probably the victim of child abuse, and the parents are travelling in the ambulance. It is preferable that the family are not privy to that assessment because they may stop being cooperative and/or become aggressive. In fact, it is best not to be sitting right next to the patient when transmitting your report to the emergency department.

For a code to be of any use, everyone using the radio must know the meaning of the code words. When codes are used, therefore, they should be simple and standardised within a given region, and a copy of the code should be posted at every radio terminal.

When and if you use codes, remember that one of their main purposes is to shorten air time.

Whenever codes are used, they should be kept simple and reserved for cases in

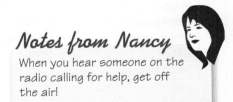

Notes from Nancy

When you hear someone on the radio calling for help, get off the air!

which they are really needed. During MIs, when personnel unfamiliar with the codes may be staffing radios and when everyone is apt to be anxious, it is usually best to abandon codes and use words that all understand. Most services use standard terms rather than codes for regular day-to-day operations as well.

Dispatching

There are two essential roles when it comes to dispatching, the emergency medical dispatcher and the call taker. The call taker obtains as much information as possible about the emergency and provides the caller with whatever advice may be needed to manage the situation until help arrives. The EMD directs the appropriate vehicle to the scene, monitors and coordinates communication with the scene and maintains accurate records of events.

Information Gathering

There are two main methods used in the UK to gather information from the caller and prioritise the call. These are the Advanced Medical Priority Dispatching System (AMPDS) and Criterion Based Dispatching system (CBD). When a call for the ambulance service comes in, the call taker will elicit the following information as a minimum:

- The exact location of the patient (s), including the street name and number; the proper geographic designation (such as whether the street is Green Street or Green Close) and the name of the community (adjacent towns may have streets by the same name). If the call comes from a rural area, the call taker should try to establish landmarks (such as the nearest pub, church, or shop).
- The telephone number (call-back number) of the caller, in case the call is disconnected or there is a need to phone the caller back for more information. It is not uncommon for

paramedics not to be able to find the address and to ask for help from the original caller. Asking for the caller's telephone number also helps discourage nuisance calls to the ambulance service because hoax callers are reluctant to supply their phone numbers. Finally, the caller's telephone exchange may help to pinpoint his or her location if the caller is unfamiliar with the region, as is often the case of a traveller calling from the road. In services equipped with an enhanced 999 system, a lot of the information mentioned—such as the phone number and location of the caller—is recorded automatically through sophisticated telephone technology, and the EMD need only confirm the information on the screen.

- The caller's perception of the nature of his or her or the patient's problem.
- Specific information concerning the patient's condition that will help evaluate the urgency of the situation and the call taker's need to provide the caller with prearrival instructions by phone. The call taker should ask specifically:
  - Is the patient conscious?
  - If not, is the patient breathing?
  - Is the patient bleeding badly?
- If the emergency is a motor vehicle collision, further important information should be obtained:
  - The kinds of vehicles involved (that is, cars, lorries, motorcycles, buses). If a lorry is involved, is there any indication of the cargo it is carrying? A lorry carrying dynamite requires a different approach from one carrying bananas!
  - The number of people injured and an estimate of the extent of injuries. This information will enable the EMD to estimate the magnitude of the problem.
  - Apparent hazards at the scene, such as heavy traffic, fallen power lines, fire, spilled chemicals, and peculiar odours.

You are the Paramedic Part 3

The glucometer reads "1.6". You immediately tell your partner, who draws up a bolus of glucose 10%. As you give the glucose, your patient's level of consciousness begins to improve. She remains somewhat confused but can provide her name and states that she has type 2 diabetes. You provide supplemental oxygen at 15 l/min via nonrebreathing mask, and her ECG indicates sinus tachycardia.

Reassessment	Recording Time: 10 Minutes
Level of consciousness	Alert, with a Glasgow Coma Scale score of 14
Skin	Pale, warm, slightly perspiring
Pulse	120 beats/min, strong and regular
Blood pressure	128/86 mm Hg
Respirations	20 breaths/min
SpO_2	95%
Blood glucose	1.6 mmol/l

7. As your patient's level of consciousness improves, what issues do you foresee?
8. How does your ability to communicate effectively impact upon patient care?

Information about such hazards enables the EMD to contact other agencies that may have to be involved, such as the electricity board to take care of fallen wires or a highways agency to deal with spilled fuel. In most modern communication centres, the EMD has visual prompts with the key questions to ask on the computer screen.

Dispatch

As soon as the address and phone number is confirmed, a vehicle will be dispatched if available. The EMD is responsible for ensuring that the appropriate vehicle is dispatched to the caller, taking into account the type of incident. While this is taking place, the call taker will continue to question the caller and then the EMD can update the crew while en route if necessary. This is important for two reasons:

- So that you may know if the response requires travel under emergency conditions, using emergency warning devices
- So that while en route you may anticipate and prepare for tasks to be performed at the scene: assembling the equipment to deliver a baby or transmitting cardiac information to the receiving hospital

Advice to the Caller

If the call taker suspects your patient has a life-threatening emergency, that call taker should provide instructions to the caller in very simple terms about emergency care techniques (such as airway maintenance, Heimlich manoeuvre, CPR, haemorrhage control). The caller is likely to be in an agitated state, so instructions must be clear and simple.

Ongoing Communications With the Field

It is important for your EMD to monitor the communications of the ambulance and to be aware of what is occurring in the prehospital environment. Your EMD must coordinate communications between the ambulance and the hospital and contact any other agencies (such as fire and police) whose presence may be required at the scene. The EMD should also receive and record communications from you when you are in the field regarding the following:

- The time the ambulance departed for the scene
- The time the ambulance arrived at the scene
- The time the crew made contact with the patient
- The time the ambulance left the scene
- The time the ambulance arrived at the hospital
- The time the ambulance went back in service

Much of this information is now collected electronically. The roles of the EMD are summarised in **Table 16-2**.

Documenting Times

In general, it is routine practice to use standard military time when documenting times for calls. Most EMDs use this format when providing times over the radio as well.

Factors That May Affect Communications

In communication, many things may go wrong, and not all of them are equipment failures. You need to be prepared for such situations. Radio communication is very technical and technology-driven. At times, systems may have problems, such as damage to a radio mast, computer crashes, and audio problems, and you may have to adapt to necessary changes. Follow your local guidelines regarding radio failure.

You have learned how important communication skills are in previous chapters. (Chapter 10 includes a detailed discussion on communication skills.) You can be faced with a number of problems, including patients who do not speak your primary language or patients with communication disorders. Ask "those in the know" about telephone interpreters, people on your service who speak more than one language, and learn what you can do before you see your patients. Review your patient assessment skills for patients with impaired hearing.

Documentation

What do you call the report in your trust setting? Here is a list of different terms used to describe the written documentation or report for calls:

- Patient Clinical Record (PCR)

Documentation and Communication

Cultural diversity is found in prehospital care every day. If you are not familiar with the various cultures present in your community, consider a training session in which leaders from various cultural organisations in your community are invited to meet members of your organisation. This could open up dialogue for both groups and could create an avenue for growth and development to reduce communication barriers in ambulance service calls. In addition, training members of your ambulance service organisation to speak other languages that are spoken in your area may also be of significant benefit to your community.

Table 16-2	Phases of Dispatch	
Call Taker	**EMD**
Answers telephone promptly. Obtains address of incident, call-back number, perceived problem, patient's name.	Dispatches (first) ambulance.
Gives first aid advice if required. Obtains more information about patient condition. For a road accident, will try to identify the number of vehicles, kinds of vehicles, number of victims.	
Identifies any hazards at the scene.	Notifies responding ambulances of special circumstances. Dispatches additional ambulances as needed. Liaises with other agencies (fire, police, hospitals). Monitors communications from the field. Keeps accurate records of events.

- Prehospital patient report (PPR)
- Patient report form (PRF)

Whatever you call it, do you know and understand the importance of it? The adage, "If you didn't write it down it didn't happen" is very true in the ambulance service. Your written report, most commonly referred to as the PCR, is the only written record of the events that transpired during the call for service. It needs to be one of the most important skills you learn as a paramedic. It will be the legal record for the call and a part of the patient's medical record and the hospital's A&E chart. The PCR provides for a continuum of patient care on arrival at the receiving facility. Time will not allow you to relay all of the information obtained through patient assessment and findings in a radio report or the verbal report on arrival. Your verbal report should be a brief summary of the assessment findings and the event, but your written report should be a more detailed account from the very moment the call began until it concluded. The written report should accurately reflect, or paint a picture, of the events of the call.

Although you may include subjective information from the patient, such as statements from him or her about symptoms, no bias or personal opinions (subjectivity) of yours should be contained within your written report. Poorly written, inappropriately documented PCRs could have adverse implications for patient care and for your career. Omissions or errors in your report could lead to further errors in care. Improper and inadequate reports also could result in litigation, loss of job or registration, a negative reflection on one's reputation as an ambulance clinician, and more.

No matter what your particular writing style, your report should be complete, well-written, legible, professional, and your sole source of information about the call. Your report may also be used in legal proceedings. In some cases, it may be your only defence against a complaint about a call—if you document what happened, you will have solid evidence of your conduct and what transpired on the call. Your memory may not serve you well 3 years from now, but your written report will remain the same. If it is well written, it will jog your memory and should provide a picture of the events of the call to all who read it. As a health care professional, it is important that you use proper spelling, proper grammar, and accurate terminology in your report. Do not attempt to use medical terms and abbreviations if you do not fully understand their meaning. Never make up your own abbreviations because they will only be meaningful to you and could confuse others. Doing so could result in patient care errors and leave your professional character at stake if the report is called into question.

In addition, you should write every PCR as if your medical director were reading it, such as in a quality assurance review. Your report is the only record (unless your medical director was on the call with you) of why you performed a certain procedure or why you administered a particular medication to a patient. Reports that your medical director and trust can read and understand will help them evaluate your performance accurately.

On occasion, ambulance service reports may be requested for medical audits and other educational settings. Run incident reviews, or sessions in which peers and other medical professionals review care reports for adherence to clinical guidelines, quality assurance, and quality monitoring, may occur. Your written and computer-based reports may be used to calculate the number of times you have performed a specific skill, such as medication administration or endotracheal intubation. Always accurately document all skills attempted and performed with patient care.

You are the Paramedic Part 4

As your patient becomes alert and oriented, she tells you that she was riding her bike home from work when she became shaky. She says that she thought she had some chocolate in her backpack but was unable to find it. She decided to continue home, and the next thing she remembered she was lying on the ground surrounded by strangers.

Reassessment	Recording Time: 15 Minutes
Level of consciousness	Alert, with a Glasgow Coma Scale score of 15
Skin	Pale, warm, slightly perspiring
Pulse	110 beats/min, strong and regular
Blood pressure	126/82 mm Hg
Respirations	18 breaths/min
SpO_2	98%
Blood glucose	6.7 mmol/l

9. How do body language and tone of voice communicate as much or more than words?
10. How does total patient care enter into this scenario?
11. What is the purpose of documentation?
12. Who is your documentation audience?

Do you know if the procedures you are performing are making a difference to your patient's outcome? Your careful documentation of procedures is the basis of research and evaluation of their effectiveness. Research is very difficult to do without accurate data and information from your written report.

Medical Terminology

Using medical terminology correctly is essential to ambulance service communications. You should learn the established and accepted medical terms and abbreviations for your ambulance service operations. Some ambulance service systems have specific approved lists of medical abbreviations and terms that must be used.

Medical terminology may seem to be a foreign language. Well, it is! Most terminology comes from the ancient Roman language, Latin. In addition, some common words used in the ambulance service such as "packaging a patient for transport" or "bagging the patient during airway management" might be used. Make sure you know acceptable terms and words used in your trust. An ongoing review of the anatomy and physiology chapter can help you become familiar with medical terminology. Let's take a more in-depth look at commonly used medical terms and their meanings.

Medical Abbreviations

Medical abbreviations can be very useful for documentation purposes, but you must be certain the abbreviations you are using are consistent with approved medical abbreviations in your ambulance service system. Incorrect or inappropriate medical abbreviations can cause confusion and, in the worst cases, could lead to medication and treatment errors. You should learn the approved medical abbreviations for your service area before you use them in a report. Each ambulance service system should have a list of approved medical abbreviations available for use and documentation purposes. Once again, accuracy, neatness, and completeness reflect a professional writing style. Common medical abbreviations are listed in the student workbook and web site for this text. Note that many abbreviations have more than one meaning, so extreme care is needed when using them.

Documenting Incident Times

Keeping good records of time is essential to all ambulance service operations. The role of timekeeper falls to the control centre. You must also keep track of time during your documentation of the incident. You should compare your times with those of the EMD to ensure accuracy and proper timekeeping. Several times are absolutely vital to be kept and documented for accurate report writing.

- **Time of call.** The time when the call for help is placed or requested
- **Time of dispatch.** Time when the ambulance service vehicle is alerted to respond to the call
- **Time of arrival at the scene.** Time when the ambulance service vehicle arrives on scene

- **Time with patient.** Time recorded when patient contact is made (this may not be the same time of arrival, for example, a patient at the top of a block of flats; should include the time it takes to physically get to the patient)
- **Time of medication administration.** Time when medications are administered for adherence to guidelines
- **Time of departure from scene.** Time recorded when the ambulance service vehicle leaves the scene
- **Time of arrival at hospital.** Time when arriving at hospital (if a patient is transported)
- **Time back in service.** Time when the ambulance service vehicle and crew are ready for return to service

Notes from Nancy

Symptoms belong in the history. Signs belong in the physical examination.

General Documentation Considerations

Paramedics must know and understand that ambulance service documentation is a required and necessary element of patient care. Paramedics should pride themselves not only on their patient care skills, but also on their documentation skills.

Documentation of the narrative portion of the PCR should be a detailed segment indicating the elements of the call. It should be written in a format accepted by your trust and should be accurate and complete. Simply writing "followed ACLS guidelines" may not be sufficient documentation for your trust or medical director. Specifics of the call should be recorded such as "the patient was intubated with a 7.5 ETT and ventilatory assistance provided with supplementary oxygen at 15 l/min. ETT placement was confirmed by breath sounds, chest rise, and a tube check, before securing the ETT at the mark of 26 at the teeth. The end-tidal CO_2 detector and pulse oximeter were placed immediately and their readings were: _____ and _____ [Be sure to clarify which is which.]".

Many methods for narrative documentation exist. Your trust or medical director may prefer a specific method to be used when documenting PCRs. Be familiar with the approved methods and all required elements for report writing for your trust. Some examples of narrative writing styles for reports are as follows:

- **Chronological order.** This is telling the narrative in a story format from the time of the initial dispatch until the call was completed. If used regularly, this format allows you to explain the call from start to finish.
- **SOAP method: Subjective, Objective, Assessment, and Plan (for treatment).** Simple and logical method used to document various aspects of the patient care encounter

- **CHARTE method: Chief complaint, History, Assessment, Treatment (Rx), Transport, and Exceptions.** Similar to the SOAP format for report writing but allows you to break the narrative down into logical sections similar to that of your ambulance service assessment
- **Body systems approach.** Documenting each body system from head to toe. This method of report writing may be difficult to apply in prehospital care and may be too time-consuming for paramedics.

Regardless of the style of narrative report writing you and your service agree on, be sure to follow it routinely. Switching from one format to another or attempting to change formats during report writing may lead you to forget certain elements or essential details that should have been included. Proper grammar and spelling are essential when writing reports. You might consider carrying a pocket guide, reference, or medical terminology book in your ambulance to avoid spelling errors.

Notes from Nancy

Always report your findings in the same sequence, regardless of the sequence in which they were actually obtained.

Pertinent negatives should be documented when writing your ambulance service report. This is a record of negative findings that warrant no care or intervention but indicate that a thorough and complete examination and history were performed. For example, "The patient denies any shortness of breath with his chest pain, patient denies any radiation of the chest pain to other parts of the body". This would indicate that you not only obtained the information about the chest pain, but also inquired about shortness of breath and radiation of the pain.

The use of pertinent spoken accounts made by your patient and others on scene may be essential to the continuum of patient care. If you use any spoken accounts made by the patient or others, be sure to indicate who made the statement and place the exact words in quotations. This may include statements about the patient's behaviour, the mechanism of injury, safety-related information such as the use of weapons, information that may be useful to criminal investigators as a part of their investigation, disposition of valuables, admissions of suicidal intentions made by a patient, or any first aid interventions provided by bystanders before the arrival of the ambulance service.

Report Writing

You should also document the use of mutual aid services such as helicopters, specialised rescue teams, and other agencies called in to assist. Unusual occurrences should be documented as well, including having to use the police for securing a patient with restraining devices for safe transport or other situations in which unusual circumstances arise. If you need to summon an additional crew for lifting a heavy patient or if you will have an extended scene time owing to a prolonged extrication, this information should be clearly documented to explain why "something out of the ordinary" occurred.

Elements of a Properly Written Report

Documentation accuracy depends on all information being provided, such as times, narrative information, and checkboxes, and it must be comprehensive and precise. All sections should show that you have completed them, even if a section was not applicable to the call. For example, if your PCR has a section of check boxes for specific information on cardiac arrest calls but the call you are documenting was not a cardiac arrest call, note that on the report in a manner that is approved by your trust. Simply leaving the boxes blank may raise questions about the completeness of the report.

All reports should be legible and written in ink. Black ink should be used to complete the PCR. Handwriting, especially in the narrative portion of the report, needs to be neat and easily read by others. In addition, take great care to not contaminate your written reports with any liquid found in the field. Evidence of your own rehydration activities should not appear on your written report! Place all your completed reports in a secure location agreed on by you and your partner that protects the patient's privacy, until they can be secured in the proper place at your trust or headquarters.

The PCR needs to be timely, even in ambulance service systems where call volume is high. If you respond to multiple calls without accurately completing PCRs before proceeding to the next call, details may be forgotten and important information left out, or worse, inaccurate information may be written. Your trust should allow you a reasonable amount of time to complete your reports, replenish supplies, and clean and disinfect vehicles *before* returning them to service.

All reports should be reviewed by the paramedic who authors them before submitting them to the receiving hospital and to the paramedic's trust. Reviewing for completeness, accuracy, grammar, spelling, and proper use of medical terminology and abbreviations will help ensure a well-written and well-documented report.

Too often, we ignore the importance of report writing and documentation in the ambulance service. Negative sentiments are often associated with report writing, but you should not let them "get to you". Be positive; report writing reflects on the paramedic who authors the report. When you file a complete, well-documented, legible report, you have done the most important part of the completion of your call.

Documenting Patient Care Refusal

Legal aspects of patient care were discussed in Chapter 4, but here we will discuss the necessary documentation in more depth. Refusal of care is one of the most difficult elements of patient care documentation. Competent adult patients have the right to refuse medical care or to consent to treatment. You must know and understand the rights of your patients. You

Prep Kit

■ Ready for Review

- You must be able to communicate rapidly, efficiently, and effectively when responding to a call to fulfill your role as a paramedic.
- The phases of communication include notification, potential prearrival instructions for the caller, dispatch, communication during on-scene care, and communication with the receiving facility while en route.
- The call taker communicates with people who call in an emergency and passes the details to the EMD.
- The EMD identifies the exact location of the patient, the telephone number, the nature of the problem, and specific information about the patient's condition and emergency, such as the types of vehicles involved in a car crash or hazards at the scene.
- The EMD is responsible for monitoring communications with the ambulance, coordinating communication with other agencies, and recording the times when the various phases of the call occurred.
- Call taking requires special training which teaches staff to provide basic medical instructions to emergency callers over the phone. Updates resulting from this prearrival care can be communicated to the ambulance service crew as they are en route.
- Radio is one of the main methods of communication in the ambulance service. The most commonly used bands for medical communications are the very high frequency (VHF) band and ultrahigh frequency (UHF) band. The higher the band, the less interference there is, but the shorter the transmission range.
- Trunking is the ability for multiple agencies or systems to share frequencies. This allows the EMD to reprogramme radios so that agencies which do not normally talk to each other are able to, if necessary, such as in a mass-casualty incident.
- Biotelemetry (often referred to as telemetry) is used to transmit vital life signs to a distant terminal. In the ambulance service it is usually used for transmitting an ECG. This can be useful in diagnosing myocardial infarction and can allow the hospital to prepare to administer fibrinolytic therapy.
- Mobile telephones are becoming more common in ambulance service communications systems. Many newer mobile phones have global positioning systems built in which aide the enhanced 999 operator to determine exactly where the call is being made.
- Systems used for radio transmission include simplex, duplex, and multiplex. Simplex operates on one frequency and only allows transmission to go one way. Duplex operates on two frequencies and allows simultaneous transmission and reception. Multiplex operates on two or more frequencies and allows for more than one transmission simultaneously.
- An ambulance service communications system consists of a base station, mobile and portable transmitters or receivers, a repeater, a remote console, and a landline or backup communications system.
- Keep radio communication simple, brief, and direct. One of the main goals is clarity. Use the international phonetic alphabet to aid transmission of spellings.
- Remember that your words can be heard by anyone who is listening. Keep your communications professional at all times. Do not transmit the patient's name or personal information over the radio.
- Most ambulance systems use plain English in radio communications, but some use radio codes. If your trust uses codes, be sure to learn them.
- When reporting medical information, include the patient's age and sex, chief complaint, brief history, level of consciousness, degree of distress, vital signs, physical findings, ECG findings, and treatment.
- Your written report, or patient clinical record, is the only record of events that transpired during the call and serves as a legal record. It should be complete, well-written, legible, and professional. Proper use of terminology is essential. Learn common medical abbreviations.
- You will need to write a narrative in your patient clinical record. There are many methods, including chronological order, the SOAP method, the CHARTE method, and the body systems approach. Learn the method used by your system.
- The patient care report needs to be filled out promptly. Be sure to fill it out directly after the call.
- If a patient refuses care, ensure that you have obtained vital signs and a complete history, fully inform the patient of the situation and thoroughly document the situation.
- If you must revise or correct your patient clinical record, note the date, time, and purpose for the correction. Place a single line through the error and write the correct information next to it.
- Inaccurate or poor documentation could lead to subsequent caregivers providing inappropriate care to the patient. It could also work against you in a lawsuit, and negatively affect your reputation.

■ Vital Vocabulary

base station Assembly of radio equipment consisting of at least a transmitter, receiver, and antenna connection at a fixed location.

biotelemetry Transmission of physiological data, such as an ECG, from the patient to a distant point of reception (commonly referred to in the ambulance service as "telemetry").

computer-aided dispatch An automated computer system that processes the information received and assists the EMD with multiple functions and tasks.

dispatch To send to a specific destination or to send on a task.

duplex Radio system using more than one frequency to permit simultaneous transmission and reception.

emergency medical dispatcher (EMD) A person who receives information from a call taker regarding an emergency call and dispatches the most appropriate resource to respond in a timely manner, as well as receiving incident information from ambulance crews who are travelling or already at the scene.

encoded A message is put into a code before it is transmitted.

enhanced 999 system An emergency call-in system in which additional information such as the phone number and location of the caller is recorded automatically through sophisticated telephone technology and the EMD need only confirm the information on the screen.

frequency In radio communications, the number of cycles per second of a signal, inversely related to the wavelength.

hertz (Hz) Unit of frequency equal to 1 cycle per second.

landline Communications system linked by wires, usually in reference to a conventional telephone system.

mobile telephones Low-power portable radios that communicate through an interconnected series of repeater stations called "cells".

multiplex Method by which simultaneous transmission of voice and ECG signals can be achieved over a single radio frequency.

noise In radio communications, interference in a radio signal.

push-to-talk Commonly abbreviated as PTT, a method for communicating on a half-duplex communications system by pushing a button on the communication device to send and releasing the button to receive.

repeater Miniature transmitter that picks up a radio signal and rebroadcasts it, extending the range of a radio communications system.

simplex Method of radio communication using a single frequency that enables transmission or reception of voice or an ECG signal but is incapable of simultaneous transmission and reception.

transceiver A radio transmitter and receiver housed in a single unit; a two-way radio.

trunking Sharing of radio frequencies by multiple agencies or systems.

ultrahigh frequency (UHF) band The portion of the radio frequency spectrum between 300 and 3,000 mHz.

very high frequency (VHF) band The portion of the radio frequency spectrum between 30 and 150 mHz.

wavelength The distance in a propagating wave from one point to the corresponding point on the next wave.

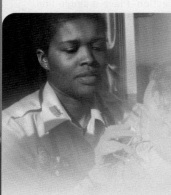

Assessment in Action

You are dispatched to a care home for a patient in respiratory distress. When you arrive, you find the patient with agonal respirations, and he is cold to the touch and grossly perspiring. His heart rate is 50 beats/min; his rhythm on the monitor is junctional. He has no palpable radial pulses and a palpable systolic blood pressure of 70 mm Hg. The staff stated he was "just fine" 30 minutes before they called 999. He was found slumped in his chair.

Your treatment for this patient includes IV atropine, a bolus dose of normal saline, and endotracheal intubation with a 7.5 ET tube. You transport and transfer the patient to the accident and emergency department. You now need to prepare the PCR.

1. **Which of the following statements is true for a PCR?**
   A. It is the only written record of the prehospital events.
   B. Documentation in the PCR is one of the most important skills learned as a paramedic.
   C. It is a legal record and part of the patient's medical record.
   D. All of the above.

2. **When a paramedic intubates a patient, all of the following should be documented, EXCEPT:**
   A. the size of the tube.
   B. the brand of the tube.
   C. who intubated the patient.
   D. the confirmation devices used.

3. **There are several charting "systems" a paramedic can use when documenting. They include all of the following, EXCEPT:**
   A. SOAP.
   B. CHARTE.
   C. body system approach.
   D. SOPE.

4. **How should you document a patient's words?**
   A. Document using quotes on the PCR.
   B. Write down what the patient stated.
   C. Rephrase what the patient said.
   D. Use a special incident report to state what the patient said.

5. **True or false? Pertinent negatives should be documented when writing your PCR.**
   A. True
   B. False

6. **Ensuring that documentation is complete, accurate, and legible is part of the _____ of paramedics.**
   A. standing orders
   B. medical director responsibilities
   C. professional responsibility
   D. department of health requirements

7. **The best time for a paramedic to write the PCR is:**
   A. en route to the hospital.
   B. after a verbal patient report to the receiving hospital.
   C. after returning to headquarters.
   D. while waiting to transfer the patient at the receiving hospital.

Introduction

Trauma has emerged to become the primary cause of death and disability in people 1 to 34 years of age. With improvements in health care and management of chronic diseases, death rates due to conditions such as heart disease, neoplasms, cerebrovascular events, and respiratory illnesses have decreased significantly in younger age groups. During the last 40 years, unintentional trauma, which excludes suicide, was the fifth leading cause of death in all age groups, accounting for 10,000 deaths reported in the United Kingdom each year.

Basic concepts of the mechanics and biomechanics of trauma will help you analyse and manage your patient's injuries. Analysing a trauma scene is a vital skill because you are the eyes and ears of the accident and emergency department at the scene of the trauma. Your paramedic-written patient history is the *only* source for hospital staff to understand the events and mechanisms that led to your trauma patient's chief complaint. Your information is critical as a foundation to visualise and search for injuries that may not be apparent on physical examination.

Trauma, Energy, Biomechanics, and Kinematics

Trauma is the acute physiological and structural change (injury) that occurs in a patient's body when an external source

At the Scene

The top five causes of trauma death are road traffic collisions, falls, poisonings, burns, and drownings.

of energy dissipates faster than the body's ability to sustain and dissipate it   Figure 17-1 ▾ .

If a body in a motor vehicle—your patient's body—smashes into a wall, the energy delivered by an external source—the moving motor vehicle—is released when the car is stopped by the wall. Your patient's body is moving at the same rate of speed as the car, and his or her body does not have bumpers to absorb the energy from stopping. If the energy is not absorbed in other ways, the patient's body absorbs it, often with bones that break and internal organs that rupture—what you see as trauma injuries.

Different forms of energy produce different kinds of trauma. These external energy sources can be mechanical, chemical, thermal, electrical, and barometric.

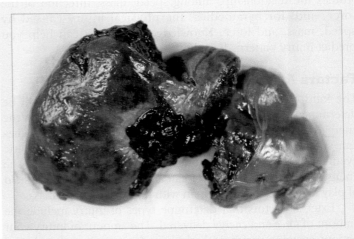

Figure 17-1 Traumatic injury occurs when the body's tissues are exposed to energy levels beyond their tolerance. Some traumatic injuries may not be visible. This photo shows a ruptured spleen.

You are the Paramedic Part 1

You are dispatched to 239a High Road for "man fallen from a roof". This address is located in the business district of your patch. En route to the call, you learn that this man had been running from police and had come from a building in that area. The patient is in police custody, and the scene is considered safe.

You arrive but are unable to assess much because the patient is combative and unwilling to answer your questions. You can see that his skin is slightly moist and a bit pale.

Initial Assessment	Recording Time: 0 Minutes
Appearance	Grimacing, screaming, punching
Level of consciousness	A (Alert to person, place, and day)
Airway	Patent
Breathing	Rapid and deep
Circulation	Unable to assess owing to patient combativeness

1. What initial information about the fall gives rise for concern?
2. What deductions may you draw based on the reported location of this incident?
3. Given the location, what other conditions are you worried about?

Mechanical energy is energy from motion (kinetic energy ie, a moving vehicle) or energy stored in an object (potential energy—a concrete bridge abuttment). Kinetic energy would be found in two moving vehicles colliding. Potential energy would be present in a fall from a height. In that case, gravity would be the *potential* source of energy that can cause the object to fall. Chemical energy can be found in an explosive or an acid or even from a reaction to an ingested or medically delivered agent or drug. Electrical energy comes in the form of high voltage electrocution or a lightning strike. Barometric energy can result from sudden and radical changes in pressure, often occurring during diving or flying.

Biomechanics is the study of the physiology and mechanics of a living organism using the tools of mechanical engineering. Biomechanics provides a way of analysing the mechanisms and results of trauma sustained by the human body. Kinetics studies the relationships among speed, mass, direction of the force, and, for paramedics, the physical injury caused by speed, mass, and force. Knowledge of kinetics can help you predict injury patterns found in a patient.

Factors Affecting Types of Injury

The kind of injury resulting after trauma is sustained will be determined by the ability of the patient's body to disperse the energy delivered by the traumatic event. Some patients' bodies can stretch and bend to absorb the energy of the traumatic event. But other patients' bone and tissue cannot absorb the energy. A healthy rugby player can absorb a "tackle" on the field of play better than an older man with diminished bone mass.

External factors that determine types of injury include the amount of *force* and *energy* delivered. The amount of injury your patient sustains varies with the size (or mass) of the objects delivering the force and energy, with the change in velocity (how fast your patient is travelling), with acceleration or deceleration (how much the object or your patient speeds up or slows down), and with the body area of the application of force. The primary reasons for the extent of trauma your patients sustain are the amount of energy in the object and the mechanism by which the object is delivered to the body. The body receives wider-spread trauma from a cannon ball (more energy inside) than it does from a bullet, although both are often lethal. (Proving, if proof were needed, that size does matter.)

Duration and *direction* of the force of application are also important. In vehicle collisions, paramedics learn to recognise the directional patterns in injuries from front-end, side, and rear-end collisions. The larger the area of force dissipation, the more pressure is reduced to a specific spot on the body, often without making a visible cut. Bullet impact is less if the energy in the bullet is dissipated over the ceramic plate inside a bulletproof vest than if all the force of the bullet is applied at a small location on the skin.

In trauma medicine, this spreading of impact is described as *blunt trauma*. Ambulance service providers at all levels quickly learn in the prehospital environment that blunt trauma is difficult to diagnose because there is usually no evidence of cutting on the skin. Paramedics study kinetics to find this lethal, but almost invisible trauma.

At the Scene

Suspect a spinal injury when you see a cracked windscreen, steering wheel or dashboard damage, intrusion into a vehicle, or fractured feet or ankles after a fall. It will make a difference in how you handle the ABCs. Lack of airbag deflation is not always a positive sign.

The *rate of force application* affects trauma because rapidly applied amounts of energy are less tolerated than a similar amount of energy delivered over a longer period. Rapidly delivered energy causes broken wrists, whereas longer term energy delivery might show up as repetitive stress injuries—even though the amount of force ultimately might be exactly the same.

The position of the trauma victim—how he or she is standing or sitting—at the time of the event is an external factor. Seatbelts have done a great deal to effect the reduction in lethal injuries by keeping occupants in positions least likely to cause fatal injuries.

Internal injuries sustained when the break point of an organ is exceeded are easier to diagnose. In the skin, they include contusions, abrasions, lacerations, punctures, and degloving injuries. Bones will fracture or buckle. The viscera covering structures of internal organs will have ruptures, or disruptions.

The *impact resistance of body parts* will also have a bearing on types of tissue disruption. Impact resistance is often determined by what is inside your patient's organs: gas, liquid, or solid.

Biomechanical engineers would measure the *densities of tissues* that are damaged. Paramedics need to know that organs that have gas inside, such as in the lungs and intestinal tract, will scatter energy more than liquid or solid boundaries. This means that the organ around the gas will be easily compressed, so look for lung and intestinal trauma first. Water-bearing organs include the vascular system, the liver, spleen, and muscle. Water-bearing tissues are less compressible than gas-containing tissues. Solid density interfaces occur mostly in bones such as in the cranium, spine, and long bones.

Because many injuries are not obvious on first presentation, understanding the effects of forces and energy transfer patterns will help in the assessment of the mechanism of injury (MOI), which in turn can help predict the type of injuries you are most likely to see when you are in the field **Figure 17-2 ▶**. Paramedic students need to learn to have a *high index of suspicion* for injuries that otherwise might be undetected for several hours. Anticipate the possibility of specific types of injury: you will help your patient and the trauma team who will need your assessment of the scene. Sometimes, you will find you need to be aggressive with your initial assessment "ABC" interventions to prevent further problems for your patient.

▋Trauma Centres

Paramedics need a good working knowledge of the hospital resources with a reasonable idea of how long transport will

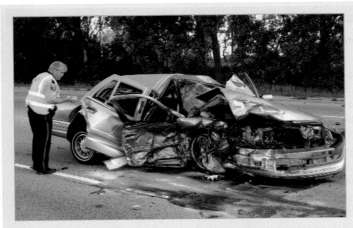

Figure 17-2 The appearance of the car can provide you with critical information about the severity of the crash and the possible injuries to the occupants.

Documentation and Communication

So much emphasis is placed on the MOI because obtaining a complete and accurate history of the incident can help identify as many as 95% of the injuries present. After ensuring your personal safety and maintaining the ABCs, the mechanism of injury is key information to obtain from the trauma scene. You must relay what you suspect as the MOIs by radio and by written report to the receiving trauma centre. You are the eyes and ears of the trauma team in the accident and emergency department.

take. Frequently, you will be the decision maker about where your patient should be transported. Before you even get to the scene, you should know what is available in your area.

The Royal College of Surgeons of England and the British Orthopaedic Association are the governing bodies responsible for the designation of trauma centres. There are four separate categories of verification as described by The Royal College of Surgeons of England and the British Orthopaedic Association (Level 1, 2, 3, and minor injuries units). The guidelines in Table 17-1 ▶ are an overview of the verification criteria.

Criteria for Referral to a Trauma Centre

Paramedics are responsible for determining whether a patient should go to a trauma centre—and at what level. You might even have to determine whether air transport is required to a Level I centre. *The criteria for transport to a trauma centre vary from system to system.* However, the criteria for transport to a trauma centre as defined by the American College of Surgeons in its ATLS protocols are summarised below:

1. If one of the following is present, the patient should be referred to a trauma centre:
   – GCS (Glasgow Coma Scale score) < 14
   – RR (respiratory rate) < 10 or > 29
   – SBP (systolic blood pressure) < 90
   – RTS (revised trauma score) < 11
   – PTS (paediatric trauma score) < 9
2. If one of the following is diagnosed in the prehospital environment, the trauma centre is a more appropriate triage endpoint:
   – Flail chest
   – Two or more proximal long bone fractures
   – Amputation proximal to wrist or ankle
   – All penetrating trauma to head, neck, torso, or extremities proximal to elbow or knee
   – Any limb paralysis
   – Pelvic fractures
   – Combination of trauma with burns
   – Open and depressed skull fractures
3. Evaluate at this point the MOI and examine the trauma scene for evidence of high-energy trauma. If one of the following is present, refer to a trauma centre:
   – Ejection from a motor vehicle
   – Traumatic death in same passenger compartment
   – Pedestrian thrown or run over or car-pedestrian injury at > 5 mph
   – High-speed car on car collision (> 40 mph)
   – Intrusion into passenger compartment of > 30 cm
   – Major vehicle deformity > 45 cm
   – Vehicle rollover with unrestrained passenger
   – Extrication time > 20 minutes
   – Falls > 6 m
   – Motorcycle crash at > 20 mph or with separation of rider and bike
4. If none of the above criteria are met, then consider transfer to trauma centre if:
   – Patient of age < 5 or > 55 years
   – Known immunosuppressed patients
   – Known cardiac disease or respiratory disease comorbidity
   – Type 1 diabetes, cirrhosis, morbid obesity, or coagulopathy

Patients suffering from burns alone will benefit from being transferred directly to a burns unit. Similarly, patients who are pregnant beyond 20 weeks should be taken to a unit with obstetric facilities.

At the Scene

In addition to being trauma centres, some hospitals specialise in neurology, burns, paediatric trauma, cardiac care (centres for heart transplantation, coronary catheter labs), microsurgery (hand and limb reimplantation), or hyperbaric therapy. When you work with a service, you must know or have access to this information for your patients' sake.

The prehospital assessment of trauma patients is key to the management of and transport to the appropriate definitive care facility.

Transport Considerations

When making a decision to transport a patient, several options must be considered. What are the needs of the patient? What is

Table 17-1 Key Elements for Trauma Centres

Level	Definition	Key Elements
Level 1	**The Major Acute Hospital** 1. This will be a designated large acute hospital. 2. There should be only one major acute hospital in each system. 3. The major acute hospital will receive all trauma from its immediate catchment population. 4. The major acute hospital will receive patients directly from any part of the trauma system, even though this may mean bypassing other hospitals when appropriate. 5. The major acute hospital will receive secondary transfers from other hospitals in the system. 6. The major acute hospital will provide prehospital advice to ambulance personnel. 7. The major acute hospital will receive trauma patients from other hospitals in the system when the standards of care cannot be met by an acute general hospital.	1. A 24-hour resuscitative trauma team, led by a consultant with current ATLS certification or equivalent, must be in place. 2. A 24-hour fully staffed Accident and Emergency (A&E) department, supported by on-call A&E consultants, supported by specialist registrars. 3. Intensive care unit (ICU) beds on the same site as the A&E department. 4. On-site 24-hour X-ray and CT scanning with appropriate staffing and immediate reporting facilities. 5. The equivalent of four to eight whole-time consultants exclusively dealing with orthopaedic trauma. 6. A dedicated trauma theatre and daily consultant orthopaedic trauma lists. 7. A helicopter pad close to the A&E department is mandatory. There should be no additional secondary journey by road. The helicopter landing site should allow landing throughout the 24 hours. 8. There must be on-site departments of Orthopaedic Trauma, Neurosurgery, General and Vascular Surgery, Plastic Surgery, Cardiothoracic or Thoracic Surgery, Head and Neck Surgery, Urology, Anaesthesia with intensive care, Interventional Radiology, Paediatric Surgery, and intensive care beds for children. 9. A named consultant director of trauma.
Level 2	**The Acute General Hospital** 1. These hospitals will inevitably vary in size and will not have all of the major surgical disciplines on site. 2. They will often be at some distance from the major acute hospital. 3. They will act in partnership with the major acute hospital. 4. They must be able to resuscitate the severely injured. 5. Audit will scrutinise whether hospitals receiving few severely injured patients would be able to retain sufficient expertise to deal with them.	1. A 24-hour resuscitative trauma team, led by a consultant with current ATLS certification or equivalent, must be in place. 2. A 24-hour fully staffed A&E department supported by A&E consultants with specialist registrars. 3. ICU beds and trauma beds on the same site as the A&E department. 4. On-site 24-hour X-ray and CT scanning with appropriate staffing and immediate reporting facilities. CT scanning linked to neurosurgery centre allows optimum management of head injuries and transfer where necessary. 5. At least six consultants in orthopaedics with a special interest in trauma taking part in an emergency rota. 6. A dedicated trauma theatre and daily consultant orthopaedic trauma lists. 7. A helicopter landing pad close to the A&E department is mandatory. There should be no additional secondary journey by road. The helicopter landing site should allow landing throughout the 24 hours. 8. A named consultant director of trauma.
Level 3	**The Acute General Hospital** 1. It should be emphasised that the role of some acute general hospitals, whether in thinly populated rural areas or in conurbations, will change little but these hospitals are less likely to meet the standards required. 2. Some acute general hospitals do not receive sufficient numbers of major trauma patients to retain the skills of the staff and to justify the expensive resources required for the reception and resuscitation of major injuries. 3. Patients with severe injuries or multiple injuries should bypass these level 3 hospitals and be taken directly to the major acute hospital (level 1) or an acute general hospital (level 2), even if they are further from the scene of the incident than the level 3 hospital.	1. A 24-hour staffed A&E department with dedicated resident medical staff. 2. 24-hour X-ray facilities including CT scanning. 3. At least six consultant surgeons dealing with trauma taking part in an emergency rota. 4. Daily consultant orthopaedic trauma lists. 5. Orthopaedic surgery, general surgery, and general medicine on-site. 6. Pre-agreed arrangements for immediate (blue light) inter-hospital transfer to a level 1 or 2 facility. 7. A named consultant should direct the trauma service.

Table 17-1	Key Elements for Trauma Centres (continued)

Level   **Definition**

Minor Injuries Units

1. Minor Injuries Units (MIUs) have no role in the management of severely injured patients and explicit bypass policies must be implemented such that these units never receive blue light ambulances.

2. An MIU is defined as a unit offering open access and self-referral for minor injuries and ailments in ambulatory patients. These units may also see patients referred by family doctors and pre-agreed patients with minor injuries arriving by ambulance.

3. Consultants in A&E medicine should be closely involved in the MIUs. The staff of such units, in order to retain skills, should rotate through large A&E departments.

4. It is recognised that the contribution general practitioners make to minor injuries units is considerable.

Adapted from: Royal College of Surgeons and British Orthopaedic Association. *Better Care for the Severely Injured.* 2000: 42-46.

the level of the hospital? The patient should be transported to the closest, most appropriate hospital to receive optimal care. You must also decide on the mode of transport that will offer the greatest benefit. Should you call for air transport, or is ground transport sufficient?

When making the decision to transport by ground, several factors should be taken into consideration. Can the appropriate facility be reached within a reasonable timeframe by ground? What is the extent of injuries? If in a congested area, can the patient be transported to a more accessible landing zone for air medical transport?

Air transport must be considered in several situations: (1) when there is extended transport time by ground, (2) when there are multiple casualties, (3) when extrication times are prolonged and patients are critically injured, and (4) when there are long distances to an appropriate facility as opposed to the closest accident and emergency department. There also may be other times that air transport is appropriate Figure 17-3 ▶ . If the patient can be transported to definitive care within a reasonable amount of time by ground, there is no need to call for air transport. Take into consideration the time it will take for the aircraft to lift off, travel, and land, just to reach the scene. By weighing the timeframe against transport by ground, you will be able to make an informed decision. Also take into account the terrain. Is there an adequate area for landing? If not, how far will the patient need to be transported to reach a landing zone? If there is a great distance, ground transport may be a more reasonable option. It is important to remember that most helicopter emergency medical services are restricted to flying during daylight hours. Once the decision is made to call for air medical transport, contact your dispatcher to request a unit, or follow local protocols regarding contacting air support.

Helicopter Triage Criteria

All levels of prehospital providers should recognise the need for and the criteria used in making the decision to use aeromedical transport in their own service. The key to success is recognising the need for the aeromedical transport of patients and activating the service as early as possible. The trauma triage guidelines in this chapter should be used as a guideline.

A Little Physics

Although drivers might not obey traffic laws, they must—whether they want to or not—obey the laws of physics that govern all objects on our planet. A little familiarity with these

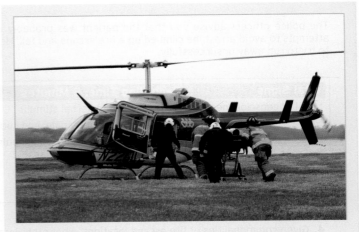

Figure 17-3 A helicopter may be used to transport patients quickly to the proper trauma centre.

At the Scene

The Platinum Ten Minutes refers to the goal of the maximum time spent at a scene for a critical trauma patient. Scene times should be limited as much as possible to get the patient to more definitive care at a trauma centre. Trauma, more often than not, means that onsite stabilisation is a questionable paramedic procedure. However, other problems may be better handled by onsite paramedic stabilisation. One of your major tasks as a student paramedic is to learn the difference between the two.

Controversies

Some situations may have contraindications or relative contraindications for aeromedical transport. These situations include traumatic cardiac arrest, inclement weather conditions, extremely combative patients, morbidly obese patients, patients with baro-trauma (diving injuries may necessitate lower flying altitudes), and situations in which ground transport and appropriate level of care are available and would permit quicker care.

laws will help you understand more about the mechanisms of trauma.

Velocity (V) is the distance an object travels per unit time. The difference between velocity and speed is that velocity is also defined by moving in a specific direction. Acceleration (a) of an object is the rate of change of velocity that an object is subjected to, whether speeding up or slowing down. Gravity (g) is the downward acceleration that is imparted to any object on earth by the effect of the earth's mass. During each second of a fall, the velocity or speed of the falling object increases by 9.8 m/sec^2.

The kinetic energy (KE) of an object is the energy associated with that object in motion. It reflects the relationship between the weight (mass) of the object and the velocity at which it is travelling and is expressed mathematically as:

$$\text{Kinetic energy} = \frac{\text{Mass}}{2} \times \text{Velocity}^2$$
$$\text{or, } KE = \frac{m}{2} \times V^2$$

Thus, velocity has a much greater effect on KE than weight because it is squared   Figure 17-4 ▶ .

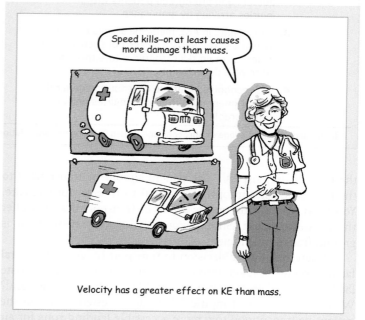

Speed kills—or at least causes more damage than mass.

Velocity has a greater effect on KE than mass.

Figure 17-4

You are the Paramedic Part 2

The police officers advise you that the patient was probably under the influence of PCP (phencyclidine hydrochloride), and in his attempts to avoid arrest, he climbed up a fire escape and fell. He landed on his hands and feet, stumbled for a few steps, and continued to try to run away unsuccessfully.

Vital Signs	Recording Time: 5 Minutes
Level of consciousness	V (Responsive to verbal stimuli)
Skin	Slightly moist, slightly pale, and cool
Pulse	Carotid (unable to access radial pulses because patient is being restrained); rapid
Blood pressure	168 by palpation
Respirations	60 breaths/min
SpO$_2$	99% while breathing room air

4. Given commonalities of fire escape locations, what other information do you have?
5. How does your patient's condition hinder your assessment techniques?
6. How do you compensate for this hindrance?

In other words, an object increases its kinetic energy more by increasing its velocity than by increasing its mass. The kinetic energy of an object involved in a collision must be *dissipated* as the object comes to rest. The kinetic energy of a car in motion that stops suddenly must be somewhere Figure 17-5 ▸ . In a car, kinetic energy can be dissipated by braking, transforming to heat (another form of energy). If all the energy is not transformed into heat, however, the KE is transformed into deformed metal (potential energy), which results in damage to the car and its occupants. The mechanics of dissipation can result in injury. For example, a car travelling at 35 mph hits a wall, which stops the car, but the driver is still travelling at 35 mph until stopped by the seatbelts or the air bag, or, if not wearing a seatbelt, the steering wheel, dashboard, or windscreen.

Speed kills exponentially: look what happens when velocity increases 10 mph versus when the person weighs in at 10 kg heavier.

- 154 lb (70 kg) person at 10 mph = 7,700 KE units
- 154 lb (70 kg) person at 20 mph = 30,800 KE units
- 154 lb (70 kg) person at 30 mph = 69,300 KE units
- 154 lb (70 kg) person at 40 mph = 123,200 KE units
- 176 lb (80 kg) person at 40 mph = 140,800 KE units
- 154 lb (70 kg) person at 55 mph = 232,925 KE units
- 154 lb (70 kg) person at 65 mph = 325,325 KE units

Note that when weight increases by 10 kg but velocity remains the same, there is not much change in the kinetic energy. However, when the velocity increases from 55 to 65 mph (a difference of only 10 mph), the KE (remember, that's energy in motion!) increases by 92,400 KE units!

Modern cars are designed to have crumple zones to maximise the amount of energy dissipated by deformation before the passenger compartment is involved. Because the motor vehicle damage so often shows just how fast the car was going, the amount of damage provides information to help in your decision about patient destination.

In addition to the velocity at which the car (and its passengers) are travelling, the vehicle's angle of impact (front collision versus side impact, or how your patient hit the inside of a motor vehicle), the differences in the sizes of the two vehicles, and the restraint status and protective gear of the occupants will affect the amount of energy dissipation that affects your patients in a crash.

Remember the laws of physics that no driver can break? Here's a quick review in physics-ese. The law of conservation of energy states that energy can be neither created nor destroyed, it can only change form. Energy generated from a sudden stop or start must be transformed to one of the following energy forms: thermal, electrical, chemical, radiant, or mechanical (as discussed earlier).

Energy dissipation, as you know, is the process by which KE is transformed into one of these forms of mechanical energy. When a car stops slowly, its KE is converted to thermal energy—heat—by friction of the braking action. If the car crashes, KE is also dissipated into mechanical energy as the car body crumples in a collision. Mechanical energy is further dis-

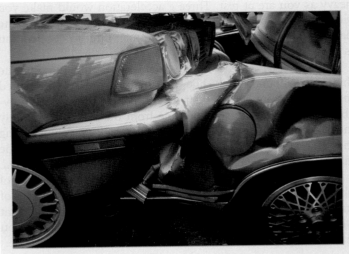

Figure 17-5 The kinetic energy of a speeding car is converted into the work of stopping the car, usually by crushing the car's exterior.

sipated in the form of injury as the occupants sustain fractures or other bodily harm.

Protective devices such as seatbelts, air bags, and helmets are designed to *manipulate* the way in which energy is dissipated into injury. For example, a seatbelt converts kinetic energy of the occupants into a seatbelt to body-pressure force rather than into a steering wheel deformation against the torso or a windscreen shattering against the head.

Newton's first law of motion states that a body at rest will remain at rest unless acted on by an outside force. Similarly, a body in motion tends to remain in motion at a constant velocity, travelling in a straight line, unless acted on by an outside force. Most bodies in motion (without the assistance of a motor or other propulsion device) tend to stop eventually, owing to the action of forces of friction, wind resistance, or other force resulting in deceleration.

Newton's second law of motion states that the force that an object can exert is the product of its mass times its acceleration:

Force = Mass (Weight) × Acceleration (or Deceleration)

The higher an object's mass and acceleration, the higher the *force* that needs to be applied to make a change of course or stop the object. Remember our cartoon? Force equals mass × acceleration or deceleration. Deceleration is slowing to a stop. Rapid deceleration, as may occur in a collision, dissipates tremendous forces and, therefore, major injuries. Deceleration and acceleration can also be measured in numbers of *g* forces. One *g* force is the normal acceleration of gravity. A two or three *g* acceleration or deceleration force is, logically enough, two or three times the force associated with the acceleration of gravity. A two *g* deceleration would make you feel as if you are twice as heavy as you are at rest. Three g acceleration would make you feel three times heavier. High-speed collisions can generate decelerations in *hundreds* of g. The human limit to deceleration is about 30 g.

In a *head-on collision* with two vehicles travelling in opposite directions along a straight line, transferred energy is represented in part as the sum of both their speeds. If a car strikes an immovable object, forces generated come from the speed of the only moving object. In a *rear impact* of two vehicles travelling along the same line, the energy potential is lessened because it is the difference in speed between them, also known as the *closing speed*.

It is important to have an understanding of these laws of physics because they help define the types and patterns of trauma you will see in the field. You are the most important witness the hospital trauma team has—the information you learn from physics will affect the outcome of your patient's life.

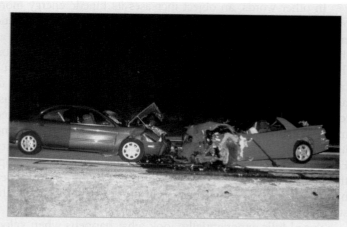

Figure 17-6 Blunt trauma typically occurs in road traffic collisions.

Types of Trauma

Injuries are generally described as the consequence of blunt or penetrating trauma. Blunt trauma refers to injuries in which the tissues are not penetrated by an external object Figure 17-6 ▸ . Blunt trauma typically occurs in road traffic collisions, in pedestrians hit by a vehicle, in motorcycle crashes, in falls from heights, in serious sports injures, and in blasts when no shrapnel is involved and the pressure wave is the primary cause of the injuries.

Penetrating trauma results when tissues are penetrated by single or multiple objects Figure 17-7 ▸ . Penetrating trauma results from gunshot wounds caused by a single or multiple projectiles, stab wounds, and blasts with shrapnel or secondary projectiles. Penetrating trauma may also occur in combination with blunt injuries such as in implement injuries during a road traffic collision or a fall out of a tree and onto a fence.

At the Scene

As a general rule for ballistic trauma, the entrance wound is smaller than the exit wound. Assume that cavitation involves internal structures that are not readily visible on your clinical examination.

Injuries Caused by Deceleration

Abrupt deceleration injuries are produced by a sudden stop of a body's forward motion. Whether from a fall, shaking a baby, or a high-speed vehicle crash, decelerating forces can induce shearing, avulsing, or rupturing of organs and their restraining fascia, vasculature, nerves, and other soft tissues. These injuries are often invisible during examination, so every paramedic needs to understand how such injuries are sustained.

You are the Paramedic Part 3

The police officers restrain the patient so that you can perform your initial assessment and a rapid trauma assessment, all while taking spinal precautions. You are able to apply a cervical collar and minimise his movement on a longboard. During your rapid trauma assessment, you find that he has deformity of both legs below the knees. He also has some abrasions to both hands and arms. It appears as though the majority of force was absorbed by the legs during the fall.

Reassessment	Recording Time: 10 Minutes
Level of consciousness	V (Responsive to verbal stimuli)
Skin	Slightly moist, slightly pale, and cool
Pulse	Carotid (unable to access radial pulses as patient is being restrained); rapid
Blood pressure	168 by palpation
Respirations	60 breaths/min
SpO2	98% while breathing room air; patient noncompliant with nonrebreathing mask

7. Given this information, what other injuries do you suspect?

8. How can a patient who is under the influence of drugs be difficult to manage?

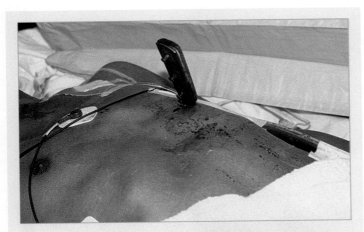

Figure 17-7 Injuries from low-energy penetrations, such as a stab wound, are caused by the sharp edges of the object moving through the body.

At the Scene

According to the Department for Transport, Transport Statistics 2005, there were:

- 271,017 reported casualties on roads in Great Britain, 3% fewer than in 2004.
- 3,201 people were killed, 1% fewer than in 2004.
- 28,954 were seriously injured, 7% fewer than in 2004.
- 238,862 were slightly injured, 3% fewer than in 2004.
- 198,735 road accidents involving personal injury, 4% fewer than in 2004. Of these, 27,942 involved death or serious injury. Child casualties fell by 9%. There were 141 child fatalities, 15% fewer than in 2004.
- 3,472 children killed or seriously injured, 11% fewer than in 2004. Of those, 2,134 were pedestrians, 9% fewer than in 2004.
- 178,302 car user casualties, 3% fewer than in 2004. Although fatalities remained at the same level.
- 16,561 pedal cyclist casualties, 1% fewer than in 2004. 2,212 seriously injured casualties, 2% higher than in 2004. The number of pedal cyclists killed went up by 10% from 134 to 148.
- Two wheeled motor vehicle user casualties were lower than the 2004 level at 24,824. The number killed fell 3% to 569 and the number of seriously injured also fell by 2% to 5,939.
- Over 300,000 people are hurt in road traffic accidents, 5% of them children. It is the leading cause of death amongst children aged 0 to 14 years.
- Over half a million accidents result in hospital admission.

The head is particularly vulnerable to deceleration injuries. The brain is a fairly heavy organ that lies in fluid inside the skull. Any trauma that will jerk the patient's head causes the brain to hit the inside of the skull, causing bleeding, bruising, tearing, and crush injuries. All of these injuries are extremely dangerous and might not show up on a cursory examination. Your paramedic index of suspicion should be on high alert for these injuries.

The chest is vulnerable to aorta injury. The *aorta*, the large blood vessel near the heart, is the most common site of deceleration injury in the chest. The aorta is often torn away from its points of fixation in the body. Shearing of the aorta can result in rapid loss of all the body's blood and immediate death.

Abdominal blunt trauma results as the forward motion of the body stops and internal organs continue their forward motion, resulting in tearing at their points of attachment, in shearing injuries, and tearing in abdominal walls. Organs that can be affected include the liver, kidneys, small intestine, large intestine, pancreas, and spleen.

Kidneys are injured as forward motion produces tears to the organ or to points of attachment with the abdominal aorta or through the renal arteries. Also, as forward motion is restrained by the large bowel, the small bowel can tear and result in free air in the abdomen. Trauma can also do damage without tearing by causing an insufficient supply of blood to the bowel. The spleen can also be torn, sometimes resulting in life-threatening internal bleeding.

Injuries Caused by External Forces

Crush and compression injuries are the result of forces applied to the body by things external to the body at the time of impact. Crush and compression injuries occur *at* the time of impact, unlike deceleration injuries, which occur *before* impact. Crush and compression injuries are often caused by dashboards, windscreens, the floor, and heavy objects falling on the body.

Compression head injuries, which may result in skull fractures, are often associated with cervical spine injury. Therefore, you need to assume spinal cord injuries and severe injury to the brain. Brain tissue does not compress; it swells within the enclosed area of the skull. As the brain swells inside the skull, it is crushed, causing a catastrophic injury.

Compression injuries of the chest may produce *fractured ribs*, which can lead to internal injuries of the lungs and heart. One of the signs of a lung injury is a *flail chest*, a condition in which the chest wall moves paradoxically with respirations (moves opposite of normal). Fractured ribs may also cause blood or air to seep into the chest space, which would require decompression and placement of a chest tube. Blunt cardiac injury can compress the heart between bones in the chest, causing arrhythmias and direct injury to the heart muscle. If the lungs are compressed, causing fulminant interstitial and alveola oedema, acute respiratory distress syndrome (ARDS) can result, although this usually manifests 12 to 48 hours after an initial trauma.

Almost all abdominal organs can be affected by hitting an external object. Organs often injured are the pancreas, spleen, liver, and, occasionally, kidneys. Compression against the seatbelt may result in *bowel rupture, bladder rupture, diaphragm tearing,* and *spinal injuries*. The abdomen has its own large blood-carrying vessel called the aorta. A common injury is the rupture of a valve in this vessel, caused by blood going the wrong way in the abdominal aorta.

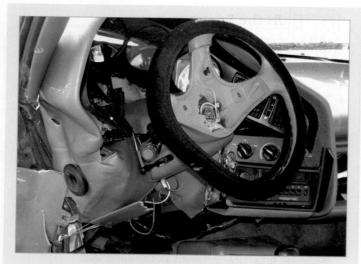

Figure 17-8 Deceleration of the occupant starts during sudden braking and continues during impact and collision. The appearance of the interior of the car can provide you with information about the severity of the patient's injuries.

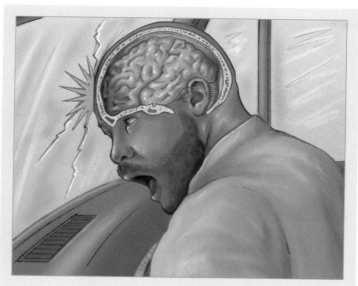

Figure 17-9 Deceleration of internal organs involves the body's supporting structures and movable organs that continue their forward momentum until stopped by anatomical restraints. In this illustration, the brain continues its forward motion and strikes the inside of the skull, resulting in a compression injury to the anterior portion of the brain and stretching of the posterior portion.

Pelvic fractures also result from external compressive trauma, potentially injuring the bladder, vagina, rectum, lumbar plexus, and pelvic floor and leading to severe bleeding in the large arteries near the hip bones.

Road Traffic Collisions

When a motor vehicle collides with another object, trauma in the collision is composed of *five phases* tied to the affects of progressive deceleration. The first phase, *deceleration of the vehicle,* occurs when the vehicle strikes another object and is brought to an abrupt stop. The forward motion of the car continues until its KE is dissipated in the form of mechanical deformation and damage to the vehicle and occupant or until the restraining force of the object is removed (for example, sheared off pole, yielding of a guard rail) and the vehicle motion continues until its KE is gently dissipated by drag or continued braking. The second phase is *deceleration of the occupant,* which starts during sudden braking and continues during impact and collision. This results in deceleration, compression, and shear trauma to the occupants **Figure 17-8 ▲** . The effects on vehicle occupants will vary depending on the mass of each occupant, protective mechanisms in the vehicle such as restraints and air bags, body parts involved, and points of impact. The third phase, *deceleration of internal organs,* involves the body's supporting structures (skull, sternum, ribs, spine, and pelvis) and movable organs (brain, heart, liver, spleen, and intestine) that continue their forward momentum until stopped by anatomical restraints **Figure 17-9 ▶** . Energy is dissipated by internal organs as they are injured. Movement of fixed and nonfixed parts may result in tears and shearing injuries. The fourth phase is the result of *secondary collisions,* which occur when a vehicle occupant is hit by objects moving within the car such as packages, animals, or other passengers. These objects may continue to travel at the car's initial speed and then hit a passenger who has come to rest.

At the Scene

Don't forget that the collision of internal organs striking against the body can result in severe damage, though this may not always be obvious.

These types of collisions have been known to cause severe spine and head trauma. The final phase is the result of *additional impacts* that the vehicle may receive, as when it is hit and deflected into another vehicle, tree, or another object. This may increase the seriousness of original injuries or cause further injury. For example, a frontal collision may cause a posterior hip dislocation and an acetabular fracture via a dashboard mechanism and a subsequent side impact from another vehicle may add a lateral compression pelvic ring injury, resulting in complex pelvic and acetabular trauma. **Table 17-2 ▶** shows the structural clues, body clues, and resulting injuries for different types of collisions.

Notes from Nancy

When the windscreen is cracked or broken, the front seat occupant has a cervical spine injury until proved otherwise.

Predicting Types of Injury by Examining the Scene

Important clues to predict injury types can be obtained by paying attention to the history of the collision and by an examination of the scene. Using your new-found knowledge

pulmonary blast injuries Pulmonary trauma resulting from short-range exposure to the detonation of high explosives.

shearing An applied force or pressure exerted against the surface and layers of the skin as tissues slide in opposite but parallel planes.

spalling Delaminating or breaking off into chips and pieces.

trauma Acute physiological and structural change that occurs in a victim as a result of the rapid dissipation of energy delivered by an external force.

tympanic membrane The eardrum; a thin, semi-transparent membrane in the middle ear that transmits sound vibrations to the internal ear by means of the auditory ossicles.

velocity The speed of an object in a given direction.

Waddell triad A pattern of motor vehicle-pedestrian injuries in children and people of short stature in which (1) the bumper hits pelvis and femur, (2) the chest and abdomen hit the grille or low bonnet, and (3) the head strikes the ground.

whiplash An injury to the cervical vertebrae or their supporting ligaments and muscles, usually resulting from sudden acceleration or deceleration.

◼ Points to Ponder

You and your partner are dispatched as a second paramedic unit to assist in a two-car road traffic collision. You arrive on scene and are directed to a vehicle approximately 90 metres from the initial impact. Witnesses state that this vehicle was struck on the passenger side at a high rate of speed and slid out of control through a metal fence and the driver's side is now resting against a large tree. You are told that the other vehicle involved in the collision drove through a red light, driving approximately 50 mph. The passenger side has an intrusion of more than 60 cm. There are two women inside the vehicle. They are conscious, alert, and orientated and very upset, crying hysterically. The fire and rescue service are extricating the patients from the wreckage.

What is the mechanism(s) of injury to the vehicle? What type of injuries would you suspect the patients may have? What are major concerns and thoughts you must have during your assessment and treatment of these trauma patients? What level trauma hospital would you take these patients to?

Issues: Understanding Kinematics of Trauma, Predicting Injury Patterns, Examining the Scene and Patients, Knowledge of Receiving Hospital Specialities.

Assessment in Action

You are dispatched for a single-vehicle road traffic collision and encounter a wet, slippery road. The driver of the vehicle is slumped in the driver compartment. Witnesses tell you that she was driving and then suddenly lost control of her vehicle, struck a post box, and then drove head on into a pole.

1. **What is Newton's first law of motion?**
   A. The force that an object can exert is the product of its mass times its acceleration.
   B. A body at rest will remain at rest and a body in motion will remain in motion unless acted on by an outside force.
   C. Energy cannot be created or destroyed but can be changed in form.
   D. Kinetic energy is a function of an object's weight and speed.

2. **Trauma in a collision is composed of how many phases, which represent the effects of progressive deceleration?**
   A. 2
   B. 3
   C. 4
   D. 5

3. **A patient's ability to dissipate the energy determines the pattern of injury.**
   A. True
   B. False

4. **What type of impact would you suspect in the preceding scenario?**
   A. Lateral
   B. Rear
   C. Frontal
   D. Rotational

5. **Injuries are generally categorised as:**
   A. head and spinal trauma.
   B. extremity and body trauma.
   C. blunt and penetrating trauma.
   D. closed and open trauma.

6. **The role of air bags is to:**
   A. cushion forward movement of the occupant.
   B. protect the occupant from ejection.
   C. accelerate the occupant away from the point of impact.
   D. block the occupant's view of the impact.

Challenging Questions

You are dispatched to a woman who has fallen. On arrival, you find a 38-year-old woman supine on the ground. Initially, she is responsive to deep painful stimuli.

7. **The severity of injuries will depend on a number of factors that will be in important in assessing the patient. List these factors.**

18 Haemorrhage and Shock

Objectives

Cognitive

- Describe the epidemiology, including the morbidity/mortality and prevention strategies, for shock and haemorrhage.
- Discuss the anatomy and physiology of the cardiovascular system.
- Predict shock and haemorrhage based on mechanism of injury.
- Discuss the various types and degrees of shock and haemorrhage.
- Discuss the pathophysiology of haemorrhage and shock.
- Discuss the assessment findings associated with haemorrhage and shock.
- Identify the need for intervention and transport of the patient with haemorrhage or shock.
- Discuss the treatment plan and management of haemorrhage and shock.
- Discuss the management of external haemorrhage.
- Differentiate between controlled and uncontrolled haemorrhage.
- Differentiate between the administration rate and amount of IV fluid in a patient with controlled versus uncontrolled haemorrhage.
- Relate internal haemorrhage to the pathophysiology of compensated and decompensated hypovolaemic shock.
- Relate internal haemorrhage to the assessment findings of compensated and decompensated hypovolaemic shock.
- Discuss the management of internal haemorrhage.
- Define shock based on aerobic and anaerobic metabolism.
- Describe the incidence, morbidity, and mortality of shock.
- Describe the body's physiological response to changes in perfusion.
- Describe the effects of decreased perfusion at the capillary level.
- Discuss the cellular ischaemic phase related to hypovolaemic shock.
- Discuss the capillary stagnation phase related to hypovolaemic shock.
- Discuss the capillary washout phase related to hypovolaemic shock.
- Discuss the assessment findings of hypovolaemic shock.
- Relate pulse pressure changes to perfusion status.
- Relate orthostatic vital sign changes to perfusion status.
- Define compensated and decompensated hypovolaemic shock.
- Discuss the pathophysiological changes associated with compensated shock.
- Discuss the assessment findings associated with compensated shock.
- Identify the need for intervention and transport of the patient with compensated shock.
- Discuss the treatment plan and management of compensated shock.
- Discuss the pathophysiological changes associated with decompensated shock.
- Discuss the assessment findings associated with decompensated shock.
- Identify the need for intervention and transport of the patient with decompensated shock.
- Discuss the treatment plan and management of the patient with decompensated shock.
- Differentiate between compensated and decompensated shock.
- Relate external haemorrhage to the pathophysiology of compensated and decompensated hypovolaemic shock.
- Relate external haemorrhage to the assessment findings of compensated and decompensated hypovolaemic shock.
- Differentiate between the normotensive, hypotensive, or profoundly hypotensive patient.
- Differentiate between the administration of fluid in the normotensive, hypotensive, or profoundly hypotensive patient.
- Apply epidemiology to develop prevention strategies for haemorrhage and shock.
- Integrate the pathophysiological principles to the assessment of a patient with haemorrhage or shock.
- Synthesise assessment findings and patient history information to form an initial impression for the patient with haemorrhage or shock.
- Develop, execute and evaluate a treatment plan based on the initial impression for the haemorrhage or shock patient.

Affective

None

Psychomotor

- Demonstrate the assessment of a patient with signs and symptoms of hypovolaemic shock.
- Demonstrate the management of a patient with signs and symptoms of hypovolaemic shock.
- Demonstrate the assessment of a patient with signs and symptoms of compensated hypovolaemic shock.
- Demonstrate the management of a patient with signs and symptoms of compensated hypovolaemic shock.
- Demonstrate the assessment of a patient with signs and symptoms of decompensated hypovolaemic shock.
- Demonstrate the management of a patient with signs and symptoms of decompensated hypovolaemic shock.
- Demonstrate the assessment of a patient with signs and symptoms of external haemorrhage.
- Demonstrate the management of a patient with signs and symptoms of external haemorrhage.
- Demonstrate the assessment of a patient with signs and symptoms of internal haemorrhage.
- Demonstrate the management of a patient with signs and symptoms of internal haemorrhage.

Introduction

After managing the airway, recognising bleeding and understanding how it affects the body are perhaps the most important skills you will learn as a paramedic. Any kind of bleeding is potentially dangerous because it may first cause weakness and then lead to shock. Uncontrolled bleeding may eventually lead to significant hypervolaemia and, ultimately, death.

Bleeding is also the most common cause of shock. As used in this chapter, shock describes a state of collapse and failure of the cardiovascular system in which blood circulation slows and eventually ceases. Shock is actually a normal compensatory mechanism used by the body to maintain systolic blood pressure (BP) and brain perfusion during times of distress. This response can accompany a broad spectrum of events, ranging from heart attacks to falls to allergic reactions to road traffic collisions. If not treated promptly, shock will injure the body's vital organs and ultimately lead to death. Your early and rapid actions can help significantly reduce the morbidity and mortality rates from bleeding and shock.

Anatomy and Physiology of the Cardiovascular System

The cardiovascular system is designed to carry out one crucial job: keep blood flowing between the lungs and the peripheral tissues. In the lungs, blood sheds the gaseous waste products of metabolism—chiefly carbon dioxide—and picks up life-sustaining oxygen. In the peripheral tissues, the process is reversed: Blood unloads oxygen and picks up wastes. If blood flow were to stop or slow significantly, the results would be catastrophic. The cells of the brain, heart, and other organs of the body would have nowhere to eliminate their wastes and would be rapidly engulfed by the toxic by-products of their own metabolism. Oxygen delivery to the tissues also would be disrupted. For a few minutes, the cells could switch to an emergency metabolic system—one that does not require oxygen (anaerobic metabolism), but that form of metabolism produces even more acids and toxic wastes. Within a few minutes of circulatory failure, cells throughout the body would begin to suffocate and die, leading to the state known as *shock*.

To keep the blood moving continuously through the body, the circulatory system requires three intact components Figure 18-1 ▶ :

- A functioning pump: the heart
- Adequate fluid volume: the blood and body fluids
- An intact system of tubing capable of reflex adjustments (constriction and dilatation) in response to changes in pump output and fluid volume: the blood vessels

All three components must interact effectively to maintain life. If any one becomes damaged or is deficient, the whole system is in jeopardy.

Structures of the Heart

The heart is a muscular, cone-shaped organ whose function is to pump blood throughout the body. Located approximately

You are the Paramedic Part 1

You and your colleague have just finished a meal break on what has been a quiet night shift. Suddenly, the station phone rings and you are called to a shooting at a local petrol station. The dispatcher alerts you that police on the scene are requesting "an ambulance urgently".

As you park in front of the garage, you notice a crowd gathering on the pavement. Police officers are establishing a cordon. You grab your primary response bag and head inside as your colleague pulls out the stretcher with the help of a police officer.

As you enter the shop, a detective informs you, "There was a robbery; the clerk was shot and the robber has left the scene". You observe a 22-year-old man sitting on the floor behind the counter and leaning against the wall. He is holding his left upper abdominal quadrant with his bloody hand. The patient appears to weigh about 70 kg. Although he is conscious, alert, and in obvious pain, he tells you that the shooting occurred just as the clock struck 23:00. It is now 23:10. As you begin to talk to the patient, you reach down to palpate his radial pulse but cannot feel it.

Initial Assessment	Recording Time: 0 Minutes
Appearance	Awake and anxious
Level of consciousness	A (Alert to person, place, and day)
Airway	Open and clear
Breathing	Rapid, shallow, and laboured
Circulation	Unpalpable radial pulse

1. Do the lack of significant visible bleeding and the fact that he is alert indicate that this patient is not bleeding seriously?
2. What is the significance of time in this type of incident?

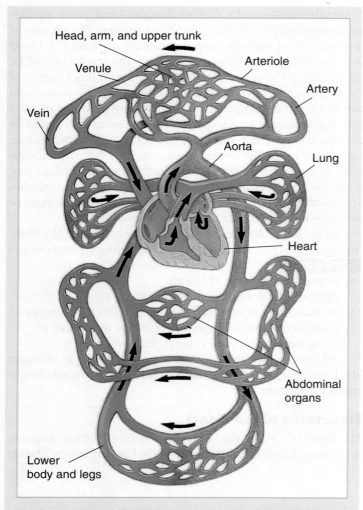

Figure 18-1 The circulatory system requires continuous operation of its three components: the heart, the blood and body fluids, and the blood vessels.

Blood Flow Within the Heart

Two large veins, the superior vena cava and the inferior vena cava, return deoxygenated blood from the body to the right atrium Figure 18-2 ▶ . Blood from the upper part of the body returns to the heart through the superior vena cava; blood from the lower part of the body returns through the inferior vena cava (the larger of the two veins). From the right atrium, blood passes through the tricuspid valve into the right ventricle. The right ventricle then pumps the blood through the pulmonary valve into the pulmonary artery and then on to the lungs.

In the lungs, oxygen is returned to the blood and carbon dioxide and other waste products are removed from it. The freshly oxygenated blood returns to the left atrium through the pulmonary veins. Blood then flows through the bicuspid (mitral) valve into the left ventricle, which pumps the oxygenated blood through the aortic valve, into the aorta (the body's largest artery), and then to the entire body (systemic circulation).

The Cardiac Cycle

The cardiac cycle is the repetitive pumping process that begins with the onset of cardiac muscle contraction and ends with the beginning of the next contraction. Myocardial contraction results in pressure changes within the cardiac chambers, causing the blood to move from areas of high pressure to areas of low pressure.

The pressure in the aorta against which the left ventricle must pump blood is called the afterload. The greater the afterload, the harder it is for the ventricle to eject blood into the aorta. A higher afterload, therefore, reduces the stroke volume, or the amount of blood ejected per contraction.

Cardiac Output = Stroke Volume × Heart Rate

The amount of blood pumped through the circulatory system in 1 minute is referred to as the cardiac output. Cardiac output is expressed in litres per minute (l/min). The cardiac output equals the heart rate multiplied by the stroke volume. Factors that influence the heart rate, the stroke volume, or both will affect cardiac output and, therefore, oxygen delivery (perfusion) to the tissues.

Increased venous return to the heart stretches the ventricles somewhat, resulting in increased cardiac contractility. This relationship, which was first described by the British physiologist Ernest Henry Starling, is known as Starling's law of the heart. Starling noted that if a muscle is stretched slightly before it is stimulated to contract, it would contract with greater force. Thus, if the heart is stretched, the muscle contracts more forcefully.

Although the amount of blood returning to the right atrium varies somewhat from minute to minute, a normal heart continues to pump the same percentage of blood returned, a measure called the ejection fraction. If more blood returns to the heart, the stretched heart pumps harder rather than allowing the blood to back up into the veins. As a result, more blood

behind the sternum, the heart is about the size of a closed fist. It weighs 300 to 350 g in men and 250 to 300 g in women. Roughly two thirds of the heart lies to the left of the mediastinum, the area between the lungs that also contains the great vessels.

The human heart consists of four chambers: two atria (upper chambers) and two ventricles (lower chambers). Each atrium receives blood that is returned to the heart from other parts of the body; each ventricle pumps blood out of the heart. The upper and lower portions of the heart are separated by the atrioventricular valves, which prevent backward flow of blood. The semilunar valves, which serve a similar function, are located between the ventricles and the arteries into which they pump blood. Blood enters the right atrium via the superior and inferior vena cava and the coronary sinus, which consists of veins that collect blood returning from the walls of the heart. Blood from four pulmonary veins enters the left atrium.

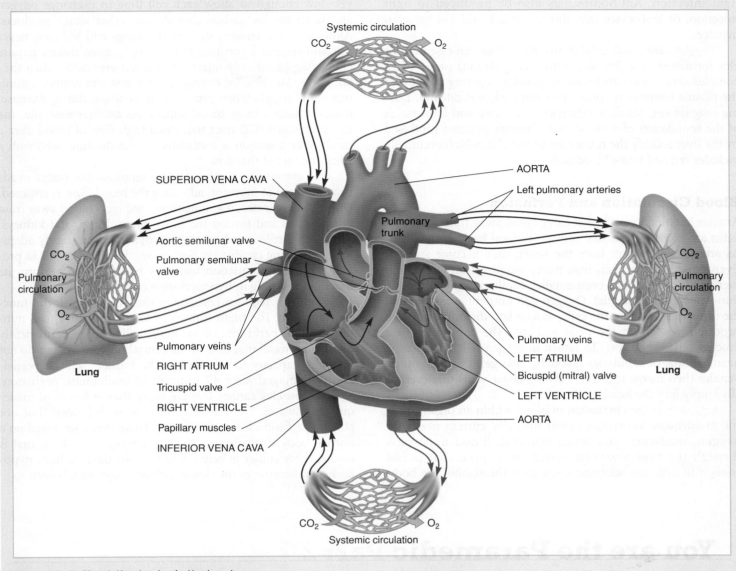

Figure 18-2 Circulation begins in the heart.

is pumped with each contraction, yet the ejection fraction remains unchanged: The amount of blood that is pumped increases, but so does the amount of blood returned. This relationship maintains normal cardiac function when a person changes positions, coughs, breathes, or moves.

Blood and Its Components

Blood consists of plasma and formed elements or cells that are suspended in the plasma. These cells include red blood cells (RBCs), white blood cells (WBCs), and platelets. The purpose of blood is to carry oxygen and nutrients to the tissues and cellular waste products away from the tissues. In addition, the formed elements serve as the mainstay of numerous other body functions, such as fighting infections and controlling bleeding.

Plasma is a watery, straw-coloured fluid that accounts for more than half of the total blood volume. It consists of 92% water and 8% dissolved substances such as chemicals, minerals, and nutrients. Water enters the plasma from the digestive tract, from fluids between cells, and as a by-product of metabolism.

The disc-shaped RBCs (erythrocytes) are the most numerous of the formed elements. Erythrocytes are unable to move on their own; instead, the flowing plasma passively propels them to their destinations. RBCs contain haemoglobin, a protein that gives them their reddish colour. Haemoglobin binds oxygen that is absorbed in the lungs and transports it to the tissues where it is needed.

Several types of WBCs (leucocytes) exist, each of which has a different function. The primary function of all WBCs is to fight infection. Antibodies may also be produced to fight infection, or leucocytes may directly attack and kill bacterial invaders.

Platelets are small cells in the blood that are essential for clot formation. The blood clotting (coagulation) process is a complex series of events involving platelets, clotting proteins in the plasma (clotting factors), other proteins, and calcium. During coagulation, platelets aggregate in a clump and form much of the foundation of a blood clot. Clotting proteins produced by the liver solidify the remainder of the clot, which eventually includes red and white blood cells.

Blood Circulation and Perfusion

Arteries are blood vessels that carry blood away from the heart. Veins are blood vessels that transport blood back to the heart. As arteries get further from the heart, they become smaller. Eventually, they branch into many small arterioles, which themselves divide into even smaller capillaries (microscopic, thin-walled blood vessels). Oxygen and nutrients pass through the capillaries and into the cells, and carbon dioxide and waste products pass from the cells and into the capillaries in a process called diffusion. To return deoxygenated blood to the heart, groups of capillaries gradually enlarge to form venules. Venules then merge together, forming larger veins that eventually empty into the heart.

Perfusion is the circulation of blood within an organ or tissue in adequate amounts to meet the cells' current needs for oxygen, nutrients, and waste removal. Blood must pass through the cardiovascular system at a speed that is fast enough to maintain adequate circulation throughout the body, yet slow enough to allow each cell time to exchange oxygen and nutrients for carbon dioxide and other waste products. Although some tissues, such as the lungs and kidneys, never rest and require a constant blood supply, most tissues require circulating blood only intermittently, but especially when they are active. Muscles, for example, are at rest and require a minimal blood supply when you sleep. In contrast, during exercise, muscles need a large blood supply. As another example, the gastrointestinal (GI) tract requires a high flow of blood after a meal. After digestion is completed, it can do quite well with a small fraction of that flow.

The autonomic nervous system monitors the body's needs from moment to moment, adjusting the blood flow as required. During emergencies, it automatically redirects blood away from other organs and toward the heart, brain, lungs, and kidneys. Thus, the cardiovascular system is dynamic, constantly adapting to changing conditions. Sometimes, however, it fails to provide sufficient circulation for every body part to perform its function, resulting in hypoperfusion or shock.

The heart requires constant perfusion, or it will not function properly. The brain cannot go for more than 4 to 6 minutes without perfusion, or the nerve cells will be permanently damaged—recall that cells of the central nervous system do not have the capacity to regenerate. The kidneys will be permanently damaged after 45 minutes of inadequate perfusion. Skeletal muscles cannot tolerate more than 4 hours of inadequate perfusion. The GI tract can exist with limited (but not absent) perfusion for several hours. These times are based on a normal body temperature (36.8°C). An organ or tissue that is considerably colder is better able to resist damage from hypoperfusion because of the slowing of the body's metabolism.

You are the Paramedic Part 2

Additional help arrives on the scene as you complete your initial assessment. Your colleague has brought in the stretcher and is beginning to administer supplemental oxygen via a nonrebreathing mask at 15 l/min. Police inform you that the robber's weapon may have been a "sawn-off shotgun" that was fired at a fairly close range. The patient tells you a single shot was fired after he told the robber that he would not open the till.

You give the patient some gauze and tell him to hold it firmly against the wound. When you complete your initial assessment of the patient, you decide to perform the rapid physical examination in the back of the ambulance and the SAMPLE history as you have limited time, given the higher priorities and need for rapid transport.

Initial Assessment	Recording Time: 3 Minutes
Breathing	Rapid, laboured, but mechanically intact (no flail segment, punctures, or impaled objects). Oxygen has been started.
Circulation	A rapid, weak carotid pulse can be felt, the external bleeding is easily controlled with direct pressure and gauze. The skin is pale, cool, and moist.

3. On the basis of the information you have so far, and remembering that the patient weighs approximately 70 kg, how much blood did he have before the incident? How much could he have lost so far?

4. What phase or stage of shock is this patient in?

5. Which BLS and ALS interventions would be most appropriate for this patient at this time? Should you insert an intravenous (IV) line at the scene?

Pathophysiology of Haemorrhage

Haemorrhage simply means bleeding. Bleeding can range from a "nick" to a capillary while shaving, to a severely spurting artery from a deep cut with a knife, to a ruptured spleen from striking the steering wheel during a road traffic collision. External bleeding (visible haemorrhage) can usually be controlled by using direct pressure or a pressure bandage. Internal bleeding (haemorrhage that is not visible) is usually not controlled until a surgeon locates the source and sutures it closed. Because internal bleeding is not as obvious, you must rely on signs and symptoms to determine the extent and severity of the haemorrhage.

External Haemorrhage

External bleeding is usually due to a break in the skin. Its extent or severity is often a function of the type of wound and the types of blood vessels that have been injured. (Wound types are discussed in detail in Chapter 19). Bleeding from a capillary usually oozes, bleeding from a vein flows, and bleeding from an artery spurts.

These descriptions are not infallible. For example, considerable oozing from capillaries is possible when a patient gets a very large abrasion (such as the road rash when a cyclist slides along the road surface without protective clothing). Likewise, varicose veins on the leg can produce copious bleeding.

Arteries may spurt initially, but as the patient's BP decreases, often the blood simply flows. In addition, an artery that is incised directly across or in a transverse manner will often recoil and attempt to slow its own bleeding. By contrast, if the artery is cut on an angle, it does not recoil and continues to bleed.

Some injuries that you might expect to be accompanied by considerable external bleeding do not always have serious haemorrhaging. For example, a person who falls off the platform at the railway station and is run over by a train may have amputations of one or more extremities, yet experience little bleeding because the wound was cauterised by the heat of the train's wheels on the rail. Conversely, a person who pulled over on the hard shoulder of the road and was removing the jack from his car's boot when another motorist slammed into the rear of the car, pinning him between the two vehicles, may have severely crushed legs. In such a case, bleeding may be severe, with immediate haemorrhage control required.

Internal Haemorrhage

Internal bleeding as a result of trauma may appear in any portion of the body. A fracture of a bone (such as humerus, ankle, or tibia) produces a somewhat controlled environment in which a relatively small amount of bleeding can occur. By contrast, bleeding into the trunk (that is, thorax, abdomen, or pelvis), because of its much larger space, tends to be severe and uncontrolled. Nontraumatic internal haemorrhage usually occurs in cases of GI bleeding from the upper or lower GI tract, ruptured ectopic pregnancies, ruptured aneurysms, or other conditions.

Any internal bleeding must be treated promptly. The signs of internal haemorrhage (such as discolouration and haematoma) do not always develop quickly, so you must rely on other signs and symptoms and an evaluation of the mechanism of injury (MOI) to make this diagnosis. Pay close attention to patient complaints of pain or tenderness, development of tachycardia, and pallor. In addition to evaluating the MOI, be alert for the development of shock when you suspect internal bleeding.

Management of a patient with internal haemorrhaging focuses on the treatment of shock, minimising movement of the injured or bleeding part or region, and rapid transport. In time, it is likely that the patient will need a surgical procedure to stop the bleeding. In recent years, ultrasound has been used to locate bleeding in the accident and emergency (A&E) department before transferring the patient to the theatre for the surgical resolution of the problem.

Controlled Versus Uncontrolled Haemorrhage

Bleeding that you can control (such as external bleeding that responds to a pressure bandage) and bleeding that you cannot control (such as a bleeding peptic ulcer) are serious emergencies. As a consequence, the initial assessment of the patient includes a search for life-threatening bleeding. If found, the haemorrhage must be controlled; if the haemorrhage cannot be controlled in the prehospital environment, all of your efforts should concentrate on attempting to control the bleeding as you transport the patient as quickly as possible to the A&E.

Most external bleeding can be managed with direct pressure, although arterial bleeding may take 5 or more minutes of direct pressure to form a clot. (Remember this if you accidentally cannulate the brachial artery instead of the vein in the arm!) Military experience has shown that the use of pressure points is not as effective as previously thought and is difficult to manage while trying to evacuate a person rapidly from the battlefield. For this reason, most military medical training calls for use of a tourniquet for external bleeding to an extremity that cannot be controlled with direct pressure and a pressure bandage.

Because most cases of internal bleeding are rarely fully controlled in the prehospital setting, a patient with this type of injury needs rapid transport to the A&E department. Some strategies may be effective in the prehospital environment depending on the cause of the bleeding. For example, the external circumferential pressure of a pelvic splint may help control the massive bleeding that accompanies a pelvic fracture.

The Significance of Bleeding

When patients have serious external haemorrhage, it is often difficult to determine the amount of blood loss. Blood looks different on different surfaces, for example when it is absorbed in clothing compared to when it has been diluted by being mixed in water. Although you should attempt to determine the amount of external blood loss, the patient's presentation and your assessment will ultimately direct your care and treatment plan.

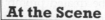

At the Scene

Not every person has the same amount of blood, so you must be able to estimate the patient's blood volume *before* the trauma occurred. Blood volume is relative to weight—it accounts for 6% to 8% of the total body weight. One litre of blood weighs approximately 1 kg.

The adult male body contains approximately 70 ml of blood per kilogram of body weight, whereas adult female bodies contain approximately 65 ml/kg. For a typical adult weighing 80 kg (13 st 5 lb), the total blood volume is approximately 6 litres (10 to 12 units). The body cannot tolerate an acute blood loss of more than 20% of this total blood volume. Thus, if the typical adult loses more than 1 litre (approximately 2 units) of blood, significant changes in vital signs will occur, including increasing heart and respiratory rates and decreasing BP. An isolated femur fracture, for example, can easily result in the loss of 1 litre or more of blood in the soft tissues of the thigh.

Because infants and children have less blood volume than their adult counterparts, they may experience the same effect with smaller amounts of blood loss. For example, a 1-year-old child has a total blood volume of about 800 ml, so significant symptoms of blood loss may occur after only 100 to 200 ml of blood loss. To put this in perspective, remember that a soft drink can holds roughly 330 ml of liquid **Figure 18-3 ▾**.

How well people compensate for blood loss is related to how rapidly they bleed. A healthy adult can comfortably donate one unit (500 ml) of blood in a period of 15 to 20 minutes without having ill effects from this decrease in blood volume. If a similar blood loss occurs in a much shorter period, hypovolaemic shock, a condition in which low blood volume results in inadequate perfusion and even death, may develop rapidly.

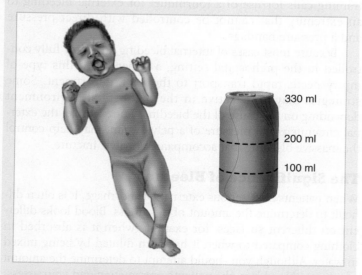

330 ml

200 ml

100 ml

Figure 18-3 A soft drink can holds roughly 330 ml of liquid.

Consider bleeding to be serious if any of the following conditions are present:

- A significant MOI, especially when the MOI suggests that severe forces affected the abdomen or chest
- Poor general appearance of the patient
- Signs and symptoms of shock
- Significant amount of blood loss
- Rapid blood loss
- Uncontrollable bleeding

Physiological Response to Haemorrhage

Typically, bleeding from an open artery is bright red (because of the high oxygen content) and spurts in time with the pulse. The pressure that causes the blood to spurt also makes this type of bleeding difficult to control. As the amount of blood circulating in the body drops, so does the patient's BP and, eventually, the arterial spurting diminishes.

Blood from an open vein is much darker (low oxygen content) and flows steadily. Because it is under less pressure, most venous blood does not spurt and is easier to manage. Bleeding from damaged capillary vessels is dark red and oozes from a wound steadily but slowly. Venous and capillary bleeding is more likely to clot spontaneously than arterial bleeding.

On its own, bleeding tends to stop rather quickly, within about 10 minutes, in response to internal clotting mechanisms and exposure to air. When vessels are lacerated, blood flows rapidly from the open vessel. The open ends of the vessel then begin to narrow (vasoconstrict), which reduces the amount of bleeding. Platelets aggregate at the site, plugging the hole and sealing the injured portions of the vessel, a process called haemostasis. Bleeding will not stop if a clot does not form, unless the injured vessel is completely cut off from the main blood supply. Direct contact with body tissues and fluids or the external environment commonly triggers the blood's clotting factors.

Despite the efficiency of this system, it may fail in certain situations. A number of medications, including anticoagulants such as aspirin and warfarin, interfere with normal clotting. With a severe injury, the damage to the vessel may be so extensive that a clot cannot completely block the hole. Sometimes, only part of the vessel wall is cut, preventing it from constricting. In these cases, bleeding will continue unless it is stopped by external means. In a case involving acute blood loss, the patient might die before the body's haemostatic defences of vasoconstriction and of clotting can help.

Assessment of a Bleeding Patient

The assessment of any patient begins with a good scene assessment and proceeds to your general impression and initial assessment. Once the scene is deemed safe to enter, you will need to take the appropriate level of universal precautions. Depending on the severity of bleeding and your general impression, this will entail gloves, mask, eyeshield/goggles, and, when the patient is very bloody or blood is spurting, a plastic apron **Figure 18-4 ▸**.

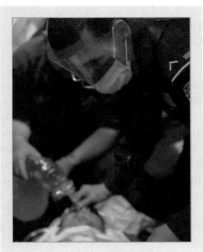

Figure 18-4 Depending on the severity of bleeding and your general impression, universal precautions will entail gloves, mask, eyeshield, and, in some cases, a plastic apron.

During the initial assessment, after determining the patient's mental status with AVPU, you must locate and manage immediate threats to life involving the airway, breathing, and circulation. Ensure that the patient has a patent airway. If you observe bleeding from the mouth or facial areas, keep the suction unit within reach.

If the patient has minor external bleeding, you can note it and move on with the initial assessment; management of this problem can wait until the patient has been properly assessed and prioritised. Do not get sidetracked by applying dressings and bandages to a patient who has much more serious problems. If major external bleeding is present, you should deal with it during the initial assessment. If you suspect internal bleeding, begin management by keeping the patient warm and administering supplemental oxygen by a nonrebreathing mask at 15 l/min.

At the Scene

When you are dealing with a bleeding patient, be sure to take necessary precautions to protect yourself from splashing or splattering. Wear appropriate PPE, including gloves, apron, mask, and eye protection. This is especially essential when arterial bleeding is present. Also remember that frequent, thorough handwashing between patients and after every call is mandatory.

Carefully assess the MOI in trauma patients because it may be your best indicator that the patient has sustained an internal injury and may be bleeding. **Table 18-1 ▸** lists some MOIs that can give clues about internal bleeding.

During your focused history, elaborate on the patient's chief complaint using the OPQRST mnemonic, and obtain a history of the present illness using SAMPLE. Ask the patient if

At the Scene

Consider any patient exhibiting signs and symptoms of shock without obvious injury to have probable internal bleeding, usually in the abdominal cavity.

Table 18-1	The MOI: Indicators of Internal Bleeding
Mechanism of Injury	**Potential Internal Bleeding Sources**
Fall from a ladder striking head	Head injury or haematoma
Fall from a ladder striking extremities	Possible fractures; consider chest injury
Child struck by car (Waddell's triad)	Head trauma, chest and abdomen injuries, leg fractures
Fall on outstretched arm	Possible broken bone or joint injury
Child thrown or falls from height	Children usually have a head-first impact, causing head injury
Unrestrained driver in head-on collision (up-and-over route)	Head and neck, chest, abdomen injuries
Unrestrained driver in head-on collision (down-and-under route)	Knees, femur, hip, and pelvis injuries
Unrestrained front-seat passenger, side impact collision with intrusion into vehicle	Humeral fracture exposing the chest wall (possible flail chest); pelvis and acetabular injuries
Unrestrained driver crushed against steering column	Chest and abdomen injuries, ruptured spleen, neck trauma
Road bike or mountain bike (over the handlebars)	Fractured clavicle, abrasions (road rash), head trauma if no helmet
Abrupt motorcycle stop, causing rider to catapult over the handlebars	Fractured femurs, head and neck injuries
Diving into the shallow end of a swimming pool	Head and neck injuries
Assault or fight	Punching or kicking injury to chest and abdomen and the face
Blast or explosion	Injury from direct strike with debris; indirect and pressure wave in enclosed space

he or she experiences any dizziness or syncope. Are there any signs and symptoms of hypovolaemic shock? Ask the patient about current medications that may thin the blood and about any history of clotting insufficiency. Is there any pain, tenderness, bruising, guarding, or swelling? These signs and symptoms may indicate internal bleeding.

During the physical examination (rapid or focused, depending on the MOI), note the colour of bleeding and try to determine its source. Bright red blood from a wound or the mouth, rectum, or other orifice indicates fresh arterial bleeding. Coffee-ground coloured emesis is a sign of upper GI bleeding; this kind of blood is old and looks like used coffee grounds.

Melaena, the passage of dark, tarry stools, indicates lower GI bleeding. Haematochezia, by contrast, is the passage of stools containing bright red blood and may indicate bleeding near the external opening of the colon. Haemorrhoids in the lower colon tend to cause haematochezia (bleeding from the anus). Haematuria (blood in the urine) may suggest serious renal injury or illness. Nonmenstrual vaginal bleeding is always significant as well.

Management of a Bleeding Patient

Always take universal precautions when treating bleeding patients. As with all patient care, ensure that the patient has an open airway and is breathing adequately. Provide high-flow supplemental oxygen, and assist ventilation if needed, paying special attention to cervical spine control in trauma patients.

Managing External Haemorrhage

To control external haemorrhaging, follow these steps:

1. Apply direct pressure over the wound.
2. Elevate the injury above the level of the heart if no fracture is suspected.
3. Apply a pressure dressing.
4. Apply pressure at the appropriate pressure point while maintaining direct pressure.

A tourniquet is generally used only as a last resort, when arterial bleeding is uncontrolled by all other methods.

Bleeding From the Nose, Ears, and Mouth

Bleeding from the nose (epistaxis) or bleeding from the ears following a head injury may indicate a skull fracture. In such a case, you should not attempt to stop the blood flow. Applying excessive pressure to the injury may force the blood leaking through the ear or nose to collect within the head, ultimately increasing intracranial pressure and possibly causing permanent damage. If you suspect a skull fracture, cover the bleeding site loosely with a sterile gauze pad to collect the blood and help keep contaminants away from the site—there is always a risk of infection to the brain with a skull fracture. If blood contains cerebrospinal fluid, the dressing will show a characteristic staining of the dressing that resembles a bull's-eye target with cerebrospinal fluid forming a halo around the blood.

Bleeding From Other Areas

Haemorrhages from other areas of the body should be controlled through use of direct pressure and elevation, if appropriate. Apply pressure dressings, especially at pressure points for the upper and lower extremities. In addition, use splints (or inflatable splints) as necessary, always following your local guidelines. Reserve the tourniquet for use as a last resort with bleeding when all else has failed.

Once bleeding is controlled and a sterile dressing and pressure bandage have been applied, keep the patient warm and in the appropriate position. Allow the patient's condition to dictate the mode of transport.

Special Management Techniques for External Haemorrhage

Much of the bleeding associated with broken bones occurs because the sharp ends of the bones lacerate vessels, muscles, and other tissues. As long as a fracture remains unstable, the bone ends will move and continue to damage tissues and vessels. They may also break up clots that have partially formed, resulting in ongoing bleeding. For these reasons, immobilising a fracture is a priority in the prompt control of bleeding. Often, simple splints will quickly control the bleeding associated with a fracture. If not, you may need to use a different splinting device.

Inflatable Splints

Inflatable splints can control the bleeding associated with severe soft-tissue injuries, such as massive or complex lacerations, or with simple fractures. They also stabilise the simple fracture itself. An inflatable splint acts like a pressure dressing applied to an entire extremity rather than to a small, local area.

Once you have applied an inflatable splint, monitor circulation in the distal extremity. Because an inflatable splint is typically inflated to approximately 50 mm Hg (so you can still dent the splint with your fingertips), it would not be appropriate to use on arterial bleeding because the splint would not actually control the bleeding until the patient's systolic BP dropped to the pressure of the splint. Use only PPE-approved, clean, or disposable valve stems when orally inflating the splint. The use of inflatable splints in the UK is very rare and seldomly encouraged due to the potential tourniquet effect and adverse side effects of this.

Forceps

Forceps may be helpful when a vessel has been severed, especially if it has retracted into the surrounding tissue. Simply apply forceps to the ends of the vessel. Be sure to check your local guidelines about the use of forceps in your area.

Tourniquets

The tourniquet is useful if a patient is bleeding severely from a partial or complete amputation and other methods of bleeding control have proved ineffective. The paramedic should realise that its application can cause permanent damage to nerves, muscles, and blood vessels, resulting in the loss of an extremity. The procedure for tourniquet application is shown in Skill Drill 19-2 in Chapter 19. Whenever applying a tourniquet, make sure you observe the following precautions:

- Do not apply a tourniquet directly over any joint. Where possible use a commercially available device or blood pressure cuff inflated above the patient's systolic blood pressure.
- If the above is not available, use the widest bandage possible. Make sure that it is tightened securely.
- Never use wire, rope, a belt, or any other narrow material as the tourniquet; it could cut into the skin.

- Use wide padding under the tourniquet, if possible, to protect the tissues and help with arterial compression.
- Make a note of the time the tourniquet was applied.
- Never cover a tourniquet with a bandage or let clothing slide over and hide it. Leave it in full view.
- Do not loosen the tourniquet after you have applied it. Hospital clinicians will loosen it once they are prepared to manage the bleeding.

Managing Internal Haemorrhage

The definitive management of a patient with internal haemorrhage occurs in the hospital. Prehospital management of suspected internal bleeding involves treating for shock and splinting injured extremities:

1. Keep the patient supine (on blankets), open the airway, and check breathing and pulse.
2. Administer high-flow supplemental oxygen and assist ventilation if needed.
3. Splint broken bones or joint injuries. If a pelvic fracture is suspected, you may consider use of a pelvic splint (if available).
4. Place blankets under the patient to maintain body heat.
5. If no fractures are suspected, elevate the legs 30 cm.
6. Insert a large-bore (14- or 16-gauge) IV cannula if the systolic blood pressure falls below 90 mm Hg, and administer a fluid challenge of 250 ml (provided the lungs are clear) en route to hospital. Insert an IV cannula at the scene only if transport is delayed (such as if the patient is trapped). Whenever possible, use pre-warmed IV fluids to prevent the patient from becoming chilled.
7. Consider giving analgesia if required and the vital signs are stable.
8. Monitor the serial vital signs, and watch diligently for developing shock.

If the patient shows any signs of shock (hypoperfusion), transport rapidly while providing aggressive management en route. Because a patient in shock is usually emotionally upset, you should provide psychological support as well.

Transport of Patients With Haemorrhage

In case of haemorrhage, the issue is not whether the patient will be transported, but rather how fast the transport decision should be made and where the patient should be taken for definitive care. There are a few exceptions to this rule—for example, if you are standing by at a sporting event or concert and are asked by a "first responder" to evaluate a minor wound that has been bleeding. The decision to transport a patient with even a relatively minor wound should take into consideration factors such as the need for stitches, whether the patient has had a tetanus injection in the past 10 years, where the patient lives, the location of a local A&E department, and whether the patient or his or her companion is reliable and will follow up properly. (Wounds are discussed in more detail in Chapter 19.)

Most patients with internal or external haemorrhage will need to be transported to hospital for further care. Consideration for the priority of the patient and the availability of a regional trauma centre should be your concerns when making a transport decision in such cases. Patients who have severe internal or external bleeding, especially if uncontrolled, will usually be candidates for surgical interventions and should be transported to a hospital with those capabilities. Patients with specific causes of bleeding such as major trauma or specific devastating wounds (such as leg amputation, glove avulsion) should be taken to a hospital that is fully prepared to care for the patient. In ambulance services with helicopters available, it may be appropriate to consider this method of transport for a patient with suspected severe internal or uncontrollable external bleeding, where time or distance is a major factor.

Pathophysiology of Shock

Hypoperfusion occurs when the level of tissue perfusion decreases below normal. Early decreased tissue perfusion may result in subtle changes, such as altered mental status, long before a patient's vital signs (blood pressure, pulse, respiratory rate) appear abnormal. Shock refers to a state of collapse and failure of the cardiovascular system that leads to inadequate circulation, creating inadequate tissue perfusion. Like internal bleeding, shock cannot be seen. It is not a specific disease or injury, but rather a dangerous condition that results in inadequate flow of blood to the body's cells and failure to rid the body of metabolic wastes.

Notes from Nancy

Don't wait until the BP falls before you suspect shock and begin treatment!

Evaluation of a patient's level of organ perfusion is important in diagnosing shock. If the conditions causing shock are not promptly addressed, the patient will soon die. When the body senses tissue hypoperfusion, compensatory mechanisms are set into action. In some cases, this is enough to stabilise the patient's condition. In other cases, the severity of disease or injury overwhelms the normal compensatory mechanisms, leading to progressive deterioration in the patient's condition. Perfusion depends on cardiac output, systemic vascular resistance (SVR), and transport of oxygen:

Cardiac Output = Heart Rate × Stroke Volume

Blood Pressure = Cardiac Output × Systemic Vascular Resistance

Because the heart cannot pump out what is not in its holding chambers, BP varies directly with cardiac output, SVR, and blood volume. Hypoperfusion, therefore, can result from inadequate cardiac output, decreased SVR, or the inability of RBCs to deliver oxygen to tissues.

At the Scene

Remember that BP may be the last measurable factor to change in shock. The body has several automatic mechanisms to compensate for initial blood loss and to help maintain BP. Thus, by the time you detect a drop in BP, shock is well developed. This is particularly true in infants and children, who can maintain their BP until they have lost close to half their blood volume.

Mechanisms of Shock

Recall that normal tissue perfusion requires three intact mechanisms: a pump (heart), fluid volume (blood and body fluids), and tubing capable of reflex adjustments (constriction and dilatation) in response to changes in pump output and fluid volume (blood vessels). If any one of those mechanisms is damaged, tissue perfusion may be disrupted, and shock will ensue.

When shock arises because of failure of the heart, it is called cardiogenic shock (*cardio* = heart + *genic* = causing). Cardiac arrest is the most drastic form of cardiogenic shock, but not the only form. Cardiogenic shock may occur secondary to myocardial infarction, cardiac arrhythmias, pulmonary embolism, severe acidosis, or a variety of other conditions. All of these conditions have one thing in common: They interfere with the heart's ability to pump normally.

Shock may also occur because of a loss of fluid volume; perfusion cannot take place if there isn't enough fluid to propel through the system. When shock comes about because of inadequate volume, it is termed hypovolaemic shock (*hypo* = deficient + *vol* = volume + *aemia* = in the blood). Volume can be lost through bleeding, plasma (as in burns), or electrolyte solution (as in vomiting, diarrhoea, and sweating). Suspect a hypovolaemic component of shock in any patient with unexplained shock, and treat the patient for hypovolaemia first.

Notes from Nancy

Suspect a hypovolaemic component in any patient with unexplained shock, and treat for hypovolaemia first.

Failure of vasoconstriction (that is, a decrease in the peripheral vascular resistance [PVR]) may lead to neurogenic shock, so called because the sympathetic nervous system ordinarily controls the dilatation and constriction of blood vessels. In a healthy person, the diameter of the blood vessels constantly changes in response to signals from the nervous system, allowing the body to adapt to changes in position, fluid volume, and so forth. When you stand up, for example, blood vessels in your legs reflexively constrict to divert the circulation toward more vital areas, like the brain. Similarly, when you donate blood or sweat a litre of fluid, your blood vessels constrict to accommodate a smaller fluid volume. In certain situations, nervous system control over the diameter of blood vessels becomes deranged—for example, after spinal cord injury or in some cases of pul-

monary embolism or gastric overdistension—and the blood vessels lose their tone and dilate. A given blood volume then has to be accommodated quite suddenly in a much larger container. The net effect is a relative hypovolaemia (the volume in the container is now inadequate relative to the increased size of the container), which the body experiences as shock.

More than one component of the circulatory system may be affected in case of shock. For example, a patient in shock after a myocardial infarction is likely to have an element of cardiogenic shock, because the damaged heart can no longer pump efficiently, and an element of hypovolaemic shock, if the patient has been vomiting, sweating, or is too nauseated to take in fluids. Some types of shock always result from combined deficits from both fluid leakage into the interstitial space as well as vasodilatation.

Certain categories of patients are at high risk to develop shock. They include patients known to have had trauma or bleeding; elderly people, but especially elderly men with urinary tract infections; patients with massive myocardial infarction; pregnant women; and patients with a possible source for septic shock (such as burned patients and people with diabetes or cancer).

Compensation for Decreased Perfusion

Central among the homeostatic mechanisms that regulate cardiovascular dynamics are those that maintain BP. When any event results in decreased perfusion (such as in blood loss, myocardial infarction, loss of vasomotor tone, or tension pneumothorax), the body must respond immediately to preserve the vital organs. Baroreceptors located in the aortic arch and carotid sinuses sense the decreased blood flow and activate the vasomotor centre, which oversees changes in the diameter of blood vessels, to begin constriction of the vessels.

Stimulation typically occurs when the systolic pressure is between 60 and 80 mm Hg in adults or even lower in children. A decrease in systolic pressure to less than 80 mm Hg stimulates the vasomotor centre to increase arterial pressure by constricting vessels. The drop in arterial pressure decreases the stretching of the arterial walls, thereby decreasing baroreceptor stimulation. Normally, baroreceptor stimulation inhibits the vasoconstrictor centre of the medulla and excites the vagal centre, leading to vasodilatation in the peripheral circulatory system and a decrease in heart rate and contractility, causing a concomitant decrease in arterial pressure. The sympathetic nervous system is also stimulated as the body recognises a potential catastrophic event.

In response to hypoperfusion, the renin-angiotensin-aldosterone system is activated and antidiuretic hormone is released from the pituitary gland. Together, these mechanisms trigger salt and water retention and peripheral vasoconstriction. The result is an increase in the patient's BP and cardiac output. Depending on the severity of the insult, variable amounts of fluid will shift from the interstitial tissues into the vascular compartment. The spleen also releases some RBCs that are normally stored there to augment the blood's oxygen-carrying capacity. The overall response of the initial compensatory mechanisms is to increase the preload, stroke volume, and heart rate, which usually results in an increase in cardiac output.

As hypoperfusion persists, the myocardial oxygen demand continues to increase. Eventually, the accelerated compensatory mechanisms are no longer able to keep up with the body's demand. Myocardial function then worsens, with decreased cardiac output and ejection fraction. Tissue perfusion decreases, leading to impaired cell metabolism. Often, the systolic BP decreases, especially in progressive hypoperfusion or "decompensated" shock. Fluid may leak from the blood vessels, causing systemic and pulmonary oedema. Other signs of hypoperfusion may also be present, such as dusky skin colour, oliguria, and impaired thinking.

The body produces its own "medicine", adrenaline and noradrenaline, in the adrenal glands in response to hypoperfusion. These substances are released by the body as part of the global compensatory state. Adrenaline is also administered by health care professionals in cases of anaphylaxis, severe airway disease, and cardiac arrest.

Release of adrenaline improves cardiac output by increasing the heart rate and strength. The alpha-1 response to its release includes vasoconstriction, increased peripheral vascular resistance, and increased afterload from the arteriolar constriction. Alpha-2 effects ensure a regulated release of alpha-1. Beta responses from the release of adrenaline primarily affect the heart and lungs. Increases in heart rate, contractility, conductivity, and automaticity occur in tandem with bronchodilation.

Effects of noradrenaline are primarily alpha-1 and alpha-2 in nature and centre on vasoconstriction and increasing PVR. This vasoconstriction allows the body to shunt blood from areas of lesser need to areas of greater need; that is, it serves to keep the brain and other vital organs perfused in the early phases of shock. In an effort to maintain circulation to the brain, the body will shunt blood away from the following tissues, in this order: placenta, skin, muscles, gut, kidneys, liver, heart, lungs. The skin and muscles can survive with minimal blood flow from vasoconstriction for a much longer period than can major organs such as the kidneys, liver, heart, and lungs. If the blood supply is inadequate to the major organs for more than 60 minutes, they often develop complications that will lead to death, such as renal failure and respiratory distress syndrome. This concept has been traditionally referred to as the "golden hour of trauma", and it explains why it is so important to address the cause of the shock in as timely a manner as possible.

Failure of compensatory mechanisms to preserve perfusion leads to decreases in preload and cardiac output. Myocardial blood supply and oxygenation decrease, reducing myocardial perfusion. As cardiac output further decreases, coronary artery perfusion also decreases, leading to myocardial ischaemia.

Types of Shock

The inadequate oxygen and nutrient delivery to the metabolic apparatus of the cell experienced in shock results in impaired cellular metabolism. Once a certain level of tissue hypoperfusion is reached, cell damage proceeds in a similar manner, regardless of the type of initial insult. Impairment of cellular metabolism results in the inability to use oxygen and glucose properly at the

You are the Paramedic Part 3

You decide that the patient does not require spinal immobilisation. He reports that he was not blown to the ground, but rather felt dizzy and sat down on his own. You and your colleague decide to quickly pick the patient up and load him onto the stretcher, rather than spending the time for immobilisation to a longboard. You also decide to insert the IV cannula en route to hospital.

The patient is starting to become confused as you place him supine with legs elevated and head out the door. He states that he is nauseated and thirsty and asks your colleague, "Am I going to die"? When closing the back of the ambulance, you note on your watch that 7 minutes have elapsed on the scene. Your plan for the next few minutes is to reassess, get IV fluids running, pre-alert the A&E department, and do the rapid trauma assessment and SAMPLE history.

Vital Signs	Recording Time: 5 Minutes
Mental status	V (Responsive to verbal stimuli), confused about place and day
Respirations	26 breaths/min, shallow and laboured
Pulse	120 beats/min, thready (core only, not peripheral)
Blood pressure	106/80 mm Hg
Skin	Pale, cool, and moist
SpO_2	95% on nonrebreathing mask at 15 l/min of supplemental oxygen
ECG	Sinus tachycardia with no ectopic

6. For this patient, is the SpO_2 a helpful indicator?

7. Why weren't the baseline vital signs taken at the scene?

cellular level. The cell converts to anaerobic metabolism, which causes increased lactic acid production and metabolic acidosis, decreased oxygen affinity for haemoglobin, decreased adenosine triphosphate (ATP) production, changes in cellular electrolytes, cellular oedema, and release of lysosomal enzymes. Glucose impairment leads to an elevated blood glucose level due to release of catecholamines and cortisol. In addition, fat breakdown (lipolysis) with ketone formation may occur.

Shock can occur due to inadequacy of the central circulation (the heart and great vessels) or the peripheral circulation (the remaining vessels and the microscopic circulation, such as arterioles, venules, and capillaries). The Weil-Shubin classification considers shock from a mechanistic point of view. From this perspective, two types of shock are distinguished: central shock, which consists of cardiogenic shock and obstructive shock, and peripheral shock, which includes hypovolaemic shock and distributive shock.

Regardless of type, shock is characterised by reduced cardiac output, circulatory insufficiency, and rapid heartbeat (tachycardia). Most types of shock also include pallor, except for spinal shock and sepsis. The patient's mental status may be altered. Low BP, although classically associated with shock, is a late sign, especially in children.

Cardiogenic Shock

Cardiogenic shock occurs when the heart is unable to circulate sufficient blood to maintain adequate peripheral oxygen delivery. Circulation of blood throughout the vascular system requires the constant pumping action of a normal and vigorous heart muscle. Many diseases can cause destruction or inflammation of this muscle. Within certain limits, the heart can adapt to these problems. If too much muscular damage occurs, however, the heart no longer functions effectively. Filling is impaired because of a lack of pressure to return blood to the heart (preload), or outflow is obstructed by a lack of pumping function. In either case, direct pump failure is the cause of shock. In the case of ischaemic heart disease, pump failure is generally due to a loss of 40% or more of the functioning myocardium.

The most common cause of cardiogenic shock is extensive infarction of the left ventricle, diffuse ischaemia, or decompensated congestive heart failure resulting in primary pump failure. The heart damage may be due to a single massive event or result from cumulative damage. Other forms of cardiac dysfunction may result in cardiogenic shock as well—for example, large ventricular septal defect, cardiomyopathy, or significant cardiac arrhythmias.

Patients have a poor prognosis when more than 40% of the left ventricle is destroyed. Historically, in about 7.5% of patients with acute myocardial infarction, cardiogenic shock develops, and mortality rates range as high as 80%, even with appropriate therapy.

Obstructive Shock

Obstructive shock occurs when blood flow in the heart or great vessels becomes blocked. In pericardial tamponade, diastolic filling of the right ventricle is impaired, leading to a decrease in cardiac output. Aortic dissection leads to a false lumen (aortic opening) with loss of normal blood flow. A left atrial tumour may obstruct flow between the atrium and ventricle, thereby decreasing cardiac output. Obstruction of the superior or inferior vena cava (such as vena cava syndrome as in third-trimester pregnancy) decreases cardiac output by decreasing venous return. A large pulmonary embolus or tension pneumothorax may prevent adequate blood flow to the lungs, resulting in inadequate venous return to the left side of the heart.

Hypovolaemic Shock

Hypovolaemic shock occurs when the circulating blood volume does not deliver adequate oxygen and nutrients to the body. It is subdivided into two types, exogenous and endogenous, depending on where the fluid loss occurs.

The most common cause of exogenous hypovolaemic shock is external bleeding. Haemorrhage is most prevalent in trauma patients due to blunt or penetrating injuries to vessels or organs, long bone or pelvic fractures, major vascular injuries (as in traumatic amputation), and multisystem injury. The organs and organ systems with a high incidence of exsanguination from penetrating injuries include the heart, thoracic vascular system, abdominal vascular system (such as abdominal aorta, superior mesenteric artery), venous system (such as inferior vena cava or portal vein), and liver.

Endogenous hypovolaemic shock occurs when the fluid loss is contained within the body, as in dehydration, burn injury, and crush injury. With severe thermal burns, for example, intravascular plasma leaks from the circulatory system into the burned tissues that lie adjacent to the injury. By comparison, crushing injuries may result in the loss of blood and plasma from damaged vessels into injured tissues.

Abnormal losses of fluids and electrolytes (that is, dehydration) may occur through a variety of mechanisms:

- GI losses, especially through vomiting and diarrhoea
- Increased loss as a consequence of fever, hyperventilation, or high environmental temperatures (through the lungs)
- Increased sweating
- Internal losses ("third-space" losses), as in peritonitis, pancreatitis, and ileus
- Plasma losses from burns, drains, and granulating wounds

Other causes of body fluid deficits include ascites, diabetes insipidus, acute renal failure, and osmotic diuresis secondary to hyperosmolar states (such as diabetic ketoacidosis).

In each case, the fluid lost has a unique electrolyte composition, and long-term therapy aims to restore the deficient body chemicals. For treatment in the prehospital environment, however, all excessive fluid losses can be considered to lead to dehydration.

Symptoms of dehydration include loss of appetite (anorexia), nausea, vomiting, and sometimes fainting when standing up (postural syncope). Physical examination of a dehydrated patient reveals poor skin turgor (the skin over the forehead or sternum will "tent" when pinched); a shrunken, furrowed tongue; and sunken eyes. The pulse will be weak and rapid, rising more than 20 beats/min when the patient is raised from a recumbent to a sitting position (a manoeuvre that may cause the patient to feel faint). When fluid and electrolyte depletion are severe, shock and coma may be present.

A dehydrated patient needs replacement of fluid and electrolytes and should be given an IV infusion of normal saline or Hartmann's solution at a rate of 100 to 200 ml/h for an adult, depending on the circumstances. Keep the patient flat to optimise circulation to the brain.

Distributive Shock

Distributive shock occurs when there is widespread dilation of the resistance vessels (small arterioles), the capacitance vessels (small venules), or both. As a result, the circulating blood volume pools in the expanded vascular beds and tissue perfusion decreases. The three most common types of distributive shock are septic shock, neurogenic shock, and anaphylactic shock.

Septic Shock

Sepsis comes from the Greek word meaning "to putrefy". Septic shock is defined as the presence of sepsis syndrome plus a systolic BP of less than 90 mm Hg or a decrease from the baseline BP of more than 40 mm Hg.

Sepsis occurs as a result of widespread infection, usually due to gram-negative bacterial organisms; gram-positive bacteria, fungi, viruses, and rickettsia can also be causative agents. Complex interactions occur between the pathogen and the body's defence systems. Initially, the body's defence mechanisms may keep the infection at bay. The infection activates the inflammatory-immune response, which invokes humoral, cellular, and biochemical pathways. This response results in increased microvascular permeability (leaky capillaries), vasodilation, third-space fluid shifts, and microthrombi formation. In some patients, an uncontrolled and unregulated inflammatory-immune response occurs, resulting in hypoperfusion to the cells owing to opening of AV shunts, tissue destruction, and organ death. Left untreated, the result is multiple-organ dysfunction syndrome and, often, death.

Septic shock is a complex problem. First, there is an insufficient volume of fluid in the container, because much of the blood has leaked out of the vascular system (hypovolaemia). Second, the fluid that leaks out often collects in the respiratory system, interfering with ventilation. Third, a larger-than-normal vascular bed is asked to contain the smaller-than-normal volume of intravascular fluid.

Neurogenic Shock

Neurogenic shock usually results from spinal cord injury. Less commonly, it may derive from medical causes such as brain conditions, tumours, pressure on the spinal cord, or spina bifida. The effect of these conditions is loss of normal sympathetic nervous system tone and vasodilation.

In neurogenic shock, the muscles in the walls of the blood vessels are cut off from the nerve impulses that cause them to contract. As a consequence, all vessels below the level of the spinal injury dilate widely, increasing the size and capacity of the vascular system and causing blood to pool. The available 5 to 6 litres of blood in the body can no longer fill this enlarged vascular system. Perfusion of organs and tissues becomes inadequate, even though no blood or fluid has been lost, and shock occurs. The patient experiences relative hypovolaemia, which leads to hypotension (systolic BP usually between 80 and 100 mm Hg). In addition, relative bradycardia occurs because the sympathetic nervous system is not stimulated to release catecholamines. The skin is pink, warm, and dry because of cutaneous vasodilation. There is no release of adrenaline and noradrenaline, which would otherwise produce the classic sign of pale, cool, perspiring skin. Instead, a characteristic sign of neurogenic shock is the absence of sweating below the level of injury.

The term *spinal shock* refers to the local neurological condition that occurs immediately after a spinal injury produces motor and sensory losses (which may not be permanent). Damage to the spinal cord, particularly at the upper cervical levels, may cause significant injury to the autonomic nervous system, which controls the size and muscular tone of the blood vessels. Swelling and oedema of the cord begin within 30 minutes after an insult, creating a "physiological" transaction with nerve conduction disruption. Severe pain may be present just above the level of injury owing to a zone of heightened sensitivity. Spinal shock is characterised by flaccid paralysis, flaccid sphincters, and absent reflexes. There is an absence of all pain, temperature, touch, proprioception, and pressure below the level of the lesion; absent or impaired thermoregulation; absent somatic and visceral sensations below the lesion; bowel distension; and loss of peristalsis.

Anaphylactic Shock

Anaphylaxis occurs when a person reacts violently to a substance to which he or she has been sensitised. Sensitisation means developing a heightened reaction (becoming allergic) to a substance. An allergic reaction typically does not occur, or occurs in a milder form, during sensitisation. Do not be misled by a patient who reports no history of allergic reaction to a substance following a first or second exposure: Each subsequent exposure after sensitisation tends to produce a more severe reaction.

In anaphylactic shock, there is no loss of blood, no vascular damage, and only a slight possibility of direct cardiac muscular injury. Instead, the patient experiences widespread vascular dilation, resulting in relative hypovolaemia. In other words, relative to the now larger container, the normal blood volume is less. The combination of poor oxygenation and poor perfusion, however, may easily prove fatal.

In anaphylaxis, immune system chemicals, such as histamine and other vasodilator proteins, are released on exposure to an allergen. Their release causes the severe bronchoconstriction that accounts for wheezing if the patient is actually moving enough air. Anaphylaxis is also accompanied by urticaria (hives). The results are widespread vasodilation, which causes distributive shock, and blood vessels that continue to leak. Fluid leaks out of the blood vessels and into the interstitial spaces, resulting in hypovolaemia and potentially causing significant swelling. In some cases, this swelling may occlude the upper airway, resulting in a life-threatening condition **Figure 18-5 ▶** .

Recurrent large areas of subcutaneous oedema of sudden onset, usually disappearing within 24 hours and mainly seen in young women (frequently as a result of allergy to food or drugs), is called angio-oedema.

Shock-Related Events at the Capillary and Microcirculatory Levels

As perfusion decreases, cellular ischaemia occurs. Minimal blood flow passes through the capillaries, causing the cells to switch from aerobic metabolism to anaerobic metabolism, which can lead rapidly to metabolic acidosis. With less circulation, the blood stagnates in the capillaries. The precapillary sphincter relaxes in response to the buildup of lactic acid, vasomotor centre failure, and increased amounts of carbon dioxide. The postcapillary sphincters remain constricted, causing the capillaries to become engorged with fluid.

The capillary sphincters—circular muscular walls that constrict and dilate—regulate blood flow through the capillary beds. These sphincters are under the control of the autonomic nervous system, which regulates involuntary functions such as sweating and digestion. Capillary sphincters also respond to other stimuli such as heat, cold, increased demand for oxygen, and the need for waste removal. Thus, regulation of blood flow is determined by cellular need and is accomplished by vessel constriction or dilation, working in tandem with sphincter constriction or dilation.

The body can tolerate anaerobic metabolism for only a limited time. Anaerobic metabolism is much less efficient than aerobic metabolism and leads to systemic acidosis and depletion of the body's normally high energy reserves (ATP). Although hypoxia decreases the rate of ATP synthesis in the cells, it will not damage the mitochondria unless it is sustained, severe, and associated with ischaemia.

During anaerobic metabolism, incomplete glucose breakdown leads to an accumulation of pyruvic acid. Pyruvic acid cannot be converted to acetyl coenzyme A without oxygen, however, it is transformed in greater amounts to lactate and other acid by-products. Acidosis develops because ATP is hydrolyzed to adenosine diphosphate and phosphate with the release of a proton. Hydrogen ion accumulates, decreasing the pool of bicarbonate buffer. Lactate also buffers protons, and lactic acid accumulates in the body.

At the same time, ischaemia stimulates increased carbon dioxide production by the tissues. The higher the body's metabolic rate, the higher the carbon dioxide level in hypoperfused states. The excess carbon dioxide combines with intracellular water to produce carbonic acid. Increased tissue acids will, in turn, react with other buffers to form more intracellular acidic substances. Thus, acidosis serves as an indirect measure of tissue perfusion. The acidic condition of the blood inhibits haemoglobin in the RBCs from binding with and carrying oxy-

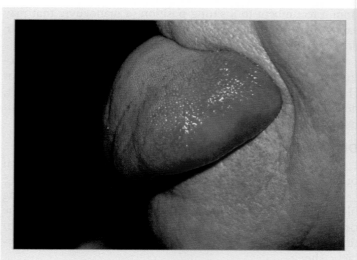

Figure 18-5 In anaphylaxis, interstitial fluid may cause significant swelling. In some cases, this swelling may occlude the upper airway, resulting in a life-threatening condition.

gen. This adds to the cellular oxygen debt, shifting the oxyhaemoglobin dissociation curve to the right.

Meanwhile, sodium, which is usually more abundant outside the cells than inside them, is naturally inclined to diffuse into the cells. Normally the sodium-potassium pump acts like a "buffer" at the cell membrane, sending the sodium back out against the concentration gradient. This mechanism involves active transport and requires an ample supply of ATP to fuel the buffer. Reduced levels of ATP, however, result in a dysfunctional sodium-potassium pump and alter the cell membrane function. Excessive sodium begins to diffuse into the cells, along with water, which ultimately depletes the interstitial compartment.

The intracellular enzymes that usually help digest and neutralise bacteria introduced into a cell are bound in a relatively impermeable membrane. Cellular flooding explodes that membrane and releases these lysosomal enzymes, which then autodigest the cell. If enough cells are destroyed in this way, organ failure will become evident. The release of the lysosomes opens the floodgates for the onset of the last phase of shock, called irreversible shock.

To compound these problems, accumulating acids and waste products act as potent vasodilators, further decreasing venous return and diminishing blood flow to the vital organs and tissues. The arterial pressure falls to the point at which even the "protected organs" such as the brain and heart are no longer being perfused. When aortic pressures fall below a mean arterial pressure (MAP) of 60 mm Hg, the coronary arteries no longer fill, the heart is weakened, and the cardiac output falls. Myocardial depressant factor is released from an ischaemic pancreas, further decreasing the pumping action of the heart and slowing the cardiac output.

Eventually, the reduced blood supply to the vasomotor centre in the brain results in slowing and then stopping of sympathetic nervous system activity. The metabolic wastes are released into the slower-flowing blood. The blood's sluggish flow coupled with its acidity leads to platelet agglutination and formation of microthrombi. Because the capillary walls are stretched, they lose their ability to retain large molecules, allowing them to leak into the surrounding interstitial spaces. Hydrostatic pressure forces plasma into the interstitial spaces, further increasing the distance from the capillaries to the cells. In turn, oxygen transport decreases, increasing cellular hypoxia.

The continuing buildup of lactic acid and carbon dioxide acts as a potent vasodilator, leading to relaxation of the postcapillary sphincters. The accumulated hydrogen, potassium, carbon dioxide, and thrombosed (clotted) RBCs wash out into the venous circulation, increasing the metabolic acidosis. This has been referred to as the capillary "washout phase". The result is an even greater drop in cardiac output. Ischaemia and necrosis ultimately lead to multiple-organ dysfunction syndrome, in which the various organ systems fail, like falling dominos.

Multiple-Organ Dysfunction Syndrome

Multiple-organ dysfunction syndrome (MODS) is a progressive condition characterised by combined failure of several organs, such as the lungs, liver, and kidney, along with some clotting mechanisms, which occurs after severe illness or injury. First described in 1975, MODS has a mortality rate of 60% to 90%. It is the major cause of death following septic, traumatic, and burn injuries. MODS is classified as primary or secondary. Primary MODS is a direct result of an insult, such as a pulmonary contusion from striking the chest on the steering wheel during a collision. Secondary MODS encompasses the organ dysfunction that occurs as an integral component to the host's response (such as renal failure following trauma).

MODS occurs when injury or infection (as in septic shock) triggers a massive systemic immune, inflammatory, and coagulation response, resulting in the release of numerous inflammatory mediators and activation of the following systems:

- **Activation of the complement system.** Normally, this group of plasma proteins functions to eliminate invading bacteria—that is, these components are part of the immune response. In MODS, an overactive complement system activates phagocytes and induces further inflammation and damage to cells.
- **Activation of the coagulation system.** Endothelial damage and coagulation, especially in the microscopic venules and arterioles, become uncontrolled in MODS, which results in microvascular thrombus formation and tissue ischaemia.
- **Activation of the kallikrein-kinin system.** The release of bradykinin, a potent vasodilator, leads to tissue hypoperfusion and may contribute to hypotension.

The net outcome of overactivity in these systems is maldistribution of systemic and organ blood flow. Often tissues attempt to compensate by accelerating their metabolism. The result is an oxygen supply-demand imbalance that leads to tissue hypoxia, tissue hypoperfusion, exhaustion of the cells' fuel supply (ATP), metabolic failure, lysosome breakdown, anaerobic metabolism, and acidosis and impaired cellular function. As MODS progresses, various organs begin to malfunction as a result of the cell and tissue hypoxia.

MODS typically develops within hours to days following resuscitation. In a 14- to 21-day period, renal and liver failure can develop, along with collapse of the GI and immune systems. If the patient does not respond to treatment of the underlying condition, cardiovascular collapse and death typically occur within days to weeks of the initial insult.

MODS affects specific organs and organ systems in the following ways:

- **Heart.** Hypoperfusion may stun a healthy heart and result in arrhythmias, muscle ischaemia, infarction, and pump failure with ejection fractions falling far below 40%. Peripheral pulses are weak or absent. Extremities become cyanotic and cold.
- **Lungs.** Failure is evidenced by adult respiratory distress syndrome or noncardiogenic pulmonary oedema. Hypoxic vasoconstriction of pulmonary beds increases pulmonary arterial pressures and produces pulmonary hypertension, putting a strain on the right ventricle. Pulmonary capillary blood flow reduction results in impaired gas exchange, a reduced pO_2 level, and an increased pCO_2 level. Alveolar cells become ischaemic and slow their production of surfactant, resulting in massive atelectasis and a reduction in pulmonary compliance. At the same time, pulmonary capillaries become permeable to water, resulting in interstitial and intra-alveolar oedema at low wedge pressures (< 18 mm Hg). The net results are respiratory failure, severe hypoxaemia, and respiratory acidosis.
- **Central nervous system.** Decreased cerebral perfusion pressure and cerebral blood flow result in confusion, reduced responses to verbal and painful stimuli, and, ultimately, unresponsiveness.
- **Kidneys.** A reduction in renal blood flow produces acute tubular necrosis, which in turn leads to oliguria (urine output, < 20 ml/h). Toxic waste products cannot be excreted, so they are retained in the blood. Metabolic acidosis worsens as the kidneys become unable to excrete acids or retain bicarbonate.
- **Liver.** Impaired metabolic function and alterations in clotting factors produce coagulopathies such as disseminated intravascular coagulation, in which clotting and bleeding occur at the same time. The liver fails to filter bacteria, leaving the patient vulnerable to infections. Failure to metabolise waste products, such as ammonia and lactate, causes markedly increased blood levels of these toxins. Cell death is evidenced by an increase in enzyme levels (including lactate dehydrogenase, aspartate aminotransferase, and alanine aminotransferase) when the patient's blood is tested at the hospital. The net result is ischaemic hepatitis, hypoxic hepatitis, or shock liver.

- **GI tract.** Hypoperfusion results in ischaemic gut syndrome. Release of vasodilating endotoxins contributes to the progression of shock.

Signs and symptoms of MODS include hypotension, insufficient tissue perfusion, uncontrollable bleeding, and multisystem organ failure caused mainly by hypoxia, tissue acidosis, and severe local alterations of metabolism. Patients can have a pyrexia fever from the inflammatory response and are tachycardic and dyspnoeic. They may prove difficult to oxygenate owing to the presence of adult respiratory distress syndrome.

Phases of Shock

Shock occurs in three successive phases (compensated, decompensated, and irreversible). Your goal is to recognise the clinical signs and symptoms of shock in its earliest phase and begin immediate treatment before permanent damage occurs. To do so, you must be aware of the subtle signs exhibited while the body is compensating effectively (Table 18-2) and treat the patient aggressively. Anticipate the potential for shock from the scene assessment and evaluation of the MOI. Recognise the signs of poor perfusion that precede hypotension, and do not rely on any one sign or symptom to determine the phase of shock the patient is going through. Always remain cautious when treating a potential shock patient. Rapid assessment and immediate transport are essential to preserve any chance of survival.

Table 18-2 Compensated Versus Decompensated Hypoperfusion

Compensated Hypoperfusion	Decompensated Hypoperfusion
Agitation, anxiety, restlessness	Altered mental status (verbal to unresponsive)
Sense of impending doom	Hypotension
Weak, rapid (thready) pulse	Laboured or irregular breathing
Clammy (cool, moist) skin	Thready or absent peripheral pulses
Pallor with cyanotic lips	Ashen, mottled, or cyanotic skin
Short of breath	Dilated pupils
Nausea, vomiting	Diminished urine output (oliguria)
Delayed capillary refill in infants and children	Impending cardiac arrest
Thirst	
Normal BP	

At the Scene

Regardless of the type of bleeding—whether hidden in the body cavities or visible on the kitchen floor—all patients will proceed through the phases of shock if their bleeding is not controlled. In hypovolaemic shock, the specific phase of shock is a function of the percentage of blood volume lost. Because internal bleeding is more likely to be uncontrolled, stay alert for the subtle signs of shock and be aggressive in your management of its early phase to avoid the slippery downward slope of shock's later phases.

Compensated Phase of Shock

The earliest stage of shock, in which the body can still compensate for blood loss, is called compensated shock. In this phase, the patient's level of responsiveness is a better indicator of tissue perfusion than most other vital signs. Release of chemical mediators by the autonomic nervous system as it recognises a potential catastrophic event causes the arterial BP to remain normal or slightly elevated. There is an increase in the rate and depth of respirations as the body attempts to bring in more oxygen and remove more carbon dioxide. This effort helps to maintain the acid-base balance by creating respiratory alkalosis to offset the metabolic acidosis.

During the compensated phase of shock, BP is maintained. Blood loss in hypovolaemic shock can be estimated at 15% to 30% at this point. A narrowing of the pulse pressure (the difference between the systolic and diastolic pressures) also occurs. The pulse pressure reflects the tone of the arterial system and is more sensitive to changes in perfusion than the systolic or diastolic BP alone. Patients in the compensated phase will also have a positive orthostatic tilt test result.

Treatment at this stage of shock will typically result in recovery.

At the Scene

The term *orthostatic* has to do with positioning. Orthostatic hypotension, for example, is a drop in systolic BP when moving from a sitting to a standing position. An *orthostatic tilt test* is used to determine dehydration or hypovolaemia. Blood pressure and pulse are measured as patients are lying, seated, and standing. A positive tilt test result occurs if the patient becomes dizzy, has a pulse increase of at least 20 beats/min, or has a systolic BP decrease of at least 20 mm Hg.

Decompensated Phase of Shock

The next stage of shock, when BP is falling, is decompensated shock (also called uncompensated shock or progressive shock). It occurs when blood volume drops by more than 30%. The compensatory mechanisms begin to fail, and signs and symptoms become much more obvious. The cardiac output falls dramatically, leading to further reductions in BP and cardiac function. The signs and symptoms become more obvious as blood is shunted to the brain, heart, and kidneys. At this point, vasoconstriction can have a disastrous effect if allowed to continue. Cells in the nonperfused tissues become hypoxic, leading to anaerobic metabolism. Treatment at this stage will sometimes result in recovery.

Blood pressure may be the last measurable factor to change in shock. The body has several automatic mechanisms to compensate for initial blood loss and to help maintain BP. Thus, by

Prep Kit

Ready for Review

- The cardiovascular system is designed to carry out one crucial job: keep blood flowing between the lungs and the peripheral tissues.
- Haemorrhage simply means bleeding.
  - Bleeding can range from a "nick" to a capillary while shaving, to a severely spurting artery from a deep slash with a knife, to a ruptured spleen from striking the steering column during a road traffic collision.
  - External bleeding can usually be easily controlled by using direct pressure or a pressure bandage.
  - Internal bleeding is usually not controlled until a surgeon locates the source and sutures it closed.
- The assessment of any patient begins with a good scene assessment and proceeds to your general impression and initial assessment.
  - Once the scene is deemed safe to enter, you will need to take the appropriate level of universal precautions.
  - Depending on the severity of bleeding and your general impression, this will entail gloves, mask, eyeshield, and, when the patient is very bloody or blood is spurting, an apron.
- In case of haemorrhage, the issue is not whether the patient will be transported, but rather how fast the transport decision should be made and where the patient should be taken for definitive care.
- Hypoperfusion occurs when the level of tissue perfusion decreases below normal.
  - Early decreased tissue perfusion may result in subtle changes, such as aberrant mental status, long before a patient's vital signs (that is, BP, pulse, respiratory rate) appear abnormal.
  - Shock refers to a state of collapse and failure of the cardiovascular system that leads to inadequate circulation, creating inadequate tissue perfusion.
- As with any patient, airway and ventilatory support take top priority when treating a patient with suspected shock.
- If a patient is suspected to be in shock, transport is inevitable; the questions to be asked are simply when and where.
  - Consideration for the priority of the patient and the availability of a regional trauma centre should be your concerns, and local transport guidelines may specifically deal with these issues.
  - Patients who have suspected shock, whether compensated or decompensated, will benefit from early surgical intervention and should be transported to a hospital with those capabilities.
- Prevention of shock and its deadly effects begins with your immediate assessment of the MOI, initial assessment findings, and the patient's clinical picture.
  - Be alert, and search for early signs of shock.

Vital Vocabulary

aerobic metabolism Metabolism that can proceed only in the presence of oxygen.

afterload The pressure in the aorta against which the left ventricle must pump blood.

anaerobic metabolism Metabolism that takes place in the absence of oxygen.

anaphylaxis An unusual or exaggerated allergic reaction to foreign protein or other substances.

angio-oedema Recurrent large areas of subcutaneous oedema of sudden onset, usually disappearing within 24 hours, which is seen mainly in young women, frequently as a result of allergy to food or drugs.

blood The fluid that is pumped by the heart through the arteries, veins, and capillaries and consists of plasma and formed elements or cells, such as red blood cells, white blood cells, and platelets.

capacitance vessels The smallest venules.

cardiac output The amount of blood pumped through the circulatory system in 1 minute.

cardiogenic shock A condition caused by loss of 40% or more of the functioning myocardium; the heart is no longer able to circulate sufficient blood to maintain adequate oxygen delivery.

cardiovascular collapse Failure of the heart and blood vessels; *shock*.

central shock A condition that consists of cardiogenic shock and obstructive shock.

compensated shock The early stage of shock, in which the body can still compensate for blood loss. The systolic blood pressure and brain perfusion is maintained.

decompensated shock The late stage of shock, when blood pressure is falling.

distributive shock A condition that occurs when there is widespread dilation of the resistance vessels, the capacitance vessels, or both.

ejection fraction The portion of the blood ejected from the ventricle during systole.

epistaxis A nosebleed.

erythrocytes Red blood cells.

haematochezia Passage of stools containing bright red blood.

haemoglobin The oxygen-carrying pigment in red blood cells.

haemorrhage Bleeding.

haemostasis Stopping haemorrhage.

hypoperfusion A condition that occurs when the level of tissue perfusion decreases below that needed to maintain normal cellular functions.

hypovolaemic shock A condition that occurs when the circulating blood volume is inadequate to deliver adequate oxygen and nutrients to the body.

irreversible shock The final stage of shock, resulting in death.

leucocytes White blood cells.

melaena Passage of dark, tarry stools.

multiple-organ dysfunction syndrome (MODS) A progressive condition usually characterised by combined failure of several organs, such as the lungs, liver, and kidney, along with some clotting mechanisms, which occurs after severe illness or injury.

neurogenic shock Circulatory failure caused by paralysis of the nerves that control the size of the blood vessels, leading to widespread dilation; seen in spinal cord injuries.

obstructive shock Shock that occurs when there is a block to blood flow in the heart or great vessels, causing an insufficient blood supply to the body's tissues.

orthostatic hypotension A drop in systolic blood pressure when moving from a sitting to a standing position.

perfusion The delivery of oxygen and nutrients to the cells, organs, and tissues of the body.

peripheral shock A condition that consists of hypovolaemic shock and distributive shock.

plasma The fluid portion of the blood from which the cells have been removed.

platelets Small cells in the blood that are essential for clot formation.

pulse pressure The difference between the systolic and diastolic pressures.

resistance vessels The smallest arterioles.

sensitisation Developing sensitivity to a substance that initially caused no allergic reaction.

septic shock Shock caused by severe infection, usually a bacterial infection.

shock An abnormal state associated with inadequate oxygen and nutrient delivery to the metabolic apparatus of the cell.

stroke volume The amount of blood that the left ventricle ejects into the aorta per contraction.

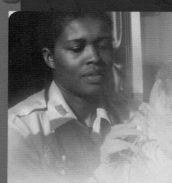

Assessment in Action

You are called to a shopping centre by security on a Friday night for a person who was assaulted. When you arrive, you see a man in his late 20s who is sitting on a bench holding a towel to his face. There is a trail of blood from the men's toilets, and the towel is dripping with blood. According to the security officer, there was a fight in the toilet and they found this man, Henry, stumbling and drenched in blood. Apparently, a couple of gang members beat him up and slashed his face and neck with razors.

You quickly don PPE and ensure that the scene is safe. The police are just arriving behind you. The initial assessment reveals an alert and orientated but anxious patient who has an open and clear airway, has 26 shallow breaths/min and has a very weak and thready radial pulse. He has external bleeding from the face and neck, which your colleague is attempting to control with direct pressure. His carotid pulse is 120 beats/min, and his skin is pale, cool, and clammy. You begin to administer supplemental oxygen with a nonrebreathing mask at 15 l/min and lie the patient down with his feet raised so you can do a rapid trauma assessment.

Meanwhile, a second ambulance arrives and the crew brings the stretcher so the patient can be rapidly removed from the scene. The assessment reveals that there may also be potential for internal bleeding because the patient was kicked in the ribs and abdomen when he was down on the floor. You quickly load the patient and decide to insert two IV lines en route to the regional trauma centre. Your colleagues join you in your ambulance so you can have plenty of personnel working on your patient en route to the A&E department because there is much to do to save his life.

1. **This patient has one very obvious injury involving:**
   A. a flail chest.
   B. the facial and neck lacerations.
   C. a ruptured spleen.
   D. an injured left kidney.

2. **With a patient who has so much obvious external bleeding, you should don which PPE?**
   A. Disposable gloves
   B. An eye shield
   C. A disposable mask
   D. All of the above

3. **An example of an injury that is potentially life threatening yet difficult to see in this patient would be:**
   A. internal bleeding.
   B. the facial laceration.
   C. the neck laceration.
   D. head trauma.

4. **What is the significance of the weak radial pulse in this patient?**
   A. It demonstrates he is generally physically fit.
   B. It demonstrates that his bleeding is actually minimal.
   C. It indicates that his systolic blood pressure is already dropping.
   D. It indicates that his body is compensating well for the injuries.

5. **What is the significance of the pale, cool, and clammy skin in this patient?**
   A. It demonstrates that he was on a cold floor.
   B. It shows that the vessels in the skin have been constricting.
   C. It shows that the vessels in the skin have been dilating.
   D. It shows that he has an adequate supply of blood to the brain.

6. **With the patient alert and orientated at this point, how serious is his condition?**
   A. Not very serious at all once a bandage is applied to the face and neck.
   B. The lacerations are serious and will need to be sutured in A&E.
   C. Very serious owing to the combination of external and internal bleeding.
   D. Very serious owing to the symptoms of a head injury.

7. **With deep lacerations to the face and neck, how should the bleeding be controlled?**
   A. Pressure point
   B. Tourniquet
   C. Cold application
   D. Direct pressure

8. **What phase of shock is this patient in at this point?**
   A. Terminal
   B. Decompensated
   C. Compensated
   D. Guarded

9. **What type of shock does this patient potentially have?**
   A. Septic
   B. Neurogenic
   C. Hypovolaemic
   D. Anaphylactic

10. **Aside from controlling the external bleeding, giving supplemental oxygen, and using the Trendelenburg position, what other treatment would be appropriate for this patient en route to the regional trauma centre?**
    A. Two large-bore IV lines for normal saline
    B. Perform a needle chest decompression
    C. Cooling the patient with chilled IV fluid
    D. Administer adrenaline, titrated to effect

Challenging Question

11. **If the patient weighed 100 kg and you obtained a BP of 86/60 on palpation en route to the A&E department, what phase of shock is he in, how much blood did he have (roughly) before the assault, and how much blood has he already lost?**

Points to Ponder

You respond to the scene of a single-car road traffic collision in which a 45-year-old woman is walking around the scene. It is obvious from the bull's-eyed windscreen and her forehead laceration that she struck the glass with her head. She is nervous that she will get in trouble and states she was wearing a seatbelt and did not hit the windscreen. You also note the smell of alcohol on her breath, and she denies any medical history. She allowed you to feel her weak rapid radial pulse but now is refusing to let you do any further assessment. Her head lacerations are no longer bleeding, although she has plenty of blood on her white blouse. She is refusing to go to hospital, stating there is nothing wrong with her. The police officer, who has been dealing with the traffic congestion, states he is going to administer a breathalyser test.

How should you deal with this patient's refusal to go to hospital?

Issues: MOI for Internal Injury, Recognition of Shock, Estimating Phases of Shock, Compensation Versus Decompensation During Shock, Treatment Plan for a Patient With Suspected Shock, and Patient Refusal.

19 Soft-Tissue Injuries

Objectives

Cognitive

- Describe the incidence, morbidity, and mortality of soft-tissue injuries.
- Describe the layers of the skin, specifically:
  - Epidermis and dermis (cutaneous)
  - Superficial fascia (subcutaneous)
  - Deep fascia
- Identify the major functions of the integumentary system.
- Identify the skin tension lines of the body.
- Predict soft-tissue injuries based on mechanism of injury.
- Discuss the pathophysiology of wound healing, including:
  - Haemostasis
  - Inflammation phase
  - Epithelialisation
  - Neovascularisation
  - Collagen synthesis
- Discuss the pathophysiology of soft-tissue injuries.
- Differentiate between the following types of closed soft-tissue injuries:
  - Contusion
  - Haematoma
  - Crush injuries
- Discuss the assessment findings associated with closed soft-tissue injuries.
- Discuss the management of a patient with closed soft-tissue injuries.
- Discuss the pathophysiology of open soft-tissue injuries.
- Differentiate between the following types of open soft-tissue injuries:
  - Abrasions
  - Lacerations
  - Major arterial lacerations
  - Avulsions
  - Impaled objects
  - Amputations
  - Incisions
  - Crush injuries
  - Blast injuries
  - Penetrations/punctures
- Discuss the incidence, morbidity, and mortality of blast injuries.
- Predict blast injuries based on mechanism of injury, including:
  - Primary
  - Secondary
  - Tertiary
- Discuss types of trauma including:
  - Blunt
  - Penetrating
  - Barotrauma
  - Burns
- Discuss the pathophysiology associated with blast injuries.

- Discuss the effects of an explosion within an enclosed space on a patient.
- Discuss the assessment findings associated with blast injuries.
- Identify the need for rapid intervention and transport of the patient with a blast injury.
- Discuss the management of a patient with a blast injury.
- Discuss the incidence, morbidity, and mortality of crush injuries.
- Define the following conditions:
  - Crush injury
  - Crush syndrome
  - Compartment syndrome
- Discuss the mechanisms of injury in a crush injury.
- Discuss the effects of reperfusion and rhabdomyolysis on the body.
- Discuss the assessment findings associated with crush injuries.
- Identify the need for rapid intervention and transport of the patient with a crush injury.
- Discuss the management of a patient with a crush injury.
- Discuss the pathophysiology of haemorrhage associated with soft-tissue injuries, including:
  - Capillary
  - Venous
  - Arterial
- Discuss the assessment findings associated with open soft-tissue injuries.
- Discuss the assessment of haemorrhage associated with open soft-tissue injuries.
- Differentiate between the various management techniques for haemorrhage control of open soft-tissue injuries, including:
  - Direct pressure
  - Elevation
  - Pressure dressing
  - Pressure point
  - Tourniquet application
- Differentiate between the types of injuries requiring the use of an occlusive versus non-occlusive dressing.
- Identify the need for rapid assessment, intervention, and appropriate transport for the patient with a soft-tissue injury.
- Discuss the management of the soft-tissue injury patient.
- Define and discuss the following:
  - Dressings
    - Sterile
    - Non-sterile
    - Occlusive
    - Non-occlusive
    - Woven
    - Low adherence

Although not the permanent repair, the plug temporarily stops the blood loss and is the beginning of blood clot formation.

Inflammation

In inflammation (the next stage of wound healing), additional cells move into the damaged area to begin repair. White blood cells migrate to the area to combat pathogens that have invaded exposed tissue. Chemicals and proteins known as chemotactic factors are released and call repairing cells into the area. Granulocytes and macrophages, among the first restoration cells to arrive, engulf bacteria through phagocytosis, which involves ingestion of damaged cellular parts. Foreign products and bacteria can also be removed from the body by phagocytosis. Similarly, lymphocytes (a type of white blood cell) destroy bacteria and other pathogens.

Mast cells release histamine as part of the body's response in the early stages of inflammation. Histamine causes dilation of blood vessels, increasing blood flow to the injured area and resulting in a reddened, warm area immediately around the site. Histamine makes capillaries more permeable, and swelling may occur as fluid seeps out of these "leaky" capillaries.

Inflammation ultimately leads to the removal of foreign material, damaged cellular parts, and invading microorganisms from the wound site. Reconstruction of the injured region through epithelialisation, neovascularisation, and collagen synthesis can then begin.

Epithelialisation

In the outer layer of skin, epithelial cells are stacked in layers. To replace the area damaged in a soft-tissue injury, a new layer of epithelial cells must be moved into this region—a process known as epithelialisation. Cells from the stratum germinativum quickly multiply and redevelop across the edges of the wound. Except in cases of clean incisions, the appearance of the restructured area seldom returns to the preinjury state. For example, large wounds or injuries that result in significant disruption of the skin will often have incomplete epithelialisation. In individuals with lightly pigmented skin, a pink line of scar tissue may signal the presence of collagen, a structural protein that has reinforced the damaged tissue. Despite the changed appearance, the function of the area may be restored to near normal.

Neovascularisation

In neovascularisation, new blood vessels form as the body attempts to bring oxygen and nutrients to the injured tissue. New capillaries bud from intact capillaries that lie adjacent to the damaged skin. These vessels provide a conduit for oxygen and nutrients and serve as a pathway for waste removal. Because they are new and delicate, bleeding might result from a very minor injury. It may take weeks to months for the new capillaries to be as stable as preexisting vessels.

Collagen Synthesis

Collagen is a tough, fibrous protein found in scar tissue, hair, bones, and connective tissue. This vital structural repair unit is synthesised by fibroblasts, repair cells that migrate into damaged tissue. In wound healing, collagen provides stability to the damaged tissue and joins wound borders, thereby closing the open tissue. Unfortunately, collagen cannot restore the damaged tissue to its original strength.

Alterations of Wound Healing

Wound healing does not always follow the pattern described above. Infection or an abnormal scar may develop, excessive bleeding may occur, or healing may be slow. This section discusses altered wound healing and potential complications.

Anatomical Factors

Areas of the body subjected to repeated motion throughout the day, such as the fingers, tend to heal slowly. One strategy used to speed healing in such cases is to splint the affected part, preventing movement. The arrangement of an open wound in relation to skin tension lines also affects how the wound will heal and determines whether an abnormal scar will form.

You are the Paramedic Part 2

After bandaging and splinting the patient's leg, you assess pulse, motor, and sensory functions; they are grossly intact. The remainder of your focused physical examination is unremarkable. After placing the patient onto the stretcher and loading him into the ambulance, your partner gathers SAMPLE history information from the patient while you obtain a set of baseline vital signs.

Vital Signs	Recording Time: 8 Minutes
Skin	Pink and perspiring
Pulse	120 beats/min; strong and regular at the radial artery
Blood pressure	148/88 mm Hg
Respirations	24 breaths/min; adequate depth
SpO2	98% on room air
Pain scale	10 on a scale of 0 to 10

3. Is this patient in shock?

4. What additional care should you provide to this patient?

Some medications can delay healing—namely, corticosteroids, nonsteroidal anti-inflammatory drugs, penicillin, anticoagulants, and anti-neoplastic agents. Likewise, a variety of medical conditions may interfere with normal healing—advanced age, severe alcoholism, acute uraemia, diabetes, hypoxia, severe anaemia, peripheral vascular disease, malnutrition, advanced cancer, hepatic failure, and cardiovascular disease.

High-Risk Wounds

Wounds that carry a high risk for developing infection include human and animal bites. Because the mouth is warm and constantly moist, it offers a hospitable environment for growth of bacteria. Injection of human saliva into tissue can result in significant infection. In particular, rabies is a serious infection that can develop from the bite of an infected animal (such as dogs and cats).

Cases in which a foreign body or organic matter is embedded in an open wound are considered high-risk injuries because of the likelihood that the material involved is impregnated with microorganisms. Once the material breaches the skin barrier, the pathogen has easy entry into the rest of the body. A foreign body that remains in place on evaluation should be left in place because a lacerated blood vessel may not be bleeding freely because of the foreign body's position. *Do not remove an impaled object in the prehospital environment unless it interferes with the airway.*

Other high-risk wounds include injection wounds, wounds with significant devitalised tissue, crush wounds, wounds in immunocompromised patients, and injuries to patients with poor peripheral circulation.

Abnormal Scar Formation

Excessive collagen formation can occur if the healing process is not balanced between the building up and breaking down phases of healing. A hypertrophic or keloid scar may develop from the excess protein. Hypertrophic scar formation occurs in areas subject to high tissue stress, such as the elbow and knee. Such a scar does not extend past the borders of the wound margins and tends to form in people with lightly pigmented skin. In contrast, a keloid scar typically develops in people with darkly pigmented skin. It grows over the wound margins and can become larger than the wound area. Keloid scars tend to form on the ears, upper extremities, lower abdomen, and sternum.

Pressure Injuries

Pressure injuries may occur when a patient is bedridden or when pressure is applied for a prolonged period in an unconscious patient or a patient immobilised on a longboard. The involved tissues are deprived of oxygen, which leads to localised hypoxia and cell deterioration. Prevention involves determining the risk and providing a mechanism to reduce or release the pressure on the skin.

Early recognition and treatment is also a key determinant in dealing with pressure injuries (also referred to as pressure sores). Commonly, the injury is classified into four stages:

- **Stage 1.** Skin appears red or discoloured but is not broken. This remains for more than 30 minutes following pressure removal.
- **Stage 2.** The epidermis becomes broken and a superficial open sore develops.
- **Stage 3.** This sore continues down through the dermis and subcutaneous fat tissue.
- **Stage 4.** The sore continues down and penetrates the underlying muscle and may even go as far as the bone. Profound tissue necrosis will be present, accompanied by discharge from the site.

This type of injury is most commonly found on the heels, toes, sacrum, hips, elbows, shoulders, back of head, and any area that is subjected to routine friction.

Wounds Requiring Closure

Many open wounds heal without intervention from healthcare professionals, but some require closure with sutures, staples, adhesive paper tapes, or tissue adhesive (medical glue). Closure involves bringing the wound edges together to allow for optimal healing. Open injuries that require closure include those that affect cosmetic areas, such as the lips, face, or eyebrows. Such injuries should be considered for closure because scarring often has psychological implications. Gaping wounds and those over tension lines also require closure. Degloving injuries require substantial irrigation and debridement before closing by a surgeon. Closure is also indicated for ring injuries and skin tears.

Open injuries should be closed within 6 hours of the injury, although there is some variation based on body region. Initial hospital management for open wounds involves assessment for foreign material followed by irrigation. The practitioner can then determine appropriate wound closing options.

Three types of wound closure are performed: primary closure, secondary intention, and tertiary closure. In primary closure, the wound margins are brought together as neatly and evenly as possible. Secondary intention entails dressing high-risk wounds and allowing them to heal through normal body processes. Tertiary closure, also known as delayed primary closure, is applied to wounds that would have a poor cosmetic appearance if treated by secondary intention.

Patients who receive sutures need appropriate follow-up care to determine whether healing is normal or abnormal. Serious complications, including localised or systemic infection, can arise without adequate follow-up care. In some cases, sutures may need to be removed early to allow a wound to drain infectious material.

Infection

Because the skin serves as an initial barrier against microorganisms, any break can lead to infection. Larger openings and deeper penetrations result in a higher level of risk for developing an infection. Not only will there be a delay in healing from the infection, but additional complications or systemic infection can result.

Once in the body tissues, pathogens begin to grow and multiply, although clinical signs of infection may not appear for several days. Visible clues of infection include erythema, pus, warmth, oedema, and local discomfort. Because an inflammatory response is part of the normal healing process, some redness is normal. However, red streaks adjacent to the wound indicate that the patient has developed lymphangitis, an inflammation of the lymph channels. More serious infections can cause systemic signs, such as fever, shaking, chills, joint pain, and hypotension.

Gangrene

Approximately 3,300 cases of <u>gangrene</u> occur in the United Kingdom each year, of which 72% require hospital admission. *Clostridium perfringens* is an anaerobic, toxin-producing bacterium that leads to the development of gas gangrene. Once it enters deeply into tissue, it causes the production of a foul-smelling gas. If the gangrene is not treated, the skin will become necrotic and the infection may lead to sepsis. Prompt recognition and early, aggressive hospital therapy offer the best chance for reducing morbidity and mortality.

Tetanus

Tetanus is caused by infection with an anaerobic bacterium, *Clostridium tetani* (a member of the same family that causes gangrene). This bacterium produces a potent toxin, which results in painful muscle contractions that are strong enough to fracture bones. Muscle stiffness may be noted first in the jaw ("lockjaw") and neck, with progression down the remainder of the body. Early recognition is important because conventional therapy does not result in rapid recovery.

Of the total number of tetanus cases reported to the Health Protection Agency in England and Wales from 1984 to 2003, the highest incidence was in adults over 65 years of age, with no cases of tetanus reported in infants or children less than 5 years of age. Over the last 10 years, the number of cases of tetanus has been consistently low, with an average of just six cases each year. Most cases of tetanus now occur in older people who would not have been routinely immunised as children. Infection usually occurs following injury outdoors (eg, in the garden). In virtually every case, the person was unimmunised or incompletely immunised. Tetanus used to be more common in women than in men because many men had been immunised when doing National Service. In the last few years this difference has largely disappeared, and men and women are equally at risk. According to the latest guidance from the Department of Health, patients who have received a full course (five doses) of tetanus vaccine are considered to have life-long immunity. Therefore these individuals do not require a booster dose, *even in the presence of a tetanus prone wound.*

The following wounds are considered to be a high risk of contamination by tetanus spores in patients who have *not* received a full course (five doses) of tetanus vaccine:

- Wounds received more than 6 hours prior to commencement of treatment
- Puncture wounds
- Dirty and contaminated wounds, especially those containing soil, compost, or manure
- Wounds showing signs of infection
- Wounds with a large amount of devitalised tissue
- Animal bites

Necrotising Fasciitis

Necrotising fasciitis involves the death of tissue from bacterial infection. This disease is caused by more than one infecting organism—most commonly, haemolytic streptococci and *Staphylococcus aureus*. Although necrotising fasciitis is rare, the mortality rate ranges from 70% to 80%. Surgical debridement and antibiotic therapy are among the available treatments.

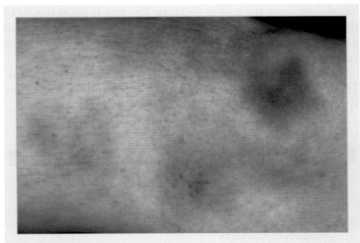

Figure 19-2 A contusion, or bruise, produces characteristic black-and-blue discolouration (bruising).

Closed Versus Open Wounds

Closed Wounds

In a <u>closed wound</u>, soft tissues beneath the skin surface are damaged, but there is no break in the epidermis. The characteristic closed wound is a <u>contusion</u> **Figure 19-2 ▲**. In a contusion (bruise), the skin is intact, but damage has occurred beneath the epidermis. Trauma to the nerve endings produces pain, and leakage of fluid into spaces between the damaged cells produces swelling (oedema). If small blood vessels in the dermis are disrupted, a black-and-blue mark (<u>bruising</u>) will cover the injured area; if large blood vessels are torn beneath the contused area, a <u>haematoma</u>—a collection of blood beneath the skin—will be evident as a lump with a bluish discolouration **Figure 19-3 ▲**.

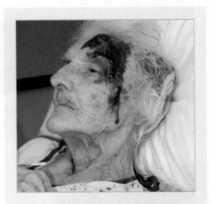

Figure 19-3 A haematoma.

Open Wounds

An <u>open wound</u> is characterised by a disruption in the skin. Open wounds are potentially much more serious than closed wounds for two reasons. First, they are vulnerable to infection. An open wound is <u>contaminated</u>—that is, microorganisms enter it. Whether the contamination produces infection depends in large measure on how the wound is managed. Second, open wounds have a greater potential for serious blood loss. When the skin is unbroken, bleeding from a disrupted blood vessel is limited. Although a significant volume of blood—up to about 2 units—can be lost into the soft tissues of the leg, eventually the increasing pressure within the leg will prevent further bleeding. In an open wound, the patient's entire blood volume may be lost.

Certain wounds should always be evaluated by a doctor. The injuries in (**Table 19-1** ▾) require transport, even if they appear minor.

Table 19-1	Conditions That Require Transport

- Compromise of:
  - Nerves
  - Vessels
  - Muscles
  - Tendons or ligaments
- Foreign body or cosmetic complications
- Heavy contamination

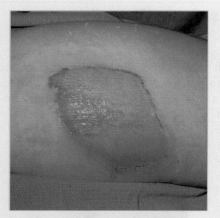 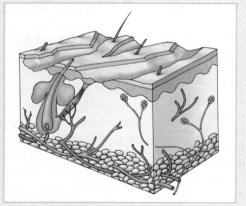

Figure 19-4 Abrasions usually do not penetrate completely through the dermis, but blood may ooze from the capillaries. These wounds are typically superficial and result from rubbing or scraping across a hard, rough surface.

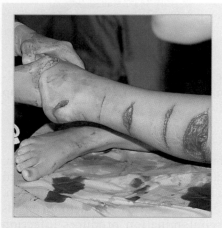 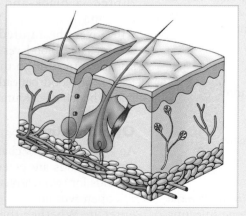

Figure 19-5 Lacerations can vary in depth and can extend through the skin and subcutaneous tissue to the underlying muscles, nerves, and blood vessels. These wounds can be smooth or jagged as a result of a cut by a sharp object or a blunt force that tears the tissue.

Abrasions

An abrasion (**Figure 19-4** ▾) is a superficial wound that occurs when the skin is rubbed or scraped over a rough surface and part of the epidermis is lost. So-called brush burns or friction burns are good examples. Abrasions typically ooze small amounts of blood and may be quite painful. They may also be contaminated with dirt and debris—for example, from "road rash" caused by sliding on the road surface in a motorcycle accident. Because the skin has been disrupted, infection is a danger.

Don't try to clean an abrasion in the prehospital environment; you don't have the means to do so properly. If you feel compelled to do *something,* cover the wound lightly with a sterile dressing.

Lacerations

A laceration (**Figure 19-5** ▾) is a cut inflicted by a sharp instrument, such as a knife or razor blade, that produces a clean or jagged incision through the skin surface and underlying structures. Sometimes the word *laceration* is reserved for jagged or irregular cuts, and incision is used to refer to a clean (linear) cut. Incisions tend to heal better than lacerations because of their relatively even wound margins. The seriousness of a laceration will depend on its depth and the structures that have been damaged. Lacerations may be the source of significant bleeding if they disrupt the wall of a blood vessel, particularly in regions of the body where major arteries lie close to the surface (as in the wrist). The first priority in treating a laceration is to control bleeding, initially by applying direct manual pressure over the wound. Laceration of a major artery can be fatal due to the severe bleeding that can occur.

A wound caused by broken glass should be assumed to have a retained glass foreign body until proved otherwise. Such patients need to be transported, as they need an X-ray.

Puncture Wounds

A puncture wound (**Figure 19-6** ▸) is a stab from a pointed object, such as a nail or a knife. Technically speaking, a bullet wound is a puncture wound. Most puncture wounds do not cause significant external bleeding, but they may produce extensive—even fatal—internal bleeding and wreak other havoc that cannot be seen from the outside of the body.

A special case of the puncture wound is the impaled foreign object (**Figure 19-7** ▸). When the instrument that caused the injury remains embedded in the wound, immobilise the object, and transport the patient.

Avulsions

An avulsion occurs when a flap of skin is torn loose, partially (**Figure 19-8** ▸) or completely. Depending on where the avulsion

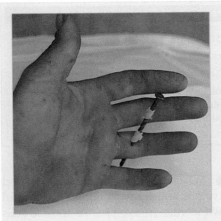
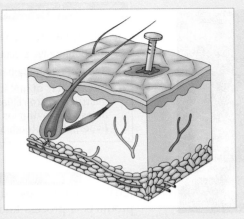

Figure 19-6 Penetrating wounds may cause very little external bleeding but can damage structures deep in the body.

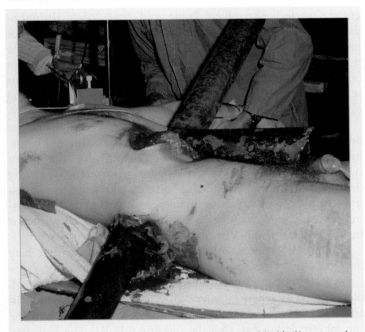

Figure 19-7 An impaled object remains embedded in the wound.

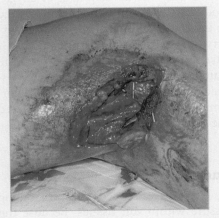
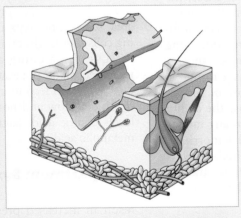

Figure 19-8 Avulsions are characterised by complete separation of tissue or tissue hanging as a flap. Significant bleeding is common.

occurs, it may or may not be accompanied by profuse bleeding. The principal danger in this type of injury—besides blood loss and contamination—is loss of the blood supply to the avulsed flap. If the part of the flap that connects it to the body (the pedicle) is folded back or kinked, circulation to the flap will be compromised and that piece of skin will die if the circulation is not restored quickly.

Amputations

An amputation is an avulsion involving the complete loss of a body part, typically one or more of the extremities. If the amputation was produced by a sharp object, blood loss is often much less than expected because the blood vessels retain the ability to constrict. In contrast, a crushing or tearing amputation can result in exsanguination (excessive blood loss due to haemorrhage) if the paramedic does not intervene rapidly.

Wound edges in an amputation are commonly jagged, and sharp bone edges may protrude Figure 19-9 ▶. During wound care, be aware of any sharp bone protrusions that may lead to an exposure. Large, thick dressings should be used to cover the site. In some cases, the body part will be completely detached. In a partial amputation, soft tissues remain attached. A degloving injury is a specific form of amputation that involves unravelling of skin from the hand, much like partial removal of a glove.

Crush Injuries

When a body part is crushed between two solid objects, a crush injury may occur to the underlying soft tissues and bones Figure 19-10 ▶. Such injuries range from an innocuous finger injury to a life-threatening entrapment of the torso. The latter is likely to be encountered in cases involving structural collapse (such as in collapse of masonry or steel structures, construction accidents, mudslides, road traffic collisions, and industrial accidents). A crush injury can also occur when an unconscious patient has an upper extremity pinned between the body and the floor.

The forces involved in a crush injury may be great enough to rupture internal organs. You must rapidly assess the mechanism of injury and determine the likelihood for massive internal trauma. Also, note that the longer an injured area remains compressed, the greater the chance for systemic complications.

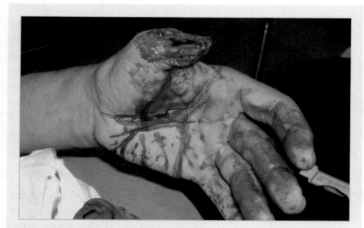

Figure 19-9 An amputation involving the thumb.

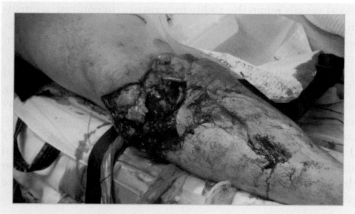

Figure 19-10 A crush injury is characterised by extensive tissue damage and deformity that is often accompanied by swelling and extreme pain.

Table 19-2	The Progression of Crush Syndrome

1. A body part is trapped for more than 4 hours.
2. Rhabdomyolysis occurs.
3. The trapped body part is freed.
4. By-products of metabolism and harmful products from tissue destruction are released, possibly resulting in cardiac arrest, dysrhythmias, kidney damage, hyperkalaemia, and hyperphosphataemia.

In a crush injury, the external appearance may not adequately represent the level of internal damage. An upper extremity that merely appears swollen may, in fact, have enough muscle destruction to cause systemic problems, especially if the extremity has been trapped for longer than 4 hours, which is enough time to develop crush syndrome. In other cases, the injured region may be mangled beyond recognition. Remember that grotesque injuries may not necessarily be the primary problem. Always concentrate on threats to life before addressing injured extremities, no matter how bad the initial appearance.

One of the body's first responses to a vessel injury is localised vasoconstriction that reduces the flow of blood. When vessels are crushed and torn, they often lose the ability to constrict, resulting in a free flow of blood from any unnatural opening. Crush injuries tend to result in haemorrhage that cannot easily be controlled by standard methods. Inability to precisely locate bleeding or massive extremity trauma may also lead to difficulty in controlling haemorrhage.

Crush Syndrome

When an area of the body is trapped for longer than 4 hours and arterial blood flow is compromised, <u>crush syndrome</u> can develop Table 19-2 ▲. When muscles are crushed beyond repair, tissue necrosis develops and leads to release of harmful products, a process known as <u>rhabdomyolysis</u>. As muscle cells are destroyed, they experience an influx of water, sodium chloride, and calcium from extracellular fluid. In addition, the body develops an efflux of potassium, purines (from disintegrating nuclei), phosphate, lactic acid, <u>myoglobin</u>, thromboplastin, creatine, and creatine kinase. The oppressing force prevents the return of blood from the injured body part, so the release of these products into the systemic circulation does not occur until *after* the limb is freed from entrapment. For this reason, rescuers must intervene *before* lifting the crushing object off the body.

Freeing the limb or other body part from entrapment not only results in release of by-products of metabolism and harmful products of tissue destruction, but also involves the potential for cardiac arrest. In prolonged entrapment, "smiling death" may occur if paramedics do not take proactive measures. In this situation, the trapped person is alert and conversing with rescuers; however, when the entrapped body part is freed, cardiac arrest is almost instantaneous.

Renal failure is another serious complication that may develop after release of the crushing force. <u>Glomerular filtration</u> can be impaired when the kidneys do not receive enough blood, such as when hypotension develops from bleeding. In addition, the release of large quantities of myoglobin into the central circulation can clog the filtering tubules. The high levels of acids and phosphates can directly damage the kidneys. This problem is compounded by the development of oxygen free radicals. These products travel throughout the affected area, scavenging oxygen molecules and damaging and destroying cells that might otherwise survive the initial injury.

Life-threatening arrhythmias may also develop from increased blood potassium levels (<u>hyperkalaemia</u>). <u>Hyperphosphataemia</u> can lead to calcifications that can interfere with normal blood flow and normal nervous tissue function. Increased levels of uric acid, lactic acid, and potassium may also cause metabolic acidosis.

Compartment Syndrome

<u>Compartment syndrome</u> develops when oedema and swelling result in increased pressure within soft tissues. Because the skin can stretch only so far, pressure begins to increase within the compartment, which in turn leads to compromised circulation. Compartment syndrome commonly develops in the

extremities and may occur in conjunction with open or closed injuries (although it is more likely with closed injuries due to the buildup of pressure inside the body). As pressure develops, delivery of nutrients and oxygen is impaired and by-products of normal metabolism accumulate. The longer this situation persists, the greater the chance for tissue necrosis.

Compartment syndrome presents with the six Ps: Pain, Paraesthesia, Paresis, Pressure, Passive stretch pain, and Pulselessness. Many of these signs may be delayed or nonspecific. Distal perfusion, sensation, and motor function may be intact.

Compartment syndrome that persists for more than 8 hours carries a serious risk for death of local tissues. In such cases, disfiguring wound debridement that can leave visible and psychologic scars is required. There is also a risk of sepsis. In-hospital intervention includes <u>fasciotomy</u>, or incision of the skin and underlying soft tissue with a scalpel. This limb-saving procedure also prevents a <u>Volkmann contracture</u>—a deformity of the hand, fingers, and wrist resulting from damage to forearm muscles—and preserves cutaneous sensation.

Blast Injuries

In recent years the UK has seen numerous bombings as a result of domestic and international terrorism. The London Underground bombs on 7th July 2005 killed 56 and injured thousands. In 1984, the Brighton Bombing killed five people Figure 19-11 ▶ . Although this attack clearly illustrated the devastating power of an explosive force, many other circumstances can lead to an explosion—dust buildup in grain silos, sawdust in wood factories, and explosive products transported by rail, sea, or air. You must be mentally and physically prepared to respond to an incident involving an explosion.

Blast injuries occur in four phases: primary, secondary, tertiary, and quaternary.

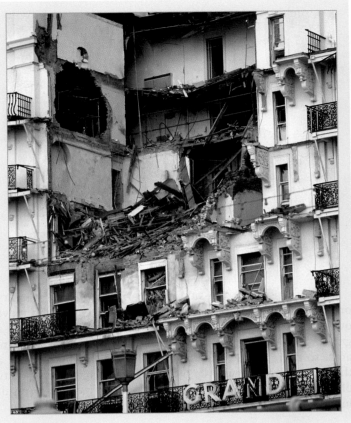

Figure 19-11 The Brighton Bombing at the Grand Hotel on 12 October 1984 killed five people.

Primary Phase

When an explosion occurs, a pressure wave rapidly develops; this tremendous but concentrated pressure results from air displacement and heat originating from the centre of the blast. The pressure wave damages air-filled cavities (such as the ears and lungs). Burns may occur.

You are the Paramedic Part 3

After establishing an IV line of normal saline and administering further treatment, you begin transport to a hospital located approximately 15 miles away. The patient remains conscious and alert and states that his pain is not as severe as it was initially. With an estimated time of arrival at the hospital of 15 minutes, you reassess the patient.

Reassessment	Recording Time: 15 Minutes
Skin	Pink and perspiring
Pulse	94 beats/min; strong and regular at the radial artery
Blood pressure	122/68 mm Hg
Respirations	18 breaths/min; adequate depth
S$_P$O$_2$	99% on room air
Pain scale	5 on a scale of 0 to 10

5. What is compartment syndrome and is this patient at risk for it?

6. What are the signs and symptoms of compartment syndrome?

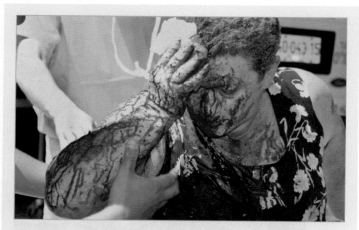

Figure 19-12 Nails, wood splinters, and glass shards can impale victims of a blast explosion.

All origins of the pressure wave carry a high risk of injury or death. Explosions from a bomb start at the centre and move outward, so people closer to the device will be affected to a greater extent. Explosions from fumes or dust involve an entire area, so there is no "safe" region. Underwater blasts have a three times greater range because of the near incompressibility of water. Explosions that occur within a confined space result in more force applied to the body.

Secondary Phase

A blast wind occurs as combustible gases move across the affected area. Although less forceful than the pressure wave, the blast wind is longer lasting. Projectiles also present serious hazards—flying debris may cause blunt and penetrating injuries. With bombs, the casing fragments rip apart with monumental force, spreading in all directions. Structural elements can break apart and travel at high rates of speed. Nails, wood splinters, and glass shards can impale victims located in the area of the blast Figure 19-12 ▲ .

Tertiary Phase

Victims may be injured from displacement away from the blast site or from collapse of the surrounding structure. Displacement occurs when a person is in proximity to the explosion; survival in this circumstance is highly unlikely. Falling structural beams, walls, and other heavy items may lead to crush injuries that compound the conditions already present. Injuries develop when the person is thrown against rigid surfaces, such as the ground, walls, or other rigid objects. There is also a risk for entrapment that can be prolonged for days. In addition, there may be multiple victims.

Quaternary Phase

Injuries result from the miscellaneous events that occur during an explosion. For example, the heat generated during an explosion may cause burns, ranging from superficial flash burns to full-thickness burns involving the entire or large areas of the body.

▌ Assessment of Soft-Tissue Injuries

Although skin trauma is often dramatic, it rarely is immediately life threatening. It is important to stay focused on the assessment format used throughout this book to first identify threats to you and your crew using the scene evaluation and then identify threats to the patient's life using the initial assessment.

The skin is more than just a wrapper; it performs important functions that are altered by trauma. When conducting your initial assessment, you need to determine the nature and mechanism of the injury. The severity of the injury may not be initially apparent, but it will be revealed as you do your rapid trauma assessment or focused physical examination.

Scene Safety and Evaluation

The first aspect to address in any scenario is safety. If you are responding to a vehicle collision, ensure that traffic is controlled and personnel are operating with protective measures in place. When responding to a reported explosion, wait for police personnel to secure the scene and declare it safe before you approach any victims. When a blast seems to be intentional, look for possible secondary devices. Responders have been injured and killed by other explosive devices planted away from the original detonation site.

Once you have determined that the scene is safe, begin evaluating the mechanism of injury. Maintain a high index of suspicion whenever a significant mechanism of injury is present, even if external injuries appear minor. Consider carefully the forces involved as you determine the likelihood of internal damage.

Next, determine how many patients are involved. Diligently search for ejected patients in the case of a significant vehicle collision.

As a part of your scene evaluation, be aware that skin injuries typically result in a risk of exposure to blood and other bodily fluids. Significant exposures include contact with body fluids through open wounds or mucous membranes. Less worrying exposures include body fluid contact with intact skin. Be sure to protect yourself and the patient, and review Chapters 2 and 36 regarding infection control procedures.

Initial Assessment

When the scene has been secured and universal precautions have been taken, rapidly determine whether threats to life are present. First, note your general impression as you approach the patient. Much information can be obtained from simply looking at the patient and the immediate surroundings. For example, a patient who is lying prone on the ground in a large pool of blood is clearly in worse shape than a patient who meets you at the door with a cut finger.

Many patients have potential injuries to the neck or spine. In such cases, you should assign a crew member to manually immobilise the head and neck. This is an important step because it will determine which manoeuvres are used to open the airway.

Assess the airway as soon as you arrive at the patient's side. Determine whether air is moving from the nose, mouth, or

Control of External Bleeding

External bleeding is bleeding that can be seen coming from a wound when the integrity of the skin has been violated. Theoretically, bleeding can be characterised according to the type of blood vessel that has been damaged **Figure 19-15 ▾**. Arterial bleeding occurs in spurts, and the blood is usually bright red because of the fully saturated haemoglobin. Venous bleeding is more likely to be slow and steady, and the colour of the blood is darker. In reality, most open wounds show a combination of arterial and venous bleeding. Capillary bleeding is characterised by a slow, even flow of bright or dark red blood and is present in minor injuries, such as abrasions or superficial lacerations.

Five methods are used in the prehospital environment to control external bleeding: direct pressure, elevation, pressure point control, immobilisation, and a tourniquet.

Direct Pressure

Application of pressure over a bleeding wound stops blood from flowing into the damaged vessels, allowing the platelets to seal the vascular walls.

Notes from Nancy

Steady, direct pressure against the bleeding site is the most effective way of controlling bleeding.

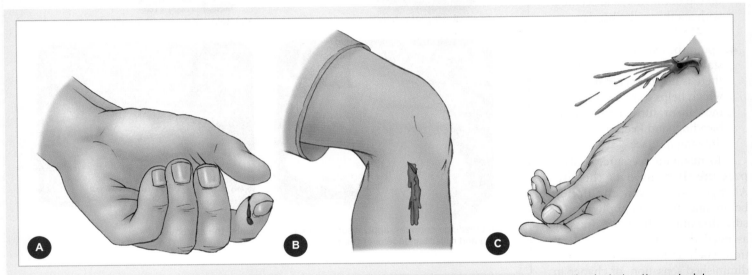

Figure 19-15 A. Capillary bleeding is dark red and oozes from the wound slowly but steadily. **B.** Venous bleeding is darker than arterial bleeding and flows steadily. **C.** Arterial bleeding is characteristically brighter red and spurts in time with the pulse.

You are the Paramedic Part 4

The patient remains haemodynamically stable throughout transport; however, he tells you that his leg is still hurting. You reassess his vital signs and consider the need for additional treatment. Your estimated time of arrival at hospital is 5 minutes.

Reassessment	Recording Time: 20 Minutes
Skin	Pink and perspiring
Pulse	100 beats/min; strong and regular at the radial artery
Blood pressure	124/70 mm Hg
Respirations	18 breaths/min; adequate depth
SpO₂	98% on room air
Pain scale	5 on a scale of 0 to 10

7. Is further treatment indicated for this patient?

8. Are there any special considerations regarding the treatment you have provided to this patient?

If possible, use a sterile dressing to exert pressure, and then use your gloved hand to apply pressure over the bleeding site. The steps for controlling bleeding are shown in **Skill Drill 19-1 ▶** :

1. Apply a dry, sterile dressing over the entire wound. Apply pressure to the dressing with your gloved hand **Step 1**.

2. Maintain the pressure, and secure the dressing with a roller bandage **Step 2**.

3. If bleeding continues or recurs, leave the original dressing in place. Apply a second dressing on top of the first, and secure it with another roller bandage **Step 3**.

4. Splint the extremity to stabilise the injury, even if there is no suspected fracture, which helps to minimise movement, further control the bleeding, and keep the dressing in place **Step 4**.

To maintain pressure, apply a pressure dressing over the site. Always assess distal circulation before and after you apply a pressure dressing. Adjust the dressing as needed in case of a complication, such as loss of distal pulse, diminished sensation, or change in skin colour and temperature distal to the dressing.

Skill Drill 19-1: Controlling Bleeding From a Soft-Tissue Injury

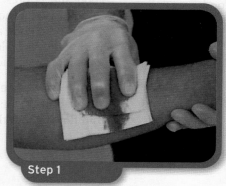

Step 1

Apply direct pressure with a sterile bandage.

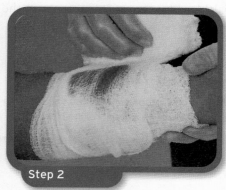

Step 2

Maintain pressure with a roller bandage.

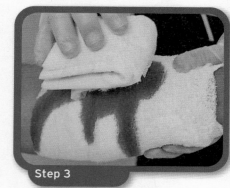

Step 3

If bleeding continues, apply a second dressing and roller bandage over the first.

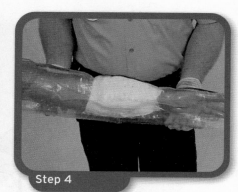

Step 4

Splint the extremity.

Elevation

In cases of venous bleeding from an extremity, the rate of bleeding can be substantially slowed by elevating the extremity above the level of the heart. This measure alone will not control bleeding, but it may be helpful in conjunction with other measures, such as direct pressure.

Pressure Point Control

When direct pressure is not sufficient to control bleeding or when the same artery is associated with a number of bleeding points, pressure point control **Figure 19-16 ▶** may help slow the bleeding. The artery chosen must be fairly superficial and overlie a hard structure against which it can be compressed. Three pressure points are typically used: (1) the temporal artery, which overlies the temporal bone of the skull and is used to control bleeding from the scalp; (2) the brachial artery, which overlies the humerus and is used to control bleeding from the forearm; and (3) the femoral artery, which can be compressed against the pelvis and is used to control bleeding from the leg.

Immobilisation

Any movement of an extremity, even an uninjured extremity, promotes blood flow within that extremity. When the extremity is also injured, motion may disrupt the clotting process and lacerate more blood vessels. It follows that preventing motion of an injured extremity will have the opposite effects. Advise the patient to make every effort to minimise movement. If that is not possible and conditions warrant, apply a splint to prevent motion.

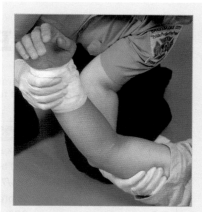

Figure 19-16 Applying pressure at the appropriate pressure point while holding direct pressure may slow difficult-to-control bleeding.

An inflatable splint or padded box splint works well to keep an upper or lower extremity immobilised. Use of an inflatable splint gives a double benefit—splinting *and* direct pressure. Remember to assess distal pulses, motor function, and sensation distal to the splint before and after application.

Tourniquet

In the civilian setting, it is rarely, if ever, necessary to use a tourniquet for control of external haemorrhage. Bleeding control can almost always be achieved by one or more of the four methods already described. Furthermore, use of a tourniquet is associated with potential hazards, including damage to nerves and blood vessels and, when the tourniquet is in place for an extended period, loss of the distal extremity. A tourniquet applied too loosely, by contrast, may increase bleeding if it occludes venous return without hampering arterial inflow. *Use a tourniquet only as a last resort, when it is the only way to save the patient's life.*

In military settings, application of a tourniquet would occur more often owing to the nature of injuries experienced during battle. In addition, rapid transport to a medical facility is typically more difficult on the battlefield than in civilian situations. In such a scenario, a tourniquet may be lifesaving, particularly in patients with a traumatic partial amputation of a limb.

Some tourniquets can be applied with one arm Figure 19-17 ▶ , although you may not have access to them. If a tourniquet is required, observe the following application guidelines Skill Drill 19-2 ▶ :

1. Use wide, flat materials, such as a cravat or folded triangular bandage. Never use rope, wire, or other narrow materials that might cut into the skin and damage underlying tissues. A blood pressure cuff inflated above the systolic reading works well for upper extremities.
2. Apply a pad over the artery to be compressed.
3. Wrap the tourniquet twice around the extremity, at a point about 4 inches distal to the axilla or groin, and tie a half-knot Step 1 .
4. Place a stick, pencil, or similar object on top of the half knot, and complete the square knot above the stick Step 2 .
5. Twist the stick to tighten the tourniquet just until the bleeding stops Step 3 .
6. Secure the stick in that position so that it will not unwind. Never cover a tourniquet with a bandage or anything else, lest it escape notice when the patient arrives at the hospital. To make doubly sure that the tourniquet is not overlooked, write "TK" and the exact time you applied the tourniquet on a piece of adhesive tape, and fasten the tape to the patient's forehead Step 4 .
7. Do not remove a tourniquet because removal can result in release of an embolus, significant rebleeding, or tourniquet shock.
8. Record on the patient clinical record the time at which the tourniquet was applied.

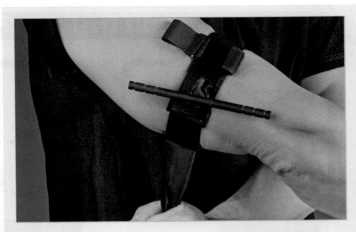

Figure 19-17 A tourniquet that can be applied using only one arm has been developed.

Pain Control

Application of a cold compress will help reduce pain and diminish blood flow to an open wound. Once the dressing is in place, apply the cold pack. Avoid placing the compress directly on the site because excessively cold temperature may do further harm. A pressure dressing may alleviate pain and minimise swelling.

If basic pain control measures fail to relieve pain, consider administering morphine sulphate or other agents as allowed by guidelines. As with all medications, assess the patient carefully for allergies, and document pertinent information.

Managing an Avulsion

In treating a partially avulsed piece of skin (or skin flap), irrigate any earth or debris out of the wound and then gently fold the skin flap back onto the wound so that it is more or less normally aligned. Unless you are competent in primary closure techniques, the wound should be temporarily covered with a non-adhesive dressing to hold the flap in place and referred to a suitably qualified clinician.

Preservation of Amputated Parts

When a part of the body is completely avulsed (ie, amputated)—whether a section of skin or an entire limb—it is important to try to preserve the amputated part in optimal condition to maximise the chances of it being successfully reimplanted. Once the patient's injuries have been stabilised, turn your attention to the amputated part, which will also require meticulous care. Follow these guidelines:

1. Note the time of the amputation.
2. Rinse the amputated part free of debris with cool sterile saline.
3. Wrap the part loosely in saline moistened gauze. The amputated part should not be placed directly in water or directly on ice, as this can cause further cellular damage.

Skill Drill 19-2: Applying a Tourniquet

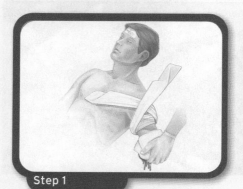

Step 1

Create a 4″, multilayered bandage. Wrap the bandage twice around the extremity, just above the bleeding site, and tie a half-knot.

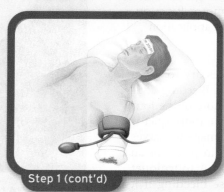

Step 1 (cont'd)

You can also use a blood pressure cuff as an effective tourniquet.

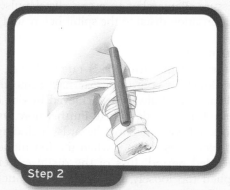

Step 2

Place a stick on top of the half-knot and tie a square knot over the stick.

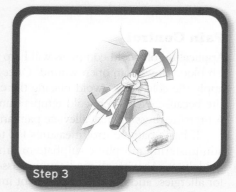

Step 3

Twist the stick until the bleeding stops.

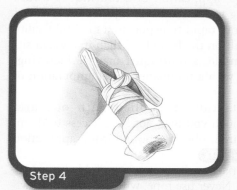

Step 4

Secure the stick so that it will not unwind. Write "TK" and the exact time you applied the tourniquet on a piece of adhesive tape, fasten the tape to the patient's forehead, and notify hospital personnel on arrival.

4. Subsequently, the amputated part should be securely wrapped and sealed in a plastic bag, which should be placed in a second plastic bag and sealed.

5. The double wrapped part should then be kept cool in an ice-water mix.

Transport the patient and the amputated part as expeditiously as possible. When the amputated part is a limb or part of a limb, notify A&E staff in advance of the type of case you are transporting and your estimated time of arrival so that a surgical team can be paged and mobilised while you are en route.

Managing Impaled Objects

The following are basic points regarding management of an impaled object:

- Do not try to remove an impaled object. Efforts to do so may precipitate uncontrolled internal haemorrhage, which may lead to exsanguination or further injury to underlying structures.

At the Scene

Never place an amputated part directly on ice because this may cause frostbite and prevent reattachment.

- Control haemorrhage by direct compression, but do not apply pressure on the impaled object itself or on immediately adjacent tissues.
- Do not try to shorten an impaled object unless it is extremely cumbersome (such as a fence post impaled in the chest); any motion of the object may damage surrounding tissues.
- Stabilise the object in place with a bulky dressing, and immobilise the extremity (if the object is impaled in an extremity) with a splint to prevent motion.

The goal for prehospital care is to limit motion of the impaled object as soon as possible to minimise additional damage. One technique that is effective for thin objects is to use gauze pads cut midway through the centre. Stack several pads vertically, and arrange the cut portions so that each stack of pads overlaps. Once it is determined that enough pads are in place for stabilising, tape or bandage them securely. This technique has the dual benefits of providing stabilisation and aiding in bleeding control. Larger objects that are impaled in the body can be secured with rolled towels or splinting materials.

Impaled objects in the eye can be managed using gauze pads, a Styrofoam cup, and bandage material. Do not apply pressure to the eye because pressure may cause vital fluids (the vitreous humour) to leak out. First, stabilise the object by hand. Once that is accomplished, use gauze pads cut midway into the centre as outlined previously. Place the cup on top of the stacked pads after the height is sufficient. Bandage or tape the cup into place. It is important to cover both eyes because consensual movement may cause additional damage Figure 19-18 ▼ . In such cases, it is particularly important to continually provide reassurance to the patient, who may be anxious because of the object and the blocked vision.

Whatever presentation you may encounter, it is important to avoid causing additional harm. Secure the object as best as possible, and be creative in using securing materials. Provide reassurance to the patient and family. Constantly assess the risk for developing threats to life, such as airway compromise, breathing inadequacy, and uncontrolled haemorrhage.

On rare occasions, removal of an impaled object may be the best course of action. If the object directly interferes with airway control and the patient's condition is deteriorating rapidly, medical direction may authorise removal. It may also be necessary to remove an object that interferes with chest compressions in a patient who is in cardiac arrest and deemed viable. In severe cases, it may be impossible to leave the object in place, such as when the patient is impaled on an immovable object.

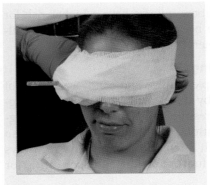

Figure 19-18 Stabilise an object impaled in the eye using gauze pads, a paper or Polystyrene cup, and bandage material.

Managing Wound Healing and Infection

In the prehospital setting, management of altered wound healing and infection entails basic measures. Wounds that are not healing properly or show signs of infection should be dressed and bandaged appropriately. In severe cases, pain control measures may be indicated.

Dressing Specific Anatomical Sites

Dressing and bandaging wounds is not the same for every part of the body. This section describes the various factors that need to be considered for a given body region.

Scalp Dressings

Scalp injuries tend to bleed profusely owing to their rich blood supply. When bleeding is present, application of direct pressure is often effective owing to the rigid skull that lies under the scalp. Be careful to accurately determine the extent of the injury because significant trauma may lead to skull damage. In that case, control of bleeding must be balanced against the issue of not causing additional damage. When the skull has been compromised and bleeding must be controlled, apply pressure to the areas around the break. Use a bulky dressing that assists in stopping blood loss and helps prevent excessive direct pressure on the already fractured cranium.

The shape of the skull is a consideration when dressing wounds that involve the scalp. Improperly applied dressings can easily slide up or down the scalp, becoming ineffective. In addition, hair may interfere with securing dressings in place.

Facial Dressings

Facial injuries tend to cause significant anxiety for patients and family. While tending to the clinical needs, take the time to reassure the patient. Application of direct pressure is an effective means to control bleeding from soft-tissue disruption along the face. If an avulsed piece of tissue is present, attempt to replace the pedicle to its normal anatomical location as closely as possible. Note that bleeding tends to be quite heavy owing to the rich blood supply in this area.

Assess the patient for the presence of or potential for airway compromise early in your encounter. Blood pouring into an unprotected airway is a recipe for disaster. Be prepared to suction and position the patient to facilitate drainage. Do not allow a gruesome facial injury to distract you from attending to life threats. Burns to the face can be covered in a commercial dressing, such as Water-Jel, that allows the patient to breathe and speak through suitably positioned holes.

Ear or Mastoid Dressings

Trauma to the ear is commonly external, although internal injury is a possibility. Never place a dressing in the ear canal, but loosely apply it along the entire length of the external ear. Gauze swabs work well to aid in stopping blood loss. If blood is flowing from the ear canal, do not attempt to control it directly. Cerebrospinal fluid may be leaking, and halting the blood flow may increase pressure within the skull. Place a bulky dressing to the external ear, and transport the patient rapidly.

Neck Dressings

Important anatomical structures in the neck include large blood vessels, the airway, and the cervical spine. There is little room for error when trauma is present in this area. A minor neck laceration can lead to an air embolism, a small puncture can penetrate the spinal canal, and an anterior open wound

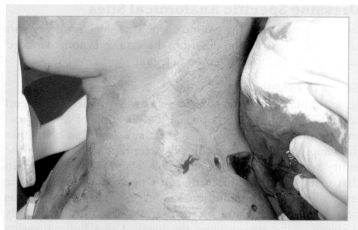

Figure 19-19 Neck wounds can lead to other serious situations such as air embolism and airway problems. Seal with an occlusive dressing right away.

can disrupt the airway   Figure 19-19 ▲ . Pay close attention to the clinical signs that accompany the external trauma.

Open injuries to the neck require use of an occlusive dressing to prevent the drawing of air into the circulatory system. Apply dressings carefully so that they do not interfere with blood flow or movement of air through the trachea.

Shoulder Dressings

The shoulder is relatively easy to dress and bandage. Apply direct pressure to control external haemorrhage in this region. If immobilisation is indicated, a sling will prevent motion of the shoulder girdle.

Torso Dressing

Injuries to the torso require vigilant assessment for underlying internal trauma. A seemingly innocuous hole may be the only indication that a gunshot wound is present. Cover open wounds with an occlusive dressing that is taped on three sides. Assessment of breath sounds becomes a high priority when you find an open chest wound because a pneumothorax or haemothorax may develop from penetrating trauma to the thorax. Continually reassess a patient with thoracic soft-tissue injuries.

The best choice for securing a truncal dressing in place is medical tape. Wrapping the entire torso may interfere with chest movement.

Groin and Hip Dressings

Soft-tissue injuries to the groin and hip do not present a significant challenge to paramedics. Typically, application of a dressing and bandage in combination with direct pressure work well to control blood loss in this region. Injuries to the genitalia are best managed by a clinician of the same sex, whenever feasible. In many cases, it is possible to provide the patient with a dressing and allow self-directed care. This makes an uncomfortable scenario easier for patient and clinician. If proper care cannot

be accomplished by working directly with the patient, you must be exceedingly professional and respect the patient's modesty in all but the most serious of cases.

Hand, Wrist, and Finger Dressings

The hands, wrists, and fingers are among the easiest sites to dress and bandage properly. A dressing is applied over any open wound, and bandage material is wrapped completely around the affected area. When possible, the hand should be placed in the position of function. This is accomplished by placing a roll of gauze in the patient's hand   Figure 19-20 ▼ . If limited motion is necessary, the hand and wrist can be easily splinted.

Elbow and Knee Dressings

Joints are not difficult to dress and bandage, but movement may cause the materials to shift from their original position. It is a good practice to provide immobilisation of the elbow or the knee when a larger wound is present. Even smaller wounds may be difficult to manage because of skin tension lines and high tissue stress in these areas. When either of these joints is injured, it becomes very important to assess dis-

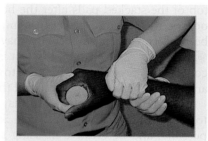

Figure 19-20 The position of function for the hand.

tal neurovascular status. Elbow injuries have a higher risk for neurovascular compromise because of the limited space available for blood vessels and nerves.

Ankle and Foot Dressings

The ankle and foot are simple to dress and bandage. Control of bleeding is accomplished by direct pressure and may be augmented by elevation and pressure points in cases involving significant bleeding. Application of a bandage must not be so tight that it interferes with circulation or sensation. Always assess distal neurovascular function before and after caring for the wound.

Crush Syndrome Management

Crush syndrome has been widely studied in recent years. In January 1995, a massive earthquake shook the southern part of Hyogo Prefecture, Japan, producing 41,000 casualties and 5,500 deaths. When researchers evaluated 372 patients who were diagnosed with crush syndrome, they found that most had lower extremity injuries that led to development of crush syndrome. Upper extremity injuries and trunk entrapment also caused some cases of crush syndrome, albeit to a much lesser extent.

Paramount to the issue of managing a case involving crush syndrome is making every effort to treat the patient before removing the crushing object   Figure 19-21 ▶ . Fail-

Prep Kit

Ready for Review

- The skin is a complex organ that fulfils several crucial roles, including maintaining homeostasis, protecting tissue from injury, and regulating temperature.
- The main layers of the skin are the epidermis and the dermis. The epidermis, the outer layer, serves as the principal barrier. The dermis, the inner layer, includes collagen, elastin, and ground substance, which contribute to the skin's strength. It also contains nerve endings, blood vessels, sweat glands, hair follicles, and sebaceous glands.
- The subcutaneous layer lies beneath the dermis and contains adipose tissue. Below the subcutaneous layer is the deep fascia, which offers support and protection to underlying structures such as muscle and bone.
- The skin is arranged in patterns of tautness known as tension lines. Wounds that occur parallel to skin tension lines may remain closed. Wounds that run opposite to tension lines may remain open.
- Soft-tissue injuries may be dramatic but are seldom the most serious. Don't let them distract you from thorough initial assessment!
- The first stage of wound healing is cessation of bleeding. The body uses several mechanisms to control bleeding, such as constricting the size of vessels and releasing platelets to form a blood clot.
- The second stage of healing is inflammation, in which additional cells enter the damaged area in an effort to repair it. Epithelialisation (creation of a new layer of epithelial cells) occurs, followed by neovascularisation (formation of new vessels).
- Wound healing is affected by factors such as the amount of movement the part is subjected to, medications, and medical conditions. A wound is more likely to become infected if it is caused by a human or an animal bite or if a foreign body has been impaled. Pressure injuries can develop when a patient is bedridden or remains on a backboard for too long.
- Signs of infection include redness, pus, warmth, oedema, and local discomfort. Gangrene, tetanus, and necrotising fasciitis are serious infection-related conditions that must be recognised early.
- In a closed wound, the skin is not broken but soft tissues beneath the skin are damaged. An example is a bruise. A haematoma (collection of blood beneath the skin) can also form.
- In an open wound, the skin is broken. Such an injury can become infected and can result in serious blood loss. Open wounds include abrasions, lacerations, puncture wounds, avulsions, and amputations.
- In a crush injury, a body part is crushed between two solid objects, resulting in damage to soft tissues and bone. The patient's external appearance may not adequately represent the level of internal damage.
- Crush syndrome may develop after a body part has been trapped for more than 4 hours. Necrosis occurs in crushed muscles, and harmful products are released in a process called rhabdomyolysis. Freeing the trapped body part can cause these harmful products to be released into the circulation, which can prove fatal. Kidney damage, cardiac arrest, and arrhythmias can also result.
- Compartment syndrome results when pressure increases in the injured area. Tissue necrosis and sepsis may then develop. Patients present with the six Ps: Pain, Paresthaesia, Paresis, Pressure, Passive stretch pain, and Pulselessness.
- Blasts (explosions) can result in soft-tissue injuries. A blast wind from the gases released can be very forceful, and projectiles can impale victims; both cause injuries. Falling structures can injure patients, and burns can also occur.
- Observe scene safety before assessing patients with soft-tissue injuries; hazards that caused the injury may still be present. Regardless of the grotesqueness of the injury, assess the ABCs first.
- While taking the history, ask about the event that caused the injury, such as whether a weapon was used or whether the patient lost consciousness. Find out when the patient last had a tetanus booster. Pay attention to whether the patient is taking any medications that may affect haemostasis.
- Depending on whether the mechanism of injury is significant or not, complete your physical examamination en route or at the scene, respectively. Direct your attention to the chief complaint and area of injury, and perform frequent reassessments.
- Be empathetic to patients with soft-tissue injuries.
- Managing soft-tissue injuries includes controlling bleeding. With closed injuries, follow the RICE mnemonic: Rest, Ice, Compression, and Elevation.
- When managing open wounds, control bleeding and keep the wound as clean as possible by irrigating and using sterile dressings. Try to determine the colour and type of bleeding and the amount of blood the patient has lost.
- Dressings and bandages are used to cover the wound, control bleeding, and limit motion. Types of dressings include sterile and nonsterile, occlusive and nonocclusive, adherent and nonadherent, and wet and dry. Types of bandages include roller and gauze, absorbent gauze sponges, elastic, and triangular bandages.
- Medical tape may be used to secure a bandage in place, except for patients with thin skin such as older patients because it can cause damage on removal. Do not apply dressings too tightly.
- Methods of bleeding control include direct pressure, elevation, pressure point control, immobilisation, and tourniquets. Cold compresses may help reduce pain. IV medications may be administered if basic measures do not relieve pain.
- Tourniquets are rarely needed in the civilian setting but may be used as a last resort. They can damage nerves and blood vessels and lead to loss of an extremity.
- Management of an avulsion includes irrigation, gently folding the flap back onto the wound, and applying a dry, sterile compression dressing. If the wound is an amputation, preserve the amputated part and transport it.
- Do not remove impaled objects in the prehospital environment. Instead, stabilise the object in place with a bulky dressing. Control bleeding with direct compression, but do not apply pressure on the object or on the immediately adjacent tissues.
- Dressing and bandaging techniques vary for different parts of the body. For example, the shape of the skull and the presence of hair make dressing the scalp challenging.
- Trapped patients must be managed before being freed from the crushing object because this approach improves their chances of survival after experiencing crush syndrome. Aggressive fluid therapy can help prevent kidney failure. Normal saline should be infused. Once the patient has been freed, transport him or her as quickly as possible.
- Blast injuries can include pulmonary damage such as tension pneumothorax and pulmonary contusion, abdominal trauma such as ruptured organs and internal haemorrhage, damage to the ears, and penetrating wounds. Use the DCAP-BTLS mnemonic to assess the patient rapidly.
- Soft-tissue injuries of the face, neck, thorax, and abdomen deserve special attention because these areas contain vital structures. Do not underestimate the seriousness of these injuries, and maintain a high index of suspicion.
- Document scene findings, including vehicle damage or the calibre of weapon used and patient presentation and position; size, location, depth, and complications of injuries; assessment findings; and interventions.

Vital Vocabulary

abrasion An injury in which a portion of the body is denuded of epidermis by scraping or rubbing.

adipose Referring to fat tissue.

amputation An injury in which part of the body is completely severed.

avulsion An injury that leaves a piece of skin or other tissue partially or completely torn away from the body.

bandage Material used to secure a dressing in place.

bruising Extravasation of blood under the skin to produce a "black-and-blue" mark.

chemotactic factors The factors that cause cells to migrate into an area.

closed wound An injury in which damage occurs beneath the skin or mucous membrane but the surface remains intact.

collagen Protein that gives tensile strength to the connective tissues of the body.

compartment syndrome A condition that develops when oedema and swelling result in increased pressure within soft tissues, causing circulation to be compromised, possibly resulting in tissue necrosis.

contaminated Containing microorganisms.

contusion A bruise; an injury that causes bleeding beneath the skin but does not break the skin.

crush injury An injury in which the body or part of the body is crushed, preventing tissue function and, possibly, resulting in permanent tissue damage.

crush syndrome Significant metabolic derangement that can lead to renal failure and death. It develops when crushed extremities or other body parts remain trapped for prolonged periods.

deep fascia A dense layer of fibrous tissue below the subcutaneous tissue; composed of tough bands of tissue that ensheath muscles and other internal structures.

degloving A traumatic injury that results in the soft tissue of the hand being drawn downward like a glove being removed.

degranulate To release granules into the surrounding tissue.

dermis The inner layer of skin, containing hair follicle roots, glands, blood vessels, and nerves.

dressing Material used to directly cover a wound.

elastin A protein that gives the skin its elasticity.

epidermis The outermost layer of the skin.

epithelialisation The formation of fresh epithelial tissue to heal a wound.

erythema Reddening of the skin.

fasciotomy A surgical procedure that cuts away fascia to relieve pressure.

gangrene An infection commonly caused by *C perfringens*. The result is tissue destruction and gas production that may lead to death.

glomerular filtration The first step in the formation of urine; calculated to determine renal function.

granulocytes Cells that contain granules.

ground substance Material between cells.

haematoma A localised collection of blood in the soft tissues as a result of injury or a broken blood vessel.

homeostasis The tendency to constancy or stability in the body's internal environment.

hyperkalaemia An increased level of potassium in the blood.

hyperphosphataemia An increased level of phosphate in the blood.

hypertrophic scar An abnormal scar with excess collagen that does not extend over the wound margins.

impaled object An object that has caused a puncture wound and remains embedded in the wound.

incision A wound usually made deliberately, as in surgery; a clean cut, as opposed to a laceration.

integument The skin.

keloid scar An abnormal scar commonly found in people with darkly pigmented skin. It extends over the wound margins.

laceration A wound made by tearing or cutting tissues.

lymphangitis Inflammation of a lymph channel.

lymphocytes White blood cells that function to remove invading pathogens.

macrophages Cells that are responsible for protecting the body against infection.

melanin The pigment that gives skin its colour.

mucopolysaccharide gel A key component of ground substance that is a polysaccharide that forms complexes with proteins.

myoglobin A protein found in muscle that is released into the circulation after crush injury or other muscle damage and whose presence in the circulation may produce kidney damage.

neovascularisation Development of vessels to aid in healing an injured soft tissue.

open wound An injury in which there is a break in the surface of the skin or the mucous membrane, exposing deeper tissue to potential contamination.

pedicle A narrow strip of tissue by which an avulsed piece of tissue remains connected to the body.

puncture wound A stab injury from a pointed object, such as a nail or a knife.

rhabdomyolysis The destruction of muscle tissue leading to a release of potassium and myoglobin.

scar revision A surgical procedure to improve the appearance of a scar, reestablish function, or correct disfigurement from soft-tissue damage, surgical incision, or lesion.

sebaceous gland The gland located in the dermis that secretes sebum.

sebum An oily substance secreted by the sebaceous glands.

subcutaneous Beneath the skin.

tension lines The pattern of tautness of the skin, which is arranged over body structures and affects how well wounds heal.

Volkmann contracture Deformity of the hand, fingers, and wrist resulting from damage to forearm muscles; develops from muscle ischaemia and is associated with compartment syndrome.

Points to Ponder

You are dispatched to the site of a motorcycle accident on the slip road of a motorway. When you arrive on scene, you see a man lying on his right side. You've carried your longboard and cervical collar with you, so you begin to provide full cervical-spine stabilisation. You note a tremendous amount of "road rash" and numerous lacerations. While you are placing the board and collar on this patient, your partner begins to attend to the obvious wounds. After you log roll the patient onto the longboard, you note copious amounts of blood in the patient's airway and determine that he has agonal respirations at about 8 breaths/min. You do not feel a radial pulse; however, you are able to obtain a weak and thready carotid pulse at about 110 beats/min. The patient is nonverbal. Your colleague is cleaning the patient's arm of debris and glass.

What are your priorities supposed to be in this situation? What do you need to do for this patient?

Issues: Priorities Regarding Life-Threatening Injuries and Wound Closure, The Value of the Written Report.

Assessment in Action

You are dispatched to the outside of a house for a dog bite. When you arrive, you notice that the patient is sitting upright, speaking in full sentences. She is conscious, alert, orientated, and complaining of pain in both of her arms and head. The family has wrapped towels over both arms and one over her head.

When you unwrap the right arm, you note two large lacerations greater than 10 cm and multiple puncture wounds. When you examine the upper arm, you notice white material that looks like muscle fascia. You control the bleeding with bandages. The left arm is not as bad, but it is bleeding. When you begin to check out the head, you notice that a piece of the scalp is missing. The family hands you a plastic bag with the missing piece.

1. **A "wound" is defined as:**
   A. any injury to the soft tissues, with or without involvement of the subcutaneous tissues and muscle beneath.
   B. any injury to the soft tissues that requires special care to stop the bleeding.
   C. any injury to the soft tissues, with involvement of the subcutaneous tissues and muscle beneath.
   D. any injury to the soft tissues that extends into the bone.

2. **What are the two types of wound classifications?**
   A. Open wounds and lacerations
   B. Lacerations and incisions
   C. Contusions and closed wounds
   D. Closed and open wounds

3. **A laceration is defined as:**
   A. a superficial wound that occurs when the skin is rubbed or scraped over a rough surface so that part of the epidermis is lost.
   B. a cut inflicted by a sharp instrument, such as a knife or razor blade, that produces a clean or jagged incision through the skin surface and underlying structure.
   C. a clean (linear) cut.
   D. a stab from a pointed object, such as a nail or a knife.

4. **A puncture wound is defined as:**
   A. a superficial wound that occurs when the skin is rubbed or scraped over a rough surface so that part of the epidermis is lost.
   B. a cut inflicted by a sharp instrument, such as a knife or razor blade, that produces a clean or jagged incision through the skin surface and underlying structure.
   C. a clean (linear) cut.
   D. a stab from a pointed object, such as a nail or a knife.

5. **An avulsion is defined as:**
   A. a superficial wound that occurs when the skin is rubbed or scraped over a rough surface so that part of the epidermis is lost.
   B. a cut inflicted by a sharp instrument, such as a knife or razor blade, that produces a clean or jagged incision through the skin surface and underlying structure.
   C. a flap of skin that has been torn loose, partially or completely.
   D. a complete loss of a body part, typically involving the extremities.

6. **Evaluation of the skin involves:**
   A. inspection and auscultation.
   B. auscultation and circulation.
   C. inspection and palpation.
   D. palpation and auscultation.

7. **Bleeding may be controlled by using:**
   A. direct pressure.
   B. elevation.
   C. pressure point control.
   D. all of the above.

8. **It is important to preserve the amputated part because this:**
   A. maximises the chances of its being successfully reimplanted.
   B. allows it to be donated.
   C. minimises the chances of it being unsuccessfully reimplanted.
   D. all of the above.

9. **Scalp injuries tend to bleed more because:**
   A. there is no blood supply to this area.
   B. there is a rich blood supply in this area.
   C. there is an excessive number of veins in the scalp.
   D. these are life-threatening injuries.

10. **Written documentation must be completed for every patient contact. It should include all of the following, EXCEPT:**
   A. ABCs.
   B. relevant scene findings.
   C. interventions and how the patient responded to them.
   D. paraphrasing of the patient's statements.

Challenging Questions

You are dispatched to a scene involving a man caught between a car and a low-end loader. When you arrive, you see that the man is pinned between the two vehicles. He complains of pain in his lower abdomen and pelvic region.

11. **What type of injury is this?**

12. **What treatment do you need to administer?**

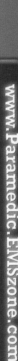

20 Burns

Objectives

Cognitive

- Describe the anatomy and physiology pertinent to burn injuries.
- Describe the epidemiology, including incidence, mortality/morbidity, risk factors, and prevention strategies for the patient with a burn injury.
- Describe the pathophysiological complications and systemic complications of a burn injury.
- Identify and describe types of burn injuries, including a thermal burn, an inhalation burn, a chemical burn, an electrical burn, and a radiation exposure.
- Identify and describe the depth classifications of burn injuries, including a superficial burn, a partial-thickness burn, and a full-thickness burn.
- Identify and describe methods for determining body surface area percentage of a burn injury including the "rule of nines", the "rule of palms", and other methods described by local guidelines.
- Identify and describe the severity of a burn including a minor burn, a moderate burn, a severe burn, and other severity classifications described by local guidelines.
- Differentiate criteria for determining the severity of a burn injury between a paediatric patient and an adult patient.
- Describe special considerations for a paediatric patient with a burn injury.
- Discuss considerations which impact management and prognosis of the burn injured patient.
- Discuss mechanisms of burn injuries.
- Discuss conditions associated with burn injuries, including trauma, blast injuries, airway compromise, respiratory compromise, and potential abuse.
- Describe the management of a burn injury, including airway and ventilation, circulation, pharmacological, non-pharmacological, transport considerations, psychological support/communication strategies, and other management described by local guidelines.
- Describe the epidemiology of a thermal burn injury.
- Describe the specific anatomy and physiology pertinent to a thermal burn injury.
- Describe the pathophysiology of a thermal burn injury.
- Identify and describe the depth classifications of a thermal burn injury.
- Identify and describe the severity of a thermal burn injury.
- Describe considerations which impact management and prognosis of the patient with a thermal burn injury.
- Discuss mechanisms of burn injury and conditions associated with a thermal burn injury.
- Describe the management of a thermal burn injury, including airway and ventilation, circulation, pharmacological, non-pharmacological, transport considerations, and psychological support/communication strategies.
- Describe the epidemiology of an inhalation burn injury.
- Describe the specific anatomy and physiology pertinent to an inhalation burn injury.
- Describe the pathophysiology of an inhalation burn injury.

- Differentiate between supraglottic and infraglottic inhalation injuries.
- Identify and describe the depth classifications of an inhalation burn injury.
- Identify and describe the severity of an inhalation burn injury.
- Describe considerations which impact management and prognosis of the patient with an inhalation burn injury.
- Discuss mechanisms of burn injury and conditions associated with an inhalation burn injury.
- Describe the management of an inhalation burn injury, including airway and ventilation, circulation, pharmacological, non-pharmacological, transport considerations, and psychological support/communication strategies.
- Describe the epidemiology of a chemical burn injury and a chemical burn injury to the eye.
- Describe the specific anatomy and physiology pertinent to a chemical burn injury and a chemical burn injury to the eye.
- Describe the pathophysiology of a chemical burn injury, including types of chemicals and their burning processes and a chemical burn injury to the eye.
- Identify and describe the depth classifications of a chemical burn injury.
- Identify and describe the severity of a chemical burn injury.
- Describe considerations which impact management and prognosis of the patient with a chemical burn injury and a chemical burn injury to the eye.
- Discuss mechanisms of burn injury and conditions associated with a chemical burn injury.
- Describe the management of a chemical burn injury and a chemical burn injury to the eye, including airway and ventilation, circulation, pharmacological, non-pharmacological, transport considerations, and psychological support/communication strategies.
- Describe the epidemiology of an electrical burn injury.
- Describe the specific anatomy and physiology pertinent to an electrical burn injury.
- Describe the pathophysiology of an electrical burn injury.
- Identify and describe the depth classifications of an electrical burn injury.
- Identify and describe the severity of an electrical burn injury.
- Describe considerations which impact management and prognosis of the patient with an electrical burn injury.
- Discuss mechanisms of burn injury and conditions associated with an electrical burn injury.
- Describe the management of an electrical burn injury, including airway and ventilation, circulation, pharmacological, non-pharmacological, transport considerations, and psychological support/communication strategies.
- Describe the epidemiology of a radiation exposure.
- Describe the specific anatomy and physiology pertinent to a radiation exposure.
- Describe the pathophysiology of a radiation exposure, including the types and characteristics of ionising radiation.
- Identify and describe the depth classifications of a radiation exposure.

- Identify and describe the severity of a radiation exposure.
- Describe considerations which impact management and prognosis of the patient with a radiation exposure.
- Discuss mechanisms of burn injury associated with a radiation exposure.
- Discuss conditions associated with a radiation exposure.
- Describe the management of a radiation exposure, including airway and ventilation, circulation, pharmacological, non-pharmacological, transport considerations, and psychological support/communication strategies.
- Integrate pathophysiological principles to the assessment of a patient with a thermal burn injury.
- Integrate pathophysiological principles to the assessment of a patient with an inhalation burn injury.
- Integrate pathophysiological principles to the assessment of a patient with a chemical burn injury.
- Integrate pathophysiological principles to the assessment of a patient with an electrical burn injury.
- Integrate pathophysiological principles to the assessment of a patient with a radiation exposure.
- Synthesise patient history information and assessment findings to form an initial impression for the patient with a thermal burn injury.
- Synthesise patient history information and assessment findings to form an initial impression for the patient with an inhalation burn injury.
- Synthesise patient history information and assessment findings to form an initial impression for the patient with a chemical burn injury.
- Synthesise patient history information and assessment findings to form an initial impression for the patient with an electrical burn injury.
- Synthesise patient history information and assessment findings to form an initial impression for the patient with a radiation exposure.
- Develop, execute, and evaluate a management plan based on the initial impression for the patient with a thermal burn injury.
- Develop, execute, and evaluate a management plan based on the initial impression for the patient with an inhalation burn injury.
- Develop, execute, and evaluate a management plan based on the initial impression for the patient with a chemical burn injury.
- Develop, execute, and evaluate a management plan based on the initial impression for the patient with an electrical burn injury.
- Develop, execute, and evaluate a management plan based on the initial impression for the patient with a radiation exposure.

Affective

- Value the changes of a patient's self-image associated with a burn injury.
- Value the impact of managing a burn injured patient.
- Advocate empathy for a burn injured patient.
- Assess safety at a burn injury incident.
- Characterise mortality and morbidity based on the pathophysiology and assessment findings of a patient with a burn injury.
- Value and defend the sense of urgency in burn injuries.
- Serve as a model for universal precautions and body substance isolation (BSI).

Psychomotor

- Take body substance isolation procedures during assessment and management of patients with a burn injury.
- Perform assessment of a patient with a burn injury.
- Perform management of a thermal burn injury, including airway and ventilation, circulation, pharmacological, non-pharmacological, transport considerations, psychological support/communication strategies, and other management described by local guidelines.
- Perform management of an inhalation burn injury, including airway and ventilation, circulation, pharmacological, non-pharmacological, transport considerations, psychological support/communication strategies, and other management described by local guidelines.
- Perform management of a chemical burn injury, including airway and ventilation, circulation, pharmacological, non-pharmacological, transport considerations, psychological support/communication strategies, and other management described by local guidelines.
- Perform management of an electrical burn injury, including airway and ventilation, circulation, pharmacological, non-pharmacological, transport considerations, psychological support/communication strategies, and other management described by local guidelines.
- Perform management of a radiation exposure, including airway and ventilation, circulation, pharmacological, non-pharmacological, transport considerations, psychological support/communication strategies, and other management described by local guidelines.

Introduction

Approximately 82% of all civilian fire-related deaths occur in residential buildings **Figure 20-1 ▾** . The incidence of burn injuries and death in the United Kingdom has decreased somewhat with the advent of stricter building regulations and widespread use of smoke detectors. Other effective burn prevention techniques include reducing domestic water heater temperatures to 49°C to prevent severe scalds and making disposable lighters child-safe. According to the Department for Communities and Local Government, 491 people died of fire-related causes in the United Kingdom during 2005. Children younger than 5 years and elderly people are at particularly high risk of dying in fires.

Just as building regulation and smoke detectors have decreased fire-related deaths, our ability to treat large burns effectively has steadily improved. Before the medical advances of the 20th century, death was "almost inevitable" when more than one third of the body was burned. Now, however, better understanding of "burn shock", advances in the use of fluid therapy and antibiotics, improved ability to excise dead tissue, and the use of biological dressings to aid early wound closure have vastly improved burn care. The formation of specialised teams to resuscitate patients from burn shock, delay infection, and achieve wound closure has resulted in impressive gains in survival rates.

Deaths and serious injuries also occur from electrical and chemical burns. As a consequence, numerous public safety campaigns have focused on the use of smoke detectors and the dangers that surround the use of flammable liquids, petroleum products, solvents, propane, and fireworks.

Although you probably won't see moderate or severe burns on a daily basis, you will encounter some serious burn injuries during your career, and you might encounter serious electrical, chemical, and radiation injuries as well. Accurate recognition of the severity of burn injuries can dramatically enhance the care of burned patients by allowing you to institute proper emergency care and notify the receiving hospital so personnel can be better prepared to care for the patient, and by allowing triage to or consultation with a specialised burn centre.

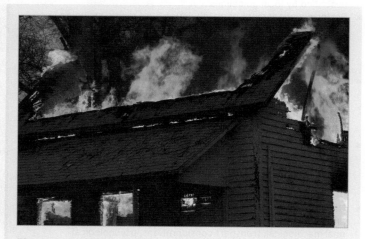

Figure 20-1 Of all civilian fire fatalities, 82% occur in the home.

Anatomy and Function of the Skin

The human skin is much more than a wrapping that keeps the inside of the body from falling out. The skin, also known as the integument, is the largest and one of the most complex organs in the body. It has a crucial role in maintaining homeostasis (balance) within the body. The skin is durable, flexible, and usually able to repair itself. It varies in thickness from almost 1 cm on the heel to 1 mm on the eyelid. The skin has four functions:

- It acts as an all-purpose fortress to protect the underlying tissue from injury and exposure from extremes of

You are the Paramedic Part 1

You are dispatched to assist the fire service with a fire at 56 Hitherwell Drive. Within a few minutes, you are briefed by the fire officer at scene indicating they have found a fire victim. He points out which side of the structure the fire fighters will exit, and you take your equipment and wait for them there.

Within a few moments, the fire fighters emerge with a child who appears to be approximately 8 years old. She is crying, coughing, and holding up her forearm. As you approach, you can see that the young girl has what seems to be a partial-thickness burn to her right arm.

Initial Assessment	Recording Time: 0 Minutes
Appearance	Tearful and upset
Level of consciousness	A (Alert to person, place, and day)
Airway	Patent, loud crying
Breathing	Tachypnoeic but with good tidal volume
Circulation	Not yet assessed, skin covered with soot

1. What are your patient care priorities?
2. What are patient care concerns when dealing with victims of a structure fire?

At the Scene

Many fires generate toxic compounds such as cyanides (thiocyanate), which are produced as a result of the combustion of synthetic fabrics and furniture.

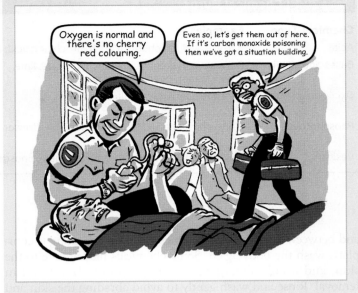

Figure 20-10

by the burning process), and tissue damage and toxic effects caused by chemicals in the smoke. Such problems are particularly common when a person is caught in a burning building, stands up, and breathes in superheated gases.

Carbon Monoxide Intoxication

The combustion process produces a variety of toxic gases. The less efficient the combustion process, the more toxic the gases—such as carbon monoxide (CO) and carbon dioxide (CO_2)—that may be created. When boilers, kerosene heaters, and other heating devices are in poor repair, they may emit unsafe levels of these toxic gases. Internal combustion engines may emit many of the same gases and, consequently, should always have their exhaust vented to the outdoors. A common cause of CO exposure is running a small engine in an enclosed space like a garage or basement. Fire fighters who are performing a clean up after a fire may be exposed to high levels of CO, as may people who are exposed to large amounts of car exhaust (such as road construction workers and car mechanics). Methylene chloride (found in some paint removers) may also produce CO gas.

CO intoxication should be considered whenever a group of people in the same place all complain of headache or nausea (a malfunctioning boiler or car exhaust being sucked into the air-handling system can cause CO intoxication in groups of people). Similarly, you should be suspicious when people complain of feeling sick at home but not when they go to work or school.

CO can displace oxygen from the alveolar air and the blood haemoglobin. Because CO binds to receptor sites on haemoglobin at least 240 times more easily than oxygen (O_2), the patient's haemoglobin may become saturated with the wrong chemical. Being exposed to relatively small concentrations of CO (such as in cigarette smoke) will result in progressively higher blood levels of CO. Most people have approximately 2% CO attached to their haemoglobin, but these levels may be as high as 4% to 8% in heavy smokers. Levels of 50% or higher may be fatal.

Traditional wisdom tells us that patients with CO intoxication will appear "cherry red". Most practitioners agree that this cherry red skin is most likely to be seen in people who have died, not living people. So, never rule out CO intoxication because the patient's skin isn't cherry red.

Patients with severe CO intoxication usually present with an O_2 saturation of normal or better. For this reason, you should never trust a pulse oximeter when dealing with a suspected CO poisoning case **Figure 20-10**. New devices that

can measure CO levels will soon be common in prehospital care; they will allow us to find and treat low-level CO intoxication far more readily than we can today.

At the Scene

Regardless of the cause, hyperbaric oxygen therapy for CO inhalation may be beneficial because it decreases the time it takes for haemoglobin to become saturated with oxygen. The treatment of patients with fairly low levels of CO may also be helpful.

Chemical Burns

Chemical burns occur when the skin comes in contact with strong acids, alkalis or bases, or other corrosive materials **Table 20-1**. The burn progresses as long as the corrosive substance remains in contact with the skin. The cornerstone of therapy is, therefore, removal of the chemical from contact with the patient's body.

Skin destruction is determined by the chemical's concentration and duration of contact. Systemic toxicity is determined by the degree of absorption. Immediately removing the patient's clothing will often remove the majority of the chemical from skin contact. Most chemicals are most efficiently removed by washing with copious amounts of low-pressure water (such as in a shower, sink, or eye-wash station). Have the patient bend over when washing the hair and head to avoid allowing residual chemicals to run over the rest of the body. Chemicals can collect in skin folds, where they remain in contact with the tissue and continue to cause more severe damage. Care must be taken to wash the skinfolds meticulously at joints

Table 20-1	Chemical Burns	
Chemical Type	**Examples**	**Injury**
Acids	Battery acid (sulphuric acid), hydrochloric acid, hydrofluoric acid	Coagulative necrosis
Bases and alkalis	Potassium hydroxide, sodium hydroxide, lime, drain cleaner, oven cleaner, lye	Liquefactive necrosis
Oxidising agents	Hydrogen peroxide, sodium chlorate	Exothermic (heat) reaction in addition to tissue destruction; could cause systemic poisoning
Phosphorous	White phosphorous, tracer ammunition, fireworks	Burns when exposed to air; could cause systemic poisoning
Vesicants	Lewisite, sulphur mustard (mustard gas), phosgene oxime	Blister agents; respiratory compromise if inhaled

and between fingers and toes. Once you think washing is complete, wash the body again. Some chemicals may adhere to the skin, and a mild detergent (washing-up liquid) will aid in removal. Rinse and wash gently to avoid abrading the skin and exacerbating the injury or absorption of the chemical.

Some chemicals react violently with water, which obviously precludes irrigation. Such chemicals are usually powders, so it is reasonable to brush off as much dry powder as possible before irrigating any chemical exposure.

At the Scene

Continue the irrigation until the patient experiences absence of or a significant decrease in pain or burning in the wound.

Injuries From Chemical Burns

Six mechanisms of injury may damage the body's tissues in case of chemical burns:

- **Reduction.** Protein denaturation caused by the reduction of the amide linkages following exposure to a reducing agent (such as alkyl mercuric compounds, diborane, lithium aluminum hydride and other metallic hydrides)
- **Oxidation.** Caused when a chemical inserts oxygen, sulphur, or a halogen (such as chlorine) atoms (such as from sodium hypochlorite, potassium permanganate, peroxides, chromic acid) into the body's proteins
- **Corrosion.** Chemicals that corrode the skin and cause massive protein denaturing (such as phenols, hydroxides, sodium, potassium, ammonium, and calcium)
- **Protoplasmic poisons.** Chemicals that form esters with proteins (such as formic acid and acetic acid) or that bind or inhibit the inorganic ions needed for the body's normal functions (such as oxalic acid and hydrofluoric acid)
- **Desiccation.** Desiccants that damage the body by extracting water from tissues (such as concentrated or fuming

At the Scene

Hydrofluoric acid is a corrosive, inorganic acid used in the manufacture of plastics, pottery glazing, and rust removers. Pain and erythema at the site of exposure are the symptoms of exposure to this chemical.

sulphuric acid); reaction often causes heat (exothermic), which adds insult to the injury

- **Vesication.** Vesicants rapidly produce cutaneous blisters and typically are referred to as chemical warfare agents or weapons of mass destruction (such as mustard gas).

With a chemical burn injury, it is difficult to estimate the extent of the burn—it may have penetrated deep into the body's tissues. By using the rule of nines, estimate the body surface area affected, but be aware that the extent of the injury may be much more severe. Do not underestimate the power of a small quantity of chemical. Chemicals such as phenols and highly corrosive acids can cause considerable damage to the skin and its underlying tissues very quickly. Flush, flush, and then flush some more!

When contacting a local poisons centre for medical advice on handling specific chemical substances, you will need to identify the chemical and estimate the depth (superficial, partial thickness, or full thickness) of the chemical burn injury.

At the Scene

Prolonged contact with petroleum products such as petrol or diesel fuel may produce a chemical injury to the skin that is actually a full-thickness burn but initially appears to be only a partial-thickness injury. Sufficient absorption of the hydrocarbon may cause organ failure and even death.

Initial Assessment

As you approach a burn trauma patient, simple clues may help identify how serious the injuries are and how quickly you need to assess and treat the patient. If the patient greets you with a hoarse voice and a chief complaint of "trouble breathing", your general impression might be that the patient has a potential airway and/or breathing problem. In the absence of hypoxia or other trauma, a patient with a severe burn may be conscious and is often able to hold a conversation. Although burns are often painful, the more serious burns may present with little or no pain. Indeed, the chief complaint is often "I'm cold". What may first appear to be tattered clothing could turn out to be sheets of the patient's own skin hanging from his burned limbs. Recently burned patients may appear dazed or disconnected from events around them.

Despite what the injuries may look or smell like, you must use compassion when approaching the patient. Burns are obviously traumatic for the patient; if the person survives, he or she may face significant hospitalisation and years of rehabilitation. But burns are also traumatic for you, the provider.

Ensure an Open Airway

As in any other seriously ill or injured patient, airway management is a priority in a patient with a burn. The airway may be in particular jeopardy because the same heat and flames that caused the external burn may have produced potentially life-threatening damage to the airway.

Although rare, laryngeal oedema can develop with alarming speed in burn patients, especially in infants and children. Early endotracheal intubation—before the airway has closed off—could be lifesaving in such cases and should be performed by the most confident and experienced paramedic on your team. To intervene early, however, you need to spot the problem early. Airway management is discussed in greater detail later in this chapter.

Assess for Adequate Breathing

Listen to lung sounds, with special attention to stridor, which may be a sign of impending upper airway compromise. Note that patients with preexisting lung disease may have bronchospasm after even relatively minor exposure to smoke; they may respond well to inhaled beta-2 agonists.

Anyone suspected of having a burn to the upper airway may benefit from humidified, cool oxygen. If you do not carry a high-output humidifier, consider using a nebuliser to administer nebulised normal saline. This approach will not provide a high concentration of oxygen, so you will need to balance the need for a high O_2 concentration against the desire for cool humidity. Keep in mind that the patient's oxygen saturation may be suspect if there is the possibility of CO intoxication.

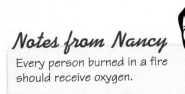

Notes from Nancy

Every person burned in a fire should receive oxygen.

Ensure Adequate Circulation

During the first 24 to 48 hours of a patient's burn care, a great deal of emphasis is placed on fluid resuscitation to prevent burn shock. Burn shock is caused by fluid shifts that typically occur 6 to 8 hours after the burn. Severely burned patients will ultimately require large volumes of fluid, but they don't need it during the first minutes of prehospital care unless their burn injury occurred some time ago. Most patients will ultimately require central venous access, and most intravenous (IV) lines placed in the prehospital setting will be removed owing to tissue swelling and infection risk. If the patient is not grossly hypotensive, do not delay transport by making multiple attempts at vascular access. Of course, if the patient has an obvious peripheral vessel, your early vascular access will be put to good use by hospital or burn centre staff for continued fluid replacement and pain management.

Patients with other trauma may require immediate vascular access just like any other trauma patient. Although it is preferable to avoid starting IV lines through burned tissue, it isn't contra-indicated. Burn patients may challenge your vascular access skills. New options for intra-osseous access may provide you with more choices than were available to your paramedic predecessors.

Notes from Nancy

If a burned patient is in shock in the prehospital phase, look for another injury as the source of shock.

Evaluate Mental Status

Patients with a burn injury may demonstrate varied mental status responses. Combative patients should be considered hypoxic until proven otherwise. Because partial-thickness burns are extremely painful, a patient with this type of injury may be awake and in pain. Even patients with excessive burns will often be awake and attempting to communicate. Isolated burns do not cause unconsciousness (although toxic inhalations can). Unresponsive burn patients must be carefully assessed for the presence of other deadly injuries.

Burn Severity

The burn wound is categorised by the degree of injury. Historically, such an injury has been described by three pathological progressions or zones, which radiate from the central zone of greatest damage. Skin nearest the heat source suffers the most profound cellular changes. The central area of the skin, which suffers the most damage, is called the zone of coagulation. There is little or no blood flow to the injured tissue in this area. The peripheral area surrounding the zone of coagulation has decreased blood flow and inflammation; it is known as the zone of stasis. This area may undergo necrosis within 24 to 48 hours after the injury, particularly if perfusion is compromised by burn shock. Last, the zone of hyperaemia is the area least affected by the thermal injury. In this area, cells will typically recover in 7 to 10 days.

How Deep Is the Burn?

During your initial assessment, your goal is to identify and manage life threats, as well as to determine the level of care the patient requires (burn centre, trauma centre, local A&E department). This means you will need to get an idea of the burn's size and severity to report to the receiving hospital. The nature of the patient's burns will evolve during the next 24 hours, and estimations of their size and severity will inevitably change, so little is to be gained by conducting a comprehensive and time-consuming evaluation of every inch of the patient's body at the scene. Nevertheless, a reasonably accurate estimation of the scope of the patient's injuries is helpful for determining the appropriate care.

The traditional labels given to burns were first, second, and third degree. Many centres have expanded that concept, describing burns as fourth, fifth, and sixth degree as tissue destruction goes into the deeper tissues, muscle, and bone. Prehospital providers should limit their assessment to superficial, partial and full-thickness burns (described later) to simplify the process and avoid confusion and miscommunication. The hospital staff need to know, for example, that they are getting an x-year old male with approximately x% full-thickness and x% mixed partial-thickness burns with possible airway decompensation.

Quickly assess the burns while considering the presence or absence of pain, swelling, skin colour, capillary refill time, moisture and blisters, the appearance of the wound edges, the presence of foreign bodies, debris and contaminants, bleeding, and circulatory adequacy. Make sure you assess for concomitant soft-tissue injury.

Determination of burn depth is a subjective assessment that depends on provider judgement. Based on this assessment, the burn injury should be classified as superficial, partial thickness, or full thickness Figure 20-13 ▶ .

A superficial burn involves the epidermis only. The skin is red and, when touched, the colour will blanch and return. Usually blisters are not present. Patients will experience pain because nerve endings are exposed to the air. Such a burn will heal spontaneously in 3 to 7 days. The most common example is a sunburn.

A partial-thickness burn involves the epidermis and varying degrees of the dermis. This category can be subdivided into superficial partial-thickness and deep partial-thickness burns. With a *superficial partial-thickness burn,* the skin is red; when touched, the colour will blanch and return. Usually there are blisters or moisture present, and the patient may experience extreme pain. Hair follicles remain intact. A superficial partial-thickness burn will heal spontaneously but may scar or have a changed appearance. In contrast, a *deep partial-thickness burn* extends into the dermis, damaging the hair follicle and sweat and sebaceous glands. Hot liquids, steam, or grease are often to blame for these injuries. In the prehospital setting, the delin-

eation between deep partial thickness and full thickness may be difficult to determine.

A full-thickness burn involves destruction of both layers of the skin, including the basement membrane of dermis that produces new skin cells. In such an injury, the skin is white and pale, brown and leathery, or charred. Dry and leathery skin is referred to as eschar. No capillary refill occurs with this type of burn because the capillaries have been destroyed. Sensory nerves are destroyed as well, so there may be no pain in the full-thickness section. Because patients usually have mixed depths of burns, they will often experience significant pain in the areas surrounding the full-thickness burns. Treatment of a full-thickness burn will usually require skin grafting because the dermis has been destroyed.

How Much Surface Area Is Burned?

While evaluating the patient's burns, you must approximate the total body surface area (TBSA) burned. Most paramedics advocate counting only the areas of partial- and full-thickness burns (ignoring the areas of superficial burns). The most universal mechanism of calculating the area burned is the rule of nines, which is based on dividing the body into 9% segments. The provider adds the portions of the body to obtain a total of the body area affected by the burn injury. Because our proportions change as we grow, different rules of nines apply to infants, children, and adults Figure 20-14 ▶ .

Another mechanism of assessing the TBSA is the rule of palm. This assessment uses the size of the patient's palm (excluding the fingers) to represent about 1% of the patient's body surface area. This calculation is helpful when the burn covers less than 10% of the body surface area or is irregularly shaped. The Lund and Browder chart is an even more specific method used to estimate the burned area by dividing the body into even smaller and more specific regions, but is seldom used prehospital Figure 20-15 ▶ .

You must balance the need for accuracy against the time required to make an estimate of the TBSA. The prehospital estimation is used to guide the patient to the correct place for treatment. The A&E department estimation of burned area may be used to initiate fluid therapy. The burn centre's estimation of injured area will undoubtedly be more accurate and specific.

Focused History and Physical Examination

With burn patients, proceed through the steps of physical assessment in the usual sequence, starting with the general appearance and moving on to the vital signs. Obtaining vital signs may be challenging if the patient has extensive burns on the arms. Nevertheless, you should try to document vital signs accurately because the management of shock, airway compromise, and pain control depends on them to some degree. It is worth remembering that blood pressure, pulse, and capillary refill time can still be taken on the lower limbs, whilst not desirable in the first instance it will help to produce a baseline set of observations.

When you have finished your brief inspection of the patient's skin, you have only just begun the head-to-toe exami-

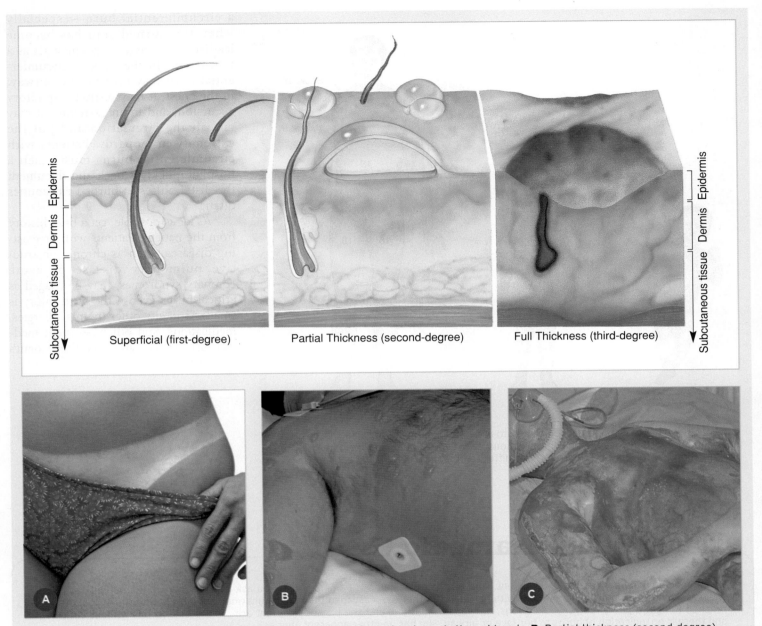

Figure 20-13 Classification of burns. **A.** Superficial (first-degree) burns involve only the epidermis. **B.** Partial-thickness (second-degree) burns involve some of the dermis but do not destroy the entire thickness of the skin. The skin is mottled, white to red, and often blistered. **C.** Full-thickness (third-degree) burns extend through all layers of the skin and may involve subcutaneous tissue and muscle. The skin is dry, leathery, and often white or charred.

nation. The detailed physical examination is intended to make sure that no other injuries have higher priority for treatment. Often such injuries may be obscured by the burn itself, so you need to pay attention to the circumstances of the burn and the possible mechanisms of injury. If the patient jumped from a second-floor window, for example, there may be fractures beneath the obvious burns on the legs.

Look for injuries to the eyes, and cover injured eyes with moist, sterile pads. Check the neck, chest, and extremities for <u>circumferential burns</u>. Progressive oedema beneath

At the Scene

Signs and symptoms of vascular compromise in a burned extremity that may necessitate an escharotomy include cyanosis, pallor, deep tissue pain, progressive paraesthesia, progressive decrease or absence of the pulse, or sensation of a cold extremity.

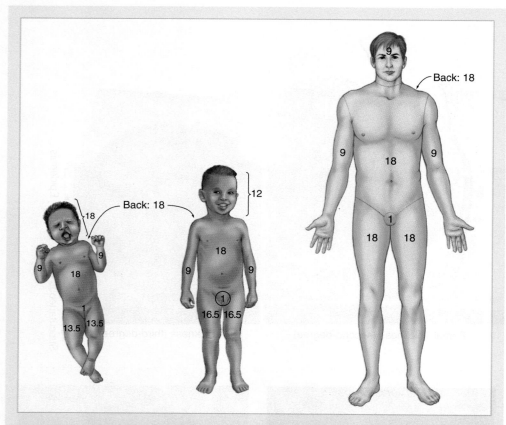

Figure 20-14 The rule of nines is a quick way to estimate the amount of surface area that has been burned. It divides the body into sections, each representing approximately 9% of the total body surface area. The proportions differ for infants, children, and adults.

a circumferential burn—especially when the burned skin has become leathery and unyielding—may act as a tourniquet. In the neck, a circumferential burn may obstruct the airway; in the chest, it may restrict respiratory excursion; and in an extremity, it may cut off the circulation and put the extremity in jeopardy. Patients with circumferential burns must reach a hospital quickly. Check and document the distal pulses in burned extremities often.

As far as possible, get a brief history from the patient. Patients with preexisting diseases, such as chronic obstructive pulmonary disease or acute coronary syndromes, may be triaged as critical burns even if the burn injury is small. As in any other trauma, allergies, medications, and other pertinent medical history may influence the patient's care plan.

You are the Paramedic Part 2

You immediately begin treating your patient, who tells you her name is Pamela. When you ask what happened, the patient says that she was playing with petrol and matches with her older brother (who escaped the house unharmed and now is with the police). As she reached to light a pile of petrol-soaked rags, the vapours flashed, and she burned her right arm. She is able to talk without difficulty, and there is no indication of burns to her face or airway. She has no other apparent injuries.

By using the rule of palm, you estimate the size of Pamela's burn to be approximately 4% to 5% involving her right arm and hand. You administer supplemental oxygen. Your colleague initiates an IV line in the unburned arm while you assess the injured right arm and apply a gel-based dressing. Pulse and motor and sensory functions are present.

Vital Signs	Recording Time: 5 Minutes
Level of consciousness	Alert, with a Glasgow Coma Scale score of 15
Skin	Warm, pink, dry with some soot on skin and clothing
Pulse	Radial pulse, 120 beats/min, strong and regular
Blood pressure	116 by palpation
Respirations	36 to 42 breaths/min, clear and equal breath sounds bilaterally
SpO_2	100% while breathing room air

3. Why is pulse oximetry unreliable in these circumstances?

4. Are your transport considerations affected by the location of her burn?

5. What are common complications of burns?

Region	%
Head	
Neck	
Ant. Trunk	
Post. Trunk	
Right arm	
Left arm	
Buttocks	
Genitalia	
Right leg	
Left leg	
Total burn	

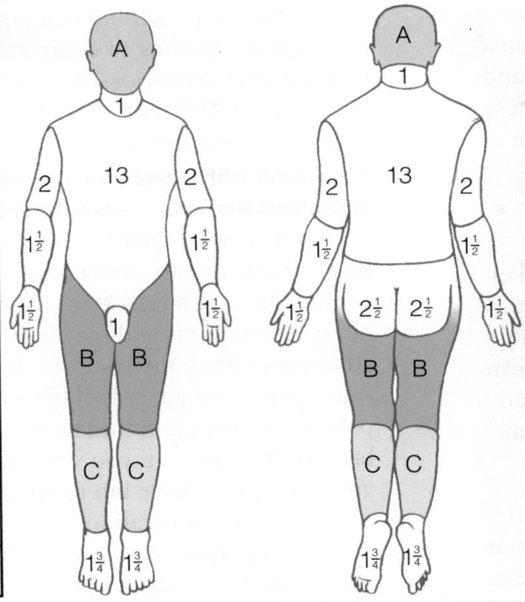

Relative percentages of body surface area affected by growth

Age (years)	A ($\frac{1}{2}$ of head)	B ($\frac{1}{2}$ of one thigh)	C ($\frac{1}{2}$ of one leg)
0	$9\frac{1}{2}$	$2\frac{3}{4}$	$2\frac{1}{2}$
1	$8\frac{1}{2}$	$3\frac{1}{4}$	$2\frac{1}{2}$
5	$6\frac{1}{2}$	4	$2\frac{3}{4}$
10	$5\frac{1}{2}$	$4\frac{1}{4}$	3
15	$4\frac{1}{2}$	$4\frac{1}{2}$	$3\frac{1}{4}$
Adult	$3\frac{1}{2}$	$4\frac{3}{4}$	3

Figure 20-15 The Lund and Browder chart.

At the Scene

Heat loss is a critical problem for burn patients. Take immediate steps to prevent hypothermia, such as heating the ambulance until it's uncomfortable for the crew and using warm blankets and fluids.

Detailed Physical Examination and Ongoing Assessment

If the patient is considered to have a significant mechanism of injury, en route to the hospital, you should perform a detailed physical examination and the ongoing assessment (see Chapters 13 and 14). Reassessment of vital signs to establish trends is done every 5 minutes for critical patients and every 15 minutes for lower priority patients (in stable condition).

Assessment of Radiation Burns

First and foremost, the assessment of a patient who may have been exposed to radiation involves a scene assessment to determine if the scene is safe for rescuers to enter. In some cases, it may be appropriate to contact the hazardous materials response team so they may determine the appropriate precautions, including exposure-limiting suits, and the most appropriate A&E department for the patient's treatment. Not all A&E departments are set up to handle a patient who has been exposed to radiation, so learn the capabilities of your hospitals before an incident occurs! The ambulance service that operates in an area where there is a nuclear power plant or other research facility typically has additional training offered by the facility and regularly practise responding to radiation-related emergencies.

Once the scene is deemed safe, you may proceed with your initial assessment of the patient. Assess the patient's mental status and ABCs, and then prioritise the patient's care. Unfortunately, patients who have sustained a significant radiation exposure and a major burn are unlikely to survive, even with major resources expended to keep them alive (a burn of > 70% of the TBSA is probably fatal by itself; a burn and radiation of > 30% of the TBSA are probably fatal). When confronted with large numbers of patients who have been exposed to radiation and simultaneously received thermal burns, keep the 30% rule in mind when triaging and making transport decisions. In the prehospital environment, it is difficult to determine the extent of the patient's internal injuries because radiation can "cook from the inside out" (like the microwave ovens we are all too familiar with).

Management of Burns

Definitive burn care can be divided into four phases. While paramedics will be most heavily involved in the first phase, it is important to appreciate the magnitude of care that a patient with a severe, or even moderate, burn must receive. Early actions of the paramedic may dramatically affect the patient's long-term outcome. Paramedics may also find themselves transporting patients to specialised rehabilitation facilities at later stages of their care.

Unlike many emergencies you will encounter, burn patient care is measured in weeks, not hours. Burns are devastating multi-system traumatic injuries that dramatically alter a person's life. You should recognise not only the massive physical trauma caused by burns, but also the emotional, psychological, and financial burdens these horrific injuries impose. Once these costs are appreciated, it is easy to understand the importance of teaching injury prevention strategies to the people we serve.

General Management

Management of a burned patient begins with the steps taken during the scene assessment and initial assessment to extinguish the fire and ensure adequate ABCs. Only when the ABCs are under control should you turn your attention to the burn itself. It is important to have all resuscitative equipment ready for use when treating a burn patient, including advanced airway equipment and heart monitors.

Immediate Management

Stop the burning. When a person burns a hand on a hot oven at gas mark 8, the person will usually stick the hand under cool running water for a few seconds. Is that long enough to cool the tissues and stop the burning? Usually not. It often takes several minutes to completely cool the burned area and achieve some pain relief. The fire needs to be put out, and the burned areas need to be cooled. All jewellery, metal buttons, zips, and hooks should be cool to the touch as well. Of course, never use ice on a burn. En-route to hospital apply a gel-based dressing.

After cooling the burns, *keep the patient warm.* This seems like a contradiction, because it is. The trick is to put out the fire without making the patient hypothermic. Remember, people with large burned areas have lost their primary mechanism for thermoregulation. Keep the patient covered and move him or her into the ambulance as soon as possible to minimise hypothermic stress.

Don't forget other injuries. If the patient is at risk for spinal trauma from a fall or explosion, address this injury the same way you would in any other trauma patient. The same is true for gross bleeding and other traumatic injuries. Burns can also exacerbate a patient's underlying medical conditions, such as chronic obstructive pulmonary disease, asthma, and cardiac conditions. Follow the same priorities for these emergencies as you would for any other patient.

Airway Management

Many burn patients will ultimately require intubation, even though they were talking to you and in no distress. Although it is obviously preferable to have such patients intubated in a controlled environment with a full complement of anaesthesia agents, a few patients will absolutely require an emergency advanced airway in the prehospital setting. Burn patients fall into four general categories for airway management.

1. **The patient with an acutely decompensating airway who requires prehospital intubation.** This group includes burn patients who are in cardiac or respiratory arrest and conscious patients whose airways are swelling before your eyes. In these chaotic and difficult situations, you need to plan for the possibility that you cannot intubate. Supraglottic swelling or complete obstruction can occur in some burn scenarios. Surgical airways or rescue devices may be necessary if intubation is not possible and bag-valve-mask ventilation fails.

2. **The patient with a deteriorating airway from burns and toxic inhalations who might require intubation.** It is obviously better for the patient to defer treatment of this airway problem to hospital teams with anaesthesia, surgery, specialised equipment, and a fully stocked pharmacy. Patients will often be conscious and may become combative with attempts to place them supine, let alone intubate them. Attempt to intubate only if left with no other choice. If the patient's airway continues to swell and intubation will become impossible if you wait for arrival at the hospital, you have little choice but to attempt intubation.

   Serious consideration should be made toward performing rapid-sequence intubation if you have been trained in this procedure, carry the appropriate medications, and have authorisation. The procedure for rapid-sequence intubation is discussed in Chapter 11. It is also advised that the "most experienced" intubator perform this procedure because the swelling can make for a difficult intubation.

   The choice of endotracheal (ET) tube may present another conundrum. It would obviously be beneficial to use the largest tube possible. Sometimes the ET tube will clog with soot from the patient's airway, causing complete occlusion. At the same time, a smaller than usual ET tube may be necessary owing to airway oedema. Select the largest ET tube that will not cause additional trauma during insertion. Never cut the ET tube down to make it shorter. Oedema of the face can actually cause ET tube dislodgement on postburn day 2 or 3.

3. **The patient whose airway is currently patent but who has a history consistent with risk factors for eventual airway compromise.** Cool, humidified oxygen from a high-output nebuliser is appropriate. The patient will probably *not* require acute interventions at the scene, but make sure you report the patient's history to hospital personnel. Many patients will ultimately undergo elective intubation.

4. **The patient with no signs of or risk factors for airway compromise who is in no distress.** It is reasonable to provide supplemental oxygen to burn patients, even if they are not in distress. It is safe to oxygenate until you are comfortable with the situation surrounding the burn and have completed a full assessment.

Fluid Resuscitation

An IV line may be inserted to administer fluids and/or pain medications. A 14 gauge IV cannula should be inserted as early as possible in any patient who has been severely burned. Do not delay transport to do so, but try to get a large-bore IV cannula into a large vein, and give normal saline. You can use the burned extremity for the IV site if you cannot find another site—an IV line in a burned upper extremity is still preferable to an IV line in a lower extremity.

Approximate the amount of fluid the burned patient will need by using the Parkland formula, which states that *during the first 24 hours,* the burned patient will need:

> 4 ml × body weight (in kg) × percentage of body surface burned

Half of that amount needs to be given during the first 8 hours. For example, if a 70-kg man has sustained burns to 30% of his body, his fluid needs during the first 24 hours will be:

> 4 ml × 70 kg × 30 = 8,400 ml

Half of the 8,400 ml—that is, 4,200 ml—should be administered during the first 8 hours.

As aggressive as the Parkland formula may seem, current trends actually lean toward delivering *more* fluid than the Parkland formula indicates (**Table 20-2** ▾). Of course, you do not need to attempt to deliver the entire initial amount in the prehospital environment. Most seriously burned patients will need central venous access, and IV lines placed in the prehospital setting will most often be lost as peripheral swelling begins.

At the Scene

The adequacy of resuscitation is based on monitoring the vital signs, the patient's mental state, and the urine output.

Pain Management

With any patient with burns, you should provide aggressive pain management. Assess the patient's pain before administering any analgesia. Reassessment should be completed using the same scale (for example, 1 to 10) every 5 minutes.

Burn patients may require higher than usual doses of pain medications to achieve relief. Their metabolism rates are accelerated, which creates the need for higher than normal doses of analgesics. Consult your clinical guidelines or contact the receiving hospital for guidance in administering analgesics.

Management of Superficial Burns

Although superficial burns can be very painful, they rarely pose a threat to life unless they involve nearly the entire surface of the body. If you reach a patient with superficial burns within the first hour after the injury occurred, immerse the burned area in cool water or apply cold compresses to the burn. Burned hands or feet may be soaked directly in cool water; and towels soaked in cold water may be applied to burns of the face or trunk.

The objectives of this exercise are twofold: stop the burning process and relieve pain. Commercial products are available that meet both objectives (**Figure 20-16** ▶). However you cool the burn, take care not to cool the whole body—don't let the patient become chilled. A dry sheet or blanket applied over the wet dressings will help prevent systemic heat loss.

Table 20-2	Parkland Formula Chart									
% Burn	**10 kg**	**20 kg**	**30 kg**	**40 kg**	**50 kg**	**60 kg**	**70 kg**	**80 kg**	**90 kg**	**100 kg**
10	25	50	75	100	125	150	175	200	225	250
20	50	100	150	200	250	300	350	400	450	500
30	75	150	225	300	375	450	525	600	675	750
40	100	200	300	400	500	600	700	800	900	1,000
50	125	250	375	500	625	750	875	1,000	1,125	1,250
60	150	300	450	600	750	900	1,050	1,200	1,350	1,500
70	175	350	525	700	875	1,050	1,225	1,400	1,575	1,750
80	200	400	600	800	1,000	1,200	1,400	1,600	1,800	2,000
90	225	450	675	900	1,125	1,350	1,575	1,800	2,025	2,250
20 ml/kg	200	400	600	800	1,000	1,200	1,400	1,600	1,800	2,000

This table represents the fluid recommended in the *first hour* (⅛ of the initial 8-hour dose) by the Parkland formula. The final row represents the amount of a 20-ml/kg bolus.

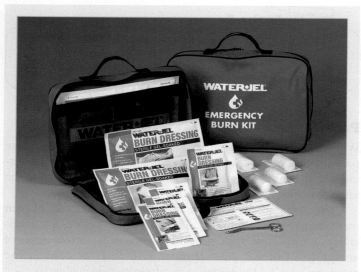

Figure 20-16 Sample burn dressing (Water-Jel).

Do not use salves, ointments, creams, sprays, or any similar non water soluble materials on any type of burn. They will just have to be scrubbed off in the A&E department or burns unit, causing the patient further pain. Never apply ice to burns because it can exacerbate the tissue injury.

No further treatment should be necessary at the scene for an uncomplicated, superficial burn. Simply transport the patient in a comfortable position to the hospital.

Management of Partial-Thickness Burns

Treatment of partial-thickness burns in the prehospital environment is similar to that of superficial burns. Cooling the burned area with water or application of wet or gel-based dressings within the first hour can diminish oedema and provide significant pain relief. Burned extremities should be elevated to minimise oedema formation.

Do not attempt to rupture blisters over the burn; they initially act as a physiological burn dressing. Establish IV fluids with normal saline as dictated by local guidelines. Pain in partial-thickness burns may be severe, so complete a pain assessment and administer pain medication as allowed by your guidelines.

Management of Full-Thickness Burns

Although full-thickness burns may not cause pain, most patients will have varying degrees of burns within the affected region of injury. For this reason, a pain assessment should be completed and pain medication should be administered as described earlier. Gel-based dressings can be applied to up to 12.5% of the body. Special care can be applied to face and hands with specific dressings. Ensure the patient is sufficiently "secondarily" wrapped to ensure he or she is not overcooled.

At the Scene

Pain medication is best given via the IV route. Owing to changes in fluid volume and tissue blood flow, absorption of any intramuscular or subcutaneous drug is unpredictable. Accurately measure and assess the patient's pain, and continuously monitor response to pain medication.

You are the Paramedic Part 3

As you are en route to the appropriate hospital, your partner works with the local police service in an attempt to contact the patient's parents. One relative is found—the patient's grandmother, who consents to Pamela's treatment and transport and adds that she is a normally healthy child with no medications or allergies. You address the patient's pain by providing morphine, elevate her arm with pillows, cover her with a blanket, and place her in a comfortable position. You also reassess the affected extremity for the presence of pulse and motor and sensory functions throughout transport.

Reassessment	Recording Time: 10 Minutes
Level of consciousness	Alert, with a Glasgow Coma Scale score of 15
Skin	Warm, pink, and dry
Pulse	Radial pulse, 118 beats/min, strong and regular
Blood pressure	116 by palpation
Respirations	28 to 36 breaths/min
SpO2	100%
Blood glucose	5.0 mmol/l
ECG	Sinus tachycardia

6. What is appropriate fluid resuscitation for a paediatric patient?
7. Given the nature of burns, what is another important consideration regarding burn care?

Management of Chemical Burns

Speed is essential when treating chemical burns. Begin flushing the exposed area of the patient's body immediately with copious quantities of water **Figure 20-17 ▶**. If the patient is in or near the home, the shower is ideal. In an industrial setting, use the decontamination shower. While flushing, rapidly remove the patient's clothing, especially shoes and socks that may have become contaminated with the offending agent, taking care not to get any of the hazardous chemicals on your own clothing or skin.

Do not waste time looking for specific antidotes; copious flushing with water is more effective and more immediately available **Figure 20-18 ▶**. Flushing is preferable for 30 minutes before moving the patient; for chemical burns caused by strong alkalis (such as oven and drain cleaners), 1 to 2 *hours* of flushing has been recommended. Paramedics must weigh the realities of flushing on the scene for long periods against the benefits of transport and their ability to continue flushing en route. After flushing, limit hypothermia by keeping the patient covered and warm.

Special Cases of Chemical Burns

If you do not know the identity of the chemical that caused the burn, assume it is *not* a special case, and flush the burn wound with copious water as described.

In alkali burns caused by dry lime, combination with water will produce a highly corrosive substance. For that reason, when a patient has been in contact with dry lime, *first* remove the patient's clothing and *brush* as much lime as you can from the skin (you need to wear gloves!). *Then* start flushing copiously with a garden hose or shower. Your intention is to completely overwhelm any damaging chemical reaction with a deluge of water.

Sodium metals produce considerable heat when mixed with water and may explode. Cover this type of burn with oil, which will stop the reaction by preventing the sodium from coming in contact with the atmosphere.

Hydrofluoric (HF) acid is used in drain cleaners in the home and for etching glass and plastic in industrial settings. HF acid burns that exceed 3% to 5% of the TBSA can be fatal. The patient will complain bitterly of pain (caused by the HF acid sucking calcium out of the body), and the pain will not improve even with continuous flushing—a sign that the process of tissue destruction is ongoing. Calcium chloride (CaCl) jelly may be available in an industrial setting that uses HF acid; this jelly is placed on small-area HF acid burns (small burns from splashing or pinholes in gloves) to help reduce continued pain and injury.

Hot tar burns are, strictly speaking, thermal burns, not chemical burns, although they tend to be classified with chemical burns. The most important step in the prehospital phase is to immerse the affected area in cold water to dissipate the heat from the tar and speed up the hardening process. Once the tar has cooled, it will not do further damage, and there is no need to try to remove it.

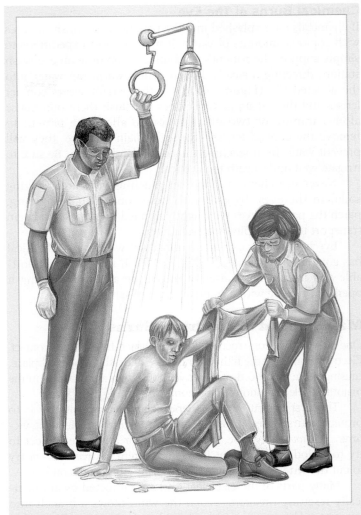

Figure 20-17 Flush the burned area with large amounts of tepid water.

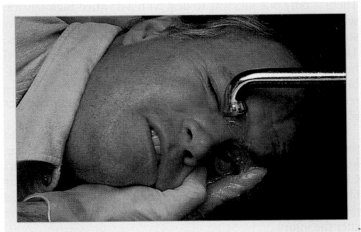

Figure 20-18 Flood the affected eye with a gentle stream of water. Hold the eyelids open—a challenging task because the patient's reflex is to keep the eye shut. Take care to prevent the chemical from getting into the other eye during the flushing.

Chemical Burns of the Eye

If chemicals have splashed into the patient's eyes, flush the eyes with copious amounts of water. It may be most expeditious to simply support the patient's head under a tap or at an eye-wash station, directing a steady stream of lukewarm tap water into the affected eye (Figure 20-18). If the patient wears contact lenses and the stream of water does not flush them out, pause after a minute or two of irrigation to allow the patient to remove the contact lenses—if they remain in place, they will prevent water from reaching the cornea underneath. Be sure to irrigate well underneath the eyelids.

Never use chemical antidotes (such as vinegar or baking soda) in the eyes. Irrigate with water only. After irrigating, patch the patient's eyes with lightly applied dressings and begin transport to the hospital for evaluation.

Eye irrigation is extremely important whenever a chemical has gone into the eye Figure 20-19 ▶. It may be uncomfortable and inefficient to attempt to irrigate an eye by prying it open and rinsing with a standard normal saline IV set.

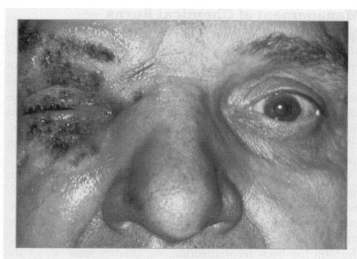

Figure 20-19 The eyes are particularly vulnerable to chemical burns.

Management of Electrical Burns

One of every five construction deaths is caused by electrical contact. Electrical contact is the fifth leading cause of death in the workplace, causing more than 40 deaths per year. Children are involved in the majority of electrocutions in the home Figure 20-20 ▶.

The first priority at the scene of an electrical injury is to protect yourself and bystanders from becoming the next victims. Do *not* use a rope, wooden pole, or any other object to try to dislodge the patient from the current source. Do *not* try to cut the wire. Do *not* go anywhere near a high-tension line.

Many parts of the electrical grid are protected by automatically resetting breakers. When the wind blows a branch into wires or a cheeky squirrel bridges the gap between two wires, it is desirable to have the breaker reset after a few moments to avoid power outages. As a consequence, a downed wire that "looks dead" can jump back to life, perhaps several times. There is only one safe way to deal with a downed high-tension wire: Call the local electric board. Wait until a qualified person has shut off the power before you approach the patient. This can be a traumatic event for paramedics, who will feel helpless waiting for the power to be shut down while a possibly critical patient lies on the ground nearby. But remember—*rescuers die in these situations.* You can help the greatest number of people by being cautious and safe in this circumstance.

Once the electric hazard has been neutralised, proceed to the ABCs. Open the airway using the jaw-thrust manoeuvre, keeping in mind the possibility of cervical spine injury. Start CPR as indicated, and attach the monitor to identify ventricular fibrillation. If the patient is not in cardiac arrest, dysrhythmias remain a risk, and cardiac monitoring is indicated for 24 hours after the injury.

Make careful note of the patient's state of consciousness, and record his or her vital signs. Try to determine the path the current has taken through the body by looking for entrance and exit wounds and by carefully palpating the skin and soft

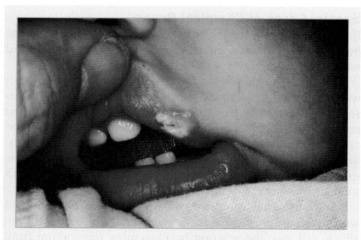

Figure 20-20 Children often sustain electrical burns.

tissues. When deep tissues have been seriously damaged by heat, the surrounding muscle may swell and become rock-hard. Thus, a rigid abdomen or rigid extremity may indicate a serious internal injury. Be alert for fractures or dislocations, and check the distal pulses in all four extremities.

Electrical burns may produce devastating internal injuries with little external evidence. The degree of tissue injury is related to the resistance of the body tissues, the intensity of current that passes through the victim, and the duration of exposure.

When a person comes in contact with an electrical source, the amount of current delivered to the inside of the body depends to some extent on the resistance of the skin. Wet, thin, clean skin offers less resistance than dry, thick, dirty skin; thus a moist inner surface of the forearm will have much less resistance than a dry, callused palm.

As electric current travels from the contact site into the body, it is converted to heat, which follows the current flow—usually along blood vessels and nerves—causing extensive damage to the tissues in its path. The greater the current flow, the greater the heat generated. When the voltage is low (< 1,000 volts, as in household sources), current follows the path of least resistance, generally along blood vessels, nerves, and muscles. When the voltage is high (as from high-tension lines), current takes the shortest path.

Alternating current is considerably more dangerous than direct current because the alternations cause repetitive muscle contractions, which may "freeze" the victim to the conductor until the current source is turned off. Furthermore, alternating current is more likely than direct current to induce ventricular fibrillation. The direction of current flow is also significant. Current moving from one hand to the other is particularly dangerous because current may then flow across the heart; a current of only 0.1 amp to the heart can provoke ventricular fibrillation.

If the patient has life-threatening injuries, begin related care and prepare to transport the patient as soon as practical. Generally, aside from the fluid therapy for the care of a burn injury, no specific pharmacological interventions are indicated, other than the normal medications used to manage a cardiac dysrhythmia or extreme pain. Early oxygen therapy is helpful, as is managing the patient for impending shock. Transport decisions should be made early and take into consideration the regional resources for the care of a patient with a severe (electrical) burn. Contact ambulance control for advice in making a transport decision or regarding the need to use helicopter evacuation directly to the burn centre. The patients will be very anxious and scared, so be sure to talk with them calmly and explain what you are doing and how you plan to obtain the best care for them.

Management of Lightning-Related Injuries

When you reach the scene of a lightning strike, all the usual priorities apply, but there are two special considerations to keep in mind.

First, if the electrical storm is still going on, your first priority is to get any patients and rescuers to a safe place, preferably indoors, or at least inside the ambulance. Lightning **can** strike twice in the same place. There is, however, no hazard in touching the victim of a lightning strike—contrary to what your grandmother may have told you, electricity does not remain within the body of a person who has been hit by lightning.

Second, be aware that a lightning strike is apt to injure more than one person. Therefore, the first thing you need to do on arrival at the scene—before you leave the safety of the ambulance—is a rapid assessment of the entire scene to determine the number of patients.

Notes from Nancy

In a lightning strike with multiple victims, priority goes to the victims who are not breathing.

Carry out the initial assessment as usual, and start CPR when necessary. When establishing an airway, bear in mind the possibility of cervical spine injury, and do not hyperextend the neck; use the jaw-thrust manoeuvre.

Patients with cardiac arrest caused by a lightning strike deserve aggressive, continuing CPR. The chances of a successful resuscitation in such a case are good, even when the patient appears beyond help initially and even when there is a long delay in the return of spontaneous breathing. Minimise the interruption in compressions, and push hard and fast with full chest recoil!

Treatment of lightning injuries is similar to that of injuries sustained from high-voltage lines:

- Make sure the scene is safe. Move the victim to a safer location if necessary.
- Priority for treatment goes to patients who are not breathing.
- Establish an airway, with cervical spine precautions. Perform CPR as needed.
- Administer supplemental oxygen.
- Monitor cardiac rhythm.
- Insert a large-bore IV cannula and run in normal saline solution wide open to keep the kidneys flushed out.
- Cover any surface burns with dry, sterile dressings.
- Splint fractures.
- If the patient has fallen, immobilise the cervical spine.

Management of Radiation Burns

Patients with radiation burns may be contaminated with radioactive material, so they should be decontaminated before transport. The majority of contaminants can be removed by simply disrobing the patient.

Irrigate open wounds. Washing should be gentle to avoid further damage to the skin, which could result in additional internal radiation absorption. The head and scalp should be irrigated the same way. The A&E department should be notified as soon as practical if you are transporting a potentially contaminated patient. In contrast with other types of contamination, radioactive particulate matter probably poses a relatively small risk to the rescuer. Consider providing basic care to the patient before decontamination if you are wearing protective clothing.

Radiation injury follows the "inverse square law": Exposure drops exponentially as distance is increased. Increasing your (and your patient's) distance from the source by even a few metres may dramatically decrease your exposure, so it is important to identify the radioactive source and the length of the patient's exposure to it. You must try to limit your duration of exposure, increase your distance from the source, and attempt to place shielding between yourself and sources of gamma radiation.

With contact radiation burns, decontaminate the wound as if it were a chemical burn to remove any radioactive particulate matter. You may then treat it as a burn.

Notes from Nancy

Don't give up quickly on a patient in cardiac arrest due to a lightning strike.

Many radioactive isotopes are used in medicine and industry, some of which can be absorbed or have their toxic effects blunted by another substance. Like their radioactive effects, the toxic effects of these isotopes vary. Antidotes may help bind an isotope, enhance its elimination from the body, or reduce the toxic effects on other organs. Such antidotal therapy should be considered only under the guidance of a knowledgeable doctor or public health agency.

Management of Burns in Paediatric Patients

Escaping from a fire can be difficult for children. More than half of the fire-related deaths and injuries involve preschool children. Research suggests that young children are not awakened as effectively by smoke detectors, and they are often disorientated immediately after waking. The "reliable waking rate" in children younger than 15 years may be as low as 6%. Young children are also more likely to sustain severe scald injuries. Children's thin skin and delicate respiratory structures are more easily damaged by thermal insults than are those of older children and adults.

In children, fluid resuscitation may be more challenging because of their increased body surface/weight ratio. As a consequence, children may require more fluid per kilogram than adults. You may start with the Parkland formula in children. Because of poor glycogen stores, children may require glucose-containing solutions earlier than adults. Blood glucose monitoring should be routinely performed in seriously ill children.

Burns may raise the suspicion of abuse. Pay careful attention to the mechanism of injury, and pass this information onto the hospital staff.

Management of Burns in Elderly Patients

Approximately 120 older adults die of fire-related causes each year, making it the sixth leading cause of death in this population. Some 13% of older adults smoke, and smoking is the leading cause of fires that lead to death of elderly people. Burns from fires caused by smoking while wearing supplemental oxygen are the leading sentinel event in home care. Cooking fires represent another distinct hazard to elderly people, who may be less able to smell a gas leak or a fire in the kitchen. Relatively small fires can produce toxic fumes before detection or suppression devices are activated.

Elderly patients may also have poor glycogen stores, so their blood glucose levels should be checked to assess for hypoglycaemia. Cardiac monitoring should, of course, be implemented. Although fluid resuscitation is important, pulmonary oedema is more likely to develop in older patients. Routinely assess lung sounds.

■ Transfer to a Burn Specialty Centre

Patients with the following injuries should ideally be transferred to a burn specialty centre. If this is not possible due to time or distance etc., then the patient should be taken to the nearest A&E department to be stabilised before onward transfer to the special burns unit.

- Partial-thickness burns of more than 10% of the body surface area
- Burns that involve the face, hands, feet, genitalia, perineum, or major joints

You are the Paramedic Part 4

As you arrive at hospital, the patient seems much more comfortable. She is no longer crying as vigorously and occasionally gives you a glimpse of a smile. The grandmother meets you at the hospital and informs you that Pamela's mother is nowhere to be found. You provide a report including the history of events (including the home situation) to the A&E department staff.

Reassessment	Recording Time: 20 Minutes
Level of consciousness	Alert, with a Glasgow Coma Scale score of 15
Skin	Warm, pink, and dry
Pulse	Radial pulse, 98 beats/min, strong and regular
Blood pressure	108/58 mm Hg
Respirations	24 breaths/min
SpO_2	100%
Temperature	37°C
ECG	Normal sinus rhythm

8. What is burn shock, and how does it relate to the prehospital setting?
9. What other considerations must be made when dealing with a paediatric burn patient?

- Full-thickness burns of more than 5% in any age group
- Electrical burns, including lightning
- Chemical burns
- Inhalation burns
- Burn injuries in conjunction with preexisting medical conditions that could complicate management, prolong recovery, or affect mortality
- Burns and concomitant trauma in which the burn injury poses the greatest risk of morbidity or mortality
- Burn injury that requires special social, emotional, or long-term rehabilitation
- Circumferential burns of the limbs or chest
- Burns at the extremes of age (children and the elderly)
  Burn severity classifications are accepted as:
- **Minor burns**
  - Superficial—body surface area less than 50% (such as sunburns)
  - Partial thickness—body surface area less than 15%
  - Full thickness—body surface area less than 2%
- **Moderate burns**
  - Superficial—body surface area greater than 50%
  - Partial thickness—body surface area less than 30%
  - Full thickness—body surface area less than 10%
- **Critical burns**
  - Partial thickness—body surface area greater than 30%
  - Full thickness—body surface area greater than 10%
  - Inhalation injury
  - Partial- or full-thickness burns involving hands, feet, joints, face, or genitalia

All patients with critical burns should be transported to a specialty burn centre.

Consequences of Burns

The Patient

Serious burn injuries are devastating events that leave patients with long-term physical and psychological challenges. People with major injuries average about 1 day of inpatient treatment for each 1% of the TBSA burned. Extensive rehabilitation may also be necessary to regain function. Survivors of serious burns are left with a host of long-term consequences, including problems with thermoregulation, motor function, and sensory function. Although tremendous improvements in the care of critical burn patients have made long-term survival possible for many who would have died of their injuries a decade ago, large surface area burns remain a critical care challenge on par with other forms of severe multi-system trauma.

The Paramedic

Caring for patients with severe burn emergencies can be one of the most horrifying tasks undertaken by paramedics. Fire scenes are chaotic and dangerous. Patients are often in severe pain. The smell of burned hair and flesh permeates your clothes and equipment. Sheets of tissue may peel off the patient when you perform simple tasks like attempting to take vital signs or moving the patient. Despite the traumatic circumstances, with the proper training and the right mix of confidence and courage, you can make a tremendous impact in the treatment and overall survival of burn patients.

You are the Paramedic Summary

1. What are your patient care priorities?

Your patient care priorities, after ensuring the safety of the scene, are the ABCs. For fire victims, issues of maintaining a patent airway with good ventilation and oxygenation can present a particular challenge for prehospital providers.

2. What are patient care concerns when dealing with victims of a structure fire?

Superheated gases and by-products of combustion can cause airway irritation and severe oedema. It is essential to act quickly if you believe your patient has inhalation burns—time is of the essence in obtaining and maintaining a patent airway. The presence of soot or burns around the nose or mouth, singed facial hair, wheezing, and stridor are ominous signs. Be prepared to provide advanced airway management.

3. Why is pulse oximetry unreliable in these circumstances?

By-products of incomplete combustion include noxious gases such as CO, formaldehyde, sulphur dioxide, nitrogen dioxide, hydrogen sulphide, cyanide, and particulates. Inhalation of these gases (particularly CO) can be deadly because haemoglobin's affinity for CO is roughly 240 times greater than its affinity for oxygen. The excess CO causes severe tissue hypoxia despite the possibility of acceptable or relatively normal readings on the pulse oximeter.

4. Are your transport considerations affected by the location of her burn?

Yes. This child should be taken to a burn centre because her right hand is burned. Accepted criteria for transport to a burn centre include partial-thickness burns on greater than 10% of the TBSA; any full-thickness burns; burns involving the hands, feet, face, major joints, or groin; burns involving the airway; circumferential burns (especially involving the chest or neck); electrical burns (including lightning and high-voltage electricity injuries); chemical burns; underlying medical conditions and/or traumatic injuries that could be exacerbated; or the lack of facilities necessary for treating burn patients appropriately.

5. What are common complications of burns?

Depending on the area affected (usually when an area greater than 10% of the TBSA is involved) and the thickness of the burn, patients may experience difficulties with thermoregulation. For this reason, you should take steps to preserve body temperature.

6. What is appropriate fluid resuscitation for a paediatric patient?

The Parkland formula provides guidelines for fluid resuscitation of burn patients. During the first 24 hours, the burn patient will receive 4 ml × body weight (in kilograms) × percentage of body surface burned. Half of that amount needs to be given during the first 8 hours. However, paediatric patients may need more fluids than their adult counterparts, so be prepared to make adjustments accordingly.

7. Given the nature of burns, what is another important consideration regarding burn care?

Beyond estimating the extent of the burn and cooling and covering the area, be aware that burns are extremely painful. As health care professionals, we must be prepared to provide appropriate pain management. Morphine sulphate is highly effective with repeated doses as needed.

8. What is burn shock, and how does it relate to the prehospital setting?

Burn shock occurs because of fluid loss through the damaged skin and a series of volume shifts within the body. Capillaries become leaky, so intravascular fluid oozes out of the circulation and into the interstitial spaces. Meanwhile, cells of normal tissues take in increased amounts of salt and water from the fluid around them. This process occurs during a 6- to 8-hour period. Therefore, if a burned patient is in shock in the prehospital phase, look for another injury as the source of shock. In particular, make sure that you auscultate lung sounds before administration of fluid therapy.

9. What other considerations must be made when dealing with a paediatric burn patient?

Monitor the patient's blood glucose level, and be prepared to administer glucose as needed. Also, when dealing with minors or older people, be aware of the potential for abuse. It is your responsibility to report suspected abuse or neglect to the proper authorities.

Prep Kit

Ready for Review

- Although you probably won't see moderate or severe burns on a daily basis, you will encounter some serious burn injuries during your career.
- The skin has four functions:
  - Protects the underlying tissue from injury and exposure
  - Regulates temperature
  - Prevents excessive loss of water from the body
  - Acts as a sense organ
- Significant damage to the skin may make the body vulnerable to bacterial invasion, temperature instability, and major disturbances of fluid balance.
- Burns are diffuse soft-tissue injuries created from destructive energy transferred via radiation, thermal, or electrical energy.
- The many types of burns, coupled with the many possible presentations of burn patients, can challenge your assessment skills. Address a burned patient in a consistent, efficient, and systematic manner so you don't develop tunnel vision for the major burn trauma and miss other occult injuries that could affect the patient's outcome.
- Although you will be most heavily involved in the first phase of burn care, it is important to appreciate the magnitude of care that a patient with a severe or even moderate burn must receive. Early actions of paramedics may dramatically affect the patient's long-term outcome.
- Serious burn injuries are devastating events that leave patients with long-term physical and psychological challenges.

Vital Vocabulary

acute radiation syndrome The clinical course that usually begins within hours of exposure to a radiation source. Symptoms include nausea, vomiting, diarrhoea, fatigue, fever, and headache. The long-term symptoms are dose-related and are haematopoietic and gastrointestinal.

adipose tissue Fat tissue.

anaerobic metabolism The metabolism that takes place in the absence of oxygen; the principal product is lactic acid.

burn shock The shock or hypoperfusion caused by a burn injury and the tremendous loss of fluids.

circumferential burns A burn that encircles a particular area whose subsequent swelling may cause additional problems.

collagen A protein that gives tensile strength to the connective tissues of the body.

comedo A noninflammatory acne lesion.

contact burn A burn produced by touching a hot object.

cutaneous Pertaining to the skin.

dermis The inner layer of skin containing hair follicle roots, glands, blood vessels, and nerves.

desquamation The continuous shedding of the dead cells on the surface of the skin.

elastin A protein that gives the skin its elasticity.

epidermis The outermost layer of the skin.

escharotomy A surgical cut through the eschar or leathery covering of a burn injury to allow for swelling and minimise the potential for development of compartment syndrome in a circumferentially burned limb or the thorax.

flame burn A thermal burn caused by flames touching the skin.

flash burn An electrothermal injury caused by arcing of electric current.

full-thickness burn A burn that extends through the epidermis and dermis into the subcutaneous tissues beneath; previously called a third-degree burn.

homeostasis A tendency to constancy or stability in the body's internal environment.

integument The skin.

Lund and Browder chart A detailed version of the rule of nines chart that takes into consideration the changes in body surface area brought on by growth.

melanin The pigment that gives skin its colour.

mucopolysaccharide gel One of the complex materials found, along with the collagen fibres and elastin fibres, in the dermis of the skin.

Parkland formula A formula that recommends giving 4 ml of normal saline for each kilogram of body weight, multiplied by the percentage of body surface area burned; sometimes used to calculate fluid needs during lengthy transport times.

partial-thickness burn A burn that involves the epidermis and part of the dermis, characterised by pain and blistering; previously called a second-degree burn.

rule of nines A system that assigns percentages to sections of the body, allowing calculation of the amount of skin surface involved in the burn area.

rule of palm A system that estimates total body surface area burned by comparing the affected area with the size of the patient's palm, which is roughly equal to 1% of the patient's total body surface area.

scald burn A burn produced by hot liquids.

sebaceous gland A gland located in the dermis that secretes sebum.

sebum An oily substance secreted by sebaceous glands.

steam burn A burn that has been caused by direct exposure to hot steam exhaust, as from a broken pipe.

subcutaneous layer Beneath the skin.

superficial burn A burn involving only the epidermis, producing very red, painful skin; previously called a first-degree burn.

supraglottic Located above the glottic opening, as in the upper airway structures.

thermal burn An injury caused by radiation or direct contact with a heat source on the skin.

thermoregulation The ability of the body to maintain temperature through a combination of heat gain by metabolic processes and muscular movement and heat loss through respiration, evaporation, conduction, convection, and perspiration.

total body surface area (TBSA) Used in the calculation of a burn injury to determine the percentage of the surface of the patient's body that has been injured. This is commonly estimated by using the rule of palm or the rule of nines.

zone of coagulation The reddened area surrounding the leathery and sometimes charred tissue that has sustained a full-thickness burn.

zone of hyperemia In a thermal burn, the area that is least affected by the burn injury.

zone of stasis The peripheral area surrounding the zone of coagulation that has decreased blood flow and inflammation. This area can undergo necrosis within 24 to 48 hours after the injury, particularly if perfusion is compromised due to burn shock.

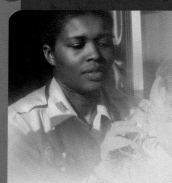

Assessment in Action

You arrive on scene to find an 81-year-old woman outside being attended to by fire service. The fire fighters report that the patient was found on the floor in the kitchen by her grandson. The kitchen was full of smoke, and the grandson carried her outside. The patient is conscious but combative and asking repetitive questions. You and your colleague transfer the patient to the ambulance, where you begin your assessment. The patient's respirations are 18 breaths/min, pulse oximeter is 95% on room air, her blood pressure is 150/90 mm Hg, and she has a heart rate of 110 beats/min. You notice a significant amount of soot around the patient's face, especially in the nostrils, mouth, and oral airway. The patient remains conscious but does not recognise her family and continues to ask repetitive questions. You place the patient on high flow oxygen, cannulate her, and begin your transport to the local burn centre, which is approximately 20 minutes away.

1. **What type of burn is described in this scenario?**
   A. Thermal burn
   B. Scald burn
   C. Contact burn
   D. Airway burn

2. **Anyone exposed to smoke from a fire may have _____ burns.**
   A. thermal
   B. scald
   C. contact
   D. radiation

3. **_____ damage is more often associated with the inhalation of superheated gases.**
   A. Upper airway
   B. Lower airway
   C. Upper and lower airway
   D. None of these

4. **In the lower airway, _____ and _____ may result from heat inhalation.**
   A. laryngospasm, pulmonary damage
   B. pulmonary damage, bronchospasm
   C. laryngospasm, bronchospasm
   D. mild, severe damage

5. **True or false? If your patient greets you with a hoarse voice and a chief complaint of "trouble breathing", your general impression should be that there is probably nothing wrong with this patient.**
   A. True
   B. False

6. **Combative patients should be considered:**
   A. as having head trauma.
   B. intoxicated.
   C. diabetic.
   D. hypoxic.

7. **_____ can develop with alarming speed in burn patients, especially in infants and children.**
   A. Laryngeal oedema
   B. A pulmonary injury
   C. An inhalation burn
   D. Bronchial oedema

8. **After listening to lung sounds, you hear _____. This may be a sign of impending upper airway compromise.**
   A. wheezing
   B. stridor
   C. rhonchi
   D. rales

9. **Burn patients fall into several general categories for airway management. They include:**
   A. the patient with the acutely decompensating airway who requires prehospital intubation.
   B. the patient with the deteriorating airway from burns and toxic inhalations.
   C. the patient with no signs of or risk factors for airway compromise who is in no distress.
   D. all of the above.

10. **Approximately _____ older adults die of fire-related causes each year, making it the sixth leading cause of death in this population group.**
    A. 120
    B. 10
    C. 20
    D. 110

Challenging Questions

It is 14:00 hours and you are sent to a house. On arrival, you hear the members of the fire service calling you, stating they have a victim. The patient was inside the burning house and was standing on the roof when the fire fighters arrived. Fire fighters had the patient drop and roll. The patient is still smouldering and is in a great deal of pain. You call for a medical helicopter and transfer the patient to the landing zone. You estimate that the burn involves 30% of the TBSA.

11. **What is your treatment while you are driving to the landing zone?**

12. **How do you assess the TBSA burned?**

13. **How much fluid will this patient require?**

Points to Ponder

You and your crew are called to the scene of a fire at a block of flats in which two to three vehicles are involved. When you arrive, you find three other patients being treated by fire fighters for minor inhalation injuries. The patient in the worst condition seems to be a man in his mid 30s. He has dark, discoloured patches of skin on his chest, lower right arm, and lower back. He also has a circumferential burn on his left upper arm. His voice is slightly hoarse, and twice he coughs up dark-coloured sputum. However, he denies having difficulty breathing or having much pain. He is sitting up at the scene, watching all that is going on around him.

Why is this patient of particular concern? What must you make sure to do in treating this patient?

Issues: The Impact of Managing a Burn-Injured Patient, Mortality and Morbidity Based on Pathophysiology and Assessment Findings.

21 Head and Maxillofacial Injuries

Objectives

Cognitive

- Describe the incidence, morbidity, and mortality of facial injuries.
- Explain facial anatomy and relate physiology to facial injuries.
- Predict facial injuries based on mechanism of injury.
- Predict other injuries commonly associated with facial injuries based on mechanism of injury.
- Differentiate between the following types of facial injuries, highlighting the defining characteristics of each:
  - Eye
  - Ear
  - Nose
  - Throat
  - Mouth
- Integrate pathophysiological principles to the assessment of a patient with a facial injury.
- Differentiate between facial injuries based on the assessment and history.
- Formulate an initial impression for a patient with a facial injury based on the assessment findings.
- Develop a patient management plan for a patient with a facial injury based on the initial impression.
- Explain the pathophysiology of eye injuries.
- Relate assessment findings associated with eye injuries to pathophysiology.
- Integrate pathophysiological principles to the assessment of a patient with an eye injury.
- Formulate an initial impression for a patient with an eye injury based on the assessment findings.
- Develop a patient management plan for a patient with an eye injury based on the initial impression.
- Explain the pathophysiology of ear injuries.
- Relate assessment findings associated with ear injuries to pathophysiology.
- Integrate pathophysiological principles to the assessment of a patient with an ear injury.
- Formulate an initial impression for a patient with an ear injury based on the assessment findings.
- Develop a patient management plan for a patient with an ear injury based on the initial impression.
- Explain the pathophysiology of nose injuries.
- Relate assessment findings associated with nose injuries to pathophysiology.
- Integrate pathophysiological principles to the assessment of a patient with a nose injury.
- Formulate an initial impression for a patient with a nose injury based on the assessment findings.
- Develop a patient management plan for a patient with a nose injury based on the initial impression.
- Explain the pathophysiology of throat injuries.
- Relate assessment findings associated with throat injuries to pathophysiology.
- Integrate pathophysiological principles to the assessment of a patient with a throat injury.
- Formulate an initial impression for a patient with a throat injury based on the assessment findings.
- Develop a patient management plan for a patient with a throat injury based on the initial impression.
- Explain the pathophysiology of mouth injuries.
- Relate assessment findings associated with mouth injuries to pathophysiology.
- Integrate pathophysiological principles to the assessment of a patient with a mouth injury.
- Formulate an initial impression for a patient with a mouth injury based on the assessment findings.
- Develop a patient management plan for a patient with a mouth injury based on the initial impression.
- Explain anatomy and related physiology of the CNS to head injuries.
- Predict head injuries based on mechanism of injury.
- Distinguish between head injury and brain injury.
- Explain the pathophysiology of head/brain injuries.
- Explain the concept of increasing intracranial pressure (ICP).
- Explain the effect of increased and decreased carbon dioxide on ICP.
- Define and explain the process involved with each of the levels of increasing ICP.
- Relate assessment findings associated with head/brain injuries to the pathophysiological process.
- Classify head injuries (mild, moderate, severe) according to assessment findings.
- Identify the need for rapid intervention and transport of the patient with a head/brain injury.
- Describe and explain the general management of the head/brain injury patient, including pharmacological and non-pharmacological treatment.
- Analyse the relationship between carbon dioxide concentration in the blood and management of the airway in the head/brain injured patient.
- Explain the pathophysiology of diffuse axonal injury.
- Relate assessment findings associated with concussion, moderate and severe diffuse axonal injury to pathophysiology.
- Develop a management plan for a patient with a moderate and severe diffuse axonal injury.
- Explain the pathophysiology of skull fracture.
- Relate assessment findings associated with skull fracture to pathophysiology.
- Develop a management plan for a patient with a skull fracture.

- Relate assessment findings associated with cerebral contusion to pathophysiology.
- Develop a management plan for a patient with a cerebral contusion.
- Explain the pathophysiology of intracranial haemorrhage, including:
  - Extradural
  - Subdural
  - Intracerebral
  - Subarachnoid
- Relate assessment findings associated with intracranial haemorrhage to pathophysiology, including:
  - Extradural
  - Subdural
  - Intracerebral
  - Subarachnoid
- Develop a management plan for a patient with an intracranial haemorrhage, including:
  - Extradural
  - Subdural
  - Intracerebral
  - Subarachnoid

- Describe the various types of helmets and their purposes.
- Relate priorities of care to factors determining the need for helmet removal in various prehospital situations including sports related incidents.
- Develop a management plan for the removal of a helmet for a head injured patient.
- Integrate the pathophysiological principles to the assessment of a patient with head/brain injury.
- Differentiate between the types of head/brain injuries based on the assessment and history.
- Formulate an initial impression for a patient with a head/brain injury based on the assessment findings.
- Develop a patient management plan for a patient with a head/brain injury based on the initial impression.

Affective

None

Psychomotor

None

Head and Face Injuries

As a paramedic, you will encounter many patients with injuries to the head, neck, and face, ranging in severity from a broken nose to traumatic brain injury. The first part of this chapter provides a detailed review of the anatomy and physiology of the head and face. The second part discusses head and face injuries, including their respective signs and symptoms and appropriate prehospital care: maxillofacial injuries, eye and ear injuries, oral and dental injuries, injuries to the anterior part of the neck, and head and traumatic brain injuries.

The Skull and Facial Bones

The Scalp

The brain—the most important organ in the body—requires maximum protection from injury. The human body ensures that it receives this protection by housing the brain within several layers of soft and hard wrappings.

Starting from the outside and proceeding inward toward the brain, the first protective layer is the scalp, which consists of the following layers, listed in descending order:

- Skin, with hair
- Subcutaneous tissue, which contains major scalp veins that bleed profusely when lacerated.
- Galea aponeurotica, a tendon expansion that connects the frontal and occipital muscles of the cranium
- Loose connective tissue (alveolar tissue), which is easily stripped from the layer beneath in "scalping" injuries. The looseness of the alveolar layer also provides room for blood to accumulate after blunt trauma between the scalp and skull bone (subgaleal haematoma).
- Periosteum, the dense fibrous membrane covering the surface of bones

The Skull

At the top of the axial skeleton is the skull, which consists of 28 bones in three anatomical groups: the auditory ossicles, the cranium, and the face. The six auditory ossicles function in hearing and are located, three on each side of the head, deep

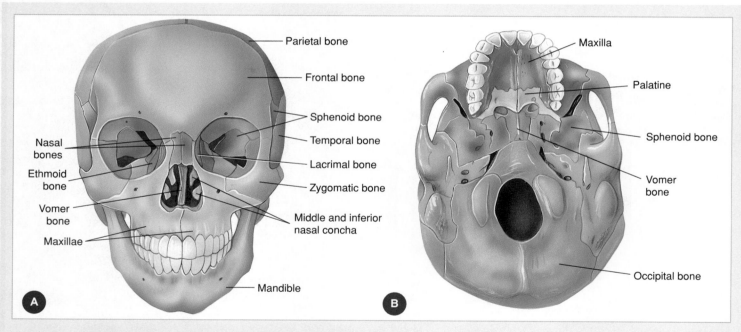

Figure 21-1 The skull and its components. **A.** Front view. **B.** Bottom view.

You are the Paramedic Part 1

You respond to the scene of a motorcycle collision. The patient, a young male, was thrown from his bike when it struck a tree; he was not wearing a helmet. The scene is safe, and two police officers are at the scene directing the flow of traffic. As you approach the patient, you note that he is lying in a supine position. His eyes are closed, and he is not moving.

1. What should be your initial concern about this patient?
2. How should you direct your initial care of this patient?

within the cavities of the temporal bone. The remaining 22 bones constitute the cranium and the face (Figure 21-1 ◄).

The cranial vault consists of eight bones that encase and protect the brain: the parietal, temporal, frontal, occipital, sphenoid, and ethmoid bones. The brain connects to the spinal cord through a large opening at the base of the skull called the foramen magnum.

The bones of the skull are connected at special joints known as sutures (Figure 21-2 ▼). The paired parietal bones join together at the sagittal suture. The parietal bones abut the frontal bone at the coronal suture. The occipital bone attaches to the parietal bones at the lambdoid suture. Fibrous tissues called fontanelles, which are soft in infants, link the sutures. The tissues felt through the fontanelles are layers of the scalp and thick membranes overlying the brain. Under normal conditions, the brain may not be felt through the fontanelles. By the time a child is 18 months old, the sutures should have solidified and the fontanelles closed.

At the base of each temporal bone is a cone-shaped section of bone known as the mastoid process. This area is an important site for attachment of various muscles. In addition, a portion of the mastoid process contains hollow mastoid air cells (Figure 21-3 ▼).

The Floor of the Cranial Vault

Viewed from above, the floor of the cranial vault is divided into three compartments: the anterior fossa, middle fossa, and posterior fossa (Figure 21-4 ►). The crista galli forms a prominent bony ridge in the centre of the anterior fossa and is the point of attachment of the meninges, the three layers of membranes that surround the brain and spinal cord. On the other side of the crista galli is the cribriform plate of the ethmoid bone, a horizontal bone that is perforated with numerous openings (foramina) allowing the passage of the olfactory nerve filaments from the nasal cavity. The olfactory nerves, the cranial nerves for smell, send projections through the foramina in the cribriform plate and into the nasal cavity, the chamber inside the nose that lies between the floor of the cranium and the roof of the mouth.

The Base of the Skull

When the mandible is removed, the base of the skull appears amazingly complex, with numerous foramina visible (Figure 21-5 ►). The occipital condyles on the occipital bone, which are the points of articulation between the skull and the vertebral column, lie on either side of the foramen magnum. Portions of the maxilla and the palatine bone, the irregularly shaped bone in the posterior nasal cavity, form the hard palate, which is the bony anterior part of the palate, or roof, of the mouth. The zygomatic arch is the bone that extends along the front of the skull below the orbit.

The Facial Bones

The frontal and ethmoid bones are part of the cranial vault and the face. The

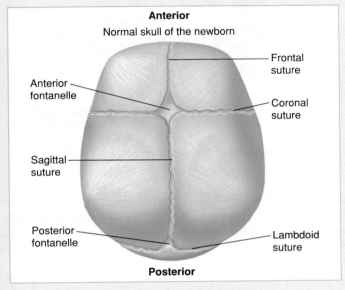

Anterior
Normal skull of the newborn

- Frontal suture
- Anterior fontanelle
- Coronal suture
- Sagittal suture
- Posterior fontanelle
- Lambdoid suture

Posterior

Figure 21-2 The sutures of the skull in a newborn.

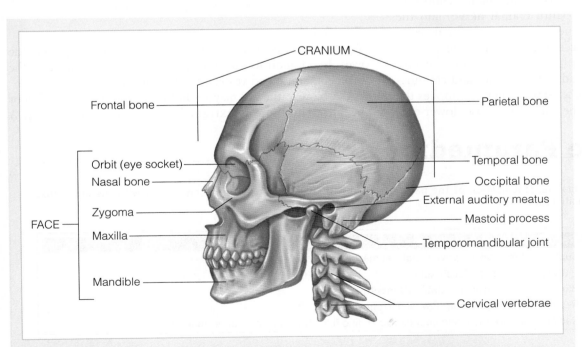

- CRANIUM
- Frontal bone
- Orbit (eye socket)
- Nasal bone
- Zygoma
- Maxilla
- Mandible
- FACE
- Parietal bone
- Temporal bone
- Occipital bone
- External auditory meatus
- Mastoid process
- Temporomandibular joint
- Cervical vertebrae

Figure 21-3 The mastoid air cells are located in the mastoid process. Just anterior to the mastoid is the external auditory meatus, which is associated with the ear canal.

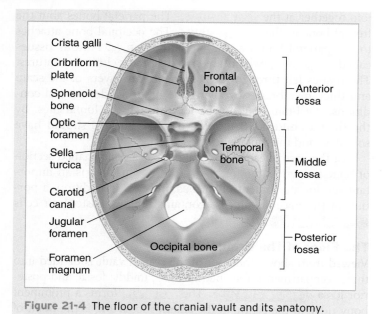

Figure 21-4 The floor of the cranial vault and its anatomy.

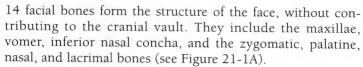

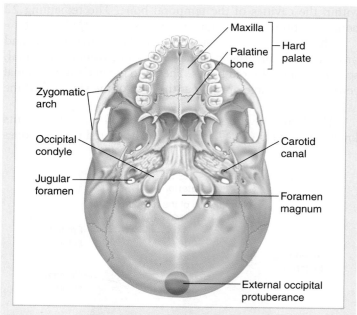

Figure 21-5 The base of the skull from below.

14 facial bones form the structure of the face, without contributing to the cranial vault. They include the maxillae, vomer, inferior nasal concha, and the zygomatic, palatine, nasal, and lacrimal bones (see Figure 21-1A).

The facial bones protect the eyes, nose, and tongue; they also provide attachment points for the muscles that allow chewing. The zygomatic process of the temporal bone and the temporal process of the zygomatic bone form the zygomatic arch Figure 21-6 ▸ , which lends shape to the cheeks.

Two major nerves provide sensory and motor control to the face: the trigeminal nerve (fifth cranial nerve) and the facial nerve (seventh cranial nerve). The trigeminal nerve branches into the ophthalmic nerve, maxillary nerve, and mandibular nerve. The ophthalmic nerve (a sensory nerve) supplies the skin of the forehead, upper eyelid, and conjunctiva. The maxillary nerve (another sensory nerve) supplies the skin on the posterior part of the side of the nose, lower eye-

lid, cheek, and upper lip. The mandibular nerve (a sensory and motor nerve) supplies the muscles of chewing (mastication) and skin of the lower lip, chin, temporal region, and part of the external ear. The facial nerve supplies the muscles of facial expression.

Blood supply to the face is provided primarily through the external carotid artery, which branches into the temporal, mandibular, and maxillary arteries. Because the face is highly vascular, it tends to bleed heavily when injured.

The Orbits

The orbits are cone-shaped fossae that enclose and protect the eyes. In addition to the eyeball and muscles that move it, the orbit contains blood vessels, nerves, and fat.

A blow to the eye may result in fracture of the orbital floor because the bone is extremely thin and breaks easily. A

You are the Paramedic Part 2

As your partner maintains manual stabilisation of the patient's head and simultaneously opens his airway with the jaw-thrust manoeuvre, you perform an initial assessment.

Initial Assessment	Recording Time: 0 Minutes
Appearance	Supine, not moving, massive facial trauma
Level of consciousness	P (Responsive to painful stimuli)
Airway	Blood is draining from the patient's mouth
Breathing	Respirations are gurgling, slow, and irregular
Circulation	Radial pulses are rapid and bounding; bleeding from the mouth; no other major bleeding

3. How will you manage this patient's airway?

4. Would it be appropriate to intubate this patient? If so, when?

blowout fracture (**Figure 21-7** ▼) results in transmission of forces away from the eyeball itself to the bone. Blood and fat then leak into the maxillary sinus.

The Nose

The nose is one of the two primary entry points for oxygen-rich air to enter the body. The nasal septum—the separation between the nostrils—is located in the midline. Often, it bulges slightly to one side or the other. The external portion of the nose is formed mostly of cartilage.

Several bones associated with the nose contain cavities known as the paranasal sinuses (**Figure 21-8** ▶) . These hollowed sections of bone, which are lined with mucous membranes, decrease the weight of the skull and provide resonance for the voice. The contents of the sinuses drain into the nasal cavity.

The Mandible and Temporomandibular Joint

The mandible is the large moveable bone forming the lower jaw and containing the lower teeth. Numerous muscles of chewing attach to the mandible and its rami. The posterior condyle of the mandible articulates with the temporal bone at the temporomandibular joint (TMJ), allowing movement of the mandible (see Figure 21-3).

The Hyoid Bone

The hyoid bone "floats" in the superior aspect of the neck just below the mandible. While it is not actually part of the skull, it supports the tongue and serves as a point of attachment for many important neck and tongue muscles.

▌The Eyes, Ears, Teeth, and Mouth

The Eye

The globe, or eyeball, is a spherical structure measuring about 2.5 cm in diameter that is housed within the eye socket, or orbit. The eyes are held in place by loose connective tissue and several muscles. These muscles also control eye movements. The oculomotor nerve (third cranial nerve) innervates the muscles that cause motion of the eyeballs and upper eyelids. It also carries parasympathetic nerve fibres that cause constriction of the pupil and accommodation of the lens. The optic nerve (second cranial nerve) provides the sense of vision (**Figure 21-9** ▶) .

The structures of the eye (**Figure 21-10** ▶) include the following:

- The sclera ("white of the eye") is a tough, fibrous coat that helps maintain the shape of the eye and protect the contents of the eye. In some illnesses, such as hepatitis, the sclera become yellow (icteric) from staining by bile pigments.
- The cornea is the transparent anterior portion of the eye that overlies the iris and pupil. Clouding of the cornea during ageing results in a condition known as cataract.
- The conjunctiva is a delicate mucous membrane that covers the sclera and internal surfaces of the eyelids but not the iris. Cyanosis can be detected in the conjunctiva when it is not easily assessed on the skin of dark-skinned patients.

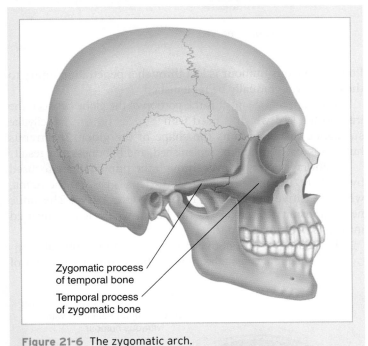

Zygomatic process of temporal bone

Temporal process of zygomatic bone

Figure 21-6 The zygomatic arch.

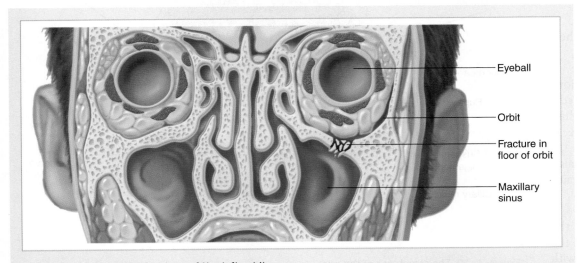

Eyeball

Orbit

Fracture in floor of orbit

Maxillary sinus

Figure 21-7 A blowout fracture of the left orbit.

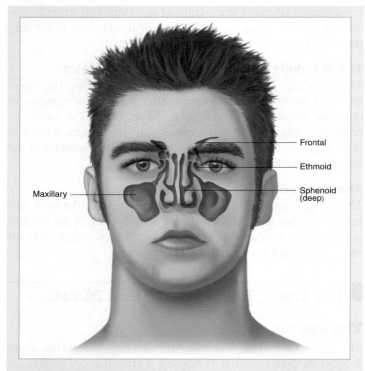

Figure 21-8 The paranasal sinuses.

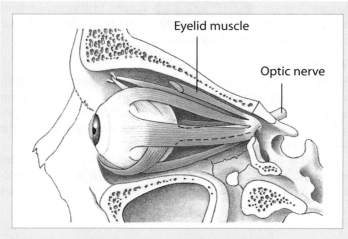

Figure 21-9 The optic nerve.

- The <u>iris</u> is the pigmented part of the eye that surrounds the pupil. It consists of muscles and blood vessels that contract and expand to regulate the size of the pupil.
- The <u>pupil</u> is the circular adjustable opening within the iris through which light passes to the lens. A normal pupil dilates in dim light to permit more light to enter the eye and constricts in bright light to decrease the light entering the eye.
- Behind the pupil and iris is the <u>lens</u>, a transparent structure that can alter its thickness to focus light on the retina at the back of the eye.
- The <u>retina</u>, which lies in the posterior aspect of the interior globe, is a delicate, 10-layered structure of nervous tissue that extends from the optic nerve. It receives light impulses and converts them to nerve signals that are conducted to the brain by the optic nerve and interpreted as vision.

The <u>anterior chamber</u> is the portion of the globe between the lens and the cornea. It is filled with <u>aqueous humour</u>, a clear watery

fluid. If aqueous humour is lost through a penetrating injury to the eye, it will gradually be replenished.

The <u>posterior chamber</u> is the portion of the globe between the iris and the lens which is filled with <u>vitreous humour</u>, a jellylike substance that maintains the shape of the globe. If vitreous humour is lost, it cannot be replenished, and blindness may result.

Light rays enter the eyes through the pupil and are focused by the lens. The image formed by the lens is cast on the retina, where sensitive nerve fibres form the optic nerve. The optic nerve transmits the image to the brain, where it is converted into conscious images in the <u>visual cortex</u>.

There are two types of vision: central and peripheral. <u>Central vision</u> facilitates visualisation of objects directly in front of

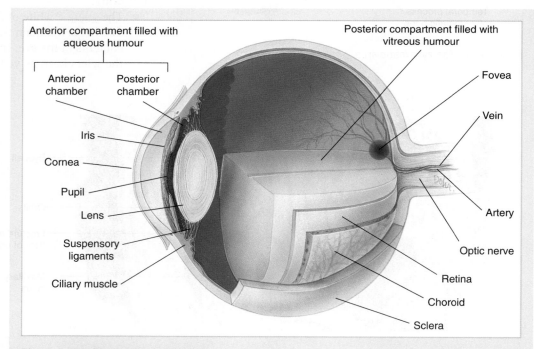

Figure 21-10 The structures of the eye.

you, and is processed by the macula, the central portion of the retina. The remainder of the retina processes peripheral vision, which gives us visualisation of lateral objects while looking forward.

The lacrimal apparatus secretes and drains tears from the eye. Tears produced in the lacrimal gland drain into lacrimal ducts, then into lacrimal sacs that pass into the nasal cavity via the nasolacrimal duct. Tears moisten the conjunctivae **Figure 21-11 ▼**.

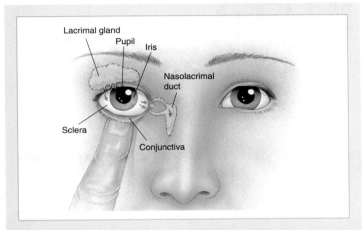

Figure 21-11 The lacrimal system consists of tear glands and ducts. Tears act as lubricants and keep the anterior part of the eye from drying.

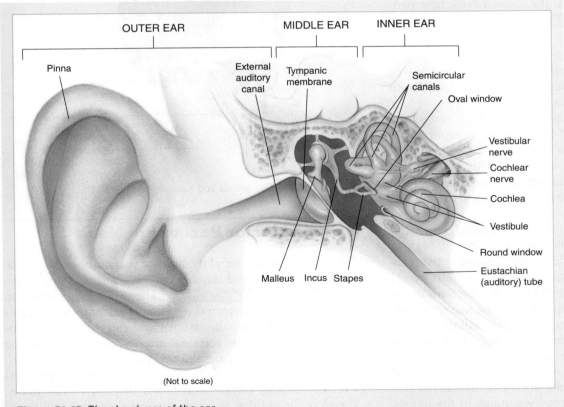

Figure 21-12 The structures of the ear.

The Ear

The ear is divided into three anatomical parts: external, middle, and inner **Figure 21-12 ▼**. The external ear consists of the pinna, external auditory canal, and the exterior portion of the tympanic membrane or what is commonly known as the eardrum. The middle ear consists of the inner portion of the tympanic membrane and the ossicles while the inner ear consists of the cochlea and semicircular canals.

Sound waves enter the ear through the auricle, or pinna, the large cartilaginous external portion of the ear. They then travel through the external auditory canal to the tympanic membrane. Vibration of sound waves against the tympanic membrane sets up vibration in the ossicles, the three small bones on the inner side of the tympanic membrane. These vibrations are transmitted to the cochlear duct at the oval window, the opening between the middle ear and the vestibule. Movement of the oval window causes fluid within the cochlea, a shell-shaped structure in the inner ear, to vibrate. Within the cochlea at the organ of Corti, vibration stimulates hair movements that form nerve impulses that travel to the brain via the auditory nerve. The brain then converts these impulses into sound.

The Teeth

The normal adult mouth contains 32 permanent teeth. The primary or deciduous teeth are lost during childhood. Adult teeth are distributed about the maxillary and mandibular arches. The teeth on each side of the arch are mirror images of each other and form four quadrants: right upper, left upper, right lower, and left lower. Each quadrant contains one central incisor, one lateral incisor, one canine, two premolars, and three molars **Figure 21-13A ▶**. The third molars or what are called wisdom teeth (which have nothing to do with wisdom) do not appear until late adolescence.

The top portion of the tooth, external to the gum, is the crown, containing one or more cusps. Below the crown lie the neck and the root. The pulp cavity fills the centre of the tooth and contains blood vessels, nerves, and specialised connective tissue, called pulp. Dentine and enamel surround the pulp cavity and protect the tooth from damage. Dentine,

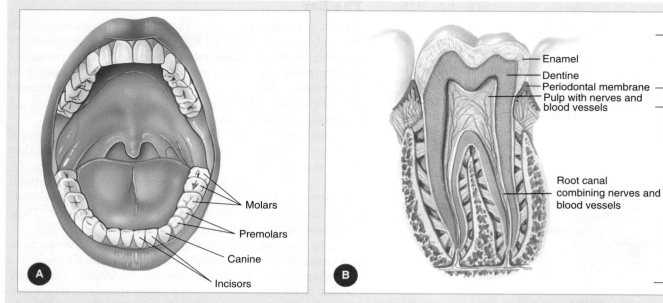

Figure 21-13 The teeth of the adult mouth. **A.** The incisors are used for biting. Canines are used for tearing food. The premolars and molars are used for grinding and crushing. **B.** Each tooth contains nerves and blood vessels.

which forms the principal mass of the tooth, is much denser and stronger than bone. The bony sockets for the teeth that reside in the mandible and maxilla are called alveoli. The ridges between the teeth, the alveolar ridges, are covered by the gingiva, or gums, which are thickened connective tissue and epithelium. Teeth are attached to the alveolar bone by a periodontal membrane Figure 21-13B ▲ .

The Mouth

Digestion begins in the mouth with mastication, or the chewing of food by the teeth. During mastication, food is mixed with secretions from the salivary glands.

The tongue, a muscular process in the floor of the mouth, is the primary organ of taste; it is also important in the formation of speech and in chewing and swallowing of food. The tongue is attached at the mandible and hyoid bone, is covered by a mucous membrane, and extends from the back of the mouth upward and forward to the lips Figure 21-14 ▶ .

The hypoglossal, glossopharyngeal, trigeminal, and facial nerves supply the mouth and its structures. The hypoglossal nerve (12th cranial nerve) provides motor function to the muscles of the tongue. The glossopharyngeal nerve (ninth cranial nerve) provides taste sensation to the posterior portions of the tongue and carries parasympathetic fibres to the salivary glands on each side of the face. The mandibular branch of the trigeminal nerve (fifth cranial nerve) provides motor innervation to the muscles of mastication. The facial nerve (seventh cranial nerve), in addition to supplying motor activity to all muscles of facial expression, provides the sense of taste to the anterior two thirds of the tongue and cutaneous sensations to the tongue and palate.

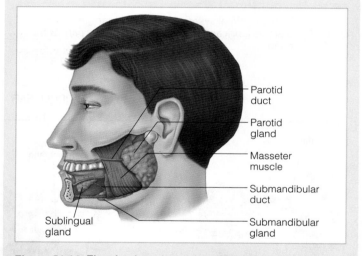

Figure 21-14 The glands and muscles of the mouth.

The Anterior Part of the Neck

The principal structures of the anterior part of the neck include the thyroid and cricoid cartilage, trachea, and numerous muscles and nerves Figure 21-15 ▶ . The major blood vessels in this area are the internal and external carotid arteries Figure 21-16 ▶ and the internal and external jugular veins Figure 21-17 ▶ . The vertebral arteries run laterally to the cervical vertebrae in the posterior part of the neck.

The major arteries of the neck—the carotid and vertebral arteries—supply oxygenated blood directly to the brain. Therefore, in addition to causing massive bleeding and hypovolaemic shock, injury to any of these major vessels can pro-

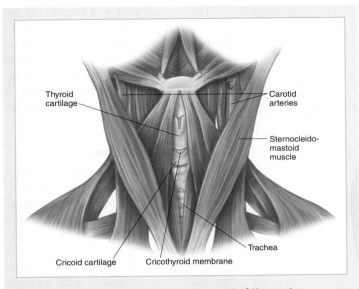

Figure 21-15 Anatomy of the anterior part of the neck.

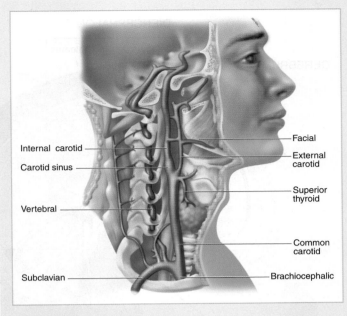

Figure 21-16 The arteries of the neck.

duce cerebral hypoxia, infarct, air embolism and/or permanent neurological impairment.

Other key structures of the anterior part of the neck that may sustain injury from blunt or penetrating mechanisms include the vagus nerves, thoracic duct, oesophagus, thyroid and parathyroid glands, lower cranial nerves, brachial plexus (which is responsible for function of the lower arm and hand), soft tissue and fascia, and various muscles.

The Brain

The brain, which occupies 80% of the cranial vault, contains billions of neurones (nerve cells) that serve a variety of vital functions   Figure 21-18 ▶ . The major regions of the brain are the cerebrum, diencephalon (thalamus and hypothalamus), brain stem (medulla, pons, midbrain [mesencephalon]), and the cerebellum. The remaining intracranial contents include cerebral blood (12%) and cerebrospinal fluid (8%).

The brain accounts for only 2% of the total body weight, yet it is the most metabolically active and perfusion-sensitive organ in the body. The brain metabolises 25% of the body's glucose, burning approximately 60 mg/min, and consumes 20% of the total body oxygen (45 to 50 ml/min). Because the brain has no storage mechanism for oxygen or glucose, it is totally dependent on a constant source of both fuels via cerebral blood flow provided by the carotid and vertebral arteries. As such, the brain will continually manipulate the physiology

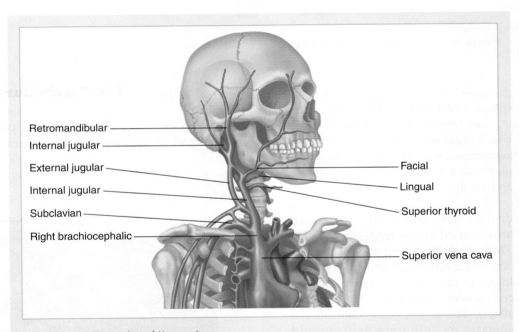

Figure 21-17 The veins of the neck.

as needed to guarantee that a ready supply of oxygen and glucose are available.

The Cerebrum

The largest portion of the brain is the cerebrum, which is responsible for higher functions, such as reasoning. The cerebrum is divided into right and left hemispheres by a longitudinal fissure. The hemispheres of the cerebrum are not entirely equivalent functionally. In a right-handed person, for example,

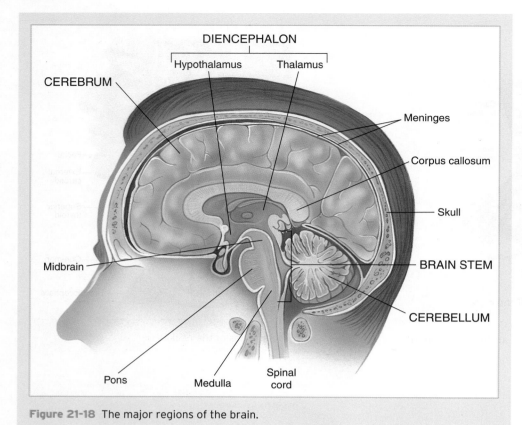

Figure 21-18 The major regions of the brain.

The speech centre is located in the temporal lobe. In approximately 85% of the population, the speech centre is located on the left side of the temporal lobe. The temporal lobe also controls long-term memory, hearing, taste, and smell. It is separated from the rest of the cerebrum by a lateral fissure.

The Diencephalon

The diencephalon, which is located between the brain stem and the cerebrum, includes the thalamus, subthalamus, hypothalamus, and epithalamus Figure 21-20 ▶ . The thalamus processes most sensory input and influences mood and general body movements, especially those associated with fear and rage. The subthalamus controls motor functions. The functions of the epithalamus are unclear. The most inferior portion of the diencephalon, the hypothalamus, is vital in the control of many body functions, including heart rate, digestion, sexual development, temperature regulation, emotion, hunger, thirst, vomiting, and regulation of the sleep cycle.

The Cerebellum

The cerebellum is located beneath the cerebral hemispheres in the inferoposterior part of the brain. It is sometimes called the "athlete's brain" because it is responsible for the maintenance

the speech centre is usually located in the left cerebral hemisphere, which is then said to be the dominant hemisphere.

The largest portion of the cerebrum is the cerebral cortex, which regulates voluntary skeletal movement and the level of awareness. Injury to the cerebral cortex may result in paresthesia, weakness, and paralysis of the extremities.

Each cerebral hemisphere is divided functionally into specialised areas called lobes Figure 21-19 ▶ . The frontal lobe is important for voluntary motor action and personality traits. Injury to the frontal lobe may result in convulsions or placid reactions (flat affect). The parietal lobe controls the somatic or voluntary sensory and motor functions for the opposite (contralateral) side of the body, as well as memory and emotions; it is separated from the frontal lobe by the central sulcus. Posteriorly, the occipital lobe, from which the optic nerve originates, is responsible for processing visual information. After a blow to the back of the head, a person may "see stars" which results when the occipital poles of the brain (the vision centres) bang against the back of the skull.

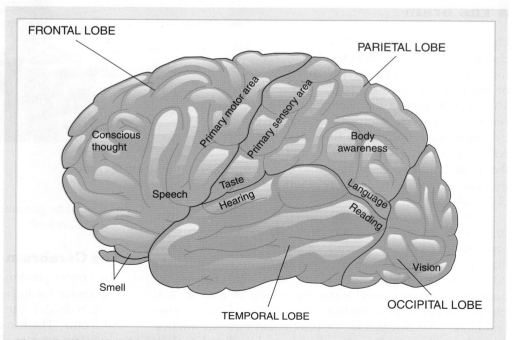

Figure 21-19 Lobes of the cerebrum.

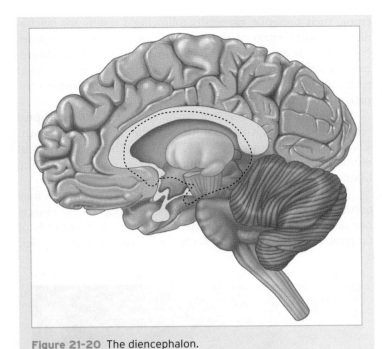

Figure 21-20 The diencephalon.

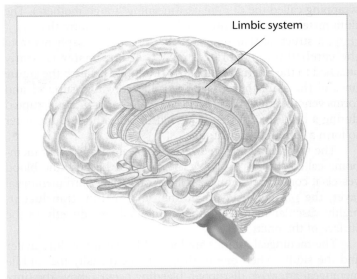

Figure 21-21 The limbic system is the seat of emotions, instincts, and other functions.

of posture and equilibrium and the coordination of skilled movements.

The Brain Stem

The brain stem consists of the midbrain, pons, and the medulla. It is located at the base of the brain and connects the spinal cord to the remainder of the brain. The brain stem houses many structures that are critical to the maintenance of vital functions. High in the brain stem, for example, is the reticular activating system (RAS), which is responsible for maintenance of consciousness, specifically one's level of arousal. The centres that control basic but critical functions—heart rate, blood pressure, and respiration—are located in the lower part of the brain stem. Damage to this area can easily result in cardiovascular compromise, respiratory arrest, or death.

The midbrain lies immediately below the diencephalon and is the smallest region of the brain stem. Deep within the cerebrum, diencephalon, and midbrain are the basal ganglia, which have an important role in coordination of motor movements and posture. Portions of the cerebrum and diencephalon constitute the limbic system, which influences emotions, motivation, mood, and sensations of pain and pleasure Figure 21-21 ▶ .

The oculomotor nerve (third cranial nerve) originates from the midbrain; it controls pupillary size and reactivity.

The pons, which lies below the midbrain and above the medulla, contains numerous important nerve fibres, including those for sleep, respiration, and the medullary respiratory centre.

The inferior portion of the midbrain, the medulla, is continuous inferiorly with the spinal cord (see Figure 21-18). It serves as a conduction pathway for ascending and descending nerve tracts. It also coordinates heart rate, blood vessel diameter, breathing, swallowing, vomiting, coughing, and sneezing. The vagus nerve (tenth cranial nerve), a bundle of nerves that primarily innervates the parasympathetic nervous system, originates from the medulla.

The Meninges

The meninges are protective layers that surround and enfold the entire central nervous system—specifically the brain and spinal cord Figure 21-22 ▾ . The outermost layer is a strong, fibrous

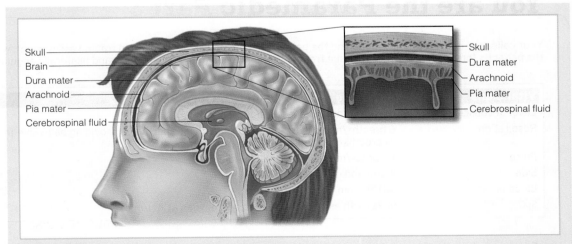

Skull
Brain
Dura mater
Arachnoid
Pia mater
Cerebrospinal fluid

Skull
Dura mater
Arachnoid
Pia mater
Cerebrospinal fluid

Figure 21-22 The meninges.

wrapping called the dura mater (meaning "tough mother"). The dura mater covers the entire brain, folding in to form the tentorium, a structure that separates the cerebral hemispheres from the cerebellum and brain stem. The dura mater is firmly attached to the internal wall of the skull. Just beneath the suture lines of the skull the dura mater splits into two surfaces and forms venous sinuses. When those venous sinuses are disrupted during a head injury, blood can collect beneath the dura mater to form a subdural haematoma.

The second meningeal layer is a delicate, transparent membrane called the arachnoid. It is so named because the blood vessels it contains resemble a spider's web. The third meningeal layer, the pia mater ("soft mother"), is a thin, translucent, highly vascular membrane that firmly adheres directly to the surface of the brain.

The meningeal arteries are located between the dura mater and the skull. When one of these arteries (usually the middle meningeal artery) is disrupted, bleeding occurs above the dura mater, resulting in an extradural haematoma.

The meninges are bathed in cerebrospinal fluid (CSF), which is manufactured in the ventricles of the brain. CSF flows in the subarachnoid space, located between the pia mater and the arachnoid.

CSF is manufactured by cells within the choroid plexus in the ventricles, hollow storage areas in the brain. These areas normally are interconnected, and CSF flows freely between them. CSF is similar in composition to plasma. The meninges and CSF form a fluid-filled sac that cushions and protects the brain and spinal cord.

Face Injuries

Soft-Tissue Injuries

Although open soft-tissue injuries to the face—lacerations, abrasions, and avulsions—by themselves are rarely life threatening, their presence, especially following a significant mechanism of injury, suggests the potential for more severe injuries (eg, closed head injury, cervical spine injury). Furthermore, massive soft-tissue injuries to the face, especially if associated with oropharyngeal trauma and bleeding, can compromise the patient's airway and lead to ventilatory inadequacy.

Maintain a high index of suspicion when a patient presents with closed soft-tissue injuries to the face, such as contusions and haematomas **Figure 21-23** ▾. These indicators of blunt trauma suggest the potential for more severe underlying injuries.

Impaled objects in the soft tissues or bones of the face may occur in association with facial trauma. Although these objects can damage facial nerves, the risk of airway compromise is of far greater consequence. This is especially true when an impaled

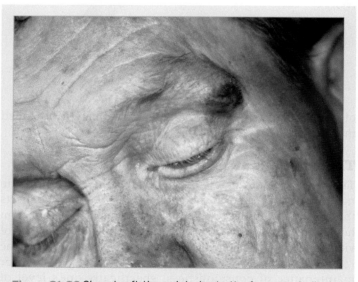

Figure 21-23 Closed soft-tissue injuries to the face may indicate more severe underlying injuries.

You are the Paramedic Part 3

Your colleague is appropriately managing the patient's airway. You perform a rapid trauma assessment, which reveals a haematoma to the patient's forehead, massive soft-tissue trauma to the face, unstable facial bones, and bilaterally angulated femurs.

Vital Signs	Recording Time: 5 Minutes
Level of consciousness	Glasgow Coma Scale score of 6
Respirations	6 breaths/min and irregular (baseline); your partner is providing bag-valve-mask ventilation at a rate of 10 breaths/min and supplemental oxygen
Pulse	110 beats/min; regular and bounding
Skin	Warm and dry
Blood pressure	140/90 mm Hg
S$_P$O$_2$	96% (with assisted ventilation and oxygen at 15 l/min)

5. How can facial trauma complicate airway management?
6. Is this patient in hypovolaemic shock? Why or why not?

At the Scene

Be careful when assessing the patient with soft-tissue injuries to the face, especially if he or she has experienced a significant mechanism of injury. Although facial lacerations and avulsions are often the most obvious and dramatic, they are usually not life threatening.

object penetrates the cheek, because massive oropharyngeal bleeding can result in airway obstruction, aspiration, and ventilatory inadequacy. In addition, blood is a gastric irritant. For many people, just swallowing 10 to 20 ml of blood can make them vomit, further increasing the likelihood of aspiration.

Maxillofacial Fractures

Maxillofacial fractures commonly occur when the facial bones absorb the energy of a strong impact. The forces involved may be massive. For example, a force up to 150g (g = acceleration of the body due to gravity) is required to fracture the maxilla; a force of that magnitude will be likely to produce closed head injuries and cervical spine injuries as well. Therefore, when assessing a patient with a suspected maxillofacial fracture, you should protect the cervical spine and monitor the patient's neurological signs, specifically their level of consciousness.

The first clue to the presence of a maxillofacial fracture is usually bruising, so a black-and-blue mark on the face should alert you to this possibility. A deep facial laceration should likewise increase your index of suspicion that the underlying bone may have been fractured, and pain over a bone tends to support the suspicion of fracture. General signs and symptoms of maxillofacial fractures include bruising, swelling, pain to palpation, crepitus, dental malocclusion, facial deformities or asymmetry, instability of the facial bones, impaired ocular movement, and visual disturbances.

Nasal Fractures

Because the nasal bones are not as structurally sound as the other bones of the face, nasal fractures are the most common facial fracture. These fractures are characterised by swelling, tenderness, and crepitus when the nasal bone is palpated. Deformity of the nose, if present, usually appears as lateral displacement of the nasal bone from its normal midline position.

Nasal fractures, like any maxillofacial fracture, are often complicated by the presence of an anterior or a posterior nosebleed (epistaxis), which can compromise the patient's airway.

Mandibular Fractures and Dislocations

Second only to nasal fractures in frequency, fractures of the mandible typically result from massive blunt trauma to the lower third of the face; they are particularly common following an assault injury. Because significant force is required to fracture the mandible, this structure may be fractured in more than one place and, therefore, unstable to palpation. The fracture site itself is most commonly located at the angle of the jaw.

Mandibular fractures should be suspected in patients with a history of blunt trauma to the lower third of the face who present with dental malocclusion (misalignment of the teeth), numbness of the chin, and inability to open the mouth. There is likely to be swelling and bruising over the fracture site, and teeth may be partially or completely avulsed.

Although temporomandibular joint (TMJ) dislocations may occur as the result of blunt trauma to the lower third of the face, this outcome is rare. Mandibular dislocations are usually the result of yawning extravagantly or otherwise opening the mouth very widely. The patient commonly feels a "pop" and then cannot close his or her mouth; it is locked in a wide-open position. The jaw muscles eventually go into spasm, causing severe pain.

Maxillary Fractures

Maxillary fractures to the midface area are commonly associated with mechanisms that produce massive blunt facial trauma, such as road traffic collisions, falls, and assaults. They produce massive facial swelling, instability of the midfacial bones, malocclusion, and an elongated appearance of the patient's face. Midfacial structures include the maxilla, zygoma, orbital floor, and nose.

Le Fort fractures **Figure 21-24 ▾** are classified into three categories:

- **Le Fort I fracture.** A horizontal fracture of the maxilla that involves the hard palate and inferior maxilla

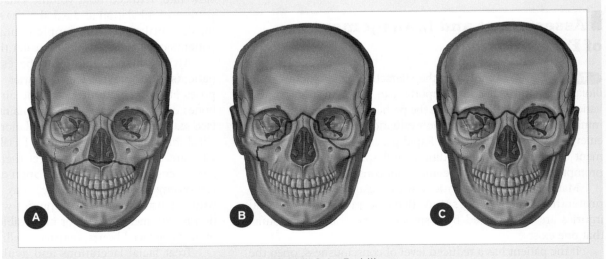

Figure 21-24 Le Fort fractures. **A.** Le Fort I. **B.** Le Fort II. **C.** Le Fort III.

- **Le Fort II fracture.** A pyramidal fracture involving the nasal bone and inferior maxilla
- **Le Fort III fracture** (craniofacial disjunction). A fracture of all midfacial bones, separating the entire midface from the cranium.

Le Fort fractures can occur as isolated fractures (Le Fort I) or in combination (Le Fort I and II), depending on the location of impact and the amount of trauma.

Orbital Fractures

The patient with an orbital fracture (such as a blowout fracture [see Figure 21-7]) may complain of double vision (diplopia) and lose sensation above the eyebrow or over the cheek secondary to associated nerve damage. Massive nasal discharge may occur, and vision is often impaired. Fractures of the inferior orbit are the most common type and can cause paralysis of upward gaze (the patient's injured eye will not be able to follow your finger *above* the midline).

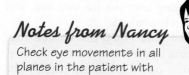

Notes from Nancy

Check eye movements in all planes in the patient with possible facial fractures.

Zygomatic Fractures

Fractures of the zygomatic bone (cheek bone) commonly result from blunt trauma secondary to road traffic collisions and assaults. When the zygomatic bone is fractured, that side of the patient's face appears flattened, and there is loss of sensation over the cheek, nose, and upper lip; paralysis of upward gaze may also be present. Other injuries commonly associated with zygomatic fractures include orbital fractures, ocular injury, and epistaxis.

Notes from Nancy

Any patient with significant head injury also has cervical spine injury until proved otherwise.

Assessment and Management of Face Injuries

Table 21-1 ▶ summarises the characteristics of various maxillofacial fractures. It is not important to distinguish among the various maxillofacial fractures in the prehospital setting; this determination requires radiographic evaluation in the collision and emergency (A&E) department. Rapid patient assessment, management of life-threatening conditions, full spinal precautions, and prompt transport are far more important considerations.

Management of the patient with facial trauma begins by protecting the cervical spine. Because many severe facial injuries are complicated by a spinal injury, you must assume that one exists.

If the patient has a reduced level of consciousness, open the airway with the jaw-thrust manoeuvre while simultaneously

Table 21-1 — Summary of Maxillofacial Fractures

Injury	Signs and Symptoms
Multiple facial bone fractures	· Massive facial swelling · Dental malocclusion · Palpable deformities · Anterior or posterior epistaxis
Zygomatic and orbital fractures	· Loss of sensation below the orbit · Flattening of the patient's cheek · Paralysis of upward gaze
Nasal fractures	· Crepitus and instability · Swelling, tenderness, lateral displacement · Anterior or posterior epistaxis
Maxillary (Le Fort) fractures	· Mobility of the facial skeleton · Dental malocclusion · Facial swelling
Mandibular fractures	· Dental malocclusion · Mandibular instability

maintaining manual stabilisation of the head in the neutral position unless the patient complains of severe pain or discomfort upon movement. Should that occur, the head/neck should be immobilised in the position found. Inspect the mouth for fragments of teeth, dentures, or any other foreign bodies that could obstruct the airway, and remove them immediately. Suction the oropharynx as needed to keep the airway clear of blood and other liquids.

Insert an airway adjunct as needed to maintain airway patency. However, *do not insert a nasopharyngeal airway or attempt nasotracheal intubation in any patient with suspected nasal fractures or in patients with CSF or blood leakage from the nose.* After establishing and maintaining a patent airway, assess the patient's breathing and intervene appropriately. Apply 100% oxygen via nonrebreathing mask if the patient is breathing adequately. Patients who are breathing inadequately (ie, fast or slow rate, reduced tidal volume [shallow breathing], irregular pattern of inhalation and exhalation) should receive bag-valve-mask ventilation with supplemental oxygen. Maintain the patient's oxygen saturation at greater than 95%.

Airway management can be especially challenging in patients with massive facial injuries. Oropharyngeal bleeding poses an immediate threat to the airway, and unstable facial bones can hinder your ability to maintain an effective mask-to-face seal for bag-valve-mask ventilation. Therefore, perform tracheal intubation of patients with facial trauma, especially those who are unconscious, to protect their airway from aspiration and to ensure adequate oxygenation and ventilation. Cricothyroidotomy (surgical or needle) may be required for patients with extensive maxillofacial injuries when endotracheal intubation is extremely difficult or impossible to perform (eg, in cases of unstable facial bones, massive swelling, severe oral bleeding).

Treat facial lacerations and avulsions as you would any other soft-tissue injury. Control all bleeding with direct pres-

At the Scene

Blood or CSF drainage from the nose (cerebrospinal rhinorrhoea) suggests a skull fracture. Do not make any attempt to control this bleeding: doing so may increase intracranial pressure (ICP) if the patient has a concomitant brain injury. Furthermore, the insertion of nasal airway adjuncts and nasotracheal intubation should be avoided in patients with suspected nasal fractures, especially if rhinorrhoea is present. A nasally inserted airway device could enter the cranial vault through an occult fracture (such as a cribriform plate fracture) and penetrate the brain, further worsening the situation.

sure as appropriate, and apply sterile dressings. If you suspect an underlying facial fracture, apply just enough pressure to control the bleeding. Leave impaled objects in the face in place and appropriately stabilise them, unless they pose a threat to the airway (such as an object impaled in the cheek). When removing an object from the cheek, carefully remove it from the same side that it entered. Next, pack the inside of the cheek with sterile gauze and apply counterpressure with a dressing and bandage firmly secured over the outside of the wound. If profuse bleeding continues, position the patient on his or her side—while maintaining stabilisation of the cervical spine—to facilitate drainage of secretions from the mouth and suction the airway as needed.

For severe oropharyngeal bleeding in patients with inadequate ventilation, suction the airway for 15 seconds and provide ventilatory assistance for 2 minutes; continue this alternating pattern of suctioning and ventilating until the airway is cleared of blood or secured with an endotracheal (ET) tube. Monitoring the pulse oximeter during this process can further serve to keep the patient from becoming hypoxic.

Epistaxis following facial trauma can be severe and is most effectively controlled by applying direct pressure to the nares. If the patient is conscious and spinal injury is not suspected, instruct the patient to sit up and lean forward as you pinch the nares together. Unconscious patients should be positioned on their side, unless contraindicated by a spinal injury. Proper positioning of the patient with epistaxis is important to prevent blood from draining down the throat and compromising the airway either by occlusion or by vomiting and then aspirating gastric contents. If the conscious patient with severe epistaxis is immobilised on a longboard, you should consider rapid-sequence intubation (RSI) to gain definitive control of the airway, if authorised.

Although facial lacerations and avulsions can contribute to hypovolaemic shock, they are rarely the sole cause of this condition in adults. Severe epistaxis, however, can result in significant blood loss. To counter this problem, you should carefully assess the patient for signs of haemorrhagic shock and administer intravenous (IV) crystalloid fluid boluses as needed to maintain adequate perfusion.

If the facial fracture is associated with swelling and bruising, cold compresses may help minimise further swelling and alleviate pain. Do not apply a compress to the eyeball (globe) if you suspect that it has been injured following an orbital fracture; doing so may increase the intraocular pressure (IOP) and further damage the eye. Other than protecting the airway, little can be done to treat facial instabilities; however, firmly applying a self-adhering roller bandage can stabilise the mandible. Make sure that you do not compromise the airway when stabilising the mandible.

After addressing all life-threatening injuries and conditions, you should attempt to ascertain the events that preceded the injury and determine whether the patient has any significant medical problems. The incident that caused the injury may have been preceded by exacerbation of an underlying medical condition (such as acute hypoglycaemia, cardiac dysrhythmia, convulsion). For unconscious patients, medications that the patient is taking may provide information about his or her medical history. Determine the approximate time that the injury occurred, and ask about any drug allergies and the last oral intake during your SAMPLE history **Figure 21-25 ▼** .

Special Considerations

Relative to younger, healthy adults, elderly patients are at high risk for severe epistaxis following even minor facial injuries, especially in those with a history of hypertension or anticoagulant medication use (such as warfarin). This bleeding often originates in the posterior nasopharynx and may not be grossly evident during your assessment.

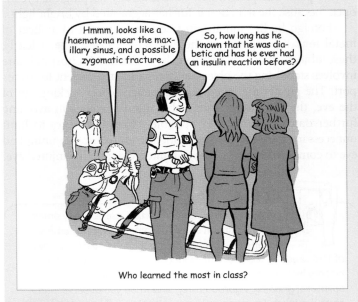

Figure 21-25

Eye Injuries

Because trauma to the eyes is so common and the potential consequences are so serious, you must know how to assess and manage ocular injuries.

Eye injuries are frequently caused by blunt trauma, penetrating trauma, or burns. Blunt mechanisms of injury may include road traffic collisions, motorcycle crashes, falls, and assaults. Penetrating injuries are often secondary to foreign bodies on the surface of the eye (such as sand) or an object impaled in the globe. Burns to the eye can result from a variety of corrosive chemicals or during industrial accidents (such as welding burns).

Lacerations, Foreign Bodies, and Impaled Objects

Lacerations of the eyelids require meticulous repair to restore appearance and function. Bleeding may be heavy, but it usually can be controlled by gentle, manual pressure. *If there is a laceration to the globe itself, apply no pressure to the eye;* compression can interfere with the blood supply to the back of the eye and result in loss of vision from damage to the retina. Furthermore, excess pressure may squeeze the vitreous humour, iris, lens, or even the retina out of the eye and cause irreparable damage or blindness Figure 21-26 ▸ .

The protective orbit prevents large objects from penetrating the eye. However, moderately sized and smaller foreign objects can still enter the eye and, when lying on the surface of the eye, produce severe irritation Figure 21-27 ▸ . The conjunctiva becomes inflamed and red—a condition known as conjunctivitis—almost immediately, and the eye begins to produce tears in an attempt to flush out the object Figure 21-28 ▸ . Irritation of the cornea or conjunctiva causes intense pain. The patient may have difficulty keeping the eyelids open, because the irritation is further aggravated by bright light.

Foreign bodies ranging in size from a pencil to a sliver of metal may be impaled in the eye Figure 21-29 ▸ . Clearly, these objects must be removed by a doctor. Prehospital care involves stabilising the object and preparing the patient for transport. The greater the length of the foreign object sticking out of the eye, the more important stabilisation becomes in avoiding further damage. Whenever possible, cover both eyes to limit unnecessary movement as the patient tries to use the uninjured eye to compensate for the loss or limited vision of the injured eye.

At the Scene

Large and small foreign bodies, particularly small metal fragments, can become completely embedded in the globe. The patient may not even be aware of the cause of the problem. Suspect such an injury when the history includes metal work (such as hammering, exposure to splinters, grinding, vigorous filing) and when you observe signs of ocular injury (such as redness, irritation, inflammation).

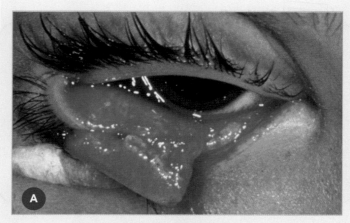
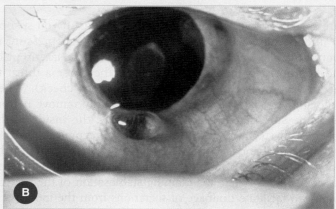

Figure 21-26 Eye lacerations are serious injuries that require prompt transport. **A.** Although bleeding can be heavy, never exert pressure on the eye. **B.** Pressure may squeeze the vitreous humour, iris, lens, or retina out of the eye.

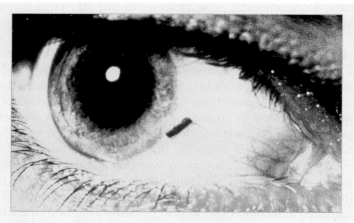

Figure 21-27 A foreign object on the surface of the eye.

Blunt Eye Injuries

Blunt trauma can cause serious eye injuries, ranging from swelling and bruising Figure 21-30 ▸ to rupture of the globe. Hyphaema is bleeding into the anterior chamber of the eye that obscures vision, partially or completely

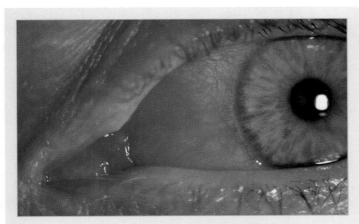

Figure 21-28 Conjunctivitis is often associated with the presence of a foreign object in the eye.

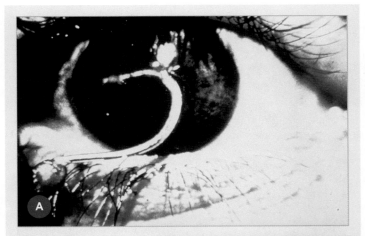

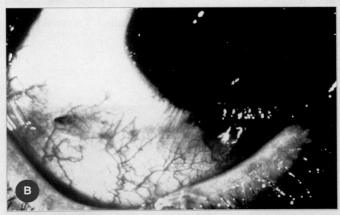

Figure 21-31 ▸ . It often follows blunt trauma and may seriously impair vision. Approximately 25% of hyphaemas are associated with globe injuries.

In orbital blowout fractures, the fragments of fractured bone can entrap some of the muscles that control eye movement, causing double vision (diplopia) **Figure 21-32 ▸** . Any patient who reports pain, double vision, or decreased vision following a blunt injury about the eye should be assumed to have a blowout fracture and should be promptly transported to an appropriate medical facility.

Another potential result of blunt eye trauma is retinal detachment, or separation of the inner layers of the retina from the underlying choroid (the vascular membrane that nourishes the retina). Retinal detachment is often seen in sports injuries, especially boxing. This painless condition produces flashing lights, specks, or "floaters" in the field of vision and a cloud or shade over the patient's vision. Because it can cause devastating damage to vision, retinal detachment is an ocular emergency and requires *immediate* medical attention.

Burns of the Eye

Chemicals, heat, and light rays can all burn the delicate tissues of the eye, often causing permanent damage. Your role is to stop the burning process and prevent further damage.

Chemical burns, which are usually caused by acid or alkali solutions, require immediate emergency care **Figure 21-33 ▸** . Flush the eye with water or a sterile saline solution. If sterile saline is not available, you can use any clean water. Specific techniques for irrigating the eyes are discussed later in this chapter.

Thermal burns occur when a patient is burned in the face during a fire, although the eyes usually close rapidly because of the heat. This reaction is a natural reflex to protect the eyes from further injury. However, the eyelids remain exposed and are frequently burned **Figure 21-34 ▸** .

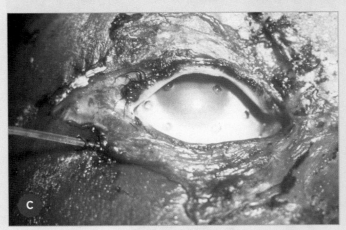

Figure 21-29 Any number of objects can be impaled in the eye. **A.** Fishhook. **B.** Sharp, metal sliver. **C.** Knife blade.

Infrared rays, eclipse light (if the patient has looked directly at the sun), and laser burns can cause significant damage to the sensory cells of the eye when rays of light become focused on the retina. Retinal injuries that are caused by exposure to extremely bright light are generally not painful but may result in permanent damage to vision.

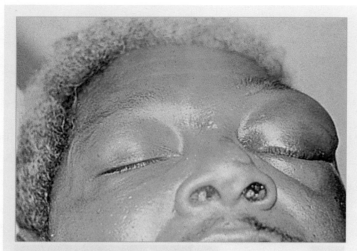

Figure 21-30 Swelling and bruising are hallmark findings associated with blunt trauma to the eye.

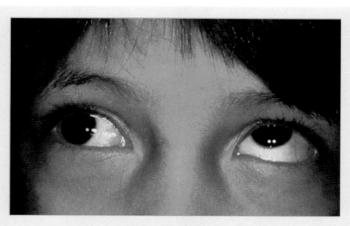

Figure 21-32 In a patient with a blowout fracture, the eyes may not move together because of muscle entrapment, so the patient sees double images of any object.

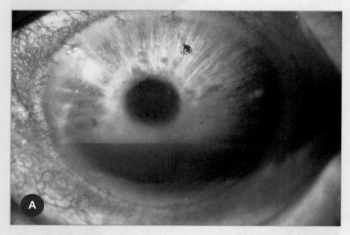

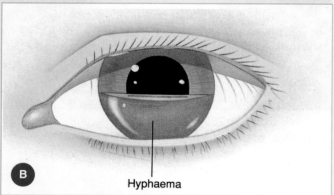

Hyphaema

Figure 21-31 A hyphaema, characterised by bleeding into the anterior chamber of the eye, can occur following blunt trauma to the eye. This condition should be considered a sight-threatening emergency. **A.** Actual hyphaema. **B.** Illustration.

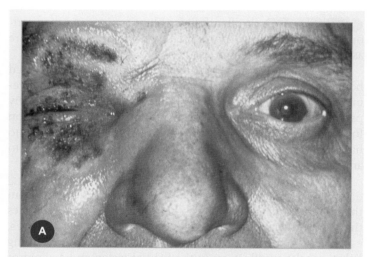

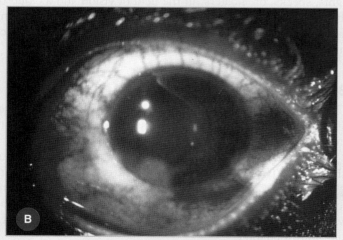

Figure 21-33 **A.** Chemical burns typically occur when an acid or alkali is splashed into the eye. **B.** A chemical burn from lye, an alkaline solution.

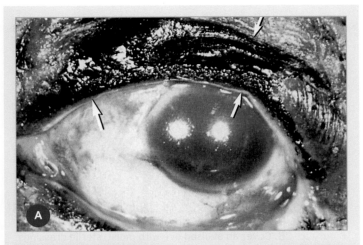

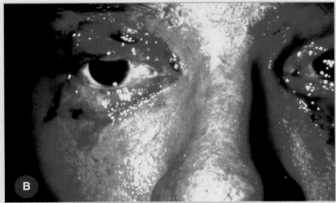

Figure 21-34 Thermal burns occasionally cause significant damage to the eyelids. **A.** Arrows show some full-thickness burns. **B.** Burns of the eyelids require immediate hospital care.

Superficial burns of the eye can result from ultraviolet rays from an arc welding unit, prolonged exposure to a sunlamp, or reflected light from a bright snow-covered area (snow blindness). This kind of burn may not be painful initially but may become so 3 to 5 hours later, as the damaged cornea responds to the injury. Severe conjunctivitis usually develops, along with redness, swelling, and excessive tear production.

Assessment and Management of Eye Injuries

The first step in assessing a patient with an eye injury is to note the mechanism of injury (ie, blunt or penetrating trauma, burn). If it suggests the potential for a spinal injury, use spinal motion restriction precautions. Ensure a patent airway and adequate breathing, and control any external bleeding. If the mechanism of injury is significant, or if the patient's clinical status dictates it, perform a rapid trauma assessment.

When obtaining the history, determine how and when the injury happened, when the symptoms began, and what symptoms the patient is experiencing. Were both eyes affected? Does the patient have any underlying diseases or conditions of the eye (such as glaucoma)? Does the patient take medications for his or her eyes?

A variety of symptoms may indicate serious ocular injury:

- *Visual loss* that does not improve when the patient blinks is the most important symptom of an eye injury. It may indicate damage to the globe or to the optic nerve.
- *Double vision* usually points to trauma involving the extraocular muscles, such as a fracture of the orbit.
- *Severe eye pain* is a symptom of a significant eye injury.
- A *foreign body sensation* usually indicates superficial injury to the cornea or the presence of a foreign object trapped behind the eyelids.

During the physical examination of the eyes, evaluate each of the visible ocular structures and ocular function:

- **Orbital rim:** for bruising, swelling, lacerations, and tenderness
- **Eyelids:** for bruising, swelling, and lacerations
- **Corneas:** for foreign bodies
- **Conjunctivae:** for redness, pus, inflammation, and foreign bodies
- **Globes:** for redness, abnormal pigmentation, and lacerations
- **Pupils:** for size, shape, equality, and reaction to light
- **Eye movements in all directions:** for paralysis of gaze or discoordination between the movements of the two eyes (dysconjugate gaze)
- **Visual acuity:** Make a rough assessment by asking the patient to read a newspaper or a hand-held visual acuity chart. Test each eye separately and document the results.

At the Scene

Anisocoria, a condition in which the pupils are not of equal size, is a significant finding in patients with ocular injuries or closed head trauma. However, simple or physiological anisocoria occurs in approximately 20% of the population. Usually, the patient's pupils differ in size by less than 1 mm; however, approximately 4% of people have pupils that vary in size by more than 1 mm. This is not a clinically significant finding.

Unilateral cataract surgery may also cause inequality of pupil size. The pupil of the eye affected by cataract will be nonreactive to light.

Treatment for specific eye injuries begins with a thorough examination to determine the extent and nature of any damage. Always perform your examination using universal precautions, taking great care to avoid aggravating the injury.

Although isolated eye injuries are usually not life threatening, they should be evaluated by a doctor. More severe eye injuries often require evaluation and treatment by an ophthalmologist.

Injuries to the eyelids—lacerations, abrasions, and contusions—require little in the way of prehospital care other than bleeding control and gentle patching of the affected eye. No eyelid injury is trivial, so every patient with eyelid trauma should be transported to the hospital.

Most injuries to the globe—including contusions, lacerations, foreign bodies, and abrasions—are best treated in the A&E department, where specialised equipment is available. Aluminum eye shields (not gauze patches) applied over *both* eyes are generally all that are necessary in the prehospital environment. Follow these three important guidelines in treating penetrating injuries of the eye:

1. *Never exert pressure* on or manipulate the injured globe in any way.
2. If part of the globe is exposed, gently apply a moist, sterile dressing to prevent drying.
3. *Cover the injured eye* with a protective metal eye shield, cup, or sterile dressing. Apply soft dressings to both eyes, and provide prompt transport to the hospital.

If hyphaema or rupture of the globe is suspected, take spinal motion restriction precautions. Such injuries indicate that a significant amount of force was applied to the face and, thus, may include a spinal injury. Elevate the head of the longboard approximately 40° to decrease IOP and discourage the patient from performing activities that may increase IOP (eg, coughing).

On rare occasions following a serious injury, the globe may be displaced (avulsed) out of its socket Figure 21-35 ▶ . Do not attempt to manipulate or reposition it in any way! Cover the protruding eye with a moist, sterile dressing and stabilise it along with the uninjured eye to prevent further injury due to sympathetic eye movement, the movement of both eyes in unison. Place the patient in a supine position to prevent further loss of fluid from the eye, and provide prompt transport to the hospital.

Burns to the eye that are caused by ultraviolet light are most effectively treated by covering the eye with a sterile, moist pad and an eye shield. The application of cool compresses *lightly* over the eye may afford the patient pain relief if he or she is in extreme

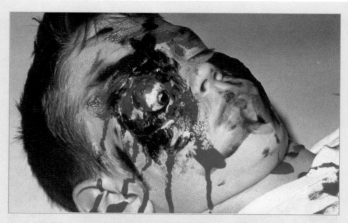

Figure 21-35 Cover an avulsed eye with moist, sterile dressings and protect it from further injury.

distress. Place the patient in a supine position during transport, and protect the patient from further exposure to bright light.

Chemical burns to the eye—acid or alkali—can rapidly lead to total blindness if not immediately treated. The most important prehospital treatment in such cases is to begin immediate irrigation with sterile water or saline solution. *Never use any chemical antidotes (such as vinegar, baking soda) when irrigating the patient's eye; use sterile water or saline only.*

The goal when irrigating the eye is to direct the greatest amount of solution or water into the eye as gently as possible. Because opening the eye spontaneously may cause the patient pain, you may have to force the lids open to irrigate the eye adequately. Ideally, you should use a bulb or irrigation syringe, a nasal cannula, or some other device that will allow you to control the flow Figure 21-36 ▶ . In some circumstances, you may have to pour water into the eye by holding the patient's head under a gently running tap. You can have the patient immerse his or her face in a large pan or basin of water and rapidly blink the affected eyelid. If only one eye is affected, take care to avoid contaminated water getting into the unaffected eye.

Irrigate the eye for at least 5 minutes. If the burn was caused by an alkali or a strong acid, irrigate the eye continuously for 20 minutes because these substances can penetrate deeply. One common possibility occurs where anhydrous ammonia is used during the process of cooking methamphetamine. If the eyes are not irrigated promptly and efficiently, permanent damage is likely. Whenever you have to irrigate the eye(s), continue to irrigate the eye en route to the hospital if possible.

Irrigation with a sterile saline solution will frequently flush away loose, small foreign objects lying on the surface of the eye. Always flush from the nose side of the eye toward the outside to avoid flushing material into the other eye. After its removal, a foreign body will often leave a small abrasion on the surface of the conjunctiva, which leads to continued irritation; for this reason, you should transport the patient to the hospital for further assessment and treatment.

At the Scene

As soon as you cover both of the patient's eyes, he or she can no longer see. Therefore, you will have to serve as the patient's eyes, keeping him or her constantly reassured and oriented to your location and what you are doing.

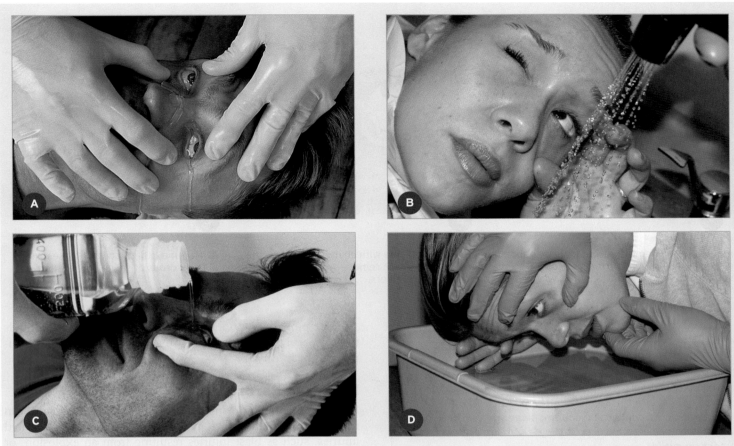

Figure 21-36 Four ways to effectively irrigate the eye: **A.** Nasal cannula. **B.** Shower. **C.** Bottle. **D.** Basin. Always protect the uninjured eye from the irrigating solution to prevent exposure to the substance.

Gentle irrigation usually will not wash out foreign bodies that are stuck to the cornea or lying under the upper eyelid. To examine the undersurface of the upper eyelid, pull the lid upward and forward. If you spot a foreign object on the surface of the eyelid, you may be able to remove it with a moist, sterile, cotton-tipped applicator. *Never attempt to remove a foreign body that is stuck or imbedded in the cornea.*

When a foreign body is impaled in the globe, *do not remove it!* Stabilise it in place. Cover the eye with a moist, sterile dressing; place a cup or other protective barrier over the object, and secure it in place with bulky dressing Figure 21-37 ▸ . Cover the unaffected eye to prevent further damage caused by sympathetic eye movement, and promptly transport the patient to the hospital.

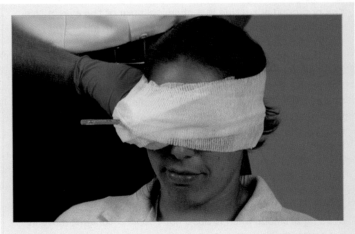

Figure 21-37 Securing an impaled object in the eye with a protective barrier and bulky dressing.

Ear Injuries

Injuries to the ear may be isolated, or they may occur in conjunction with other injuries to the head or face. Although isolated ear injuries are typically not life threatening, they can result in sensory impairment and permanent disfigurement.

Soft-Tissue Injuries

Lacerations, avulsions, and contusions to the external ear can occur following blunt or penetrating trauma. The pinna can be contused, lacerated, or partially or completely avulsed. Trauma to the earlobe can result in similar injuries.

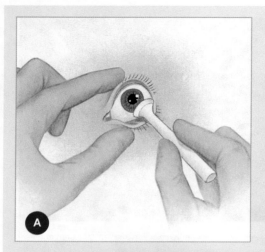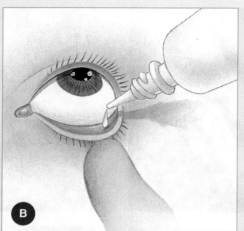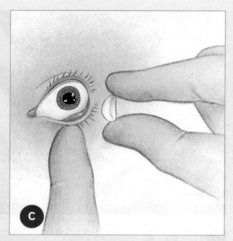

Figure 21-38 Removing contact lenses should be limited to patients with chemical burns to the eye. **A.** To remove hard contact lenses, use a specialised suction cup moistened with sterile saline solution. **B.** To remove soft contact lenses, instill 1 or 2 drops of saline or irrigating solution. **C.** Pinch off the lens with your gloved thumb and index fingers.

Special Considerations

Contact Lenses and Artificial Eyes

There are three types of contact lenses: hard, rigid gas-permeable, and soft (hydrophilic). Small, hard contact lenses usually are tinted, making them relatively easy to see. Large, soft contact lenses are clear and can be very difficult to see even more so if they "float" up or down under an eyelid.

In general, you should not attempt to remove contact lenses from a patient with an eye injury, lest you aggravate the injury. The only indication for removing contact lenses in the prehospital setting is a chemical burn of the eye. In this situation, the lens can trap the offending chemical and make irrigation difficult thus worsening the injury.

To remove a hard contact lens, use a small suction cup, moistening the end with saline (Figure 21-38A ▲). To remove soft lenses, place one to two drops of saline in the eye (Figure 21-38B ▲), gently pinch the lens between your gloved thumb and index finger, and lift it off the surface of the eye (Figure 21-38C ▲). Place the contact lens in a container with sterile saline solution. Always advise emergency department staff if a patient is wearing contact lenses.

Occasionally, you may care for a patient who is wearing an eye prosthesis (artificial eye). You should suspect an eye of being artificial when it does not respond to light, move in concert with the opposite eye, or appear quite the same as the opposite eye. If you are unsure as to whether the patient has an eye prosthesis, ask him or her. Although no harm will be done if you care for an artificial eye as you would a normal one, you need to be totally clear about the patient's eye function. In addition, it can be quite embarrassing to pass on information during your radio report that the patient has a nonreactive pupil only to find out at the A&E department that the patient has a prosthetic eye.

The pinna has an inherently poor blood supply, so it tends to heal poorly. Healing of the cartilaginous pinna is often complicated by infection.

Ruptured Eardrum

Perforation of the tympanic membrane (ruptured eardrum) can result from foreign bodies in the ear or from pressure-related injuries, such as blast injuries resulting from an explosion, or diving-related injuries that result in barotrauma to the ear. Signs and symptoms of a perforated tympanic membrane include loss of hearing and blood drainage from the ear. Although the injury is extremely painful for the patient, the tympanic membrane typically heals spontaneously and without complication. Nevertheless, a careful assessment should be performed to detect and treat other injuries, some of which may be life threatening.

▮ Assessment and Management of Ear Injuries

Assessment and management of the patient with an ear injury begins by ensuring airway patency and breathing adequacy. If the mechanism of injury suggests a potential for spinal injury, apply full spinal motion restriction precautions.

An adequate assessment of the external ear canal and middle ear cannot be performed out of hospital. In general, the ears' poor blood supply limits the amount of external bleeding. If manual direct pressure does not control this bleeding, first place a soft, padded dressing between the ear and the scalp since bandaging the ear against the tender scalp can be extremely painful. Then apply a roller bandage to secure the dressing in place (Figure 21-39 ▶). An icepack can also help reduce swelling and pain.

If the pinna is partially avulsed, carefully realign the ear into position and gently bandage it with sufficient padding that has been slightly moistened with normal saline. If the pinna is completely avulsed, attempt to retrieve the avulsed part, if possible, for reimplantation at the hospital. If the detached part of the ear is recovered, treat it as any other amputation; wrap it in saline-moistened gauze, place it in a plastic bag, and place the bag on ice. If a chemical icepack is used, it is recommended to shield the avulsed part with several 10 cm × 10 cm gauze pads to diffuse the cold, as chemical icepacks are actually colder than ice and inadvertent freezing of the part can occur. Better to use a cool pack.

If blood or CSF drainage is noted, apply a loose dressing over the ear—taking care *not* to stop the flow—and assess the patient for other signs of a basilar skull fracture.

Do not remove an impaled object from the ear. Instead, stabilise the object and cover the ear to prevent gross movement and minimise the risk of contamination of the inner ear.

Because isolated ear injuries are typically not life threatening, you must perform a careful assessment to detect or rule out potentially more serious injuries. You may then proceed with specific care of the ear, provide emotional support, and transport the patient to an appropriate medical facility.

Oral and Dental Injuries

Oral and dental injuries are commonly associated with trauma to the face. Blunt mechanisms are commonly the result of road traffic collisions or direct blows to the mouth or chin. Penetrating mechanisms are commonly the result of lacerations, and puncture wounds.

The primary risk associated with oral and dental injuries is airway compromise from oropharyngeal bleeding, occlusion by a displaced dental appliance such as a bridge or partial plate, or possibly by the aspiration of avulsed or fractured teeth. Any patient with significant facial trauma should be carefully assessed for injuries to the mouth and teeth.

Soft-Tissue Injuries

Lacerations and avulsions in and around the mouth are associated with a risk of intraoral haemorrhage and subsequent airway compromise. Therefore, your assessment of any patient with facial trauma should include a careful examination of the mouth, including the teeth. Fractured or avulsed teeth and lacerations of the tongue may cause profuse bleeding into the upper airway Figure 21-40 . A conscious patient with severe oral bleeding is often unable to speak unless he or she is leaning forward—this position facilitates drainage of blood from the mouth.

Patients may swallow blood from lacerations inside the mouth, so the bleeding may not be grossly evident. Because blood irritates the gastric lining, the risks of vomiting and aspiration are significant. Objects that are impaled in or through

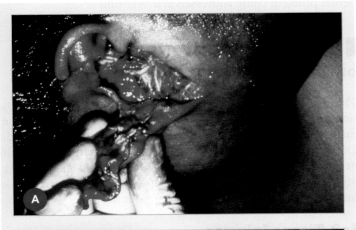

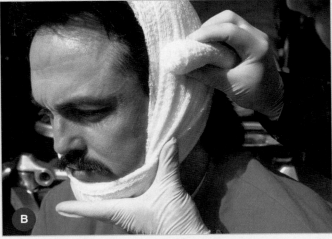

Figure 21-39 A. A major laceration of the ear. **B.** Place a soft, sterile pad behind the ear, between it and the scalp. Then wrap a roller gauze bandage around the head to include the entire ear.

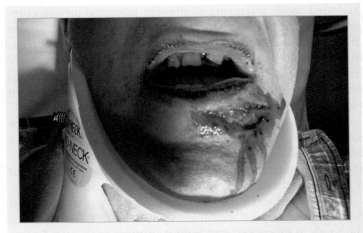

Figure 21-40 Soft-tissue injuries around the mouth can be associated with profuse oral bleeding and airway compromise.

the soft tissues of the mouth (such as the cheek) can also result in profuse bleeding and once again, the threat of vomiting with aspiration.

Dental Injuries

Fractured and avulsed teeth—especially the anterior teeth—are common following facial trauma. Dental injuries may be associated with mechanisms that cause severe maxillofacial trauma (such as road traffic collisions), or they may occur in isolation (such as a direct blow to the mouth from an assault).

You should always assess the patient's mouth following a facial injury, especially in cases of fractured or avulsed teeth. Teeth fragments (or even whole teeth) can become an airway obstruction and should be removed from the patient's mouth immediately.

At the Scene

When assessing a patient with fractured or avulsed teeth following an assault, you should also assess the individual who struck the patient, if it is safe to do so. The human mouth is filled with bacteria and other microorganisms, and lacerations to the person's hands or knuckles can easily become infected without proper care.

Assessment and Management of Oral and Dental Injuries

Ensuring airway patency and adequate breathing are the priorities of care when managing patients with oral or dental trauma. Suction the oropharynx as needed, and remove fractured tooth fragments to prevent potential airway compromise. Apply spinal motion restriction precautions as dictated by the mechanism of injury. If profuse oral bleeding is present and the patient cannot spontaneously control his or her own airway (such as with a decreased level of consciousness), pharmacologically assisted intubation (such as RSI) may be necessary.

Impaled objects in the soft tissues of the mouth should be stabilised in place unless they interfere with the patient's breathing or your ability to manage the patient's airway. In those cases, remove the impaled object from the direction that it entered, and control bleeding with direct pressure.

An avulsed tooth may be successfully reimplanted even if it has been out of the mouth for up to 1 hour. Carefully place the tooth in its socket, and hold it in place with your fingers or have the patient gently bite down **Table 21-2 ▶**.

Table 21-2	Care for an Avulsed Tooth

- Handle the tooth by the crown only. Avoid touching the root surface of the tooth.
- Gently rinse the tooth with sterile saline or water. Avoid the use of soap or chemicals, and do not scrub the tooth!
- Do not allow the tooth to dry. Place it in one of the following:
  - A break-resistant storage container with soft inner walls and a pH-balanced solution that nourishes and preserves the tooth
  - Cold whole milk
  - Sterile saline solution (for storage periods of less than 1 hour)
- Transport the tooth with the patient, and notify the hospital of the situation.

Retrieval and reimplantation or storage of an avulsed tooth is a low priority if the patient is in a clinically unstable condition (such as compromised airway or shock). In such cases, aggressive airway management, spinal precautions, and rapid transport of the patient are obviously more important with the dental problem being addressed at a later time.

Injuries to the Anterior Part of the Neck

The neck is a very vulnerable stretch of anatomy because it houses a critical portion of the airway (ie, larynx, trachea), the major blood vessels to and from the head, and the spinal cord. Other structures contained within the neck that are also vulnerable to injury include muscles, nerves, and glands. Any injury to the anterior part of the neck—blunt or penetrating—must be considered critical until proved otherwise.

Soft-Tissue Injuries

Blunt and penetrating mechanisms can damage the soft tissues of the anterior part of the neck and its associated structures. In both cases, you must be alert for the possibility of cervical spine injury and airway compromise.

Common mechanisms of blunt trauma include road traffic collisions, direct trauma to the neck, and hangings. Such injury often results in swelling and oedema; injury to the various structures such as the trachea, larynx, or oesophagus; or injury to the cervical spine. Less commonly, blunt injuries may damage the vasculature of the anterior part of the neck. Because blunt trauma to the neck is associated with a high incidence of airway compromise and ventilatory inadequacy, you must carefully assess the patient and be prepared to initiate aggressive management.

Common mechanisms of penetrating trauma include stabbings and impaled objects. The lacerations or puncture wounds produced may be superficial and involve only the fas-

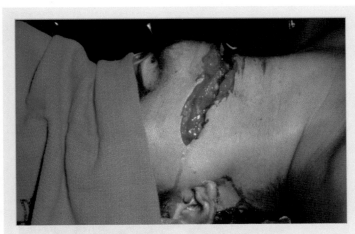

Figure 21-41 Open injuries to the neck can be very dangerous. If veins are exposed to the environment, they can suck in air, resulting in a potentially fatal air embolism.

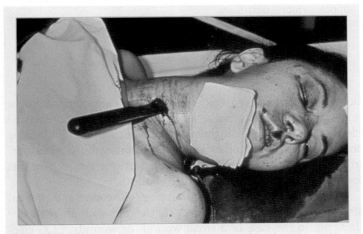

Figure 21-42 Impaled objects in the neck can cause profuse bleeding, if the major blood vessels are damaged, and direct injury to the larynx, trachea, oesophagus, or cervical spine.

cia or fatty tissues of the neck, or they may be deep and involve injury to the larynx, trachea, oesophagus, nerves, or major blood vessels. The primary threats from penetrating neck trauma are massive haemorrhage from major blood vessel disruption and airway compromise secondary to soft-tissue swelling or direct damage to the larynx or trachea.

A special danger associated with open neck injuries is the possibility of a fatal air embolism. If the jugular veins of the neck are exposed to the environment, they may entrain air into the vessel and occlude the flow of blood to the lungs **Figure 21-41 ▲**. As such, open neck wounds should be sealed with an occlusive dressing immediately.

Impaled objects in the neck can present several life-threatening problems for the patient—namely, injury to major blood vessels with massive haemorrhage; damage to the larynx, trachea, or oesophagus; or injury to the cervical spine **Figure 21-42 ▲**. Impaled objects should not be removed but

rather stabilised in place and protected from movement. The *only* exception is if the object is obstructing the airway or impeding your ability to effectively manage the airway. In some cases, an emergency cricothyroidotomy may be necessary to establish and maintain airway patency.

Injuries to the Larynx, Trachea, and Oesophagus

A variety of life-threatening injuries can result if the structures of the anterior part of the neck are crushed against the cervical spine following blunt trauma or if they are penetrated by a knife or similar object. The larynx and its supporting structures (ie, hyoid bone, thyroid cartilage) may be fractured, the trachea may be separated from the larynx (tracheal transection), or the oesophagus may be perforated. Many injuries to the larynx, trachea, and oesophagus are occult; because they are not as obvious and dramatic as penetrating neck injuries, they can be easily overlooked. Therefore, you must maintain a high index of suspicion and perform a careful assessment of *any* patient with blunt trauma to the anterior part of the neck.

Significant injuries to the larynx or trachea pose an *immediate* risk of airway compromise due to disruption of the normal passage of air, soft-tissue swelling, or aspiration of blood into the lungs. In addition, oesophageal perforation can result in mediastinitis, an inflammation of the mediastinum often due to leakage of gastric contents into the thoracic cavity. Mediastinitis is associated with a high mortality rate if not surgically repaired in a timely manner.

At the Scene

Any force that is powerful enough to disrupt the larynx, trachea, or oesophagus is powerful enough to injure the cervical spine, so the use of spinal motion restriction precautions is important. Carefully assess the patient for signs of a spinal injury: vertebral deformities (step-offs), paralysis, paresthesia, and signs of neurogenic shock (hypotension, normal or slow heart rate, lack of diaphoresis). Even a grunt or groan, or withdrawal by the patient during palpation, should be assumed to be a positive finding; therefore, spinal motion restriction precautions should be implemented.

Patients with injuries to the anterior part of the neck may experience concomitant maxillofacial fractures, which can make bag-valve-mask ventilation difficult (usually because of an inadequate mask-to-face seal). Likewise, endotracheal intubation may be extremely challenging, if not impossible, owing to distortion of the normal anatomical structures of the upper airway. If basic and advanced techniques to secure the patient's airway are unsuccessful or impossible, a surgical or needle cricothyroidotomy may be your only means of establishing a patent airway and ensuring adequate oxygenation and ventilation. Prior to deciding to perform a surgical airway, use of a gum elastic bougie may get the airway secured in a timely fashion while avoiding more risky procedures.

Assessment and Management of Injuries to the Anterior Part of the Neck

Begin your assessment by noting the mechanism of injury and maintaining a high index of suspicion, especially if the patient has experienced blunt or penetrating trauma between the upper part of the chest and head. Fractures of the first rib are associated with close to 50% mortality, not because of the rib fracture, but because the force it takes to fracture such a short, stout bone takes so much force that significant face, head, and neck trauma are almost always present as well. Remember that obvious and dramatic-appearing soft-tissue injuries may mask occult injuries to the larynx, trachea, or oesophagus. Also, the patient may have experienced trauma to multiple body systems, especially following a significant mechanism of injury.

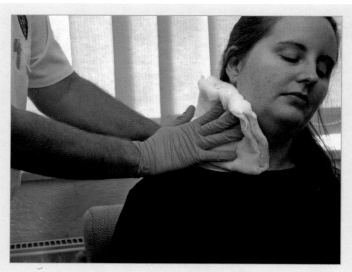

Figure 21-43 Cover open neck wounds with an occlusive dressing, and apply manual pressure to control bleeding. Do not compress both carotid arteries simultaneously because this may impair cerebral perfusion.

At the Scene

On any 999 call, ensure that the scene is safe before entering it. If the patient's injury is the result of an assault, be aware that the assailant may still be present. Check with ambulance control that police are on the scene, and do not enter the scene until they state that it is safe to do so.

As you begin your initial assessment, manually stabilise the patient's head in a neutral in-line position and simultaneously open the airway with the jaw-thrust manoeuvre if the patient has a reduced level of consciousness. Use suction as needed to clear the airway of blood or other liquids. Assess the patient's breathing—rate, regularity, and depth—and intervene immediately. If the patient is breathing adequately, apply a nonrebreathing mask at 15 l/min. If breathing is inadequate (ie, reduced tidal volume, fast or slow respirations), assist with bag-valve-mask ventilation and supplemental oxygen.

Your primary focus is always treating the injuries that will be the *most rapidly fatal*. Because death following trauma to the anterior part of the neck is usually the result of airway compromise or massive bleeding, aggressive airway management and external bleeding control are the highest priorities of care. After addressing any life-threatening or other serious problems with the ABCs during the initial assessment, you may perform a rapid trauma assessment to detect and treat other injuries.

To control bleeding from an open neck wound and prevent air embolism, immediately cover the wound with an occlusive dressing. In the case of a small wound, or wounds, ECG electrodes can be fast and effective ways to seal a small hole or holes. Apply manual direct pressure over the occlusive dressing with a bulky dressing. As a last resort, you can secure a pressure dressing over the wound by wrapping roller gauze loosely around the neck and then firmly through the opposite axilla 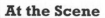 . *Do not* circumferentially wrap bandages around the neck to secure the dressing in place. This is contraindicated and could even be fatal, because they may impair cerebral perfusion by occluding both carotid arteries or interfere with the patient's breathing. Monitor the patient's pulse for reflex bradycardia, which indicates parasympathetic nervous stimulation due to excessive pressure on the carotid artery.

Bruising, redness to the overlying skin, and palpable tenderness are common signs associated with all injuries to the anterior part of the neck. **Table 21-3 ►** summarises the signs and symptoms of specific injuries.

If signs of shock are present, keep the patient warm, establish vascular access with at least one large-bore IV en route to the hospital if possible, or on-scene if indicated and infuse an isotonic crystalloid solution (such as Hartmann's or normal saline) as needed to maintain adequate perfusion.

At the Scene

Never use a flow-restricted, oxygen-powered ventilation device (ie, a manually triggered ventilator) on a patient with trauma to the anterior part of the neck and signs of laryngeal or tracheal injury. The high pressure delivered by such devices can cause barotrauma and potentially exacerbate the patient's injury. If ventilatory support is necessary, use bag-valve-mask ventilation.

Table 21-3	Signs and Symptoms of Injuries to the Anterior Part of the Neck
Injury	**Signs and Symptoms**
Laryngeal fracture, tracheal transection	• Laboured breathing or reduced air movement • Stridor • Hoarseness, voice changes • Haemoptysis (coughing up blood) • Subcutaneous emphysema • Swelling, oedema
Vascular injury	• Gross external bleeding • Signs of shock • Haematoma, swelling, oedema • Pulse deficits
Oesophageal perforation	• Dysphagia (difficulty swallowing) • Haematemesis • Haemoptysis (suggests aspiration of blood)
Neurological impairment	• Signs of a stroke (suggests air embolism or cerebral infarct) • Paralysis or paraesthesia • Cranial nerve deficit • Signs of neurogenic shock

If the patient has experienced an open tracheal wound, you may be able to pass a cuffed ET tube directly through the wound to establish a patent airway. Use caution, however: The trachea may be perforated anteriorly *and* posteriorly, which would increase the risk of false passage of the ET tube outside the trachea. It is critical to use *multiple* techniques for confirming correct tube placement: frequently monitor breath sounds, use capnometry, assess for adequate chest rise, and assess for vapour mist in the ET tube during exhalation.

Controversies

Some clinicians advocate aiming for air bubbles, which indicate the *general location* of the glottis, when attempting to intubate a patient with a head, face, or neck injury and severe oropharyngeal bleeding. While this practice is dangerous, it can also be both practical and potentially the best approach! A common mechanism that might require this tactic is a failed suicide with a shotgun. As the patient attempts to pull the trigger with the toe, the gun shifts slightly and subsequent physical devastation to the front of the face, though not fatal, results in significant bleeding along with difficult airway management challenges. Whenever possible, suction the airway as needed to facilitate an adequate view of the vocal cords. If this is unsuccessful, you should consider performing a cricothyroidotomy without delay if the "tube the bubbles" approach doesn't work or doesn't seem practical.

Head Injuries

A head injury is a traumatic insult to the head that may result in injury to soft tissue, bony structures, or the brain. More than 50% of all traumatic deaths result from a head injury. When head injuries are fatal, the cause is invariably associated injury to the brain.

Road traffic collisions are the most common cause of injury, with more than two thirds of people involved in such collisions experiencing a head injury. Head injuries also occur commonly in victims of assault, when elderly people fall, during sports-related incidents, and in a variety of incidents involving children.

There are two general types of head injuries: open and closed. A closed head injury (the most common type) is usually associated with blunt trauma. Although the dura mater remains

You are the Paramedic Part 4

You apply full spinal motion restriction precautions and quickly load the patient into the ambulance. You and your colleague agree that the patient should be intubated as he has lost his gag reflex and is not responsive. Subsequently, the ET tube is successfully placed and confirmed by auscultation.

Reassessment	Recording Time: 10 Minutes
Level of consciousness	Glasgow Coma Scale score of 3
Respirations	Intubated and ventilated at a rate of 10 breaths/min
Pulse	70 beats/min; regular and bounding
Skin	Warm and dry
Blood pressure	160/100 mm Hg
SpO_2	98% (intubated and ventilated with oxygen at 15 l/min)

7. What do the patient's vital signs indicate?
8. What else should you assess for in this patient?

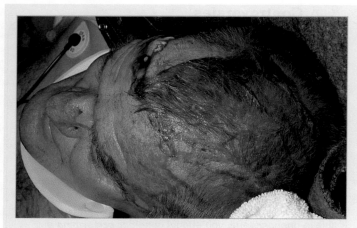

Figure 21-44 The scalp has a rich blood supply, so even small lacerations can lead to significant blood loss.

intact and brain tissue is not exposed to the environment, closed head injuries may result in skull fractures, focal brain injuries, or diffuse brain injuries. Furthermore, these injuries are often complicated by increased ICP.

With an open head injury, the dura mater and cranial contents are penetrated, and brain tissue is open to the environment. Gunshot wounds have a high mortality rate, and for those who survive there is almost always significant neurological impairment and a decreased quality of life.

Scalp Lacerations

Scalp lacerations can be minor or very serious. Because of the scalp's rich blood supply, even small lacerations can quickly lead to significant blood loss (**Figure 21-44 ▲**). Hypovolaemic shock in adults is rarely caused by scalp lacerations alone; this is more common in children. However, bleeding from the scalp can contribute to hypovolaemia in any patient, especially one with multiple injuries. In addition, because scalp lacerations usually result from direct blows to the head, they often indicate deeper, more severe injuries.

Skull Fractures

Four types of skull fractures are distinguished: linear, depressed, basilar, and open (**Figure 21-45 ▶**). The significance of a skull fracture is directly related to the type of fracture, the amount of force applied, and the area of the head that suffered the blow. Skull fractures are most commonly seen following road traffic collisions and significant falls. They may or may not be associated

with soft-tissue scalp injuries. Potential complications of any skull fracture include intracranial haemorrhage, cerebral damage, and cranial nerve damage, among others.

Linear Skull Fractures

Linear skull fractures (nondisplaced skull fractures) account for approximately 80% of all fractures to the skull; approximately 50% of linear fractures occur in the temporal-parietal region of the skull (see Figure 21-45A). Radiographic evaluation is required to diagnose a linear skull fracture because there are often no gross physical signs (such as deformity, depression). If the brain is uninjured and the scalp is intact, linear fractures are relatively benign. However, if a scalp laceration occurs in conjunction with a linear fracture—making it an open fracture—there is a risk of infection. In addition, if the fracture occurs over the temporal region of the skull, injury to the middle meningeal artery may result in extradural bleeding.

Depressed Skull Fractures

Depressed skull fractures result from high-energy direct trauma to a small surface area of the head with a blunt object (such as a baseball bat to the head) (see Figure 21-45B). The frontal and parietal regions of the skull are most susceptible to these types

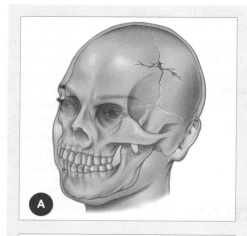
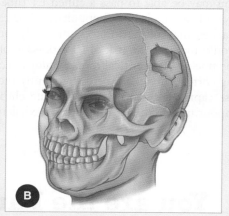
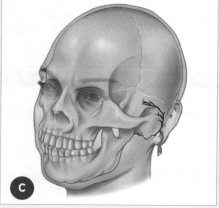
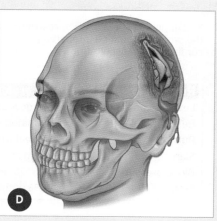

Figure 21-45 Types of skull fracture. **A.** Linear. **B.** Depressed. **C.** Basilar. **D.** Open.

of fractures because the bones in these areas, compared with other bones of the skull, are relatively thin. As a consequence, bony fragments may be driven into the brain, resulting in underlying injury. The overlying scalp may or may not be intact. Patients with depressed skull fractures often present with neurological signs (such as loss of consciousness).

Basilar Skull Fractures

Basilar skull fractures also are associated with high-energy trauma, but they usually occur following diffuse impact to the head (eg, falls, road traffic collisions). These injuries generally result from extension of a linear fracture to the base of the skull and can be difficult to diagnose with radiography (X-ray) (see Figure 21-45C).

Signs of a basilar skull fracture include CSF drainage from the ears **Figure 21-46 ▾**, which indicates rupture of the tympanic membrane and freely flowing CSF through the ear. Patients with leaking CSF are at risk for bacterial meningitis.

Other signs of a basilar skull fracture include periorbital bruising that develops under or around the eyes,

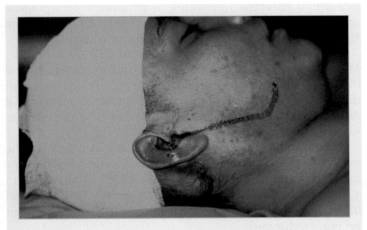

Figure 21-46 Blood draining from the ear after a head injury may contain CSF and suggests a basilar skull fracture.

which is also known as raccoon eyes **Figure 21-47A ▾**, or bruising behind the ear over the mastoid process known as Battle's sign **Figure 21-47B ▾**. Depending upon the extent of the damage, raccoon eyes and Battle's sign may appear relatively quickly, but in many cases, they may not appear until up to 24 hours following the injury, so their absence in the prehospital setting does not rule out a basilar skull fracture.

Open Skull Fractures

Open fractures of the cranial vault result when severe forces are applied to the head and are often associated with trauma to multiple body systems (see Figure 21-45D). Brain tissue may be exposed to the environment, which significantly increases the risk of a bacterial infection (such as bacterial meningitis). Open cranial vault fractures have a high mortality rate.

Traumatic Brain Injuries

The Medical Disability Society Working Party Report on the Management of Traumatic Brain Injury defines traumatic brain injury (TBI) as, 'Brain injury caused by trauma to the head (including the effects upon the brain of other possible complications of injury, notably hypoxaemia and hypotension, and intracerebral haematoma).' Traumatic brain injuries are classified into two broad categories: primary (direct) injury and secondary (indirect) injury. Primary brain injury is injury to the brain and its associated structures that results instantaneously from impact to the head. Secondary brain injury refers to the "after effects" of the primary injury; it includes abnormal processes such as cerebral oedema, intracranial haemorrhage, increased ICP, cerebral ischaemia and hypoxia, and infection. Secondary brain injury can occur anywhere from a few minutes to several days following the initial injury.

The brain can be injured directly by a penetrating object, such as a knife, bullet, or other sharp object. More commonly,

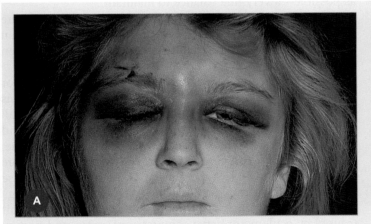
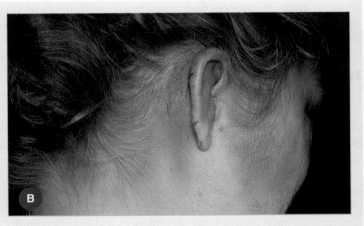

Figure 21-47 Suspect a basilar skull fracture if a head trauma patient has bruising. **A.** Bruising under or around the eyes (raccoon eyes). **B.** Bruising behind the ear over the mastoid process (Battle's sign).

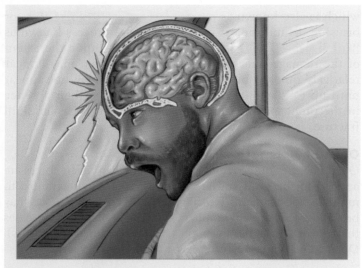

Figure 21-48 For the unrestrained victim in a road traffic collision, the brain continues its forward motion and strikes the inside of the skull, resulting in compression injury to the anterior portion of the brain and stretching of the posterior portion.

such injuries occur indirectly, as a result of external forces exerted on the skull. Consider the most common cause of brain injury, the road traffic collision. When the passenger's head hits the windscreen on impact with a fixed object, the brain continues to move forward until it comes to an abrupt stop by striking the inside of the skull. This rapid deceleration results in compression injury (or bruising) to the anterior portion of the brain along with stretching or tearing of the posterior portion of the brain (Figure 21-48 ▲). As the brain strikes the front of the skull, the body begins its path of moving backward. The head falls back against the headrest and/or seat, and the brain slams into the rear of the skull. This type of front-and-rear injury is known as a coup-contrecoup injury. The same type of injury may occur on opposite sides of the brain in a lateral collision.

The injured brain starts to swell, initially because of cerebral vasodilation. An increase in cerebral water (cerebral oedema) then contributes to further brain swelling. Cerebral oedema may not develop until several hours after the initial injury, however.

Intracranial Pressure

For adults the skull is a rigid, unyielding globe that allows little, if any, expansion of the intracranial contents. It also provides a hard and somewhat irregular surface against which brain tissue and its blood vessels can be injured when the head suffers trauma.

Accumulations of blood within the skull or swelling of the brain can rapidly lead to an increase in intracranial pressure (ICP), the pressure within the cranial vault. Increased ICP squeezes the brain against bony prominences within the cranium.

Normal ICP in adults ranges from 0 to 10 mm Hg. An increase in ICP (such as from cerebral oedema or intracranial

At the Scene

The brain accounts for 80% of the intracranial contents, the cerebral blood volume accounts for 12%, and the CSF volume accounts for the remaining 8%.

haemorrhage) decreases cerebral perfusion pressure and cerebral blood flow. Cerebral perfusion pressure (CPP), the pressure of blood flow through the brain, is the difference between the mean arterial pressure (MAP), the average (or mean) pressure against the arterial wall during a cardiac cycle, and ICP (CPP = MAP − ICP). Obviously, decreasing cerebral blood flow is a potential catastrophe because the brain depends on a constant supply of blood to furnish the oxygen and glucose it needs to survive.

The critical minimum threshold, or minimum CPP required to adequately perfuse the brain, is 60 mm Hg in the adult. A CPP of less than 60 mm Hg will lead to cerebral ischaemia, potentially resulting in permanent neurological impairment or even death. A *single* drop in CPP below 60 mm Hg *doubles* the brain-injured patient's chance of death!

The body responds to a decrease in CPP by increasing MAP, resulting in cerebral vasodilation and increased cerebral blood flow; this process is called autoregulation. However, an increase in cerebral blood flow causes a further increase in ICP. As ICP continues to increase, CSF is forced from the cranium into the spinal cord.

Clearly, the patient with increased ICP is caught in the midst of a vicious cycle. As ICP increases, cerebral blood flow increases secondary to autoregulation, which in turn leads to a potentially fatal increase in ICP. Conversely, if cerebral blood flow decreases, CPP decreases as well, and the brain becomes ischaemic.

CPP cannot be calculated in the prehospital setting. Therefore, prehospital treatment must focus on maintaining CPP (and cerebral blood flow), while mitigating ICP as much as possible—a very fine balance to maintain.

If increased ICP is not treated promptly in a definitive care setting, cerebral herniation may occur. In herniation, the brain is forced from the cranial vault, either through the foramen magnum or over the tentorium.

You must closely monitor the head-injured patient for signs and symptoms of increased ICP. The exact clinical signs encountered depend on the amount of pressure inside the skull and the extent of brain stem involvement. Early signs and symptoms include vomiting (often without nausea), headache, an altered level of consciousness, and convulsions. Later, more ominous signs include hypertension (with a widening pulse pressure), bradycardia, and irregular respirations (Cushing's triad), plus a unilaterally unequal and nonreactive pupil (caused by oculomotor nerve compression), coma, and posturing. Decorticate (flexor) posturing is characterised by flexion of the arms and extension of the legs; decerebrate (extensor) pos-

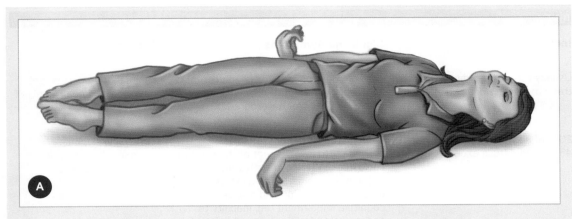

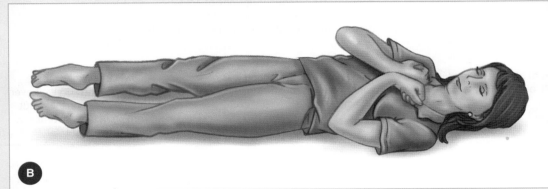

Figure 21-49 Posturing indicates significant ICP. **A.** Decerebrate (extensor) posturing. **B.** Decorticate (flexor) posturing. You can remember this by thinking of the arms being pulled into the "core" of the body.

Diffuse Axonal Injury

Diffuse axonal injury (DAI) is associated with or similar to a concussion. Unlike a concussion, however, this more severe diffuse brain injury is often associated with a poor prognosis. DAI involves stretching, shearing, or tearing of nerve fibres with subsequent axonal damage. An axon is a long, slender extension of a neurone (nerve cell) that conducts electrical impulses away from the neuroneal soma (cell body) in the brain.

DAI most often results from high-speed, rapid acceleration-deceleration forces (such as road traffic collisions, significant falls). The severity and, thus, the prognosis of DAI depends on the degree of axonal damage (ie, stretching versus shearing or tearing); DAI is classified as being mild, moderate, or severe Table 21-4 ▶ .

turing is characterised by extension of the arms and legs Figure 21-49 ▲ .

Diffuse Brain Injuries

Brain injuries are broadly classified as diffuse or focal. A diffuse brain injury is any injury that affects the entire brain. These injuries include cerebral concussion and diffuse axonal injury.

Cerebral Concussion

A cerebral concussion occurs when the brain is jarred around in the skull. This kind of mild diffuse brain injury is usually caused by rapid acceleration-deceleration forces (coup-contrecoup), such as those seen following road traffic collisions or falls.

A concussion injury results in transient dysfunction of the cerebral cortex; its resolution is usually spontaneous and rapid and is not associated with structural damage or permanent neurological impairment. Signs of a concussion range from transient confusion and disorientation to confusion that may last for several minutes. Loss of consciousness may or may not occur. Retrograde amnesia, a loss of memory relating to events that occurred before the injury, or anterograde (posttraumatic) amnesia, a loss of memory relating to events that occurred after the injury, may follow a concussion.

Focal Brain Injuries

A focal brain injury is a specific, grossly observable brain injury (ie, it can be seen on a CT scan). Such injuries include cerebral contusions and intracranial haemorrhage.

Cerebral Contusion

In a cerebral contusion, brain tissue is bruised and damaged in a local area. Because a cerebral contusion is associated with physical damage to the brain, greater neurological deficits (such as prolonged confusion, loss of consciousness) are more commonly observed than with a concussion. The same mechanisms of injury that cause concussions—acceleration-deceleration forces and direct blunt head trauma—also cause cerebral contusions.

The area of the brain most commonly affected by a cerebral contusion is the frontal lobe, although multiple areas of contusion can occur, especially following coup-contrecoup injuries. As with any bruise, the reaction of the injured tissue will be to swell. This swelling inevitably leads to increased ICP and the negative consequences that accompany it.

Intracranial Haemorrhage

The closed box of the skull has no extra room for accumulation of blood, so bleeding inside the skull also increases ICP. Bleeding can occur between the skull and dura mater, beneath the

Table 21-4	Diffuse Axonal Injury		
Pathophysiology	**Incidence**	**Signs and Symptoms**	**Prognosis**
Mild DAI			
Temporary neuroneal dysfunction; minimal axonal damage	Usually the result of blunt head trauma; concussion is an example	Loss of consciousness (brief, if present); confusion, disorientation, amnesia (retrograde and/or anterograde)	Minimal or no permanent neurological impairment
Moderate DAI			
Axonal damage and minute petechial bruising of brain tissue; often associated with a basilar skull fracture	20% of all severe head injuries; 45% of all diffuse axonal injuries	Immediate loss of consciousness: secondary to involvement of the cerebral cortex or the reticular activating system of the brain stem; Residual effects: persistent confusion and disorientation; cognitive impairment (eg, inability to concentrate); frequent periods of anxiety; uncharacteristic mood swings; sensory/motor deficits (such as altered sense of taste or smell)	Survival likely, but permanent neurological impairment common
Severe DAI			
Severe mechanical disruption of many axons in both cerebral hemispheres with extension into the brain stem; formerly called "brain stem injury"	16% of all severe head injuries; 36% of all diffuse axonal injuries	Immediate and prolonged loss of consciousness; posturing and other signs of increased ICP	Survival unlikely; most patients who survive never regain consciousness but remain in a persistent vegetative state

At the Scene

It is generally not possible, or necessary, to distinguish between a cerebral contusion and intracranial haemorrhage in the prehospital setting. Instead, you should recognise the signs of increasing ICP and appreciate that those signs represent a critically injured patient who needs immediate treatment and prompt transport to an appropriate facility.

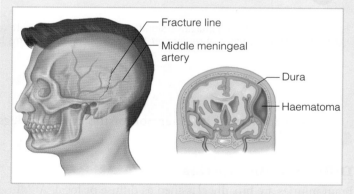

Figure 21-50 An extradural haematoma is usually the result of a blow to the head that produces a linear fracture of the temporal bone and damages the middle meningeal artery. Blood accumulates between the dura mater and the skull.

dura mater but outside the brain, within the parenchyma (tissue) of the brain itself (intracerebral space), or into the CSF (subarachnoid space).

Extradural Haematoma

An extradural haematoma is an accumulation of blood between the skull and dura mater; it occurs in approximately 0.5% to 1% of all head injuries Figure 21-50 ▸ . An extradural haematoma is nearly always the result of a blow to the head that produces a linear fracture of the thin temporal bone. The middle meningeal artery courses along a groove in that bone, so it is prone to disruption when the temporal bone is fractured. In such a case, brisk arterial bleeding into the extradural space will result in rapidly progressing symptoms.

Often, the patient loses consciousness immediately following the injury; this is often followed by a brief period of consciousness ("lucid interval"), after which the patient lapses back into unconsciousness. Meanwhile, as ICP increases, the oculomotor nerve (third cranial nerve) is compressed against the tentorium, and the pupil on the side of the haematoma becomes fixed and dilated. Death will follow very rapidly without surgery to evacuate the haematoma.

Subdural Haematoma

A subdural haematoma is an accumulation of blood beneath the dura mater but outside the brain Figure 21-51 ▸ . It usually occurs after falls or injuries involving strong deceleration forces and occurs in approximately 5% of all head injuries. Subdural haematomas are more common than extradural haematomas and may or may not be associated with a skull fracture. Bleeding within the subdural space typically results from rupture of the veins that bridge the cerebral cortex and dura.

A subdural haematoma is associated with venous bleeding, so this type of haematoma—and the signs of increased ICP—typically develops more gradually than with an extradural haematoma. The patient with a subdural haematoma often

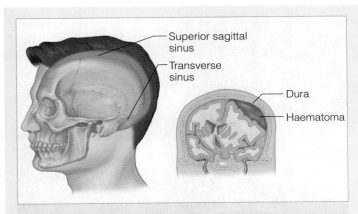

Figure 21-51 In a subdural haematoma, venous bleeding occurs beneath the dura mater but outside the brain.

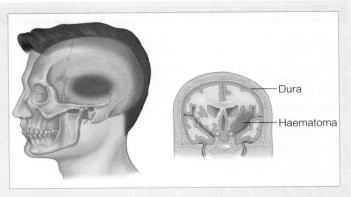

Figure 21-52 An intracerebral haematoma involves bleeding within the brain tissue itself.

experiences a fluctuating level of consciousness, focal neurological signs (such as unilateral hemiparesis), or slurred speech.

Subdural haematomas are classified as acute (clinical signs developing within 24 hours following injury) or chronic (symptoms may not appear for as long as 2 weeks). Chronic subdural haematomas are more common in elderly patients, patients with alcoholism, patients with bleeding diathesis (such as haemophilia), and patients taking anticoagulants (such as warfarin).

Intracerebral Haematoma

An intracerebral haematoma involves bleeding within the brain tissue itself **Figure 21-52 ▶**. This type of injury can occur following a penetrating injury to the head or because of rapid deceleration forces.

Many small, deep intracerebral haemorrhages are associated with other brain injuries, such as DAI. The progression of increased ICP and neurological deficit depends on several factors, including the presence of other brain injuries, the region of the brain involved (frontal and temporal lobes are most common), and the size of the haemorrhage. Once symptoms appear, the patient's condition often deteriorates quickly. Intracerebral haematomas have a high mortality rate, even if the haematoma is surgically evacuated.

Subarachnoid Haematoma

In a subarachnoid haematoma, bleeding occurs into the subarachnoid space, where the CSF circulates. It results in bloody CSF and signs of meningeal irritation (such as nuchal rigidity, headache). Common causes of a subarachnoid haematoma include trauma or rupture of an aneurysm or arteriovenous malformation.

The patient with a subarachnoid haematoma typically presents with a sudden, severe headache. This headache is often localised initially but later becomes diffuse secondary to increased meningeal irritation. As bleeding into the subarachnoid space increases, the patient experiences the signs and symptoms of increased ICP: decreased level of consciousness, pupillary changes, posturing, vomiting, and convulsions.

You are the Paramedic Part 5

Your patient's condition is clearly critical, so you ask another ambulance colleague from another vehicle to drive your ambulance to the A&E located approximately 5 miles away to free up your colleague to work in the back with you. En route, you establish two large-bore IV lines with normal saline running to keep vein open (TKVO) and apply the cardiac monitor. The patient's pupils are bilaterally dilated and sluggish to react.

Reassessment	Recording Time: 15 Minutes
Level of consciousness	Glasgow Coma Scale score of 3
Respirations	Intubated and ventilated at a rate of 10 breaths/min
Pulse	50 beats/min; regular and bounding
Skin	Warm and dry
Blood pressure	180/90 mm Hg
SpO₂	98% (intubated and ventilated with oxygen at 15 l/min)

9. Should this patient receive IV fluid boluses? When are IV fluid boluses indicated in a head-injured patient?

10. When is hyperventilation indicated for a head-injured patient? What ventilation rate defines hyperventilation in an adult?

Table 21-5	Signs and Symptoms of Head Injury

- Lacerations, contusions, or haematomas to the scalp
- Soft area or depression noted on palpation of the scalp
- Visible fractures or deformities of the skull
- Battle's sign or raccoon eyes
- CSF rhinorrhoea or otorrhoea
- Pupillary abnormalities
  - Unequal pupil size
  - Sluggish or nonreactive pupils
- A period of unresponsiveness
- Confusion or disorientation
- Repeatedly asking the same question(s) (perseveration)
- Amnesia (retrograde and/or anterograde)
- Combativeness or other abnormal behavior
- Numbness or tingling in the extremities
- Loss of sensation and/or motor function
- Focal neurological deficits
- Convulsions
- Cushing's triad: hypertension, bradycardia, and irregular or erratic respirations
- Dizziness
- Visual disturbances, blurred vision, or double vision (diplopia)
- Seeing "stars"
- Nausea or vomiting
- Posturing (decorticate and/or decerebrate)

At the Scene

Ensure that any scene is safe before you enter it, regardless of the nature of the call, and take appropriate universal precautions before making physical contact with the patient. Once patient care begins, you must remain constantly aware of your surroundings and appreciate the fact that even the most docile scene can quickly turn dangerous.

A sudden, severe subarachnoid haematoma usually results in death. People who survive often have permanent neurological impairment.

Assessment and Management of Head and Brain Injuries

Prehospital assessment and management of the head-injured patient should be guided by factors such as the severity of the injury and the patient's level of consciousness. As with any patient, your treatment priorities must be based on what will kill the patient *first*.

Assessment of Head and Brain Injuries

Road traffic collisions, direct blows, falls from heights, assault, and sports-related injuries are common causes of head and traumatic brain injuries. A patient who has experienced any of these events should immediately elevate your index of suspicion and prompt a search for signs and symptoms of these types of injuries Table 21-5 ▲ . A deformed windscreen or

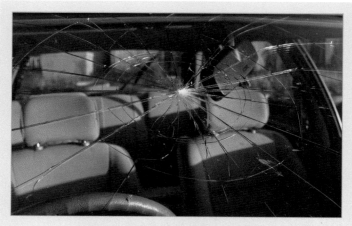

Figure 21-53 The classic "bulls-eye" on the windscreen after a road traffic collision is a significant indicator of injury. Be alert for the signs and symptoms of head and cervical spine injury.

dented or cracked helmet indicates a major blow to the head Figure 21-53 ▲ .

Level of Consciousness

A change in the level of consciousness is the single most important observation that you can make when assessing the severity of brain injury. The level of consciousness usually indicates the

Notes from Nancy

The most important single sign in the evaluation of a head-injured patient is a changing state of consciousness.

extent of brain dysfunction. Whenever you suspect a head injury, you should perform a baseline neurological assessment using the AVPU scale (Alert; responsive to Verbal stimuli; responsive to Pain; Unresponsive) and record the time.

Use the more detailed Glasgow Coma Scale (GCS) when performing serial neurological assessments of a head-injured patient Figure 21-54 ▶ . The GCS—a widely accepted method of assessing level of consciousness—is based on three independent measurements: eye opening, verbal response, and motor response. The GCS score is used to classify the severity of the patient's brain injury and is a reliable predictor of the brain-injured patient's outcome Table 21-6 ▶ .

Documentation and Communication

A single assessment of the patient's GCS score cannot reliably capture his or her clinical progression. Obtain a baseline GCS score and frequently (at least every 5 minutes if possible) reassess it in a head-injured patient. Document all GCS scores and the times they were obtained on the patient report form. The doctor will compare his or her neurological assessment with those you performed in the prehospital environment.

GLASGOW COMA SCALE

Eye Opening

Spontaneous	4
To Voice	3
To Pain	2
None	1

Verbal Response

Oriented	5
Confused	4
Inappropriate Words	3
Incomprehensible Words	2
None	1

Motor Response

Obeys Command	6
Localises Pain	5
Withdraws (pain)	4
Flexion (pain)	3
Extension (pain)	2
None	1
Glasgow Coma Score Total	**15**

Figure 21-54 Glasgow Coma Scale scores should be assessed frequently in head-injured patients. The lower the score, the more severe the extent of brain injury.

Table 21-6	Brain Injury Classification Based on the GCS

- **13 to 15.** Mild traumatic brain injury
- **8 to 12.** Moderate traumatic brain injury
- **3 to 8.** Severe traumatic brain injury

Pupillary Assessment

Frequently monitor the size, equality, and reactivity of the patient's pupils. The nerves that control dilation and constriction of the pupils are very sensitive to ICP. When you shine a pentorch into the eye, the pupil should briskly constrict. A pupil that is slow (sluggish) to constrict is a relatively early sign of increased ICP; a sluggish pupil could also indicate cerebral hypoxia. Unequal or bilaterally fixed and dilated ("blown") pupils are later, more ominous signs of increased ICP and indicate pressure on one or both oculomotor nerves 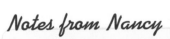 Figure 21-55 ▶.

Notes from Nancy

The most important aspect of neurological assessment is whether the patient's findings are changing and in what direction.

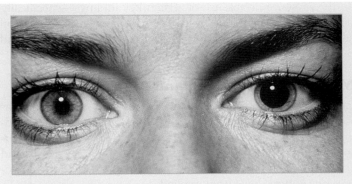

Figure 21-55 Unequal (shown above) or bilaterally fixed and dilated pupils in a head-injured patient are ominous signs and indicate a significantly increased ICP.

Table 21-7	Levels of ICP
Mild elevation	• Increased blood pressure; decreased pulse rate • Pupils still reactive • Cheyne-Stokes respirations (respirations that are fast and then become slow, with intervening periods of apnoea) • Patient initially attempts to localise and remove painful stimuli; this is followed by withdrawal and extension • Effects are reversible *with prompt treatment*
Moderate elevation	• Widened pulse pressure and bradycardia • Pupils are sluggish or nonreactive • Central neurogenic hyperventilation (deep, rapid respirations; similar to Kussmaul, but without an acetone breath odour) • Decerebrate posturing • Survival possible but not without permanent neurological impairment
Marked elevation	• Ipsilaterally fixed and dilated ("blown") pupil • Ataxic respirations (Biot respirations; characterised by irregular rate, pattern, and volume of breathing with intermittent periods of apnoea) or absent respirations • Flaccid paralysis • Irregular pulse rate • Changes in the QRS complex, ST segment, or T wave • Fluctuating blood pressure; hypotension common • Most patients do not survive this level of ICP

Assessing ICP

Although ICP cannot be quantified (assigned a numeric value) in the prehospital setting, the severity of increase can be estimated based on the patient's clinical presentation Table 21-7 ▲. Critical treatment decisions for brain-injured patients are based on the presence or absence of certain key findings—specifically, posturing, hypotension or hypertension, and abnormal pupil signs. Use serial assessments of the patient's GCS scores and pupillary assessment as indicators of the progression of ICP.

Management of Head and Brain Injuries

Patients with head injuries often have cervical spine injuries as well. Therefore, as you begin your initial assessment of a head-injured patient, manually stabilise the cervical spine in a neutral, in-line position. Avoid moving the neck unnecessarily, and continue manual stabilisation until full spinal motion restriction precautions have been applied.

Managing Airway and Breathing

The most important step in the treatment of any type of head injury is to establish and maintain a patent airway. Open the airway with the jaw-thrust manoeuvre if the patient has a reduced level of consciousness or is otherwise unable to maintain his or her own airway spontaneously.

Patients with a head injury often vomit (especially children). Therefore, after opening the airway, you must be prepared to roll the patient to the side—while maintaining spinal stabilisation—to prevent aspiration. If it is safe to do so, manually remove any large debris from the patient's mouth by sweeping the oropharynx with your freshly gloved finger. Use suction to clear secretions, such as blood or thin secretions from the oropharynx. *Mortality increases significantly if aspiration occurs.*

If the patient has a decreased level of consciousness, insert a basic airway adjunct (ie, oral or nasal airway). *Do not insert a nasal airway if CSF or bloody rhinorrhoea is present or if you suspect a nasal fracture.*

After you have cleared the airway, assess the patient's ventilatory status. Cerebral oedema and ICP are aggravated by hypoxia and hypercarbia; therefore, you must constantly ensure adequate oxygenation and ventilation in any patient with a head injury.

Administer 100% oxygen via nonrebreathing mask if the patient is breathing adequately (ie, adequate rate and depth [tidal volume], regular respiratory pattern). An injured brain is even less tolerant of hypoxia than a healthy one, and research has demonstrated that prompt administration of supplemental oxygen can reduce the amount of brain damage and improve neurological outcome.

If the respiratory centre of the brain (pons, medulla) has been injured, the rate, depth, or regularity of breathing may be ineffective. Ventilation may also be impaired by concomitant chest injuries or, if the spinal cord is injured, by paralysis of some or all of the respiratory muscles. Patients with inadequate ventilation, especially if associated with a decreased level of consciousness, should receive bag-valve-mask ventilation and supplemental oxygen. Ventilate a brain-injured adult at a rate of 10 breaths/min or as dictated by local protocols. *Avoid routine hyperventilation of brain-injured patients.* Although hyperventilation causes cerebral vasoconstriction, which will shunt blood from the cranium and lower ICP, this outcome will merely provide additional room for the injured brain to swell or for more blood to accumulate in the skull. Most importantly, cerebral vasoconstriction shunts oxygen away from the brain, resulting in a drop in CPP and bringing on cerebral ischaemia. Hyperventilation (20 breaths/min for adults) is recommended *only* if signs of cerebral herniation are present ▐ **Table 21-8 ▾** ▌. In such brain-injured patients, brief periods of hyperventilation may be beneficial. If available, end-tidal carbon dioxide

Table 21-8	Signs of Cerebral Herniation

Unresponsive patient with both of the following:

- Asymmetric (unequal) pupils *or* bilaterally fixed and dilated pupils
- Decerebrate (extensor) posturing *or* no motor response to painful stimuli

You are the Paramedic Part 6

Your estimated time of arrival at A&E is 5 minutes. Without time to perform a detailed physical examination, you reassess the patient's vital functions and make an ASHICE call to the hospital.

Reassessment	Recording Time: 20 Minutes
Level of consciousness	Glasgow Coma Scale score of 3
Respirations	Intubated and ventilated at a rate of 10 breaths/min
Pulse	70 beats/min; regular and bounding
Skin	Warm and dry
Blood pressure	170/80 mm Hg
SpO_2	98% (intubated and ventilated with oxygen at 15 l/min)

11. Should you be concerned with the exact aetiology of this patient's head injury? Why or why not?

12. What are the most important interventions you can perform to maintain cerebral perfusion in this patient?

cerebral contusion A focal brain injury in which brain tissue is bruised and damaged in a defined area.

cerebral cortex The largest portion of the cerebrum; regulates voluntary skeletal movement and one's level of awareness—a part of consciousness.

cerebral oedema Cerebral water; causes or contributes to swelling of the brain.

cerebral perfusion pressure (CPP) The pressure of blood flow through the brain; the difference between the mean arterial pressure (MAP) and intracranial pressure (ICP).

cerebrospinal fluid (CSF) Fluid produced in the ventricles of the brain that flows in the subarachnoid space and bathes the meninges.

cerebrospinal rhinorrhoea Cerebrospinal fluid drainage from the nose.

cerebrum The largest portion of the brain; responsible for higher functions, such as reasoning; divided into right and left hemispheres, or halves.

Cheyne-Stokes respirations The respirations that are fast and then become slow, with intervening periods of apnoea; commonly seen following brain stem injury.

choroid plexus Specialised cells within the hollow areas in the ventricles of the brain that produce CSF.

cochlea The shell-shaped structure within the inner ear that contains the organ of Corti.

cochlear duct A canal within the cochlea that receives vibrations from the ossicles.

conjunctiva A thin, transparent membrane that covers the sclera and internal surfaces of the eyelids.

conjunctivitis An inflammation of the conjunctivae that usually is caused by bacteria, viruses, allergies, or foreign bodies; should be considered highly contagious; also called pink eye.

cornea The transparent anterior portion of the eye that overlies the iris and pupil.

coronal suture The point where the parietal bones join with the frontal bone.

coup-contrecoup injury Dual impacting of the brain into the skull; coup injury occurs at the point of impact; contrecoup injury occurs on the opposite side of impact, as the brain rebounds.

cranial vault The bones that encase and protect the brain, including the parietal, temporal, frontal, occipital, sphenoid, and ethmoid bones; also called the cranium or skull.

craniofacial disjunction A Le Fort III fracture; involves a fracture of all of the midfacial bones, thus separating the entire midface from the cranium.

cribriform plate A horizontal bone perforated with numerous foramina for the passage of the olfactory nerve filaments from the nasal cavity.

crista galli A prominent bony ridge in the centre of the anterior fossa and the point of attachment of the meninges.

critical minimum threshold Minimum cerebral perfusion pressure required to adequately perfuse the brain; 60 mm Hg in the adult.

crown The part of the tooth that is external to the gum.

Cushing's triad Hypertension (with a widening pulse pressure), bradycardia, and irregular respirations; classic trio of findings associated with increased ICP.

cusps Points at the top of a tooth.

decerebrate (extensor) posturing Abnormal posture characterised by extension of the arms and legs; indicates pressure on the brain stem.

decorticate (flexor) posturing Abnormal posture characterised by flexion of the arms and extension of the legs; indicates pressure on the brain stem.

dentine The principal mass of the tooth, which is made up of a material that is much more dense and stronger than bone.

depressed skull fractures Result from high-energy direct trauma to a small surface area of the head with a blunt object (such as a baseball bat to the head); commonly result in bony fragments being driven into the brain, causing injury.

diencephalon The part of the brain between the brain stem and the cerebrum that includes the thalamus, subthalamus, and hypothalamus.

diffuse axonal injury (DAI) Diffuse brain injury that is caused by stretching, shearing, or tearing of nerve fibres with subsequent axonal damage.

diffuse brain injury Any injury that affects the entire brain.

diplopia Double vision.

dura mater The outermost layer of the three meninges that enclose the brain and spinal cord; it is the toughest meningeal layer.

dysconjugate gaze Paralysis of gaze or lack of coordination between the movements of the two eyes.

dysphagia Difficulty swallowing.

epistaxis Nosebleed.

external auditory canal The area in which sound waves are received from the auricle (pinna) before they travel to the eardrum; also called the ear canal.

external ear One of three anatomical parts of the ear; it contains the pinna, the ear canal, and the external portion of the tympanic membrane.

extradural haematoma An accumulation of blood between the skull and dura.

facial nerve The seventh cranial nerve; supplies motor activity to all muscles of facial expression, the sense of taste, and anterior two thirds of the tongue and cutaneous sensation to the external ear, tongue, and palate.

focal brain injury A specific, grossly observable brain injury.

fontanelles The soft spots in the skull of a newborn and infant where the sutures of the skull have not yet grown together.

foramen magnum The large opening at the base of the skull through which the spinal cord exits the brain.

foramina Small natural openings, perforations, or orifices, such as in the bones of the cranial vault; plural of foramen.

frontal lobe The portion of the brain that is important in voluntary motor actions and personality traits.

galea aponeurotica Tough, tendinous layer of the scalp.

Glasgow Coma Scale (GCS) A widely accepted method of assessing level of consciousness that is based on three independent measurements: eye opening, verbal response, and motor response.

globe The eyeball.

glossopharyngeal nerve Ninth cranial nerve; supplies motor fibres to the pharyngeal muscle, providing taste sensation to the posterior portion of the tongue, and carrying parasympathetic fibres to the parotid gland.

haemoptysis Coughing up blood.

hard palate The bony anterior part of the palate, which forms the roof of the mouth.

head injury A traumatic insult to the head that may result in injury to soft tissue, bony structures, or the brain.

herniation Process in which tissue is forced out of its normal position, such as when the brain is forced from the cranial vault, either through the foramen magnum or over the tentorium.

hyoid bone A bone at the base of the tongue that supports the tongue and its muscles.

hyperpyrexia A very high body temperature.

hyphaema Bleeding into the anterior chamber of the eye; results from direct ocular trauma.

hypoglossal nerve Twelfth cranial nerve; provides motor function to the muscles of the tongue and throat.

hypothalamus The most inferior portion of the diencephalon; responsible for control of many body functions, including heart rate, digestion, sexual development, temperature regulation, emotion, hunger, thirst, and regulation of the sleep cycle.

inner ear One of three anatomical parts of the ear; it consists of the cochlea and semicircular canals.

intracerebral haematoma Bleeding within the brain tissue (parenchyma) itself; also referred to as an intraparenchymal haematoma.

intracranial pressure (ICP) The pressure within the cranial vault; normally 0 to 10 mm Hg in adults.

iris The coloured portion of the eye.

lacrimal apparatus The structures in which tears are secreted and drained from the eye.

lambdoid suture The point where the occipital bones attach to the parietal bones.

Le Fort fractures Maxillary fractures that are classified into three categories based on their anatomical location.

lens A transparent body within the globe that focuses light rays.

limbic system Structures within the cerebrum and diencephalon that influence emotions, motivation, mood, and sensations of pain and pleasure.

linear skull fractures Account for 80% of skull fractures; also referred to as nondisplaced skull fractures; commonly occur in the temporal-parietal region of the skull; not associated with deformities to the skull.

malocclusion Misalignment of the teeth.

mandible The moveable lower jaw bone.

mandibular nerve A sensory and motor nerve that supplies the muscles of chewing and skin of the lower lip, chin, temporal region, and part of the external ear.

mastication The process of chewing with the teeth.

mastoid process A cone-shaped section of bone at the base of the temporal bone.

maxillary nerve A sensory nerve; supplies the skin on the posterior part of the side of the nose, lower eyelid, cheek, and upper lip.

mean arterial pressure (MAP) The average (or mean) pressure against the arterial wall during a cardiac cycle.

mediastinitis Inflammation of the mediastinum, often a result of the gastric contents leaking into the thoracic cavity after oesophageal perforation.

medulla Continuous inferiorly with the spinal cord; serves as a conduction pathway for ascending and descending nerve tracts; coordinates heart rate, blood vessel diameter, breathing, swallowing, vomiting, coughing, and sneezing.

meninges A set of three tough membranes, the dura mater, arachnoid, and pia mater, that encloses the entire brain and spinal cord.

middle ear One of three anatomical parts of the ear; it consists of the inner portion of the tympanic membrane and the ossicles.

nasal cavity The chamber inside the nose that lies between the floor of the cranium and the roof of the mouth.

nasal septum The separation between the right and left nostrils.

nasolacrimal duct The passage through which tears drain from the lacrimal sacs into the nasal cavity.

neuroneal soma The body of a neurone (nerve cell).

occipital condyles Articular surfaces on the occipital bone where the skull articulates with the atlas on the vertebral column.

occipital lobe The portion of the brain that is responsible for the processing of visual information.

oculomotor nerve Third cranial nerve; innervates the muscles that cause motion of the eyeballs and upper eyelid.

olfactory nerves Participates in the transmission of scent impulses.

ophthalmic nerve A sensory nerve that supplies the skin of the forehead, the upper eyelid, and conjunctiva.

optic nerve Either of the second cranial nerves that enter the eyeball posteriorly, through the optic foramen.

orbits Bony cavities in the frontal part of the skull that enclose and protect the eyes.

organ of Corti A structure located in the cochlea that contains hairs that are stimulated by vibrations to form nerve impulses that travel to the brain and are perceived as sound.

ossicles The three small bones in the inner ear that transmit vibrations to the cochlear duct at the oval window.

oval window An oval opening between the middle ear and the vestibule.

palatine bone An irregularly shaped bone found in the posterior part of the nasal cavity.

paranasal sinuses The sinuses, or hollowed sections of bone in the front of the head, that are lined with mucous membrane and drain into the nasal cavity.

parietal lobe The portion of the brain that is the site for reception and evaluation of most sensory information, except smell, hearing, and vision.

periorbital bruising Bruising under or around the orbits that is commonly seen following a basilar skull fracture; also called raccoon eyes.

peripheral vision Visualisation of lateral objects while looking forward.

pia mater The innermost and thinnest of the three meninges that enclose the brain and spinal cord; rests directly on the brain and spinal cord.

pinna The large outside portion of the ear through which sound waves enter the ear; also called the auricle.

pons Lies below the midbrain and above the medulla and contains numerous important nerve fibres, including those for sleep, respiration, and the medullary respiratory centre.

posterior chamber The posterior area of the globe between the lens and the iris.

primary brain injury An injury to the brain and its associated structures that is a direct result of impact to the head.

pulp Specialised connective tissue within the pulp cavity of a tooth.

pupil The circular opening in the centre of the eye through which light passes to the lens.

raccoon eyes Bruising under or around the orbits that is commonly seen following a basilar skull fracture; also called periorbital bruising.

reticular activating system (RAS) Located in the upper brain stem; responsible for maintenance of consciousness, specifically one's level of arousal.

retina A delicate 10-layered structure of nervous tissue located in the rear of the interior of the globe that receives light and generates nerve signals that are transmitted to the brain through the optic nerve.

retinal detachment Separation of the inner layers of the retina from the underlying choroid, the vascular membrane that nourishes the retina.

retrograde amnesia Loss of memory relating to events that occurred before the injury.

sagittal suture The point of the skull where the parietal bones join.

sclera The white part of the eye.

secondary brain injury The "after effects" of the primary injury; includes abnormal processes such as cerebral oedema, increased intracranial pressure, cerebral ischaemia and hypoxia, and infection; onset is often delayed following the primary brain injury.

skull The structure at the top of the axial skeleton that houses the brain and consists of 28 bones that comprise the auditory ossicles, the cranium, and the face.

subarachnoid haematoma Bleeding into the subarachnoid space, where the cerebrospinal fluid (CSF) circulates.

subarachnoid space The space located between the pia mater and the arachnoid mater.

subdural haematoma An accumulation of blood beneath the dura but outside the brain.

subthalamus The part of the diencephalon that is involved in controlling motor functions.

sympathetic eye movement The movement of both eyes in unison.

temporal lobe The portion of the brain that has an important role in hearing and memory.

temporomandibular joint (TMJ) The joint between the temporal bone and the posterior condyle that allows for movements of the mandible.

tentorium A structure that separates the cerebral hemispheres from the cerebellum and brain stem.

thalamus The part of the diencephalon that processes most sensory input and influences mood and general body movements, especially those associated with fear or rage.

tracheal transection Traumatic separation of the trachea from the larynx.

traumatic brain injury (TBI) A traumatic insult to the brain capable of producing physical, intellectual, emotional, social, and vocational changes.

trigeminal nerve Fifth cranial nerve; supplies sensation to the scalp, forehead, face, and lower jaw and innervates the muscles of mastication, the throat, and the inner ear.

tympanic membrane A thin membrane that separates the middle ear from the inner ear and sets up vibrations in the ossicles; also called the eardrum.

ventricles Specialised hollow areas in the brain.

visual cortex The area in the brain where signals from the optic nerve are converted into visual images.

vitreous humour A jellylike substance found in the posterior compartment of the eye between the lens and the retina.

zygomatic arch The bone that extends along the front of the skull below the orbit.

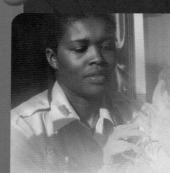

Assessment in Action

Your ambulance is dispatched to a house for an assault. You respond in 7 minutes. When you arrive, a police officer advises you that the scene is safe to enter and he escorts you to the patient, a man in his late 30s. According to witnesses, the patient was struck in the side of the head with a steel pipe during an altercation with his neighbour. As you approach the patient, you note that he is lying in a supine position and is not moving; there is no gross bleeding. The neighbour is in police custody.

1. **After your partner manually stabilises the patient's cervical spine, you should:**
   A. vigorously shake the patient to determine his level of consciousness.
   B. open his airway with the head tilt–chin lift manoeuvre or tongue jaw lift.
   C. suction his oropharynx for 30 seconds to ensure that it is clear of blood.
   D. determine his level of consciousness, and ensure that his airway is clear.

2. **Your initial assessment reveals that the patient is unconscious and unresponsive. You insert an oropharyngeal airway and assess his respirations, which are slow and shallow. His radial pulses are slow and bounding. What must you do next?**
   A. Perform immediate endotracheal intubation.
   B. Provide bag-valve-mask ventilation and supplemental oxygen.
   C. Apply a nonrebreathing mask, and reassess him.
   D. Start an IV line and administer atropine sulphate.

3. **The patient's BP is 170/100 mm Hg, his pulse rate is 50 beats/min and bounding, and his baseline respirations are 6 breaths/min and have now become irregular. What is the pathophysiology of this patient's vital signs?**
   A. An increase in mean arterial pressure, cerebral vasodilation, and pressure on the brain stem
   B. Cerebral vasoconstriction, shunting of blood from the brain, and complete brain stem herniation
   C. A decrease in mean arterial pressure, cerebral vasodilation, and a decrease in cerebral perfusion pressure
   D. Cerebral vasodilation, a decrease in cerebral blood flow, and increased parasympathetic tone

4. **All of the following are clinical signs of pressure on the upper brain stem, EXCEPT:**
   A. Cheyne-Stokes respirations.
   B. an increase in the patient's BP.
   C. a marked increase in heart rate.
   D. bilaterally fixed and dilated pupils.

5. **Which of the following are indications for hyperventilation of a brain-injured patient?**
   A. A systolic BP that exceeds 200 mm Hg
   B. Bilaterally dilated and slowly reactive pupils
   C. An absent motor response to painful stimuli
   D. Withdrawal from pain with flexor posturing

6. **Your patient has been intubated and ventilations are continuing. Further assessment reveals that the patient is unresponsive to all stimuli, has unequal pupils, and shows extensor posturing. How many ventilations per minute should this patient receive?**
   A. 10
   B. 20
   C. 25
   D. 30

7. **Which of the following is the most appropriate IV fluid regimen for a head-injured patient with a BP of 70/50 mm Hg?**
   A. An amount sufficient to maintain a systolic BP of at least 90 mm Hg
   B. 1,000 ml to 2,000 ml followed by a reassessment of the patient's BP
   C. A crystalloid solution infusion set to run at approximately 120 ml/h
   D. Set the IV line(s) to keep the vein open because fluids will worsen cerebral oedema

8. **Which of the following drugs would you be *least* likely to use when treating a patient with a severe head injury?**
   A. Lorazepam (Ativan)
   B. Lignocaine
   C. Glucose 10%
   D. Normal saline

9. **Which of the following parameters does the Glasgow Coma Scale (GCS) measure?**
   A. Pupil size, eye opening, verbal response
   B. Eye opening, motor response, heart rate
   C. Verbal response, pupil size, motor response
   D. Eye opening, verbal response, motor response

10. **You have arrived at the hospital and have transferred patient care to the attending doctor. You later learn that the patient had bleeding between the outer meningeal layer and the skull. This is called a(n):**
    A. subdural haematoma.
    B. extradural haematoma.
    C. subarachnoid haemorrhage.
    D. intraparenchymal haematoma.

Challenging Questions

A 27-year-old highly intoxicated male was riding on the back of a flat bed lorry, when he fell off and struck his head on the pavement. Your assessment reveals that the patient is unconscious and unresponsive. His respirations are slow and irregular and his pulse rate is slow and bounding. The only visible injuries are a non-bleeding laceration to his right temporal region and blood draining from his right ear. Your partner manually stabilises the patient's c-spine and begins ventilation assistance with a bag-valve-mask device and supplemental oxygen. Suddenly, the patient begins regurgitating massive amounts of liquid.

11. **What is the most effective way to initially manage this patient's airway?**

12. **What is the pathophysiology of the patient's vital signs? What would you expect his blood pressure to be?**

Points to Ponder

You are conveying a 30-year-old woman with blunt head trauma. She is conscious but persistently confused. You have applied 100% oxygen via nonrebreathing mask, started an IV line of normal saline and set the flow rate to keep vein open, and applied the cardiac monitor. Because of the mechanism of injury, full spinal motion restriction precautions have been applied. The patient's BP is 138/88 mm Hg, pulse rate is 100 beats/min, and respirations are 20 breaths/min and regular. As you are conversing with the patient, you note that her level of consciousness is progressively decreasing. You reassess her airway, which is still patent, but her respirations are now slow. The patient's pupils have increased in size but are still equal and reactive to light. She responds to pain by pushing your hand away. Noting these changes, you insert an airway adjunct and begin hyperventilating by bag-valve-mask ventilation at a rate of 24 breaths/min and continue to do so until you arrive at hospital 20 minutes later. After delivering the patient to hospital and returning to service, you learn that the patient experienced an anoxic brain injury.

Why did this occur? Could you have done something to prevent it?

Issues: Recognising Clinical Signs of the Different Levels of Intracranial Pressure, Knowing the Appropriate Ventilation Rates for Head-Injured Patients, Understanding the Importance of Maintaining Cerebral Perfusion Pressure.

Objectives

Cognitive

- Describe the incidence, morbidity, and mortality of spinal injuries in the trauma patient.
- Describe the anatomy and physiology of structures related to spinal injuries.
  - Cervical
  - Thoracic
  - Lumbar
  - Sacrum
  - Coccyx
  - Head
  - Brain
  - Spinal cord
  - Nerve tract(s)
  - Dermatomes
- Predict spinal injuries based on mechanism of injury.
- Describe the pathophysiology of spinal injuries.
- Explain traumatic and non-traumatic spinal injuries.
- Describe the assessment findings associated with spinal injuries.
- Describe the management of spinal injuries.
- Identify the need for rapid intervention and transport of the patient with spinal injuries.
- Integrate the pathophysiological principles to the assessment of a patient with a spinal injury.
- Differentiate between spinal injuries based on the assessment and history.
- Formulate an initial impression based on the assessment findings.
- Develop a patient management plan based on the initial impression.
- Describe the pathophysiology of traumatic spinal injury related to:
  - Spinal shock
  - Spinal neurogenic shock
  - Quadriplegia/paraplegia
  - Incomplete cord injury/cord syndromes:
    - Central cord syndrome
    - Anterior cord syndrome
    - Brown-Sequard syndrome
- Describe the assessment findings associated with traumatic spinal injuries.
- Describe the management of traumatic spinal injuries.
- Integrate pathophysiological principles to the assessment of a patient with a traumatic spinal injury.
- Differentiate between traumatic and non-traumatic spinal injuries based on the assessment and history.
- Formulate an initial impression for traumatic spinal injury based on the assessment findings.
- Develop a patient management plan for traumatic spinal injury based on the initial impression.
- Describe the pathophysiology of non-traumatic spinal injury, including:
  - Low back pain
  - Herniated intervertebral disc
  - Spinal cord tumours

- Describe the assessment findings associated with non-traumatic spinal injuries.
- Describe the management of non-traumatic spinal injuries.
- Integrate pathophysiological principles to the assessment of a patient with non-traumatic spinal injury.
- Differentiate between traumatic and non-traumatic spinal injuries based on the assessment and history.
- Formulate an initial impression for non-traumatic spinal injury based on the assessment findings.
- Develop a patient management plan for non-traumatic spinal injury based on the initial impression.

Affective

- Advocate the use of a thorough assessment when determining the proper immobilisation management for spine injuries.
- Appreciate the implications of failing to properly immobilise a spine injured patient.

Psychomotor

- Demonstrate a clinical assessment to determine the proper immobilisation management for a patient with a suspected traumatic spinal injury.
- Demonstrate a clinical assessment to determine the proper management for a patient with a suspected non-traumatic spinal injury.
- Demonstrate immobilisation of the urgent and non-urgent patient with assessment findings of spinal injury from the following presentations:
  - Supine
  - Prone
  - Semi-prone
  - Sitting
  - Standing
- Demonstrate documentation of suspected spinal cord injury to include:
  - General area of spinal cord involved
  - Sensation
  - Dermatomes
  - Motor function
  - Area(s) of weakness
- Demonstrate preferred methods for stabilisation of a helmet from a potentially spine injured patient.
- Demonstrate helmet removal techniques.
- Demonstrate alternative methods for stabilisation of a helmet from a potentially spine injured patient.
- Demonstrate documentation of assessment before spinal immobilisation.
- Demonstrate documentation of assessment during spinal immobilisation.
- Demonstrate documentation of assessment after spinal immobilisation.

Introduction

Spinal cord injury (SCI) is one of the most devastating injuries encountered by prehospital providers. Unfortunately, treatment options for SCIs are currently limited, with therapy relying heavily on rehabilitation over acute intervention. Preventive measures directed toward reducing the incidence of primary and secondary SCIs are the health care provider's best option for decreasing the morbidity and mortality associated with SCI.

In the United Kingdom, an estimated 800 new cases of SCI occur each year. Around 160 of these are related to illnesses such as polio or spina bifida. The remainder can be classified into four major categories: road traffic collisions (44%), acts of violence (3%), falls (41%), and sporting activities—especially diving (12%).

The overall in-hospital mortality rate is 7% for isolated SCI. In the first few months after injury, the mortality is as high as 20%, a rate that increases with age. The leading causes of death for SCI patients who are discharged from the hospital are pneumonia, pulmonary embolism, and septicaemia.

Anatomy and Physiology

An understanding of the form and function of spinal anatomy coupled with a high level of suspicion for SCI is required to decipher the often subtle findings associated with SCI.

The Spine

The spine consists of 33 irregular bones (vertebrae) articulating to form the vertebral column, which is the major structural component of the axial skeleton   Figure 22-1 ▶ . These skeletal components are stabilised by both ligaments and muscle. Together these components support and protect neural elements while allowing for fluid movement and erect stature.

Vertebrae are identified according to their location as cervical, thoracic, lumbar, sacral, or coccyx. The vertebral body, the anterior weight-bearing structure, is made of bone that provides support and stability. Components of the vertebra include the lamina, pedicles, and spinous processes   Figure 22-2 ▶ . Each vertebra is unique in appearance and, with the exception of the atlas and axis (C1 and C2)   Figure 22-3 ▶ , shares basic structural characteristics.

The inferior border of each pedicle contains a notch forming the intervertebral foramen. This space in the middle of the

At the Scene

Patients with SCI face dramatic changes in lifestyle. A simple walk in the park, a trip to the shopping centre, or the commute to work becomes, much more difficult. Caring for the SCI patient also brings significant financial costs.

You are the Paramedic Part 1

On your first day of work as a paramedic, you are dispatched to a location just off the M5 for an "aircraft crash". En route to the scene, the emergency communications centre informs you that a witness saw a single-passenger aircraft fly into some power lines, then plummet to the ground.

You arrive to find a small aircraft that has crashed in the middle of a large field of wheat. You see power lines lying across the aeroplane and an entrapped occupant who is slightly pale.

Initial Assessment	Recording Time: 0 Minutes
Appearance	Eyes open, anxious, holding lower back
Level of consciousness	A (Alert to person, place, and day)
Airway	Patent; calling for help
Breathing	Rapid and deep
Circulation	Not yet obtained

1. What is your primary concern?
2. What additional resources (if any) would you request and when?
3. How can you immediately assess and communicate with this patient in a safe manner?

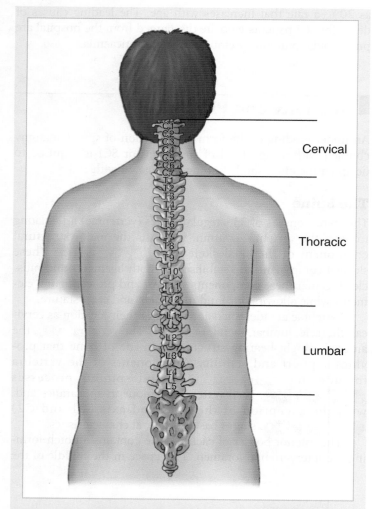

Figure 22-1 The spinal column consists of 33 bones divided into three sections. Each vertebra is numbered and referred to by a letter corresponding to the section of the spine where it is located plus its number. For example, the fifth thoracic vertebra is referred to as T5.

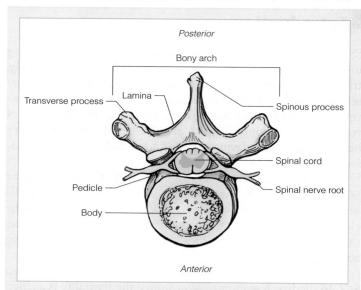

Figure 22-2 The human vertebra. Vertebrae in different sections of the spinal column vary in shape; this is a general representation. The space through which the spinal cord passes is called the vertebral foramen, and the space through which a nerve root passes is called an intervertebral foramen.

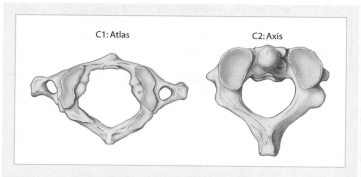

Figure 22-3 Structure of the atlas and axis.

vertebra allows the exit of a peripheral nerve root and spinal vein as well as the entrance of a spinal artery on both sides at each vertebral junction.

The transverse processes comprise the junction of each pedicle and lamina on each side of a vertebra. They project laterally and posteriorly and form points of attachments for muscles and ligaments. The posterior process is formed by the fusion of the posterior lamina and serves as an attachment site for muscles and ligaments.

The cervical spine includes the first seven bones of the vertebral column and its supporting structures. In addition to protecting the vital cervical spinal cord, the cervical spine supports the weight of the head and permits a high degree of mobility in multiple planes. The atlas (C1) and axis (C2) are uniquely suited to allow for rotational movement of the skull.

The thoracic spine consists of 12 vertebrae in addition to the supporting muscles and ligaments found in the vertebral column; the thoracic spine is further stabilised by the rib attachments. The spinous processes are slightly larger, reflecting their role as attachment points for muscles that hold the upper body erect and assist with the movement of the thoracic cavity during respiration.

The lumbar spine includes the five largest bones in the vertebral column, and is integral in carrying a large portion of the upper body weight. The lumbar spine is especially susceptible to injury because of this weight-bearing capacity.

The sacrum is composed of five fused vertebrae that form the posterior plate of the pelvis. The coccyx is made up of small fused vertebrae. Coccyx injuries, although often extremely painful, are typically clinically insignificant.

Each vertebra is separated and cushioned by intervertebral discs that limit bone wear and act as shock absorbers. As the body ages, these discs lose water content and become thinner, causing the height loss associated with ageing. Stress

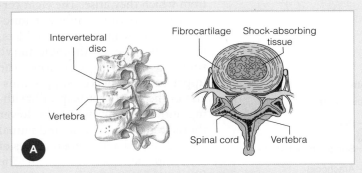
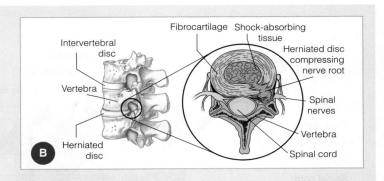

Figure 22-4 A. Normal, uninjured vertebral disc. **B.** Herniated disc.

At the Scene

The lumbar spine is a common site of injury. Many of these injuries involve muscle spasm and do not threaten the integrity of the spinal cord and its roots. Nonetheless, low back pain is a common problem, as well as a major cause of impairment and disability.

on the vertebral column may cause a disc to herniate into the spinal canal, resulting in a spinal cord or nerve root injury Figure 22-4 ▲ .

The muscles, tendons, and ligaments that connect the vertebrae allow the spinal column a degree of flexion and extension, limited to an extent by the stabilisation they must provide to the spinal column. The vertebral column can sustain normal flexion and extension of 60% to 70% without stressing the spinal cord. Flexion or extension beyond those limits may damage structural ligaments and allow excess vertebral movement that could expose the spinal cord to injury.

The Brain and Meninges

The central nervous system (CNS) consists of the brain and the spinal cord, both of which are encased in and protected by bone. The brain, located within the cranial cavity, is the largest component of the CNS. It contains billions of neurones that serve a variety of vital functions.

The brain stem, which consists of the medulla, pons, and midbrain, connects the spinal cord to the remainder of the brain. The brain stem is vital for numerous basic body functions. Damage to this critical structure can easily result in death. All but two of the 12 cranial nerves exit from the brain stem.

The entire CNS is enclosed by a set of three membranes collectively known as the meninges Figure 22-5 ▶ . The outer membrane, called the dura mater, is tough and fibrous. The middle layer, called the arachnoid, contains blood vessels that give it the appearance of a spider web. The innermost layer, resting directly on the brain or spinal cord, is the pia mater. The subarachnoid space (the space between the arachnoid and pia mater) contains cerebrospinal fluid (CSF). The meninges and CSF form a fluid-filled cushion that protects the brain and spinal chord.

You are the Paramedic Part 2

You request additional resources to aid you in safely treating and transporting the patient. After the known hazards have been addressed, you approach the patient, who says her name is Lorna, to begin your hands-on assessment. As you near her, you notice a strong odour of fuel and the patient says, "I stink! I've got fuel all over me"!

Reassessment	Recording Time: 10 Minutes
Level of consciousness	A (Alert to person, place, and day)
Skin	Cool, slightly pale, and dry
Pulse	110 beats/min, strong and regular
Blood pressure	140 by palpation
Respirations	36 breaths/min
S_PO_2	98% on 15 l/min via nonrebreathing mask

4. Given the information your patient has provided, have your priorities changed?
5. Given the mechanism of injury and other factors, what injuries do you suspect?

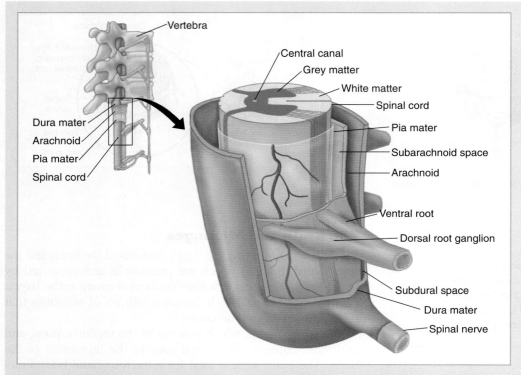

Figure 22-5 The spinal cord and its layers. The meninges enclose the brain and spinal cord.

from which they arise. The eight cervical roots perform different functions in the scalp, neck, shoulders, and arms. The 12 thoracic nerve roots have varying functions; the upper thoracic nerves supply muscles of the chest that help in breathing and coughing, while the lower thoracic nerves provide abdominal muscle control and contain nerves of the sympathetic nervous system. The five lumbar nerve roots supply hip flexors and leg muscles, as well as providing sensation to the anterior legs. The five sacral nerves provide for bowel and bladder control, sexual function, and sensation in the posterior legs and rectum. The coccyx has a single nerve root.

Nerve roots occasionally converge in a cluster called a <u>plexus</u> that permits peripheral nerve roots to rejoin and function as a group **Figure 22-6 ▸** . For example, the cervical plexus includes C1 through C5; the phrenic nerve (C3–C5) arises from this plexus and innervates the diaphragm. The brachial plexus (C5–T1) joins nerves controlling the upper extremities; the main nerves arising from this plexus are the axillary, median, musculocutaneous, radial, and ulnar. The lumbar plexus (L1–L4) supplies the skin and muscles of the abdominal wall, external genitalia, and part of the lower limbs. The sacral plexus (L4–S4) gives rise to the pudendal

The Spinal Cord

The <u>spinal cord</u> transmits nerve impulses between the brain and the rest of the body. Originating at the base of the brain, it represents the continuation of the CNS. This bundle of nerve fibres leaves the skull through a large opening at its base called the <u>foramen magnum</u>. The spinal cord extends from the base of the skull to L2; here it separates into the <u>cauda equina</u>, a collection of individual nerve roots. Thirty-one pairs of spinal nerves arise from the different segments of the spinal cord; each pair is named according to its corresponding segment.

A cross-section of the spinal cord (see Figure 22-5) reveals a butterfly-shaped central core of grey matter that is composed of neural cell bodies and synapses. This grey matter is divided into posterior (dorsal) horns, which carry sensory input, and anterior (ventral) horns, which innervate the motor nerve of that segment. Surrounding the grey matter on each side are three columns of peripheral white matter composed of myelinated ascending and descending fibre pathways. Messages are relayed to and from the brain through these spinal tracts.

Specific groups of nerves are named based on their source of origin and point of termination. Ascending tracts carry information to the brain, and descending tracts carry information to the rest of the body **Table 22-1 ▸** .

Spinal Nerves

The 31 pairs of spinal nerves emerge from each side of the spinal cord and are named for the vertebral region and level

Table 22-1	Major Spinal Tracts	
Anterior Spinal Tracts	
Anterior spinothalamic tracts (ascending)	Carry sensation of crude touch and pressure sensation to the brain
Lateral spinothalamic tracts (ascending)	Carry pain and temperature
Spinocerebellar tracts (ascending)	Coordinate impulses necessary for muscular movements by carrying impulses from muscles in the legs and trunk to the cerebellum
Corticospinal tracts (descending)	Voluntary motor commands
Reticulospinal tracts (descending)	Muscle tone and sweat gland activity
Rubrospinal tracts (descending)	Muscle tone
Posterior Spinal Tracts	
Fasciculus gracilis and cuneatus	<u>Proprioception</u>, vibration, light touch, deep pressure, two-point discrimination, and stereognosis

vessels and bronchioles, and have chronotropic and inotropic effects on myocardial cells. The sympathetic nervous system is also responsible for sweating, pupil dilation, and temperature regulation, as well as the shunting of blood from the periphery to the core—the "flight or fight" responses.

A spinal cord injury at or above the level of T6 may disrupt the flow of sympathetic communication. Loss of sympathetic stimulation can disrupt homeostasis and leave the body poorly equipped to deal with changes in its environment. Stimulation of sympathetic nerves without parasympathetic input can cause sympathetic overdrive, resulting in autonomic dysreflexia; this complication of SCI is discussed later in this chapter.

The Parasympathetic Nervous System

The parasympathetic nervous system includes fibres arising from the brain stem and upper spinal cord that carry signals to organs of the abdomen, heart, lungs, and the skin above the waist. The vagus nerve travels from its origins outside of the medulla to the heart via the carotid arteries, thus vagal tone remains intact following a spine injury. When the sympathetic nerves are stimulated and produce autonomic dysreflexia, the parasympathetic nerves attempt to control the rapidly increasing blood pressure by slowing the heart rate. Parasympathetic nerves that supply the reproductive organs, pelvis, and leg begin at the sacral level (S2–S4). Disruption of the lower parasympathetic nerves in the sacrum results in the loss of bowel/bladder tone and sexual function.

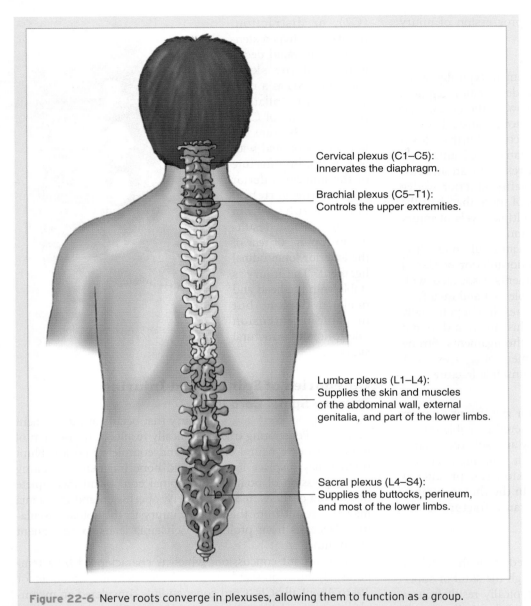

Figure 22-6 Nerve roots converge in plexuses, allowing them to function as a group.

Cervical plexus (C1–C5): Innervates the diaphragm.

Brachial plexus (C5–T1): Controls the upper extremities.

Lumbar plexus (L1–L4): Supplies the skin and muscles of the abdominal wall, external genitalia, and part of the lower limbs.

Sacral plexus (L4–S4): Supplies the buttocks, perineum, and most of the lower limbs.

and sciatic nerves and supplies the buttocks, perineum, and most of the lower limbs.

The Sympathetic Nervous System
The sensory (afferent) and motor (efferent) nerves are responsible for the somatic functions of the spinal cord and often overshadow the role of the spinal cord in the involuntary autonomic nervous system. The sympathetic nervous system is controlled by the brain's hypothalamus. Information from the brain is transmitted through the brain stem and the cervical spinal cord and then exits at the thoracic and lumbar levels of the spine to reach target structures. The thoracolumbar system provides sympathetic stimulation to the periphery largely through alpha and beta receptors. Alpha receptor stimulation induces smooth muscle contraction in blood vessels and bronchioles. Beta receptors respond with relaxation of smooth muscles in blood

Pathophysiology

Mechanism of Injury
Acute injuries of the spine are classified according to the associated mechanism, location, and stability of the injury. Vertebral fractures can occur with or without associated SCI. Because stable fractures do not involve the posterior column, they pose less risk to the spinal cord. Unstable injuries involve the posterior column of the spinal cord and typically include damage to portions of the vertebrae and ligaments that directly protect the spinal cord and nerve roots. Unstable injuries carry

a higher risk of complicating SCI and progression of injury without appropriate treatment.

Flexion Injuries

Flexion injuries result from forward movement typically of the head, and typically as the result of rapid deceleration (eg, in a road traffic collision) or from a direct blow to the occiput. At the level of C1–C2, these forces can produce an unstable dislocation with or without an associated fracture. Further down the spinal column, flexion forces are transmitted anteriorly through the vertebral bodies and can result in an anterior wedge fracture. Depending on their severity, anterior wedge fractures can be stable or unstable. Loss of more than half the original size of the vertebral body or multiple levels of injury suggest involvement of the posterior column.

Hyperflexion injuries of greater force can result in teardrop fractures—avulsion fractures of the anterior-inferior border of the vertebral body. The injuries to ligaments associated with teardrop fractures raise concern for possible SCI and qualify as unstable fractures. Severe flexion can also result in a potentially unstable dislocation of vertebral joints. This situation does not involve fracture but can severely injure the ligaments. Strong forces can result in the anterior displacement of facet joints. A bilateral facet dislocation is an extremely unstable fracture.

Rotation with Flexion

The only area of the spine that allows for significant rotation is C1–C2. Injuries to this area are considered unstable due to its high cervical location and scant bony and soft-tissue support. Rotation-flexion injuries often result from high acceleration forces. Rotation with abrupt flexion can produce a stable dislocation in the cervical spine. In the thoracolumbar spine, rotation-flexion forces typically cause fracture rather than dislocation.

Vertical Compression

Vertical compression forces are transmitted through vertebral bodies and directed either inferiorly through the skull or superiorly through the pelvis or feet. They typically result from a direct blow to the crown (parietal region) of the skull or rapid deceleration from a fall through the feet, legs, and pelvis. Forces transmitted through the vertebral body cause fractures, ultimately shattering and producing a "comminuted" or compression fracture without associated SCI **Figure 22-7 ▸** . Compression forces can cause the herniation of discs, subsequent compression on the spinal cord and nerve roots, and fragmentation into the canal.

Although most fractures resulting from these injuries are stable, primary SCI can occur when the vertebral body is shattered and fragments of bone become embedded in the cord. Some compression injuries may be associated with significant retropharyngeal oedema, and serious airway compromise is a consideration.

Hyperextension

Hyperextension of the head and neck can result in fractures and ligamentous injury of variable stability. The hangman's fracture (C2), or distraction, results from hyperextension due to rapid deceleration of the skull, atlas, and axis as a unit. The resulting bilateral pedicle fracture of C2 is an unstable fracture but is rarely associated with SCI. A teardrop fracture of the anterior-inferior edge of the vertebral body results from hyperextension, resulting in rupture or tear of the anterior longitudinal ligament. The injury is stable with the head and neck in flexion, but unstable in extension due to loss of structural support.

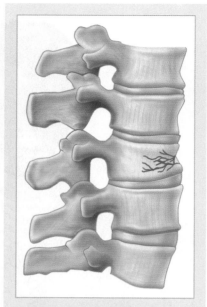

Figure 22-7 A compression fracture.

Categories of Spinal Cord Injuries

Primary Spinal Cord Injury

Primary spinal cord injury is injury that occurs at the moment of impact. Penetrating trauma typically results in transection of nonregenerative neural elements and complete injuries. Blunt trauma may displace ligaments and bone fragments, resulting in compression of points of the spinal cord or an incomplete dislocation of the vertebral body. Hypoperfusion and ischaemia may also result from this type of injury to the spinal vasculature. Necrosis from prolonged ischaemia leads to permanent loss of function.

Spinal cord concussion, which is characterised by a temporary dysfunction that lasts from 24 to 48 hours, accounts for 3% to 4% of all SCIs. Cord concussion is considered an incomplete injury and may present in patients with simple compression fractures or in those without radiologic evidence of a fracture. The temporary dysfunction may be due to a short-duration shock or pressure wave within the cord.

Spinal cord contusions are caused by fracture, dislocation, or direct trauma. They are associated with oedema, tissue damage, and vascular leakage. Haemorrhagic disruption may cause temporary to permanent loss of function despite normal X-rays.

Cord laceration usually occurs when a projectile or bone enters the spinal canal. Such an injury is likely to result in haemorrhage into the cord tissue, swelling, and disruption of some portion of the cord and its associated communication pathways.

Secondary Spinal Cord Injury

Secondary spinal cord injury occurs when multiple factors permit a progression of the primary SCI; the ensuing cascade of inflammatory responses may result in further deterioration. These effects can be exacerbated by exposing neural elements to further hypoxaemia, hypoglycaemia, and hypothermia. Although some SCI may be unavoidable, the prehospital provider should minimise further injury through stabilisation—that is, through spinal motion restriction. In addition, minimising heat loss and maintaining oxygenation and perfusion are key elements in the care of a patient with a possible SCI.

Regardless of the mechanism of injury, all SCIs are classified as complete or incomplete depending on the degree of damage. Complete spinal cord injury involves complete disruption of all tracts of the spinal cord, with permanent loss of all cord-mediated functions below the level of transection. When the injury affects the patient high in the cervical spine, quadriplegia results. A similar injury in the high thoracic area would result in paraplegia. In an incomplete spinal cord injury, the patient retains some degree of cord-mediated function. The degree of SCI is best determined 24 hours after the initial injury; the initial dysfunction may be temporary, and there is some potential for recovery.

Anterior cord syndrome results from the displacement of bony fragments into the anterior portion of the spinal cord, often due to flexion injuries or fractures. The anterior spinal artery provides blood to the anterior two thirds of the spinal cord; disruption of this flow will present as an anterior cord syndrome. Physical findings include paralysis below the level of the insult with loss of sensation to pain, temperature, and touch.

In central cord syndrome, hyperextension injuries to the cervical area present with haemorrhage or oedema to the central cervical segments. This type of damage is rarely associated with fractures or bone disruption but more often occurs in conjunction with tears to the anterior longitudinal ligament. Central cord syndrome is frequently seen in older patients, who may already have a significant degree of cervical spondylosis and stenosis due to arthritic changes. A brief episode of hyperextension can exert pressure on the spinal cord within the relatively diminished spinal canal. Within the central cord, motor (efferent) fibres are distributed in a unique fashion, with more cervical and thoracic motor and sensory tracts than in the periphery of the cord. The patient with central cord syndrome will present with greater loss of function in the upper extremities than in the lower extremities, with variable loss of sensation to pain and temperature. The patient may also have some bowel and bladder dysfunction. The prognosis for central cord syndrome is typically good; many patients regain all motor function or have only some residual weakness in the hands.

Posterior cord syndrome is associated with extension injuries. This relatively rare syndrome produces dysfunction of the dorsal columns, presenting as decreased sensation to light touch, proprioception (the ability to perceive the position and movement of one's body), and vibration, while most other motor and sensory functions remain intact. Recovery of function is less prevalent than with central cord syndrome, but the overall prognosis remains good with therapy and rehabilitation.

Brown-Sequard syndrome occurs when penetrating trauma is accompanied by hemitransection of the cord and complete damage to all spinal tracts on the involved side. Injury to the corticospinal motor tracts causes motor loss on the same side as the injury, but below the lesion. Damage to the dorsal column causes loss of sensation to light touch, proprioception, and vibration on the same side as the injury (below it). Disruption of the spinothalamic tracts causes loss of sensation to pain and temperature on the opposite side of injury, below the lesion.

Spinal shock refers to the temporary local neurological condition that occurs immediately after spinal trauma. Swelling and oedema of the cord begin within 30 minutes of the initial insult and can lead to a physiological transection, mechanically disrupting all nerve conduction distal to the injury. The patient may present with variable degrees of acute spinal injury, potentially with flaccid paralysis, flaccid sphincters, and absent reflexes. Sensory function below the level of injury will be impaired, as will thermoregulation and visceral sensation below the lesion, resulting in bowel distention from a loss of peristalsis. Spinal shock usually subsides in hours to weeks, depending on the severity of injury.

Neurogenic shock results from the temporary loss of autonomic function, which controls cardiovascular function, at the level of injury. Marked haemodynamic and systemic effects are seen: hypotension occurs due to absent or impaired peripheral vascular tone with the loss of alpha receptor stimulation; blood pools in the enlarged vascular space, causing a relative hypovolaemia and making the patient extremely sensitive to sudden position changes; and cardiac preload decreases, resulting in decreased stroke volume and cardiac output. Bradycardia results as well. The adrenal gland loses its sympathetic stimulation and does not produce adrenaline or noradrenaline. Hypothermia and absence of sweating are also seen because of the loss of sympathetic stimulation. The classic case of neurogenic shock is a hypotensive, bradycardic patient whose skin is warm, flushed, and dry below the level of the spinal lesion.

Patient Assessment

Limiting the progression of secondary SCI is a major goal of prehospital management of SCI. You should be familiar with the circumstances that commonly produce SCI and try to determine, through history-taking and examination of the scene, whether any of these circumstances exist.

Special Considerations

Spinal cord injury without X-ray abnormalities (SCIWORA) can occur in children because their articular facets are more horizontal Figure 22-8 ; in adults, the vertebrae are more curved. A child's vertebrae can easily dislocate and quickly relocate back into their normal positions. The X-ray of a child who has experienced SCIWORA may have no evidence of fracture and will show a perfectly aligned vertebral column, yet the cord itself has been compressed or transected. SCIWORA cannot be diagnosed in the prehospital setting. Even in the accident and emergency (A&E) department, sophisticated studies such as MRI may be required.

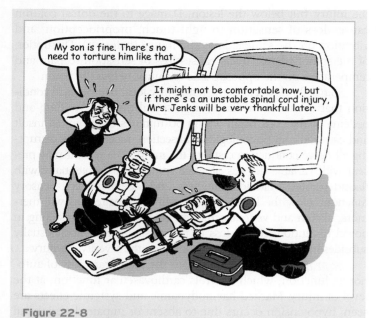

Figure 22-8

When to Suspect a Spinal Cord Injury

The history of present illness typically provides most of the information necessary to reach a diagnosis. Maintain a high index of suspicion in any case for which the mechanism of injury suggests the possibility of SCI. Associated injuries, especially those that reflect involvement of massive forces, may also provide clues of the presence of SCI. Treat all patients who experience multiple trauma or those who are found unconscious after trauma as if a spine injury exists, because the majority of cervical spine injuries are associated with head injury. Patients with evidence of major trauma above the clavicle should be considered at risk for an associated spine injury.

The following high-risk mechanisms of injury strongly suggest spine injury:

- High-velocity road traffic collision (> 40 mph) with severe vehicle damage

- Unrestrained occupant of moderate- to high-speed road traffic collision
- Vehicular damage with compartmental intrusion (30 cm) into the patient's seating space
- Fall from three times the patient's height
- Penetrating trauma near the spine
- Ejection from a moving vehicle
- Motorcycle crash at greater than 20 mph with separation of rider from vehicle
- Diving injury
- Car-pedestrian or car-bicycle collision with greater than 5 mph impact
- Death of occupant in the same passenger compartment
- Rollover accident (unrestrained)

Mechanisms of uncertain risk for spine injury include the following events:

- Moderate- to low-velocity road traffic collision (< 40 mph)
- Patient involved in a road traffic collision has an isolated injury without positive assessment findings for SCI
- Isolated minor head injury without positive mechanism for spine injury
- Syncopal event in which the patient was already seated or supine
- Syncopal event in which the patient was assisted to a supine position by a bystander

Determine as precisely as possible the circumstances of the incident and types of energy imparted to the patient, including the degree of force and the speed and trajectory of impact. Was there blunt or penetrating trauma? Was it a flexion injury, such as the classic diving accident? Was there torsion on the neck? In the case of a fall, estimate the height of the fall and determine whether anything was struck on the way down, how the patient landed, and what the patient landed on. In road traffic

> **Notes from Nancy**
> Any patient with significant head injury also has cervical spine injury until proved otherwise.

You are the Paramedic Part 3

Fire fighters aid you in decontaminating the patient as well as applying spinal precautions. Lorna finds it difficult to lie flat on the board, and tells you that her back hurts a lot. She reports, "It feels better if I hold it". She denies any weakness, numbness, or tingling in her extremities.

Reassessment	Recording Time: 15 Minutes
Level of consciousness	A (Alert to person, place, and day)
Skin	Cool, slightly pale, and dry
Pulse	110 beats/min, strong and regular
Blood pressure	140 by palpation
Respirations	36 breaths/min
SpO2	100% on 15 l/min via nonrebreathing mask

6. What other factors can impact a patient's ability to handle the stress of trauma?

7. What other information beyond the history of events should you obtain from your patient?

8. If you must decontaminate a patient in the open, how can you preserve patient modesty?

collisions, note the use and positioning of restraints, the patient's position in the vehicle, and the degree of damage to the vehicle. Find out the exact time of the initial injury and record any times and changes in the patient's presentation throughout the prehospital phase.

Special Considerations

The indications for longboard spinal immobilisation of infants and toddlers are unknown. Infants and young children cannot verbally communicate symptoms such as weakness, numbness, or pain, so the threshold for immobilisation must be lower than for older children and adults. However, restraining a conscious child on a longboard will cause pain and agitation in a short time. Reassure nervous children that the immobilisation is necessary but only temporary. Try distraction techniques.

Always give consideration to other techniques; the most important thing is to immobilise the patient, not just use a piece of immobilisation equipment. In extreme circumstances, allowing a parent to hold an upset and very mobile child still will produce the desired result.

Modify the physical examination of any patient with suspected SCI based on the patient's level of consciousness, reliability as a historian, and mechanism of injury. In cases of high- or intermediate-risk mechanisms, whenever possible complete the physical examination with the patient in a neutral position without any movement of the spine. Apply manual stabilisation while asking the patient not to move unless specifically asked to do so. The neck and trunk must not be flexed, extended, or rotated. Frequent reassessments are necessary to determine whether the patient is stabilising, improving, or deteriorating. Also, be sure to document suspected spinal cord injury, noting the area involved, sensation, dermatomes (discussed in the next section), motor function, and areas of weakness.

Scene Assessment

After donning personal protective equipment (PPE), the initial step of any assessment should be a determination of scene safety and the need for any additional resources. Decide whether additional resources should be activated (eg, air evacuation of the patient to a hospital with spinal injury management facilities). Note the general age and gender of the patient. Observe the position in which the patient is found and determine if the patient's condition is life-threatening. While maintaining the head and neck in a neutral position through manual stabilisation, determine the level of consciousness, using AVPU ini-

Notes from Nancy

The most important single sign in the evaluation of a head-injured patient is a changing state of consciousness.

tially and then the Glasgow Coma Scale (GCS score—a standardised method of relaying information regarding a patient's overall level of consciousness) as time allows. A cervical collar may be applied as soon as the assessment of the airway and neck are complete. Sedation or rapid sequence intubation (RSI) procedures, depending on local guidelines, may be required for a combative patient to ensure the patient's protection and spine stabilisation.

Initial Assessment

Airway

After confirming that the scene is safe and determining the patient's mental status, the next priority is to ensure an open airway. Stertorous or noisy respirations usually indicate a positional problem, while gurgling respirations often indicate a need for suction. The oropharynx may become occluded by the tongue, secretions, blood, vomitus, foreign bodies, or improperly inserted airways. A retropharyngeal haematoma associated with injury of the upper cervical spine (C2) may also impinge on the airway.

While maintaining the head and neck in neutral alignment, clear the mouth and carefully but quickly suction if necessary. Use a jaw-thrust manoeuvre to open the airway; if this technique is successful, insert an oropharyngeal airway or a nasopharyngeal airway as appropriate. An intact gag reflex is a contraindication for an oropharyngeal airway, because vomiting will increase the likelihood of airway compromise and increase the risk of aspiration. Facial fractures and physical findings or suspicion for a basilar skull fracture are relative contraindications for a nasopharyngeal airway.

A definitive airway with in-line endotracheal intubation should follow the placement of any temporary airway device. If the patient is awake with an impaired airway or has a deteriorating GCS score (8 or less), consider drug-assisted orotracheal intubation with in-line stabilisation (ie, RSI). Turn the patient to the side to allow gravity to assist in evacuation of the airway while secured to a longboard or while you maintain manual in-line stabilisation of the head and neck. Follow up with suction to remove the minor secretions. Local guidelines may include sedation or RSI.

Breathing

Evaluate the patient's breathing, noting the rate, depth, and symmetry of each respiration. The diaphragm is innervated by the phrenic nerve (C3–C5). Lesions occurring at or above C3–C4 may consequently lead to diaphragmatic paralysis, which is seen clinically as abdominal breathing with use of the accessory muscles of the neck. An injury involving the lower cervical or upper thoracic spinal cord (T2) may result in paralysis of the intercostal muscles, leaving the patient dependent on the diaphragm and accessory muscles of the neck for breathing. Inadequate respirations with or without evidence of decreased oxygenation will require assisted ventilation with a bag-valve-mask device with 12 to 15 l/min of supplementary oxygen flowing, at 10 to 12 breaths/min. If a head injury is suspected, use $ETCO_2$ monitoring to maintain CO_2 levels at 35 to 45 mm Hg.

Circulation

To assess perfusion, compare the radial and carotid pulses for their presence, rate, quality, regularity, and equality, and examine the patient's skin colour, temperature, and moisture. Patients with significant sensory loss from SCI may equilibrate to the surrounding environmental temperature due to the lack of input from the periphery for temperature control. In neurogenic shock, the skin is usually warm, dry, and flushed due to vasodilation and the absence of sweating. These findings should be correlated with the patient's mental status.

In the absence of a pulse, immediately initiate CPR. Control any external bleeding with direct pressure or pressure dressings. Volume resuscitation may be necessary in patients with absent or diminished pulses, especially in the setting of multi-system trauma with hypovolaemic shock. Patients with SCI in pure neurogenic shock may not require large amounts of volume resuscitation but may need vagolytic drugs (eg, atropine) to reverse the uninhibited vagal stimulation and alpha receptor blockade associated with this type of shock.

Transport Decision

Early on in the initial assessment, you must decide whether to complete the focused history and physical examination on scene or to transport the patient immediately with interventions en route. The unstable or potentially unstable patient should be transported as soon as possible to the most appropriate hospital.

Focused History and Physical Examination

An accurate history and physical examination are critical for directing management of patients with potential SCIs. A patient's reliability as a historian must always be assessed before performing a focused or detailed assessment. The patient must appear calm, cooperative, nonimpaired, and able to perform cognitive functions appropriately. Patients who present with an acute stress reaction, distracting injuries (eg, long-bone fractures, rib fractures, pelvic fractures, or clinically significant abdominal pain), or an alteration in mental status due to brain injury or intoxication from drugs and/or alcohol must be considered unreliable in terms of the neurological examination. These patients should have continuous spine protection until the presence of an injury can be excluded using an X-ray at the receiving hospital.

The focused physical examination should begin with baseline vital signs and a SAMPLE history. In case of potential spine injuries, the examination includes rapid inspection and palpation of the head, neck, chest, abdomen, pelvis, extremities, and back for injuries. Use the mnemonic DCAP-BTLS—Deformity, Contusion, Abrasion, Puncture/penetration wounds, Bruising, Tenderness, Laceration, and Swelling—to help you remember specific points. An evaluation of neurovascular integrity should include distal PMS (pulse, motor, and sensory function) for all four extremities. Any deficits in the neurological examination must be noted and monitored.

In addition to evaluating responsiveness with AVPU during your initial assessment, also obtain a GCS score because it provides more specific clinical information. Assess the pupils for their size, shape, equality, and reactivity to light. If possible, obtain a glucose level in patients who show evidence of alterations in sensation. Perform a brief motor and sensory examination, including PMS in all four extremities, in patients with potential SCI.

You will need to expose the patient for your examination. Cut away the clothes to minimise motion of the spine during examination or treatment. Directly observe the back to assess

You are the Paramedic Part 4

As soon as Lorna is packaged, you begin transport. You initiate IV therapy, apply the cardiac monitor, and reassess your patient for any signs and symptoms of spinal cord compromise. Her mental status and vital signs remain stable throughout transport, and you transfer patient care to the hospital staff without incident.

Reassessment	Recording Time: 20 Minutes
Level of consciousness	A (Alert to person, place, and day)
Skin	Warm, pink, and dry
Pulse	106 beats/min, strong and regular
Blood pressure	138/70 mm Hg
Respirations	30 breaths/min
SpO$_2$	100% on 15 l/min via nonrebreathing mask

The patient experienced compression fractures of her lumbar spine, but no spinal cord damage. She underwent surgery and made a recovery that did not limit her quality of life, including her ability to function as a pilot.

9. What is the standard for maximum on-scene time for any significant trauma patient?

10. How does prompt, appropriate care affect the patient beyond immediate survival of the injuries sustained?

for penetrating trauma. Palpate the spine to assess for deformity or displacement (step off) of vertebral bodies. Once the examination is completed, recover the patient with a blanket to maintain normal body temperature. Hypothermia will impair the patient's ability to unbind oxygen from haemoglobin and increase the risk of mortality and morbidity. In colder climates, move the patient to a warmer environment, such as the ambulance, as quickly as possible without compromising the spine further.

Placement on the Longboard

Before you immobilise a patient, be sure you have documented your assessment thus far. It will also be important to document your findings during the immobilisation process, and after the patient has been immobilised.

Most patients can be log rolled with visualisation for deformity or injury as well as palpation over each posterior spinous process for pain, deformity, or step off. The absence of pain or tenderness along the spine, coupled with a normal neurological examination and low-risk mechanism of injury, may eliminate the need for manual in-line spinal immobilisation. In contrast, paralysed limbs should always be protected with appropriate longboard and stretcher immobilisation.

Patients in severe pain may require an alternative method of transfer to a longboard. Use of a scoop stretcher often results in less movement of the patient. Once the scoop is in place, another paramedic or EMT can slide the longboard or air mattress underneath the patient. Although the patient can still be palpated with this method, inability to conduct visual inspection of the area is a disadvantage of this procedure.

Time on a longboard should be kept to a minimum because skin breakdown can be a major complication of SCI **Figure 22-9 ▶**. This problem occurs as a result of excessive pressure over the bones of the buttocks, the scapular ridges, and the base of the occiput. These five areas are the primary points supporting the patient's weight. The initial stages of pressure lesions may occur in a matter of hours; 32% of patients with SCI develop a skin lesion within 24 hours of injury. Blood distribution shifts to the skin and subcutaneous tissues, and decreased muscle tone and sensation predispose the SCI patient to these injuries.

Several new devices have been developed to enhance patient comfort. The extrication vest takes pressure off specific areas of the back and fills voids that may otherwise allow patient movement. This low-profile air mattress fits under the patient from the shoulders to the waist **Figure 22-10 ▶**. Slightly flexing the knees with towel rolls or a blanket and slightly separating the legs with a pillow or blanket increases patient comfort and decreases the likelihood of post immobilisation problems, yet still provides adequate immobilisation of the patient **Figure 22-11 ▶**. Concave longboards also conform more closely to a patient's anatomy than do flat boards. Spider straps should be used to properly immobilise a patient. Although quick clip straps are easier to use, they do not restrict movement as effectively as the spider strap.

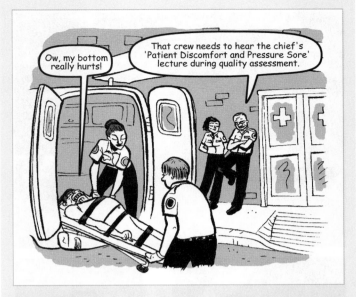

Figure 22-9

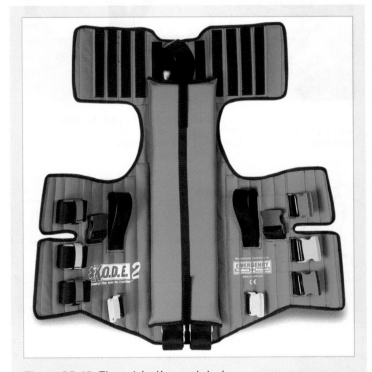

Figure 22-10 The extrication vest device.

Detailed Physical Examination

A detailed physical examination for a trauma patient with a significant MOI should take place while en route to the hospital.

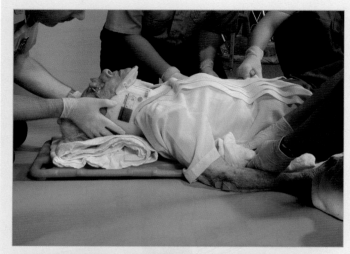

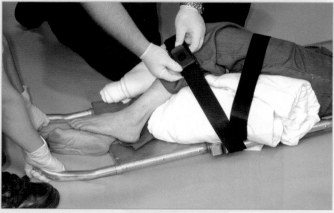

Figure 22-11 Using towel rolls or blankets to pad the longboard will increase patient comfort and can minimise problems resulting from immobilisation of the older patient.

At the Scene

Always palpate over the spinous process before concluding that a patient "has no neck pain".
Some providers simply ask the patient and never perform a physical examination.

Closely examine the head, neck, chest, abdomen, pelvis, extremities, back, and buttocks. A detailed head-to-toe examination can often reveal significant findings, especially in patients with questionable reliability, unclear mechanisms, or multi-system trauma.

Thoroughly assess the head and neck, as many SCI patients will have associated head and facial injuries; a complaint of pain is most predictive of a spine injury. Examination of the neck should include gentle palpation of the cervical spine for pain, deformity, or dislocation.

Evaluate the chest and abdomen for both internal and external injuries. Fractures of the ribs, sternum, clavicle, scapula, or pelvis are often associated with SCI in patients with multi-system trauma. Visualisation and palpation are the mainstays of this evaluation. Bear in mind that the physical examination in the SCI patient may be distorted due to potentially decreased sensation below the level of the spine injury. Assess the chest wall visually for symmetry of chest wall movement, work of breathing, and use of accessory muscles. Auscultation to assess breath sounds may reveal a shortened inspiratory phase. Inadequate ventilation, accessory muscle use, or paradoxical ventilations may indicate diaphragmatic impairment due to SCI.

Continually monitor the cardiovascular system for signs of shock. Neurogenic shock may require pharmacologic management and/or transcutaneous pacing.

Examination of the gastrointestinal system may be unreliable in the presence of a neurological deficit. First, inspect the abdomen for evidence of trauma, noting its contour. Severe gastric distention may impair respiration and lead to airway compromise due to vomiting. Palpate all four quadrants for tenderness, guarding, or rigidity, but remember that patients may be insensitive to pain and may not develop a rigid abdomen because of absence of muscle tone. Lower abdominal distention with or without suprapubic tenderness may be due to urinary retention. In men, assess the ureteral meatus for evidence of blood, scrotal swelling, and scrotal ecchymosis, which may be present with pelvic fractures. Assess for priapism as well.

Inspect all extremities for deformity, contusion, abrasions, punctures, lacerations, and oedema. Palpate for deformity, tenderness, instability, or crepitus. Look for any abnormal posturing, and assess the patient for potential long bone or other significantly distracting painful injuries that may mask a potential spine or cord injury.

Neurological Examination

The focused neurological evaluation in the prehospital environment is intended to establish a baseline level of the lesion for later comparison—that is, to determine the completeness of the lesion and to identify cord syndromes if the lesion is incomplete. A normal neurological examination does not rule out the possibility of SCI. Patients who experienced vehicular trauma have been known to walk away from the crash only to become totally paralysed hours later, when an incautious nod of the head squeezed an unstable vertebral column down against the spinal cord. The neurological assessment is intended not only to determine whether the patient should be immobilised, but also to furnish data to the hospital about the precise initial presentation of the patient so that personnel there may evaluate any changes in condition and determine if immediate surgery is necessary.

The initial step of any neurological assessment is a determination of the level of consciousness. First note the patient's AVPU in the initial assessment, and then address the GCS level during further assessment. When assigning the GCS, do not score the patient as having no motor response if limbs are paralysed. Ask the patient to blink or move some facial muscles that would be innervated by a cranial nerve. Remember that an unconscious patient is always at risk for having a spinal injury.

Table 22-2	Landmark Myotomes		
Nerve Root	**Muscle Group**	**Nerve Root**	**Muscle Group**
C3-C5	Diaphragm	L2	Hip flexors: iliopsoas
C5	Elbow flexors: biceps, brachialis, brachioradialis	L3	Knee extensors: quadriceps
C6	Wrist extensors	L4	Ankle dorsiflexors: tibialis anterior
C7	Elbow extensors: triceps	L5	Long toe extensors: extensor hallucis longus
C8	Finger flexors: flexor digitorum profundus to middle finger	S1	Ankle plantar flexors (gastronemius, soleus)
T1	Hand intrinsics: interossei, small finger abductors	S4-S5	Anus, bowel, bladder
T2-T7	Intercostal muscles		

Table 22-3	Landmark Dermatomes		
Nerve Root	**Anatomical Location**	**Nerve Root**	**Anatomical Location**
C2	Occipital protuberance	T10	Umbilicus
C3-C4	Supraclavicular fossa	L1	Inguinal line
C5	Lateral side of antecubital fossa	L2	Mid anterior thigh
C6	Thumb and medial index finger (6-shooter)	L3	Medial aspect of the knee
C7	Middle finger	L5	Dorsum of the foot
C8	Little finger	S1-S3	Back of leg
T2	Apex of axilla	S4-S5	Perianal area
T4	Nipple line		

Motor components of spinal nerves innervate discrete tissues and muscles of the body in regions called myotomes Table 22-2 ▲. The examination of these myotomes should take place in the typical head-to-toe fashion, starting with an assessment of the cranial nerves. Cranial nerve assessment is especially important in circumstances suggestive of a high cervical injury. Observe the patient for drooping of the upper eyelid and a small pupil (Horner's syndrome) that would indicate an injury to C3.

Bilaterally assess each major motor group from the top down to identify the lowest spinal segment associated with normal voluntary motor function. Because of the possibility of incomplete spinal cord lesions, it is important to determine the extent of function in segments below this level. Monitor for possible ascending lesions, paying special attention to alterations in respiratory patterns with cervical lesions.

Ask the patient to flex (C5) and extend (C7) both elbows and then both wrists (C6). Have the patient abduct the fingers and keep them open against resistance, and then adduct the fingers and attempt to open them against resistance (T1) Figure 22-12 ▶. As an alternative manoeuvre, have the patient curl all four fingers while the examiner applies opposing pull with his or her fingers to determine strength against resistance. This will test the finger flexors (C8).

To evaluate the lower extremities, ask the patient to bend and extend the knees. Next ask the patient to plantar flex the feet and ankles as if pressing down on the accelerator pedal of a car (S1–S2) and to dorsiflex the toes to gravity and against resis-tance (L5) Figure 22-13 ▶.

Assessment of motor integrity in an unconscious patient is largely based on the patient's response to a painful stimulus. Spine injury with loss of motor function is likely if an uncon-scious patient grimaces, vocalises, or opens his or her eyes to a painful response above the level of the neurological deficit but does not move the limbs. Pain responses should be tested at several locations before assuming an absence of response. If the motor examination cannot be completed due to local injury, the examination is considered unreliable and spine motion restriction is necessary.

Sensor components of spinal nerves innervate specific and discrete areas of the body surface called dermatomes Table 22-3 ▲. In addition to testing a general loss of sensation, ask the patient about abnormal sensations in these areas such as "pins and needles", electric shock, or hyperacute pain to touch (hyperaesthesia). As with the motor examination, sensory integrity must be assessed bilaterally but from the feet up. Determine the lowest level of normal sensation and any areas of intact or "spared" sensation below this level. In the conscious patient, a thorough evaluation will include perception of light touch, temperature, and position (proprioception).

Reflexes are usually not assessed on scene but can provide valuable information regarding sensory input, especially in the unconscious patient. In significant SCIs, reflexes are usually absent but return several hours to several weeks after injury. If reflexes are intact, the preservation of motor and sensory activity in the same spinal cord segments is likely. A positive Babinski reflex occurs when the toes move upward in response to stimulation of the sole of the foot. Under normal circumstances, the toes move downward.

Notes from Nancy

The most important aspect of neurological assessment is whether the patient's findings are changing and in what direction.

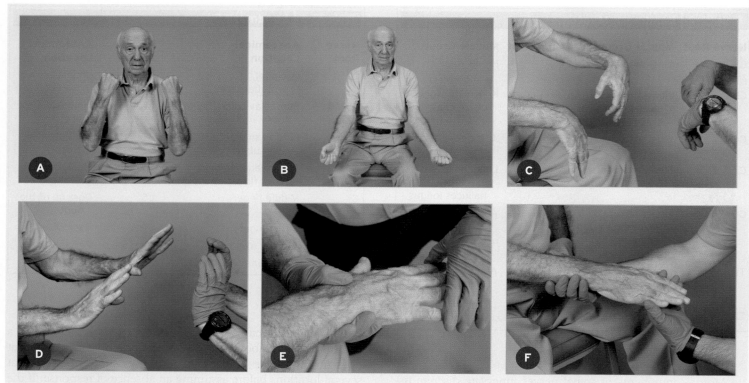

Figure 22-12 Neurological evaluation of the upper extremities. Ask the patient to flex (**A**) and then extend (**B**) both elbows. Ask the patient to flex (**C**) and then extend (**D**) both wrists. Have the patient abduct the fingers and keep them open against resistance (**E**). Have the patient adduct the fingers and attempt to open them against resistance (**F**).

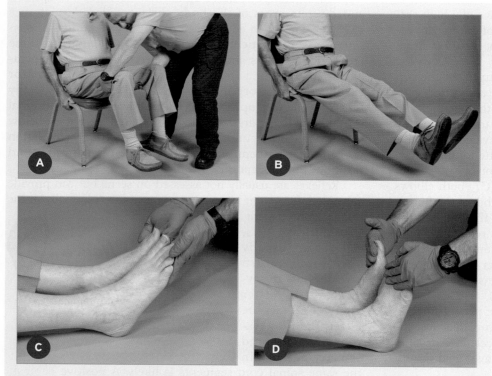

Figure 22-13 Neurological evaluation of the lower extremities. Ask the patient to bend (**A**) and extend (**B**) the knees. Ask the patient to flex the feet and ankles downward (**C**) and flex the toes upward (**D**).

Ongoing Assessment

Vital signs should be monitored every 5 minutes (unstable patients) to 15 minutes (stable patients), with special attention to the patient's cardiovascular status. Be alert for hypotension without other signs of shock. The combination of hypotension with a normal or slow pulse and warm skin is highly suggestive of neurogenic shock. The SCI responsible for neurogenic shock also generally produces a flaccid paralysis and complete loss of sensation below the level of the injury. In contrast to neurogenic shock, hypovolaemic shock is associated with pale, cold, clammy skin and tachycardia.

Check interventions such as oxygen flow and spinal immobilisation to ensure that they are still effective. Some ambulance services may administer an antiemetic or corticosteroid in accordance with medical advice. Repeat the physical examination and reprioritise the patient as necessary.

Prep Kit

Ready for Review

- SCIs are among the most devastating injuries encountered by pre-hospital providers.
- In order to decipher the often subtle findings associated with SCI, you need to understand the form and function of spinal anatomy.
- Acute injuries of the spine are classified according to the associated mechanism, location, and stability of injury.
- Vertebral factures can occur with or without associated SCI.
- Stable fractures do not involve the posterior column and pose lower risk to the spinal cord.
- Unstable injuries involve the posterior column of the spinal cord and typically include damage to portions of the vertebrae and ligaments that directly protect the spinal cord and nerve roots.
- Primary SCI occurs at the moment of impact.
- Secondary SCI occurs when multiple factors permit a progression of the primary SCI. The ensuing cascade of inflammatory responses may result in further deterioration.
- Limiting the progression of secondary SCI is a major goal of pre-hospital management of SCI.
- Current principles of spine trauma management include recognition of potential or actual injury, appropriate immobilisation, and reduction or prevention of the incidence of secondary injury.
- Short-acting, reversible sedatives are recommended for the acute patient after a correctible cause of agitation has been excluded.
- The use of corticosteroids in the acute phase of SCI remains controversial.
- The complications of SCI are a consistent cause of the high morbidity and mortality associated with this type of injury.
- Back pain is one of the most common physical complaints to present to A&E departments. Most cases of low back pain are idiopathic and difficult to diagnose precisely.

Vital Vocabulary

anterior cord syndrome A condition that occurs with flexion injuries or fractures resulting in the displacement of bony fragments into the anterior portion of the spinal cord; findings include paralysis below the level of the insult and loss of pain, temperature, and touch sensation.

arachnoid The middle membrane of the three meninges that enclose the brain and spinal cord.

autonomic dysreflexia A potentially life-threatening late complication of spinal cord injury in which massive, uninhibited uncompensated cardiovascular response occurs due to stimulation of the sympathetic nervous system below the level of injury. Also known as autonomic hyperreflexia.

Babinski reflex When the toe(s) moves upward in response to stimulation to the sole of the foot. Under normal circumstances, the toe(s) moves downward.

brain Part of the central nervous system, located within the cranium and containing billions of neurones that serve a variety of vital functions.

brain stem The portion of the brain that connects the spinal cord to the rest of the brain, and contains the medulla, pons, and midbrain.

Brown-Sequard syndrome A condition associated with penetrating trauma with hemisection of the spinal cord and complete damage to all spinal tracts on the involved side.

cauda equina The location where the spinal cord separates, composed of nerve roots.

central cord syndrome A condition resulting from hyperextension injuries to the cervical area that cause damage with haemorrhage or oedema to the central cervical segments; findings include greater loss of function in the upper extremities with variable sensory loss of pain and temperature.

central nervous system (CNS) The system containing the brain and spinal cord.

cerebrospinal fluid (CSF) Fluid produced in the ventricles of the brain that flows in the subarachnoid space and bathes the meninges.

complete spinal cord injury Total disruption of all tracts of the spinal cord, with all cord mediated functions below the level of transection lost permanently.

dermatomes Areas of the body innervated by sensor components of spinal nerves.

dura mater The outermost of the three meninges that enclose the brain and spinal cord, it is the toughest membrane.

facet joint The joint on which each vertebra articulates with adjacent vertebrae.

flexion injury A type of injury that results from forward movement of the head, typically as the result of rapid deceleration, such as in a car crash, or with a direct blow to the occiput.

foramen magnum A large opening at the base of the skull through which the spinal cord exits the brain.

hyperaesthesia Hyperacute pain to touch.

hyperextension Extension of a limb of other body part beyond its usual range of motion.

incomplete spinal cord injury Spinal cord injury in which there is some degree of cord-mediated function; initial dysfunction may be temporary and there may be potential for recovery.

lamina Arise from the posterior pedicles and fuse to form the posterior spinous processes.

myotomes Regions of the body innervated by the motor components of spinal nerves.

neurogenic shock Shock caused by massive vasodilation and pooling of blood in the peripheral vessels to the extent that adequate perfusion cannot be maintained.

parasympathetic nervous system Subdivision of the autonomic nervous system, involved in control of involuntary, vegetative functions, mediated largely by the vagus nerve through the chemical acetylcholine.

pedicles Thick lateral bony struts that connect the vertebral body with spinous and transverse processes and make up the lateral and posterior portions of the spinal foramen.

pia mater The innermost of the three meninges that enclose the brain and spinal cord, it rests directly on the brain and spinal cord.

plexus A cluster of nerve roots that permits peripheral nerve roots to rejoin and function as a group.

posterior cord syndrome A condition associated with extension injuries with isolated injury to the dorsal column; presents as decreased sensation to light touch, proprioception, and vibration while leaving most other motor and sensory functions intact.

posterior process Formed by the fusion of the posterior lamina, this is an attachment site for muscles and ligaments.

primary spinal cord injury Injury to the spinal cord that is a direct result of trauma, for example transection of the spinal cord from penetrating trauma or displacement of ligaments and bone fragments, resulting in compression of the spinal cord.

proprioception The ability to perceive the position and movement of one's body or limbs.

rotation-flexion injury A type of injury typically resulting from high acceleration forces; can result in a stable unilateral facet dislocation in the cervical spine.

secondary spinal cord injury Injury to the spinal cord, thought to be the result of multiple factors that result in a progression of inflammatory responses from primary spinal cord injury.

spinal cord The part of the central nervous system that extends downward from the brain through the foramen magnum and is protected by the spine.

spinal shock The temporary local neurological condition that occurs immediately after spinal trauma; swelling and oedema of the spinal cord begin immediately after injury, with severe pain and potential paralysis.

sympathetic nervous system Subdivision of the autonomic nervous system that governs the body's fight-or-flight reactions by inducing smooth muscle contraction or relaxation of the blood vessels and bronchioles.

transverse process The junction of each pedicle and lamina on each side of a vertebra; these project laterally and posteriorly and form points of attachment for muscles and ligaments.

vertebral body Anterior weight-bearing structure in the spine made of cancellous bone and surrounded by a layer of hard, compact bone that provides support and stability.

vertical compression A type of injury typically resulting from a direct blow to the crown of the skull or rapid deceleration from a fall through the feet, legs, and pelvis, possibly causing a burst fracture or disc herniation.

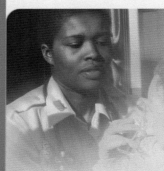

Assessment in Action

You and your partner respond to a patient who has fallen. On arrival, you find a 42-year-old man lying conscious and supine on the ground outside a home. A ladder is lying beside him, with paint spilled on the lawn. Neighbours say the patient fell at least 8 metres while painting the second-floor windows. On initial assessment, he complains of pain in his neck area and lower back. His respirations are 22 breaths/min; pulse, 58 beats/min; and blood pressure, 94/58 mm Hg. The skin is warm, red, and dry. He has no sensation below the navel. He cannot move his lower extremities and has no reflexes below the hip.

1. **After the initial assessment reveals adequate ABCs, you should:**
   A. inquire about history.
   B. notify the local hospital.
   C. apply manual in-line cervical spine immobilisation.
   D. perform a neurological examination.

2. **You apply oxygen and apply a longboard and rigid cervical collar. Now you must decide whether to treat on scene or transport. Which factor should you base your decision on?**
   A. Distance of fall
   B. Patient preference
   C. Vital signs
   D. Mechanism of injury

3. **You are beginning the transport. Where should the patient be transported to?**
   A. The closest hospital
   B. An A&E department with trauma facilities
   C. A local medical centre
   D. None of the above

4. **What is the maximum scene time for this patient?**
   A. 5 minutes
   B. 10 minutes
   C. 15 minutes
   D. However long it takes to immobilise the patient safely

5. **Based on the vital signs and mechanism, what should you suspect is causing the hypotension?**
   A. Blood loss
   B. Head injury
   C. Neurogenic shock
   D. All of the above

6. **What should your treatment actions be?**
   A. Continue assessment and seek out other injuries.
   B. Determine the Glasgow Coma Scale score.
   C. Initiate IV therapy.
   D. All of the above

7. **Based on the level of sensation, what area of the spine may be injured?**
   A. C7
   B. L3
   C. T10
   D. S1

Challenging Questions

You respond to a road traffic collision. The vehicle struck a bridge pillar on the motorway, resulting in substantial damage to the car. The driver is unconscious and slumped over the steering wheel. He is breathing with difficulty. You suspect partial airway obstruction by his tongue. Smoke is coming from the car's engine compartment.

8. **What should you do?**

■ Points to Ponder

You respond to a call about a fall. On arrival, you find the patient at the foot of a staircase at the local community college. The patient reports that he slipped while running up the steps, and fell backwards from the top to the bottom. The patient is conscious, alert, and orientated, complaining only of pain in his left leg. He has several bruises on the head, legs, and arms. No serious bleeding is noted, and the patient denies loss of consciousness. You immediately secure the cervical spine and begin a neurological assessment. The patient's pupils are equal and reactive. He has good pulse, motor, and sensation in all extremities, and his reflexes are normal. You find no neurological abnormalities.

Should you immobilise this patient?

Issues: Thorough Assessment, Proper Management of Spine Injuries.

Objectives

Cognitive

- Describe the incidence, morbidity, and mortality of thoracic injuries in the trauma patient.
- Discuss the anatomy and physiology of the organs and structures related to thoracic injuries.
- Predict thoracic injuries based on mechanism of injury.
- Discuss the types of thoracic injuries.
- Discuss the pathophysiology of thoracic injuries.
- Discuss the assessment findings associated with thoracic injuries.
- Discuss the management of thoracic injuries.
- Identify the need for rapid intervention and transport of the patient with thoracic injuries.
- Discuss the pathophysiology of specific chest wall injuries, including:
  - Rib fracture
  - Flail segment
  - Sternal fracture
- Discuss the assessment findings associated with chest wall injuries.
- Identify the need for rapid intervention and transport of the patient with chest wall injuries.
- Discuss the management of chest wall injuries.
- Discuss the pathophysiology of injury to the lung, including:
  - Simple pneumothorax
  - Open pneumothorax
  - Tension pneumothorax
  - Haemothorax
  - Haemopneumothorax
  - Pulmonary contusion
- Discuss the assessment findings associated with lung injuries.
- Discuss the management of lung injuries.
- Identify the need for rapid intervention and transport of the patient with lung injuries.
- Discuss the pathophysiology of myocardial injuries, including:
  - Cardiac tamponade
  - Myocardial contusion
  - Myocardial rupture
- Discuss the assessment findings associated with myocardial injuries.
- Discuss the management of myocardial injuries.
- Identify the need for rapid intervention and transport of the patient with myocardial injuries.
- Discuss the pathophysiology of vascular injuries, including injuries to:
  - Aorta
  - Vena cava
  - Pulmonary arteries/veins
- Discuss the assessment findings associated with vascular injuries.
- Discuss the management of vascular injuries.
- Identify the need for rapid intervention and transport of the patient with vascular injuries.

- Discuss the pathophysiology of diaphragmatic injuries.
- Discuss the assessment findings associated with diaphragmatic injuries.
- Discuss the management of diaphragmatic injuries.
- Identify the need for rapid intervention and transport of the patient with diaphragmatic injuries.
- Discuss the pathophysiology of oesophageal injuries.
- Discuss the assessment findings associated with oesophageal injuries.
- Discuss the management of oesophageal injuries.
- Identify the need for rapid intervention and transport of the patient with oesophageal injuries.
- Discuss the pathophysiology of tracheobronchial injuries.
- Discuss the assessment findings associated with tracheobronchial injuries.
- Discuss the management of tracheobronchial injuries.
- Identify the need for rapid intervention and transport of the patient with tracheobronchial injuries.
- Discuss the pathophysiology of traumatic asphyxia.
- Discuss the assessment findings associated with traumatic asphyxia.
- Discuss the management of traumatic asphyxia.
- Identify the need for rapid intervention and transport of the patient with traumatic asphyxia.
- Integrate the pathophysiological principles to the assessment of a patient with thoracic injury.
- Differentiate between thoracic injuries based on the assessment and history.
- Formulate a working diagnosis based on the assessment findings.
- Develop a patient management plan based on the working diagnosis.

Affective

- Advocate the use of a thorough assessment to determine a differential diagnosis and treatment plan for thoracic trauma.
- Advocate the use of a thorough scene survey to determine the forces involved in thoracic trauma.
- Value the implications of failing to properly diagnose thoracic trauma.
- Value the implications of failing to initiate timely interventions to patients with thoracic trauma.

Psychomotor

- Demonstrate a clinical assessment for a patient with suspected thoracic trauma.
- Demonstrate the following techniques of management for thoracic injuries:
  - Needle decompression
  - Fracture stabilisation
  - Elective intubation
  - ECG monitoring
  - Oxygenation and ventilation

Introduction

Thoracic (chest) trauma is not a disease of modern society. For as long as humans have been capable of falling or injuring one another, damage to the thoracic cavity has been a significant concern in the management of the trauma patient Figure 23-1 ▾ . As more rapid forms of transportation and more lethal weapons continue to evolve, the incidence and severity of thoracic trauma is not likely to diminish, nor is the need for its rapid assessment and treatment.

Only head trauma and traumatic brain injuries account for more deaths among trauma victims. An estimated one in four trauma deaths is directly due to thoracic injuries, and thoracic trauma is a contributing factor in another 25% of trauma patients who die of their injuries.

Given the specific organs that are housed within the thoracic cavity, it is not surprising that these injuries can be so deadly. In addition, the mechanism producing these injuries often involves a great deal of force transmitted to the body, with road traffic collisions accounting for seven in every ten patients with blunt thoracic trauma.

At the Scene

Thoracic injuries, whether severe or seemingly minor, often give rise to elusive findings that are overshadowed by associated injuries.

Anatomy

The thorax consists of a bony cage overlying some of the most vital organs in the human body. The dimensions of the thorax are defined posteriorly by the thoracic vertebrae and ribs, inferiorly by the diaphragm, anteriorly and laterally by the ribs, and superiorly by the thoracic inlet Figure 23-2 ▸ .

The dimensions of this area of the body are of great importance in the physical assessment of the patient. Although the thoracic cavity extends to the 12th rib posteriorly, the diaphragm inserts into the anterior thoracic cage just below the fourth or fifth rib. With the movement of the diaphragm during respiration, the size and dimensions of the thoracic

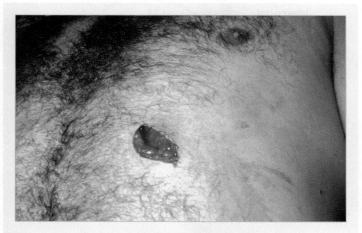

Figure 23-1 Thoracic trauma is a significant concern in the management of the trauma patient.

You are the Paramedic Part 1

While you are working as a paramedic for a local ambulance service, you and your colleague are sent to a nearby town to assist with an RTC. En route, you are informed that it is a head-on collision on a dual carriageway. Two people have already been pronounced dead at the scene.

You arrive to find an 18-year-old male passenger who was partially ejected from the vehicle; he was not wearing a seatbelt. Fire service personnel have extricated the patient from the vehicle, placed him in full cervical spine precautions, and are currently assisting his ventilations with a bag-valve-mask device.

Initial Assessment	Recording Time: 0 Minutes
Appearance	Secured to a longboard
Level of consciousness	U in AVPU (Unresponsive)
Airway	Patent with an oropharyngeal airway
Breathing	Assisted ventilations at a rate of 10 to 12 breaths/min
Circulation	Pale skin

1. What will your initial priorities be when assessing and managing this patient?
2. Given the mechanism of injury for an unrestrained passenger in a car and this patient's vital signs, what kinds of injuries should you think about during your assessment?

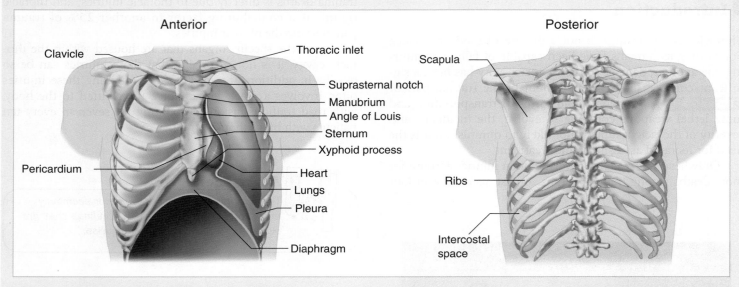

Figure 23-2 The thorax, anterior and posterior views.

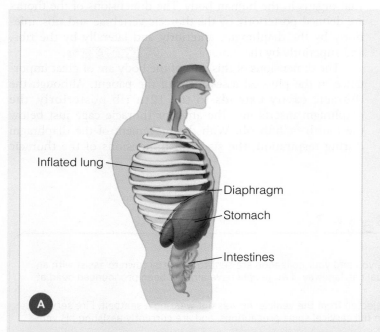

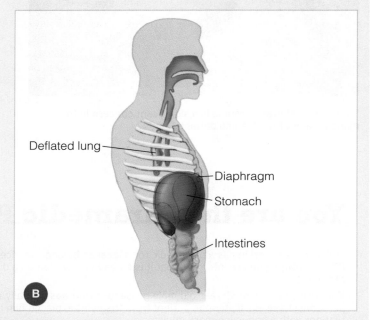

Figure 23-3 The anatomy of the thoracic cavity during inspiration (**A**) and expiration (**B**).

cavity will vary **Figure 23-3 ▲**, which could in turn affect the organs or cavities (thoracic versus abdominal) in case of blunt or penetrating injury.

The bony structures of the thorax include the sternum, clavicle, scapula, thoracic vertebrae, and 12 pairs of ribs. The sternum consists of three separate portions: the superior manubrium, the central sternal body, and the inferior xyphoid process. The space superior to the manubrium is termed the suprasternal notch; the junction of the manubrium and sternal body is referred to as the angle of Louis.

The clavicle is an elongated, S-shaped bone that connects to the manubrium medially and overlies the first rib as it proceeds laterally toward the shoulder. Beneath the clavicle lies the subclavian artery and vein. Laterally, the clavicle connects to the acromion process of the scapula, the triangular bone that overlies the posterior aspect of the upper thoracic cage.

Each of the 12 matched pairs of ribs attach posteriorly to the 12 thoracic vertebrae. Anteriorly, the first seven pairs of ribs attach directly to the sternum via the costal cartilage. The costal cartilage then continues inferiorly from the seventh ribs and provides an indirect connection between the anterior portions of the eighth, ninth, and tenth ribs and the sternum. The eleventh and twelfth ribs have no anterior connection and, therefore, are known as the "floating ribs".

Between each rib lies an intercostal space. These spaces are numbered according to the rib superior to the space (ie, the space between the second and third ribs is the second intercostal space). These spaces house the intercostal muscles and the neurovascular bundle, which consists of an artery, vein, and nerve.

The central region of the thorax is the mediastinum, which contains the heart, great vessels, oesophagus, lymphatic channels, trachea, mainstem bronchi, and paired vagus and phrenic nerves. The heart resides within a tough fibrous sac called the pericardium. Much like the pleura, the pericardium has two surfaces—the inner (visceral) layer, which adheres to the heart and forms the epicardium, and the outer (parietal) layer, which comprises the sac itself. The pericardium that covers the inferior aspect of the heart is directly attached to the diaphragm. The heart is positioned so that the most anterior portion is the right ventricle, which has relatively thin chamber walls. The pressure within the right ventricle is approximately one quarter of the pressure within the left ventricle. Most of the heart is protected anteriorly by the sternum. With each beat, the apex of the heart can be felt in the fifth intercostal space along the midclavicular line, a phenomenon known as cardiac impulse (apical beat). The average cardiac output for an adult (heart rate times the stroke volume) is $70 \times 70 = 4,900$ ml/min, though it varies depending on the patient's size.

The aorta is the largest artery in the body. As it exits the left ventricle, it ascends toward the right shoulder before turning to the left and proceeding inferiorly toward the abdomen. This artery has three points of attachment—the anulus at its origin from the aortic valve, the ligamentum arteriosum, and the aortic hiatus. These attachments represent sites of potential injury when the vessel is subject to significant shearing forces, such as those seen during sudden deceleration mechanisms.

The lungs occupy most of the space within the thoracic cavity. Like the pericardium, the lungs are lined with a dual layer of connective tissue known as the pleura. The parietal pleura lines the interior of each side of the thoracic cavity. The visceral pleura lines the exterior of each lung.

A small amount of viscous fluid separates the two layers of pleura. This fluid allows the two layers of connective tissue to move against each other without friction or pain. It creates a surface tension that holds the layers together, thereby keeping the lung from collapsing away from the thoracic cage on exhalation. If this space becomes filled with air, blood, or other fluids, the surface tension is lost and the lung collapses.

The diaphragm, the primary muscle of breathing, forms a barrier between the thoracic and abdominal cavities. It works in conjunction with the intercostal muscles to increase the size of the thoracic cavity during inspiration, creating the negative pressure that pulls air in via the trachea. In times of distress, this breathing effort can be aided by other accessory muscles of the thoracic cavity, including the trapezius, latissimus dorsi, rhomboids, pectoralis, and sternocleidomastoid Figure 23-4 ▶ .

You are the Paramedic Part 2

As you assume patient care, you begin by assessing the patient's airway. As the bag-valve-mask ventilations continue, you find the patient has a patent airway without stridor. His mental status remains unresponsive with a quickly estimated Glasgow Coma Scale score of 5 and some decorticate posturing. You and your colleague decide to manage the patient's airway with endotracheal intubation, while still maintaining manual in-line immobilisation of the cervical spine.

The patient is intubated without difficulty, the placement of the endotracheal tube is confirmed by multiple methods, and assisted ventilation is continued. You prepare for transport, as your colleague starts an IV to administer a fluid bolus of normal saline. After moving the patient, you reassess his ventilation and note that his breath sounds are absent on the right side. His neck reveals jugular vein distension, and you're not really sure if the trachea is deviated to the left side.

Vital Signs	Recording Time: 10 Minutes
Level of consciousness	U (Unresponsive) with a Glasgow Coma Scale score of 5
Pulse	Radial pulse, 128 beats/min
Blood pressure	70/38 mm Hg
Respirations	Intubated; ventilating with 100% supplemental oxygen
Skin	Cool, pale, and perspiring
SpO_2	88% on room air

3. Why does the patient remain hypoxic despite confirmed airway management and the delivery of high-concentration oxygen?

4. Do his vital signs and physical examination suggest any threats to his breathing that may be correctable?

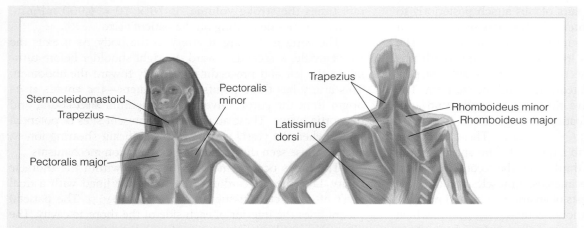

Figure 23-4 The muscles of the thoracic cavity include the trapezius, latissimus dorsi, rhomboid, pectoralis, and sternocleidomastoid muscles.

Physiology

The primary physiological functions of the thorax and its contents are to maintain oxygenation and ventilation and (via the heart) to maintain circulation.

The process of breathing includes both the delivery of oxygen to the body and the elimination of carbon dioxide from the body. While these processes are often accomplished simultaneously, they are, in fact, different aspects of the breathing process.

First, however, the brain must stimulate the person to breathe. This stimulation occurs via chemoreceptors that are located in the carotid sinus and aortic arch. These receptors are in essence "little chemists" that analyse the arterial blood. When the level of carbon dioxide gets too high, the receptors send a message to the brain, which responds by increasing the respiratory rate in an effort to "blow off the CO_2". Some patients with end-stage chronic obstructive pulmonary disease (COPD) may employ a secondary mechanism called hypoxic drive for this function because they retain excess CO_2 on a chronic basis.

As the diaphragm contracts downward, the intercostal and accessory muscles pull the chest wall out and away from the centre of the body. The resulting negative pressure within the thoracic cavity draws air in through the mouth and nose, down the trachea, passing through smaller and smaller bronchioles until finally it reaches the alveolar spaces. The new air both mixes with and replaces the air contained within the alveoli.

While respiration is occurring, blood is being delivered via the pulmonary circulation to the capillaries that lie adjacent to the alveoli. This blood has returned to the heart after traversing the body, having delivered its oxygen to the cells and removed the cellular waste products such as CO_2. As a result, the blood entering the capillaries adjacent to the alveoli has a low O_2 concentration and a high CO_2 concentration.

The process of oxygenation includes the delivery of oxygen from the air to the blood, where it is carried to cells and tissues throughout the body. Because the air entering the alveoli contains a higher concentration of O_2 (ranging from 21% in room air to as much as 100% in a nonrebreathing mask or bag mask under ideal circumstances) than the blood in the nearby capillaries, the oxygen will follow its concentration gradient and enter the blood. Most of the oxygen binds to haemoglobin within the red blood cells, and the oxygen returns to the heart with the blood, where it is then pumped throughout the body.

Ventilation is the process by which CO_2 is removed from the body. The air in our environment contains very little CO_2 (0.033%). As a result, when air enters the alveoli, it contains very little CO_2 compared to the blood in the nearby capillaries. The CO_2 diffuses down its concentration gradient, leaving the blood and entering the air within the alveoli.

As the diaphragm and the chest wall relax, positive pressure is created within the thorax. The air from which oxygen has been absorbed and into which carbon dioxide has been diffused is then exhaled. With each subsequent respiration (inhalation and exhalation), the process is repeated.

Proper functioning of the heart is essential to the delivery of blood to the body's tissues. As blood returns from the body via the inferior and superior vena cavae, it is pumped from the right side of the heart to the lungs, where the processes of oxygenation and ventilation take place. As oxygenated blood returns from the lungs, it enters the left side of the heart and is then pumped out to the body.

The ability to pump blood depends on having a functional pump (the heart), an adequate volume of blood to be pumped, and a lack of resistance to the pumping mechanism (afterload)—properties that are collectively known as cardiac output. Cardiac output is the volume of blood delivered to the body in 1 minute. The volume is identified by counting the number of times the heart beats in a minute (heart rate) and determining the amount of blood delivered to the body with each beat (stroke volume). Thus cardiac output equals the heart rate (beats/min) multiplied by the stroke volume (millilitres of blood per beat). Any injury that limits the heart's pumping ability, the delivery of blood to the heart, the blood's ability to leave the heart, or the heart rate will affect cardiac output.

Pathophysiology of Thoracic Injuries

Traumatic injury to the thoracic cavity presents the possibility of compromise of ventilation, oxygenation, or circulation. Accordingly, the assessment of the thoracic cavity becomes an integral part of the overall assessment of the patient's ABCs, the initial assessment, and the continuing assessment. These injuries, if missed or inappropriately treated, could contribute significantly to the patient's morbidity or even cause death.

The patient's ventilation may be affected by both mechanical and functional impairments. Air or blood entering the pleural space may result in the loss of airspace in which ventilation normally occurs. Similarly, injuries to the chest wall or diaphragm may limit the movement of the thorax, thereby constraining the patient's ability to ventilate. Finally, ventilation may be affected simply by a painful injury that limits the patient's ability or willingness to fully ventilate his or her lung tissue with each breath.

Within the lung itself, loss of alveolar space may result in the inability to exchange gases such as oxygen, ultimately leading to clinical hypoxaemia. This problem may be caused by alveolar collapse (atelectasis) due to incomplete chest wall and lung expansion, haemorrhage into the lung tissue itself, or airway obstruction.

Within the cardiovascular structures of the thoracic cavity, acute blood loss from vascular injury may result in systemic hypoperfusion. In such a case, localised blood loss within the pericardium may result in immediate cardiovascular collapse.

Chest Wall Injuries
Flail Chest

Flail chest Figure 23-5 ▾, a major injury to the chest wall, may result from a variety of blunt force mechanisms such as falls, road traffic collisions, assaults, and even birth trauma. Mortality rates are directly related to the underlying and associated injuries. Patients are more likely to suffer a fatal injury

if they are elderly, have seven or more rib fractures or three or more associated injuries, present with shock, or have associated head trauma.

A flail segment is defined as two or more adjacent ribs that are fractured in two or more places. The segment between those two fracture sites becomes separated from the surrounding chest wall, leaving it free to succumb to the underlying pressures—hence the name "free-floating segment." Both the location and the size of the segment can affect the degree to which the flail segment impairs chest wall motion and subsequent air movement. In a flail sternum (the most extreme case), the sternum is completely separated from the ribs because of fractures or ruptured costal cartilage. This type of injury results in mechanical dysfunction of both sides of the chest and more severe respiratory impairment.

Once a flail segment has occurred, the underlying physiological pressures cause paradoxical movement of the segment when compared to the rest of the chest wall. Expansion of the chest wall on inspiration results in negative pressure within the thoracic cavity, which in turn draws the flail segment in toward the centre of the chest. As the chest relaxes or is actively contracted (depending on the degree of dyspnoea), the resulting positive pressure forces air from the lungs and also forces the flail segment out away from the thoracic cavity. Because of these movements, the lung tissue beneath the flail segment is not adequately ventilated. Clearly, a flail segment can quickly become life-threatening, which explains why it is managed in the initial assessment of the patient. Typical management involves pressing down on the segment as the patient exhales so that the free-floating segment conforms with the rest of the chest wall. Some providers still use a bulky dressing to stabilise the segment; 5 cm adhesive tape can also be used as a functional binder to tape the ribs so that they move in tandem.

At the Scene

Pulmonary contusion is the main cause of hypoxaemia seen with flail chest injuries.

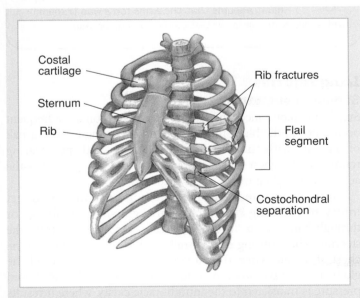

Figure 23-5 In flail chest injuries, two or more adjacent ribs are fractured in two or more places. A flail segment will move paradoxically when the patient breathes.

The blunt force trauma that causes the flail segment can also produce a pulmonary contusion Figure 23-6 ▸, an injury to the underlying lung tissue that inhibits the normal diffusion of oxygen and carbon dioxide. Three physics principles contribute to the formation of a pulmonary contusion: the Spalding effect, inertial effects, and implosion. With the Spalding effect, the pressure waves generated by either penetrating or blunt trauma disrupt the capillary-alveolar membrane, resulting in haemorrhage. Inertial effects are created by tissue density differences between the alveoli and the larger bronchioles. These tissues accelerate and decelerate at different rates, causing them to tear and haemorrhage. Finally, the positive pressure created by the trauma compresses the gases within the lung, which quickly re-expand.

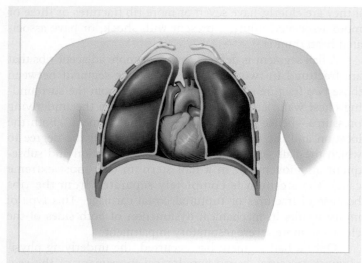

Figure 23-6 Pulmonary contusion.

In blunt trauma, the force applied to the thoracic cage results in a fracture of the rib in one of three areas: the point of impact, the edge of the object, or the posterior angle of the rib (weak point). Because they are less well protected by other bony and muscular structures, ribs from 4 to 9 inclusive are the most commonly fractured.

The ribs are part of a ring that helps to expand and contract the thoracic cavity. Because a fracture of one or more ribs destroys the integrity of this ring, the patient's ability to adequately ventilate is diminished. Just as importantly, the patient will attempt to limit the pain caused by these injuries by using shallow breathing. This tendency results in atelectasis and may lead to hypoxia or pneumonia.

The presence of rib fractures is also suspicious for other associated injuries. When the clinical examination suggests a fracture of ribs from 4 to 9, you should be concerned about associated aortic injury, tracheobronchial injury, pneumothorax, vascular injury, or other more serious injuries. Similarly, fractures of the lower ribs (from 9 to 11) should raise your concern for an associated intra-abdominal injury.

Sternal Fractures

Approximately one in 20 patients with blunt thoracic trauma will suffer a sternal fracture. Although this injury is of little consequence by itself, it is associated with other injuries that cause more than one quarter of patients with this fracture to die. Specifically, findings of myocardial contusions, flail sternum, pulmonary contusions, head injuries, intra-abdominal injuries, and myocardial rupture increase the likelihood of death.

If this re-expansion is too great, the lung tissue will suffer an implosion injury.

If the blunt force that fractures the ribs drives those bone fragments further into the body, a pneumothorax or haemothorax may result. In addition, the pain associated with the fractures may prevent the patient from taking in adequate tidal volume because he or she is consciously trying to minimise the movement of that segment of the chest. This "self-splinting" action uses the intercostal muscles and purposefully limited chest wall movement to minimise pain. Unfortunately, it further limits the pulmonary system's ability to compensate for the injury.

Rib Fractures

Rib fractures—the most common thoracic injuries—are seen in more than half of all thoracic trauma patients. Even when the patient experiences no underlying or associated injury, the pain produced by the broken ribs can result in significant morbidity as it contributes to inadequate ventilation, self-splinting, atelectasis, and the possibility of infection (pneumonia) due to inadequate respiration.

When you are examining the chest of a patient who has sustained either blunt or penetrating injury, palpate for subcutaneous emphysema (air under the skin), which can indicate a potential pneumothorax. It has been described as a "snap, crackle, pop" sensation under the skin or a feeling like popping the plastic bubbles in the wrap used to protect fragile items sent in the post.

At the Scene

The sternum is a very thick bone. If the thorax receives enough force to fracture the sternum, you must assume that the same force was transmitted to the heart, great vessels, lungs, and diaphragm.

Lung Injuries

Simple Pneumothorax

Small pneumothoraces that are not under tension are a frequent occurrence in the blunt trauma patient, occurring in almost half of patients with thoracic trauma. Patients with penetrating trauma to the chest almost always have a pneumothorax—the accumulation of air or gas in the pleural cavity.

Injuries may result in pneumothoraces either by direct injury to the lung (ie, rib fracture, gunshot, stabbing) or through barotrauma. In the latter case, pressure (eg, from the steering wheel during a road traffic collision) is applied to the chest at a time when the patient has inhaled and closed the glottis in anticipation of the trauma and/or pain. This increased pressure is translated to the intrathoracic cavity, where it results in rupture of the lung. In both direct injury and barotrauma, air is allowed to escape into the pleural space, causing a pneumothorax Figure 23-7 ▶.

Special Considerations

The incidence of rib fractures varies with age. The ribs of children are pliable, so they may injure underlying structures without being fractured. In older patients, the frail nature of the bones makes the ribs more likely to fracture.

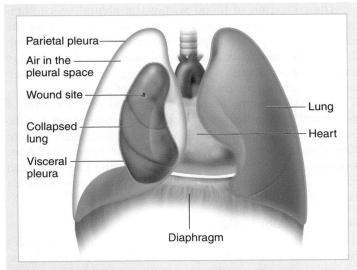

Figure 23-7 Pneumothorax occurs when air leaks into the space between the pleural surfaces from an opening in the chest or the surface of the lung. The lung collapses as air fills the pleural space.

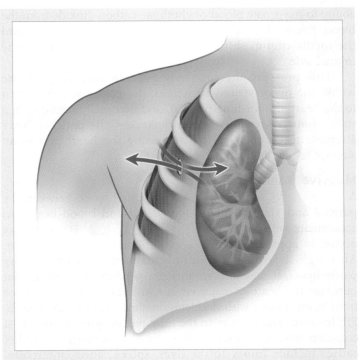

Figure 23-8 With a sucking chest wound, air passes from the outside into the pleural space and back out with each breath, creating a sucking sound. The size of the defect does not need to be large to compromise ventilation.

Open Pneumothorax

An open pneumothorax occurs when a defect in the chest wall allows air to enter the thoracic space. It results from penetrating chest trauma—for example, gunshot/knife wounds or other impaled objects. The penetrating injury creates a link between the external environment and the pleural space. With each inspiration, the negative pressure created within the thoracic cavity draws more air into the pleural space, resulting in a pneumothorax. As the pneumothorax increases in size, the lung on the involved side loses its ability to expand. Also, if the "hole" is larger than the glottic opening, the air is more likely to enter the chest wall rather than entering via the trachea. As a consequence, the respiratory effort moves air in through the chest wound rather than through the lung, creating the "sucking chest wound" **Figure 23-8 ▸**.

The collapse of the involved lung creates a mismatch between ventilation and perfusion. If you assume that the pulmonary vasculature on the involved side remains intact, the heart will continue to perfuse the involved lung while the pneumothorax prevents adequate ventilation. The result is an inability to deliver oxygen to the involved lung (hypoxia) and an inability to eliminate carbon dioxide (hypercarbia).

Tension Pneumothorax

A tension pneumothorax **Figure 23-9 ▸** is a life-threatening condition that results from continued air accumulation within the intrapleural space. Air may enter the pleural space from an open thoracic injury, an injury to the lung parenchyma due to blunt trauma (the most common cause of tension pneumothorax), barotrauma due to positive-pressure ventilation, or tracheobronchial injuries due to shearing forces.

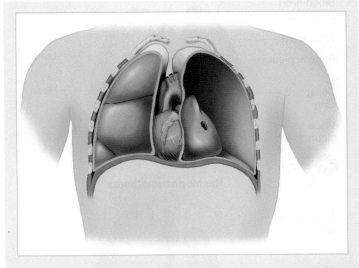

Figure 23-9 In a tension pneumothorax, air accumulates in the pleural space, eventually causing compression of the heart and great vessels.

An injury to the lung can cause a one-way valve to develop, allowing air to move into the pleural space but not to exit from it. As it continues to accumulate, the air exerts increasing pressure against the surrounding tissues. This growing pressure compresses the involved lung, diminishing its ability to oxygenate blood or eliminate carbon dioxide from the blood. Eventually, the lung will both collapse and push toward the mediastinum, shifting the mediastinum away from the injured side.

This pressure increase may even exceed the pressure within the major venous structures, decreasing venous return to the heart, diminishing preload, and eventually resulting in a shock state. As venous return decreases, the patient's body attempts to compensate by increasing the heart rate in an attempt to maintain cardiac output.

Massive Haemothorax

A haemothorax occurs when the potential space between the parietal and visceral pleura is violated and blood begins to accumulate within this space Figure 23-10 ▾ . Haemothorax occurs in approximately 25% of patients with chest trauma. Although it is most commonly caused by tears of lung parenchyma, it may also result from penetrating wounds that puncture the heart or major vessels within the mediastinum or from blunt trauma with deceleration shearing of major vessels. Rib fractures and injuries to the lung parenchyma are the most common sources of injury in the case of a haemothorax. Other causes include injury to the liver, spleen, aorta, intercostal arteries (which can lose up to 50 ml of blood per minute), and other intrathoracic vessels.

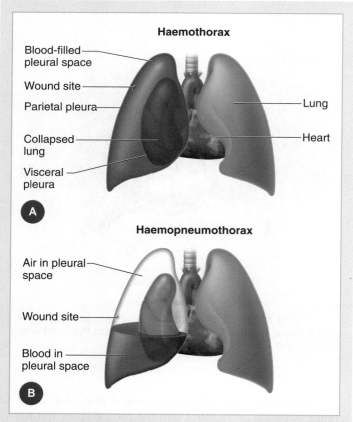

Figure 23-10 A. A haemothorax is a collection of blood in the pleural space produced by bleeding within the chest. **B.** In a haemopneumothorax, both blood and air are present.

The collection of blood within the pleural space compresses and displaces the surrounding lung, limiting the patient's capacity for adequate oxygenation and ventilation. Unlike a pneumothorax, this injury has the added potential of causing hypovolaemia. A haemopneumothorax occurs when both blood and air are present in the pleural space.

A massive haemothorax is defined as accumulation of more than 1,500 ml of blood within the pleural space. For the average adult, this amount represents approximately 25% to 30% blood volume loss, meaning that the patient will have progressed to decompensated shock. Because each lung can hold up to 3,000 ml, it is possible for a patient to completely bleed out into the thoracic cavity.

Pulmonary Contusion

The position of the lungs just beneath the thoracic cage places them at increased risk for injury with thoracic trauma. As the lung tissue is compressed against the chest wall by force or by the positive pressure within the chest during a thoracic injury, alveolar and capillary damage results. It leads immediately to a loss of fluid and blood into the involved tissues, followed by white blood cell migration into the area, and, eventually, local tissue oedema.

This local tissue injury and oedema dilute the local surfactant in the alveoli, diminishing their compliance and causing alveolar collapse (atelectasis). The oedema also reduces the delivery of oxygen across the capillary-alveolar interface, resulting in hypoxia. The hypoxia then worsens the situation by thickening the mucus produced, which may in turn lead to bronchiolar obstruction and further atelectasis.

If the contusion is large, the body compensates by vaso-constricting pulmonary blood flow and increasing cardiac output. This is an attempt to shunt blood from the injured area and increase its delivery to pulmonary tissue that may be able to oxygenate the blood. This pulmonary shunting decreases the functional reserve capacity and leads to mixed venous blood being returned to the heart, further worsening the hypoxaemia.

Myocardial Injuries

Cardiac Tamponade

Cardiac tamponade Figure 23-11 ▸ is defined as excessive fluid in the pericardial sac, causing compression of the heart and decreased cardiac output. The haemodynamic effects of cardiac tamponade are determined by the size of the perforation in the pericardium, the rate of haemorrhage from the cardiac wound, and the chamber of the heart involved. The injury may be caused by a blunt or (more commonly) penetrating mechanism. Very few patients with blunt thoracic trauma experience cardiac tamponade, whereas almost all patients with cardiac stab wounds develop this condition.

The mortality associated with tamponade varies, with high-velocity injuries (gunshots) carrying a higher risk of death than low-velocity injuries (stabbings). If cardiac tamponade is the only injury, mortality is greatly reduced.

Cardiac tamponade can occur in both medical and trauma patients. In the medical setting, inflammatory processes (ie, pericarditis, uraemia, myocardial infarction) lead to the slow collection of fluid within the pericardial sac and the gradual distension of the parietal pericardium. During this process, 1,000 to 1,500 ml of fluid may accumulate in the pericardial sac. Conversely, the bleeding in the trauma patient can be rapid, with blood loss from the coronary vasculature or the myocardium itself quickly collecting between the visceral and parietal pericardium. Because the parietal pericardium is not able to stretch in such a case, as little as 50 ml of blood may lead to cardiac tamponade.

As the pericardium fills, the continued bleeding increases the pressure within the pericardium. The more pliable structures within the pericardium—namely, the atria and the vena cavae—become compressed, which drastically reduces the preload being delivered to the heart and thereby diminishes stroke volume. The heart initially attempts to compensate for this reduction in preload by increasing the heart rate. This attempt to maintain cardiac output is only temporary, as the continued bleeding will further restrict preload and diastolic filling. The pressure within the pericardial sac will also reduce the perfusion in the myocardium, resulting in global myocardial dysfunction. The combination of these two processes leads to the development of hypotension.

Myocardial Contusion

The heart's anterior position just behind the sternum puts it in a potentially precarious position during a blunt force mechanism. At speeds of greater than 20 to 35 miles per hour, the sudden deceleration of the chest wall may cause the heart to move forward until it collides with the posterior aspect of the sternum, leading to the blunt cardiac injury known as myocardial contusion. This type of injury is characterised by local tissue contu-

sion and haemorrhage, oedema, and cellular damage within the involved myocardium. Direct damage to the epicardial vessels (coronary arteries and veins) may compromise the blood flow to the heart. Damage to the myocardium tissue at a cellular level may result in ectopic electrical activity, re-entry pathways, and arrhythmias.

Complications of myocardial contusions are similar to the complications seen in patients who experience a myocardial infarction. Arrhythmias may occur (although they are uncommon in children) due to cellular membrane injury and changes in the myocardial action potential. Structural changes may include the development of a ventricular septal defect, myocardial rupture or aneurysm formation, and coronary artery occlusion.

Myocardial Rupture

Myocardial rupture is an acute perforation of the ventricles, atria, intraventricular septum, intra-atrial septum, chordae, papillary muscles, or valves. The application of severe blunt force to the chest compresses the heart between the sternum and the vertebrae, which can rupture the myocardium. In penetrating trauma, a foreign object or bony fragment may be propelled into the heart, resulting in a laceration of the myocardial wall. Whether it occurs from a penetrating injury or blunt trauma, a ruptured myocardium is a life-threatening condition that accounts for 15% of fatal chest injuries.

Commotio Cordis

If the thorax receives a direct blow during the critical portion of the heart's repolarisation period, the result may be immediate cardiac arrest. This phenomenon, termed commotio cordis, has been documented to have occurred after patients were struck with footballs, cricket balls or bats, snowballs,

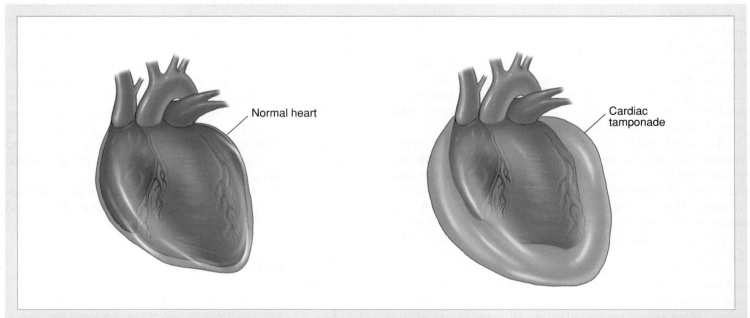

Normal heart

Cardiac tamponade

Figure 23-11 Cardiac tamponade is a potentially fatal condition in which fluid builds up within the pericardial sac, compressing the heart's chambers and dramatically impairing its ability to pump blood.

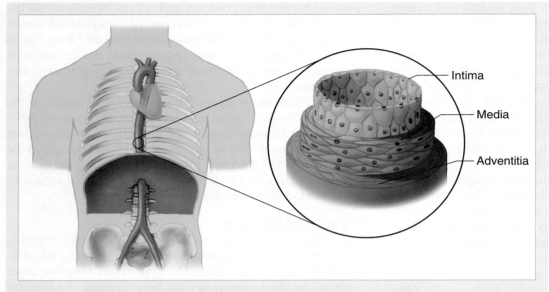

Figure 23-12 The aortic arch, descending aorta, and layers of the aorta.

fists, and even kicks during kickboxing. Such a patient may present with ventricular fibrillation that responds positively to early defibrillation if provided within the first 2 minutes. For this reason, public access to defibrillators in schools and sports venues is essential.

Vascular Injuries

Thoracic Aortic Dissection/Transection

One in every five deaths due to blunt trauma includes a transection of the aorta; the most common causes are high-speed road traffic collisions and falls from a height. Given that the body's entire blood volume passes through this vessel, the high mortality associated with such an injury comes as no surprise. Of those patients who experience an aortic injury, only a few will survive until an ambulance arrives; most of the individuals reached by ambulance service personnel can survive with prompt management including surgical intervention.

The most widely accepted theory of how this injury evolves holds that the aorta is injured at its fixed points due to shearing forces. The high-velocity, high-energy impacts that result in these injuries cause the aortic arch to swing forward. The resulting tension, along with rotation and torque on the area, causes the descending aorta to rupture at its point of attachment to the posterior thoracic wall **Figure 23-12 ▲**.

The aorta includes three layers—the intima, the media, and the adventitia. If the injury tears the intima, the high pressure within the aorta allows the blood to dissect along the media. More severe injuries damage all three layers of the aorta, allowing blood to leak from the aorta into the surrounding tissues. If these tissues can't stop the bleeding, the patient may survive only with prompt intervention. Otherwise, the injury will be fatal.

Great Vessel Injury

With the exception of the aorta, the great vessels are located in areas that offer protection from adjacent bony structures and other tissues. As a consequence, injury to these vessels is much more likely with penetrating trauma. In rare instances, blunt trauma may damage the overlying structures or produce a severe rotational injury (such as that caused by machinery).

Some great vessel injuries may result in occlusion or spasm of the involved artery. These injuries will present with ischaemic changes (pain, pallor, paresthesias, pulselessness, paralysis) in the area with a blood supply coming from the involved artery.

Other Thoracic Injuries

Diaphragmatic Injuries

Diaphragmatic injury occurs in a relatively small percentage of all trauma patients, yet the potential for this injury has prompted a change in the management of penetrating trauma in recent years. For example, some surgeons manage penetrating trauma between the midaxillary lines, below the clavicle, and above the iliac crests by undertaking surgical exploration to ensure that the diaphragm is intact. This conservative approach reflects the possibility that a missed diaphragmatic injury may result in significant complications in the years following the injury.

Injury to the diaphragm may result from direct penetrating injury or blunt force trauma leading to diaphragmatic rupture. Because the diaphragm is protected by the liver on the right side, most diaphragmatic injuries (particularly those due to blunt trauma) occur on the left side. Once the diaphragm has been injured, the healing process is inhibited by the natural pressure differences between the abdominal and thoracic cavities.

Injury to the diaphragm and the associated physical findings have been separated into three phases: acute, latent, and

At the Scene

Blunt disruptions of the diaphragm are usually associated with herniation of all or part of the liver into the right side of the chest and the stomach into the left side of the chest.

obstructive. The acute phase begins at the time of injury and ends with recovery from other injuries (which may overshadow the diaphragmatic injury and serves to explain why less than one quarter of these injuries are identified during the acute phase). In the latent phase, the patient experiences intermittent abdominal pain due to the periodic herniation or entrapment of abdominal contents in the defect. The obstructive phase occurs when any abdominal contents herniate through the defect, cutting off their blood supply (infarct) in the process.

A very rare but ultimate complication of a diaphragmatic injury is the herniation of sufficient abdominal contents into the thoracic cavity. The resulting increased intrathoracic pressure both compresses the lung on the affected side and compromises circulatory function; this finding is called a tension gastrothorax.

Oesophageal Injuries

Oesophageal injuries are some of the most rapidly fatal injuries to the gastrointestinal tract, particularly if the diagnosis is not made early. Fortunately, even with penetrating trauma, such injuries are rare. Because of the location of the oesophagus, however, it is often associated with other significant injuries.

Tracheobronchial Injuries

Injuries to the major airways are rare. In most instances, they are caused by penetrating injuries, but they may occasionally be seen in severe deceleration injuries. Tracheobronchial injuries have high mortality due to the associated airway obstruction.

As with aortic injuries, the site of a tracheobronchial injury is often close to a point of attachment—namely, the carina. The injury to the trachea or mainstem bronchi allows for rapid movement of air into the pleural space, resulting in a pneu-

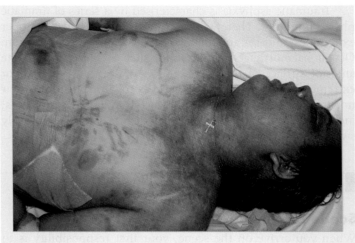

Figure 23-13 Traumatic asphyxia.

mothorax. As this injury progresses to a tension pneumothorax, a needle thoracentesis is often insufficient because the rate of air entry into the pleural space exceeds the rate at which the air can escape from the inserted angiocath.

Traumatic Asphyxia

Traumatic injuries that suddenly and forcefully compress the thoracic cavity may induce traumatic asphyxia Figure 23-13 ▲ . The sudden compression of the chest causes pressure to be translated into the major veins of the head, neck, and kidneys. This massive increase in pressure then passes into the capillary beds, resulting in their rupture.

You are the Paramedic Part 3

After determining that the patient has a tension pneumothorax, you perform a needle chest decompression. You hear a rapid "rush" of air as the needle cannula enters the thoracic cavity. You place the patient on a cardiac monitor and reassess the vital signs.

Reassessment	Recording Time: 15 Minutes
Skin	Cool, pale, perspiring extremities with a pinker core
Pulse	114 beats/min, somewhat irregular
Blood pressure	98/54 mm Hg
Respirations	Intubated; ventilating with 100% supplemental oxygen
SpO₂	95%
Electrocardiogram	Sinus tachycardia with occasional premature ventricular contractions and premature atrial contractions

5. What further injuries within the thorax could account for the patient's persistent hypotension and tachycardia?

6. Are there interventions that you can provide in the prehospital environment if such injuries are identified?

Traumatic asphyxia is characterised by a series of dramatic physical findings. There will be cyanosis of the head, the upper extremities, and the torso above the level of the compression. Ocular haemorrhage may be mild, such as bleeding into the anterior surface of the eye (subconjunctival haematoma), or extremely dramatic, causing the eyes to protrude from their normal position (exophthalmos). Other facial structures, including the tongue and lips, may also become dramatically swollen and cyanotic.

General Assessment

Scene Assessment

When you arrive on the scene, your first responsibility is to ensure the safety of both you and your partner. Make sure that the scene is safe to enter and that you are using the appropriate personal protective equipment. After you identify the number of patients, triage those patients, and request any additional resources needed, you should begin assessment of your assigned patient.

Initial Assessment

As with any patient, your initial assessment begins with an assessment of his or her mental status, airway, breathing, and circulation. Pay special attention to the identification and management of any injuries that may jeopardise the patient's vital functions. Such injuries present an immediate threat to the life of the patient and must be managed as soon as they are identified.

Mental Status and the Airway

The initial assessment begins with evaluation of the patient's mental status using AVPU. Assess the patient's level of consciousness and airway status while providing manual in-line immobilisation of the cervical spine.

While considering the mechanism of injury and its contribution to the thoracic injuries (ie, the unrestrained passenger who strikes the anterior part of the neck on the dashboard of the vehicle), you should assess for injuries that may result in either obstruction or impairment of the airway. The most common cause of airway obstruction is the tongue's posterior displacement in the setting of altered mental status. Other foreign bodies that may obstruct the airway include the patient's teeth, dentures, blood, mucus, or vomitus. Additionally, the trauma may either directly injure the airway or result in secondary obstruction due to inflammation or oedema.

Patients with airway compromise may present in a variety of ways, depending on the severity of the impairment, its duration, and other associated injuries. The airway itself may manifest signs of obstruction—for example, stridor, hoarseness or other changes in the voice, gurgling or snoring respirations, or coughing. Patients may also demonstrate signs of either hypoxia or hypercarbia. Alterations in mental status may range from anxiety to stupor to unresponsiveness. Abnormal respira-

tory findings may include tachypnoea, coughing, haemoptysis, accessory muscle use, and recession.

When a patient has airway impairment, you must take immediate action to remedy the situation. Any patient with an airway issue should be assumed to have a simultaneous cervical spine injury and should be manually immobilised. Because of the potential for compromising the cervical spine, the head tilt–chin lift should be avoided in favour of the jaw-thrust manoeuvre. Suction, basic airway adjuncts (ie, oropharyngeal or nasopharyngeal airways), advanced airway adjuncts (ie, endotracheal intubation, laryngeal mask airway, or a Combitube), or surgical airway management should be used as needed to ensure adequate airway management and protection.

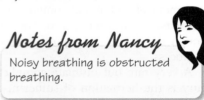

Notes from Nancy

Noisy breathing is obstructed breathing.

Breathing

Once the airway has been assessed and managed appropriately, the assessment should turn to the patient's breathing. The goal here is to identify and manage any impairment of the patient's oxygenation and ventilation **Figure 23-14 ▾**. Such problems may result from deficiencies in diffusion due to pulmonary injuries, preexisting disease, or deficiencies in air movement due to pulmonary, musculoskeletal, or neurological impairments.

To assess the patient's breathing adequately, the patient's clothing must be removed to expose the chest. A systematic approach to assessment will then help to identify both obvious and subtle injuries or impairments.

The breathing assessment begins with an inspection of the patient's thorax. Consider the contour, appearance, and symmetry of the chest wall. Signs of soft-tissue injury (contusions,

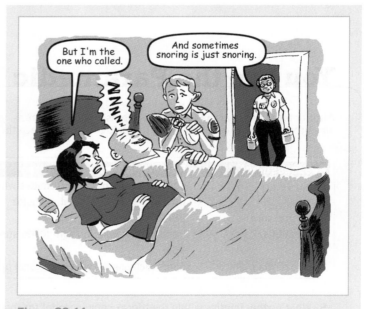

Figure 23-14

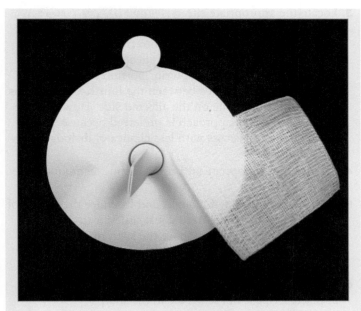

Figure 23-16 An Ascherman chest seal. A sucking chest wound can be covered with a large airtight dressing that seals three sides.

An open pneumothorax rarely progresses to a tension pneumothorax. If it does, you should remove the patient's occlusive dressing to allow the pneumothorax to "vent" through the opening in the thoracic cavity. If this measure does not relieve this life-threatening condition, treatment should progress as described in the next section.

Tension Pneumothorax

The classic signs of a tension pneumothorax are an absence of breath sounds on the affected side, tachycardia, jugular vein distension, and tracheal deviation. While tachycardia may not be a unique finding in the trauma patient, tension pneumothorax induces this change—not because of a hypovolaemic state, but rather because of the inability of blood to return easily to the heart from the venous system. The increasing pressure within the thoracic cavity leads to the accumulation of blood within the great vessels just outside the thoracic cavity. As the pressure is translated into the most superficial of these veins—the jugular veins—they become distended with blood. Such jugular vein distension is usually a late sign of tension pneumothorax.

The jugular veins, which exit the thoracic cavity from beneath the clavicles and cross over the sternocleidomastoid muscles as they move superiorly, are considered to be distended when they are engorged to a level 1 to 2 cm above the clavicle. This assessment is properly done with the patient in a 45° recumbent position, however—something that can't be accomplished during the initial assessment of the patient in the prehospital environment.

Because of the mediastinal shift caused by the increasing pressure, palpation or visualisation of the trachea may manifest in a deviation of the trachea away from the affected side. Nevertheless, this late finding in a tension pneumothorax may not be present despite the rapid decompensation of the patient's clinical status. For this reason, you must be vigilant in watching for the cardiopulmonary findings associated with a tension pneumothorax and not rely on the presence of all the classic physical findings in making the diagnosis.

You are the Paramedic Part 4

An assessment of the patient's circulation reveals no evidence of muffled heart sounds, jugular vein distension, dullness to chest percussion, or evidence of traumatic asphyxia. After loading the patient into the ambulance, you complete a detailed physical examination and continue fluid resuscitation.

Your physical assessment reveals crepitus and palpable deformity over the ninth and tenth ribs on the left, as well as a rigid abdomen. Deformity of the left lower leg is evident, and the patient has multiple soft-tissue injuries on all extremities.

Reassessment	Recording Time: 20 Minutes
Skin	Cool, pale extremities with a pink core
Pulse	108 beats/min
Blood pressure	104/58 mm Hg
Respirations	Intubated; ventilating with 100% supplemental oxygen
SpO₂	98%
Electrocardiogram	Sinus tachycardia without further ectopics

7. What additional injuries might your physical findings suggest?
8. What additional treatments may be needed for this patient?

The accumulation of air within the pleural space decreases the lung volume and diminishes the breath sounds on the affected side when you auscultate the chest. Because air causes the loss of breath sounds on that side, the chest will be resonant (like a bell) when percussed, as opposed to the dull sensation expected with fluid or blood.

Due to the injury and the collapsing lung, a patient with a tension pneumothorax often complains of pleuritic chest pain and dyspnoea. The resulting hypoxia may cause the patient to become anxious, tachycardic, tachypnoeic, and even cyanotic.

Hypotension, as a late finding of tension pneumothorax, should not be used either to confirm or exclude the possibility of a tension pneumothorax. Its presence may suggest that the pneumothorax has produced such significant pressure as to severely impede preload, or it may represent a simultaneous shock state due to other injuries. Normal blood pressure suggests that, when other signs of a tension pneumothorax are present, the heart is adequately compensating for the diminished venous return.

At the Scene

Shock (a late sign), decreased breath sounds, and hyperresonance to percussion on the same side of the chest mean a tension pneumothorax until proven otherwise.

All patients presenting with signs of a tension pneumothorax should immediately be placed on high-flow supplemental oxygen (12 to 15 l/min) via a nonrebreathing mask. Immediate relief of the elevated pressures must then be accomplished through a needle decompression, also referred to as a "needle thoracentesis." The steps for performing a needle decompression are described below (**Skill Drill 23-1 ▸**):

1. Assess the patient to ensure that the presentation matches that of a tension pneumothorax (**Step 1**):
   - Difficult ventilation despite an open airway
   - Jugular vein distension (may not be present with associated haemorrhage)
   - Absent or decreased breath sounds on the affected side
   - Hyperresonance to percussion on the affected side
   - Tracheal deviation away from the affected side (this late sign is not always present)
2. Prepare and assemble the necessary equipment (**Step 2**):
   - Large-bore IV cannula, preferably 14-gauge and at least 5 cm long
   - Alcohol or povidone iodine (Betadine) preps
   - Adhesive tape

3. Locate the appropriate site (**Figure 23-17 ▾**) (**Step 3**). Find the second or third rib, as you'll need to insert the needle just above the third rib into the intercostal space at the midclavicular line on the affected side. If there is significant trauma to the anterior portion of the chest, use the intercostal space between the fourth and fifth ribs at the midaxillary line on the affected side. However, the midclavicular line approach is preferred because it's usually easier to access with less chance of dislodging the needle.
4. Cleanse the appropriate area using aseptic technique (**Step 4**).
5. Insert the needle at a 90° angle, and listen for the release of air (**Step 5**). Insert the needle just superior to the third rib, midclavicular, or just above the sixth rib, midaxillary. (The nerves, arteries, and veins run along the inferior borders of each rib.)
6. Withdraw the needle, leaving the catheter/cannula in place. Dispose of the needle in the sharps bin (**Step 6**).

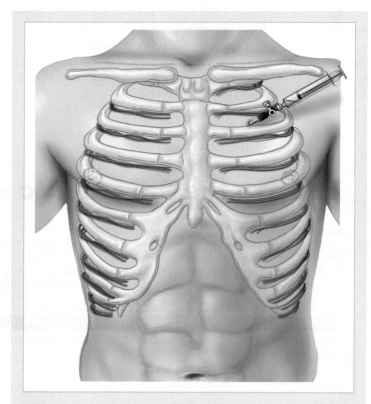

Figure 23-17 Correct placement of needle for decompression. The position of nerves, arteries, and veins are shown in relation to the ribs.

Skill Drill 23-1: Needle Decompression (Thoracentesis) of a Tension Pneumothorax

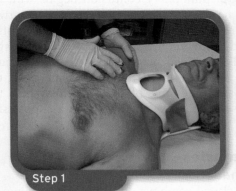

Step 1

Assess the patient.

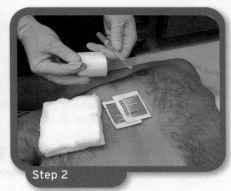

Step 2

Prepare and assemble all necessary equipment.

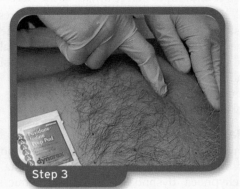

Step 3

Locate the appropriate site between the second and third rib.

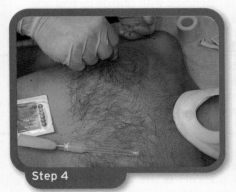

Step 4

Cleanse the appropriate area using aseptic technique.

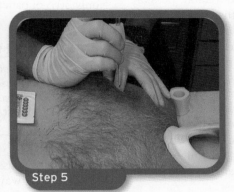

Step 5

Insert the needle at a 90° angle.

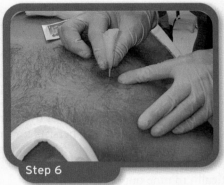

Step 6

Remove the needle, leaving the catheter/cannula in place, and listen for release of air. Dispose of the needle properly in the sharps bin.

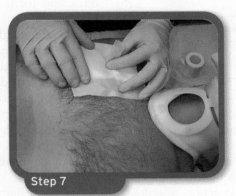

Step 7

Secure the catheter/cannula in place. Monitor the patient closely for recurrence of the tension pneumothorax.

7. Secure the catheter/cannula in place in the same manner you would use to secure an impaled object (**Step 7**).

8. Monitor the patient closely for recurrence of the tension pneumothorax. This procedure may need to be repeated several times before arrival at the A&E department.

The performance of a needle decompression is not without risk. If the needle is improperly placed (ie, not inserted over the top of the rib), injury to the intercostal vessels may result in significant haemorrhage. Similarly, passing the needle into the chest may injure the lung parenchyma. Failure to treat this condition will cause the patient to progress to pulseless electrical activity and cardiopulmonary arrest.

Massive Haemothorax

Physical assessment of the massive haemothorax will reveal signs of both ventilatory insufficiency (hypoxia, agitation, anxiety, tachypnoea, dyspnoea) and hypovolaemic shock (tachycardia, hypotension, pale and clammy skin). The physical findings that help to differentiate this haemothorax from other injuries include the lack of JVD, the lack of tracheal deviation, possible bloody sputum (haemoptysis), and dullness that may be noted on percussion of the affected side of the chest.

The prehospital management of a suspected haemothorax is supportive. If the airway does not require intervention, place the patient on high-flow supplemental oxygen via a nonrebreathing mask. Initiate two large-bore peripheral IVs, with fluid resuscitation being guided by local guidelines and directed at limiting the duration of hypotension. Hypovolaemic shock with hypotension that persists for more than 30 minutes raises the mortality from one in ten patients to as high as one in two. For individuals older than age 65, that risk jumps dramatically, to nine out of ten patients.

At the Scene

The major problem following a massive haemothorax is the development of hypovolaemic shock and respiratory compromise.

Pulmonary Contusion

The assessment of the patient with a pulmonary contusion may not initially reveal the presence or severity of the injury as it may take 24 hours before the severity of the injury becomes clinically evident. Because not every trauma patient presents immediately (eg, cases involving domestic violence, assaults, injuries that occur while intoxicated, patients in remote areas who are not immediately located, or search and rescue operations), it is important to be familiar with the clinical presentation of this injury.

Hypoxia and carbon dioxide retention lead to respiratory distress, dyspnoea, tachypnoea, agitation, and restlessness. Due to the capillary injury and the haemorrhage into the pulmonary parenchyma, the patient may present with haemoptysis (coughing up blood). Evidence of overlying injury may include contusions, tenderness, crepitus, or paradoxical motion. Auscultation may reveal wheezes, crackles or rales, or diminished lung sounds in the affected area. In severe cases, cyanosis and low oxygen saturations may be found.

The treatment of pulmonary contusion begins with the assessment and, as needed, management of the patient's airway. Both high-concentration oxygen and positive-pressure ventilation may be used to overcome the pathological changes described earlier. Because oedema may exacerbate the injury, use caution when administering IV fluids. In some cases, the administration of small amounts of analgesics may help the patient to maximise ventilatory function without suppressing ventilatory drive.

Myocardial Injuries
Cardiac Tamponade

Beck's triad is the classic combination of physical findings in patients with cardiac tamponade: muffled heart sounds, hypotension, and jugular vein distension. Even so, this triad is seen in only 30% of patients diagnosed with cardiac tamponade.

At the Scene

Hypotension and distended neck veins in the presence of normal lung sounds (which rules out pneumothorax), combined with an appropriate history, suggest cardiac tamponade.

Another classic finding in cardiac tamponade (albeit one that is not always present) is the ECG finding of <u>electrical alternans</u>. As fluid accumulates within the pericardial sac, the heart begins to oscillate with each beat. As the heart swings back and forth within the pericardium, its electrical axis changes. Electrical alternans is not commonly seen in acute cardiac tamponade and must be differentiated from bigeminal ectopy, but it is a classic sign of cardiac tamponade.

The reduced cardiac output, hypoperfusion, and hypotension observed in cardiac tamponade produce the findings typical of a patient in shock: weak or absent peripheral pulses, diaphoresis, dyspnoea, cyanosis, altered mental status, tachycardia, tachypnoea, and agitation. Although these symptoms by themselves do not suggest or exclude the presence of cardiac tamponade, identifying them can flesh out the physical assessment.

Physical findings in a patient with cardiac tamponade are not significantly different to those of a tension pneumothorax—namely, hypotension, jugular vein distension, tachycardia, altered mental status, and signs of tissue hypoperfusion. **Table 23-2 ▸** compares the physical findings of these two emergencies.

The treatment of the patient with cardiac tamponade begins by ensuring adequate oxygen delivery and establishing intravenous access. Giving IV fluids might appear to slow the patient's deterioration by momentarily increasing preload. The

Table 23-2	Physical Findings of Cardiac Tamponade Versus Tension Pneumothorax	
Physical Finding	Cardiac Tamponade	Tension Pneumothorax
Presenting sign/symptom	Shock	Respiratory distress
Neck veins	Distended	Distended
Trachea	Midline	Deviated
Breath sounds	Equal on both sides	Decreased or absent on side of injury
Chest percussion	Normal	Hyperresonant on side of injury
Heart sounds	Muffled	Normal

patient with a cardiac tamponade should be transported rapidly to an A&E department for a pericardiocentesis—a procedure in which blood is removed from the pericardial sac via an intracardiac needle inserted through the chest wall. Definitive management occurs in the operating theatre, in the hands of a cardiothoracic surgeon.

Myocardial Contusion

Sharp, retrosternal chest pain is the most common complaint among patients with myocardial contusion. Inspection of the area may reveal soft tissue or bony injury in the area. Crackles or rales (due to pulmonary oedema from left ventricular dysfunction) may be heard on auscultation.

At the Scene

Many patients with myocardial contusion are relatively asymptomatic, at least initially. Accompanying injuries may present more dramatically. Helpful signs are ECG changes and persistent sinus tachycardia without obvious hypovolaemia.

The ECG in a patient with a myocardial contusion is often abnormal. Sinus tachycardia is the most common ECG abnormality seen in cardiac contusion patients. Additional ECG changes may include atrial fibrillation or flutter, premature atrial contractions (PACs) or premature ventricular contractions (PVCs), a new right bundle branch block, AV blocks, nonspecific ST-segment and T-wave changes, and ventricular tachycardia or fibrillation. In the event of a coronary artery injury (likely the right coronary artery), ischaemic changes consistent with those seen in myocardial infarction may also occur.

The treatment of patients with possible myocardial contusion begins with nonspecific, supportive care, including oxygen administration, frequent assessment of vital signs, cardiac monitoring, and establishing IV access. Fluid resuscitation should be instituted as needed to maintain the patient's blood pressure. The administration of antiarrhythmic agents to trauma patients should be given in accordance with local guidelines.

Notes from Nancy

If the mechanisms of injury suggest pulmonary contusion, be sparing with IV fluids unless there are signs of shock.

Myocardial Rupture

Remember that myocardial rupture is life-threatening. Patients may present with acute pulmonary oedema or signs of cardiac tamponade. Unless the latter is present and a pericardiocentesis can be done, patients with myocardial rupture should receive supportive care and be rapidly transported to a facility where a thoracotomy can be performed.

Vascular Injuries
Thoracic Aortic Dissection/Transection

Depending on the exact nature of the injury, the symptoms and physical examination in cases of thoracic aortic dissection or transection will vary from an unstable patient to one with no

You are the Paramedic Part 5

The patient's vital signs are monitored en route to hospital with no further deterioration. You administer IV fluids to prevent further hypotension. With a police officer driving, you and your colleague care for the patient's injuries en route to the A&E department.

When you arrive, the trauma team takes over the patient's care. You and your partner provide a concise, complete report to the team, including the mechanism of injury, the deaths of two other passengers, your initial physical assessment, the interventions you undertook, and the patient's response to those treatments.

During the A&E department evaluation, the patient is found to have a right-sided pneumothorax, a left-sided pulmonary contusion, fractures of left ribs 8 through 11, a lacerated spleen, a fractured left tibia and fibula, and multiple soft-tissue injuries. A chest drain is inserted in the A&E department, and your needle thoracotomy is removed. The patient is taken to theatre for repair of his abdominal and orthopaedic injuries and, after a 15-day hospitalisation, is discharged home with no permanent disability.

physical complaints. However, most patients will have a complaint of pain behind the sternum or in the scapula. Other findings may include signs of hypovolaemic shock, dyspnoea, and altered mental status. If a haematoma forms in the area of the oesophagus, trachea, or larynx, the patient may present with dysphagia, stridor, and hoarseness, respectively. A harsh murmur may be noted due to the turbulence created as the blood passes the site of the injury to the intima in the aorta.

Assessment of the patient's pulses in all extremities is an important key to the identification of these injuries. As the dissection or rupture compresses the aorta and progresses along its branch vessels, blood flow to the extremities may be compromised. This phenomenon results in diminished pulses compared to those closer to the injury. On examination, you will note a stronger pulse (and higher blood pressure) in the right arm than in the left arm or the lower extremities.

Because of the high energy involved with aortic injuries, associated injuries are to be expected. They may include multiple rib fractures, flail segment, sternal or scapular fracture, cardiac tamponade, haemothorax or pneumothorax, and clavicle fracture.

Controversies

It has long been taught that first or second rib fractures (which are often an X-ray finding rather than a physical examination finding) are indicative of aortic injuries, but this association has lately come into question.

The prehospital management of potential aortic injuries is symptomatic. After assessment and management of the ABCs, the patient should receive gradual IV hydration for the treatment of hypotension. Aggressive fluid administration may result in sudden changes in the intra-aortic pressure that could worsen the injury. Expedited transport to a trauma centre with an available cardiothoracic surgeon is essential.

Notes from Nancy

Suspect aortic rupture in any collision involving powerful deceleration forces.

Great Vessel Injury

If the vessel is not injured in such a way that bleeding is prevented, the patient will present with signs and symptoms of hypovolaemic shock, haemothorax, or cardiac tamponade. If the bleeding results in formation of a haematoma, the compression of adjacent structures (ie, oesophagus, trachea) may produce additional signs and symptoms.

The management of potential injuries to the great vessels is no different from the management of any other form of acute blood loss. Establish IV hydration en route to the A&E department, and treat cardiac tamponade immediately if it is found.

Other Thoracic Injuries
Diaphragmatic Injuries

Although diaphragmatic injuries are not likely to be identified in the prehospital setting, you should still maintain clinical suspicion for such injuries **Figure 23-18**. It is likely you will be caring for the patient during the acute phase, but delayed presentations in the obstructive phase are also possible.

In the acute phase, the patient may present with hypotension, tachypnoea, bowel sounds in the chest, chest pain, or absence of breath sounds on the affected side. These signs indicate a large diaphragmatic injury that may be followed by herniation of the abdominal contents into the thoracic cavity.

In the obstructive phase, as the blood supply to the herniated organs becomes compromised, symptoms will include nausea, vomiting, abdominal pain, constipation, dyspnoea, and abdominal distension. In many cases, these symptoms are severe and unrelenting. The most severe findings may be consistent with a tension gastrothorax.

In both the acute and obstructive phases, management of diaphragmatic injury focuses on maintaining adequate oxygenation and ventilation and rapid transport to the hospital. In prehospital systems that allow for such procedures, nasogastric tube placement may improve the patient's condition by decompressing the involved gastrointestinal organs.

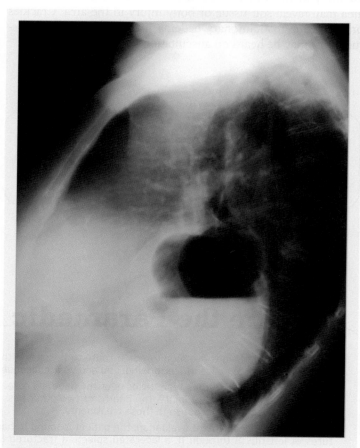

Figure 23-18 X-ray of a diaphragmatic rupture.

Oesophageal Injuries

Oesophageal injuries often present with other thoracic and spinal injuries due to the location of the oesophagus within the thorax. The patient may experience pleuritic chest pain, and particularly pain that is made worse by swallowing or flexion of the neck. Subcutaneous emphysema may occur, but more than half of oesophageal injury patients with this finding have an associated tracheal injury.

No specific therapy for oesophageal injuries is possible in the prehospital setting. Definitive care occurs once the patient is evaluated in the hospital and an appropriate surgical consultation is achieved. In the meantime, ensuring that the patient is given nothing orally will help to minimise complications related to this injury.

Tracheobronchial Injuries

The clinical presentation of tracheobronchial injuries may vary from mildly symptomatic to severe respiratory compromise. Expected physical findings include hoarseness, dyspnoea and tachypnoea, respiratory distress, and haemoptysis. Look for findings of a pneumothorax or tension pneumothorax.

The treatment of a patient with a suspected tracheobronchial injury centres on adequate assessment and management of the patient's ABCs. The patient with a tenuous airway who can be managed with bag-valve-mask ventilation should not be intubated, because introducing an endotracheal tube may complete a partial tracheal injury and result in complete airway obstruction. Similarly, because of the rapid loss of air into the pleural space, high ventilatory pressures should be avoided when providing positive-pressure ventilation (bag the patient gently and slowly).

Traumatic Asphyxia

Although the term "asphyxia" implies a uniformly fatal outcome for patients, this is not always the case. Given the significant force required to produce traumatic asphyxia, however, your suspicion for associated injuries should be quite high. Don't let the dramatic physical findings in the head and neck, which are not immediately life-threatening, distract you from those injuries that are.

After other life-threatening injuries are managed, the treatment of patients exhibiting traumatic asphyxia is relatively brief. In the absence of intubation, provide high-flow supplemental oxygen via a nonrebreathing mask. Take cervical spine precautions, including spinal immobilisation. IV access should be obtained with two large-bore IVs. Transport to the nearest A&E department or other facility as dictated by local guidelines should then be expedited.

You are the Paramedic Summary

1. What will your initial priorities be when assessing and managing this patient?

Assessment of airway, breathing, and circulation with interventions to correct any life-threatening conditions are the assessment and treatment priorities of all prehospital providers. You can't have good ALS without good BLS. The skills and priorities you learnt as a technician will continue to apply to the care you provide as a paramedic.

2. Given the mechanism of injury for an unrestrained passenger in a car and this patient's vital signs, what kinds of injuries should you think about in your assessment?

This case involves a significant mechanism of injury, given the head-on collision and dual carriageway speeds, plus the presence of other fatalities. If your patient outwardly appeared to be uninjured, you would still be extremely suspicious of internal bleeding and injuries. Because the patient is unconscious and was unrestrained and partially ejected, you should suspect significant head, chest, abdominal, pelvic, and long bone injuries.

3. Why does the patient remain hypoxic despite confirmed airway management and the delivery of high-concentration oxygen?

The patient remains hypoxic because he has developed a tension pneumothorax. This life-threatening condition must be recognised and corrected immediately. The presence of JVD and tracheal deviation are late signs of tension pneumothorax.

4. Do his vital signs and physical examination suggest any threats to his breathing that may be correctable?

His hypotension, tachycardia, decreased breath sounds, JVD, and tracheal deviation all point to tension pneumothorax. This requires emergency needle thoracocentesis.

5. What further injuries within the thorax could account for the patient's persistent hypotension and tachycardia?

The patient has hypotension and tachycardia due to increased intrathoracic pressures induced by a tension pneumothorax. This pressure prevents adequate cardiac preload, and therefore decreased cardiac output with resultant hypotension and tachycardia.

6. Are there interventions that you can provide in the prehospital environment if such injuries are identified?

A tension pneumothorax is a correctable condition that requires the release of built-up pressures through the introduction of a large-bore needle into the intercostal space between the second and third ribs, at the midclavicular line of the affected side.

7. What additional injuries might your physical findings suggest?

Given the location of the rib fractures, hypotension, and rigid abdomen, you should be highly suspicious of injury to the spleen. Splenic injuries are one of the most common forms of abdominal injury and can result in significant, life-threatening blood loss.

8. What additional treatments may be needed for this patient?

Obviously, once the major life-threatening conditions are addressed, then injuries such as lower extremity fractures can be addressed. Splinting and management of the affected lower extremity as well as managing any soft-tissue injuries would be appropriate at this time.

Prep Kit

Ready for Review

- The thorax contains the ribs, thoracic vertebrae, clavicle, scapula, sternum, heart, lungs, diaphragm, great vessels (including the aorta), oesophagus, lymphatic channels, trachea, mainstem bronchi, and nerves.
- Oxygenation and ventilation (delivery of oxygen and removal of carbon dioxide) take place within the thorax, as well as some aspects of circulation.
- Injuries to the thorax can cause air or blood to enter the lungs, or may prevent the organs from being able to move properly, inhibiting oxygenation and ventilation.
- Chest wall injuries include flail chest, rib fractures, and sternal fractures.
- In flail chest, two or more ribs are broken in two or more places. It can result in a free-floating segment of rib that can move paradoxically in comparison to the rest of the chest wall. The lung tissue beneath the flail segment is not adequately ventilated as a result.
- Rib fractures produce significant pain and can prevent adequate ventilation. Sternal fractures are also problematic in that they are usually associated with other serious injuries.
- Lung injuries include simple pneumothorax, open pneumothorax, tension pneumothorax, massive haemothorax, and pulmonary contusion.
- A pneumothorax occurs when air leaks into the space between the pleural surfaces from an opening in the chest or the surface of the lung. The lung collapses as air fills the pleural space. The result is a mismatch between ventilation and perfusion.
- A tension pneumothorax is life-threatening and results from collection of air in the pleural space. The air exerts increasing pressure on surrounding tissues as it accumulates, compromising ventilation, oxygenation, and circulation.
- A haemothorax is the accumulation of blood between the parietal and visceral pleura. It results in compression of structures around the collection of blood and compromises ventilation, oxygenation, and circulation.
- A haemopneumothorax is the collection of both blood and air in the pleural space.
- Pulmonary contusion occurs from compression of the lung. It results in alveolar and capillary damage, oedema, and hypoxia.
- Myocardial injuries include cardiac tamponade, myocardial contusion, myocardial rupture, and commotio cordis.
- Cardiac tamponade occurs when excessive fluid builds up in the pericardial sac around the heart. The heart becomes compressed and stroke volume is compromised.
- Myocardial contusion is essentially blunt trauma to the heart. Haemorrhage, oedema, and cellular damage result. Arrhythmias may occur.
- Myocardial rupture is perforation of one or more elements of the anatomy of the heart, such as the ventricles, atria, or valves. It can occur from blunt or penetrating trauma.
- Commotio cordis occurs from a direct blow to the chest during a critical portion of the heart's repolarisation period, resulting in possible cardiac arrest.
- Vascular injuries include thoracic aortic dissection/transaction and great vessel injury. Thoracic aortic dissection/transaction is literally ripping of the aorta. Injuries to other great vessels may cause similar problems of potentially fatal bleeding.
- Other thoracic injuries include diaphragmatic injuries (abdominal contents may herniate through the injury and cut off the blood supply); oesophageal injuries, which can be rapidly fatal; tracheobronchial injuries (injury to the airways); and traumatic asphyxia (sudden compression of the chest leading to pressure on the head, neck, and kidneys, causing capillary beds to rupture).
- Begin the assessment of a thoracic trauma patient as you would any other patient—with a scene assessment and assessment of the ABCs.
- In assessing breathing, note any signs of injury to the thorax, which could indicate additional underlying injuries. Look for paradoxical motion, retractions, subcutaneous emphysema, impaled objects, or penetrating injuries.
- Consider adequacy of ventilation and oxygenation. Watch for signs of hypoxia, an irregular pulse, changes in blood pressure, and JVD.
- Because the mechanism of injury that caused the thoracic problem may have been traumatic, always consider cervical spine stabilisation in such cases.
- Several chest injuries may have similar signs and symptoms, such as hypoxia, pain, tachycardia, cyanosis, and shock. Managing the various chest injuries involves several common steps: maintaining the airway, ensuring oxygenation and ventilation, supporting circulatory status, and transporting quickly. Learning the subtle differences between various chest injuries can help you manage them more specifically.
- The one exception to airway management in patients with thoracic trauma is the decision to endotracheally intubate a patient with a possible tracheal injury. Such a decision could further tear the trachea. These patients should be managed with minimal invasion to the airway.
- Management of flail chest includes airway management and possibly positive-pressure ventilation, if the patient experiences respiratory failure. Intubation may also be necessary.
- Management of rib fractures should focus on the ABCs and gentle splinting of the patient's chest by having the patient hold a pillow or blanket against the area.
- Management of a pneumothorax begins with the ABCs and high-concentration oxygen. Cover a sucking chest wound with an occlusive dressing secured on three sides.
- Patients with a tension pneumothorax should be placed on high-flow supplemental oxygen by nonrebreathing mask, and a needle decompression should be performed.
- For patients with pulmonary contusions or cardiac tamponade, follow general management (ABCs) and consider administering IV fluids.
- Management of patients with myocardial contusion should be supportive, but also includes cardiac monitoring and intravenous access.
- Care for patients with thoracic aortic dissection focuses on symptom control. Management of patients with great vessel injuries is no different from those with acute blood loss.
- Care for patients with tracheobronchial injuries entails assessment and management of the ABCs.
- Don't be distracted by the dramatic appearance of patients with traumatic asphyxia. Care for the ABCs, obtain IV access, and transport.
- Management of these chest injuries is supportive only: sternal fractures, haemothorax, and myocardial rupture.

Vital Vocabulary

angle of Louis Prominence on the sternum that lies opposite the second intercostal space.

atelectasis Alveolar collapse that prevents use of that portion of the lung for ventilation and oxygenation.

cardiac output The volume of blood delivered to the body in 1 minute.

cardiac tamponade A condition in which the atria and right ventricle are collapsed by a collection of blood or other fluid within the pericardial sac, resulting in a diminished cardiac output.

clavicle An S-shaped bone, also called the collarbone, that articulates medially with the sternum and laterally with the shoulder.

commotio cordis An event in which an often fatal cardiac arrhythmia is produced by a sudden blow to the thoracic cavity.

crepitus A grating sensation made when two pieces of broken bone are rubbed together or subcutaneous emphysema is palpated.

diaphragm Large skeletal muscle that plays a major role in breathing and separates the chest cavity from the abdominal cavity.

electrical alternans An ECG pattern in which the QRS vector changes with each heart beat. This pattern is pathognomonic for cardiac tamponade.

exophthalmos Protrusion of the eyes from the normal position within the socket.

flail chest An injury that involves two or more adjacent ribs fractured in two or more places, allowing the segment between the fractures to move independently of the rest of the thoracic cage.

haemopneumothorax A collection of blood and air in the pleural cavity.

haemothorax The collection of blood within the normally closed pleural space.

intercostal space The space between two ribs, named according to the number of the rib above it, that contains the intercostal muscles and neurovascular bundle.

jugular vein distension (JVD) A prominence of the jugular veins due to increased volume or increased pressure within the central venous system or the thoracic cavity.

manubrium The superior segment of the sternum; its lower border defines the angle of Louis.

mediastinum Space within the chest that contains the heart, major blood vessels, vagus nerve, trachea, and oesophagus; located between the two lungs.

myocardial contusion Blunt force injury to the heart that results in capillary damage, interstitial bleeding, and cellular damage in the area.

myocardial rupture An acute traumatic perforation of the ventricles, atria, intraventricular septum, intra-atrial septum, chordae, papillary muscles, or valves.

needle decompression Also referred to as a needle thoracentesis, this procedure introduces a needle or angiocath into the pleural space in an attempt to relieve a tension pneumothorax.

neurovascular bundle A closely placed grouping of an artery, vein, and nerve that lies beneath the inferior edge of a rib.

open pneumothorax The result of a defect in the chest wall that allows air to enter the thoracic space.

oxygenation The process of delivering oxygen to the blood by diffusion from the alveoli following inhalation into the lungs.

pericardial sac The potential space between the layers of the pericardium.

pericardiocentesis A procedure in which a needle or angiocath is introduced into the pericardial sac to relieve cardiac tamponade.

pericardium Double-layered sac containing the heart and the origins of the superior vena cava, inferior vena cava, and the pulmonary artery.

pleura Membrane lining the outer surface of the lungs (visceral pleura), the inner surface of the chest wall, and the thoracic surface of the diaphragm (parietal pleura).

pneumothorax The collection of air within the normally closed pleural space.

pulmonary contusion Injury to the lung parenchyma that results in capillary haemorrhage into the tissue.

scapula A large, flat, triangular bone along the posterior thorax that articulates with the clavicle and humerus.

sternum Also known as the breastbone, this bony structure along the midline of the thorax provides a point of anterior attachment for the thoracic cage.

subconjunctival haematoma The collection of blood within the sclera of the eye, presenting as a bright red patch of blood over the sclera but not involving the cornea.

subcutaneous emphysema A physical finding of air within the subcutaneous tissue.

suprasternal notch The indentation formed by the superior border of the manubrium and the clavicles, often used as a landmark for procedures such as subclavian vein access.

tension pneumothorax A life-threatening collection of air within the pleural space; the volume and pressure have both collapsed the involved lung and caused a shift of the mediastinal structures to the opposite side.

thoracic inlet The superior aspect of the thoracic cavity, this ring-like opening is created by the first vertebral vertebra, the first rib, the clavicles, and the manubrium.

thorax The part of the body between the neck and the diaphragm, encased by the ribs.

traumatic asphyxia A pattern of injuries seen after a severe force is applied to the thorax, forcing blood from the great vessels and back into the head and neck.

ventilation The process of eliminating carbon dioxide from the blood by diffusion into the alveoli and exhalation from the lungs.

xyphoid process An inferior segment of the sternum often used as a landmark for CPR.

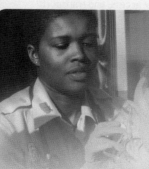

Assessment in Action

You are dispatched to an office building for a patient who has fallen from a ladder. On arrival, you find a 34-year-old man who is in a left lateral recumbent position. He complains of chest pain and shortness of breath. While maintaining in-line stabilisation, you notice some bruising to his upper back that extends into his left flank area. Looking at the ladder, you note that he fell at least 8 m.

1. **In a patient who has sustained blunt trauma to the chest, you may find:**
   A. pulmonary contusion.
   B. fractured rib(s).
   C. sternal fracture.
   D. all of the above.

2. **With a fall victim who is complaining of shortness of breath and chest pain, you should suspect which of the following injuries?**
   A. Tension pneumothorax
   B. Flail segment
   C. Pulmonary contusion
   D. All of the above

3. _____ is the most common cause of a tension pneumothorax.
   A. Barotrauma
   B. Blunt force trauma
   C. Tracheobronchial injuries
   D. Open thoracic injury

4. Traumatic injury to the thoracic cavity presents the possibility of compromise of:
   A. ventilation.
   B. oxygenation.
   C. circulation.
   D. all of the above.

5. Which injuries must be identified and treated during assessment of the patient's breathing?
   A. Flail chest, tension pneumothorax, and cardiac tamponade
   B. Open pneumothorax, tension pneumothorax, and flail chest
   C. Aortic injuries, open pneumothorax, and flail chest
   D. Open pneumothorax, tension pneumothorax, and myocardial contusion

6. All of the following are classic signs of a tension pneumothorax, EXCEPT:
   A. absence of breath sounds on the affected side.
   B. absence of breath sounds on the unaffected side.
   C. tachycardia.
   D. jugular vein distension.

7. Traumatic injuries that result in the sudden and forceful compression of the thoracic cavity may cause:
   A. traumatic asphyxia.
   B. traumatic pneumothorax.
   C. exophthalmos.
   D. haematoma.

8. The pathology of a tension pneumothorax includes all of the following, EXCEPT:
   A. the lung collapses on the affected side with mediastinal shift to the opposing side.
   B. a serious reduction in cardiac output by the deformation of the vena cava, reducing preload.
   C. the lung collapse leads to right-to-left intrapulmonary shunting and hypoxia.
   D. the lung collapse leads to left-to-right intrapulmonary shunting and hypercarbia.

9. Muffled heart sounds, hypotension, and jugular vein distension—a classic combination of findings in patients with cardiac tamponade—are collectively called:
   A. Beck's triad.
   B. Circle of Wills.
   C. pulsus paradoxus.
   D. myocardial contusion.

10. The pathology of a myocardial contusion may include any of the following, EXCEPT:
    A. development of a cardiac tamponade when the epicardium or endocardium is lacerated.
    B. clear demarcation of the areas of contusion.
    C. undefined areas of contusion.
    D. conduction defects on the ECG caused by the areas of contusion.

Challenging Question

You are dispatched to the home of a 45-year-old woman. The call came in as a stabbing. At the scene, you perform a scene assessment and determine that it's safe to enter the house. The patient is located upstairs in the bedroom, where she is lying prone on the floor. She is not breathing, and a small quantity of blood is pooling beneath her. She has no pulse.

Maintaining in-line stabilisation, you roll the patient over on a longboard (after examining her back for any obvious injuries). You open her airway and begin ventilating with 100% oxygen. You immediately begin high-quality CPR (pushing hard, fast, and allowing full chest recoil). Your partner successfully intubates the patient, and you hear good breath sounds on the right side. There is no tracheal deviation, but there is jugular vein distension. The monitor shows a narrow-complex pulseless electrical activity at a rate of 100 beats/min.

The police tell you that the patient was in a verbal argument with her husband, who then stabbed her with a 30 cm steak knife. The knife is by her side. You notice a wound just under her left clavicle and feel some subcutaneous emphysema surrounding the wound. When you intubate the patient, you don't hear any breath sounds on the left side. You believe she has a tension pneumothorax.

You properly perform a chest decompression. You hear a rush of air exit the cannula.

11. What type of injury is this?

12. What other injuries should you expect?

■ Points to Ponder

You are dispatched to a local motorway for a road traffic collision—a car has run into a wall. When you arrive, the fire service is in the process of extricating the patient. During your initial scene assessment, you determined that it was safe to enter the zone. You also noticed a midsize car with severe front-end damage and damage to the top of the roof. The A-post was completely bent down. You have no real access to the patient other than to see that he is unconscious, has agonal respirations, and is grossly perspiring. Blood is coming out of his mouth.

You ask witnesses if they saw anything. They tell you that the car was moving at a high rate of speed (in excess of 70 miles per hour). When it was going around the bend, the car slid on an ice patch and the driver lost control of the vehicle. He drove into the cement abuttment head on. The vehicle then flipped up and its roof struck the wall. The vehicle landed on its wheels. There is significant damage to the driver's compartment, including the steering wheel.

The patient is finally extricated from the vehicle, and the fire service assist you to provide full spinal precautions.

What will you as the paramedic do for this patient?

Issues: Thorough Assessment to Determine Diagnosis and Treatment Plan, Thorough Scene Assessment to Determine Forces Involved, Proper Treatment of a Patient With Thoracic Trauma.

www.Paramedic.EMSzone.com/UK/

24 Abdominal Injuries

Objectives

Cognitive

- Describe how the epidemiology of abdominal injuries influences prevention strategies.
- Describe the anatomy and physiology of organs and structures related to abdominal injuries.
- Differentiate between the injury patterns of blunt and penetrating abdominal trauma.
- Describe open and closed abdominal injuries.
- Describe the assessment findings associated with abdominal injuries.
- Identify the need for rapid intervention and transport of the patient with abdominal injuries based on assessment findings.
- Describe the prehospital management of abdominal injuries.
- Describe how the assessment and history inform the initial diagnosis.
- Formulate a treatment plan based on the initial diagnosis.
- Differentiate between the assessment findings of solid and hollow organ injury.
- Describe the mechanism of injury, history, signs, and symptoms that would lead you to suspect abdominal vascular injury.
- Describe the treatment plan and management of abdominal vascular injuries.
- Describe the epidemiology, including the morbidity/mortality and prevention strategies for pelvic fractures.
- Describe the mechanism of injury, history, signs and symptoms that would lead you to suspect abdominal pelvic fracture.
- Describe the treatment plan and management of pelvic fractures.
- Describe the assessment findings associated with other related abdominal injuries.
- Formulate an initial diagnosis based upon the assessment findings for a patient with abdominal injuries.
- Develop a patient management plan for a patient with abdominal injuries, based upon the initial diagnosis.

Affective

- Advocate the use of a thorough evaluation of the mechanism of injury, full history, and methodical assessment to determine a differential diagnosis and treatment plan for abdominal trauma.
- Advocate the use of a thorough scene survey to determine the forces involved in abdominal trauma.
- Value the implications of failing to properly diagnose abdominal trauma and initiate timely interventions for patients with abdominal trauma.

Psychomotor

- Demonstrate a clinical assessment to determine the proper treatment plan for a patient with suspected abdominal trauma.

Introduction

The abdominal cavity is the largest cavity in the body. It extends from the diaphragm to the pelvis, making the evaluation and management of patients with abdominal trauma challenging for the paramedic. There is great variability in the presentation of conditions, which are rarely resolved in the prehospital setting. Abdominal injuries may be life threatening, and assessment should be rapid so management and transport to an appropriate hospital can be started.

The abdominal cavity contains several vital organ systems such as the digestive, urinary, and genitourinary systems. These organ systems are vulnerable to trauma partly because of their location but they also lack some of the protective structures afforded by the skeletal system. Abdominal trauma may be caused by blunt or penetrating forces and range from minor single-system injuries to the more complicated and potentially devastating multi-system injuries. Abdominal injuries can be difficult to prevent, as that would involve avoiding collisions and other forms of trauma! An empty bladder and toned abdominal muscles can help decrease potential damage should trauma occur to the abdomen.

Because of the broad spectrum of abdominal injuries, assessments and interventions should be made quickly and cautiously. Delays in the recognition and management of abdominal injuries can have disastrous consequences. Assessments in the prehospital environment can be difficult because of other system injuries that may lead to changes in a patient's mental status and sensation. For example, an unconscious patient or a patient who does not feel pain after spinal trauma may not be able to communicate, leaving the determination of existing injuries to be based solely on presenting signs and the mechanism of injury.

According to the Royal Society for the Prevention of Accidents (ROSPA), trauma is the leading cause of death in people aged 1 to 44 years. Blunt abdominal trauma is the leading cause of morbidity and mortality in all age groups. In recent years, there has been a concerted effort to reduce morbidity and mortality resulting from abdominal trauma. This process has taken shape at several different levels. The education of prehospital providers in recognising the need for rapid transport has made a significant reduction in the time from injury to definitive care. The advances in hospital care, such as improved diagnostic equipment (eg, ultrasound), surgical techniques, and postoperative care have also improved patient outcomes. Furthermore, trauma system development has played a large role in providing advanced interventions and detection of traumatic injuries.

The purpose of this chapter is to supply the information necessary to assess and begin managing the trauma patient as quickly and with as much confidence as possible. This chapter provides the concepts and vocabulary for the effective understanding and communication of critical data that will improve patient assessment and understanding of the mechanism of

At the Scene

Late recognition of abdominal trauma can be a fatal mistake. Abdominal trauma often goes unrecognised because the mechanism of injury is often not fully appreciated or noticed.

You are the Paramedic Part 1

As you walk into the ambulance station for the start of your shift, you hear the front doorbell. When you answer the door, you find a child who tells you that, while he was waiting across the street for the school bus, he saw a man lying in the alleyway. You alert your colleague, grab a response bag, and follow the child, who takes you directly to the man.

As you approach, you see a man lying in the alleyway between two houses, curled in a ball and holding his left ankle. He appears dirty, dishevelled, and pale, and you recognise him as a homeless man, Mr. Campbell (Stan), you've seen on previous calls involving drugs, alcohol, and abusive behaviour. When you ask him what is wrong, he mutters something about tripping and hurting his leg.

Initial Assessment	Recording Time: 0 Minutes
Appearance	Eyes closed; fetal position
Level of consciousness	V (Responsive to verbal stimuli)
Airway	Patent; patient is moaning
Breathing	Rapid and shallow
Circulation	Rapid radial pulse

1. What are your immediate concerns?
2. What about this patient immediately grabs your attention?
3. At this point, what are your treatment priorities?

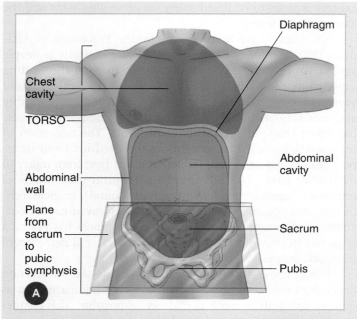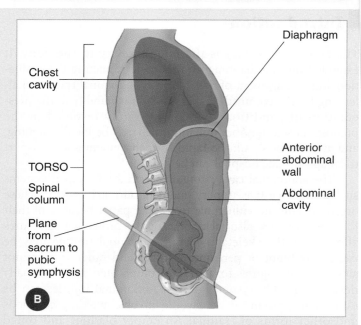

Figure 24-1 The external abdomen consists of the anterior abdomen, the flanks, and the back (retroperitoneal area). The boundaries of the abdomen are the anterior and posterior abdominal cavity walls, the diaphragm, and an imaginary plane from the pubic symphysis to the sacrum. **A.** Anterior view. **B.** Lateral view.

injury. Your initial diagnosis from the scene is the only source for doctors and surgeons to understand the events and mechanism that led to any given trauma presentation. This information is critical in visualising and searching for injuries that may not be obviously apparent on physical examination, as is often the case with abdominal injuries.

Anatomy Review

Knowledge of the anatomic boundaries of the abdomen is important as we discuss potential injury patterns, such as hollow organ injury, vascular injury, solid organ injury, or injuries to the retroperitoneal area. The oval-shaped abdominal cavity extends from the dome-shaped diaphragm, a large muscle separating the thoracic cavity from the abdomen, to the pelvic brim. The pelvic brim stretches at an angle from the intervertebral disks between L5 and S1 to the pubic symphysis.

Knowledge of the anatomical boundaries of the abdomen is an important factor when discussing potential injury patterns. Historically the abdomen has been divided in to either four quadrants or nine regions (Figure 24-1 ▲), the purpose of both methods is to enable health care professionals to report on findings which can be related to the underlying structures in a consistent and readily understood manner.

Superiorly the upper regions of the abdominal cavity are protected by the lower rib cage; inferiorly protection is afforded by a ring formed by the sacrum and bones of the pelvis. The posterior abdomen is protected by the lumbar, lower thoracic spine, and the inferior ribs. Thus some of the organs contained

within the abdomen are protected by the lower thoracic cage and depending on which phase of the respiratory cycle can be as high as the fourth intercostal space. This point is significant when determining whether thoracic or abdominal insults also intrude in to another cavity or organ(s). The flanks are identified by the anterior and posterior axillary lines, which extend from the sixth intercostal space to the iliac crest.

To describe a location in the abdomen, or a source of pain found when conducting your assessment, either the ninths or the quadrant system are generally used (Figure 24-2 ▶). If you were to place a large imaginary "+" sign with the centre directly on the umbilicus (navel) with the vertical axis extending from the pubic symphysis to the xiphoid process and the horizontal axis extending to both flanks, this would create four quadrants. These four regions are as follows: the right upper quadrant (RUQ), the right lower quadrant (RLQ), the left lower quadrant (LLQ), and the left upper quadrant (LUQ). The area around the umbilicus is referred to as the periumbilical area.

The abdominal cavity is lined with a membrane called the peritoneum, which is similar to the pleura that line the thoracic cavity. The mesentery is a membranous double fold of tissue in the abdomen that attaches various organs to the body wall. The internal abdomen is structurally divided into three regions: the peritoneal space, the retroperitoneal space, and the pelvis (Figure 24-3 ▶). Intraperitoneal structures, encased in the peritoneum, include the liver, spleen, stomach, small bowel, colon, gallbladder, and, in women, the female reproductive organs. The retroperitoneal space contains the aorta, vena cava, pancreas, kidneys, ureters, and portions of the duodenum and large intestine. The rectum, ureters, pelvic vascular plexus,

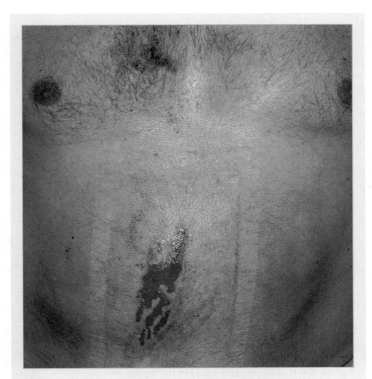

Figure 24-9 Remember that abdominal injury can be severe even in the absence of symptoms. Contamination of the intra-abdominal space may not produce pain or fever for hours or even days.

At the Scene

All trauma patients should be assumed to have a full stomach, even if they deny having taken any food or liquids recently.

tising the patient. Many of these patients live through the initial assessment; their more subtle signs and symptoms are uncovered in the focused history and physical examination.

Focused History and Physical Examination

The first step in the physical examination is inspection of the abdomen. This means you will need to expose the abdomen and inspect for signs of trauma (such as DCAP-BTLS). Often the injury to the abdomen involves ecchymosis, abrasions, or lacerations.

Blood, gastrointestinal contents, and urine that have spilled into the peritoneum may produce peritonitis that could result in decreased or absent abdominal sounds, but auscultation of bowel sounds is not a useful assessment tool in the prehospital setting. The next steps in the abdominal examination are percussion and palpation. With these manoeuvres, look for tenderness and signs of peritonitis (such as the patient guarding his or her abdomen or experiencing pain while being gently moved to the stretcher). Carefully palpate the entire abdomen while assessing the patient's response and noting abdominal masses and deformities.

Controversies

Listening to bowel sounds in the prehospital environment may not be helpful. To properly auscultate bowel sounds, it is necessary to listen for several minutes. This is not practical in the prehospital environment, and the ambient noise may be too great to determine the presence or absence of bowel sounds.

A common misconception is that patients without abdominal pain or abnormal vital signs are unlikely to have serious intra-abdominal injuries. Keep in mind that peritonitis can take hours or even days to develop. Similarly, nonspecific symptoms such as hypotension, tachycardia, and confusion may not develop until the patient has lost more than 40% of his or her circulating blood volume. Always maintain a high index of suspicion in any patient who has a mechanism of injury consistent with abdominal trauma, regardless of the examination findings.

Special Considerations

Because older people usually have a more flaccid abdominal wall (containing less muscle and more fat) than younger people, apply increased pressure when palpating the abdomen to assess for injury. You should suspect that any older trauma patient who complains of abdominal pain has an internal organ injury.

initial assessment. The abdomen should be examined closely for bruising, road rash, localised swelling, lacerations, distention, or pain. Clues to intra-abdominal trauma will include symptoms of hypovolaemia not proportional to obvious external evidence or estimated blood loss. Retroperitoneal haemorrhage may be present because of damaged muscle, lacerated or avulsed kidneys, and injuries to the vessels of the supporting mesentery. All abdominal organs have a generous blood supply, making them susceptible to significant bleeding as a result of blunt forces causing a shearing-type injury. An injury to the abdomen can be fatal primarily because of haemorrhage. The injury can be slow to develop, and may be subtle and difficult to locate and assess.

Scene Assessment

As with all other aspects of prehospital care, scene safety remains the priority before providing any patient care. It is always important to remember that if a patient has penetrating or blunt trauma, some external force caused this injury (such as a gun, knife, or the cricket bat in the corner of the room!). These cases could also be potentially dangerous to the paramedic.

Initial Assessment

Once you have sized up the scene and determined that it is safe, the first patient priorities are those of the initial assessment: mental status, airway, breathing, circulation, and priori-

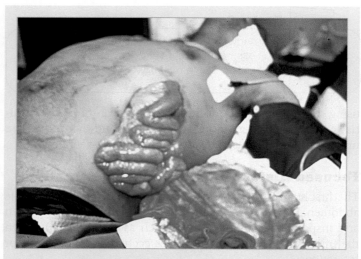

Figure 24-10 An abdominal evisceration is an open abdominal wound from which internal organs or fat protrude.

Abdominal distention is a late indication of abdominal trauma. Patients must have a significant volume of blood enter the abdominal cavity to fill it and produce distention.

Try to obtain as many details about an injury as possible, keeping in mind that trauma patients should be transported to the hospital quickly. In other words, in addition to getting information about the patient (such as the SAMPLE history), it is important to obtain details on how the injury occurred, whether from the patient, witnesses, police, or other ambulance service providers.

In blunt trauma caused by a road traffic collision, determine the types of vehicles involved, the speed at which they were travelling, and how they collided. You should also try to find out other information about the event, such as the use of seatbelts, the deployment of air bags, and the patient's position in the vehicle.

In penetrating trauma, it's helpful to identify the type of weapon used. However, this is often impossible because assailants usually leave with their weapon. In a gunshot case, determine the type of gun and the number of shots, if possible. Providers should try to ascertain an estimated distance between the victim and the assailant whenever possible. In stab wounds, determine the type of knife, possible angle of the entrance wound, and number of stab wounds.

As part of the focused history and physical examination of a trauma patient, you may be faced with a number of challenges associated with abdominal trauma. You may discover the presence of an abdominal evisceration—displacement of an organ outside the body   Figure 24-10 ▲ . This is where the abdominal organs are found protruding through a wound in the abdominal wall. Generally, little pain is associated with this type of injury; do not apply any material that will adhere to the abdominal structures. Providers may also be confronted with impaled objects   Figure 24-11 ▶ . Impaled objects are stabilised and transported in the position they were found. Stabilisation of impaled objects can be impractical in some prehospital environments, but effective stabilisation and safe transportation

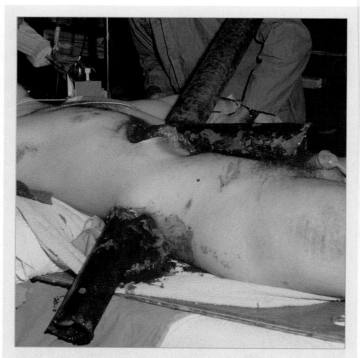

Figure 24-11 An object impaled in the abdomen.

At the Scene

Always examine the back of the patient as carefully as you examine the front. Gunshot wounds or stab wounds can easily be missed in creases of the body, especially if the patient is obese or has large quantities of body hair.

can help reduce serious tissue damage. Additionally, significant infection often develops in this type of wound, so early intervention with sterile techniques should be employed.

If you suspect injury to the diaphragm, focus on the airway, breathing, and circulatory status of the patient. Remember that the diaphragm plays a large role in the mechanical process of breathing. Examine the patient's neck and chest, paying particular attention to the trachea (tracheal deviation due to mediastinal shift), symmetry of the chest during expansion, and absence of breath sounds.

At the Scene

Cullen's sign is a black-and-blue discolouration (bruising) in the umbilical region caused by peritoneal bleeding. Grey Turner's sign includes bruising present in the lower abdominal and flank regions. They are both caused by intra-abdominal bleeding found 12 to 24 hours after the initial injury. The presence of these signs is helpful, but their absence does not rule out life-threatening abdominal haemorrhage.

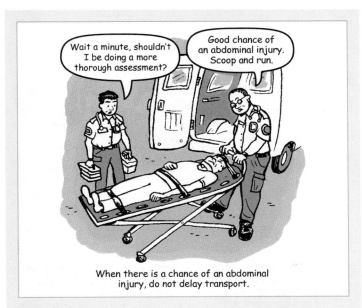

Figure 24-12

Detailed Physical Examination

Perform a detailed physical examination on a patient who has abdominal trauma and was found to have a significant MOI. Because, at this point, you will have completed the initial assessment as well as the rapid trauma examination, the detailed physical examination should be conducted en route to the A&E department to avoid any unnecessary delays **Figure 24-12 ▲**. Basically, the detailed physical examination assesses the same structures as the rapid trauma examination, except more methodically. Close examination may uncover additional findings that were either not picked up during the rapid trauma examination or are only now starting to develop (such as haematoma, bruises, or tender areas). As long

Notes from Nancy

An injury to the chest anywhere below the nipples is also an injury to the abdomen.

Documentation and Communication

Pertinent documentation of the abdominal trauma assessment should include the following: whether or not seatbelts were worn, which type, and their position on the patient; the location, intensity, and quality of pain; whether or not nausea or vomiting is present; the contour of the abdomen; any bruising or open areas present on the soft-tissue inspection; the presence or absence of rebound tenderness, guarding, rigidity, spasm, or localised pain; any changes in the level of consciousness and serial vital signs; other injuries found; the presence or absence of alcohol, opioids, or any type of analgesic; and the results of your ongoing assessment.

as you can ensure that the problems found in the initial assessment have been attended to, and there is time en route, perform a very thorough detailed physical examination on your patient.

Ongoing Assessment

The ongoing assessment includes reassessment of the initial assessment as well as retaking vital signs and checking interventions on the patient.

Management Overview

In general, the prehospital management of patients who have abdominal trauma is straightforward. As always, ensuring an open airway while taking spinal precautions is the first step. Administer high-concentration oxygen to the patient via a nonrebreathing mask.

In the United Kingdom, current guidelines suggest that the use of fluid therapy is less aggressive than it was in previous years. To these ends, if there is visible external blood loss greater than 500 ml, fluid replacement should be commenced with a 250 ml bolus of crystalloid.

- If the central pulse and radial pulse are absent, it is an absolute indication for urgent fluid.
- If the patient has a carotid pulse but no radial pulse, then other clinical factors should also be considered before making a decision on fluid administration.
- If the central pulse is present but the radial pulse is absent, there is a relative indication for urgent fluid depending on other indications including tissue perfusion and blood loss.
- If the central pulse and radial pulse are both present, do not commence fluid replacement unless there are other signs of poor central tissue perfusion (eg, altered mental state, cardiac rhythm disturbance).

Do not delay transport to initiate IV therapy; establish IV lines whenever possible during transport. Minimise external haemorrhage by applying pressure dressings. Apply a cardiac monitor. Transport the patient to the appropriate hospital, depending on your local transport protocols. Note that the assessment should also not delay patient care and transport. Repeated abdominal examinations are the key to discovering a patient's worsening condition before vital signs change. Perform your examinations en route during the ongoing assessment.

In some cases of penetrating injury, part of an abdominal organ may protrude outside of the body (evisceration). If this occurs, do not attempt to place the organ back into the body. Rather, cover it with a sterile dressing moistened with saline, and protect the organ from damage during transport.

Notes from Nancy

A distended, tender abdomen after injury means internal bleeding. Treat for shock and transport immediately.

At the Scene

There is an old medical school scenario of a patient who was shot in the head who is hypotensive. The puzzle is, "What's wrong with the patient?" The answer, as we have learned in this chapter, is that the patient was probably shot in the belly with a second bullet! Always remember that haemorrhaging will continue until controlled in the operating room under "bright lights and cold steel." Survival may be determined by the length of time from the injury to definitive surgical control of the haemorrhage. Delays may negatively impact the patient's long-term survival. So, if you are not the solution to this patient's problem, don't add to the problem. Get the patient to definitive care!

Administering pain medication often is contraindicated because of the patient's hypotension.

Pelvic Fractures

The pelvis is best thought of as a ring, with its sacral, iliac, ischium, and pubic bones held together by ligaments. Large forces are required to damage this ring. The majority of pelvic fractures are a result of blunt trauma from road traffic collisions or from vehicles striking pedestrians.

Because of the forces required to break the pelvis, suspect multi-system trauma if your patient has a pelvic injury (until proven otherwise). Commonly associated injuries are urethral disruptions, bladder rupture, and abdominal, thoracic, and head trauma **Figure 24-13 ▶**. Signs and symptoms of blunt trauma to the pelvis include pain in the pelvis, groin, or hips; haematomas or contusions to the pelvic region; obvious external bleeding; or hypotension without obvious external bleeding.

Anteroposterior compression, which can result from a head-on collision, may lead to an "open-book" pelvic fracture in which the pubic symphysis spreads apart. The subsequent increase in volume of the pelvis means a patient with internal pelvic bleeding may lose a much larger amount of blood than someone without an open-book fracture. Such patients will

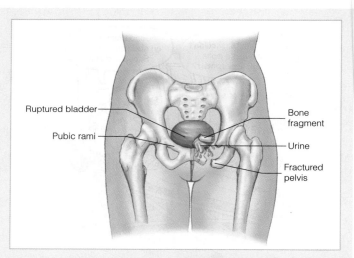

Figure 24-13 Pelvic fractures occasionally cause laceration of the bladder as a result of penetration by bony fragments. Externally, pelvic fractures can cause severe bruising and swelling.

Special Considerations

Paediatric trauma patients are less likely to have pelvic fractures than adults.

require IV fluids with Hartmann's or normal saline but may still remain hypotensive on the scene.

Lateral compression of the pelvis results from a side impact. It generally does not result in an unstable pelvis. Because the volume in the pelvis is reduced, not increased, life-threatening haemorrhage is less of a concern in such cases.

Vertical shear is seen in falls from heights. It results in one side of the pelvis moving superiorly or inferiorly compared to the other, disrupting the bony or ligamentous structures. This unstable fracture results in an increased pelvic volume.

Saddle injuries result from falling on an object. They may result in fractures of the bones that are directly under the female and male genitalia (pubic rami fractures).

Although penetrating trauma to the pelvis may result in bony fractures, the more worrisome injury is to the major vascular structures, which can cause life-threatening haemorrhage.

You are the Paramedic Part 4

Upon your arrival at hospital, the patient's condition is immediately evaluated and he is taken to the operating theatre. You later learn that he had significant blood loss from liver lacerations and a ruptured spleen. He also had multiple fractures of his left distal tibia and fibula as a result of several blows from a cricket bat.

10. How can age and medical problems make traumatic injuries worse?

Open fractures (not to be confused with open-book fractures) may result from either penetrating or blunt trauma and frequently result in chronic pain and disability that persist for years after the initial injury.

Assessment and Management

Properly evaluating and treating the patient is more important than identifying the specific type of pelvic fracture. A search for entry and exit wounds for a penetrating trauma is helpful but an extended search should never delay quick transport and treatment of hypotension. In both blunt and penetrating trauma, the presence of thoracic trauma may result in a life-threatening tension pneumothorax. In addition, if you suspect an open-book pelvic fracture in a patient with hypotension, tie a sheet around the patient's hips at the level of the superior anterior iliac crests, thereby decreasing the pelvic volume. There are several devices specific to the management of this type of injury that provide superior immobilisation and are faster to apply. One device, the SAM Sling, has a patented "autostop" buckle to provide the correct circumferential force to close and stabilise open-book pelvic fractures.

You are the Paramedic Summary

1. What are your immediate concerns?

Your first priority is always scene safety. Given your previous exposure to the patient and your knowledge of his history of drugs, alcohol, and assaultive behaviour, you should discreetly request police response as well as ask one of your colleagues to locate the child's parents. If the child's parents are not available, liaise with the police who will arrange an appropriate place of safety for the child until his parents or his legal guardian can be contacted.

2. What about this patient immediately grabs your attention?

The patient's location, his level of consciousness, and his body position are immediate causes for concern. Given the time of day, question how long he has been lying in this location. You should also wonder about the possibilities of alcohol and/or drug use and their effects in limiting your patient's ability to accurately perceive pain and injury.

3. At this point, what are your treatment priorities?

Assessing and managing life-threatening conditions is always your top priority. A patient who exhibits a decreased level of consciousness, tachycardia, and tachypnoea should be treated swiftly and appropriately.

4. What do these signs indicate to you?

Given the patient's decreased level of consciousness, skin signs, tachycardia, and hypotension in the presence of abdominal guarding, he is likely to have lost a significant amount of blood.

5. What does abdominal guarding usually indicate?

Abdominal guarding usually indicates peritonitis, an inflammation of the lining of the abdomen that results from either blood or hollow organ contents spilling into the abdominal cavity.

6. Is this condition an early or late finding?

Peritonitis is a late finding: It can take hours or even days to develop. Blood loss significant enough to produce signs and symptoms of hypovolaemia may not develop until 30% or more of the patient's blood volume is lost. For this reason, you should be highly suspicious of injuries resulting from significant blunt or penetrating trauma. Patients with these injuries can appear to have normal vital signs in the presence of significant injuries in the early stages.

7. Why is it important to provide rapid transport and interventions such as IVs en route to hospital?

Definitive care for the trauma patient is available at the nearest appropriate trauma centre. To delay transport so as to initiate IVs, splint fractures, and the like would delay the care the patient ultimately needs. Be aware of scene times, striving to keep these to 10 minutes or less. Obviously, if extra time has to be spent on the scene for issues such as extrication, provide interventions as required and document the reasons for the delayed transport.

8. Are patients' chief complaints and primary problems always identical?

Your patients may or may not complain of pain or discomfort associated with the source of their primary problem. In this scenario, the patient is more concerned about his leg and ankle pain; you should be more concerned about the internal bleeding in his abdomen. This is an important lesson for any paramedic—don't allow yourself to become consumed with the outward, most obvious injuries, as they may or may not be life threatening.

9. Which organs are at risk of injury given the apparent location of this patient's injury?

You should be worried that the liver and spleen could have significant damage given the patient's skin condition and vital signs. Injury to one or both of these organs can produce significant bleeding. The liver can suffer lacerations as well as contusions in blunt trauma, and the spleen is at great risk of rupture.

10. How can age and medical problems make traumatic injuries worse?

Elderly and paediatric patients do not have the same compensatory mechanisms that healthy young and middle-aged adults possess. Extremes of age (and disease processes such as diabetes, heart conditions, and high blood pressure, along with their accompanying medicines) can mask signs and symptoms in otherwise healthy patients. Also, mechanisms of injury and their associated damage can change with age. Children who are struck by vehicles have different injury patterns than those of adults. Older patients on beta blockers are not able to compensate for blood loss with increased heart rates in the same way that younger patients can. For this reason, whenever possible, you should obtain a trauma patient's medical history, including medications and allergies.

Prep Kit

Ready for Review

- Unrecognised abdominal trauma is the leading cause of unexpected death in trauma patients. Recognising abdominal injuries and providing rapid transport is one of the best contributions you can make to a patient who has these injuries.
- The abdomen contains many vital organs and structures, including the kidneys, liver, spleen, pancreas, diaphragm, small and large intestines, stomach, bladder, and several great vessels.
- The quadrant system is generally used to describe a location in the abdomen. These are the right upper quadrant (RUQ), the right lower quadrant (RLQ), the left lower quadrant (LLQ), and the left upper quadrant (LUQ).
- The peritoneum is a membrane that lines the abdominal cavity. Abdominal trauma can lead to peritonitis, an inflammation of the peritoneum that results from either blood or hollow organ contents spilling into the abdominal cavity. This is a life-threatening infection.
- The retroperitoneal space is the area behind the peritoneum and contains the aorta, vena cava, pancreas, kidneys, ureters, and portions of the duodenum and large intestine.
- When a patient has experienced trauma to the chest or abdomen, suspect that he or she also has additional internal abdominal injuries. Also suspect abdominal trauma in patients who have unexplained symptoms of shock.
- Injury to the abdomen can be slow to develop, and can be fatal. An injury may be subtle and difficult to locate and assess.
- Solid organs such as the liver and spleen have a large blood supply and can easily be crushed by blunt trauma. The abdomen and retroperitoneum can accommodate large amounts of blood but produce few signs and symptoms.
- Injury to hollow organs can cause the release of toxins such as urine, bile, or stomach acid into the abdominal cavity, causing major peritonitis.
- At least two thirds of all abdominal injuries involve blunt trauma, occurring mostly during road traffic collisions. Blunt trauma can often lead to a closed abdominal injury.
- Penetrating trauma most commonly results from stab wounds or low-velocity gunshot wounds. Penetrating trauma causes open abdominal injury.
- During the assessment, try to obtain as many details about an injury as possible. Also note the use of seatbelts, deployment of air bags, and the patient's position in the vehicle. If a weapon was involved, note the type of weapon if this information is available.
- Peritonitis can take hours to days to develop. Shock, tachycardia, and confusion may not develop until the patient has lost a significant amount of blood. Maintain a high index of suspicion for a patient who has a mechanism of injury consistent with abdominal trauma, regardless of vital signs and other findings.

- Generally, management of patients with abdominal trauma is straightforward:
  - Ensure a secure airway.
  - Establish intravenous access and fluid replacement without delaying transport.
  - Minimise haemorrhaging with pressure dressings.
  - Apply a cardiac monitor and oxygen therapy, and then transport.
- Assessment should never delay patient care and transport!
- Pelvic fractures can result in damage to the major vascular structures, which can cause life-threatening haemorrhage.
- Because of the forces required to break the pelvis, if the patient has a pelvic fracture, suspect multi-system trauma.

Vital Vocabulary

blunt trauma Injury resulting from compression or deceleration forces, potentially crushing an organ or causing it to rupture.

closed abdominal injury An injury in which there is soft-tissue damage inside the body, but the skin remains intact.

duodenum The first part of the small intestine.

ecchymosis Black-and-blue discolouration.

evisceration Displacement of an organ outside the body.

haemoperitoneum The presence of extravasated blood in the peritoneal cavity.

Kehr's sign Left shoulder pain that may indicate a ruptured spleen.

mesentery A membranous double fold of tissue in the abdomen that attaches various organs to the body wall.

open abdominal injury An injury in which there is a break in the surface of the skin or mucous membrane, exposing deeper tissue to potential contamination.

penetrating trauma An injury in which the skin is broken; direct contact results in laceration of the structure.

peritoneum A membrane in the abdomen encasing the liver, spleen, diaphragm, stomach, and transverse colon.

peritonitis Inflammation of the peritoneum (the lining around the abdominal cavity) that results from either blood or hollow organ contents spilling into the abdominal cavity.

periumbilical Pertaining to the area around the umbilicus.

pylorus A circumferential muscle at the end of the stomach that acts as a valve between the stomach and duodenum.

retroperitoneal space The area in the abdomen containing the aorta, vena cava, pancreas, kidneys, ureters, and portions of the duodenum and large intestine.

Assessment in Action

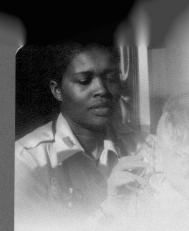

You are dispatched to a road traffic collision at a major road junction. When you arrive, you find two vehicles, one of which has been crashed into on the driver's side. The driver is still in the vehicle and the fire and rescue service is in the process of extricating her. You notice that the damage to the driver's side door is significant. There is approximately a 46 cm intrusion.

The driver is conscious, alert, and orientated. She is complaining only of pain in the right upper quadrant of her abdomen, just below her rib cage. Her vital signs are: respirations, 20 breaths/min; pulse, 130 beats/min; blood pressure, 100/60 mm Hg; and pulse oximetry, 98% on room air. The patient's c-spine is immobilised and she is removed from the vehicle. In the ambulance, you perform a complete assessment. Everything is unremarkable except she has pain on palpation to her right upper quadrant and pain in her left shoulder. Her abdomen is soft, and she is not guarding it. You initiate two large-bore IVs, apply oxygen, and transport the patient to the nearest appropriate hospital.

1. **What type of injury should you suspect?**
   A. Lacerated liver
   B. Ruptured spleen
   C. Contusion of the heart
   D. Ruptured appendix

2. **What type of impact did this patient receive?**
   A. Frontal impact
   B. Rear impact
   C. Lateral or side impact
   D. Rotational impact

3. **Which are solid organs of the abdomen?**
   A. Liver, spleen, kidneys, and pancreas
   B. Liver, spleen, and pancreas
   C. Large intestine, small intestine, and kidneys
   D. Liver, spleen, kidneys, and intestines

4. **On-scene care of a patient who has signs of shock from abdominal injury should include which of the following?**
   A. Comprehensive physical examination
   B. Initiation of IV fluid therapy
   C. Ongoing assessment
   D. Oxygen administration

5. **When the spleen ruptures, blood spills into the:**
   A. duodenum.
   B. peritoneum.
   C. stomach.
   D. pylorus.

6. **Some patients who have a splenic injury may report only left shoulder pain. This is called:**
   A. Cullen's sign.
   B. Grey Turner's sign.
   C. Peritoneal's sign.
   D. Kehr's sign.

7. **The abdominal cavity is lined with a membrane called the:**
   A. retroperitoneal space.
   B. pylorus.
   C. peritoneum.
   D. periumbilical.

8. **The spleen is a highly vascular organ that lies in the _____ quadrant.**
   A. right upper
   B. left lower
   C. left upper
   D. right lower

9. **Rupture of an organ can lead to haemorrhage and:**
   A. peritoneum.
   B. peritonitis.
   C. haemoperitoneum.
   D. internal bleeding.

10. **True or false? Patients without abdominal pain or abnormal vital signs are unlikely to have serious intra-abdominal injuries.**
    A. True
    B. False

Challenging Questions

You are dispatched to the local pub for an assault victim. On arrival you find a 38-year-old man on the ground, conscious, and alert and orientated to person, place, and time. He is in the right lateral recumbent position. You notice a large pool of blood under him. He has a weak radial pulse and his skin is cool, pale, and perspiring. His vital signs are: respirations, 40 breaths/min; pulse, 120 beats/min with sinus tachycardia on the monitor; systolic blood pressure, 80 mm Hg; and pulse oximetry, 92% on room air. He is complaining of pain to his stomach and is becoming very agitated. There is a 30-cm long knife lying next to him. You check his back for wounds and then quickly log roll him onto a longboard and provide c-spine precautions. On examination of the abdomen, you see a stab wound to the upper right quadrant. You immediately move the patient to your ambulance.

11. **What type of injury should you suspect?**

12. **What are the major complications of a lacerated liver?**

13. **What is your further treatment for this patient?**

■ Points to Ponder

You are called to the scene of a minor traffic collision in which a car has hit a telephone pole. When you arrive, you immediately notice that the driver is not inside the vehicle. The air bag has deployed, but the windscreen appears intact. The steering wheel appears slightly deformed. Bystanders say the vehicle was not travelling very fast when it hit the pole. They do not think the driver was wearing a seatbelt.

You approach the driver to ask him about the collision. He is sitting on the grass, with no apparent external injuries. Even though it is early afternoon, you smell what you think is alcohol as you speak with him. He tells you he doesn't know how the collision happened, but he insists he is fine and doesn't want to be examined or questioned. Though you can see no injuries, he is guarding his abdomen, and gri-

maces as though he's in pain as you're speaking. The more you try to encourage him to be examined by either you or a doctor, the more defensive and angry he gets. You tell him the risks of not being examined, and tell him he can sign a consent form to not be treated. He agrees to let you take his vital signs and then signs the consent form to refuse treatment. His blood pressure is 80/60 mm Hg; pulse, 130 beats/min; and respirations, 27 breaths/min.

When you find this, what do you do?

Issues: Thorough Scene Assessment, Thorough Assessment, Patient Refusal of Treatment.

25 Musculoskeletal Injuries

Objectives

Cognitive

- Describe the incidence, morbidity, and mortality of musculoskeletal injuries.
- Discuss the anatomy and physiology of the musculoskeletal system.
- Predict injuries based on the mechanism of injury, including:
  - Direct
  - Indirect
  - Pathologic
- Discuss the types of musculoskeletal injuries:
  - Fracture (open and closed)
  - Dislocation/fracture
  - Sprain
  - Strain
- Discuss the pathophysiology of musculoskeletal injuries.
- Discuss the assessment findings associated with musculoskeletal injuries.
- List the 6 Ps of musculoskeletal injury assessment.
- List the primary signs and symptoms of extremity trauma.
- List other signs and symptoms that can indicate less obvious extremity injury.
- Discuss the need for assessment of pulses, motor, and sensation before and after splinting.
- Identify the need for rapid intervention and transport when dealing with musculoskeletal injuries.
- Discuss the management of musculoskeletal injuries.
- Discuss the general guidelines for splinting.
- Explain the benefits of cold application for musculoskeletal injury.
- Explain the benefits of heat application for musculoskeletal injury.
- Describe age-associated changes in the bones.
- Discuss the pathophysiology of open and closed fractures.
- Discuss the relationship between volume of haemorrhage and open or closed fractures.
- Discuss the assessment findings associated with fractures.
- Discuss the management of fractures.
- Describe the special considerations involved in femur fracture management.
- Discuss the pathophysiology of dislocations.

- Discuss the assessment findings of dislocations.
- Discuss the out-of-hospital management of dislocation/fractures, including splinting and realignment.
- Explain the importance of manipulating a knee dislocation/fracture with an absent distal pulse.
- Describe the procedure for reduction of a shoulder, finger, or ankle dislocation/fracture.
- Discuss the pathophysiology of sprains.
- Discuss the assessment findings of sprains.
- Discuss the management of sprains.
- Discuss the pathophysiology of strains.
- Discuss the assessment findings of strains.
- Discuss the management of strains.
- Discuss the pathophysiology of a tendon injury.
- Discuss the assessment findings of tendon injury.
- Discuss the management of a tendon injury.
- Integrate the pathophysiological principles to the assessment of a patient with a musculoskeletal injury.
- Differentiate between musculoskeletal injuries based on the assessment findings and history.
- Formulate an initial diagnosis of a musculoskeletal injury based on the assessment findings.
- Develop a patient management plan for the musculoskeletal injury based on the initial diagnosis.

Affective

- Advocate the use of a thorough assessment to determine a working diagnosis and treatment plan for musculoskeletal injuries.
- Advocate for the use of pain management in the treatment of musculoskeletal injuries.

Psychomotor

- Demonstrate a clinical assessment to determine the proper treatment plan for a patient with a suspected musculoskeletal injury.
- Demonstrate the proper use of immobilisation, soft and traction splints for a patient with a suspected fracture.

Introduction

Musculoskeletal injuries are one of the most common reasons for patients to seek medical attention. Complaints related to the musculoskeletal system lead to about 1.7 million patients requiring visits to hospitals in the United Kingdom each year. Many more with multiple trauma will also have musculoskeletal injuries. The cost to the taxpayer for these admissions is significant—the ever-increasing pressures on NHS budgets and resulting losses from absences at work cost millions of pounds every year. An estimated 70% to 80% of all patients with multiple system trauma have one or more musculoskeletal injuries. Some areas of public policy, legislative changes, and public education have been effective in reducing the injury problem. For example, efforts related to mobile phone use by drivers, child safety seat use and availability, and falls in older people have had positive impacts.

Injuries related to the musculoskeletal system are usually easily identifiable because of the associated pain, swelling, and deformity. Although these injuries are rarely fatal, they often result in short- or long-term disability. By providing prompt temporary measures, such as splinting and analgesia, paramedics may help reduce the period during which patients are disabled. However, despite the sometimes dramatic appearance of these injuries, you should not focus on the musculoskeletal injury without first determining that no life-threatening injury exists. *Never forget the ABCs!*

Anatomy and Physiology of the Musculoskeletal System

The musculoskeletal system gives the body its shape and allows for its movement. It is essential that you understand its basic anatomy and physiology.

Functions of the Musculoskeletal System

The musculoskeletal system performs many important functions within the body. Bones help *support* the soft tissues of the body and form a framework that gives the human body its shape and allows it to maintain an erect posture. *Movement* is generated because muscles are attached to bones by <u>tendons</u>. (Reminder: Muscles-To-Bones [MTB] means Muscles–Tendons–Bones.) When a muscle contracts, the force generated by the muscle is transferred to a bone on the opposite side of the <u>joint</u> from the muscle, leading to motion. Bones also offer *protection* to the more fragile organs and structures beneath them—for example, the skull's protection of the brain, the rib cage's protection of the heart and lungs, and the spinal column's protection of the spinal cord.

Another important function of the musculoskeletal system is <u>haematopoiesis</u>—the process of generating blood cells. In adults, it most commonly occurs in the red bone marrow of the sternum, ribs, vertebral bodies, pelvis, and the proximal portions of the femur and humerus. Each day, the body produces new red blood cells, white blood cells, and platelets from the stem cells that are present in the bone marrow, thereby replacing those that have been lost or that are no longer functional.

The Body's Scaffolding: The Skeleton

The integrated structure formed by the 206 bones of the body is called the skeleton. It may be divided into two distinct portions: the <u>axial skeleton</u> and the <u>appendicular skeleton</u>. The axial skeleton is composed of the bones of the central part, or axis, of the body; its divisions include the vertebral column, skull, ribs, and sternum. The skull is composed of the cranium, basilar skull, face, and inner ear   **Figure 25-1 ▶** .

The spine is composed of 33 spinal vertebrae: 7 cervical, 12 thoracic, 5 lumbar, 5 sacral, and 4 coccygeal. Moving anteriorly, the thorax is formed by the sternum and 12 pairs of

You are the Paramedic Part 1

You have been sent to a private house for a man who has fallen off a ladder. On the way to the scene, ambulance control advises you that a neighbour had witnessed the incident, and estimated the fall to be between 5 and 6 metres in height.

On arrival, you find a 63-year-old man on the ground next to a ladder that is leaning against the house. He complains of pain in his left leg and left wrist, is slow to respond to your questions, but remembers what happened.

Initial Assessment	Recording Time: 0 Minutes
Appearance	Wincing and holding his left arm
Level of consciousness	A (Alert to person, place, and day)
Airway	Patent
Breathing	Rapid with adequate tidal volume
Circulation	Blood-soaked left sleeve, rapid radial pulse

1. What are your initial assessment and treatment priorities?
2. What other information should be obtained about the patient and the incident?

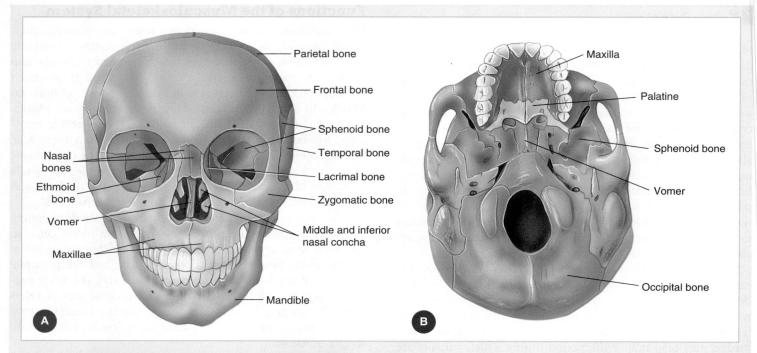

Figure 25-1 The skull and its components. **A.** Front view. **B.** Bottom view.

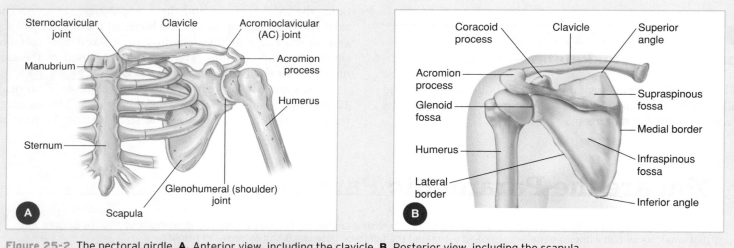

Figure 25-2 The pectoral girdle. **A.** Anterior view, including the clavicle. **B.** Posterior view, including the scapula.

ribs. The appendicular skeleton is divided into the pectoral girdle, the pelvic girdle, and the bones of the upper and lower extremities.

Shoulder and Upper Extremities

The pectoral girdle (Figure 25-2 ▲), also referred to as the shoulder girdle, consists of two scapulae and two clavicles. The scapula (shoulder blade) is a flat, triangular bone held to the rib cage posteriorly by powerful muscles that buffer it against injury. The clavicle (collarbone) is a slender, S-shaped bone

attached by ligaments at the medial end to the sternum and at the lateral end to the raised tip of the scapula, called the acromion. The clavicle acts as a strut to keep the shoulder propped up; however, because it is slender and very exposed, this bone is vulnerable to injury.

The upper extremity (Figure 25-3 ▶) joins the shoulder girdle at the glenohumeral joint. The proximal portion contains the humerus, a bone that articulates proximally with the scapula and distally with bones of the forearm—the radius and ulna—to form the hinged elbow joint.

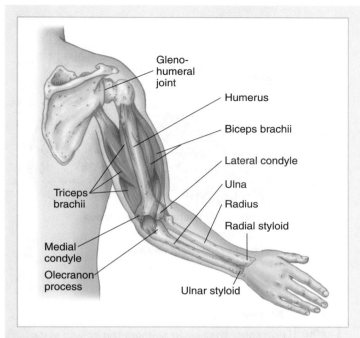

Figure 25-3 The anatomy of the arm.

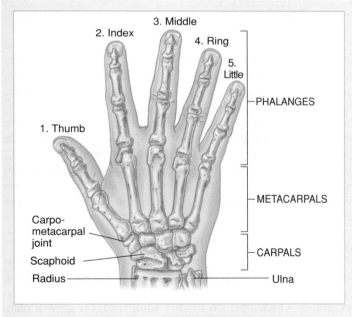

Figure 25-4 The anatomy of the wrist and hand.

The radius and ulna make up the forearm. The radius, the larger of the two forearm bones, lies on the *thumb* side of the forearm. Distally, the ulna is narrow and is on the little-finger side of the forearm. It serves as the pivot around which the radius turns at the wrist to rotate the palm upward (supination) or downward (pronation). Because the radius and the ulna are arranged in parallel, when one is broken, the other is often broken as well.

The hand Figure 25-4 ▲ contains three sets of bones: wrist bones (carpals), hand bones (metacarpals), and finger

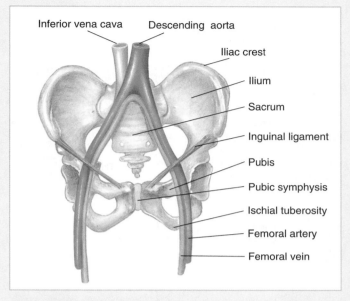

Figure 25-5 The pelvic girdle.

At the Scene

To remember the difference between supination and pronation, think of soup. The SUPinated hand can hold a cup of SOUP.

bones (phalanges). The carpals, especially the scaphoid, are vulnerable to fracture when a person falls on an outstretched hand. Phalanges are more apt to be injured by a crushing injury, such as being slammed in a car door.

Pelvis and Lower Extremities

The pelvic girdle Figure 25-5 ▲ is actually three separate bones—the ischium, ilium, and pubis—fused together to form the innominate bone. The two iliac bones are joined posteriorly by tough ligaments to the sacrum at the sacroiliac joints; the two pubic bones are connected anteriorly by equally tough ligaments to one another at the pubic symphysis. These joints allow very little motion, so the pelvic ring is strong and stable.

The lower extremity consists of the bones of the thigh, leg, and foot Figure 25-6 ▶ . The femur (thigh bone) is a long, powerful bone that articulates proximally in the ball-and-socket joint of the pelvis and distally in the hinge joint of the knee. The *head* of the femur is the ball-shaped part that fits into the acetabulum. It is connected to the *shaft,* or long tubular portion of the femur, by the femoral *neck.* The femoral neck is a common site for fractures, generally referred to as hip fractures, especially in the older population.

The lower leg consists of two bones, the tibia and the fibula. The tibia (shin bone) forms the inferior component of the knee joint. Anterior to this joint is the patella (kneecap), a bone that is important for knee extension. The tibia runs down the front of

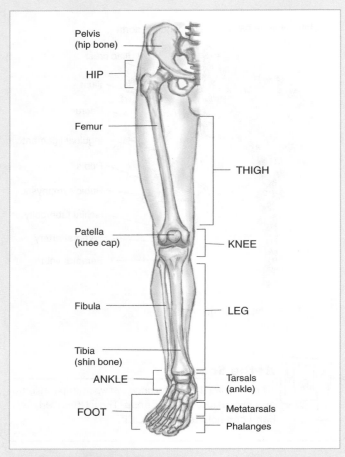

Figure 25-6 The bones of the leg.

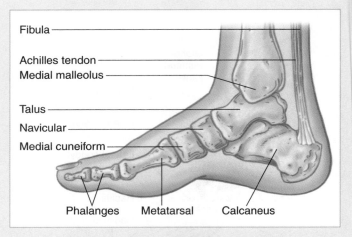

Figure 25-7 The bones of the foot and ankle.

At the Scene

Here's a tip to help remember which bones are carpal (hand bones) and which bones are tarsal (foot bones): "I steer my CAR (pal) with hands and walk through TAR (sal) with my feet".

the lower leg, where it is vulnerable to direct blows, and can be felt just beneath the skin. The much smaller fibula runs posteriorly and laterally to the tibia. The fibula is not a component of the knee joint, but it does make up the lateral knob of the ankle joint (lateral malleolus) at its distal articulation.

The foot consists of three classes of bones: *ankle bones* (tarsals), *foot bones* (metatarsals), and *toe bones* (phalanges) Figure 25-7 ▶ . The largest of the tarsal bones is the heel bone, or calcaneus, which is subject to injury when a person jumps from a height and lands on the feet.

Characteristics and Composition of Bone
Bone Shapes
Bones may be classified based on their shape. Long bones are longer than they are wide; examples include the femur,

At the Scene

Fractures that occur through the growth plate in a bone of a child may affect the future growth of that bone.

humerus, tibia, fibula, radius, and ulna. Short bones are nearly as wide as they are long; they include the phalanges, metacarpals, and metatarsals. Flat bones are thin, broad bones; they include the sternum, ribs, scapulae, and skull. Irregular bones do not fit into one of the other categories but rather have a shape that is designed to perform a specific function, such as the bones of the vertebral column and the mandible. Round bones are generally found in proximity to a joint and help with movement. They are often referred to as sesamoid bones because of their location within a tendon. The patella is the largest of these bones.

Typical Long Bone Architecture
Long bones have several distinct regions and anatomical features Figure 25-8 ▶ . These bones can grow to such long lengths because of the presence of the growth plate, or physis, in children. Once a person reaches adulthood, the growth plate closes and the mature adult bone is complete. The long bone is divided into three regions: the diaphysis, the epiphysis, and the metaphysis.

The articular surfaces of a long bone come in contact with other bones to form articulations (joints). These regions of the bone are covered by articular cartilage, a substance that acts as a cushion to protect the bone from damage and wear.

The portion of bone that is not covered by articular cartilage is, instead, covered by the periosteum. This dense, fibrous membrane contains capillaries and cells that are important for bone repair and maintenance. In the inner portion of the long bone, blood comes from the nutrient artery of the bone. Once

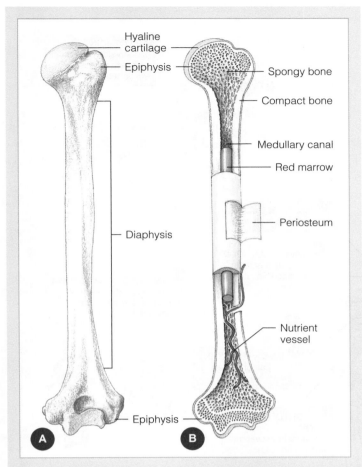

Figure 25-8 Anatomy of the long bone. **A.** The humerus. Notice the long shaft and dilated ends. **B.** Longitudinal section of the humerus showing compact bone, spongy bone, and marrow.

Labels on figure: Hyaline cartilage, Epiphysis, Spongy bone, Compact bone, Medullary canal, Red marrow, Periosteum, Diaphysis, Nutrient vessel, Epiphysis

Special Considerations

Splinting an injured extremity, eg, a fractured forearm, is best done when the injured limb is in a straightened position. However, in some older patients, straightening the injured limb may not be possible and may, in fact, cause further injury. This is particularly true in patients who suffer from arthritis—a degenerative condition that causes a reduction in motion of the joints. In these cases, should the patient complain of increasing pain while an attempt to straighten is being made, you should stop and splint the limb in the position in which it is resting. Use of vacuum splints is recommended in these circumstances.

increasing the risk of disc herniation. In some joints, the cartilage may become degraded, leading to arthritis and pain; in others, the cartilage becomes calcified, leading to restricted motion.

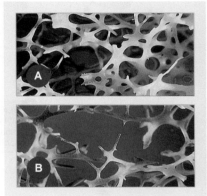

Figure 25-9 The structural difference between normal and osteoporotic bone. **A.** Normal bone in a 29-year-old woman. **B.** Osteoporotic bone in a 92-year-old-woman.

Joints

When two bones come together, they articulate with one another to form a joint. Some joints are fused and allow for no motion, such as the joints of the skull. Other joints allow for motion by permitting movement between the two bones, typically within a certain plane of motion that is defined by the structure of the bones that form it. The various motions that a joint may allow include flexion, extension, abduction, adduction, rotation, circumduction, pronation, and supination Figure 25-10 ▶.

Types of Joints

The three general types of joints are fibrous, cartilaginous, and synovial Figure 25-11 ▶. Fibrous joints, also referred to as synarthroses or fused joints, contain dense fibrous tissue that does not allow for movement. Examples include the bones of the skull and the distal tibiofibular joint.

Cartilaginous joints, also called amphiarthroses, allow for very minimal movement between the bones. The pubic symphysis and the joints connecting the ribs to the sternum are examples of this type of joint.

Synovial joints, or diarthroses, are the most mobile joints of the body. They are surrounded by an extension of the periosteum called the joint capsule, with the bones that form them being held in place by very strong ligaments. Within the joint are the articular cartilage and the synovial membrane, which secretes synovial fluid into the joint cavity to lubricate it.

it penetrates the bone's outer cortex, the artery enters the medullary canal, the hollow inner portion of the shaft that is lined by the endosteum (similar to the periosteum, but on the inside) and contains yellow (fatty) marrow in adults.

Age-Associated Changes in Bone

Bone ages just like any other tissue of the body, decreasing in density after the age of 35 years, leading to a loss of height, and producing changes in facial structure. In women, this decrease in density is further accelerated once menopause is reached because of the loss of oestrogen, a hormone that helps promote bone formation. A significant decrease in bone density, called osteoporosis Figure 25-9 ▶, is associated with a higher risk of fracture. People with osteoporosis are at risk for incurring a fracture, especially in the hip, spine, and wrist.

Other changes associated with ageing of bone include ageing of muscles, cartilage, and other connective tissues that may also lead to degradation of joints and disc herniation. For example, the water content of the intervertebral discs decreases,

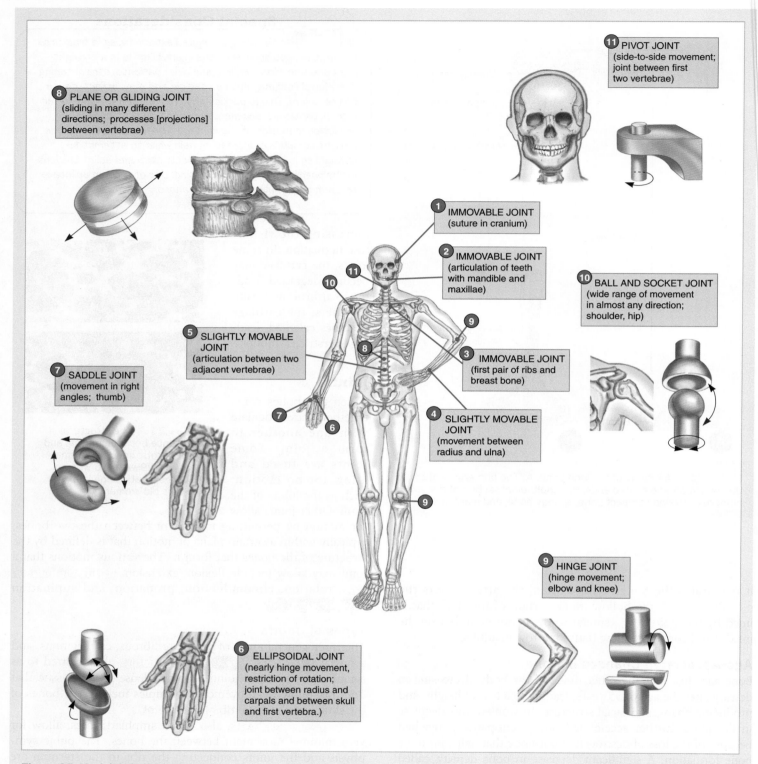

Figure 25-10 Joints in the body.

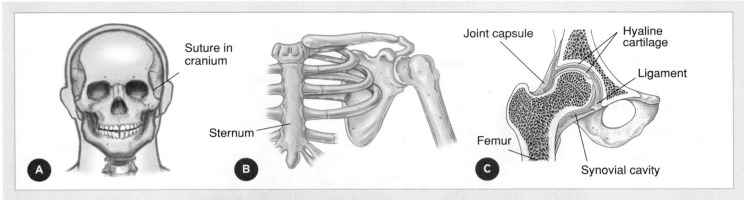

Figure 25-11 Types of joints. **A.** Fibrous. **B.** Cartilaginous. **C.** Synovial.

Bursa

A bursa is a padlike sac or cavity located within the connective tissue, usually in proximity to a joint. It may be lined with a synovial membrane and typically contains fluid that helps reduce the amount of friction between a tendon and a bone or between a tendon and a ligament. Examples include the olecranon bursa of the elbow and the prepatellar bursa of the knee. Bursitis is inflammation of a bursa.

Skeletal Connecting and Supporting Structures

Tendons connect muscle to bone. These flat or cordlike bands of connective tissue are white and have a glistening appearance.

Ligaments connect bone to bone and help maintain the stability of joints and determine the degree of joint motion. These inelastic bands of connective tissue have a structure similar to that of tendons.

Cartilage consists of fibres of collagen embedded in a gelatinous substance. This flexible connective tissue forms the smooth surface over bone ends where they articulate, provides cushioning between vertebrae, gives structure to the nose and external ear, forms the framework of the larynx and trachea, and serves as the model for the formation of the skeleton in children. Cartilage has a very limited neurovascular supply—it receives nutrients through diffusion from the outer covering of the cartilage or from the synovial fluid—so it does not heal well if it is injured.

The Moving Forces: Muscles

Muscles are composed of specialised cells that contract (shorten) when stimulated to exert a force on a part of the body. Three types of muscle are found in the body: smooth muscle, cardiac muscle, and skeletal muscle (**Figure 25-12 ▸**).

Skeletal Muscle

Skeletal muscle (**Figure 25-13 ▸**) is also called voluntary muscle, because its contractions are largely under voluntary control, or striated muscle, because striations can be seen in it during microscopic examination. Skeletal muscle includes all

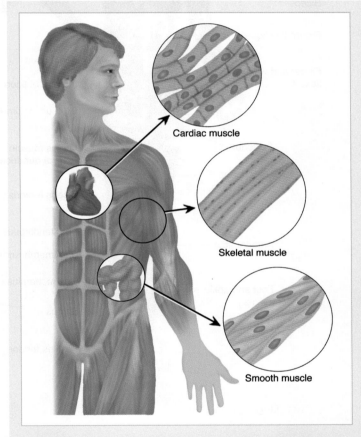

Figure 25-12 The three types of muscle are skeletal, smooth, and cardiac.

of the muscles attached to the skeleton and forms the bulk of the tissue of the arms and legs. It is also found along the spine and buttocks. By maintaining a state of partial contraction, this type of muscle allows the body to maintain its posture and to sit or stand. It varies greatly in size and shape, from thin strands to the large muscles of the thigh and back. It also constitutes the muscles of the tongue, soft palate, scalp, pharynx, upper oesophagus, and eye. About 40% to 50% of normal

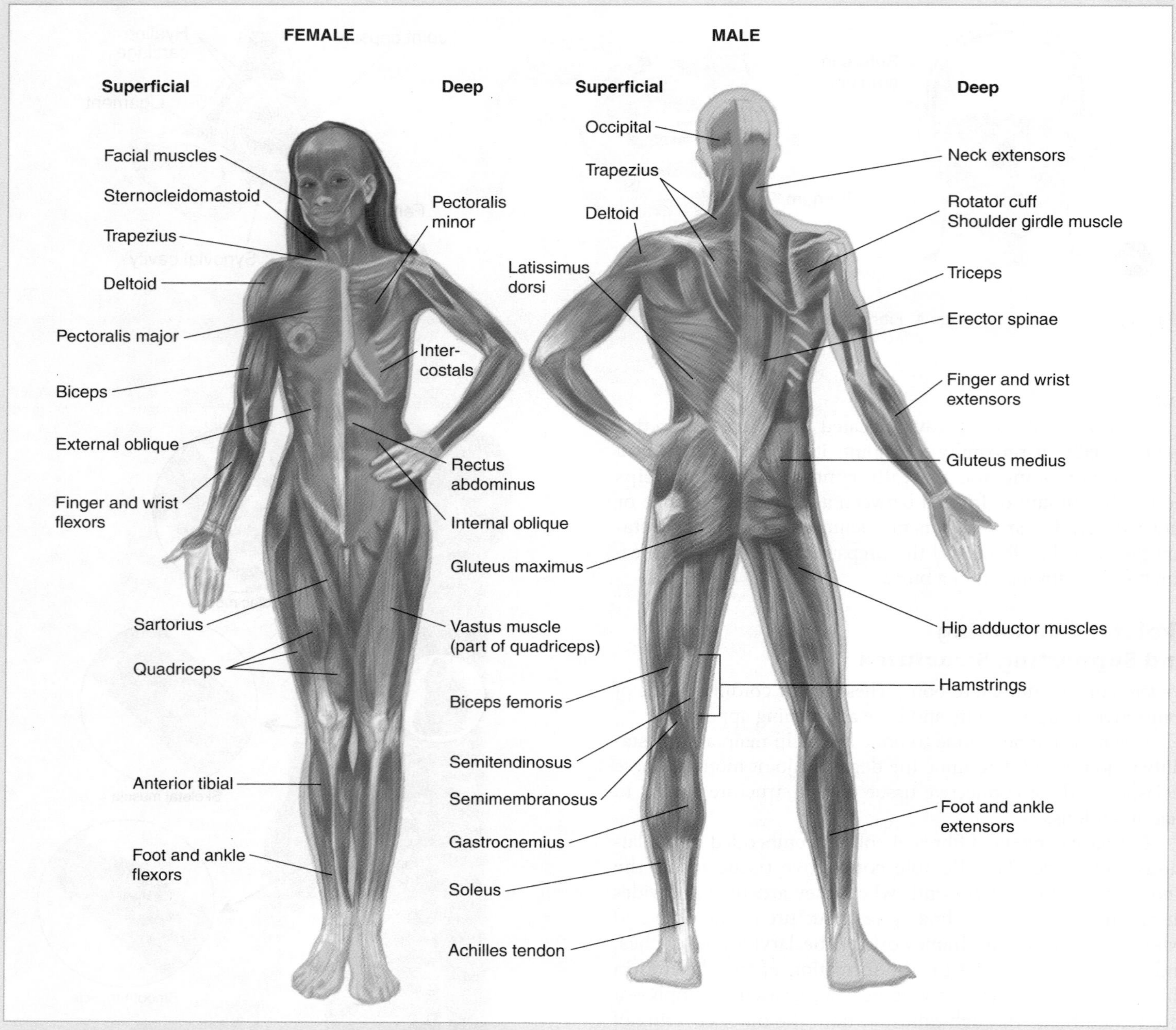

Figure 25-13 Muscles in humans.

body weight is skeletal muscle, as it has a high water content. In addition, because of its high metabolic rate and demand for energy and oxygen, skeletal muscle has a very rich blood supply, which causes it to bleed significantly when injured.

Skeletal muscles are profoundly affected by the amount of training and work to which they are subjected. Unused muscles tend to atrophy (shrink or waste away), whereas physical training promotes hypertrophy (increase in size).

Skeletal muscles are attached to bones by tendons. Tendons cross joints to create a pulling force between two bones

when a muscle contracts. The biceps muscle, for example, has its origin on the scapula; the biceps tendon passes over the head of the humerus, where it fuses with the body of the biceps muscle; at the distal end of the biceps, a tendon passes over the anterior surface of the elbow and inserts on the radius. Thus, when the biceps muscle contracts, the force causes the elbow to bend (flex).

Muscle contraction requires energy. This energy is derived from the metabolism of glucose and results in the production of lactic acid (lactate). Lactic acid, in turn, must be converted

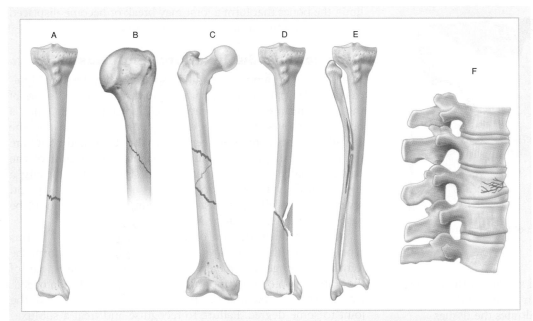

Figure 25-17 Types of fractures. **A.** Transverse fracture of the tibia. **B.** Oblique fracture of the humerus. **C.** Spiral fracture of the femur. **D.** Comminuted fracture of the tibia. **E.** Greenstick fracture of the fibula. **F.** Compression fracture of a vertebral body.

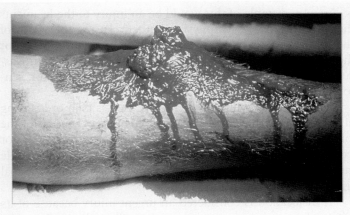

Figure 25-18 An open fracture.

fracture, the increased interstitial pressure within the haematoma compresses the blood vessels, limiting the size of the haematoma. In a closed femur fracture, the blood loss may exceed 1 litre before enough pressure develops to tamponade the bleeding. In contrast, open fractures allow much of the blood to escape, so tamponade does not occur as readily or at all.

Signs and Symptoms of a Fracture

The primary symptom of a fracture is *pain* that is usually well localised to the fracture site. In addition, the patient may report hearing a snap or feeling a break. Signs of fracture detected on physical examination include the following:

- *Deformity* is one of the most reliable signs of a fracture. The limb may be found in an unnatural position or show motion at a place where there is no joint. Compare the deformed limb with the extremity on the other side Figure 25-19 ▶.
- *Shortening* occurs in fractures when the broken ends of a bone override one another. It is characteristic of femur fractures, for example, because the broken femur can no longer serve as a strut to oppose spasm in the powerful thigh muscles.

 At the Scene

The ends of a fractured bone are sharp. Use caution whenever bone ends are exposed to prevent a puncture injury to yourself, your crew, or the splint.

Table 25-3	Fracture Classification Based on Displacement	
Type of Fracture	**Description**	**Common Causes**
Nondisplaced fracture	Bone remains aligned in its normal position, despite the fracture.	Low-energy injury
Displaced fracture	Ends of the fracture move from their normal positions.	High-energy injury
■ Overriding	Muscles pull the distal fracture fragment alongside the proximal one, leading them to overlap; the limb becomes shortened.	Only occurs when a fracture is fully displaced and there is no bone contact
■ Distraction injury	A powerful tensile force is rapidly applied to a bone, causing it to fracture—the bone ends are pulled apart.	Industrial equipment, machinery
■ Impacted fracture (impaction injury)	A massive compressive force is applied to a bone, causing it to become wedged into another bone.	More likely to happen in cancellous bone
■ Avulsion fracture	A powerful muscle contraction causes the insertion site of the muscle to be fractured off of the bone.	Sudden "jerking" of a body part
■ Depression fracture	Blunt trauma to a flat bone (such as the skull) causes the bone to be pushed inward.	Blunt injury

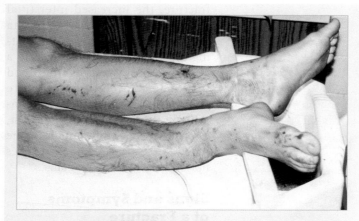

Figure 25-19 Obvious deformity is a sign of bone fracture.

- Visual inspection will usually reveal *swelling* at the fracture site due to bleeding from the broken bone and the accumulation of fluid. As blood infiltrates the tissues around the broken bone ends, *bruising* will become apparent.
- *Guarding* and *loss of use* characterise most fractures. The patient will try to keep a fractured bone still and will avoid putting any stress on it. Sometimes the measures a patient takes to protect a fractured bone from movement are so characteristic that one can almost diagnose the fracture without examining the extremity. A patient who walks to the ambulance holding the dorsum of one wrist in the other hand, for example, almost certainly has a Colles fracture. A patient standing with the head cocked toward a "knocked-down shoulder" probably has a fracture of the clavicle on the side to which the head is leaning.
- A fractured bone is almost invariably *tender to palpation* over the fracture site.
- Palpation may reveal crepitus, a grating sensation, over the broken bone ends. Crepitus may be noted as an incidental finding during splinting attempts. Do *not* try to elicit this sign, because your efforts may result in further injury to the bone and surrounding soft tissues, not to mention severe pain.

Notes from Nancy

The best way to detect deformity or any other abnormality in an extremity is to compare it to the extremity on the other side.

- In an open fracture, *exposed bone ends* may be visible in the wound.

Ligament Injuries and Dislocations

The shapes of the bones that form a joint and the tightness of the ligaments that hold them in place are key factors in determining a joint's range of motion. When forced beyond their normal limit, the bones that form a joint may break or become displaced and the supporting ligaments and joint capsule may tear.

Dislocations, Subluxations, and Diastasis

In a dislocation, a bone is totally displaced from the joint. Typically, at least part of the supporting joint capsule and some of the joint's ligaments are disrupted. Dislocations occur when a body part moves beyond its normal range of motion and the articular surfaces are no longer intact. The dislocated bones are then locked in place by muscle spasms. Evaluation of the patient usually reveals an obvious and significant deformity, a significant decrease in the joint's range of motion (ROM), and severe pain. In all cases of a dislocation, a fracture should be suspected until ruled out by X-rays.

The partial dislocation of a joint is a subluxation. In this type of injury, the articular surfaces of the bones that form the joint are no longer completely in contact. In some cases, part of the joint capsule and supporting ligaments may be damaged. Despite the subluxation, the patient may be able to move the joint to some degree. Failure to recognise and treat a subluxation may lead to persistent joint instability and pain.

When the ligaments that hold two bones in a fixed position with respect to one another are disrupted and the space between them increases, a situation known as a diastasis occurs. An example of this would be an injury to the ligaments that hold the pubic symphysis together, causing the width of the joint to increase (diastasis of the pubic symphysis). For these reasons, you should always assess the patient's neurovascular status distal to the site of dislocation (check motor, sensory and circulatory functions [MSC]).

The principal symptom of a dislocation is pain or a feeling of pressure over the involved joint, plus loss of motion of the joint. A patient with a posterior dislocation of the shoulder, for example, is unable to raise the arm but holds it against the side instead. Sometimes the joint will seem "frozen". The principal sign of dislocation is deformity.

A dislocation is considered an urgent injury because of its potential to cause neurovascular compromise distal to the site of injury. If the dislocated bone presses on a nerve, there may be numbness or weakness distally; if an artery is compressed, there may be absent distal pulses (such as in a knee dislocation). For these reasons, you should always assess the patient's neurovascular status distal to the site of dislocation (check pulse and motor and sensory functions [PMS]).

Sprains

Sprains are injuries in which ligaments are stretched or torn. They usually result from a sudden twisting of a joint beyond its normal range of motion that also causes a temporary subluxation. The majority of sprains involve the ankle or the knee because most occur after a person misjudges a step or landing. Evasive moves, like those done during a sporting event, commonly cause sprains in athletes. Sprains are typically characterised by pain, swelling, and discolouration over the injured joint and unwillingness to use the limb. In contrast with fractures and dislocations, sprains usually do not involve deformity and joint mobility is

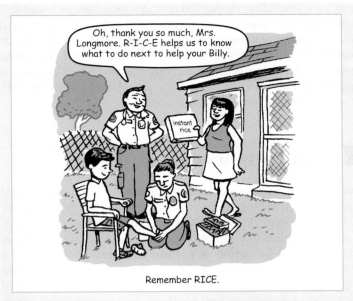

Remember RICE.

Figure 25-20

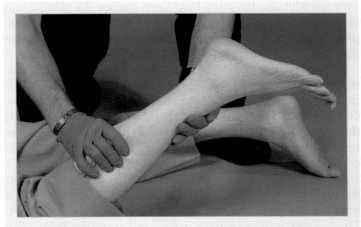

Figure 25-21 The Thompson test or Simmons test.

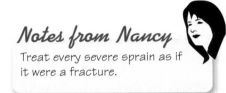

Notes from Nancy

Treat every severe sprain as if it were a fracture.

usually limited by pain, not by joint incongruity.

Because it may be difficult to differentiate among the various types of injuries in the prehospital environment, it is best to err on the side of caution and treat every severe sprain as if it were a fracture. General treatment of sprains is similar to that of fractures and includes the following (numbers 1 through 4 form the mnemonic RICE) **Figure 25-20 ▲** :

1. **Rest.** Immobilise or splint injured area
2. **Ice** or cold pack over the injury
3. **Compression** with an elastic bandage (usually applied at hospital once an X-ray has ruled out a fracture)
4. **Elevation**
5. Reduced or protected weight bearing
6. Pain management as soon as practical

Muscle and Tendon Injuries

Strains

A strain (pulled muscle) is an injury to a muscle and/or tendon that results from a violent muscle contraction or from excessive stretching. Often no deformity is present and only minor swelling is noted at the site of injury. Some patients may complain of increased pain with passive movement of the injured extremity.

Achilles Tendon Rupture

A rupture of the Achilles tendon is common in athletes older than 30 years who are involved in stop and start sports such as football,

rugby, or basketball, etc. The most immediate indications are pain from the heel to the calf and a sudden inability for plantar flexion of the foot. As time passes, the calf muscles begin to contract proximally and a deformity within the calf may develop. The Thompson test or Simmons test can be performed in the prehospital environment to identify an Achilles tendon rupture. To perform this test, have the patient assume a prone position and then squeeze the calf muscles of the injured leg **Figure 25-21 ▲** . If the foot plantar flexes while squeezing, the tendon is probably intact. If there is no movement of the foot, the Achilles tendon has likely been torn. Management of an Achilles tendon injury includes RICE and pain control. These injuries are treated with surgery or multiple casts and can require up to 6 months for recovery.

Inflammatory Processes

When a muscle is subjected to frequent and repetitive use, its tendon or nearby bursa are at risk for becoming inflamed. When inflammation of the tendon causes pain, the patient is said to have tendinitis. There will typically be point tenderness on the inflamed tendon with pain often increasing if the person performs the movement that led to the inflammation. When a bursa becomes painful and inflamed, it is called bursitis. Patients with bursitis often complain of pain in the region of the inflamed bursa, especially with motions that cause the space where the bursa sits to become smaller. Examination of the site may reveal tenderness, swelling, erythema, and warmth. Tendinitis and bursitis are treated with RICE, analgesia, and, in many cases, steroid injections.

Arthritis

Arthritis means inflammation of a joint. The three most common types of arthritis are osteoarthritis, rheumatoid arthritis, and gout.

Osteoarthritis (OA) is a disease of the joints that occurs as they age and begin to wear. It is characterised by pain and stiffness, which typically get worse with use, and "cracking" or "crunching" of the affected joints. The spine, hands, knees, and hips are the most commonly affected sites. In general, the risk of developing OA increases with age, but other factors also increase the risk, such as obesity and prior joint injury. Treatment of OA involves low-impact physical therapy, pain control, anti-inflammatory medications, joint injections, and, in severe cases, joint replacement surgery.

Rheumatoid arthritis (RA) is a systemic inflammatory disease that affects joints and other body systems. In RA, significant bone erosion at the affected joints makes them more susceptible to fractures and dislocations. Of particular concern is the cervical spine, which is at high risk of subluxating following trauma or during intubation. Give extra attention to the cervical spine of a patient with RA to prevent further injury.

Gout is a condition in which the body has difficulty eliminating uric acid. When the concentration of uric acid in the blood becomes too great, the uric acid may crystallise within a joint. The patient will then have a hot, red, swollen joint with decreased range of motion. Prehospital treatment involves immobilisation, pain relief, and transport to an A&E department where the fluid in the joint can be aspirated to search for the characteristic crystals of gout.

Injuries That May Signify Fractures

Amputations

An amputation is the separation of a limb or other body part from the remainder of the body Figure 25-22 ▾ . The amputation may be incomplete, leaving only a small segment of tissue connecting the part, or it may be complete, causing the part to be fully separated. Haemorrhage from complete or incomplete amputations can be severe and life threatening. Fractures may also be present with amputations. Amputations are discussed in more detail in Chapter 19.

Lacerations

A laceration is a smooth or jagged cut caused by a sharp object or a blunt force that tears the tissue. The depth of the injury

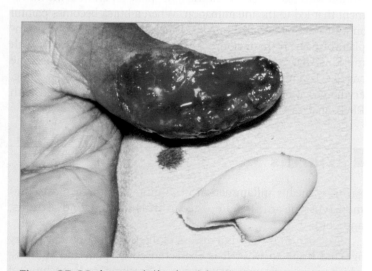

Figure 25-22 An amputation involving the thumb.

can vary, extending through skin and subcutaneous tissue and even into the underlying muscles and adjacent nerves and blood vessels. Lacerations involved in damaged arteries or veins may result in severe bleeding. The presence of lacerations may also be a sign of an underlying fracture. Deep lacerations may injure the muscle nerves, or vasculature, so distal PMS functions should always be evaluated.

Vascular Injuries

When blood vessels are damaged following a musculoskeletal injury, devascularisation of the body part that is supplied by the vessel may occur. The types of injuries that a vessel may sustain include a contusion of the vessel wall, laceration, kinking or bending, and formation of pseudoaneurysms. In addition, a blood vessel may thrombose (become occluded by a clot) when the injury causes blood flow to become very slow. Regardless of the type of vascular injury involved, it is important to assess and reassess pulses, control bleeding, and maintain adequate intravascular volume by using intravenous (IV) fluid.

General Principles of Assessment and Management

When assessing an injured patient, *do not be distracted by visually impressive injuries!* It is essential to complete the initial assessment of the patient before focusing on the extremities. In cases of musculoskeletal injuries, patients may be classified based on the presence or absence of associated injuries:

- Life- or limb-threatening injury or condition, including life- or limb-threatening musculoskeletal trauma
- Life-threatening injuries and only simple musculoskeletal trauma
- Life- or limb-threatening musculoskeletal trauma and no other life-threatening injuries
- Isolated, non–life- or non–limb-threatening injuries

Notes from Nancy

Musculoskeletal injuries are rarely, if ever, an immediate threat to life. A fracture can wait. The airway cannot.

Volume Deficit Due to Musculoskeletal Injuries

Fractures may lead to significant blood loss from damage to vessels within the bone and musculature around the bone and, in some cases, from damage to large blood vessels in the region of the fracture. When caring for patients with fractures, undertake interventions such as applying direct pressure, splinting,

General Interventions

The overall goal in the treatment of a musculoskeletal injury is to identify the type and extent of the injury and to create a biological environment that maximises the normal healing process of the injured structure. This process begins at the scene with a thorough assessment of the patient and proper immobilisation of injuries to prevent further harm.

Pain Control

A patient who has sustained a musculoskeletal injury may experience pain for a number of reasons. Pain may be caused by a fracture or continued movement of an unstable fracture, muscle spasm, soft-tissue injury, nerve injury, or muscle ischaemia. Orthopaedic injuries are often extremely painful, so the goal of prehospital pain control should be to diminish the patient's pain to a tolerable level.

A number of interventions may be performed in the prehospital environment to control pain from a musculoskeletal injury. The first step is to assess the level of pain. Establishing a baseline level of pain, and reassessing it after each intervention, allows you to determine the effectiveness of the treatment being provided. Simple methods for controlling pain include splinting, resting and elevating the injured part, and applying ice or heat packs.

When simple procedures do not control a patient's pain effectively, consider the administration of an analgesic. Analgesics used in the prehospital environment include: Entonox (a 50-50 mix of nitrous oxide and oxygen) and morphine. These agents should be reserved for patients in haemodynamically stable condition who have an isolated musculoskeletal injury. It is important to obtain vital signs before and after administering any medication for pain and to monitor the patient's respiratory status for signs of respiratory depression. After pain medication is administered, reassess the patient's pain to ensure that pain relief is adequate.

Administering pain medication before splinting may allow the extremity to be immobilised more effectively. Remember, *it hurts* to have an injured extremity held in the proper position for splinting. Analgesia may make it possible for the patient to tolerate that position longer and allow the splint to be applied properly.

Cold and Heat Application

Cold packs are useful for treating patients during the initial 48 hours following an injury and are very effective at decreasing pain and swelling. Cooling the injured area causes vasoconstriction of the blood vessels in the region and decreases the release of inflammatory mediators. As a result, swelling and inflammation are reduced when ice packs are used during the acute stage of an injury.

Conversely, heat therapy should not be used during the initial 48 to 72 hours following an injury because it may actually increase pain and swelling during this period. Once the

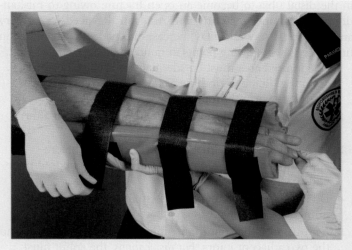

Figure 25-23 Splinting reduces pain and helps prevent additional damage to the extremity.

acute phase of the injury ends and the damaged blood vessels become clotted, heat is useful for increasing blood flow to the region to decrease stiffness and to promote healing. As a consequence, heat packs may be beneficial for patients who have had an injury for several days before calling for help.

Splinting

Splinting is intended to provide support to and prevent motion of the broken bone ends (Figure 25-23 ▲). Correctly splinting an injured extremity not only decreases the pain a patient experiences, but also reduces the risk of further damage to muscles, nerves, blood vessels, and skin. In addition, splinting helps to control bleeding by allowing clots to form where vessels were damaged.

When a patient with multiple orthopaedic injuries must be transported immediately, you will not have time to splint each fracture one by one. The best way to stabilise multiple fractures when the patient's overall condition is critical is to splint the axial skeleton by using a longboard and straps or an alternative device, such as a vacuum mattress. This will serve two purposes: (1) It will protect against a spinal injury. (2) It will reduce the movement of injured extremities by securing them to the board.

> *Notes from Nancy*
>
> When a patient with multiple fractures requires immediate transport, immobilise the whole patient on a longboard or vacuum mattress.

Principles of Splinting

Splinting is one of the most crucial skills to learn when caring for patients with musculoskeletal injuries. Failure to properly splint an injured extremity leads to unnecessary discomfort and the possibility of further injury or harm. Allowing a closed fracture in the distal tibia to become an open fracture owing to mishandling or improper splinting will result in the need for surgery and a hospital stay and may increase the patient's rehabilitation time. Keep the following points in mind when applying a splint:

1. The injured area must be adequately visualised before splinting. Remove clothing as necessary so that you can inspect the area thoroughly.

2. Assess and *record* distal PMS functions before and after splinting.

3. Cover all wounds with a dry, sterile dressing before applying the splint. Do not attempt to push exposed bone ends back under the skin.

4. Do not move the patient before splinting unless an immediate hazard exists.

5. *For fractures,* the splint must immobilise the bone ends and the two adjacent joints. *For dislocations,* the splint must extend along the entire length of the bone above and the entire length of the bone below the dislocated joint.

6. Pad the splint well to prevent local pressure and to provide optimal motion restriction.

7. Support the injured site manually with one hand above and one hand below the injury, and minimise movement until the splint is applied and secured.

8. If a long bone fracture is severely angulated, gently apply longitudinal traction (tension) to attempt to realign the bone and improve circulation. Use a smooth, firm grip to apply manual traction, and take care to avoid any sudden, jerky movements of the limb. *Do not attempt to straighten fractures involving joints without first obtaining medical direction.* In fact, there is no need to straighten or manipulate the joint unless it has no distal pulse.

9. Splint the knee straight if not directly injured and angulated; splint the elbow at a right angle. (The patient may not be able to tolerate this procedure, and rapid transport should be initiated.)

10. If the patient complains of severe pain or offers resistance to movement, discontinue applying traction, splint in the position of deformity, and carefully monitor the distal neurovascular status (PMS).

11. Splint firmly, but not so tightly as to occlude the distal circulation.

12. If possible, do not cover fingers and toes with the splint to allow for monitoring of skin CTC (colour, temperature, and condition).

13. If possible, apply cold packs and elevate the splinted limb to minimise swelling.

Notes from Nancy

Always check the pulses, strength, and sensation distal to a musculoskeletal injury.

14. When the patient has a life-threatening injury, individual splint application for possible fractures must not delay transport and might not be accomplished.

Documentation and Communication

Document the neurovascular examination and distal PMS functions before and after splinting.

Types of Splints

Any device used to immobilise a fracture or dislocation is considered a splint. Commercially available splints include board splints, inflatable or vacuum splints, and traction splints. Lack of a commercially made splint should never prevent proper immobilisation of an injured patient; multiple casualties may tax the resources of even the best-equipped ambulance, requiring improvisation.

Rigid Splints

A rigid splint is any inflexible device that may be attached to a limb to maintain stability—a padded board, a piece of heavy cardboard, or an aluminum "ladder" or SAM splint moulded to fit the extremity. More elaborate rigid splints are designed to quickly fit around two or three sides of an extremity and be secured with Velcro straps or triangular bandages. Some rigid splints are made of a radiolucent material that allows X-rays to be obtained without removal of the splint. Whatever its construction, the splint must be generously padded to ensure even pressure along the extremity and long enough to be secured well above and below the fracture site (beyond the proximal and distal joints).

When applying a rigid splint, grasp the extremity above and below the fracture site, and apply gentle traction. Another provider should then place the splint alongside the limb. While one provider maintains traction, the other wraps the limb and splint in self-adhering bandages that are tight enough to hold the splint firmly to the extremity but not so tight as to occlude circulation Figure 25-24 ▾ . (If the splint has its own straps

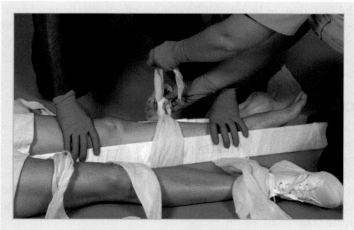

Figure 25-24 In applying a rigid splint, wrap the limb and splint so that the splint is firmly in place but does not cut off circulation.

that are used to secure it to the extremity, this step is not required.) Leave the fingers or toes out of the bandage so that distal circulation can be monitored.

Sling and Support Bandage

An arm sling may be fashioned from a triangular bandage and is useful to immobilise injuries that involve the shoulder or as an adjunct to a rigid splint of the upper extremity. The sling holds the injured part against the chest wall and takes some of the weight off the injured area.

To apply a sling, place the splinted extremity in a comfortable position across the chest and lay the long edge of a triangular bandage along the patient's side opposite the injury. Bring the bottom edge of the bandage up and over the forearm, and tie it *at the side* of the neck to the other end. Tie or pin the pointed end of the sling, at the elbow, to form a cradle. Secure the sling so that the hand is carried higher than the elbow and the fingers are visible for checking peripheral circulation Figure 25-25 ▾ .

An arm that is splinted with a sling can be further immobilised by adding a support bandage. Create a support bandage by using one or more triangular bandages to secure the arm firmly to the chest wall. This technique is particularly useful for injuries to the clavicle and for anterior dislocations of the shoulder. Do not use a sling if the patient has a neck injury.

Pneumatic Splints

Pneumatic splints (also known as air splints or inflatable splints) are useful for immobilising fractures involving the lower leg or forearm. They are not effective for angulated fractures or for fractures that involve a joint because they will forcefully attempt to straighten the fracture or joint. Likewise, air splints should not be used on open fractures in which the bone ends are exposed.

Air splints offer two distinct advantages: They can help slow bleeding and minimise swelling by applying pressure over fracture sites to decrease small-vessel bleeding.

The method of application for an air splint depends on whether it is equipped with a zip. If it is not, gather the splint on your own arm so that its proximal edge is just above your wrist. Grasp the patient's hand or foot while an assistant maintains proximal countertraction, then slide the air splint over your hand and onto the patient's extremity. Position the air splint so that it is free of wrinkles. Then, while you continue to maintain traction, instruct your assistant to inflate the splint with a commercially available device that is compatible with the splint system—do *not* use a compressed air tank to inflate an air splint. If the air splint has a zip, apply it to the injured area while an assistant maintains traction proximally and distally; then zip it up and inflate Figure 25-26 ▸ . In either case, inflate the splint just to the point at which finger pressure will make a slight dent in the splint's surface.

You must watch air splints carefully to ensure that they do not lose pressure or become overinflated. Overinflation is particularly likely when the splint is applied in a cold area and the patient is subsequently moved to a warmer area because the air inside the splint will expand as it gets warmer. Air splints will also expand when going to a higher altitude if the patient compartment is unpressurised, a factor that must be considered when patients are transported by air ambulance.

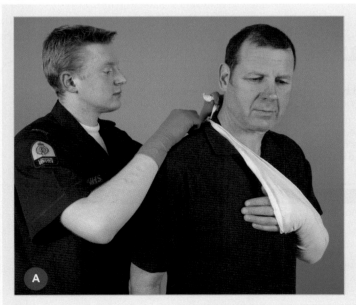
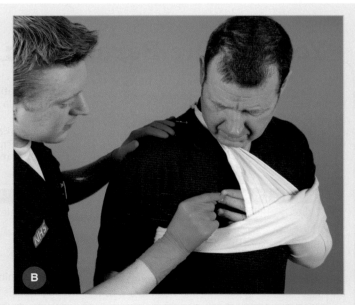

Figure 25-25 **A.** Apply the sling so that the knot is tied at one side of the neck. **B.** Secure the sling. Leave the fingers exposed to allow for circulation checks.

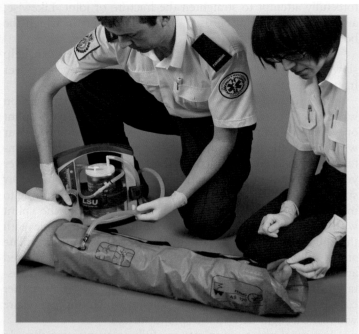

Figure 25-26 Positioning a vacuum splint on a lower limb.

Vacuum Splints

A vacuum splint consists of a sealed mattress that is filled with air and thousands of small plastic beads. The mattress is laid out on the stretcher, and the patient is placed on top of it and allowed to settle into a comfortable position. A suction pump attached to the mattress is then used to evacuate the air from inside the mattress. The resulting vacuum inside the mattress compresses the beads in such a way that the whole splint becomes rigid, much like a plaster cast that has been moulded to conform to the contours of the patient's entire posterior surface.

The vacuum mattress is an excellent splint, but there are a few factors that may limit its broad appeal. The splint is quite bulky, so it not only takes up a lot of storage room in the vehicle, but also can be difficult to work with in cramped quarters. Furthermore, like all vacuum splints, it requires a mechanical suction pump, yet another piece of equipment to grab.

A smaller vacuum splint is available to splint individual limbs. This type of splint is applied by positioning the injured limb on the splint and then evacuating the air from inside of it. The result is a splint that is moulded to the extremity. This type of vacuum splint requires less space than a mattress-style vacuum splint but is still relatively expensive compared with standard rigid splints.

Pillow Splints

A pillow is an effective means to immobilise an injured foot or ankle. Simply mould an ordinary pillow around the affected foot and ankle in a position of comfort, then secure the pillow in place with several support bandages. Pillows can also be moulded around an injured knee or elbow and are invaluable for padding longboards when they are used to immobilise patients with dislocated hips.

Special Considerations

Because vacuum mattresses conform to the body, they may be the best choice for immobilising older patients who have abnormal curvatures of the spine and are suspected of having spinal column injuries.

You are the Paramedic Part 3

You have assessed the patient's airway, breathing, and circulation and have controlled significant bleeding found on the left arm. During this time, your partner has inserted a large-bore IV cannula in the right arm. She has also noted that the patient's lung sounds are clear and initiated a bolus of 250 ml bolus normal saline.

As you continue your rapid trauma examination, you find that the left pedal pulse is absent. When you expose the leg, you see significant deformity of the knee consistent with a posterior dislocation. The patient has difficulty feeling his foot and moving his toes. You recognise that this is a true emergency. With the patient correctly immobilised on a longboard, you decide to move him to your ambulance.

Reassessment	Recording Time: 7 Minutes
Skin	Pink, warm, and slightly moist; pale and cool left foot
Pulse	110 beats/min, full and regular
Blood pressure	140 by palpation
Respirations	40 breaths/min
SpO2	100% on 15 l/min via nonrebreathing mask
ECG	Sinus tachycardia with no ectopics

6. Why would this dislocation be considered a true emergency?

7. What is an important consideration before manipulating a dislocation?

Traction Splints

Following a femur fracture, the strong muscles of the thigh go into spasm and often lead to significant pain and deformity. Traction splints provide constant pull on a fractured femur, thereby preventing the broken bone ends from overriding as a result of unopposed muscle contraction. In addition, these splints help maintain alignment of the fracture pieces and provide effective immobilisation of the fracture site. As a result, patients are likely to experience less pain.

Traction splints also reduce blood loss. Normally, the thigh is shaped like a cylinder. In a femur fracture, the thigh is shortened and becomes spherical. The volume of a sphere can be substantially greater than that of a cylinder, so a person with an untreated femur fracture can accumulate more blood in the thigh than a person whose thigh is pulled out to length by a traction splint.

Traction splints are indicated for the treatment of most femur fractures. They should not be used when the patient has an additional fracture below the knee on the same extremity. The most commonly used traction splints are the Sager and the Hare traction splints. The basic principles of application are the same for both. After assessing the injured extremity for distal PMS functions, place the splint next to the uninjured leg to determine the proper length. The traction splint should extend 15 to 25 cm beyond the foot.

Support and stabilise the leg to minimise movement while another member of the ambulance crew applies the ankle hitch. When the hitch is secure, the second crew member will apply gentle longitudinal traction using enough force to realign the extremity. The initial paramedic can then place the splint into position and connect the upper attachment point of the splint and then the ankle hitch Figure 25-27 ▾ . After applying the splint, reassess PMS functions before securing the patient and splint for transport.

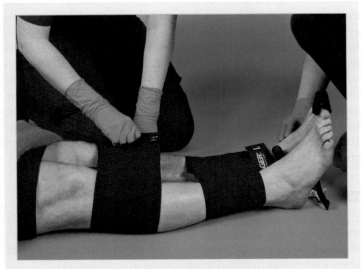

Figure 25-27 A Hare traction splint is shown here. One paramedic connects the straps and another checks distal pulse, motor function, and sensation.

Buddy Splinting

Buddy splinting is used to splint injuries that involve the fingers or toes. With this technique, an adjacent uninjured finger or toe serves as a splint to the injured one. To buddy splint, tape the injured digit to an uninjured one. Place a gauze pad between the digits that are taped together, and ensure that the tape does not pass over joints.

Complications of Musculoskeletal Injuries

Musculoskeletal injuries can lead to numerous complications—not just those involving the musculoskeletal system, but also systemic changes or illness. It is essential to not focus all of your attention on the musculoskeletal injury: Keep in mind that there is a patient attached to the injured extremity!

The likelihood of having a complication is often related to the strength of the force that caused the injury, the injury's location, and the patient's overall health. Any injury to a bone, muscle, or other musculoskeletal structure is likely to be accompanied by bleeding. In general, the greater the force that caused the injury, the greater the haemorrhage that will be associated with it.

Following a fracture, the sharp ends of the bone may damage muscles, blood vessels, arteries, and nerves, or the ends may penetrate the skin and produce an open fracture. A significant loss of tissue may occur at the fracture site if the muscle is severely damaged or if the bone's penetration of the skin causes a large defect. To prevent infection following an open fracture, you should brush away any obvious debris on the skin surrounding an open fracture before applying a dressing. Do not enter or probe the open fracture site in an attempt to retrieve debris because this may lead to further contamination.

Long-term disability is one of the most devastating consequences of a musculoskeletal injury. In many cases, a severely injured limb can be repaired and made to look almost normal. Unfortunately, many patients cannot return to work for long periods because of the extensive rehabilitation required and because of chronic pain. Paramedics have a critical role in mitigating the risk of long-term disability. By preventing further injury, reducing the risk of wound infection, minimising pain by the use of cold and analgesia, and transporting patients with musculoskeletal injuries to an appropriate hospital with specialist fracture management facilities, they help reduce the risk or duration of long-term disability.

Neurovascular Injuries

The skeletal system normally protects the neurovascular structures within the limbs from injury. These critical structures typically lie deep within the limb and close to the skeleton. For example, the brachial plexus is situated within the axilla and the inner aspect of the arm, shielded from injury by the shoulder girdle. When the shoulder girdle or proximal humerus is fractured, displaced fracture fragments may lacerate or impale the nerves of the plexus, leading to a neurological deficit. Neurovascular injuries are also likely to occur following a joint dislocation because the nerves and vessels in the region of a joint tend to be more securely tethered to the soft tissues and are less likely to escape injury.

Compartment Syndrome

Within a limb, groups of muscles are surrounded by an inelastic membrane called fascia. Thus, the muscles are confined to an enclosed space, or compartment, that can accommodate only a limited amount of swelling. When bleeding or swelling occurs within a compartment as the result of a fracture or severe soft-tissue injury, the pressure within it rises. Too-high pressure may impair circulation and lead to pain, sensory changes, and progressive muscle death. This condition, known as compartment syndrome, is one of the most devastating consequences of a musculoskeletal injury.

External and internal factors can lead to the development of compartment syndrome. External factors include bandages, splints, or casts that are applied too tightly and restrict circulation. A number of internal factors can also increase the amount of material within a compartment. For example, bleeding within a compartment may occur because of a fracture, dislocation, crush injury, vascular injury, soft-tissue injury, or bleeding disorder. Alternatively, fluid leakage or oedema may occur secondary to ischaemia, excessive exercise, trauma, burns, or any condition associated with the leakage of proteins and fluid from vessels into the interstitial space. A common misconception is that open fractures are safe from compartment syndrome—a notion that is not true.

Signs and symptoms of compartment syndrome include early and late findings. Typically, the first complaint will be of a searing or burning *pain* that is localised to the involved compartment and out of proportion to the injury. This pain is often severe and typically not relieved with analgesics, including opioids. When examining the patient, passive stretching of an ischaemic muscle will result in severe pain. In the lower extremities, test for this condition by flexing and extending the big toe and by dorsiflexion and plantar flexion of the foot. In the upper extremity, use finger and hand flexion and extension.

During examination of the patient, the affected area may feel very firm and there may be skin pallor. Typical neurological changes include paraesthesias, such as a burning sensation, numbness, or tingling, and paralysis of the involved muscles, which occurs late in the condition. Another late sign of compartment syndrome is pulselessness. By the time the pressure within the compartment reaches the point where it totally occludes the artery passing through it, significant muscle necrosis has probably occurred.

The goal of pre-hospital care is to deliver the patient to a suitable A&E department before the extremity becomes pulseless. Thus, management should include elevating the extremity to heart level (not above!), placing ice packs over the extremity, loosening any tight clothing or constricting splinting material, and considering transfer to hospital as an emergency.

Crush Syndrome

Crush syndrome occurs because of a prolonged compressive force that impairs muscle metabolism and circulation—actually, following the extrication or release of an entrapped limb. This condition happens not only in trauma patients, but also in patients who have been lying on an extremity for an extended period (4–6 hours of compression)—for example, when a drug overdose or stroke victim is not found for an extended period.

After a muscle is compressed for 4 to 6 hours, the muscle cells begin to die and release their contents into the localised vasculature. When the force compressing the region is released, blood flow is reestablished and the material from the cells that was released into the local vasculature quickly returns to the systemic vasculature. The primary substances that are of concern are lactic acid, potassium, and myoglobin. In particular, the return of myoglobin is likely to result in decreased blood pH, hyperkalaemia, and renal dysfunction.

Treatment of crush syndrome, which aims to prevent complications due to toxin release, should always be performed with medical direction. A number of steps must be taken before releasing the compressing force. As with all patients, assess the ABCs in case of suspected crush syndrome. Ensure that the patient is being given high-flow supplemental oxygen, and then administer a bolus of crystalloid solution to increase the intravascular volume and to protect the kidneys from the forthcoming myoglobin load. Establish cardiac monitoring to evaluate for electrocardiographic (ECG) changes related to hyperkalaemia (such as peaked T waves, widening QRS complex, prolonged P-R interval, arrhythmia). Many patients who suffer a prolonged crush injury will benefit from interventions that are beyond the scope of UK paramedic practice. This may include the use of salbutamol to protect against potassium surges, treatments for hyperkalaemia, and other interventions. To this end medical advice should be sought for all prolonged crush injuries prior to attempting release.

Thromboembolic Disease

Thromboembolic disease, including deep vein thrombosis (DVT) and pulmonary embolism, is a significant cause of death following musculoskeletal injuries, especially injuries to the pelvis and lower extremities that lead to prolonged immobilisation.

Signs and symptoms of DVT include disproportionate swelling of an extremity, discomfort in an extremity that worsens with use, and warmth and erythema of the extremity.

At the Scene

A patient who shows evidence of compartment syndrome must be transported on an emergency basis to the hospital. There is no treatment for this syndrome other than surgery—do not delay transport.

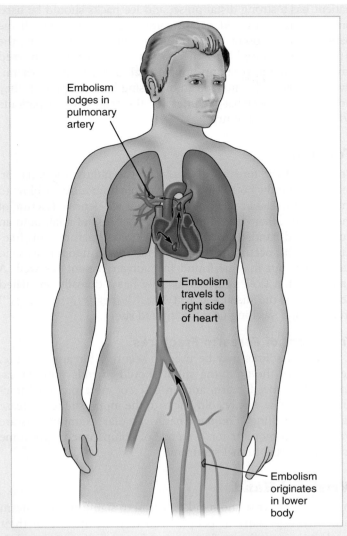

Figure 25-28 When a portion of a DVT dislodges, it may travel to the pulmonary arteries and inhibit blood flow from the heart to the lungs.

When a DVT dislodges, it may cause a pulmonary embolism—a blood clot that occludes a portion or all of the pulmonary arteries **Figure 25-28 ▲** . Signs and symptoms of a pulmonary embolism include a sudden onset of dyspnoea, pleuritic chest pain, dyspnoea, tachypnoea, tachycardia, right-sided heart failure, hypovolaemia, and, in some cases, cardiac arrest.

In addition to the risk of DVT, patients with long bone or pelvic fractures are at risk for developing a fat embolism. In this condition, fat droplets become lodged in the vasculature of the lungs. Affected patients have inflammation of the vasculature of the lungs and other blood vessels where fat is deposited. Generally, symptoms begin within 12 to 72 hours of injury; they include tachycardia, dyspnoea, tachypnoea, pulmonary congestion, fever, petechiae, change in mental status, and organ dysfunction.

Treatment for throboembolic disease in the prehospital environment is limited to maintaining a clear airway, providing adequate oxygenation, ensuring adequate intravascular volume, and rapid transport to an A&E department of an appropriate hospital.

Specific Fractures

Shoulder Girdle
The shoulder girdle consists of the clavicle, shoulder, and scapula.

Clavicle
Clavicle fractures are very common and often occur in children. In most cases, the clavicle fractures in the middle third of the bone, typically from a fall onto an outstretched hand or from direct lateral trauma to the shoulder (as in contact sports and cycling). Patients have pain in the region of the shoulder, swelling, unwillingness to raise the arm, and tilting of the head toward the injured side.

Shoulder
Fractures of the shoulder include those that involve the glenoid fossa of the scapula, the humeral head, and the humeral neck. Most shoulder fractures are caused by a fall onto an outstretched hand and usually occur in elderly patients (younger patients tend to dislocate the shoulder because they have stronger bones). Patients with a shoulder fracture rarely have evidence of a significant deformity, but instead have considerable swelling, bruising, and pain with movement of the arm. In some cases, an associated injury to the brachial plexus may be identified during the neurological examination.

Scapula
Injuries to the scapula usually result from violent, direct trauma. Therefore, when a scapular injury is suspected, it is essential to look for associated injuries—particularly intrathoracic injuries, such as pneumothorax, haemothorax, and fractured ribs. Signs and symptoms of a scapular fracture include pain that increases with arm abduction and swelling in the region of the scapula. Potential complications include axillary artery or nerve injury, brachial plexus injury, pulmonary contusion, and clavicle fractures.

Treatment of Shoulder Girdle Fractures
Fractures in the shoulder region may usually be treated by using a sling and support bandage. These bindings should be applied to maintain the extremity in the position of comfort, often keeping the arm against the chest wall to allow the body to act as a splint. In cases of suspected scapula fractures, full spinal immobilisation is usually warranted given the amount of force required to cause a fracture.

Midshaft Humerus
Fractures of the shaft of the humerus usually occur in younger patients secondary to high-energy injuries, such as road traffic collisions. Unlike fractures that occur more proximally, these

injuries typically have substantial deformity. Examination of the extremity usually reveals a significant amount of swelling, bruising, gross instability of the region, and crepitus. If the force that caused the injury is severe enough, the nerves and blood vessels in the upper arm may also be damaged. Of particular concern is the radial nerve, which may be injured by the force itself or could become entrapped within the fracture site. The classic sign of a radial nerve injury is wrist drop.

Treatment of Midshaft Humerus Fractures
If the fracture is angulated, longitudinal traction may be applied to correct the deformity, but efforts should be halted if the patient's pain is too severe or if neurovascular status worsens. Once the extremity is in the desired position, apply a rigid splint that extends from the axilla to the elbow. Next, apply a sling and support bandage to immobilise the arm to the chest wall, and place cold packs over the fracture site to decrease the patient's pain and swelling.

Elbow
Distal Humerus
Supracondylar fractures of the humerus occur most often in children. The typical mechanism is a fall onto an outstretched hand with the elbow in extension, thereby breaking the distal humerus; as a result, the distal fragment of the humerus is pushed posteriorly and the humeral shaft is pulled anteriorly, where it compresses the brachial artery and the radial and median nerves. If the brachial artery is compromised, the patient could develop compartment syndrome in the forearm. When this complication occurs, the patient is at risk for a Volkmann ischaemic contracture, a condition in which muscles of the forearm degenerate from prolonged ischaemia. The patient's muscles that allow for movement of the fingers become contracted and nonfunctional, and the patient loses the ability to use the hand. Patients with a distal humerus fracture will complain of pain in the area of the elbow and typically have a significant degree of swelling and bruising.

Proximal Radius and Ulna
Radial head fractures may result from a fall onto an outstretched hand or from a direct blow to the bone. This injury causes the patient to have significant pain when he or she attempts supination or pronation. In either case, the patient is likely to have pain and bruising in the region of the injury. Similar to distal humerus fractures, these injuries may lead to an injury of the nerves or blood vessels in proximity to the fracture site. Therefore, a careful neurovascular examination should be performed.

Treatment of Elbow Fractures
Treatment of injuries in the region of the elbow is the same regardless of the exact location of the injury. The injured extremity must be repeatedly assessed for evidence of compartment syndrome. Before splinting the extremity, it is mandatory to document a neurovascular examination. The injured extremity should be splinted in the position that it is found if the patient has a strong distal pulse, and ice packs should be used only if there is no evidence of compartment syndrome. If the patient has an absent distal pulse or neurological deficits, the limb is threatened and the patient must be transported urgently to the nearest appropriate A&E department for definitive treatment. This may mean bypassing local hospitals if they do not offer specialist facilities for the treatment of patients with these types of injury.

Forearm
Fractures of the forearm may involve the radius, the ulna, or, more commonly, both. Injury may result from a direct blow to the bone, the classic example of which is a defensive fracture of the ulna. In other cases, injury occurs because of a fall onto an outstretched hand, as in the case of a Colles fracture. This fracture typically occurs in older patients with osteoporosis who have fallen but may be found in younger patients as well. A patient with a Colles fracture usually has a dorsally angulated deformity of the distal forearm (the "dinner fork deformity") and pain and swelling near the injured site.

Treatment of Forearm Fractures
A variety of splints may be used to secure a forearm fracture. Regardless of the type, the splint should provide immobilisation of the entire forearm and, in cases of more proximal fractures, the elbow. Apply cold packs to the injury site to decrease pain and swelling. Frequent neurovascular examinations are warranted to monitor for evidence of compartment syndrome and acute carpal tunnel syndrome.

Wrist and Hand
Injuries to the wrist and hand may lead to significant long-term disability, especially in people who rely on the use of their hands to earn a living. Sometimes these injuries occur while working at the job or at home; in other cases they result from a fall or during a sporting event. Careful splinting of the injured site is essential to help reduce the risk of long-term disability.

Scaphoid
The scaphoid, also called the carpal navicular, is located just distal to the radius. It may be injured from a fall onto an outstretched hand, for which the classic finding is pain and tenderness in the anatomical snuffbox. To identify the anatomical snuffbox on yourself, extend your thumb. Two tendons will be visible at the base of the thumb on the radial aspect of the wrist. The region between these two tendons is the snuffbox Figure 25-29 ▶ . The major complication of a scaphoid fracture is avascular necrosis of the bone, or poor fracture healing because of the limited blood supply to this bone.

Boxer's Fracture
A boxer's fracture is a fracture of the neck of the fifth metacarpal (little finger). It commonly occurs after punching a hard object, such as a wall or a door. The patient typically has pain over the ulnar aspect of the hand and may have noticeable swelling.

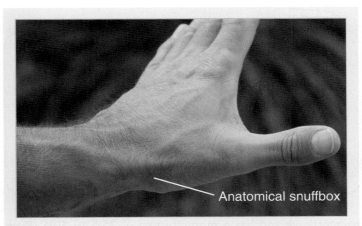

Figure 25-29 The region between the two tendons shown is the anatomical snuffbox.

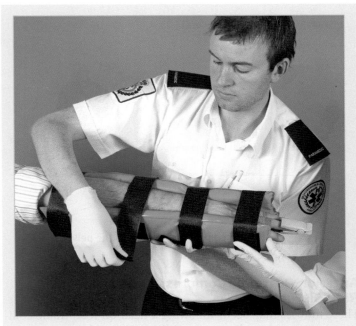

Figure 25-30 Splinting the wrist.

Metacarpal Shaft

Fractures of the metacarpals may result from a crush injury or from direct trauma. Assessment of the injured hand may reveal abnormal rotation or alignment of the fingers, swelling of the palm, with pain and tenderness in the region of injury. You should assess the neurovascular function of the hand and fingers following a crush injury, because development of compartment syndrome is possible within the hand.

Mallet Finger

A mallet finger occurs when a finger is jammed into an object, such as a cricket ball or basketball, resulting in an avulsion fracture of the extensor tendon. The patient will not be able to extend the distal phalynx and will maintain it in a flexed position.

Treatment of Wrist and Hand Fractures

Splint the injured hand in the position of function by placing the wrist in about 30° of dorsiflexion with fingers slightly flexed (a roll of gauze approximately 5 to 8 cm in diameter accomplishes this nicely). Next, secure the extremity to a rigid splint that extends proximally to the elbow and is slightly elevated to help reduce swelling **Figure 25-30 ▶**. For injuries that are isolated to the digits, use a foam-padded flexible aluminum splint to splint the injured digit, if available. In the case of penetrating injuries, regardless of whether a fracture is present, apply bulky dressings to the site of injury and splint the injured hand in the position of function.

Pelvis

Pelvic fractures are relatively uncommon injuries, accounting for fewer than 3% of all fractures. Despite their low incidence, these injuries are responsible for a significant number of deaths in blunt trauma patients. The risk of death following a pelvic fracture ranges from 8% to 50%, depending on the severity of the injury; when the fracture is open, the mortality rate rises to 25% to 50%. Death after a pelvic fracture commonly results from massive haemorrhage caused by damage to the arteries and veins of the pelvis.

Disruptions of the pelvic ring occur in secondary to high-energy trauma such as crush injuries, motorcycle collisions, and falls from a significant height. A number of structures within the pelvis are at risk for injury when it is fractured—the bladder, urethra, rectum, vagina, and sacral nerve plexus. The blood vessels that are most prone to damage are the veins within the pelvis, but there may be damage to the internal or external iliac and arteries in the lumbar region. The nerves at greatest risk of injury are those in the lumbar and sacral regions and the sciatic and femoral nerves.

Patients with pelvic ring disruptions who have a stable injury, such as a minimal lateral compression injury, may complain of pain in the pelvis and difficulty bearing weight. Patients with a more severe injury may show evidence of profound hypovolaemia, gross pelvic instability, and diffuse pelvic and lower abdominal pain. There may also be bruising or lacerations in the perineum, scrotum, groin, suprapubic region, and flank and haematuria (blood in the urine) or blood coming from the meatus of the penis, vagina, or rectum.

Lateral Compression Pelvic Ring Disruptions

Lateral compression injuries result from an impact on the side of the body (such as being struck by a car from the side or falling from a significant height and landing on one side of the body). The side of the pelvis that sustains the impact becomes internally rotated around the sacrum, and the actual volume within the pelvis decreases **Figure 25-31 ▶**. Although this injury is not commonly associated with massive haemorrhage into the pelvis, it is often associated with injuries in other regions of the body.

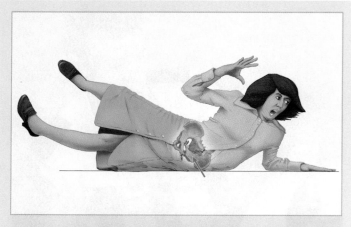

Figure 25-31 A lateral compression injury to the pelvis.

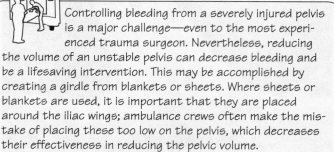

At the Scene

Controlling bleeding from a severely injured pelvis is a major challenge—even to the most experienced trauma surgeon. Nevertheless, reducing the volume of an unstable pelvis can decrease bleeding and be a lifesaving intervention. This may be accomplished by creating a girdle from blankets or sheets. Where sheets or blankets are used, it is important that they are placed around the iliac wings; ambulance crews often make the mistake of placing these too low on the pelvis, which decreases their effectiveness in reducing the pelvic volume.

Anterior-Posterior Compression Pelvic Ring Disruptions

These injuries may occur following a head-on road traffic collision, motorcycle collision, or fall or in a pedestrian who is struck head-on by a vehicle. The force of the impact compresses the pelvis in the anterior-to-posterior direction, causing the pubic symphysis and posterior supporting ligaments to be disrupted and tear apart. The pelvis then spreads apart and opens like a book—hence the name open book pelvic fracture. Such an injury has the potential for massive blood loss because the volume of the pelvis is greatly increased.

Vertical Shear

Vertical shear injuries occur when a major force is applied to the pelvis from above or below, such as when a person falls from a significant height and lands on the feet. On landing, the force is transmitted through the legs to the pelvis, leading to the complete displacement of one or both sides of the pelvis toward the head. Thus, this kind of injury has anterior and posterior components. The anterior component involves a fracture of the rami or disruption of the symphysis pubis. The posterior component involves a fracture of the ilium or sacrum or a disruption of the sacroiliac joint. The patient is likely to have significant shortening of the limb on the affected side and is at risk for massive haemorrhage into the pelvis.

Straddle Fracture

A straddle fracture occurs after a fall when a person lands in the region of the perineum and sustains bilateral fractures of the inferior and superior rami. This injury does not interfere with weightbearing, but it does carry a risk owing to its associated complications, particularly those of the lower genitourinary system.

Open Pelvic Fractures

Open pelvic fractures are life-threatening injuries. Such an injury is defined by the presence of a laceration of the skin in the pelvic region, vagina, or rectum. This uncommon fracture is caused by a high-velocity injury with subsequent massive haemorrhage and has a mortality rate of 25% to 50%. Even small amounts of blood found during a vaginal or rectal examination should raise your suspicion for an open fracture.

Treatment of Pelvic Fractures

Assessment of the patient with a possible pelvic fracture should begin as in any other trauma patient—with an initial assessment of the mental status and ABCs, taking spinal precautions. During the rapid trauma examination of the patient, you should search for injuries typically associated with pelvic fractures. Assess the pelvis for bleeding, lacerations, bruising, and instability. Formal assessment for instability by pressing the iliac wings toward the midline and then posteriorly should be avoided in the prehospital environment. It can lead to exanguinating haemorrhage, and clinical suspicion should be high based on the mechanism of injury alone. Where an unstable pelvis is suspected, manipulation of the iliac wings should be avoided until definitive care is immediately available.

Treatment should include careful monitoring of the ABCs, spinal immobilisation, and IV access with at least one (if not two) large-bore cannulas. Management of the pelvic injury is aimed at reducing the amount of bleeding and decreasing the degree of instability. It is often appropriate to seek medical direction for the management of these patients, especially for determining how to best stabilise the pelvis. Methods used to accomplish this may include application of a pelvic binder or simply tying a sheet around the pelvis. Applying pressure to the iliac wings and forcing them to shift toward the midline reduces the potential space within the pelvis, which may allow for tamponade of the bleeding vessels. Once packaged, the patient should be rapidly transported to an appropriate A&E department, and IV fluid should be administered to maintain adequate tissue perfusion but avoiding hypertension.

Hip

A hip fracture involves a fracture of the femoral head, femoral neck, intertrochanteric region, or proximal femoral shaft. Fractures of the femoral head are uncommon injuries that are usually associated with a hip dislocation. Femoral neck and intertrochanteric fractures typically occur in older patients with osteoporosis who have fallen and sustained direct trauma to the hip. They may occur in younger patients with healthy the digit is dislocated to the dorsal side, extend the digit; if it is dislocated to the palmar side, flex the digit. Next, use gentle longitudinal traction to bring the digit back into its normal position. It may be helpful to apply pressure at the dislocated joint to push the distal part into position. Following reduction, the neurovascular status of the digit should be reassessed and the digit should be fully immobilised to prevent it from dislocating again.

Hip Dislocation

More than 90% of all hip dislocations involve posterior dislocation. The majority of these occur due to deceleration injuries, in which a flexed knee strikes an immobile object with a great degree of force **Figure 25-37 ▾** . When a patient has a posterior hip dislocation, the leg of the affected side is typically found in flexion, adduction, and internal rotation, and it is noticeably shorter. Patients complain of severe pain and inability to move the leg, and significant soft-tissue swelling may be evident. Complications arising from such injuries include sciatic nerve injury, avascular necrosis of the hip, and associated fractures of the acetabulum.

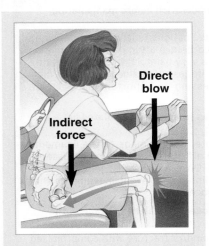

Figure 25-37 When a flexed knee strikes a dashboard, the force may be transmitted to the femur causing it to be driven posteriorly. The hip may dislocate, and the acetabulum may fracture.

Anterior hip dislocations usually follow a forceful spreading injury that occurs while the hip is flexed. The affected leg is usually flexed, abducted, and externally rotated, and the patient complains of severe pain. Major complications of this type of injury include injury to the femoral artery or nerve and avascular necrosis of the hip.

Treatment of Hip Dislocation

Because the majority of hip dislocations are associated with a high-energy mechanism, a full trauma assessment should be conducted and the patient fully immobilised. Splint the injured extremity in the position in which it is found by using blankets and pillows. Perform regular neurovascular checks and record these on your patient report form. Having arrived at hospital, the patient generally requires sedation and muscle relaxants to allow the hip to be reduced.

Knee Dislocation

Dislocations of the knee are true emergencies that may threaten the limb. When the knee is dislocated, the ligaments that provide support to it may be damaged or torn. The knee may be dislocated by high-energy trauma (as in road traffic collisions), or it may dislocate secondary to powerful twisting forces (as when athletes attempt to avoid another player). In most cases, the knee will spontaneously reduce following the injury and there may be no obvious evidence of injury.

The direction of dislocation refers to the position of the tibia with respect to the femur. Anterior knee dislocations, which result from extreme hyperextension of the knee, are the most common, occurring in almost half of all cases. Commonly, the anterior and posterior cruciate ligaments are damaged, but there is also a high risk of injury to the popliteal artery.

In posterior dislocations, a direct blow to the knee forces the tibia to shift posteriorly. There is also the possibility of damage to the cruciate ligaments and injury to the popliteal artery.

Medial dislocations result from a direct blow to the lateral part of the leg. Because the deforming force causes the medial aspect of the knee to stretch apart, there is a high likelihood of injury to the medial collateral and cruciate ligaments. When the force is applied from the medial direction, a lateral dislocation occurs and the lateral part of the knee is stretched apart, injuring the lateral collateral ligament. Lateral and medial dislocations happen less commonly and have a lesser risk of injuring the popliteal artery.

Patients with a knee dislocation will typically complain of pain in the knee and report that the knee "gave way". If the knee did not spontaneously reduce, there may be evidence of significant deformity and decreased range of motion. Complications may include limb-threatening popliteal artery disruption; injuries to the popliteal, peroneal, and tibial nerves; and joint instability. Do not confuse this injury with a relatively minor patella dislocation.

Treatment of Knee Dislocation

In all cases of knee dislocation, distal neurovascular function must be assessed frequently and will often guide the management. If a pulse is palpable in the foot, splint the knee in the position in which it is found. If there is no palpable pulse, you may need to reduce the knee to restore circulation. A number of factors, including time to the hospital and duration of dislocation, will affect this decision, so you should always seek medical direction before reducing a dislocated knee.

To reduce a dislocated knee, apply longitudinal traction to the tibia in the direction of the foot. While one crew member is applying traction, a second crew member should apply pressure to the distal femur and proximal tibia. If the knee is dislocated anteriorly, apply pressure to the femur in the anterior direction and to the tibia in the opposite direction. In the case of a posterior dislocation, apply pressure in the opposite manner, with the tibia pressed anteriorly and the femur pressed posteriorly. Once the reduction has been accomplished, check the patient's neurovascular status and splint the leg securely. If the attempt at reduction fails, splint the knee in the position in which it is found and undertake rapid transport to an appropriate hospital.

You are the Paramedic Summary

1. What are your initial assessment and treatment priorities?

As with any trauma patient, after assuring that the scene is safe, the initial assessment priorities for this patient are the mental status, the ABCs, and prioritising the patient. Then proceed with a rapid trauma examination to identify the patient's injuries. Because this patient fell from a significant height, it is also important to protect his spine. During the initial assessment, you note that he has a site of bleeding from his arm; this bleeding should be controlled. Once this is accomplished, IV access should be obtained and the assessment should continue in a systematic and orderly manner.

2. What other information should be obtained about the patient and the incident?

Obtain information about the events that led the patient to fall, such as how he felt before falling and why he thought he fell. It is also important to learn details about the fall, such as how his extremities were positioned when he landed or whether he struck any other objects while falling. Obtain any other information related to the patient's status after the fall, such as loss of consciousness, mental status, and movement of extremities, from the patient or anyone who witnessed the fall. Also obtain information about any allergies the patient may know he has, any medication he takes, and the last time he had anything to eat or drink.

3. What are the potential complications of an open fracture?

One of the most significant complications following an open fracture is infection of the bone or soft tissues. To reduce the risk of infection, do not probe open fractures, brush away any debris on the surface of the skin, and cover the wound with a sterile dressing. Other complications of open fractures include poor healing of the fracture, soft-tissue loss, neurovascular injury, and long-term disability.

4. Why are open fractures prone to bleeding more than closed fractures?

In general, open fractures are higher-energy injuries than closed fractures, so they are likely to have more soft-tissue damage and, hence, more bleeding. Also, because the fracture is open, the blood that would normally accumulate within the closed fracture site is allowed to escape, so there is no tamponade of the bleeding vessels.

5. Would your treatment priorities change if the patient complained of abdominal pain in the presence of hypotension?

If the patient were found to be in unstable condition with evidence of an intra-abdominal injury, immediate and rapid transport to an A&E department with the appropriate facilities would

be warranted. For a trauma patient in unstable condition who has a fracture, place the patient on a longboard and fully immobilise the patient. While immobilising the spine, the injured extremities may be immobilised as well by securing them to the board. The result is a compromise: The injured extremity is secured in place and protected from further movement without dedicating precious time to applying a formal splint.

6. Why would this dislocation be considered a true emergency?

When a patient with a dislocated knee has a pulseless foot, medical direction should be obtained and consideration should be given to manipulating the dislocation. Some ambulance services may have practice guidelines to deal with this type of situation. Factors that will influence this decision include the duration of the dislocation, time to the hospital, the patient's vital signs, and the patient's overall condition.

7. What is an important consideration before manipulating a dislocation?

If the patient has no contraindications (such as hypotension), sedation should be considered before attempting manipulation of the extremity. This can be a very painful procedure, and without determining the appropriateness of analgesics such as morphine, you will not be addressing an important patient care issue—comfort.

8. Why should a joint that has just been manipulated be splinted immediately?

A dislocation is often associated with damage to the ligaments and capsule that support the affected joint, making it susceptible to recurrent dislocations. Once a dislocated joint has been manipulated, it should be splinted to prevent movements that may allow for it to dislocate once again.

9. What facts should be included in an alert message to the A&E department?

The presence of a dislocation and/or fracture with compromised neurovascular status should be relayed immediately to the receiving hospital. Any attempts to correct the impairment should be explained, along with any changes or responses to treatment. Paint a clear picture of the mechanism of injury and the patient's condition. Remember, the only information the A&E department staff have to plan for your arrival is based on your brief radio report.

Prep Kit

Ready for Review

- Injuries and complaints related to the musculoskeletal system are one of the most common reasons that patients seek medical attention.
- Musculoskeletal injuries are sometimes very dramatic, but attention should not be focused on them until life-threatening conditions have been excluded.
- You have a vital role in reducing the complications associated with musculoskeletal injuries by promptly and effectively splinting injured extremities.
- Assume the existence of a fracture whenever a patient who complains of a musculoskeletal injury has deformity, bruising, decreased range of motion, or swelling.
- Always perform and record an accurate neurovascular examination before and after splinting an injured extremity.
- When a dislocation is associated with absent distal pulses, obtain medical direction to determine whether the injury should be reduced.
- Look for injuries to the chest and abdomen, and fully immobilise the spine when patients have evidence of a high-energy injury, such as a femoral shaft or scapular fracture.
- Because fractures may be associated with significant blood loss, resuscitation with IV fluid may be necessary.
- Pelvic fractures are potentially lethal injuries owing to the massive potential for blood loss.
- *Never forget the ABCs!* Do not become distracted; the fracture can wait, if airway, breathing, or circulation problems are noted.

Vital Vocabulary

6 Ps of musculoskeletal assessment Pain, Paralysis, Parasthesias, Pulselessness, Pallor, and Pressure.

abduction Movement *away* from the midline of the body.

acetabulum The cup-shaped cavity in which the rounded head of the femur rotates.

acromion Lateral extension of the scapula that forms the highest point of the shoulder.

adduction Movement *toward* the midline of the body.

amputation Severing of a part of the body.

angulation The presence of an abnormal angle or bend in an extremity.

anterior tibial artery The artery that travels through the anterior muscles of the leg and continues to the foot as the dorsalis pedis.

appendicular skeleton The part of the skeleton comprising the upper and lower extremities.

arthritis Inflammation of the joints.

articulations The locations where two or more bones meet; *joints*.

atrophy Wasting away of a tissue.

avascular necrosis Tissue death resulting from the loss of blood supply.

avulsion fracture A fracture that occurs when a piece of bone is torn free at the site of attachment of a tendon or ligament.

axial skeleton The part of the skeleton comprising the skull, spinal column, and rib cage.

axilla The armpit.

axillary artery The artery that runs through the axilla, connecting the subclavian artery to the brachial artery.

bowing fracture An incomplete fracture typically occurring in children in which the bone becomes bent as the result of a compressive force.

boxer's fracture A fracture of the head of the fifth metacarpal that usually results from striking an object with a clenched fist.

brachial artery The artery that runs through the arm and branches into the radial and ulnar arteries.

buckle fracture A common incomplete fracture in children in which the cortex of the bone fractures from an excessive compression force.

buddy splinting Securing an injured digit to an adjacent uninjured one to allow the intact digit to act as a splint.

bursa A fluid-filled sac located adjacent to joints that reduces the amount of friction between moving structures.

bursitis Inflammation of a bursa.

calcaneous The heel bone; the largest of the tarsal bones.

cancellous bone Trabecular or spongy bone.

carpals The eight small bones of the wrist.

cartilage Tough, elastic substance that covers opposable surfaces of moveable joints and forms part of the skeleton.

cartilaginous joints Joints that are spanned completely by cartilage and allow for minimal motion.

clavicle The collar bone.

closed fracture A fracture in which the skin is not broken.

comminuted fracture A fracture in which the bone is broken into three or more pieces.

compartment syndrome An increase in tissue pressure in a closed fascial space or compartment that compromises the circulation to the nerves and muscles within the involved compartment.

complete fracture A fracture in which the bone is broken into two or more completely separate pieces.

compound fracture An open fracture; a fracture beneath an open wound.

crepitus A grating sensation felt when moving the ends of a broken bone.

crush syndrome A condition that arises after a body part that has been compressed for a significant period is released, leading to the entry of potassium and other metabolic toxins into the systemic circulation.

deep vein thrombosis (DVT) The formation of a blood clot within the larger veins of an extremity, typically following a period of prolonged immobilisation.

depression fracture A fracture in which the broken region of the bone is pushed deeper into the body than the remaining intact bone.

devascularisation The loss of blood to a part of the body.

diaphysis The shaft of a long bone.

diastasis An increase in the distance between the two sides of a joint.

digital arteries The arteries that supply blood to the fingers and toes.

dinner fork deformity The dorsal deformity of the forearm that results from a Colles fracture.

dislocation The displacement of a bone from its normal position within a joint.

distraction injury An injury that results from a force that tries to increase the length of a body part or separate one body part from another.

dorsal Referring to the back or posterior side of the body or an organ.

dorsiflex To bend the foot or hand backward.

endosteum The inner lining of a hollow bone.

fascia A strong, fibrous membrane that covers, supports, and separates muscles.

fatigue fractures Fractures that result from multiple compressive loads.

femoral artery The main artery supplying the thigh and leg.

femoral shaft fractures A break in the diaphysis of the femur.

femur The proximal bone of the leg that extends from the pelvis to the knee.

fibrous joints The joints that contain dense fibrous tissue and allow for no motion.

fibula The smaller of the two bones of the lower leg.

flat bones Bones that are thin and broad, such as the scapula.

fracture A break or rupture in the bone.

glenoid fossa Socket in the scapula in which the head of the humerus rotates.

gout A painful disorder characterised by the crystallisation of uric acid within a joint.

greenstick fracture A type of fracture occurring most frequently in children in which there is incomplete breakage of the bone.

haematopoiesis The generation of blood cells.

humerus The bone of the upper arm.

hypertrophy An increase in size.

ilium The broad, uppermost bone of the pelvis.

impacted fracture A broken bone in which the end of one bone becomes wedged into another bone, as could be the case in a fall from a significant height.

incomplete fracture A fracture in which the bone does not fully break.

indirect injury An injury that results from a force that is applied to one region of the body but leads to an injury in another area.

intertrochanteric fractures Fractures that occur in the region between the lesser and greater trochanters.

irregular bones Bones with unique shapes that allow them to perform a specific function and that do not fit into the other categories based on shape.

ischium The lowermost dorsal bone of the pelvis.

joint The point at which two or more bones articulate, or come together.

joint capsule A saclike envelope that encloses the cavity of a synovial joint.

lactic acid A metabolic end product of the breakdown of glucose that accumulates when metabolism proceeds in the absence of oxygen.

lateral compression A force that is directed from the side toward the midline of the body.

ligaments Tough bands of tissue that connect bone to bone around a joint or support internal organs within the body.

linear fracture A fracture that runs parallel to the long axis of a bone.

long bones Bones that are longer than they are wide.

malleolus The large, rounded bony protuberance on either side of the ankle joint.

mallet finger An avulsion fracture of the extensor tendon of the distal phalynx caused by jamming a finger into an object.

march fractures *See* fatigue fractures.

medullary canal The hollow centre portion of a long bone.

metacarpals The five bones that form the palm and back of the hand.

metaphysis The region of the long bone between the epiphysis and diaphysis.

metatarsals The five long bones extending from the tarsus to the phalanges of the foot.

muscle fatigue The condition that arises when a muscle depletes its supply of energy.

neurovascular compromise The loss of the nerve supply, blood supply, or both to a region of the body, typically distal to a site of injury; characterised by alterations in sensation, including numbness and tingling, or by a loss or decrease of motor function; vascular compromise is indicated by weak or absent pulses, poor skin colour, and cool skin.

nondisplaced fracture A break in which the bone remains aligned in its normal position.

nursemaid's elbow The subluxation of the radial head that often results from pulling on an outstretched arm.

oblique fracture A fracture that travels diagonally from one side of the bone to the other.

olecranon The proximal bony projection of the *ulna* at the elbow.

open book pelvic fracture A life-threatening fracture of the pelvis caused by a force that displaces one or both sides of the pelvis laterally and posteriorly.

open fracture Any break in a bone in which the overlying skin has been damaged.

osteoarthritis (OA) The degeneration of a joint surface caused by wear and tear that leads to pain and stiffness.

osteoporosis A condition characterised by decreased bone density and increased susceptibility to fractures.

overriding The overlap of a bone that occurs from the muscle spasm that follows a fracture, leading to a decrease in the length of the bone.

palmar Pertaining to the palm or sole of the hand.

paraesthesias Abnormal sensations such as burning, numbness, or tingling.

patella The kneecap.

pathologic fracture A fracture that occurs in an area of abnormally weakened bone.

pectoral girdle The shoulder girdle.

pelvic girdle The large bone that arises in the area of the last nine vertebrae and sweeps around to form a complete ring.

periosteum The fibrous tissue that covers bone.

phalanges The bones of the fingers or toes.

physis The growth plate in long bones.

plantar Referring to the sole of the foot.

plantar flexion Bending of the foot toward the ground.

point tenderness The tenderness that is sharply localised at the site of the injury, found by gently palpating along the bone with the tip of one finger.

popliteal artery The artery in the area or space behind the knee joint.

posterior tibial artery The artery that travels through the calf muscles to the plantar aspect of the foot.

pronation The act of turning the palm of the hand backward or downward, performed by internal rotation of the forearm.

pubic symphysis The midline articulation of the pubic bones.

pubis One of two bones that form the anterior portion of the pelvic ring.

pulmonary embolism Obstruction of a pulmonary artery or arteries by solid, liquid, or gaseous material swept through the right side of the heart into the lungs.

radial artery The artery pertaining to the wrist.

radius The bone on the thumb side of the forearm.

range of motion (ROM) The arc of motion of an extremity at a joint in a particular direction.

recruitment The process of signaling additional muscle fibres to contract to create a more forceful contraction.

rheumatoid arthritis (RA) An inflammatory disorder that affects the entire body and leads to degeneration and deformation of joints.

round bones The small bones that are found adjacent to joints that assist with motion.

sacroiliac joints The points of attachment of the *ilium* to the sacrum.

scaphoid The wrist bone that is found just beyond that most distal portion of the radius.

scapula The shoulder blade.

segmental fracture A bone that is broken in more than one place.

short bones The bones that are nearly as wide as they are long.

skeletal muscle Muscle that is attached to bones and usually crosses at least one joint; striated or voluntary muscle.

snuffbox The region at the base of the thumb where the scaphoid may be palpated.

somatic motor neurones The nerve fibres that transmit impulses to a muscle.

spiral fracture A break in a bone that appears like a spring on an X-ray.

sprains Injuries, including a stretch or a tear, to the ligaments of a joint that commonly lead to pain and swelling.

straddle fracture A fracture of the pelvis that results from landing on the perineal region.

strain Stretching or tearing of a muscle by excessive stretching or overuse.

stress fracture A fracture that results from exaggerated stress on the bone caused by unusually rapid muscle development.

striated muscle Skeletal muscle that is under voluntary control.

subclavian artery The artery that travels from the aorta to each upper extremity.

subluxation A partial or incomplete dislocation.

supination To turn the forearm laterally so that the palm faces forward (if standing) or upward (if lying supine).

supracondylar fractures Fractures of the distal humerus that occur just proximal to the elbow.

synovial joints Joints that permit movement of the component bones.

synovial membrane The lining of a joint that secretes synovial fluid into the joint space.

talus The bone of the foot that articulates with the tibia.

tarsals The ankle bones.

tendinitis Inflammation of a tendon that usually results from overuse.

tendons The fibrous portions of muscle that attach to bone.

Thompson test Squeezing of the calf muscle to evaluate for plantar flexion of the foot to determine whether the Achilles tendon is intact. Also called the Simmons test.

thromboembolic disease The condition in which a patient has a DVT or pulmonary embolism.

tibia The shin bone.

torus fracture See buckle fracture.

transverse fracture A fracture that runs in a straight line from one edge of the bone to the other and that is perpendicular to each edge.

twisting injuries Injuries that commonly occur during athletic activities in which an extremity rotates around a planted foot or hand.

ulna The larger bone of the forearm, on the side opposite the thumb.

ulnar artery The artery of the forearm that travels along its medial aspect.

vertical shear The type of pelvic fracture that occurs when a massive force displaces the pelvis superiorly.

Volkmann ischaemic contracture Contraction of the fingers and, sometimes, the wrist, with loss of muscular power, that sets in rapidly after severe injury around the elbow joint.

voluntary muscle Muscle that can be controlled by a person.

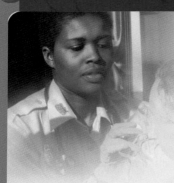

Assessment in Action

You have been sent to the home of a 13-year-old boy with pain in his foot. When you arrive, the boy is sitting in his mother's car complaining of severe pain in his left foot, ankle, and leg. On assessment, he has a distal pulse; his foot is cold and has limited range of motion. There is swelling noted in ankle region. There is no discolouration or obvious deformity. The remainder of his vital signs are within normal limits.

He tells you that he was skateboarding. He went down a hill when suddenly, a lamp-post was in the way. He struck the lamp-post with the bottom of his left foot (travelling approximately 20 mph). He felt immediate pain in his foot and then began to feel a burning sensation up his left leg. His mother drove him back to their house, approximately 45 minutes away. He had no pain while travelling, but when he attempted to step out of the vehicle, the pain soared through him. You provide comfort care for the young man and transport him to hospital. He tells you that his pain is about 7 on a 1 to 10 scale. You follow-up at the hospital and are told that he has a comminuted fracture in his heel and a fractured ankle.

1. **What type of injury force did this young man sustain?**
   A. Tapping injury force
   B. Crush injury force
   C. Penetrating injury force
   D. Indirect injury force

2. **With the complaint of pain in his left leg, what other type of injury should have been suspected?**
   A. Indirect injury
   B. Direct injury
   C. Twisting injury
   D. March fracture

3. **The foot consists of three classes of bones. Which are they?**
   A. Tarsals, metatarsals, and calcaneus
   B. Tarsals, metatarsals, and phalanges
   C. Tarsals, calcaneus, and tibia
   D. Tibia, fibula, and malleolus

4. **Signs and symptoms of extremity trauma that have a high urgency include which of the following?**
   A. Absent distal pulses
   B. Crepitus
   C. Decreased range of movement
   D. Swelling and deformity

5. **Flexion, extension, abduction, and circumduction are all movements allowed by what type of joint?**
   A. Hinge
   B. Synovial
   C. Saddle
   D. Ball and socket

6. **Muscles are composed of specialised cells that contract when stimulated to exert a force on a part of the body. Three types of muscles found in the body are:**
   A. smooth, cardiac, and skeletal.
   B. smooth, cardiac, and striated.
   C. ligaments, cartilage, and smooth.
   D. cardiac, skeletal, and cartilage.

7. **When a person sustains a musculoskeletal injury, the arteries that supply the injured region may be damaged as well. What arteries supply the ankle and the foot?**
   A. Tibial artery; anterior tibial artery
   B. Popliteal artery; anterior tibial artery
   C. Anterior tibial artery; posterior tibial artery
   D. Popliteal artery; posterior tibial artery

8. **What is the _primary_ symptom of a fracture?**
   A. Pain
   B. Deformity
   C. Shortening
   D. Loss of use

9. **When assessing the patient's pain, you should use the mnemonic:**
   A. PQRST.
   B. OPRST.
   C. OPQRST.
   D. OPRST.

Challenging Questions

You have been sent to the home of a 60-year-old man found by neighbours. On your arrival, you find the man in a right lateral recumbent position and he is moaning. You're not sure how long he has been on the ground, but there is 4 days' worth of post on the floor. You apply a longboard and cervical collar because you are not sure of the reason the patient is on the ground. His blood pressure is 100/60 mm Hg and the heart rate is 120 beats/min with sinus tachycardia, he has strong radial pulses, and his respirations are 12 breaths/min. He is verbally responsive by moaning. He is unable to tell you what happened or if anything hurts.

You provide supportive and comfort care en route to hospital. His body is very stiff and you have difficulty manipulating his extremities. When you perform an assessment, you note that there is a coin embedded in his head. There are large areas of bruising along his right pelvic area and his right leg. His right shoulder has open wounds. He is incontinent of urine and faeces. This man was admitted to the intensive care unit with a diagnosis of acute sepsis and crush syndrome.

10. **What signs and symptoms would you recognise for the crush syndrome?**

11. **How would you treat this type of injury?**

12. **What will be the concerns of the hospital staff for this patient?**

Points to Ponder

You have been sent to an old people's home for a lady who has fallen out of bed while trying to get up. When you arrive, the woman is still on the floor next to her bed. She tells you that her left leg and back hurt, but she is mentally alert and denies any other symptoms. She is sitting up, and it does not appear that she has bumped her head or injured herself in any other way besides the fall. Your physical examination reveals tenderness and pain in her left leg and crepitus and instability in her left hip. The staff tells you that the woman has osteoporosis but no other major medical problems.

How would you best treat this patient?

Issues: Thorough Assessment of Musculoskeletal Injuries, Pain Management.

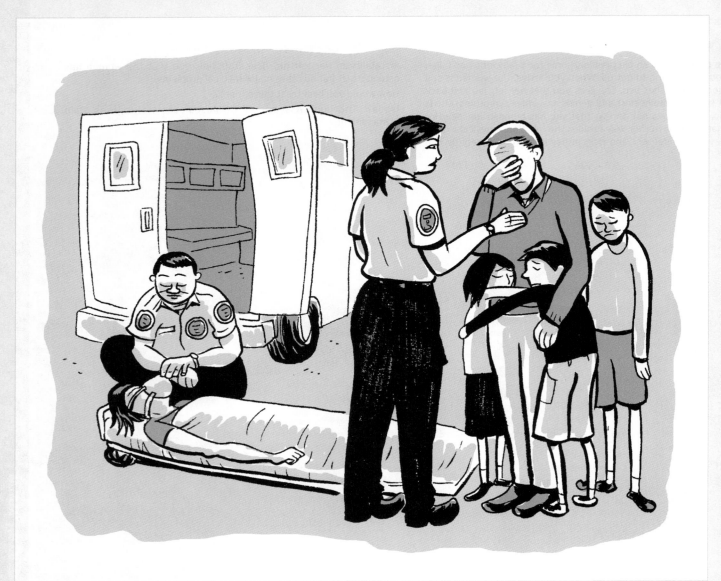

Medical Emergencies

Section Editor: David Whitmore

Section 5

26 Respiratory Emergencies

Objectives

Cognitive

- Discuss the epidemiology of pulmonary diseases and conditions.
- Identify and describe the function of the structures located in the upper and lower airway.
- Discuss the physiology of ventilation and respiration.
- Identify common pathological events that affect the pulmonary system.
- Discuss abnormal assessment findings associated with pulmonary diseases and conditions.
- Compare various airway and ventilation techniques used in the management of pulmonary diseases.
- Review the pharmacological preparations that paramedics use for management of respiratory diseases and conditions.
- Review the pharmacological preparations used in managing patients with respiratory diseases that may be prescribed by physicians.
- Review the use of equipment used during the physical examination of patients with complaints associated with respiratory diseases and conditions.
- Identify the epidemiology, anatomy, physiology, pathophysiology, assessment findings, and management for the following respiratory diseases and conditions:
  - Adult respiratory distress syndrome
  - Asthma
  - Chronic bronchitis
  - Emphysema
  - Pneumonia
  - Pulmonary oedema
  - Pulmonary thromboembolism
  - Neoplasms of the lung
  - Upper respiratory infections
  - Spontaneous pneumothorax
  - Hyperventilation syndrome

Affective

- Recognise and value the assessment and treatment of patients with respiratory diseases.
- Indicate appreciation for the critical nature of accurate initial impressions of patients with respiratory diseases and conditions.

Psychomotor

- Demonstrate proper use of airway and ventilation devices.
- Conduct a history and patient assessment for patients with pulmonary diseases and conditions.
- Demonstrate the application of a CPAP/BiPAP unit.

Introduction

There are few incentives to dial 999 more powerful than the feeling of being unable to breathe (dyspnoea). In the majority of cases, that distressing feeling is caused by a problem in the respiratory system itself. In this chapter, we examine some of the respiratory problems that produce dyspnoea. We begin by reviewing the anatomy and physiology of the respiratory system. We next consider the assessment of a patient whose chief complaint is dyspnoea—namely, which aspects to emphasise in taking the history and carrying out the physical examination. Then we look at some of the problems that may assault each component of the respiratory system—from the respiratory control centres in the brain to the alveolus, the smallest functional unit of respiration in the lung.

Review of Respiratory Anatomy and Function

The primary components of the respiratory system are often compared to an inverted tree, with the trachea representing the tree's trunk and the alveoli resembling the tree's leaves. That is a nice analogy to get things started, but in reality a respiratory tree would have to branch 24 times and have nearly a billion leaves   **Figure 26-1 ▾** . Imagine attempting to pull fluid from the ground into those leaves by exerting a negative pressure at the leaf ends, and you may begin to appreciate the complexities of breathing.

The Upper Airway

Air enters the upper airway primarily through the nares (nostrils) of the nose. Nares are lined with nasal hairs. The hairs serve as filters that catch particulate matter in the air we breathe. The external nares are separated by the nasal septum.

At any given time, one nostril is usually more open than the other and would be the better choice for the insertion of a nasogastric (NG) tube or a nasopharyngeal airway. Occlude one nostril and have the patient inhale, and repeat the procedure with the other nostril. It is usually easy to tell which one is less obstructed.

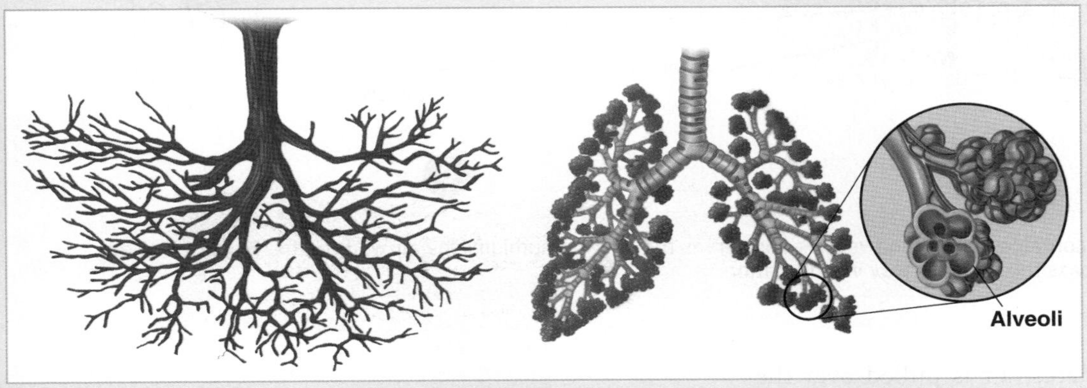

Figure 26-1 The tracheobronchial tree branches in much the same way as a tree, except that even the most branched tree has only half as many branchings as those inside the lung.

You are the Paramedic Part 1

You are dispatched to 275 Thomas Lane to help an older man who is having difficulty breathing. You arrive to find a 65-year-old man sitting in the tripod position at his kitchen table. As you speak with him, you notice that he is struggling to breathe and can give you only one- or two-word responses. His extremities are pale and his face is flushed. As you attempt to obtain more information regarding his medical history, the patient grabs your arm and says, "I'm so tired"!

Initial Assessment	Recording Time: 0 Minutes
Appearance	Anxious, tired
Level of consciousness	V (Responsive to verbal stimuli)
Airway	Open
Breathing	Rapid and laboured; accessory muscle use
Circulation	Weak radial pulse

1. What about this patient's presentation gives you cause for concern?
2. What are your assessment and treatment priorities?
3. If you are unable to gather much information from your patient about his medical history, in what other ways can you obtain this information?

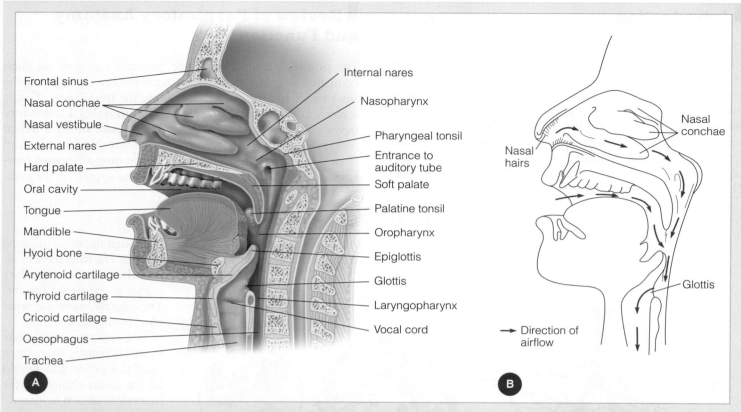

Figure 26-2 **A.** The upper airway contains many blood vessels and serves to heat and humidify the air we breathe. **B.** Note that an important filter is lost when we bypass the upper airway via intubation.

After passing through the nares, air is pulled over the turbinates. These ridges of tissue are covered with a mucous membrane and contain many blood vessels. The mucous membrane traps more particulate matter, and the large surface area of the turbinates warms and humidifies the air we breathe as the air passes over it. Processes such as intubation or a tracheostomy allow inhaled air to skip this trip through the nose, bypassing the humidification and filtering. Because the turbinates contain many blood vessels, they easily swell (causing a stuffy nose) or bleed (epistaxis).

Anyone with hay fever can attest to the severe swelling that can occur in the nasal cavity. In children, foreign bodies such as pencil rubbers, sweets, and beans frequently obstruct a nostril. These items often sit in the nose for a day or two before the child presents with pain and a foul-smelling nasal discharge. Don't try to remove the obstruction yourself. Accident and emergency (A&E) departments are skilled in performing "beanectomies".

Quiet breathing typically allows air to flow through the nose (**Figure 26-2 ▲**). Even people who breathe through their mouth usually have some nasal airflow. It is typically not necessary to tell patients that they must breathe through their nose when you apply a nasal cannula. Unless the nasal passages are actually swollen shut from oedema or trauma, the cannula will function well.

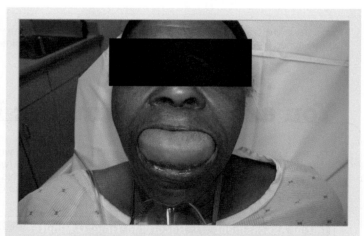

Figure 26-3 Angio-oedema is an acute swelling, usually of the lips and tongue, secondary to an allergic reaction. Some medications cause angio-oedema after the first or second dose.

The mouth and oropharynx also contain many blood vessels and are covered by a mucous membrane. Swelling can be extreme, and potentially dangerous. Bee stings to the lips or tongue can cause profound swelling. Angio-oedema (**Figure 26-3 ▲**) is an allergic reaction that may cause severe swelling of the tongue and lips. Always ask patients who may be experiencing an allergic reaction if their tongue "feels thick". Monitor their speech for symptoms (such as low volume or a raspy voice) of oral or laryngeal swelling.

The oropharynx and nasopharynx meet in the back of the throat at the hypopharynx (sometimes called the posterior pharynx). The gag reflex is most profound in this area. Triggering the gag reflex, on purpose or by accident, can cause vagal bradycardia (a slow heartbeat caused by stimulation of the vagus nerve), vomiting, and increased intracranial pressure. A gag reflex may make the use of many devices difficult or inappropriate 　Figure 26-4 ▸ 　. Conversely, patients with a diminished or absent gag reflex may require endotracheal intubation to help isolate and protect the airway from foreign materials.

The larynx (voicebox) 　Figure 26-5 ▾ 　 and glottis (opening at the top of the trachea) are typically considered the dividing line between the upper airway and the sterile lower airway. The thyroid cartilage is the most obvious external landmark of the larynx. The glottis and vocal cords are found in the middle of the thyroid's cartilaginous structure.

Several cartilages that may be visible when intubating the patient support the vocal cords. The arytenoid cartilages appear as two pearly white lumps at the distal end of each vocal cord. In some people, the cuneiform and corniculate cartilages may also be visible during laryngoscopy. On either side of the glottis, tissue forms a pocket called the piriform fossa 　Figure 26-6 ▸ 　. Sometimes NG tubes or endotracheal (ET) tubes will get stuck here during placement, causing "tenting" that is visible externally on the neck. Any device stuck in a piriform fossa must be withdrawn a few inches and reinserted.

The glottic opening is covered by the epiglottis. Most of us were taught that the epiglottis covers the glottis like a trap door when we swallow, keeping food and liquid from entering the trachea. In reality, many people aspirate around their epiglottis, but others seem to swallow effectively even after their epiglottis has been surgically removed. Because the epiglottis can make it difficult to see the vocal cords, one of your primary tasks during

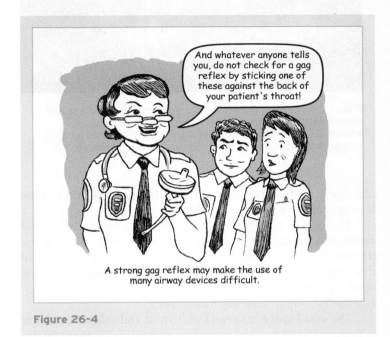

A strong gag reflex may make the use of many airway devices difficult.

Figure 26-4

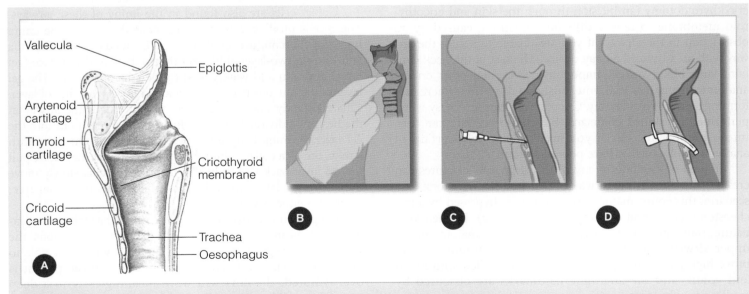

Figure 26-5 It is imperative that you completely understand the anatomy of the larynx in order to perform a number of airway management skills. **A.** Anatomy of the larynx. **B.** Applying pressure to the cricoid cartilage, which compresses the oesophagus while keeping the trachea open (Sellick manoeuvre). **C.** An IV cannula is inserted into the cricothyroid membrane. **D.** A tracheostomy tube is inserted below the cricoid cartilage.

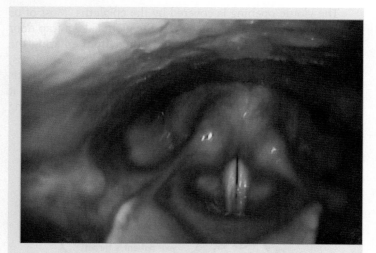

Figure 26-6 The arytenoid cartilages and piriform fossae are sometimes the only landmarks visible during a difficult intubation. The arytenoid cartilages are a pair of small pyramid-shaped cartilages to which the vocal cords are attached.

endotracheal intubation is to identify the epiglottis and use the laryngoscope to move it out of the way.

The cricoid cartilage can be palpated just below the thyroid cartilage in the neck. It forms a complete ring and maintains the trachea in an open position. Pressing on the anterior portion of this ring compresses the oesophagus while keeping the trachea open. Applying pressure to the cricoid cartilage (Sellick manoeuvre) may be helpful in airway maintenance.

The small space between the thyroid and cricoid cartilages is the cricothyroid membrane. The membrane doesn't contain many blood vessels and is covered only by skin and minimal subcutaneous tissue. It is a potential site for performing a cricothyroidotomy (an incision through the skin and cricothyroid membrane to relieve difficulty breathing caused by an obstruction in the airway) if you are unable to secure the airway with an advanced airway device. The rest of the neck contains large blood vessels, important nerves, and other critical anatomic structures that you must avoid cutting when performing a cricothyroidotomy. Cricothyrotomies look easy when performed by skilled clinicians, but this procedure can turn into a bloody disaster if you aren't absolutely certain of anatomic landmarks, or have poor technique.

Trauma or swelling of any of the laryngeal structures can create a life-threatening airway obstruction. In the worst-case scenario, this entire anatomic region may be bypassed by a tracheostomy (a surgical opening into the trachea). By their very nature, traumatic injuries may alter the typical anatomy of the upper airway. Procedures such as a cricothyroidotomy can prove highly challenging when the airway is filled with blood and vomit, and the anatomic landmarks are obscured by swelling or subcutaneous air.

The Lower Airway

Inspired gas is distributed to the millions of alveoli by a network of conducting airways. Gas in these tubes does not come into close contact with capillaries, so it does not participate in ventilation. This wasted ventilation is called anatomic dead space. Typically, anatomic dead space is about 2 ml per kilo of ideal body weight (a 70 kilo person has about 150 ml of anatomic dead space). This dead space remains relatively constant. If a 70 kilo patient took an average breath (tidal volume [V_T] of 700 ml, about 550 ml would participate in ventilation at the alveolar level; the other 150 ml would fill the tubes and would never be exposed to blood flow. If the same patient were to drop his or her V_T to 500 ml, only 350 ml would participate in ventilation, because 150 ml would be stuck in the tubes.

The trunk of these tubes—the tracheobronchial tree—is the trachea. It is about 10 to 13 cm long and extends from the level of the sixth cervical vertebra to its point of bifurcation (carina) at roughly the fifth thoracic vertebra (approximately nipple level) **Figure 26-7 ▸** . At this point, it forks into the right and left mainstem bronchi. In adults, the right mainstem bronchus typically branches at a less acute angle than the left. Thus, if you advance an ET tube too far into an adult, it almost always goes down the right mainstem bronchus. Similarly, aspirated foreign bodies often end up in the right mainstem bronchus.

The mainstem bronchi branch into lobar bronchi, segmental bronchi, subsegmental bronchi, and bronchioles. These structures account for approximately 15 branchings of the airway and are lined with ciliated epithelium. Cilia are little hair-like structures that rhythmically wave in a pattern that helps move particulate matter up and out of the airway **Figure 26-8 ▸** . If a particle gets deeper into the lungs than level 15, there is no mechanism to get it back out.

Goblet cells are also found in the lining of these airways. These cells produce a blanket of mucus that covers the entire lining of the conducting airways. The mucus covers the cilia and forms a two-layered blanket that is thick at the surface (gel layer) and thin and watery next to the cilia (sol layer). The gel layer of the mucous blanket is thick and floats over the sol layer. Cilia constantly push the gel layer up and out of the airway in the healthy individual. As the cilia beat, they reach out into the gel layer, pushing it up and toward the glottis. On the return stroke, the cilia collapse into the sol layer, so that they don't pull the gel layer back down. In this manner, the cilia slowly move the entire gel layer up and out of the tracheobronchial tree, where it is either swallowed or expectorated.

If a person is dehydrated, or if he or she has taken medications such as antihistamines that dry the normal secretions, the sol layer will begin to dry up, and the cilia will not be able to move secretions effectively. The same is true if the patient is overhydrated: the cilia will wave meaninglessly in a deep watery layer without ever affecting the thick gel layer.

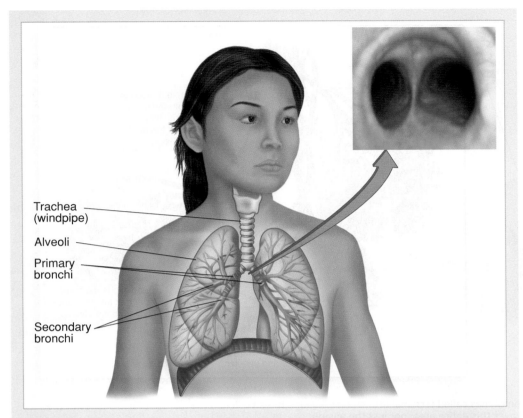

Figure 26-7 The carina is the point of bifurcation of the right and left mainstem bronchi. In an adult, it is located at roughly the fifth intercostal space.

Labels in figure:
- Trachea (windpipe)
- Alveoli
- Primary bronchi
- Secondary bronchi

Smooth muscle surrounds the conducting airways down to the subsegmental level. Bronchospasm occurs when the smooth muscle constricts around these larger airways. Below this level, bronchodilator medications have little effect upon the airways. Wheezing that is resolved with bronchodilator medication was probably caused by constriction of the smooth muscles. Wheezing that is not resolved with these medications may be caused by a variety of pathological conditions deeper in the tracheobronchial tree.

The terminal airways and alveoli include branches 16 through 24 of the tracheobronchial tree, the so-called terminal bronchioles. The tracheobronchial tree ends with the alveoli, but the transfer of oxygen and carbon dioxide can nevertheless take place across both the alveoli and the terminal bronchioles. It is often helpful to think of alveoli as little balloons at the end of a straw. Alveoli cluster around the terminal bronchioles, and capillaries cover the alveoli and

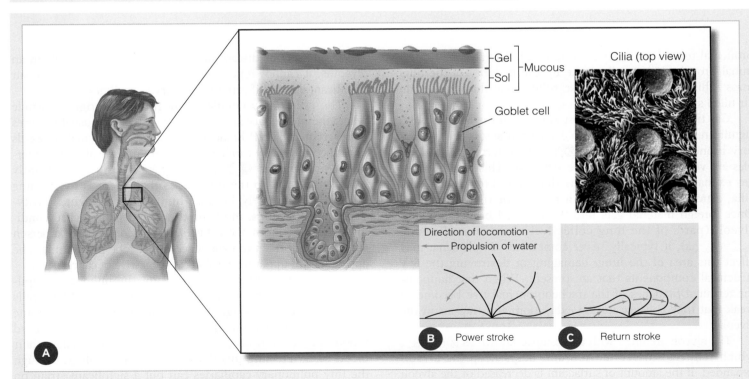

Labels in figure:
- Gel
- Sol
- Mucous
- Goblet cell
- Cilia (top view)
- Direction of locomotion
- Propulsion of water
- **B** Power stroke
- **C** Return stroke
- **A**

Figure 26-8 Cilia line the larger airways of the respiratory tract (**A**). Their regular pattern of movement between the gel and sol layers of mucus helps move foreign material out of the tracheobronchial tree (**B** and **C**).

Inset photo: © Dr. Kessel & Dr. Kardon/Tissue & Organs/Visuals Unlimited

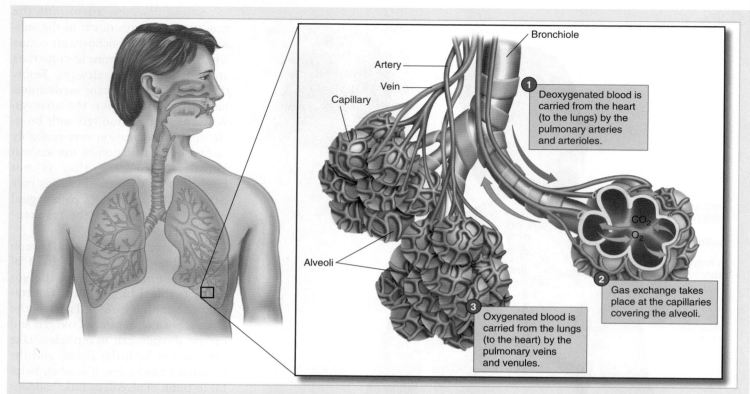

Bronchiole

Artery

Vein

Capillary

① Deoxygenated blood is carried from the heart (to the lungs) by the pulmonary arteries and arterioles.

CO_2
O_2

Alveoli

② Gas exchange takes place at the capillaries covering the alveoli.

③ Oxygenated blood is carried from the lungs (to the heart) by the pulmonary veins and venules.

Figure 26-9 The respiratory bronchioles, sometimes called terminal bronchioles, include the alveoli and the last several branches of the tracheobronchial tree. Gas exchange occurs over this entire area, not just the alveoli.

bronchial tubes from level 16 to level 24. The alveoli and terminal bronchioles actually make up the majority of the lung mass. This tissue feels more like solid tissue than it does an air-filled sponge.

Gas transfer is probably most efficient in the alveoli, but a significant amount of gas is also exchanged across the respiratory bronchioles (**Figure 26-9** ▲). These terminal bronchioles are very thin and have little structure. This is helpful for gas exchange, but it also means that these bronchioles lack cilia, a mucous blanket, smooth muscle, or rigid structures. Once foreign material gets into the terminal bronchioles and alveoli (parts of the lung collectively known as the lung parenchyma), it typically never comes out. Emphysema may affect this area of the lung, damaging or destroying the few structural components that are present. When that happens, the terminal branches of the tracheobronchial tree become so weak that they collapse during exhalation, and trap air in the alveoli.

The alveoli are lined with a substance known as surfactant, which reduces surface tension and helps keep the alveoli expanded. If the amount of surfactant is decreased or the alveoli are not inflated, the alveoli collapse, which results in a condition known as atelectasis.

If smoking or disease destroys certain types of cells in an alveolus, it cannot repair itself. Conversely, alveoli can repair significant damage if certain cells survive an illness.

The pulmonary circulation begins at the right ventricle where the pulmonary artery (the only artery that usually carries deoxygenated blood) branches into increasingly smaller vessels until the pulmonary capillary bed surrounds the alveoli and terminal bronchioles (**Figure 26-10** ▶). There is significantly more circulation to the lung bases than there is to the lung apices. Unfortunately, because humans are upright, gravity-dependent creatures, most infections and pathological conditions affect the bases of our lungs. It is uncommon for a person who isn't bedridden to experience upper lobe pneumonia. The appearance of upper lobe lesions is suggestive of cancer.

Like all the capillaries in the body, the pulmonary capillaries are very narrow, and typically allow only red blood cells to pass through in single-file fashion. People with chronic lung disease and chronic hypoxia often make a surplus of red blood cells over time (polycythaemia), which makes their blood thick. Pushing this thicker-than-normal blood through the tiny pulmonary capillaries can put a significant strain on the right side of the heart. When alveoli are distended by COPD, they push against the capillary bed, further narrowing the capillaries and straining the right side of the heart. Right heart failure secondary to chronic lung disease is known as <u>cor pulmonale</u>.

Airway Problems Versus Breathing Problems

From your first cardiopulmonary resuscitation (CPR) lesson, the differences between maintaining the airway and breathing for the patient are highlighted. Unfortunately, a paramedic can still easily become confused between pathological conditions that affect one versus the other. Many patients present with an airway that can use a little assistance. No one should be snoring, gurgling, squeaking, or using accessory muscles to inhale. You must remain vigilant that secretions, soft tissue,

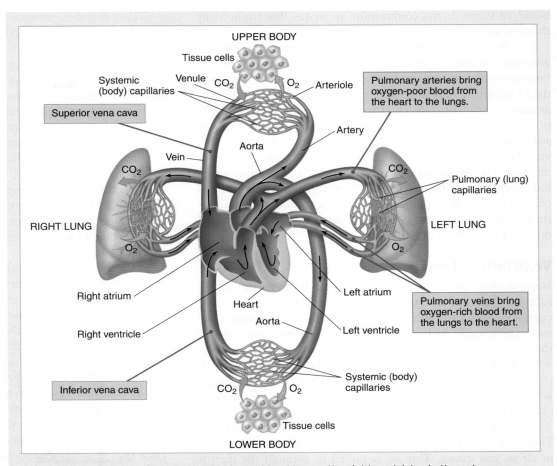

Figure 26-10 Pulmonary circulation begins as blood leaves the right ventricle via the pulmonary artery. The pulmonary capillary bed brings red blood cells very close to the terminal bronchioles. There is more perfusion to the bases of the lungs than to the apices. After picking up oxygen, the blood returns to the left atrium via the pulmonary veins.

You are the Paramedic Part 2

As you apply oxygen and obtain vital signs, you notice that the nail beds and oral mucosa of your patient are bluish (cyanosis). You adjust the sensor location of the pulse oximeter and obtain a reading. The patient's wife tells you that her husband has been running a fever, has experienced progressive weakness, and has had a productive cough (with thick, yellowish green sputum) for the past 4 to 5 days. She also tells you that her husband has been up all night struggling to breathe. He also has COPD and has smoked two packs of cigarettes a day since he was 15 years old. On auscultation of the chest, you note crackles in all lung fields on both inspiration and expiration.

Vital Signs	Recording Time: 5 Minutes
Level of consciousness	A (Alert to person, place, and day)
Skin	Pale, cool extremities, perspiring
Pulse	110 beats/min, weak; occasionally irregular
Blood pressure	108/54 mm Hg
SpO_2	75% (receiving oxygen via nonrebreathing mask at 15 l/min)
Temperature	39°C
ECG	Sinus tachycardia with occasional premature ventricular contractions

4. Given the patient's presentation, which assessment tools should you use to obtain a greater understanding of the patient's medical condition?

5. What other treatments could you consider?

blood, or vomit do not compromise an airway that you initially thought was open.

At the same time, an open airway does not ensure that an adequate volume of gas is moving in and out of the lungs. Proper ventilation is necessary to provide adequate oxygen to the bloodstream and to remove carbon dioxide. Increasing the amount of available oxygen ensures that even a patient who is not moving adequate volumes of gas (eg, hypoventilating) can still maintain adequate oxygen saturation. Unfortunately, if ventilation remains inadequate, carbon dioxide levels will increase. Hypoventilating patients become hypercapnic (have too much carbon dioxide in their blood) and acidotic (the pH of their arterial blood falls too low). Both conditions can interrupt important body systems and, if uncorrected over a period of time, can result in death.

Ventilation Revisited

Many airway problems can be bypassed by inserting an ET tube. By contrast, alterations in breathing can be much more complex. They can involve problems with the conducting airways (branches), such as asthma or bronchitis; difficulties at the alveolar level, such as pneumonia or emphysema; problems with the muscles and nerves that make breathing work, as in Guillain-Barré syndrome or spinal cord injury; or problems with the rigid structure of the thorax that allows the pressure changes that make breathing work, such as flail chest.

We are usually negative-pressure breathers (air suckers). Think about a vacuum cleaner at the base of the lungs sucking in air as you inhale. This air is pulled in through the mouth and the nose, over the turbinates, and around the complex terrain of the epiglottis and glottis. Air typically does not enter the oesophagus and stomach because it is preferentially sucked into the trachea (**Figure 26-11** ▾).

This negative-pressure vacuum effect occurs because the thorax is essentially an airtight box with a flexible diaphragm (the major muscle of breathing) at the bottom and an open tube (the trachea) at the top. During quiet breathing, when the diaphragm flattens, the overall size of the container increases, and air is sucked in through the tube at the top to fill the increasing space inside the thorax. You can increase the amount of air you move each minute (minute ventilation) by dropping the diaphragm more aggressively (deep breathing, or hyperpnoea) or by breathing more rapidly (tachypnoea). To breathe even more deeply, you can use additional muscles to pull the ribs up and out, further increasing both the size of the thoracic cavity as well as increasing the negative-pressure environment and moving larger volumes of air. Clearly, disruptions of the thoracic cage will hinder your ability to move air by this mechanism.

Holes in the thorax provide another place for air to be sucked in, resulting in a sucking chest wound (**Figure 26-12** ▾). When multiple ribs are broken in more than one place (flail chest), free-floating sections of the thorax get pulled in when you breathe, limiting the amount of air that can be sucked in through the trachea. Infants and small children have a lot of elastic cartilage in their chest wall; when they use a lot of muscle to breathe, the sternum or ribs often collapse, causing recession.

When you ventilate someone with positive-pressure (eg, with a pocket mask or bag-valve-mask ventilation), air is forced into the upper airway and flows into both the trachea and oesophagus unless steps are taken to help direct it into the trachea (**Figure 26-13** ▸). Indeed, positive-pressure ventilation with bag-valve-mask ventilation or a pocket mask is physiologically the opposite of normal (negative-pressure) ventilation.

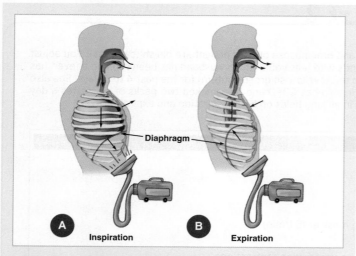

Figure 26-11 Normal ventilation is negative-pressure ventilation, meaning that we suck air into our lungs, much as a vacuum cleaner sucks in air. The diaphragm flattens, creating a negative pressure in the chest which causes the lungs to fill (**A**). When the diaphragm relaxes, the pressure increases and the lungs empty (**B**). Compare with positive-pressure ventilation, shown in Figure 26-13.

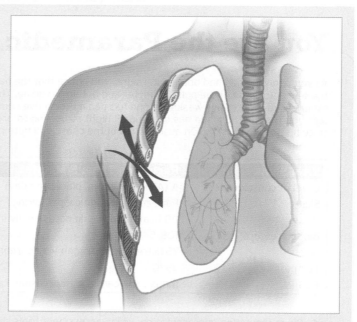

Figure 26-12 A sucking chest wound reduces ventilation by allowing air to enter the thorax during the inspiratory or negative-pressure phase of ventilation.

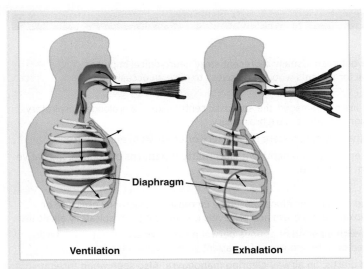

Figure 26-13 Positive-pressure ventilation is physiologically the opposite of normal ventilation. Air is pushed into the respiratory tract with bag-valve-mask ventilation and can go into the oesophagus and stomach unless careful technique is applied. Compare with negative-pressure ventilation, shown in Figure 26-12.

Exhalation is usually a passive process. After the size of the thorax has increased during inhalation, the components of the respiratory system return to their original places, and air is pushed out of the trachea under positive pressure. When a patient has trouble exhaling, for example, in asthma, reactive airway disease, or COPD, he or she may need to use the abdominal muscles to push air out. When this occurs, exhalation is no longer a passive process. Watch your patient work as he or she breathes. Is the patient having trouble pulling air in or pushing air out? Difficulty in exhalation usually indicates obstructive disease; difficulty in inhalation may indicate upper airway obstruction.

The neurological control of respiration is complex. At least four parts of the brain are responsible for the smooth, rhythmic respirations that we take for granted—one area helps control rate, another depth, another inspiratory pause, and yet another rhythmicity. Patients with traumatic brain injuries may exhibit bizarre respiratory patterns when one or more of these respiratory centres are damaged or deprived of adequate blood flow. Table 26-1 ► summarises the various breathing patterns.

Most of these respiratory centres are in and around the brain stem Figure 26-14 ▼ . Patients who suffer serious trauma to the upper cerebral hemispheres (such as from a gunshot wound) are often still breathing despite mortal wounds. Apneustic breathing results from damage to the apneustic centre in the brain, which regulates inspiratory pause. A patient exhibiting apneustic respirations will have a short, brisk inhalation with a long pause before exhalation. This pattern is indicative of severe pressure within the cranium or direct trauma to the brain. Similarly, Biot respirations are seen when the centre that controls breathing rhythm is damaged. This respiratory pattern is grossly irregular, sometimes with lengthy apnoeic periods.

Cheyne-Stokes respirations are more of a high-brain function. Many deep sleepers or intoxicated people will exhibit this type of respiratory pattern. The depth of breathing (or volume of snoring) gradually increases, then decreases (crescendo-decrescendo), followed by an apnoeic period. The apnoeic period is usually brief in the relatively healthy patient. Exaggerated Cheyne-Stokes respirations may be seen in patients who have a severe brain injury, where the crescendo-decrescendo is much more prominent. The apnoeic period may last 30 to 60 seconds.

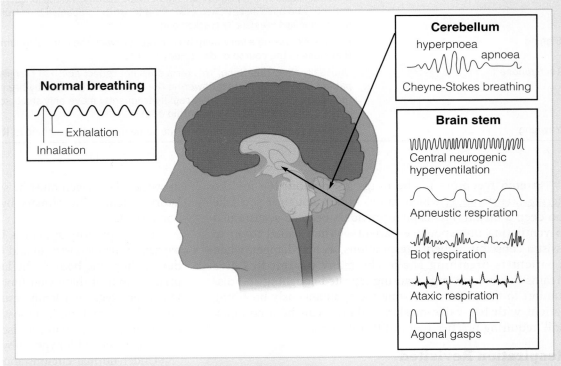

Figure 26-14 The neurological control of respiration is complex, and many variations in the respiratory pattern may be noted in the scenario of brain injury. The respiratory patterns shown have been documented using an end-tidal carbon dioxide detector. Note that most irregular breathing patterns are controlled by the brain stem.

Table 26-1	Breathing Patterns
Pattern	**Comments**
Agonal	Irregular gasps that are few and far between. Usually represent stray neurological impulses in the dying patient. It is not unusual for patients who are pulseless to have an occasional agonal gasp.
Apneustic	When the pneumotaxic centre in the brain is damaged, the apneustic centre causes a prolonged inspiratory hold (fish breathing). This ominous sign indicates severe brain injury.
Ataxic	Completely irregular respirations that indicate severe brain injury or brain-stem herniation.
Biot respirations	Respirations with an irregular pattern, rate, and depth with intermittent patterns of apnoea. Indicative of severe brain injury or brain-stem herniation.
Bradypnoea	Unusually slow respirations.
Central neurogenic hyperventilation	Tachypnoeic hyperpnoea. Rapid and deep respirations caused by increased intracranial pressure or direct brain injury. Drives carbon dioxide levels down and pH levels up, resulting in respiratory alkalosis.
Cheyne-Stokes respirations	Crescendo-decrescendo breathing with a period of apnoea between each cycle. It is not considered ominous unless grossly exaggerated or in the context of a patient who has brain trauma.
Cough	Forced exhalation against a closed glottis; an airway-clearing manoeuvre. Also seen when foreign substances irritate the airways. Controlled by the cough centre in the brain. Antitussive medications work on the cough centre to reduce this sometimes-annoying physiological response.
Eupnoea	Normal breathing.
Hiccup	Spasmodic contraction of the diaphragm causing short exhalations with a characteristic sound. Sometimes seen in cases of diaphragmatic (or phrenic nerve) irritation from acute myocardial infarction, ulcer disease, or endotracheal intubation.
Hyperpnoea	Unusually deep breathing. Seen in various neurological or chemical disorders. Certain drugs may stimulate this type of breathing in patients who have overdosed. It does not reflect respiratory rate—only respiratory depth.
Hypopnoea	Unusually shallow respirations.
Kussmaul respirations	The same pattern as central neurogenic hyperventilation, but caused by the body's response to metabolic acidosis; the body is trying to rid itself of blood acetone via the lungs. Kussmaul respirations are seen in patients who have diabetic ketoacidosis, and are accompanied by a fruity (acetone) breath odour. The mouth and lips are usually cracked and dry.
Sighing	Periodically taking a very deep breath (about twice the normal volume). Sighing forces open alveoli that close in the course of day-to-day events.
Tachypnoea	Unusually rapid breathing. This term does not reflect depth of respiration, nor does it mean that the patient is hyperventilating (lowering the carbon dioxide level by breathing too fast and too deep). In fact, patients who breathe very rapidly frequently move only small volumes of air and are *hypo*ventilating (much like a panting dog).
Yawning	Yawning seems to be beneficial in the same manner that sighing is. It also appears to be contagious!

Stretch receptors in the lungs are responsible for the Hering-Breuer reflex, which causes you to cough if you take too deep a breath. Prehospital providers become accustomed to ventilating unresponsive patients. When called upon to assist a conscious patient's respirations, as may happen when a patient is breathing shallowly, many paramedics give breaths that are too large, causing repeated coughing and discomfort to the patient. Assisting the spontaneously breathing patient with bag-valve-mask ventilation can be a complex skill, requiring practice that is difficult to find.

Respiration Revisited

Respiration is the process by which oxygen is taken into the body, distributed to the cells, and used by the cells to make energy. Respiration takes place in each cell. It involves using oxygen and glucose to make energy that allows the cell to do

its work. The oxygen must be supplied by the lungs and circulatory systems. The primary byproduct of this process is carbon dioxide.

The respiratory system is involved in the delivery of the oxygen to the bloodstream and the removal of the waste carbon dioxide from the body. If the lungs are not functioning appropriately, both of these vital functions may be impaired. Failure to deliver oxygen efficiently results in cellular hypoxia. Hypoxia kills cells by making it impossible for them to make enough energy to do their work; it also causes acidosis. We can often help the patient with hypoxia by providing additional oxygen.

Under normal circumstances, the carbon dioxide evolved during cellular respiration is returned to the lungs by the circulatory system, where it is exhaled during ventilation. When the lungs are not working adequately, carbon dioxide is not efficiently disposed of and accumulates in the blood. This carbon dioxide infarctions present as congestive heart failure, as do renal crises. Tachypnoea can signal anxiety, diabetes, or shock. In addition, the vast majority of chronically ill patients have a respiratory component to their disease. A whole host of pathological conditions can masquerade as respiratory distress, especially in patients who have underlying respiratory disease. Don't be too quick to conclude that your patient's *only* problem is a relatively straightforward respiratory issue. Always dig deeper to determine what else may be triggering or worsening the patient's respiratory distress.

The Focused Physical Examination

By the time you have elicited the history of a patient who has respiratory complaints, you should already have some important information about the patient's physical signs. In particular, you should have observed the patient's level of consciousness, position, degree of distress, and so forth. This section presents the components of the physical examination in sequence, noting at each step the points of particular relevance to the dyspnoeic patient.

Neck Examination

In the neck, look for <u>jugular venous distention</u> when a patient is in a semi-sitting position. Jugular venous distention is a condition in which the jugular veins are engorged with blood. It is common in cardiac patients but may also be present in patients with COPD. Healthy young adults often demonstrate jugular venous distention when they are supine (lying on their back), and it is common to see gross jugular venous distention when people are laughing or singing Figure 26-18 ◄ . When jugular venous distention is present in patients who are sitting upright, it can provide a rough measure of the pressure in the right atrium of the heart. Distended neck veins may implicate cardiac failure as the source of the patient's dyspnoea. Jugular venous distention may also indicate high pressure in the thorax, which keeps the blood from draining out of the head and neck. Cardiac tamponade, pneumothorax, heart failure, and COPD can all cause jugular venous disten-

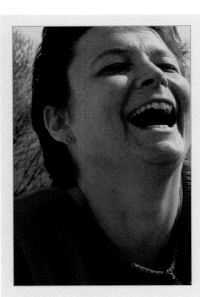

Figure 26-18 Jugular venous distention may be a normal finding in a healthy young adult who is supine or laughing. But in an adult who is sitting upright, it may indicate blood backing up as it tries to enter the thorax or the right atrium.

tion. The abdominojugular test (hepatojugular reflux) is positive when the jugular veins engorge during pressure on the abdomen for 10 seconds; it often indicates left-sided heart disease.

Obviously, jugular venous distention must be interpreted in light of the patient's position and other vital signs. The trauma patient who demonstrates grossly distended jugular veins despite a blood pressure of 80/40 mm Hg should cause considerable concern. A healthy 20 year old who has jugular venous distention when lying flat (but not while sitting) is of little concern.

While looking at the neck, note the trachea. Tracheal deviation is a classic—albeit late—sign of a tension pneumothorax Figure 26-19 ▼ . Tension pneumothorax is very difficult to see except in extreme cases. On an X-ray, the trachea can clearly be seen deviating because of a tension pneumothorax. Consider

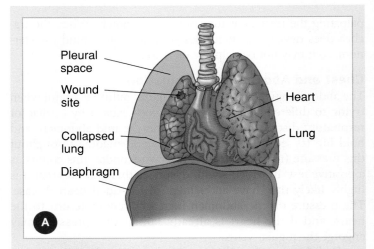

A

Pleural space
Wound site
Collapsed lung
Diaphragm
Heart
Lung

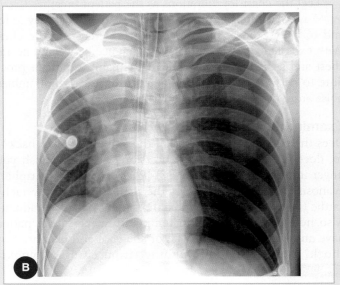

B

Figure 26-19 A pneumothorax occurs when air leaks into the pleural space between the lung and the chest wall (**A**). The X-ray image (**B**) shows a collapsed lung on the right, which appears darker.

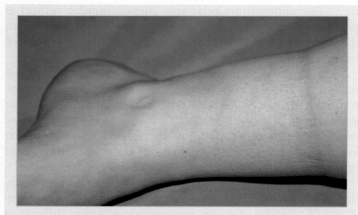

Figure 26-20 Pitting oedema is present when you palpate the area, and your fingers leave temporary depressions in the tissue.

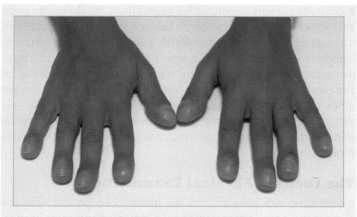

Figure 26-21 Digital clubbing is often a sign of chronic hypoxia. It usually accompanies chronic respiratory conditions, but sometimes it can be hereditary or be caused by heart or other disease.

palpating the trachea at the suprasternal notch. When the trachea does deviate, it often does so at a point behind the sternum, so it may not be palpable or visible.

Chest and Abdominal Examination

The abdominojugular test (hepatojugular reflux) is useful when trying to differentiate between dyspnoea caused by cardiac or respiratory disease. Apply pressure on the mid-abdomen, and hold for 10 seconds. If the jugular veins engorge throughout this pressure (not just for the first few seconds), this counts as a positive test. In patients with dyspnoea this indicates that it is highly likely they have an element of left-sided heart disease. The pressure on the abdomen increases venous return to the heart, and if the heart is already failing that pressure may engorge the jugular veins.

Feel the chest for vibrations as the patient breathes (tactile fremitus); secretions in the large airways are usually easy to feel and to hear. Some people recommend percussing the chest. With experience, you can tell the difference between a normal chest and a pneumothorax, but this remains a difficult procedure to perform in the prehospital setting because of ambient noise around you and the patient.

Examination of the Extremities

Does the patient have oedema of the ankles or lower back? If so, does it pit, and leave a depression, when you push your finger into the oedema Figure 26-20 ▲ ? Is there peripheral cyanosis? Check the pulse. Is the patient profoundly tachycardic (from exertion or hypoxia)? Is there pulsus paradoxus? Also note the patient's skin temperature. Does the patient have an obvious fever, or is he or she cool and clammy from shock? Is there digital clubbing (from chronic hypoxia) Figure 26-21 ▶ ?

Data Collection

As appropriate to your patient care plan, attach any monitors that are immediately available to you. Repeated vital signs, ECG, and pulse oximetry readings are the data most commonly

collected. In some situations, depending on available equipment, you might also record peak expiratory flow, end-tidal carbon dioxide, or even transcutaneous carbon monoxide levels. (Monitoring devices are discussed later in the chapter.)

The Stethoscope

As far as stethoscopes go, the following guideline applies: the longer the tubing, the more extraneous the noise you will probably hear. Avoid overly long stethoscopes. Higher-quality stethoscopes have a tubing-within-the-tubing design that limits external noise interference. Although the Sprague-Rappaport design is popular Figure 26-22 ▼ , its two parallel tubes often bang against each other while moving, which can create extra noise.

Practically speaking, your stethoscope, if you buy one for yourself, is the single most important investment you will make as a paramedic. Buy the best you can afford and take good care of it. Periodically check to make sure the earpieces are clean and clear of earwax. Stethoscopes have been shown to carry a wide range of bacteria, so on a regular basis wipe it with 70% alcohol swabs even if it appears to be clean; this also helps maintain it in good condition. It is

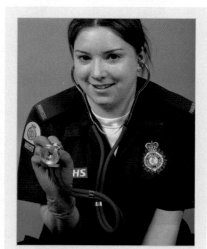

Figure 26-22 Earpieces should follow the normal (forward) slant of your ear canals. Note the Sprague-Rappaport–style stethoscope.

not good practice to share stethoscopes with colleagues.

The diaphragm of the stethoscope is for high-pitched sounds (breath sounds); the bell (if present) is for low-pitched sounds (some heart tones). If you press the bell firmly against the skin, it stretches the skin beneath it and makes it act like a diaphragm. Hence, the bell should be placed lightly against the skin if you hope to hear the lower-pitched sounds. Some newer stethoscopes take advantage of this principle, allowing a single head to help transmit high- and low-pitched sounds based upon the pressure exerted by the operator. In older style stethoscopes, the bell rotates, allowing you to better hear the sounds you are trying to assess.

Your ear canals tend to point anteriorly in your skull (toward your eyes). You may wish to tilt the earpieces on your stethoscope more forward for a better fit. But be careful: you may hear little or nothing if you accidentally place your stethoscope in your ears backward, causing the earpieces to hit the sides of your ear canal.

Auscultation

Whenever possible, auscultate the lungs systematically. While we tend to compare the left and right sides, the lungs are not symmetrical. The right lung has three lobes: right upper lobe (RUL), right middle lobe (RML), and right lower lobe (RLL). The left lung has only two lobes: left upper lobe (LUL) and left lower lobe (LLL). Understand where you must listen to hear the various lobes **Figure 26-23 ▶**. Some of the pathological conditions you will listen for are gravity-dependent, meaning most pneumonias and congestive heart failure will tend to be found in the lung bases. In the case of wheezing, it may be diffuse and spread throughout the lung fields. The bases are almost exclusively heard by listening to the patient's back or at least their axillae. The upper lobes, which rarely have abnormalities, are heard by listening to the anterior part of the chest. The right middle lobe can best be heard by listening just beneath, or lateral to, the right breast. The best left-right differentiation can be appreciated in the midaxillary line; this is the best place to listen for ET tube placement. If you listen to the anterior part of the chest, you are very close to the noisemaker (the endotracheal tube), whether it is in the trachea or the oesophagus.

Specific Breath Sounds

The breath sounds you hear are made by turbulent airflow in the large airways, which are transmitted through the remainder of the lungs and chest wall to your stethoscope. Normal breath sounds can be broadly grouped into 2 main types. Tracheobronchial sounds are loud, harsh and heard over the trachea and main bronchi; they have an expiratory phase as long as the inspiratory phase. Vesicular sounds are more common, they are quiet, soft and heard over all areas of the chest distal to the central large airways; importantly the expiratory sound is much shorter than inspiration (about one-third of the length). In small areas near but not over the central airways you may identify sounds between these two extremes. You will want to listen to a large number of healthy lungs to become familiar with the different sounds **Figure 26-24 ▶**. Pathological conditions may cause you to hear some normal breath sounds in abnormal places!

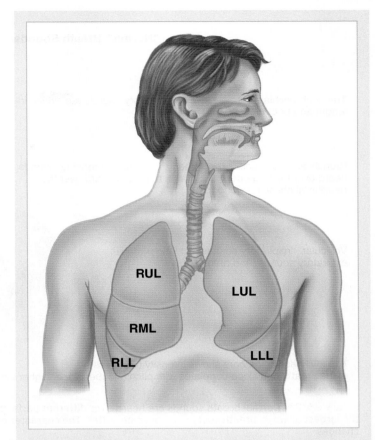

Figure 26-23 The lungs are not symmetrical. Most acute pathological conditions are best heard in the lung bases, requiring you to listen to the patient's back or axillae. The right middle lobe is best heard beneath the right breast, or just lateral to it. LUL, left upper lobe; LLL, left lower lobe; RUL, right upper lobe; RML, right middle lobe; RLL, right lower lobe.

Sound moves better through fluid than it does through air. Thus, the more air that is present in a patient's chest (as in COPD or asthma), the quieter the breath sounds will be in the periphery. Conversely, in a dense lung, the breath sound will be louder and harsher (as long as air is entering the bronchus), with the expiratory sound transmitted more clearly. Hence, if an area of lung has consolidation (as in pneumonia, where the inflamed alveoli are filled with pus), then the breath sounds will be tracheobronchial in nature. They are loud, harsh and with equally long inspiratory and expiratory phases. If heard away from the large airways (when they are normal) these are called bronchial breath sounds, because you appear to be listening over the main bronchi, when in fact you are on the periphery of the chest wall over an area of consolidation. They may also occur in atelectasis, when large areas of lung collapse.

Breath sounds will be diminished (quiet) if there is generalised reduced airflow (obstructive lung disease, poor respiratory effort), or localised reduced airflow (pus or mucus plug in a bronchus). An increased distance between the lung and the stethoscope (obesity, pleural effusion), particularly if that area is filled with air (pneumothorax), will also cause reduced breath sounds. Because breath sounds vary between individuals, it is

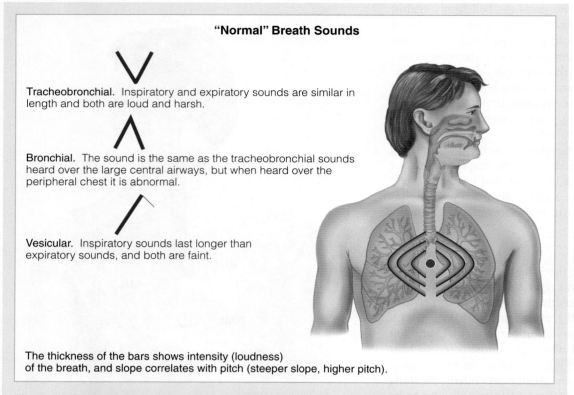

"Normal" Breath Sounds

Tracheobronchial. Inspiratory and expiratory sounds are similar in length and both are loud and harsh.

Bronchial. The sound is the same as the tracheobronchial sounds heard over the large central airways, but when heard over the peripheral chest it is abnormal.

Vesicular. Inspiratory sounds last longer than expiratory sounds, and both are faint.

The thickness of the bars shows intensity (loudness) of the breath, and slope correlates with pitch (steeper slope, higher pitch).

Figure 26-24 Normal breath sounds are heard over different parts of the chest. As you move away from the largest airways, breath sounds will become softer. The character of inspiration versus exhalation also changes.

useful to compare sounds from the same location on both sides of the chest. This enables you to identify one-sided pathological conditions.

Both breath sounds and vocalisations travel more efficiently through a firm, fluid-filled lung than through a healthy lung, but travel poorly through a hyperinflated lung. If a patient speaks while you are auscultating the chest, you cannot usually understand what he or she is saying through your stethoscope. If you can, it may mean consolidation from pneumonia or atelectasis. You will likely hear these sounds directly only over the consolidated lobe. **Table 26-2 ▶** lists tests that indicate consolidation.

Adventitious (abnormal) breath sounds are the extra noises that you may hear on top of the breath sounds described previously. Continuous sounds (for example, a wheeze) can be heard across some portion of each breath. Discontinuous sounds are the instantaneous pops, snaps, and clicks that we often identify as crackles **Figure 26-25 ▶** .

Wheezes are high-pitched, whistling sounds made by air being forced through narrowed airways, which makes them vibrate, much like the reed in a musical instrument. Wheezing may be diffuse, as in asthma and congestive heart failure, or localised, as when a foreign body obstructs a bronchus. Pathological conditions such as asthma rarely cause one-sided wheezing. Ask the patient to cough and listen again if you hear a sound on only one side; it could be caused by the movement

of secretions. Wheeze indicates obstruction of the lower airways, usually from bronchospasm, secretions, or inflammation. Wheeze is often an expiratory noise, as the shrinking lung compresses already narrowed bronchioles. The volume of the wheeze is not associated with the severity, but some evidence suggests the more prolonged the wheeze the more severe the narrowing. Rhonchi are low-pitched wheezes (also described as rattling or snoring), caused by secretions in the larger bronchi narrowing the airways. Stridor is a harsh, high pitched wheeze normally heard on inspiration, it indicates upper airway obstruction.

Crackles (also called crepitations or rales) are any discontinuous noises heard on auscultation. They are caused by the popping open of small airways that have closed on expiration (fine crackles) or the bubbling of air through fluid (coarse crackles). They are usually associated with increased fluid in the lungs, or disease effecting lung compliance such as atelectasis, fibrosis, or COPD. Fine crackles are often inspiratory noises, but the coarse, gurgling crackles of excessive secretions tend to spread over expiration as well.

The most ominous breath sounds are no breath sounds at all. They mean the patient is not moving enough air to ventilate the lungs. *Silence means danger!*

Table 26-2	Signs of Consolidation
Sign	**Test**
Bronchophony	When the patient says "99" repeatedly, it should sound like a hum. Through consolidated lung, you can understand the words.
Egophony	The patient says "eeeeee" while you are auscultating, and you hear "aaaaaa".
Whispered pectoriloquy	The patient whispers while you are auscultating, and you can understand what is said.
Bronchial breath sounds	Peripheral loud, harsh sound with equally long inspiratory and expiratory phases.

Table 26-4	Infections That Can Impair the Upper Airway
Infection	**Comments**
Croup	Viral infection of area around glottis. Most common in children between 6 months and 3 years of age. Usually occurs in middle of night when air gets cool (in spring and autumn). Child has classic seal-bark cough. May be distressing but is not typically fatal. Also called laryngotracheobronchitis. Do not manipulate the airway.
Epiglottitis	Severe, rapidly progressive infection of epiglottis and surrounding tissues that may be fatal because of sudden respiratory obstruction. Most common infectious organism is *Haemophilus influenzea* type b. Vaccination has helped make acute epiglottitis rare. Unlike croup, patients may present at any age and at any time of year. Patients typically drool and have a fever, hoarse voice, and purposeful hyperextension. Epiglottitis is a true emergency. Do not manipulate airway.
Peritonsillar abscess (quinsy)	Uncommon in children (more common in young adults). Abscess forms behind palatine tonsil on one side. Patient has fever and sore throat. May be mistaken for epiglottitis until you look in throat and see lateral abscess (unilateral tonsillar swelling). Do not manipulate the airway.
Retropharyngeal abscess	Most common in children, in whom infections from retropharyngeal lymph nodes can flourish. May also be caused by direct trauma to pharynx. Patient may have fever and sudden stridor. May be mistaken for epiglottitis until laryngoscope examination reveals huge retropharyngeal pus sack (instead of cherry-red epiglottis). Do not manipulate the airway.
Diphtheria	Causative bacterium attacks and kills layer of epithelial tissue, creating pseudomembrane that is often seen in tonsillar area. Membrane (and swelling of upper airway caused by disease) can obstruct upper airway. Most children receive diphtheria, tetanus, and pertussis (DTP) immunisation and receive boosters. Do not manipulate the airway.
Enormous tonsils	Palatine tonsils can swell excessively, resulting in fever, difficulty swallowing, and throat pain. Tonsils can grow to golf-ball size in some individuals. Severely swollen tonsils rarely compromise the airway but can cause snoring or stridor. Do not manipulate the airway.

have had trauma or who overdosed. Follow these guidelines when treating such patients:

1. Aggressively reduce the risk of aspiration by avoiding gastric distention when ventilating. The stomach may need decompressing with an NG tube in hospital.

2. Aggressively monitor the patient's ability to protect his or her own airway, and seek to protect the patient's airway with an advanced airway if this is impossible.

3. Aggressively treat aspiration with suction and airway control if steps 1 and 2 fail!

If basic life-support manoeuvres fail to clear an obstructed airway, use laryngoscopy and Magill forceps and, if necessary, perform a needle or surgical cricothyroidotomy.

Aspiration could also refer to foreign body airway obstruction. Remember that most adults choke when they are intoxicated or traumatised or have a reduced gag reflex from stroke or ageing. Chronic aspiration of food is also a common cause of pneumonitis in older patients. Make sure you don't make the situation worse by allowing these patients to eat when they are having difficulty breathing.

Obstructive Airway Diseases

Obstructive airway diseases are characterised by diffuse obstruction to airflow within the lungs. The most common obstructive airway diseases are emphysema and chronic bronchitis (chronic diseases), and asthma (an acutely episodic syndrome). Emphysema and chronic bronchitis are collectively classified as COPD because the changes in pulmonary structure and function are chronic, progressive, and irreversible. Asthma is often considered a separate entity because it is usually a condition of *reversible* airway narrowing; however, some types of chronic asthma are a form of COPD.

Obstructive disease occurs when the positive pressure of exhalation causes the small airways to pinch shut, trapping gas in the alveoli. The harder the patient tries to push air out, the more it gets trapped in the alveoli Figure 26-32 ▶ . Hence, patients with obstructive disease end up with large amounts of gas trapped in their lungs that they can't effectively expel. Patients with obstructive disease learn that if they push the gas out slowly at a low pressure, they can exhale more than if they try to push it out hard and fast.

Patients with obstructive airway disease may demonstrate a variety of physical findings that can alert you to the nature of their disease:

■ **Pursed-lip breathing.** Breathing in this way allows patients to push a breath out slowly under controlled pressure.

■ **Increased inspiratory-to-expiratory (I:E) ratio.** The I:E ratio is typically 1:2 in healthy people breathing quietly (it takes about twice as long to exhale as it does to inhale). Patients who are very sick with obstructive disease may have an I:E ratio of 1:6 or 1:8.

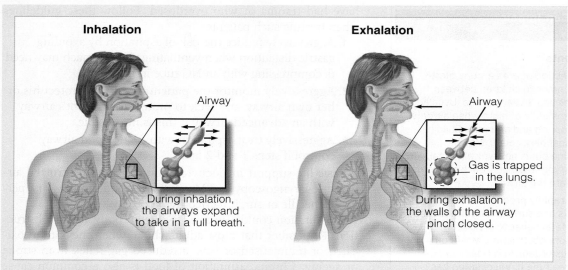

Inhalation

Airway

During inhalation, the airways expand to take in a full breath.

Exhalation

Airway

Gas is trapped in the lungs.

During exhalation, the walls of the airway pinch closed.

Figure 26-32 Obstructive disease involves changes to the smaller airways that cause them to pinch closed during exhalation, trapping air inside the patient's lungs. Healthy airways narrow during exhalation but not to the extent that causes obstruction or air trapping.

- **Abdominal muscle use.** We use abdominal muscles to push air out (exhalation). Patients with obstructive disease must work to push air out with every breath. Patients who have asthma often complain of abdominal pain after an attack. They do the equivalent of hundreds of sit-ups as they force each exhalation.
- **Jugular venous distention.** The diseased lung creates pulmonary hypertension. This increases the pressure in the right side of the heart and from there blood may back up into the jugular veins, causing jugular venous distension.

Asthma

The name asthma (from Greek, meaning "panting") was first given to this disease by the second-century Greek physician Aretaeus "because in the paroxysms, the patients also pant for breath". Bronchial asthma is characterised by an increased reactivity of the trachea, bronchi, and bronchioles to a variety of stimuli. That hyperreactivity results in widespread, reversible narrowing of the airways, or bronchospasm **Figure 26-33 ▸** . Sometimes we refer to this condition as reactive airway disease to indicate that the patient experiences bronchospasm when exposed to certain triggers, such as dust, cold, or smoke. In addition, oedema (swelling, or inflammation) of the airways and increased mucus production can cause significant airway obstruction.

At the Scene

Asthma is a term describing a triad of airway problems, which can result in: acute air trapping, increased work of breathing, and ultimately fatigue (Figure 26–33).

Asthma characteristically occurs in acute attacks of variable duration. Between attacks, the patient may be relatively asymptomatic.

Of 5.2 million people receiving treatment for asthma in the UK in 2002, 1.1 million were children. One in 5 households contains someone with asthma; the incidence has risen over the last 20 years but it is unclear why. In 2002 in the UK, 69,000 people where admitted to hospital with asthma, and over 1,400 people died from the disease. Two-thirds of these deaths were in those aged over 65, usually (but not exclusively) in those with previous severe disease. Women are more likely to die from the disease than men. Twenty-eight of the deaths were children.

Hospital admission and death rates show little improvement over the last 20 years. Deaths could have been prevented by better routine and emergency treatment, reducing delays in getting help and by taking prescribed medication. At particular risk of death are those who comply poorly with treatment, those with mental health problems, and those with poor socio-economic status.

Bronchospasm

Bronchospasm is caused by the constriction of smooth muscle that surrounds the larger bronchi in the lungs **Figure 26-34 ▸** . This may occur because of stimulation by an allergen or irritants such as dust, perfume, cat dander, or

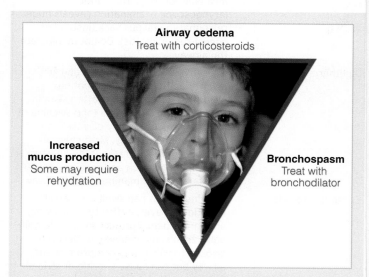

Airway oedema
Treat with corticosteroids

Increased mucus production
Some may require rehydration

Bronchospasm
Treat with bronchodilator

Figure 26-33 The asthma triad demonstrates the three primary components of asthma, and the corresponding treatments for each component. Asthma presents differently in different people, so individual treatments will need to vary as well.

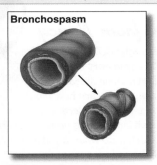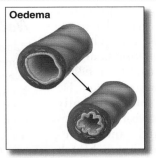

Bronchospasm

With bronchospasm, the muscle contracts, causing the entire tube to narrow.

Oedema

With oedema, the wall of the tube swells, causing only the lumen to narrow.

Figure 26-34 Bronchospasm is a constriction (narrowing) of the entire airway, whereas bronchial oedema is a swelling of the airway wall. Both cause the functional diameter of airways to be reduced.

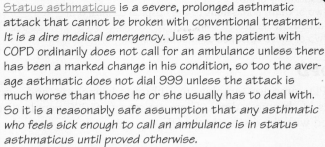

Notes from Nancy

Status asthmaticus is a severe, prolonged asthmatic attack that cannot be broken with conventional treatment. It is a dire medical emergency. Just as the patient with COPD ordinarily does not call for an ambulance unless there has been a marked change in his condition, so too the average asthmatic does not dial 999 unless the attack is much worse than those he or she usually has to deal with. So it is a reasonably safe assumption that any asthmatic who feels sick enough to call an ambulance is in status asthmaticus until proved otherwise.

On examining the patient in status asthmaticus, you will find him or her fighting desperately to move air through the obstructed airways, with prominent use of accessory muscles of respiration. The chest is maximally hyperinflated. Breath sounds and wheezes may be entirely inaudible because air movement is negligible, and the patient is usually exhausted, severely acidotic, and dehydrated.

cold temperatures or by other stimuli such as exercise or stress. When air is forced through the constricted tubes, it causes them to vibrate, which creates wheezing. Bronchospasm and turbulent airflow will often reduce the peak expiratory flow. The primary treatment of bronchospasm is a breathing treatment for the administration of bronchodilator medication.

Bronchial Oedema

Swelling of the bronchioles also creates turbulent airflow, wheezing, and air trapping. Bronchodilator medications do little to reduce bronchial oedema. If a patient takes such a medication and the peak flow does not improve dramatically, you should suspect some degree of bronchial oedema, the primary treatment of which is corticosteroids. Unlike a breathing treatment which can improve breathing immediately, steroids take a few hours to reduce inflammation.

Increased Mucous Production

Thick secretions may plug the distal airways and contribute to air trapping. People who have asthma may be significantly dehydrated because of their increased fluid loss from tachypnoea and their often-poor fluid intake. Dehydration makes secretions even thicker, further worsening the air trapping event. Taking antihistamine medications may further thicken secretions. The primary approach to dealing with secretions in asthma is to improve hydration.

In the United Kingdom, asthma is classified according to its severity. This enables prehospital professionals to plan and implement the most appropriate treatment and transport regime for each patient. The patient will be classified as having either moderate, severe, or life-threatening asthma.

Moderate

- Able to talk normally
- Respiratory rate of < 25 breaths/min
- Some accessory muscle use
- Peak expiratory flow reading (PEFR) > 50% of predicted best
- Pulse < 110 beats/min

Severe

- Unable to complete a sentence in one breath
- Increased dyspnoea and wheeze
- Respiratory rate increases ≥ 25 breaths/min (> 50 breaths/min 2 to 5 years and > 30 breaths/min 5 to 18 years)
- Reticent to move around
- PEFR < 50% of predicted best
- Tachycardia ≥ 110 beats/min (> 130 beats/min 2 to 5 years and > 120 beats/min 5 to 18 years)

Life-threatening

- Severe wheeze or "silent chest"
- PEFR < 33% of predicted best
- Bradycardia
- Cyanosis
- Confusion, agitation, and restlessness leading to unconsciousness

Most people who have asthma have a combination of these three pathological conditions, although their predominance varies in individual patients. The condition of a person who has asthma whose primary issue is bronchoconstriction would respond very well to inhaled bronchodilators. The condition of a person who has asthma whose primary issue is bronchial oedema would respond much less to inhaled bronchodilators, and probably would not show significant improvement until administered corticosteroids have taken effect (typically several hours after their administration).

Potentially Fatal Asthma

Patients who have potentially fatal asthma often have severely compromised ventilation all of the time. Such patients are at serious risk if something triggers acute bronchospasm or if they get an infection. A patient who has asthma is at high risk of respiratory arrest if he or she has a history consistent with any of the factors in Table 26-5 ▶. Medication noncompliance, psychiatric disorders, and poor socio-economic status are risk factors for potentially fatal attacks.

Table 26-5	Potentially Fatal Asthma

- Previous intubation for respiratory failure or respiratory arrest
- Respiratory acidosis
- Two or more admissions to the hospital despite oral corticosteroid use
- Two or more episodes of pneumothorax

COPD

COPD comprises emphysema, chronic bronchitis, and some cases of chronic asthma. There are over 900,000 people diagnosed with the disease in the UK.

Notes from Nancy

All that wheezing is not asthma.

Among the other causes of diffuse wheezing are acute left heart failure ("cardiac asthma"), smoke inhalation, chronic bronchitis, and acute pulmonary embolism. Localised wheezing reflects an obstruction, by foreign body or tumour, in a specific area. Only a careful history and physical examination will enable you to reach the correct diagnosis. It is particularly important to distinguish the wheezing of asthma from that caused by left heart failure, because the treatment of the two conditions is markedly different.

In the acute asthmatic attack, silence is not golden—it's deadly!

Emphysema

Emphysema is a chronic weakening and destruction of the walls of the terminal bronchioles and alveoli. Some people have emphysema caused by a congenital enzyme deficiency (alpha$_1$-antitrypsin deficiency), but the most common cause of emphysema in the UK is cigarette smoking.

In pure emphysema, the breakdown of the connective tissue structure of the terminal airways results in groups of alveoli merging into large blebs or bullae, which are far less efficient and collapse far more easily (causing obstruction) than does normal lung tissue. Although little can be done in the prehospital environment to help this condition, many patients have associated bronchospasm, oedema, fluid, or infections that can be relieved, helping improve the patient's overall situation. Many patients who have emphysema have a barrel chest caused by chronic lung hyperinflation. These patients are often tachypnoeic, as they attempt to maintain a normal carbon dioxide level despite their dysfunctional lungs. They often use extreme amounts of energy attempting to breathe, cannibalising their own muscle mass in the process.

Chronic Bronchitis

Chronic bronchitis is officially defined as sputum production most days of the month for 3 or more months out of the year for more than 2 years. The hallmark of this disease is excessive mucous production in the bronchial tree, which is nearly always accompanied by a chronic or recurrent productive cough (a cough that produces phlegm). The typical patient who has chronic bronchitis is almost invariably a heavy cigarette smoker. He or she is usually somewhat obese, congested, and sometimes has a bluish complexion. His or her blood gases tend to be abnormal, with elevated $_pCO_2$ (hypercapnia) and decreased $_pO_2$ (hypoxaemia) levels. Often he or she has associated heart disease and right heart failure (cor pulmonale).

The pink puffing emphysemic and the obese cyanosed chronic bronchitic represent two extremes of the COPD spectrum. In reality, as the disease progresses, most patients with COPD fall somewhere between these two clinical extremes, showing signs and symptoms of both disease processes.

Notes from Nancy

Patients with COPD ordinarily come to some sort of modus vivendi with their disease. Over the years, they learn how much exertion they can tolerate, in what position sleep is possible, and so forth. So when a patient with COPD calls for an ambulance, it nearly always means that something has changed—and changed for the worse.

Typical Presentations of COPD

Patients who have COPD are often very sick people, with little or no respiratory reserves to help them deal with any additional respiratory insults. You must actively search for what has pushed them over the edge from a relatively stable state to the insufficiency that caused them to call 999. The following are some common issues that conspire to cause the patient who has COPD to decompensate.

COPD With Pneumonia

Because they are chronically ill, have poor secretion clearance, and sometimes have excessive mucous production (which acts like a culture medium for nasty bugs), these patients often get infections in their bronchi and lungs. Do they have a fever? Has the colour or amount of their sputum production changed? Do they have other signs of infection (such as body aches, general malaise, or pain when breathing)? Are auscultated breath sounds (such as bronchial breath sounds and crackles) consistent with pneumonia?

COPD With Right Heart Failure

It is very difficult for the right side of the heart to push the patient's thick blood—thick because of polycythaemia—through capillaries that are being squashed by hyperinflated alveoli. This commonly causes right heart failure secondary to the patient's lung disease (cor pulmonale). If patients take in too much salt or fluid, or if they do not get rid of fluid (because of renal failure or insufficient diuretic use), they may have an episode of congestive heart failure. Do they have peripheral oedema? Jugular venous distention with abdomino-jugular test? End inspiratory crackles? (It may be difficult to tell the difference between the crackles of congestive heart failure and the crackles that these patients always have secondary to their COPD.) Do they say they have had a progressive increase in dyspnoea over several days? Have they taken in more fluid than usual, or run out of their diuretics?

COPD With Left Heart Failure

Patients with COPD are at high risk of having a sudden cardiac event. Any sudden left ventricular dysfunction such as an AMI or cardiac rhythm disturbance (arrhythmia) can cause them to have sudden-onset left heart failure. Don't allow your initial impression of COPD to prevent you from identifying the patient who is also having an acute myocardial infarction!

Acute Exacerbation of COPD

In the acute exacerbation, no co-pathological condition such as congestive heart failure or pneumonia clearly accounts for the patient's sudden decompensation. Instead, the patient's condition suddenly becomes worse, often because of some environmental change such as weather, humidity, or sudden activation of the heating or cooling system. An acute exacerbation can also be prompted by the inhalation of trigger substances. Did your patient decide to go through some old boxes today? Did a neighbour just visit with a cat? Is someone painting in the next room?

End-Stage COPD

Patients with severe COPD will eventually reach a point when their lungs simply cannot support oxygenation and ventilation any longer. You may come to know these patients well as their calls to 999 become more frequent. Some will be in hospice care. In the end stages of the disease, it can be difficult to determine whether a patient has an exacerbation that can be resolved or if he or she has reached the end of the disease process. Unfortunately, endotracheal intubation may result in a situation where the patient cannot make his or her wishes known. In addition, the more frequently the patient has to be intubated and placed on a ventilator, the more difficult it becomes to wean the patient off the ventilator. Having this knowledge increases the anxiety level of the patient, thus increasing his or her cardiac workload and cardiac oxygen consumption—a potentially lethal combination for the end-stage COPD patient.

All ambulance services have their own ways of dealing with do-not-resuscitate orders. It is important to secure documentation of the patient's wishes as the terminal phase of the disease begins. Follow local protocol or your control centre as needed regarding such issues.

Oxygen and Hypoxic Drive

Hypoxic drive has been much written about and much misunderstood. It is a theory that suggests COPD patients depend on hypoxia as their primary stimulus to breathe, and that relieving this hypoxia (and therefore removing the stimulus) may cause respiratory depression and eventually apnoea. In practice it is unknown whether oxygen reduces ventilation to any significant degree, either through this mechanism or any other.

Providing excessive levels of oxygen to some COPD patients can still be dangerous. It has been shown that oxygen can cause hypercapnic respiratory failure (CO_2 retention and respiratory acidosis). This complicates hospital treatment and makes patients more likely to need intensive care. The dominant (but not isolated) cause for this effect is probably a mismatch between the ventilation of the alveoli and the perfusion of the alveolar capillaries with blood. Administering oxygen raises the pO_2 in the alveoli, which in turn causes pulmonary blood vessels to dilate and so increase blood flow. This is normally matched with a rise in ventilation to blow off the increased CO_2 returning to the lungs. Some COPD patients are unable to compensate in this way, and the increased CO_2 ends up in the venous blood leaving the lungs. This can result in hypercapnia, which in turn can cause electrolyte abnormalities, acidosis, and a diminished level of consciousness or even coma.

The paramedic is in a position of balancing the risks of hypoxia with the risks of oxygen induced CO_2 retention and acidosis. In making this decision, the following points should be considered:

1. Oxygen saturations down to 90% (hypoxaemia) are tolerated well in COPD with minimal risks.
2. There is increasing recognition of the potential damage of hyperoxaemia (too much oxygen in the blood) and subsequent serious hypercapnic respiratory failure. This affects a significant minority of patients and you cannot tell who they are just by looking at them.
3. Much expert opinion in the UK now believes that for COPD patients oxygen therapy should be started at a low rate, such as 2 l/min via a nasal cannula (or if available a 28% Venturi mask) and kept at the minimum level required to obtain an oxygen saturation of between 90 and 92–93% (no higher).
4. If the patient becomes apnoeic, it is probably due to exhaustion; provide artificial ventilation with supplemental oxygen as normal and consider intubation.
5. Oxygen saturation (SpO_2) is a valuable tool to aid your decisions, but it does not tell you about the carbon dioxide levels. End-tidal carbon dioxide monitoring may be increasingly available in the future.

At the Scene

Bagged to Death

Not everyone should be ventilated the same way.

If you are ventilating a patient who has severe obstructive disease such as those with either decompensated asthma or COPD, remember that these patients have difficulty exhaling. If each breath is not allowed to come back out before the delivery of the next, then pressures in the thorax will continually go up. This phenomenon, which is called auto-PEEP (positive end-expiratory pressure), can eventually cause a pneumothorax or cardiac arrest. If the pressure in the chest exceeds the pressure of blood returning to the heart, thus limiting venous return, cardiac arrest may occur.

Such patients should be ventilated as little as four to six breaths per minute to avoid "bagging them to death". This is very difficult to do when your partner, bystanders, another crew, and your own adrenaline release are all telling you to hyperventilate the patient, but it is an absolute necessity if you hope to avoid the dire consequences of raising the thoracic pressure more with each breath. Seek guidance from your medical director and local protocols when you encounter patients who have severe COPD or asthma who are in cardiac arrest or near-arrest. However, also remember that the standard ventilation rate for adults is only 10 to 12 breaths/min.

Common Respiratory Presentations

Asthma With Fever

When patients with reactive airways begin wheezing, their inhalers usually will help for only a little while before their symptoms return. The typical asthma attack that responds to treatment but occurs again in a few hours is sometimes caused by an underlying infection (such as pneumonia or bronchitis) that continually triggers the asthma like symptoms. The asthma attack won't go away until the patient receives treatment of the trigger. Does your patient have a fever or chills? Is he or she coughing up colourful sputum?

Failure of a Metered-Dose Inhaler

Metered-dose inhalers indicate how many actuations (puffs) they are designed to deliver, but most patients don't keep track of their usage very well. Often the medication may be exhausted even though some propellant remains in the canister. The patient may have been sucking nothing but propellant for days, which explains why their wheezing isn't getting better. Similar problems can occur when patients use grossly outdated medications or medications that have been overheated (left in a hot car or similar environment). In this case, your bronchodilator may work well, even though theirs has failed. Another problem that can occur is that patients who do not fully understand how to use the device do not inhale at an appropriate point and then end up spraying the medicine on the inside of their mouths. This is one reason why physicians often prescribe a spacer device to be added to the metered-dose inhaler for children and for adults who have difficulty using the device.

Travel-Related Problems

Some patients present with significant pulmonary oedema after a lengthy journey. The reason: they didn't want to take their diuretics while travelling. Who wants to have to look for a toilet every half hour while on the road? Don't forget to ask the obvious: "What medications do you use"? Which should always be followed by: "And did you take them today"?

Dyspnoea Triggers

Just because someone knows that their reactive airways are triggered by cats, perfume, cigarette smoke, cold, or pollen doesn't mean that they can always avoid these triggers. Sometimes a social or family situation is sufficiently important for patients to be willing to risk experiencing an episode of dyspnoea. Sometimes people who are allergic to cats will hold a cat, and people who are on strict fluid restriction will drink like a fish.

Seasonal Issues

You can expect an increase in calls from chronically ill respiratory patients when excessive heat, humidity, cold, pollen, dust or air pollution conspire to push them over the edge so they experience an attack or exacerbation of their disease.

Noncompliance With Therapy

Many patients who have chronic respiratory disease will rebel against their therapy as a means of seeming to regain some control over their lives. Sometimes, the long-term nature of their therapy isn't fully understood, and they attempt to wean themselves off of their medications, oxygen, or respiratory support devices. Unfortunately, this may cause them to have a crisis.

Many patients have been prescribed home oxygen, metered-dose inhalers, nebulisers, continuous positive airway pressure (CPAP), bilevel positive airway pressure (BiPAP), and a variety of medications that they refuse to use or use only sporadically. Some medications, such as longer term oral corticosteroids, can cause dangerous complications if their use is terminated abruptly.

Failure of Technology/Running Out of Medicine

Advances in technology have allowed patients who have chronic respiratory disease much more freedom to get out of the house and to travel. This creates the risk that you will be called to assist someone whose oxygen tank has run dry, whose portable ventilator has suddenly malfunctioned, or whose medications were left behind.

Complications of General-Sales-List Medications

Few feelings are worse than not being able to breathe. Dyspnoeic patients will often resort to using—and sometimes misusing—general-sales-list (GSL) medications in addition to their prescribed medications. The following is a list of GSL medications that a patient may be using in conjunction with his or her prescribed medication:

- *Antihistamines* dry secretions and are not a good idea for people who have asthma. Unfortunately, antihistamines are a common ingredient in many GSL cough and cold medications.
- *Antitussives* are used to suppress coughs. Of course, coughing helps clear secretions from the airways. Sometimes it might be best not to suppress that normal bodily function.

Clots may also form when patients are immobile for long periods of time. Sudden pulmonary embolisms sometimes occur in people after long car trips or lengthy aeroplane flights. Bedridden patients are often prescribed anticoagulants or wear special stockings or other devices to reduce the formation of blood clots in the legs. Patients at high risk, who are unsuitable for anticoagulation therapy, may have a vena cava filter inserted. This device, which opens like a mesh umbrella in the main vein that returns blood to the heart, is intended to catch any clots that break loose and travel from the legs.

Very large pulmonary emboli can lodge at the bifurcation of the right and left pulmonary arteries. These are called a saddle embolus and may be immediately fatal. Cardiac arrest caused by a large pulmonary embolus is a very difficult situation that few patients survive. You may note cape cyanosis—deep cyanosis of the face, neck, chest, and back—despite good-quality CPR and ventilation with 100% supplemental oxygen in this scenario.

Disorders of Ventilation

Ventilation is the movement of air in and out of the lungs. With the use of supplemental oxygen, reasonable and even high oxygen levels are easy to maintain in patients who have healthy lungs, even if ventilation is severely compromised. The best measurement of ventilation, however, is the carbon dioxide level. Under normal circumstances, the volume of ventilation (minute volume) is regulated by the need to maintain the $_pCO_2$ in the range of 35 to 45 mm Hg. In a person at rest, that goal is usually accomplished by breathing a tidal volume of around 500 ml at a rate of 12 to 16 breaths/min—that is, with a minute volume in the range of 6 to 8 l. During deep sleep, a smaller minute volume may suffice, while the muscular exertion associated with exercise may require a larger minute volume. As long as the $_pCO_2$ remains in the normal range, ventilation is considered normal.

The carbon dioxide level is also directly related to pH (acid-base balance). Patients who are hypoventilating usually have respiratory acidosis. As their carbon dioxide level goes up, their pH level goes down. Patients who are hyperventilating are usually in respiratory alkalosis. As their carbon dioxide level goes down, their pH level goes up.

Respiratory Failure Resulting From Hypoventilation

Many different problems can cause patients to hypoventilate:
- Conditions that impair lung function
- Conditions that impair the mechanics of breathing
- Conditions that impair the neuromuscular apparatus
- Conditions that reduce respiratory drive

In these circumstances, you must often provide aggressive treatment to help the patient's respiratory efforts.

Conditions That Impair Lung Function
When the patient is breathing but gas exchange is impaired, carbon dioxide levels rise. This can happen in severe cases of atelectasis, pneumonia, pulmonary oedema, asthma, or COPD. Oxygen therapy may result in increased alveolar perfusion, but in some COPD patients there is insufficient alveolar ventilation to match; this may also raise carbon dioxide levels.

Conditions That Impair the Mechanics of Breathing
A high cervical fracture, flail chest, diaphragmatic rupture, severe recession, an abdomen full of air or blood, abdominal or chest binding (such as seat belts or immobilisation straps), or anything else that impairs the pressure changes that allow breathing can result in reduced gas flow.

Pickwickian syndrome is the name given to respiratory compromise secondary to extreme obesity. One of the earliest descriptions of the combination of obesity, respiratory compromise, and sleep apnoea can be found in the character of "Joe the fat boy" in Charles Dickens's *Pickwick Papers*. Poor Joe would fall asleep in midsentence, snore loudly, and generally exhibit signs of hypercapnia. This syndrome does not seem to be on the decline in today's society given the almost constant media coverage of obesity.

Conditions That Impair the Neuromuscular Apparatus
Patients who have had head trauma, intracranial infections, or brain tumours may have damage to the respiratory centres of the brain, which in turn may compromise ventilation. Serious injury to the spinal cord (above C5) may block the nerve impulses that cause breathing to occur. Guillain-Barré syndrome causes progressive muscle weakness and paralysis that moves up the body from the feet. If the paralysis reaches the diaphragm, the patient will be unable to breathe effectively. Amyotrophic lateral sclerosis also causes progressive muscle weakness. This disease is fatal, with death usually coming from respiratory failure as the muscles of respiration become unable to maintain adequate ventilation. Botulism is caused by the bacterium *Clostridium botulinum*. Though somewhat rare, it is usually the result of food poisoning or from an unknowing mother giving her infant or young child raw honey. Botulism can cause muscle paralysis and is typically fatal when it reaches the muscles of respiration.

Conditions That Reduce Respiratory Drive
Perhaps the most common hypoventilation crisis seen by ambulance staff is the acute heroin overdose. Intoxication with alcohol, narcotics, and a host of other drugs or toxins can reduce the respiratory drive. Head injury, or asphyxia can all present with grossly low respiratory rates and volumes. Of course, the ultimate expression of hypoventilation is respiratory and then cardiac arrest.

Hyperventilation

Hyperventilation occurs when people breathe in excess of metabolic need. This typically occurs when they breathe so much by either increasing the rate at which they breathe, the depth they breathe, or both, that their carbon dioxide level begins to fall. Interestingly, a falling carbon dioxide level may make the patient feel short of breath, so they tend to become anxious and breathe even more rapidly and deeply. In acute hyperventilation syndrome, patients usually feel as if they cannot breathe at all. The continued fall in their carbon dioxide level leads to a rise in their pH level, which results in respiratory alkalosis that in turn causes numbness or tingling in the hands and feet and around the mouth. If this continues, patients may complain of chest pain and will ultimately experience carpopedal spasm, during which the hands and feet lock up in a clawlike position. These symptoms frighten the patient even further, and usually make him or her hyperventilate even more. The hysterical hyperventilator may eventually lose consciousness, but not before undergoing extreme distress. If the patient doesn't calm down and stop hyperventilating upon awakening, the process could repeat itself.

The traditional therapy for hyperventilation called for patients to rebreathe their own carbon dioxide by breathing into a paper bag, or by applying a partial rebreather mask at 21% oxygen. This a very dangerous practice for important reasons:

■ Patients quickly exhaust the oxygen in the gas they are breathing (and rebreathing). Remember, hyperventilation does not mean that the patient has too much oxygen, but rather that he or she is blowing off too much carbon dioxide. Do not cause the patient to become hypoxic while trying to stop a relatively benign hyperventilation episode.

■ Any patient who is acidotic might be hyperventilating in an attempt to drive their pH level down to normal levels. In diabetic ketoacidosis, for example, the patient's body is making too much acid because of inadequate glucose metabolism, so the body attempts to compensate for the acidosis by hyperventilating (Kussmaul respirations). It would be a grave error to force such a patient to breathe into a paper bag. A variety of overdoses, toxic exposures, and metabolic abnormalities can also result in acidosis and

compensatory hyperventilation, and none of them have the kind of hyperventilation that should be treated by rebreathing carbon dioxide. You should never come to the conclusion that your patient is just hyperventilating until you have ruled out all other potential causes for their presentation, which may be very difficult to do in the prehospital environment.

Ultimately, treatment may include sedating the truly hysterical hyperventilator once in the hospital. Frequently, hyperventilation will follow some emotional stressor, ie, after a family fight, finding out about an unexpected pregnancy in a teen, or being notified that you are having a tax audit. More often than not, a variety of psychological support techniques will help. Probably the single most important part of your patient care is to make the patient understand that if the behaviour that precipitated the hyperventilation is repeated, almost without fail, they will hyperventilate again. Contacting social services or a teen pregnancy counsellor will provide the patient with confidence to confront the situation. Other techniques include breathing *with* the patient, having the patient count to two between each breath (increasing to higher numbers as he or she is successful), and various distraction techniques (such as asking the patient to recite his or her life stories). Hyperventilation that is not caused by some metabolic crisis is usually self-limiting. At the very least, try not to feed into the patient's anxieties and make things worse, and don't let them do that either.

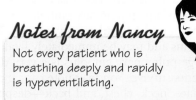

Notes from Nancy

Not every patient who is breathing deeply and rapidly is hyperventilating.

You are the Paramedic Part 4

Your patient continues to deteriorate despite your treatment. In the ambulance he is now unresponsive, floppy, and cyanosed; his spontaneous respiratory rate begins to fall. He easily accepts an OP airway. You choose to intubate the patient, and you successfully pass the tube and confirm correct placement. You continue to ventilate your patient on the way to hospital.

Reassessment	Recording Time: 20 Minutes
Level of consciousness	U (Unresponsive); Glasgow Coma Scale score, 3
Skin	Pale, cyanosis improving
Pulse	120 beats/min
Blood pressure	115/60 mm Hg
Respirations	Intubated; ventilated at 10 breaths/min
SpO_2	82% with bag-valve-mask ventilation and supplemental oxygen
Capnography	45 mm Hg
ECG	Sinus tachycardia

8. Beyond inadequate ventilation and oxygenation, what must you take into consideration before attempting intubation?

9. If capnography, pulse oximetry, and other similar pieces of assessment equipment are unavailable, how can you determine whether your interventions are improving the patient's condition?

10. What other techniques can you use to improve ventilation and oxygenation?

pressure during exhalation). Because this type of positive airway pressure is a little more like normal breathing, it is often more comfortable for the patient. It causes a pressure variation in the chest, which allows for more normal blood flow. It is also a more complex and expensive device, and one that is not commonly used in the prehospital environment.

Automated Transport Ventilators

Automated transport ventilators are essentially flow-restricted oxygen-powered ventilation devices (FROPVDs) with timers on them. They can be set to deliver a particular volume at a particular rate, which can be very helpful when you need an extra pair of hands   Figure 26-42 ▸ . They are particularly good for replacing the role of bag-valve-mask ventilation when the patient who is in cardiac or respiratory arrest has been intubated. Basic automated transport ventilators may lack any alarms, the ability to control flow rate, or the ability to provide various modes of ventilatory support. They are *not* little ventilators and are *not* intended to ventilate patients without direct observation and attention by a skilled paramedic. These types of ventilator are usually only appropriate for intubated patients who are unresponsive and who are not breathing spontaneously. Some ventilators lack the ability to have the tidal volume and respiratory rate altered independently; this

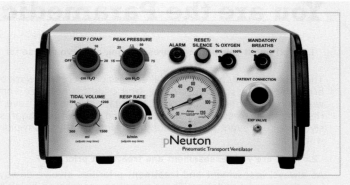

Figure 26-42 Automated transport ventilators are flow-restricted oxygen-powered ventilation devices. They can be very helpful during a cardiac arrest, but the preset flow of 40 l/min is not appropriate for conscious patients.

may result in hyperventilation, which has been demonstrated to be harmful in cardiac arrest. Remember that current resuscitation guidelines recommend a tidal volume of 6–7 mls/kg (about 400–500 mls for an average adult), and a rate of 10 breaths/min. Any ventilator used in these situations should be capable of being set to these levels.

You are the Paramedic Summary

1. What about this patient's presentation gives you cause for concern?

The patient's body position, facial expression, increased work of breathing, accessory muscle use, and cries for help are very worrying. All of these signs point to a patient who is in severe respiratory distress. This patient will need appropriate, aggressive care to prevent his condition from significantly and rapidly worsening.

2. What are your assessment and treatment priorities?

As always, assessment and treatment priorities involve airway, breathing, and circulation. These priorities are learned in initial ambulance technician training. No matter how advanced you become in your education and knowledge as a medical professional, you must always remember that the fundamentals of emergency medicine are built upon the principles of basic life support—that is, assessment and treatment of life-threatening illness and injury inherently related to a problem with airway, breathing, and circulation.

3. If you are unable to gather much information from your patient about his medical history, in what other ways can you obtain this information?

Utilise the scene or—better yet—the patient's family members or friends. Significant others are usually highly aware of acute changes in the patient's condition. They may be the first to offer information that can clarify the patient's condition or provide new insight that the patient had not noticed. If no family member is available, you should look for medical identification tags or bracelets and prescription bottles, and assess the scene to gain a better understanding of your patient's medical history. Use resources wisely to avoid delaying lifesaving patient care by searching throughout the home.

4. Given the patient's presentation, which assessment tools should you use to obtain a greater understanding of the patient's medical condition?

Listening to lung sounds is a given and, as a well-trained medical professional, you are likely to have many other assessment tools at your disposal. It is critical that you understand when and how to use tools such as tactile fremitus, egophony, bronchophony, whispered pectoriloquy, and percussion. It is rarely wise to spend precious minutes using these assessment tools on a patient whose condition is deteriorating rapidly. As a paramedic, you must determine how to best use your time and your resources in accordance with your patient's condition. For example, to delay transport to check the function of all 12 cranial nerves in the presence of an obvious cerebrovascular accident is inappropriate and could cost the patient his or her life.

5. What other treatments could you consider?

In an acute exacerbation of COPD you can administer 5 mg of nebulised salbutamol. If the patient does not respond, you can repeat the salbutamol dose and simultaneously add 500 mcg of ipratropium bromide to the nebuliser. Unfortunately, this means you are then unable to alter the concentration of oxygen you are administering. A COPD patient often only needs low concentrations of oxygen to maintain a saturation above 90%, and an oxygen driven nebuliser runs the small risk of causing hypercapnic respiratory failure. Alternatively, you may be unable to provide high concentrations of oxygen to a severely hypoxic patient (like this one). If possible, keep the nebuliser treatment short, and then apply an appropriate level of oxygen.

6. Is your patient ventilating and oxygenating adequately?

Given the information regarding his level of consciousness; his respiratory rate, depth, and quality; his skin signs; and the oximetry reading, it is obvious that this patient is not ventilating or oxygenating adequately.

7. What options do you have available to maintain this patient's airway?

The most important skills for successfully maintaining a patient's airway are basic life support measures—specifically, bag-valve-mask ventilation and use of airway adjuncts. The importance of these skills becomes painfully obvious in the event of failed intubations or failure of alternative airways.

In the UK (out of hospital) it is very unusual to have access to someone trained and qualified to perform rapid sequence induction. In the United States some paramedics use drugs to induce anaesthesia and paralysis, in order to allow intubation in someone who is conscious, partly conscious, or who still has any gag reflex. This practice is still controversial, and carries significant risks. Without the aid of drugs a patient must have no gag reflex, and be deeply unconscious or be in cardiac arrest in order for intubation to be successful, and to avoid causing laryngospasm and vomiting.

If intubation is inappropriate, then oropharyngeal, nasopharyngeal and laryngeal mask airways are all potential airway adjuncts to be considered. Ventilate the patient using a bag-valve-mask and supplemental oxygen, and continually monitor the airway for the need to suction secretions.

8. Beyond inadequate ventilation and oxygenation, what must you take into consideration before attempting intubation?

Consider the patient's level of consciousness, the presence of any remaining gag reflex, and the journey time to hospital. You should also consider the patient's anatomy and your ability to place the ET tube correctly. Patients with small mouths or short necks or who are obese can be quite difficult to intubate.

9. If capnography, pulse oximetry, and other similar pieces of assessment equipment are unavailable, how can you determine whether your interventions are improving the patient's condition?

Almost anyone who has worked with an experienced partner is likely to have heard that new staff are too dependent on gadgets. Some of this disdain could be rooted in fear of change, but it still makes a valid point. Prehospital providers can become overly dependent on equipment to provide information that can and should be validated in the patient's signs and symptoms. Reassess the patient for signs of improvement.

10. What other techniques can you use to improve ventilation and oxygenation?

Another advantage of obtaining a definitive airway is the potential to provide tracheal suctioning. This patient definitively would benefit from the removal of secretions, which may or may not be performed prehospital.

Prep Kit

■ Ready for Review

- The primary components of the respiratory system are like an inverted tree, with the trachea representing the tree's trunk and the alveoli resembling the tree's leaves.
- The mouth and oropharynx are very vascular and are covered by a mucous blanket. Swelling can be profound and potentially dangerous.
- The larynx and glottis are typically considered the dividing line between the upper airway and the lower airway. The thyroid cartilage is the most obvious external landmark of the larynx. The glottis and vocal cords are found in the middle of the thyroid cartilage.
- The cricoid cartilage can be palpated just below the thyroid cartilage in the neck. It forms a complete ring and maintains the trachea in an open position. Applying cricoid pressure or Sellick manoeuvre may be helpful with intubation.
- The small space between the thyroid and cricoid cartilages is the cricothyroid membrane. It is a good choice for inserting a large IV cannula or a small breathing tube.
- Cilia line the larger airways and help move foreign material out of the tracheobronchial tree. If a patient is dehydrated or has taken medications that dry secretions (such as antihistamines), the cilia will not be able to effectively move secretions. The same is true if the patient is overhydrated.
- Pulmonary circulation begins at the right ventricle, where the pulmonary artery branches into increasingly smaller vessels until it reaches the pulmonary capillary bed, which surrounds the alveoli and terminal bronchioles.
- Patients who have traumatic brain injuries may exhibit bizarre respiratory patterns, including agonal gasps; apneustic and ataxic patterns; and Biot, Cheyne-Stokes, and Kussmaul respirations; as well as central neurogenic hyperventilation, bradypnoea, hyperpnoea, hypopnoea, and tachypnoea.
- The respiratory system delivers oxygen to the body and removes the primary waste product of metabolism, carbon dioxide. If the lungs are not functioning appropriately, both of these vital functions may be impaired. Hypoxia, cell death, and acidosis can then occur.
- The brain is very sensitive to reduced levels of oxygen. It requires a regular supply of both oxygen and glucose to function, but can store neither. Alteration in level of consciousness could represent respiratory compromise.
- A patient who has respiratory disease may not be able to talk because he or she is having difficulty breathing. You may have to obtain the history from a family member or from only a few clues.
- It is critical to evaluate how hard your patient is working to breathe. Patients in respiratory distress may be able to compensate at first, but will eventually become sleepy, have a decreased respiratory rate and depth, and then, decompensate.
- Patients who have chronic respiratory disease are often knowledgeable about their disease and may have tried several potential treatment options already. Ask them about these efforts and what results, if any, they produced.
- Onset and duration of distress are important considerations in determining the underlying cause. Find out if the problem happened suddenly or gradually worsened over time.
- Assessing the patient's position of comfort and difficulty speaking may help you gauge the patient's degree of distress. A patient sitting completely upright and speaking only in two- or three-word statements is probably in considerable distress.
- Patients in respiratory distress tend to seek the tripod position. The condition of a patient in respiratory distress who is willing to lie flat may be quickly deteriorating. Head bobbing is also an ominous sign.

- Find out if the patient's condition is a recurrence of a past condition. If so, compare the current situation with other episodes.
- Note any audible abnormal respiratory noises. Noisy breathing is obstructed breathing.
- Snoring indicates partial obstruction of the upper airway by the tongue. Stridor indicates narrowing of the upper airway, usually as a result of swelling (laryngeal oedema).
- Assessing the level of consciousness is enormously important in dyspnoeic patients.
- Assess the patient's mucous membranes for cyanosis (a bluish or dusky colour), pallor, and moisture.
- Look for jugular venous distention in the neck, with the patient in a semi-sitting position. Distended neck veins may be caused by cardiac failure.
- Feel the chest for vibrations as the patient breathes. Check for oedema of the ankles or lower back. Check for peripheral cyanosis. Check the pulse and note the patient's skin temperature. Attach any available monitors.
- Auscultate the lungs whenever possible. Adventitious breath sounds are the extra noises that you may hear; they include wheezing or crackles.
- Crackles are any discontinuous noises heard on auscultation of the lungs. They are caused by the popping open of air spaces and are usually associated with increased fluid in the lungs.
- Wheezes are high-pitched, whistling sounds made by air being forced through narrowed airways, which makes them vibrate. Wheezing may be diffuse in conditions such as asthma and congestive heart failure or localised when caused by a foreign body obstructing a bronchus.
- *Silence means danger!* If you don't hear anything with your stethoscope, the patient is not moving enough air to ventilate the lungs.
- Note whether the patient is coughing up colourful sputum, if the colour or amount of sputum has changed, and if it contains blood or pus.
- A pulse oximeter indicates what percentage of the patient's haemoglobin has oxygen attached to it. An oxygen saturation of 95% or more is considered normal.
- The peak flow is the maximum flow rate at which the patient can expel air from the lungs. Normal peak flows run from about 300/650 l/min. A peak flow of less than 150 l/min is very low and signals significant distress.
- A variety of infections can cause swelling in the upper airway. Croup is one of the most common, though it usually occurs only in small children.
- Pulmonary aspiration of stomach contents is very dangerous. Avoid causing gastric distention when bagging the patient, and monitor the patient's ability to protect his or her airway. If you determine that the patient can't protect his or her airway, one of your primary jobs is to protect it for them.
- Common obstructive airway diseases include emphysema, chronic bronchitis, and asthma. Emphysema and chronic bronchitis are collectively classified as COPD, along with some cases of chronic asthma.
- Asthma is caused by allergens or irritants and is characterised by widespread, reversible narrowing of the airways (bronchospasm), oedema of the airways, and increased mucous production. It can cause significant airway obstruction.
- Primary treatment of bronchospasm is bronchodilator medication. Primary treatment of bronchial oedema is corticosteroids, which may be administered in the prehospital setting.

■ Status asthmaticus is a severe, prolonged asthmatic attack that cannot be broken with conventional treatment. It is a dire medical emergency. Any person with asthma who feels sick enough to call an ambulance is in status asthmaticus until proved otherwise.

■ When a patient has recurring asthma attacks, his or her inhaler could be empty or the medication could no longer be effective. Try administering a new bronchodilator.

■ Emphysema is a chronic weakening and destruction of the walls of the terminal bronchioles and alveoli. A patient with emphysema classically has a barrel chest, muscle wasting, and pursed-lip breathing. Such patients are often tachypnoeic.

■ Chronic bronchitis is characterised by excessive mucous production in the bronchial tree, nearly always accompanied by a chronic or recurrent productive cough. A patient with chronic bronchitis tends to be sedentary and obese, sleep in an upright position, use many tissues, have copious secretions, and be cyanotic.

■ In assessing patients who have COPD, search for what pushed them over the edge. Look for signs of infection, peripheral oedema, jugular venous distention with or without a positive abdominojugular test, and crackles. Find out if the onset of dyspnoea was sudden or gradual.

■ Not everyone should be ventilated the same way. Allow each breath to come back out before the delivery of the next breath. If you don't, pressures in the thorax will rise, eventually causing pneumothorax or cardiac arrest. Patients with severe obstructive diseases should be ventilated as little as 4 to 6 breaths/min.

■ Noncompliance could trigger an asthma attack. Ask what the patient was doing when the asthma attack began. Ask if the patient took his or her medications today. Ask if movement worsens the dyspnoea.

■ Pneumonia may be caused by a variety of bacterial, viral, and fungal agents. The patient with pneumonia usually reports weakness, productive cough, fever, and sometimes chest pain that worsens with coughing. Supportive care includes oxygenation, suctioning, and transport to an appropriate facility.

■ Pulmonary oedema occurs when fluid migrates into the lungs. The patient expectorating pink and foamy secretions probably has severe pulmonary oedema.

■ When a patient has a pneumothorax, air collects between the visceral pleura and the parietal pleura. Administer high concentration oxygen and monitor the patient's respiratory status closely.

■ Pleural effusion will make the patient dyspnoeic. Supportive care, including proper positioning and aggressive oxygen administration, should be given.

■ A pulmonary embolism occurs when a blood clot breaks off in the circulation and travels to the lungs, blocking blood flow and nutrient exchange. Bedridden patients, those with cancer, and people who have had major surgery are at risk of pulmonary embolism. The hallmark of pulmonary embolus is cyanosis that does not resolve with oxygen therapy.

■ Respiratory failure, or insufficient ventilation, can occur from a multitude of pathological conditions, from injuries to the lungs, heart, and neurological system to overdoses. Care includes providing supplemental oxygen.

■ In hyperventilation syndrome, ventilation is excessive. If it continues, the patient may experience chest pain and carpopedal spasm. Psychological support techniques such as counting breaths, and distraction work best and help calm the patient.

■ In managing the condition of a patient who is in respiratory distress, begin by ensuring that there is an open and maintainable airway. Suction if necessary and keep the airway optimally positioned. Remove constricting clothing. Reduce the patient's effort to breathe.

■ Patients in respiratory failure may ultimately need to be intubated. There are major drawbacks and risks to intubating in the prehospital environment, but it can also be lifesaving. Weigh these issues along with guidelines, medical direction, and the patient's wishes.

■ Metered-dose inhalers deliver medication as a nebuliser treatment. They are usually the delivery method of choice for both bronchodilators and corticosteroids in the home setting. Improper technique may result in little or no medication actually getting into the lungs.

■ Nebulisers deliver liquid medications in the form of a fine mist to the respiratory tract. Weigh the potential benefits of nebuliser therapy against the lower FiO_2 delivered during the treatment.

■ Drug administration methods that require the patient to inhale the medication may become unreliable or ineffective when the patient's airways are severely compromised. Some cases may warrant delivering medications intramuscularly or subcutaneously instead.

■ Medications can be instilled directly into the tracheobronchial tree when patients are intubated or have a tracheostomy.

■ Continuous positive airway pressure (CPAP) is used as therapy for acute cardiogenic pulmonary oedema. Within several minutes of application, the patient's oxygen saturation should increase, and the respiratory rate should decrease.

■ Bilevel positive airway pressure (BiPAP) is CPAP that delivers one pressure during inspiration and a different pressure during exhalation. It is more like normal breathing and is often more comfortable for the patient.

■ Automated transport ventilators are essentially flow-restricted oxygen-powered breathing devices with timers on them. They are particularly good choices for filling the role of the bag-valve-mask ventilator when the intubated patient is in cardiac or respiratory arrest, but are not intended to ventilate patients without direct observation and attention from a skilled practitioner.

■ Vital Vocabulary

abscess A collection of pus in a sac, formed by necrotic tissues and an accumulation of white blood cells.

adventitious A type of breath sound that occurs in addition to the normal breath sounds; examples are crackles and wheezes.

alveoli Sac-like units at the end of the bronchioles where gas exchange takes place (singular: alveolus).

angio-oedema An allergic reaction that may cause profound swelling of the tongue and lips.

arytenoid cartilages One of the paired, pitcher-shaped cartilages at the back of the larynx, at the upper border of the cricoid cartilage.

atelectasis Collapse of the alveolar air spaces of the lungs.

beta-2 agonist Pharmacological agent that stimulates the beta-2 receptor sites found in smooth muscle; include common bronchodilators like salbutamol and terbutaline.

botulism Poisoning from eating food containing botulinum toxin.

bronchospasm Severe constriction of the bronchial tree.

bronchial breath sounds A loud, harsh breath sound with equally long inspiratory and expiratory phases; heard over the peripheral chest (where vesicular sounds should be heard), indicating lung consolidation.

cape cyanosis Deep cyanosis of the face and neck and across the chest and back; associated with little or no blood flow after a large pulmonary embolism; it is particularly ominous.

carina Point at which the trachea bifurcates into the right and left mainstem bronchi.

carpopedal spasm Contorted position of the hand in which the fingers flex in a clawlike attitude and the thumb curls toward the palm.

chronic bronchitis Chronic inflammatory condition affecting the bronchi that is associated with excess mucous production that results from overgrowth of the mucous glands in the airways.

cilia Hairlike microtubule projections on the surface of a cell that can move materials over the cell surface.

cor pulmonale Heart disease that develops secondary to a chronic lung disease, usually affecting primarily the right side of the heart.

crackles Abnormal breath sounds that have a fine, crackling quality; previously called rales.

cricoid cartilage Ringlike cartilage forming the lower and back part of the larynx.

cricothyroid membrane Membrane between the cricoid and thyroid cartilages of the larynx.

croup Common disease of childhood characterised by swelling of the larynx and resulting upper airway obstruction.

dead space The portion of the tidal volume that does not reach the alveoli and thus does not participate in gas exchange.

diuresis Secretion of large amounts of urine by the kidney.

emphysema Infiltration of any tissue by air or gas; a chronic obstructive pulmonary disease characterised by distention of the alveoli and destructive changes in the lung parenchyma.

end-tidal carbon dioxide The numeric partial pressure of carbon dioxide contained in the last few millilitres of the patient's exhaled air.

epistaxis Nosebleed.

glottis Opening between the vocal cords.

goblet cells Cells that produce a protective mucous lining.

Guillain-Barré syndrome A disease of unknown aetiology that causes paralysis that progresses from the feet to the head (ascending paralysis). If the paralysis reaches the diaphragm, the patient may require respiratory support.

haemoglobin Oxygen-carrying pigment of the red blood cells. When haemoglobin has absorbed oxygen in the lungs, it is bright red and is called oxyhaemoglobin. After haemoglobin has given up its oxygen in the tissues, it is purple and is called reduced haemoglobin.

haemoptysis Coughing up blood.

Hering-Breuer reflex The nervous system mechanism that terminates inhalation and prevents lung overexpansion.

hypoventilate To not move adequate volumes of gas; underventilate.

hypoxic drive A theory that suggests in COPD a person's stimulus to breathe comes from a fall in arterial pO_2 rather than the normal stimulus, a rise in arterial pCO_2.

jugular venous distention The visible bulging of the jugular veins when the patient is in semi-recumbent or completely upright position. This is indicative of raised right atrial pressure due to heart failure, narrowed heart valves, or lung disease.

Kussmaul respirations A respiratory pattern characteristic of the person with diabetes who is in ketoacidosis, with marked hyperpnoea and tachypnoea.

larynx The organ of voice production.

metastasis Change in location of a disease from one organ or part of the body to another. Often used to describe a cancer that has migrated to other parts of the body.

oedema A condition in which excess fluid accumulates in tissues, manifested by swelling.

oropharynx The area behind the base of the tongue between the soft palate and the upper portion of the epiglottis.

orthopnoea Severe dyspnoea experienced when recumbent and relieved by sitting or standing up.

palatine tonsils One of three sets of lymphatic organs that comprise the tonsils; located in the back of the throat, on each side of the posterior opening of the oral cavity; help protect the body from bacteria introduced into the mouth and nose.

parenchyma The functional part of an organ, rather than the supporting tissue.

paroxysmal nocturnal dyspnoea Severe shortness of breath occurring at night after several hours of recumbency, during which fluid pools in the lungs.

piriform fossa Hollow pockets on the lateral sides of the glottic opening.

pleural effusion Excessive accumulation of fluid in the pleural space.

pneumonitis Inflammation of the lung. Implies lung inflammation from an irritant such as a chemical, dust, or radiation, or from aspiration. When lung inflammation is caused by an infectious agent, it would typically be called pneumonia.

polycythaemia The production of more red blood cells over time, making the blood thick; a characteristic of people who have chronic lung disease and chronic hypoxia.

pseudomembrane A false membrane formed by a dead tissue layer. Seen in the posterior pharynx of patients with diphtheria.

pulsus paradoxus Weakening or loss of a palpable pulse during inhalation, characteristic of cardiac tamponade and severe asthma.

purulent Full of pus; having the character of pus.

rales Old terminology for abnormal breath sounds that have a fine, crackling quality; now called crackles.

reactive airway disease A term used to describe any condition that causes hyperreactive bronchioles and bronchospasm.

recession Drawing in the intercostal muscles and the muscles above the clavicles in respiratory distress.

rhonchi (singular: rhonchus) Low-pitched wheezes also described as rattling or snoring. Caused by secretions in the larger bronchi narrowing the airways.

Sellick manoeuvre Pressure applied over the cricoid to seal off the oesophagus and prevent reflux of gastric contents.

shunt Situation in which a portion of the output of the right side of the heart reaches the left side of the heart without being oxygenated in the lungs; may be caused by atelectasis, pulmonary oedema, or a variety of other conditions. In haemodialysis, an anastomosis between a peripheral artery and vein.

smooth muscle Nonstriated involuntary muscle found in vessel walls, glands, and the gastrointestinal tract.

snoring Noise made on inhalation when the upper airway is partially obstructed by the tongue.

spacer A device that collects medication as it is released from the canister of a metered-dose inhaler, allowing more to be delivered to the lungs and less to be lost to the environment.

status asthmaticus A severe, prolonged asthma attack that cannot be broken with conventional treatment.

stridor Harsh, high pitched wheeze normally heard on inspiration, indicating upper airway obstruction, such as that from infection, burns, or a foreign body.

surfactant A liquid protein substance that coats the alveoli in the lungs.

tactile fremitus Vibrations in the chest as the patient breathes.

tidal volume The amount of air inhaled or exhaled during one breath.

tracheostomy Surgically opening in the trachea to create an airway.

tuberculosis A chronic bacterial disease caused by *Mycobacterium tuberculosis* that usually affects the lungs but can also affect other organs such as the brain or kidneys.

turbinates A set of bony convolutions on the sides of the nasal cavity, also called conchae, covered with a mucous membrane to warm and humidify inspired air.

vena cava filter A mesh filter placed in the inferior vena cava to catch blood clots in patients who are at high risk of pulmonary embolus.

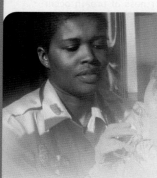

Assessment in Action

You arrive on the scene and find a 63-year-old woman in moderate respiratory distress. She is in the tripod position, using some accessory muscles, and is speaking in three- to four-word sentences. The patient is conscious, alert, and orientated to person, place, and time. Her blood pressure is 134/70 mm Hg; heart rate is 118 beats/min and regular; and her respiratory rate is 28 breaths/min. The pulse oximeter reads 90%. The patient's skin is warm and her nail beds are slightly cyanotic. She has been taking her salbutamol inhaler all day and it hasn't worked. She states this all began 2 days ago and has not got any better. She is wheezing in all lung fields.

1. **Which of the following is essential for normal ventilations to occur?**
   A. Functional diaphragm and intercostal muscles
   B. Interstitial space that is not filled with fluid
   C. Adequate blood volume
   D. Pulmonary capillaries that are not occluded

2. **What is chronic obstructive pulmonary disease?**
   A. A recurring condition of partially reversible airflow obstruction
   B. An acute inflammation of the lungs
   C. An absence of breath sounds on one side
   D. A progressive and irreversible disease of the airway

3. **What might bring about an exacerbation in an underlying respiratory condition?**
   A. Stress and infections
   B. Cigarette smoking
   C. Exercising
   D. All of the above

4. **What are important questions to ask this patient?**
   A. Has this happened before?
   B. Have you ever been intubated in the past?
   C. Is breathing uncomfortable when you lie down (more comfortable when you are sitting up or standing)?
   D. All of the above.

5. **What is usually the most reliable indicator of the patient's severity of respiratory distress?**
   A. One-word sentences
   B. Gross perspiring and pale colour
   C. Patient's description of respiratory distress
   D. Tachycardia

6. **What are wheezes?**
   A. High-pitched, whistling sounds
   B. Noises heard on auscultation of lungs, caused by popping open of air spaces
   C. Absent breath sounds
   D. Bubbling sounds heard at bases of the lungs

7. **What is emphysema?**
   A. Reversible narrowing of the airways
   B. Chronic weakening and destruction of the walls of the terminal bronchioles and alveoli
   C. An acute inflammatory condition of the lungs
   D. The leading cause of respiratory illnesses in children

8. **What may cause hypercapnic respiratory failure?**
   A. Hypoxia in a COPD patient
   B. Excessive oxygen in a patient with pulmonary oedema
   C. Excessive oxygen in a COPD patient
   D. All of the above

9. **You can never do any harm by giving high concentration oxygen to a patient with COPD.**
   A. True
   B. False

10. **What is peak expiratory flow?**
    A. Maximum flow rate at which patients can expel air from their lungs
    B. Partial obstruction of the upper airway by the tongue
    C. Adventitious breath sounds when auscultating the lungs
    D. Silent lung fields

Challenging Questions

You are dispatched to the railway station. Arriving on the scene, you find a 54-year-old man in respiratory distress. Upon auscultation of his lungs, you note wheezing in all lung fields. The patient is unable to talk to you.

11. **Is this patient having an asthma attack?**

■ Points to Ponder

It's a cold winter evening, your shift is just beginning and you are dispatched to the home of a 90-year-old man who has respiratory problems. You enter the house and immediately hear audible crackles coming from the next room. You place the patient on high concentration oxygen via nonrebreathing mask. The patient is conscious, alert, and orientated to person, place, and time. Blood pressure is 220/110 mm Hg, respiratory rate is 40 breaths/min, heart rate is 85 beats/min, pulse oximetry is 91%. The patient has jugular venous distention and peripheral oedema.

The patient appears to be in severe respiratory distress, using accessory muscles, speaking in one-word sentences, and grossly perspiring.

Family states that this all began while he was watching TV approximately 45 minutes ago, and has become progressively worse. The patient's medications include bisoprolol, pravastatin, furosemide, captopril, and digoxin. The family cannot tell you much about his medical history.

What do you know about this patient, based on his presentation and medications?

Issues: Recognising a Respiratory Emergency, Prompt and Correct Treatment, Determining Medical History Based on Medications.

27 Cardiovascular Emergencies

Objectives

Cognitive

- Describe the incidence, morbidity, and mortality of cardiovascular disease.
- Discuss prevention strategies that may reduce the morbidity and mortality of cardiovascular disease.
- Identify the risk factors most predisposing to coronary artery disease.
- Describe the anatomy of the heart, including the position in the thoracic cavity, layers of the heart, chambers of the heart, and location and function of cardiac valves.
- Identify the major structures of the vascular system.
- Identify the factors affecting venous return.
- Identify and define the components of cardiac output.
- Identify phases of the cardiac cycle.
- Identify the arterial blood supply to any given area of the myocardium.
- Compare and contrast the coronary arterial distribution to the major portions of the cardiac conduction system.
- Identify the structure and course of all divisions and subdivisions of the cardiac conduction system.
- Identify and describe how the heart's pacemaking control, rate, and rhythm are determined.
- Explain the physiological basis of conduction delay in the AV node.
- Define the functional properties of cardiac muscle.
- Define the events comprising electrical potential.
- List the most important ions involved in myocardial action potential and their primary function in this process.
- Describe the events involved in the steps from excitation to contraction of cardiac muscle fibres.
- Describe the clinical significance of Starling's law.
- Identify the structures of the autonomic nervous system (ANS).
- Identify the effect of the ANS on heart rate, rhythm, and contractility.
- Define and give examples of positive and negative inotropism, chronotropism, and dromotropism.
- Discuss the pathophysiology of cardiac disease and injury.
- Identify and describe the details of inspection, auscultation, and palpation specific to the cardiovascular system.
- Define pulse deficit, pulsus paradoxus, and pulsus alternans.
- Identify the normal characteristics of the point of maximal impulse (PMI).
- Identify and define the heart sounds.
- Relate heart sounds to haemodynamic events in the cardiac cycle.
- Describe the differences between normal and abnormal heart sounds.
- Identify and describe the components of the focused history as it relates to the patient with cardiovascular compromise.
- Explain the purpose of electrocardiograph (ECG) monitoring.
- Describe how ECG wave forms are produced.
- Correlate the electrophysiological and haemodynamic events occurring throughout the entire cardiac cycle with the various ECG wave forms, segments, and intervals.
- Identify how heart rates, durations, and amplitudes may be determined from ECG recordings.
- Relate the cardiac surfaces or areas represented by the ECG leads.
- Given an ECG, identify the arrhythmia.
- Identify the limitations to the ECG.
- Differentiate among the primary mechanisms responsible for producing cardiac arrhythmias.
- Describe a systematic approach to the analysis and interpretation of cardiac arrhythmias.
- Describe the arrhythmias originating in the sinus node, the atrioventricular (AV) junction, the atria, and the ventricles.
- Describe the arrhythmias originating or sustained in the AV junction.
- Describe the abnormalities originating within the bundle branch system.
- Describe the process of differentiating wide QRS complex tachycardias.
- Recognise the pitfalls in the differentiation of wide QRS complex tachycardias.
- Describe the conditions of pulseless electrical activity.
- Describe the phenomena of re-entry, aberration, and accessory pathways.
- Identify the ECG changes characteristically produced by electrolyte imbalances and specify the clinical implications.
- Identify patient situations where ECG rhythm analysis is indicated.
- Recognise the changes on the ECG that may reflect evidence of myocardial ischaemia and injury.
- Recognise the limitations of the ECG in reflecting evidence of myocardial ischaemia and injury.
- Correlate abnormal ECG findings with clinical interpretation.
- Identify the major therapeutic objectives in the treatment of the patient with any arrhythmia.
- Identify the major mechanical, pharmacological, and electrical therapeutic interventions.
- Based on your initial diagnosis, identify the need for rapid intervention for the patient in cardiovascular compromise.
- Describe the incidence, morbidity, and mortality associated with myocardial conduction defects.
- Identify the clinical indications for transcutaneous and permanent artificial cardiac pacing.
- Describe the components and the functions of a transcutaneous pacing system.
- Explain what each setting and indicator on a transcutaneous pacing system represents and how the settings may be adjusted.
- Describe the techniques of applying a transcutaneous pacing system.
- Describe the characteristics of an implanted pacemaking system.
- Describe artifacts that may cause confusion when evaluating the ECG of a patient with a pacemaker.
- List the possible complications of pacing.
- List the causes and implications of pacemaker failure.
- Identify additional hazards that interfere with artificial pacemaker function.

- Recognise the complications of artificial pacemakers as evidenced on ECG.
- Describe the epidemiology, morbidity and mortality, and pathophysiology of angina pectoris.
- List and describe the assessment parameters to be evaluated in a patient with angina pectoris.
- Identify what is meant by the OPQRST of chest pain assessment
- List other clinical conditions that may mimic signs and symptoms of coronary artery disease and angina pectoris.
- Identify the ECG findings in patients with angina pectoris.
- Identify the paramedic responsibilities associated with management of the patient with angina pectoris.
- Based on the pathophysiology and clinical evaluation of the patient with chest pain, list the anticipated clinical problems according to their life-threatening potential.
- Describe the epidemiology, morbidity, and mortality of myocardial infarction.
- List the mechanisms by which an acute myocardial infarction (AMI) may be produced by traumatic and non-traumatic events.
- Identify the primary haemodynamic changes produced in myocardial infarction.
- List and describe the assessment parameters to be evaluated in a patient with a suspected myocardial infarction.
- Identify the anticipated clinical presentation of a patient with a suspected acute myocardial infarction.
- Differentiate the characteristics of the pain/discomfort occurring in angina pectoris and acute myocardial infarction.
- Identify the ECG changes characteristically seen during evolution of an acute myocardial infarction.
- Identify the most common complications of an acute myocardial infarction.
- List the characteristics of a patient eligible for thrombolytic therapy.
- Describe the "window of opportunity" as it pertains to reperfusion of a myocardial injury or infarction.
- Based on the pathophysiology and clinical evaluation of the patient with a suspected acute myocardial infarction, list the anticipated clinical problems according to their life-threatening potential.
- Specify the measures that may be taken to prevent or minimise complications in the patient suspected of myocardial infarction.
- Describe the most commonly used cardiac drugs in terms of therapeutic effect and dosages, routes of administration, side effects, and toxic effects.
- Define the principle causes and terminology associated with heart failure.
- Identify the factors that may precipitate or aggravate heart failure.
- Describe the physiological effects of heart failure.
- Define the term "acute pulmonary oedema" and describe its relationship to left ventricular failure.
- Define preload, afterload, and left ventricular end-diastolic pressure and relate each to the pathophysiology of heart failure.
- Differentiate between early and late signs and symptoms of left ventricular failure and those of right ventricular failure.
- Explain the clinical significance of paroxysmal nocturnal dyspnoea.
- Explain the clinical significance of oedema of the extremities and sacrum.
- List the interventions prescribed for the patient in acute congestive heart failure.

- Describe the most commonly used pharmacological agents in the management of congestive heart failure in terms of therapeutic effect, dosages, routes of administration, side effects, and toxic effects.
- Define the term "cardiac tamponade".
- List the mechanisms by which cardiac tamponade may be produced by traumatic and non-traumatic events.
- Identify the limiting factor of pericardial anatomy that determines intrapericardiac pressure.
- Identify the clinical criteria specific to cardiac tamponade.
- Describe how to determine if pulsus paradoxus, pulsus alternans, or electrical alternans is present.
- Identify the paramedic responsibilities associated with management of a patient with cardiac tamponade.
- Describe the incidence, morbidity, and mortality of hypertensive emergencies.
- Define the term "hypertensive emergency".
- Identify the characteristics of the patient population at risk for developing a hypertensive emergency.
- Explain the essential pathophysiological defect of hypertension in terms of Starling's law of the heart.
- Identify the progressive vascular changes associated with sustained hypertension.
- Describe the clinical features of the patient in a hypertensive emergency.
- Rank the clinical problems of patients in hypertensive emergencies according to their sense of urgency.
- From the priority of clinical problems identified, state the management responsibilities for the patient with a hypertensive emergency.
- Correlate abnormal findings with clinical interpretation of the patient with a hypertensive emergency.
- Define the term "cardiogenic shock".
- Describe the major systemic effects of reduced tissue perfusion caused by cardiogenic shock.
- Explain the primary mechanisms by which the heart may compensate for a diminished cardiac output and describe their efficiency in cardiogenic shock.
- Differentiate progressive stages of cardiogenic shock.
- Identify the clinical criteria for cardiogenic shock.
- Describe the characteristics of patients most likely to develop cardiogenic shock.
- Correlate abnormal findings with clinical assessment of the patient in cardiogenic shock.
- Identify the paramedic responsibilities associated with management of a patient in cardiogenic shock.
- Define the term "cardiac arrest".
- Identify the characteristics of patient population at risk for developing cardiac arrest from cardiac causes.
- Identify non-cardiac causes of cardiac arrest.
- Describe the arrhythmias seen in cardiac arrest.
- Identify the critical actions necessary in caring for the patient with cardiac arrest.
- Explain how to confirm asystole using the 3-lead ECG.
- Define the terms defibrillation and synchronised cardioversion.
- Specify the methods of supporting the patient with a suspected ineffective implanted defibrillation device.
- Describe the most commonly used pharmacological agents in the managements of cardiac arrest in terms of therapeutic effects.
- Identify resuscitation.

- Identify circumstances and situations where resuscitation efforts would not be initiated.
- Identify and list the inclusion and exclusion criteria for termination of resuscitation efforts.
- Identify communication and documentation guidelines with medical direction and police used for termination of resuscitation efforts.
- Describe the incidence, morbidity, and mortality of vascular disorders.
- Describe the pathophysiology of vascular disorders.
- List the traumatic and non-traumatic causes of vascular disorders.
- Define the terms "aneurysm", "claudication", and "phlebitis".
- Identify the peripheral arteries most commonly affected by occlusive disease.
- Identify the major factors involved in the pathophysiology of aortic aneurysm.
- Recognise the usual order of signs and symptoms that develop following peripheral artery occlusion.
- Identify the clinical significance of claudication and presence of arterial bruits in a patient with peripheral vascular disorders.
- Describe the clinical significance of unequal arterial blood pressure readings in the arms.
- Recognise and describe the signs and symptoms of dissecting thoracic or abdominal aneurysm.
- Describe the significant elements of the patient history in a patient with vascular disease.
- Identify the haemodynamic effects of vascular disorders.
- Identify the complications of vascular disorders.
- Identify the paramedic's responsibilities associated with management of patients with vascular disorders.
- Develop, execute, and evaluate a treatment plan based on the initial diagnosis for the patient with vascular disorders.
- Differentiate between signs and symptoms of cardiac tamponade, hypertensive emergencies, cardiogenic shock, and cardiac arrest.
- Based on the pathophysiology and clinical evaluation of the patient with chest pain, characterise the clinical problems according to their life-threatening potential.
- Apply knowledge of the epidemiology of cardiovascular disease to develop prevention strategies.
- Integrate pathophysiological principles into the assessment of a patient with cardiovascular disease.
- Apply knowledge of the epidemiology of cardiovascular disease to develop prevention strategies.
- Integrate pathophysiological principles into the assessment of a patient with cardiovascular disease.
- Synthesise patient history, assessment findings, and ECG analysis to form an initial diagnosis for the patient with cardiovascular disease.
- Integrate pathophysiological principles to the assessment of a patient in need of a pacemaker.
- Synthesise patient history, assessment findings, and ECG analysis to form an initial diagnosis for the patient in need of a pacemaker.
- Develop, execute, and evaluate a treatment plan based on your initial diagnosis for the patient in need of a pacemaker.
- Based on the pathophysiology and clinical evaluation of the patient with chest pain, characterise the clinical problems according to their life-threatening potential.
- Integrate pathophysiological principles to the assessment of a patient with chest pain.
- Synthesise patient history, assessment findings, and ECG analysis to form an initial diagnosis for the patient with angina pectoris.
- Develop, execute, and evaluate a treatment plan based on the initial diagnosis for the patient with chest pain.

- Integrate pathophysiological principles to the assessment of a patient with a suspected myocardial infarction.
- Synthesise patient history, assessment findings, and ECG analysis to form an initial diagnosis for the patient with a suspected myocardial infarction.
- Develop, execute, and evaluate a treatment plan based on the initial diagnosis for the suspected myocardial infarction patient.
- Integrate pathophysiological principles to the assessment of the patient with heart failure.
- Synthesise assessment findings and patient history information to form an initial diagnosis of the patient with heart failure.
- Develop, execute, and evaluate a treatment plan based on the initial diagnosis for the heart failure patient.
- Integrate pathophysiological principles to the assessment of a patient with cardiac tamponade.
- Synthesise assessment findings and patient history information to form an initial diagnosis of the patient with cardiac tamponade.
- Develop, execute, and evaluate a treatment plan based on the initial diagnosis for the patient with cardiac tamponade.
- Integrate pathophysiological principles to the assessment of the patient with a hypertensive emergency.
- Synthesise assessment findings and patient history information to form an initial diagnosis of the patient with a hypertensive emergency.
- Develop, execute, and evaluate a treatment plan based on the initial diagnosis for the patient with a hypertensive emergency.
- Integrate pathophysiological principles to the assessment of the patient with cardiogenic shock.
- Synthesise assessment findings and patient history information to form an initial diagnosis of the patient with cardiogenic shock.
- Develop, execute, and evaluate a treatment plan based on the initial diagnosis for the patient with cardiogenic shock.
- Integrate the pathophysiological principles to the assessment of the patient with cardiac arrest.
- Synthesise assessment findings to formulate a rapid intervention for a patient in cardiac arrest.
- Synthesise assessment findings to formulate the termination of resuscitative efforts for a patient in cardiac arrest.
- Integrate pathophysiological principles to the assessment of a patient with vascular disorders.
- Synthesise assessment findings and patient history to form an initial diagnosis for the patient with vascular disorders.
- Integrate pathophysiological principles to the assessment and prehospital management of a patient with chest pain.

Affective

- Value the sense of urgency for initial assessment and intervention in the patient with cardiac compromise.
- Value and defend the sense of urgency necessary to protect the window of opportunity for reperfusion in the patient with suspected myocardial infarction.
- Defend patient situations where ECG rhythm analysis is indicated.
- Value and defend the application of transcutaneous pacing system.
- Value and defend the urgency in identifying pacemaker malfunction.
- Based on the pathophysiology and clinical evaluation of the patient with acute myocardial infarction, characterise the clinical problems according to their life-threatening potential.
- Defend the measures that may be taken to prevent or minimise complications in the patient with a suspected myocardial infarction.

- Defend the urgency based on the severity of the patient's clinical problems in a hypertensive emergency.
- From the priority of clinical problems identified, state the management responsibilities for the patient with a hypertensive emergency.
- Value and defend the urgency in rapid determination of and rapid intervention of patients in cardiac arrest.
- Value and defend the possibility of termination of resuscitative efforts in the out-of-hospital setting.
- Based on the pathophysiology and clinical evaluation of the patient with vascular disorders, characterise the clinical problems according to their life-threatening potential.
- Value and defend the sense of urgency in identifying peripheral vascular occlusion.
- Value and defend the sense of urgency in recognising signs of aortic aneurysm.

Psychomotor

- Demonstrate how to set and adjust the ECG monitor settings to varying patient situations.
- Demonstrate a working knowledge of various ECG lead systems.

- Demonstrate how to record an ECG.
- Perform, document, and communicate a cardiovascular assessment.
- Set up and apply a transcutaneous pacing system.
- Given the model of a patient with signs and symptoms of heart failure, position the patient to afford comfort and relief.
- Demonstrate how to determine if pulsus paradoxus, pulsus alternans, or electrical alternans is present.
- Demonstrate satisfactory performance of psychomotor skills of basic and advanced life support techniques according to the current European Resuscitation Council standards and guidelines, including:
  - Cardiopulmonary resuscitation
  - Defibrillation
  - Synchronised cardioversion
  - Transcutaneous pacing
- Complete appropriate documentation used for ROLE and, if required, liaise with police.
- Demonstrate how to evaluate major peripheral arterial pulses.

Introduction

Cardiovascular disease (CVD) has been the number one killer in Europe almost every year since 1900. It was for the purpose of providing early, definitive treatment for patients with acute myocardial infarction (AMI) that the primary role of a paramedic first came into being 40 years ago. Even with paramedic availability, more than 110,000 people in England die every year of coronary heart disease; approximately half die in an accident and emergency (A&E) department or before reaching hospital, during the first minutes and hours after the onset of symptoms. It is easy to see why the recognition and management of cardiovascular emergencies continue to receive strong emphasis in paramedic education.

This chapter is intended to prepare you to integrate pathophysiological principles and assessment findings to formulate an initial diagnosis and implement the treatment plan for patients with CVD. We begin by looking at the epidemiology of CVD in terms of its prevalence, mortality and morbidity, risk factors, and prevention strategies. After reviewing the anatomy and function of the cardiovascular system, we examine some of the clinical manifestations of CVD. Considerable emphasis is given to the interpretation of cardiac arrhythmias and their management within the context of the patient's overall clinical condition. Finally, we examine the pharmacological and other treatment modalities that make up advanced cardiac life support (ACLS).

Epidemiology

The many risk factors for coronary artery disease (CAD) include age, family history, hypertension, elevated cholesterol level, and smoking. It was previously thought that CAD was a man's disease, but we now realise that more women die of a cardiac event than men. Other factors contributing to CAD include diet, obesity, oral contraceptive use, sedentary lifestyle, stress, and personality type.

A healthy lifestyle may be all a person with a low risk needs to ward off CAD. High-risk people may be treated by using a combination of drug and nondrug therapies. Patients classified as being at intermediate risk may benefit from further testing for signs of atherosclerosis, which is an indicator of heart disease.

Education and early recognition are also important prevention strategies. Making people aware of the risk factors and signs and symptoms of CVD may decrease its prevalence. This is an area of interest for ambulance service providers who are involved in community heath promotion. ▐ Table 27-1 ▾ ▌ lists goals for decreasing CVD risks.

Cardiovascular Anatomy and Physiology

Structure and Function

The cardiovascular system is composed of the heart and blood vessels. Its primary function is to deliver oxygenated blood and nutrients to every cell in the body. It is also responsible for delivering chemical messages (hormones) within the body and

Table 27-1	Goals for Decreasing CVD Risks

- Quit smoking
- Lower and control blood pressure
- Lower total cholesterol level
- Lower LDL cholesterol level
- Increase HDL cholesterol level
- Lower weight, if overweight
- Increase aerobic exercise

LDL indicates low-density lipoprotein; and HDL, high-density lipoprotein.

You are the Paramedic Part 1

You are called to Mrs Beresford, a 65-year-old woman who has been struggling with her breathing for the past 6 hours. Once on scene, you find the patient sitting on the edge of her bed. She is pale, sweaty, and clearly gasping for breath. There is a bowl on the bedside cabinet with copious amounts of frothy sputum and you notice that her ankles are swollen.

Initial Assessment	Recording Time: 0 minutes
Appearance	Looks exhausted, leaning forward in a tripod position.
Level of consciousness	A (Alert, but can only manage single words between gasps)
Breathing	Rapid, shallow, and dyspnoeic.
Circulation	Rapid radial pulses with pale, perspiring skin

1. Which body system do you think is the primary cause for this patient's signs and symptoms?
2. What questions would you like to ask your patient at this time?

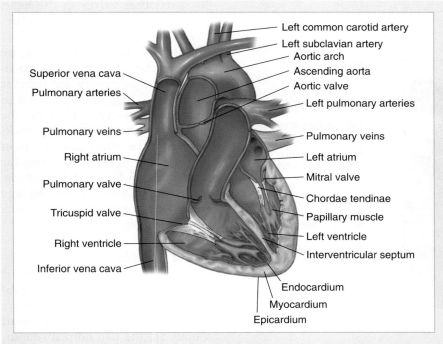

Figure 27-1 Anatomy of the heart.

At the Scene

Three components are necessary for adequate tissue perfusion: pump (heart), container (vessels) and fluid (blood).

for transporting the waste products of metabolism from the cells to sites of recycling or waste disposal.

The Heart

The driving force behind this extensive pickup and delivery service is the heart (Figure 27-1 ▲), a remarkable little pump that sits in the chest, above the diaphragm, behind and slightly to the left of the lower sternum (retrosternal). The heart is not much larger than a man's fist and weighs only 250 to 300 g. Despite its relatively small size, it is big and strong enough to move 7,000 to 9,000 litres of blood around the body every day of our lives!

On visualisation of the chest, one may be able to see the apical thrust or point of maximal impulse (PMI). The PMI is normally located on the left anterior part of chest, in the midclavicular line, at the fifth intercostal space. This thrust occurs when the heart's apex rotates forward with systole, gently beating against the chest wall and producing a pulsation.

Surrounding the heart is a tough, fibrous sac called the pericardium. The pericardium normally contains about 30 ml of serous fluid, which serves as a lubricant—that is, it enables

the heart muscle, as it contracts and relaxes, to slide easily within the pericardial sac. The pericardium does not stretch readily, so it cannot accommodate sudden accumulations of fluid.

The wall of the heart consists of three layers:

- The epicardium, the outermost surface layer, is a thin serous membrane.
- The endocardium is the innermost smooth layer of connective tissue.
- The myocardium is the muscular layer of the cardiac wall found between the epicardium and endocardium.

Like all cells in the body, myocardial cells require an uninterrupted supply of oxygen and nutrients. Indeed, the cardiac demand for oxygen is particularly unremitting because the heart never stops to rest (not without catastrophic consequences), so it is essential for the heart to have an absolutely reliable blood supply. Oxygenated blood reaches the heart through the coronary arteries Figure 27-2 ▶ , which branch off the aorta at the coronary ostia, just above the leaflets of the aortic valve. There are two main coronary arteries—left and right. The left main coronary artery subdivides into the left anterior descending and circumflex coronary arteries, both of which branch widely to supply the more muscular left ventricle of the heart along with the interventricular septum and part of the right ventricle. The right coronary artery (RCA) supplies the right atrium and ventricle and part of the left ventricle. The numerous connections (anastomoses) between the arterioles of the various coronary arteries allow for the development of alternative routes of blood flow (collateral circulation) in case of blockage. Unfortunately, the coronary arteries are also vulnerable to narrowing in atherosclerotic heart disease. When the lumen (channel) of one of those arteries becomes so narrowed that blood flow through it is impeded, the symptoms of angina occur.

The arteries and the main coronary vein cross the heart in a groove, called the coronary sulcus, that separates the atria from the ventricles. Venous blood empties into the coronary sinus, a large vessel in the posterior part of the coronary sulcus, which in turn ends in the right atrium of the heart.

Structurally, the heart consists of four chambers (see Figure 27-2). The upper chambers of the heart, or atria, are separated from their respective lower chambers, or ventricles, by atrioventricular (AV) valves, which prevent backflow during ventricular contraction. The tricuspid valve separates the right atrium from the right ventricle; the mitral valve (also called bicuspid) separates the left atrium from the left ventricle. Anatomical guide wires, called chordae tendineae, attached to papillary muscles within the heart anchor those two valves and keep them from inverting (prolapsing) during ventricular contraction. Injury or disease, however, may disrupt the chordae tendineae and permit a valve to prolapse, allowing blood to regurgitate from the ventricle into the atrium.

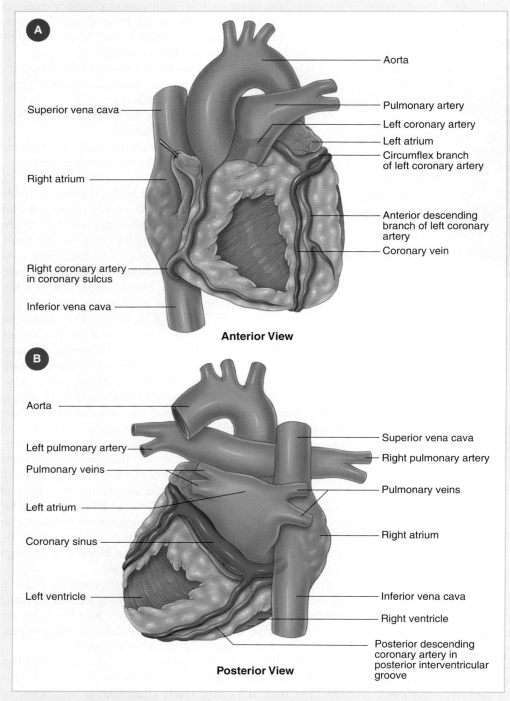

Figure 27-2 Coronary arteries. **A.** Anterior view, showing takeoff point of left and right main coronary arteries from the aorta. **B.** View from below and behind, showing the coronary sinus.

Two other valves in the heart **Figure 27-3 ▶**, which are collectively known as semilunar valves because of their half-moon shape, are found at the junction of the ventricles and the pulmonary and systemic circulation. The pulmonic valve separates the right ventricle from the pulmonary artery, preventing backflow from the artery into the right ventricle. The aortic valve serves the same function for the left ventricle, preventing blood that has already entered the aorta from flowing back into the left ventricle.

Heart Sounds

The purpose of listening to heart sounds is to identify the "lub-dub" that indicates the cardiac valves are operating properly. The major heart sounds are the two normal sounds, S_1 and S_2 **Figure 27-4 ▶**, and the two abnormal sounds, S_3 and S_4 **Figure 27-5 ▶**.

S_1 occurs near the beginning of ventricular contraction (systole), when the tricuspid and mitral valves close. The closing of these two valves should occur simultaneously as the pressure within the ventricles increases. Any delay in the closing of these two valves, heard as a split sound, is considered abnormal.

S_2 occurs near the end of ventricular contraction (systole), when the pulmonary and aortic valves close. As the ventricles relax, these valves close because of backward flow in the pulmonary artery and aorta. The two valves can close simultaneously or with a slight delay between them under normal physiological circumstances.

S_3 is the result of the end of the rapid filling period of the ventricle during the beginning of diastole. An S_3 sound should occur 120 to 170 milliseconds (ms) after S_2, if it is heard at all. S_3 is generally heard in children and young adults. When it is heard in older adults, it often signifies heart failure.

S_4, if heard, coincides with atrial contraction at the end of ventricular diastole. If heard at any other time, it usually occurs in patients who have resistance to ventricular filling, as in a weak left ventricle.

At the Scene

The mitral valve is on the left side of the heart. The left side has higher pressure than the right. Because the mitral valve is involved in the higher pressure side, remember it as the "mighty" valve.

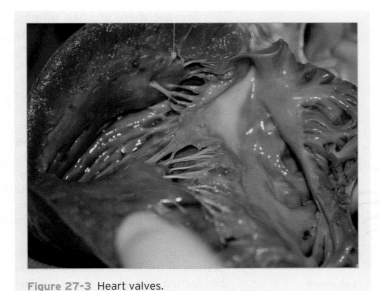

Figure 27-3 Heart valves.

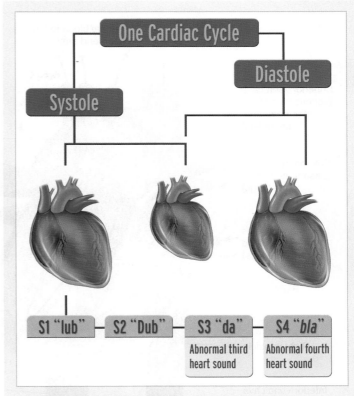

Figure 27-5 The abnormal S₃ and S₄ heart sounds.

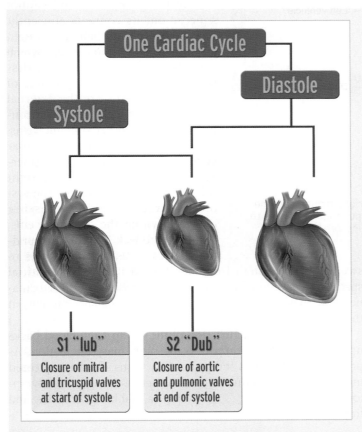

Figure 27-4 The normal S₁ and S₂ heart sounds.

The Cardiac Cycle

The cardiac cycle comprises one complete phase of atrial and ventricular relaxation (diastole), followed by one atrial and ventricular contraction (systole).

During the relatively longer relaxation phase (normally 0.52 second [s]), the left atrium fills passively with blood,

At the Scene

Atrial kick describes approximately 20% of blood flow that comes from the atria to the ventricles by contraction. The other 80% gets from the atria to the ventricles passively via gravity.

under the influence of venous pressure. Approximately 80% of ventricular filling also occurs during this time as blood flows through the open tricuspid and mitral valves.

With atrial contraction (normally both atria contract at the same time), the contents of each atrium are squeezed into the respective ventricle to complete ventricular filling. The contribution to ventricular filling made by contraction of the atrium is referred to as atrial kick—it is the amount of blood "kicked in" by the atrium. At the beginning of ventricular contraction, the AV valves snap shut, the two ventricles contract (ventricular systole), and the semilunar valves are forced open. Blood squeezed out of the right ventricle moves forward, through the pulmonic valve, and into the pulmonary arteries. Blood from the left ventricle is pushed through the aortic valve and out into the aorta. Systole is usually accomplished in a little more than half the time it takes to fill the ventricles, about 0.28 s.

Two Pumps in One

Although we called the heart a pump, that description is not entirely accurate. Functionally, the heart is actually *two*

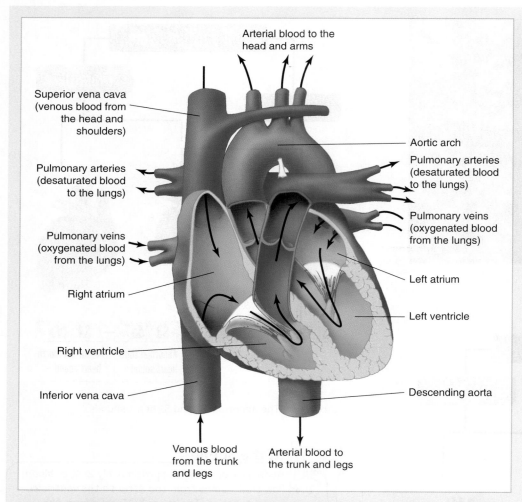

Arterial blood to the
head and arms

Superior vena cava
(venous blood from
the head and
shoulders)

Aortic arch

Pulmonary arteries
(desaturated blood
to the lungs)

Pulmonary arteries
(desaturated blood
to the lungs)

Pulmonary veins
(oxygenated blood
from the lungs)

Pulmonary veins
(oxygenated blood
from the lungs)

Left atrium

Right atrium

Left ventricle

Right ventricle

Inferior vena cava

Descending aorta

Venous blood
from the trunk
and legs

Arterial blood to
the trunk and legs

Figure 27-6 Blood flow through the heart. Desaturated blood enters the right atrium from the vena cavae, proceeds to the right ventricle, and from there moves via the pulmonary arteries to the lungs. Oxygenated blood enters the left atrium from the pulmonary veins, proceeds to the left ventricle, and then goes out to the body via the aorta.

pumps—a right pump and a left pump, separated by a thin wall (the interventricular septum)—that just happen, for purposes of efficiency, to be housed in one organ and to work in parallel Figure 27-6 ▲.

The right side of the heart, which is composed of the right atrium and right ventricle, is a *low-pressure* pump: It pumps against the relatively low resistance of the pulmonary circulation. The right atrium collects oxygen-poor venous blood from the vena cavae and the coronary sinus and pumps it into the right ventricle, which pumps the blood into the pulmonary artery for distribution to the alveoli and oxygenation.

The pulmonary veins collect the now oxygen-rich blood and return it to the left side of the heart—specifically, to the left atrium, which pumps it into the powerful left ventricle. The left side of the heart is a *high-pressure* pump: It drives blood out of the heart against the relatively high resistance of the systemic arteries.

Because there are two pumps, there must be two sets of tubing into which the pumps empty. Thus, the human body, in effect, has two circulations. The systemic circulation Figure 27-7A ▸ consists of all blood vessels beyond the left ventricle up to the right atrium, which receive the output of the left side of the heart. The pulmonary circulation Figure 27-7B ▸ comprises the blood vessels between the right ventricle and left atrium, which receive the output of the right side of the heart.

At any given time, a major proportion of the body's blood flow may be shunted into one of these two circulations. If, for example, the right side of the pump fails and cannot squeeze out its contents efficiently, blood will back up behind the right atrium into the systemic veins, which then become engorged and distended. The most readily visible of the systemic veins are the external jugular veins, which reflect the condition of all the other systemic veins. Distension of the external jugular veins signals that there is considerable back pressure from the right side of the heart throughout the systemic circulation. As pressure increases within the systemic veins, fluid starts to leak into the surrounding tissues, causing the tissues to swell. When enough fluid has leaked into the interstitial spaces, that swelling becomes visible as oedema in the subcutaneous tissues; it is less readily visible, but equally present, in the liver, walls of the intestine, and other internal tissues.

By contrast, if the left side of the pump fails, blood backs up behind the left atrium into the pulmonary circulation. As pressure builds up in the pulmonary veins, fluid is squeezed into the alveoli, producing the characteristic signs and symptoms of pulmonary oedema: dyspnoea, bubbling, crackles, and frothy sputum.

The Blood Vessels

Besides the "cardio" component (the heart), the cardiovascular system includes a second, "vascular" component—that is, the blood vessels. There are two principal types of blood vessels in the human body—arteries and veins—both of which share a common structure Figure 27-8 ▸. A protective outer layer of fibrous tissue, the tunica adventitia, provides blood vessels with the strength needed to withstand high pressure against their

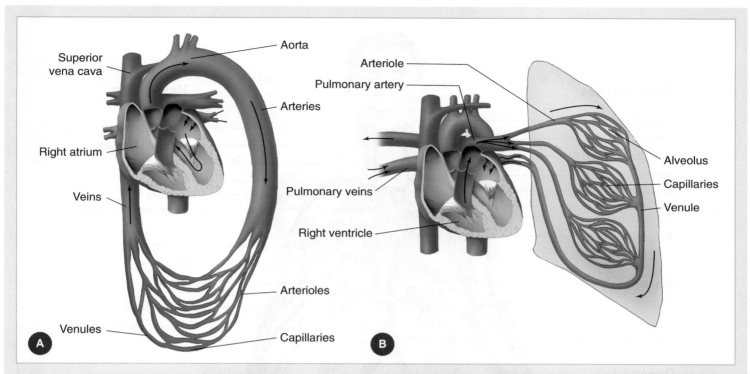

Figure 27-7 Dual human circulation. **A.** The systemic circulation consists of all blood vessels distal to the left ventricle. **B.** The pulmonary circulation consists of all blood vessels between the right ventricle and the left atrium.

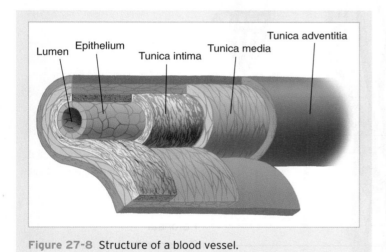

Figure 27-8 Structure of a blood vessel.

walls. A middle layer of elastic fibres and muscle, the tunica media, gives strength and contractility to blood vessels. This medial layer is much thicker and more powerful in arteries than in veins. The innermost layer of the blood vessel, the tunica intima, is a smooth inner lining that is only one cell thick. The opening within the blood vessel is referred to as the lumen.

Arteries are thick-walled, muscular vessels—befitting pipes operating in a high-pressure system—that carry blood away from the heart. Usually, arteries carry *oxygenated* blood; the only exceptions are the pulmonary arteries, which carry

oxygen-depleted blood from the right ventricle to the lungs (they carry blood away from the heart). Arteries range in size from the largest artery in the body, the aorta, to the tiniest arterial branch, or arteriole. (**Figure 27-9** ▸) depicts the major arteries in the body.

Arterial walls are highly sensitive to stimulation from the autonomic nervous system. Indeed, in response to that stimulation, their diameter may change significantly as the arteries contract and relax. In that manner, the arteries help to regulate blood pressure—that is, the pressure exerted by the blood against the arterial walls. Blood pressure is generated by repeated forceful contractions of the left ventricle, which keep blood flowing through the body. The magnitude of the blood pressure is influenced not only by the output of the heart and the volume of blood present in the system, but also by the relative constriction or dilatation of arteries.

Veins, which operate on the low-pressure side of the system, have thinner walls than arteries and, consequently, less capacity to decrease their diameter. The thinner walls also make the veins much more likely to distend when exposed to small increases in "backpressure". Veins carry blood to the heart—as a rule, oxygen-poor blood. The only exceptions are the pulmonary veins, which carry oxygenated blood to the left side of the heart. The smallest veins, or venules, gradually empty into larger and larger veins, terminating in the two largest veins of the body, the inferior and superior vena cavae. Veins also contain valves (which are unnecessary in arteries); these valves keep the blood flowing in the forward direction only.

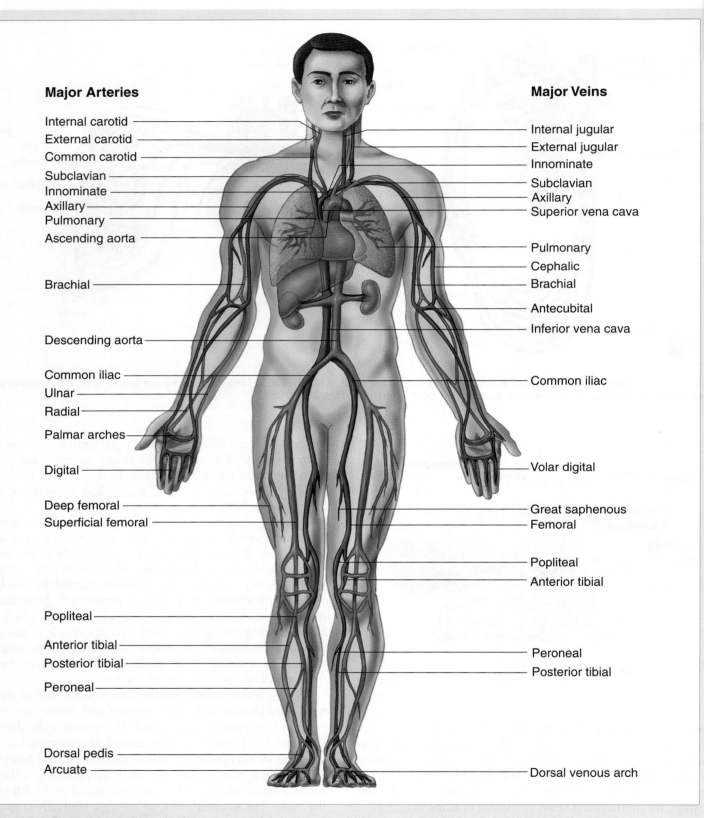

Major Arteries

Internal carotid
External carotid
Common carotid
Subclavian
Innominate
Axillary
Pulmonary
Ascending aorta
Brachial
Descending aorta
Common iliac
Ulnar
Radial
Palmar arches
Digital
Deep femoral
Superficial femoral
Popliteal
Anterior tibial
Posterior tibial
Peroneal
Dorsal pedis
Arcuate

Major Veins

Internal jugular
External jugular
Innominate
Subclavian
Axillary
Superior vena cava
Pulmonary
Cephalic
Brachial
Antecubital
Inferior vena cava
Common iliac
Volar digital
Great saphenous
Femoral
Popliteal
Anterior tibial
Peroneal
Posterior tibial
Dorsal venous arch

Figure 27-9 The major arteries and veins.

Between the tiny arterioles and venules at the tissue level is a network of microscopic blood vessels called <u>capillaries</u>. The walls of capillaries are extremely thin—only one cell thick—enabling the exchange of gases and nutrients across them; the capillary diameter is so small that red blood cells must pass through them in single file.

The Pump at Work

To understand how the heart functions as a pump, it is necessary to learn some technical terms:

- <u>Cardiac output (CO).</u> The amount of blood that is pumped out by either ventricle. The left and right ventricles are approximately equal in interior size, so the two ventricles have relatively equivalent outputs. Normal CO for an average adult is 5 to 6 litres per minute.
- <u>Stroke volume (SV).</u> The amount of blood pumped out by either ventricle in a single contraction (heartbeat). Normally, the SV is 60 to 100 ml, but the healthy heart has considerable spare capacity and can easily increase SV by at least 50%.
- <u>Heart rate (HR).</u> The number of cardiac contractions (heartbeats) per minute—in other words, the pulse rate. The normal HR for adults is 60 to 100 beats/min.

The volume of blood that either ventricle pumps out per minute equals the volume of blood it pumps out in a single contraction times the number of contractions per minute:

$$CO = SV \times HR$$

To meet changing demands, the heart must be able to increase its output several times over in response to the body's increased demand for oxygen—for example, during exercise. The CO equation tells us that the heart can increase its output by increasing its SV, increasing its rate, or both.

In a mechanical piston pump, the SV is a fixed quantity related to the distance travelled by the piston and the size of the cylinder. The heart, by contrast, has several ways of increasing SV. One characteristic of cardiac muscle is that, when it is stretched, it contracts with greater force to a limit—a property called the Frank-Starling mechanism. If an increased volume of blood is returned from the systemic veins to the right side of the heart or from the pulmonary veins to the left side of the heart, the muscle surrounding the cardiac chambers must stretch to accommodate the larger volume. The more the cardiac muscle stretches, the greater the force of its contraction, the more completely it empties, and, therefore, the greater the SV. From the CO equation, it is clear that any increase in SV, with the HR held constant, will cause an increase in the overall CO.

The pressure under which a ventricle fills is called the <u>preload</u> and is influenced by the volume of blood returned by the veins to the heart. In situations of increased oxygen demand, the body returns more blood to the heart (preload increases), and CO consequently increases through the Frank-Starling mechanism. In a diseased heart, the same mechanism is used

At the Scene

The Frank-Starling mechanism is named after the two men who first described it. In the late 19th century, Otto Frank discovered that in the frog heart, the strength of ventricular contraction was increased when the ventricle was stretched before contraction. In the 20th century, Ernest Starling expounded on this information with studies finding that increasing venous return, and, therefore, the filling pressure of the ventricle, led to increased SV in dogs.

to achieve a normal resting CO (which explains why some diseased hearts become enlarged).

The heart can also vary the degree of contraction of its muscle *without* changing the stretch on the muscle—a property called <u>contractility</u>. Changes in contractility may be induced by medications that have a positive or negative inotropic effect. The ventricles are never completely emptied of blood with any single beat. However, if the heart squeezes into a tighter ball when it contracts, a larger percentage of the ventricular blood will be ejected, thereby increasing SV and overall CO. Nervous controls regulate the contractility of the heart from beat to beat. When the body requires increased CO, nervous signals increase myocardial contractility, thereby augmenting SV.

The heart can also increase its CO, given a constant SV, by increasing the number of contractions per minute—that is, by increasing the HR (positive <u>chronotropic</u> effect). As an example, consider a heart that has a resting SV of 70 ml/beat and a resting rate of 70 beats/min:

$$CO = 70 \text{ ml} \times 70 \text{ beats/min} = 4,900 \text{ ml}$$

Suppose that the owner of that heart begins to exercise. Oxygen demand increases, and nervous mechanisms stimulate the heart to increase its rate. If, for example, the HR increases to 110 beats/min without any change in the SV, the CO would increase as follows:

The Frank-Starling mechanism is an intrinsic property of heart muscle—that is, it is not under nervous system control. By contrast, contractility and changes in HR are regulated by the nervous system.

$$CO = 70 \text{ ml/beat} \times 110 \text{ beats/min} = 7,700 \text{ ml/min}$$

The Electrical Conduction System of the Heart

Heart muscle is unique among body tissues because it can generate its own electric impulses without stimulation from nerves, a property known as <u>automaticity</u>. In addition, the heart is endowed with specialised conduction tissue that can rapidly propagate electrical impulses to the muscular tissue of the heart. The area of conduction tissue in which the electrical activity arises at any given time is called the pacemaker, because it sets the pace (that is, rate) for cardiac contraction. This system as a whole is termed the electrical conduction system.

The Dominant Pacemaker: The Sinoatrial Node

Theoretically, any cell within the heart's electrical conduction system can act as a pacemaker. In the normal heart, however, the dominant pacemaker is the sinoatrial (SA) node, which is located in the right atrium, near the inlet of the superior vena cava (**Figure 27-10 ▾**). The SA node receives blood from the right coronary artery (RCA). If the RCA is occluded, as in an acute myocardial infarction (AMI), the SA node will become ischaemic. The subsequent death of the conduction cells will prevent the SA node from firing.

The SA node is the fastest pacemaker in the heart. Electric impulses generated in this node spread across the two atria through internodal pathways (including the Bachman bundle) in the atrial wall in about 0.08 s, causing the atrial tissue to depolarise as they pass. From there, they move to the atrioventricular (AV) node in the region of the AV junction (which includes the AV node and its surrounding tissue along with the bundle of His). The AV node serves as a "gatekeeper" to the ventricles. In 85% to 90% of humans, its blood supply comes from a branch of the RCA; in 10% to 15%, it comes from a branch of the left circumflex artery. The conduction of the impulse is delayed in the AV node for about 0.12 s so that the atria can empty into the ventricles. Approximately 70% to 90% of the blood in the atria fills the ventricles by gravity; the remaining 10% to 30% comes from atrial contraction (atrial kick).

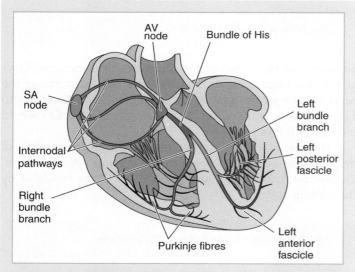

Figure 27-10 Electrical conduction system of the heart. Impulses that originate in the SA node spread through the atria and along the internodal pathways to the AV node. From the AV node, they travel down the bundle of His and right and left bundle branches and into the Purkinje network of the ventricles.

When the atrial rate becomes very rapid, not all atrial impulses can get through the AV junction. Normally, however, impulses pass through it into the bundle of His and then move rapidly into the right and left bundle branches located on either side of the interventricular septum. Next, they spread into the Purkinje fibres, thousands of fibrils distributed through the ventricular muscle. It takes about 0.08 s for an electric impulse to spread across the ventricles, during which time the ventricles contract simultaneously. The effect on the velocity of conduction is referred to as the dromotropic effect.

Depolarisation and Repolarisation

Depolarisation—the process by which muscle fibres are stimulated to contract—comes about through changes in the concentration of electrolytes across cell membranes (**Figure 27-11A ▸**). Myocardial cells, like all cells in the body, are bathed in an electrolyte solution. Chemical pumps inside the cell maintain the concentrations of ions within the cell, in the process creating an electric gradient across the cell wall. As a consequence, a resting (polarised) cell normally has a net charge of −90 millivolts (mV) with respect to the outside of the cell (Figure 27-11, part A1). When the myocardial cell receives a stimulus from the conduction system (Figure 27-11, part A2), the permeability of the cell wall changes through opening of specialised channels in such a way that sodium ions (Na^+) rush into the cell, causing the inside of the cell to become more positive. Calcium ions (Ca^{++}) also enter the cell—albeit more slowly and through a different set of specialised channels—helping to maintain the depolarised state of the cell membrane and supplying calcium ions for use in contraction of the cardiac muscle tissue. This reversal of electric charge—depolarisation—starts at one spot in the cell and spreads in a wave along the cell until the cell is completely depolarised (Figure 27-11, part A3). As the cell depolarises and calcium ions enter, mechanical contraction occurs.

If the cell were to remain depolarised, it could never contract again! Fortunately, the cell is able to recover from depolarisation through a process called repolarisation (**Figure 27-11B ▸**). Repolarisation starts with the closing of the sodium and calcium channels, which stops the rapid inflow of these ions. Next, special potassium channels open, allowing a rapid escape of potassium ions (K^+) from the cell. This helps restore the inside of the cell to its negative charge; the proper electrolyte distribution is then reestablished by pumping sodium ions out of the cell and potassium ions back in. After the potassium channels close, this sodium-potassium pump helps move sodium and potassium ions back to their respective locations. For every three sodium ions this pump moves out of the cell, it moves two potassium ions into the cell, thereby maintaining the polarity of the cell membrane. To accomplish this task, the sodium-potassium pump moves ions against the natural gradient by a process called active transport, which requires the expenditure of energy.

Table 27-7	Responses to Sympathetic Stimulation
Organ	**Sympathetic Stimulation**
Heart	Increased HR (positive chronotropic effect) (beta-1)
	Increased force of contraction (positive inotropic effect) (beta-1)
	Increased conduction velocity (positive dromotropic effect) (beta-1)
Arteries	Constriction (alpha)
Lungs	Bronchial muscle relaxation (beta-2)

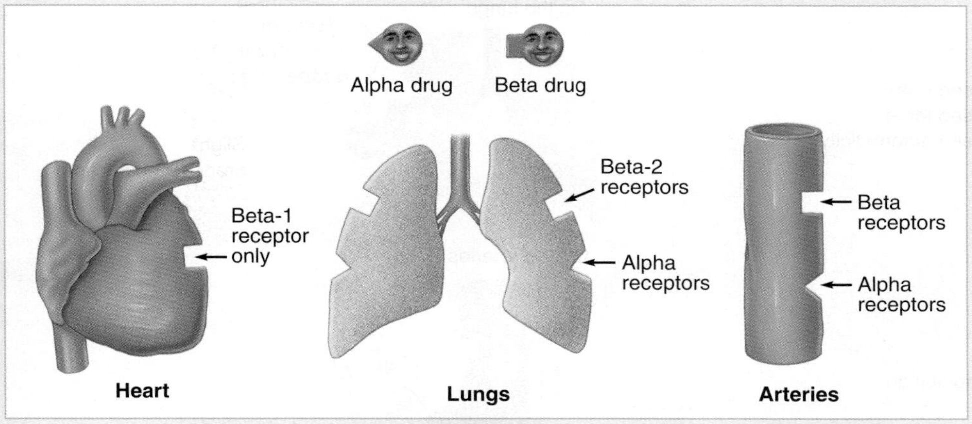

Figure 27-14 Receptor sites of the sympathetic nervous system in the heart, lungs, and arteries.

drug receptor can be visualised as analogous to the ignition switch in a car. When the proper key is inserted into the car's ignition and turned, a predictable sequence of events follows: The battery sends a current to the starter and the spark plugs, which fire; combustion of petrol and air occurs; and the engine starts. Although many keys may fit into a specific car's ignition, not every key that fits will turn and start the car—but all that do turn cause the same reaction. Likewise, the organs of the body have a number of "ignition switches". In the sympathetic nervous system, those switches, or receptors, are labelled alpha and beta. Whenever one of those switches is activated by a "key" (a drug or hormone), a predictable sequence of responses will occur Table 27-7 .

The heart has only one ignition switch for a beta agent. Any beta agent will have the same effect on the heart—that is, it will increase the heart's rate, force, and automaticity. The arteries, by contrast, have receptors for alpha and beta agents. An alpha drug will turn on the switch that causes vasoconstric-

At the Scene

To remember the difference between beta-1 and beta-2, ask yourself, "How many hearts do I have"? One heart—beta-1. "How many lungs do I have"? Two lungs—beta-2.

tion; a beta agent will activate the switch that causes vasodilation. Similarly, the lungs have alpha and beta receptors. Alpha agents don't have much effect on the lungs; at most, they cause minor bronchoconstriction. By contrast, beta agents (such as drugs used to treat asthma) trigger significant bronchodilation. Figure 27-14 represents these concepts schematically.

Drugs that have alpha or beta sympathetic properties are called sympathomimetic drugs because they imitate (mimic) the actions of naturally occurring sympathetic chemicals. If we know whether a sympathomimetic drug is an alpha or beta agent, we can predict the response by the heart, lungs, and arteries.

Consider isoproterenol. It is a pure beta agent. Armed with this knowledge, we can recognise immediately that isoproterenol acts in the manner shown in Figure 27-15 —it stimulates the heart, dilates the bronchi, and dilates the arteries.

Phenylephrine by contrast, is a pure alpha agent. It has no direct effect on the heart but causes slight bronchoconstriction and marked vasoconstriction Figure 27-16 .

In reality, things are not always so simple. Although isoproterenol and phenylephrine are pure beta and alpha agents, respectively, most other sympathomimetic drugs have varying degrees of alpha and beta activity Figure 27-17 . Noradrenaline is chiefly an alpha agent, and its alpha effects predominate; because it also has some beta activity, however, it will have effects on the heart. Conversely, adrenaline is chiefly a beta agent, and its beta effects predominate; nevertheless, when administered in high doses, adrenaline will produce some alpha effects, especially on the arteries.

Table 27-8 lists several sympathomimetic agents that are commonly encountered in the prehospital environment. Two of the drugs, noradrenaline and adrenaline, are also naturally occurring chemicals of the sympathetic nervous system. Their actions are the same whether they are produced in the body and released from the nervous system or manufactured in a factory and injected.

Beta sympathetic agents can be classified into two groups based on the subtle differences between the beta receptors in the heart and the lungs. Drugs that act primarily on cardiac beta receptors are called beta-1; those that act chiefly on pulmonary beta receptors are called beta-2. Some newer bronchodilators—such as salbutamol and terbutaline—are selective beta-2 agents, so they provide effective bronchodilation with far fewer cardiac side effects.

Another class of drugs that acts on the sympathetic nervous system comprises the sympatholytic or sympathetic blockers. As their name implies, they block the action of sympathetic

Table 27-8	Common Sympathomimetic Agents
Alpha	**Phenylephrine**
Alpha	Noradrenaline bitartrate
↓	Dopamine
Beta	Adrenaline
Beta	Salbutamol
	Isoproterenol

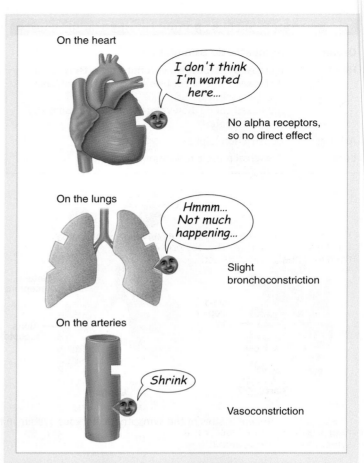

Figure 27-16 Alpha agents have no direct effect on the heart; they cause slight bronchoconstriction and marked vasoconstriction.

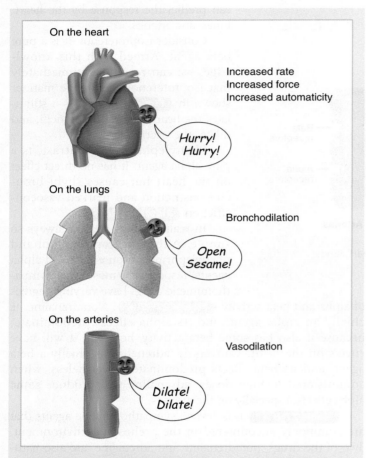

Figure 27-15 Beta sympathetic agents increase the rate, force, and automaticity of the heart; dilate the bronchi; and dilate peripheral arteries.

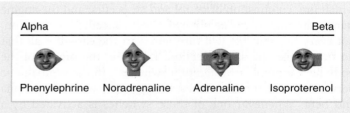

Figure 27-17 Many sympathomimetic agents have alpha and beta properties.

agents by beating them to the receptor sites and preventing these agents from turning on the ignition. The receptor sites, which aren't very smart, cannot distinguish a blocker from a stimulator until it is too late. With the blocker occupying the receptor site, the stimulating agent cannot get in to turn on the switch (Figure 27-18 ▸).

Beta blockers occupy beta receptors in the heart, lungs, and arteries, as well as elsewhere in the body (Figure 27-19 ▸). Thus beta agents, whether released from sympathetic nerve endings or given intravenously, cannot exert their full effects when a beta blocker such as propranolol has been administered previously (Figure 27-20 ▸).

The indications for the major autonomic stimulating and blocking agents can be deduced once we know the properties of the drugs and the manner in which they interact with the autonomic nervous system:

- **Atropine.** Parasympathetic blocker, opposing the vagus nerve. It is used to speed the heart when excessive vagal firing has caused bradycardia.
- **Noradrenaline.** Sympathetic agent (primarily alpha), causing vasoconstriction. It is used to increase the blood pressure when hypotension is caused by vasodilation (as in neurogenic shock).

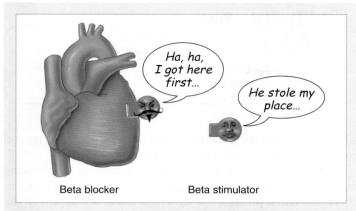

Figure 27-18 A sympathetic blocker occupies the receptor site for the stimulating drug, thereby preventing the stimulating drug from exerting its usual effect.

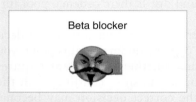

Figure 27-19 A beta blocker is a sympathetic blocking agent.

- **Isoproterenol.** Sympathetic agent (almost pure beta), causing a strong increase in HR and dilation of bronchi. It is used in extreme cases to increase CO and to dilate bronchi in asthma.
- **Adrenaline.** Sympathetic agent (predominantly beta), with actions similar to those of isoproterenol, but having an additional, primarily peripheral vasoconstrictor effect. Indications for adrenaline are similar to those for isoproterenol, but also include asystole, pulseless electrical activity (PEA), and ventricular fibrillation (to increase the automaticity of the heart and vasoconstriction); and anaphylactic shock (for all of its effects—bronchodilation, vasoconstriction, increased CO).
- **Dopamine.** Sympathetic agent, used at low (beta) doses to increase the force of cardiac contractions in cardiogenic shock. Its dilation (beta) effects on renal and mesenteric arteries mean that dopamine may help maintain urine flow and good perfusion to abdominal organs.
- **Salbutamol, isoetharine, terbutaline.** Sympathetic beta-2 agents that act on the lungs. These agents are used to induce bronchodilation in asthma, chronic obstructive pulmonary disease, and other bronchospastic conditions.
- **Propranolol.** Sympathetic beta blocker, opposing the actions of beta-stimulating agents. It is used clinically to slow the HR in certain tachyarrhythmias, to decrease the pain of chronic angina (by decreasing the work of the heart), and to depress irritability in the heart (by decreasing the tendency of the heart to fire automatically). Its use is contraindicated in asthma.

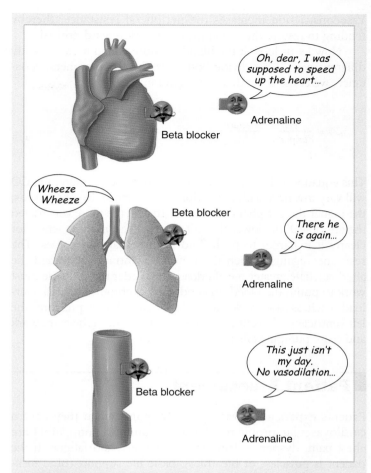

Figure 27-20 By occupying beta receptor sites, the beta blocker prevents adrenaline from exerting its usual effects on the heart, lungs, and blood vessels.

The Sympathetic Nervous System and Blood Pressure Regulation

The body attempts to maintain a fairly constant blood pressure to ensure perfusion of vital organs. At any given moment, the blood pressure is influenced by the CO and the resistance (degree of constriction) of the arterioles:

$$Blood\ Pressure = CO \times Peripheral\ Resistance$$

Thus, the blood pressure can be increased by increasing the CO, the peripheral resistance, or both.

Under normal circumstances, the body balances flow and resistance to maintain a stable blood pressure. That is, alterations in one variable bring about compensatory changes in the other variable to restore blood pressure toward normal. Consider, for example, a situation in which CO decreases suddenly, as in haemorrhage. The fall in CO will inevitably lead to a fall in blood pressure unless the peripheral resistance is altered. The falling CO activates the sympathetic nervous system, however, which in turn causes the arterioles to constrict.

Vasoconstriction increases the peripheral resistance, thereby tending to restore the blood pressure back toward normal.

Now let us look at the blood pressure equation in a slightly different way. If we divide both sides by the peripheral resistance, we come up with a new equation:

$$CO = \frac{Blood\ Pressure}{Peripheral\ Resistance}$$

This equation tells us that, for any given blood pressure, the CO will vary inversely with the peripheral resistance. In other words, the higher the peripheral resistance (that is, the more constricted the arterioles), the lower the CO. That makes intuitive sense, for clearly it is harder to push fluid through narrower pipes. The resistance against which the ventricle contracts is termed the afterload. The greater the afterload, the harder the ventricle must work to pump the blood. In conditions of chronically high afterload, such as arteriosclerosis-induced high blood pressure, the left ventricle may eventually grow exhausted from the extra work and cease pumping efficiently or even fail.

Patient Assessment

Patients experience a variety of symptoms when they have a cardiovascular problem. The most common complaints are chest pain, dyspnoea, fainting, palpitations, and fatigue. If the patient is pulseless or breathless, basic life support (BLS) measures may be used. In some cases, advanced cardiac life support (ACLS) procedures may be necessary. This section reviews the organised approach to assessing patients by focusing on their cardiac and pulmonary systems. For this assessment, we will assume the patient is conscious and breathing and has a pulse.

Scene Assessment
The initial assessment begins with assessing the scene and ensuring scene safety. In addition, you should try to anticipate the need for other resources such as extra personnel.

Initial Assessment
Observe the patient's general appearance as you approach him or her, and assess for apparent life threats. The initial assessment is fairly consistent for all patients, but this discussion has a cardiac focus. Sometimes assessing the ABCs can be accomplished easily by merely greeting the patient and introducing yourself, assuming that the patient can answer you, is conscious, has an open airway, is breathing, and has a pulse. Determine the patient's level of consciousness (LOC) based on his or her response to your greeting, and use the AVPU scale.

Determine the patency of the patient's airway. If the patient is talking to you, the airway is patent. The patient may be able to maintain an open airway or, depending on the LOC, may need help with clearing obstructions (debris, blood, or teeth) by your properly positioning the head and/or placing an airway

At the Scene

Just by shaking someone's hand and introducing yourself, you can learn a lot about the patient. It's a great way to check the ABCs as long as the person is conscious.

adjunct. Note the rate, quality, and effort of the breathing, and consider initiating oxygen therapy at this time.

Assessment of circulation is done primarily by checking the patient's pulse. For a conscious patient, you will typically check the radial pulse; if the patient is unconscious, check the carotid pulse. While checking the pulse, note the rate, regularity, and overall quality. Is it weak, bounding, or irregular?

While holding the patient's hand in yours, assess the skin colour and condition. The skin is the largest organ of the body, so a good indication that the rest of the body is getting adequate circulation is that the skin and mucous membranes are pink and the skin is warm and dry. Is there oedema, poor turgor, or skin "tenting"?

The initial assessment ends with making a transport decision for your patient. Based on your findings to this point, you should be able to determine whether the patient requires immediate transport. If you are unsure, continue with the focused assessment, and the correct decision may become more apparent.

Focused History and Physical Examination
During the focused history and physical examination, you will perform a focused assessment. This inquiry into the patient's medical history and a physical examination are based on the patient's chief complaint; the inquiry is also referred to as the history of present illness. The SAMPLE history is included in this assessment. In patients with acute coronary syndromes (ACSs), the most common chief complaints are chest pain, dyspnoea, fainting, palpitations, and fatigue.

Symptoms
Chest pain is often the presenting symptom of an AMI. The patient's description of the pain is important for assessing its significance. The OPQRST format can be used to elaborate on the patient's chief complaint:

O   What is the *Onset* or origin of the pain—that is, how did it begin (suddenly or gradually)? Has anything like this ever happened before?

P   What *Provoked* the pain—that is, what, if anything, brought it on? Is it exertional or nonexertional? What was the patient doing at the time? Sitting in a chair? Changing a tyre? Having an argument with the boss? Does anything make it worse? What palliates the pain—that is, does anything make it better? Patients with chronic coronary artery disease (CAD) may take glyceryltrinitrate (GTN) for episodes of chest pain. Ask whether the patient did so and, if so, whether it helped.

Q What is the *Quality* of the pain—that is, what does it feel like? Get the patient's narrative description. Dull? Sharp? Crushing? Heavy? Squeezing? Note the exact words the patient uses to describe the pain, and observe the patient's body language as he or she does so. Try not to lead the patient's description unless he or she is unable to describe the pain. In such cases, try to give alternatives, such as "Is it sharp or dull"?

R Does the pain *Radiate*? From where to where? To the jaw? Down the left arm? Into the back?

S What is the *Severity* of the pain—that is, how bad is it? Use the pain scale of 1 to 10, with 10 being the worst. If the patient has chronic angina, ask him or her to compare the pain with the usual angina pain.

T What was the *Timing* of the attack—that is, when did it start? How long did it last? What time did it get worse or better? Was it continuous or intermittent?

Another chief complaint among patients with an acute coronary syndrome (ACS) is dyspnoea. In the context of ACSs, dyspnoea may be the first clue to failure of the left side of the heart. To explore this possibility, ask the following questions:

- When did the dyspnoea start? Did it awaken the patient from sleep? Paroxysmal nocturnal dyspnoea (PND) is an acute episode of shortness of breath in which the patient suddenly awakens from sleep with a feeling of suffocation. Often the patient will report going to a window to get "more air" or will move from the bed to a chair. PND is one of the classic signs of left-sided heart failure, although it may also occur in chronic lung diseases.
- Did the dyspnoea come on gradually or suddenly?
- Is it continuous or intermittent?
- Does it happen during activity or while at rest?
- Does any position make the dyspnoea better or worse? The dyspnoea of pulmonary oedema usually worsens when the patient is lying down (orthopnoea), because blood pools in the lungs when the body is horizontal. Patients with significant orthopnoea will often sleep with several pillows, or even sitting in a chair, to maintain a semi-upright position.
- Has the patient ever had dyspnoea like this before? If so, under what circumstances?
- Does the patient have a cough? Is it dry or productive?
- Were there any associated symptoms?

Fainting (syncope) occurs when CO suddenly declines, leading to a reduction in cerebral perfusion. Cardiac causes of syncope include arrhythmias, increased vagal tone, and heart lesions. There are also numerous noncardiac causes of syncope (discussed in Chapter 28). As part of taking a history from someone who has fainted, try to sort out whether the patient fainted from cardiac or noncardiac causes:

- Under what circumstances did the syncopal episode occur? What was the patient doing at the time? A 20-year-old who faints at the sight of blood is unlikely to have significant underlying cardiac disease; a 60-year-old who faints after feeling some "fluttering" in the chest may have a dangerous cardiac arrhythmia.

- Were there any warning feelings before the episode, or did the fainting spell occur suddenly and unexpectedly?
- What position was the patient in when he or she fainted? Standing? Sitting? Lying down? Losing consciousness while sitting or lying down has more ominous implications than fainting while standing up.
- Has the patient fainted before? If so, under what circumstances?
- Were there any associated symptoms, such as nausea, vomiting, urinary incontinence, or convulsions?

Finally, patients with cardiac problems may present with a chief complaint of palpitations. Palpitations refer to the sensation of an abnormally fast or irregular heartbeat—except after extreme exertion, a person normally remains blissfully unaware of his or her heartbeat. The cause of palpitations is often a cardiac arrhythmia, such as premature ventricular contractions (PVCs) or paroxysmal supraventricular tachycardia (PSVT). The patient may not use the word "palpitations" but may report feeling the heart "skip a beat" or use words to that effect. In such a case, inquire about the onset, frequency, and duration of this symptom and previous episodes of palpitations. Also ask about the presence of associated symptoms (such as chest pain, dizziness, and dyspnoea).

Patients may report a variety of other related symptoms as you explore their history of present illness. They may have a "feeling of impending doom" or a sense that they will soon experience a life-changing event. Some patients relate feeling nauseous or having vomited. Listen carefully for indications that trauma may be involved or that their activity has been limited as a result of their condition. Observe their faces as you listen to them tell their stories. Do you see a look of fear or anguish? Are they holding their chest? Most of the other associated complaints your patients may have are related to hypoxia or poor perfusion resulting from inadequate CO—for example, decreased LOC, perspiring, restlessness and anxiety, fatigue, headache, behavioural changes, and syncope.

After exploring the patient's chief complaint, inquire briefly about pertinent aspects of the patient's other medical history:

- Is the patient under treatment for any serious illnesses or conditions? Ask specifically whether he or she has ever been diagnosed with any of the following:
  - Coronary artery disease
  - Atherosclerotic heart disease: angina, previous acute myocardial infarction (AMI), hypertension, congestive heart failure (CHF)
  - Valvular disease
  - Aneurysm
  - Pulmonary disease
  - Diabetes
  - Renal disease
  - Vascular disease
  - Inflammatory cardiac disease
  - Previous cardiac surgery (such as coronary artery bypass graft or valve replacement)
  - Congenital anomalies
- Is the patient taking any medications regularly? The focused history is a great opportunity to ask about which

drugs have been prescribed and whether the patient is taking them as instructed. Be sure to ask when the patient took the medications last. Is he or she taking medications that were prescribed for someone else (borrowed)? Also ask about any general-sales-list medications or any herbal supplements the patient uses. It may be appropriate to ask about recreational drug use. Take particular note of the groups of medications prescribed for the treatment of cardiac problems listed in **Table 27-9 ▸**. If you are unfamiliar with any medication, ask the patient what it was prescribed for. It is also a good idea to ask if the patient takes any medication for each medical condition he or she reports as part of the history and to verify these medical conditions match the medications the patient is actually taking.

- Does the patient have known allergies to foods or medications? If so, ask what kind of reaction the patient has with each one.

- Ask the patient when he or she last had anything to eat or drink, and note the time that occurred. This information will prove helpful later in many situations.

- If you haven't asked already, find out the history of the current event. Get any extra information about what was happening when the problem started and what was done before your arrival.

Vital Signs
Pulse
When you take the vital signs, make a careful assessment of the patient's pulse. Is it regular or irregular? Abnormally fast or slow? Strong or weak? An irregular pulse signals a disturbance in cardiac rhythm. A very rapid pulse (tachycardia) may simply indicate anxiety, but it can also occur secondary to severe pain, CHF, or a cardiac arrhythmia. A weak, thready pulse suggests a reduction in CO.

You should be familiar with the potentially abnormal pulse findings. For example, the patient may have a pulse deficit. A deficit occurs when the palpated radial pulse rate is less than the apical pulse rate; it is reported numerically as the difference between the two. To assess for a deficit, check the peripheral radial pulse while listening to an apical pulse.

Another abnormal pulse finding is pulsus paradoxus. Pulsus paradoxus is an excessive drop (> 10 mm Hg) in the systolic blood pressure with each inspired breath. Pulsus paradoxus can sometimes be palpated as a decrease in the amplitude of the pulse waveform, which makes the affected pulse beats feel weaker than the others. This observation can best be made when the rhythm is regular. If the variation is slight, it can be detected only by use of a blood pressure cuff and stethoscope.

Finally, you might recognise pulsus alternans. This pulse alternates in strength from one beat to the next.

Blood Pressure
In patients older than 50 years, a systolic blood pressure of more than 140 mm Hg is a much more important risk factor for CVD than the diastolic pressure. Patients with a systolic

Table 27-9	Medicines Prescribed to Treat or Prevent Heart Disease
Category	**Drug**
Angiotensin-converting enzyme inhibitors	Captopril, enalapril lisinopril, benazepril, fosinopril, ramipril, quinapril, perindopril, trandolapril, moexipril
Calcium channel blockers	Amlodipine, felodipine, diltiazem, verapamil, nifedipine, nicardipine, nisoldipine, bepridil
Angiotensin II receptor blockers	Losartan, valsartan, irbesartan, candesartan
Cholesterol-lowering drugs	Statins: lovastatin, fluvastatin, pravastatin, atorvastatin, simvastatin Niacins: nicotinic acid, extended-release niacin, Bile acid resins: colestipol, cholestyramine, cholesevelam,Fibrates: clofibrate, gemfibrozil, fenofibrate
Anti-arrhythmics	Amiodarone, sotalol
Cardiac glycoside	Digoxin
Anti-platelet agents	Clopidogrel, ticlopidine, aspirin
Diuretics	Furosemide, bumetanide, torsemide, hydrochlorothiazid, metolazone, spironolactone
Beta blockers	Acebutolol, bisoprolol, esmolol, propranolol, atenolol, labetalol, carvedilol, metoprolol
Vasodilators	Isosorbide dinitrate*, isosorbide, mononitrate, hydralazine*
Coumarin anti-coagulant	Warfarin

*Isosorbide dinitrate and hydralazine are given together.

blood pressure of 120 to 139 mm Hg or a diastolic blood pressure of 80 to 89 mm Hg are considered "prehypertensive" and need to adopt a healthier lifestyle to prevent CVD.

In emergency situations, an elevated blood pressure may reflect the patient's anxiety or pain. A systolic blood pressure of less than 90 mm Hg might suggest serious hypotension and shock, depending on the patient's overall condition and chief complaint. The pulse pressure (the difference between the systolic and diastolic pressures) gives a rough indication of the elasticity of the arterial walls and the SV. In patients with arteriosclerosis, the arterial walls are stiffened, and the pulse pressure is increased. In cardiogenic shock or cardiac tamponade, the SV is reduced because the heart cannot pump effectively, so the pulse pressure is narrowed accordingly.

It may be beneficial to take the blood pressure in both arms and compare the readings. Some conditions such as stroke or aortic aneurysm may cause blood pressures to vary from the right to the left side.

Respirations
Note the rate and quality of the patient's respirations. Is the respiratory rate abnormally rapid (tachypnoea)? Is the patient

labouring to breathe? Respiratory distress in a cardiac patient suggests the possibility of CHF, with fluid in the lungs. Remember the old saying, "Look, listen, and feel"? In this physical examination, it is called inspection, auscultation, and palpation.

Cardiac Monitoring and Pulse Oximetry

As part of taking the vital signs, attach the cardiac monitor and pulse oximeter if you have not done so already. Use the ECG interpretation and oxygen saturation measurement just as you do other vital signs—that is, as tools to help you in your assessment and not as the only guide to treatment (treat the patient, not the monitor). When caring for a patient in relatively stable condition who does not require rapid assessment, the physical examination may be done at this point.

Focused Physical Examination

The focused physical examination is similar for many medical patients. Nevertheless, certain aspects warrant greater emphasis in the patient whose chief complaint suggests a cardiac problem.

When observing the patient's general appearance, pay particular attention to the LOC, which is an excellent indicator of the adequacy of cerebral perfusion. If a patient is alert and orientated, the brain is getting enough oxygen, which in turn means the heart is doing its job as a pump. Conversely, stupor or confusion may indicate poor CO, which may be the result of myocardial damage or dysfunction. Skin colour and temperature are also valuable indicators of the state of the patient's circulation: The cold, sweaty skin of many patients with AMI reflects massive peripheral vasoconstriction.

Physical Examination

In continuing the physical examination, begin by inspecting the neck and tracheal position. Is the trachea midline and mobile to gentle manipulation? Press down with your finger in the patient's suprasternal notch to verify that the trachea is midline.

What about the adjacent structures such as the neck veins? The external jugular veins reflect the pressure within the patient's systemic circulation. Normally, they are collapsed when a person is sitting or standing. If the function of the right side of the heart is compromised, however, blood will back up into the systemic veins behind the right side of the heart and distend those veins. To estimate the patient's venous pressure, place the patient in a semi-sitting position (45° angle) with the head slightly rotated away from the jugular vein you are examining; observe the height of the distended fluid column within the vein, and note how far up the distension extends above the sternal angle.

Continue the assessment by inspecting and palpating the chest. Look for surgical scars that might indicate previous cardiac surgery. Is there a GTN patch on the patient's skin? Is there a bulge under the patient's skin indicating a pacemaker or an implanted cardioverter defibrillator (ICD)? These devices are implanted just below the right or left clavicle and are about the size of a small matchbox **Figure 27-21 ▶**. Is the anterior-posterior diameter of the chest enlarged, as in a barrel-chested patient with COPD? On palpation, do you observe any sign of crepitus?

Listen carefully to the chest with your stethoscope. Crackles or wheezes may be suggestive of left-sided heart failure with pulmonary oedema. Listen for a third heart sound ("lub da-da" instead of "lub-dub"), known as an S_3 gallop, which again gives evidence of CHF. Examine the extremities and back for oedema, a sign of failure of the right side of the heart.

Ongoing Assessment

Once the history and vital signs have been taken and the physical examination has been completed, treatment of the patient should be continued and transport initiated. The ongoing assessment is accomplished en route to hospital. It begins with a repeated initial assessment (LOC and ABCs). The vital signs should be taken every 5 to 15 minutes during this time as well. A repeated physical examination should be accomplished to see if any changes have occurred or if any conditions were missed in the initial physical examination. Finally, all the effectiveness of interventions implemented should be assessed. For

You are the Paramedic Part 2

Although the history is difficult to obtain, you learn that Mrs Beresford has been getting increasingly short of breath on exertion and waking at night gasping for breath. You also review her prescribed medication and note that she is taking aspirin, ramipril, furosemide, bisoprolol, and digoxin. On examination, there is widespread wheeze and basal crackles in both lungs. In addition, you find a raised JVP and pitting oedema to the level of her sacrum.

Vital Signs	Recording Time: 5 minutes
Skin	Pale, cool, and perspiring
Pulse	140 beats/min, irregular
Blood pressure	195/115 mm Hg
Respirations	43 breaths/min, shallow and laboured
SpO_2	87% on supplemental oxygen at 15 l/min

3. Why does the patient wake at night gasping for breath?
4. What types of medication is the patient taking? How does this help you with the patient's medical history?

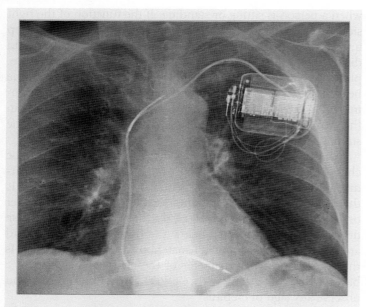

Figure 27-21 An ICD is attached directly to the heart and continuously monitors heart rhythm, delivering shocks as needed. The electricity from the ICD is so low that it has no effect on rescuers.

example, is the IV fluid still flowing or has the pain diminished after GTN administration?

Pathophysiology and Management of Cardiovascular Problems

CAD and Angina

Coronary artery disease (CAD) is the most common form of heart disease and the leading cause of death in European adults. The coronary arteries supply oxygen and nutrients to the myocardium. If one of these blood vessels becomes blocked, the muscle it supplies will be deprived of oxygen (ischaemia). If this oxygen supply is not quickly restored, the ischaemic area of heart muscle will eventually die (undergo infarction).

Atherosclerosis is of particular concern because it affects the inner lining of the aorta and cerebral and coronary blood vessels, leading to the narrowing of those vessels and reduction of blood flow through them. The atherosclerotic process begins, probably in childhood, when small amounts of fatty material are deposited along the inner wall (intima) of arteries, usually at points of turbulent blood flow (such as where the arteries bifurcate or where the arterial wall has been damaged). As the streak of fat enlarges, it becomes a mass of fatty tissue, an atheroma, which gradually calcifies and hardens into a plaque. The atheromatous plaque infiltrates the arterial wall and decreases its elasticity. At the same time, it narrows the arterial lumen and interferes with blood flow through the lumen. The narrowed, roughened area of the arterial intima

provides a locus for the formation of a fixed blood clot, or thrombus, which may then obstruct the artery altogether (when in a coronary artery is known as a coronary thrombosis). In addition, calcium may precipitate from the bloodstream into the arterial walls, causing arteriosclerosis, which greatly reduces the elasticity of the arteries.

Risk Factors for Atherosclerosis

Although atherosclerosis is widespread in industrialised countries, certain factors increase the risk of developing atherosclerosis and CAD: hypertension (high blood pressure), cigarette smoking, diabetes, high serum cholesterol levels (which may be related to a high dietary intake of saturated fats and calories), lack of exercise, obesity, family history of heart disease or stroke, and male sex. Clearly, these risk factors include some things we can't do anything about (other than thank our parents). We cannot, for example, select our parents and grandparents or choose to be born female. Nevertheless, we can do something about nearly half the risk factors for CAD, which are, therefore, called modifiable risk factors:

- Cigarette smoking is the most significant cause of preventable death in Europe, and a smoker's chances of sudden death are several times greater than those of a non-smoker. The good news is that smokers who quit return very rapidly to the same risk level as non-smokers.

- Hypertension cannot be prevented or cured, but it can be controlled with changes in diet and with medications. A person with uncontrolled hypertension has two to three times the risk of CAD as a person with normal blood pressure.

- The levels of serum cholesterol are at least in part a consequence of dietary intake of saturated fats. In populations with low fat intake, the incidence of CAD is also low. Furthermore, lowering the serum cholesterol levels has been shown to reduce the incidence of heart attacks and other dangerous cardiac events. Cholesterol may also be controlled with medications, if necessary.

- One behaviour that may have a role in elevating serum cholesterol is lack of exercise, which also has a variety of other untoward effects on the body. Exercise improves overall fitness, cardiac reserve, and collateral coronary circulation.

- Obesity may go hand in hand with several other risk factors (such as diabetes and hypertension). But obesity by itself also may contribute to an increased risk of CAD. Weight reduction, through consumption of a sensible diet and increased physical exercise, can reap several lifelong and life-extending benefits. Normalising body weight will lower elevated blood pressure, elevated serum cholesterol levels, elevated blood glucose levels, and the risk of CAD.

Peripheral Vascular Disorders

Although atherosclerosis is rarely the primary cause of medical emergencies, it is a major contributor to other conditions that may become medical emergencies. For example, arterial bruits or "swishing" sounds (heard with a stethoscope placed over the carotid arteries) signal the presence of atherosclerosis and contra-indicate the use of carotid sinus massage. Atherosclerosis can also contribute to claudication, a severe pain in the calf muscle caused by narrowing of the arteries in this muscle and leading to a painful limp. Finally, atherosclerosis may be associated with phlebitis—swelling and pain along the veins that can lead to the formation of blood clots (thrombophlebitis). If dislodged, these thrombi become emboli that could travel to the heart and through its right side, lodging in the pulmonary arterial tree and causing a pulmonary embolism.

An estimated 1 in 20 people in the United Kingdom are affected by significant peripheral vascular disorders annually. The most dangerous complication of these disorders is pulmonary embolism. Risk factors for peripheral vascular disorders include age, oral contraceptive use, smoking, recent surgery, repeated IV drug use, trauma, and extended immobilisation. Identification of these risk factors has a significant role in diagnosing peripheral vascular occlusions. Signs of peripheral vascular occlusion may include pain, redness, swelling, warmth, and tenderness in the extremity; these signs are present in only about half of all cases, however. The presence of claudication indicates a significant narrowing of the peripheral arteries associated with peripheral vascular disorders. Arterial bruits are another sign of vascular narrowing that can contribute to ischaemia or stroke.

Because peripheral vascular disorders can have serious consequences, such as pulmonary embolism or loss of limb through arterial occlusions, you must be familiar with the signs, symptoms, and risk factors for these conditions. Unfortunately, prehospital treatment of peripheral vascular conditions is limited. Beyond supplementary oxygen, IV access, and, possibly, aspirin administration, little can be done in the prehospital environment if you suspect a peripheral vascular disorder.

Acute Coronary Syndrome

Acute coronary syndrome (ACS) is the term used to describe any group of clinical symptoms consistent with acute myocardial ischaemia. Acute myocardial ischaemia typically presents as chest pain due to insufficient blood supply to the heart muscle, which itself is a result of CAD. The life-threatening ACS disorders are responsible for much of the prehospital care and hospitalisation in Europe.

Patients experiencing symptomatic, acute myocardial ischaemia should receive a 12-lead ECG to determine whether they have ST-segment elevation. Most patients whose ECG displays ST-segment elevation will ultimately develop a "Q-wave AMI" (heart attack), also known as STEMI (ST-elevation myocardial infarction). Patients who have ischaemic discomfort (chest pain) without ST-segment elevation are having unstable angina or a non–ST-segment elevation AMI that usually leads to a non–Q-wave AMI; these conditions are collectively known as UAP/NSTEMI (unstable angina pectoris/non–ST-elevation myocardial infarction). Patients who experience angina may also present with ST-segment depression. Finally, some patients experiencing angina or AMI may have *no* changes indicated by the ECG.

Angina Pectoris

The principal symptom of CAD is angina pectoris (literally "choking in the chest"). Angina occurs when the supply of oxygen to the myocardium is insufficient to meet the demand. As a result, the cardiac muscle becomes ischaemic, and a switch to anaerobic metabolism leads to the accumulation of lactic acid and carbon dioxide. The concept of "supply and demand" is critical here. When at rest, a person with heart disease may have an adequate supply of oxygen to the heart to meet these sedentary needs, despite some narrowing of the coronary arteries. When the same person exercises or experiences some other stress, however, the blood flow to the myocardium may not be able to satisfy the heart's increased demand for oxygen; in that case, angina will result. Clearly, the patient who experiences angina at rest, when oxygen needs are minimal, has more severe CAD than a person who experiences angina only with vigorous exercise.

When taking the history from a patient with chest pain, it is important to distinguish between stable angina and unstable angina. Stable angina follows a recurrent pattern: A person with stable angina experiences pain after a certain, predictable amount of exertion, such as climbing one flight of stairs or walking for three streets. The pain also has a predictable location, intensity, and duration. The patient may report, for example, "Every time I walk up the hill to the bus stop, I get a squeezing pain under my breast bone, and I have to sit down for 2 or 3 minutes until it goes away".

At the Scene

Other names for unstable angina include pre-infarction angina, crescendo angina, and ACS.

Patients with chronic, stable angina often take GTN or some other form of "nitrate" for relief of anginal pain. In its usual formulation, GTN is supplied as a white tablet, which is placed under the tongue (sublingual) and allowed to dissolve there, or in a spray form that is sprayed under the tongue. It may also be given as sustained-release capsules taken two or three times a day, as a cream rubbed into the skin (topical), or as a patch worn on the skin. Regardless of which form is used, GTN will have a predictable effect in stable angina, producing relief of symptoms within a few minutes.

Unstable angina is much more serious than stable angina and indicates a greater degree of obstruction of the coronary arteries. It is characterised by noticeable changes in the frequency, severity, and duration of pain and often occurs without predictable stress. The patient may report that the anginal attacks have grown more frequent and severe during the past several days or weeks or that they awaken him or her from sleep or occur when otherwise at rest. Such attacks are often warning signs of an impending AMI.

Management Considerations

Of course, not all chest pain is caused by cardiac ischaemia or injury. Many other conditions—such as pulmonary embolism, pneumothorax, pneumonia, pericarditis, aortic dissection, indigestion, and peptic ulcer—may cause chest pain that can be mistaken for angina or an AMI. It is important to perform a thorough physical examination, including a focused history, to determine whether the cause of the complaint is likely to be cardiac in origin.

> **Notes from Nancy**
>
> When a patient with chest pain calls for an ambulance, it means that the patient never had chest pain before or that his or her chronic chest pain has changed. Either way, it's serious.

As a general rule, it is safe to assume that any patient who has called for an ambulance because of chest pain has, at the least, unstable angina and perhaps an evolving AMI. Patients with chronic, stable angina rarely call for help unless something has changed—often dramatically—for the worse. Because it is difficult and sometimes impossible to differentiate between angina and an AMI in the prehospital environment, the treatment of angina should be the same as for an AMI. It is far better to overtreat angina as an AMI than to undertreat an AMI by assuming it is angina.

Acute Myocardial Infarction

An acute myocardial infarction (AMI), or heart attack, occurs when a portion of the cardiac muscle is deprived of coronary blood flow long enough to cause portions of the muscle to die (undergo necrosis or infarct). Several things can diminish flow through coronary vessels, especially if the vessels are already narrowed by atherosclerotic disease: occlusion of a coronary artery by a blood clot (thrombus), spasm of a coronary artery, or reduction of overall blood flow from any cause (such as shock, arrhythmias, or pulmonary embolism).

The location and size of a myocardial infarct depend on which coronary artery is blocked and where along its course the blockage occurred. The majority of infarcts involve the left ventricle. When the anterior, lateral, or septal walls of the left ventricle are infarcted, the source is usually occlusion of the left coronary artery or one of its branches. Inferior wall infarcts are usually the result of RCA occlusion. When the ischaemic process affects only the inner layer of muscle, the infarct is referred to as subendocardial. When the infarct extends through the

> **Notes from Nancy**
>
> For purposes of treatment outside the hospital, the patient with chest pain must be assumed to be suffering an acute myocardial infarction until proven otherwise and should therefore be treated as any other patient with a suspected AMI.

entire wall of the ventricle, it is a transmural AMI giving a Q wave. The infarcted tissue is invariably surrounded by a ring of ischaemic tissue—an area that is relatively deprived of oxygen but still viable. That ischaemic tissue tends to be electrically unstable and is often the source of cardiac arrhythmias.

Acute myocardial infarction is the leading cause of death in the United Kingdom, accounting for approximately 115,000 deaths per year; of those deaths, around 50% occur outside of hospital, during the first 2 to 3 hours after the onset of symptoms. Of all deaths from AMI, 90% are due to arrhythmias, usually ventricular fibrillation, which typically occur during the early hours of the infarct. Arrhythmias can be prevented or treated, so *most deaths from AMI are preventable.*

Symptoms of AMI

Although there is no "typical AMI patient", when most Europeans think about the symptoms of an AMI, they envision the classic pain presentation usually associated with men. In fact, AMIs can occur in younger and older people and in men and women. The patient may be slightly overweight and may have recently overindulged at the dinner table or perhaps on the tennis court. Nevertheless, many heart attacks occur at rest or just after getting up in the morning.

The most common symptom of AMI is chest pain. This pain is similar to that of angina but can be much more severe and last more than 15 minutes. A patient with chronic angina will be aware that something very different from previous anginal attacks is happening. The pain of AMI is typically felt just beneath the sternum and is variously described as heavy, squeezing, crushing, or tight. Often the patient unconsciously clenches a fist when describing the pain (Levine's sign) to convey in body language the squeezing nature of the pain. In 25% of cases, the pain radiates to the arms (most often the left arm) and into the fingers; it may also radiate to the neck, jaw, upper back, or epigastrium. Occasionally, a patient will mistake the pain of AMI for indigestion and may take antacids in an attempt to relieve the discomfort. The pain of AMI is not influenced by coughing, deep breathing, or other body movements.

Not every AMI patient has chest pain, however. In fact, 10% to 20% of patients with AMI *do not experience any chest pain.* People with diabetes, older people, and heart transplant patients, for example, generally do not present with chest pain, a condition referred to as "silent AMI". Instead, these patients may present with symptoms related to a drop in CO. It is not unusual for them to develop sudden dyspnoea, progressing rapidly to pulmonary oedema, a sudden loss of consciousness, an unexplained drop in blood pressure, an apparent stroke, or simply confusion.

Women with an AMI may present differently from men with the same condition. Women may experience nausea, lightheadedness, epigastric burning, or sudden onset of weakness or unexplained tiredness. Because they are not experiencing the typical chest pain expected with an AMI, many women ignore their symptoms. Unfortunately, CVD is the number one cause of death for women in the United States.

At the Scene

More men have heart disease, but more women die of heart disease, in part because their symptoms are less clear-cut.

When obtaining the history from a patient whose chief complaint is chest pain, ask the usual OPQRST questions to elaborate on the chief complaint, but also ask whether the patient has taken anything for the pain and, if so, whether it helped. If the patient reports having taken GTN without relief, it is important to establish *why* the patient did not obtain relief.

Two reasons might explain this failure. One possibility is that the patient is, indeed, having an AMI, for which GTN would not provide complete pain relief. The other possibility is that the GTN has simply gone stale. To retain its potency, GTN must be stored in a dark, air-tight container; if it is left out in the open for any period (for example, if the patient stores the medicine on the window sill above the kitchen sink), it loses its therapeutic effectiveness. To distinguish between the two explanations, ask the patient whether the GTN had the usual effects. GTN tablets that are therapeutically active cause a slight burning under the tongue, may make the patient feel flushed, or may give the patient a transient throbbing headache. If the patient confirms that he or she felt one of those effects but the chest pain still wouldn't go away, then you know there was nothing wrong with the GTN but there may be something very wrong with the patient.

Notes from Nancy

Start treatment immediately for any patient with chest pain.

As soon as you have elicited a chief complaint of a cardiac nature, you will need to start treating the patient; obtaining a focused history and physical examination can wait. For purposes of discussion, though, we shall continue here to proceed through the history and physical examination. Besides pain (or, sometimes, instead of pain), a number of other symptoms are associated with AMI:

- Diaphoresis (sweating), often profuse, is principally the result of massive discharge by the autonomic nervous system. The patient may soak through his or her clothing and complain of a cold sweat.
- Dyspnoea may be a warning of impending left-sided heart failure.
- Anorexia (loss of appetite), nausea, vomiting, or belching frequently accompanies AMI. Hiccups may occasionally occur as well, due to irritation of the diaphragm by an inferior wall AMI.
- Weakness may be profound, and the patient may describe this feeling with phrases such as "a limp rag".
- If CO is significantly diminished, dizziness may reflect the reduced circulation to the brain.

- Palpitations are sometimes experienced by patients with cardiac arrhythmias as a sensation that the heart has skipped a beat.
- A feeling of impending doom is common among patients having an AMI. The patient is frightened, looks frightened, and expresses his or her fear to other people—all of which adds to a general atmosphere of panic and dread.

Signs of AMI

Although patients with AMI often have abnormalities in the physical examination, many have relatively normal physical examination findings, and the diagnosis in the prehospital environment (and, indeed, in the A&E department) depends chiefly on the history. Nevertheless, it is important to take note of a few specific things during the physical examination to detect the development of complications following AMI, such as heart failure or cardiogenic shock.

- Pay attention to the patient's general appearance. Does the patient appear anxious? Frightened? In obvious pain?
- What is the patient's state of consciousness? Is he or she fully alert? Confused? Remember: Poor perfusion creates confusion. If the patient does not seem "all there", it may be because the heart is giving out and not enough oxygenated blood is reaching the brain.
- Is the skin pale, cold, and clammy?
- Assess the patient's vital signs. Is the pulse strong or weak? Regular or irregular? Is the respiratory rate abnormally rapid? Is the blood pressure abnormally high or low?
- Are there signs of left-sided heart failure (wheezes or crackles)? Signs of right-sided heart failure (distended neck veins, pedal or presacral oedema)?

A typical patient with an AMI is very apprehensive, with an ashen-grey pallor and cold, wet skin. He or she *looks* scared. The pulse may be rapid unless heart block has occurred. The blood pressure may be decreased, reflecting decreased CO from the damaged heart, or it may be elevated from pain and anxiety.

Prehospital Management of ACSs

On your arrival at the scene, start treatment at once for any middle-aged or older patient with chest pain, even before you complete the history and physical examination. The longest delay in treatment seems to be the phase from onset of symptoms to patient recognition, so your care must begin immediately. The goals of treatment are to limit the size of the infarct, to decrease the patient's fear and pain, and to prevent the development of serious cardiac arrhythmias.

Place the Patient at Physical and Emotional Rest

The stress response causes the adrenal glands to squeeze out a surge of catecholamines (adrenaline and noradrenaline), which in turn can send the damaged heart racing. At the same time, the massive discharge throughout the fight-or-flight system puts the peripheral circulation in a state of severe vasoconstriction; thus, not only is the heart being flogged to go faster and faster, but it also has to work harder and harder against the increased afterload.

The heart's need for oxygen, therefore, soars precisely when it is already in a state of marked oxygen deprivation. This cycle can lead quickly to arrhythmias and death. Prehospital deaths are related to arrhythmias (often ventricular fibrillation), and most occur during the first 4 hours after onset of symptoms. Nevertheless, this deadly cycle can be interrupted by community education programmes designed to assist the public in the early recognition of symptoms, early activation of the ambulance service, and, if needed, cardiopulmonary resuscitation (CPR) and early access to an automated external defibrillator (AED).

To begin your treatment, put the patient physically at ease. Recall that one goal of treatment is to try to limit the size of the infarct; one way to do so is to decrease the amount of work that the heart must do, which will begin to decrease the patient's myocardial oxygen requirements immediately. The position in which cardiac work is minimal is the semi-recumbent position—that is, reclining on the stretcher with the back of the stretcher raised about 30°. Of course, the patient has to get to the stretcher and must not be permitted to do so alone. From the time you arrive, the patient must not do anything, including walking to the ambulance.

Administer Oxygen and Aspirin

The mnemonic MONA is used to help remember the supportive treatments of Morphine, Oxygen, Nitrates (GTN), and Aspirin for a patient with an ACS—but these treatments are not to be given in that order. MONA is administered in the following order, provided these measures are not contraindicated by hypotension: (1) oxygen, (2) aspirin, (3) GTN, and (4) morphine.

Oxygen may limit ischaemic myocardial injury and reduce the amount of ST-segment elevation. Its effects on morbidity and mortality in acute infarction are unknown. The recommendation is to initiate high-flow oxygen at a rate of 12 to 15 l/min via nonrebreathing mask. Monitor the SpO_2 and titrate until the patient is in stable condition or the hypoxaemia is corrected (that is, $SpO_2 > 90\%$).

In most ambulance services, as long as the patient has no aspirin allergy or gastrointestinal bleeding, dispatchers may advise patients to chew aspirin (300 mg). If this has not been done before your arrival or the patient has not already taken aspirin on his or her own, then give the patient 300 mg of non–enteric-coated aspirin to chew.

Provide Pain Relief

Some form of pain relief must be provided because the pain of AMI is very severe and places enormous stress on the patient's autonomic nervous system—stress that may contribute to complications. GTN is a good place to start, but make sure the patient's blood pressure is adequate before its administration.

At the Scene
Oxygen is the first drug in the treatment of AMI.

In particular, before giving this medication, it is imperative that you ascertain whether the patient is taking phosphodiesterase-5 (PDE-5) inhibitors (eg, Viagra) for erectile dysfunction **Table 27-10 ▾**. These drugs may worsen certain medical conditions and interact with a number of drugs, especially nitrate medications (such as GTN) prescribed to prevent or treat acute angina. Both types of medication dilate blood vessels, and their combined effects can cause dizziness, low blood pressure, and loss of consciousness.

Place a 400-mcg tablet (or spray) of GTN under the patient's tongue. If the patient is experiencing an AMI and not simply angina, this medication is unlikely to relieve his or her pain, but it may help to reduce the size of the infarction. Do *not* give GTN if there is hypotension or bradycardia. GTN may be repeated every 5 to 10 minutes, however the patient's blood pressure should be monitored and administration stopped if the blood pressure falls below 90 mm Hg (systolic).

If GTN provides no relief of pain, morphine sulphate may be titrated in IV doses according to local guidelines. Be sure to reassess the patient's blood pressure, pulse, and respiratory rate after each dose, until the patient experiences relief of pain or experiences a drop in pulse or blood pressure. If bradycardia occurs, notify the doctor immediately. Remember that morphine should *not* be given to patients with low blood pressure (less than about 90 mm Hg systolic or according to local guidelines). At least half of all patients with AMI of the inferior wall will also experience a right ventricular infarction; as a consequence, they may already be hypotensive or the administration of GTN and morphine may cause hypotension.

Perform Cardiac Monitoring

Apply the basic 3-lead ECG monitor, and run a strip to document the initial rhythm. As long as you are applying electrodes to the chest, also place your anterior chest leads in anticipation of doing a 12-lead ECG. The ear is far more sensitive than the eye to slight irregularities in rhythm, so the chances are that you will *hear* the beginning of a cardiac arrhythmia much sooner than you will see it on the monitor. Keep the other cardiac drugs that you carry close at hand so you can reach them quickly if a cardiac arrhythmia develops.

At the Scene
Patients may not be forthcoming about taking medications. They may omit something from their list of home medications if they do not take the medicine daily. Be sure to ask.

Table 27-10	PDE-5 Inhibitors	
Generic Name		**Duration of Effect**
Sildenafil citrate		Up to 4 h
Vardenafil		Up to 4 h
Tadalfil		24 to 36 h

Record the Vital Signs

Obtain vital signs, including pulse, respirations, blood pressure, and oxygen saturation. Measure the blood pressure, and repeat that measurement at least every 5 minutes. Measure the pulse. The ECG monitor provides information only about the electrical activity of the heart; it gives no information about the strength of the heartbeat (muscular activity) or even about whether the heart is beating at all! It is, therefore, necessary to monitor the patient's pulse to assess peripheral blood flow, especially during transport, when blood pressure measurements are difficult and unreliable.

Perform a Detailed History and Physical Examination

After you have completed the preceding steps (as appropriate), you should obtain a more detailed history and perform a physical examination. Find out if the patient has a history of cardiac disease; takes any heart medications, such as beta-blockers, angiotensin-converting enzyme inhibitors, diuretics, or GTN (nitrates); or has had a previous heart attack or any heart surgery (such as coronary artery bypass graft). Also obtain a more complete description of the present symptoms, especially regarding their onset. Gathering that information should not, however, delay transport to hospital. Once you have taken the necessary precautions to stabilise the patient's condition (aspirin, oxygen, IV saline, monitor/12-lead ECG, analgesia), there is no reason to remain at the scene any longer, unless a cardiac arrest or arrhythmia requires immediate treatment. Take the rest of the history en route to hospital. Remember that "time is muscle". Heart cells are being destroyed during the infarction before angioplasty reperfusion therapy is started in hospital.

Transport the Patient

Once the patient is in stable condition, transport him or her to an appropriate hospital in a semi-recumbent position (unless the patient is in shock, in which case he or she should be supine). Do all you can to ensure that the patient is as relaxed and as comfortable as possible. En route, some additional treatment measures may be worthwhile, especially when transport will take a long time.

If a serious arrhythmia occurs during transport, consider stopping the vehicle, institute treatment immediately, and notify the receiving hospital. Except under unusual circumstances, treatment of life-threatening situations should not be attempted in a moving ambulance. Whenever possible, the driver should pull over to the side of the road and go to the back of the vehicle to help the other practitioner. However, it is possible to insert an IV if the paramedic carries this out on a straight road and informs the driver so that they can work together.

Reperfusion Techniques for ACSs

The majority of AMIs occur as a result of thrombus (fixed blood clot) formation at the site of a pre-existing atherosclerotic plaque. The thrombus occludes the coronary artery, preventing further blood flow through it. Thus, it seems reasonable to try to restore circulation through the occluded coronary artery, thereby restoring perfusion to the ischaemic myocardium. Simply put, that is reperfusion.

The most immediate forms of reperfusion are thrombolytic therapy and percutaneous intervention (PCI). All paramedics should be alert for patients who are good candidates for reperfusion, should know which hospitals in their area carry out thrombolytic therapy and/or PCI, and should provide early notification (along with 12-lead ECG results) to the A&E or coronary care unit that a candidate for such therapy is en route.

Thrombolysis

One way in which to reperfuse the blocked coronary artery is to try to dissolve the occluding blood clot, thereby restoring circulation to the ischaemic heart. That idea is the essence of thrombolytic therapy.

In fact, this concept is not altogether new. Attempts to use thrombolytic agents in the treatment of AMI were reported at least 40 years ago, albeit without success. In retrospect, we realise that one reason the early attempts failed was that thrombolytic therapy was started too late, after irreversible damage to the myocardium had already occurred. With that realisation came the concept that "time is myocardium". The longer a segment of myocardium remains unperfused, the smaller the chances of salvaging that tissue and restoring its normal function. The obvious corollary is that the sooner thrombolytic therapy can begin with respect to the onset of the blockage, the better the chances for saving the affected distal myocardium. Indeed, thrombolytic treatment given within 30 to 60 minutes of the onset of symptoms can sometimes abort the AMI altogether.

In the 1980s, providers began to start thrombolytic treatment as soon as possible after the patient with an AMI reached the A&E department, rather than waiting until he or she was admitted to the coronary care unit. Inevitably, applying the doctrine that time is myocardium led to the idea of starting thrombolytic treatment even earlier, in the prehospital phase of care.

At the Scene

Time is muscle (myocardium)!

Recent clinical trials have shown the benefit of starting thrombolysis as soon as possible after the onset of ischaemic-type chest pain in patients with STEMI or new or presumably new left bundle branch block. Several prospective studies have also documented reduced time to administration of thrombolytics and decreased mortality rates when out-of-hospital thrombolytics were given to patients with STEMI and no contraindications to thrombolytics. Some

| **Table 27-11** | **ST-Segment Elevation or New or Presumably New LBBB: Evaluation for Reperfusion** |

Step 1: Assess time and risk

- Time since onset of symptoms
- Risk of STEMI
- Risk of thrombolysis
- Time required to transport to skilled PCI catheterisation suite

Step 2: Select reperfusion (thrombolysis or invasive) strategy

Note: If presentation < 3 hours and no delay for PCI, then no preference for either strategy.

Thrombolysis is generally preferred if:	**An invasive strategy is generally preferred if:**
■ Early presentation (≤ 3 hours from symptom onset) ■ Invasive strategy is not an option (eg, lack of access to skilled PCI facility or difficult vascular access) or would be delayed —Medical contact-to-balloon or door-balloon > 90 min —(Door-to-balloon) minus (door-to-needle) is > 1 hour ■ No contraindications to thrombolysis	■ Late presentation (symptom onset > 3 hours ago) ■ Skilled PCI facility available with surgical backup ■ Medical contact-to-balloon or door-balloon < 90 min ■ (Door-to-balloon) minus (door-to-needle) is < 1 hour ■ Contraindications to thrombolysis, including increased risk of bleeding and ICH ■ High risk from STEMI (CHF, Killip class is ≥ 3) ■ Diagnosis of STEMI is in doubt

Modified from ACC/AHA 2004 Update Recommendations.

ambulance services may opt to start thrombolytic treatment in the prehospital environment, and in rural areas with very long transport times, prehospital initiation of thrombolytic therapy may make a lot of sense. Even in ambulance services in which paramedics do not give thrombolytic therapy, their ability to identify candidates for such therapy has a decisive role in helping A&E personnel administer thrombolytic therapy early enough to make a difference. For these reasons, all paramedics should thoroughly understand the principles of thrombolytic therapy for AMI.

Thrombolytic therapy seeks to administer, during the early hours of AMI, an agent that will activate the body's own internal system for dissolving clots, the thrombolytic system. Once activated, that system can begin to dissolve the clot that has formed within the coronary artery, thereby reopening the artery (recanalisation) and allowing the resumption of blood flow through it (reperfusion). Unfortunately, if an agent capable of promoting clot dissolution is given intravenously, its effects cannot be limited to the clot in the coronary artery; it can also act anywhere else in the body where clots are being formed and, therefore, may lead to bleeding. Thus, the benefit of thrombolytic therapy—the possible salvage of myocardium—must always be weighed against its risks—principally, the risk of bleeding.

To determine the appropriate candidates for thrombolytic agents, we need to be as certain as possible that we are really dealing with a patient who is having an AMI. A patient having chest pain from another source would receive no potential benefit from thrombolytic therapy—so he or she would be subjected to this therapy's risks for no reason. Although it is difficult in the early hours of an AMI to be certain of the diagnosis, inclusion criteria have been established to help select patients most likely to be having an AMI. At the same time, exclusion criteria are used to identify patients for whom the risk of thrombolytic therapy is unacceptably high—for example, patients most likely to experience haemorrhagic complications. **Table 27-11 ▲** summarises the inclusion and exclusion criteria for thrombolytic therapy.

Most treatment regimes for thrombolysis include: alteplase, tenecteplase, streptokinase, or reteplase. All of them work by converting, in one way or another, the body's own clot-dissolving enzyme from its inactive form, plasminogen, to its active form, plasmin.

According to the ERC's 2005 guidelines, the key to realising the benefits of thrombolysis is to start early. A prehospital thrombolytic program is recommended only in systems with well-established guidelines, checklists, experience in ACLS, ability to communicate with the receiving institution, and a medical director with training and experience in the management of STEMI.

Percutaneous Intervention

As an alternative to thrombolysis, many institutions perform a PCI on a 24-hour basis with direct admission to the unit for the ambulance service. Patients with complex, multivessel disease or ACSs may benefit from PCI. In this therapy, balloons, stents, or other devices are passed through a 2-mm-diameter catheter via a peripheral artery to recanalise and keep the blocked coronary artery open. The success rate is high, and the risks are low. PCI is often used for patients who are not candidates for thrombolytic therapy, or for rescue angioplasty when thrombolysis has been unsuccessful.

Congestive Heart Failure

Congestive heart failure (also known as chronic heart failure) occurs when the heart is unable, for any reason, to pump powerfully enough or fast enough to empty its chambers; as a result, blood backs up into the systemic circuit, the pulmonary circuit, or both. Although CHF may develop in situations other than AMI—for example, in a patient with chronic high blood pressure—the basic principles of diagnosis and treatment are similar, whatever the precipitating factors.

Left-Sided Heart Failure

The left ventricle is usually damaged during an AMI. Likewise, in chronic hypertension, the left ventricle tends to suffer the

Table 27-12	Differentiation and Treatment of Asthma and Left-Sided Heart Failure	
	Asthma	**Left-Sided Heart Failure**
History	Often a younger patient May have allergic history or family history of allergy Previous attacks of acute, episodic dyspnoea May have had recent respiratory infection Unproductive cough Medications may include: ■ Inhalers: isoproterenol, salbutamol, adrenaline, isoetharine, isoproterenol ■ Pills: calcium carb/glycine chew, pseudoephedrine, theophylline and guaifenesin, triprolidine and pseudoephedrine, theophylline/ephedrine/hydroxyaine-oral	Often an older patient May have history of heart problems, hypertension Dyspnoea worse when lying down (orthopnoea) Recent rapid weight gain Cough with watery or frothy sputum Medications may include: ■ Digitalis glycosides: digoxin, digitoxin ■ Diuretics: chlorothiazide, furosemide, hydrochlorothiazide, ethacrynic acid, trichlormethiazide
Possible physical findings	Wheezing Chest hyperinflated and hyperresonant Use of accessory muscles to breathe If bronchospasm severe, chest may be silent	Wheezing Crackles S_3 gallop Distended neck veins Pedal or presacral oedema
Treatment	Oxygen (humidified) Intermittent positive-pressure breathing Monitor Selective beta-2 adrenergic medications	Oxygen Intermittent positive-pressure breathing Monitor IV: normal saline to keep vein open (TKVO) Morphine Diuretics (furosemide) GTN

long-term effects of having to pump against an increased afterload (constricted peripheral arteries). In both cases, the right side of the heart continues to pump relatively normally and to deliver normal volumes of blood to the pulmonary circulation. By comparison, the left side of the heart may no longer be able to pump the blood being delivered from the pulmonary vessels. As a result, blood backs up behind the left ventricle, and the pressure in the left atrium and pulmonary veins increases. As the pulmonary veins become engorged with blood, serum is forced out of the pulmonary capillaries and into the alveoli. The serum mixes with air in the alveoli to produce froth (pulmonary oedema).

When fluid occupies the alveoli, oxygenation is impaired. The patient experiences that impairment as shortness of breath (dyspnoea), particularly in the recumbent position (orthopnoea). If left ventricular failure is the result of chronic overload (as opposed to AMI), the patient is likely to give a history of a week or two of PND. To compensate for the impairment in oxygenation, the patient's respiratory rate increases (tachypnoea); even so, if the patient's condition is advanced enough, cyanosis may become evident. In some patients with pulmonary oedema, especially elderly patients, Cheyne-Stokes respirations may be present.

Fluid from the pulmonary vessels also leaks into the interstitial spaces in the lungs, and increasing interstitial pressure causes narrowing of the bronchioles. Air passing through the narrowed bronchioles creates wheezing noises, whereas air bubbling through the fluid-filled alveoli produces crackles. Furthermore, the patient may cough up the oedema fluid in the form of frothy, blood-tinged sputum. As the airways narrow

and the lungs grow heavier from the accumulation of fluid, the work of breathing increases, which puts an even greater strain on the already floundering heart. Dyspnoea and hypoxaemia produce a state of panic, which induces the release of adrenaline from the adrenals. The heart is pushed even harder, and its oxygen demand is increased precisely when fluid in the alveoli is reducing the amount of oxygen available.

To make matters worse, the sympathetic nervous system response produces peripheral vasoconstriction: Peripheral resistance (afterload) increases, and the weakened, hypoxic heart finds itself trying to push blood out into smaller and smaller pipes. Clinically, peripheral vasoconstriction is apparent as pallor and elevated blood pressure. The massive sympathetic discharge also produces sweating of the pale, cold skin.

It is not unusual for a patient with left-sided heart failure to become frantic from air hunger. He or she may pace or thrash about or may even be combative and struggle with the paramedics. Furthermore, hypoxaemia results in inadequate oxygen supply to the brain, often manifested as confusion or disorientation. If hypoxaemia is severe, cardiac arrest may follow quickly.

Signs and Symptoms of Left-Sided Heart Failure

The signs and symptoms of left-sided heart failure include extreme restlessness and agitation, confusion, severe dyspnoea and tachypnoea, tachycardia, elevated blood pressure, crackles and possibly wheezes, and frothy, pink sputum. Sometimes, it may be difficult to distinguish the wheezing of asthma from that of left-sided heart failure. Table 27-12 ▲ presents some of the features that can help you differentiate the two conditions.

Management of Left-Sided Heart Failure

Prehospital treatment of left-sided heart failure is aimed at improving oxygenation and decreasing the workload of the heart, chiefly by reducing the volume of venous blood returned to the heart (the preload), so that the left ventricle is less overburdened.

Administer high-flow supplemental oxygen, preferably by demand valve or bag-valve-mask device with positive end-expiratory pressure, because positive pressure is helpful in driving fluid out of the alveoli. If the patient will not tolerate either of those modalities, use the nonrebreathing mask. Monitor oxygenation with pulse oximetry.

Sit the patient up, with the feet dangling. That position encourages venous pooling in the legs, thereby reducing venous return to the heart. The sitting position also makes breathing easier for a patient in respiratory distress.

Start an IV with normal saline at a keep-vein-open rate. Also, attach monitoring electrodes because patients in CHF are prone to arrhythmias.

Pharmacological therapy of left-sided heart failure may vary slightly from place to place, but the mainstays of drug therapy include the drugs mentioned below. Refer to your usual guidelines, have the appropriate medications drawn up, and be ready to administer them. Remember to monitor the blood pressure constantly because many of these medications lower it. Aspirin may be given. Check that the patient is not allergic and then get the patient to chew the tablet and then swallow.

GTN, 400 mcg sublingually, may be ordered as a vasodilator to create venous pooling, thereby reducing the volume of blood returned from the periphery to the heart.

Furosemide is a diuretic that has two positive effects in left-sided heart failure. Initially (within the first 5 to 10 minutes), it has a venodilating effect, increasing peripheral pooling of blood. Subsequently, it removes excess fluid from the body by promoting its excretion by the kidneys. Furosemide is given by IV bolus.

Morphine sulphate has long been part of the standard treatment of cardiogenic pulmonary oedema. Like GTN, morphine works as a vasodilator, increasing the pooling of blood in the periphery, but it also has a substantial calming effect on a frantic patient. If morphine is ordered, first check the patient's blood pressure (do not give morphine if the patient is hypotensive). Then give 2.5 mg slowly by IV bolus, and recheck the blood pressure. If the blood pressure remains stable, another 2.5 mg may be given.

The presence of wheezing indicates that bronchoconstriction has developed from the excessive fluid. In such a case, bronchodilator drugs such as salbutamol, metaproterenol sulphate, or ipratropium may be used.

Transport the patient to the hospital in a sitting position, with legs dangling down, if possible.

Right-Sided Heart Failure

Right-sided heart failure is most likely to occur as a result of left-sided heart failure. As blood backs up from the left side of the heart into the lungs, the right side has to work increasingly harder to pump blood into the engorged pulmonary vessels.

Eventually, the right side of the heart is unable to keep up with the increased workload, and it, too, fails. Right-sided heart failure may also occur as a result of pulmonary embolism or long-standing COPD, especially chronic bronchitis.

When right-sided heart failure occurs, blood backs up behind the right ventricle and increases the pressure in the systemic veins, causing them to become engorged. Distension can be seen in the veins visible on the surface of the body, such as the external jugular veins. Over time, as the pressure within the systemic veins increases, serum is forced out of the veins and into the surrounding tissues, producing oedema. Oedema is most likely to be visible in dependent parts of the body, such as the feet in a person who is sitting or standing or the lower back in a bedridden patient. Oedema is also present in parts of the body that are *not* visible; a painful liver easily palpable in the right upper quadrant, for example, signals engorgement and swelling within that organ (hepatomegaly).

The development of right-sided heart failure can actually improve left-sided heart failure because the failing right side of the heart can no longer pump as much blood into the lungs. The decrease in output from the right side, in essence, amounts to a decrease in preload for the left side of the heart and may lessen pulmonary congestion.

Right-sided heart failure, by itself, is seldom a life-threatening emergency. Usually it develops gradually over days to weeks; likewise, it requires days to weeks to reverse the process by slowly ridding the body of excess salt and water. Treatment in the prehospital environment of a patient with right-sided heart failure, therefore, is simply to make the patient comfortable, preferably in the semi-recumbent position. Monitoring is always indicated in any patient with significant cardiac disease. If signs of associated left-sided heart failure are present, treat them as outlined in the previous section.

Cardiac Tamponade

The pericardium is a tough, fibrous membrane with the ability to stretch only up to a point. Normally, a small amount of pericardial fluid separates the pericardium and the outer surface of the heart. Cardiac tamponade occurs when excessive fluid accumulates within the pericardium, limiting the heart's ability to expand fully after each contraction and resulting in reduced CO. If unrecognised and untreated, this condition will reduce cardiac filling to the point that the heart is unable to circulate the blood.

Signs and Symptoms of Cardiac Tamponade

Cardiac tamponade can occur as a result of tumours, pericarditis, or trauma to the chest. Pericarditis, for example, can cause excessive amounts of fluid to accumulate in the pericardial space. Blunt or penetrating trauma can cause bleeding from blood vessels on the surface of the heart, allowing accumulation of blood in the pericardial space.

Signs and symptoms of cardiac tamponade vary depending on its cause. If the onset is gradual (as with pericarditis), the initial complaints might be dyspnoea and weakness. If the cause is traumatic, the chief complaint might be chest pain. As the volume of fluid increases in the pericardium, the SV decreases, causing an initial drop in the systolic blood pressure. Eventually, the diastolic pressure will slowly rise, resulting in the classic symptom of narrowing pulse pressure. The initial drop in blood pressure is usually followed by an increase in HR, which leads to tachycardia. The heart sounds may be muffled or quieter than usual owing to the buildup of fluid, although this sign may be difficult to identify in the prehospital environment. The patient may experience jugular vein distension as well, owing to the backup of blood from the right side of the heart. The combination of narrowing pulse pressure (hypotension) along with jugular vein distension and muffled heart sounds is commonly known as Beck's triad.

The ECG is of limited value in identifying cardiac tamponade. Aside from tachycardia, you might see electrical alternans (alternating small- and large-amplitude QRS complexes). In addition, you might identify pulsus alternans (alternating strong and weak pulses). Pulsus paradoxus—a drop in systolic blood pressure of more than 10 mm Hg with the patient's inhalation that may be associated with a weakening pulse during inhalation—may also be present.

Identification of cardiac tamponade requires a thorough assessment. Changes in blood pressure can be recognised only after at least three values have been obtained, usually 5 to 10 minutes apart. Muffled heart sounds, pulsus alternans, electrical alternans, and pulsus paradoxus are not common signs and so may easily be overlooked. Occasionally, you may have difficulty distinguishing between cardiac tamponade and tension pneumothorax. One way to differentiate between the two is to remember that in cardiac tamponade, the breath sounds will be equal and the trachea will be midline because the lungs are not affected.

Management of Cardiac Tamponade

The ultimate treatment for cardiac tamponade is pericardiocentesis, which involves inserting a needle attached to a syringe into the chest far enough to penetrate the pericardium and then withdrawing fluid. Often, withdrawal of as little as 50 ml of fluid will result in significant improvement in the patient's condition. This technique is risky, however, and it is not performed by paramedics. The one treatment that will significantly enhance the patient's survival is rapid transport to a hospital that can perform this procedure.

Supporting the patient's airway, breathing, and oxygenation during transport are essential. When giving your pre-alert call, make sure that you identify all signs and symptoms that led you to believe the patient has cardiac tamponade so that the receiving hospital will be prepared to perform the pericardiocentesis.

Cardiogenic Shock

Cardiogenic shock occurs when the heart is so severely damaged that it can no longer pump a volume of blood sufficient to maintain tissue perfusion. An AMI nearly always produces some impairment of left ventricular function. When 25% of the left ventricular myocardium is involved in the AMI, left-sided heart failure usually develops. When 40% or more of the left ventricle has been infarcted, cardiogenic shock occurs. Thus, cardiogenic shock indicates extensive injury to the myocardium; accordingly, there is a high mortality rate. Transient cardiogenic shock can occur after resuscitation. Patients recovering from defibrillation for ventricular fibrillation, for example, often have signs of cardiogenic shock.

Signs and Symptoms of Cardiogenic Shock

The signs and symptoms of cardiogenic shock are similar to those of most other kinds of shock. Because of the reduced cerebral perfusion, the patient is often confused or even comatose; if awake, he or she is likely to be restless and anxious. Massive peripheral vasoconstriction results in pale, cold skin, and poor renal perfusion is reflected in minimal or absent urine output. Respirations are rapid and shallow, with a possibility of adventitious breath sounds, and the pulse is racing and thready.

As these compensatory mechanisms begin to fail, the blood pressure will fall, sometimes to less than 90 mm Hg systolic. This vital sign may be deceptive, however: In patients with pre-existing hypertension, systolic pressures higher than 90 mm Hg may still be associated with cardiogenic shock. The goal in treatment of cardiogenic shock is to identify and support the patient before the blood pressure drops to the point where the shock becomes irreversible.

Management of Cardiogenic Shock

Treatment of cardiogenic shock focuses on improving oxygenation and peripheral perfusion without adding to the work of the heart. Secure the patient's airway, and administer high-flow supplemental oxygen by mask or bag-valve-mask device. An advanced airway (that is, endotracheal tube or laryngeal mask airway) will be necessary if the patient is comatose. Place the patient in a supine position unless pulmonary oedema is present; in that case, the patient should be placed in the semi-recumbent position.

Start an IV with normal saline at a keep-vein-open rate. Apply monitoring electrodes and obtain a 12-lead ECG. Arrhythmias may bring about hypotension by causing severe disturbances in CO; thus, until major arrhythmias are corrected, you cannot be certain that the patient's hypotension is due to cardiogenic shock.

Transport the patient expeditiously to hospital. Except for the correction of life-threatening arrhythmias, there are no measures that can stabilise the condition of a patient in cardiogenic shock in the prehospital environment. Thus, there is nothing to be gained by delaying at the scene.

Aortic Aneurysm

The word aneurysm comes from a Greek word meaning a widening; it refers to the dilatation or outpouching of a blood vessel. The aneurysms of greatest concern to you are those that involve the aorta, particularly acute dissecting aneurysms of the thoracic aorta and expanding or ruptured aneurysms of the abdominal aorta.

Acute Dissecting Aneurysm of the Aorta

The proximal aorta is subject to enormous haemodynamic forces. Anywhere from 60 to 100 times a minute, 60 minutes an hour, 24 hours a day—that is, around 40 million times a year—pulsatile waves of blood come pounding out of the left ventricle against the aortic walls. Over the years, that pounding takes its toll, producing degenerative changes in the media (the middle layer) of the aorta, especially the ascending aorta (the part of the aorta that rises from the heart toward the aortic arch). The degenerative changes are more pronounced with advancing age and in people with chronic high blood pressure, and their effect is to "unglue" the layers of the aortic wall from one another.

Eventually, the degenerative changes in the aortic media may lead to a disruption of the underlying intima (innermost layer of the artery). Tearing of the intima is most likely to occur in the portions of the thoracic aorta that are under the greatest stress—specifically, the ascending aorta just distal to the aortic valve (approximately 65% of cases) and the descending aorta just beyond the takeoff point of the left subclavian artery.

Once the intima is torn, the process of dissection, or separation of the arterial wall, often begins. With each ventricular systole, a jet of blood is forced into the torn arterial wall, creating a false channel between the intimal and medial layers of the wall. This channel is propagated distally and sometimes proximally along the length of the wall. If the dissection progresses back into the aortic valve, it may prevent the valve from closing, so that blood regurgitates back from the aorta into the left ventricle during systole. Recall that the coronary arteries branch off from the aorta just above the leaflets of the aortic valve; thus, if the valve is affected, coronary blood flow is likely to be affected as well. If the dissection involves the takeoff point of the innominate, left common carotid, or left subclavian artery, blood flow through the affected artery or arteries will be compromised.

Signs and Symptoms of Acute Dissecting Aneurysm of the Aorta

The typical patient with a dissecting aneurysm is a middle-aged or older man with chronic hypertension, although dissection may occur during pregnancy and in younger patients with Marfan syndrome. By far, the most common chief complaint is chest pain, which is usually described as "the worst pain I have ever experienced", or as "ripping", "tearing", "sharp", or "like a knife". This pain comes on very suddenly and is located in the anterior part of the chest or in the back between the shoulder blades.

On the basis of the patient's description, it may be difficult to differentiate the chest pain of a dissecting aneurysm from that of an AMI, but a number of distinctive features may help. The pain of an AMI is often preceded by other symptoms— nausea, "indigestion", weakness, and sweating—and tends to

Table 27-13	AMI Versus Dissecting Aortic Aneurysm	
	AMI	**Dissecting Aneurysm**
Onset of pain	Gradual, with prodromal symptoms	Abrupt, without prodromal symptoms
Severity of pain	Increases with time	Maximal from the outset
Timing of pain	May wax and wane	Does not abate once it has started
Location of pain	Substernal; back is rarely involved	Back is often involved, between the shoulder blades
Clinical signs	Peripheral pulses equal	Blood pressure discrepancy between arms or decrease in a femoral or carotid pulse

come on gradually, getting more severe with time and often being described as "pressure" rather than "stabbing". By contrast, the pain of a dissecting aneurysm usually comes on full force from one minute to the next, without prodromal symptoms. **Table 27-13 ▲** summarises the differences in the clinical presentations of AMI and dissecting aortic aneurysm.

Other signs and symptoms of dissecting aneurysm will depend on the site of the intimal tear and the extent of the dissection. In dissections of the ascending aorta, which tend to occur in younger patients previously in good health, one or more of the vessels of the aortic arch are usually compromised. Disruption of flow through the innominate artery, for example, is likely to produce a difference in blood pressure between the two arms. (If you don't routinely check the blood pressure in both arms, you'll never pick up that sign!) You may also find that one femoral or carotid pulse is missing or weak. Disruption of blood flow into the left common carotid artery may produce signs and symptoms of a stroke. When the dissection extends proximally to the ostia of the coronary arteries, coronary blood flow is apt to be compromised, and ECG changes of myocardial ischaemia are likely. Death from dissection of the ascending aorta is nearly always a result of aortic rupture into the pericardium and resultant cardiac tamponade. In such a case, you will see the characteristic signs of cardiac tamponade: distended neck veins, hypotension, narrow pulse pressure, and muffled heart sounds.

Dissection of the descending aorta occurs more commonly in older patients, especially those with a history of hypertension. The pain is apt to be somewhat less severe when the descending aorta is involved; indeed, the patient may wait a few days before seeking help. The dissection usually proceeds distally, so the aortic arch is spared, which means that blood pressure discrepancies between the two arms are not part of the picture. The pulses in the lower extremities, however, may be affected.

Management of Acute Dissecting Aneurysm of the Aorta

The goal of prehospital management in a suspected dissecting aneurysm is primarily to provide adequate pain relief. In the hospital, medications will be given to lower the patient's blood pressure and reduce myocardial contractility to take some of the haemodynamic load off the aorta.

The steps of prehospital management in suspected dissecting aneurysm are as follows:

- Calm and reassure the patient.
- Administer high-flow supplemental oxygen by nonrebreathing mask at 15 litres per minute.
- Insert an IV, and give a crystalloid solution, if no radial pulse is present or if there are problems with perfusion.
- Apply monitoring electrodes and obtain an ECG rhythm strip.
- If the patient is not hypotensive, administer IV morphine sulphate, 2.5 mg at a time, up to a total dose of 10 mg.
- Transport without delay. Nothing can be done to stabilise the patient's condition in the prehospital environment. He or she will need aggressive therapy in the intensive care unit and possibly surgery, so don't dawdle!

Expanding and Ruptured Abdominal Aortic Aneurysms

Abdominal aortic aneurysms (AAAs) affect approximately 6,000 to 10,000 people in England and Wales each year, with only around 20% surviving to discharge. Most commonly, the aneurysm is located just distal to the renal arteries. An expanding aneurysm is, as the name implies, an aneurysm that is getting larger and producing symptoms by compressing on adjacent structures, although the aortic wall remains intact. When an aneurysm starts expanding and producing symptoms, one can assume that rupture is imminent.

Signs and Symptoms of Expanding and Ruptured AAAs

The typical patient with an AAA is a man in his late 50s or 60s. So long as the aneurysm is stable, the patient will usually be asymptomatic. When the aneurysm starts to expand, however, the patient becomes symptomatic, with the sudden onset of abdominal or back pain. When the pain is principally in the abdomen, it tends to centre on the umbilicus. Often, the pain may be located solely in the lower back, leading the patient to think he or she has "pulled a muscle" or otherwise injured the back. The pain is constant and moderate to severe; it cannot be relieved by changes in position. It tends to radiate into the thigh and groin. If the aneurysm is leaking blood into the retroperitoneal space, the patient may complain of an urge to defecate. In some patients, an episode of syncope heralds the onset of symptoms.

The most characteristic physical finding in an AAA is a pulsatile mass palpable in the abdomen. The patient is likely to be normotensive when first seen, but signs of shock, with or without hypotension, may develop rapidly if the aneurysm has ruptured.

Management of Expanding and Ruptured AAAs

Prehospital management of an expanding or ruptured aortic aneurysm is aimed at getting the patient to hospital as expeditiously as possible because the definitive treatment requires urgent surgery. The key is to maintain a high index of suspicion whenever a middle-aged or older man presents with sudden back pain and a pulsatile abdominal mass. The more likely problem in the prehospital environment in a conscious patient is a leaking aneurysm that has yet to rupture.

The steps of prehospital management in expanding or ruptured aortic aneurysm are as follows:

- Administer supplemental oxygen.
- Transport without delay.
- Insert an IV line en route, and give normal saline. Use a large-gauge cannula, but maintain the flow to keep the vein open unless signs of shock appear. If there are signs of shock, treat as for any other case of shock, with IV fluids.

Hypertensive Emergencies

Hypertension (high blood pressure) afflicts over 10 million people in the UK, that is 1 in every 5 people. It is further estimated that around half of the people over the age of 65 years have a condition linked to hypertension. In addition, it is a major contributing cause in many cases of AMI, CHF, and stroke. Most hypertension is the result of advanced atherosclerosis or arteriosclerosis, which decreases the lumen of the arteries and reduces their elasticity. The resulting high afterload on the heart leads to an increase in filling volume and stimulates the Frank-Starling reflex, which raises the pressure behind the blood leaving the heart.

Hypertension is present when the blood pressure at rest is consistently greater than about 140/90 mm Hg. Many conditions, such as anxiety or pain, can transiently elevate a person's blood pressure (especially the systolic blood pressure), so a single blood pressure measurement taken during an emergency scarcely constitutes adequate grounds for telling a patient that he or she is hypertensive. Instead, one may say something like this: "Sir, your blood pressure is a little high right now. That may be because of the stress you are under and may not have any real significance. To be safe, you should have your blood pressure rechecked a couple of times in the next few months under less stressful circumstances".

Persistent elevation of the diastolic pressure, by contrast, is indicative of hypertensive disease. If left untreated, hypertension significantly shortens the life span and predisposes the patient to a variety of other medical problems. The most common complications of hypertension include renal damage, stroke, and heart failure—the last a result of the left ventricle having to pump for years against a markedly increased afterload.

Signs and Symptoms of Hypertensive Disease

In the majority of cases, hypertension is entirely asymptomatic and is detected by chance during routine examination. By the time symptoms start to occur, hypertension is already in a more advanced stage and has probably produced at least some damage to organs such as the heart, kidneys, and brain.

The symptoms that occur in advanced hypertensive disease may be related to the elevated blood pressure or to secondary complications. Headache is the most common symptom directly related to blood pressure elevation; hypertensive headache is usually localised to the occipital region of the head and occurs when the patient first awakens in the morning, then subsides gradually over the next few hours. Other symptoms of moderately severe hypertension include dizziness, weakness, epistaxis, and blurring of vision. Often a patient with these hypertension-related signs and symptoms has already been prescribed medication for hypertension but is not taking it as prescribed.

Management of Hypertensive Diseases

Hypertensive emergencies occur in about 1% of all hypertensive patients. A hypertensive emergency is defined as an acute elevation of blood pressure with evidence of end-organ damage. That last phrase is important, because it is the evidence of end-organ dysfunction that determines the urgency of the situation, not the reading on the sphygmomanometer. Two end-organ emergencies that may result from uncontrolled hypertension were discussed earlier in this chapter: left-sided heart failure and dissecting aortic aneurysm. A rare but much more devastating complication of hypertension is hypertensive encephalopathy.

Hypertensive encephalopathy (also known as acute hypertensive crisis) may complicate any form of hypertension. Hypertensive crisis is usually signalled by a sudden, marked rise in blood pressure to levels greater than 200/130 mm Hg. The determining factor for hypertensive encephalopathy is usually the mean arterial pressure (MAP). The MAP is calculated by adding one third of the difference between the systolic blood pressure (SBP) and diastolic blood pressure (DBP) to the diastolic blood pressure.

$$MAP = DBP + \frac{1}{3}(SBP - DBP)$$

When the MAP exceeds 150 mm Hg, the pressure breaches the blood-brain barrier and fluid leaks out, increasing intracranial pressure. Usually the first symptoms noticed are severe headache, nausea, and vomiting. They are followed by convulsions and alternations in mental status (that is, confusion to unresponsiveness). Sometimes patients may show focal neurological signs, such as sudden blindness, aphasia (disturbances in speech production or comprehension), or hemiparesis. Widespread neuromuscular irritability may be signalled by muscle twitching.

The goal of treatment in hypertensive encephalopathy is to lower the blood pressure in a gradual, controlled manner during a 30- to 60-minute period so that cerebral blood flow is restored to normal. That is best accomplished under controlled conditions in hospital. Thus, provide supportive treatment only:

- Secure the airway, and administer supplemental oxygen by nasal cannula or nonrebreathing mask.
- Establish an IV.
- Apply monitoring electrodes, and run an ECG rhythm strip (consider running a second 12-lead ECG en route to the A&E department).
- Transport without delay. Be prepared to deal with convulsions en route, and have diazepam ready.

▌ Cardiac Arrhythmias

Cardiac rhythm disturbances or arrhythmias **Table 27-14 ▶** may arise from a variety of causes; they are not solely caused by AMI. A cardiac arrhythmia is simply a disturbance in the normal cardiac rhythm, which may or may not be clinically significant. Sometimes arrhythmias are caused by ischaemia, electrolyte imbalances, disturbances or damage in the electrical conduction system resulting in escape beats, circus re-entry, or enhanced automaticity. Thus, it is always necessary to evaluate the arrhythmia in the context of the patient's overall clinical condition. Indeed, it is the patient's clinical condition—not the lines and squiggles on a piece of paper—that should ultimately determine whether treatment is necessary. Treat the patient, not the monitor!

You are the Paramedic Part 3

You diagnose the patient as having acute pulmonary oedema secondary to exacerbation of her congestive heart failure. You administer a 400-mcg spray of sublingual GTN every 5 to 10 minutes, 50 mg of furosemide IV, and monitor the patient closely for any deterioration. You complete another set of observations, noting an irregular pulse and run off a 3-lead ECG rhythm strip.

Reassessment	Recording Time: 10 minutes
Skin	Pale, cool, and perspiring
Pulse	135 beats/min, irregular
Blood pressure	180/105 mm Hg
Respirations	37 breaths/min, shallow and laboured
SpO_2	90% on 100% supplemental oxygen

5. How do these two drugs help in acute pulmonary oedema?
6. What rhythm do you expect to find on the ECG given the rhythm of the pulse and knowing that the patient is on digoxin?

Table 27-14	Causes of Cardiac Arrhythmias

- Myocardial ischaemia or infarction
- Other forms of heart disease
- Rheumatic heart disease
- Cor pulmonale
- Generalised hypoxaemia from any cause
- Autonomic nervous system imbalance
- Increased vagal tone
- Increased sympathetic output
- Distension of cardiac chambers (as in heart failure)
- Electrolyte disturbances, especially those involving

- potassium, calcium, or magnesium
- Drug toxicity
- Certain poisons (such as organophosphate insecticides)
- Central nervous system damage
- Hypothermia
- Metabolic imbalance
- Normal variations
- Trauma (such as cardiac contusions)

One of the most important tasks in the prehospital care of a patient with an AMI is to anticipate, recognise, and treat life-threatening arrhythmias. Arrhythmias develop after an AMI for two principal reasons. First, irritability of the ischemic heart muscle surrounding the infarct may cause the damaged muscle to generate abnormal currents of electricity that cause abnormal cardiac contractions. When the arrhythmia arises from irritable spots in the myocardium (ectopic foci), it is usually a rapid arrhythmia (tachyarrhythmia), such as (VT), premature atrial contractions, or PVCs. Second, arrhythmias may occur after an AMI because the infarct damages the conduction tissues. In such a case, the abnormal rhythm is usually a heart block or a bradyarrhythmia.

Very slow HRs (< 40 to 50 beats/min) lead to inadequate CO and often precede electrical instability of the heart. Furthermore, when the sinus rate becomes very slow, ectopic pacemakers in the AV node or ventricles may fire and produce escape beats to assist in maintaining CO.

Conversely, very rapid HRs (> 120 to 140/min) increase the work of the heart, causing further myocardial ischaemia and damage. Tachycardias may also be associated with decreased CO secondary to decreased SV because the ventricles have less time to fill between beats. Hypoxia, metabolic alkalosis, hypokalaemia, and hypocalcaemia can lead to electrical instability; cells with no automaticity property may then begin to fire impulses. This kind of enhanced automaticity may occur with the use of drugs such as digitalis or atropine and is manifested by ectopic beats anywhere in the heart. The result is the potential for tachycardias, flutters, and fibrillations in the atria or ventricles, heralding grave rhythms such as VT and VF. Circus re-entry can also be a serious problem Figure 27-22 ▸ . The AV node may be bombarded by more than one impulse—potentially blocking the pathway for one impulse and allowing the other to stimulate cardiac cells that have already depolarised. The danger here comes when these impulses get "stuck" in a pattern of repetition, causing multiple ectopic beats or VF.

ECG analysis is indicated in any patient who might have a cardiac-related condition. Any patient with a chest pain should certainly undergo ECG analysis, but this monitoring should also be instituted for any patient with a history of heart problems. Given that age is a contributing factor to heart disease, ECG analysis is appropriate for elderly patients in many situations. Indeed, the ECG should be thought of as another vital sign, similar to the blood pressure or pulse oximetry.

ECG Monitoring: Placement of Leads and Electrodes

How reliable would ECG tracings or 12 leads be if the electrodes were placed anywhere on the patient? To maintain consistency in monitoring and obtaining a useful and consistent ECG, there are predetermined locations to place electrodes and leads.

Electrodes used in the prehospital setting are generally adhesive and have a gel centre to aid in skin contact. Some manufacturers offer a "diaphoretic" electrode that sticks to a

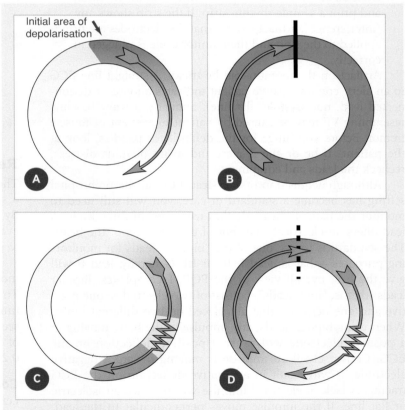

Figure 27-22 A. The original impulse site fires and triggers a depolarisation wave that spreads throughout the rest of the cells in the direction shown. **B.** By the time the depolarisation wave reaches the original site (represented by the black line) the original site is still refractory and cannot accept the new impulse. The depolarisation wave essentially dies at this point. **C.** The area in yellow represents an area of slow conduction. The depolarisation wave slows down as it traverses this area. **D.** By the time the depolarisation wave reaches the original site (represented by the dotted black line) the original site is now ready to receive a new impulse. The result is a circular movement that is self-perpetuating.

sweating patient more effectively. Whichever type is used, certain basic principles should be followed to achieve the best skin contact and minimise artifact in the signal:

- To maintain the correct lead placement, it may be necessary to shave body hair from the electrode site. Don't be fooled by a hairy chest. It may appear that you have great skin contact initially, but the electrode will rise off the skin and stick to the hair. Shaving should also be done when using hands-free adhesive defibrillation pads.
- To remove oils and dead tissues from the surface of the skin, rub the electrode site briskly with an alcohol swab or skin adhesive tape before application. Wait for the alcohol to dry before electrode application or dry it with a quick wipe of a gauze pad.
- Another trick of the trade to provide excellent skin contact is to gently scrape the electrode site with the disposable plastic backing of the electrode to "rough up" the skin cells before application. This is often overlooked.
- Attach the electrodes to the ECG cables before placement.
- Once all electrodes are in place, switch on the monitor, and print a sample rhythm strip. If the strip shows any "interference" (artifact), verify that the electrodes are firmly applied to the skin and the monitor cable is plugged in correctly.

Artifact on the monitor can be tricky. A straight-line ECG in an alert, communicative patient indicates a loose or disconnected lead, not asystole (flat line). Similarly, a wavy baseline resembling VF may be caused by patient movement or muscle tremor. Before you lunge for the defibrillator paddles, look at the patient! If he or she is alert and in no obvious distress, recheck the leads and equipment.

Although acquisition of a 12-lead ECG in the prehospital setting has become a standard of care, you will still need to monitor the patient's heart rhythm using one of three leads. A lead offers an electrical snapshot of certain parts of the heart. The standard is to use one of the "bipolar" leads for monitoring purposes—that is, lead I, II, or III. Generally, lead II will give the best overall view of the PQRST complexes. Bipolar leads (that is, "limb leads") consist of two electrodes, one positive and one negative, that are placed on two different limbs. When using bipolar leads, any impulse in the body moving to a positive electrode will cause a positive deflection on the ECG. Conversely, if an impulse is moving toward a negative electrode, it will result in a negative deflection on the ECG tracing. A lack of electrical impulse will produce an isolectric or flat line. If the impulse moves perpendicular to the lead, the result will be a "biphasic" waveform, which is above and below the isoelectric baseline.

When correctly positioned on the chest, these leads form a triangle around the heart, called the Einthoven triangle **Figure 27-23 ▸**. Today, it is not necessary to change the electrical poles of the electrodes to get a different lead. ECG monitors have the ability to change the polarity of the leads so that we can view leads I, II, and III by turning a knob or pressing a soft key.

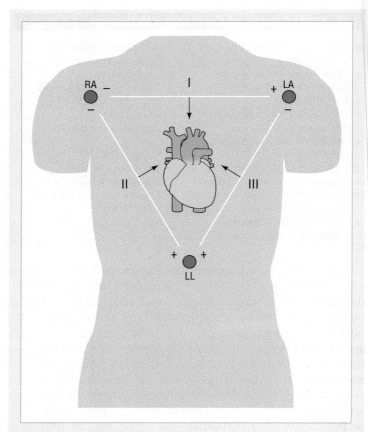

Figure 27-23 The Einthoven triangle.

Reading an ECG Rhythm Strip

The most reliable method of analysing a rhythm strip is to use a systematic approach and examine every strip the same way. By using such an approach, you will find in most cases that even the most complex-appearing arrhythmias can be reduced to simple terms and correctly identified.

ECGs are recorded on standardised graph paper, which is moved past a heated stylus at a standardised speed (25 mm/s). Thus, a given distance on the graph paper represents a given time. Specifically, one small (1 mm) box is equivalent to 0.04 second (1/25th of a second), and one large box (which consists of five small boxes) is equivalent to 0.20 second (0.04 × 5 = 0.20) **Figure 27-24 ▸** .

Components of an ECG Complex

Let's break down the ECG waveforms into their individual components.

P Wave

The P wave is normally a small, upright waveform (in leads I and II). It immediately precedes the QRS. The P wave is formed as the impulse is generated by the SA node in the right atrium and spreads over the atria, causing depolarisation. Lasting only 0.06 to 0.11 s, P waves can give clues to the pacemaker site if they are missing or do not have a uniform appearance.

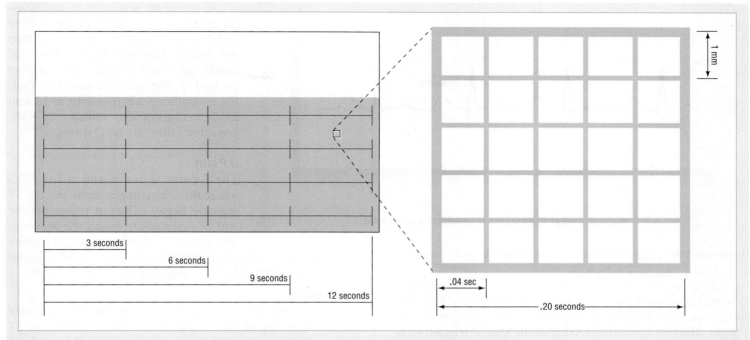

Figure 27-24 ECG paper. Height (amplitude) is measured in millimetres (mm) and width in milliseconds (ms).

If there are no P waves, the pacemaker for the heart is not in the SA node, and one must consider the possibility of atrial fibrillation or a junctional or ventricular rhythm. If a QRS complex is not preceded by a P wave, the pacemaker site for that beat is not in the SA node, but rather in some ectopic focus (a location other than the SA node). If a P wave is present but not followed by a QRS complex, a block is present somewhere in the AV junction or below and is preventing conduction from the atria to the ventricles. P waves that vary in size and configuration mean that there are several pacemaker sites at different locations throughout the atria.

P-R Interval
The P-R interval (PRI) includes atrial depolarisation and the conduction of the impulse through the AV junction. It includes the slight delay that normally occurs when the impulse is held in the AV node, allowing time for ventricular filling **Figure 27-25 ▸** .

The PRI is measured from the start of the P wave to the point at which the QRS complex begins. Although it normally lasts 0.12 to 0.20 s (three to five small boxes on the ECG strip), the PRI may be prolonged and give clues that the AV node is diseased or damaged, as in an AMI **Figure 27-26 ▸** . A PRI that exceeds 0.20 s (five small boxes), for example, is called first-degree AV block and may indicate injury to the AV junction. A PRI may also be shorter than 0.12 s in cases of Wolff-Parkinson-White syndrome, when the AV node is bypassed altogether.

QRS Complex
The QRS complex, which consists of three waveforms, represents depolarisation of two simultaneously contracting ventri-

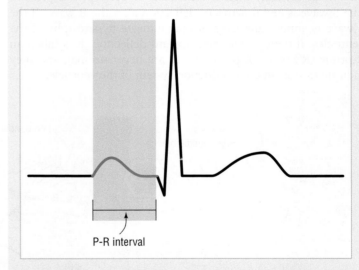

Figure 27-25 The normal P-R interval is 0.12 to 0.20 s.

cles. It is measured from the beginning of the Q wave to the end of the S wave and should follow each P wave in a consistent manner.

In healthy people, the QRS complex is narrow, with sharply pointed waves, and has a duration of less than 0.12 s (three small boxes on the ECG strip). Such a complex indicates that conduction of the impulse has proceeded normally from the AV junction, through the bundle of His, left and right bundles, and the Purkinje system. If abnormal, the complex has a bizarre appearance and a duration longer than 0.12 s. It signifies some

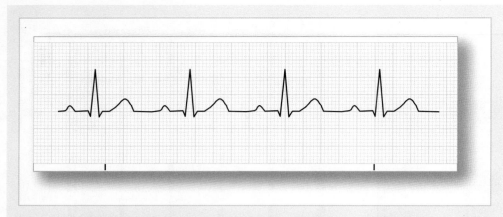

Figure 27-26 A P-R interval greater than 0.20 s is considered prolonged.

abnormality in conduction through the ventricle as in a bundle branch block **Figure 27-27 ▾**.

The first downward deflection in the QRS is called a Q wave; this wave represents conduction through the ventricular septum. The electricity spreads from right to left through the septum. The first upward deflection of the QRS is referred to as the R wave. Most of both ventricles are depolarised during the R wave. The R wave may be wide if the ventricle is enlarged and may be abnormally high if ventricular hypertrophy is present. The S wave is any downward deflection after the R wave. If the S wave is abnormally large, it may indicate hypertrophy of the ventricles. If there is a second upward deflection, it is called an R-prime (R′) wave. R-prime waves are never normal, and they indicate trouble in the conduction system of the ventricle.

Q waves are abnormal or pathological if they are one small square (0.04 s) wide on the ECG strip. Likewise, if they are deeper than one third of the total height (amplitude) of the QRS complex (in lead II), they are abnormal. This finding is significant when looking at 12-lead ECGs because it may indicate an AMI. Sometimes there are no Q waves.

J Point

The J point is the point in the ECG where the QRS complex ends and the ST segment begins. Thus, it represents the end of depolarisation and the apparent beginning of repolarisation. In some cases, the J point may be easier to locate than the ST segment when you are looking for elevation (another clue to an AMI).

ST Segment

The ST segment, which is the line between the QRS complex and the beginning of the T wave, is normally isolectric. An ST segment that is significantly (> 1 mm or one small box) above or below the isoelectric line is highly suggestive of myocardial ischaemia or injury, although a full 12-lead ECG is required to determine the precise significance of ST segment elevation or depression.

T Wave

A T wave represents ventricular repolarisation, but may also show abnormalities such as those found with electrolyte disturbances. In hyperkalaemia, for example, the T wave may be tall and sharply peaked.

For the most part, the T wave remains in a state of relative refractoriness, which means that the cells are partially repolarised. Early in the T wave, the cells will not accept another impulse. However, on the down slope (the vulnerable period), a strong impulse could cause depolarisation, overpowering the primary pacemaker to take over the pacemaker control. The supernormal phase is the time near the end of the T wave (the last one third), just before the cells become completely repolarised. During this period, a stimulus weaker than normally required can cause depolarisation, resulting in a dangerous heart rhythm.

This behaviour of the T wave is the main reason there are "synch" (synchronise) buttons on monitors and defibrillators.

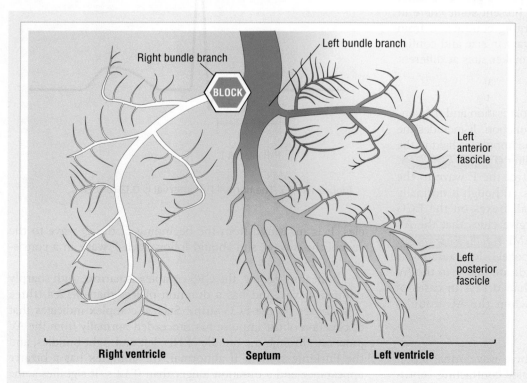

Figure 27-27 Bundle branch block.

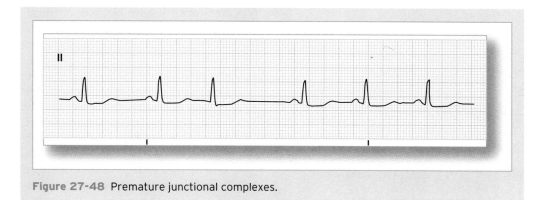

Figure 27-48 Premature junctional complexes.

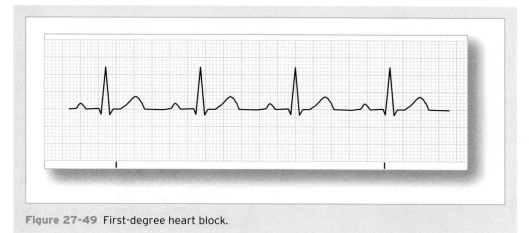

Figure 27-49 First-degree heart block.

Premature Junctional Complex

Premature junctional complex (PJC) is not, strictly speaking, an arrhythmia (just as PAC is not), but rather the existence of a particular complex within another rhythm **Figure 27-48 ▲**. Premature junctional complexes are also known as ectopic complexes, meaning that they occur out of the normal location. A PJC also occurs earlier in time than the next expected sinus complex, causing the R-R interval to be less between it and the previous complex.

The rate depends on the underlying rhythm, and the PJC will make the rhythm irregular. The P wave, if present, will be inverted or upside down, and it may precede or follow the QRS complex. The P-R interval, if present, will measure less than 0.12 s. The QRS complex will measure 0.04 to 0.12 s.

Premature junctional complexes can be caused by many of the same problems that cause premature atrial contractions. They are rarely treated in the prehospital setting but may be a predictor of future cardiac arrhythmias.

Heart Blocks

After the SA node initiates impulses, the impulses proceed through the atria and ventricles and result in contraction of the heart. When they reach the AV node, the impulses are delayed to allow the atria to contract and fill the ventricle. This delay is a normal function of the AV node and usually causes no prob-lems. Occasionally, however, the impulses travelling through the AV node are delayed more than usual, resulting in heart blocks.

Heart blocks are classified into different degrees based on the seriousness of the block and the amount of myocardial damage. The least serious heart block is a first-degree heart block; the most serious is a third-degree block. In between are two types of second-degree block.

First-Degree Heart Block

A first-degree heart block occurs when each impulse reaching the AV node is delayed slightly longer than is expected and results in a P-R interval greater than 0.20 s. Because each impulse eventually passes through the AV node and causes a QRS complex, this block is considered the least serious. Nevertheless, it is often the first indication of damage that has occurred to the AV node.

Because it originates from the normal pacemaker of the heart, first-degree heart block usually has an intrinsic rate of 60 to 100 beats/min, although it typically occurs at the low end of this range **Figure 27-49 ◀**. The rhythm is regular, with minimal variation between R-R intervals. The P wave is present and upright, and it precedes each QRS complex. The P-R interval will measure greater than 0.20 s. The QRS complex will measure 0.04 to 0.12 s. The only difference between first-degree heart block and normal sinus rhythm is the prolonged P-R interval.

First-degree heart block is rarely treated in the prehospital setting unless it is associated with bradycardia that results in significantly reduced CO.

Second-Degree Heart Block: Mobitz Type I (Wenckebach)

A second-degree heart block occurs when an impulse reaching the AV node is occasionally prevented from proceeding to the ventricles and causing a QRS complex. Second-degree heart block, Mobitz type I (Wenckebach), occurs when each successive impulse is delayed a little longer, until finally one impulse is not allowed to continue.

Because it begins from the normal pacemaker of the heart, second-degree heart block, type I, usually has an intrinsic rate of 60 to 100 beats/min, although it typically occurs at the low end of this range **Figure 27-50 ▶**. The rhythm is irregular, with a prolonged R-R interval occurring between the last QRS complex before the blocked P wave and the QRS complex after the first unblocked P wave. The P wave is present and upright, and it precedes most QRS complexes. The P-R interval starts out within the normal limits of 0.12 to 0.20 s but, with each

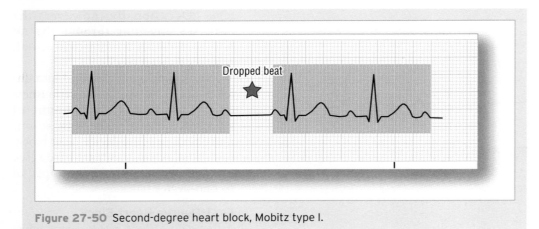

Figure 27-50 Second-degree heart block, Mobitz type I.

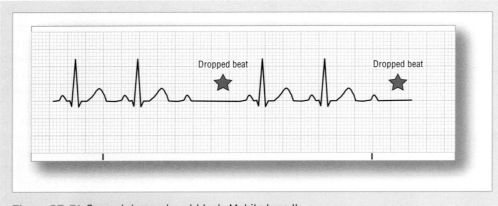

Figure 27-51 Second-degree heart block, Mobitz type II.

every other P wave blocked, or irregular, with a prolonged R-R interval between the last QRS complex before the blocked P wave and the QRS complex after the first unblocked P wave. The P wave is present and upright, and it precedes some QRS complexes. The P-R interval is always constant. In fact, this is the easiest way to identify a second-degree type II heart block. If you see a rhythm with some nonconducted P waves, but the P-R interval is constant among all conducted P waves and their corresponding QRS complexes, you have identified a second-degree type II heart block.

It is important to remember that this block can be regular or irregular. Sometimes several normal beats will occur without a nonconducted P wave; sometimes two or more nonconducted P waves may appear before one P wave is conducted. In other situations, a pattern develops that consists of one conducted P wave followed by one nonconducted P wave.

Second-degree type II heart blocks are treated in the prehospital setting only if they are associated with bradycardia that results in significantly reduced CO.

successive P wave, grows longer. It finally results in a P wave that is followed not by a QRS complex, but by another P wave; this P wave is then followed by a QRS complex with a normal P-R interval. This pattern repeats over and over in the rhythm. The QRS complex will measure 0.04 to 0.12 s.

The key to identification of second-degree type I heart block is the recognition of the increasing P-R interval followed by the P wave without a QRS complex. This rhythm is always irregular, and you can often easily see the wide R-R interval with the "extra" P wave located there.

Second-degree type I heart blocks are treated in the prehospital setting only if they are associated with bradycardia that results in significantly reduced CO.

Second-Degree Heart Block: Mobitz Type II (Classical)

Second-degree heart block, Mobitz type II, occurs when several impulses are not allowed to continue. It is sometimes called classical because it was well known before the Wenckebach heart block was discovered.

Because it originates from the normal pacemaker of the heart, second-degree heart block, type II, usually has an intrinsic rate of 60 to 100 beats/min, although it typically occurs at the low end of this range Figure 27-51 ▲. The rhythm may be regular, with

Third-Degree Heart Block (Complete Heart Block)

A third-degree heart block occurs when all impulses reaching the AV node are prevented from proceeding to the ventricles and causing a QRS complex. Unlike in first- and second-degree heart blocks, in a third-degree heart block *all* impulses from the atria are prevented from travelling to the ventricles. As a consequence, this block is also known as a complete heart block. Because all impulses from the atria are blocked, the ventricles will develop their own pacemaker to continue circulation of blood, albeit at a greatly reduced rate.

Because it originates from the normal pacemaker of the heart, third-degree heart block usually has an intrinsic atrial rate of 60 to 100 beats/min, but the ventricular rate—which depends on the activity of a ventricular pacemaker—is less than 60 beats/min Figure 27-52 ▶. The rhythm is usually regular, with the P-P and R-R intervals being consistent. The P wave is present and upright. The P-R interval in this type of heart block is nonexistent.

The classic way of identifying a third-degree heart block is to identify the presence of nonconducted P waves and then to be unable to identify a relationship between the P waves and the QRS complexes. Because the ventricular rate depends on the presence of a ventricular pacemaker, it is common to see

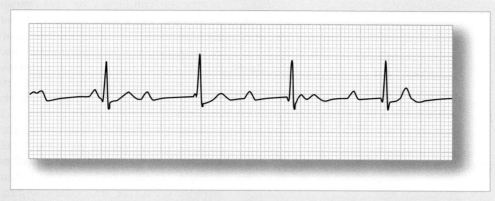

Figure 27-52 Third-degree heart block.

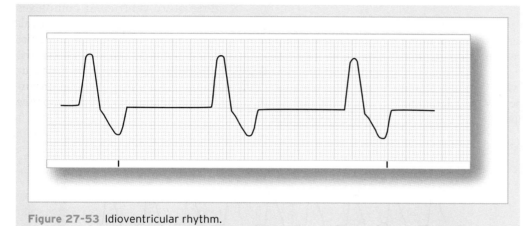

Figure 27-53 Idioventricular rhythm.

the QRS complexes in a third-degree heart block that are wider than 0.12 s. When you see a rhythm with wide QRS complexes (and no narrow QRS complexes) along with P waves, you should suspect a third-degree heart block. If the rhythm is regular and the P-R interval is not constant, it is almost certainly a third-degree heart block. The major issue with looking for third-degree heart blocks to be regular is the fact that if a premature ventricular complex (described later) occurs within the block, it will make the block appear irregular.

Third-degree heart blocks are treated in the prehospital setting only if they are associated with bradycardia that results in significantly reduced CO.

Rhythms of the Ventricles

If the SA node fails to initiate an impulse, the AV node will usually take over as pacemaker. If the AV node cannot perform this duty, however, the ventricles may begin to originate their own impulses and become the pacemaker of the heart. Such ventricular rhythms will have missing P waves and wide QRS complexes.

If an impulse is generated in the ventricles, it must travel through the ventricles in a cell-to-cell manner because the cell originating the impulse is unlikely to be located on the conduction system. Because impulses travel more slowly via

cell-to-cell transmission than when they travel on the conduction system, ventricular-initiated impulses result in very wide QRS complexes—more than 0.12 s in duration. Because the intrinsic rate of the ventricles is 20 to 40, ventricular rhythms normally demonstrate rates of 20 to 40 beats/min.

Idioventricular Rhythm

An idioventricular (meaning only the ventricles or produced by the ventricles) rhythm occurs when the SA and AV nodes fail, and the ventricles must take over pacing the heart **Figure 27-53 ◄**. It has a rate of 20 to 60 beats/min owing to the intrinsic rate of the ventricles as pacemakers. An idioventricular rhythm is usually regular, with little variation between R-R intervals. P waves are absent owing to the failure of the SA and AV nodes. Because there is no P wave, there is no P-R interval. The QRS complex will measure greater than 0.12 s because it originates in the ventricles.

Idioventricular rhythms are serious and may or may not result in a palpable pulse. Treatment is geared toward improving the CO by increasing the rate and, if possible, treating the underlying cause. In such a case, the patient's condition is usually severely compromised.

Accelerated Idioventricular Rhythm

Occasionally, an idioventricular rhythm exceeds its normal upper rate of 60 beats/min but remains less than 100 beats/min. Because the rhythm is greater than 60 beats/min, it cannot be considered a "normal" ventricular rhythm; because it is less than 100 beats/min, it cannot be called tachycardia either. In this case, the rhythm is called accelerated idioventricular rhythm.

An accelerated idioventricular rhythm is also regular, with little variation between R-R intervals. The P waves are absent, so the P-R interval does not exist **Figure 27-54 ►**. The QRS complex will measure greater than 0.12 s.

Accelerated idioventricular rhythms are serious, but they are seldom treated in the prehospital setting.

Ventricular Tachycardia

Ventricular rhythms occur when the SA and AV nodes fail as the pacemakers of the heart. Occasionally, a ventricular rhythm has a rate that exceeds 100 beats/min. Any rhythm that results in a ventricular rate greater than 100 beats/min is considered tachycardia. In this case, the rhythm is termed ventricular tachycardia.

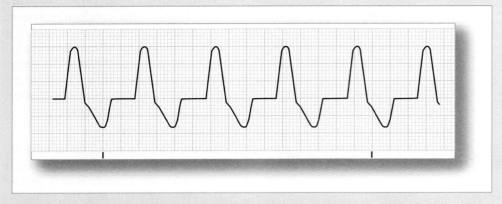

Figure 27-54 Accelerated idioventricular rhythm.

ventricular complexes are also known as ectopic complexes, meaning that they occur out of the normal location. A premature ventricular complex also occurs earlier than the next expected sinus complex, causing the R-R interval to be less between it and the previous complex.

Because the rate depends on the underlying rhythm, the premature ventricular complex will make the rhythm irregular. There is no P wave associated with the premature ventricular complex, so there is no P-R interval. The QRS complex will measure more than 0.12 s.

Premature ventricular complexes may also be further distinguished as unifocal or multifocal. Unifocal premature ventricular complexes originate from the same spot or "focus" within the ventricle and will appear the same on the ECG **Figure 27-58 ▶**. Two premature ventricular complexes with different appearances are multifocal, meaning there is more than one focus initiating ventricular impulses **Figure 27-59 ▶**.

Ventricular tachycardia is regular, with no variation between R-R intervals. The P waves are absent, so the P-R interval also does not exist. The QRS complex will measure greater than 0.12 s.

Ventricular tachycardia usually presents with QRS complexes that have uniform tops and bottoms; this type of VT is referred to as monomorphic (having one common shape of QRS complex) **Figure 27-55 ▶**. Occasionally, VT will present with QRS complexes that vary in height in an alternating pattern; this type of VT is called polymorphic VT **Figure 27-56 ▶**. The most common polymorphic VT is torsade de pointes, which is usually seen in patients who have a condition of a prolonged Q-T interval. Torsade de pointes may be normal for the patient or it may be induced by medications or drugs such as quinidine. Polymorphic VT is usually considered worse than monomorphic VT and converts spontaneously back to a normal rhythm or degenerates into VF.

Ventricular tachycardia is extremely serious, and it may require treatment in the prehospital setting because the rate is usually too fast to maintain adequate CO. This reduced CO, in conjunction with the increased workload of the heart due to the tachycardia, usually leads to ventricular failure or fibrillation if not treated promptly.

Premature Ventricular Complex

Premature ventricular complex is not, strictly speaking, an arrhythmia (just as premature atrial and junctional complexes are not), but rather the existence of a particular complex within another rhythm **Figure 27-57 ▶**. Premature

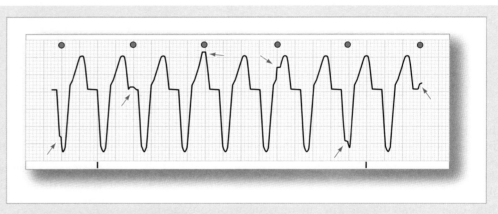

Figure 27-55 Monomorphic ventricular tachycardia.

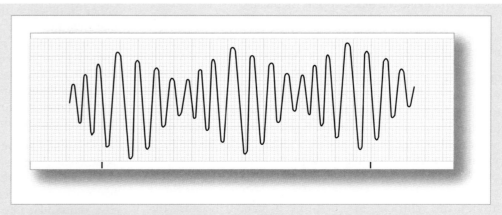

Figure 27-56 Polymorphic ventricular tachycardia.

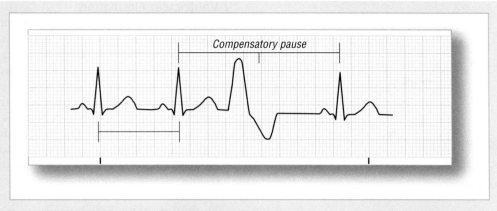

Figure 27-57 Premature ventricular complex.

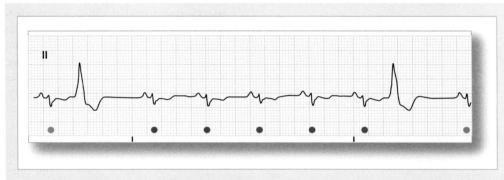

Figure 27-58 Unifocal premature ventricular complexes.

Sometimes two premature ventricular complexes may occur together without any pause between them. This pair of complexes is referred to as a couplet **Figure 27-60 ▸**. If three or more premature ventricular complexes occur in a row, they constitute a "run" of ventricular tachycardia. Occa-

sionally, these complexes will become so frequent that they alternate with normal complexes. This pattern is called bigeminy of premature ventricular complexes **Figure 27-61 ▸**. If every third beat is a premature ventricular complex, the pattern is called trigeminy.

Premature ventricular complexes can be caused by many of the same problems that cause premature atrial and junctional contractions, but they usually originate on account of ischaemia in the ventricular tissue. They are generally considered more serious than premature atrial or junctional complexes. Multifocal, couplet, and bigeminy premature ventricular complexes are considered more serious than unifocal premature ventricular complexes. One of the principal hazards of premature ventricular complexes is that they might occur at a time when the ventricles are not fully repolarised (as indicated by the T wave). This so-called R-on-T phenomenon often results in VF. For this and other reasons, premature ventricular complexes are considered serious and an indication of serious underlying heart conditions. Nevertheless, this condition is not usually treated in the prehospital setting, unless it is significantly affecting CO, and even then it must be treated with caution.

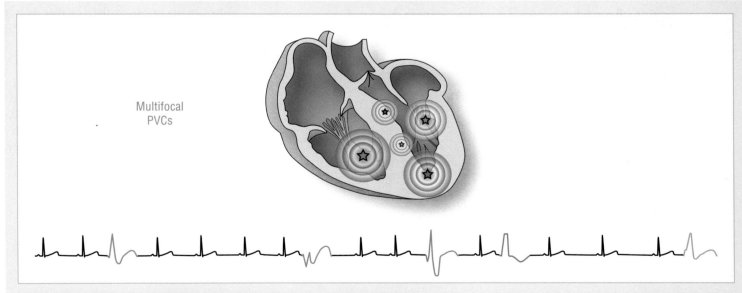

Figure 27-59 Multifocal premature ventricular complexes.

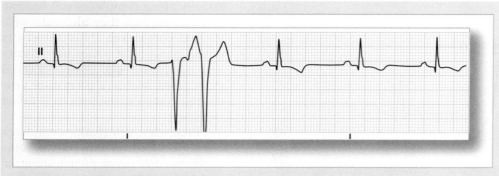

Figure 27-60 Couplet premature ventricular complexes.

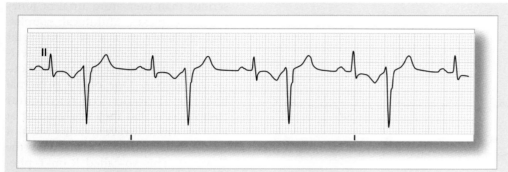

Figure 27-61 Bigeminy premature ventricular complexes.

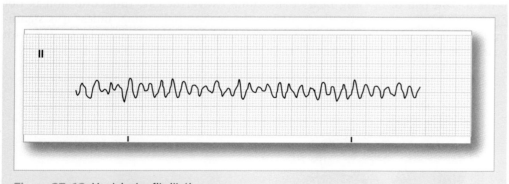

Figure 27-62 Ventricular fibrillation.

Ventricular Fibrillation

Ventricular fibrillation is a rhythm in which the entire heart is no longer contracting but rather fibrillating or quivering without any organised contraction. It occurs when many different cells in the heart become depolarised independently rather than in response to an impulse from the SA node Figure 27-62 ◄ . The result of this random depolarisation is a fibrillating or chaotic baseline without indication of organised activity. As opposed to atrial fibrillation, there are no P waves, no P-R interval, and no QRS complexes.

Early in VF, the cardiac cells have energy reserves that allow a considerable amount of electrical energy to be expended and cause the height of the chaotic waves to be large. These large waves are sometimes referred to as "coarse" VF Figure 27-63 ▼ . As the ventricles continue to go without circulation, the energy reserves of the cardiac cells are gradually used up, leading to a great reduction of the height of the chaotic waves. This phenomenon is sometimes called "fine" VF Figure 27-64 ► .

Ventricular fibrillation is the rhythm most commonly seen in adults who go into cardiac arrest. Fortunately, it responds well to defibrillation performed with an automated or manual defibrillator within the first 4 to 5 minutes of an arrest. If the collapse is not witnessed, provide 2 minutes of CPR prior to defibrillation.

Asystole

Asystole ("flat line") is a rhythm in which the entire heart is no longer contracting but rather is sitting still within the thorax without any organised activity Figure 27-65 ► . It occurs when

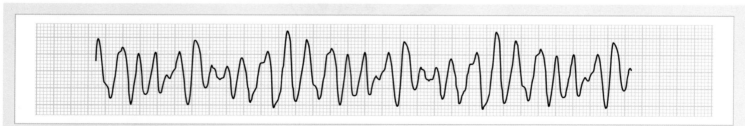

Figure 27-63 Coarse ventricular fibrillation.

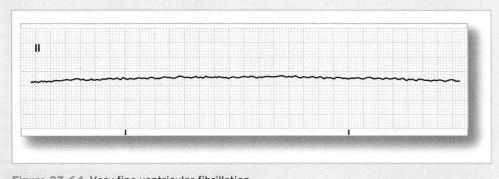

Figure 27-64 Very fine ventricular fibrillation.

ing from the impulse travelling through the ventricles. Another type of pacemaker is attached to the atria and the ventricle; it produces a pacemaker spike that is followed by a P wave and another pacemaker spike followed by a wide QRS complex. Many of the newer pacemakers are equipped with sensors that can identify the rate of spontaneous depolarisation of the heart. These "demand" pacemakers begin to generate pacing impulses only when they sense that the natural pace of

many cells of the heart have been hypoxic for so long that they no longer have any energy for any kind of contraction. Asystole presents with a complete absence of electrical activity: no P waves, no P-R intervals, no QRS complexes, and no T waves.

In one variation of asystole, the flat baseline associated with asystole is interrupted by a small sinusoidal complex. This condition, which is termed agonal rhythm, is probably a result of residual electrical discharge from a dead heart. Agonal rhythm should not be confused with an idioventricular rhythm **Figure 27-66 ▶** . An idioventricular rhythm may result in a palpable pulse, but an agonal rhythm will not.

Artificial Pacemaker Rhythms

Many of your patients will have experienced problems with their cardiac conduction systems and had artificial pacemakers implanted in their chest. When these patients are connected to the heart monitor, the presence of the artificial pacemaker is obvious. The firing of an artificial pacemaker causes a unique vertical spike on the ECG tracing **Figure 27-67 ▶** . When you attach the cardiac monitor to a patient and see these sharp vertical spikes on the ECG, you can assume the patient has an artificial pacemaker **Figure 27-68 ▶** .

Many types of artificial pacemakers exist, and more are being developed. The most common type in the past has been the ventricular pacemaker, which is attached to the ventricles only; it causes a sharp pacemaker spike followed by a wide QRS complex result-

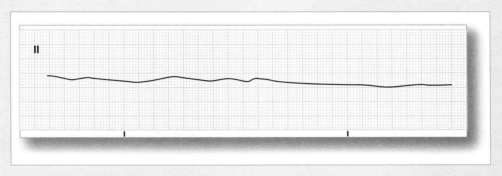

Figure 27-65 Asystole.

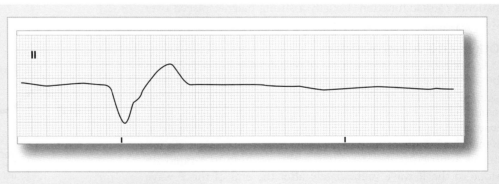

Figure 27-66 Agonal rhythm.

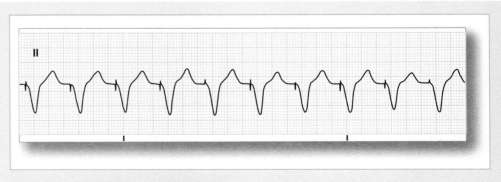

Figure 27-67 Artificial pacemaker rhythm.

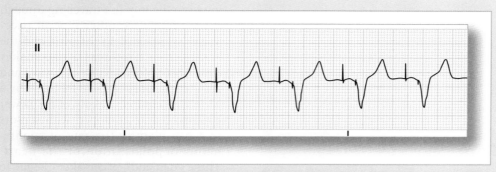

Figure 27-68 Artificial pacemaker rhythm (AV sequential).

cardiac impulses has slowed below a specific number (usually 60 per minute) Figure 27-69 ▾.

Occasionally, a patient may experience a problem with his or her pacemaker. If the patient's pacemaker is failing (eg, due to battery failure), the pacemaker spikes may still be visible, but they will not be followed by a QRS complex. This loss of capture indicates the pacemaker is not operating properly. A loss of capture may also occur if the wire connecting the pacemaker to the patient's heart becomes dislodged. In either of these cases, the patient's heartbeat now depends on the natural pacemaker (usually the ventricles), resulting in greatly reduced CO. In such cases, patients need trancutaneous pacing (TCP) instituted as quickly as possible.

Another type of pacemaker failure involves a "runaway" pacemaker. A runaway pacemaker presents as a very tachycardic pacemaker rhythm that must be slowed to preserve the patient's cardiac function. Usually a strong magnet placed over the pacemaker will "reset" a runaway pacemaker.

Other ECG Abnormalities

A few other ECG abnormalities are not identified as arrhythmias but are indicative of significant cardiac conditions. For example, a delta wave is an indication of Wolff-Parkinson-White (WPW) syndrome. Patients with WPW syndrome have an accessory pathway between the atria and the ventricles called the bundle of Kent. This bundle of conductive tissue bypasses the AV node and begins ventricular depolarisation early, resulting in a rapid up slope to the R wave immediately after the end of the P wave Figure 27-70 ▸. This early up slope can be interpreted as a widened QRS complex (more than 0.12 s), which would seem

to indicate a ventricular pacemaker. This situation, which is referred to as aberrant conduction, can lead to the misinterpretation of SVTs (narrow complex tachycardias) as ventricular in origin. Patients with WPW syndrome are highly susceptible to SVTs (narrow complex tachycardias).

Another important abnormality is an Osborne, or J, wave. It occurs in cases of hypothermia and presents as what appears to be a P wave at the end of the QRS complex Figure 27-71 ▾. The J wave may also be accompanied by ST-segment depression and T-wave inversion. Generally, the more serious the hypothermia, the larger the J wave. Evidence of a J wave should be considered only an indication of hypothermia; it is not enough to make a definitive diagnosis.

Electrolyte imbalances can also cause changes in the ECG that are not arrhythmias but can be indicators of serious conditions. The two most common of these electrolyte imbalances are hyperkalaemia and hypokalaemia. Hyperkalaemia often presents with very tall, pointed T waves; these T waves may be as tall or taller than the QRS complex Figure 27-72 ▸. By contrast, hypokalaemia usually presents with flat or apparently absent T waves along with the

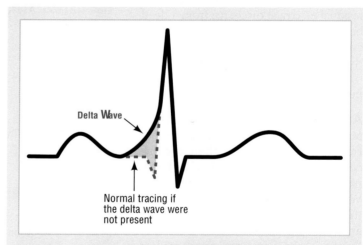

Figure 27-70 Delta wave: WPW syndrome.

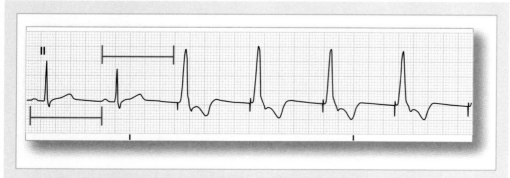

Figure 27-69 Artificial pacemaker rhythm (demand pacemaker).

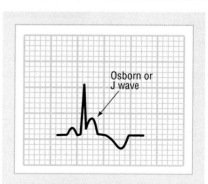

Figure 27-71 Osborne (J) wave.

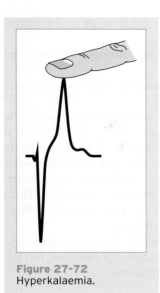

Figure 27-72
Hyperkalaemia.

development of a U wave. The U wave is a small wave (smaller even than a P wave) that occurs after a T wave but before the next P wave. U waves are very uncommon and may often be mistaken for extra P waves or another unknown abnormality Figure 27-73 ▾ .

Other electrolyte imbalances do not cause such obvious changes in the ECG. Hypercalcaemia may cause a shortened Q-T interval, for example, whereas hypocalcaemia may slightly lengthen the Q-T interval. These changes would likely not be obvious in the prehospital environment.

Bedtime Stories: Tragic Tales of Arrhythmias

Cast

Sidney Sinus. Sidney, the SA node, is boss of the heart. He ordinarily dispatches messengers 70 to 80 times per minute; the messengers are supposed to dash down the atria, slip through the AV junction, and depolarise the ventricles. Sidney is not terribly bright but is usually conscientious and reliable.

Albert and Alice Atria. Albert and Alice are the right and left atria. These somewhat temperamental little pouches normally contract in response to the messages sent by Sidney and squeeze their blood into the ventricles, providing the ventricles with an atrial kick. Their contraction is represented on the ECG by the P wave.

AV Abe. Abe, the AV node, is a lower-level pacemaker who secretly yearns to be boss of the heart. Unfortunately, because of his lower intrinsic rate, he rarely gets the opportunity to run the show. Abe stands at the threshold of the ventricles and checks out every messenger sent by Sidney Sinus. Normally, Abe lets the messengers pass into the ventricles after a brief security check (P-R interval).

However, as the node in charge of traffic control into the ventricles, Abe does regulate the flow of messengers and occasionally closes a few southbound lanes, especially when the traffic gets very heavy or when he's not feeling well.

Vance and Virginia Ventricle. Vance and Virginia are big, tough, muscular types, also not very bright, who are charged with the enormous responsibility of pumping blood to the whole body. Normally, they take their orders from the messengers sent by Sidney Sinus, but sometimes the Ventricles grow irritable and contract without orders, especially when they run a little short on oxygen. They also tend to be impatient when they don't hear from Sidney on time; under that circumstance, they sometimes contract on their own.

Montgomery, Mimi, Mortimer, Millicent, et al. These messengers consist of tiny electric impulses. Earnest and dedicated, their job is to carry the orders for depolarisation from Sidney's headquarters all the way to the ventricles.

First-Degree AV Block, or "The Little Messenger That Could"

One fine day, Sidney Sinus dispatched Mortimer Messenger with the usual order: "Depolarise the ventricles". Mortimer scampered down the atria without difficulty but arrived at the AV node to find a pile of debris blocking the entrance to the ventricles. "Sorry", said AV Abe, "we're closed for repairs".

"But I *have* to get through", said Mortimer.

"Impossible", said Abe.

But Mortimer was brave and determined. "I think I can. I think I can. I know I can", he said, gathering his few milliamps of strength. Finally, after a long struggle (prolonged P-R interval), Mortimer crashed through the AV junction into the ventricles and breathlessly issued the order to contract Figure 27-74 ▸ . The ventricles were depolarised, and everyone lived happily ever after, until . . .

Second-Degree AV Block, Type I

When Montgomery Messenger left for work that day, there was no sign there would be trouble. He took his first set of orders from Sidney Sinus, whistled down the atria, zipped through the AV node, and smartly ordered the ventricles to depolarise.

On the next trip down, however, Montgomery felt just a bit tired and slowed slightly as he crossed the AV junction. "Why break my neck"? he thought. "So, the P-R interval will be a tiny bit prolonged. Who'll notice, anyway"?

On his third trip, Montgomery encountered several roadblocks in the region of the AV junction and had to pick his way around them. Glancing at his watch as he reached the ventricles, he scowled. "Nuts", he said, "0.24 s. Boy, is Sidney going to be mad".

Making his fourth trip from the SA node, Montgomery found the gates to the ventricles closed and locked. Frantically, he banged on the gates. "Come on, Abe, I know you're around somewhere. Let me through". To no avail. The gates remained tightly shut. Defeated, Montgomery returned to the SA node, leaving a lonely P wave to chronicle his struggle Figure 27-75 ▸ .

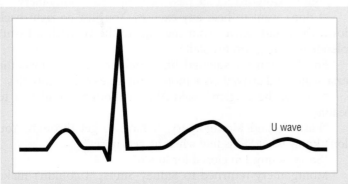

U wave

Figure 27-73 Hypokalaemia.

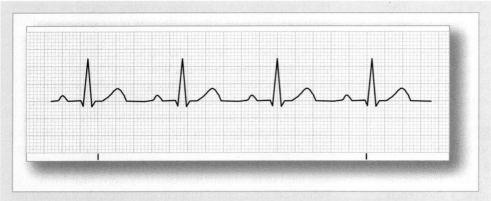

Figure 27-74 First-degree AV block. When there is trouble at the AV junction, it may take the messengers from the SA node longer to get through.

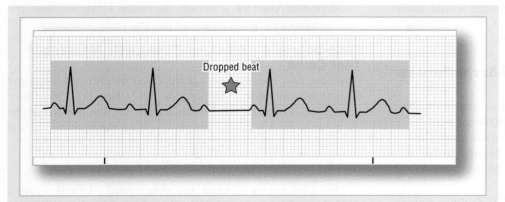

Dropped beat

Figure 27-75 Second-degree AV block, type I (Wenckebach). Each transit through the AV junction is a bit slower, until finally the messenger cannot get through, and a beat is dropped.

"What do you mean, you couldn't get through"? Sidney Sinus demanded.

"I couldn't get through", Montgomery said. "I'm telling you the gates were locked tight".

"Okay", said Sid, "off to the showers. You've had it for the day". So Sidney called Mimi Messenger. "Now look", he told her, "I want you to go straight down to the ventricles and give them this message, and no fooling around at the AV junction, understand"?

"Oh, yes sir", said Mimi, always eager to please. So off Mimi went, sailing down the atria, through the AV junction, and into the ventricles. "Hmm, 0.14 s", she noted to herself. "Sid can't complain about that". On her second run, however, Mimi tripped over a shoelace and barely made it in under 0.2 s. On the third trip, some highway construction held her up for 0.24 s. But the fourth trip south was the worst, for she arrived at the AV junction to find that once again Abe had locked the gates. Mimi banged and banged on the gates. "Come on, Abe, open up. I'm going to lose my job". No response. Crestfallen, Mimi returned to the SA node.

"And what happened to you"? Sid demanded.

"I couldn't get through to the ventricles this time".

"Couldn't get through? Did you get lost, maybe"?

"But at least I made a nice P wave", Mimi ventured.

"A nice P wave! A nice *P wave,* she says. What good's a P wave without a QRS complex? Do you think the atria are going to supply blood to the whole body? They're strictly small-time, sweetheart. The big guns are in the ventricles. That's why I sent you to depolarise them. Now you get to the showers".

And so it went. Messenger after messenger faltered at the AV junction, but the worst was yet to come.

Second-Degree AV Block, Type II

It just wasn't Montgomery's week. Reporting for work the next day, he received the usual order from Sidney to depolarise the ventricles. Montgomery set out full of confidence and vigour, traversing the atria without difficulty. But when he arrived at the threshold of the ventricles, he found his path blocked by AV Abe.

"Let me through", Montgomery said. "I have an important message for the ventricles".

"Get lost", said Abe, who was feeling rather dyspeptic that day.

"But I have to get through. I've already used up 0.19 s".

"Beat it, sonny. I'm the boss around here".

Montgomery returned to Sidney Sinus disgraced. "What happened to you"? Sidney wanted to know. "You were supposed to order the ventricles to contract".

"I couldn't get past Abe", Montgomery replied.

"What do you mean, you couldn't get past Abe? I just sent your friend, Mimi Messenger down there, and she got through without any problem".

"But he wouldn't let me pass", whimpered Montgomery.

"I don't want to hear any excuses. You just go right back down there and deliver your message to the ventricles. I can't tolerate weaklings on my staff".

So Montgomery squared his shoulders, sailed down the atria again, and arrived once more at the gate of the ventricles.

"Are you here again"? said Abe. "I thought I told you to beat it".

"Please", said Montgomery, "I have to get through. You don't know what Sid is like when he gets upset".

"Sorry, sonny, I'm closed for lunch".

Montgomery returned to Sidney Sinus. "I couldn't make it", he said.

"Look, Montgomery", said Sidney, "Millicent Messenger just breezed by Abe right after you left. Now you march back down there and do your job".

"Yes, sir", said Montgomery.

Arriving again at the threshold of the ventricles, Montgomery once more found Abe blocking his path.

"Listen, Abe, I'm not kidding this time. If you don't let me through, I'm going to use some atropine and blast the gate open".

"Those are big words, sonny", said Abe, "but I'm not scared of a little atropine".

"The last time they used atropine, you were zonked for hours", Montgomery reminded him.

"I'll take my chances".

And so it went. Each time Montgomery reached the gate to the ventricle, AV Abe barred his path. Yet the messenger coming right after Montgomery kept getting through (2:1 block) Figure 27-76 ▸.

"Montgomery", cautioned Sidney, "if this keeps up, they're going to put in a pacemaker, and we'll all be out of a job. Shape up".

But the worst was yet to come.

Complete Heart Block (Third-Degree AV Block)

The next day was even worse for Sidney's operation. It was bad enough, Montgomery not getting through. "Every second P wave not followed by a QRS complex", wailed Sidney. "My reputation is being ruined"! But then, suddenly, the situation became even worse. Sidney had just sent Mildred Messenger down to the ventricles, and she arrived at the AV junction to find the gate shut and bolted. A sign tacked to the gate read: "Closed until further notice".

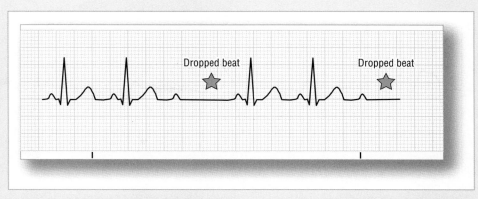

Figure 27-76 Second-degree AV block, type II. Every second impulse from the SA node is blocked at the AV junction.

"That's impossible", said Sidney when he heard the story. "Abe can't do that to me". So he sent another messenger, Marvin, to depolarise the ventricles. Marvin charged down the atria and ran smack into the closed gate. He banged and shouted, but there was no response.

"Impossible", said Sidney. "Abe must be sleeping". So he dispatched Melvin Messenger. Again the door was bolted tight.

"Oh, what I'd give for a bolus of atropine", sighed Sidney.

Meanwhile, the ventricles were starting to get nervous, and Vance, the right ventricle, said to Virginia, the left ventricle, "Have you heard anything from the atria lately"?

"Not a thing".

"Funny. Those messengers are usually pretty prompt".

"Must have run into some problems with Abe".

"Yeah. Every time that guy has a little too much digitalis, he gets delusions of grandeur and starts hassling the messengers".

"How long do you suppose we ought to wait"?

You are the Paramedic Part 4

You arrive at hospital and wheel the patient straight into the resuscitation room. You hand-over the patient to the waiting staff and notice that the doctor orders 5 mg of diamorphine and 50 mg of furosemide to be administered. The nursing staff are preparing the kit to administer continuous positive airway pressure (CPAP). You return with another patient 90 minutes later and drop by to check on Mrs Beresford. She looks much better and even manages a wave of recognition.

Reassessment	Recording Time: 20 minutes
Skin	Pale, cool, and perspiring.
Pulse	110 beats/min, irregular
Blood pressure	165/90 mmHg
Respirations	35 breaths/min, shallow, and laboured.
SpO_2	92% on supplemental oxygen at 15 l/min

7. Why did the doctor administer morphine? Should you have done this en route to hospital?

8. How does administering positive airways pressure help the patient?

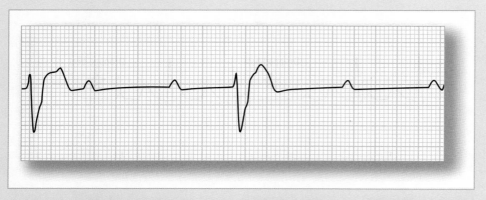

Figure 27-77 Third-degree AV block. The atria and ventricles are marching to the beat of different drummers.

"I don't know. It's already been more than a second, and the brain is starting to complain about not getting enough oxygen".

"The brain is always complaining about something".

"Yeah, but the kidneys don't sound very happy either".

"Okay, okay. Let's go ahead and contract. I hate to do it without authorisation from above".

So Vance and Virginia set off on their own, contracting slowly (about 30 times per minute) so as not to attract much attention, little appreciating that back in the atria Sidney was frantically sending messenger after messenger, all in vain, to assault the closed gate (**Figure 27-77** ▲).

"What's happened to Sidney"? Virginia said to Vance, as they plodded along slowly.

"I wish I knew", said Vance.

12-Lead ECGs

Up to now, we have considered ECG rhythm strips obtained from monitoring a single lead. For purposes of rhythm interpretation, a single lead (usually lead II) is usually sufficient. To localise the site of injury to heart muscle, however, we must be able to look at the heart from several angles. That is precisely the purpose of a 12-lead ECG.

What Is a 12-Lead ECG?

Suppose you wanted to check out the condition of a used car you were thinking of buying. If you needed to know only whether the motor was running, you could stand anywhere near the car and listen (just as you can use any one lead to monitor the cardiac rhythm). But if you wanted to know what kind of shape the car body is in, you would have to walk around the car and look at it from all sides. The driver's side might be in mint condition, but if you stroll around to the passenger's side, you might see that the entire door frame is caved in from a road accident.

Similarly, each ECG lead looks at the heart from a different angle. Although one lead may see a normal myocardium, another may be looking at major damage.

What Do ECG Leads Record?

What does a lead "see" when it looks at the heart? The word *lead*, as it is used in electrocardiography, can be somewhat confusing. Sometimes the word is used to refer to one of the cables and monitoring electrodes that connect the ECG machine to the patient (such as the "right arm lead"). A lead provides an electrical picture of the heart taken from a specified vantage point. Lead I, for example, "looks" at the heart from the left, so it "sees" the left side of the heart. Lead aVF looks up at the heart from the feet (F stands for "foot"), so it "sees" the bottom of the heart. In the standard ECG, we record 12 leads—that is, 12 different pictures of the electrical activity of the heart.

Six of the leads—I, II, III, aVR, aVL, and aVF—are called limb leads because the pictures taken by those leads are derived from attaching cables to the patient's limbs. The limb leads look at the heart from the sides and from the feet, in the vertical plane. (**Figure 27-78** ▶) shows the viewpoint of each of the limb leads. For example, lead II has a direct view of the bottom of the heart (the inferior or diaphragmatic wall of the heart), whereas aVL (L stands for "left") looks at the heart from the vantage point of the left shoulder.

In addition to the limb leads, there are six precordial leads (V_1 to V_6), also called chest leads, anterior leads, or V leads. The six precordial leads are placed on the anterior and lateral chest walls, usually with adhesive electrodes, in the positions shown in (**Figure 27-79** ▶). These leads look at the heart in the horizontal plane (as shown in the inset to Figure 27-79), so they provide a picture of the heart taken from the front (anterior wall of the heart) and from the left side (anterolateral). More specifically, leads V_1 and V_2 look at the septum; V_3 and V_4 look at the anterior wall of the left ventricle; and V_5 and V_6 look at the lateral wall of the left ventricle.

12-Lead ECG Lead Placement

How reliable would 12-lead ECGs be if you could place the electrodes anywhere on the chest? When a 12-lead ECG is read, it is assumed that the person who performed the recording placed the electrodes correctly on the chest. Correct placement is important because the 12-lead ECGs are compared with previous ECGs. For the comparison to be reliable for identifying existing problems or highlighting the appearance of new problems (such as ST-segment elevation), the electrodes must be placed consistently. (**Table 27-15** ▶) outlines where the different leads look.

When a current is moving toward a lead, it creates a positive (upright) deflection on the ECG tracing of that lead. Thus,

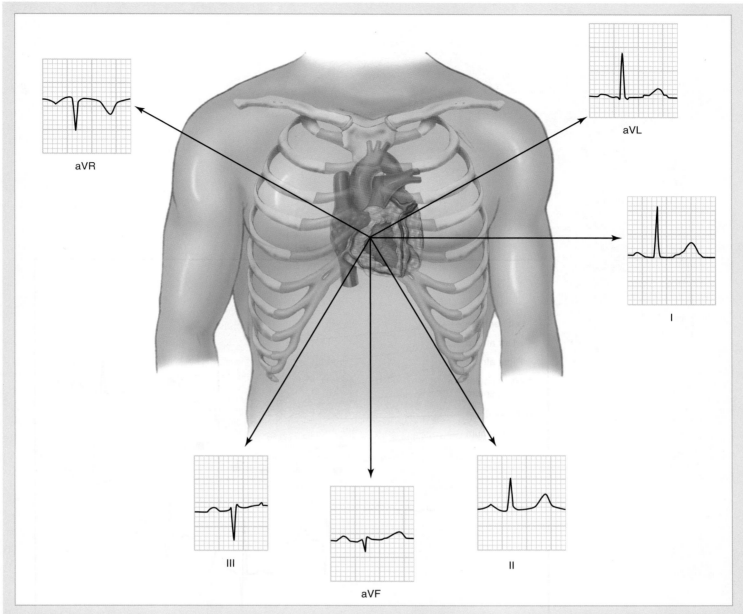

Figure 27-78 Limb leads look at the heart in the vertical plane. Leads II, III, and aVF give us a picture of the wall of the heart that rests on the diaphragm, the inferior wall.

in **Figure 27-80 ▸**, the current depolarising the ventricles is moving toward lead II, so what we see in lead II is an upright QRS complex (recall that the QRS complex is produced by depolarisation of the ventricles). If the depolarising current is moving toward lead II, then it must be moving away from lead aVR, so we would expect to see a negative deflection in aVR. And, indeed, the QRS complex in aVR is a downward deflection. That makes intuitive sense. If you and a friend are standing facing each other at opposite ends of a football pitch, a ball kicked toward your friend will look bigger and bigger to the friend as it approaches; the same ball will meanwhile look smaller and smaller to you as it travels the same course. Simi-

larly, leads II and aVR, being nearly opposite each other, will present nearly opposite pictures of the same wave of electrical depolarisation. If a depolarising wave is coming toward lead II, it will be going away from aVR.

 At the Scene

If the PQRST configuration is upright in lead aVR, the limb leads are on wrong! Specifically, the red and white leads have been switched.

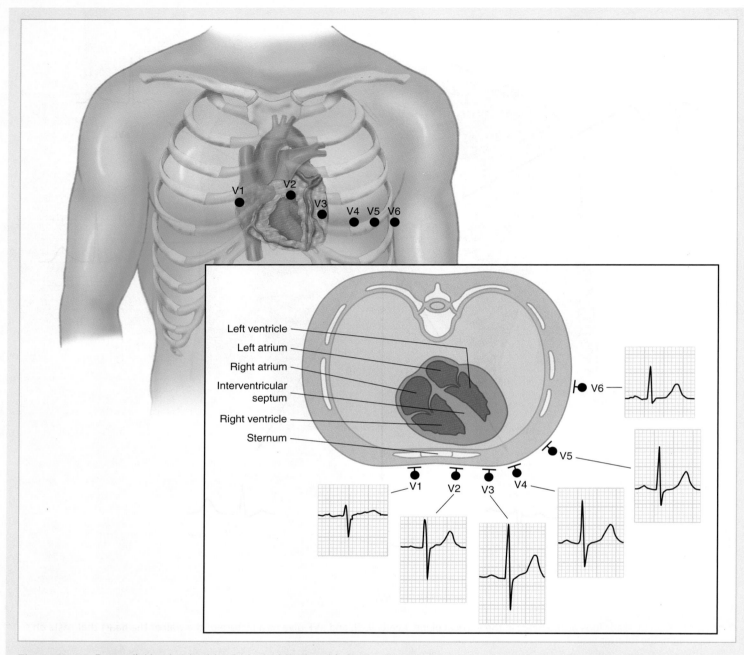

Figure 27-79 Precordial leads (chest leads) look at the heart in the horizontal plane. Inset: V_1 and V_2 look at the right ventricle. V_3 and V_4 "see" the interventricular septum. V_5 and V_6 see the anterior and lateral left ventricle.

Table 27-15	Focus of ECG Leads		
Leads	**Area of Damage**	**Coronary Artery Involved**	**Possible Complications**
II, III, and aVF	Inferior wall LV	RCA: posterior descending	Hypotension, LV dysfunction
V_1 and V_2	Septum	LCA: LAD, septal	Infranodal blocks and BBBs
V_3 and V_4	Anterior wall LV	LCA: LAD, diagonal	LV dysfunction, CHF, BBBs, complete heart block, PVCs
V_5, V_6, I, and aVL	Lateral wall LV	LCA: circumflex	LV dysfunction, AV nodal block in some
V_4R (II, III, aVF)	RV	RCA: proximal	Hypotension, supranodal and AV nodal blocks, atrial fibrillation, PACs

LV indicates left ventricle; LAD, left anterior descending; BBB, bundle branch block; RV, right ventricle; RCA, right coronary artery; LCA, left coronary artery; PAC, premature atrial contraction; PVC, premature ventricular contraction.

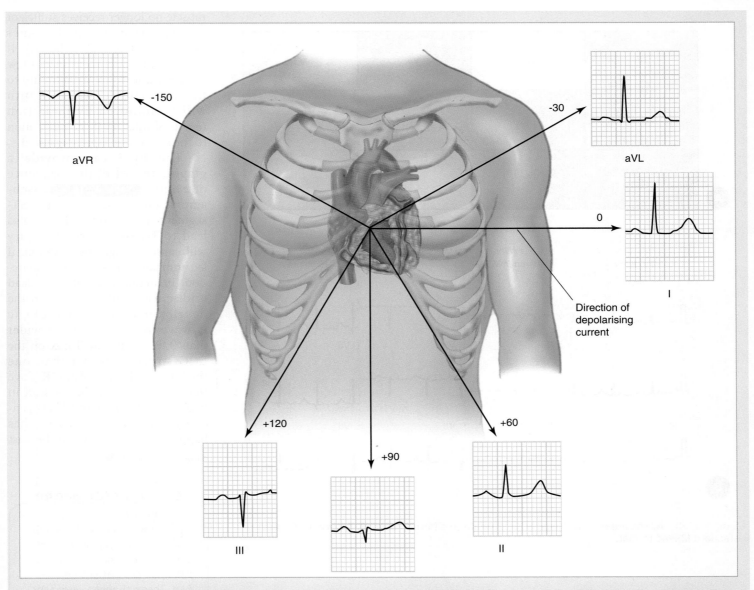

Figure 27-80 The morphology of QRS complexes varies based on the lead position and the direction of the electrical impulse movement within the heart. If the electrical impulses are moving primarily toward lead II, it will be upright as shown, while lead aVR will be inverted since the impulse is moving away from it.

The 12-Lead ECG in a Normal Heart

The gold standard for multilead ECGs is the 12-lead ECG. Cardiac catheterisation laboratories, especially electrophysiology catheterisation laboratories, may perform 15- or 18-lead ECGs! Any ECG that is recorded electronically always has the same layout on the paper, meaning that the leads will be plotted out in the same manner every time Figure 27-81 ▶

Each of the colours in Figure 27-82A ▶ has a purpose; that is, each colour represents the leads that look at a particular wall of the heart. Lead aVR is not used for this purpose, so no colour is assigned to it.

 Figure 27-82B ▶ depicts an ECG. (Some information has been added to help you out.) Notice that the specific wall of the left ventricle is listed along with the coronary artery that supplies that wall for each lead. The left ventricle is the

stronger and more muscular of the two ventricles; it will be the first to let its owner know that it is not getting enough oxygen. If the left ventricle becomes damaged, in addition to pain, the patient may develop deadly arrhythmias such as ventricular fibrillation. Each wall requires 2 to 4 leads or views to see its image completely. Those leads are anatomically contiguous—that is, the leads look at the same general area of the heart. When we are looking for evidence of injury to the heart and we must see it in 2 or more contiguous leads, then the following information will be important:

Contiguous Inferior Leads

- Lead II is contiguous with lead III.
- Lead III is contiguous with leads II and aVF.
- Lead aVF is contiguous with lead III.

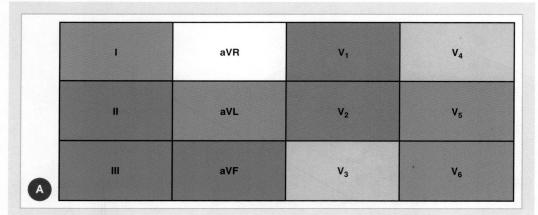

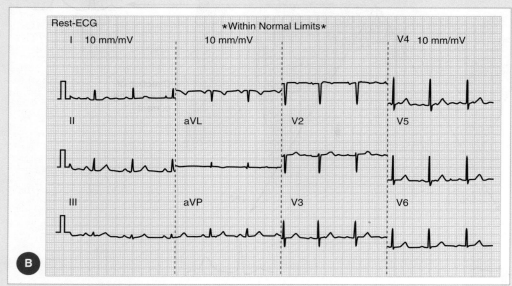

Figure 27-81 **A.** The areas on a 12-lead ECG correlate to different leads. **B.** A normal ECG with standard 12-lead format.

muscle no longer receives sufficient oxygen; that is, it becomes ischaemic (deprived of blood). If ischaemia persists more than a few minutes, it leads to actual injury to the heart muscle, which in turn will be followed by infarction (death of muscle) if the circulation to the area is not rapidly restored.

The ECG can provide a graphic record of that sequence of events (Table 27-16 ▶). Ischaemia commonly causes ST-segment depression and may also lead to T-wave inversion. Injury will cause ST-segment elevation; if left untreated, it will lead to infarction. Infarction (indicative of dead cardiac tissue) often results in the development of a pathologic Q wave. A Q wave that is wider than 0.04 s (one small box on the ECG strip) or deeper than one third of the height of the R wave that follows it and that is seen in two or more contiguous leads generally indicates an infarction has happened at some time in the past (Figure 27-83 ▶).

 At the Scene

When a doctor reads an ECG and sees pathological Q waves, he or she will usually ask when the patient had his AMI. These changes represent an evolved AMI of unknown age.

Contiguous Septal-Anterior-Lateral Leads

- V_1 is contiguous with V_2.
- V_2 is contiguous with V_1 and V_3.
- V_3 is contiguous with V_2 and V_4.
- V_4 is contiguous with V_3 and V_5.
- V_5 is contiguous with V_4 and V_6.
- V_6 is contiguous with V_5 and lead I.
- Lead I is contiguous with V_6 and aVL
- aVL is contiguous with lead I.

The 12-Lead ECG in a Damaged Heart

The ECG tells the practitioner many things about a patient's heart. For our purposes in the prehospital environment, we will keep it simple and look for any evidence that the patient is having an AMI. To do so, we must focus on three parts of the ECG: the ST segment, the Q wave, and the T wave.

Recall the sequence of events in an AMI. As the blood supply to the affected area of heart muscle slows to a trickle, the

In 40% of patients who experience an inferior wall AMI, a right ventricular AMI will eventually develop as well. To verify this, an electrode can be placed in the fifth intercostal space at the midclavicular line on the right side of the chest (V_4R). Unsnap the original V_4 on the left side of the chest and snap it onto the new lead on the right side, leaving all the other electrodes in place. Now press "acquire" on the 12-lead ECG monitor. If you see ST-segment elevation of greater than 1 mm in the V_4R lead on this second ECG, there is a high likelihood that you have identified a right ventricular AMI. Of course, the ECG monitor does not know that this V_4 is a right-sided one, so on printing this ECG tracing, you should add an "R" next to the "V_4", and circle the V_4R to make it stand out.

Patients who are experiencing an AMI of the right ventricle may already be hypotensive or may become extremely

Generally speaking, wide QRS complexes are presumed to be ventricular in origin, whereas narrow QRS complexes (< 0.12 s) are presumed to be supraventricular in origin. SVTs (narrow complex tachycardias) may originate in the SA node, elsewhere else in the atria, or in the AV node (junctional rhythms). The differentiation among these three pacemaker sites requires examining the P wave. In tachycardias with rates exceeding 150 beats/min, however, the P waves (if present) are usually "buried" within the T wave of the preceding beat. The inability to see P waves limits us to labelling these tachycardias as supraventricular rather than giving a specific site of origin.

Occasionally, aberrant conduction of a supraventricularly originated beat will make it difficult to identify a tachycardia as truly ventricular or supraventricular. In either case, you should administer oxygen and establish an IV line.

In SVTs (narrow complex tachycardias), you should attempt to stimulate the patient's vagus nerve. Many vagal stimulation techniques exist, including carotid sinus massage, but the most common is having the patient bear down against a closed glottis. The patient is instructed to perform this technique as if attempting to have a bowel movement. The stimulation of the vagal nerve in turn stimulates the parasympathetic nervous system to slow the heart. If this technique is successful, the patient should still be transported for hospital evaluation because the condition is likely to recur. If it reappears, instruct the patient to repeat the vagal manoeuvre.

If the patient is in stable condition but the rhythm is ventricular in origin, the patient should be transported to hospital while you watch carefully for the development of serious signs and symptoms.

Any patient with a tachycardic rhythm should be monitored carefully Figure 27-88 ▶ . A heart that is stressed by the requirements of excessive tachycardia is very likely to become ischaemic and is at high risk for arrest.

Techniques of Management in Cardiac Emergencies

This section profiles some of the devices and methods used in the treatment of patients with cardiac emergencies. Not all of the techniques or devices described are used in every ambulance service, and not all are required for certification as a paramedic. Direct your attention to the material that is relevant to your local practice.

Defibrillation

Defibrillation is the process by which a surge of electric energy is delivered to the heart. Recall that when the heart fibrillates, its individual muscle fibres get "out of synch" with one another and begin contracting individually. As a result, the heart as a whole ceases any useful movement. Indeed, if you were to look at a fib-

rillating heart, you would see movement resembling that of a bag of energetic worms. The idea behind defibrillation is to deliver a current to the heart that is powerful enough to depolarise all of its component muscle cells; ideally, when those cells repolarise after the shock, they will respond to an impulse from the SA node and begin organised depolarisation, leading to cardiac contraction.

Defibrillation needs to be carried out as soon as possible in VF or pulseless VT because the likelihood of its success declines rapidly with time. If the arrest is not witnessed and CPR is not in progress, immediately start CPR and continue for at least 2 minutes before delivering the first shock. If the patient's rhythm converts to VF or pulseless VT and the defibrillator is already attached, perform CPR only long enough to charge the defibrillator and then defibrillate. Defibrillation is *not* useful in asystole because there is no evidence that the myocardial cells are spontaneously depolarising. Defibrillation of asystole is unlikely to be beneficial and may be harmful. Thus, if you are unsure about asystole after checking more than one lead, resume CPR and follow the asystole pathway in the pulseless arrest algorithm until the next pulse and rhythm check.

Defibrillation Algorithm

To perform defibrillation, attach the adhesive defibrillation pads to the chest as instructed on the package. As with ECG electrode placement, you may have to dry the skin before placing the defibrillation pads. Once they are in place, turn the main power switch on. Set the energy level to 200 J (for biphasic defibrillation of unknown type), or follow the defibrillator manufacturer's recommendations regarding the appropriate energy level. Monophasic monitors should be charged to 360 J for the first and all successive shocks. Charge the defibrillator.

If using paddles instead of adhesive hands-free pads, it will be necessary to reduce the resistance of the patient's skin to passage of electric current by applying a conductive medium to the paddles; otherwise, the energy will be delivered largely to the skin itself, resulting in burns to the skin and ineffective energy delivery to the heart. Use electrode paste or saline gel pads to make good electric contact between the paddles and the skin. Apply about 12 kg of pressure to hold the paddles in contact with the chest.

Whichever method you choose—saline pads or electrode paste—take care to prevent contact (bridging) between the two conductive areas on the chest wall. If the saline or paste from one paddle comes into contact with that from the other paddle, the electric current will simply pass along the skin from one paddle to the other. Effective current will thus bypass the heart, causing superficial burns of the skin instead.

If there is a GTN patch on the patient's chest, remove it and wipe the skin dry before you apply the defibrillator paddles. Although GTN does not—contrary to popular legend—explode, the backing used on some GTN patches can support electrical arcing during defibrillation, producing smoke, noise, and burns to the patient.

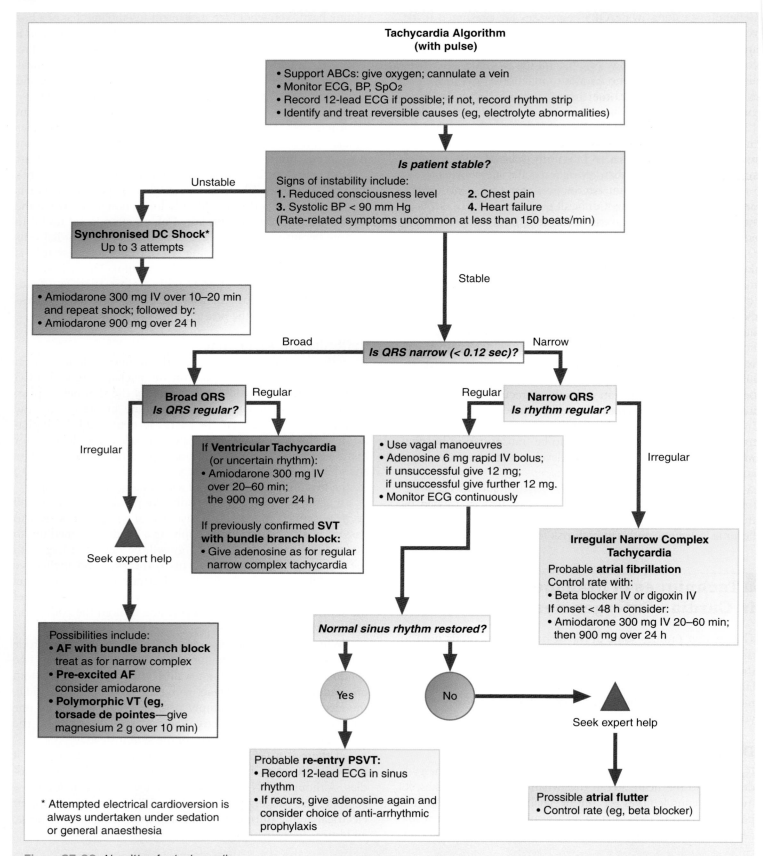

Figure 27-88 Algorithm for tachycardia.

Reproduced from *Tachycardia Algorithm.* © European Resuscitation Council.

Position the paddles so that the negative (sternum) paddle is just to the right of the upper part of the sternum below the right clavicle and the positive (apex) paddle is just below and to the left of the left nipple **Figure 27-89 ▾** . Exert firm pressure (10 to 12 kg) on each paddle to make good skin contact. Inadequate contact is another cause of burns and ineffective countershock.

When the defibrillator is charged, clear the area so that no one—including the operator—is in contact with the patient or stretcher. The operator should then announce, "Stand clear"! At this point, discharge the defibrillator by pressing the button on each handle simultaneously or pressing the button on the machine if using a hands-free system. If current has reached the patient, contraction of the chest and other muscles will be evident. If you do not see contraction, check the defibrillator to be certain the synchronising switch is off and the battery is charged.

Immediately after delivering the defibrillating current, resume CPR. Continue CPR for 2 minutes or 5 cycles, and then pause to check for a pulse and reevaluate the rhythm. If at any point you see an organised rhythm on the monitor, check for a pulse.

An implanted artificial pacemaker—which you may detect from the pacemaker-produced spikes on the ECG or the bulge where its battery pack has been implanted under the patient's skin—is *not* a contraindication to defibrillation. Just make certain that you do not place the electrode paddles or pads directly over the pacemaker battery. Should you mix up the apex and sternum pads, the defibrillation will start to work, but according to the manufacturer it is not as efficient.

The defibrillator should be inspected at the beginning of each shift, using a checklist to cover all aspects of the appara-tus and its gear. Inspection should include the paddles, cables and connectors, power supply, monitor, ECG recorder, and any ancillary supplies (such as electrode gel, pads, spare battery). Conscientious use of the checklist should significantly reduce the incidence of defibrillator accidents and failures.

The following list summarises the procedures for defibrillation:

1. Turn the main power on, and make sure the synchronise switch is off.
2. Set the energy level at 200 J (or the appropriate setting for your defibrillator).
3. Lubricate the paddles and position them on the chest, or place the hands-free pads on the chest.
4. Charge the paddles.
5. Clear the area.
6. Discharge the defibrillator.
7. Resume CPR, and recheck the rhythm in 2 minutes.

Automated External Defibrillator

The AED is a "smart" defibrillator that can—thanks to sophisticated computer chips—analyse the patient's ECG rhythm and determine whether a defibrillating shock is needed. AEDs may be fully automatic or semi-automatic. The fully automatic versions assess the patient's rhythm and—if VF is present—charge the paddles and deliver countershocks, without any intervention by the rescuer. By contrast, the semi-automatic AEDs require decisions by the rescuer. That is, the semi-automatic AED identifies the rhythm and then instructs the rescuer what to do about it. If, for example, the AED detects VF, a voice prompt may say, "Shock advised. Press to shock". The rescuer must then depress the shock button to defibrillate the patient. Thus the "A" in AED is *automated* and not *automatic*.

Whether the AED is fully automatic or semi-automatic, the basic sequence of steps for using an AED is the same:

1. Expose the patient's chest.
2. Attach the two self-adhesive electrode pads firmly to the patient's chest—the sternal pad at the junction of the right clavicle and upper border of the sternum; the apex pad along the left lower rib margin at the anterior axillary line.
3. Turn on the AED.
4. Stop CPR, and instruct everyone to stand clear of the patient.
5. The AED assesses the rhythm (for 6 s) and determines whether it is "shockable" (that is, whether the rhythm is one that will respond to defibrillation).
6. If the AED detects a shockable rhythm, it will instruct the rescuer to press the charge button, which takes 5 to 10 seconds.
7. Defibrillating shocks are then delivered by the rescuer pressing the shock button, after a visual safety check and loud verbal "stand clear" command.

New AEDs appear on the market all the time, and each model comes with its own operating manual. If you will be using an AED, train with the specific apparatus carried by your service, using the manufacturer's instructions for that machine.

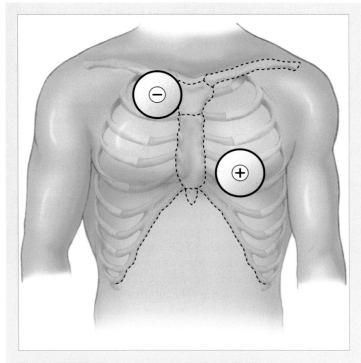

Figure 27-89 Position the paddles for defibrillation.

Cardioversion

Cardioversion is the use of the defibrillator to terminate arrhythmias other than VF. In cardioversion, unlike defibrillation, the current is synchronised with the ECG so that it will not be delivered during the vulnerable period (that is, on top of the T wave). Electrical cardioversion is performed just as defibrillation except that the synchronise setting on the defibrillator is selected first. When the defibrillator is "fired" in the synchronise mode, the machine monitors the R waves of the QRS complexes and delivers the shock at a time when the R-on-T phenomenon is least likely to occur. The R-on-T phenomenon occurs when the defibrillator fires at the top of the T wave and usually results in the rhythm changing to VF. Although this can happen with the synchroniser on, it is much less likely to occur when the shock is "synchronised".

Emergency cardioversion is indicated for rapid ventricular and supraventricular rhythms that are associated with severely compromised CO—such as rapid VT or SVT (narrow complex tachycardia).

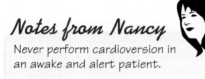

Notes from Nancy

Never perform cardioversion in an awake and alert patient.

When cardioversion is performed electively on a conscious patient, the patient *must* be sedated first; cardioversion is a painful and terrifying experience for an awake patient. Medications commonly used for sedation in these circumstances include benzodiazepines such as diazepam or midazolam.

The following is the procedure for cardioversion:

1. Turn the main power on, and then turn the synchronise switch on the machine to the on position (unlike for defibrillation).
2. Prepare and apply the pads or paddles as described for defibrillation.
3. Set the energy level. Energy levels required for cardioversion vary depending on the type of arrhythmia and the type of defibrillator. Supraventricular tachycardia, for example, can often be converted with energy levels as low as 100 J; by contrast, VT will usually require at least 100 J. In emergencies, if an initial attempt to convert a rapid rhythm with a low energy level fails, immediately turn the setting up (stepwise to 100, 200, 300, and then 360 J) and repeat the shock as needed.
4. Charge the paddles.
5. Clear the area by announcing, "Stand clear"!
6. Depress the shock buttons, and keep them depressed until the defibrillator discharges. That may take a few seconds because the charge is synchronised to fire about 10 ms after the peak of the R wave.
7. Reassess the patient's condition (ECG rhythm and pulse). Repeat the cardioversion if necessary.

8. If a cardioversion shock produces VF, immediately:
   - Recharge the defibrillator to the setting for defibrillation.
   - Turn the synchroniser circuit to the off position if it has not defaulted to that position.
   - Deliver the defibrillation.

Transcutaneous Cardiac Pacing

Artificial pacemakers deliver repetitive electric currents to the heart. Like the tiny electric currents generated by natural pacemakers, the current from an artificial pacemaker can cause the myocardial tissue to depolarise. In this way, the artificial pacemaker can substitute for a natural pacemaker that has become blocked or nonfunctional.

The artificial pacemakers first developed for emergency use consisted of a small battery pack and a wire that had to be threaded through a vein into the right ventricle of the heart. Insertion of one of those transvenous pacemakers was a tricky and often time-consuming job, usually best undertaken in a coronary care unit. Recently, however, effective transcutaneous pacemakers—that is, pacemakers that deliver their current through the skin of the chest—have been developed and have come into widespread use. Indeed, most prehospital monitor-defibrillators now come equipped with TCP capability.

In TCP, a small electrical charge is passed through the patient's skin across the heart between one externally placed pacing pad and another. The pacer is set for a specific rate, and the energy is increased until the heart just begins to respond to the stimulus. This phenomenon, which is termed "capture", is usually associated with depolarisation of the ventricles, which appears as a wide QRS complex on the ECG and results in a corresponding pulse.

TCP may have several useful applications in prehospital care:
- Interhospital transfer of patients needing pacemaker implantation (for example, a patient with complete heart block admitted to a small community hospital that does not have the facilities to implant a permanent pacemaker)
- Symptomatic patients with artificial pacemaker failure
- Patients with bradyarrhythmias or blocks associated with severely reduced CO and that are unresponsive to atropine, before cardiac arrest

In any of those circumstances, TCP may buy time for the patient and enable him or her to reach the hospital in a state of optimal perfusion rather than in or near cardiac arrest.

Many brands of transcutaneous external cardiac pacemakers are available, and you must become familiar with the particular pacemaker used in your local ambulance service. In general, the steps in initiating TCP are as follows:

1. Apply the pacing electrodes. Often the defibrillation position is used when the same pads can be used for defibrillation and pacing. The alternative is to place one pad anteriorly left of the lower sternum and the other pad posteriorly just below the left scapula.

2. Switch the pacer power on.

3. Set the pacing rate (60 to 80 beats/min is commonly chosen).

4. Start increasing the current. Raise the current by 10 to 20 milliamps every few seconds.

5. Check for capture; that is, look for every pacemaker spike being followed by a (usually wide) QRS complex **Figure 27-90 ▾** . If the QRS is not present, the pacemaker current is not depolarising the ventricles. Increase the current gradually until there is consistent capture.

6. Once capture is achieved, briefly lower the current until capture is lost, and then increase it by the smallest amount possible to restore capture. The purpose of this action is to find the lowest energy setting that achieves consistent capture.

7. Immediately transport the patient.

Transcutaneous pacemakers depolarise not only cardiac muscle, but also muscles in the chest wall beneath the pacing electrode. As a result, patients who are conscious when TCP is initiated (or who regain consciousness during pacing) usually experience chest discomfort and sometimes severe pain from the procedure. Some form of analgesia and sedation (such as diazepam or morphine) should be given to conscious patients when transcutaneous pacemakers are used.

Medications Commonly Prescribed to Patients With Cardiovascular Diseases

Patients with diseases affecting the cardiovascular system may be taking a wide variety of medications, including aspirin, for a variety of reasons, and it is not always possible to identify the patient's specific problem on the basis of a medication that he or she is taking. Beta blockers, for example, are prescribed for

relief of angina, to lower blood pressure in hypertension, and to prevent recurrence of AMI. Similarly, diuretic medications may be given simply to help rid the body of excess fluid in CHF or because of their effects in lowering blood pressure. Thus, one needs to look at any given medication the patient is taking in the context of the patient's clinical history and the other medications he or she is taking **Figure 27-91 ▸** .

Digitalis Preparations

Digitalis preparations are prescribed for the treatment of chronic CHF or for certain rapid atrial arrhythmias (such as rapid atrial flutter, atrial fibrillation, supraventricular arrhythmias). Digitalis acts by increasing the strength of cardiac contractions, thereby improving CO, and slowing conduction through the AV junction (such as in atrial fibrillation or flutter, allowing fewer impulses to be conducted through to the ventricles so the overall HR slows). In at least 30% of patients taking digitalis, some symptoms of toxic effects of the drug develop—for example, loss of appetite, nausea, vomiting, headache, blurred vision, yellow vision, or various cardiac arrhythmias. *Virtually any cardiac arrhythmia may be caused by the toxic effects of digitalis,* so it is important to ask all patients with disturbances in cardiac rhythm to determine whether they are taking digitalis.

Patients taking digitalis are very sensitive to calcium preparations. They are also highly sensitive to a decline in the serum potassium level, so caution must be exercised in giving agents that might reduce the body's potassium stores (such as diuretics or large quantities of sodium bicarbonate). Commonly used digitalis preparations include digoxin and digitoxin.

Anti-anginal Agents

Three major classes of drugs are used to relieve the pain of angina: nitrates, beta blockers, and calcium channel blockers. All of them work exclusively or primarily on the demand side of the oxygen supply-demand equation; that is, all of them diminish, in one way or another, myocardial oxygen demand.

Nitrates

Nitrates were the first drugs to be used for the relief of angina. The prototype of this group is GTN, which comes as rapid-acting sublingual tablets, sustained-release oral tablets, topically applied ointment, and skin patches **Table 27-20 ▸** . If a patient reports that he or she takes a medicine that is put under the tongue, that medicine is likely to be GTN.

GTN is thought to exert its therapeutic effect by decreasing the work of the heart. The heart's need for oxygen is, therefore, decreased, as is the anginal pain that results from insufficient

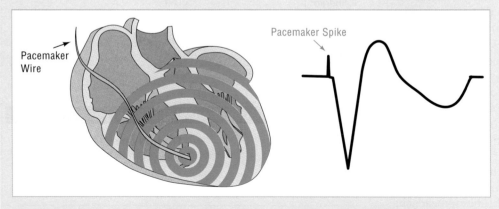

Figure 27-90 Pacemaker spike followed by QRS complex.

Pacemaker Wire

Pacemaker Spike

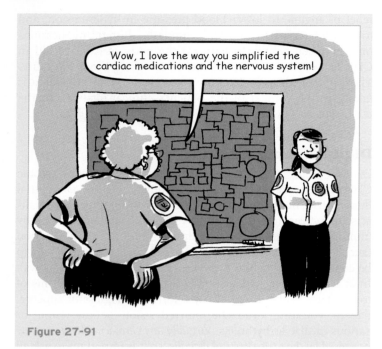

Figure 27-91

a burning sensation under the tongue; and a bitter taste. If the patient did not find the pill bitter or did not experience a headache when he or she took the GTN, chances are the drug was outdated or ineffective. If the patient experienced a throbbing headache but still got no relief from the chest pain, suspect that the patient is having an AMI.

Beta Blockers

Drugs that block beta sympathetic receptors are also prescribed for the relief of angina **Table 27-21 ▾**. They work by decreasing the rate and strength of cardiac contractions, thereby decreasing the heart's demand for oxygen. Taking beta-blocking drugs on a regular basis usually leads to resistance to the action of beta-stimulating agents, such as adrenaline. When such patients have a cardiac arrest, therefore, the administration of adrenaline during resuscitation attempts may not have the desired effect because the action of adrenaline may be blocked.

Calcium Channel Blockers

Calcium channel blockers, as their name implies, block the influx of calcium ions into cardiac muscle. These agents relieve angina in two ways: (1) by preventing spasm of the coronary arteries and (2) by weakening cardiac contraction, thereby decreasing myocardial oxygen demand. Hypotension may be a significant side effect. **Table 27-22 ▾** lists calcium channel blockers.

Table 27-20	Commonly Prescribed Nitrates
Generic Name	**Trade Name**
Glyceryl trinitrate	GTN, Nitromin, Glytrin Spray, Coro-Nitro Spray, Suscard
Isosorbide dinitrate	Isosorbide Dinitrate, Angitak
Isosorbide mononitrate	Isosorbide Mononitrate, Elantan

Table 27-21	Beta blockers
Generic Name	**Trade Name**
Acebutolol	Sectral
Atenolol	Tenormin
Bisoprolol	Cardicor
Carvedilol	Carvedilol
Esmolol	Brevibloc
Labetalol	Labetalol Hydrochloride, Trandate
Metoprolol	Lopressor, Betaloc
Nadolol	Corgard
Pindolol	Visken
Propranolol	Inderal
Sotalol	Sotalol, Sotacor, Beta-Cardone
Timolol	Betim

Table 27-22	Calcium Channel Blockers
Generic Name	**Trade Name**
Diltiazem	Diltiazem
Nifedipine	Adalat
Verapamil	Verapamil

oxygenation. GTN usually takes effect within 3 to 5 minutes of administration.

GTN also causes significant vasodilation. For that reason, it is sometimes used in the prehospital environment as an adjunctive therapy in the treatment of pulmonary oedema secondary to left-sided heart failure. Used in that circumstance, GTN produces an "internal phlebotomy"—that is, a pooling of blood within the venous vessels that reduces the blood volume in the pulmonary vasculature just as if blood had been physically withdrawn from the body (phlebotomy).

When a patient reports taking GTN for chest pain, you need to find out the answers to two questions: (1) How many GTN tablets did the patient take? (2) Did the GTN relieve the pain? Failure of GTN to relieve anginal pain can occur for one of two reasons—the pain is of extraordinary severity, such as that associated with an AMI, or the GTN has been open too long and is no longer effective. Fresh, potent GTN has certain distinct side effects, including a transient, throbbing headache;

Anti-arrhythmic Drugs

Anti-arrhythmic drugs are used to control chronic disturbances in cardiac rhythm. Thus, when you encounter a patient taking one of these agents, you know the patient has had significant arrhythmias in the past, which justifies particular surveillance for recurrent rhythm disturbances. Patients taking anti-arrhythmic drugs should be monitored while under your care.

Some of the drugs mentioned under other categories are also used for their anti-arrhythmic activity. Digitalis preparations, for example, are used to suppress atrial arrhythmias. Beta blockers are sometimes prescribed for their suppressive effect on myocardial excitability, as are some of the calcium channel blockers. Finally, the seizure medication, phenytoin sodium, is occasionally used for cardiac arrhythmias, particularly for arrhythmias due to the toxic effects of digitalis. **Table 27-23 ▸** lists commonly used anti-arrhythmic drugs.

Diuretics

Diuretics ("water tablets") are prescribed to patients with chronic fluid overload, principally patients with chronic CHF, but are also used as primary or adjunctive therapy in the treatment of hypertension. Diuretics trick the kidneys into excreting more sodium and water than usual (the desired effect). The kidneys also tend to dump out potassium along with the sodium (an undesired effect). Thus, patients taking diuretics often become depleted of potassium if they are not given potassium supplements. Patients in whom potassium deficits (hypokalaemia) develop are prone to cardiac arrhythmias—especially if they are also taking digitalis. **Table 27-24 ▸** lists commonly prescribed diuretics.

Anti-hypertensive Drugs

As the name implies, anti-hypertensive agents are used to treat hypertension (high blood pressure). Many of the diuretic agents already mentioned are also used as anti-hypertensives or in combination with anti-hypertensives for a synergistic effect. Similarly, beta blockers are used in the treatment of hypertension.

It is often difficult to regulate the dosage of anti-hypertensives so that the patient's blood pressure is lowered enough but not too much. As a consequence, some patients taking these agents may have symptoms of hypotension, including weakness and dizziness. Many will experience a feeling of giddiness with a change in position (such as when moving from a recumbent to a sitting or standing position); this phenomenon is termed orthostatic hypotension. Every patient taking anti-hypertensive drugs, therefore, should have his or her blood pressure checked in the recumbent and sitting positions to detect orthostatic hypotension. **Table 27-25 ▸** lists commonly prescribed anti-hypertensive agents.

Table 27-23 Commonly Used Anti-arrhythmic Drugs

Generic Name	Trade Name	Indications
Amiodarone	Cordarone	Ventricular tachycardia and other life-threatening ventricular arrhythmias
Digoxin	Lanoxin	Atrial flutter or fibrillation
Flecainide	Tambocor	Life-threatening ventricular arrhythmias
Mexiletine	Mexitil	Ventricular arrhythmias
Procainamide	Pronestyl	Ventricular arrhythmias
Verapamil	Cordilox, Securon	Ventricular tachycardias

Table 27-24 Commonly Prescribed Diuretics

Generic Name	Trade Name
Bumetanide	Bumex
Furosemide	Lasix
Hydralazine	Apresoline

Thiazides
  cyclothiazide
  chlorothiazide
  hydrochlorothiazide
  hydroflumethiazide
	Anhydron
	Diuril
	HydroDIURIL
	Saluron

Triamterene	Dytac

Table 27-25 Commonly Prescribed Anti-hypertensive Agents

Generic Name	Trade Name
Captopril	Capoten
Clonidine	Catapres
Enalapril	Innovace
Labetalol*	Trandate
Lisinopril	Zestril
Propranolol*	Inderal

*Beta blocker.

Anti-coagulant Drugs

Anti-coagulant drugs ("blood thinners") diminish the ability of the blood to clot. They are prescribed to patients who have had recurrent problems with blood clots (such as patients who have had pulmonary emboli) and to patients who might be prone to develop clots (such as some patients who have had an AMI in the past; patients with artificial heart valves or valvular heart disease; patients whose normal heart rhythm is atrial fibrillation). Patients who take anti-coagulants are apt to bleed excessively from minor trauma or even venepuncture, so you should be alert to that possibility. The principal oral anti-coagulant drug is warfarin. Patients undergoing home dialysis may be taking the IV anti-coagulant, heparin, during their dialysis cycle.

You are the Paramedic Summary

1. Which body system do you think is the primary cause of the patient's signs and symptoms?

Your first instinct might be to say the respiratory system as the patient is having breathing difficulties. However, there are a few clues that should make you look elsewhere. Difficulty breathing, lots of frothy sputum, and swollen ankles are a good sign that your patient may have congestive heart failure. It is the cardiovascular system that is the culprit this time.

2. What questions would you like to ask your patient at this time?

SAMPLE! SAMPLE! SAMPLE! Did we mention SAMPLE? Specific questions you need to ask in relation to the patient's history include asking about waking at night gasping for breath and breathlessness lying flat. See how many pillows your patient needs to sleep with at night. Don't forget to find out about previous episodes, especially those that resulted in hospital admission. Patients who have had previous AMIs or who are hypertensive are at increased risk.

3. Why does the patient wake at night gasping for breath?

The medical term for this is paroxysmal nocturnal dyspnoea (PND). It occurs because left ventricular filling pressures rise due to nocturnal fluid redistribution and enhanced renal reabsorption. Patients often describe waking suddenly feeling as if they were suffocating and it is associated with difficulty breathing, cough, and frothy sputum.

4. What types of medication is the patient taking? How does this help you with the patient's medical history?

The patient is taking aspirin (anti-platelet), ramipril (ACE inhibitor), furosemide (loop diuretic), bisoprolol (beta blocker), and digoxin (cardiac glycoside). The patient's medications can give clues about their past medical history. For example, ACE inhibitors, diuretics, and beta blockers are commonly used together to treat heart failure. Take time to recognise the names of commonly prescribed drugs and the conditions they are used to treat.

5. How do these two drugs help in acute pulmonary oedema?

In acute pulmonary oedema, there is a need to reduce both the amount of blood returning to the heart (preload) and the pressure that the heart has to overcome in order to pump blood around the arteries (afterload). The drug of choice for this is GTN, which lowers both preload and afterload with its potent vasodilatory action. The evidence base for the use of furosemide is not so good, but it is still in common use. It causes venodilation first and then diuresis later on, both of which decrease preload.

6. What rhythm do you expect to find on the ECG given the rhythm of the pulse and knowing that the patient is on digoxin?

As well as treating heart failure, digoxin is also commonly prescribed for patients who have atrial fibrillation (AF). However, you don't always need an ECG to work this out. Just by palpating the patient's pulse, you should be able to pick up the irregularly irregular rhythm that is AF.

7. Why did the doctor administer morphine? Should you have done this en route to hospital?

Morphine is another drug that is commonly used to treat heart failure, despite the fact that there is little evidence to support its use. It works by venodilation (reducing preload) and decreases anxiety. At present, paramedics in the UK are only allowed to administer morphine for pain relief, so it would not have been appropriate for you to have administered morphine to this patient en route to hospital.

8. How does administering positive airways pressure help the patient?

Continuous positive airways pressure (CPAP) provides a continuous level of positive pressure throughout the breathing cycle. This is useful in heart failure as it splints the alveoli open, which increases oxygen exchange. There is evidence that this intervention works well in the prehospital setting, especially in the treatment of acute left ventricular failure.

Prep Kit

■ Ready for Review

- Cardiovascular disease has been the number one killer in Europe almost every year since 1900.
- The cardiovascular system is composed of the heart and blood vessels. Its primary function is to deliver oxygenated blood and nutrients to every cell.
- Patients experience a variety of symptoms when they have a cardiovascular problem.
- Coronary artery disease is the most common form of heart disease and the leading cause of death in adults in Europe.
- Cardiac rhythm disturbances or arrhythmias may arise from a variety of causes—they are not solely caused by AMI.
- Most cardiac arrest victims have evidence of atherosclerosis or other underlying cardiac disease. However, cardiac arrest can also occur secondary to electrocution, submersion, and other types of trauma. Indeed, many cardiac arrest victims have no warning before the event occurs.
- A patient who presents with or develops symptomatic bradycardia needs to be treated in a manner that will increase the HR and improve CO.
- A patient who presents with or develops tachycardia presents a more complicated situation than one in bradycardia. Tachycardia can have a supraventricular pacemaker site or may be ventricular in origin. In addition, the patient may be mildly or severely symptomatic owing to the tachycardia or another condition. Because of the many possible variations in tachycardic patients, several judgements must be made before treatment is begun.
- Patients with diseases affecting the cardiovascular system may be taking a wide variety of medications for a variety of reasons, and it is not always possible to identify the patient's specific problem on the basis of a medication that he or she is taking.

■ Vital Vocabulary

aberrant conduction The abnormal conduction of the electrical impulse through the heart.

absolute refractory period The early phase of cardiac repolarisation, wherein the heart muscle cannot be stimulated to depolarise.

acetylcholine A chemical mediator of the parasympathetic nervous system.

acute coronary syndrome Term used to describe any group of clinical symptoms consistent with acute myocardial ischaemia.

acute myocardial infarction (AMI) A condition present when a period of cardiac ischaemia caused by sudden narrowing or complete occlusion of a coronary artery leads to death (necrosis) of myocardial tissue.

afterload The resistance against which the ventricle contracts.

agonal rhythm A cardiac arrhythmia seen just before the heart stops altogether; essentially asystole with occasional QRS complexes that are not associated with cardiac output.

aneurysm A sac or bulge resulting from the weakening of the wall of a blood vessel or ventricle.

angina pectoris The sudden pain from myocardial ischaemia, caused by diminished circulation to the cardiac muscle. The pain is usually substernal and often radiates to the arms, jaw, or abdomen and usually lasts 3 to 5 minutes and disappears with rest.

aorta The largest artery in the body, originating from the left ventricle.

aortic valve The valve between the left ventricle and the aorta.

arrhythmias Disturbances in cardiac rhythm.

arteries The muscular, thick-walled blood vessels that carry blood away from the heart.

arteriole A small blood vessel that carries oxygenated blood, branching into yet smaller vessels called capillaries.

arteriosclerosis A pathological condition in which the arterial walls become thickened and inelastic.

artifact An artificial product; in cardiology, is used to refer to noise or interference in an ECG tracing.

asystole The absence of ventricular contractions; a "straight-line ECG".

atrial kick The addition to ventricular volume contributed by contraction of the atria.

atropine A parasympathetic blocker; opposes the action of acetylcholine on the heart and elsewhere, thereby allowing the body's natural sympathetic system to speed up the heart rate.

atrioventricular (AV) node A specialised structure located in the AV junction that slows conduction through the AV junction.

atrioventricular (AV) valves The mitral and tricuspid valves.

atherosclerosis A common type of arteriosclerosis affecting the coronary and cerebral arteries.

autonomic nervous system A subdivision of the nervous system that controls primarily involuntary body functions. It comprises the sympathetic and parasympathetic nervous systems.

AV junction The atrioventricular junction; the portion of the electric conduction system of the heart located in the upper part of the interventricular septum that conducts the excitation impulse from the atria to the bundle of His.

automaticity Spontaneous initiation of depolarising electric impulses by pacemaker sites within the electric conduction system of the heart.

bigeminy An arrhythmia in which every other heartbeat is a premature contraction.

blood pressure The pressure exerted by the pulsatile flow of blood against the arterial walls.

bradycardia A slow heart rate, less than 60 beats/min.

bronchoconstriction Narrowing of the bronchial tubes.

bronchodilation Widening of the bronchial tubes.

bundle of His The portion of the electric conduction system in the interventricular septum that conducts the depolarising impulse from the atrioventricular junction to the right and left bundle branches.

bundle branch block A disturbance in electric conduction through the right or left bundle branch from the bundle of His.

capillaries Extremely narrow blood vessels composed of a single layer of cells through which oxygen and nutrients pass to the tissues. Capillaries form a network between arterioles and venules.

cardiac cycle The period from one cardiac contraction to the next. Each cardiac cycle consists of ventricular contraction (systole) and relaxation (diastole).

cardiac output (CO) Amount of blood pumped by the heart per minute, calculated by multiplying the stroke volume by the heart rate per minute.

cardiopulmonary arrest The sudden and often unexpected cessation of adequate cardiac output.

cardiac tamponade Restriction of cardiac contraction, failing cardiac output, and shock, caused by the accumulation of fluid or blood in the pericardium.

cardioversion The use of a synchronised direct current (DC) electric shock to convert tachyarrhythmias (such as atrial flutter) to normal sinus rhythm.

chordae tendineae Fibrous strands shaped like umbrella stays that attach the free edges of the leaflets, or cusps, of the atrioventricular valves to the papillary muscles.

chronotropic effect The effect on the rate of contraction of the heart.

circumflex coronary artery One of the two branches of the left main coronary artery.

Prep Kit

collateral circulation The mesh of arteries and capillaries that furnishes blood to a segment of tissue whose original arterial supply has been obstructed.

contractility The strength of heart muscle contractions.

coronary arteries The blood vessels of the heart that supply blood to its walls.

coronary artery disease (CAD) A pathological process caused by atherosclerosis that leads to progressive narrowing and eventual obstruction of the coronary arteries.

coronary sinus A large vessel in the posterior part of the coronary sulcus into which the coronary veins empty.

coronary sulcus The groove along the exterior surface of the heart that separates the atria from the ventricles.

couplet Two premature ventricular contractions occurring sequentially.

defibrillation The use of an unsynchronised direct current (DC) electric shock to terminate ventricular fibrillation.

delta wave The slurring of the upstroke of the first part of the QRS complex that occurs in Wolff-Parkinson-White syndrome.

depolarisation The process of discharging resting cardiac muscle fibres by an electric impulse that causes them to contract.

diastole The period of ventricular relaxation during which the ventricles fill passively with blood.

digitalis preparations The drugs used in the treatment of congestive heart failure and certain atrial arrhythmias.

dissection In references to blood vessels, an aneurysm, or bulge, formed by the separation of the layers of an arterial wall.

dromotropic effect The effect on the velocity of conduction.

electrical conduction system In the heart, the specialised cardiac tissue that initiates and conducts electric impulses. The system includes the SA node, internodal atrial conduction pathways, atrioventricular junction, atrioventricular node, bundle of His, and the Purkinje network.

endocardium The thin membrane lining the inside of the heart.

epicardium The thin membrane lining the outside of the heart.

first-degree heart block A partial disruption of the conduction of the depolarising impulse from the atria to the ventricles, causing prolongation of the P-R interval.

heart rate (HR) The number of heart contractions per minute.

hyperkalaemia An excessive amount of potassium in the blood.

hypertension High blood pressure, usually a diastolic pressure greater than 90 mm Hg.

hypokalaemia An abnormally low concentration of potassium in the blood.

hypocalcaemia A low level of calcium in the blood.

infarction Death (necrosis) of a localised area of tissue caused by the cutting off of its blood supply.

internodal pathways The three pathways of the electrical conduction system found in the atria that transmit the impulse from the SA node to the AV node.

interventricular septum A thick wall that separates the right and left ventricles.

ischaemia Tissue anoxia from diminished blood flow to tissue, usually caused by narrowing or occlusion of the artery.

isoelectric line The baseline of the ECG.

junctional rhythm An arrhythmia arising from ectopic foci in the area of the atrioventricular junction; often shows an absence of the P wave, a short P-R interval, or a P wave appearing after the QRS complex.

lead Any one of the conductors, composed of two or more electrodes, in the ECG that shows the electrical conduction in the heart.

left atrium The upper left chamber of the heart; receives blood from the pulmonary veins.

left ventricle The thick-walled, muscular, lower left chamber of the heart; receives blood from the left atrium and pumps it out through the aorta into the systemic arteries.

limb leads The ECG leads attached to the limbs and that form the hexaxial system, dividing the heart along a coronal plane into the anterior and posterior segments.

lumen The inside diameter of an artery or other hollow structure.

mitral valve The valve located between the left atrium and the left ventricle of the heart.

monomorphic Having one common shape of QRS complex.

multifocal Arising from or pertaining to many foci or locations.

myocardium The cardiac muscle.

necrosis The death of tissue, usually caused by a cessation of its blood supply.

noradrenaline A neurotransmitter and drug sometimes used in the treatment of shock; produces vasoconstriction through its alpha stimulator properties.

normal sinus rhythm The normal rhythm of the heart, wherein the excitation impulse arises in the SA node, travels through the internodal pathways to the atrioventricular junction, down the bundle of His, through the bundle branches, and into the Purkinje network without interference.

orthopnoea Severe dyspnoea experienced when lying down and relieved by sitting up.

orthostatic hypotension A fall in blood pressure when changing to an erect position.

P wave The first wave of the ECG complex, representing depolarisation of the ventricles.

pacemaker The specialised tissue within the heart that initiates excitation impulses; an electronic device used to stimulate cardiac contraction when the electric conduction system of the heart is malfunctioning, especially in complete heart block. An electronic pacemaker consists of a battery-powered pulse generator and a wire that transmits the electric impulse to the ventricles.

palpitations A sensation felt under the left breast of the heart "skipping a beat", usually caused by a premature ventricular contraction.

papillary muscles Protrusions of the myocardium into the ventricular cavities to which the chordae tendineae are attached.

parasympathetic nervous system A subdivision of the autonomic nervous system that is involved in control of involuntary, vegetative functions, mediated largely by the vagus nerve through the chemical acetylcholine.

paroxysmal nocturnal dyspnoea (PND) Severe shortness of breath occurring at night after several hours of recumbency, during which fluid pools in the lungs; the person is forced to sit up to breathe. PND is caused by left heart failure or decompensation of chronic obstructive pulmonary disease.

pericardium The double-layered sac containing the heart and the origins of the superior vena cava, inferior vena cava, and pulmonary artery.

phlebitis Inflammation of the wall of a vein, sometimes caused by an IV line, manifested by tenderness, redness, and slight oedema along part of the length of the vein.

phlebotomy The withdrawal of blood from a vein.

plaque In cardiology, the white to yellow lesion found in atherosclerosis that is made up of lipids, cell debris, and smooth muscles cells; in older people, may also include calcium.

plasmin A naturally occurring clot-dissolving enzyme, usually present in the body in its inactive form, plasminogen.

point of maximal impulse (PMI) The palpable beat of the apex of the heart against the chest wall during ventricular contraction; normally palpated in the fifth left intercostal space in the midclavicular line.

precordial leads Another term used to describe the chest leads in an ECG.

preload The pressure under which the ventricle fills.

pulmonary artery One of two arteries that carry deoxygenated blood from the right ventricle to the lungs.

pulmonary circulation The flow of blood from the right ventricle through the pulmonary arteries and all of their branches and capillaries in the lungs and back to the left atrium through the venules and pulmonary veins; also called the lesser circulation.

pulmonary oedema Congestion of the pulmonary air spaces with exudate and foam, often secondary to left heart failure.

pulmonary veins The vessels that carry oxygenated blood from the lungs to the left atrium.

pulmonic valve The valve between the right ventricle and the pulmonary artery.

pulsus paradoxus A weakening or loss of a palpable pulse during inhalation, characteristic of cardiac tamponade and severe asthma.

Purkinje fibres A system of fibres in the ventricles that conducts the excitation impulse from the bundle branches to the myocardium.

P-R interval The period between the beginning of the P wave (atrial depolarisation) and the onset of the QRS complex (ventricular depolarisation), signifying the time required for atrial depolarisation and passage of the excitation impulse through the atrioventricular junction.

QRS complex Deflections of the ECG produced by ventricular depolarisation.

R-R interval The period between the onset of one QRS complex and the onset of the next QRS complex.

recanalisation The opening up of new channels through a blocked artery.

receptors Specialised areas in tissues that initiate certain actions after specific stimulation.

refractory period A short period immediately after depolarisation in which the myocytes are not yet repolarised and are unable to fire or conduct an impulse.

relative refractory period That period in the cell-firing cycle at which it is possible but difficult to restimulate the cell to fire another impulse.

reperfusion The resumption of blood flow through an artery.

retrosternal Situated or occurring behind the sternum.

right atrium The upper right chamber of the heart; receives blood from the venae cavae and supplies blood to the right ventricle.

right ventricle The lower right chamber of the heart; receives blood from the right atrium and pumps blood out through the pulmonic valve into the pulmonary artery.

ST segment The interval between the end of the QRS complex and the beginning of the T wave; often elevated or depressed with respect to the isoelectric line when there is significant myocardial ischaemia.

semilunar valves The two valves, the aortic and pulmonic, that divide the heart from the aorta and pulmonary arteries.

sinoatrial (SA) node The dominant pacemaker of the heart, located at the junction of the superior vena cava and the right atrium.

sinus arrhythmia A slight irregularity of the heart rate caused by changes in parasympathetic tone during breathing.

sinus bradycardia A sinus rhythm with a heart rate less than 60 beats/min.

sinus tachycardia A sinus rhythm with a heart rate greater than 100 beats/min.

stable angina Angina pectoris characterised by periodic pain with a predictable pattern.

stroke volume (SV) The volume of blood pumped forward with each ventricular contraction.

sympathetic nervous system A subdivision of the autonomic nervous system that governs the body's fight-or-flight reactions, stimulating cardiac activity.

syncope Fainting; brief loss of consciousness caused by transiently inadequate blood flow to the brain.

systemic circulation The flow of blood from the left ventricle through the aorta, to all of its branches and capillaries in the tissues, and back to the right atrium through the venules, veins, and venae cavae; also called the greater circulation.

systole The period during which the ventricles contract.

T waves The upright, flat, or inverted wave following the QRS complex of the ECG, representing ventricular repolarisation.

tachycardia A rapid heart rate, more than 100 beats/min.

thrombolytic therapy The therapy that uses medications that act to dissolve blood clots.

tricuspid valve The valve between the right atrium and right ventricle of the heart.

trigeminy A premature complex in every third heartbeat.

tunica adventitia The outer layer of tissue of a blood vessel wall, composed of elastic and fibrous connective tissue.

tunica intima The smooth, thin, inner lining of a blood vessel.

tunica media The middle and thickest layer of tissue of a blood vessel wall, composed of elastic tissue and smooth muscle cells that allow the vessel to expand or contract in response to changes in blood pressure and tissue demand.

U wave A small flat wave sometimes seen after the T wave and before the next P wave.

unifocal Arising from a single site.

unstable angina Angina pectoris characterised by a changing, unpredictable pattern of pain, which may signal an impending acute myocardial infarction.

vagus nerve The 10th cranial nerve, the chief mediator of the parasympathetic nervous system.

Valsalva manoeuvre Forced exhalation against a closed glottis, the effect of which is to stimulate the vagus nerve and, thereby, slow the heart rate.

vasoconstriction Narrowing of the diameter of a blood vessel.

vasodilation Widening of the diameter of a blood vessel.

veins The blood vessels that carry blood to the heart (except pulmonary).

vena cavae The largest veins of the body; they return blood to the right atrium.

venules Very small veins.

Wolff-Parkinson-White (WPW) syndrome A syndrome characterised by short P-R intervals, delta waves, nonspecific ST-T wave changes, and paroxysmal episodes of tachycardia caused by the presence of an accessory pathway.

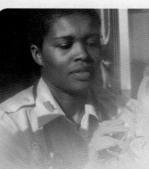

Assessment in Action

You are dispatched to the home of an 88-year-old man who is complaining of shortness of breath. When you arrive on scene, you find the patient in severe respiratory distress, speaking in two- to three-word sentences. He is grossly perspiring and complains of chest tightness. The patient tells you that he has no medical problems and does not take any medications. His vital signs are as follows: respiratory rate, 42 breaths/min with a room air pulse oximetry of 88%; blood pressure, 220/110 mm Hg; heart rate, 130 beats/min. The ECG monitor shows rapid atrial fibrillation.

1. **What differential diagnosis can you make?**
   A. Angina
   B. Angina pectoris
   C. Congestive heart failure
   D. Acute myocardial infarction

2. **Cardiac output is:**
   A. the amount of blood that is pumped out by either ventricle, measured in litres per minute.
   B. the pressure exerted by the blood against the arterial walls.
   C. the contribution to ventricular filling made by contraction of the atrium.
   D. one complete phase of atrial and ventricular relaxation.

3. **What is the most common form of heart disease and is the number one killer of men and women?**
   A. Angina
   B. Pulmonary oedema
   C. Myocardial infarction
   D. Coronary artery disease

4. **What is the principal symptom of CAD?**
   A. Pulmonary oedema
   B. Myocardial infarction
   C. Angina pectoris
   D. Unstable myocardium

5. **The term that describes when a portion of the cardiac muscle is deprived of coronary blood flow long enough that the muscle dies is:**
   A. unstable angina.
   B. stable angina.
   C. CAD.
   D. acute myocardial infarction.

6. **The mnemonic _____ is used to help remember the supportive treatments of a patient with acute coronary syndrome.**
   A. MONA
   B. MEMA
   C. NOMO
   D. OANE

7. **The most immediate methods of reperfusion for an AMI are:**
   A. GTN and oxygen.
   B. thrombolytic therapy and percutaneous intervention.
   C. thrombolytic therapy and intravenous therapy.
   D. percutaneous intervention alone.

8. **What term describes the situation when the heart is so severely damaged that it can no longer pump a volume of blood sufficient to maintain tissue perfusion?**
   A. Acute myocardial infarction
   B. Cardiogenic shock
   C. Unstable angina
   D. Pulmonary oedema or congestive heart failure

9. **Given the patient's age, are there any special considerations that you should keep in mind?**

Points to Ponder

You are dispatched to a care home for a 78-year-old woman who is feeling weak, dizzy, and nauseous. When you arrive, you find the patient resting comfortably. She tells you that while she was trying to open her bowels, she suddenly became very dizzy. There was no perspiration or shortness of breath. Her vital signs are as follows: respiratory rate, 18 breaths/min with a room air pulse oximetry reading of 97%; blood pressure, 90/58 mm Hg; pulse rate, 40 beats/min. When you apply the ECG to monitor her pulse rate, you notice a third-degree block. The patient's medical history includes hypertension, congestive heart failure, and renal failure secondary to type 1 diabetes. Her medications consist of metoprolol, furosemide, potassium, digoxin, and insulin. She tells you that she has taken all of her medicines this morning as prescribed.

What steps should you take to manage this patient's condition?

Issues: Understanding the Importance of a Complete Physical Examination, Understanding the Importance of ECG Rhythm Analysis.

Objectives

Cognitive

- Describe the incidence, morbidity and mortality of neurological emergencies.
- Identify the risk factors pertaining to the nervous system.
- Discuss the anatomy and physiology of the organs and structures related to the nervous system.
- Discuss the pathophysiology of non-traumatic neurological emergencies.
- Discuss the assessment findings associated with non-traumatic neurological emergencies.
- Identify the need for rapid intervention and the transport of the patient with non-traumatic emergencies.
- Discuss the management of non-traumatic neurological emergencies.
- Discuss the pathophysiology of coma and altered mental status.
- Discuss the assessment findings associated with coma and altered mental status.
- Discuss the management/treatment plan of coma and altered mental status.
- Describe the epidemiology, including the morbidity/mortality and prevention strategies, for convulsions.
- Discuss the pathophysiology of convulsions.
- Discuss the assessment findings associated with convulsions.
- Define convulsion.
- Describe and differentiate the major types of convulsions.
- List the most common causes of convulsions.
- Describe the phases of a generalised convulsion.
- Discuss the pathophysiology of syncope.
- Discuss the assessment findings associated with syncope.
- Discuss the management/treatment plan of syncope.
- Discuss the pathophysiology of headache.
- Discuss the assessment findings associated with headache.
- Discuss the management/treatment plan of headache.
- Describe the epidemiology, including the morbidity/mortality and prevention strategies, for neoplasms.
- Discuss the pathophysiology of neoplasms.
- Describe the types of neoplasms.
- Discuss the assessment findings associated with neoplasms.
- Discuss the management/treatment plan of neoplasms.
- Define neoplasms.
- Recognise the signs and symptoms related to neoplasms.
- Correlate abnormal assessment findings with clinical significance in the patient with neoplasms.
- Differentiate among the various treatment and pharmacological interventions used in the management of neoplasms.
- Integrate the pathophysiological principles and the assessment findings to formulate a working diagnosis and implement a treatment plan for the patient with neoplasms.
- Describe the epidemiology, including the morbidity/mortality and prevention strategies, for abscess.
- Discuss the pathophysiology of abscess.
- Discuss the assessment findings associated with abscess.
- Discuss the management/treatment plan of abscess.
- Define abscess.

- Recognise the signs and symptoms related to abscess.
- Correlate abnormal assessment findings with clinical significance in the patient with abscess.
- Differentiate among the various treatment and pharmacological interventions used in the management of abscess.
- Integrate the pathophysiological principles and the assessment findings to formulate a working diagnosis and implement a treatment plan for the patient with abscess.
- Describe the epidemiology, including the morbidity/mortality and prevention strategies, for stroke and intracranial haemorrhage.
- Discuss the pathophysiology of stroke and intracranial haemorrhage.
- Describe the types of stroke and intracranial haemorrhage.
- Discuss the assessment findings associated with stroke and intracranial haemorrhage.
- Discuss the management/treatment plan of stroke and intracranial haemorrhage.
- Define stroke and intracranial haemorrhage.
- Recognise the signs and symptoms related to stroke and intracranial haemorrhage.
- Correlate abnormal assessment findings with clinical significance in the patient with stroke and intracranial haemorrhage.
- Differentiate among the various treatment and pharmacological interventions used in the management of stroke and intracranial haemorrhage.
- Integrate the pathophysiological principles and the assessment findings to formulate a working diagnosis and implement a treatment plan for the patient with stroke and intracranial haemorrhage.
- Describe the epidemiology, including the morbidity/mortality and prevention strategies, for transient ischaemic attack.
- Discuss the pathophysiology of transient ischaemic attack.
- Discuss the assessment findings associated with transient ischaemic attack.
- Discuss the management/treatment plan of transient ischaemic attack.
- Define transient ischaemic attack.
- Recognise the signs and symptoms related to transient ischaemic attack.
- Correlate abnormal assessment findings with clinical significance in the patient with transient ischaemic attack.
- Differentiate among the various treatment and pharmacological interventions used in the management of transient ischaemic attack.
- Integrate the pathophysiological principles and the assessment findings to formulate a working diagnosis and implement a treatment plan for the patient with transient ischaemic attack.
- Describe the epidemiology, including the morbidity/mortality and prevention strategies, for degenerative neurological diseases.
- Discuss the pathophysiology of degenerative neurological diseases.
- Discuss the assessment findings associated with degenerative neurological diseases.
- Discuss the management/treatment plan of degenerative neurological diseases.

- Define the following:
  - Muscular dystrophy
  - Multiple sclerosis
  - Dystonia
  - Parkinson's disease
  - Trigeminal neuralgia
  - Bell's palsy
  - Amyotrophic lateral sclerosis
  - Peripheral neuropathy
  - Myoclonus
  - Spina bifida
  - Poliomyelitis
- Recognise the signs and symptoms related to degenerative neurological diseases.
- Correlate abnormal assessment findings with clinical significance in the patient with degenerative neurological diseases.
- Differentiate among the various treatment and pharmacological interventions used in the management of degenerative neurological diseases.
- Integrate the pathophysiological principles and the assessment findings to formulate a working diagnosis and implement a treatment plan for the patient with degenerative neurological diseases.
- Integrate the pathophysiological principles of the patient with a neurological emergency.
- Differentiate between neurological emergencies based on assessment findings.
- Correlate abnormal assessment findings with the clinical significance in the patient with neurological complaints.
- Develop a patient management plan based on working diagnosis in the patient with neurological emergencies.

Affective

- Characterise the feelings of a patient who regains consciousness amongst strangers.
- Formulate means of conveying empathy to patients whose ability to communicate is limited by their condition.

Psychomotor

- Perform an appropriate assessment of a patient with coma or altered mental status.
- Perform a complete neurological examination as part of the comprehensive physical examination of a patient with coma or altered mental status.
- Appropriately manage a patient with coma or altered mental status, including the administration of oxygen, oral glucose, glucose 10%, and narcotic reversal agents.
- Perform an appropriate assessment of a patient with syncope.
- Appropriately manage a patient with syncope.
- Perform an appropriate assessment of a patient with convulsions.
- Appropriately manage a patient with convulsions, including the administration of diazepam or lorazepam.
- Perform an appropriate assessment of a patient with stroke and intracranial haemorrhage or TIA.
- Appropriately manage a patient with stroke and intracranial haemorrhage or TIA.
- Demonstrate an appropriate assessment of a patient with a chief complaint of weakness.

Introduction

Many paramedics love the challenge of trauma and the excitement of dealing with its sudden nature. Trauma injuries can be graphic and attract your attention easily. By contrast, the medical patient is an entirely different animal. These patients require a keen eye, sharp assessment skills, and—above all—critical thinking to determine the nature of the problem. Medical patients can be very challenging as they often have complaints that are not apparent.

Neurological patients can be extremely vulnerable or even helpless. Many of the reflexes that protect an awake person may not function when the nervous system is depressed. The eyelids don't blink away dust and irritants. The larynx doesn't gag and cough in reaction to secretions oozing down the airway. The body doesn't seek a more comfortable position in response to compression of a limb in an awkward position. The tongue goes slack. The airway is at risk.

In this chapter, the anatomy and physiology of the nervous system are reviewed first. Then the general pathology of neurological conditions is explored, laying the proper foundation for discussion of their assessment and treatment.

Anatomy and Physiology

The nervous system is the most complex organ system within the human body. It consists of two major structures, the brain and spinal cord, plus thousands of nerves that allow every part of the body to communicate. This system is responsible for fundamental functions such as controlling breathing, heart rate, and blood pressure. But the real beauty of the nervous system is found in its higher level activity. Reading a good book (like this one), enjoying music, having a discussion with a friend, and even watching television requires the brain to engage memory, understanding, and thought. Here is where the true complexity of this system can be seen.

Figure 28-1 ▶ shows the basic structure of the nervous system. The major structures are divided into two main categories: the central nervous system (CNS), which is responsible for thought, perception, feeling, and autonomic body functions; and the peripheral nervous system (PNS), which transmits commands from the brain to the body and receives feedback from the body.

Consider the case of Justin—a child riding a bicycle. This common and seemingly simple activity is rich with both conscious and unconscious functions. It's a beautiful summer morning, so Justin goes to the garage to get his bike. Already the brain is hard at work. As Justin enters the garage, the brain must determine which object is a bike. Justin scans the garage. The images produced by his eyes are transmitted via the optic nerve to the occipital lobe of the brain Figure 28-2 ▶ . There the image, which is transmitted upside down, is reorientated. The occipital lobe then pores through tens of thousands of stored images. Has this image been seen before?

Once the image is recognised, an existing pathway is accessed to the temporal lobe, where language and speech are stored. Now, as Justin walks through the garage, he is able to put names to what he sees—a car, a workbench, a bike. When Justin was learning to speak, he often became confused about the names of objects. As he practised, he received reinforcement for the correct names and redirection for the incorrect names. In his brain, more pathways were established between the image of an object with two wheels, a seat, and pedals, which was stored in the occipital lobe, and the word for that object (bike), which was stored in the temporal lobe.

As Justin retrieves his helmet, the frontal lobe of his brain springs into action. The frontal lobe, which controls voluntary motion, sends signals out of the CNS along efferent nerves to the arms, shoulders, chest, and hands to perform

You are the Paramedic Part 1

You are dispatched to 16 Courage Court for an elderly man who has fallen. You arrive to find Mr Harris, an 81-year-old man, lying on the floor. His two sons explain that they visited their father last night and left around 19:00 hrs. When they returned this morning, they found the patient lying on the floor next to the chair in which he was sitting when they last saw him. He has been unable to explain what happened and, because he lives alone, no one is sure how long he's been on the floor.

The patient is awake and responding to his sons, but they say he is "not acting right". They describe him as "very sharp", but today he keeps getting their names confused. They say this only happens when his blood glucose level is low. The patient has type 2 diabetes.

Initial Assessment	Recording Time: 0 Minutes
Appearance	Lying on the floor, appears clean
Level of consciousness	V (Responsive to verbal stimuli), orientated to person and place, but not day
Airway	Patent
Breathing	Non-laboured
Circulation	Strong radial pulse

1. What do you suspect as the reason(s) why Mr Harris is on the floor?
2. How would you prioritise those reasons?

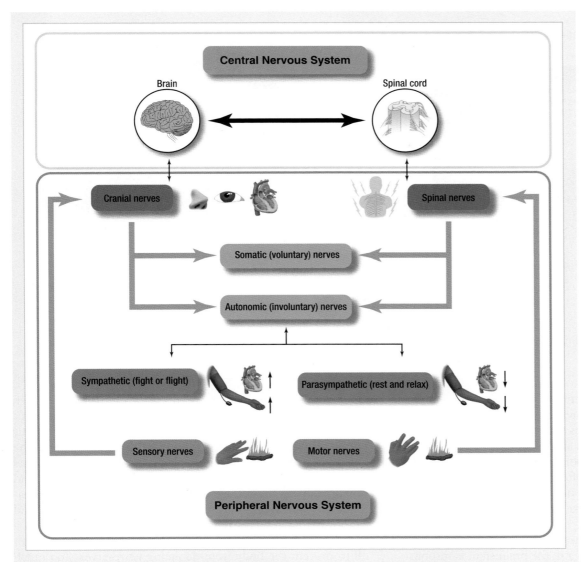

Figure 28-1 Organisation of the nervous system.

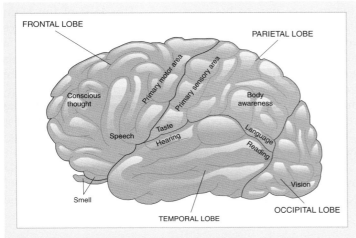

Figure 28-2 Lobes of the brain.

the task of picking up the helmet. The efferent nerves leave the brain through the PNS and convey commands to other parts of the body.

Which way should the helmet be applied? This motor memory is stored in the frontal lobe; the brain stores memories in the areas that are initially stimulated. As he places the helmet on his head, Justin needs to make fine adjustments to its position. His brain is receiving impulses from nerves within the skull and muscles of his head, indicating that the helmet is uncomfortable. Justin senses pressure and possibly pain from the improperly positioned helmet. The afferent nerves (that send information to the brain) transmit signals of discomfort to the parietal lobe, where the body's sense of touch and pain perception are found. Signals sent from the parietal lobe to the frontal lobe make the body adjust the helmet until the pressure signals have stopped.

As you have been reading this tale, huge amounts of information have been pouring from your PNS into your CNS. Signals are sent from organs, muscles, and areas of the skin to the spinal cord until they reach the lower portions of the CNS. The position of your legs, the distribution of your body weight, the sensation of the pages in your fingers, the state of your renal arteries—all of these data are being sent to the CNS. How does the brain manage this massive amount of information without confusion and misdirection? By using the <u>diencephalon</u> and <u>brain stem</u> **Figure 28-3 ▶**.

One major role of the diencephalon is to filter out unneeded information from the cerebral cortex. Imagine if you had to "think" about shifting your weight on a chair when it became uncomfortable. The signals of pressure or pain being sent via the peripheral nerves initially stop in the diencephalon. The body's administrative assistant then decides whether the big boss (the cerebral cortex) needs to be bothered with this information. In the case of an uncomfortable bottom, the diencephalon simply sends commands so that you move

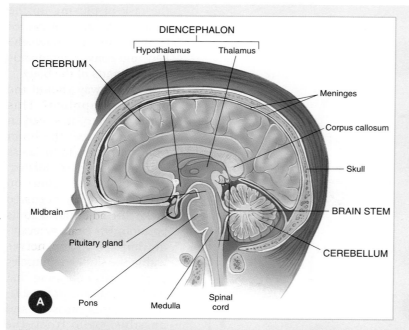

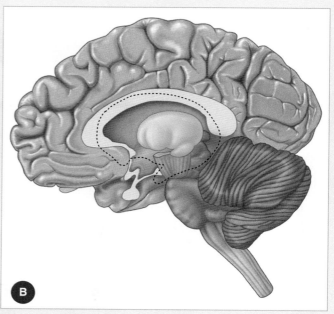

Figure 28-3 **A.** Areas of the brain, including the brain stem. **B.** The diencephalon.

slightly. Unless you were concentrating on how you were sitting, you would never even know that you moved.

How did Justin know it was time to get up this morning? His internal alarm clock went off, of course. The midbrain (part of the brain stem) is responsible for regulating the level of consciousness (LOC). You often get tired at the same time each day due to the functions of the reticular activating system (RAS). Justin is wide awake and thinking clearly thanks to his RAS.

How are blood pressure, heart rate, respiratory rate, and breathing pattern controlled? Again, the brain stem is responsible. The pons **Figure 28-4 ▶**, which is located just inferior to the midbrain, regulates your respiratory pace and the depth at which you breathe. The medulla oblongata controls the blood pressure and heart rate. Of course, these functions need to occur constantly, but Justin couldn't ride his bike if he needed to spend time and energy consciously controlling his pulse. The brain stem frees the cerebral cortex up to engage in higher level activities.

Justin now mounts his bike and begins to ride. The smile on his face reveals that he is having fun. Emotions come from two main areas within the brain: the limbic system **Figure 28-5 ▶**, where rage and anger are generated; and the hypothalamus (a part of the diencephalon), where pleasure, thirst, and hunger are found. All emotions are then mediated by the prefrontal cortex so people can choose how they are going to act in relation to how they feel.

Justin begins to pick up speed. As he approaches a corner, he must turn or risk crashing into a tree. The excitement increases his heart rate and blood pressure. The hypothalamus communicates to the pituitary gland, a member of the endocrine system. The pituitary gland, in turn, sends chemical commands to the adrenal glands to release adrenaline and noradrenaline. The release of these chemicals by the sympathetic nervous system gives Justin the increased strength and cardiovascular reserves that he needs to handle the bike in a tight turn. Just as quickly as these chemicals act, they are shut off to prevent the body from depleting its reserves. Too much adrenaline and noradrenaline can also be damaging over the long term.

Justin shifts his weight and makes the turn successfully, due in large part to his cerebellum. This lobe of the brain (located in the posterior, inferior area of the skull) manages complex motor activity. When Justin first learned to ride a bike, he had to think about what to do, where to shift his weight, and how to hold his upper body. Eventually, the frontal lobe of the brain got tired of sending the same commands again and again, so this task was transferred to the cerebellum. This lobe keeps track of Justin's body position at all times and helps to manage activities such as walking, swimming, and riding a bike.

All of this wonderfully complex activity is made possible by the synapses. Nerve cells don't actually come in direct contact with one another. Instead, a slight gap separates the

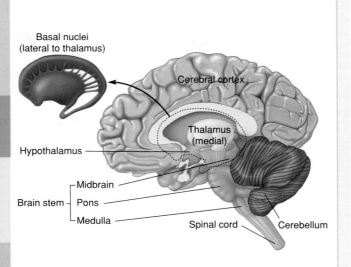

Cerebral cortex
• Receives sensory information from skin, muscles, glands, and organs
• Sends messages to move skeletal muscles
• Integrates incoming and outgoing nerve impulses
• Performs associative activities such as thinking, learning, and remembering

Basal nuclei
• Plays a role in the coordination of slow, sustained movements
• Suppresses useless patterns of movement

Thalamus
• Relays most sensory information from the spinal cord and certain parts of the brain to the cerebral cortex
• Interprets certain sensory messages such as those of pain, temperature, and pressure

Hypothalamus
• Controls various homeostatic functions such as body temperature, respiration, and heartbeat
• Directs hormone secretions of the pituitary

Cerebellum
• Coordinates subconscious movements of skeletal muscles
• Contributes to muscle tone, posture, balance, and equilibrium

Brain stem
• Origin of many cranial nerves
• Reflex centre for movements of eyeballs, head, and trunk
• Regulates heartbeat and breathing
• Plays a role in consciousness
• Transmits impulses between brain and spinal cord

Basal nuclei (lateral to thalamus)
Cerebral cortex
Thalamus (medial)
Hypothalamus
Midbrain
Brain stem — Pons
Medulla
Spinal cord
Cerebellum

Figure 28-4 The pons.

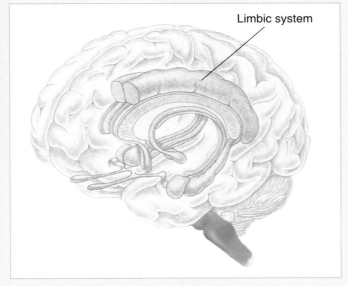

Limbic system

Figure 28-5 The limbic system is the seat of emotions, instincts, and other functions.

cells, which allows for a far greater level of fine control. The synapse, which is present wherever a nerve cell terminates, "connects" to the next cell via chemicals called <u>neurotransmitters</u>. A host of neurotransmitters are present in the brain and throughout the body. Dopamine, acetylcholine, adrenaline, and serotonin are all examples of neurotransmitters. These chemicals take the electrically conducted signal from one nerve cell (a neuron) and relay it to the next cell. Nerve cells respond to these signals in an "all or nothing" fashion: They either fire or they don't. A neuron can't fire weakly.

How do the neurotransmitters achieve a greater degree of control than that permitted by simply wiring the cells together? The answer lies in the connections made as the signal travels from the cell to the synapse Figure 28-6 ▸.

1. The first neuron fires and sends a signal along its <u>axon</u> to the axon terminal.

2. The impulse reaches the axon terminal, where neurotransmitters are released and trickle across the synapse.

3. Dendrites detect these chemicals and are triggered to send the signal to the cell's nucleus, which then transmits it down that axon, and so on.

4. Dendrites release neurotransmitter deactivators so that one impulse from cell 1 generates one response from cell 2.

The complexity in the system derives from how the cells are connected. In Figure 28-6, each cell is connected in a straight-line fashion. Although this is a reliable method of getting a signal from point A to point B, gaining more control requires more complexity. In Figure 28-7 ▸, three cells are brought together to connect with the same cell. Cell 4 will not respond unless it receives simultaneous stimulation from cells 1, 2, and 3. The same concept can be extended to the situation in which one cell sends signals to many different cells. In Figure 28-7, for example, cell 4 stimulates cells 5 and 6. As a consequence of this joint action, Justin is able to see his bike, recognise the object, know its name, instantly know how to use it, know how to make the muscles of his mouth say the word "bike", and appreciate how it will feel to ride the bike.

Neurons may or may not have <u>myelin</u> around their axons. Myelin is a type of "insulation" that allows the cell to consistently send its signal along the axon without "shorting out" or losing electricity to surrounding fluids and tissues. Myelin also increases the speed of conduction. Where speed is important, neurons have myelin. Where speed is less crucial, neurons don't have myelin. Most of the neurons within the body have myelin.

Table 28-1 ▸ summarises the structures of the nervous system and their functions.

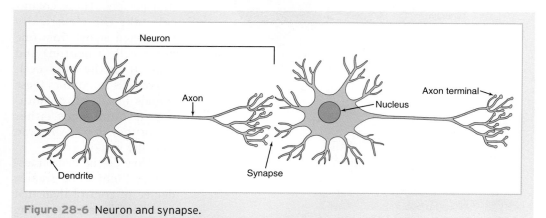

Figure 28-6 Neuron and synapse.

Pathophysiology

The pathophysiology of the nervous system can be examined from several angles. Discussion of cancerous, degenerative, developmental, infectious, vascular, and multifactorial causes of neurological conditions will be followed by a review of increased intracranial pressure and its effects on the nervous system.

Neoplastic (Cancerous) Causes

<u>Neoplasms</u> (the medical term for new growth) are caused by errors that occur during mobile reproduction, especially during the unwinding and reproduction of the DNA during cell duplication. If the error is critical, the cell will not be able to survive; it will die, and the damaged DNA will die with it. If the error is subtler, however, the cell may survive. In this case, the daughter cell is not identical to the parent. The altered cell may then reproduce and copy the error to its daughter cells. The magnitude of the cancer depends on how effectively the altered cells get sufficient nutrients for their growth and reproduction.

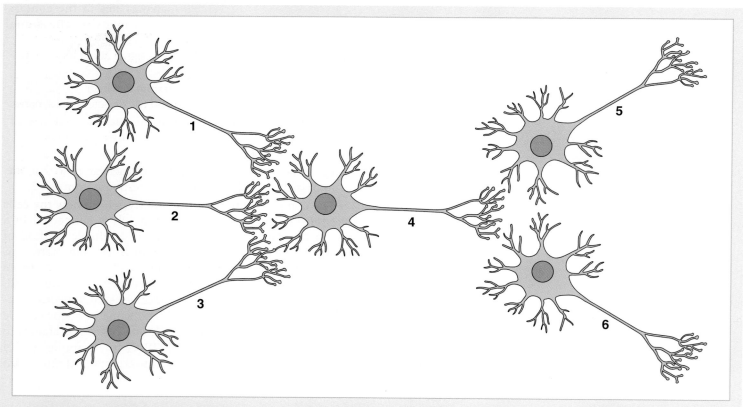

Figure 28-7 Complex synapse. Many cells (1, 2, 3) are brought together to connect with one cell (4). Cell 4 then connects with cells 5 and 6.

Table 28-1	Structures of the Nervous System and General Functions	
Major Structure	**Subdivision**	**General Function**
Central nervous system		
Brain	Occipital	Vision and storage of visual memories
	Parietal	Sense of touch and texture; storage of those memories
	Temporal	Hearing and smell; language; storage of sound and odour memories
	Frontal	Voluntary muscle control; storage of those memories
	Prefrontal	Judgement and predicting consequences of actions; abstract intellectual functions
	Limbic system	Basic emotions; basic reflexes (eg, chewing, swallowing)
	Diencephalon (thalamus)	Relay centre; filters important signals from routine signals
	Diencephalon (hypothalamus)	Emotions; temperature control; interaction with endocrine system
Brain stem	Midbrain	LOC; RAS; muscle tone and posture
	Pons	Respiratory patterning and depth
	Medulla oblongata	Heart rate; blood pressure; respiratory rate
Spinal cord		Reflexes; relays information to and from body
Peripheral nervous system		
Cranial nerves		Brain to body part communication; special peripheral nerves that connect directly to body parts
Peripheral nerves		Brain to spinal cord to body part communication; receive stimuli from body; send commands to body

Neoplasms can be categorised as either benign (noncancerous) or malignant (cancerous). Essentially, benign neoplasms are not very aggressive. They tend to remain within a capsule, so their growth is limited. In addition, these tumours are usually relatively easy to remove. By contrast, malignant neoplasms may forcefully take over blood supplies, grow unchecked, and move to other sites within the body (metastasis). They create finger-like projections into surrounding tissue, spreading and invading new areas. This growth without regard to other cells explains why many malignancies are fatal.

Degenerative Causes

Degenerative conditions result when a normal structure is altered over time. Such damage can occur in several ways—for example, due to wear and tear. Consider the effects of osteoarthritis on the knee joint. Every time a person falls on the knee, a small amount of damage is done to this joint. If the damage is not completely repaired, it may continue to accumulate until the patient experiences pain. With enough damage, the patient experiences limited mobility and pain to the joints.

Degenerative conditions may also occur through autoimmune effects. The body has the ability to determine which proteins are "self" and which are "nonself". This recognition enables the immune system to attack the bacteria in a cut yet leave the surrounding skin cells alone. In autoimmune disorders, the body begins to attack its own cells. The immune system is no longer able to distinguish friend from foe.

Under normal conditions, myelin coats the axons of most nerve cells and allows for smooth transmission of signals to their target cell Figure 28-8 ▾ . In multiple sclerosis (MS), however, the body believes that the proteins making up this insulation are foreign. It therefore attacks the myelin, creating gaps in the insulation that produce the signs and symptoms of MS.

Developmental Causes

Developmental conditions arise when portions of the nervous system are not formed correctly. Such an error can occur at any point in the development from embryo to fetus. The earlier the error occurs, the more severe the damage. In the case of spina bifida, embryonic growth does not proceed correctly.

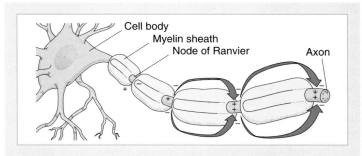

Figure 28-8 The myelin sheath normally allows impulses to jump from node to node, greatly accelerating the rate of transmission.

Soon after conception, the fetus is a ball of cells—each cell identical to all the others. Within just 8 days, however, the once uniform ball of cells is ready to give rise to an embryo. One of the critical changes that must occur is the formation of the neural tube. Around days 15 to 20, a layer of cells will fold in and form a hollow tube that will eventually become the entire nervous system. In spina bifida, some cells do not fold correctly and remain outside the neural tube. This creates an outcropping of nervous system cells that expands as the embryo grows. The ultimate result is a child born with part of its nervous system outside the body.

Even if the fetus is formed correctly, other problems may occur. If an infection or chemical agent is able to gain access to the growing fetus, it may damage areas of the brain. Likewise, a temporary decrease in oxygen may lead to brain damage. These mechanisms are postulated as the causes of cerebral palsy.

Genetics appear to play a role in many diseases, which has implications for developmental causes of neurological disorders. DNA provides the recipe for building every part of the body and outlining every process that should occur. If the recipe is perfect, then the body part will function normally. If the recipe is only slightly off, the final product may function normally but may not be able to handle stress or wear and tear as easily. However, if the recipe is very wrong, a person has an obvious disease.

This concept helps to explain why some people seem to get diseases very easily while others do not. Consider a man who has been smoking for many years. Although smoking often leads to cardiovascular disease, this man lives to be 90 years old. Another man who eats correctly, exercises every day, and never smokes dies of a heart attack at age 45. Why?

Some of the answer lies in how their coronary arteries were created. Perhaps the smoker had larger, more resilient arteries than those of the 45-year-old heart attack victim. Even though the first man makes many unhealthy lifestyle choices, he benefits from the greater capacity of his coronary arteries, which prevents them from narrowing dramatically. The second man, even though he follows a much healthier lifestyle, has narrower arteries at the beginning, so even a small amount of narrowing has a more profound impact on coronary perfusion. This basic concept is becoming more important in understanding disease incidence and severity.

Infectious Causes

Infectious diseases result when bacteria, viruses, fungi, or prions (a certain type of protein) gain access to the body, where they reproduce and cause damage. These organisms have the same basic goal as humans do—to continue to live. When they begin to attack the body, they are simply looking for fuel so that they can create the next generation of bacteria, viruses, or other organisms. The damage that these invaders inflict occurs due to one of two mechanisms—the body's reaction to the infection or the activities of the attacking organisms.

The most common sign of infectious disease is the presence of a fever. Many organisms prefer to grow in a very narrow temperature range, so even a 1° or 2°C increase in body temperature can slow down the reproduction of some viruses or bacteria. This

allows the immune system to get the upper hand. It also provides valuable time for neutrophils (the body's soldiers) to find and kill the invading organisms. Finally, it signals the rest of the body that an attack is under way. In response, more white blood cells are produced and chemical mediators are released to improve the body's effectiveness at finding and eliminating the organisms.

If the temperature of the body becomes too high, however, the brain can be affected. The increased temperature may make a person's thinking dull, make it difficult to concentrate, and lead to a headache. Neurons are highly sensitive to temperature changes. As the temperature rises, the effects on the neurons can become more profound. Eventually, a person may hallucinate, become delusional, or lose consciousness. The random firing of neurons might also produce a febrile convulsion.

Infectious agents may also damage the body by destroying cells. These organisms may produce endotoxins or exotoxins that alter living cells. Endotoxins are proteins that are released by gram-negative bacteria when they die. Exotoxins are proteins that are secreted by some bacteria or fungi to aid in the death and digestion of other cells. In poliomyelitis, for example, the virus responsible for the disease attacks the axons directly and destroys them. This virus shows a preference for motor axons—the neurons responsible for making muscles contract. Without these axons, the patient can experience weakness, paralysis, and respiratory arrest.

Vascular Causes

Blood vessels are needed to supply nutrients and oxygen to cells and to remove waste products **Figure 28-9 ▾** . If a blood vessel suddenly becomes blocked, as in an embolism, the cells

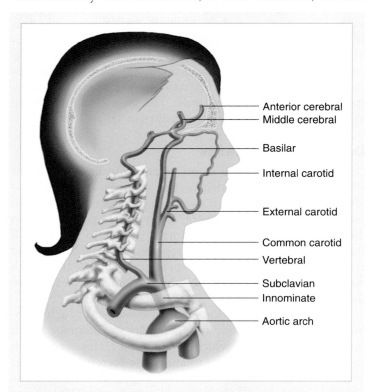

Figure 28-9 Blood supply to the brain.

- Anterior cerebral
- Middle cerebral
- Basilar
- Internal carotid
- External carotid
- Common carotid
- Vertebral
- Subclavian
- Innominate
- Aortic arch

Notes from Nancy

Once brain cells are destroyed, from whatever cause, they cannot be regenerated. Clearly, then, it is of enormous importance to provide the brain with maximum protection from harm.

beyond the blockage may become ischaemic. As oxygen and glucose levels drop, brain cells resort to anaerobic metabolism to stay alive. Unfortunately, this mechanism is only a stop-gap measure. Anaerobic metabolism creates minuscule amounts of energy for the cell and produces acidic by-products. If circulation is not restored quickly, the cell will not have enough fuel to survive.

Vascular emergencies may occur either suddenly or gradually over time. Sudden occurrences typically result from emboli or aneurysms. Emboli are insoluble objects that float in the bloodstream until they reach a point in the artery that is too narrow for them to pass through. Common types of emboli include pieces of a thrombus that have broken off or small clots that are produced by turbulent blood flow within the heart. Patients with atrial fibrillation, for example, need to have their heart rhythm controlled and take anticoagulants to prevent clots from forming in the heart and travelling to the brain, which could cause a stroke. Other types of emboli include globules of fat from long bone fractures, air bubbles infused from an IV, or a portion of an IV cannula that has been sheared off during insertion. These objects stop blood flow distal to the blockage, causing ischaemia and necrosis of tissue Figure 28-10 ▾ .

Artery walls consist of three layers of tissue. Aneurysms, which are weaknesses in those walls, occur in the following circumstances:

1. A small tear or defect occurs within the wall of an artery.
2. Blood penetrates between the layers of the artery.
3. Pressure builds up and the initial small tear increases in size.
4. If the buildup continues, the wall will become so damaged that it can no longer withstand the normal pressure of blood within it. A bulge may then develop. If the weakness is severe, the bulge may leak or fail catastrophically, causing an intracranial haemorrhage.

Gradual processes occur as plaque accumulates in blood vessels over the years. This buildup creates turbulence within the artery, allowing small clots (called thrombi) to form on its walls. The amount of plaque buildup reflects a combination of lifestyle choices (how we eat, exercise, and relieve stress) and family history (how we process food, manage fats, and the elasticity of our blood vessels). Over time, the buildup narrows the diameter of the arterial lumen. Eventually, the narrowing becomes so severe that blood flow is either diminished or cut off.

Even the blood vessel itself may cause difficulties for some patients. In trigeminal neuralgia, the normal functioning of facial blood vessels produces severe pain. As the blood vessels change in diameter to meet the needs of the surrounding tissue, their pulsations can irritate the trigeminal nerve. This nerve is responsible for receiving signals related to pain, temperature, and pressure on the face.

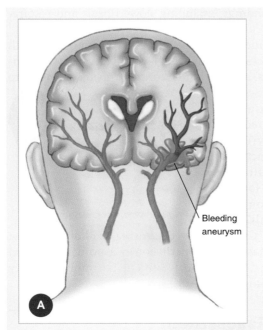
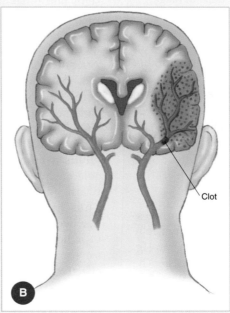
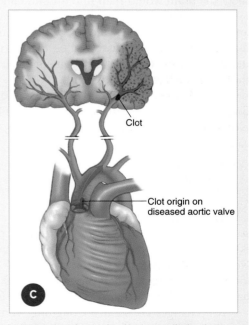

Figure 28-10 Vascular causes of neurological conditions. **A.** Aneurysms are areas of weakness in the walls of arteries that can dilate (bulge out) and eventually rupture or leak. **B.** Atherosclerosis can damage the wall of a cerebral artery, producing narrowing and/or a clot. When the vessel is completely blocked, blood flow may be blocked and cells begin to die. **C.** An embolus, a blood clot usually formed on a diseased heart valve, can travel through the body's vascular system, lodge in a cerebral artery, and cause a stroke.

Multifactorial Causes

Most diseases or conditions are multifactorial, meaning that they have multiple causes. Just because a person gets an infection, that doesn't mean that the individual will experience tissue damage. Just because someone eats unhealthy foods, it doesn't mean that his or her arteries will definitely become blocked. The following factors explain why many people get diseases:

- How well the body system was created during development as an embryo/fetus
- How effective the body's defence and repair mechanisms are
- How severe or prolonged the factors trying to damage the body are

Thus a health-conscious person may have a body that is less effective at repair and maintenance. In contrast, a person who smokes, drinks alcohol, and does not pursue a healthy lifestyle may have a body that is very effective at repair, which can help minimise the impact of those unhealthy activities.

Intracranial Pressure

Haemorrhagic strokes that cause bleeding into the brain place patients at risk for increased intracranial pressure (ICP). Treatment of these patients is directed at providing some degree of control over this potentially deadly effect.

The skull (cranial vault) is filled with three substances: brain, blood, and cerebrospinal fluid (CSF). These substances exert a pressure (ICP) against the skull, and the skull in turn exerts a reflected pressure. This balanced exchange allows the brain to fit snugly within the skull without permitting any voids. If the skull contained empty spaces, with head movement the brain would slam into the skull and cause damage.

When the pressure within the cranial vault begins to climb and remains high, it creates two major problems. The brain may either become ischaemic due to lack of blood supply or herniate (push through the ligaments that compartmentalise the brain, such as the tentorium).

As ICP rises, the amount of blood available to the brain decreases. Cerebral perfusion pressure (CPP), the pressure of blood within the cranial vault, then begins to fall. CPP can be calculated by the following equation:

$$CPP = MAP - ICP$$

The mean arterial pressure (MAP) is the average (mean) pressure within the blood vessels. The average pressure is typically 80 to 90 mm Hg. Normal ICP usually ranges from 1 to 10 mm Hg. Normal CPP is, therefore, in the range of 70 to 80 mm Hg. The lower end of normal CPP is around 50 to 60 mm Hg. With CPP below 50 mm Hg, the brain begins to become ischaemic.

ICP changes constantly. Coughing, vomiting, and bearing down, for example, will increase ICP. These momentary spikes in ICP are not harmful. By contrast, if there is blood, swelling, pus, or a tumour within the cranial vault, ICP will increase and remain high. Because the volume of the cranial vault is limited and inflexible, pressure increases as more substances squeeze into this space. As long as there is no significant drop in blood pressure or significant rise in ICP, the heart will still be able to get blood into the brain. However, if ICP rises sharply or blood pressure falls critically, patients may experience serious problems.

Consider a patient with meningitis (an infection of the membranes that cover the brain and spinal cord). The battle between the infecting organism and the immune system causes fluid to accumulate around the brain, which in turn causes ICP to climb. As long as the increase remains moderate, the brain will continue to receive adequate oxygen and nutrients. If the infection goes unchecked and travels to the general circulatory system, however, septicaemia occurs. Then, as the organism continues to grow and feed, capillaries may begin to leak. Eventually, the blood pressure will decline and the MAP will fall. At a certain point, CPP may drop so low that the brain starts to become ischaemic.

This concept dictates the priorities for treatment. Given how critical normal perfusion of the brain is, blood pressure must be closely monitored in any patient with a potential ICP problem. Frequent assessment becomes even more essential when a decrease in blood pressure is also present. For any patient at risk for ICP, the paramedic needs to ensure a blood pressure of at least 110 to 120 mm Hg systolic.

Another potential outcome of ICP is herniation, or displacement of the brain out of the cranial vault. Herniation results when pressure increases within the skull and the brain is pressed down through the foramen magnum (the "large hole" at the inferior portion of the skull where the spinal cord exits). Pressure on the medulla oblongata (located directly superior to the spinal cord) can result in rather bizarre vital signs and other findings, including slowed heart and respiratory rates.

Carbon dioxide and oxygen levels are important with increased ICP. Excessively high O_2 levels will cause vasoconstriction of cerebral arteries, which further impairs perfusion to the brain and causes cerebral hypoxia. Conversely, lowered CO_2 levels will decrease ICP, which yields a more suitable environment for brain perfusion. Thus hyperventilation will decrease CO_2 (thereby decreasing ICP) and increase O_2 (thereby decreasing brain perfusion)—a no-win situation for the paramedic. Prehospital treatment is simply not very effective at decreasing ICP.

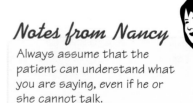

Notes from Nancy

Always assume that the patient can understand what you are saying, even if he or she cannot talk.

General Assessment

The brain is the organ that is most sensitive to fluctuating levels of oxygen, glucose, and temperature; it responds to alterations in these levels with changes in its function. The difficulty for the paramedic is that the brain is relatively resilient to internal environmental changes: It doesn't simply shut down when oxygen levels fall. The key to identifying a neurological problem is to look for both the gross or obvious changes and the subtle, sometimes hidden changes that can indicate disease.

This section reviews the assessment process for the neurological patient. As with all patients, begin with the scene assessment.

Scene Assessment

Body substance isolation (BSI) precautions are taken for granted in many ambulance services. Its purpose is to protect the provider from exposure to potentially harmful organisms or environments. Patients having tonic/clonic convulsions, for example, may be incontinent.

Some unconscious patients may be suffering from overdoses. With the use of illegal drugs, the presence of weapons, money, and crime increases. This potentially places the paramedic close to armed criminals.

Patients with altered levels of consciousness may not be able to walk, may be combative, or may be completely unresponsive. You may need additional assistance with lifting and moving these patients. Special circumstances can be overcome more easily if additional resources—such as helicopter transportation, rescue equipment, the fire service—are requested early in the call.

Examine the scene to ascertain the number of patients. Clues can be obtained from the dispatch information. Also consider the mechanism of injury or history of present illness. Road traffic collisions typically involve more than one vehicle and, therefore, more than one patient. If many patients exhibit similar signs and symptoms, you should be very cautious. One

patient with a headache does not stand out. If an entire family in the same house complains of a headache, then you should consider the possibility of carbon monoxide exposure. In such a case, the house may be an unsafe scene, so ensure that you have the correct personal protective equipment (PPE).

Weapons of mass destruction can follow similar patterns. If you encounter several patients who all exhibit the same signs and symptoms, all within the same general time frame and geographic location, you should consider immediate evacuation, donning appropriate PPE and contacting ambulance control to begin a more in-depth investigation.

Initial Assessment

Begin assessing the neurological patient as you would any other patient. Assess and secure the ABCs. Use the AVPU system to determine LOC. If the patient does not respond to verbal stimuli, consider whether he or she may be displaying some abnormal posturing; these unconscious movements may indicate severe brain dysfunction. There are two main abnormal postures that the patient may demonstrate with painful stimulation—decorticate and decerebrate. If you see either posture, you should immediately consider the patient to be critical.

In decorticate posturing, the patient flexes the arms and curls them toward the chest. At the same time, he or she points her toes. Finally, the wrists are flexed. This posture, which is also called abnormal flexion, may indicate damage to the area directly below the cerebral hemispheres Figure 28-11 ▶ .

In decerebrate posturing, the patient again points the toes, but now extends the arms outward and rotates the lower arms in a palms-down manner (called pronation). The wrists are again flexed. This posture is a more severe finding than

You are the Paramedic Part 2

You obtain the patient's vital signs. As your partner obtains his blood glucose level, you continue your assessment and determine that he is quite confused. He is alert and orientated to person and place, but is unsure as to what day it is and cannot describe the events leading up to your arrival.

The patient shows no signs of trauma. During your assessment of his pupils, however, he takes your penlight and tries to shave his face with it. He also seems to use inappropriate words for common, household objects and appears frustrated that you can't understand him.

Vital Signs	Recording Time: 5 Minutes
Level of consciousness	Verbal, orientated to person and place, but not day, with a Glasgow Coma Scale score of 14
Skin	Pale, warm, and dry
Pulse	90 beats/min and irregular
Blood pressure	142/86 mm Hg
Respirations	26 breaths/min
SpO2	98% on 15 l/min via nonrebreathing mask
Blood glucose	6.1 mmol/l

3. Given the information you have now, what do you think could be this patient's underlying illness, injury, or condition?

4. Do your assessment and treatment priorities ever change?

5. What are appropriate interventions?

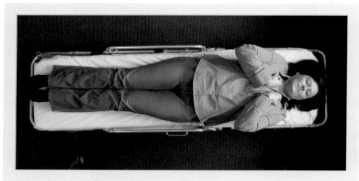

Figure 28-11 Decorticate posturing.

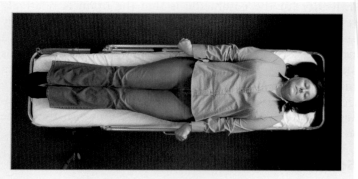

Figure 28-12 Decerebrate posturing.

decorticate posturing, as the level of damage is within or near the brain stem (diencephalon/pons/midbrain) Figure 28-12 ▶ .

Airway

The trigeminal, glossopharyngeal, vagus, and hypoglossal nerves are responsible for airway control. These nerves allow for swallowing, controlling the tongue, and ensuring that the muscles in the hypopharnyx are slightly contracted. Alteration in the signals from these nerves can produce too much relaxation or too much constriction of the airway Figure 28-13 ▶ .

Trismus, in which the teeth are clenched closed, can make managing the airway very difficult. Trismus can occur in conscious or unconscious patients. In an unconscious patient, it can indicate a convulsion in progress, severe head injury, or cerebral hypoxia.

Breathing

As part of your assessment of the neurological patient, you need to check the rate and rhythm of breathing. Rhythms can have subtle changes or be dramatically different from normal. Generally, the greater the deviation from normal, the more severely the nervous system is affected.

Circulation

Evaluate the peripheral and central pulse pressures. Are they the same? The absence of a peripheral pulse with a central pulse present should cause the paramedic to suspect shock. What is the characteristic of the skin? Do you see evidence of gross bleeding? Is the pulse bounding? Remember, shock is rarely caused solely by a neurological problem.

If a patient suffers from increased pressure within the cranium, the vital signs may provide evidence of this problem. Table 28-2 ▶ shows the vital signs associated with increased ICP. Notice how the blood pressure rises, the heart/respiratory rates fall, and the pulse pressure widens (systolic hypertension) in increased ICP. This set of conditions—known as Cushing's triad—are the opposite of what is expected in shock.

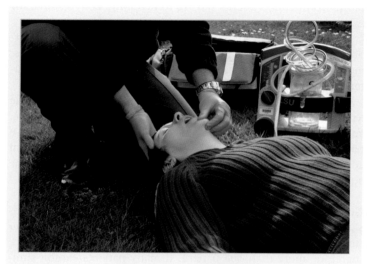

Figure 28-13 Securing and maintaining the airway in a patient who is unconscious is critical. Be sure to have suction readily available in the event that the patient vomits.

Table 28-2	Vital Signs for Shock Versus Increased ICP			
	Heart Rate	Respiratory Rate	Blood Pressure	Pulse Pressure
Shock	↑	↑	↓	Narrowed
Increased ICP	↓	↓	↑	Widened

As ICP rises, blood flow to the brain diminishes. To compensate, the medulla oblongata sends signals to the heart to increase the force of contraction. This causes systolic pressure to rise. If the ICP continues to increase, downward forces on the brain stem begin to damage the medulla's ability to send signals to the body. The diastolic blood pressure falls as the blood vessels relax or dilate, which in turn results in a widened pulse pressure. Finally, this pressure damages the ability to control respiratory and heart rate; consequently, both decrease.

Transport Decision

At this point in the examination, the paramedic may make a broad decision about whether to "load and go" or "stay and play". Critical patients—those with alterations in their initial assessment or significant mechanism of injury (MOI) and history of present illness—should be transported urgently to an accident and emergency (A&E) department. Defer gathering very detailed information about these patients; instead, focus on stabilising and maintaining ABCs. With stable patients—those with normal initial assessments and minor MOI/history of present illness—you have more time to gather detailed information at the scene. You can question family and bystanders to gain valuable insight into your patient's complaint.

Special Considerations

When you are working with older patients, take their past medical history into account. Patients with a history of dementia will be very complicated to manage. The primary question is: How much change has occurred in the patient's LOC? Don't assume that the patient's baseline LOC is what you would consider "normal"; speak to family, friends, or other parents to determine the patient's baseline LOC. Document that level clearly, using active language.

Focused History and Physical Examination

Rapid Trauma Assessment

Once the initial assessment is complete, you need to decide how to proceed. Is the patient stable or unstable? Do you suspect a major problem just below the surface? How should you transport this patient? At this point, you have two choices:

- Complete a rapid assessment using a full head-to-toe approach
- Perform a focused history and physical examination (ie, evaluate only the area of patient complaint)

You should perform a rapid assessment for any patient who has an abnormal initial assessment, has a significant MOI/history of present illness, or whom you suspect may have a major problem. Examples would include individuals who are unconscious, are having a convulsion, or experience a sudden loss of movement of the body. The focused history and physical examination is done on patients who are stable and have narrow complaints. These individuals have a completely normal initial assessment and a minor MOI/history of present illness, and you suspect a very local problem. Examples would include patients with headaches or nontraumatic back pain.

Be cautious. If a patient has a headache, stress may not be the cause. Stroke patients can also experience headaches. If you suspect a more complicated problem, perform a rapid assessment to ensure that you give the patient the best possible care.

Documentation and Communication

Avoid using terms that can have multiple meanings, such as "lethargic", "sleepy", "sluggish", or "out of it". Instead, describe the patient using active language.

Potentially confusing: "Arrive to find male patient who is out of it".

Better: "Arrive to find a male patient disorientated to place and day".

Potentially confusing: "Caring for a 43-year-old sluggish male".

Better: "Caring for a 43-year-old male who is very slow to respond to painful stimulation".

History

History taking in the patient with a potential neurological complaint should follow the same process followed for any other medical or trauma patient. For example, if weakness is a symptom found in a medical patient with no trauma, use the OPQRST mnemonic to elaborate on the complaint of general body weakness. The physical examination for this complaint should investigate potential cardiac, neurological, respiratory, metabolic, or infectious causes. Appropriate tests and serial vital signs such as blood glucose levels, ECG, vital signs, lung sounds, and temperature will also help you rule out potential causes of the weakness.

Special Considerations

In the paediatric population, consider the developmental stage of the child. A 1-year-old should cry when assessed; that's a normal reaction to strangers. A 5-year-old who normally talks freely may be rather tight-lipped with a stranger.

Detailed Physical Examination

The detailed physical examination examines all of the areas covered within the rapid assessment, but looks at them more closely.

Head

The head is the area where you will spend the most time, gathering critical information on the functioning of the nervous system. Of course, you want to assess the head for trauma. Deformities, Contusion, Abrasions, Penetrations, Burns, Tenderness, Lacerations, and Swelling (DCAP-BTLS) are the trauma assessment components you should assess on every body area.

There are many shades of LOC and many ways to evaluate LOC. A patient may be interacting appropriately with the environment or not at all. **Figure 28-14 ▾** shows a continuum that ranges from what most would consider to be normal behaviour to no response whatsoever. The point on the extreme right side of the continuum is coma, a state in which the patient does not respond to verbal or painful stimuli. The points in between (guide markings) are not intended to imply that every patient will stop at every point as his or her LOC increases or decreases, but rather illustrate the relationships between various levels of consciousness. While the extremes are easy to understand, the points in the middle (the shades of grey) can be more confusing.

One tool to assist with the consistent evaluation of LOC is the Glasgow Coma Scale (GCS) **Table 28-3 ▸** . This assessment tool provides a basis to determine a patient's degree of illness or injury. It is used to determine the patient's LOC and evaluate responses to eye opening as well as verbal

Notes from Nancy

A patient in a coma is a patient in danger. Institute the ABCs immediately.

Table 28-3	Glasgow Coma Scale	
	Adult	**Paediatric Patient (< 5 y)**
Eye opening	4. Spontaneous	4. Spontaneous
	3. Voice	3. To shout/voice
	2. Pain stimulation	2. Pain stimulation
	1. None	1. None
Verbal	5. Orientated	5. Cry, smile, coo, words correct for age
	4. Disorientated	4. Cries, inappropriate words for age
	3. Inappropriate words	3. Inappropriate scream or cry
	2. Incomprehensible	2. Grunts
	1. None	1. None
Motor	6. Obeys	6. Spontaneous
	5. Localises pain	5. Localises pain
	4. Withdraws from pain	4. Withdraws from pain
	3. Decorticate	3. Decorticate
	2. Decerebrate	2. Decerebrate
	1. None	1. None

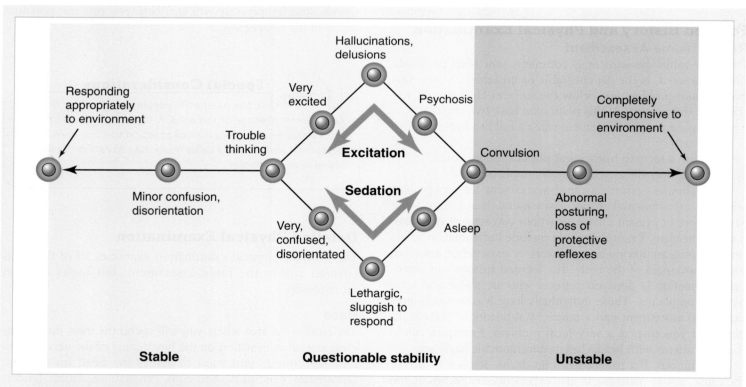

Figure 28-14 Level of consciousness continuum.

and motor skills Figure 28-15 ▾ . To determine the GCS score, add the three numbers together from each of the subsections of the GCS.

The GCS score can provide information as to what care should be given and where the patient should be transported. Table 28-4 ▸ provides general guidelines for using these scores. Patients with mild conditions need standard care; usually the paramedic can honour their request to be transported to a particular hospital. Patients with moderate conditions are very difficult to manage. They are not stable enough for you to relax, and not critical enough to completely get your attention. With this group, close assessment and transport to the nearest appropriate hospital are prudent. Critical patients need airway management and rapid transport to the closest appropriate hospital.

Changes in the patient's mood or tempo of the nervous system should alert you to changes in neurological status. Oxygen levels or blood pressure could be falling. Body temperature could be climbing. A psychiatric condition could be escalating. Blood glucose levels could be too high or too low. Regardless of the underlying cause, your observation of a change should prompt further evaluation to ensure the appropriate level of care. Mood or affect is another attribute that provides insight into the patient's condition. Ask the patient how he or she feels. Frustration, anger, or aggression can be caused by low glucose or oxygen levels.

Ask the patient how easy it is for him or her to think. Patients who have decreased blood glucose levels or who are taking opiates can experience difficulty concentrating. Lower

Table 28-4	Interpretations of Glasgow Coma Scale Scores		
GCS Score	**Interpretation**	**Treatment**	**Hospital**
13–15	Mild	Standard care	Patient/family choice
9–12	Moderate	Close airway assessment, watch for decreasing consciousness	Closest appropriate hospital
8 or less	Severe	Intubation, decrease scene time (less than 8, intubate)	Closest appropriate hospital

blood glucose levels and narcotics tend to produce sedation of the nervous system. In contrast, patients who are taking cocaine may experience difficulty concentrating due to excitement or mania. Cocaine, a sympathomimetic, increases nervous system activity, causing thoughts to come very quickly. If the speed of nervous system activity continues to increase, the patient may hallucinate or become delusional or psychotic.

Visual Findings

Perform the DCAP-BTLS assessment. Look at the symmetry of the face. Is there an obvious facial droop? Look at the eyes. Are the eyelids bilaterally even? Ptosis (drooping eyelids) can indicate Bell's palsy or a stroke. Figure 28-16 ▸ demonstrates what happens when such a patient is asked to smile; weakness to one side of the face causes facial droop and slight ptosis.

Assess the cranial nerves, the peripheral nerves that control various portions of the body (see Chapter 13). Look for the ability to respond, strength of response, and symmetry. Patients with stroke, trigeminal neuralgia, myasthenia gravis, or other neurological conditions may demonstrate abnormal cranial nerve functioning.

Speech

Listen to the quality of the speech. Is it slurred? Slurring is a classic finding with stroke. Is the speech appropriate? Focus on not only the quality of the words that are spoken, but also the appropriateness of those words. Sometimes speech may be clear but word choice is incorrect. Assess the patient's object recognition abilities.

Patients may be able to speak clearly, yet have subtle knowledge deficits. In agnosia (*a* = without, *gnosis* = knowledge), patients will be unable to name common objects because connections between visual interpretation of objects and the words that name them have become damaged. Apraxia (*a* = without, *praxia* = movement) refers to the inability to know how to use a common object.

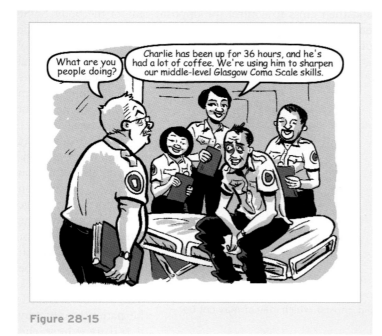

Figure 28-15

To test for these signs, simply show the patient your pen, scissors, or a set of keys. Ask the patient to name the object. If the individual responds correctly, hand the object to the patient and ask him or her to demonstrate the object's use. The patient should write with the pen, cut with the scissors, and turn a lock with the keys. Patients may have one of these signs without the other. One is not a more severe finding than the other. They simply indicate that some degree of misfiring of neurons is occurring between the occipital lobe and the temporal lobe (agnosia) or between the temporal lobe and the frontal lobe (apraxia).

Language can be affected by injury or disease. In dysphasia, speech is affected. There are three main forms of dysphasia:

- **Receptive dysphasia.** The patient cannot understand (receive) speech, but is able to speak clearly. This form of dysphasia indicates damage to the temporal lobe. Ask patients questions to which both you and they know the answer: "Who is the Prime Minister"? "What month is it"? Do not ask yes/no questions. If the patient speaks clearly but gives incorrect answers, he or she may have receptive dysphasia.
- **Expressive dysphasia.** The patient can't speak (express themselves) clearly, but is able to understand speech. This form of dysphasia indicates damage to the frontal lobe, which controls the motor portion of speech. Ask patients to raise an arm. If they respond correctly, they can understand you. Ask patients their name. If they can't respond or their responses are slurred, they have expressive dysphasia.
- **Global dysphasia.** This form of dysphasia is a combination of expressive and receptive dysphasia. In this setting, the patient will not follow commands and can't answer your questions. Nevertheless, patients with global dysphasia can often think clearly. They have

needs, anxieties, and discomforts, but no way to express them. This can be incredibly frightening for patients who can't understand anything that you're saying and can't speak to you. Be sensitive to this state. Move slowly and purposely. Use therapeutic touch and good eye contact to reassure the patient.

Pupils

Pupillary shape can be changed by trauma, glaucoma, or increased ICP. Cocaine, methamphetamines, and hallucinogens tend to cause dilation of the pupils. Depressants usually lead to constriction of the pupils.

Equality of pupils is an important observation. Unequal pupils, called anisocoria, can be a sign of increased ICP **Figure 28-17 ▸** . Many people have a slight inequality in pupillary size. Anything greater than a 1-mm difference is worth noting, however. As pressure increases within the skull, the brain stem can be squeezed. This squeezing can interrupt signals to one pupil, resulting in dramatically different-size pupils.

Finally, determine whether the eyes are twitching. Nystagmus (the involuntary, rhythmic movement of the eyes) can be caused by convulsions, vertigo, and MS.

Movement of the Body

Observe how the patient moves. Does the body move equally on both sides? Patients with strokes may suffer from weakness (hemiparesis) or paralysis (hemiplegia) of one side of the body. Sometimes you may discover patients with weakness on one side of their body but facial droop on the other side. This condition may be caused by decussation, in which nerves cross as they leave the cerebral cortex, move through the brain stem, and arrive at the spinal cord. Nerves that decussate start on one side of the brain and then cross to control the opposite side of the body. Some nerves do not decussate—facial nerves, for example. The left side of the brain controls the right side of the body, but the left side of the face. A left cerebral stroke would therefore result in right-sided arm and leg weakness, but left-sided facial droop.

Examining the function of the cerebellum can also allow you to gather information about potential damage to the brain. Ask the patient to close his or her eyes and hold out the arms in front of the body at the same level. With the eyes closed, the patient's only way of telling where the

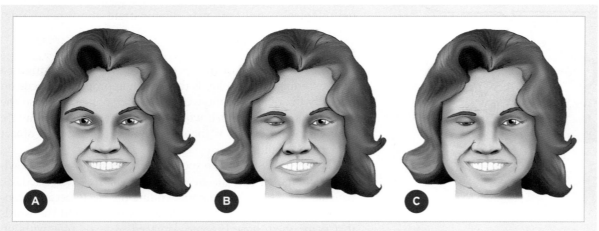

Figure 28-16 **A.** A normal smile. **B.** Facial droop, including a drooping eyelid (ptosis), which may or may not be present. **C.** A normal smile with ptosis present.

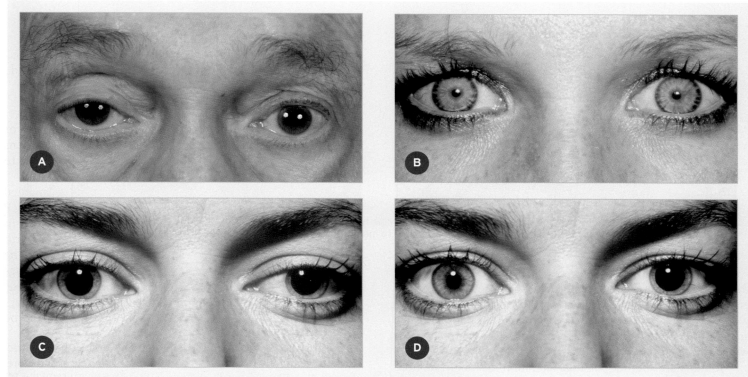

Figure 28-17 Pupil responses. **A.** Normal. **B.** Constricted (pinpoint). **C.** Dilated. **D.** Unequal.

arms are located is from the sensations being processed by the cerebellum. If the individual has suffered a stroke, one of the arms may drift away from the other **Figure 28-18 ▶**.

Ask the patient to walk for several steps (unless some medical reason rules the activity out). Assessing gait (walking patterns) is another way to test the activity of the cerebellum. Walking is really a controlled fall. As your centre of gravity moves forward, you must move a leg forward to catch yourself. Once you learn how to walk, your cerebellum controls these mechanics, so you can focus on where you want to walk, not how to walk. Damage to the cerebellum may be manifested as erratic walking, stumbling, or even losing the ability to walk.

Several medical conditions cause alterations in the patient's gait. Ataxia is the term used to describe changes in a person's ability to perform coordinated motions like walking. Patients with Parkinson's disease exhibit a classic gait in which they place their feet very close together and shuffle. Their stride is short, and they have great difficulty changing direction. Such a patient will shuffle-walk in a straight line and, when asked to turn, will take very small steps until the turn is complete. With this kind of bradykinesia, routine motions may slow dramatically. In contrast, patients with cerebral palsy may walk with a scissors gait. In the spastic form of this disease, the person will point the toes inwardly, have a stiff gait, and nearly touch the knees together while walking.

In addition to the patient's gait, you should assess the posture. Ask the individual to stand straight. Place one hand on the patient's chest and the other hand behind the back (to catch the patient in the event that he or she can't do so), and then push on the chest. Normally, as you push backward, the patient will compensate quickly and take a step forward to prevent a fall. In Parkinson's disease, the patient's posture is so rigid that they can't compensate quickly enough and will fall over.

Bizarre movements may indicate a disruption within the nervous system. Myoclonus is a type of involuntary contraction of the muscles that is rapid and jerky in nature. Most people have suffered myoclonic jerks at some point. Have you ever seen a seated person who is very tired? As the person gets closer to falling sleep, the head will begin to sag. Often the person will involuntarily jerk the head upward (myoclonic jerk) and wake up.

Another form of bizarre movement is dystonia, in which a part of the body contracts and remains contracted. A foot cramp where the great toe extends while the other toes curl under is an example of a common dystonia. Alternatively, the face may become extremely distorted as one side contracts. The head can twist to one side. An arm or leg can become frozen in a contracted position. Dystonia can be caused by brain injuries or medication reactions.

When you are watching the patient, does he or she move smoothly? This kind of motion requires proper functioning of

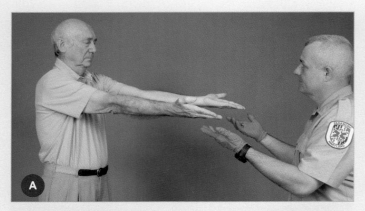 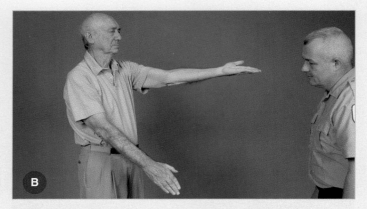

Figure 28-18 A. A person who has not experienced a stroke will be able to hold both hands in front of the body and maintain them there. **B.** If a person has had a suspected stroke, he or she may not be able to maintain this position. Instead, one arm will drift down and turn toward the body.

the frontal lobe, cerebellum, brain stem, spinal cord, and peripheral nerves. When they are functioning correctly, muscle groups will alternately contract and relax, allowing the body to move smoothly. Patients with Parkinson's disease suffer from rigidity in which this fine balance is upset, so they move in fits and spurts.

Tremors are another potential alteration in smooth motion. These fine oscillating (back-and-forth) movements are usually found in the hands and head.

- **Rest tremors**—occur with the patient at rest and not in motion. They are common in Parkinson's disease.
- **Intension tremors**—occur when the patient tries to reach out and grab an object. These tremors may increase as the patient gets closer to the object to be grabbed. Intension tremors are common in MS.
- **Postural tremors**—occur when a body part is required to maintain the same position for a long period of time. Most people have experienced this type of tremor when they were working hard for a long time. As they tire, their worked body parts begin to shake. A postural tremor can also occur when a person is standing and the head oscillates back and forth. Patients with Parkinson's disease also experience these tremors.

Convulsions may appear very similar to tremors. Generally, tremors are fine movements while convulsions are larger, less focused types of movement. There are two basic types of movements that patients can perform while having a convulsion:

- **Tonic activity** is a very rigid, contracted body posture. The arms, legs, neck, and back can contract so tightly that the body part will shake slightly from the intensity of the contraction.
- **Clonic activity** is a rhythmic contraction and relaxation of muscle groups. It may appear as bizarre, non-purposeful movements of any body part. Arms and legs may flail, teeth may clench, the head may bob, and the torso may move wildly.

Sensation

Many neurological conditions can alter the ability to feel pain, temperature, pressure, or light touch. A sensation of numbness or tingling is called paraesthesia. If the patient can feel nothing within a body part, the condition is called anaesthesia.

Blood Glucose Level

Glucose is the fuel that runs the brain. The brain uses glucose faster than any other part of the body, but it has no means to store glucose. For this reason, all patients with a change in LOC should have their blood glucose level checked. A normal blood glucose reading is 3.34 to 6.66 mmol/l. As glucose levels fall below 3.34 mmol/l, LOC begins to decrease. LOC can also be affected by a high blood glucose level, although a significant increase is required before LOC is altered. Glucose levels below 0.5 mmol/l are incompatible with brain functioning and typically lethal. Generally, if levels are below 1.6 or above 16.7 mmol/l, confusion or unconsciousness will occur. Blood glucose monitoring is standard care for the patient with an altered LOC.

Chest

Evaluate the chest for DCAP-BTLS. Look for symmetry in its shape. Does the chest rise and fall equally? Apply the cardiac monitor and evaluate the ECG. Many cardiac arrhythmias can cause neurological disorders by decreasing the blood supply to the brain. Perform a 12-lead ECG in all patients with sudden loss of consciousness. How much effort must the patient make to breathe? Do you observe any degree of respiratory distress? Listen to lung sounds. Evaluate for the presence of adventitious sounds and equality of sounds. Determine the pulse oximeter reading, remembering that normal readings are 95% to 100% on air and that this number is affected by the amount of haemoglobin within the body and the presence of carbon monoxide or supplemental oxygen.

Abdomen

Examine the abdomen for DCAP-BTLS. Do you note any masses? Are there any pulsations within the abdomen? Does the patient have any complaints related to the abdomen? Signs of nausea and vomiting are common with some neurological conditions, such as headaches or increased ICP.

Pelvis

Examine the pelvis for DCAP-BTLS. Is it stable to stress? If the patient is able to walk without assistance, the pelvis should be stable. Does the patient have any incontinence? Urinary or faecal incontinence are common findings with convulsions or syncope. Incontinence also serves as a relatively objective marker for the severity of the unconsciousness. When we sleep, we are not incontinent. Thus if incontinence is present, the LOC has decreased below that of sleep.

Extremities

Examine the limbs for DCAP-BTLS. Do you see any signs of oedema? Look for venepuncture marks and note whether these marks are at various stages of healing. Such marks may indicate recent illegal drug use.

Ongoing Assessment

The ongoing assessment is intended to monitor patients for changes. Talk with them. Ask them how they're feeling. Ask about their children. Ask if they caught the game last night. Casual conversation will allow you to closely monitor brain functions. It also communicates a caring environment. If the patient is non-verbal, keep a close eye on respiratory patterns and eye and body movements, and monitor for convulsion activity.

Routine monitoring should include heart rate, ECG, blood pressure, respiratory rate and pattern, pulse oximetry, and repeat glucose checks (if the level was low and sugar was given to the patient). Continue oxygenation and ventilation support. Monitor IVs closely to ensure that accidental fluid overload does not occur. If the patient's condition undergoes a sudden dramatic change, repeat the rapid assessment and detailed physical examination as if this were a new patient. This will give you a chance to modify your care so as to manage the new development.

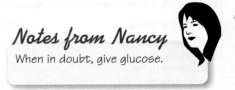

Notes from Nancy

When in doubt, give glucose.

General Management

This management guideline should be followed with all patients who experience a change in LOC. The focus of care for neurological patients is directed at ensuring that the body has an adequate internal environment to allow for optimal brain function. The three major elements that the brain needs to function are *oxygen, glucose,* and *normal temperature.* The general management techniques discussed in this section—the standard care—serve as the foundation on which additional care for specific neurological problems is built.

As always, provide for universal precautions and scene safety. Ensure that you and your partner are safe and you have universal precautions in place.

Evaluate the patient's airway and effectiveness of breathing. If necessary, secure the airway, and provide ventilatory support to make sure oxygen saturation remains higher than 90%. Routine hyperventilation of neurological patients can be harmful, so provide hyperventilation only to those patients with documented unconsciousness *and* signs of increased ICP.

You are the Paramedic Part 3

In the interest of time, you place your patient on the trolley, obtain IV access and administer normal saline TKVO, and perform an ECG. In addition, you complete a thrombolysis checklist whilst en route to hospital. You ask one of the patient's sons to accompany you and provide more information regarding his medical history. The patient's son tells you that his medical history includes atrial fibrillation (which you confirm on the monitor) and that the patient takes aspirin, diltiazem, warfarin, and metformin. The patient has no known drug allergies, has no recent history of illness, and has been compliant with his medications and diet.

Reassessment	Recording Time: 10 Minutes
Level of consciousness	Alert, with a Glasgow Coma Scale score of 14
Skin	Pale, warm, and dry
Pulse	92 beats/min, strong and irregular
Blood pressure	140/84 mm Hg
Respirations	24 breaths/min
SpO2	100% on 15 l/min via nonrebreathing mask

6. Would you choose to place this patient in manual in-line spinal precautions?

7. What places this patient at greater risk for cerebrovascular event?

Table 28-5	Hallmarks of Increased ICP	
Cushing's Triad	**Other Signs**	
■ Bradycardia ■ Bradypnoea ■ Widened pulse pressure (systolic hypertension)	■ Decorticate posturing ■ Decerebrate posturing ■ Anisocoria	■ Biot respirations ■ Apneustic respirations ■ Cheyne-Stokes respirations

Establish IV access, and then administer normal saline. Consider drawing blood samples for later analysis at the hospital, if your service advocates this. Check the patient's blood pressure and heart rate. Support hypotension to ensure adequate CPP; the target is a systolic blood pressure of 110 to 120 mm Hg.

Continuously monitor the patient on an ECG.

Check the blood glucose level. If it's low, administer 10 g (100 ml) of glucose 10% IV. Be very cautious when you can't check the patient's blood glucose level. If the patient is unresponsive or has a decreased LOC and no blood glucose monitor is available, administer 5 g (50 ml) and then reassess the response. Proceed with additional glucose cautiously, based on responses to previous doses. Hyperglycaemia can increase the morbidity rate among stroke patients.

Look for the hallmarks of increased ICP   Table 28-5 ▲ . In patients who are unconscious *and* demonstrate other signs of increased ICP, ensure a systolic blood pressure of 110 to 120 mm Hg. Administer fluids as needed. Unless you are concerned about possible cervical spine fracture, elevate the head 30°. Provide ventilatory support at 16 to 20 breaths/min. Don't increase the rate any higher than 30 breaths/min, as hyperventilation will cause vasoconstriction and decrease perfusion to the brain. Ensure that the airway is clear, but don't suction vigorously. Stimulating the cough and gag reflexes will increase ICP.

A patient with increased ICP may be bradycardic. Atropine and pacing are not indicated, however, due to the systolic hypertension that accompanies the bradycardia. The ICP is causing the bradycardia, not the reverse. Instead, notify the hospital and provide rapid transport.

Check for drug use. If the patient may have taken a narcotic, administer naloxone, 0.4 to 2 mg IV. Watch for convulsions. If the convulsion is prolonged, administer diazepam or lorazepam.

Special Considerations

When assessing for ICP in infants, consider the quality of the cry. As ICP increases, the pitch of the cry will increase until a shriek similar to that of a cat can be heard. At the same time, the shape of the pupils can change from round to more oval. These two findings lead to the saying related to infants and ICP: "cats' eyes and cats' cries".

Documentation and Communication

You may be the only provider to witness some patient activity, so good documentation is critical to ensure continuity of care.

Evaluate the patient's temperature. If it is low, cover the patient, turn on the heat, and prevent heat loss. If it is high, remove clothing, cover the naked patient in a sheet, and turn the heat off in the patient compartment.

Provide emotional support for the patient and family. Neurological emergencies can produce confusion, fear, anger, and helplessness. Consider giving a therapeutic gentle touch on the shoulder. Touch can communicate compassion. Use a calm, reassuring voice to show that you're there to help. Try to reorientate the patient, as confusion is often present in these cases.

Administration of Glucose

Consult your local guidelines to determine whether the blood glucose reading is considered low. If the blood glucose level is below 4.0 mmol/l, then glucose is needed. Three medications are available for prehospital treatment of hypoglycaemia: Hypostop, glucose 10%, and glucagon. When administering glucose, you must establish an IV line. This access site should be within a large vessel (18-gauge or larger is preferred) because glucose is quite thick. Ensure that the IV is patent *before* you attempt to give the glucose. Extravasation of glucose into the interstitial space can cause severe damage to muscles, nerves, and skin or even death. The effects from glucose typically begin in 30 seconds to 2 minutes.

Patients who are severely malnourished, such as chronic alcoholics, may have insufficient supplies of vitamin B1 (thiamine) to metabolise glucose adequately. (Thiamine allows the body to convert its store of glycogen into glucose as part of the Krebs cycle.) If you cannot obtain vascular access, administer 1 mg of glucagon IM. The LOC and blood glucose levels should increase within 20 minutes after administration.

There is currently no safe way to lower high blood glucose levels in the prehospital environment. Trials are underway to administer insulin in the prehospital setting. Administration of insulin can be very problematic and can easily overshoot the mark, sending the patient into a hypoglycaemic state. For these patients, provide standard care and ensure adequate blood pressure. Hyperglycaemic patients are often dehydrated and usually need volume support.

Oral glucose administration (Hypostop) is another option for patients with a decreased LOC who can swallow safely. Assess these patients carefully, confirming that they are sufficiently awake to follow commands. Administer oral glucose 23 g (one tube of Hypostop). Alternatives to oral glucose include cake icing, a plain chocolate bar (without nuts), or orange juice with sugar added. Administration of sugar by mouth will take longer to raise blood glucose levels. Constantly supervise patients as they consume the sugar. Make sure they don't aspirate.

Airway Management

Sometimes patients may not be able to protect the airway adequately or ventilate themselves. The use of a bag-valve-mask, laryngeal mask airway, or endotracheal intubation should be initiated to provide sufficient oxygen, ventilation, and airway protection in such cases. Endotracheal intubation is the most effective means by which you can isolate and protect the trachea from aspiration. Ensure that the pulse oximeter reading is higher than 90%. Provide oxygen via nasal cannula or mask as necessary. Provide ventilatory assistance as needed.

If the patient has trismus, determine how effectively the patient can be ventilated with a bag-valve-mask. If this is unsuccessful, consider using a paralytic agent to relax the mouth and allow for airway management. If paralytics are not available or are contraindicated and the patient can't be ventilated, transtracheal airway management is the only option of preventing hypoxia and death.

Administration of Naloxone

Naloxone (Narcan) is used for the treatment of unconscious patients or those with suspected narcotic overdose. The initial dose is 0.4 to 2.0 mg IV. You may repeat this dose until you reach 10 mg. This narcotic antagonist will compete with any circulating narcotic, displacing it from its receptors and allowing the LOC to increase. Naloxone can have quite a dramatic effect: Patients with a GCS score of 3 can move to a score of 15 within 30 seconds. This rapid change in LOC may cause patients to become fearful and potentially angry or aggressive. Make sure that you have the ability to leave the scene quickly *before* you administer naloxone. It may be advisable to push the drug in small increments until an improvement in LOC or respiration is noted, or administer some amounts via the IM route.

Airway management in relation to the narcotic overdose can also be tricky. Airway and ventilation are the focus of much of the care provided to unconscious patients. When you encounter a severely bradypnoeic, cyanotic patient, you reflexively want to establish an airway and intubate the patient quickly. When considering administering naloxone, however, a slightly different approach is recommended.

Ensure airway control and adequate ventilation but don't immediately intubate the patient. As you are oxygenating the patient, establish an IV and administer the naloxone carefully. Given the drug's quick onset of action and the potential for a dramatic response, an intubated patient may quickly wake up after the naloxone, grab the endotracheal tube, and yank it out.

The result of this violent extubation may be vocal cord or tracheal trauma. If the medication doesn't produce a response, then intubation may be needed.

Temperature Assessment

The patient's temperature can be difficult to determine in the prehospital environment. If you suspect hypothermia or hyperthermia, the standard of care is to use a thermometer to establish the patient's temperature. Oral, otic, transdermal, or rectal temperature can be measured. Avoid using the axillary method of measurement due to its inaccuracy.

Not all but most ambulance services have the ability to check a patient's temperature. In such a situation, you can still gather information about the history of present illness that can lead to a conclusion of temperature alteration. Was the patient in water for a long period of time? Has the patient been out in the snow? Did the patient fall and lie on the floor of a cold home, unable to get up for several days? In these cases, hypothermia should be considered. It would be reasonable to cover the patient in blankets and turn the heat up in the patient compartment.

Has the patient been out in the hot sun for several hours? Is the skin hot and dry? Is there a history of fever? In these cases, it would be prudent to remove the patient's clothing, place a sheet over the individual, and at least turn the heat off in the patient compartment.

Assessment and Management of Specific Injuries and Illnesses

Table 28-6 ▶ will help you better classify specific neurological conditions based first on the part of the nervous system they affect and then on the type of condition.

One way to manage these conditions is to try to create a patient profile that describes the circumstances that typically characterise a particular disease. How old is the typical patient? What sex and race is the patient? What are the common signs and symptoms of the condition? Are any unusual signs present that are uncommon in other conditions? How does the condition develop over time? If the patient profile indicates that men are more likely to be affected by the condition, remember that females may also suffer from it.

The patient profile is intended to distil the condition down to its core elements. You can use this valuable system to create flash cards that you can study. This summary of typical age, sex, race, history of present illness, signs and symptoms, and treatment will be provided for each condition discussed in the remainder of this chapter.

Stroke

Cerebrovascular events (CVEs) or strokes represent a serious medical condition in which the blood supply to areas of the brain becomes interrupted, resulting in ischaemia. Today

Table 28-6	Neurological Disease by Type of Condition	
Major System	**Disease**	**Type of Condition**
Central nervous system	Neoplasm	Cancer (malignant or benign)
	Alzheimer's disease	Degenerative
	Amyotrophic lateral sclerosis	Degenerative
	Parkinson's disease	Degenerative
	Cerebral palsy	Developmental
	Spina bifida	Developmental
	Abscess	Infectious
	Poliomyelitis	Infectious
	Dystonia	Various causes
	Headaches	Various causes
	Convulsions	Various causes
	Cerebral vascular events	Vascular
	Transient ischaemic events	Vascular
Peripheral nervous system	Bell's palsy	Infectious
	Guillain-Barré syndrome	Degenerative
	MS	Degenerative
	Myasthenia gravis	Degenerative
	Trigeminal neuralgia	Various
Muscles	Muscular dystrophy	Degenerative

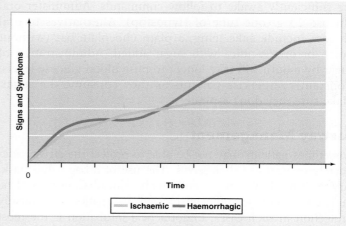

Figure 28-19 Symptom patterns for haemorrhagic versus ischaemic CVE.

nearly half of all patients who suffer from brain attacks or strokes deny their symptoms. Many will not activate ambulance services and subsequently delay seeking care. The goal of treatment is early recognition and rapid, appropriate intervention. The longer the CVE continues without intervention, the less likely the patient will have a promising outcome. "Time is neurons".

Two basic types of strokes are distinguished: ischaemic and haemorrhagic. **Figure 28-19 ▸** provides some insight into the evolution of strokes.

In 75% of cases, strokes are ischaemic rather than haemorrhagic. In ischaemic stroke, a blood vessel is blocked, so the tissue distal to the blockage becomes ischaemic. Eventually that tissue will die if blood flow is not restored. This pathology is self-limiting; only the tissue beyond the blockage is affected, so the areas of the brain involved are limited. The signs and symptoms eventually stop increasing and then plateau, indicating that the area of the brain involved is no longer working. The extent and severity of the stroke will be dictated by which artery is involved and which portion of the brain is denied oxygen. An ischaemic CVE to the brain stem is life-threatening.

In contrast, haemorrhagic CVEs tend to worsen over time due to bleeding within the cranium. This bleeding increases ICP and leads to herniation of the brain stem. One hallmark of

a haemorrhagic CVE is the "worst headache of my life" complaint. If the patient complains of a very severe headache, later cannot speak, becomes difficult to arouse, and finally shows signs of increased ICP, you should strongly consider a diagnosis of haemorrhagic CVE.

Patients with a suspected stroke or transient ischaemic attack (TIA; discussed in the next section) are usually older than age 65. Although men have more strokes, women die from them more often. Afro-Caribbeans experience twice as many incidences of stroke as Caucasians.

Presentation

Patients with stroke can exhibit a variety of signs and symptoms. Language effects may include slurred speech, dysphasia, agnosia, and apraxia. Movement effects—hemiparesis, hemiplegia, arm drifting, facial droop, ptosis, and ataxia—may be observed as well. Sensation effects may include headache (in haemorrhagic CVE), sudden blindness, and sudden unilateral paraesthesia. Consciousness problems, such as decreasing LOC, difficulty thinking, convulsions, and coma, may be noted. The patient may also develop hypertension.

Documentation and Communication

Patients with strokes can present a wide range of communication difficulties.
- Patients who are multilingual may lose understanding of only one language.
- Patients may be able to visually understand the written word but not the spoken word.
- Patients may not be able to understand any form of communication.
- Be open to trying various ways to communicate. Remember, communication problems do not indicate that the patient is not thinking, just that the patient can't get you to understand those thoughts.

Controversies

Traditionally within the United Kingdom patients are transported to the nearest receiving hospital. This is not always in the best interest of the patient. The CVE patient provides an excellent example of this potential dilemma.

Suppose a 62-year-old woman is having a stroke. Your assessment reveals left-sided weakness, slurred speech, and an arm drift (she has a positive FAST Score). These changes began around 08:15. It's now 08:45, and you are caring for the patient, who says that she has the worst headache of her life. She's getting very sleepy and becoming more difficult to arouse. You place the patient in the ambulance and begin transport to the local hospital, but the patient begins to have decorticate posturing. What should you do?

Appropriate care for this patient should include excellent airway management, initial hyperventilation, and rapid transport. But transport to where? Given the patient history, physical findings, and rapid deterioration of LOC, this patient appears to be suffering from a haemorrhagic CVE. If your working diagnosis is correct, she will ultimately need a facility capable of neurosurgery. Her family wants her to go to the closest hospital, which is 15 minutes away but does not have neurosurgery capability. The closest facility with immediate neurosurgery capability is 50 minutes away. Which is better for the patient: immediate transfer to a facility that may not be able to completely manage the patient or a lengthened transport time?

Your main objective is to provide quality care, which includes acting as a patient advocate. One way to advocate for quality patient care is to engage in discussions with your ambulance service's clinical director about the idea of triaging patients to appropriate hospitals. Before your discussion, you need to do your homework:

- Gather information about how different types of strokes present.
- Research haemorrhagic stroke and its care.
- Identify the capabilities of the local hospitals.
- Create a template guideline to be discussed with the clinical director.

During the conversation with the clinical director, control your emotions and be prepared to compromise. Speak from facts. Speak from good patient care. Whatever guideline or template you create, ensure that it leaves room for later modification. If you present yourself well, you'll pave the way for more responsibility as a paramedic and increased respect for the profession. You will also improve patient care.

When faced with a potential diagnosis of stroke, consider following the algorithm for management of patients with suspected stroke (**Figure 28-20 ▶**). The hospital will take different paths of care for each type of stroke. In any event, speedy treatment is essential. For ischaemic strokes, thrombolytics must be administered within 3 hours of onset of symptoms. In haemorrhagic stroke, the more the patient bleeds into the cranium, the greater the potential for increased ICP and brain stem damage.

Prehospital Management

Ambulance clinicians need to be involved in educating the community about stroke signs and symptoms, the effects of strokes, and the ambulance service. Too many patients deny their complaints or drive themselves to A&E departments. Reinforce with the public the common signs and symptoms of a stroke and how to activate the ambulance service in their community.

Prehospital care of the stroke patient should begin with the standard care outlined previously. Ensure adequate ABCs and blood pressure. Establish the patient's oxygen and glucose level. Establish IV access in case fluids or medications are needed.

During the assessment phase, use a stroke assessment tool such as the Face Arm Speech Test (FAST) (**Table 28-7 ▶**) to increase the accuracy of your working diagnosis. Rapid identification is imperative.

Complete a thrombolysis checklist. Focus on when the signs and symptoms started or when the patient was last seen without new complaints. In some cases, pinning down the exact time the stroke began can be very difficult, such as with patients who live alone. In those cases, ask family or care providers when the patient last seemed "normal". This checklist will allow you to gather information that the A&E department doctor will need before thrombolytics can be considered. Thrombolytics need to be administered within 3 hours of stroke onset. Don't administer aspirin in the prehospital environment; it will help the ischaemic CVE but compromise the haemorrhagic CVE. Aspirin should be administered only after a computed tomography (CT) scan or magnetic resonance imaging (MRI) has been completed in the hospital.

Protect any impaired limbs from injury. Patients may not be able to feel or move their arms or legs if they begin to get injured.

Identify an appropriate facility for transport—namely, a hospital with a stroke team that's trained in the administration of thrombolytics. Contact the facility to ensure that its CT/MRI scanner is operational. Some facilities will need to contact technicians to operate the scanners during night hours or weekends, so early hospital notification to the A&E department can decrease the time until the patient gets scanned. If the patient

Documentation and Communication

Stroke documentation points:
- When did the patient last seem "normal"?
- When did the signs and symptoms begin?
- Was there any change in the patient during transport?
- Document the reason for the choice of hospital.

Recognition of Stroke/TIA Symptoms

i.   Every opportunity should be taken to raise awareness of stroke symptoms, particularly in high risk groups, eg, people with: hypertension, atrial fibrillation, previous vascular events and diabetes.
ii. For suspected stroke call an emergency ambulance.
iii. Stroke classically presents with the **SUDDEN** onset of neurological loss eg, one or more of: limb weakness, difficulty speaking or understanding speech, loss of vision, clumsiness or numbness of arms or legs. For suspected stroke, use the **FAST** test (Table 28-7).

Prehospital Management of Stroke

i.   Assess **A**irway, **B**reathing, **C**irculation, and **D**isability.
ii.   If conscious sit up.
iii. Patients should be nil by mouth.
iv.   An informant should be encouraged to accompany the patient.
v.   All medication should be brought with the patient.
vi.   Give oxygen to maintain saturation over 95%.
vii. Blood glucose should be measured, and if < 3 mmol/l, 100 ml 10% glucose (Dextrose) should be administered via IV cannula.
viii. Repeat FAST.
ix.   Actively manage hypotension by giving saline and/or raising the foot of the trolley.
x.   Perform 12-lead ECG.
xi.   History of event, including time of onset, signs and symptoms and previous medical, drug, and social history, should be taken from patient and/or informant.
xii. If patient suitable for thrombolysis, pre-alert the nearest specialist centre.

Investigation and Management of Patients With Suspected TIA

The risk of developing a stroke after a hemispheric TIA can be as high as 30% within the first month, with the greatest risk being within the first 72 hours.

i.   Patients first seen in the community with TIA, or with a stroke but having made a good recovery when seen, should be assessed and investigated in a specialist service (eg, neurovascular clinic), as soon as possible and certainly within 7 days of the incident
ii. Patients likely to have a diagnosis of TIA should be prescribed an antiplatelet regime immediately.
iii. Patients likely to have a diagnosis of TIA should be advised not to drive until assessed by a specialist.
iv. Patients should be advised to go to hospital immediately should the symptoms return.
v.   **Immediate admission** to a specialist stroke service is vital for those with a greater than 20% risk of developing a completed stroke. These are patients with more than one TIA in 7 days or who have three or more of the following characteristics: blood pressure greater than 140/90 mm Hg; unilateral weakness or speech disturbance; symptoms lasting 60 minutes or more; or those who have diabetes.

Figure 28-20 Algorithm for management of patients with suspected stroke.

Modified from the Royal College of Physicians: Recognition and Emergency Management of Suspected Stroke and TIA. Used with permission.

Table 28-7	Face Arm Speech Test (FAST)		
Facial movements	Ask the patient to smile or show teeth.	Look for *new* lack of symmetry.
Arm movements	Ask the patient to lift their arms together and hold.	Does one arm drift or fall down?
Speech	If the patient attempts a conversation.	Look for *new* disturbances of speech.
Test all three	If one or more is abnormal.	Suspect stroke.

is rapidly decompensating or you suspect a potential CVE, consider transport to a hospital that can do neurosurgery.

Transient Ischaemic Attack

Transient ischaemic attacks (TIAs) are episodes of cerebral ischaemia that do not inflict any permanent damage. Any of the typical presentations associated with a CVE can occur with TIAs, but the TIA signs and symptoms resolve within 24 hours without any residual damage to brain tissue. These ministrokes are often signs of a serious vascular problem that requires medical evaluation. More than one third of patients with TIAs will suffer a CVE soon afterward.

As with strokes, management of TIAs begins with standard care. Follow the same management guidelines as for CVE. Close neurological assessment is needed. Patients may experience multiple TIAs in a short timeframe—coming and going.

Strongly encourage the patient to let you take him or her to hospital. If the individual refuses transportation, appeal to the patient's family for assistance. Encourage the patient to seek medical care very soon. It is important to reinforce the message that the TIA is a warning sign of a very serious and potentially deadly problem with the blood vessels within the brain. In fact, hypertension is the number one preventable cause of strokes and TIAs. Encourage the patient to talk with his or her doctor about blood pressure control and to take any anti-hypertensive medications prescribed.

Notes from Nancy

Just because the patient is a known alcoholic or because his breath smells of alcohol, it does not mean that he cannot be in a coma from other causes.

Special Considerations

Many medications can alter LOC. Explore all medications that the patient is taking, including prescription, non-prescription, herbal, supplements, homeopathic substances, and illegal drugs. Older patients may have many doctors, many conditions, and many medications. Combinations of medications can result in unexpected neurological effects.

You are the Paramedic Part 4

During transport, the patient's condition did not change. You continue to monitor his mental state, vital signs, and deficits while en route to hospital. You provide a pre-alert call to the receiving hospital, and deliver your patient to the A&E department without incident.

Reassessment	Recording Time: 15 Minutes
Level of consciousness	Alert, with a Glasgow Coma Scale score of 14
Skin	Pale, warm, and dry
Pulse	88 beats/min, strong and irregular
Blood pressure	140 by palpation
Respirations	24 breaths/min
SpO_2	100% on 15 l/min via nonrebreathing mask

8. What other important considerations relate to total patient care?

Altered Level of Consciousness/Coma

Altered mental status has many possible causes, so these calls are relatively common. One way to remember the most common causes is to use the mnemonic AEIOU-TIPS (Alcohol/acidosis, Epilepsy, Insulin, Overdose, Uraemia, Trauma, Infection, Psychosis, and Stroke). As with most medical complaints, the history of present illness is vital to identifying the underlying cause of the patient's complaints. An easy approach is to determine when the patient was last seen functioning normally.

Presentation

Evaluate the speed of onset for the altered LOC; this may help distinguish its cause. It is very rare that a person would be absolutely healthy one minute and be unresponsive from infection the next, for example. By contrast, convulsions can cause unresponsiveness almost instantly. The common signs and symptoms for altered LOC/coma are thought effects (decreasing LOC, confusion, hallucinations, delusions, psychosis, difficulty thinking, being unusually sleepy), speech effects (slurred speech, agnosia, apraxia, dysphasia), movement effects (ataxia, convulsions, posturing), and total unresponsiveness or coma.

Prehospital Management

In the case of altered LOC, care proceeds in two stages. First, the paramedic needs to support vital functions, including securing and maintaining ABCs. Second, the paramedic needs to gather information about the possible cause of the altered LOC. Determine past medical history, evaluate medications, look for signs of trauma, and determine the history of present illness. Does the patient have a medic alert bracelet? Was drug paraphernalia found near the patient? How was the patient acting before you were called?

In-hospital care will focus on supporting ABCs and attempting to discover the underlying problem. Patients will routinely need blood and urine specimens, radiographs, and CT/MRI scans.

Convulsion

Convulsions involve sudden, erratic firing of neurons. Patients who have epilepsy commonly have convulsions, for example. Patients may experience a wide array of signs and symptoms when having convulsions, ranging from one hand shaking or having a taste of pennies in the mouth to movement of every limb or the complete loss of consciousness. They may be aware of the convulsion, or they may wake up afterward not knowing what happened.

The paramedic should try to determine the cause of the convulsion. In particular, ask about medication compliance. Phenytoin, lorazepam, carbamezapine, and valproate are common anti-convulsant medications, but patients may be taking them at insufficient strengths to prevent convulsions. Patients may feel that they are cured because they haven't suffered a convulsion in many months, and stop taking their medications. Children may outgrow their anti-convulsant dosage. Older patients may be unable to afford the medication.

Infants who have a fever may suffer a febrile convulsion. Diabetics may have low blood glucose levels which can cause convulsions. Knowing the cause will help direct management. Table 28-8 ▾ lists many of the causes of convulsions.

Classification of Convulsions

Convulsions can be classified as generalised (affecting large portions of the brain) or partial (affecting a limited area of the brain). The classifications of convulsions are outlined in Table 28-9 ▸ .

Within the category of generalised convulsions are the grand mal and petit mal types. Grand mal convulsions, normally called tonic/clonic convulsions, present the paramedic with the most challenges. Most tonic/clonic convulsions follow a pattern, travelling through each of the following steps in order, although sometimes skipping a step:

1. **Aura.** A sensation the patient experiences before the convulsion occurs (eg, muscle twitch, funny taste, seeing lights, hearing a high-pitched noise).
2. **Loss of consciousness.**
3. **Tonic phase.** Body-wide rigidity.
4. **Hypertonic phase.** Arched back and rigidity.
5. **Clonic phase.** Rhythmic contraction of major muscle groups. Arm, leg, head movement; lip smacking; biting; teeth clenching.
6. **Post-convulsion.** Major muscles relax, nystagmus may still be occurring. Eyes may be "rolled back".
7. **Postictal.** Reset period of the brain. This can take several minutes to hours before the patient gradually returns to the pre-convulsion LOC Figure 28-21 ▸ . During this time patients are often initially aphasic (unable to speak), confused or unable to follow commands, very emotional, and tired or sleeping. They may present with a headache. Gradually the brain will begin to function normally.

During the convulsing process, respirations may become very erratic, loud, and obviously abnormal. Alternately, the patient may stop breathing and become cyanotic. These periods

Table 28-8	Causes of Convulsions
■ Abscess	■ Idiopathic (no known cause)
■ AIDS	■ Inappropriate medication dosage
■ Alcohol	
■ Birth defect	■ Organic brain syndromes
■ Brain infections (meningitis, encephalitis)	■ Recreational drugs
	■ Stroke or TIA
■ Brain trauma	■ Systemic infection
■ Diabetes mellitus	■ Tumour
■ Fever	■ Uraemia (kidney failure)

Table 28-9 | Convulsion Classifications

Generalised Convulsions	Characteristics
Absence (petit mal) convulsion	■ Staring episodes or "absence spells", during which the patient's activity ceases; loss of motor control is uncommon, although eye blinking or lip smacking may occur. ■ Most common in children between 4 and 12 years of age; rarely occurs after age 20. ■ Typically lasts less than 15 seconds, after which the child's LOC immediately returns to normal.
Tonic/clonic (grand mal) convulsion	■ Characterised by a loss of consciousness, followed by generalised (entire-body) muscle contraction (tonic phase) alternating with rhythmic "jerking" movements (clonic phase). ■ Often preceded by an aura—a strange taste, smell, or other abnormal sensation—that warns the patient of the impending convulsion. ■ Can occur at any age. ■ Often lasts several minutes; may progress to status epilepticus—a prolonged convulsion or two consecutive convulsions without an intervening lucid interval. ■ Typically followed by a postictal phase, during which the patient is confused, appears sleepy, and may be agitated or combative.

Partial (Focal) Convulsions	Characteristics
Simple partial convulsion	■ Also referred to as focal motor or "Jacksonian March" convulsions. ■ Characterised by tonic/clonic activity localised to one part of the body; may spread and progress to a generalised tonic/clonic convulsion. ■ No aura or associated loss of consciousness.
Complex partial convulsion	■ Also referred to as temporal lobe or psychomotor convulsions. ■ Manifests as changes in behaviour (mood changes, abrupt bouts of rage). ■ Often preceded by an aura. ■ Usually lasts less than 1 to 2 minutes, after which patient quickly regains normal mental status (no postictal phase).

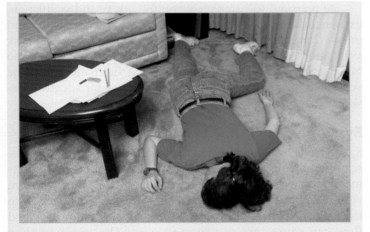

Figure 28-21 A patient who has had a convulsion may be found in the postictal state when you arrive. In such a case, ask family members or bystanders to verify that a convulsion has occurred and describe how the convulsion developed.

of apnoea are usually very short-lived and do not require assistance. If the patient is apnoeaic for more than 30 seconds, immediately begin ventilatory assistance. Another disconcerting aspect of convulsions, particularly for the patient, is incontinence.

In contrast to tonic/clonic convulsions, petit mal or absence convulsions present with little movement. The typical patient with absence convulsions is a child. Classically the child will simply stop moving; he or she may be walking and just stop, may be speaking and stop mid-sentence, or may be playing and freeze with a toy in the hand. The child will rarely fall. These convulsions usually last no more than several seconds. There is no postictal period and no confusion. These may be brought on by flashing lights or hyperventilation.

Partial convulsions may be classified as either simple partial or complex partial. Such convulsions involve only a limited portion of the brain. They may be localised to just one spot within the brain or they may begin in one spot and move in wave-like fashion to other locations. Such a Jacksonian March wave is akin to the ripples that occur from dropping a pebble in a still pond.

Simple partial convulsions involve either movement of one part of the body (frontal lobe) or altered sensations in one part of the body (parietal lobe). An example of a Jacksonian March in a simple partial convulsion would be shaking of the left hand, which moves to the left arm, then to the shoulder, then to the head, then to the right arm, then to the right hand, and finally stops. Complex partial convulsions involve subtle LOC changes. The patient may become confused, lose alertness, suffer hallucinations, or be unable to speak. The head or eyes may make small movements. Patients typically do not become unresponsive.

Prehospital Management

Most convulsions are self-limiting, so you simply need to monitor and protect patients from injuring themselves. Prehospital management of patients with convulsion begins with standard care. Quickly determine whether trauma is a concern.

- Where was the patient before the convulsion?
- What was the patient doing before the convulsion?
- How did the patient get to the current position?
- If the situation is unclear or there is confirmed trauma, perform manual in-line immobilisation.

Care during the convulsion includes calmness on your part. Don't restrain the patient or try to stop the convulsing movement. Prevent the patient from striking objects and becoming injured. Place nothing within the patient's mouth while the convulsion is ongoing. If bystanders have placed objects (eg, spoons, butter knives) in the mouth, remove them.

Provide ventilatory assistance only if the convulsion or apnoea is prolonged. Ventilation of the actively seizing patient will be very difficult. Oral or nasotracheal intubation will be next to impossible during a convulsion.

In the post-convulsion phase, emotional support is very important. Provide privacy. Speak calmly and slowly. Be prepared to repeat yourself. Reorientate the patient to place and time. If a child is febrile, encourage parents to administer an antipyretic (paracetamol or ibuprofen).

Unless a clear and easily reversible cause for the convulsion is found, all patients should be transported because convulsions can be a warning sign of more serious nervous system problems. If the patient has a known history of convulsions, he or she may not wish to go to the hospital. Advise the patient to follow up with the family doctor within 24 hours. A person with diabetes who is awakened after glucose administration may not wish to go to hospital. Advise this patient to eat a good meal and follow up with the family doctor.

Any patient who you suspect could develop convulsions should have the following care.

- Establish IV access. Diazepam and lorazepam are the drugs of choice to stop convulsions. In patients who are having a convulsion and in whom IV access cannot be established, diazepam can be administered rectally.
- Place blankets over the rails of the trolley.
- Place blankets over hard surfaces near the patient.
- Ensure that the patient's trolley straps are not too tight.

In-hospital management will seek to identify the cause of the convulsion. Blood studies, including drug and blood glucose determinations, will be done. CT or MRI scans may be performed.

Status Epilepticus

Status epilepticus is a convulsion that lasts for longer than 5 minutes or consecutive convulsions that occur without consciousness returning between convulsion episodes. This time frame is arbitrary, however, and some authors suggest that status epilepticus does not occur until 20 minutes of uninterrupted convulsing. Refer to your local guidelines for advice on how long a convulsion can continue before you should intervene.

During a convulsion, neurons are in a hypermetabolic state (using huge amounts of glucose and producing lactic acid). For a short period, this state does not produce long-term damage. If the convulsion continues, however, the body can't remove the waste products effectively or ensure adequate glucose supplies. Such a hypermetabolic state can result in neurons being damaged or killed. The goal of prehospital care is to stop the convulsion and ensure adequate ABCs.

Management of status epilepticus begins with standard care. Administer benzodiazepines (diazepam, 10 mg IV or PR). You may repeat diazepam after 5 minutes to a total dose of 20 mg. If you are unable to obtain IV access, you may give diazepam rectally.

Be prepared to completely control airway and ventilation, as benzodiazepines can cause respiratory depression and arrest. Continue to use airway positioning and bag-valve-mask ventilations until the convulsion stops. If benzodiazepines do not quickly control the convulsion and the patient can't be ventilated, paralytics may be needed to allow for adequate airway management.

Syncope

Syncope (fainting) is the sudden and temporary loss of consciousness with accompanying loss of postural tone. It affects mainly adults and accounts for nearly 3% of all A&E department visits. The brain uses glucose at a high rate and has no ability to store glucose, so even a 3- to 5-second interruption in blood flow can cause loss of consciousness. The question then becomes, What caused the sudden decrease in cerebral perfusion? **Table 28-10 ▶** lists the common causes of syncope.

Presentation

Classically, the patient with syncope is in a standing position when the event occurs. With young adults, the pattern is usually one of vasovagal syncope. The person will experience fear, emotional stress, or pain. Suddenly the room will seem to spin, and the individual will pass out. (This is why you should always seat a patient before drawing blood or starting an IV.) In older adults, cardiac arrhythmia is a more typical cause of syncope. The patient experiences a sudden run of ventricular tachycardia, the blood pressure drops, and the person falls to

Table 28-10	Causes of Syncope
Category	**Causes**
Cardiac rhythm	Bradycardia of any type Sick sinus syndrome Supraventricular tachycardia Torsade de pointes Transient asystole Transient ventricular fibrillation Ventricular tachycardia
Cardiac muscle	Cardiomyopathy Myocardial infarction
Others	Dehydration Hypoglycaemia Vasovagal

Table 28-11	Differentiating Syncope from Convulsion	
Characteristic	**Syncope**	**Convulsion**
Position of patient before event	Standing	Any position
Prodromal signs and symptoms	Dizziness, visual changes, shortness of breath, weakness	Aura: funny taste, seeing lights, hearing sound, twitching
Activity during event	Relaxed	Generalised body movement
Response after event	Quick return of orientation	Slow return of orientation

the floor. The rhythm terminates, the blood pressure rises, and the individual regains consciousness. In either case, the whole process takes less than 60 seconds.

Patients with syncope usually experience prodrome, signs or symptoms that precede a disease or condition. For syncope, prodromal complaints include feelings of dizziness, weakness, shortness of breath, chest pain, headache, or visual disturbances. Incontinence is possible with syncope, though uncommon. Convulsions and syncope can be difficult to differentiate; Table 28-11 provides some guidelines for making this distinction.

Prehospital Management
Begin with standard care. Determine whether the patient may have experienced trauma during the fall, and take cervical spine precautions as needed. Focus on blood glucose level and likely cardiac causes. Obtain orthostatic vital signs if possible.

Provide emotional support, as syncope can be very embarrassing. Syncope can be a sign of life-threatening cardiac arrhythmias, stroke, or another serious medical condition. However, most syncope cases will result in the patient being discharged at scene.

Headache
Almost everyone has suffered a headache at one time or another. What exactly is hurting? The brain and skull don't have pain receptors. Headache pain originates from the nerves within the scalp, face, blood vessels, and muscles of the neck and head.

Several types of headaches may be identified. Muscle tension headaches—the most common type—are caused by life stress (tension) that results in residual muscle contractions within the face and head. The pain tends to occur on both sides of head and travels from back to front; it is a dull ache or squeezing in nature. The jaw, neck, or shoulders may be stiff or sore.

Migraine headaches are thought to be caused by changes in blood vessel size within the base of the brain. The patient may experience an aura (eg, seeing bright lights) and unilateral, focused pain that then spreads over time. The pain is throbbing, pounding, or pulsating in nature. Nausea or vomiting may be present. These patients prefer dark, quiet environments. Migraines can last several days.

Cluster headaches are rare vascular headaches that start in the face. They occur in groups or clusters. They last only 30 to 45 minutes, but a patient may have several each day. The headaches may recur for days and then stop entirely. They may return the next month. The pattern consists of minor pain around one eye, pain that quickly intensifies and spreads to one side of the face, and a feeling of anxiety.

Sinus headaches are caused by inflammation or infection within the sinus cavities of the face. The pain, which is located in the superior portions of the face, increases with bending the head forward. It's worse when first waking. The patient may have a sore throat and nasal discharge.

Other, rare types of headaches include those caused by tumours, inflammation of the temporal artery, strokes, CNS infections, or hypertension. Their presentations vary depending on the underlying cause.

Headaches can be frustrating calls for ambulance clinicians. Many may feel that such calls are a waste of ambulance resources—at least, until they experience a migraine of their own Figure 28-22 . One problem faced by paramedics is that the complaint is entirely subjective; there is no way to "prove" the person is or is not having a severe headache. Try to determine the patient's level of stress, possible infections, and history of headaches. The patient can have various locations and intensity of pain, and may have nausea, vomiting, or light and sound phobia.

The majority of patients have real pain and need assistance from the ambulance service. Others, however, may be drug-seeking, addicted, or abusing medications. Here are some clues to drug-seeking behaviour:

- Does the patient have a history of calling 999 for headaches?
- Do the patient's allergies limit him or her to a small number of narcotic medications?
- Is the patient very reluctant to try other pain management options besides narcotics?
- Does the patient suddenly relax after being told that narcotics are on the way?

No single presentation characteristic should lead you to classify the patient as drug-seeking. Instead, consider the entire

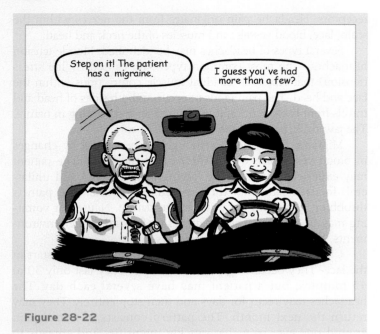

Step on it! The patient has a migraine.

I guess you've had more than a few?

Figure 28-22

environment. What has the patient done to manage this headache? When did it start? How bad is it? Even if you suspect drug-seeking behaviour, it would be inappropriate to withhold medication from the patient. Upon arrival at the hospital, relay your concerns to A&E department personnel in a fact-based conversation. Point out specifics of behaviour, comments, history, and other factors that have led you to suspect possible drug-seeking.

Be cautious, as headaches can indicate a more serious problem. Give standard care. Consider stroke, abscess, tumour, hypertension, and CNS infections. Ask which medications the patient has taken. Many patients will appreciate a darkened, quiet environment, so don't use lights and sirens if transporting. Medications for pain management may include metoclopramide and morphine. Also consider cyclizine for nausea or vomiting. In-hospital management would include analgesics and ruling out serious medical problems.

Abscess

Abscesses result when an infectious agent invades the brain or spinal cord. The bacteria or fungi then attack brain cells and destroy tissue. In response, the immune system attempts to kill the infectious agent but fails to do so. To prevent the bacteria or fungi from spreading, the body erects a barrier around the area. The area within the barrier contains the infectious agent, dead or dying brain cells, dead white blood cells, and white blood cells that continue fighting the infection. Over time, with the continued destruction of tissue and the immune system's ongoing attempts to kill the agent, swelling can occur.

The underlying cause of an infection within the brain may be an infection of the sinuses, throat, gums, or ears that has spread. The organism can also be injected during trauma to the

head. Such an infection has two major consequences: damage to the brain tissue and the presence of an abscess within the cranial vault that leads to increased ICP. These two factors may result in low- or high-grade fever, persistent headache (often localised), drowsiness, confusion, general or focal convulsions, nausea and vomiting, focal motor or sensory impairments, and hemiparesis. Abscess usually occurs in people younger than 50 years of age and has a gradual onset.

Prehospital management starts with standard care. Although no specific care is available for the abscess patient in the prehospital setting, the paramedic needs to pay close attention for evidence of increased ICP. Look for changes in LOC, respiratory patterns, and posturing. If needed, begin hyperventilation. Notify the hospital of the critical nature of your patient. Take convulsion precautions and be ready to administer diazepam if needed.

In-hospital management will likely involve antibiotics, convulsion precautions, and potentially surgical removal of the abscess.

Multiple Sclerosis

Multiple sclerosis (MS) is an autoimmune condition in which the body attacks the myelin sheath of the neurons in the brain and spinal cord, leading to areas of scarring. This disease is more prevalent in temperate regions than in tropical regions. Some evidence suggests that an environmental trigger—perhaps a virus, although none have been identified—begins to focus the attention of the immune system on the myelin. MS typically affects people between the ages of 20 and 40.

The presentation of MS follows a pattern of attacks and remissions. The attacks can vary in intensity and the remissions can vary in length. Patients may recover or have long-term complaints. In the initial attack, double vision and blurred vision are common complaints. Other symptoms include muscle weakness; impairment of pain, temperature, and touch senses; pain (moderate to severe); ataxia; intension tremors; speech disturbances; vision disturbances; vertigo; bladder or bowel dysfunction; sexual dysfunction; depression; euphoria; cognitive abnormalities; and fatigue during attacks.

Prehospital management is supportive. Give standard care. In-hospital treatment will be directed at controlling the symptoms. Anti-inflammatory medications may be administered to decrease the length of the attack. There is currently no cure for MS.

Neoplasm

For the purposes of this chapter, a neoplasm is defined as cancer within the brain or spinal cord. Two basic types of cancer are identified: primary and metastatic. Primary neoplasms begin within the nervous system. Metastatic neoplasms begin in some other part of the body, gain access to the bloodstream or lymphatic system, and then take up residence within the nervous system. Lung and breast cancers are the cancers that most commonly metastasise to the CNS. Once mature, neurons no longer divide, so only rarely do they become cancerous.

Primary CNS cancers are usually caused by mitosis errors in the support structures of the CNS.

Headache, nausea and vomiting, convulsions, changes in mental status, and stroke-like signs and symptoms are common in cases of neoplasm. The rate and intensity of these signs and symptoms depend on the cancer's growth rate and location. Patients may have months of headaches, or suddenly experience a convulsion without any prior complaints.

Prehospital management is supportive. Watch for status epilepticus and increased ICP. All patients with new-onset convulsions or chronic headaches that cannot be managed need medical evaluation. In-hospital management is complex and depends on the type of cancer and location.

Dystonia

Dystonia are marked by severe, abnormal muscle spasms that cause bizarre contortions, repetitive motions, or postures. These movements are involuntary and often painful. The initial episode usually occurs before the patient is in his or her 40s. Sudden onset may be precipitated by stress or continuous use of a muscle group. Patients tend to have normal intelligence and no psychiatric medical history.

Dystonia is both a sign and a condition. Some patients who take antipsychotic medications may suffer a sudden onset of bizarre contortions of the face or body; this is considered a secondary dystonia. Primary dystonias occur for unknown reasons, although a defect in the body's ability to process neurotransmitters is thought to lie at the heart of this problem. Spasmodic torticollis is a primary dystonia in which the neck muscles contract, twisting the head to one side and pulling it forward or backward. The head then remains painfully frozen in that position.

Prehospital management should focus on ruling out other problems such as convulsions, strokes, or psychiatric medication reaction. If you suspect a dystonic reaction to antipsychotics, benadryl is the drug of choice to stop the contraction. Unfortunately, this medication is ineffective in primary dystonias. Give standard care. Regardless of the underlying cause, dystonias are socially upsetting as patients suddenly twist and writhe uncontrollably. Providing compassionate care is critical. In-hospital management involves a variety of medication options to control the condition. There currently is no cure for dystonia.

Parkinson's Disease

In Parkinson's disease, the substantia nigra (the portion of the brain that produces dopamine) becomes damaged. Dopamine is the neurotransmitter that, among other things, ensures smooth muscular contractions. Parkinson's disease symptoms have a gradual onset that spans months to years. The initial signs are often unilateral tremors. Over time, as dopamine levels fall, more areas of the body become involved. Genetics play an important role in this disease. Parkinson-like activity can be observed in head injuries and some overdose patients, in which progression of the symptoms occurs more rapidly. The average age of onset is 60 years, and more men are affected than women.

The classic presentation of Parkinson's disease includes four characteristics: tremor, postural instability, rigidity, and bradykinesia. Rest tremors and postural tremors are also common. Other symptoms include depression, dysphagia, speech impairments, and fatigue. Prognosis is poor as the condition advances. Patients in later stages are at a much greater risk of death from aspiration, pneumonia, falls, or complications due to immobility.

Prehospital management involves standard care and emotional support. In-hospital management will include levodopa, which may temporarily restore dopamine levels. Other medications, surgery, and modification of diet and exercise are also options.

Trigeminal Neuralgia

Trigeminal neuralgia, also called tic douloureux, is an inflammation of the trigeminal nerve (fifth cranial nerve). The trigeminal nerve receives sensory information from the face. The usual cause of trigeminal neuralgia is irradiation by an artery lying too close to the nerve. Over time, as the artery changes diameter to meet blood supply needs, this motion grates the myelin sheath off the nerve. With its insulation gone, the nerve may "short out", causing pain without trauma to the area. Patients are usually older than age 50, and more women are affected than men.

Patients experience severe shock-like or stabbing pain, usually on one side of the face. These attacks can last for several minutes to several months. They may be triggered by touching the face, speaking, brushing the teeth, eating, putting on clothing, the wind—essentially any activity that stimulates the face. There is typically no loss of taste, hearing, or facial sensation with this condition. Likewise, there is no loss of motor control over the face, so facial droop, ptosis, and difficulty controlling the airway are very uncommon.

Although not life-threatening, this condition can be very debilitating. Patients experience severe pain. Some will stay indoors, eat softer foods, or stop washing their faces in an effort to prevent an attack. These patients need compassion and understanding.

You are the Paramedic Part 5

A CT scan showed a mild stroke in the parietal lobe. The patient was not a candidate for thrombolytics because the onset of his stroke couldn't be determined. He soon returned home with the support of his family and full-time nursing care. Because you were quick to recognise his stroke and transported him with the appropriate sense of urgency, the A&E department nurses and doctors were able to confirm the type of stroke promptly and begin appropriate care.

Prehospital care consists of standard care. Morphine may be indicated to help with pain management. Try to limit conversations to decrease facial movement. Administer oxygen if the patient is in respiratory distress or has a low pulse oximeter reading. Use of a nasal cannula or a nonrebreathing mask can instigate an attack. Even trying to administer blow-by oxygen could be painful to the patient. Long-term treatment for this condition is medication (carbamazepine or phenytoin) to calm the trigeminal nerve and sometimes surgery to place a barrier between the nerve and the artery.

Bell's Palsy

Bell's palsy is a temporary paralysis of the facial nerve (seventh cranial nerve). The facial nerve controls the muscles on each side of the face, including those used in eye blinking and facial expressions such as smiling and frowning. It also controls the tear glands and the saliva glands. Finally, the facial nerve transmits taste sensations from the tongue.

Patients typically experience a minor infection before Bell's palsy appears. The attack is very sudden and can easily be confused with a stroke. Signs and symptoms include ptosis, facial droop or weakness, drooling, and loss of the ability to taste. This condition strikes all races and both sexes equally. It is more common in middle-aged people (between 15 and 60 years old).

Bell's palsy will often resolve within 2 weeks. Prehospital management involves standard care. Make sure that these patients are not suffering from a stroke. Complete a full assessment. When in doubt, treat the case as if it were a stroke. In-hospital treatment for Bell's palsy includes corticosteroids (eg, prednisolone) and aciclovir, which helps manage viral infections.

Amyotrophic Lateral Sclerosis

Amyotrophic lateral sclerosis (ALS), also known as Lou Gehrig's disease, is a disease that involves the death of voluntary motor neurons, for unclear reasons. One theory suggests that the body's immune system selectively attacks and kills these motor neurons. Some evidence indicates that genetics may play a role. ALS is more common in middle-aged males of any race.

Initially, this condition is quite subtle and progresses without drawing notice. Fatigue, general weakness of muscle groups, and difficulty performing routine activities such as eating, writing, and dressing are early signs. Patients may also experience difficulty speaking. As ALS progresses, the patient loses his or her ability to walk, move the arms, eat, and speak. The speed of progression differs for every patient. Because this condition affects only the motor neurons, patients remain completely aware of their surroundings.

The average person who is diagnosed with ALS will die within 3 to 5 years. As the destruction of motor neurons continues, eventually patients are unable to breathe effectively without ventilatory assistance. Patients die of respiratory infections or other complications related to immobility.

Prehospital treatment for these patients is standard care. Assess the ability to swallow, and monitor the airway closely. Patients may be surrounded by a variety of home medical technology, including feeding pumps, IV pumps, long-term IV access ports, and ventilators. Transportation becomes complicated by the management of this technology. General guidelines include asking for guidance from the family or home health care provider related to the operation of the technology. If necessary, disconnect the patient from the technology, after consulting clinical support, and transport.

In-hospital care for ALS is geared toward supporting vital functions. Patients will undergo physical therapy to help strengthen their remaining neurons and muscles. Medications can be given to assist with some of the symptoms; however, there is no cure for ALS.

Guillain-Barré Syndrome

Guillain-Barré syndrome is a rare condition that is frightening for most patients. It begins as weakness and tingling sensations in the legs. This weakness moves up the legs and begins to affect the thorax and arms. It can quickly become severe and lead to paralysis. In fact, the transition from being able to walk and speak to needing a ventilator to breathe may take as little as several hours. Most patients will experience maximum muscle weakness and paralysis within 2 weeks.

The cause of this condition is unclear, although some degree of immune response appears to be present. Patients usually report having a minor respiratory or gastrointestinal infection prior to the onset of weakness. One theory is that the infectious agent creates a situation in which the body attacks its own neurons. This attack damages the myelin, thereby causing "shorting" of the signals travelling along the axon.

The reversal of this disease can be almost as dramatic as its onset. Some patients will have a complete recovery without residual weakness in just a few weeks. About one third retain some degree of weakness after 3 years. Some patients will require ventilatory assistance for the remainder of their lives.

Prehospital management includes standard care and close assessment of the patient's ability to protect the airway effectively and ventilate. Because of the sheer terror that patients can experience, a comforting voice and use of therapeutic touch are important.

In-hospital management includes plasmapheresis (exchanging the plasma within the blood) and immunoglobulin injections. These therapies decrease the time until recovery.

Poliomyelitis

Poliomyelitis is a viral infection that is transmitted by the faecal-oral route. Its incidence in the United Kingdom peaked in the 1950s, after which a very effective vaccine was developed. No cases of spontaneous polio infection have been reported in the United Kingdom since 1982, and polio will likely be eradicated worldwide within 10 years. The vast majority of patients who contract the virus do not become ill. Polio can occur at any age, but very young and older patients are at greatest risk. Signs and symptoms may begin as early as one week after infection. In the most severe cases, they include sore throat, nausea, vomiting, diarrhoea, stiff neck, and weakness or paralysis of muscles.

Prehospital management consists of standard care. In severe cases, patients will need ventilatory assistance. In-hospital care for patients with the acute illness is directed at hydration, ventilation, and calorie support until the immune system gains control over the infection.

The way the virus damages the nervous system places patients at risk of problems decades after the initial infection. In the initial infection, the virus attacks motor neurons within the brain and brain stem, which causes the classic signs of weakness and paralysis. The remaining neurons then begin to send out new axons to try to compensate for this loss, which allows the patient to regain function. Over time, these neurons maintain their unusually high workload. When they begin to break down and die, the patient may develop postpolio syndrome. As a consequence, some patients who suffered polio in the early part of the 20th century (most are older than 60 years) are now having difficulty swallowing, weakness, fatigue, or breathing problems. Typically, wherever patients had symptoms when they were originally infected, they experience symptoms again, albeit in a milder form. Prehospital treatment is standard care, with emphasis on possible airway obstruction due to swallowing difficulties. In-hospital treatment includes physiotherapy and experimental medications.

Cerebral Palsy

Cerebral palsy (CP) is a developmental condition in which damage occurs to the brain (often the frontal lobe). Although it was believed that perinatal (around the time of birth) hypoxia was the primary cause, research has shown that this actually accounts for less than 10% of cases. Infections, jaundice, or Rh incompatibility also appear to be possible causes. The condition is self-limiting and does not worsen over time. Babies who are low birth weight, premature, delivered breech, or from multiple births (eg, twins or triplets) are at higher risk for CP.

The presentation of CP begins in infancy. Developmental milestones such as walking or crawling may be delayed. The type and extent of damage soon become apparent. In spastic CP (70% to 80% of cases), the muscles are in a near-constant state of contraction. If both lower legs are affected, patients will have a classic scissors walk in which the lower legs turn inward, with the legs remaining stiff and the knees almost touching. Other types of CP involve slow, uncontrolled writhing movements; tremors; or difficulties with coordination.

Prehospital management is supportive. Provide standard care. Patients may have ambulatory assistive devices (eg, wheelchairs, crutches, canes, leg braces) that will need to be transported along with them. In-hospital management is based on the particular set of symptoms. There is no cure or correction for the damage. Instead, care is directed at maximising the child's abilities through surgery on affected limbs and physiotherapy and occupational therapy.

Spina Bifida

Spina bifida is a developmental condition resulting from a neural tube defect. Because the neural tube does not close (for unknown reasons), a portion of the spinal cord remains outside its normal location. The severity of the condition depends on where the defect lies on the cord and how much it is displaced from normal. In spina bifida occulta, one small section of vertebrae is malformed and slightly displaced. The mildest form of spina bifida, it rarely has any significant clinical features and patients may not even know the malformation is present. In the most severe form, known as myelomeningocele, a portion of the spinal cord remains completely outside the vertebral column and outside of the skin. There are also two intermediary forms of spina bifida.

Consequences of spina bifida can range from no complications to complete loss of motor and sensory functions below the defect. Patients may have muscle problems ranging from mild defects to paralysis, experience convulsions, or have severe neurological impairments. In the most severe forms, the defect interferes with normal movement of CSF. CSF is made within the brain, circulates, and is then reabsorbed. Hydrocephalus (water on the brain) is common in severe spina bifida because the CSF continues to be produced but cannot circulate effectively. Pressure builds within the brain, causing increased ICP problems and convulsions.

The ambulance service may be called for problems with spina bifida patients related to medical technology, convulsions, trauma, or infections. Prehospital management is standard care. Be aware that many of these patients have latex allergies. In the most severe cases of spina bifida, children are in need of multiple types of medical technology, including feeding tubes, long-term IV access, ventilatory support, ambulatory assistive devices, and intraventricular shunts (designed to drain excess CSF from within the brain's ventricles). To avoid complications, consult with family and other home health care personnel when attempting to transport the patient. In-hospital management will be supportive. It is possible to reimplant the spinal cord, even while the fetus remains within the uterus, but the damage to the nerve tissue is permanent.

Myasthenia Gravis

Acetylcholine is an important neurotransmitter needed to allow for muscular contraction. In myasthenia gravis, the body creates antibodies against the acetylcholine receptors. The thymus gland (where T-cells mature) is believed to play a role in the production of these antibodies. As acetylcholine levels fall, muscle weakness begins. This weakness most commonly affects the eyes, eyelids, and facial muscles. Some patients will have difficulty swallowing or speaking, or leg or arm weakness. Patients suffer no sensory impairment. Myasthenia gravis usually affects women younger than 40 and men older than 60.

Myasthenia crisis is a sudden increase in the destruction of acetylcholine, resulting in weakness in the respiratory muscles. As a result, patients can become hypoxic. Infections, emotional stress, or reactions to medications can trigger this crisis.

Standard care will manage these patients effectively in the prehospital environment. Be prepared to assist with ventilations in patients with crisis. In-hospital management includes removal of the thymus gland, medications to boost neurotransmitter levels, and immunosuppressants.

Alzheimer's Disease

Alzheimer's disease (discussed in more detail in Chapter 42) is the most common form of dementia. Dementia is a chronic deterioration of a person's personality, memory, and ability to think. Alzheimer's disease is a progressive organic condition in which neurons die; there is no definitive treatment for the destroyed neurons. Prehospital management is standard care.

Peripheral Neuropathy

Peripheral neuropathy comprises a group of conditions in which the nerves leaving the spinal cord become damaged. As a consequence, the signals moving to or from the brain become distorted. Causes of peripheral neuropathy include trauma, toxins, tumours, autoimmune attacks, and metabolic disorders. Trigeminal neuralgia and Guillain-Barré syndrome are examples. The remainder of this discussion focuses on the most common form, diabetic neuropathy. Diabetic neuropathy is frequently seen in diabetic patients older than age 50; more males than females are affected. Its onset is gradual, occurring over months and years.

As blood glucose levels rise, the peripheral nerves may become damaged, resulting in misfiring and shorting of signals. Affected individuals may then experience sensory or motor impairment. Loss of sensation, numbness, burning sensations, pain, paraesthesia, and muscle weakness are common. Patients may eventually lose the ability to feel their feet or other areas.

Management in the prehospital setting is supportive. Provide standard care. In-hospital management will include pain medication. The use of antidepressants and anti-convulsants seems to have a positive effect on calming the peripheral nerves.

Muscular Dystrophy

Muscular dystrophy (MD) is a nonneurological condition of genetic origin marked by the degeneration of muscular tissue. The defective DNA causes an error in muscle tissue, such that the malformed muscle cells rupture more easily. MD is diagnosed at age 2 to 5 years and occurs only in males. Its onset is gradual, with progression over months to years.

Several forms of MD exist, each distinguished by the involvement of a particular gene and a unique set of characteristics. Generally, MD presents with progressive muscle weakness, delayed development of muscle motor skills, ptosis, drooling, and poor muscle tone. The most common type of MD, Duchenne's, manifests itself in childhood and can include damage to the respiratory and cardiac muscles. These patients have a much shortened life expectancy, rarely living beyond their middle 20s. They often die from pneumonia or cardiogenic shock.

Standard care is effective in these patients. In severe cases, ventilatory support may be necessary. Blood pressure support may be required; fluids and dopamine may be needed to manage damaged heart muscle. These severely ill patients will have extensive use of home medical technology. In-hospital management is supportive, as there is no cure for MD.

Conclusion

Neurological patients can present a major challenge to the paramedic. To avoid becoming overwhelmed, follow a methodical and systematic approach to the assessment and care of these patients. Use the same format for all of your physical examinations. Focus your care on providing an environment that will facilitate optimal nervous system functioning. Reassess the patient after your interventions to note any changes. You are part of a health care team, so be aware of how your care will affect later activities within the A&E department. Know the material within this book. When you have mastered this information, you should be able to provide your patients with the highest level of care and your profession with an example of excellence.

You are the Paramedic Summary

1. What do you suspect as the reason(s) why Mr Harris is on the floor?

This patient could be on the floor for any number of reasons, including but not limited to a syncopal episode, loss of balance with a fall, sudden onset of weakness, or exacerbation of an underlying medical condition. At this point, there are many possibilities, which will require further investigation in both history-taking and physical assessment.

2. How would you prioritise those reasons?

As a paramedic, it's your job to recognise and treat life-threatening conditions. In some instances, definitive care can be provided; in other cases, treatment options are limited. With some underlying traumatic and medical emergencies, your job is to simply recognise the signs and symptoms, provide prompt transport to the nearest appropriate hospital, and initiate supportive care without delay to definitive care.

3. Given the information you have now, what do you think could be this patient's underlying illness, injury, or condition?

Given the new information obtained, you believe the patient is experiencing a CVE. This life-threatening condition requires immediate recognition and prompt transport. There is no sure way of knowing what sort of stroke this patient is experiencing, so the goal of the paramedic is to ensure the fastest possible time to the hospital.

4. Do your assessment and treatment priorities ever change?

Although concern with ABCs is first, assessment and treatment priorities must be flexible to avoid tunnel vision and misappropriate prehospital diagnosis. At first, the patient appeared to have confusion most likely as a result of a low blood glucose level. After you assessed his blood glucose level and found it to be within appropriate levels, your overall impression changed, causing you to consider other reasons for his decreased LOC.

5. What are appropriate interventions?

Appropriate care would include placing the patient on high-flow oxygen, obtaining an ECG, initiating at least one IV for the purposes of collecting blood samples and providing a port for administration of thrombolytics if deemed necessary by A&E department staff, and completing a thrombolysis checklist prior to arrival at the hospital.

6. Would you choose to place this patient in manual in-line spinal precautions?

Keeping in mind that "time is neurons", you'll have to make the determination as to whether to place the patient in spinal precautions. If the mechanism of injury indicates risk for spinal fracture, if you are unsure, or if your local guidelines dictate it, you should immobilise this patient. As with any intervention, you should consider whether this step is appropriate.

7. What places this patient at greater risk for cerebrovascular event?

His history of atrial fibrillation places your patient at greater risk for ischaemic stroke. Clots could develop in his atria and travel to the brain, resulting in stroke.

8. What other important considerations relate to total patient care?

For patients who are unable to communicate, this experience can be quite frustrating and frightening. If possible, use other forms of communication. If you are unable to obtain information or understand the patient, do everything you can to ease his or her anxiety and fear.

Prep Kit

■ Ready for Review

- The nervous system is responsible for thought, judgement, personality, memory, emotions, voluntary motor activity, interpretation of sensory stimulation, and various autonomic activities within the body.
- Blood flow to the brain is described by the equation CPP = MAP – ICP.
- The nervous system is critical in maintaining airway control.
- Two abnormal postures that indicate brain damage in an unconscious patient are decorticate posturing (moving arms toward the core) and decerebrate posturing (moving arms away from body).
- Use the Glasgow Coma Scale to help determine a patient's level of consciousness, evaluate his or her responses to eye opening and verbal and motor skills, and guide care.
- Facial droop on one side of the face or a drooping eyelid can indicate a neurological condition.
- Problems such as slurring or difficulty recognising objects can signify a neurological problem. Three forms of language problems are receptive dysphasia, expressive dysphasia, and global dysphasia.
- Pupil shape, size, motion, and reactivity are indicators of nervous system functioning.
- Ask the patient to hold the arms out in front of the body and close the eyes. If one arm drifts away, the patient may have experienced a stroke.
- Abnormal, involuntary muscle contractions, such as tremors and convulsions, can indicate a neurological problem.
- Sensation can also be affected by nervous system conditions.
- The three major elements that the brain needs to function are oxygen, glucose, and normal temperature.
- Managing the neurological patient includes administering IV solutions, monitoring the ECG, checking blood glucose levels, managing intracranial pressure, evaluating the patient's temperature, and providing emotional support.
- You may be able to administer glucose or glucagon to treat low blood glucose levels, depending on your local guideline.
- Naloxone may be given to treat unconscious patients or those with suspected narcotic overdose.
- If you can't take the patient's temperature, use patient history to determine it. Don't actively warm or cool patients.
- Stroke is a serious medical condition in which blood supply to areas of the brain is interrupted. Ischaemic stroke results from a blocked blood vessel. Haemorrhagic stroke results from bleeding within the brain.
- Patients with stroke can be affected in their language, movement, sensation, level of consciousness, and blood pressure.
- Time is essential in managing strokes. Thrombolytics can be administered for ischaemic strokes, but must be administered within 3 hours of stroke onset.
- Stroke patients should be transported to hospitals trained in the administration of thrombolytics, and to hospitals with CT or MRI equipment.
- A TIA looks like a stroke but will resolve without damage; however, one third of patients with a TIA will eventually experience a stroke.
- Management of TIAs is the same as for stroke. Encourage the patient to be transported.
- Use the AEIOU-TIPS mnemonic to assess a patient with an altered level of consciousness. Evaluate the speed and onset. Common effects of altered LOC are changes in thought, speech, and movement. Total unresponsiveness can also result.
- Care for a patient with an altered LOC includes the ABCs and gathering information about the possible cause.
- Convulsions are the sudden erratic firing of neurons, generally characterised by involuntary shaking. They are classified as generalised (affecting large areas of the brain) or partial (affecting limited areas of the brain).
- Generalised convulsions include tonic/clonic and absence convulsions. Tonic/clonic convulsions generally consist of an aura, loss of consciousness, tonic/clonic movement, and the postictal phase.

- Absence convulsions involve little or no movement. Instead, the person—usually a child—simply "freezes".
- Partial convulsions are categorised as simple or complex. Simple partial convulsions involve movement or altered sensation in one part of the body. Complex partial convulsions involve subtle changes in level of consciousness.
- When caring for a patient with a convulsion, don't try to stop the movement. Prevent the patient from injuring himself or herself. Once the convulsion has ceased, provide care and emotional support.
- Status epilepticus is a convulsion that lasts for longer than 4 or 5 minutes or consecutive convulsions without return of consciousness between events.
- Care for a patient with status epilepticus includes administration of benzodiazepines and management of airway and ventilation.
- Syncope (fainting) is the sudden loss of consciousness and postural tone. It can be caused by cardiac problems, dehydration, hypoglycaemia, or a vasovagal reaction.
- Care for patient who experienced syncope includes standard care and emotional support.
- Types of headaches include muscle tension headaches, migraines, cluster headaches, sinus headaches, and headaches caused by a tumour, stroke, infections, hypertension, or inflammation of the temporal artery.
- Care for patients with headaches includes standard care, a thorough history, potentially medication administration, and providing a dark, quiet environment.
- An abscess is a walled-off infectious area within the cranial vault. Symptoms include a fever, persistent headache, drowsiness, confusion, general or focal convulsions, nausea and vomiting, focal motor or sensory impairments, and hemiparesis. Provide standard care.
- Multiple sclerosis is an autoimmune disorder that damages myelin of the brain and spinal cord. Patients can experience attacks and remissions, muscle weakness, changes in sensation, pain, ataxia, intension tremors, and speech and vision changes. Prehospital management is supportive.
- Neoplasm, for the purposes of this chapter, is cancer in the brain or spinal cord. It can have a gradual or sudden onset. Symptoms include headaches, convulsions, change in mental status, and stroke-like signs and symptoms. Prehospital care is supportive.
- Dystonia is the sudden onset of severe, sometimes painful, abnormal muscle contractions. Prehospital care involves ruling out other causes and administering chlorphenamine if you suspect the dystonia is a result of a reaction to antipsychotics.
- In Parkinson's disease, the brain cannot produce dopamine. These patients have tremors, bradykinesia, postural instability, and rigidity. Prehospital management is standard care.
- Trigeminal neuralgia is irritation of the trigeminal nerve. Patients experience severe electric shock-like pain in the face, which can be triggered by any activity that stimulates the face. Prehospital management is standard care.
- Bell's palsy is a temporary, sudden paralysis of the facial nerve triggered by an infection. The patient may have ptosis, facial droop, facial weakness, drooling, and loss of the ability to taste. Prehospital management is standard care.
- Amyotrophic lateral sclerosis is a disease in which the motor neurons die. It has a gradual onset with fatigue, weakness, ataxia, severe body-wide weakness, and eventual immobility. Prehospital management is standard care.
- Guillain-Barré syndrome is a rare condition characterised by a sudden onset of weakness and paraesthesia ascending from the toes to the head. Patients usually have an infection prior to the attack. Prehospital management is standard care with airway management.
- Poliomyelitis is a viral infection that attacks the myelin of motor neurons in the brain and brain stem. Symptoms include a sore throat, nausea, vomiting, diarrhoea, a stiff neck, and weakness or paralysis of muscles. Prehospital management is standard care with careful attention to the airway.

- Patients who had poliomyelitis in the past may develop postpolio syndrome later in life in which they experience the same symptoms as in the original infection, only milder.
- Cerebral palsy is a developmental condition in which the frontal lobe of the brain suffers damage. Infants may have developmental delays in walking and standing, muscles in constant contraction, a scissors walking gait, and tremors. Prehospital management is supportive.
- Spina bifida is a developmental condition in which the neural tube fails to close completely and part of the spinal cord or vertebrae are damaged and misplaced outside the normal position. Prehospital management is standard care.
- Myasthenia gravis is a condition in which the body creates antibodies against acetylcholine receptors, causing acetylcholine levels to fall. Symptoms include weakness of the face and eyes, difficulty swallowing, and leg weakness. Prehospital management is standard care.
- Peripheral neuropathy is a group of conditions characterised by damage to the peripheral nerves. Diabetic neuropathy occurs from high blood glucose levels. Patients may have paraesthesia, burning sensation, and muscle weakness. Prehospital care is supportive.
- Muscular dystrophy is a group of nonneurological conditions in which muscle tissue degenerates. It generally presents with progressive muscle weakness, delayed development of muscle motor skills, ptosis, drooling, and poor muscle tone. Prehospital management is standard care, possible with ventilatory support.

■ Vital Vocabulary

abscesses Areas created as a result of infection within the brain or spinal cord, in which brain cells have been attacked and tissue destroyed. The immune system erects a wall to prevent spread of the infection, which results in a pus-filled area buried in tissue.

adrenal glands Endocrine glands located on top of the kidneys that release adrenaline when stimulated by the sympathetic nervous system.

agnosia Inability to connect an object with its correct name.

Alzheimer's disease A progressive organic condition in which neurons die, causing dementia.

amyotrophic lateral sclerosis (ALS) Also known as Lou Gehrig's disease, this disease strikes the voluntary motor neurons, causing their death. It is characterised by fatigue and general weakness of muscle groups; eventually, the patient will not be able to walk, eat, or speak.

anaesthesia Lack of feeling within a body part.

anisocoria Unequal pupils (difference greater than 1 mm).

apraxia Inability to connect an object with its proper use.

ataxia Alteration in the ability to perform coordinated motions like walking.

aura Sensations experienced before an attack occurs. Common in convulsions and migraine headaches.

axon A projection from a neuron that makes connections with adjacent cells.

Bell's palsy A temporary paralysis of the facial nerve (7th cranial nerve), which controls the muscles on each side of the face.

bradykinesia The slowing down of voluntary body movements. Found in Parkinson's disease.

brain stem The area of the brain between the spinal cord and cerebrum, surrounded by the cerebellum; controls functions that are necessary for life, such as respirations.

central nervous system (CNS) The brain and spinal cord.

cerebellum The region of the brain essential in coordinating muscle movements of the body.

cerebral palsy (CP) A developmental condition in which damage is done to the brain. It presents during infancy as delays in walking or crawling, and can take on a spastic form in which muscles are in a near constant state of contraction.

cerebrovascular event (CVE) An interruption of blood flow to the brain that results in the loss of brain function.

clonic activity Type of convulsion movement involving the contraction and relaxation of muscle groups.

coma A state in which one does not respond to verbal or painful stimuli.

decerebrate posturing Abnormal extension of the arms with rotation of the wrists along with toe pointing. This indicates brain stem damage.

decorticate posturing Abnormal flexion of the arms toward the chest with the toes pointed. This indicates lower cerebral damage.

decussation Movement of nerves from one side of the brain to the opposite side of the body.

dementia The slow onset of progressive disorientation, shortened attention span, and loss of cognitive function.

diencephalon The part of the brain between the brain stem and the cerebrum that includes the thalamus, the subthalamus, hypothalamus, and epithalamus.

dystonia Contractions of the body into a bizarre position.

endotoxin A toxin released by some bacteria when they die.

exotoxin A toxin that is secreted by living cells to aid in the death and digestion of other cells.

expressive dysphasia Damage to or loss of the ability to speak.

gait Walking pattern.

Glasgow Coma Scale (GCS) Evaluation tool used to determine level of consciousness. Effective in determining patient outcomes.

global dysphasia Damage to or loss of both the ability to speak and the ability to understand speech.

Guillain-Barré syndrome A rare condition that begins as weakness and tingling sensations in the legs and moves to the arms and thorax; it can lead to paralysis within 2 weeks.

hemiparesis Weakness of one side of the body.

hemiplegia Paralysis of one side of the body.

haemorrhagic One of the two main types of stroke; occurs as a result of bleeding inside the brain.

hypothalamus The most inferior portion of the diencephalon, it is responsible for control of many bodily functions, including heart rate, digestion, sexual development, temperature regulation, emotion, hunger, thirst, and regulation of the sleep cycle.

idiopathic Of no known cause.

intension tremors Tremors that occur when trying to accomplish a task.

ischaemic One of the two main types of stroke; occurs when blood flow to a particular part of the brain is cut off by a blockage (eg, a clot) inside a blood vessel.

Jacksonian March The wave-like movement of a convulsion from a point of focus to other areas of the brain.

limbic system Structures within the cerebrum and diencephalon that influence emotions, motivation, mood, and sensations of pain and pleasure.

medulla oblongata The inferior portion of the midbrain, which serves as a conduction pathway for both ascending and descending nerve tracts.

midbrain The part of the brain that is responsible for helping to regulate level of consciousness.

multiple sclerosis (MS) An autoimmune condition in which the body attacks the myelin of the brain and spinal cord, leading to gaps in the insulation normally provided by the myelin, causing scarring.

muscular dystrophy (MD) A nonneurological condition of genetic origin in which defective DNA causes an error in the creation of muscle tissue, resulting in the degeneration of muscular tissue. This presents with progressive muscle weakness, delayed development of muscle motor skills, ptosis, drooling, and poor muscle tone.

myasthenia gravis A condition in which the body creates antibodies against the acetylcholine receptors, causing muscle weakness, often in the face.

myelin An insulating-type substance present in some neurons that allows the cell to consistently send its signal along the axon without "shorting out" or losing electricity to surrounding fluids and tissues.

myoclonus Jerking motions of the body.

neoplasms Tumours.

neurotransmitters Chemicals produced by the body that stimulate electrical reactions in adjacent neurons.

nystagmus The rhythmic shaking of the eyes.

paraesthesia Sensation of tingling, numbness, or "pins and needles" in a body part.

Parkinson's disease A neurological condition in which the portion of the brain responsible for production of dopamine is damaged or over-used, resulting in tremors.

peripheral nervous system (PNS) The part of the nervous system that consists of 31 pairs of spinal nerves and 12 pairs of cranial nerves. These nerves may be sensory nerves, motor nerves, or connecting nerves.

peripheral neuropathy A group of conditions in which the nerves leaving the spinal cord are damaged, resulting in distortion of signals to or from the brain. One type is diabetic, in which the peripheral nerves are damaged as blood glucose levels rise, causing loss of sensation, numbness, burning, pain, paraesthesia, and muscle weakness.

pituitary gland The gland that secretes hormones that regulate the function of many other glands in the body; also called the hypophysis.

poliomyelitis A viral infection that attacks the axons, especially motor axons, and destroys them, causing weakness, paralysis, and respiratory arrest. An effective vaccine has been developed and this disease is now rare.

pons The portion of the brain stem that lies below the midbrain and contains nerve fibres that affect sleep and respiration.

postictal The period of time after a convulsion during which the brain is reorganising activity.

postpolio syndrome A result of polio in which neurons break down and die, resulting in difficulty swallowing, weakness, fatigue, or breathing problems even after the patient has healed.

postural tremors Tremors that occur as the person holds a body part still.

prodrome The early signs and symptoms that occur before a disease or condition fully appear, eg, dizziness before fainting.

pronation Turning of the lower arms in a palm-downward manner.

psychosis Breaking with common reality and existing mainly within an internal world.

ptosis Drooping of an eyelid.

receptive dysphasia Damage to or loss of the ability to understand speech.

rest tremors Tremors that occur when the body part is not in motion.

spina bifida A development defect in which a portion of the spinal cord or meninges may protrude outside of the vertebrae and possibly even outside of the body, usually at the lower third of the spine in the lumbar area.

status epilepticus A condition in which convulsions recur every few minutes, or last more than 30 minutes.

synapses Gaps between nerve cells across which nervous stimuli are transmitted.

syncope Fainting spell or transient loss of consciousness.

tonic activity Type of convulsion movement involving the constant contraction and trembling of muscle groups.

transient ischaemic attack (TIA) A disorder of the brain in which brain cells temporarily stop working because of insufficient oxygen, causing stroke-like symptoms that resolve completely within 24 hours of onset.

trismus The involuntary contraction of the mouth resulting in clenched teeth. Occurs during convulsions and head injuries.

uraemia Severe kidney failure resulting in the buildup of waste products within the blood. Eventually brain functions will be impaired.

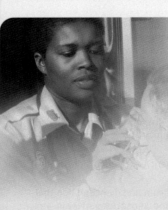

Assessment in Action

You're just walking in the door to start your shift when you are sent to a diabetic emergency. En route to the call, you are given an update: The patient is a 78-year-old man who is unconscious and unresponsive. On arrival, you find the patient supine on his bed. You notice that he has sonorous respirations; his skin is warm, dry, and normal in colour; blood pressure is 240/140 mm Hg; respirations are 24 breaths/min and shallow; pulse oximetry is 95% on room air; and heart rate is 78 beats/min. The patient has a left-side eye gaze and doesn't respond to painful or verbal stimuli.

When you speak with the family, they report that the patient woke up today with no complaints and took a shower. After the shower, he collapsed onto the bed. They called 999 at approximately 08:00 hrs. The patient has type 2 diabetes. You immediately perform a blood glucose check, which comes back as 10.6 mmol/l. The patient is unable to control his airway; however, his mouth is clenched shut and you are unable to insert an oral airway. While the patient is being transferred to the ambulance, his respiratory rate decreases, allowing you to insert an oral airway. You prepare to intubate the patient and ventilate him with 100% oxygen via a bag-valve-mask device. En route to the hospital, you successfully intubate and secure the endotracheal tube.

Arriving at the hospital, you give your report to the A&E department. When you go back to the department later that shift, you are told the patient had a "huge cerebellum bleed". His prognosis is poor and the A&E department staff is speaking with the family about removing him from the ventilator.

1. _____ is a serious medical condition in which blood supply to areas of the brain is interrupted, resulting in ischaemia.
   A. Myocardial infarction
   B. Pulmonary embolism
   C. Cerebrovascular event
   D. Bell's palsy

2. The two basic types of strokes are ischaemic and:
   A. neurological.
   B. haemorrhagic.
   C. pathologic.
   D. neoplasm.

3. A hallmark of a haemorrhagic CVE is the:
   A. "worst headache of my life".
   B. "worst chest pain of my life".
   C. "worst blurred vision of my life".
   D. "worst weakness of my life".

4. The nervous system is the most complex organ in the human body. It consists of two major structures—the_____ and_____—and thousands of nerves allowing every part of the body to communicate.
   A. brain, myocardium
   B. pulmonary, embolism
   C. brain, spinal cord
   D. spinal cord, myocardium

5. The major structures are divided into two main categories: the central nervous system and the:
   A. parasympathetic nervous system.
   B. sympathetic nervous system.
   C. peripheral nervous system.
   D. autonomic nervous system.

6. Weakness on one side of the body is called:
   A. hemiplegia.
   B. decussation.
   C. nystagmus.
   D. hemiparesis.

7. The _____ is located in the posterior, inferior area of the skull.
   A. medulla oblongata
   B. cerebellum
   C. midbrain
   D. cerebrum

8. The synapse, which is present wherever a nerve cell terminates, connects to the next cell through chemicals called:
   A. synapse.
   B. dendrites.
   C. neurotransmitters.
   D. axon terminals.

9. A hallmark of increased ICP is Cushing's triad, which means:
   A. bradycardia, bradypnoea, and widened pulse pressure.
   B. tachycardia, tachypnoea, and narrowing pulse pressure.
   C. bradycardia, tachypnoea, and widened pulse pressure.
   D. tachycardia, bradypnoea, and widened pulse pressure.

Challenging Questions

You're dispatched to a warden controlled flat for an 83-year-old woman with an altered mental status. When you arrive and the patient is speaking to you, she appears confused and repeats her statements. Her vital signs are all within normal limits: blood pressure, 130/70 mm Hg; heart rate, 84 beats/min; respiratory rate, 18 breaths/min; and pulse oximetry, 99% on room air. The staff taking care of her reports that she "hasn't been right all day". The paperwork provided to you by the staff is incomplete; however, the medication list is there and you see Aricept.

10. What type of medical history do you suspect based on this medication?

11. How should you care for this patient?

■ Points to Ponder

You and your colleague are sent to a private house for a convulsion. When you arrive on scene, you find a 24-year-old man who is responsive to verbal stimuli but is nonverbal. The family reports that the patient had a convulsion, which lasted approximately 3 minutes. It was a full-body, normal convulsion for the patient. He is in his normal postictal state as well. There is incontinence to urine and no tongue laceration. His blood pressure is 130/90 mm Hg; heart rate is 93 beats/min; respiratory rate is 16 breaths/min; and pulse oximetry is 98% on room air.

During transport to hospital, the patient slowly becomes more responsive. He appears scared and keeps asking, "What happened"? You explain that he apparently had a convulsion. You keep reassuring him throughout the transport to hospital. On arrival, he is less apprehensive and you give a hand over to the A&E department. During your follow-up, you find out he was treated and released from hospital. Apparently, the patient hasn't taken his phenytoin for several days.

How can you narrow down the cause of a convulsion in the prehospital environment? What benefits does this provide for patient care?

Issues: Understanding and Implementing Treatment of a Patient Who Experienced a Convulsion, Empathy for the Patient Who Regains Consciousness Among Strangers.

29 Endocrine Emergencies

Objectives

Cognitive

- Describe the incidence, morbidity and mortality of endocrine emergencies.
- Identify the risk factors most predisposing to endocrine diseases.
- Discuss the anatomy and physiology of organs and structures related to endocrine diseases.
- Review the pathophysiology of endocrine emergencies.
- Discuss the general assessment findings associated with endocrine emergencies.
- Identify the need for rapid intervention of the patient with endocrine emergencies.
- Discuss the management of endocrine emergencies.
- Describe osmotic diuresis and its relationship to diabetes.
- Describe the pathophysiology of type 2 diabetes.
- Describe the pathophysiology of type 1 diabetes.
- Describe the effects of decreased levels of insulin on the body.
- Correlate abnormal findings in assessment with clinical significance in the patient with a diabetic emergency.
- Discuss the management of diabetic emergencies.
- Integrate the pathophysiological principles and the assessment findings to formulate an initial diagnosis and implement a treatment plan for the patient with a diabetic emergency.
- Differentiate between the pathophysiology of normal glucose metabolism and diabetic glucose metabolism.
- Describe the mechanism of ketone body formation and its relationship to ketoacidosis.
- Discuss the physiology of the excretion of potassium and ketone bodies by the kidneys.
- Describe the relationship of insulin to serum glucose levels.
- Describe the effects of decreased levels of insulin on the body.
- Describe the effects of increased serum glucose levels on the body.
- Discuss the pathophysiology of hypoglycaemia.
- Discuss the utilisation of glycogen by the human body as it relates to the pathophysiology of hypoglycaemia.
- Describe the actions of adrenaline as it relates to the pathophysiology of hypoglycaemia.
- Recognise the signs and symptoms of the patient with hypoglycaemia.
- Describe the compensatory mechanisms utilised by the body to promote homeostasis relative to hypoglycaemia.
- Describe the management of a responsive hypoglycaemic patient.
- Correlate abnormal findings in assessment with clinical significance in the patient with hypoglycaemia.
- Discuss the management of the hypoglycaemic patient.
- Integrate the pathophysiological principles and the assessment findings to formulate an initial diagnosis and implement a treatment plan for the patient with hypoglycaemia.
- Discuss the pathophysiology of hyperglycaemia.
- Recognise the signs and symptoms of the patient with hyperglycaemia.
- Describe the management of hyperglycaemia.

- Correlate abnormal findings in assessment with clinical significance in the patient with hyperglycaemia.
- Discuss the management of the patient with hyperglycaemia.
- Integrate the pathophysiological principles and the assessment findings to formulate an initial diagnosis and implement a treatment plan for the patient with hyperglycaemia.
- Discuss the pathophysiology of nonketotic hyperosmolar coma.
- Recognise the signs and symptoms of the patient with nonketotic hyperosmolar coma.
- Describe the management of nonketotic hyperosmolar coma.
- Correlate abnormal findings in assessment with clinical significance in the patient with nonketotic hyperosmolar coma.
- Integrate the pathophysiological principles and the assessment findings to formulate an initial diagnosis and implement a treatment plan for the patient with nonketotic hyperosmolar coma.
- Discuss the management of the patient with hyperglycaemia.
- Integrate the pathophysiological principles and the assessment findings to formulate an initial diagnosis and implement a treatment plan for the patient with hyperglycaemia.
- Discuss the pathophysiology of diabetic ketoacidosis.
- Recognise the signs and symptoms of the patient with diabetic ketoacidosis.
- Describe the management of diabetic ketoacidosis.
- Correlate abnormal findings in assessment with clinical significance in the patient with diabetic ketoacidosis.
- Discuss the management of the patient with diabetic ketoacidosis.
- Integrate the pathophysiological principles and the assessment findings to formulate an initial diagnosis and implement a treatment plan for the patient with diabetic ketoacidosis.
- Discuss the pathophysiology of thyrotoxicosis.
- Recognise signs and symptoms of the patient with thyrotoxicosis.
- Describe the management of thyrotoxicosis.
- Correlate abnormal findings in assessment with clinical significance in the patient with thyrotoxicosis.
- Discuss the management of the patient with thyrotoxicosis.
- Integrate the pathophysiological principles and the assessment findings to formulate an initial diagnosis and implement a treatment plan for the patient with thyrotoxicosis.
- Discuss the pathophysiology of myxoedema.
- Recognise signs and symptoms of the patient with myxoedema.
- Describe the management of myxoedema.
- Correlate abnormal findings in assessment with clinical significance in the patient with myxoedema.
- Discuss the management of the patient with myxoedema.
- Integrate the pathophysiological principles and the assessment findings to formulate an initial diagnosis and implement a treatment plan for the patient with myxoedema.
- Discuss the pathophysiology of Cushing's syndrome.
- Recognise signs and symptoms of the patient with Cushing's syndrome.
- Describe the management of Cushing's syndrome.
- Correlate abnormal findings in assessment with clinical significance in the patient with Cushing's syndrome.
- Discuss the management of the patient with Cushing's syndrome.

- Integrate the pathophysiological principles and the assessment findings to formulate an initial diagnosis and implement a treatment plan for the patient with Cushing's syndrome.
- Discuss the pathophysiology of adrenal insufficiency.
- Recognise signs and symptoms of the patient with adrenal insufficiency.
- Describe the management of adrenal insufficiency.
- Correlate abnormal findings in assessment with clinical significance in the patient with adrenal insufficiency.
- Discuss the management of the patient with adrenal insufficiency.
- Integrate the pathophysiological principles and the assessment findings to formulate an initial diagnosis and implement a treatment plan for the patient with adrenal insufficiency.
- Integrate the pathophysiological principles to the assessment of a patient with an endocrine emergency.

- Differentiate between endocrine emergencies based on assessment and history.
- Correlate abnormal findings in the assessment with clinical significance in the patient with endocrine emergencies.
- Develop a patient management plan based on an initial diagnosis in the patient with an endocrine emergency.

Affective

None

Psychomotor

None

Introduction

Few other systems in the body share the level of responsibility assigned to the endocrine system. This system directly or indirectly influences almost every cell, organ, and function of the body. Consequently, patients with an endocrine disorder often present with a multitude of signs and symptoms that require a thorough assessment and immediate treatment to interrupt life-threatening emergencies.

Anatomy and Physiology

The endocrine system comprises a network of glands that produce and secrete chemical messengers called hormones. The main function of the endocrine system and its hormone messengers is to maintain homeostasis and promote permanent structural changes. Maintaining homeostasis requires a response to any change in the body, such as low glucose or calcium levels in the blood.

Exocrine glands (*exo* means "outside") excrete chemicals for elimination. These glands have ducts that carry their secretions to the surface of the skin or into a body cavity. Sweat glands, salivary glands, and the liver are examples of exocrine glands.

Endocrine glands (*endo* means "inside") secrete or release chemicals that are used inside the body. These glands lack ducts, so they release hormones directly into the surrounding tissue and blood. Hormones act on the body's cells by increasing or decreasing the rate of cellular metabolism. They transfer information from one set of cells to another to coordinate bodily functions, such as the regulation of mood, growth and development, metabolism, tissue function, and sexual development and function.

Whereas the nervous system—the body's major controlling system—uses nerve impulses to activate and monitor the faster processes of the body, hormones of the endocrine system—considered the body's second great controlling system—are released directly into the bloodstream and act more slowly to achieve their effects. The hormones travel in the bloodstream to target tissues **Figure 29-1 ▸**. Each target cell has specific receptor sites on the cell membrane, or inside the cell, to which the specific hormone can attach or bind. These receptors have two main functions: to recognise and bind to their particular hormones and to initiate an appropriate signal. Once the hormone has attached to the receptor site of the cell, the "message" to alter the cellular function is delivered.

Many cells contain multiple receptors and act as targets for several hormones—or for molecules introduced into the body as therapy. Agonists are molecules that bind to a cell's receptor and trigger a response by that cell; they produce some kind of action or biological effect. Antagonists are molecules that bind to a cell's receptor and block the action of agonists. Hormone antagonists are widely used as drugs.

Hormonal Regulation Mechanism

Hormones operate within feedback systems (either positive or negative) to maintain an optimal internal operating environment in the body. Release of hormones is regulated by chemical

You are the Paramedic Part 1

You are dispatched to the court for an unknown medical emergency. As you and your partner approach the court magistrates, a police officer meets you and guides you and your colleague through a sea of news vehicles and reporters to a judge's chambers where you find your patient.

Lying on the couch is a middle-aged female patient. She appears to be extremely lethargic, pale, and perspiring. A fellow member of the jury explains that as the photos of the autopsy were being shown, the woman suddenly went pale and passed out. She was immediately brought to the judge's chambers and placed on the couch. It is estimated that she was unconscious for approximately 1 to 2 minutes.

Initial Assessment	Recording Time: 0 Minutes
Appearance	Looks ill
Level of consciousness	V (Responsive to verbal stimuli)
Airway	Open
Breathing	Adequate chest rise and volume
Circulation	Weak, rapid radial pulse

1. What are some potential differential diagnoses?
2. When do symptoms of hypoglycaemia occur?

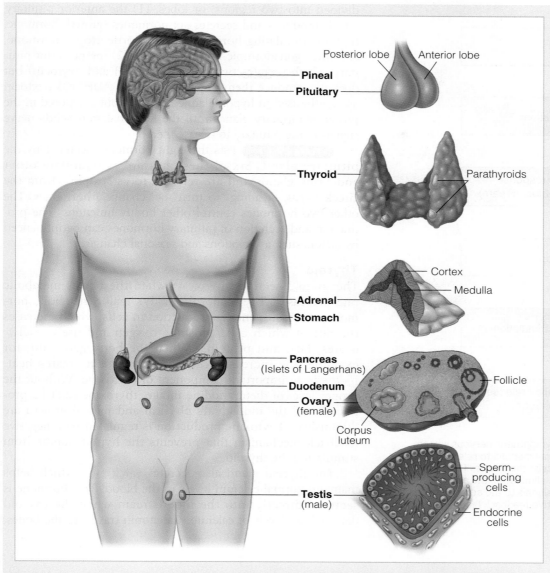

Figure 29-1 The endocrine system uses the various glands within the system to deliver chemical messages to organ systems throughout the body.

stops providing the critical negative feedback required to regulate function. Cell signalling is covered in more detail in Chapter 6.

The hypothalamic–pituitary system controls the function of multiple peripheral endocrine organs (eg, thyroid, adrenal cortex, gonads, breasts). It is often considered a part of the endocrine system, as it sends signals to the adrenal gland to release the hormones adrenaline and noradrenaline. It also produces its own hormones: antidiuretic hormone (ADH), oxytocin, and regulatory hormones. The regulatory hormones control the release of hormones by the pituitary gland.

Some of these hormones have pharmacological effects that depend on their concentration. For example, if there is a low or physiological level of ADH in the bloodstream, the renal tubules are stimulated to reabsorb sodium and water. At the same time, ADH acts as a vasopressor.

Components of the Endocrine System

The major components of the endocrine system are the hypothalamus, pituitary, thyroid, parathyroid, adrenals, and reproductive organs (gonads). The pancreas is also part of this system; it has a role in hormone production as well as in digestion.

Hypothalamus

The hypothalamus is a small region of the brain (not a gland) that contains several control centres for the body functions and emotions. It is the primary link between the endocrine system and the nervous system.

Pituitary Gland

The pituitary gland is often referred to as the "master gland" because its secretions control, or regulate, the secretions of other endocrine glands. It is located at the base of the brain and is about the size of a grape. The pituitary is attached to the hypothalamus by a very thin piece of tissue. This gland is

factors, other hormonal factors, and neural control. Endocrine regulation, through negative feedback, is the most important method by which hormonal secretion is maintained within a physiological range.

One example of this negative feedback mechanism is the release of adrenaline from the adrenal medulla in response to stress. When stress stimulates the body's neural regulation (via the sympathetic nervous system), it releases adrenaline into the bloodstream from the adrenal medulla to assist the body's response to the stress stimuli. When the stress is removed, the nervous system stimulation decreases and less adrenaline is released **Figure 29-2 ▸**.

Disease occurs when normal cell signalling is interrupted and positive feedback is given. As a consequence, the system

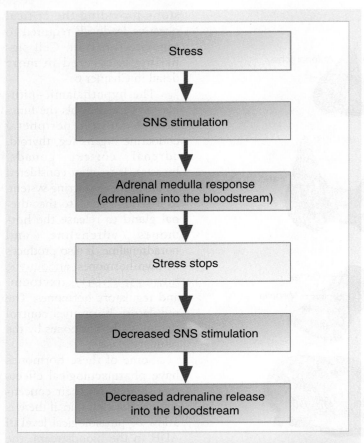

Figure 29-2 Stress stimulates the sympathetic nervous system (neural regulation) to signal the adrenal medulla to release adrenaline into the bloodstream to assist the body's "flight or fight" response. When the stimulus is eliminated, the neural regulating mechanism decreases its signals to the adrenal medulla and less adrenaline is released (negative feedback loop).

divided into two regions, or lobes: (1) the anterior pituitary, which produces and secretes six hormones (growth hormone, thyroid-stimulating hormone, adrenocorticotropin hormone, and three gonadotropic hormones); and (2) the posterior pituitary, which secretes two hormones (ADH and oxytocin) but does not produce them **Figure 29-3 ▶**. ADH and oxytocin are synthesised in hypothalamic neurones but are stored in the posterior pituitary gland until the hypothalamus sends nerve signals to the pituitary to release them.

Table 29-1 ▶ lists the eight hormones secreted by the pituitary gland. Six of these hormones stimulate other endocrine glands and are referred to as "tropic" (from the Greek *tropos,* meaning "to turn" or "change") hormones. The other two hormones control other bodily functions. The production and secretion of pituitary hormones can be influenced by factors such as emotions and seasonal changes.

Thyroid

The thyroid secretes thyroxine when the body's metabolic rate decreases. Thyroxine, the body's major metabolic hormone, stimulates energy production in cells, which increases the rate at which cells consume oxygen and use carbohydrates, fats, and proteins. When the body gets cold, for example, the increased cellular metabolism creates heat. Iodine is an important component of thyroxine. Without the proper level of dietary iodine intake, thyroxine can't be produced, and the individual's physical and mental growth are diminished. Thyroxine production is regulated by a negative feedback mechanism that prevents the hypothalamus from stimulating the thyroid.

The thyroid gland also secretes calcitonin, which helps maintain normal calcium levels in the blood. This hormone is secreted directly into the bloodstream when the thyroid detects high levels of calcium. Calcitonin travels to the bones,

You are the Paramedic Part 2

You ask your partner to obtain a set of vital signs and perform a blood glucose check while you begin your assessment of the patient. Your initial assessment reveals that she is responsive to verbal stimuli; however, she is unable to answer questions appropriately. The only other significant finding is a weak, rapid regular pulse. Your partner whispers to you that the blood glucose level came back at 1.5 mmol/l.

Vital Signs	Recording Time: 5 Minutes
Level of consciousness	Verbal
Pulse	130 beats/min, weak and regular
Blood pressure	122/68 mm Hg
Respirations	22 breaths/min, regular
Skin	Pale, cool, and perspiring
SpO$_2$	97% on room air

3. What are some of the causes of hypoglycaemia?
4. How may a person with hypoglycaemia present?

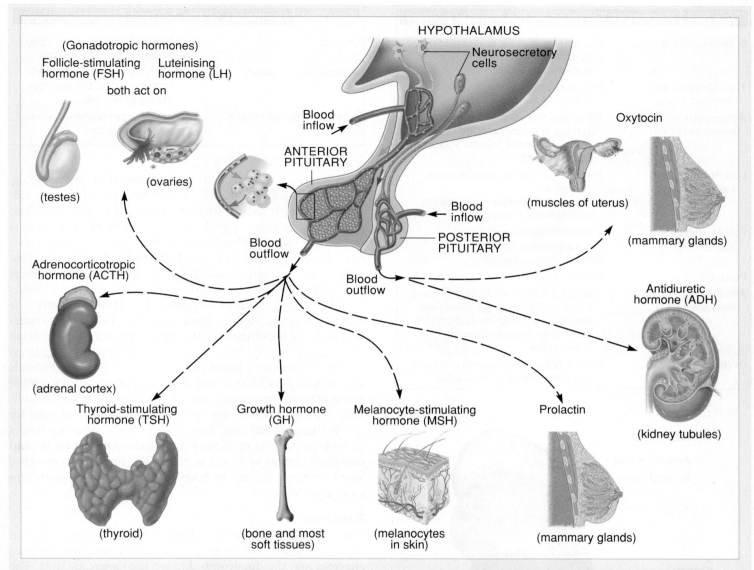

Figure 29-3 The pituitary gland secretes hormones from its two regions, the anterior pituitary lobe and the posterior pituitary lobe.

where it stimulates the bone-building cells to absorb the excess calcium. It also stimulates the kidneys to absorb and excrete excess calcium.

Parathyroid

The parathyroid gland also assists in the regulation of calcium. However, the parathyroid hormone (PTH), when secreted by the parathyroid, acts as an antagonist to calcitonin. PTH is secreted when calcium blood levels are low. It stimulates the bone-dissolving cells to break down bone and release calcium into the bloodstream. In the kidneys, PTH decreases the amount of calcium released in the urine. The secretion of PTH is regulated by the calcium level in the blood.

Adrenal Glands

The adrenal glands consist of two parts: an outer part, called the adrenal cortex, and an inner part, called the adrenal medulla Figure 29-4 ▶. Both parts produce hormones Table 29-2 ▶. The adrenal cortex produces hormones called corticosteroids, which regulate the body's metabolism, its balance of salt and water, the immune system, and sexual function. The adrenal medulla produces hormones called catecholamines (adrenaline and noradrenaline), which assist the body in coping with physical and emotional stress by increasing the heart and respiratory rates and the blood pressure.

During times of stress, the hypothalamus secretes a hormone that stimulates the anterior pituitary to release

Table 29-1	Hormones Secreted by the Pituitary Gland
Growth hormone (GH)	Regulates metabolic processes related to growth and adaptation to physical and emotional stressors
Thyroid-stimulating hormone (TSH)	Increases production and secretion of thyroid hormone
Adrenocorticotropic hormone (ACTH)	Stimulates the adrenal gland to secrete cortisol and adrenal proteins that contribute to the maintenance of the adrenal gland
Luteinising hormone (LH)	In women: ovulation, progesterone production In men: regulates spermatogenesis, testosterone production
Follicle-stimulating hormone (FSH)	In women: follicle maturation, oestrogen production In men: spermatogenesis
Prolactin	Milk production
Antidiuretic hormone (ADH)	Controls plasma osmolality; increases the permeability of the distal renal tubules and collecting ducts, which leads to an increase in water reabsorption
Oxytocin	Contracts the uterus during childbirth and stimulates milk production

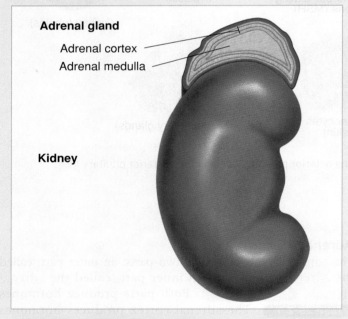

Figure 29-4 The adrenal glands, which sit on top of the kidney, consist of two parts—the adrenal cortex and the adrenal medulla.

adrenocorticotropic hormone (ACTH). ACTH targets the adrenal cortex and causes it to secrete cortisol (a glucocorticoid). Cortisol stimulates most body cells to increase their energy production.

If the body experiences a drop in blood pressure or volume, a decrease in sodium level, or an increase in the potas-

Table 29-2	Hormones of the Adrenal Glands
Cortisol	Increases metabolic rate, using fat and protein for energy
Aldosterone	Reabsorbs sodium and water from the urine, and excretes excess potassium
Adrenaline/noradrenaline	Stimulates sympathetic nervous system receptors

sium level, the adrenal cortex is stimulated to secrete aldosterone (a mineralocorticoid). Aldosterone stimulates the kidneys to reabsorb sodium from the urine and excrete potassium by altering the osmotic gradient in the blood. When sodium is reabsorbed into the blood, water follows; this action increases both blood volume and blood pressure. Aldosterone also reduces the amount of salt and water lost through the sweat and salivary glands.

The body's reaction to physical or emotional stress is referred to as the "fight or flight" response. Following stimulation from the hypothalamus, the adrenal medulla secretes small amounts of noradrenaline and large amounts of adrenaline. Noradrenaline raises blood pressure by causing blood vessels and skeletal muscles to constrict. Adrenaline stimulates sympathetic nervous system receptors throughout the body. In addition, it stimulates the liver to convert glycogen to glucose for use as energy in the cells. The action of both hormones results in increased levels of oxygen and glucose in the blood and faster circulation of blood to the brain, heart, and muscles, which in turn enables the body to respond to the short-term emergency situation.

Pancreas

The pancreas is a digestive gland that is considered both an endocrine gland and an exocrine gland. It secretes digestive enzymes into the duodenum through the pancreatic duct. The exocrine component is responsible for the secretion of the digestive enzymes. The endocrine component comprises the islets of Langerhans. These cell groups within the pancreas act like "an organ within an organ". The main hormones they secrete—glucagon and insulin—are responsible for the regulation of blood glucose levels   Figure 29-5 ▶ .

When the body's blood glucose level falls, such as between meals, glucagon (a starch form of the sugar glucose made up of thousands of glucose units) is secreted to raise the glucose level and bring the body's energy back to normal. When it enters the bloodstream, glucagon stimulates the liver to change glycogen into sugar and secrete it into the bloodstream, where cells can use it for energy.

Insulin is responsible for the removal of glucose from the blood for storage as glycogen, fats, and protein. When blood glucose levels are elevated, the islets of Langerhans secrete insulin, which is carried by the bloodstream to the cells. The cells then take in more glucose and use it to produce energy. Insulin also stimulates the liver to take in more glucose and

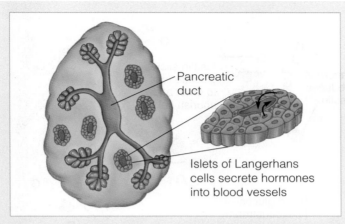

Figure 29-5 The islets of Langerhans secrete hormones into blood vessels.

Table 29-3	Hormones of the Gonads
Male	
Testosterone	Main sex hormone in males Responsible for secondary sex characteristics: voice deepening, growth of facial hair, muscle development, pubic hair, growth spurts
Female	
Oestrogen	Responsible for secondary sex characteristics: breast growth, fat accumulation at hips and thighs, pubic hair, growth spurts Involved in pregnancy Regulation of menstrual cycle
Progesterone	Involved in pregnancy Regulation of menstrual cycle Prevents maturation of additional egg during ovulation

store it as glycogen for later use by the body. Insulin is the *only* hormone that decreases the blood glucose levels. Insulin is essential in order for glucose to enter and nourish the cells. Once the blood glucose levels have returned to normal, the islets of Langerhans discontinue the secretion of insulin.

Gonads

The gonads are the main source of sex hormones (Table 29-3 ▲). In men, the gonads, or testes, are located in the scrotum and produce hormones called androgens. The most important androgen in men is testosterone. Androgens regulate body changes associated with sexual development (puberty), including growth spurts, deepening of the voice, growth of facial and pubic hair, and muscle growth and strength.

In women, the gonads are the ovaries, which release the eggs and secrete the hormones oestrogen and progesterone. Oestrogen signals the anterior pituitary gland to secrete luteinising hormone (LH) when an egg is developing in an ovarian follicle. Oestrogen and progesterone also assist in the regula-

At the Scene

Although specific pathophysiology varies for each disease, endocrine emergencies are usually due to:
- Failure of normal hormone production
- Excessive hormone production
- Failure of feedback inhibition systems involving the hypothalamus, pituitary gland, endocrine gland, and the target organ

tion of the menstrual cycle. At puberty, oestrogen also supports development of the secondary sex characteristics: enlargement of the breasts, uterine enlargement, fat deposits in the hips and thighs, and development of hair under the arms and in the pubic area.

Pathophysiology

Endocrine disorders can be caused by either hypersecretion or insufficient secretion of a gland. Hypersecretion presents as overactivity of the target organ regulated by the gland. Insufficient secretion results in underactivity of the organ controlled by the gland.

The effects of a disturbance of endocrine gland function are determined by the degree of dysfunction of the gland, as well as by the age and sex of the patient. All degrees of glandular dysfunction are possible, ranging from barely detectable variations to extreme dysfunction.

At the Scene

Despite their intricate pathophysiology, most clinically significant endocrine emergencies result in alterations of the ABCs, fluid balance, mental status, vital signs, and blood glucose level.

Diabetes Mellitus

Medically, the term "diabetes" refers to a metabolic disorder in which the body's ability to metabolise simple carbohydrates (glucose) is impaired. It is characterised by the passage of large quantities of urine containing glucose, significant thirst, and deterioration of body function. Glucose is one of the basic sugars in the body and, along with oxygen, is the primary fuel for cellular metabolism.

Diabetes mellitus means "sweet diabetes"—a reference to the presence of glucose in the urine. This disease is characterised by an inability to sufficiently metabolise glucose. It occurs either because the pancreas does not produce enough insulin or because the cells do not respond to the effects of the insulin that is produced. Both cases result in elevated glucose levels in the blood and glucose in the urine. Glucose builds up in the blood, overflows into the urine, and flows out of the body. Thus cells can starve even though the blood contains large amounts of glucose (Figure 29-6 ▶).

The prevalence of diabetes has increased in the United Kingdom (UK) over the past 9 years. The Information Centre for Heath and Social Care UK (2005–2006) estimates that over 2 million people in the UK currently live with diabetes, and over half a million more have not had their condition diagnosed.

Left untreated, diabetes leads to wasting of body tissues and death. Even with medical care, some patients with particularly aggressive forms of diabetes will die relatively young from one or more complications of the disease. The severity of diabetic complications is related to how high the average blood glucose level is and how early in life the disease begins. Although most patients live a normal life span, they must be willing to adjust their lives to the demands of the disease, especially their eating habits and activities. There is no cure for the disease, so treatment focuses on maintaining blood glucose levels within the normal range.

Two forms of diabetes exist: type 1 and type 2. Both types are serious conditions that affect many tissues and functions other than the glucose-regulating mechanism, and both require life-long medical management.

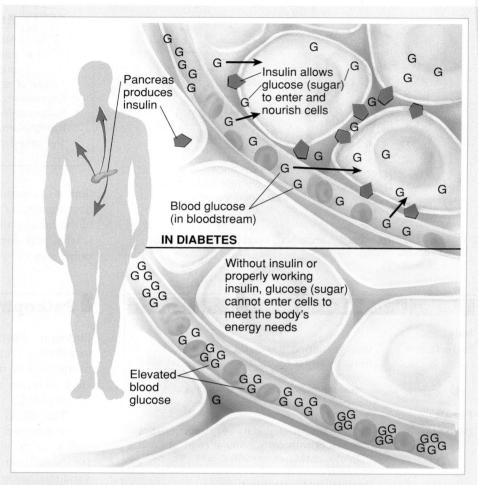

Figure 29-6 Diabetes is defined as a lack of or ineffective action of insulin. Without insulin, cells begin to "starve" because insulin is needed to allow glucose to enter and nourish the cells.

Type 1 Diabetes Mellitus

Type 1 diabetes generally strikes children as opposed to adults, so it has been referred to as "juvenile diabetes". Although type 1 diabetes has a hereditary predisposition, it is now believed that environmental factors may be part of the cause—for example, an infection that triggers an autoimmune disorder (ie, antibodies destroy the islets of Langerhans).

In type 1 diabetes, most patients do not produce insulin at all. They require daily injections of supplementary, synthetic insulin throughout their lives to control blood glucose. In addition to daily insulin injections, strict diet control must be observed; this can be difficult with young children. Increased activity and alcohol consumption can lead to low blood glucose levels (alcohol depletes glycogen stores in the liver). It is important to consider low blood sugar as a cause of altered

At the Scene

Macrovascular complications of diabetes include:
- Coronary artery disease/myocardial infarction (MI)
- Hypertension
- Dyslipidaemia
- Peripheral vascular (foot ulcers/amputations)
- Cerebrovascular (stroke)

Microvascular complications of diabetes include:
- Retinopathy
- Nephropathy (end-stage renal disease)
- Neuropathy (paraesthesias, sexual impotence, neurogenical bladder, constipation, diarrhoea)

At the Scene

The terms "juvenile onset" and "adult onset" diabetes have been replaced by type 1 and type 2 diabetes. The age of onset of the patient's symptoms is less important than whether or not the patient requires insulin to survive.

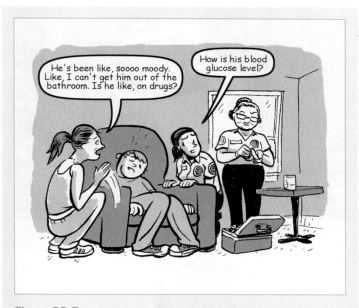

Figure 29-7

At the Scene

You are likely to encounter patients with diabetes who use insulin pumps to treat their disease. These small devices consist of an infusion set, a reservoir for insulin, and the pump itself. A promising alternative to multiple daily injections of insulin, insulin pumps provide improved control of blood glucose levels for many patients with diabetes.

mental status 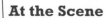 **Figure 29-7 ▲** . Complications of diabetes include kidney problems, nerve damage, blindness (diabetes is the number one cause of blindness), heart disease, and stroke.

Type 2 Diabetes Mellitus

The most common form of diabetes is type 2 diabetes (sometimes called adult-onset diabetes), in which blood glucose levels are elevated. It accounts for between 85% to 95% of all people with diabetes in the UK, and typically develops later in life, usually when the patient is middle-aged, although the disease is becoming more common in younger people. Type 2 diabetes may be related to *metabolic syndrome,* a cluster of characteristics including excessive fat in the abdominal area, elevated blood pressure, and high levels of blood lipids. Risk factors for developing metabolic syndrome include excess weight, lack of physical activity, and genetic factors.

In many people with type 2 diabetes, the pancreas actually produces enough insulin; however, for reasons not fully understood, the body cannot effectively utilise it. This condition is known as insulin resistance. One possible explanation is that the insulin receptor cells located on the target cells have changed in some way and are no longer able to receive the

Special Considerations

New-onset weakness in a pre-existing diabetes patient may be considered an MI until proven otherwise. Many type 1 and type 2 diabetes patients have an acquired dysfunction in the peripheral nervous system (neuropathy). Also, increased insulin levels result in increased blood lipid levels. This combination often leads to an earlier onset of coronary artery disease. People with diabetes don't always have typical clinical symptoms of acute coronary syndrome due to their alteration in sensation. They are more likely to present with general body weakness.

insulin when it arrives at the target cell. Type 2 diabetes can also be caused by a deficiency in insulin production.

Symptoms of type 2 diabetes may include fatigue; nausea; frequent urination; thirst; unexplained weight loss; blurred vision; frequent infections and slow healing of wounds; being cranky, confused, or shaky; unresponsiveness; and convulsions. These symptoms tend to develop gradually and usually become noticeable in middle age. In fact, the onset of type 2 diabetes may be so insidious that patients may not realise they suffer from the disorder. In some instances, the symptoms can develop over several years in overweight adults older than 40 years. A small percentage of people do not display any symptoms.

Weight loss is an important factor in helping to control type 2 diabetes. Exercise and a well-balanced, nutritious diet are key components in combating the complications of diabetes. To maintain glucose levels within the normal range, food intake must be spread throughout an entire day in coordination with daily medications/insulin injections.

Hypoglycaemia

Hypoglycaemia in the insulin-dependent person with diabetes is often the result of having taken too much insulin, too little food, or both. Unlike other tissues, which can usually metabolise fat or protein in addition to sugar, the tissues of the central nervous system (including the brain) depend entirely on glucose as their source of energy. If the level of glucose in the blood drops dramatically, the brain is literally starved. The patient will experience trembling, a rapid heart rate, sweating, and a feeling of hunger—a result of the actions of adrenaline. These symptoms reflect both the disordered function of hungry brain cells and the alarm reaction (sympathetic nervous system discharge) set off by the brain's distress. If hypoglycaemia persists, cerebral dysfunction progresses very quickly to permanent brain damage. Additional signs and symptoms associated with

At the Scene

The longer a patient remains unconscious from hypoglycaemia, the more likely there will be permanent brain damage! If more than 20 to 30 minutes go by, toxic compounds (free radicals) in the brain are produced that can cause permanent damage to the neurones.

hypoglycaemia include headache, mental confusion, memory loss, incoordination, slurred speech, irritability, dilated pupils, and convulsions and coma in severe cases.

The normal blood glucose range in a person without diabetes is maintained between 4 mmol/l and 8 mmol/l. Low blood glucose is generally defined as that less than 4 mmol/l. In the patient with diabetes, however, clinical features associated with hypoglycaemia may be present at higher blood glucose levels. Hypoglycaemia develops *very rapidly,* from minutes to a few hours. It should be suspected in any patient with diabetes who presents with bizarre behaviour, neurological signs, or coma. Often the hypoglycaemic patient appears intoxicated, because of slurred speech and lack of coordination, and may be paranoid, hostile, and aggressive.

Of course, people with diabetes are not the only individuals who are prone to episodes of hypoglycaemia. Alcoholics, patients who have ingested certain poisons or overdosed with certain drugs (notably aspirin), and patients with certain cancers, liver disease, kidney disease, and some other conditions may also suffer hypoglycaemic episodes. Don't discount the possibility of hypoglycaemia in a comatose patient just because the individual is not known to have diabetes. Conversely, don't let a known diagnosis of diabetes prevent you from considering other causes of coma. People with diabetes are not immune to head injury, stroke, convulsions, meningitis, and other traumatic injuries or conditions. Keep an open mind and assess the patient thoroughly.

Whenever you suspect hypoglycaemia, treat it *immediately:* A hungry brain is a very unhappy brain, and permanent cerebral damage may ensue if blood glucose levels are not restored rapidly. Measure the patient's blood glucose, especially if his or her age or clinical history suggests that the problem may be stroke—administration of concentrated glucose solutions in a suspected stroke situation may exacerbate cerebral damage ‣ **Figure 29-8 ▶** . Hypoglycaemia should also be excluded in any patient who has a lowered level of consciousness who is having, or has had, a convulsion.

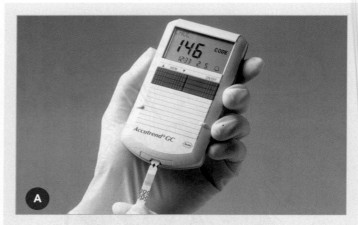

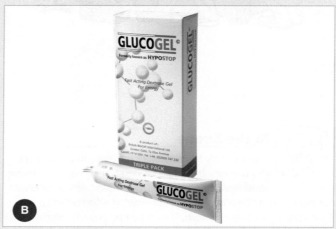

Figure 29-8 Administering glucose is appropriate in diabetic emergencies unless you have a reliable blood glucose measurement indicating normal or high blood glucose levels. Available forms include (**A**) near patient blood glucose test and (**B**) 40% glucose gel.

At the Scene

The exact value for the blood glucose is not extremely helpful. It's far more important to know the general range plus the patient's clinical presentation.

At the Scene

If uncertain of a patient's blood glucose level, always err on the "low side" and assume that hypoglycaemia is present. A period of hypoglycaemia is more dangerous to the patient than an equivalent period of hyperglycaemia.

If the patient is alert, is able to swallow, and has an intact gag reflex, administer glucose by mouth. Provide a chocolate bar, a biscuit, or sugary non-diet drink. Alternatively, where 40% glucose gel is available, this should be applied to the patient's buccal mucosa to provide a rapid source of sugar. Do *not* give anything by mouth to a patient whose level of consciousness is depressed!

If the patient is in a coma, treat him or her as any other comatose patient, with attention to the airway and supplemental oxygen. Hold off on use of an advanced airway (ie, endotracheal tube, laryngeal mask airway), until you have given the patient glucose 10% IV; if this treatment hs been successful, the patient will pull out the endotracheal tube as soon as he or she wakes up!

Cannulate the patient with a large-bore cannula, and flush with 10 to 20 ml of 0.9% NS to confirm correct placement. Glucose 10% is both hypertonic and acidic, so it can do a lot of damage if it infiltrates out of the vein and enters the surrounding tissue.

Table 29-4	Characteristics of Hyperglycaemia and Hypoglycaemia	
	Hyperglycaemia	**Hypoglycaemia**
History		
Food intake	Excessive	Insufficient
Insulin dosage	Insufficient	Excessive
Onset	Gradual (hours to days)	Rapid, within minutes
Skin	Warm and dry	Pale and moist
Infection	Common	Uncommon
Gastrointestinal tract		
Thirst	Intense	Absent
Hunger	Absent	Intense
Vomiting	Common	Uncommon
Respiratory system		
Breathing	Rapid, deep (Kussmaul respirations)	Normal or rapid
Odour of breath	Sweet, fruity	Normal
Cardiovascular system		
Blood pressure	Normal to low	Low
Pulse	Normal or rapid and full	Rapid, weak
Nervous system		
Consciousness	Restless merging to coma	Irritability, confusion, convulsion, or coma
Urine		
Sugar	Present	Absent
Acetone	Present	Absent
Treatment		
Response	Gradual, within 6 to 12 hours following medical treatment	Immediately after administration of glucose

Hyperglycaemia occurs when levels of sugar in the blood exceed normal range (4 to 8 mmol/l). Doctors tend to try to keep the glucose levels of their patients with diabetes at less than 9 mmol/l. Hyperglycaemia can be caused by excessive food intake, insufficient insulin dosages, infection or illness, injury, surgery, and emotional stress. Onset may be rapid (within minutes) or gradual (hours to days), depending on the cause. For example, excessive food intake may cause blood glucose to rise quickly, whereas an infection or illness will result in hyperglycaemia over the course of several days.

If left untreated, hyperglycaemia will progress to diabetic ketoacidosis (DKA). A life-threatening condition, DKA occurs when certain acids accumulate in the body because insulin is not available **Figure 29-9 ▶** . Patients who suffer from this condition tend to be young—teenagers and young adults. In DKA, the deficiency of insulin prevents cells from taking up the extra glucose. From the viewpoint of the cells, famine is at hand, and a distress signal goes out over the sympathetic nervous system, causing the release of various stress hormones. Because the body can't utilise glucose, it turns instead to other sources of energy—principally, fat. The metabolism of fat generates *acids* and *ketones* as waste products. (The ketones give the characteristic fruity odour to the breath of a patent in DKA.) Because glucose must be excreted in the urine in solution, the body loses excessive amounts of water and electrolytes (sodium and potassium). This may lead to disturbances in water balance and acid–base balance. Disturbances in acid–base balance and the compensatory role of the kidneys are covered in more detail in Chapter 6.

Meanwhile, glucose continues to accumulate in the blood. As the blood sugar rises, the patient undergoes massive osmotic diuresis (passing large amounts of urine because of the high solute concentration of the blood); this, together with vomiting, causes dehydration and even shock.

These processes usually progress slowly, over a period of 12 to 48 hours, with the patient's level of consciousness deteriorating only gradually. Patients in DKA are seldom deeply comatose, so if the patient is totally unresponsive, look for another source of the coma, such as head injury, stroke, or drug overdose.

If you are certain that the IV is patent, slowly administer 100 ml of glucose 10% (10 g glucose). If the cause of coma is hypoglycaemia, the patient will often waken with dramatic rapidity, although in cases of very severe hypoglycaemia you may need to administer a further 100 ml of glucose 10% after 5 minutes. Where a patient's recovery is only partial, you may need to titrate glucose 10% to a maximum of 300 ml (30 g) or until the patient regains a normal level of consciousness.

Hyperglycaemia and Diabetic Ketoacidosis

Hyperglycaemia (high blood glucose level) is one of the classic symptoms of diabetes mellitus. Common early signs include frequent and excessive thirst, accompanied by frequent and excessive urination. A hyperglycaemic condition without other classic symptoms is not dispositive of a diagnosis of diabetes mellitus, but hyperglycaemia is also an independent medical condition with other causes. The signs and symptoms of hypoglycaemia and hyperglycaemia can be quite similar **Table 29-4 ▲** .

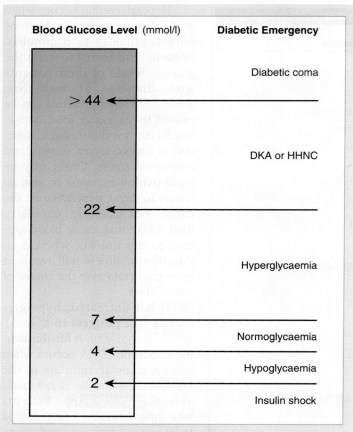

Figure 29-9 The two most common diabetic emergencies, diabetic ketoacidosis and insulin shock, develop when the patient has too much or too little glucose in the blood, respectively.

At the Scene

There is no predictable correlation between the increase in a patient's blood glucose level and the degree of ketoacidosis in the blood. Rely on the patient's clinical presentation rather than the "number".

The signs and symptoms of DKA are generally predictable from the underlying pathophysiology:

- Polyuria (excessive urine output), because of osmotic diuresis
- Polydipsia (excessive thirst), because of dehydration
- Polyphagia (excessive eating), probably related to inefficient utilisation of nutrients
- Nausea and vomiting, the latter worsening dehydration
- Tachycardia as a consequence of dehydration
- Deep, rapid respirations (Kussmaul respirations)—the body's attempt to compensate for acidosis by blowing off carbon dioxide
- Warm, dry skin and dry mucous membranes, also reflecting dehydration
- Fruity odour of ketones on the breath
- Sometimes fever, abdominal pain, and hypotension

At the Scene

Common causes of DKA include infection, injury, alcohol use, emotional discord, and illness, such as stroke or MI.

The treatment of DKA in the prehospital environment depends on making the correct diagnosis. If the patient's history and physical examination are consistent with DKA and your measurement of the patient's glucose level reveals that it is markedly elevated (more than 17 mmol/l), the doctor will probably order treatment for DKA. The goals of prehospital treatment are to begin rehydration and to correct the patient's electrolyte and acid–base abnormalities. In most instances, specific treatment with insulin should await the patient's arrival at hospital, where therapy can be closely monitored with laboratory determinations of blood glucose, ketones, etc.

Follow the procedure for any comatose patient with regard to airway maintenance and oxygen. Be particularly alert for *vomiting,* and have suction ready.

Start an IV infusion of 0.9% NS if indicated by clinical guidelines. Remember, a patient in DKA is likely to be severely dehydrated, often to the point of shock, and needs volume, usually at a rate of about 1 l/h for at least the first few hours.

Monitor cardiac rhythm. Changes in serum potassium caused by DKA can lead to marked myocardial instability. Note the contour of the T waves on the rhythm strip; if they are sharply peaked, the patient's potassium level may be dangerously high, and you may need to administer sodium bicarbonate. If ordered to do so, proceed with extreme caution—even a little too much can cause serious problems, including death.

Hyperosmolar Nonketotic Coma

Hyperosmolar nonketotic coma (HONK), also called hyperosmolar hyperglycaemic nonketotic coma (HHNC), is a metabolic derangement that occurs principally in patients with type 2 diabetes. This condition is characterised by hyperglycaemia, hyperosmolarity, and an absence of significant ketosis.

Oddly enough, coma is present in fewer than 10% of cases. Instead, most patients present with severe dehydration and focal or global neurological deficits. In addition, acute MI is frequently associated with HONK/HHNC. The clinical features of HONK/HHNC and DKA tend to overlap and are often observed simultaneously.

HONK/HHNC often develops in patients with diabetes who have some secondary illness that leads to reduced fluid intake. Although infection (in particular, pneumonia and urinary tract infection) is the most common cause, many other conditions can cause altered mental state or dehydration. In most cases, the secondary illness is not identified.

Hyperglycaemia and hyperosmolarity lead to osmotic diuresis and an osmotic shift of fluid to the intravascular space, resulting in further intracellular dehydration. Unlike patients with DKA, patients with HONK/HHNC do not develop ketoacidosis. Although most patients diagnosed with HONK/HHNC have a known history of diabetes (usually type 2), approximately 30% do not have a prior diagnosis of diabetes. The stress response to any acute illness tends to increase hormones that favour elevated glucose levels; cortisol, catecholamines (adrenaline and noradrenaline), glucagon, and many other hormones have effects that tend to counter those of insulin. Various neurological changes may be found, including drowsiness and lethargy, delirium and coma, focal or generalised convulsions, visual disturbances, hemiparesis, and sensory deficits.

The treatment of HONK/HHNC in the prehospital setting follows the pathway for dehydration and altered mental status. Airway management is the top priority. The comatose patient is

often unable to maintain and protect his or her airway. For this reason, endotracheal intubation may be indicated and should be completed as early as possible. Cervical spine immobilisation should be used for all unresponsive patients found collapsed, unless witnesses can validate that no fall occurred. Large-bore IV access should be gained as soon as possible, but do not delay transfer while initiating the IV. If necessary, obtain IV access during the transport to the accident and emergency (A&E) department. Also obtain a blood glucose level as soon as possible.

Once you have initiated the IV, a bolus of 250 ml 0.9% NS is appropriate for nearly all adults who are clinically dehydrated. In patients with a history of congestive heart failure and/or renal insufficiency, a 125 ml bolus may be a more appropriate starting point. Fluid deficits in HONK/HHNC patients may amount to 10 litres or more. These patients may receive up to 1 litre within the first hour. If the glucose level is less than 4 mmol/l, then administer glucose 10% or IM glucagon as per local guidelines.

Adrenal Insufficiency

Adrenal insufficiency is characterised by decreased function of the adrenal cortex and consequent underproduction of cortisol

You are the Paramedic Part 3

You quickly begin to look for an IV site as your colleague prepares the equipment and the glucose 10%. An IV cannula is successfully inserted into the right antecubital fossa and you administer the glucose 10%, titrated to effect. Within a few minutes, your patient becomes more alert and is confused and scared about her surroundings.

You explain to the patient what happened while she was in the courtroom. She blushes and becomes embarrassed. She admits to having diabetes and tells you that the trial has been making her stressed and as a result she has not been eating properly and trying to self-regulate her insulin. She denies any other medical history, medications, or allergies.

Reassessment	Recording Time: 11 Minutes
Skin	Pink, warm, and dry
Pulse	85 beats/min, strong and regular
Blood pressure	116/74 mm Hg
Respirations	18 breaths/min, regular
SpO_2	98% on room air
ECG	Sinus rhythm with no ectopy
Pupils	PERLA
Blood glucose	8.1 mmol/l

5. Which medications besides insulin can be used to control diabetes?

and aldosterone. A decrease in either of these adrenal hormones will result in weakness, dehydration, and the body's inability to maintain adequate blood pressure or to respond to stress properly.

Cortisol affects almost every organ and tissue in the body. Although its primary role is to assist with the body's response to stress, this adrenal hormone also helps maintain blood pressure and cardiovascular function; regulates the metabolism of carbohydrates, proteins, and fats; affects glucose levels in the blood by balancing the effects of insulin; and functions as an anti-inflammatory agent by slowing the inflammatory response.

Aldosterone regulates and maintains the salt and potassium balance in the blood. Secretion of this adrenal hormone is primarily regulated by the renin–angiotensin system, but is also stimulated by increased serum potassium concentrations.

Abnormal adrenal cortical function produces abnormalities in the metabolism of carbohydrates and protein as well as disturbances of salt and water metabolism. This condition is usually well tolerated unless there are coexisting factors (eg, infection, stress). It affects about 4.7 to 6.2 million of the UK population annually, with the peak incidence occurring in the third decade of life.

Primary Versus Secondary Adrenal Insufficiency

Adrenal insufficiency is classified as either primary or secondary. Primary adrenal insufficiency (also known as Addison's disease) is caused by atrophy or destruction of both adrenal glands, leading to deficiency of all the steroid hormones produced by these glands. A rare disease, it is most frequently the result of idiopathic atrophy, an autoimmune process in which the immune system creates antibodies that attack the adrenal cortex, which leads to its gradual destruction. This phenomenon accounts for approximately 70% of Addison's disease cases in the UK. Adrenal insufficiency occurs when at least 90% of the adrenal cortex has been destroyed. Less commonly (approximately 30% of cases), the adrenal destruction is caused by tuberculosis; bacterial, viral, or fungal infections; adrenal haemorrhage; or cancer of the adrenal glands. Patients with Addison's disease who receive treatment have a normal life expectancy.

In patients with Addison's disease, the body fails to achieve proper regulation of the amount of sodium, potassium, and water in body fluids. Blood volume and pressure fall, as does the concentration of sodium in the blood; blood potassium rises. The blood volume may become so reduced that the circulation can no longer be maintained efficiently. Patients with Addison's disease also frequently exhibit increased pigmenta-

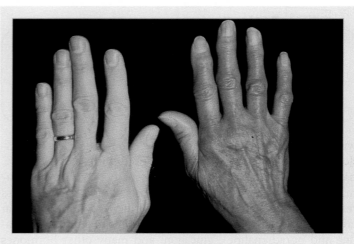

Figure 29-10 The hand of a patient with Addison's disease (right) compared with the hand of a normal subject (left).

tion of the skin, which is caused by the increased secretion of hormones **Figure 29-10 ▲**.

Secondary adrenal insufficiency (a relatively common condition) is defined as a lack of ACTH secretion from the pituitary gland. ACTH, a pituitary messenger, stimulates the adrenal cortex to manufacture and secrete cortisol. If ACTH secretion is insufficient, cortisol production is not stimulated. Patients who abruptly stop taking corticosteroids (eg, prednisolone) may also experience secondary adrenal insufficiency. Corticosteroid treatments suppress natural cortical production; however, aldosterone production is usually not affected with this form of adrenal insufficiency.

Addisonian Crisis

Signs and symptoms of acute adrenal insufficiency may appear suddenly and are referred to as an Addisonian crisis. They may result from an acute exacerbation of chronic insufficiency, usually brought on by a period of stress, trauma, surgery, or severe infection. Steroid withdrawal is the most common cause.

Although most patients with adrenal insufficiency experience symptoms that are severe enough to seek medical treatment prior to a crisis, approximately 25% of patients will develop their first symptoms during an Addisonian crisis. The primary clinical manifestation of adrenal crisis is shock. Patients may also manifest nonspecific symptoms, including weakness; lethargy; confusion or loss of consciousness; low blood pressure (vascular collapse); elevated temperature; severe pain in the lower back, legs, or abdomen; and severe vomiting and diarrhoea that leads to dehydration.

Treatment of Adrenal Insufficiency

Adrenal insufficiency is a potentially fatal disease if unrecognised and untreated. Death usually results from hypotension or cardiac arrhythmias due to hyperkalaemia. The treatment for adrenal insufficiency is based on the clinical presentation and findings, and is geared toward maintaining the airway, breathing, and circulation until arrival at the A&E department. Other goals of prehospital treatment are to begin

At the Scene

Signs of chronic adrenal insufficiency include unexplained weight loss, fatigue, vomiting, diarrhoea, anorexia, salt craving, muscle and joint pain, abdominal pain, postural dizziness, and increased pigmentation in the extensor surfaces, palm creases, and oral mucosa.

rehydration of the patient and to correct the electrolyte and acid–base abnormalities.

Follow the procedure for a patient with altered mental status or comatose patient with regard to airway maintenance and supplemental oxygen. Be alert for *vomiting*, and have suction ready.

Check and record the patient's blood glucose reading. Establish IV access and infuse an initial bolus of 250 ml of 0.9% NS, if required go to a maximum of 500 ml. Then administer 100 mg of hydrocortisone IV slowly over two minutes. If you have been unable to establish IV access, the hydrocortisone may be given IM. Fifteen minutes after giving the hydrocortisone, check the blood glucose level again. If it is less than 4 mmol/l, administer 100 ml of glucose 10%. Remember, a patient in adrenal insufficiency may be severely dehydrated, often to the point of shock and needs volume. If the patient remains hypotensive, administer further 0.9% NS in 20 ml/kg boluses, titrated to effect.

If your transport time to hospital is greater than 30 minutes, consider a further dose of 100 mg of hydrocortisone 15 minutes after the first dose. Continue to monitor the blood glucose levels and if they remain below 4 mmol/l, continue infusing 10% glucose in 100 ml boluses every 15 minutes. Monitor cardiac rhythm as changes in serum electrolytes can lead to marked myocardial instability. Pre-alert the hospital to your arrival with all details according to local guidelines.

Cushing's Syndrome

Cushing's syndrome is caused by an excess of cortisol production by the adrenal glands or by excessive use of cortisol or other similar steroid (glucocorticoid) hormones. Tumours of the pituitary gland or adrenal cortex can stimulate the production of excess hormone, for example, and lead to Cushing's syndrome. Administration of large amounts of cortisol or other glucocorticoid hormones (eg, hydrocortisone, prednisolone, methylprednisolone, or dexamethasone) for the treatment of life-threatening illnesses, such as asthma, rheumatoid arthritis, systemic lupus, inflammatory bowel disease, and some allergies, can also cause this syndrome.

Regardless of the cause, excess cortisol causes characteristic changes in many body systems. Metabolism of carbohydrate, protein, and fat is disturbed, such that the blood glucose level rises. Protein synthesis is impaired so that body proteins are broken down, which leads to loss of muscle fibres and muscle weakness. Bones become weaker and more susceptible to fracture. Other common signs and symptoms related to excess cortisol include the following:

- Weakness and fatigue
- Depression and mood swings
- Increased thirst and urination
- High blood glucose level
- Weight gain, especially on the abdomen, face ("moon face"), neck, and upper back ("buffalo hump")
- Thinning of the skin, with easy bruising and pink or purple stretch marks (striae) on the abdomen, thighs, breasts, and shoulders
- Increased acne, facial hair growth, and scalp hair loss in women, and cessation of menstrual periods
- Darkening of skin (acanthosis) on the neck
- Obesity and poor growth in height in children

The incidence of Cushing's syndrome is about 5 to 25 cases per 1 million people per year. It generally affects people between the ages of 25 and 45.

Prehospital treatment is generally supportive. Obtain a glucose level, monitor the patient's blood pressure, and treat abnormalities as they present.

Hypothyroidism and Hyperthyroidism

Thyroid hormone is secreted in response to the stimulation of the thyroid gland by the anterior pituitary gland. The anterior pituitary gland secretes thyroid-stimulating hormone (TSH) in response to the hypothalamus's secretion of thyrotropin-releasing hormone (TRH).   **Table 29-5 ▸**   summarises the major effects of hypothyroidism and hyperthyroidism.

You are the Paramedic Part 4

Concerned about the attention she has brought to herself, your patient requests not to be transported to hospital. She does not want to cause any further delays in the court proceedings or be removed from the jury. You explain to her that although her blood glucose level has returned to normal, it's still very important for her to be taken to hospital to ensure that it will remain stable. Still hesitant about going to hospital, the patient asks if she could contact her general practitioner to get his opinion. You agree and help her make the call. After much convincing from her general practitioner, she agrees to be transported to hospital for further observation.

Reassessment	Recording Time: 20 Minutes
Skin	Pink, warm, and dry
Pulse	84 beats/min, strong and irregular
Blood pressure	118/74 mm Hg
Respirations	18 breaths/min, regular
SpO₂	98% on room air
ECG	Sinus rhythm with no ectopy
Blood glucose	7.9 mmol/l

6. Does diabetes affect other organ systems?

Table 29-5	Comparison of Major Effects of Hypothyroidism and Hyperthyroidism	
	Hypothyroidism	**Hyperthyroidism**
Cardiovascular effects	Slow pulse, reduced cardiac output	Rapid pulse, increased cardiac output
Metabolic effects	Decreased metabolism, cold skin, weight gain	Increased metabolism, skin hot and flushed, weight loss
Neuromuscular effects	Weakness, sluggish reflexes	Tremor, hyperactive reflexes
Mental, emotional effects	Mental processes sluggish, personality placid	Restlessness, irritability, emotional lability
Gastrointestinal effects	Constipated	Diarrhoea
General somatic effects	Cold, dry skin	Warm, moist skin

At the Scene

Both hyperthyroidism and hypothyroidism patients are likely to require supplemental oxygen. Hyperthyroid metabolic activity increases oxygen demand. Hypothyroid conditions may lead to diminished respiratory effort that may require positive-pressure ventilation.

Myxoedema Coma

Thyroid hormones are critical for cell metabolism and organ function. If their supply becomes inadequate, organ tissues don't grow or mature (due to the decreased metabolic rate), energy production declines (a cause of the decreased metabolic rate), and the actions of other hormones are affected.

Adult hypothyroidism is sometimes called *myxoedema*. The condition is manifested by a general slowing of the body's metabolic processes due to the reduction or absence of thyroid hormone. All organ systems may exhibit symptoms in such a case, with the severity of the symptoms reflecting the degree of hormone deficiency. There are often localised accumulations of mucinous material in the skin, which gives the disease its name (*myx* = mucin; *oedema* = swelling) Figure 29-11 ◄.

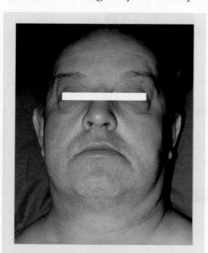

Figure 29-11 Localised accumulations of mucinous material in the neck of a hypothyroid patient.

Symptoms of hypothyroidism include fatigue, feeling cold, weight gain, dry skin, and sleepiness. Because these symptoms are often subtle and can be mistaken for other conditions, the disease may go undiagnosed. Continued decrease of the hormone levels may lead to myxoedema coma, an extreme manifestation of untreated hypothyroidism that is accompanied by physiological decompensation. When hypothyroidism is long standing, physiological adaptations occur, such as reduced metabolic rate and decreased oxygen consumption, which in turn lead to peripheral vasoconstriction. Triggers such as infection (especially lung and urine infections), exposure to cold, trauma, surgery, and certain medications are often precipitating factors in the progression to myxoedema coma.

The hallmark of myxoedema coma is deterioration of the patient's mental status. Although family members may not be overly concerned about more subtle changes, such as apathy or decreased intellectual function, more obvious changes, such as confusion, psychosis, and coma, will most certainly elicit a call for emergency assistance.

Most cases of myxoedema coma occur during the winter in women older than age 60. The condition is 4 to 8 times more common in women than in men. Just as the incidence of hypothyroidism increases with age, myxoedema coma occurs primarily in elderly patients. One consistent finding is hypothermia, and you may need to use a thermometer that records temperatures of less than 32°C in cases of myxoedema coma. Thus absence of fever in the presence of infection is a common finding.

Hypothyroidism decreases intestinal motility, and the decreased metabolic rate associated with this condition can lead to drug toxicity, especially in the elderly. A slower metabolic rate causes the levels of medications, especially those that affect the central nervous system, to rise to toxic levels in the blood. This accidental overdose in the hypothyroid patient can actually precipitate myxoedema coma.

Myxoedema coma is a metabolic and cardiovascular emergency. If not diagnosed and treated immediately, the mortality rates are approximately 50%. Thus the patient's condition must be stabilised as soon as possible.

Administer supplemental oxygen therapy to correct hypoxia. Intubation and ventilation are indicated for patients with diminished respiratory drive or those who are unable to protect their airway; these measures will help prevent respiratory failure.

Monitor the patient's cardiac status. Hypotension may respond to crystalloid therapy. If blood glucose levels are below 4 mmol/l, treat as per local guidelines depending upon the consciousness level of your patient.

At the Scene

Protrusion of the eyeballs (exophthalmos) is common in chronic hyperthyroidism.

Treat hypothermia with passive rewarming methods, as aggressive rewarming may lead to vasodilation and hypotension. Haemodynamically unstable patients with profound hypothermia, however, will require active rewarming. Avoid sedatives, narcotics, and anaesthetics because of the delayed metabolism.

Thyrotoxicosis

Thyrotoxicosis is a toxic condition caused by excessive levels of circulating thyroid hormone. Hyperthyroidism affects 2 in 100 women and 2 in 1,000 men and can cause thyrotoxicosis in some patients; however, the two conditions are not identical. Thyrotoxicosis may also be caused by goitres, autoimmune disease (Grave's disease—the most common cause of hyperthyroidism), and thyroid cancer. Grave's disease, which is most common in women aged 20 to 40 years, has a chronic course with remissions and relapses. If left untreated, it may be fatal.

At the Scene

Both hyperthyroidism and hypothyroidism can adversely affect the electrical status of the myocardium. Application of the cardiac monitor may reveal tachyarrhythmias in hyperthyroidism or bradyarrhythmias in hypothyroidism. Treat all arrhythmias according to your local protocols, while keeping in mind that these arrhythmias may be difficult to correct without first treating the underlying disorder.

A thyroid storm is a rare, life-threatening condition that may occur in patients with thyrotoxicosis. The condition is usually triggered by a stressful event or increased volume of thyroid hormones in the circulation. In addition to the normal signs and symptoms of hyperthyroidism, patients may present with fever, severe tachycardia, nausea, vomiting, altered mental status, and possibly heart failure.

General Assessment

The difficult part of assessing patients with endocrine emergencies is that their problems tend to affect many organ systems and the seriousness of their presentations varies greatly. Many of the patients will have had their conditions for some time and may already be receiving treatment. These patients or their family members may well tell you that there is a history of an endocrine problem; this information, in addition to the common signs and symptoms associated with each endocrine emergency, should help you determine the cause of the current problem. In any event, don't take these calls lightly, as poor outcomes can result very quickly. Very often patients and their relatives with these sorts of disorders are very knowledgeable about their treatment, particularly in a crisis. Listen to what they are saying and act accordingly.

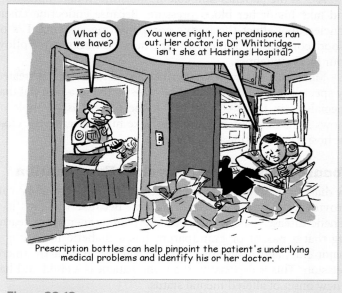

Prescription bottles can help pinpoint the patient's underlying medical problems and identify his or her doctor.

Figure 29-12

Scene Assessment

Your initial scene assessment will vary depending on the rate of the progression of deterioration and the patient's symptoms when you arrive. Regardless of the patient's condition or the cause, airway, breathing, and circulation must always be assessed first.

Your observations of the scene in which the patient is found can also furnish valuable information regarding what might have happened. Check bedside tables and medicine cabinets for medications that might give a clue as to the patient's underlying illness. If appropriate, tell the patient and relatives what you are looking for. Check the refrigerator for insulin **Figure 29-12 ▲**. Bring any medication bottles along with the patient to hospital. They can help pinpoint the patient's underlying medical problems and identify his or her doctor, who should be able to provide more information.

Initial Assessment

The initial assessment begins with the basics: airway, breathing, and circulation. Patients in the middle of any endocrine emergency may be in serious distress, so be prepared to assist them if your initial assessment reveals any of these basics to be abnormal.

When patients present with an altered level of consciousness, they may be unable to protect the airway. Many will be very ill and have chronic episodes of vomiting. Maintain the airway as needed through patient positioning, suctioning, or basic airways.

Patients with endocrine emergencies may present with a variety of breathing levels. Supplemental oxygen is recommended in all cases of suspected respiratory involvement. Although pulse oximetry is commonly used, don't let a reading at a normal or above-normal level persuade you to withhold oxygen.

Assess the patient's skin colour, moisture, and temperature, and take his or her blood pressure. Because endocrine emergencies may affect the body's compensating systems, IVs or blood component replenishment may be necessary. Follow your local guidelines.

Many patients with endocrine disorders are being treated by specialists, and they should be transported to a hospital that specialises in these conditions. If the patient is unstable or shows signs of becoming unstable, take him or her to the closest hospital for stabilisation first.

Focused History and Physical Examination

In diabetic emergencies in particular, the family history can provide very important information. Because diabetes is a genetic disease (passed down through family members), learning that a parent or grandparent has a diabetic history is a major clue, and may prove to be invaluable in your treatment decision. This is especially true if the patient is a child and has a new onset of altered mental status.

The goals of the physical examination in the comatose patient are twofold. First, you want to determine the patient's level of consciousness with precision, so that other examiners who assess him or her later can readily determine whether the patient's condition is improving or deteriorating. Second, you should look for signs that might provide clues to the source of coma.

Begin the physical assessment by observing the patient's general appearance and the position in which he or she is found. Patients found in awkward positions often have brain stem damage; conversely, a natural posture tends to be a good sign. Decorticate or decerebrate posturing should also be noted, if present; both are *bad* signs.

Your physical examination should be geared toward identifying as many atypical findings as possible. Using this information, you can make a more educated decision about treatment. Unless the patient had an endocrine emergency that caused some form of trauma, a rapid trauma assessment is usually not necessary. Always check for a medical ID medallion/bracelet on the wrist or around the neck.

Detailed Physical Examination

The detailed physical examination will reveal the finer abnormalities that will provide you with the final determining factors for your treatment.

The condition of the skin may be very informative. Cold, clammy skin is classically a sign of shock but may also signal severe hypoglycaemia, as from an insulin reaction. Cold, dry skin may indicate overdose of sedative drugs or alcohol. Hot, dry skin suggests fever or, if the circumstances are appropriate, heat stroke.

In checking the vital signs, look for the combination of hypertension and bradycardia, which suggest increased intracranial pressure. Be alert for abnormal respiratory patterns. Cheyne-Stokes breathing usually points to a nonneurological source of

the coma. More worrying are other abnormal breathing patterns, such as central neurogenic ventilation or huffing and puffing that doesn't seem to move much air. Look for "pararespiratory" motions, such as sneezing and yawning. An intact brain stem is required to produce a sneeze or a yawn, so both of those actions have positive prognostic significance. Hiccupping and coughing, by contrast, may indicate brain stem damage.

Ongoing Assessment

Once you've initiated your treatment plan, continually reassess the patient to check for obvious, and subtle, changes. For every action you take, there should be a response. No response *is* a response. Document your findings along the way.

▌General Management

Management of the ABCs should have been carried out during the initial assessment. Remember that a patient whose gag reflex is absent can't protect his or her own airway from aspiration and should be intubated at the earliest opportunity. If breathing is abnormally slow or shallow, assist breathing with bag-valve-mask ventilation. Give supplemental oxygen whether the patient is breathing spontaneously or being ventilated.

If the patient has altered mental status, establish an IV with 0.9% NS or a saline lock. Make an immediate determination of the blood glucose level and initiate treatment if the reading is less than 4 mmol/l. If the patient doesn't respond to this treatment or if you have any other reason to suspect narcotics overdosage (pinpoint pupils, needle tracks on the arms, depressed respirations), then consider administration of naloxone.

Monitor the cardiac rhythm of every comatose patient. For the neurological assessment, the most important consideration is not a single measurement at a single point in time but rather the *trend* shown by several measurements. Recheck vital signs, pupils, and level of consciousness (every 5 minutes in unstable patients and every 10 minutes in stable patients) and *record your findings* immediately.

Transport the comatose patient *supine* if he or she is intubated; otherwise, you may transport the patient in the stable side position (unless injuries preclude that position). If the patient must be supine (eg, because of suspected spine injury) and can't be intubated, keep the mouth and pharynx suctioned free of secretions, vomitus, and blood.

At the Scene

Obtaining blood specimens early is particularly important in the patient with diabetes because any administration of prehospital glucose or other medications will significantly change the chemical makeup of subsequent blood samples.

You are the Paramedic Summary

1. What are some potential differential diagnoses?

On the basis of the signs and symptoms, your patient's potential differential diagnoses can include hypotension, drug overdose, arrhythmias, and hypoglycaemia.

2. When do symptoms of hypoglycaemia occur?

Signs and symptoms of hypoglycaemia usually occur once the blood glucose level falls below 4 mmol/l. However, if the drop in glucose levels is rapid, they can be seen at higher levels.

3. What are some of the causes of hypoglycaemia?

The causes of hypoglycaemia are very diverse. The more common causes of hypoglycaemia in patients with diabetes are taking too much insulin or oral hypoglycaemic medications, not eating enough, and unusual or extreme exercise without adequate food intake. Hypoglycaemia may also be found in patients who are chronic alcoholics, suffer from malnutrition, or have pancreatic disorders, liver disease, hypothermia, cancer, or sepsis. Be on the lookout for intentional overdoses on insulin and oral hypoglycaemic medications. People with a history of eating disorders may take insulin to burn off the "extra calories" of desserts or other foods that may be considered high calorie.

4. How may a patient with hypoglycaemia present?

Why, you may actually be exhibiting signs and symptoms of hypoglycaemia as you are studying this section! Are you hungry, irritable, shaky, or have a headache? Are you having sugar cravings? These are all signs and symptoms of hypoglycaemia. Others include changes in mental status, appearance of intoxication, convulsions, and coma. Vital sign changes will include a weak, rapid pulse and pale, cool, perspiring skin.

5. Which medications besides insulin can be used to control diabetes?

Patients with type 2 diabetes may be prescribed oral hypoglycaemic agents to help regulate their glucose levels. People with type 2 diabetes are able to use these medications because they work with the body's own insulin (they have working beta cells). Examples of commonly prescribed oral hypoglycaemic agents include chlorpropamide, tolazide, tolbutamide, glipizide, and glyburide. Two newer medications include pioglitizone and metformin.

6. Does diabetes affect other organ systems?

Unfortunately, the answer to this question is yes. Patients with diabetes are at risk for developing blindness, kidney disease, peripheral neuropathy, hypertension, atherosclerosis, heart disease, and peripheral vascular disease.

Prep Kit

Ready for Review

- The endocrine system directly or indirectly influences almost every cell, organ, and function of the body.
- Patients with an endocrine disorder often present with a multitude of signs and symptoms that require a thorough assessment and immediate treatment to interrupt life-threatening emergencies.
- The endocrine system comprises a network of glands that produce and secrete hormones. The main function of the endocrine system and its hormone messengers is to maintain homeostasis and promote permanent structural changes.
- Hormones travel in the bloodstream to target tissues.
- The major components of the endocrine system are the hypothalamus, pituitary, thyroid, parathyroid, adrenals, and reproductive organs (gonads). The pancreas is also part of this system; it has a role in hormone production as well as in digestion.
- The pituitary gland is often referred to as the "master gland" because its secretions control, or regulate, the secretions of other endocrine glands.
- The thyroid secretes thyroxine when the body's metabolic rate decreases. Thyroxine, the body's major metabolic hormone, stimulates energy production in cells, which increases the rate at which cells consume oxygen and use carbohydrates, fats, and proteins. The thyroid gland also secretes calcitonin, which helps maintain normal calcium levels in the blood.
- The adrenal glands produce hormones that regulate the body's metabolism, its balance of salt and water, the immune system, and sexual function. Adrenal hormones also help the body cope with physical and emotional stress by increasing the pulse and respiratory rates and the blood pressure.
- The pancreas secretes digestive enzymes as well as the hormones glucagon and insulin, which are responsible for the regulation of blood glucose levels.
- The gonads are the main source of sex hormones (Table 29-3). In men, the gonads, or testes, are located in the scrotum and produce hormones called androgens. The most important androgen in men is testosterone. Androgens regulate body changes associated with sexual development (puberty), including growth spurts, deepening of the voice, growth of facial and pubic hair, and muscle growth and strength.
- In women, the gonads are the ovaries, which release the eggs and secrete the hormones oestrogen and progesterone.
- Diabetes is a metabolic disorder in which the body's ability to metabolise glucose is impaired. It is characterised by the passage of large quantities of urine containing glucose, significant thirst, and deterioration of body function.
- In type 1 diabetes, most patients do not produce insulin at all. They require daily injections of supplemental synthetic insulin throughout their lives to control blood glucose levels.
- The most common form of diabetes is type 2 diabetes [sometimes called adult (late)-onset diabetes], in which blood glucose levels are elevated.
- Hypoglycaemia in the patient with insulin-dependent diabetes is often the result of having taken too much insulin, too little food, or both. The patient will experience trembling, a rapid pulse rate, sweating, and a feeling of hunger—a result of the actions of adrenaline.
- Hyperglycaemia (high blood glucose level) is one of the classic symptoms of diabetes mellitus. Common early signs include frequent and excessive thirst, accompanied by frequent and excessive urination.

- If left untreated, hyperglycaemia progresses to the life-threatening condition known as diabetic ketoacidosis (DKA). DKA occurs when certain acids accumulate in the body because insulin is not available.
- Hyperosmolar nonketotic coma (HONK), also called hyperosmolar hyperglycaemic nonketotic coma (HHNC), is a metabolic derangement that occurs principally in patients with type 2 diabetes. This condition is characterised by hyperglycaemia, hyperosmolarity, and an absence of significant ketosis.
- Adrenal insufficiency is characterised by underproduction of cortisol and aldosterone, which leads to weakness, dehydration, and the body's inability to maintain adequate blood pressure or to properly respond to stress. Primary adrenal insufficiency (also known as Addison's disease) is caused by atrophy or destruction of both adrenal glands, leading to deficiency of all the steroid hormones produced by these glands. Secondary adrenal insufficiency is defined as a lack of ACTH secretion from the pituitary gland.
- Acute adrenal insufficiency is referred to as an Addisonian crisis, which may result from an acute exacerbation of chronic insufficiency, usually brought on by a period of stress, trauma, surgery, or severe infection.
- Cushing's syndrome is caused by an excess of cortisol production by the adrenal glands or by excessive use of cortisol or other similar steroid (glucocorticoid) hormones.
- Thyroid hormones are critical for cell metabolism and organ function. If their supply becomes inadequate, organ tissues don't grow or mature (due to the decreased metabolic rate), energy production declines (a cause of the decreased metabolic rate), and the actions of other hormones are affected.
- Symptoms of hypothyroidism include fatigue, feeling cold, weight gain, dry skin, and sleepiness. Continued decrease of the hormone levels may lead to myxoedema coma.
- Thyrotoxicosis is a toxic condition caused by excessive levels of circulating thyroid hormone. A thyroid storm is a rare, life-threatening condition that may occur in patients with thyrotoxicosis.
- Assessing patients with endocrine emergencies can be difficult because their conditions tend to affect many organ systems and the seriousness of their presentations varies greatly. Don't take these calls lightly, as poor outcomes can result very quickly.

Vital Vocabulary

adrenal cortex The outer part of the adrenal glands that produces corticosteroids.

adrenal glands Paired glands located above the kidneys; each adrenal gland consists of an inner adrenal medulla and an adrenal cortex.

adrenal medulla The inner part of the adrenal glands that produces catecholamines (adrenaline and noradrenaline).

adrenaline Hormone produced by the adrenal medulla that plays a vital role in the function of the sympathetic nervous system.

adrenocorticotropic hormone (ACTH) Hormone that targets the adrenal cortex to secrete cortisol (a glucocorticoid).

agonists Molecules that bind to a cell's receptor and trigger a response by that cell. Agonists produce some kind of action or biological effect.

aldosterone Hormone that stimulates the kidneys to reabsorb sodium from the urine and excrete potassium by altering the osmotic gradient in the blood.

androgens Male sex hormones that regulate body changes associated with sexual development (puberty), including growth spurts, deepening of the voice, growth of facial and pubic hair, and muscle growth and strength.

antagonist Molecules that bind to a cell's receptor and block the action of agonists. Hormone antagonists are widely used as drugs.

antidiuretic hormone (ADH) A hormone secreted by the posterior pituitary lobe of the pituitary gland, ADH constricts blood vessels and raises the blood pressure; also called vasopressin.

calcitonin The hormone secreted by the thyroid gland that helps maintain normal calcium levels in the blood.

catecholamines Hormones produced by the adrenal medulla (adrenaline and noradrenaline) that assist the body in coping with physical and emotional stress by increasing the heart and respiratory rates and the blood pressure.

corticosteroids Hormones that regulate the body's metabolism, the balance of salt and water in the body, the immune system, and sexual function.

cortisol Hormone that stimulates most body cells to increase their energy production.

Cushing's syndrome A condition caused by an excess of cortisol production by the adrenal glands or by excessive use of cortisol or other similar steroid (glucocorticoid) hormones.

diabetes mellitus Disease characterised by the body's inability to metabolise glucose sufficiently. The condition occurs either because the pancreas doesn't produce enough insulin or the cells don't respond to the effects of the insulin that's produced.

diabetic ketoacidosis (DKA) A form of acidosis in uncontrolled diabetes in which certain acids accumulate when insulin is not available.

endocrine glands Glands that secrete or release chemicals that are used inside the body. Endocrine glands lack ducts and release hormones directly into the surrounding tissue and blood.

exocrine glands Glands that excrete chemicals for elimination.

glands Cells or organs that selectively remove, concentrate, or alter materials in the blood and then secrete them back into the body.

glucagon Hormone produced by the pancreas that is vital to the control of the body's metabolism and blood sugar level. Glucagon stimulates the breakdown of glycogen to glucose.

gonads The reproductive glands; the main source of sex hormones.

hormones Chemicals secreted by the body that regulate many body functions, such as growth, reproduction, temperature, metabolism, and blood pressure.

hyperglycaemia Abnormally high blood glucose level.

hyperosmolar hyperglycaemic nonketotic coma (HHNC), also known as hyperosmolar nonketotic coma (HONK), is a metabolic derangement that occurs principally in patients with type 2 diabetes. The condition is characterised by hyperglycaemia, hyperosmolarity, and an absence of significant ketosis.

hyperosmolar nonketotic coma (HONK), also known as hyperosmolar hyperglycaemic nonketotic coma (HHNC), is a metabolic derangement that occurs principally in patients with type 2 diabetes. The condition is characterised by hyperglycaemia, hyperosmolarity, and an absence of significant ketosis.

hypoglycaemia Abnormally low blood glucose level.

hypothalamus A small region of the brain that contains several control centres for the body functions and emotions. It is the primary link between the endocrine system and the nervous system.

insulin Hormone produced by the pancreas that's vital to the control of the body's metabolism and blood sugar level. Insulin causes sugar, fatty acids, and amino acids to be taken up and metabolised by cells.

insulin resistance Condition in which the pancreas produces enough insulin but the body can't effectively utilise it.

iodine An essential element in the diet and an important component of thyroxine. Without the proper level of iodine intake, thyroxine can't be produced, and physical and mental growth are diminished.

islets of Langerhans A specialised group of cells in the pancreas where insulin and glucagon are produced.

luteinising hormone (LH) Hormone that regulates the production of both eggs and sperm, as well as production of reproductive hormones.

myxoedema coma A rare condition that can occur in patients who have severe, untreated hypothyroidism.

noradrenaline Hormone produced by the adrenal glands that is vital in the function of the sympathetic nervous system.

oestrogen One of the three major female hormones. At puberty, oestrogen brings about the secondary sex characteristics.

ovaries Female gonads; ovaries release eggs and secrete the female hormones.

pancreas The digestive gland that secretes digestive enzymes into the duodenum through the pancreatic duct. The pancreas is considered to be both an endocrine gland and an exocrine gland.

parathyroid hormone (PTH) A hormone secreted by the parathyroid gland that acts as an antagonist to calcitonin. PTH is secreted when calcium blood levels are low.

pituitary gland Gland whose secretions control, or regulate, the secretions of other endocrine glands. Often called the "master gland".

primary adrenal insufficiency Also known as Addison's disease. A rare condition in which the adrenal glands produce an insufficient amount of adrenal hormones.

progesterone One of the three major female hormones.

target tissues Tissues to which hormones are directed to act on.

testes Male gonads located in the scrotum that produce hormones called androgens.

testosterone The most important androgen in men.

thyroid Large gland located at the base of the neck that produces and excretes hormones that influence growth, development, and metabolism.

thyroid-stimulating hormone (TSH) Hormone that controls the release of thyroid hormone from the thyroid gland.

thyroid storm A rare, life-threatening condition that may occur in patients with thyrotoxicosis. The condition is usually triggered by a stressful event or increased volume of thyroid hormones in the circulation.

thyrotoxicosis A toxic condition caused by excessive levels of circulating thyroid hormone.

thyroxine The body's major metabolic hormone. Thyroxine stimulates energy production in cells, which increases the rate at which the cells consume oxygen and use carbohydrates, fats, and proteins.

type 1 diabetes The type of diabetic disease that usually starts in childhood and requires daily injections of supplemental synthetic insulin to control blood glucose. Sometimes called juvenile or juvenile-onset diabetes.

type 2 diabetes The type of diabetic disease that usually starts in later life and often can be controlled through diet and oral medications. Sometimes called adult-onset diabetes.

Assessment in Action

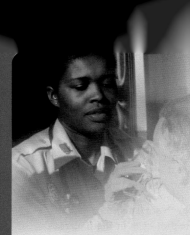

You are dispatched to a warehouse for an unconscious man. You arrive on scene and are greeted by the plant manager. He walks you through the plant and advises you that the patient has insulin-dependent diabetes and got caught up working and was unable to eat lunch on time. When you arrive to the patient's side, you find the patient unresponsive to verbal stimuli; however, he does withdraw purposefully when you attempt to perform your physical assessment. You obtain a baseline set of vital signs, which are within normal limits. You establish IV access and perform a glucose test, which gives a reading of 1.8 mmol/l. You start an infusion of glucose 10% as per local guidelines. The patient slowly responds to this and initially appears lethargic. As the glucose metabolises through his body, the patient becomes conscious, alert, orientated, and refuses transport to hospital. After you advise the patient that he should go to hospital and he still refuses, you advise him that he needs to eat a meal with carbohydrates and explain to him that the infusion you have given him can only be considered short acting.

1. **Glucagon is a hormone that:**
   A. is produced in the pancreatic alpha cells and facilitates the process of glycogenolysis.
   B. is released by the beta cells of the pancreas and facilitates the cellular uptake of glucose.
   C. causes a decrease in circulating blood glucose levels by blocking the conversion of glycogen to glucose.
   D. is typically administered by the paramedic in a dose of 25 g via rapid IV or IO push.

2. **The term diabetes mellitus refers to:**
   A. a metabolic disorder in which the body's ability to metabolise simple glucose is normal.
   B. a metabolic disorder in which the body lacks the ability to produce hormones that stimulate the sympathetic nervous system.
   C. glands that secrete or release chemicals that are utilised inside the body.
   D. a disease that is characterised by an inability to sufficiently metabolise glucose.

3. **The _____ is a digestive gland that is considered both an endocrine gland and an exocrine gland.**
   A. gonad
   B. liver
   C. kidney
   D. pancreas

4. **What is insulin responsible for?**
   A. The removal of glucose from the blood for storage as glycogen, fats, and protein
   B. The maintenance of glucose levels in the blood for storage as glycogen, fats, and protein
   C. The main source of sex hormones
   D. The hormones that regulate the body's metabolism

5. **What causes diabetes mellitus?**
   A. The liver does not produce enough insulin.
   B. There is not enough glucose in the bloodstream.
   C. The pancreas does not produce enough insulin or the cells do not respond to the effects of the insulin produced.
   D. The pancreas produces too much insulin and the cells respond appropriately to the effects of the insulin produced.

6. **What is type 1 diabetes mellitus?**
   A. The type of diabetic disease that usually starts in childhood and requires daily injections of supplemental, synthetic insulin to control blood glucose
   B. The type of diabetic disease that usually starts in later life and often requires daily injections of supplemental, synthetic insulin to control blood glucose
   C. The type of diabetic disease that usually starts later in life and often can be controlled through diet and oral medications
   D. The type of diabetic disease that usually starts in childhood and can often be controlled through diet and oral medications

7. **What is type 2 diabetes mellitus?**
   A. The type of diabetic disease that usually starts in childhood and requires daily injections of supplemental, synthetic insulin to control blood glucose
   B. The type of diabetic disease that usually starts in later life and often requires daily injections of supplemental, synthetic insulin to control blood glucose
   C. The type of diabetic disease that usually starts in later life and often can be controlled through diet and oral medications
   D. The type of diabetic disease that usually starts in childhood and can often be controlled through diet and oral medications

8. _____ in the patient with insulin-dependent diabetes is often the result of having taken too much insulin, too little food, or both and often presents with an altered mental status.
   A. Hyperglycaemia
   B. Increase in blood glucose
   C. Hypoglycaemia
   D. Hypotension

9. A normal blood glucose level is approximately:
   A. 3 to 6 mmol/l.
   B. 4 to 8 mmol/l.
   C. 5 to 9 mmol/l.
   D. 6 to 10 mmol/l.

Challenging Question

You are dispatched to the home of a person with weakness. When you arrive, the patient tells you that she has been feeling weak and fatigued for approximately 1 week. She called today because she "can't take it anymore". She states that she has been depressed recently and does not understand why. Her vital signs are within normal limits. Her medical history includes hypertension, cardiac problems (unable to specify), and lupus. Her medications include metoprolol and hydrocortisone. You question her as to whether she has had any increased thirst or urination, and she states yes.

10. What differential diagnosis can you make?

Points to Ponder

You are dispatched to the home of a patient with an altered level of consciousness. When you arrive, you are greeted by the patient's husband, who tells you that his wife is "not acting right". When you begin to assess her, she does not answer questions appropriately, and she has erratic respirations. She is hot to the touch, dry, and appears pink. Her pulse rate is 132 beats/min, with sinus tachycardia on the monitor; her blood pressure is 140/70 mm Hg. After you initiate an IV of normal saline, you perform a glucose test that reads "high" on your monitor. In your head you understand that this means her blood glucose is greater than 28 mmol/l. Her husband states that she has not been feeling well for the last 2 days, and they believed she was coming down with the flu. He called today because she appeared confused to him.

What are your priorities in this situation? What do you need to do for this patient?

Issues: Understanding the Importance of the Endocrine System, Understanding the General Assessment Findings Associated With an Endocrine Emergency.

30 Allergic Reactions

Objectives

Cognitive

- Define allergic reaction.
- Define anaphylaxis.
- Describe the incidence, morbidity, and mortality of anaphylaxis.
- Identify the risk factors most predisposing to anaphylaxis.
- Discuss the anatomy and physiology of the organs and structures related to anaphylaxis.
- Describe the prevention of anaphylaxis and appropriate patient education.
- Discuss the pathophysiology of allergy and anaphylaxis.
- Describe the common methods of entry of substances into the body.
- Define natural and acquired immunity.
- Define antigens and antibodies.
- List common antigens most frequently associated with anaphylaxis.
- Discuss the formation of antibodies in the body.

- Describe physical manifestations in anaphylaxis.
- Differentiate manifestations of an allergic reaction from anaphylaxis.
- Recognise the signs and symptoms related to anaphylaxis.
- Differentiate among the various treatment and pharmacological interventions used in the management of anaphylaxis.
- Integrate the pathophysiological principles of the patient with anaphylaxis.
- Correlate abnormal findings in assessment with the clinical significance in the patient with anaphylaxis.
- Develop a treatment plan based on initial diagnosis in the patient with allergic reaction and anaphylaxis.

Affective

None

Psychomotor

None

Introduction

Allergic reactions and anaphylaxis have been documented for many years. One of the earliest accounts may have been noted by the late 17th century clergyman Increase Mather:

> Some men also have strange antipathies in their natures against that sort of food which others love and live upon. I have read of one that could not endure to eat either bread or flesh; of another that fell into a swooning fit at the smell of a rose . . . There are some who, if a cat accidentally comes into the room, though they neither see it, nor are told of it, will presently be in a sweat, and ready to die away.

Although these cases cannot be proven to be anaphylaxis, the descriptions suggest some type of reaction was present—possibly an allergic or anaphylactic reaction given the severity and fatality of the descriptions. This chapter explores these types of reactions, including their typical signs and symptoms, and the steps you should take to manage such patients. In addition, it discusses the common causes of "swooning fit" so we can be better prepared to care for affected patients.

The first task is to clarify the many terms associated with allergic and anaphylactic reactions. An allergen is a substance that produces allergic symptoms in a patient. Most allergens are usually harmless substances that do not pose a threat to other people—for example, milk, eggs, chocolate, and strawberries. An antibody is a protein the body produces in response to an antigen. This protein (globulin) is found in the plasma—hence, its other name *immunoglobulin* (Ig). Table 30-1 ▾ lists the common antibodies, their actions, and locations.

An allergic reaction is an abnormal immune response the body develops when the person is reexposed to a substance or allergen. In most people, exposure to this substance would not be a problem; in a person with an allergic reaction, however, a local or systemic reaction may occur. In a local reaction, the body limits its response to a specific area after being exposed to a foreign substance; the swelling around an insect bite would be an example. A systemic reaction occurs throughout the body, possibly affecting multiple body systems. It is seen when a person who is allergic to strawberries, for example, has swelling and hives all over his body after eating strawberry

Table 30-1	Antibodies or Immunoglobulins	
Antibody	**Action**	**Location**
IgA	Provides localised protection to mucous membranes. Stress can lower the IgA level, making the body more susceptible to infection.	Tears, saliva, mucus, breast milk, gastrointestinal secretions, blood, and lymph
IgD	Thought to stimulate antibody-producing cells to make antibodies	Blood, lymph, and the surfaces of B cells
IgE*	Responds in allergic reactions	Located on mast and basophil cells
IgG	Provides protection against bacteria and viruses; enhances phagocytosis, neutralises toxins, triggers the complete system	Blood, lymph, intestines
IgM	One of the first to appear; causes agglutination and lysis of microbes. ABO agglutinins are IgM antibodies.	Blood, lymph, and surface of B cells

*The primary antibody you need to be concerned with during allergic and anaphylactic reactions is the IgE antibody.

You are the Paramedic Part 1

You are sent to the home of a 26-year-old patient with "trouble breathing". On arrival, you find a young man, Matthew Harris, in the living room of his home, holding his throat and working hard to breathe. You hear wheezes without the use of a stethoscope and notice that he is leaning far forward on the edge of his sofa. His wife tells you that the patient has been ill with "walking pneumonia". She had picked up a new prescription of amoxycillin for him that he took just a few minutes ago. She said her husband is normally very healthy, has no other medical history, and is not taking any other medications.

Initial Assessment	Recording Time: 0 Minutes
Appearance	Sitting on the edge of the sofa, appears very anxious
Level of consciousness	A (Alert to person, place, and day)
Airway	Coughing, hoarse voice, and audible wheezing
Breathing	Rapid and laboured
Circulation	Weak, fast radial pulse

1. How would you categorise this patient and why?
2. How would you clinically manage this patient?

Notes from Nancy

The term *anaphylaxis* is not, therefore, really accurate; for in fact the fundamental problem in an anaphylactic reaction is not lack of "protection" but overprotection. That is, anaphylaxis is a form of allergy—a very extreme and devastating form—and allergy represents the body's protective immune system gone into overdrive.

shortcake. Hypersensitivity occurs when a patient reacts with an exaggerated or inappropriate allergic symptoms after coming into contact with a substance perceived by the body to be harmful. Anaphylaxis is an extreme systemic form of an allergic reaction involving two or more body systems. This term was first used in 1902, when Portier and Richet were vaccinating

dogs with sea anemone toxin. After the second dose of the toxin, one of the dogs died. Because this response was the opposite of protection, it was referred to as anaphylaxis (meaning "without protection").

Within the UK the true incidence of anaphylaxis is unknown, but it is thought to be 10–30 cases per 100,000 head of population. The death rate from true anaphylaxis in the UK is unclear but is in the region of 20 per year for people aged over 16. Unfortunately, no exact cause for anaphylaxis can be determined in up to two thirds of patients. To anticipate anaphylaxis, of course, it would be useful to be able to identify people at greatest risk. Neither race nor sex seems to affect the incidence of anaphylaxis. The incidence of anaphylaxis resulting from an insect sting tends to be higher in men. Women have a greater incidence of anaphylactic reactions to latex, aspirin, and intravenous (IV) muscle relaxants. Anaphylactic reactions have been documented in children as young as 6 months and adults as old as 89 years. Children are more

Table 30-2	Common Causes of Anaphylactic Reactions	
General Type of Antigen	**Specific Antigen**	**Examples/Comments**
Drugs	Penicillin (antibiotic)	Causes many IgE-mediated drug interactions in the United Kingdom
	Beta-lactam antibiotics (cephalosporins)	Possibly a cross-reaction in patients allergic to penicillin
	Other antibiotics	Ampicillin
	Sulpha drugs (antibiotic)	Sulphanomide, sulphisoxazole
	Muscle relaxants, hypnotics, opioids	Paracetamol with codeine, morphine, pethidine
	Salicylates	Aspirin
	Colloids	
	Local anaesthetics	Procaine
	Enzymes	Chymotrypsin, penicillinase
	Mismatched blood transfusion	
	Iodinated radiocontrast dyes used in taking X-rays	Intravenous pyelogram
	Biological extracts and hormones	Insulin, heparin
	Vaccines	
Insect stings	Bees, hornets, wasps	0.5%–3% of the population will have a systemic reaction after being stung.
Foods (problem worldwide—most common cause of anaphylaxis)	Peanuts	As little as 100 mcg of peanut protein can cause a reaction.
	Tree nuts, fish, and shellfish	Most common to all age groups
	Some fruits	Mango, strawberries
	Egg, soya, and milk	Most common in children
Latex (may be seen in myelodysplasia, genitourinary anomalies, patients with frequent exposure to latex, and sensitised health care workers)	Gloves and other materials made from latex	The incidence rate is decreasing owing to awareness and better manufacturing practices. People with allergies to bananas, kiwi, and strawberries may have a cross-reaction to latex.
Immunotherapy	Allergen immunotherapy, skin testing (Note: Patients with atopic diseases are at greater risk for anaphylaxis.)	Rare, associated with asthma, errors in administration, overdose, and beta blocker use during immunotherapy
Animals	Dander	Long-haired animals
	Animal serum products	Horse serum, gamma globulins

Adapted from Dreskin et al, Anaphylaxis, eMedicine, www.emedicine.com/med/topic128.htm. Accessed 5/26/06.

At the Scene

It is important to be prepared for latex allergies and to consider a latex-free or latex-safe environment.

likely to have severe food allergies, whereas adults tend to have anaphylactic reactions to insect stings, anaesthetics, and radiocontrast media. **Table 30-2** lists the common substances associated with anaphylaxis.

Diseases related to allergies, such as allergic rhinitis, asthma, and atopic dermatitis increase the potential for anaphylactic reactions. One third to one half of patients with anaphylaxis have a history of atopic diseases.

The other major factors associated with anaphylaxis are the route of exposure to the allergen and time between exposures. When a substance is ingested (taken by mouth), it is less likely to cause an anaphylactic reaction, and, if a reaction occurs, it usually is not fatal. By contrast, if a substance is injected, the reaction is more likely to be severe. Also, the longer the time between exposures to a substance, the less likely a severe anaphylactic reaction will occur. This is thought to be due to the decreased production of the specific Ig (antibody) cells in the body over time.

Anatomy and Physiology

The Normal Immune Response

The immune system protects the human body from substances and organisms that are considered foreign to the body. Without our immune system for protection, life as we know it would not exist. We would be under constant attack from any bacterium, virus, or other type of invader that wanted to make our bodies their home. Luckily, for the majority of the population, the body is equipped with an amazing immune system that is on patrol 24 hours a day, 7 days a week, to detect unauthorised visits or invading attacks by foreign substances.

The body protects itself via two types of systems: cellular immunity and humoral (that is, related to the body's fluids) immunity. In cellular immunity, the body produces special white blood cells called T cells that attack and destroy invaders. In humoral immunity, the body uses the antibodies dissolved in the plasma and lymph to wage war on invading organisms. The cells producing immunity are located throughout the body in the lymph nodes, spleen, and gastrointestinal tract. Their goal is to intercept foreign forces as they enter the body, thereby limiting the invaders' spread and damage.

Routes of Entry for Allergens

Substances can invade the body through the skin, the respiratory tract, or the gastrointestinal tract. Invasion through the skin may come in the form of injection or absorption. In injection, the invading substance pierces the skin and deposits foreign material into the skin. Bees and hornets prefer this method of invasion. Absorption occurs when foreign material is deposited on the skin and slowly absorbed through the skin. Absorption invaders may take the form of lotions or therapeutic or medicinal creams to trick unsuspecting people into applying them to the skin. Invaders do not stop at the skin, but may also enter the respiratory tract as the patient quietly breathes; this type of raid is referred to as an inhalation exposure. The foreigners advance through the respiratory system and launch their attack from within the lungs. Cats, peanuts, and many plants attack in this way. The final way invading armies attack the body is through the gastrointestinal tract via ingestion. That is, invaders may camouflage themselves as some tempting delicacy such as strawberry cheesecake, a mushroom-and-cheese omlette, or a peanut butter sandwich **Figure 30-1**.

You are the Paramedic Part 2

You take Matthew's vital signs, and your colleague immediately applies high-flow oxygen (15 l/min) via nonrebreathing mask. As you begin your series of interventions, you explain to the patient what is happening to him and what you need to do to correct it. You administer 0.5 mg of adrenaline 1:1,000 via the IM route.

Vital Signs	Recording Time: 5 Minutes
Level of consciousness	Alert, with a Glasgow Coma Scale score of 14
Skin	Flushed, hives
Pulse	130 beats/min, weak and slightly irregular
Blood pressure	88/40 mm Hg
Respirations	50 breaths/min
SpO_2	90% with oxygen at 15 l/min via nonrebreathing mask

3. Why does the order of the medications matter?
4. Why is knowing all of the medication administration routes important?

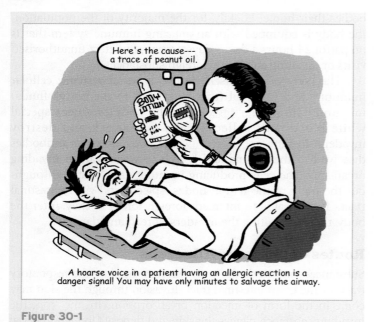

A hoarse voice in a patient having an allergic reaction is a danger signal! You may have only minutes to salvage the airway.

Figure 30-1

The basophils and mast cells produce the body's "chemical weapons"—that is, chemical mediators Table 30-3 ▸. These cells contain granules filled with a host of powerful substances that are ready to be released to fight invading forces of antigens. As long as the body is not invaded by one of the previously identified foreign substances, the granules are kept encapsulated in their protective walls and remain inactive. If an antigen invades the body and combines with one of the antibodies, however, the granules are ejected from the mast cells and detonated. The chemical mediators are then released into the surrounding tissue and the bloodstream Figure 30-2 ▾.

The chemical mediators launch and maintain the immune response. They summon more white blood cells to the area to battle the invading force. They also increase blood flow to the area under attack by dilating the blood vessels and increasing the capillary permeability. These actions are useful when a small invasion occurs to a limited area but can be extremely dangerous when they spread throughout the body. When they have systemic effects, the chemical mediators cause the signs and symptoms of the allergic and anaphylactic reactions seen in the body.

Physiology

Once a foreign substance invades the body, the body goes on alert and initiates a series of responses. The first encounter with the foreign substance begins the primary response. Cells (macrophages) immediately greet, confront, and engulf the invaders to check their papers or passports to see if they can legally be present in the body. If the body is unable to identify the substance or determines the papers are not in order, it starts a file on the outsider. It fingerprints the invader or takes a "mug shot" of the suspect for later identification by using immune cells to record the salient features of the outside substance. These cells record one or two of the proteins on the surface of the invading substance and then design specific proteins to match each substance. These proteins—called antibodies—are intended to match up with the invader—the antigen—and inactivate it.

Through the primary response, the body develops sensitivity—that is, the ability to recognise the foreigner the next time it is encountered. To determine whether the substance is "one of us", the body records enough details to assist in future identification of the substance and production of antibodies to perfectly fit the invading antigen. The body then sends out these details to the rest of the body, much like sending out "Wanted" posters to "post offices" throughout the body. The Wanted posters are distributed by placing the specific antibodies on two types of cells: basophils and mast cells. Basophils are stationed like guards in specific sites within the tissues. Mast cells are on patrol like police cruisers or bounty hunters through the connective tissues, bronchi, gastrointestinal mucosa, and other vulnerable border areas that act as barriers to foreign invaders.

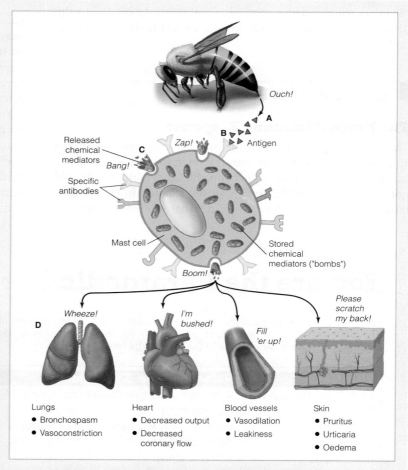

Figure 30-2 The sequence of events in anaphylaxis. **A.** The antigen is introduced into the body. **B.** The antigen-antibody reaction at the surface of a mast cell. **C.** Release of mast cell chemical mediators. **D.** Chemical mediators exert their effects on end organs.

- Recognise the signs and symptoms related to oesophageal varices.
- Describe the management for oesophageal varices.
- Integrate pathophysiological principles and assessment findings to formulate a initial diagnosis and implement a treatment plan for the patient with oesophageal varices.
- Define haemorrhoids.
- Discuss the pathophysiology of haemorrhoids.
- Recognise the signs and symptoms related to haemorrhoids.
- Describe the management for haemorrhoids.
- Integrate pathophysiological principles and assessment findings to formulate a initial diagnosis and implement a treatment plan for the patient with haemorrhoids.
- Define cholecystitis.
- Discuss the pathophysiology of cholecystitis.
- Recognise the signs and symptoms related to cholecystitis.
- Describe the management for cholecystitis.
- Integrate pathophysiological principles and assessment findings to formulate a initial diagnosis and implement a treatment plan for the patient with cholecystitis.
- Define acute hepatitis.
- Discuss the pathophysiology of acute hepatitis.

- Recognise the signs and symptoms related to acute hepatitis.
- Describe the management for acute hepatitis.
- Integrate pathophysiological principles and assessment findings to formulate a initial diagnosis and implement a treatment plan for the patient with acute hepatitis.
- Integrate pathophysiological principles of the patient with a gastrointestinal emergency.
- Differentiate between gastrointestinal emergencies based on assessment findings.
- Correlate abnormal findings in the assessment with the clinical significance in the patient with abdominal pain.
- Develop a patient management plan based on initial diagnosis in the patient with abdominal pain.

Affective

None

Psychomotor

None

Introduction

Gastrointestinal (GI) problems, in and of themselves, are rarely life-threatening. This fact does not minimise the systemic problems that can erupt from untreated or undertreated disease of the GI system. The appendix—a small, inconsequential portion of the intestine—has no known function, and its removal places the patient at no great health risk. However, an untreated infection of the appendix can have deadly consequences.

Almost everyone has suffered from abdominal pain at some point. Diarrhoea, nausea, and vomiting are also common occurrences that bring both discomfort and unpleasantness, although they are merely signs and symptoms of an underlying condition. A wide range of conditions are actually responsible for these effects, as suggested by the data in (Table 31-1 ▶) .

Certain behaviours or characteristics may predispose patients to GI disorders. For example, alcohol consumption and smoking increase a person's risk for developing stomach disorders. Both alcohol and nicotine increase the release of gastric acids within the stomach. As a result, many people will appreciate a *small* amount of wine or a beer before a meal—it primes the stomach for the food about to enter. Chronic alcohol consumption or smoking, by contrast, increases the acidity within the stomach beyond the limits of the protective mucosal layer, putting the individual at risk for ulcers within the upper GI tract. (Table 31-2 ▶) lists other activities that place patients at increased risk.

Table 31-1	Incidence and Prevalence of Gastrointestinal Disorders
Disorder	**Incidence/Prevalence**
All GI disorders	12–14 million
Constipation	2.5 million
Crohn's disease	60,000 people in the UK affected 1 in 1,000 people 3,000–6,000 new cases diagnosed per year
Diverticular disease (diverticulosis, diverticulitis)	The prevalence increases with age, affecting 50% of people by the fifth decade and 67% by the eighth decade
Gallstones	1 in 3 women and 1 in 6 men will form gallstones at some point in their lives
Gastritis	4.1 million
Gastroesophageal reflux disease	20% of UK population
Haemorrhoids	1 in 2 people in the UK will suffer with haemorrhoids at some point in their life
Hepatitis A	1 million
Hepatitis B	180,000
Hepatitis C	54,000 diagnosed, but it is believed up to 400,000 people could be suffering undiagnosed
Hepatitis D	15 million people worldwide; occurs in 5% of hepatitis B patients
Irritable bowel syndrome	1 in 3 people in the UK will suffer from symptoms at some point
Pancreatitis	10,000 cases of acute pancreatitis annually
Peptic ulcer disease	About 1 in 10 men and 1 in 15 women suffer from an ulcer at some time in their lives
Ulcerative colitis	120,000; 6,000–12,000 new cases diagnosed each year

You are the Paramedic Part 1

It's 01:00 on a busy Friday night, and you and your crewmate are finally returning to the station for the first time since starting over 8 hours ago. You have just made a cup of tea when the phone begins to ring. You are being called to a popular nightclub for a patient with uncontrolled bleeding. No other information is available at this time.

You walk into the dimly lit club that's enveloped in a haze of cigarette smoke. The barman calls you over and shouts that the patient is in the gents' toilet. You push your way through the crowd and slowly open the door. Your crewmate points to an open cubicle in the corner where a man is slumped over the toilet bowl with bright red blood trickling from the corner of his mouth. He responds appropriately but slowly when you speak to him.

Initial Assessment	Recording Time: 0 Minutes
Appearance	Ill-appearing middle-aged man
Level of consciousness	V (Responsive to verbal stimuli)
Airway	Open and clear
Breathing	Adequate chest rise and volume
Circulation	Weak, rapid radial pulse

1. What is your first priority in this situation?
2. What are some of the potential differential diagnoses?

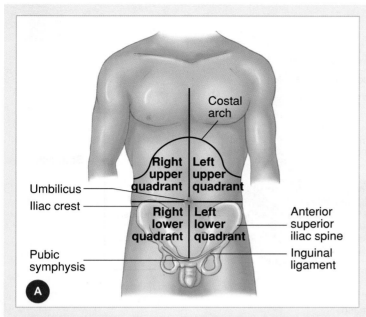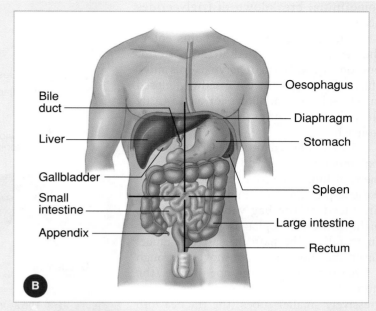

Figure 31-1 The anatomy of the abdomen. **A.** The four quadrants of the abdomen. **B.** Abdominal organs can lie in more than one quadrant.

Table 31-2	Behaviours and Corresponding Risk Factors for GI Disease
Behaviour	**Risk factor**
Smoking	Stomach/oesophageal disease
Ingestion of caustic agents	Stomach/oesophageal disease
Low-fibre diet	Colon disease/constipation
Alcohol	Stomach/oesophageal/liver disease
Ingestion of certain medications: aspirin, nonsteroidal anti-inflammatory drugs (NSAIDs), anticoagulants	Stomach/oesophageal disease
Stress	Disease throughout the GI tract

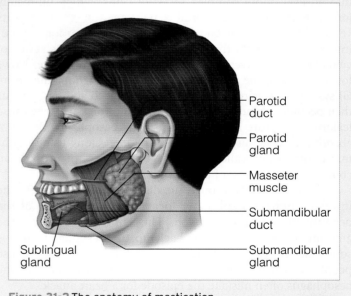

Figure 31-2 The anatomy of mastication.

Anatomy and Physiology

The main function of the GI system is to absorb the components of the diet for use by other cells in the body. Examining the journey from food intake to elimination will illustrate the normal anatomy and physiology related to the GI system **Figure 31-1 ▲**. The stages of this journey can be broken down into five elements—ingestion, propulsion, digestion, absorption, and elimination.

Ingestion begins in the mouth with the front teeth being used to tear or cut the food. At the back of the mouth, the molars pound and grind the food into a more easily swallowed consistency—a process referred to as mastication **Figure 31-2 ▲**. This mechanical activity prepares food to travel down the oesophagus more easily and prevents aspiration.

Saliva is secreted into the mouth to help lubricate food. The combination of pulverising and lubrication creates a bolus that can be easily moved. Saliva also contains enzymes that begin the chemical breakdown of foods—in particular, starches. These complex carbohydrates can be disassembled into simple sugars that are more easily absorbed. In addition, some initial breakdown of triglycerides occurs.

During swallowing, the bolus enters the oesophagus—located at the posterior portion of the laryngopharynx. This muscular tube is typically collapsed (eg, closed in on itself), which allows for air to easily flow into the lungs but not into the stomach.

This collapsed tube description also explains how gastric dilation and impairment of lung expansion can occur during positive-pressure ventilation. If the pressure produced by the bag-valve-mask is too high, then the oesophagus dilates allowing air to follow the path of least resistance. Given the choice between moving through a large tube into a large open space (the stomach) or moving down a series of progressively smaller tubes (the trachea into the right or left main bronchus), air will flow into the stomach.

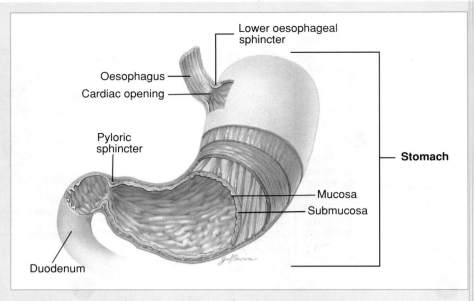

Figure 31-3 The stomach.

Intertwined around the oesophagus are veins that drain into an even more complex series of veins, which ultimately join together to form the portal vein. The portal vein transports venous blood from the GI tract directly to the liver for processing of the nutrients that have been absorbed. This series of veins lacks any valves, so if blood flow through the liver slows for any reason, the blood may back up throughout the entire GI system. The veins surrounding the stomach and oesophagus then become dilated. Even a low amount of pressure may cause leaking or rupture of these vessels. The oesophagus does not absorb nutrients but rather pushes the food along using rhythmic contractions called peristalsis, a process of propulsion common with the rest of the GI tract.

The food travels through the diaphragm and comes to the lower oesophageal sphincter located at the junction of the oesophagus and the stomach. This sphincter controls the amount of food that moves back up the oesophagus and is sometimes referred to as the cardiac sphincter. This is because people with regurgitation of acid out of the stomach into the oesophagus often mistake the episode for a heart attack.

When empty, the stomach is quite small, but it is capable of stretching many times beyond its normal size to accommodate meals **Figure 31-3 ▸**. As the food enters this muscular organ, the stomach begins to secrete hydrochloric acid, which helps to break down the food. To mix the acid with the food more evenly, the stomach also contracts, churning the acid and food mixture together until a relatively smooth consistency is achieved. The stomach absorbs some materials, such as water and fat-soluble substances.

The material that exits the pyloric sphincter at the inferior portion of the stomach, is called chyme. The stomach is designed to release only small amounts of chyme into the duo-denum, the first the portion of the small intestine, thereby enabling the small intestine to more easily manage digestion.

The duodenum is where the pancreas, liver, and gallbladder connect to the digestive system. The exocrine portion of the pancreas secretes several enzymes into the duodenum that assist with digestion of fats, proteins, and carbohydrates. In addition, pancreatic juice helps to neutralise gastric acids. The liver creates bile, which is then stored in the gallbladder. Bile is released into the duodenum, where it helps to emulsify (ie, dissolve into solution) fats.

The liver also affects the GI system indirectly, through carbohydrate metabolism. The brain cells can burn only one fuel source—glucose. If blood sugar falls, the liver can convert glycogen into glucose. Dramatic drops in sugar stores will cause the liver to convert fats and proteins into sugar. As blood flows through the liver, fat and protein metabolism continues. Without a functioning liver one would not be able to use any of the proteins that were absorbed from the GI system. In addition, the liver detoxifies drugs, completes the breakdown of dead red and white blood cells, and stores vitamins and minerals.

The real workhorse of the digestive system is the small intestine; 90% of all absorption occurs there. This 5 metre long structure is divided into three sections: the duodenum (the last section of the upper GI system), the jejunum (the first part of the lower GI system), and the ileum. The small intestine produces enzymes that work with the pancreatic enzymes to turn chyme into substances that can be directly absorbed by the capillaries of the small intestine and thereby move into the bloodstream **Figure 31-4 ▸**. Blood filled with these nutrients exits the intestinal circulation and heads to the liver, where additional metabolism of fats and proteins

Ulcerative colitis is a disease of the young; most patients are between 15 and 30 years of age. It occurs with equal incidence in men and women. There is a strong hereditary component to this disease; 20% of patients have a family member with this disease.

Crohn's Disease

Crohn's disease is similar to ulcerative colitis, but may affect the entire GI tract. In this condition, the immune system attacks the GI tract, and the activity of the white blood cells damages all layers of the portion of GI tract involved. The most likely site of inflammation is the ileum, the last portion of the small intestine before this organ joins the large intestine. The result is a scarred, narrowed, stiff, and weakened portion of the small intestine; this damaged patch is found among areas of intestine that are perfectly normal.

To date, no definitive cause for Crohn's disease has been identified. However, the presence of signs and symptoms outside the GI system supports the hypothesis that some autoimmune component is operating within this disease. Perhaps the presence of antigens within the GI tract triggers an immune response, or perhaps the immune system itself is not working correctly. Another hypothesis is that the immune system creates antibodies for an antigen that does not exist, initiating a cascade of reactions to a ghost invader.

Most patients with Crohn's disease are between the ages of 20 and 30 years. Men are diagnosed as often as women. Many of the people with this condition have a blood relative with some type of inflammatory bowel disease, suggesting that these conditions have a family/genetic component.

Acute Gastroenteritis

Acute gastroenteritis comprises a family of conditions revolving around a central theme of infection combined with diarrhoea, nausea, and vomiting. Bacterial and viral organisms that can cause this condition include *Escherichia coli, Salmonella, Shigella, Giardia,* the Norwalk virus, *Clostridium difficile,* and rotavirus. These agents typically enter the body through contaminated food or water. Patients may begin to experience upset stomach and diarrhoea as soon as several hours or several days after contact with the matter. The disease can then either run its course in 2 to 3 days or continue for several weeks.

Cholera, a type of acute gastroenteritis that is relatively unknown in the United Kingdom today, is frequently encountered in the developing world. The Norwalk virus is responsible for the majority of acute viral gastroenteritis in adults, whereas rotavirus causes the same condition in children.

Gastroenteritis

Gastroenteritis is not an infectious disease but has all of the hallmarks of its acute (infectious) cousin. Patients with this condition suffer from nausea, vomiting, and diarrhoea from a noninfectious cause, such as medications, toxins from shellfish, or chemotherapy.

Acute Hepatitis

Acute hepatitis is the result of damage to the liver caused by one of several viruses. Hepatitis viruses A, B, C, D, and E are clearly capable of damaging the liver. In the United Kingdom, the A, B, and C strains are the predominant organisms that cause this disease. Two other strains, F and G, are also being investigated for their role in causing liver damage. Other causes of acute hepatitis include the Epstein-Barr virus, cytomegalovirus, certain bacterial infections, and liver cancer. The time from the initial infection to the emergence of clinical signs and symptoms can range from 14 to 180 days with acute hepatitis.

Hepatitis viruses are transmitted in a variety of ways. Types A and E move from patient to patient by the faecal–oral route (eg, faeces from an infected person is released into the environment and then contaminates either the food or water consumed by another individual). Types B, C, and D are transmitted by person-to-person contact, typically either by sexual intercourse or parenterally (eg, blood-to-blood contact, for example by blood transfusion, accidental needle sticks, or sharing of dirty needles). IV drug users and prostitutes are at higher risk for acquiring hepatitis B, C, and D, whereas people travelling to countries where food and water safety are not adequate are at risk for developing hepatitis A and E.

Bowel Obstruction

With bowel obstruction, the underlying aetiology is decreased intestinal motility (ie, abnormally slow movement of material through the intestines). Two major reasons for this problem are paralysis of the intestines or a change in the diameter of their lumen.

Paralysis can be caused by infection, kidney disease, impaired blood flow to the intestines, or medications. In particular, narcotics and anaesthetics can paralyse the intestinal muscles. For this reason, patients who undergo major surgery often will not be released from the hospital until they have had at least one bowel movement.

Intestinal lumen diameter compromise can be caused by neoplasms (ie, tumours of the intestines), objects that the patient has swallowed, or strictures (narrowing of the lumen due to damage in the intestinal wall). Other causes include hernia, in which the intestine becomes trapped and compressed; intussusceptions, telescoping of the intestines into themselves; or twisting of the intestines (volvus). The end result is that the diameter of the intestines is narrowed or blocked.

At the Scene

All providers should have a clear understanding of the medical terms used to describe findings from a GI patient. This knowledge will avoid confusion.

■ Assessment

Scene Assessment

Scene safety is the paramount concern for all types of calls. While there are no specific concerns related to patients with GI emergencies, you need to exercise caution to ensure that all personnel remain safe. In terms of additional resources, often these patients need some type of assistance with hygiene, as GI complaints routinely involve body substances. Examples of additional resources for the GI patient include extra gloves, mask, aprons, change of uniform, suction equipment, extra linens, blankets, flannels, towels, incontinence pads.

The mechanism of injury or nature of illness, as with most medical complaints, will contribute to your initial impression. Early in the call, the only information available may have come from ambulance control. Use this information to help choose the amount of equipment you will take into the scene. Note that most calls for GI problems will not involve multiple patients. However, a call for assistance at an office building where several people are complaining about GI symptoms may lead you to suspect release of an agent. Biological or chemical agents, for example, can cause people to have abdominal pain, nausea, vomiting, diarrhoea, and other GI signs and symptoms.

At the Scene

Patients tend to assume the most comfortable position. Flexion of the hips reduces movement of the psoas muscle and decreases pain. Ask the patient whether movement, walking, or deep breathing relieves or intensifies the pain. Peritoneal pain, inflammatory in nature, intensifies with movement. Patients with colicky pain (renal, biliary, bowel) often present with restlessness.

Another important aspect of the scene assessment is the consideration of body fluid spillages. This is particularly important for GI patients. Universal precautions, including gloves, safety eyewear, and disposable aprons are required to prevent cross-infection. In addition, given that you may need to manage vomit, diarrhoea, and soiled patient clothing, additional fluid spillage management may be called upon in the form of absorbent powder spillage kits.

Initial Assessment

In forming your general impression, closely examine the location where the patient is found, as it can provide hints about what happened. Was the patient walking to

Notes from Nancy

Any severe abdominal pain that comes on suddenly and lasts more than 6 hours must be considered serious and may require surgery.

the toilet when he or she passed out? Has the patient been sick for several days and camped out on the sofa? Was the patient at work when a sudden bout of pain doubled him or her over Figure 31-6 ▾ ?

At the Scene

Remain alert to the four causes of acute abdominal pain that are immediate life threats: acute myocardial infarction (AMI), ruptured abdominal aortic aneurysm, ruptured ectopic pregnancy, and a ruptured viscus (any hollow organ).

One aspect of the general impression that is different for the GI patient is odour. What is the smell of the room or location of the patient? There are few calls that rise to the level of noxious odour as those that involve upper GI bleeding. The foul-smelling stool that accompanies these calls can make even experienced paramedics nauseous. When dealing with these strong odours, the key is to hold your ground. The sense of smell is the most acute for about 1 minute, but then more than 50% of the intensity of an odour is lost due to the olfactory nerve becoming tired of sending the same signal. If you are faced with a strong odour on a call, stay in the environment. After 2 to 5 minutes, the smell may be hardly noticeable.

Airway patency becomes a more pertinent concern with the GI patient. A patient who is vomiting has a greater chance to aspirate. Open the airway using the appropriate manoeuvres, and closely inspect it for foreign bodies. Remove or suction any obstructions that are found. While evaluating the airway, notice any unusual odours emanating from the mouth. Patients who have extremely advanced bowel obstructions can have faeculent breath, smelling of stool.

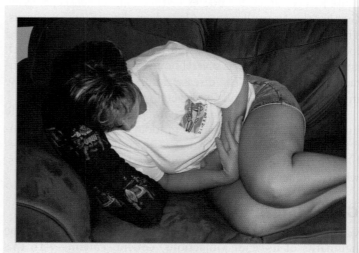

Figure 31-6 A patient experiencing abdominal pain will often curl up into a fetal position to relieve the pressure on the abdomen.

At the Scene

Ask your patient about his or her recent food intake. Fatty foods cause the gallbladder to contract, releasing bile. In the patient with gallbladder disease, this leads to distension and pain. Spicy foods act as a direct irritant on the GI tract; when eaten in large amounts, they will cause pain in most individuals. Milk products contain sugar lactose. Lactose intolerance is very common, and patients affected by it will experience bloating, pain, and often violent diarrhoea within minutes of ingestion of dairy products.

GI problems rarely affect breathing directly. If a breathing problem is encountered, it typically stems from a severe complication. Ensure that the airway is clear. In particular, if the patient has aspirated, it can affect his or her ability to oxygenate and ventilate.

The assessment of the circulatory system is essential in understanding how the GI disease is affecting the body. As with all patients, assess skin colour, temperature, and condition (ie, moisture content). Note findings consistent with shock. Determine the heart rate. Evaluate the peripheral pulses and compare them to the central pulses.

Many GI diseases involve pain and/or haemorrhage. As blood volume begins to drop, the body tries to compensate for this change by releasing catecholamines in the form of adrenaline and noradrenaline. These agents attempt to stabilise blood pressure through vasoconstriction, increased heart rate, and increased force of left ventricular contraction. Pain stimulates similar body responses. Either problem can leave the patient with tachycardia, diminished peripheral pulses, diaphoresis, and pale, cool, clammy skin.

At the Scene

Orthostatic changes usually occur when there has been a 15% to 20% loss in circulating volume. Decompensated shock is almost always present when the patient loses more than 30% of the blood volume.

Check the patient's blood pressure. To ensure this measurement's accuracy, obtain a manual pressure before you use one of the automated blood pressure machines.

Orthostatic vital signs will help you determine the extent of bleeding that has occurred. First, encourage the patient to assume a position of comfort, usually either seated or lying down. Take an accurate blood pressure and heart rate. Next, ask the patient to change positions (eg, have the patient stand or sit up). Use caution, because the patient may potentially lose consciousness with a positional change. Wait a minute or two, and then repeat the blood pressure and heart rate measurements. Normally, there should be little change in the blood

pressure or heart rate with such a positional change. When a patient has a significant loss of fluid within the vascular space, however, there may be a 10-beat increase in the heart rate and/or a 10-mm Hg drop (or more) in blood pressure.

When you examine the GI patient for gross bleeding, it is not unusual to find large amounts of blood. Take note of the amount of blood lost, focusing on being accurate. Many people grossly exaggerate the volume lost due to the emotional effects of seeing large amounts of blood. The amount of blood in a toilet is particularly difficult to estimate due to dilution. To practise volume estimation, measure the amount of water in a glass and then spill it on a carpet; note the size of the puddle. Spill another volume of water on a hard surface such as a tile floor; again note the size of the puddle.

When making your transport decision, integrate the information gathered from the initial assessment. If the patient has a positive tilt test (ie, serial vital signs change with a change in position), then thoughtfully consider how the patient will be moved. Can the patient sit up in a stair chair, or will he or she pass out? Is the patient critical, so that he or she needs to be moved urgently?

At the Scene

In females, consider possible sources such as ectopic pregnancy, spontaneous or threatened abortion, ovarian cyst, or pelvic inflammatory disease. Your history should include addressing the gynaecological system and risk factors for these patients.

In paediatrics, consider common causes such as gastroenteritis, appendicitis, and intussusception of the small bowel. Always maintain an index of suspicion for child abuse.

Older people can be poor historians, have muted symptoms, atypical pain, and low or absence of fever.

Focused History and Physical Examination

For the unstable patient, the head-to-toe examination will provide you with ample opportunities to discover clues as to the underlying problem. With a GI problem, examination of the head, neck, and chest should not reveal any major changes. Instead, the major effects from GI disease typically relate to the nervous, cardiovascular, and respiratory systems and result from pain, hypovolaemia, and infection.

Examining the abdomen can be rather embarrassing for both the patient and the paramedic. Be professional and talk calmly. As you prepare for the abdominal examination, if the patient is stable, ask him or her to lie on their back, place a pillow under his or her knees, and a pillow beneath his or her head. Have the patient relax the arms at his or her side. Maintaining straight legs and arms over the head will result in flexed abdominal muscles, which can distort your examination **Figure 31-7 ▶**. Make sure your hands are warm before you touch the abdomen. If the patient is uncomfortable with this

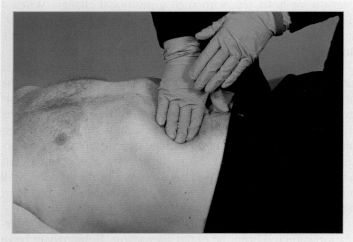

Figure 31-7 Examining a patient's abdomen.

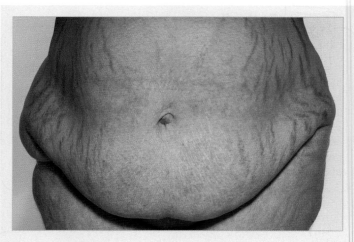

Figure 31-8 Striae.

examination, try to distract him or her by having a casual conversation. If the patient is unstable, then proceed with the examination in a quick and compassionate manner.

Examine the skin for irregularities. Do you see scars indicating trauma or past surgery? If so, ask the patient about the scarring. Do you notice stretch marks (striae)? These indicate a change in the size of the abdomen over a short period of time. Recent increases or decreases in weight, pregnancy, and severe abdominal oedema can all cause striae Figure 31-8 ▸ .

Is the abdomen symmetrical? Looking down at a supine patient, the abdomen should lie flat and gently slope from the ribs with a gentle upward slope as you approach the pelvis. Tumours, hernia, enlarged or distended organs, pregnancy, and other masses can cause asymmetry.

What is the shape of the abdomen? Is it flat, round, protuberant, or scaphoid? As people gain weight, the weight can be localised to the abdomen, producing a round abdomen. If weight becomes extreme, the abdomen may protrude (ie, become protuberant). Other causes of protuberance include fluid buildup in the abdomen (ascites), pregnancy, and organ enlargement. A scaphoid (concave) abdomen may result from decreased abdominal volume, such as would happen with an abdominal evisceration.

Listen to the abdomen before you touch it, because palpation of the abdomen can alter the bowel sound patterns. Bowel sounds are transmitted easily through the abdominal cavity. Place your stethoscope lightly on the abdominal wall and listen. Listening to one location, such as the right lower quadrant, is usually all that is needed.

Normal bowel sounds sound like gurgles and clicks and occur 5 to 30 times per minute Table 31-7 ▸ . In your examination, you are merely listening for the presence or absence of these sounds. Sometimes you may hear loud prolonged sounds. This "stomach growling" (borborygmi) indicates strong contractions of the intestines; it can be normal or it may present with diarrhoea. Interestingly, hyperperistalsis can also be heard in patients with early bowel obstruction, as the bowel contracts forcefully in an effort to overcome the obstruction.

Decreased bowel sounds—that is, listening over the right lower quadrant and not hearing anything for 15 to 20 seconds—can indicate decreased peristalsis of the intestines. This lack of movement can lead to bowel obstruction. True absent bowel sounds, which are characterised by no sounds heard for 2 minutes, are typically not practical to discover in the prehospital setting. The absence of bowel sounds means that the intestines are not contracting, so any material within them is not in motion.

At the Scene

The extraneous noise in the prehospital environment makes assessing for bowel sounds difficult. Many recommend listening for bowel sounds for anywhere from 1 to 5 minutes in each quadrant. In practice, this is rarely done. Most importantly, note whether bowel sounds are present or absent—their absence is more clinically significant than the variations in sounds that are present.

To palpate the abdomen, place your hand flat on the wall of the abdomen with your fingers together. Choose the quadrant farthest away from where the patient is having the complaint to start your assessment, and then make your way to the quadrant where the complaint is located. Such a cautious approach to an abdominal assessment will decrease the patient's anxiety, help to reveal more accurate information, and allow the patient to focus his or her attention on other portions of the abdomen that he or she may not have considered because of the current discomfort.

With your hand sitting on the wall of the abdomen, raise your wrist so that you indent the abdominal wall with your fingers about 5 cm to 10 cm. As you are palpating, assess the abdomen for the presence of a pulsatile mass. Observing a pulsatile mass may indicate an abdominal aortic aneurysm. However, it may be normal for some patients to have a degree of pulsation. Further assess for rigidity, discomfort, or masses. Sometimes patients may feel ticklish or otherwise guard the abdomen with flexed muscles, which can make it difficult to determine if the abdomen is rigid or just muscularly guarded. A rigid abdomen may indicate haemorrhage or infection.

Have the patient breathe with an open mouth. It is more difficult to hold the stomach contracted during mouth breathing, so this technique can help to relax the abdomen and allow for a more accurate assessment. You can also hold your fingers slightly depressed into the abdomen during the respiratory cycle.

When the patient exhales, the abdomen typically relaxes. You can also try to coach the patient to relax the abdomen. It isn't always possible to get the patient to relax the abdomen, however. Nevertheless, if you're going to report a rigid abdomen, you should take reasonable steps to ensure that your assessment finding is accurate.

Percussion of the abdomen at the scene is simply used to differentiate between identification of solid organs, which produce dull sounds, and any gas filled structures, such as the bowel,

At the Scene

Don't forget that cardiac pain may radiate or even originate in the abdomen. Patients typically describe the pain as aching, sharp, "gassy", or indigestion-like.

which produce more resonant sounds. The technique involves placing your left palm on the abdomen and spreading your fingers slightly apart and pressing your middle finger *firmly* against the abdomen wall. With the right hand, extend your right wrist with middle finger flexed, so that your middle finger is now at right angles to your hand. Briskly tap your flexed right middle finger onto your left middle finger. Repeat this examination over each of the abdomen's four quadrants. When percussing, listen to the noise made; in addition, feel the reverberation travelling through your finger. Various sounds can be heard; for example, percussion over the liver in the right upper quadrant will elicit a dull sound (hyporesonance) as would severe haemorrhage. The normal abdomen will sound resonant and a grossly flatus abdomen, tympanic (like a kettle-drum) or hyperresonant. One of the most common pathological causes of hyperresonance is ascites, the collection of free fluid in the abdomen. Percussion is a skill that requires lots of practise in the prehospital setting.

Pain is often a finding of importance with GI patients, because it can indicate trauma, haemorrhage, infection, or obstruction. As with the initial assessment, utilise OPQRST to elaborate on the chief complaint. **Table 31-8 ▼** describes the types of pain that may be experienced with an abdominal problem.

As with all pain evaluations, you also need to determine *when* the patient has pain. Does he or she have pain when the abdomen is not being touched? Does the palpation of the abdomen increase the pain? What is the character of the pain? Does the pain change in character or location during your palpation?

Rebound tenderness (parietal pain) may sometimes accompany abdominal pain and is a finding suggestive of a serious and potentially life-threatening pathology. It occurs when the peritoneum is irritated due to either haemorrhage or infection. The peritoneum is a thin layer within the abdominal cavity that contains most of the abdominal organs. This "bag" normally contains a small amount of fluid. Deliberately

Table 31-7	**Bowel Sounds**	
Sound Name	**Description**	**Possible Causes**
Normal	Soft gurgles or clicks occurring at 5 to 30/min	Normal movement of material through the intestines
Borborygmi	Loud gurgles, often heard without a stethoscope and occurring at greater than 30/min	Hyperperistalsis. Can be normal. If prolonged, can indicate increased intestinal contractions as with diarrhoea of any cause
Decreased	Quiet sounds occurring at less than 1 sound/15 to 20 sec	Hypoperistalsis. Can indicate impending obstruction of the intestines
Absent	No sounds after 2 min of continuous listening	Bowel obstruction/intestinal paralysis

Table 31-8	**Types of Abdominal Pain**		
Abdominal Pain Type	**Origin**	**Description**	**Cause**
Visceral pain	Hollow organs	Difficult to localise; described as burning, cramping, gnawing or aching; usually felt superficially	Organ contracts too forcefully or is distended (stretched)
Parietal pain/ rebound pain	Peritoneum	Steady, achy pain; more easy to localise than visceral. Pain increases with movement.	Inflammation of the peritoneum (blood and/or infection)
Somatic pain	Peripheral nerve tracts	Well localised pain, usually felt deeply	Irritation or injury to tissue, causing activation of peripheral nerve tracts
Referred pain	Peripheral nerve tracts	Pain originating in the abdomen and causing "pain" in distant locations; due to similar paths for the peripheral nerves of the abdomen and the distant location	Usually occurs after an initial visceral, parietal, or somatic pain

eliciting rebound tenderness in the prehospital patient is a cruel practice; this information can usually be gained from history and observing the patient's nonmovement and posture. You may also come across it in your routine palpation of the abdomen. However, the next paragraph describes the technique.

Your examination goal is to have the peritoneum vibrate. If the peritoneum is irritated, this vibration will cause a sudden increase in pain. There can also be a sudden relocation of pain to another region of the abdomen. Once you discover an area of the abdomen that is tender to the patient, depress the skin with your fingertips about 5 cm to 10 cm and then quickly pull your fingers off the abdominal wall. Speed is essential—if you pull the fingers off too slowly, you won't be able to get the desired movement of the peritoneum.

The abdomen should be quite smooth when subjected to light palpation (**Figure 31-9 ▼**). While deep palpation can determine some of the organs and structures within the cavity, this requires a level of technique rarely employed within the prehospital setting. As you palpate the abdomen, note the presence of any masses. These will feel like areas of increased density compared to the soft surrounding tissue. Masses may signal the presence of an engorged liver, bowel distension, aortic aneurysm, or cancerous tumours.

At the Scene

Be aware of common pain referral patterns:
- Biliary pain commonly radiates around to the right side of the back and angle of the scapula.
- Pancreatic pain goes straight through to the back in the midline of the lower thoracic area.
- Blood/pus under the diaphragm presents as aching pain in the top of the shoulder.
- A leaking or ruptured aneurysm causes pain in the lumbosacral area and usually in the upper thighs.
- Renal colic (kidney stones) pain radiates to the groin and external genitalia.
- Uterine and rectal pain will often be felt in the lower back.

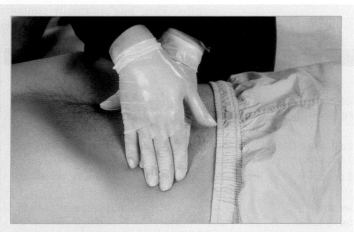

Figure 31-9 Check tenderness by gently palpating each of the four quadrants.

A positive <u>Murphy's sign</u> suggests the presence of cholecystitis. If the patient is experiencing right upper quadrant pain, ask him or her to breathe out. With the tips of your fingers, palpate deeply along the intercostal margin of the right upper quadrant. You are now applying pressure to the liver and subsequently the gallbladder. Next, ask the patient to take a deep breath in. As inspiration continues, the diaphragm will drop and eventually come in contact with the gallbladder. If the patient has cholecystitis, he or she may suddenly stop inspiring due to a sharp increase in pain; this result is reported as a positive Murphy's sign.

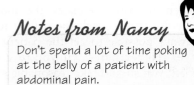

Notes from Nancy

Don't spend a lot of time poking at the belly of a patient with abdominal pain.

The SAMPLE history will help the paramedic elicit the relevant current and past medical history. When asking patients about their complaints, you will often need to discuss subjects that are not easy to describe in everyday language. It is important that you and your patient have a common frame of reference. For example, one person's "diarrhoea" may be another person's "soft stool". (**Table 31-9 ▶**) suggests ways to standardise language so that the health care providers taking over care from you will have the same understanding of the patient's condition as you do.

Ongoing Assessment

The goal of the ongoing assessment is to monitor your patient for changes en route to the hospital. Routine monitoring should include heart rate, ECG, blood pressure, respiratory rate, and pulse oximetry. If the patient is suffering from a GI bleed, continue to assess him or her for signs of shock. Equally important, you should determine what effect your treatment is having. Before giving additional fluid boluses, listen to the patient's lung sounds to determine whether he or she is developing acute pulmonary oedema.

At the Scene

When recording information about the patient's body substances, be as accurate as possible. Describe the substances in detail. Saying the patient had faeces covering the legs is adequate if melaena is not present. If you see the diarrhoea, describe how liquid it is. This information can help to determine the patient's degree of dehydration.

At the Scene

Factors that may complicate the abdominal assessment:
- **Young age.** Poor historians; fear
- **Old age.** Poor historians, muted symptoms, atypical presentations
- **Obesity/pregnancy.** A large abdomen can displace or hide abdominal organs
- **Compromised immune systems.** Don't mount a telltale response to infection or inflammatory disease.

Table 31-9	Body Substances From the GI Tract	
Substance	**Description**	**Possible Cause**
Vomit	Food and partially digested food. Strong acid odour mixed with odour of food eaten.	Influenza, food intolerance
Haematemesis or coffee-ground emesis	Dark, granular material that is the colour black or very dark red. This slurry of material may have food within it. The food and blood are indistinguishable.	Blood from the mouth, oesophagus, or stomach that has been digested by stomach acids and then vomited
Vomit with gross blood	Vomit with obvious red blood. In this setting there is distinct food and blood that are not incorporated into each other.	Bleeding from the mouth or oesophagus that has not been exposed to stomach acids
Diarrhoea	Liquid stool that is the consistency of water. It can range in colour from clear to dark brown.	Intestinal infections, bowel obstructions; usually associated with small intestinal problems; is always considered abnormal
Acholic stools	Clay-coloured, formed stools. May be softer than typical.	Liver problem; bile is released by the liver into the small intestine; bile gives stool its dark colour
Steatorrhoea	Foamy, foul-smelling, mushy, yellow to grey stools. These oily stools will usually float within water.	Liver or pancreatic disease causing excessive excretion of fat within the stool
Soft stools	Bowel movement that is the consistency of soft-serve ice cream. Can range in colour from tan to dark brown.	Normal variant for some people; caused by new foods or rapid change in diet
Haematochezia	Stool and blood that incorporated together into the same substance yet are easily distinguished from each other.	Bleeding from the lower GI tract
Melaena	Stool and blood that are blended together into one substance. You are unable to distinguish blood from stool. These are black, tarry, sticky, and very odourous.	Bleeding from the upper GI tract

Notes from Nancy

It is not necessary to diagnose the specific cause of a patient's abdominal pain in order to appreciate that the patient is in a serious condition.

Also monitor the patient's pain level. Use a recognised pain scoring system. Many patients with abdominal pain may be receiving pain medication. How effective was your treatment? Does the patient need more medication? What are the blood pressure and respiratory rate?

If the patient's condition undergoes a sudden dramatic change, repeat the rapid and detailed assessments as if this case were a new patient. This will give you the best chance of modifying your care to adequately manage this new development.

Assessment of Specific Conditions

Gastrointestinal Bleeding

Presentation of GI bleeding is variable, as it can reflect the presence of a number of diseases. Each of these conditions has its own pattern of disease progression. For example, diverticular disease has quite a gradual onset and tends to strike people in their 50s, 60s, or later decades. Mallory Weiss syndrome has a very sudden onset and affects people of all ages. Gathering the information about how the patient progressed from being healthy to needing an ambulance is critical in forming your initial diagnosis.

The patient's medical history and other possible events of abdominal pain or bleeding from the GI tract may also provide important information. Find out which medications the patient is taking; many drugs can irritate the GI tract, precipitating bleeding. Determine how long the patient has had the problem.

The most important component of the physical examination is to determine how much bleeding has occurred. Do you see evidence of bleeding in the environment? If so, estimate the amount of liquid present. Focus your assessment on evaluation for shock. Determine whether the patient is compensating for the fluid loss. Orthostatic vital signs are the key to gauging the degree of fluid loss in the prehospital setting.

Oesophageal Varices

Presentation of oesophageal varices takes two forms. Initially, the patient shows signs of liver disease—that is, fatigue, weight loss, jaundice, anorexia, oedema in the abdomen, pruritus, abdominal pain, nausea, and vomiting. This very gradual disease process takes months to years before the patient reaches a state of extreme discomfort.

By contrast, the rupture of the varices is far more sudden. The patient will complain of sudden-onset discomfort in the throat. He or she may have severe dysphagia, vomiting of bright red blood, hypotension, and signs of shock. If the bleeding is less dramatic, then haematemesis and melaena are likely. Regardless of the speed of bleeding, damage to these vessels can be life-threatening.

Mallory Weiss Syndrome

The presentation of Mallory Weiss syndrome is linked to vomiting. In women, this syndrome may be associated with hyperemesis gravidarum (ie, severe vomiting related to pregnancy). The extent of the bleeding can range from very minor, resulting in very little blood loss, to severe bleeding and extreme hypovolaemia. In extreme cases, patients may suffer from signs and symptoms of shock, epigastric abdominal pain, haematemesis, and melaena.

Haemorrhoids

Haemorrhoids present as bright red blood during defecation. This haematochezia (gross bleeding) tends to be minimal and is easily controlled. Additionally, patients may experience itching and a small mass on the rectum. Typically, this mass is a clot formed in response to the mild bleeding.

Peptic Ulcer Disease

Patients with peptic ulcers experience a classic sequence of burning or gnawing pain in the stomach that subsides or diminishes immediately after eating and then reemerges 2 to 3 hours later. Nausea, vomiting, belching, and heartburn are common as well. If the erosion is severe, gastric bleeding can occur, resulting in haematemesis and melaena.

At the Scene

Many patients who bleed from a peptic ulcer have had no prior symptoms or history of ulcer disease. When obtaining a history, ask about recent ingestion of alcohol, NSAIDS (eg, ibuprofen), or salicylates.

Cholecystitis

In the classic pattern of cholecystitis, the patient originally has no pain. He or she then eats a fatty meal and 2 to 3 hours later develops severe upper right quadrant abdominal pain. This pattern is not absolute, but may vary depending on the consistency of the food being eaten. A fatty steak will remain in the stomach longer than a vegetable dish, for example. The faster the food is emptied from the stomach, the sooner the complaints will begin after the meal.

Appendicitis

Patients with appendicitis classically present with periumbilical (around the navel) pain that migrates to the right lower quadrant. The duration of the pain is usually less than 48 hours. As the condition progresses, the pain will change characteristics. Rebound tenderness is a sign of perforation of the appendix with resultant peritonitis. Additionally, these patients often develop anorexia, nausea, and fever.

At the Scene

Missed appendicitis is more common in the young, older people, and in pregnant patients because the symptoms are often atypical.

Diverticulitis

The presentation of diverticulitis is abdominal pain, which tends to be localised to the left side of the lower abdomen. Classic signs of infection include fever, malaise, body aches, chills, nausea, and vomiting. Bleeding is rare with this condition. Due to the local infections of these pouches, adhesions may develop, narrowing the diameter of the colon and resulting in constipation and bowel obstruction.

You are the Paramedic Part 3

Your physical examination finds jaundice of the skin and eyes, jugular venous distension while sitting, and a swollen abdomen with a palpable liver. You are clearly able to smell an alcohol-like odour on the patient's breath. While completing your examination, the patient leans forward and vomits an additional 250 ml of bright red blood on the floor. You and your crewmate decide to load the patient on the stretcher and initiate treatment in the back of the ambulance. While you insert a wide-bore cannula in the right antecubital region and begin to administer normal saline, your crewmate applies 100% supplemental oxygen via a nonrebreathing mask and attaches the cardiac monitor.

Reassessment	Recording Time: 13 Minutes
Skin	Jaundiced, cool, and perspiring
Pulse	130 beats/min; weak and regular
Blood pressure	80/56 mm Hg
Respirations	26 breaths/min, regular
SpO_2	98% on nonrebreathing mask at 12 to 15 l/min of oxygen
ECG	Sinus tachycardia with no ectopy
Pupils	Pupils equal and reactive to light and accommodation

5. What does this patient need to be monitored for?

6. Is it possible that your patient has aspirated blood? Why or why not?

Pancreatitis

The pain of pancreatitis tends to be localised to the epigastric area or right upper abdomen. It can be sharp and may be quite severe. Radiation of the pain to the back is not uncommon. Patients may also experience nausea, vomiting, fever, tachycardia, hypotension, and muscle spasms in the extremities as a result of hypocalcaemia (low blood calcium).

The greatest cause for alarm with pancreatitis is internal haemorrhage. If autodigestion is advanced, blood vessels in and near the pancreas can be compromised. Severe and uncontrolled haemorrhage may then ensue. In these patients, haemodynamic instability can be present. Grey Turner's sign (bruising in the flanks) and Cullen's sign (bruising around the umbilicus) indicate that retroperitoneal bleeding may be present.

Ulcerative Colitis

The presentation of ulcerative colitis entails the gradual onset of bloody diarrhoea (haematochezia) and abdominal pain, which can range from mild to severe. Other signs and symptoms may include joint pain and skin lesions, which lends credence to the idea that this disease has an autoimmune component. Finally, patients may experience fever, fatigue, and loss of appetite as a consequence of the infections occurring within the colon.

Crohn's Disease

Crohn's disease presents with a chronic complaint of abdominal pain, often in the lower right area. This pain corresponds to the location of the ileum. Rectal bleeding, weight loss, diarrhoea, arthritis, skin problems, and fever may also be present. The bleeding tends to be small amounts over a long period of time. Acute severe haemorrhage is rare, but chronic bleeding resulting in anaemia and hypotension does occur. Patients may experience repeated episodes of mild to severe signs and symptoms.

Acute and Nonacute Gastroenteritis

The presentation of acute gastroenteritis and nonacute gastroenteritis involves diarrhoea of various types. Patients may experience large dumping-type diarrhoea or frequent small liquid stools. The diarrhoea may contain blood and/or pus, and it may have a foul odour or be odourless. Abdominal cramping is frequent as hyperperistalsis continues. Nausea, vomiting, fever, and anorexia are also present.

If the diarrhoea continues, dehydration and haemodynamic instability will result. As the volume of fluid loss increases, the likelihood of potassium and sodium imbalance increases. Watch for changes in level of consciousness and other profound signs of shock, as they indicate a critical volume loss.

Acute Hepatitis

All types of acute hepatitis, regardless of their aetiology, are associated with the same signs and symptoms. Clinically, the disease occurs in two phases. In the first phase, patients experience joint aches, weakness, fatigue, nausea, vomiting, anorexia, urticaria, and pruritus (itching). At this point in the course of the disease, the patient may be misdiagnosed as having influenza or gastroenteritis.

The second clinical phase of acute hepatitis involves damage to the liver that results in liver failure. It is characterised by acholic stools, darkening of the urine, jaundice, and icteric sclera (yellow sclera). Abdominal pain in the right upper quadrant and an enlarged liver also become apparent at this time. Depending on the disease progression, total liver failure may be only days away.

Bowel Obstruction

The presentation of bowel obstruction varies according to the underlying cause. If this condition is caused by the swallowing of some object, then obstruction can occur within hours. If it is caused by cancer, then the narrowing may take months to become apparent.

Signs of this problem include abdominal pain and fullness. Initially, diarrhoea will occur. The slowdown of stool is interpreted as a decrease in water content, so water absorption slows and peristalsis increases as the body tries to overcome the obstruction. If this effort is unsuccessful, constipation results, with decreased bowel sounds. Nausea and vomiting are common in the later stages, with both the emesis and the patient's breath having a faeculent odour. Eventually, infection may occur, leading to sepsis.

▐ Management

General Management Guidelines

Often there is little the paramedic can do about the GI disease itself, but you can care for the effects of the disease. Patients may be in extreme amount of pain; they may be suffering from severe dehydration, hypotension, or extreme nausea. Your main goals are to isolate any body fluid spillages, manage ABCs, and manage the patient's pain and nausea.

With GI patients, isolation of body fluid spillages is essential due to the high likelihood of coming in contact with infectious agents. Be prepared to deal with large amounts of vomit, faeces, and blood. The following equipment will be helpful to ensure your safety:

- Gloves/aprons/eye protection/surgical mask
- Towels and flannels
- Extra linen
- Absorbent pads
- Disposable basin
- Biohazard bags
- Sterile water for irrigation

Using this equipment to clean the patient also helps to return some degree of dignity to a person who is often quietly humiliated by the circumstances of his or her disease.

The only real airway concern for the GI patient is the potential for aspiration or obstruction of the airway due to vomit or blood. Although these complications are rare, they pose real concerns for the paramedic. Effective positioning of the patient will ensure adequate drainage of material out of the mouth. If the patient has suffered trauma, be prepared to tilt the longboard. In such a case, the patient needs to be packaged and padded well so that spinal movement is minimised during the board movement. Portable suction should be part of every primary response.

If breathing problems are present in association with GI problems, they are often associated with decreased haemoglobin due to bleeding. Be liberal in delivering oxygen to patients with GI bleeds. Don't rely on oxygen saturation readings as evidence that oxygen is not needed. A patient who has been bleeding internally may have a severely decreased haemoglobin level. Although the oxygen saturation may read 96%, if the haemoglobin is low, the patient still needs supplemental oxygen.

Oxygen masks can cause some patients to experience a sense of confinement, especially if they're experiencing nausea. The use of nasal cannulas for oxygen administration may be an alternative consideration in these cases. Monitor patients with whom you use an oxygen face mask to ensure they can get the mask off quickly if they need to vomit.

Listen to lung sounds. This baseline and continuing information is paramount to the safe administration of fluids. In patients who are suffering from dehydration, the overall goal of treatment is to refill the cellular space.

A very stable patient should receive a hypotonic solution. Giving one half of the normal saline solution will effectively move fluids from the vascular space into the interstitial space and finally into the intracellular space.

If the patient is more profoundly dehydrated, then isotonic fluid would be needed to re-expand the vascular space first. Although the cells in this setting are dehydrated, the resultant decrease in blood volume can be life-threatening, so refilling the vascular space takes priority over rehydrating the cells. This step is essential to ensure adequate perfusion to the vital organs of the body.

Care for the patient with haemorrhage is directed at maintaining perfusion of vital organs. Internal haemorrhage cannot be controlled in the prehospital setting. Although volume replacement is critical to ensure adequate circulation to the vital organs, very aggressive volume replacement can result in dramatic haemodilution (ie, dilution of the blood) and potentially death. The goal of management is to provide enough volume to keep vital organs from becoming hypoxic but not so much volume as to increase the bleeding. Maintaining peripheral perfusion at the radial artery should be adequate to allow for adequate perfusion to the brain, kidneys, and other vital organs. Once the patient arrives within the hospital, blood administration will be critical to stabilisation.

Establish secure IV lines with normal saline solution using large-bore cannulas. If the patient is hypotensive, consider a rapid bolus 250 ml and then reassess the patient's status. Listen to lung sounds before administering any fluid bolus to prevent or limit congestive heart failure, and then administer enough fluid to ensure a peripheral pulse. If the patient is suffering from dehydration, continue the fluid bolus and lung sound assessments until the systolic blood pressure is above 90 mm Hg.

There is little contemporaneous evidence to support the premise that substantial prehospital analgesia masks sinister abdomen pathology and compromises surgical assessment. Patients experiencing severe pain are often difficult to assess; pain may obscure their comprehension due to the overwhelming nature of their symptoms. Therefore, it is entirely appropriate, not to mention ethical, for paramedics to use their clinical judgement and administer titrated amounts of analgesia, in-line with local guidelines. Entonox is a consideration, but may not be effective, and should, in any case, be used with caution in patients with an obviously distended abdomen. This is due to the potential of the Entonox increasing the volume of any gas pockets within the abdomen.

The following medications provide the paramedic with the ability to manage abdominal pain. Which medications you are able to use will depend upon your guidelines and which medications you have been authorised to use.

- **Pethidine.** This synthetic opiate can cause hypotension and respiratory depression. It is often given with an anti-emetic to decrease the accompanying nausea.
- **Morphine.** This opiate can cause hypotension and respiratory depression, but is the standard analgesia for UK paramedics to administer to patients in pain.
- **Tramadol.** This is used with varying frequency in the UK and is reputed to cause fewer side effects than are associated with opioid administration.
- **Nalbuphine.** This synthetic opiate is not as strong as morphine but whilst nausea and vomiting occur less, the chance of respiratory depression is similar to that of morphine administration.
- **Fentanyl.** This is a popular opioid agonist because it is rapid-acting, very potent, and has a relatively short duration of action.

The following medications may be administered for management of nausea:

- **Metoclopramide.** A very effective anti-emetic used in patients aged 20 years and older. It acts centrally and on the gut. However, metoclopramide is contraindicated in patients suffering from phaeochromocytoma, renal failure, and acute gastrointestinal obstruction.
- **Prochlorperazine.** This is a phenothiazine which may also be used for its anti-emetic effects. It is often presented in the form of Buccastem tablets which the patient is advised to dissolve between their lip and gum.
- **Promethazine.** An antihistamine that also causes a sedative effect. Be cautious when administering this medication to patients who have taken any medication that has CNS depressive effects, as it acts synergistically to increase the CNS depression. Because this medication is formulated with phenol, promethazine has a pH between 4 and 5.5, so it produces a marked burning sensation during injection. Administer it very slowly (over 10 to 15 minutes), and dilute the drug in 10 to 20 ml of normal saline if it will be administered by the IV route.

Proper cleaning and maintenance of equipment and uniforms that become soiled during a call are essential to protecting the health of both the ambulance clinicians and their next patient. Hepatitis B, for example, can remain infectious even in dried blood for more than a week.

Gastrointestinal Bleeding

Treatment for patients with GI bleeding consists of following the general management guidelines. Fluid resuscitation is commonly needed. In most patients—even those with stable vital signs—it

Assessment in Action

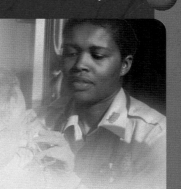

You are dispatched to a care home for someone who is "bleeding". When you arrive on scene you find the patient supine on the floor. The smell to you indicates lower GI bleeding and you immediately walk into the toilet to check out the toilet bowl, where on the floor you see approximately 200 ml of a substance that resembles coffee grounds. The patient's vital signs are as follows: pulse rate, 120 beats/min; sinus tachycardia on the cardiac monitor; blood pressure, 70 mm Hg by palpation; respiratory rate, 26 breaths/min; and pulse oximetry, 97% on room air.

1. **What are the three main conditions responsible for diseases of the GI tract?**
   A. Hypovolaemia, infection, inflammation
   B. Hypertension, hypovolaemia, tachycardia
   C. Hypovolaemia, infection, hypertension
   D. Hypovolaemia, inflammation, gallstones

2. **From what organs does an upper GI bleed originate?**
   A. Small intestine, large intestine, rectum, stomach
   B. Oesophagus, stomach, rectum
   C. Rectum, stomach, large intestine
   D. Oesophagus, stomach, small intestine

3. **An aspect of the general impression that is often different for the patient with GI bleeding is:**
   A. patient colour.
   B. patient vital signs.
   C. odour.
   D. restlessness.

4. **_____ becomes more pertinent with the GI patient.**
   A. Airway patency
   B. Breathing
   C. Circulation
   D. Bleeding

5. **As blood volume begins to drop, the body begins to compensate by releasing:**
   A. antihistamines.
   B. ketoacidosis.
   C. catecholamines.
   D. insulin.

6. **What is the dark red or black granular material called?**
   A. Haematemesis, or coffee ground emesis
   B. Vomit
   C. Diarrhoea
   D. Steatorrhoea

7. **What is the most important component of the physical examination?**
   A. The length of time the patient has been having complaints
   B. How much bleeding has occurred
   C. Where the abdominal pain, if any, is located
   D. Noting when the last bowel movement occurred

8. **_____ are the key to gauging the degree of fluid loss in the prehospital setting.**
   A. Normal vital signs
   B. Orthostatic vital signs
   C. Abnormal vital signs
   D. No vital signs

Challenging Question

You are dispatched to the home of a person with abdominal pain. When you arrive on scene, the patient is doubled over in pain and complains of point tenderness to the upper right quadrant. The patient's vital signs are as follows: pulse rate, 108 beats/min with sinus tachycardia; blood pressure, 110/70 mm Hg; respiratory rate, 24 breaths/min; and pulse oximetry, 100% on room air.

9. **What management is required for this patient with an acute abdomen?**

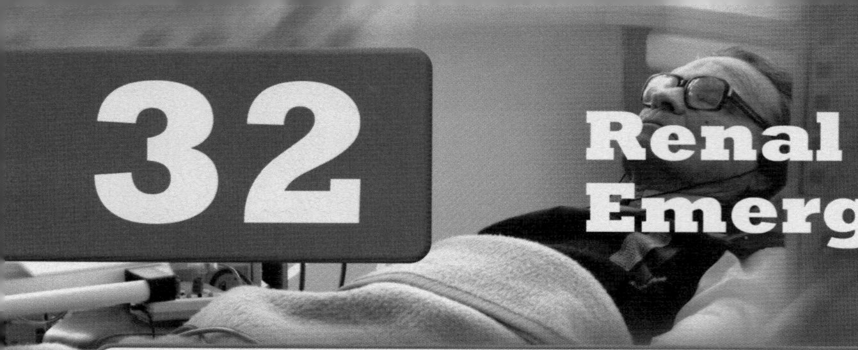

Objectives

Cognitive

- Describe the incidence, morbidity, mortality, and risk factors predisposing to urological emergencies.
- Discuss the anatomy and physiology of the organs and structures related to urogenital diseases.
- Define referred pain and visceral pain as it relates to urology.
- Describe the questioning technique and specific questions the paramedic should utilise when gathering a focused history in a patient with abdominal pain.
- Describe the technique for performing a comprehensive physical examination of a patient complaining of abdominal pain.
- Define acute renal failure.
- Discuss the pathophysiology of acute renal failure.
- Recognise the signs and symptoms related to acute renal failure.
- Describe the management for acute renal failure.
- Integrate pathophysiological principles and assessment findings to formulate a initial diagnosis and implement a treatment plan for the patient with acute renal failure.
- Define chronic renal failure.
- Discuss the pathophysiology of chronic renal failure.
- Recognise the signs and symptoms related to chronic renal failure.
- Describe the management for chronic renal failure.
- Integrate pathophysiological principles and assessment findings to formulate a initial diagnosis and implement a treatment plan for the patient with chronic renal failure.
- Define renal dialysis.
- Discuss the common complications of renal dialysis.
- Define renal calculi.
- Discuss the pathophysiology of renal calculi.
- Recognise the signs and symptoms related to renal calculi.
- Describe the management for renal calculi.
- Integrate pathophysiological principles and assessment findings to formulate a initial diagnosis and implement a treatment plan for the patient with renal calculi.
- Define urinary tract infection.
- Discuss the pathophysiology of urinary tract infection.
- Recognise the signs and symptoms related to urinary tract infection.
- Describe the management for a urinary tract infection.
- Integrate pathophysiological principles and assessment findings to formulate a initial diagnosis and implement a treatment plan for the patient with a urinary tract infection.
- Apply the epidemiology to develop prevention strategies for urological emergencies.
- Integrate pathophysiological principles to the assessment of a patient with abdominal pain.
- Synthesise assessment findings and patient history information to differentiate accurately between pain of a urogenital emergency and that of other origins.
- Develop, execute, and evaluate a treatment plan based on the initial diagnosis made in the assessment.

Affective

None

Psychomotor

None

Introduction

The urinary system performs two main functions for the body. It acts as the body's accounting firm, keeping track of the electrolytes, water content, and acids of the blood; and it acts as the blood's sewage treatment plant, removing metabolic wastes, drug metabolites, and excess fluids. The kidneys perform these functions continuously, filtering 200 l of blood each day.

According to the National Kidney Federation, recent research suggests that 1 in 10 of the UK population may have slight kidney disease. The UK Renal Registry Report published in 2005 believed that there were over 37,800 adult patients receiving Renal Replacement Therapy (RRT) in the UK. RRT is deemed as including a working transplant or dialysis. (There are approximately 1,800 kidney transplants performed per year in the UK.) Other common types of renal disease include urinary tract infections, which occur in more than 50% of all women, and noncancerous enlargement of the prostate, which 60% of men will develop by age 50. Many of these conditions can be prevented by diet and hygiene, including proper hydration.

Anatomy and Physiology

The urinary system consists of the kidneys, which filter the blood and produce urine; the urinary bladder, which stores the urine until it is released from the body; the ureters, which transport the urine from the kidneys to the bladder; and the urethra, which transports the urine from the bladder out of the body. The bean-shaped kidneys are found in the retroperitoneal space (behind the peritoneum), which extends from the twelfth thoracic vertebra to the third lumbar vertebra. The right kidney is slightly lower than the left due to the position of the liver. The medial side of the kidney is concave, forming a cleft called the hilus, where the ureters, renal blood vessels, lymphatic vessels, and nerves enter and leave the kidney   Figure 32-1 ▾ .

A fibrous capsule covers the kidney and protects it against infection. Surrounding this capsule is a fatty mass of adipose tissue, which cushions the kidney and holds it in place in the abdomen. A layer of dense fibrous connective tissue called the renal fascia anchors the kidney to the abdominal wall.

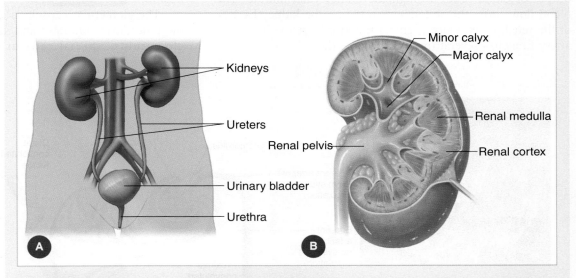

Figure 32-1 The urinary system. **A.** Anterior view showing the relationship of the kidneys, ureters, urinary bladder, and urethra. **B.** Cross-section of the human kidney showing the renal cortex, renal medulla, and renal pelvis.

You are the Paramedic Part 1

You arrive at a residence of a 71-year-old woman with severe weakness. As you enter her house, you find the patient seated in a chair in her living room. She is conscious, but somewhat confused, and she clearly appears ill. She tells you that she has missed her last few dialysis treatments because her friend—who usually takes her to and from her treatments—is out of town. Your initial assessment findings are as follows:

Initial Assessment	Recording Time: 0 Minutes
Appearance	Conscious but confused; ill appearance; skin is slightly jaundiced; hands and feet are oedematous
Level of consciousness	V (Responds to verbal stimuli), somewhat confused
Airway	Patent
Breathing	Tachypnoeic; adequate tidal volume
Circulation	Radial pulses are rapid and irregular

1. What is the purpose of dialysis?
2. What are the two types of dialysis?

The internal anatomy of the kidney can be divided into three distinct regions: the cortex, the medulla, and the pelvis. The cortex is the lighter-coloured outer region closest to the capsule. The medulla (middle layer) includes the cone-shaped renal pyramids (parallel bundles of urine-collecting tubules), and inward extensions of cortical tissue that surround the pyramids, called the renal columns. The renal pelvis is a flat, funnel-shaped tube that fills the sinus at the level of the hilus. The major and minor calyces branch off the pelvis and connect with the renal pyramids to receive the urine draining from the collecting tubules. This arrangement has been described as several strands of uncooked spaghetti (the collecting tubules) sitting in a thimble (the papilla, or tip, of the pelvis). The collected urine flows through the pelvis and into the ureter on its way to the bladder.

Approximately one quarter of the body's systemic cardiac output of blood flows through the kidney each minute. The blood flows from the abdominal aorta into the kidney by way of the renal artery. Once it enters the kidney at the hilus, the artery branches several times to become the afferent arteriole.

The afferent arteriole quickly branches into a tuft of capillaries called a glomerulus, which is the main filter for the blood in the kidney. From the glomerulus, the blood enters the efferent arteriole, which branches into the peritubular capillaries, where tubular reabsorption occurs. This secondary set of capillaries is unique to the kidney; no other organ in the body has two distinct capillary beds. The capillaries then merge, forming venules and veins, until the renal vein leaves the hilus, carrying the cleansed blood to the inferior vena cava.

Nephrons, found in the cortex, are the structural and functional units of the kidney that form urine. Each nephron is composed of the glomerulus; the glomerular (Bowman's) capsule, which surrounds the glomerulus; the proximal convoluted tubule (PCT); the loop of Henle; and the distal convoluted tubule (DCT), which connects with the kidney's collecting tubules). Each kidney contains approximately 1.25 million nephrons **Figure 32-2 ▾** .

The glomerular capsule is a double-layered cup in which the inner layer infiltrates and surrounds the capillaries of the glomerulus. Special cells in the inner membrane called

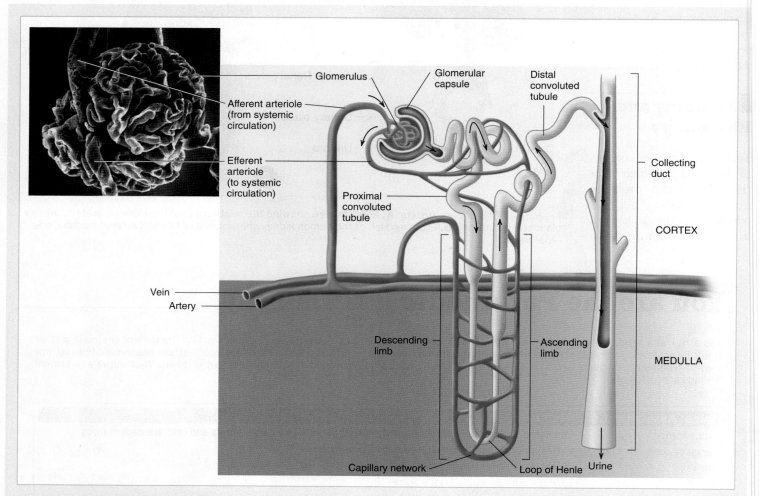

Figure 32-2 The nephrons of the kidney. Part of the nephron is located in the cortex, and part is located in the medulla. Inset at left, Electron micrograph of a glomerulus from a human nephron.

podocytes wrap around the capillaries in the glomerulus, forming filtration slits. The filtrate passes through these slits, across the filtration membrane, and into the capsule. In this manner, the filtration membrane prevents large molecules, such as proteins, from entering the capsule.

Imagine watering your garden with an open-ended hose. If you place your finger over half of the hose's opening, the same amount of water must now pass through half the space. As a consequence, the pressure increases and you can spray the water farther. The same thing happens at the glomerulus. As the blood moves from the relatively large afferent arteriole into the smaller capillaries of the glomerulus, the pressure increases. This effect, along with the smaller diameter of the efferent arteriole, causes the pressure in the glomerulus to become high enough to force the filtrate from the blood into the glomerular capsule (**Figure 32-3 ▾**).

The amount of filtrate produced, called the glomerular filtration rate (GFR), is maintained at a relatively constant rate of 125 ml/min in healthy adults. Changes in the GFR cause many of the renal emergencies encountered in the prehospital setting.

Initially, the filtrate contains everything that can pass through the filtration membrane: salts, minerals, glucose, water, and metabolic wastes. As the filtrate passes through the rest of the nephron, tubular reabsorption and tubular secretion convert the filtrate into urine. As the fluid passes through the PCT, the cells lining the PCT remove all organic nutrients and plasma proteins, as well as some ions from the filtrate.

These compounds are deposited in the interstitial fluid surrounding the PCT. As these solutes accumulate, the concentration of the surrounding fluid becomes higher than that of the filtrate. Water will then move from the filtrate by osmosis. The fluid and nutrients in the interstitial fluid, in turn, move into the peritubular capillaries around the PCT. This process re-establishes the homeostatic balance in the blood and reduces the volume of the tubular filtrate.

Additional reabsorption of water and electrolytes occurs in the loop of Henle. The loop of Henle has two sections—the descending limb, extending toward the medulla, and the ascending limb, moving toward the cortex. The cells in the descending limb are permeable to water, but impermeable to sodium and chloride ions; the cells in the ascending limb are permeable to sodium and chloride ions, but impermeable to water. As a consequence, when the sodium and chloride ions move out of the ascending limb, they increase the solute concentration of the fluid surrounding the descending limb. Water moves by osmosis from the descending limb into the surrounding tissue and eventually into the vasa recta, a series of peritubular capillaries that surround the loop of Henle. This countercurrent multiplier process allows the body to produce either concentrated or diluted urine, depending on the body's needs.

After leaving the loop of Henle, the fluid enters the DCT. At this point, approximately 80% of the water and 85% of the solutes originally forced out of the glomerulus have been reabsorbed. As the urine passes through the DCT and the collecting ducts to which it is attached (both of which are impermeable to solutes), its composition undergoes its final adjustments. Ions are actively secreted or reabsorbed, and the body alters the permeability of the DCT and collecting ducts to water as necessary, depending on the body's homeostatic needs. These adjustments to the final composition of the urine facilitate the removal of metabolic wastes while maintaining the body's fluid-electrolyte balance.

At the site where the efferent arteriole comes in contact with the DCT, a structure called the juxtaglomerular apparatus is formed. The cells in the efferent arteriole (called juxtaglomerular cells) are pressure-sensitive, and monitor the blood pressure. The cells in the DCT (called macula densa cells) are sensitive to chemical changes and monitor the concentration of the filtrate in the DCT. When triggered by changes in the blood pressure of filtrate content, the juxtaglomerular cells release renin. This enzyme initiates a cascade of reactions in the body by converting the plasma protein angiotensinogen into angiotensin I. Other enzymes present in the blood then convert angiotensin I into angiotensin II. A potent vasoconstrictor, angiotensin II promotes smooth muscle contraction in the arterioles throughout the body. This constriction raises the blood pressure by increasing peripheral resistance. Angiotensin II also increases the reabsorption of sodium from the PCT. Given that water tends to follow sodium, by increasing sodium reabsorption, the kidney increases water reabsorption and, in turn, blood pressure.

The final adjustments to the composition of the urine at the DCT and collecting duct are controlled primarily by two

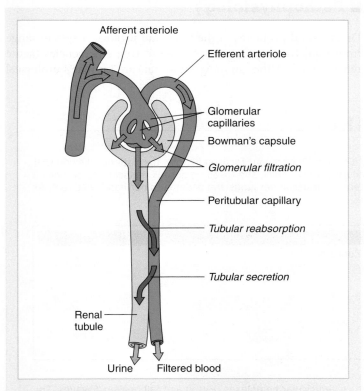

Figure 32-3 The glomerulus of the kidneys. The nephron carries out three blood-filtering processes: glomerular filtration, tubular reabsorption, and tubular secretion.

hormones: antidiuretic hormone (ADH) and aldosterone. ADH is produced by the hypothalamus and stored in the posterior lobe of the pituitary; aldosterone is produced in the adrenal glands.

Neurons in the hypothalamus monitor the solute concentration of the blood. When the solute concentration of the blood increases (eg, due to sweating or decreased fluid intake), ADH is released into the bloodstream. This hormone travels to the DCT and collecting ducts, increasing these structures' permeability to water. Water therefore leaves the DCT and collecting ducts, and reenters the bloodstream. As the solute concentration returns to normal, secretion of ADH will stop.

Aldosterone increases the rate of active reabsorption of sodium and chloride ions into the blood; a corresponding increase occurs in water reabsorption. This hormone also decreases the reabsorption of potassium ion, resulting in excess potassium being secreted in the urine.

Diuretics, chemicals that increase urinary output, work in a variety of ways. A substance that is not reabsorbed from the filtrate, for example, will increase the amount of water retained in the urine. An example of such an osmotic diuretic is glucose in a patient with diabetes mellitus. Alcohol encourages diuresis by inhibiting the production of ADH. Other diuretics, including caffeine and the diuretics commonly prescribed for hypertension and congestive heart failure (furosemide), inhibit the sodium importers in the DCT and collecting ducts.

Once the urine enters the collecting ducts (the renal pyramids of the medulla), it passes through the minor calyx, into the major calyx, and then into the renal pelvis. From there, the urine moves through the ureter (one ureter from each kidney) and is stored in the urinary bladder. Most of the bladder sits in the anterior abdominal cavity, but the dome of the bladder sits in the posterior abdominal cavity, or retroperitoneum, where the ureters and kidneys reside. When empty, the bladder collapses, and the muscular walls fold over onto themselves. In contrast, as urine accumulates, the bladder expands and becomes pear-shaped. The stretching of the bladder walls ultimately stimulates nerve impulses to produce the micturition reflex. This spinal reflex causes contraction of the bladder's smooth muscles, which in turn produces the urge to void as pressure is exerted on the internal urinary sphincter. Normally, the brain exerts control over this urge, keeping the external urinary sphincter contracted until conditions are favourable for urination. At this point, the inhibition of the external urinary sphincter is reduced and the urine passes from the urinary bladder into the urethra.

The beginning of the urethra, through which urine is expelled, sits at the inferior aspect of the bladder. In females, the urethra exits at the site of the external genitalia. The female urethra is shorter than the male urethra (4 cm versus 20 cm) **Figure 32-4 ▸** . The male urethra can be divided into three regions:

- The *prostatic urethra* begins at the bladder and extends through the prostate gland.
- The *membranous urethra* extends from the prostate gland through the abdominal wall and into the penis.
- The *spongy, or penile, urethra* passes through the penis to the external urethral opening.

Pathophysiology

Diseases and problems of the renal and urological system range from mild (urinary tract infections) to true emergencies (acute renal failure). Although the prehospital care for many urological

You are the Paramedic Part 2

You have placed the patient on oxygen via nonrebreathing mask set at 12 l/min. During your focused history, the patient tells you that she has been taking dialysis treatments for over a year for "kidney failure". Additionally, she takes numerous medications and has a history of high blood pressure. Your physical examination reveals scattered crackles in her lungs and oedema to her hands and feet. As you apply a cardiac monitor, your partner obtains baseline observations.

Vital Signs	Recording Time: 5 Minutes
Level of consciousness	V (Responds to verbal stimuli); somewhat confused
Skin	Slight jaundice; cool and dry
Pulse	110 beats/min and irregular
Blood pressure	104/58 mm Hg
Respirations	24 breaths/min; adequate tidal volume
S_PO_2	97% (on supplemental oxygen)
Blood glucose	5.8 mmol/l

The 3-lead ECG reveals sinus tachycardia at 110 beats/min with premature ventricular complexes (PVCs) and tall peaked T waves. The patient denies having any heart problems or diabetes.

3. What condition do you suspect this patient is experiencing?
4. What special concerns should you have regarding the patient's condition?

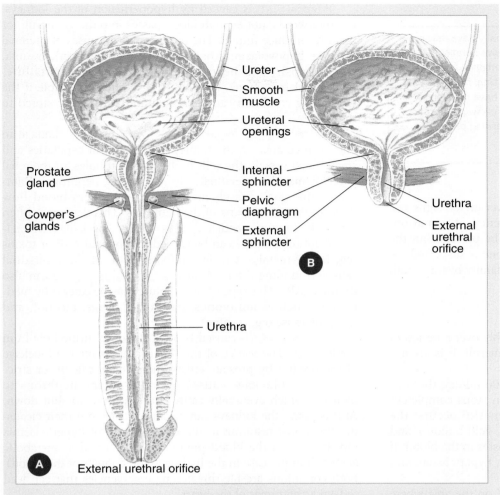

Figure 32-4 The differences in the urethras of (**A**) men and (**B**) women.

often perceived as bladder pain in women and as prostate pain in men. Sometimes the pain may be referred to the shoulder or neck. In addition, the urine will have a foul odour and may appear cloudy.

Renal Calculi (Kidney Stones)

Kidney stones originate in the renal pelvis and result when an excess of insoluble salts or uric acid crystallises in the urine (Figure 32-5 ▾). This excess of salts is typically due to water intake that is insufficient to dissolve the salts. The stones consist of different types of chemicals, depending on the precise imbalance in the urine.

The most common stones—calcium stones—occur more frequently in men than in women and may have a hereditary component. These stones also occur in patients with metabolic disorders such as gout or with hormonal disorders. Struvite stones (magnesium ammonium phosphate) are more common in women, and may be associated with chronic UTI or frequent catheterisation. Uric acid and cystine stones are the least common. Uric acid stones tend to run in families, especially those with a history of gout. Cystine stones are associated with a condition that causes large amounts of amino acids and proteins to accumulate in the urine.

diseases is supportive, your ability to recognise the signs and symptoms of the true emergencies is critical to provide your patients with the best chance of a positive outcome.

Urinary Tract Infections

Urinary tract infections (UTIs) usually develop in the lower urinary tract (urethra and bladder) when normal flora bacteria, which exist naturally on the skin, enter the urethra and grow. These infections are more common in women due to the relatively short urethra and the close proximity of the urethra to the vagina and rectum. UTIs in the upper urinary tract (ureters and kidneys) occur most often when lower UTIs go untreated. Upper UTIs can lead to pyelonephritis (inflammation of the kidney linings) and abscesses, which eventually reduce kidney function. In severe cases, untreated UTIs can lead to sepsis.

Common symptoms in patients with a lower UTI include painful urination, frequent urges to urinate, and difficulty in urination. The pain usually begins as a visceral discomfort, but then converts to an extreme burning pain, especially during urination. The pain, which remains localised in the pelvis, is

Patients who have kidney stones will almost always be in pain (many rate kidney stone pain as 11 on a scale of 1 to 10). The pain usually starts as a vague discomfort in the flank, but becomes very intense within 30 to 60 minutes. It may migrate forward and toward the groin as the stone passes through the system.

Some patients will be agitated and restless as they walk and move in an attempt to relieve the pain. Others will attempt to remain motionless and

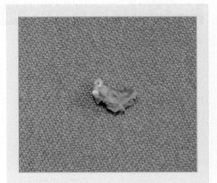

Figure 32-5 A kidney stone.

guard the abdomen. Either behaviour makes palpation of the abdomen difficult. Vital signs will vary, depending on the severity of pain. The greater the pain, the higher will be the blood pressure and pulse.

At the Scene

Patients with kidney stones usually have severe, unbearable pain, and should receive opiate analgesics (eg, morphine, consider Entonox [caution with abdominal pain]) in the prehospital setting. Because higher than usual doses are often required, have naloxone readily available if CNS depression occurs. Follow local protocols or contact the hospital as needed regarding pain relief for such patients.

If a stone has become lodged in the lower ureter, signs and symptoms of a UTI (frequency and urgency of urination, painful urination, and/or haematuria) may be present, but the patient will not have a fever. If a kidney stone is suspected, be sure to obtain both a patient history and a family history; both can supply important information.

Acute Renal Failure

Acute renal failure (ARF) is a sudden (possibly over a period of days) decrease in filtration through the glomeruli. It is accompanied by an increase of toxins in the blood.

If the urine output drops to less than 500 ml/day, the condition is called oliguria. If urine production stops completely, the condition is called anuria. Whenever ARF occurs, the patient may experience generalised oedema, acid buildup, and high levels of nitrogenous and metabolic wastes in the blood. If left untreated, ARF can lead to heart failure, hypertension, and metabolic acidosis.

ARF is classified into three types, based on the area where the failure occurs: prerenal, intrarenal, and postrenal. The signs and symptoms of each type are summarised in ▶ Table 32-1 ▾ .

Table 32-1	Signs and Symptoms of Acute Renal Failure
Prerenal acute renal failure	Hypotension Tachycardia Dizziness Thirst
Intrarenal acute renal failure	Flank pain Joint pain Oliguria Hypertension Headache Confusion Convulsions
Postrenal acute renal failure	Pain in lower flank, abdomen, groin, and genitalia Oliguria Distended bladder Haematuria Peripheral oedema

Prerenal ARF is caused by hypoperfusion of the kidneys. In other words, not enough blood passes into the glomeruli for them to produce filtrate. The most common causes of prerenal ARF are hypovolaemia (haemorrhage, dehydration), trauma, shock, sepsis, and heart failure (congestive heart failure, myocardial infarction). Prerenal ARF is often reversible if the underlying condition can be treated and perfusion restored to the kidney.

Intrarenal acute renal failure (IARF) involves damage to one of three areas in the kidney: the glomeruli capillaries and small blood vessels, the cells of the kidney tubules, or the renal parenchyma (the interstitial cells around the nephrons). Damage to the small vessels and glomeruli hinders blood flow through these vital parts of the nephrons. This damage is often caused by immune-mediated diseases (eg, type 1 diabetes mellitus). Tubule damage can be caused by prerenal ARF or toxins (eg, heavy metals). Chronic inflammation of the interstitial cells surrounding the nephrons (interstitial nephritis) can also produce IARF. This type of renal failure may be caused by medications such as antibiotics, anticancer drugs, alcohol, and drugs of abuse (eg, cocaine).

Postrenal ARF is caused by obstruction of urine flow from the kidneys. The source of this obstruction is often a blockage of the urethra by prostate enlargement, renal calculi, or strictures. This blockage causes pressure on the nephrons to increase, which eventually causes the nephrons to shut down. At this point, the kidneys can no longer carry out their cleansing functions, resulting in the development of hyperkalaemia (an increase in the blood potassium levels) and/or metabolic acidosis (an increase in the hydrogen ion content of the blood). Both conditions are life-threatening emergencies that can lead to fatal arrhythmias of the heart.

Chronic Renal Failure

Chronic renal failure (CRF) is progressive and irreversible inadequate kidney function due to permanent loss of nephrons. This disease develops over months or years. More than half of all cases are caused by systemic diseases, such as diabetes or hypertension. CRF can also be caused by congenital disorders or prolonged pyelonephritis.

As the nephrons become damaged and cease to function, scarring occurs in the kidneys. The tissue begins to shrink and waste away as the scarring progresses, leading to a loss of nephrons and renal mass. As kidney function diminishes, waste products and fluid build up in the blood. Uraemia (increased urea and other waste products in the blood) and azotaemia (increased nitrogenous wastes in the blood) develop, leading to systemic complications such as hypertension, congestive heart failure, anaemia, and electrolyte imbalances.

Patients with CRF exhibit several signs and symptoms, beginning with an altered level of consciousness due to the electrolyte imbalance and the resulting effects on nerve transmission in the brain. In the late stages, convulsions and coma are possible. The patients may also present with lethargy, nausea, headaches, cramps, and signs of anaemia.

should not be given anything by mouth because this may induce vomiting or complicate surgical procedures. Document all vital signs and report noted trends to the receiving hospital in your transfer report.

Management

The management of patients with a UTI or renal calculi centres on comfort and support. Once you have checked and established adequate airway, breathing, and circulation (ABCs), allow the patient to assume a position of comfort. Patients in severe pain may have nausea and vomiting, so be prepared to suction and be ready for the possibility of aspiration. Analgesia may be provided if necessary. Thoroughly assess and document pain before considering analgesia. Establish an IV line. If kidney function is present, administer a bolus of fluid to the patient with a UTI as well as to the patient with a kidney stone. The fluid will rehydrate the UTI patient, and increased urine will help flush the infection from the system. For the patient suffering from renal calculi, the increased urine formation will help move the stone though the system.

ARF and CRF can lead to life-threatening emergencies. Support of the ABCs is imperative. Because of the possible toxic buildup and electrolyte problems, medications to regulate acidosis and electrolyte imbalance as well as fluids for volume regulation may be required. With either of these treatments, you must monitor the patient's reaction because drastic shifts in electrolytes, although rare, may occur. Emergency transport and supportive care are often preferred over aggressive management in these patients.

The management of medical emergencies resulting from dialysis is summarised in **Table 32-2 ▶**.

Assessment and Management of Specific Emergencies

This section considers how the specifics of the more common renal and urological emergencies lead to the appropriate management plan.

Urinary Tract Infections

Patients with UTIs display a classic triad of symptoms: painful urination, frequency of urination, and difficulty of urination. They will appear restless and uncomfortable. The skin will range from pale, cool, and moist in a patient with a lower UTI to warm and dry in a patient with an upper UTI, such as pyelonephritis. Vital signs will vary with the degree of illness, but palpation of the abdomen will usually reveal tenderness over the pubis or pain in the flank, depending on the area of the infection.

Management of patients with UTIs consists mainly of supportive care of the ABCs. Mild symptoms in stable patients may

Table 32-2	Medical Emergencies in Dialysis Patients
Problem	**Prehospital Management**
Problems related to dialysis itself:	
Hypotension	Administer normal saline IV to maintain a systolic BP of 90 mm Hg
Haemorrhage from the shunt	If the shunt cannot be reconnected, clamp it off; check for signs of shock
Potassium imbalance	For hypokalaemia: treat bradycardia with atropine For hyperkalaemia: calcium and bicarbonate may be considered with medical supervision
Disequilibrium syndrome	Supportive treatment only
Air embolism	Left lateral recumbent position in about 10° of head-down tilt
Machine dysfunction	Turn off machine; clamp ends of shunt; disconnect patient from machine; transport
Problems to which dialysis patients are more vulnerable:	
Congestive heart failure	Oxygen; sitting position; rapid transport to appropriate hospital
Myocardial infarction and cardiac arrhythmias	Treat as any other patient, but use caution in administering any medications
Hypertension	Transport only; the treatment is dialysis
Pericardial tamponade	Emergency transport as soon as detected
Uraemic pericarditis	Oxygen; position of comfort; transport
Subdural haematoma	Oxygen; urgent transport

simply require general practitioner intervention. Otherwise, if there is a concern for more sinister pathology, the paramedic must transport. Allow the patient to ride in a position of comfort, but be prepared for nausea and vomiting. Analgesics will probably be needed only in severe cases of pyelonephritis. For most patients, nonpharmacological pain management with breathing and relaxation techniques is usually sufficient. Establish an IV and administer a fluid bolus, which will promote blood flow through the kidney and dilute the urine. Transport the patient to the nearest appropriate hospital for evaluation.

Kidney Stones

The prehospital management of kidney stones centres on pain relief. After ensuring the ABCs, allow the patient to assume a position of comfort. Consider analgesia, but remember that narcotics should not be given if there is a possibility of a gastrointestinal condition. Pain management may also be accomplished by using breathing techniques like those used for women during labour. Establish an IV line and administer fluids to promote movement of the stone through the system. Transport the patient to an appropriate hospital with a lithotripsy unit if possible, providing supportive care as necessary **Figure 32-15 ▶**.

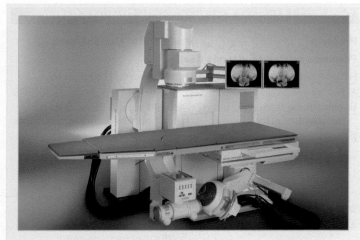

Figure 32-15 A lithotripsy unit, where kidney stones are disintegrated.

Acute Renal Failure

The toxic buildup of nitrogenous wastes and salts in the blood associated with ARF causes impaired mentation, hypotension, fluid retention, tachycardia, and increased PR and QT intervals associated with hyperkalaemia. The patient's skin will be pale, cool, and moist, and oedema will appear on the extremities and face. When inspecting the abdomen, look for any scars, bruising, or distention. If the abdomen is distended, note whether the swelling is symmetric. Palpate the abdomen for any pulsing masses, which could indicate an aortic aneurysm. A haematocrit and urinalysis (if available) may be helpful to identify such causes as acute anaemia, chronic haemorrhage, or pyelonephritis.

Because the metabolic changes caused by ARF can be life-threatening, it is imperative that the treatment plan supports the ABCs. Provide the patient with high-flow supplemental oxygen and, if necessary, provide ventilatory support with bag-mask ventilation. Place the patient in the shock position with the feet elevated to increase blood flow to the brain and vital organs. Consider an IV bolus if the patient exhibits signs of shock, but use caution to prevent pulmonary oedema. If possible, and with medical direction, you may perform a fluid lavage for patients who undergo peritoneal lavage.

The reduction of materials in cases of ARF may be toxic to the kidneys. Many medications can be nephrotoxic, including many analgesics and antibiotics. Take to appropriate hospital if you suspect ARF and are transporting a patient with antibiotic or analgesic drips.

As with any medical patient, patients with ARF need psychological support. Talk with your patient and inform him or her of what you are doing and what is occurring. Be confident and calm in your responses to questions, and reassure the patient that he or she is receiving the best care possible.

Chronic Renal Failure

Patients with CRF will exhibit an altered level of consciousness. In the late stages, convulsions and coma are possible. Patients may also present with lethargy, nausea, headaches, cramps, and signs of anaemia. The skin will be pale, cool, and moist, and may appear jaundiced with uraemic frost present around the face. Bruising of the skin and muscle twitching may also be present. Oedema in the extremities and face will be apparent, and patients will be hypotensive and tachycardic. The ECG monitor will show increasing PR and QT intervals. As hyperkalaemia increases, these arrhythmias may become an idioventricular rhythm. Pericarditis and pulmonary oedema are also common and should be evaluated during auscultation of the chest.

Management of a CRF patient is initially similar to managing an ARF patient. Support the ABCs. Provide the patient with high-flow supplemental oxygen and, if necessary, ventilatory support with bag-mask ventilation. Place the patient in the shock position with the feet elevated to increase blood flow to the brain and vital organs. If there are no signs of pulmonary oedema, consider an IV bolus if the patient shows signs of shock. Because CRF patients are prone to third-space shock (due to fluid shifts) and major electrolyte changes, treatment strategies should centre on the regulation of fluid imbalances and cardiovascular function. Ultimately, patients with CRF will require renal dialysis. After life threats are addressed, transport the patient to the appropriate hospital for treatment.

Because patients in CRF are already suffering from electrolyte imbalances in their blood, be conservative with your treatment plans for these individuals. Transport should be undertaken in a calm manner; talk quietly and confidently with the patient. If the patient has an altered mental status, be sure to assess his or her orientation frequently and record any changes.

You are the Paramedic Summary

1. What is the purpose of dialysis?

Renal dialysis is a technique for "filtering" toxic wastes from the blood, removing excess fluid, and restoring the normal balance of electrolytes. Although dialysis is most commonly used to replace the function of the kidneys in patients with acute or chronic renal failure, it is also used to remove other toxins from the blood, such as those caused by a drug overdose. Without dialysis, patients with renal failure (acute or chronic) would experience uraemia and azotaemia—conditions in which nitrogenous wastes accumulate in the blood. These conditions lead to systemic complications, such as hypertension, anaemia, electrolyte imbalances, and circulatory overload.

2. What are the two types of dialysis?

There are two types of dialysis: peritoneal and haemodialysis. With peritoneal dialysis, large amounts of specially formulated dialysis fluid are infused into (and back out of) the abdominal cavity. This fluid remains in the abdominal cavity for one to two hours, allowing equilibrium to occur. With haemodialysis, the patient's blood circulates through a dialysis machine—much in the same way that it circulates through the kidneys. Unlike peritoneal dialysis, haemodialysis utilises a shunt—a surgical connection between a vein and an artery. Patients requiring chronic dialysis usually receive treatments every 2 or 3 days for a period of 3 to 5 hours.

3. What condition do you suspect this patient is experiencing?

Given the patient's history of dialysis treatments for over a year, it is clear that her baseline problem is chronic renal failure (CRF). CRF is the progressive and irreversible failure of the kidneys due to permanent loss of nephrons—the cells that comprise the kidneys. CRF develops over months or years; hypertension—which your patient has a history of—is a common cause of CRF. Because the patient has missed her last few dialysis treatments, you should suspect that she is uraemic; this would explain her jaundiced skin colour (indicates nitrogenous waste accumulation in the blood). As evidenced by her oedematous hands and feet and crackles in her lungs, you should also suspect fluid retention. Furthermore, her severe weakness and ECG changes (ie, tall, peaked T waves) should lead you to suspect hyperkalaemia—an increased serum potassium level.

4. What special concerns should you have regarding the patient's condition?

Definitively, this patient requires dialysis to restore her body to a state of equilibrium; she will no doubt receive this in hospital. During transport, however, you should be most concerned with the fact that she is at increased risk for cardiac arrest secondary to hyperkalaemia. T waves that are tall and peaked are a classic sign of hyperkalaemia—especially in a patient with CRF who has missed dialysis treatments—and the PVCs she is experiencing indicate ventricular irritability. Close monitoring of the patient's cardiac rhythm is essential. As potassium levels continue to rise, other ECG changes may occur, such as P-R interval prolongation, disappearance of P waves, and widened QRS complexes. You must be prepared to treat this patient for ventricular fibrillation, pulseless ventricular tachycardia, asystole, or pulseless electrical activity (PEA).

5. What types of shunts are used for patients who require dialysis?

As noted earlier, a shunt is a surgical connection between a vein and an artery and is used in patients undergoing haemodialysis. There are several types of shunts used. A Scribner shunt consists of two plastic tubes—one fastened in the radial artery and the other in the cephalic vein. These two tubes are joined together near the wrist with a Teflon catheter. A Thomas shunt—similar to a Scribner shunt—is usually placed in the groin. A Haemasite is a small, button-shaped device with a rubber septum that is punctured with dialysis needles during treatment. Haemasites are usually placed in the upper arm or proximal anterior thigh. An arteriovenous (AV) fistula, an internal shunt, is an artificial connection between a vein and artery. AV fistulas are usually located in the forearm or upper arm.

6. Why should you *not* take a blood pressure in the arm that has a shunt?

A shunt can become occluded by a thrombosis (blood clot). Decreased blood flow is a common cause of thrombosis. Anything that impairs circulation to the extremity with the shunt—even for a few minutes—can result in thrombosis. For this reason, you should avoid taking a blood pressure in the arm that has a shunt.

7. What medications, if any, may be indicated for this patient in the prehospital setting?

If the patient experiences cardiac arrest, adrenaline administration is indicated. Other medications, such as amiodarone or lidocaine and atropine, may be indicated, depending on the patient's cardiac arrest rhythm. In this patient, you should suspect that severe hyperkalaemia is the underlying cause of cardiac arrest if it occurs. Hyperkalaemic cardiac arrest is treated with calcium chloride and sodium bicarbonate. Calcium chloride is used for hyperkalaemia to stabilise the cell membrane. Sodium bicarbonate is used to force potassium from the serum (blood) back into the cell, thus decreasing serum potassium levels. Depending on your transport time to hospital, the A&E consultant may order you to administer calcium chloride and sodium bicarbonate if severe hyperkalaemia is suspected (ie, frequent PVCs, widened QRS interval, P-R interval prolongation). Follow locally established protocols regarding pre-arrest pharmacological treatment for hyperkalaemia.

Prep Kit

■ Ready for Review

- Kidney disease is the most common renal disorder. Kidney stones and urinary tract infections also impact many people.
- The genitourinary system includes the kidneys, urinary bladder, ureters, urethra, male and female reproductive organs, and specific structures within the kidneys.
- Blood flows through the kidney into the afferent arteriole and then the glomerulus, the main filter. It then enters the efferent arteriole, followed by the peritubular capillaries, where it is reabsorbed.
- Urine forms in the nephrons. The nephrons are composed of the glomerulus, the glomerular capsule, the proximal convoluted tubule, loop of Henle, and the distal convoluted tubule.
- In the glomerular capsule, filtrate from the blood—which contains salts, minerals, glucose, water, and metabolic wastes—passes through a membrane. Next, it passes through the rest of the nephron; after which it is converted into urine. This urine passes through the proximal convoluted tubule and loop of Henle to be further concentrated.
- In the distal convoluted tubule, the composition of urine is further refined based on the body's needs. Two hormones, antidiuretic hormone and aldosterone, are involved in adjusting the urine composition.
- The juxtaglomerular apparatus in the kidneys can release renin, an enzyme that can cause reactions in the body such as an increase in blood pressure.
- Diuretics are chemicals that increase urinary output.
- As urine collects in the bladder, the micturition reflex causes it to contract, producing the urge to void.
- Urinary tract infections can move into the upper urinary tract when a bacterial infection in the lower urinary tract is not treated.
- The anatomy of the urethra is different in males and females. The female urethra is shorter and therefore more prone to urinary tract infection.
- Symptoms of urinary tract infection include painful urination, frequent urges to urinate, difficulty urinating, and possibly referred pain to the shoulder or neck. The urine may have a foul odour and be cloudy.
- Kidney stones result when an excess of insoluble salts or uric acid crystallises in the urine. Symptoms include severe pain in the flank that may migrate forward to the groin. The pain may cause an increased blood pressure and pulse.
- Acute renal failure is a sudden decrease in filtration through the glomeruli, resulting in a release of toxins into the blood. The three types of acute renal failure are prerenal, intrarenal, and postrenal. Signs and symptoms range from hypotension, tachycardia, dizziness, and thirst, to pain, oliguria, distended bladder, haematuria, and peripheral oedema.
- Chronic renal failure is progressive and irreversible inadequate kidney function. Nephrons become damaged, losing their functionality and causing a buildup of wastes and fluid in the blood. Symptoms include an altered level of consciousness, lethargy, nausea, headaches, cramps, anaemia, bruised skin, oedema in the extremities and face, hypotension, tachycardia, or possibly convulsions or coma. A powdery buildup of uraemic acid (uraemic frost) may appear on the skin. Hyperkalaemia may be noted on the ECG.

- Renal dialysis is a procedure for removing toxic wastes and excess fluids from the blood. Dialysis patients usually have a shunt through which they are connected to the dialysis machine. They are vulnerable to problems such as hypotension, a potassium imbalance, disequilibrium syndrome, or air embolism.
- Kidney trauma can cause flank pain and haematuria. Management is the same as for other types of abdominal trauma.
- Suspect a bladder injury in any patient who has trauma to the lower abdomen or pelvis. Symptoms include inability to urinate, blood at the urethral opening, and tenderness of the suprapubic region. Management follows basic trauma principles.
- Blunt trauma to the testicles can cause painful haematomas, testicular rupture, or testicular torsion. The scrotum may be tender and swollen. Lacerations or avulsions should be treated with gentle compression and ice packs.
- Blunt trauma to the penis can cause a large haematoma and pain. Management follows basic trauma principles.
- Vaginal trauma can cause haematomas and bruising in the lower pelvic area and on the external female genitalia, bleeding from the vagina, and tenderness on palpation of the lower pelvis.
- Assessment of renal and urological emergencies is the same as with other medical patients. It may be difficult to determine the source of pain, as it may be visceral (cramp, aching) or referred (in another area of the body). Focus on addressing life threats and providing supportive care.
- Note whether the patient seeks a particular position that reduces the pain. Determine where the pain began. Obtain a thorough history using the SAMPLE and OPQRST mnemonics. In the physical examination, use the four-quadrant system and abdominal region mapping. Perform cardiac monitoring, and do not give urological patients anything by mouth.
- Administer pain medication according to clinical need. Patients with a urinary tract infection or kidney stone should receive a bolus of IV fluid. Allow kidney stone patients to assume a position of comfort.
- For patients with acute or chronic renal failure, support the ABCs. It may be necessary to administer medications to regulate acidosis, electrolyte imbalances, and fluid volume. Provide psychological support and transport in a calm fashion.

■ Vital Vocabulary

acute renal failure (ARF) A sudden decrease in filtration through the glomeruli.

afferent arteriole The structure in the kidney that supplies blood to the glomerulus.

aldosterone One of the two main hormones responsible for adjustments to the final composition of urine, aldosterone increases the rate of active reabsorption of sodium and chloride ions into the blood and decreases reabsorption of potassium.

antidiuretic hormone (ADH) One of the two main hormones responsible for adjustments to the final composition of urine, ADH causes ducts in the kidney to become more permeable to water.

anuria A complete stop in the production of urine.

azotaemia Increased nitrogenous wastes in the blood.

calyces (singular: calyx) Large urinary tubes that branch off the renal pelvis and connect with the renal pyramids to collect the urine draining from the collecting tubules.

chronic renal failure (CRF) Progressive and irreversible inadequate kidney function due to permanent loss of nephrons.

cortex Part of the internal anatomy of the kidney; the lighter-coloured outer region closest to the capsule.

countercurrent multiplier The process in which the body produces either concentrated or diluted urine, depending on the body's needs.

distal convoluted tubule (DCT) Connects with the kidney's collecting tubules.

diuretics Chemicals that increase urinary output.

efferent arteriole The structure in the kidney where blood drains from the glomerulus.

glomerular (Bowman's) capsule A double-layered cup with the inner layer infiltrating and surrounding the capillaries of the glomerulus.

glomerular filtration rate (GFR) The rate at which blood is filtered through the glomerula.

glomerulus A tuft of capillaries located in the kidney that serve as the main filter for the blood in the kidney.

haematuria The presence of blood in the urine.

hilus A cleft where the ureters, renal blood vessels, lymphatic vessels, and nerves enter and leave the kidney.

internal shunt Also called an arteriovenous (AV) fistula, this device is an artificial connection between a vein and an artery, usually in the forearm or upper arm.

interstitial nephritis A chronic inflammation of the interstitial cells surrounding the nephrons.

intrarenal acute renal failure (IARF) A type of acute renal failure due to damage in the kidney itself, often caused by immune-mediated diseases, prerenal ARF, toxins, heavy metals, some medications, or some organic compounds.

juxtaglomerular apparatus A structure formed at the site where the efferent arteriole and distal convoluted tubule meet.

kidneys Solid, bean-shaped organs located in the retroperitoneal space that filter blood and excrete body wastes in the form of urine.

kidney stones Solid crystalline masses formed in the kidney, resulting from an excess of insoluble salts or uric acid crystallising in the urine; may become trapped anywhere along the urinary tract.

loop of Henle The U-shaped portion of the renal tubule that extends from the proximal to the distal convoluted tubule; concentrates the filtrate and converts it to urine.

medulla Part of the internal anatomy of the kidney; the middle layer.

micturition reflex A spinal reflex that causes contraction of the bladder's smooth muscles, producing the urge to void as pressure is exerted on the internal urinary sphincter.

nephrons The structural and functional units of the kidney that form urine; composed of the glomerulus, the glomerular (Bowman's) capsule, the proximal convoluted tubule (PCT), loop of Henle, and the distal convoluted tubule (DCT).

oliguria A decrease in urine output to the extent that total urine output drops below 500 ml/day.

peritubular capillaries A set of capillaries unique to the kidney that branch off from the efferent arteriole; the site of tubular reabsorption.

podocytes Special cells in the inner membrane of the glomerulus that wrap around the capillaries in the glomerulus, forming filtration slits.

postrenal ARF A type of acute renal failure caused by obstruction of urine flow from the kidneys, commonly caused by a blockage of the urethra by prostate enlargement, renal calculi, or strictures.

prerenal ARF A type of acute renal failure that is caused by hypoperfusion of the kidneys, resulting from hypovolaemia (haemorrhage, dehydration), trauma, shock, sepsis, and heart failure (congestive heart failure, myocardial infarction); often reversible if the underlying condition can be found and perfusion restored to the kidney.

proximal convoluted tubule (PCT) One of two complex sections of the nephron, the PCT includes an enlargement at the end called the glomerular capsule.

pyelonephritis Inflammation of the kidney linings.

referred pain Pain that originates in one area of the body but is interpreted as coming from a different area of the body.

renal columns Inward extensions of cortical tissue that surround the renal pyramids.

renal dialysis A technique for "filtering" the blood of its toxic wastes, removing excess fluids, and restoring the normal balance of electrolytes.

renal fascia Dense, fibrous connective tissue that anchors the kidney to the abdominal wall.

renal pelvis Part of the internal anatomy of the kidney; a flat, funnel-shaped tube filling the sinus at the level of the hilus.

renal pyramids Parallel cone-shaped bundles of urine-collecting tubules that are located in the medulla of the kidneys.

renin A hormone produced by cells in the juxtaglomerular apparatus when the blood pressure is low.

uraemia The presence of excessive amounts of urea and other waste products in the blood.

uraemic frost A powdery buildup of uric acid, especially around the face.

ureters A pair of thick-walled, hollow tubes that transport urine from the kidneys to the bladder.

urethra A hollow, tubular structure that drains urine from the bladder, passing it outside of the body.

urinary bladder A hollow, muscular sac in the midline of the lower abdominal area that stores urine until it is released from the body.

urinary tract infections (UTIs) Infections, usually of the lower urinary tract (urethra and bladder), which occur when normal flora bacteria enter the urethra and grow.

urine Liquid waste products filtered out of the body by the urinary system.

vasa recta A series of peritubular capillaries that surround the loop of Henle, into which water moves after passing through the descending and ascending limbs of the loop of Henle.

visceral pain Crampy, aching pain deep within the body, the source of which is usually hard to pinpoint; common with urological problems.

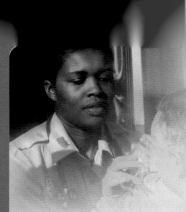

Assessment in Action

You are dispatched to the home of a 54-year-old man complaining of abdominal pain. When you arrive, you find the patient doubled over in pain and he states that this began approximately 2 hours ago. It is the worst pain he has ever had and he tells you that it "burns" when he urinates. His blood pressure is 140/90 mm Hg; pulse rate, 110 beats/min; and respiratory rate, 24 breaths/min. His rhythm on the monitor indicates sinus tachycardia. His pulse oximetry reading on room air is 100%. He has no medical problems and has no allergies.

1. **Which of the following conditions originates in the renal pelvis and is the result of an excess of insoluble salts or uric acid crystallising in the urine?**
   A. Gall stones
   B. Urinary tract infections
   C. Kidney stones
   D. Pyleonephritis

2. **What is the most common type of stone?**
   A. Struvite
   B. Calcium
   C. Uric
   D. Cystine

3. **If a stone becomes lodged in the lower ureter, signs and symptoms of a _____ may be present.**
   A. UTI
   B. uric event
   C. URI
   D. MRSA

4. **Patients who are experiencing renal problems may exhibit many of the same symptoms as a patient with other abdominal problems. These symptoms include nausea and vomiting, constipation or diarrhoea, weight loss, abdominal pain, and:**
   A. chest pain.
   B. headache.
   C. dizziness.
   D. back pain.

5. **What is the most common type of pain associated with urological problems?**
   A. Referred pain
   B. Pain in the urethra
   C. Visceral pain
   D. Pain that can be pinpointed to a specific location

6. **Pain that may be interpreted by the brain as coming from another area of the body is called:**
   A. visceral pain.
   B. urethra pain.
   C. pleurisy.
   D. referred pain.

Challenging Questions

You are dispatched to a secondary school for a rugby player who was injured. When you arrive on scene, you find the patient complaining of right flank pain. You find out that the patient was running with the ball and was tackled from the side. He was jolted and immediately felt a sharp pain in his side. He thought the pain would subside, but it hasn't. You observe his abdominal area and see a contusion in the right flank region and some bruising near his spine. You provide spinal precautions and begin transport to hospital. His vital signs appear to be within normal limits; however, he is in a great deal of pain.

7. **What do you suspect is wrong with the patient?**

8. **How would you begin treatment of this patient?**

■ Points to Ponder

You and your partner are dispatched to the dialysis centre in the local hospital for an unconscious patient. When you arrive on scene, you find a patient sitting in the chair in the dialysis centre and the staff tells you that, after the patient received dialysis, he had an episode of syncope. The patient's blood pressure is 80/40 mm Hg; pulse rate, 64 beats/min; respiratory rate, 18 breaths/min; and pulse oximetry reading on room air, 97%.

Why might a patient who had received dialysis experience syncope?

Issues: Understanding the Role of the Kidneys, Treating Patients Who Received Dialysis, Understanding Renal Dialysis.

33 Toxicology: Substance Abuse and Poisoning

Objectives

Cognitive

- Describe the incidence, morbidity, and mortality of toxicological emergencies.
- Identify the risk factors most predisposing to toxicological emergencies.
- Discuss the anatomy and physiology of the organs and structures related to toxicological emergencies.
- Describe the routes of entry of toxic substances into the body.
- Discuss the role of the National Poisons Information Service.
- List the toxic substances that are specific to your region.
- Discuss the pathophysiology of the entry of toxic substances into the body.
- Discuss the assessment findings associated with various toxidromes.
- Identify the need for rapid intervention and transport of the patient with a toxic substance emergency.
- Discuss the management of toxic substances.
- Define poisoning by ingestion.
- List the most common poisonings by ingestion.
- Describe the pathophysiology of poisoning by ingestion.
- Recognise the signs and symptoms related to the most common poisonings by ingestion.
- Correlate the abnormal findings in assessment with the clinical significance in the patient with the most common poisonings by ingestion.
- Differentiate among the various treatments and pharmacological interventions in the management of the most common poisonings by ingestion.
- Discuss the factors affecting the decision to induce vomiting in a patient with ingested poison.
- Integrate pathophysiological principles and the assessment findings to formulate a working diagnosis and implement a treatment plan for the patient with the most common poisonings by ingestion.
- Define poisoning by inhalation.
- List the most common poisonings by inhalation.
- Describe the pathophysiology of poisoning by inhalation.
- Recognise the signs and symptoms related to the most common poisonings by inhalation.
- Correlate the abnormal findings in assessment with the clinical significance in patients with the most common poisonings by inhalation.
- Differentiate among the various treatments and pharmacological interventions in the management of the most common poisonings by inhalation.
- Integrate pathophysiological principles and the assessment findings to formulate a working diagnosis and implement a treatment plan for the patient with the most common poisonings by inhalation.
- Define poisoning by injection.
- List the most common poisonings by injection.
- Describe the pathophysiology of poisoning by injection.

- Recognise the signs and symptoms related to the most common poisonings by injection.
- Correlate the abnormal findings in assessment with the clinical significance in the patient with the most common poisonings by injection.
- Differentiate among the various treatments and pharmacological interventions in the management of the most common poisonings by injection.
- Integrate pathophysiological principles and the assessment findings to formulate a working diagnosis and implement a treatment plan for the patient with the most common poisonings by injection.
- Define poisoning by surface absorption.
- List the most common poisonings by surface absorption.
- Describe the pathophysiology of poisoning by surface absorption.
- Recognise the signs and symptoms related to the most common poisonings by surface absorption.
- Correlate the abnormal findings in assessment with the clinical significance in patients with the most common poisonings by surface absorption.
- Differentiate among the various treatments and pharmacological interventions in the management of the most common poisonings by surface absorption.
- Integrate pathophysiological principles and the assessment findings to formulate a working diagnosis and implement a treatment plan for patients with the most common poisonings by surface absorption.
- Define poisoning by overdose.
- List the most common poisonings by overdose.
- Describe the pathophysiology of poisoning by overdose.
- Recognise the signs and symptoms related to the most common poisonings by overdose.
- Correlate the abnormal findings in assessment with the clinical significance in patients with the most common poisonings by overdose.
- Differentiate among the various treatments and pharmacological interventions in the management of the most common poisonings by overdose.
- Integrate pathophysiological principles and the assessment findings to formulate a working diagnosis and implement a treatment plan for patients with the most common poisonings by overdose.
- Define drug abuse.
- Discuss the incidence of drug abuse in the United Kingdom.
- Define the following terms:
  - Substance or drug abuse
  - Substance or drug dependence
  - Tolerance
  - Withdrawal
  - Addiction
- List the most commonly abused drugs (both by chemical name and street names).
- Describe the pathophysiology of commonly used drugs.

- Recognise the signs and symptoms related to the most commonly abused drugs.
- Correlate the abnormal findings in assessment with the clinical significance in patients using the most commonly abused drugs.
- Differentiate among the various treatments and pharmacological interventions in the management of the most commonly abused drugs.
- Integrate pathophysiological principles and the assessment findings to formulate a working diagnosis and implement a treatment plan for patients using the most commonly abused drugs.
- List the clinical uses, street names, pharmacology, assessment finding and management for patients who have taken the following drugs or been exposed to the following substances:
  - Cocaine
  - Marijuana and cannabis compounds
  - Amphetamines and amphetamine-like drugs
  - Barbiturates
  - Sedative-hypnotics
  - Cyanide
  - Narcotics/opiates
  - Cardiac medications
  - Caustics
  - Common household substances
  - Drugs abused for sexual purposes/sexual gratification
  - Carbon monoxide
  - Alcohols
  - Hydrocarbons
  - Psychiatric medications
  - Newer anti-depressants and serotonin syndromes
  - Lithium
  - MAO inhibitors

- Non-prescription pain medications
  - Nonsteroidal anti-inflammatory agents
  - Salicylates
  - Paracetamol
- Theophylline
- Metals
- Plants and mushrooms
- Discuss common causative agents, pharmacology, assessment findings and management for a patient with food poisoning.
- Discuss common offending organisms, pharmacology, assessment findings and management for a patient with a bite or sting.
- Integrate pathophysiological principles of the patient with a toxic substance exposure.
- Differentiate between toxic substance emergencies based on assessment findings.
- Correlate abnormal findings in the assessment with the clinical significance in the patient exposed to a toxic substance.
- Develop a patient management plan based on working diagnosis in the patient exposed to a toxic substance.

Affective

None

Psychomotor

None

Introduction

Paramedics treat patients who have taken drugs of abuse (including alcohol) on an almost daily basis. Given the nature of drug use and abuse, it is impossible to accurately identify how many "users" of such substances exist. Sometimes the abused substance is legal (licit), as in the case of alcohol and oxycodone by prescription (Figure 33-1 ▾). At other times, the substance is illegal (illicit), as in the case of heroin and ecstasy. Although research indicates that the use of street drugs has stabilised in smaller communities in recent years, larger cities have seen increases in heroin and cocaine use.

Before we actually dig into this very challenging area of paramedic practice, it is important to define some key terms. A poison is a substance that is toxic by nature, no matter how it gets into the body or in what quantities it is taken. At a minimum, a poison will make people ill; in the worst-case scenario,

it will kill them. By contrast, a drug is a substance that has some therapeutic effect (such as reducing inflammation, fighting bacteria, or producing euphoria) when given in the appropriate circumstances and in the appropriate dose. When a drug (licit or illicit) is taken in excess, the person is said to have "overdosed", which is a toxicological emergency, because the person has been "poisoned". In a nutshell, a poison is always a poison, whereas a licit or illicit substance can poison a person if it is taken to excess.

Types of Toxicological Emergencies

Toxicological emergencies usually fall under one of two general headings: intentional and unintentional. Poisoning in adults is commonly intentional. In particular, suicide is often accomplished with the use of drugs.

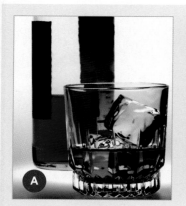 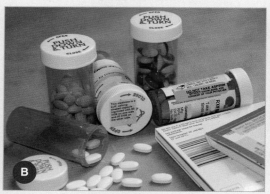 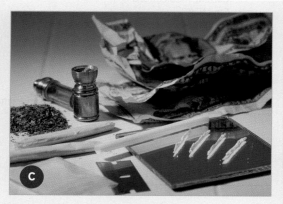

Figure 33-1 A. Alcohol is a legal substance that is a drug. **B.** Medications are legal substances that can be abused. **C.** Illegal drugs can also be abused.

You are the Paramedic Part 1

You and your colleague respond to the local secondary school for an unknown medical emergency. You are met at the school entrance by the girls' p.e. teacher, who escorts you to the sports hall. There, your attention is drawn to a group of young girls surrounding one of their peers, who is lying motionless on the floor.

Your colleague makes room for the two of you to reach the patient. You find a 14-year-old girl lying supine on the floor and unresponsive to verbal stimuli. When you apply a mild painful stimuli, she mumbles incoherently. A student steps forward and introduces herself as the patient's best friend. She says that Julie has been sleepy all morning, becoming drowsy during lunch and passing out while getting ready to play volleyball.

Initial Assessment	Recording Time: 0 Minutes
Appearance	Unconscious, no apparent distress
Level of consciousness	P (Responsive to painful stimuli), mumbles incoherently
Airway	Patent
Breathing	Adequate rate and volume
Circulation	Radial pulse present

1. What are your priorities at this point?
2. What information do you need to obtain?

An unintentional toxicological emergency can occur in many ways. For example, medication dosing errors are common problems in clinical practice. In some cases the event may be idiosyncratic: 2 mg of midazolam may simply relax one patient but cause respiratory arrest in another.

Childhood poisonings are quite common, especially in younger children who may put anything into their mouths Figure 33-2 ▾ , such as colourful berries on a house or garden plant that draw a child's attention. A parent's prescription medication may be mistaken for sweets.

Even nature is fraught with toxicological perils, as any hiker who has inadvertently wandered through a batch of nettles would attest. Wild mushrooms, once in the body, can produce a wide spectrum of results—from being a tasty treat, to being nauseating, to being deadly.

The workplace also harbours its share of toxic hazards. Unfortunately, some of these hazards aren't identified until after the exposure has occurred. For example, countless workers in the electric energy industry worked with polychlorinated biphenyls, or PCBs, on a daily basis and have developed cancer later in life. Similarly, asbestosis developed in thousands of people after continued exposure to asbestos in the workplace.

Unintentional toxicological emergencies can also occur from simple neglect or oversight. Consider an older person with diabetes, possibly combined with early-onset dementia or Alzheimer's disease, who takes his or her insulin in the morning, later cannot remember whether the dose was taken, and takes another dose. The result: a call to 999 for an "unconscious, unresponsive" person in need of assistance.

Biological warfare has drawn increasing attention in recent years owing to the heightened awareness of bioterrorism, but intentional poisoning or overdose may also commonly occur during more intimate crimes. In recent years, "date rape" drugs such as Rohypnol have been used to facilitate sexual assault. Chloral hydrate ("knockout drops") has been used to commit assault for decades, and pharmacological agents are used in murder as well.

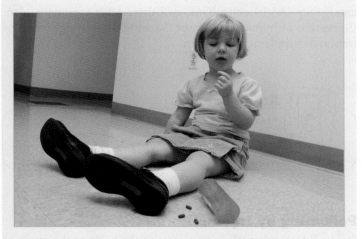

Figure 33-2 Toddlers will put anything into their mouths, including dangerous medications.

Poison Centres

Given the variety of illicit drugs coupled with the continued growth of licit drugs, even the most well-read experienced paramedic may find it difficult to keep up-to-date with the myriad drugs sold in the streets today. For this reason, National Poisons Information Service (NPIS) (0870 600 6266) may be an indispensable aid.

Suppose you are called to a home where a frantic mother is hovering over a toddler who sits beside the remains of a potted philodendron, most of which he appears to have eaten. Is the plant poisonous? How poisonous? Should you make the child vomit? Is an antidote available? In such a scenario, you can call the NPIS and get a fast rundown on the ingestion, its toxic potential, and steps to negate its effects, thereby providing proper patient care.

The NPIS is a virtual gold mine of information that you should add to your toolbox. Never hesitate to tap these resources when confronted with *any toxin* for which you have limited or no familiarity. At the same time, your call helps the centre collect data on poisonings in your region. These data may be analysed to help detect trends, spot developing public health problems, and evaluate current treatment guidelines for different poisonings.

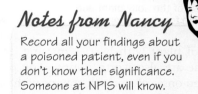

Notes from Nancy

Record all your findings about a poisoned patient, even if you don't know their significance. Someone at NPIS will know.

Routes of Absorption

As nasty as they are, toxins can't exert their effects until they enter the human body. The four primary methods of entry are ingestion, inhalation, injection, and absorption. Just as each of these methods of entry is unique, so is the rate at which a given toxin is absorbed into the body. Once a toxin is in the body, the combination of the amount of toxin and the relative speed at which it is metabolised affect the bioavailability of the toxin and the excretion rate.

Poisoning by Ingestion

Ingested poisons may produce immediate damage to tissues, or their toxic effects may be delayed for several hours. The effects of the ingestion of a caustic substance (that is, a strong acid or alkali) occurs immediately. By contrast, some poisons must be absorbed into the bloodstream before they can produce their toxic effects. Medications around the home and household chemicals (such as cleaning agents) are the most common sources of poisoning by ingestion.

Poisoning by ingestion is marked by a wide range of possibilities regarding *what* is actually ingested and *why* it was ingested. Consider, for example, a curious child who eats the bright red berries of a holly plant or the flowers of a purple foxglove Figure 33-3 ▾ . By contrast, a person who is taking paracetamol for pain relief may inadvertently increase his or her intake to a toxic level, possibly to the point of destroying the liver and leading to death. Although both of these scenarios would be considered accidental, intentional poisoning by ingestion is also possible—as when someone takes a lethal quantity or combination of drugs in a suicide attempt.

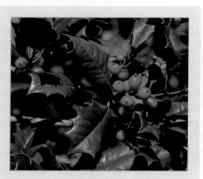

Figure 33-3 Certain berries and flowers are poisonous, such as those of the holly plant and the purple foxglove (digitalis).

Assessment clues pointing toward ingestion can be as obvious as a plant with partially chewed leaves or a section of plant with berries missing. Stained fingers, lips, or tongue are also worth noting. Any patient complaining of a sudden onset of stomach cramps with or without nausea, vomiting, or diarrhoea may have an ingestion-related problem. Empty pill bottles are another obvious clue, as is the date on which the prescription was filled. The bottle for a prescription filled 6 months ago is unlikely to have been full earlier today; an empty bottle for a prescription filled yesterday is far more ominous.

A toxin that enters the body by the oral route generally provides a more forgiving timeframe for treatment. Little absorption occurs in the stomach; indeed, the ingested substance may stay there for a variable period, with the vast majority of absorption actually taking place in the small intestine. As a consequence, much of the management of poisoning by ingestion aims to remove or neutralise the poison before it gains access to the intestines.

Poisoning by Inhalation

A person can be poisoned by inhalation if the poison is present in the surrounding atmosphere. That fact, obvious as it seems, has important implications. First, so long as the patient remains in the toxic environment, he or she will keep inhaling the poison—and so will you, if you enter that environment without the appropriate protective breathing apparatus. Second, when poisoning occurs because of a toxic environment, you are likely to encounter more than one patient at the emergency scene. Home medications and household chemical products (such as bleach and cleaning agents) are responsible for the most common types of inhalation emergencies.

Poisoning by inhalation may be accidental or intentional. Consider carbon monoxide (CO) poisoning. Leaving the garage door shut while seated in a car with the engine running and the window rolled down provides a quick, painless method of suicide. By contrast, an automatic damper on a boiler that fails to open or a bird nest that blocks a chimney may fill a house with colourless, odourless CO, quietly and efficiently poisoning those inside.

From the anatomical and physiological perspective, inhaled toxins quickly reach the alveoli, providing almost instant access to the circulation. CO, for example, binds to haemoglobin on the red blood cells (RBCs) about 240 times more readily than do oxygen molecules. As a result, rapid systemic distribution can occur with an equally rapid onset of signs and symptoms. For this reason, the window of opportunity for treatment is limited.

At the Scene

Scene safety is your primary concern when you are called to an inhalation incident. Whenever you encounter more than one patient but find no evidence of the mechanism of injury (MOI), be suspicious. Toxic fumes may be odourless and colourless, and they do not discriminate between rescuers and victims. Be suspicious of toxic fumes when encountering patients with changes in level of consciousness (LOC), especially at an industrial site or enclosed space.

Inhaled toxins produce a wide range of signs and symptoms, many of which are unique to the toxin involved. A patient with CO poisoning does not exhibit the same signs and symptoms as a person who has sniffed glue, who in turn looks nothing like a patient poisoned by a furniture stripper containing methylene chloride. Frequently, the emergency scene itself contains the clues to the identification of the toxin that is making the patient ill. That information, coupled with the assistance of the NPIS and direction from the accident and emergency (A&E) consultant, will drive your treatment plan. Correction of hypoxia is a must, so administer a high concentration of supplemental oxygen.

At the Scene

Always treat the patient despite the diagnostic evidence. Pulse oximeters may give false readings when patients have been exposed to CO.

Poisoning by Injection

Injected poisons usually gain access to the body as the result of stings or bites from a variety of unpleasant creatures. Abuse of intravenously administered drugs such as heroin, cocaine,

At the Scene

Treat all tools used to inject substances as bio-hazards. These needles or devices may have been shared with other drug users and may carry the human immunodeficiency virus or other pathogens.

At the Scene

Absorption of toxic substances through the skin is a common problem in agriculture and manufacturing. Most solvents and "cides"—insecticides, herbicides, and pesticides—are toxic and can be readily absorbed through the skin.

amphetamines, and "speedball" (heroin and cocaine together) is also common in the prehospital setting.

Depending on the geographical location, multiple possibilities for poisoning by injection may exist in the environment. Snake bites and scorpion stings have been noted in the United Kingdom due to increases in people keeping exotic pets; however, paramedics are more likely to encounter patients in coastal areas stung by jellyfish or weaver fish. Wasps and hornets have a wider geographic distribution, and stings from these insects are common occurrences throughout most of the country.

Some of these injected poisons are neurotoxic and can produce systemic reactions, whereas others may only produce localised reactions. When a bite or sting hits a vein or artery and results in a toxin immediately entering the bloodstream, the outcome is much more dangerous than when the same toxin enters a muscle mass such as the calf, which has a much slower rate of absorption and distribution.

When assessing bites and stings, physical findings will usually provide the most clues, especially local reactions such as pain at the wound site. Depending on the specific toxin, signs and symptoms can vary greatly. Frequently, the patient may be able to identify the culprit, greatly simplifying the assessment process.

Poisoning by Absorption

Some poisons gain access to the body by being absorbed through the skin. Of the poisonings that occur by absorption, those caused by pesticides such as organophosphates and similar substances are often the most serious.

Understanding and Using Toxidromes

Although the sheer number of substances of abuse may seem daunting, the good news is that many drugs, on entering the body, result in similar signs and symptoms. Consider narcotics. Irrespective of whether it is a natural product derived from opium (that is, an opiate) or a synthetic, non–opium-derived narcotic (that is, an opioid), all drugs in this group work in a similar manner, so they produce similar signs and symptoms. The syndrome-like symptoms of a poisonous agent are termed a toxic syndrome or <u>toxidrome</u>. Toxidromes are useful for remembering the assessment and management of different substances that fall under the same clinical umbrella. The major toxidromes are produced by stimulants, narcotics, cholinergics, anticholinergics, sympathomimetics, and sedative-hypnotics `Table 33-1 ▶`.

`Table 33-2 ▶` lists common signs and symptoms of poisoning. If you look at your history and physical examination findings in conjunction with the vital signs, more often than not you can develop a working diagnosis that will allow you to provide appropriate care until you can deliver the patient to the receiving hospital.

You are the Paramedic Part 2

You conduct your initial assessment of the patient. A rapid trauma assessment reveals no life-threatening conditions. As you prepare to perform a detailed physical examination, you ask the teacher to find out if the patient has any relevant medical history and to get a contact number for her mother. You also ask the patient's friend if she knows of any information that might be helpful. She says that Julie has been depressed lately over problems with her boyfriend and thinks that she might be taking some medication to help her cope. The friend seems to remember something and suddenly runs off.

Vital Signs	Recording Time: 5 Minutes
Skin	Flushed, warm, and dry
Pulse	140 beats/min, regular, and weak
Blood pressure	88/58 mm Hg
Respirations	10 breaths/min
SpO₂	93% on nonrebreathing mask at 15 l/min of supplemental oxygen

3. What are some potential differential diagnoses?

4. Which interventions should you consider at this point, if any?

Table 33-1 | Major Toxidromes

Toxidrome	Drug Examples	Signs and Symptoms
Stimulant	Amphetamine, methamphetamine, cocaine, diet aids, nasal decongestants	Restlessness, agitation, incessant talking; insomnia, anorexia; dilated pupils, tachycardia; tachypnoea, hypertension or hypotension; paranoia, convulsions, cardiac arrest
Narcotic (opiate and opioid)	Heroin, opium, morphine, hydromorphone, fentanyl, codeine-paracetamol combination (Co-codamol)	Constricted (pinpoint) pupils, marked respiratory depression; needle tracks (IV abusers); drowsiness, stupor, coma
Sympathomimetic	Pseudoephedrine, phenylephrine, phenylpropanolamine, amphetamine, and methamphetamine	Hypertension, tachycardia, dilated pupils, agitation and convulsions, hyperthermia
Sedative and hypnotic	Phenobarbital, diazepam, thiopental	Drowsiness, disinhibition, ataxia, slurred speech, mental confusion, respiratory depression, progressive central nervous system depression, hypotension
Cholinergic	Sarin, tabun, VX	Increased salivation, lacrimation, gastrointestinal distress, diarrhoea, respiratory depression, apnoea, convulsions, coma
Anticholinergic	Atropine, scopolamine, antihistamines, anti-psychotics	Dry, flushed skin, hyperthermia, dilated pupils, blurred vision, tachycardia; mild hallucinations, dramatic delirium

Table 33-2 | Common Signs and Symptoms of Poisoning

Sign or Symptom	Type	Possible Causative Agents
Odour	Bitter almonds	Cyanide
	Garlic	Arsenic, organophosphates, phosphorous
	Acetone	Methyl alcohol, isopropyl alcohol, aspirin, acetone
	Wintergreen	Methyl salicylate
	Pears	Chloral hydrate
	Violets	Turpentine
	Camphor	Camphor
	Alcohol	Alcohol
Pupils	Constricted	Narcotics, organophosphates, Jimson weed, nutmeg, propoxyphene
	Dilated	Barbiturates, atropine, amphetamine, glutethimide, lysergic acid diethylamide (LSD), cyanide, CO
Mouth	Salivation	Organophosphates, arsenic, strychnine, mercury, salicylates
	Dry mouth	Atropine, amphetamines, diphenhydramine, narcotics
	Burns in mouth	Formaldehyde, iodine, lye, toxic plants, phenols, phosphorous, pine oil, silver nitrate, acids
Skin	Pruritis	Jimson weed, belladonna, boric acid
	Dry, hot skin	Atropine (in belladonna), botulism, nutmeg
	Sweating	Organophosphates, arsenic, aspirin, amphetamines, barbiturates, mushrooms, naphthalene
Respiratory	Depressed respirations	Narcotics, alcohol, propoxyphene, CO, barbiturates
	Increased respirations	Aspirin, amphetamines, boric acid, cyanide, kerosene, methyl alcohol, nicotine
	Pulmonary oedema	Organophosphates, petroleum products, narcotics, CO
Cardiovascular	Tachycardia	Alcohol, amphetamines, arsenic, atropine, aspirin, cocaine, some anti-asthma drugs
	Bradycardia	Digitalis, petrol, nicotine, mushrooms, narcotics, cyanide, mistletoe, rhododendron
	Hypertension	Amphetamines, lead, nicotine, anti-asthma drugs
	Hypotension	Barbiturates, narcotics, tranquilisers, house plants, mistletoe, nitroglycerin, antifreeze
Central nervous system	Convulsions	Amphetamines, camphor, cocaine, strychnine, arsenic, CO, petroleum products
	Coma	All depressant drugs (such as narcotics, barbiturates, tranquilisers, alcohol), CO, cyanide
	Hallucinations	Atropine, LSD, mushrooms, organic solvents, phencyclidine (PCP), nutmeg
	Headache	CO, alcohol, disulfiram
	Tremors	Organophosphates, CO, amphetamine, tranquilisers, poisonous marine animals
	Weakness or paralysis	Organophosphates, botulism, eel, hemlock, puffer fish, pine oil, rhododendron
Gastrointestinal	Cramps, nausea, vomiting, and/or diarrhoea	Many, if not most, ingested poisons

Overview of Substance Abuse

Human beings have a long history of abusing drugs and alcohol. With the passing of time, the physiological and societal effects of alcohol abuse have become well known and thoroughly documented. Unfortunately, the area of medicine dealing with drugs of abuse is highly challenging because of uncertainty about the prevalence of the problem and the continual evolution of the substances themselves. In the 1980s, creative chemists took existing pharmacological agents and structurally manipulated them to create new or different drugs ("designer drugs") that were often far more potent than the original drugs. For example, cocaine was made into crack, a far more addictive form of the drug.

Substance abuse can be broadly defined as the self-administration of licit or illicit substances in a manner not in accord with approved medical or social practice. Part of that definition is cultural—and there is great variation in what is considered substance abuse. In our society, for example, it is acceptable to administer narcotics under medical supervision for the relief of pain; conversely, self-administration of the same drugs for the purpose of inducing euphoria is regarded as drug abuse.

Any given society's definition of abuse may have little relation to the potential harm from the abused substance. For example, our culture places no restrictions on the long-term and compulsive use of tobacco, even though it is a major contributor to cardiovascular and respiratory disease 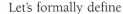 **Figure 33-4** . By comparison, use of marijuana, which has less damaging effects, may be punishable by fines or imprisonment.

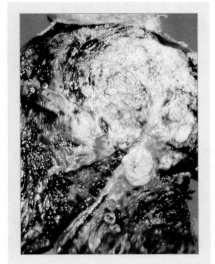

Figure 33-4 A diseased lung as a result of tobacco use.

Let's formally define some basic terms and concepts related to substance abuse:

- **Drug abuse.** Any use of drugs that causes physical, psychological, economic, legal, or social harm to the user or to others affected by the drug user's behaviour.
- **Habituation.** Psychological dependence on a drug or drugs.
- **Physical dependence.** A physiological state of adaptation to a drug, usually characterised by tolerance to the drug's effects and a withdrawal syndrome if the drug is stopped, especially if it is stopped abruptly.
- **Psychological dependence.** The emotional state of craving a drug to maintain a feeling of well-being.
- **Tolerance.** Physiological adaptation to the effects of a drug such that increasingly larger doses of the drug are required to achieve the same effect.
- **Withdrawal syndrome.** A predictable set of signs and symptoms, usually involving altered central nervous system (CNS) activity, that occurs after the abrupt cessation of a drug or after rapidly decreasing the usual dosage of a drug.
- **Drug addiction.** A chronic disorder characterised by the compulsive use of a substance resulting in physical, psychological, or social harm to the user, who continues to use the substance despite the harm.
- **Antagonist.** Something that counteracts the action of something else. In relation to drugs, a drug that is an antagonist has an affinity for a cell receptor; by binding to the receptor, the antagonist prevents the cell from responding.
- **Potentiation.** Enhancement of the effect of one drug by another drug.
- **Synergism.** The action of two substances, such as drugs, in which the total effects are greater than the sum of the independent effects of the two substances (that is, 2 + 2 = 5).

Drug abuse is not limited to members of the younger generation or to any particular stratum of society. It occurs in all age groups and at all social levels.

Alcoholism

After smoking, alcoholism kills more people in the UK than any other drug. According to government statistics one adult in 13 is dependent on alcohol. Furthermore, because of its harmful effects on organs, including the liver, stomach, heart, pancreas, brain, and CNS, alcoholism decreases a person's life span by 10 to 20 years. In addition, people with alcoholism tend to have chronic malnutrition and fall frequently, increasing the likelihood of head injury or other trauma.

Alcoholism usually consists of two distinct phases. The first phase is problem drinking, during which alcohol is used increasingly more often to relieve tensions or other emotional difficulties. Because of the disinhibition, relaxation, and sense of well-being mediated by alcohol, some degree of psychological dependence often develops with its use. Unfortunately, many people become so dependent on the psychological influences of alcohol that they become compulsive consumers. As a person becomes more dependent on drinking, his or her performance at work and relationships with friends, family, and colleagues may deteriorate. Increased absence from work, emotional disturbances, and car collisions become more frequent.

Physical dependence also results from the regular consumption of large quantities of alcohol. This becomes apparent when a person abruptly stops consuming alcohol and withdrawal symptoms result. The severity of the withdrawal can vary according to the length and intensity of

Notes from Nancy

The patient found stuporous with alcohol on his or her breath must not be assumed to be intoxicated.

the alcoholic habit. Minor withdrawal is characterised by restlessness, anxiousness, sleeping problems, agitation, and tremors.

In the second phase of alcoholism, true addiction, abstinence causes major withdrawal symptoms—for example: increased blood pressure, vomiting, and hallucinations. Delirium tremens, or alcohol withdrawal delirium, results in fever, disorientation, confusion, convulsions, and possibly death.

Alcoholism occurs in all social strata, and only a small minority of people with alcoholism fit the "skid row" stereotype. Red flags pointing to alcoholism include the following:

- Drinking early in the day
- Drinking alone or in "secret"
- Periodic binges
- Loss of memory or "blackouts"
- Tremulousness and anxiety
- Cigarette burns on clothing from falling asleep with a lit cigarette
- "Green tongue syndrome", caused by the use of chlorophyll-containing compounds to disguise the smell of alcohol on the breath
- Chronically flushed face and palms

Medical Consequences of Alcohol Abuse

Because of the toxic effects of alcohol, a person with alcoholism is considerably more prone than sober counterparts to a number of serious illnesses and injuries Table 33-3 . Chronic damage to the CNS, for example, leads to deterioration in higher mental functions, such as memory and logical thinking. Damage to the cerebellum results in problems of balance, which in turn contribute to the frequent falls experienced by people with alcoholism. Damage to the peripheral nerves leads to decreased sensation in the extremities, making the person prone to burns and similar injuries that an intact pain sense would ordinarily prevent.

As alcohol travels through the digestive system, it irritates tissue and can damage the lining of the stomach by causing acid imbalances, inflammation, and acute gastric distress. Often, the result is gastritis (an inflamed stomach) and heartburn. The more frequently consumption takes place, the greater the irritation. One of every three heavy drinkers has chronic gastritis. Heavy drinkers also have double the risk of cancer of the mouth and oesophagus. Prolonged heavy use of alcohol may cause ulcers, hiatal hernias, and cancers throughout the digestive tract.

The toxic effects of alcohol on the liver produce a variety of complications, such as coagulopathies (easy bleeding and poor clotting ability), hypoglycaemia, and gastrointestinal (GI) bleeding. In addition, people with alcoholism are at high risk of acute pancreatitis, pneumonia, and cardiomyopathy.

Table 33-3	Medical Problems to Which People With Alcoholism Are Particularly Susceptible
Condition	**Contributing Factors**
Subdural haematoma	Frequent falls; impaired clotting mechanisms
GI bleeding	Irritant effect of alcohol on the stomach lining (leading to gastritis); impaired clotting mechanisms; cirrhosis of the liver, leading to engorgement of oesophageal veins (oesophageal varices)
Pancreatitis	Indirect effect on alcohol of the pancreas
Hypoglycaemia	Damage to the liver, which normally mobilises sugar into the blood
Pneumonia	Aspiration of vomitus occurring during intoxication and coma; suppression of immune system by alcohol
Burns	Relative insensitivity to pain occurring during intoxication; falling asleep with a lit cigarette while intoxicated
Hypothermia	Insensitivity to extremes of temperatures while intoxicated; falling asleep outside in the cold
Convulsions	Effect of withdrawal from alcohol
Arrhythmias	Toxic effects of alcohol on the heart
Cancer	Mechanism not known (perhaps related to suppression of the immune system), but people with alcoholism are 10 times more likely than the general population to have cancer
Oesophageal varices (abnormally enlarged veins in the lower part of the oesophagus)	Develop when normal blood flow to the liver is blocked and blood backs up into smaller, more fragile blood vessels in the oesophagus; do not produce symptoms unless they rupture and bleed (a life-threatening condition that requires immediate medical care; can be fatal when not controlled)

Alcohol Emergencies

Any of the conditions previously mentioned may contribute to an emergency. In addition, acute consumption of and acute abstinence from alcohol may produce serious problems, including withdrawal convulsions.

Acute Alcohol Intoxication

Severe alcohol intoxication is a form of poisoning and carries the same lethal potential as poisoning with any other CNS depressant. Death from alcohol intoxication has been reported with blood alcohol levels of 400 mg/dl, which can be attained by the relatively rapid consumption of as little as a half-pint of whisky. The most immediate danger to an acutely intoxicated person is death of respiratory depression and/or aspiration of vomitus or stomach contents secondary to a suppressed gag reflex.

If an intoxicated patient is unconscious, treat him or her as you would any unconscious patient. As always, first establish and maintain the airway. With an intact gag reflex, place the patient in the recovery position with suction ready. If there is no gag reflex, the airway will need proficient management; consideration should be given to intubating the patient. In addition, give high-concentration supplemental oxygen, and assist ventilation as needed. Establish vascular access. Monitor the ECG rhythm. Assess the patient's blood glucose level, treating hypoglycaemia if it is found.

Withdrawal Convulsions

A person who has been drinking heavily for an extended period and suddenly stops drinking may have a variety of withdrawal phenomena. Convulsions usually occur within about 12 to 48 hours of the last drink. Use the same care plan described for alcohol intoxication, and consult with the A&E consultant about giving benzodiazepines for convulsion control.

Delirium Tremens

One of the most serious and lethal complications of alcohol withdrawal is delirium tremens (DTs). Symptoms usually start 48 to 72 hours after the last alcohol intake, although a week to 10 days may pass before the onset of symptoms in some cases. Delirium tremens is a serious and potentially fatal syndrome with mortality reported as high as 15%. Signs and symptoms include confusion, tremors and restlessness, fever and perspiration, hallucinations (extremely frightening—such as snakes, spiders, and rats), and hypotension, often secondary to dehydration.

The treatment for a patient in DTs is aimed at protecting him or her from injury and supporting the cardiovascular system. The often-terrifying hallucinations associated with DTs typically make for an agitated, often combative patient. Try to keep the patient calm. In addition, you should administer supplemental oxygen by nasal cannula and establish vascular access. Manage hypotension with an infusion of normal saline, and, during the ongoing assessment, reassess breath sounds. Maintain an ongoing dialogue with the patient throughout transport to help orientate and reassure the patient.

General Principles of Assessment and Management for Toxicological Emergencies

Generally, patients with toxicological emergencies are considered medical patients, although toxicological emergencies may lead to

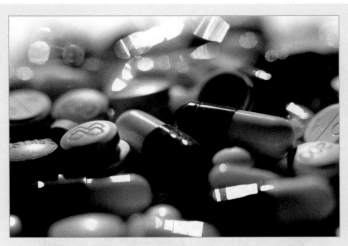

Figure 33-5 Take any bottles, containers, and their remaining contents to the A&E department.

trauma, too. The general assessment approach is the same for all patients: scene assessment, initial assessment, and then focused history and physical examination. If the mental status is altered, monitor the patient's airway and breathing diligently to ensure that he or she does not aspirate and is adequately filling the chest with air. If the patient is responsive, use the OPQRST mnemonic to elaborate on the chief complaint, take the patient's vital signs, take a SAMPLE history, and perform a focused physical examination. If the patient is not responsive, obtain vital signs and complete a rapid medical assessment; obtain the OPQRST and SAMPLE history from bystanders and family members, if possible.

To choose the appropriate course of action in a toxicological emergency, obtain at least the following specific information:

- *What is the agent?* If the patient has overdosed on a prescription drug, take the pill bottle and the remaining pills in with the patient Figure 33-5 ▲ . If the substance was a commercial product, take the container and its remaining contents to the A&E department. If the patient ingested a plant, find out what part (roots, leaves, stem, flower, or fruit) and take a sample of the plant to the A&E department for identification. If the patient vomits, save a sample of the vomitus in a clean, sealed container, and take it with you to the A&E department Figure 33-6 ▶ .
- *When was the poison ingested, injected, absorbed, or inhaled?* The decision to induce vomiting (infrequently done—check local guidelines) or to flush out (lavage) the stomach is strongly influenced by the amount of time that has elapsed since the exposure. The likelihood of retrieving significant quantities of the poison from the stomach decreases rapidly after the first 30 to 60 minutes. Also, acute-onset events often indicate a more serious patient scenario—for example, if the patient smoked crack cocaine 15 minutes ago and immediately began to have crushing chest pain.
- *How much was taken, injected, absorbed, or inhaled?* Street drugs are commonly sold in single-dose "hits" or "tabs" (tablets). If the patient says he has taken "three hits of

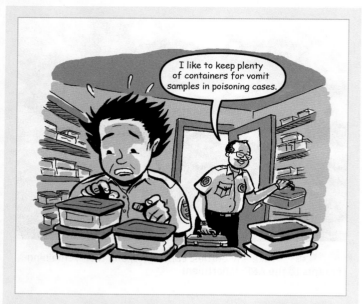

Figure 33-6

Scene Assessment

Patients who have taken an overdose may be extremely dangerous, so make sure you do a scene assessment in every case. If necessary, call for police backup.

Initial Assessment

The initial assessment of a drug-overdosed or poisoned patient begins with your general impression. It can be as simple as "a young adult man snoring in a public toilet". The initial assessment seeks for rapid identification of concerns involving mental status, airway, breathing, and circulation. Threats to life need to be managed quickly by measures such as a head tilt–chin lift, suctioning, or ventilation assistance with a bag-valve-mask device. The initial assessment may identify the MOI or nature of illness and the need for additional units and set the priority and "tone" of the call.

Focused History and Physical Examination

After completing the initial assessment, begin the focused history and physical examination. With a trauma case, you will need to classify the patient as having a significant MOI or no significant MOI. With a significant MOI, you must quickly perform a rapid trauma assessment of the major body regions—head, neck, chest, abdomen, pelvis, back, buttocks, and four extremities. Obtain a set of baseline vital signs and a SAMPLE history. This patient should also receive a detailed physical examination en route to hospital. If the patient has no significant MOI, perform a focused examination of the injured body part—that is, evaluate distal pulse, motor, and sensory functions, and range of motion.

Documentation and Communication

While at the scene, make thorough (and legible) notes about the nature of the poisoning. You can then quickly state the type and amount of substance and the time and route of exposure in your radio, verbal, and written reports. Clear notes that can be handed over on arrival will be appreciated by busy hospital staff.

acid", you know he has taken three times the "normal dose" of LSD. If the patient says that she took 4 tabs of ecstasy, that's four times a single dose. There is almost always a distinct correlation between dose and toxic effects.

- *What else was taken?* A majority of intentional self-poisonings (suicide attempts) or illicit drug overdoses involve polydrug ingestions, often with alcohol as one of the drugs. The patient may also have tried to take something as an antidote (that is, something to counteract the effect of the poison). This information can be invaluable to A&E department staff when deciding which tests to order.
- *Has the patient vomited or aspirated?* If so, how soon after the ingestion or exposure? How much?
- *Why was the substance taken?* Although you may not get a reliable answer from someone abusing illicit drugs, this is still a question worth asking. Don't assume that every patient is trying to get high. Drug use could be a coping mechanism for a person who is being abused, or it could be a suicide attempt. Put the reason in "quotation marks" on your patient clinical record (PCR).

Special Considerations

In an accidental overdose or poisoning, an older patient may have become confused about his or her drug regime. The person may have forgotten that the medication had been taken and repeat the dose one or more times. The patient could also have forgotten the doctor's instructions to discard leftover medication and might have taken the current and the older drug, resulting in increased effects or unwanted drug interactions. An older patient may also intentionally overdose in a suicide attempt.

Most poisoning and overdose cases involve patients with medical conditions, so you will need to elaborate on their chief complaint using the OPQRST questions. If the patient is not responsive, perform a rapid medical assessment (basically the same as the rapid trauma assessment), obtain baseline vital signs, and ask the SAMPLE history questions of the family or bystanders, if possible. If the patient is responsive, complete the SAMPLE history, obtain the baseline vital signs, and conduct a focused examination targeting the body system

Table 33-4	Common Caustic Substances	
Substance	**Example**	**Source**
Acids	Hydrochloric acid	Toilet bowl cleaners, swimming pool cleaners
	Sulphuric acid	Battery acid, toilet bowl cleaners (as bisulphate)
	Others	Bleach disinfectants, slate cleaners
Alkalis	Lye (sodium or potassium hydroxide)	Paint removers, washing powders, drain cleaners button-shaped batteries, Clinitest tablets
	Sodium hypochlorite	Bleach (Clorox)
	Sodium carbonate	Bleach (Purex), nonphosphate detergents
	Ammonia	Hair dyes, jewellery cleaners, metal cleaners or polishes, anti-rust agents
	Potassium permanganate	Electric dishwasher detergents

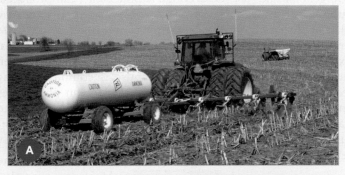

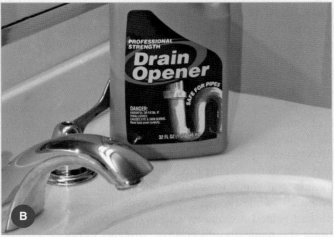

Figure 33-11 Caustic chemicals are commonly used in industry. **A.** Anhydrous ammonia tank used in agriculture. **B.** Plumbing agents used in the home.

Most patients who have swallowed caustic substances present with severe pain in the mouth, throat, or chest. Usually the airway is not a problem, nor is the patient in shock. Respiratory distress, if present, is most probably due to soft-tissue swelling in the larynx, epiglottis, or vocal cords, which means that the patient is in immediate danger of complete airway obstruction. For a caustic ingestion in an alert patient, giving milk—at least 200–250 ml for a child and 250–350 ml for an adult—may help if the NPIS or the A&E consultant agrees. Establish IV access, usually en route, because immediate transport to the A&E department is indicated.

With dermal exposure to a strong acid, the result is immediate and excruciating pain. For a strong alkali, the onset of pain is somewhat delayed, allowing more time before the patient reacts and increasing the severity of the burn. In such an injury, diluting and flushing away the caustic substance is the main goal of prehospital environment treatment. Acids tend to be more water-soluble than alkalis, so they are often diluted relatively quickly. With alkalis, it is more important to keep water continually flowing because it usually takes much longer to rinse an alkali away (compared with an acid).

Notes from Nancy

If a patient who swallowed a caustic agent is in respiratory distress, get moving without further delay to the hospital. Have your cricothyroidotomy kit ready.

At the Scene

Some chemicals react with water. Although small amounts can usually be flushed safely with large quantities of water, larger amounts of such chemicals can give off toxic fumes or explode when wet. Be sure to check the relevant warnings or placards.

For an eye exposure, cut the prong section off a nasal cannula, place it on the bridge of the patient's nose, and plug in a macro IV administration set and run it wide open to provide continuous irrigation. This also frees you up to perform other tasks. A Morgan lens may also be used after the initial gross flushing has been accomplished.

One of the most common caustic exposures in the agricultural setting involves anhydrous ammonia. The exposure usually occurs during the hook-up or disconnection of a nurse tank. Farmers often keep a small water bottle in the shirt pocket, allowing them to immediately rinse their eyes should an exposure occur. Without treatment, eye exposure to anhydrous ammonia can cause devastating damage in less than a minute, resulting in cataracts or blindness.

There are a number of significant "don'ts" for caustic ingestions:

- *Don't* give any "neutralising substances". Some product laboratories incorrectly advise neutralising the caustic agent—for example, by giving lemon juice or dilute vinegar (both weak acids) to a patient who has swallowed an alkali. Mixing an acid and an alkali produces *heat,* adding a thermal injury to the chemical injury.
- *Don't* induce vomiting—what burned on the way down will burn on the way up.
- *Don't* perform gastric lavage.
- *Don't* give activated charcoal. It is not effective in acid or alkali ingestion, and it may interfere with the patient's subsequent care by blackening the field of vision for an endoscopist who tries to inspect the oesophagus and stomach for damage.

Common Household Items

From a toxicological perspective, the average home is a nightmare. Many house plants have poisonous leaves or berries. All pesticides and herbicides used in lawn and garden care are potentially poisonous. All hydrocarbon products (such as paint thinners, solvents, gas) can cause permanent neurological damage or death if inhaled in the right amount; the same is true of glue fumes (often called "huffing"). Many household cleaning agents are also toxic if ingested.

It is not possible within the scope of this chapter to discuss all of the possibilities when it comes to household poisonings. Some of the more likely culprits are covered in several of the other sections to assist in preparing you to handle the myriad possibilities. As always, keep in mind that the NSIP is an invaluable resource.

Drugs Abused for Sexual Purposes

Drugs that are abused for sexual purposes include those that increase sexual gratification and those that are used to facilitate sexual assault.

Drugs That Increase Sexual Gratification

Drugs that increase sexual gratification constitute a long and varied list. Clearly, the most dangerous include erectile dysfunction medications such as sildenafil, which are contraindicated for patients who take nitrites for cardiac problems. Their use by people taking nitrites may result in severe hypotension or total cardiovascular collapse, ultimately leading to death. For hypotension, repeated boluses of normal saline can bring the blood pressure up to an acceptable level. If cardiac arrest occurs, follow your guidelines.

For some people, the relaxed dreamy high of marijuana is very desirable for sexual gratification. There is no overdose potential for marijuana. Supportive care is all that is required.

Cocaine and other stimulant drugs (such as amphetamines and methamphetamine) are popular choices for people seeking a more intense sexual experience. Should the patient have sustained tachycardia in such a case, hypotension can occur as a result of inadequate preload. Be alert for this possibility when the heart rate is in the range of 170 to 180 beats/min or higher, although a rate in the 160s could cause problems for a patient with an extensive cardiac history. Serial boluses of normal saline will usually stabilise the blood pressure. If fluid boluses are not effective, a vasopressor (such as dopamine or dobutamine) may be required.

Another drug that increases sexual gratification is amyl nitrite (poppers, rush, happy snaps). This organic nitrate drug can be crushed and inhaled, again producing an intense sexual experience. As with any nitrate, hypotension may result from blood pooling in the periphery owing to the drug's vasodilatory effects.

An unusual drug in this group is ecstasy. Although this so-called club drug is an analog of methamphetamine, the effects of ecstasy hardly resemble the action of methamphetamine. Ecstasy would be more correctly termed an "euphorogenic"—it creates an incredible sense of well-being.

Dextromethorphan (DXM), which is found in almost 150 general-sales-list (GSL) cough suppressants, can produce a euphoric floating sensation or out-of-body experience. At a plateau level of approximately 6 tablets (180-mg dose), DXM produces a mild stimulant effect that may enhance a sexual experience. DXM or "Robo" (Robitussin) abusers are often called "Roboheads"; this kind of abuse is common among teenagers because this drug is readily available in pharmacies and online. Consuming large quantities of DXM can lead to hallucinations, psychedelic visions, loss of motor control, confusion, blurred vision, dreamlike euphoria, and out-of-body sensations.

Drugs Used to Facilitate Sexual Assault

Drugs used to facilitate sexual assault are often administered unknowingly to a woman, frequently in an alcoholic drink. These substances are used by sexual predators, which explains why they are called "date rape" drugs. They are discussed further in Chapter 38.

Gamma-hydroxybutyrate (GHB) is an endogenous metabolite of gamma-aminobutyric acid, a neuromodulator involved with sleep cycles, memory retention, and emotional control. GHB was used as anaesthetic in Europe for about 40 years before it appeared in the United Kingdom, where it was originally sold in health food shops for body building purposes (it supposedly "burned fat" while the person was sleeping). By the late 1980s, GHB had gained popularity with young people as a club drug, earning the name "liquid ecstasy" from its euphoric effects at raves (all-night dance parties). In the mid 1990s, GHB became increasingly associated with sexual assaults. GHB is a Class C drug—illegal to have, give away, or sell. Possession can get you up to two years in jail and/or an unlimited fine. Supplying someone else, even your friends, can get you up to 14 years in jail and/or an unlimited fine.

Although GHB is available as an odourless and colourless liquid, it has a salty taste. Reportedly, it cannot be tasted when placed in a drink such as a margarita in a salt-ringed glass. Once ingested, GHB quickly crosses the blood-brain barrier, exerting its effects within 30 to 60 minutes. As little as 0.5 mg of GHB can produce a pronounced hypnotic effect along with disinhibition, severe passivity (that is, a lack of the will to resist), and antegrade amnesia. When taken with alcohol, GHB increases the risk of devastating CNS depression (culminating in coma or death); when taken with methamphetamine and similar drugs, it increases the risk of convulsions.

Treatment for GHB intoxication focuses on the CNS depression and the risks of the patient being unable to protect the airway. First, establish and maintain the airway, inserting an advanced airway as needed. Carefully monitor the patient's LOC. Assist breathing as necessary, and give high-flow supplemental oxygen. Establish vascular access. Apply the ECG monitor, pulse oximeter, and capnograph. Finally, provide rapid transport to hospital.

Poisonous Alcohols

The form of alcohol consumed by humans in alcoholic beverages is ethyl alcohol (or ethanol). It is not conventionally recognised as a poison, even though it has many properties of a poison when ingested in sufficient quantities. Instead, "poisonous alcohols" are generally considered alcohols manufactured for industrial or nongastronomic purposes, such as methyl alcohol and ethylene glycol.

Methyl Alcohol

Methyl alcohol (also known as meths) is present in paints, paint remover, windscreen washer fluids, varnishes, and antifreeze **Figure 33-12 ▸**. Methanol poisoning can occur after inadvertently drinking contaminated whisky or illegally produced alcohol or from intentional ingestion in a suicide attempt. Methanol is a popular substitute for ethanol among desperate people with alcoholism when they don't have the means to obtain ethanol. This colourless liquid has a unique odour.

Methanol itself is not harmful. Rather, its metabolic breakdown products, formaldehyde and formic acid, are responsible for the characteristic signs and symptoms of methanol poisoning. A dose of as little as 30 ml can produce toxicity and even death. Once ingested, methanol is quickly absorbed from the GI tract, with peak blood levels attained within 30 to 90 minutes. In mild toxicity, the half-life of methanol is 14 to 20 hours. As toxicity increases, the half-life increases to 24 to 30 hours. The liver eliminates 90% to 95% of the methanol.

The symptoms of methanol poisoning do not usually appear immediately but begin from 12 to 18 hours, occasionally up to 72 hours, after ingestion. As a consequence, the patient may or may not connect the symptoms to what he or she drank

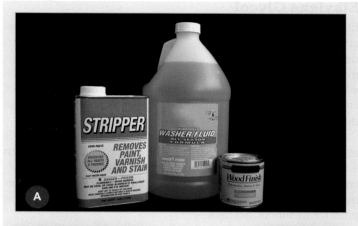
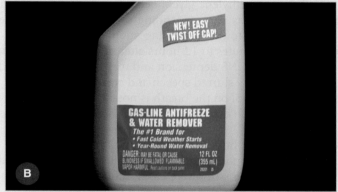

Figure 33-12 Methyl alcohol is present in paints, paint remover, windscreen washer fluids, and varnishes (**A**) and in antifreeze and canned fuels (**B**).

yesterday or several days ago. Patient complaints include nausea and vomiting (in almost 50% of cases), headache or vertigo, abdominal pain (often from pancreatitis), and blurred vision ("looks like a snowstorm") or, possibly, blindness. Findings on the physical examination may include an odour of alcohol on the breath, altered mental status ranging from drunken behaviour to convulsions or coma, dilated pupils with sluggish or no reaction, hyperpnoea and tachypnoea from metabolic acidosis, and bradycardia and hypotension (very late signs).

Prehospital environment care for methanol poisoning is primarily supportive. Establish and manage the airway, considering advanced airway placement as needed. Establish vascular access. Assess the blood glucose level, and administer glucose if the patient has hypoglycaemia. Provide immediate transport to the nearest hospital, providing a pre-alert message en route.

If the patient is alert, the ingestion took place within the last 30 minutes, and if local guideline allows it, insert a nasogastric tube and provide gastric aspiration. You should also assess the patient for other drug involvement. Administration of activated charcoal is contraindicated unless other drugs have been ingested that are adsorbable, in which case you should follow your local guideline.

Ethylene Glycol

Ethylene glycol is a colourless, odourless liquid found in a variety of commercial products, including antifreeze, coolant, deicers, polishes, and paints. Its relatively pleasant taste has made it a favourite substitute among people with alcoholism when the beverage of choice is unavailable. The lethal dose of ethylene glycol is estimated at 2 ml/kg, or as little as 150 ml in the average-size adult.

Ethylene glycol is very water-soluble. With oral intake, it is absorbed rapidly, with peak blood levels attained within 1 to 4 hours after ingestion. The liver and kidneys metabolise ethylene glycol into a number of toxic metabolites, including aldehydes, lactate, oxalate, and glycolate. In turn, these metabolites produce metabolic acidosis.

Toxicity from ethylene glycol occurs in three stages, so the signs and symptoms vary depending on when you encounter the patient relative to the time of ingestion:

- **Stage 1.** 20 minutes to 12 hours after ingestion. The patient presents with CNS depression and may appear intoxicated, as evidenced by slurred speech and ataxia, although the odour of ethanol on the breath is notably absent. The patient may also experience nausea, vomiting, convulsions, or coma.
- **Stage 2.** 12–24 hours after ingestion. Pulmonary oedema produces tachypnoea, tachycardia, mild hypertension, and rales (or crackles). In severe cases, acute respiratory distress syndrome, congestive heart failure, and cardiovascular collapse may be apparent.
- **Stage 3.** 24–72 hours after ingestion. The renal damage produced by the ethylene glycol becomes evident with patient complaints of flank pain and anuria (absence of urine formation).

The care plan for a patient with suspected ethylene glycol poisoning is the same as for methanol poisoning, with the exception of possibly getting an order from the A&E consultant to administer 10 ml of 10% calcium gluconate via slow IV push to treat the hypocalcaemia that accompanies ethylene glycol toxicity. This medication is usually ordered only after good urine flow is established and after the IV line is flushed clear of sodium bicarbonate. Once at hospital, care focuses on correction of acidosis, administration of fomepizole or ethanol (to reduce the conversion of the methanol to its toxic metabolites), and, potentially, renal dialysis.

Hydrocarbons

Hydrocarbons are compounds made up principally of hydrogen and carbon atoms, with most, but not all, obtained from the distillation of petroleum. Hydrocarbons are found in a variety of products around the home, including cleaning and polishing agents, glues, spot removers, lighter fluids, paints, paint thinners and paint removers, other fuels, and pesticides.

Hydrocarbon Inhalation

The vast majority of intentional hydrocarbon inhalations are "recreational". Frequently, people who "bag" or "huff" are young—11 to 13 years of age and, occasionally, younger children. The profile adds up with deadly simplicity: Young children who see their siblings and parents abuse alcohol or drugs may seek to emulate that behaviour but may not have the cash to make that wish a reality, so they turn to a variety of everyday products: paint thinner, solvents, paint strippers, petrol, nonstick cooking spray, and glues. The rich alveolar capillary network makes the lungs a highly efficient mechanism for providing a quick and inexpensive drug high. Unfortunately, long-term inhalant abuse can lead to permanent loss of mental function as evidenced by a variety of neuropathies, such as loss of hearing, loss of fine motor function, balance and equilibrium disorders, and occasionally death.

The modern epidemic of inhalation began in the early 1960s, when the first reports of glue sniffing and its consequences appeared. Within a short time, the number of agents being inhaled to get high had increased exponentially, as had the techniques for inhalation. Simple sniffing over the opening of a glue bottle did not provide an intense enough exposure for serious abusers. Pouring the volatile material onto a rag, placing it in a plastic bag, and holding the bag over one's face to breathe in the fumes proved far more efficient, producing a more intense high more quickly. Breathing fumes directly off a soaked rag or towel is termed huffing, whereas the use of a plastic bag is termed bagging. **Table 33-5 ▶** lists commonly abused inhaled compounds.

The primary goals when dealing with a patient who has inhaled hydrocarbons focus on removal from the noxious environment, giving high-concentration supplemental oxygen, and prompt transport to the appropriate hospital.

Hydrocarbon Ingestion

Given the ready accessibility of hydrocarbons and the high likelihood that they might be mistaken for potable beverages, it is not surprising that hydrocarbon poisonings are common among children younger than 5 years. The potential hazards of swallowing a given hydrocarbon are directly related to the viscosity of the agent: The lower the viscosity, the higher the risk of aspiration and other complications. The vast majority of hydrocarbon ingestions do *not* produce lasting damage. Patients who develop symptoms within a few minutes of ingestion are likely to have aspirated and need immediate attention.

Low-viscosity hydrocarbons (such as kerosene, naphtha, and toluene) can easily enter the lungs during swallowing. If the patient reports coughing, choking, or vomiting immediately after swallowing the substance, assume that aspiration occurred. Similarly, any signs of respiratory distress—air hunger, intercostal recessions, tachypnoea, cyanosis—must be considered danger signals.

Low viscosity also facilitates the uptake of a hydrocarbon by tissues of the CNS and, therefore, its anaesthetic effects. At first, the patient may experience excitement and euphoria, followed by weakness, incoordination, drowsiness, confusion, and coma. Some petroleum products—notably petrol—can produce hypoglycaemia and cardiac arrhythmias, so you should always monitor the patient's ECG rhythm.

Many hydrocarbon products cause gastric irritation, which results in severe abdominal pain, diarrhoea, and belching, sometimes lasting for hours after the incident. At the other end of the spectrum, just a single hydrocarbon substance exposure may cause life-threatening toxicity and, on occasion, sudden death.

If a patient who has swallowed a hydrocarbon product is asymptomatic when you arrive and remains so while you are on scene, he or she is highly unlikely to experience significant complications. In such a scenario, and after discussion with the A&E consultant, some patients may not warrant transport because they can be safely observed at home. In one study involving 211 patients suspected of hydrocarbon ingestion, fewer than 1% required doctor intervention.

By contrast, all symptomatic patients suspected of ingesting a hydrocarbon product—especially patients with respiratory symptoms—should be transported immediately to the A&E department for further evaluation and care. Management should include the following measures:

- Remove contaminated clothing and decontaminate the patient, ideally before placing the patient in the ambulance.
- Establish and maintain the airway, and ensure adequate ventilation.
- Give high-flow supplemental oxygen.
- Establish an IV.
- Continuously monitor the ECG rhythm; consider running a 12-lead.
- Administer sequential bolus infusions of normal saline to treat hypotension.
- Transport the patient to the most appropriate hospital.

Psychiatric Medications

One only needs to consider what is trying to be accomplished with psychiatric medications—altering dysfunctions of mood and affect (most commonly depression) and of thought, orientation, or perception—to appreciate the sophistication of these pharmacological agents. When patients taking psychiatric medications have toxicological emergencies, you should expect to be challenged with matters of patient care and scene management.

Tricyclic Anti-depressants

In their heyday, the tricyclic anti-depressants (TCAs) were the drugs of choice to treat depression. Unfortunately, TCAs require close attention to compliance with dosing regimes—and patients who need them have difficulty following the regime. Patients are depressed, and many also have problems with alcohol (a CNS depressant). Consequently, they are at high risk of intentional overdose.

Making matters worse, TCAs have a small therapeutic window—that is, the difference between "minimum dosing" (the least amount of drug needed for the desired effect) and "maximum dosing" (the amount at which the drug becomes toxic). With some drugs, the therapeutic window spans several thousand milligrams. With TCAs, even minimal dosing errors may produce toxic effects. Although they are no longer first-line therapy for depression, TCAs still have other applications, such as pain management.

The signs and symptoms of TCA overdose may vary dramatically among patients. One patient may present with only a mild antimuscarinic symptom such as a dry mouth, whereas

Table 33-5	Compounds Commonly Abused by Sniffing and Bagging	
Example	**Sources**	**Signs and Symptoms of Toxicity**
Halogenated hydrocarbons		
1,1,1-Trichloroethane (methylchloroform)	Cleaning solvents, typewriter correction fluid, aerosol propellant	Eye irritation, light-headedness, incoordination, CNS depression, respiratory failure, cardiac arrhythmias, sudden death
Trichloroethylene	Degreasing solvent, aerosol propellant, rubber cement, plastic cement	Euphoria, anaesthesia, weakness, vomiting, abdominal cramps, loss of coordination, neuropathy, blindness, cardiac arrhythmias, "degreaser's flush" (flushed face, neck, and shoulders when taken along with alcohol)
Tetrachloroethylene (perchloroethylene)	Solvent, dry cleaning agent	Drunken behaviour, dizziness, lightheadedness, difficulty walking, numbness, sleepiness, visual disturbances, memory impairment, eye irritation, cutaneous flushing, sudden death
Methylene chloride (dichloromethane)	Refrigerant, paint remover, aerosol propellant	Fatigue, weakness, chills, sleepiness, nausea, dizziness, incoordination, pulmonary oedema
Carbon tetrachloride	Cleaning fluid	Narcosis, sudden death
Petroleum hydrocarbons		
Benzene	Cable cleaner, industrial solvents, rubber cement	Delirium, agitation, convulsions, sudden death
Toluene	Spray paint, model and plastic cements, lacquer thinner	Narcosis, hallucinations, mania; impulsive, destructive, accident-prone behaviour; sudden death
Petrol	Petrol tank	Sudden death

another may have cardiotoxic effects, such as life-threatening or fatal arrhythmias. The most common signs and symptoms of a TCA overdose are altered mental status (drowsy, confused, slurred speech), arrhythmias (usually sinus tachycardia or supraventricular tachycardia), dry mouth, blurred vision or dilated pupils, urinary retention, constipation, and pulmonary oedema. With a more serious toxic exposure, be alert for ventricular tachycardia, hypotension, respiratory depression, QT prolongation on the ECG, and convulsions.

When TCAs exert their toxic effects, the most common cause of death is cardiac arrhythmia. A significant number of the drug overdoses involving TCAs also involve other drugs and frequently alcohol, which contributes to increased morbidity and mortality. A patient who presents with serious signs and symptoms within 6 hours of the ingestion should be considered in critical condition.

Management of patients with a TCA overdose includes the following measures:

- Maintain the airway. If the patient's mental status suddenly deteriorates, as is often the case, insert an advanced airway.
- Give high-flow supplemental oxygen.
- Establish an IV.
- Provide continuous ECG monitoring (watch for widening of the QRS).
- Manage hypotension with sequential boluses of normal saline. Be alert to the possibility of pulmonary oedema; it occurs frequently in cases of TCA overdose.
- Assess blood glucose levels. Give 10% glucose if the patient is hypoglycaemic.
- Rule out head trauma as a possible cause of decreased mental status.
- For convulsions, consider RSI and intubation.
- Provide rapid transport to an appropriate hospital.

Monoamine Oxidase Inhibitors

Monoamine oxidase inhibitors (MAOIs) are used primarily to treat atypical depression. They work by increasing norepinephrine and serotonin levels within the CNS. Unfortunately, the potential for drug interactions is a major issue for patients receiving MAOI therapy. A very tight therapeutic window also contributes to the limited popularity of MAOIs—as little as 2 mg/kg may produce a life-threatening event. In addition, MAOIs can precipitate a hypertensive crisis if taken in conjunction with tyramine-containing foods (such as beer, wine, aged cheese, chopped liver, pickled herring, sour cream, yoghurt, fava beans).

When taken in toxic levels, MAOIs can be lethal because they can produce hyperkalaemia, metabolic acidosis, and rhabdomyolysis. Symptoms of MAOI toxicity are often delayed, occurring 6 to 12 hours after ingestion and, in some cases, as long as 24 hours later. Once signs and symptoms begin to appear, you should prepare to manage a life-threatening event. When death occurs from an MAOI overdose, it is usually secondary to multiple-system organ failure.

Early signs and symptoms of MAOI overdose include hyperactivity, arrhythmias (usually sinus tachycardia), hyperventilation, and nystagmus. With increased levels of toxicity, be alert for chest pain, palpitations, hypertension, diaphoresis, agitated or combative behaviour, marked hyperthermia, and hallucinations. With a severe MAOI overdose, expect bradycardia, hypotension, convulsions, worsening hyperthermia, pulmonary oedema, coma, or cardiac arrest.

Unfortunately, there is no antidote available for an MAOI overdose. With any suspected MAOI overdose, you should establish and maintain the airway, inserting an advanced airway as needed. In addition, give high-flow supplemental oxygen. Establish large-bore vascular access. Monitor the ECG rhythm, staying alert for changes indicative of hyperkalaemia.

You are the Paramedic Part 4

Now that you have identified the substance that Julie might have taken, you contact the hospital for medical guidance. Once you establish contact with the A&E doctor, you explain what you found on arrival, your physical assessment findings (including your suspicion of amitriptyline overdose), the interventions undertaken, and the current reassessment findings.

Reassessment	Recording Time: 18 Minutes
Skin	Flushed, warm, and dry
Pulse	165 beats/min; regular and weak
ECG	Possible wide complex tachycardia
Blood pressure	88/56 mm Hg
Respirations	12 breaths/min via bag-valve-mask device
SpO₂	99% via bag-valve-mask device on 100% supplemental oxygen
Pupils	Dilated

7. Can the information you provide to hospital staff during your radio report contribute to a negative patient outcome?
8. Are there any potential complications that can arise during transport relative to the patient's condition?

With a patient in deteriorating condition, treat hypotension with sequential fluid boluses of normal saline. If convulsions occur, treat them with benzodiazepines per local guideline because persistent convulsions may contribute to the combined problems of metabolic acidosis, hyperkalaemia, and rhabdomyolysis.

Selective Serotonin Reuptake Inhibitors

A larger therapeutic window, which increases their safety margin, has helped make selective serotonin reuptake inhibitors (SSRIs) a top choice for managing depression. In addition, SSRIs have far fewer anticholinergic and cardiac effects than the TCAs. Popular SSRIs include fluoxetine, paroxetine, and sertraline.

As many as 50% of adult patients may be asymptomatic with an SSRI overdose. When symptoms are present, the most commonly seen include nausea, vomiting, arrhythmias (usually sinus tachycardia), sedation, and tremors. Other symptoms that occur much less often include dilated pupils, agitation, blood pressure changes (hypotension or hypertension), convulsions, and hallucinations, When SSRIs are taken in conjunction with alcohol, look for tachycardia, mild hypotension, and generally lethargy as the most common signs and symptoms.

A pure SSRI overdose with no other drugs or alcohol involved usually produces limited toxic effects, with the exception of convulsions or serotonin syndrome (discussed later in this section). As such, management of an SSRI overdose follows the general approach for poisoned patients:

- Establish and maintain the airway.
- Administer high-flow supplemental oxygen.
- Establish an IV.
- Provide continuous ECG monitoring.
- Transport to an appropriate hospital.

Serotonin syndrome is an idiosyncratic complication that occasionally occurs with anti-depressant therapy. This condition is not limited to patients taking SSRIs, but also can occur when patients take any combination of drugs that increase central serotonin neurotransmission. Because no laboratory test can pinpoint serotonin syndrome and the symptomatology is vague at best, it is a difficult diagnosis based on clinical suspicion after other psychiatric or medical causes have been ruled out. Lower extremity muscle rigidity is one of the few classic signs, with approximately half of patients presenting with confusion or disorientation and one third with agitation.

Although serotonin syndrome is rare, it is potentially lethal: 1 of every 10 patients dies. The primary treatment is to discontinue drug therapy, which is clearly not a prehospital intervention. In the prehospital environment, management is primarily supportive. Pay close attention to the patient's ability to protect the airway because 25% of patients with serotonin syndrome eventually require intubation.

Lithium

Despite the major advances made in many areas of psychiatric medicine, lithium remains the cornerstone drug for the treatment of bipolar disorder. In 1949, lithium salts made their debut for the treatment of mania. Eventually, they were found to be much more efficacious for the treatment of bipolar disorder, and they retain their position as first-line treatment for this condition.

Lithium is almost completely absorbed in the GI tract roughly 8 hours after ingestion. Bioelimination occurs relatively slowly, with approximately 95% of the lithium eliminated in the urine; although two thirds of the lithium dose is excreted within 12 hours after ingestion, the remainder is excreted during the next 2 weeks. Given its small therapeutic window and slow excretion process, the threat of toxic levels and overdosing is ever present.

Early signs and symptoms of lithium overdose include nausea, vomiting, hand tremors, excessive thirst, and slurred speech. With increased toxicity come increased neurological symptoms: ataxia, muscle weakness and incoordination, blurred vision, and hyperreflexia (twitching). Eventually, the patient may have convulsions and become comatose.

Management of a patient suspected of a lithium overdose is mostly supportive. Establish and maintain the airway, inserting an advanced airway as needed. Give high-flow supplemental oxygen, and ensure vascular access. If the patient experiences hypotension, administer serial boluses of normal saline. Maintain continuous ECG monitoring, being alert for AV blocks and ventricular arrhythmias. Finally, transport the patient to an appropriate hospital.

Non-prescription Pain Medications

Medications used for pain management make up a huge part of the GSL drug market. In the GSL and prescription drug markets, nonsteroidal anti-inflammatory drugs (NSAIDs) are some of the most popular options for pain relief, fever control, and anti-inflammatory action. Their convenient dosing schemes and large therapeutic windows, coupled with their safe track records relative to acute ingestion and overdose, enhance their popularity.

NSAIDs are rapidly absorbed from the GI tract before being eliminated from the body in urine and faeces. The half-lives of these agents vary widely, ranging from 2 to 4 hours for ibuprofen, to approximately 15 hours for selective cyclooxygenase-2 inhibitors, to 50 hours for some long-acting agents. Patients who take lithium and NSAIDs have slowed renal clearance of the lithium, increasing the likelihood that they will inadvertently reach a toxic lithium level.

Most of the problems associated with NSAID use involve long-term use; patients may experience GI bleeding and kidney dysfunction. Acute ingestion and overdoses are rare, with ibuprofen being the NSAID most commonly encountered in the acute setting. At toxic levels, the signs and symptoms of NSAID overdose may include headache, altered mental state (cognitive difficulties, behavioural changes), convulsions, bradyarrhythmia, hypotension, abdominal pain, nausea, and vomiting. Many patients who experience NSAID overdose remain asymptomatic, however.

For symptomatic patients, care in the prehospital setting is usually supportive. Establish and maintain the airway, inserting an advanced airway as needed. Give high-flow supplemental oxygen, and establish vascular access. If hypotension develops, administer fluid boluses of normal saline. If hypotension persists after sequential fluid boluses, consider giving a vasopressor. Treat convulsions with benzodiazepines per local guideline. Finally, transport the patient to an appropriate hospital.

A unique side effect of NSAID use is aseptic meningitis, in which a patient presents with complaints of a stiff neck, headache, and fever within several hours after taking an NSAID. Discontinuing the NSAID therapy generally resolves the problem, but patients must be evaluated at the hospital to rule out other causes.

Salicylates

Although aspirin (acetylsalicylic acid, or ASA) can be involved in a toxic event, more typically general-sales-list (GSL) products containing salicylates cause toxicity. For example, a single 30-ml dose of bismuth subsalicylate contains 261 mg of salicylate (two thirds the total dose of one aspirin). Similarly, many of the liniments used with hot-air vaporisers contain high levels of methyl salicylate. With continued use of these products for a period of days, infants or young toddlers may ingest toxic levels of the salicylate.

The clinical presentation of salicylate overdose can change based on three primary variables: the patient's age, the dose ingested, and the duration of the exposure. Ingestion of 150 mg/kg or less will usually make a person "mildly toxic". At this level, chief complaints are usually nausea, vomiting, and abdominal pain. With a dosing range of 150 to 300 mg/kg, moderate toxicity results, with signs and symptoms including vomiting, diaphoresis, hyperpnoea, ringing in the ears, pulmonary oedema, and acid-base disturbances. At levels of 300 mg/kg, severe toxicity may produce metabolic acidosis or combined respiratory alkalosis–metabolic acidosis.

When paediatric patients have an acute salicylate episode, the ingestion is usually accidental, the symptoms are mild, and they recover swiftly. A chronic event (possibly from several days of vaporiser use) is usually much more serious in paediatric patients.

By comparison, an acute salicylate event with an adult usually involves an intentional overdose, with the most common patient profile being young women with a history of drug abuse or psychiatric problems. A fatal event is possible if an adult with suspected salicylate overdose is unconscious during initial assessment and presents with a high fever, convulsions, or cardiac arrhythmias.

No salicylate antidote or antagonist is available, so prehospital management is primarily supportive. Establish and maintain the airway, inserting an advanced airway as needed. Give high-flow supplemental oxygen, and establish vascular access. If hypotension develops (from volume depletion), administer serial boluses of normal saline. Monitor carbon dioxide levels with capnometry. Finally, transport the patient to an appropriate hospital.

Paracetamol

Paracetamol is a well-tolerated drug with few side effects that is available on a GSL basis. These characteristics have made this drug one of the best-selling analgesics in the United Kingdom—and one of the most common culprits in toxic exposures. In 2000, the Toxic Drug Exposure System revealed that paracetamol was involved in 5% of all toxic exposures and produced 23% of all deaths from this cause. Its lethality is believed to stem from two sources: a widely held belief that paracetamol is not a dangerous drug and a general lack of awareness that paracetamol is an ingredient in many other preparations.

Once ingested, paracetamol is rapidly absorbed from the GI tract, producing peak serum levels in 30 to 120 minutes. Absorption slows when the drug is combined with diphenhydramine or with propoxyphene. One unique aspect of paracetamol toxicity is that the signs and symptoms appear in four distinct stages **Table 33-6 ▼**.

It is important to try to estimate accurately the time of ingestion because this information drives the decision-making process for patient care in the prehospital environment and the hospital. Although an antidote for paracetamol toxicity exists—namely, acetylcysteine—ideally this drug should be given less than 8 hours after the ingestion. Typically, however, it is administered based on the patient's laboratory results; as such, it is not a prehospital intervention.

Management of the patient in the prehospital environment first focuses on establishing and maintaining the airway, with an advanced airway being inserted as needed. Give high-flow supplemental oxygen, and establish vascular access. Finally, transport the patient to an appropriate hospital.

Theophylline

Theophylline, caffeine, and theobromine are naturally occurring alkaloids found in a variety of plants around the world; they belong to the family of drugs called methylated xanthines. It is estimated that half the world's population drinks tea, which contains caffeine and theophylline. Cocoa and chocolate contain caffeine and theobromine as well.

Table 33-6	Signs and Symptoms of Paracetamol Toxicity	
Stage	**Timeframe**	**Signs and Symptoms**
I	< 24 h	Nausea, vomiting, loss of appetite, pallor, malaise
II	24–72 h	Right upper quadrant abdominal pain; abdomen tender to palpation
III	72–96 h	Metabolic acidosis, renal failure, coagulopathies, recurring GI symptoms
IV	4–14 d (or longer)	Recovery slowly begins, or liver failure progresses and the patient dies

For many years, theophylline was used to treat patients with chronic obstructive pulmonary disease and asthma, primarily because of its bronchodilatory effects. In addition, theophylline is a potent CNS stimulant. Even when taken in normal therapeutic doses, it can cause a variety of ECG rhythm disturbances, including sinus or atrial tachycardia, frequent premature atrial contractions, atrial fibrillation, and atrial flutter. Even more problematic is the occurrence of premature ventricular contractions and ventricular arrhythmias, including ventricular tachycardia. Theophylline has a very small therapeutic window. This narrow safety range, coupled with the prevalence of CNS and cardiovascular side effects and the continued development of beta-2 agonists for chronic obstructive pulmonary disease and asthma treatment, has led to decreased use of theophylline.

Peak levels of theophylline are reached within 90 to 120 minutes after ingestion, except in the case of sustained-release preparations, which may take as long as 8 hours to produce peak serum levels. Absorption rates increase if the drug is taken on an empty stomach or with large amounts of fluids, but also can decrease when theophylline is taken with certain foods. Approximately 85% to 90% of the drug is metabolised by the liver, with the remainder excreted in the urine.

Most toxic exposures of theophylline in adults involve unintentional overdoses, usually resulting from the drug's variable absorption rate and small therapeutic window. The toxic effects may range from mild GI distress (nausea and vomiting) to life-threatening or fatal cardiac arrhythmias. Indeed, a patient taking theophylline can quickly go from being asymptomatic to a life-threatening state with little to no warning. Complaints of restlessness, insomnia, tremors, agitation, and other signs and symptoms of CNS overstimulation are common, as are cardiac arrhythmias.

Because of the rapidity with which a patient's condition may deteriorate, prompt intervention is essential, especially in regard to the use of activated charcoal, which can greatly reduce the half-life of theophylline. First, establish and maintain the airway, inserting an advanced airway as needed. Give high-flow supplemental oxygen, and establish vascular access. Continuously monitor the ECG rhythm. If hypotension develops, administer fluid boluses; if they fail to relieve the problem, administer a vasopressor. You may also consider low-dose beta blockers, per your local guideline. For symptomatic reentry supraventricular tachycardia, you may give adenosine, but stay alert for bronchospasm (a potential side effect of adenosine). Finally, treat arrhythmias per ACLS (see Chapter 27).

Metals and Metalloids

Although acute metal and metalloid toxic exposures are relatively rare, when they occur, they can produce devastating results, usually because of delayed diagnosis or misdiagnosis. The difficulty reaching the correct diagnosis may contribute to increased mortality or morbidity because of delayed or inade-

Table 33-7	Systems Affected by Lead Poisoning
System	**Signs and Symptoms**
CNS	Altered mental state, including irritability, mood changes, memory deficit, sleep disturbances; headache; convulsions; ataxia
GI	Abdominal pain (usually occurs with acute poisoning); constipation; diarrhoea
Renal	Renal insufficiency; hypertension; gout
Haematologic	Anaemia

quate treatment. Toxic exposures involving metals or metalloids usually manifest by affecting four body systems: neurological, haematological, renal, and GI.

Lead

Despite the bans on lead in petrol, paint, canning processes, and plumbing, lead poisoning remains the leading cause of chronic metal poisoning. It has long been known that elevated lead levels may significantly hamper intellectual development in children.

With inorganic lead, absorption usually occurs via the respiratory or GI tract. Once in the body, approximately 90% of the lead is stored in bone. From this site, it eventually makes its way into the bloodstream. Inorganic lead can also cross the placental barrier and negatively affective foetal development. Its excretion from the body is incredibly slow, with the half-life of lead in bone estimated at 30 years.

Most organic lead (tetraethyl lead) exposures occur in the occupational setting, although they can also occur from gas sniffing where leaded petrol is available. Once in the body, tetraethyl lead is metabolised to inorganic lead and triethyl lead, with triethyl lead the primary cause of CNS toxicity.

Lead poisoning is associated with a long list of signs and symptoms (Table 33-7 ▲). In particular, encephalopathy is a major cause of mortality and morbidity from lead poisoning.

In the prehospital environment, you have few treatment options for lead poisoning. Your most helpful move may be identification of the source of the lead, which can assist the appropriate government agency to prevent more occurrences by removing the toxin. When managing the patient, first establish and maintain the airway, inserting an advanced airway as needed. Give high-flow supplemental oxygen. Establish vascular access with a saline or heparin lock. Unless hypotension is present, don't provide fluid therapy—it may worsen cerebral oedema. Transport the patient to an appropriate hospital.

Iron

Although only a small amount of iron is required as part of a healthy diet, many adult and paediatric multivitamins contain iron. Children younger than 6 years have frequent iron exposures, usually secondary to ingesting chewable vitamins. By comparison, most toxic exposures in adults are intentional.

In the average 70-kg adult, the body's entire iron supply consists of only about 4 g. Of that total, roughly 65% is found in haemoglobin, with the remainder sequestered elsewhere. Because of its toxic potential, iron is stored in the body by several mechanisms, which permit access to the supply as needed. The body of a healthy person does not contain "free" (unbound) iron.

From a practical perspective, the toxic effects of an iron exposure reflect the amount of elemental iron ingested. With ingestion of 20 to 60 mg/kg, mild to moderate toxicity should be expected. With dosing of more than 60 mg/kg, severe and potentially lethal toxicity is a possibility.

Two broad categories of iron poisoning can be distinguished: GI and systemic. With GI toxicity, the symptoms consist of abdominal pain, vomiting (the most common sign), and diarrhoea. With systemic toxicity, patients may be hypotensive or in frank shock from coagulopathy and vomiting blood. They are commonly in metabolic acidosis and become tachypnoeic as the body attempts to adjust pH by increasing the elimination of carbon dioxide.

Children typically remain asymptomatic when they have a low-level iron exposure. However, children who ingest a large dose of iron are at risk of dying unless aggressive and timely interventions take place. Unfortunately, little can be done in the prehospital environment for iron poisoning, other than providing basic attention to the ABCs and transporting to hospital for further evaluation and laboratory studies.

Mercury

Mercury exists in a variety of organic and inorganic forms. In the human body, all forms produce toxic effects. Although accidental exposures to mercury often occur in the occupational setting, mercury can be found in the home in thermometers and in some switches used in heating and air conditioning.

Organic mercury is very lipid-soluble and quickly accumulates in the liver, CNS, and kidneys. It can also cross the placental membrane into the foetus.

Mercury poisoning can present differently depending on the type of mercury and its route of entry into the body. Most signs and symptoms involve the CNS and GI and renal systems. CNS alterations may include anxiety, depression, irritability, sleep disturbances, and memory loss. In addition, tremors, ataxia, paraesthesias, muscle weakness or rigidity, and excessive drooling may develop.

In the occupational setting, safe removal from the exposure source is the primary intervention. In all cases of suspected mercury poisoning, ambulance service management is supportive and includes basic attention to the ABCs and transport to the hospital. In the hospital setting, the patient may undergo aggressive GI decontamination and receive dimercaprol (BAL), succimer (DMSA), or other chelating agents.

Arsenic

The most common cause of acute metal poisoning and the second leading cause of chronic metal poisoning is arsenic. This metal is used in a variety of industries and appears in a variety of compounds, so it is often the source of unintentional exposures. Intentional exposures include the use of arsenic in murder and suicide.

Arsenic can enter the body by ingestion, inhalation, and absorption and dermally through a wound. It is eliminated from the body through the kidneys.

The clinical presentation of arsenic poisoning depends on the type, amount, and concentration of arsenic that enters the body and the rate of absorption and elimination. In general, symptoms appear within 30 minutes to several hours of arsenic ingestion. Arsenic poisoning should be suspected with patients who present with hypotension of unknown cause following a bout of severe gastroenteritis.

Signs and symptoms of arsenic poisoning include severe abdominal pain, nausea, explosive diarrhoea, "metal taste" in the mouth, skin rash, general malaise, weakness, hypotension secondary to fluid loss, pulmonary oedema, rhabdomyolysis, and renal failure. ECG changes and arrhythmias (usually sinus tachycardia) may be apparent, but nonspecific ST-segment and T-wave changes are also possible, as is QT prolongation. Ventricular tachycardia and torsade de pointes can occur.

A patient with acute arsenic toxicity is in critical condition and requires aggressive interventions. Establish and maintain the airway, inserting an advanced airway as needed. Give high-flow supplemental oxygen, and establish vascular access. For hypotension, administer sequential boluses of normal saline. Continuously monitor the ECG, and follow ACLS algorithms for arrhythmias—uncorrected hypotension arrhythmias may lead to death. For torsade de pointes, consider administration of magnesium after consulting with clinical support. Finally, provide rapid transport to an appropriate hospital.

Poisonous Plants

Of the thousands of plant varieties, only a few are poisonous ▶ Figure 33-13 ▶ . Oddly enough, poisonous plants represent some of the most common ornamental garden shrubs and houseplants. Perhaps for that reason, 70% to 80% of plant-related exposures involve children younger than 6 years. Thankfully, deaths from plant ingestions are rare (< 0.001% of all cases). ▶ Table 33-8 ▶ lists plants that can cause toxic results and, in some cases, death.

The ubiquitous dieffenbachia is a lovely green plant with broad, variegated leaves. It is nicknamed "dumb cane", because eating dieffenbachia can result in a person being unable to speak. All parts of the dieffenbachia plant—leaves, stems, roots—contain sharp caladium oxalate crystals. When ingested, the crystals cause burns of the mouth and tongue and, sometimes, paralysis of the vocal cords. In severe cases, oedema of the tongue and larynx may lead to airway compromise.

Caladium, with its stunning multicoloured leaves, is another hazard lurking in the flowerpot. Like dieffenbachia, it contains caladium oxalate crystals and produces the same results when ingested. Nausea, vomiting, and diarrhoea commonly occur after ingestion of either plant.

Lantana (also known as red sage or wild sage) is a perennial flowering shrub with clusters of little red berries. These berries—particularly when ripe—can lead to serious poisoning.

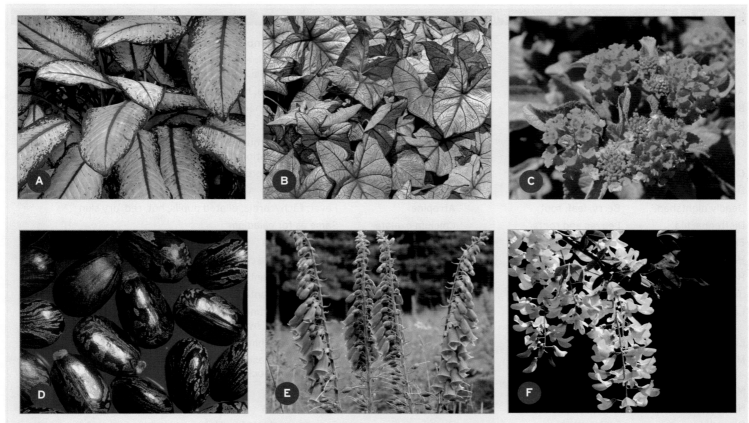

Figure 33-13 Poisonous plants. **A.** Dieffenbachia. **B.** Caladium. **C.** Lantana. **D.** Castor beans. **E.** Foxglove (digitalis). **F.** Laburnum.

Even when still green, the berries contain lantadene A, a poison that causes stomach upsets, muscle weakness, shock, and sometimes death.

Then there's the real killer in the flowerpot: castor bean. The seeds of this attractive shrub are highly poisonous—chewing on just a few seeds (and, in some cases, just one) can kill a child. Ricin, the poison in castor beans, causes a variety of toxic effects: burning of the mouth and throat; nausea, vomiting, diarrhoea, and severe stomach pains; prostration; failing vision; and kidney failure (the usual cause of death).

Foxglove, which has beautiful trumpetlike flowers, contains cardiac glycosides and is used in making the drug digitalis. Along with nausea, vomiting, diarrhoea, and abdominal cramps, ingestion of foxglove can produce hyperkalaemia and cardiac arrhythmias.

Every part of the Laburnum tree is very poisonous and worryingly they are very attractive to children. The flowers are vibrant yellow and the pea-shaped seed pods are a source of intrigue; it is proposed that just one seed can cause adverse effects in children. Symptoms of poisoning by laburnum root or seeds are intense vomiting, convulsions, drowsiness, and coma. Laburnum contains cytisine (a quinoline alkaloid), which has nicotine-like effects on the GI tract and CNS, causing GI irritation with the onset of symptoms starting after 45 minutes to 4 hours after ingestion. Respiratory failure, as in nicotine poisoning, is observed in patients with severe cases.

When you encounter a case of plant poisoning, get all the information you can from the parent, and then consult NPIS for advice:

■ *When was the plant ingested?* If it was more than 12 hours ago and the patient is still asymptomatic, chances are good that the patient will emerge unscathed. Most plant poisonings produce signs and symptoms of toxicity, if they are going to do so, within 4 hours of ingestion. One notable exception is castor bean, for which symptoms may not appear until 1 to 3 days after ingestion.

■ *What, exactly, did the child eat?* Try to find out not just what type of plant, but also what parts of the plant (leaves, root, stem, flower, or fruit) were eaten. If possible, estimate how much was ingested (such as a bite or two from a leaf, three or four leaves). If you transport the child to the hospital, take the offending plant—or whatever is left of it.

■ *What signs or symptoms, if any, does the child have?*

The vast majority of plant-related exposures require no treatment, a decision that can be made after consulting with NPIS and clinical support per local guidelines. If there is a responsible adult who can keep a close eye on the child for at least 4 to 6 hours after the ingestion, there is no need to transport the child to hospital. Conversely, a child with any signs and symptoms should be evaluated in the A&E department.

Table 33-8	Poisons in Some Common Plants		
Plant	**Poisonous Part**	**Poison**	**Signs and Symptoms of Poisoning**
Apricot	Seeds	Cyanide	Headache, dizziness, weakness, nausea, vomiting, coma, convulsions
Autumn crocus	Entire plant	Colchicine	Cramps, nausea, haematuria, diarrhoea, coma, shock
Bird of paradise	Pod	Multiple	Vomiting, diarrhoea
Buttercup	Entire plant	Protoanemonin	Gastroenteritis, convulsions
Caladium	Leaves and roots	Calcium oxalate	Burning of mucous membranes, swelling of the tongue and throat, salivation, gastroenteritis
Cherry	Bark, leaves, seed	Amygdalin	Stupor, vocal cord paralysis, convulsions, coma
Daffodil	Bulb	Multiple	Gastroenteritis
Deadly nightshade	Berry, leaf, root	Atropine	Fever; tachycardia; dilated pupils; hot, red, dry skin
Dieffenbachia	Leaves and roots	Calcium oxalate	Same as for caladium
Elderberry	Leaf, shoot, bark	Sambunigran	Gastroenteritis
Holly	Berries	Ilicin	Gastroenteritis, coma
Hyacinth	Bulb	Multiple	Severe gastroenteritis
Jack-in-the-pulpit	All parts	Calcium oxalate	Severe gastroenteritis
Laurel	All parts	Andromedotoxin	Salivation, lacrimation, rhinorrhea, vomiting, convulsions, bradycardia, hypotension, paralysis
Lily of the valley	Leaf, flowers	Glycosides	Cardiac arrhythmias, nausea
Mistletoe	All parts	Tyramine	Bradycardia, gastroenteritis, hypertension, dyspnoea, delirium, sweating, shock
Morning glory	Seeds	LSD	Hallucinations
Narcissus	Bulb	Multiple	Gastroenteritis
Oleander	Entire plant	Oleanin	Cramps, bradycardia, dilated pupils, bloody diarrhoea, coma, apnoea (one leaf is lethal)
Philodendron	Entire plant	Calcium oxalate	Oedema of tongue, throat
Poinsettia	Leaves, stem, sap	Multiple	Contact dermatitis, gastroenteritis
Potato	Green tubers, new sprouts	Solanine	Severe gastroenteritis, headache, apnoea, shock
Rhododendron	Entire plant	Andromedotoxin	Salivation
Rhubarb	Leaves only	Oxalic acid	Cramps, nausea, vomiting, anuria
Wisteria	Pods	Glycoside	Severe gastroenteritis, shock

Poisonous Mushrooms

Four groups of people are most likely to be the victims of poisoning related to mushroom ingestion: wild mushroom pickers, people looking for hallucinogenic mushrooms to get high, people attempting suicide or murder, and young children who eat them by accident. Even among educated people who like to gather their own mushrooms in the wild, mistakes can happen. Thankfully, the majority of these events result in limited or no toxic effects.

A variety of factors determine whether a mushroom ingestion will produce toxic results: the age of the mushroom, the season in which it was gathered, the amount ingested, and the preparation method. Toxic effects vary from mild GI signs and symptoms to severe cytotoxic—even lethal—effects. In the United Kingdom, almost all deaths due to mushroom ingestion involve the *Amanita* species (*Amanita phalloides, Amanita virosa,* and *Amanita verna*) Figure 33-14 ▸ .

Time of symptom onset can serve as a predictor of potential severity. If the patient presents with symptoms within approximately 2 hours of ingestion, the event is most likely to be non–life-threatening. By comparison, if symptom onset occurs 6 hours or later, there is a much greater likelihood the event will be serious and potentially fatal. The most common patient complaints involve GI signs or symptoms, including abdominal cramping and watery or bloody diarrhoea. Patients may also experience chills or headaches.

Management for a symptomatic patient with a toxic mushroom ingestion includes the usual measures. Establish and maintain the airway, and establish vascular access. For hypotension secondary to vomiting and diarrhoea, administer fluid boluses of normal saline. Contact the NPIS and an A&E consultant per local guideline, and administer activated charcoal if directed to do so. Finally, transport the patient to an appropriate hospital.

Food Poisoning

Whenever you encounter two or more people sick at the same time and at the same scene, think food poisoning or CO poisoning—your hunch is likely to be correct.

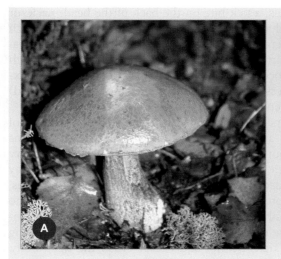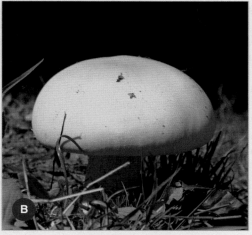

Figure 33-14 A. The deadly *Amanita* mushroom. **B.** A nonpoisonous, edible mushroom.

Arthropod Bites and Stings

If sheer numbers were the sole criterion determining such things, arthropods would rule the world. The phylum Arthropoda includes at least 1.5 million species of "joint-footed" animals, ranging from the lobster to the mite. The classes of arthropods of most medical importance, because of their ability to inject venom, are the arachnids (including spiders, scorpions, and ticks), Chilopoda (centipedes), and insects (including the Hymenoptera).

Three toxins—*Salmonella, Listeria,* and *Toxoplasma*—produce roughly 35% of all food-related deaths. Poisoning with *Clostridium botulinum,* an extremely deadly toxin, is usually the result of improper food storage or canning. In addition, the toxins produced by dinoflagellates in "red tides" may contaminate bivalve shellfish such as oysters, clams, and mussels and produce life-threatening or fatal paralytic shellfish poisoning. Cooking does not kill these toxins.

Depending on the toxin, onset of signs and symptoms can range from several hours after ingestion to days or weeks. The longer the time until symptom onset, the more difficult it will be to link the patient's problem to the event at which the toxin was ingested. Gastrointestinal complaints are the most common and include abdominal pain and cramping, nausea, vomiting, and diarrhoea. With prolonged episodes of vomiting or diarrhoea, hypotension secondary to fluid loss and electrolyte imbalance becomes likely. Respiratory distress or arrest can occur with toxins such as *C botulinum* or those found in paralytic shellfish poisoning.

Management for patients with food poisoning is usually supportive because the vast majority of cases you encounter will not be life threatening, and the signs and symptoms of acute gastroenteritis are typically self-limiting. Establish and maintain the airway, inserting an advanced airway as needed. Give high-flow supplemental oxygen, and establish vascular access. For hypotension secondary to fluid loss, administer fluid boluses of normal saline. Consider administration of chlorphenamine per local guidelines. Finally, transport the patient to an appropriate hospital.

■ Bites, Stings, and Injected Poisons

Injected poisons usually gain access to the body as the result of stings or bites from a variety of creatures. This section considers the ill effects that may result from unfriendly encounters with creatures from the land, air, and sea.

Hymenoptera Stings

The Hymenoptera family of insects includes bees, wasps, hornets, yellow jackets, and ants **Figure 33-15 ▾** . Collectively, they kill more people each year than any other venomous animals, including snakes. Death from a Hymenoptera sting usually occurs from anaphylaxis, which is covered in detail in Chapter 30.

The diagnosis of a bee sting is usually not difficult—indeed, in most cases, the patient will have already made the diagnosis. There is almost always an immediate local reaction consisting of pain (sometimes extreme), redness and swelling, and sometimes itching at the site of the sting. Honeybees sting once, usually leaving the barbed stinger and the venom sac attached to the patient's skin. By comparison, wasps and hornets can sting repeatedly until they are chased away or the patient is removed.

If the patient has no history of allergy to bee stings and does not have a systemic reaction, transport to hospital is usually unnecessary. When this decision is made, advise the patient of the warning signs of anaphylaxis and the urgency of

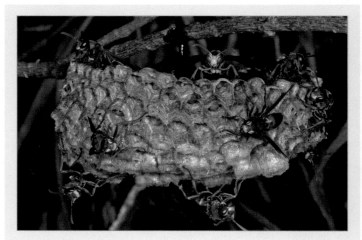

Figure 33-15 Hymenoptera stings include those from bees, wasps and hornets, and ants.

calling 999 in such an event. Instruct the patient to have the wound checked by a doctor if it does not improve markedly within 24 hours. Bee stings, especially those to the extremities, often become infected and require antibiotic treatment.

Treatment of a Hymenoptera sting focuses primarily on pain relief and minimisation of the risk of infection. First, determine whether the stinger and venom sac are still attached to the skin. If so, use a scalpel blade to gently scrape the stinger and venom sac from the wound. Do not try to pluck the stinger out with tweezers or forceps. If you squeeze the stinger or the venom sac, you will pump more venom into the wound!

After removing the stinger, clean the wound thoroughly with soap and water or an antiseptic solution such as povidone-iodine. Apply cold packs to the site for pain relief.

Tick Bites

Ticks are blood-sucking arthropods found around the world, often in rural, wooded areas. Ordinarily, tick bites are not a medical emergency, but they are of concern because ticks serve as disease vectors. Bacteria, viruses, and protozoa can be transmitted via a tick bite, and they are linked to a variety of serious illnesses, including Lyme disease.

In rare cases, a tick bite on the back of the head, neck, or spine may produce potentially life-threatening paralysis, which cannot be reversed unless the tick is removed. The clinical presentation mirrors that of Guillain-Barré syndrome. Although this is a rare occurrence, consider this possibility in unexplained weakness or paralysis after a person (especially a child) has recently been out in the woods.

The principal treatment of a tick bite is careful removal of the tick. Ticks attach themselves tenaciously to their victims using their mouth parts and a cementlike adhesive. If you try to pull the tick away from the skin, the mouth parts may remain embedded. To remove the tick, after putting on gloves, use a curved forceps to grasp the tick by the head, as close to the skin as possible, and pull straight upward using steady gentle traction. Use even pressure as you pull, and avoid twisting or jerking the tick. Do not squeeze or crush the tick's body. Dispose of the tick in a container of alcohol.

Once you have removed the tick, wash the area around the bite with soap and water. There is no reason to transport the patient if he or she remains asymptomatic. In case of tick paralysis, transport the patient with spinal immobilisation to an appropriate hospital.

You are the Paramedic Summary

1. What are your priorities at this point?

Safety is the main priority at all times. In this scenario, crowd control might be a factor. Once you are confident of scene safety, turn your attention to addressing the patient's ABCs. Additional priorities include obtaining as much pertinent information as possible and appointing someone to contact the patient's parents or parents.

2. What information do you need to obtain?

This scenario emphasises the need to obtain as much information related to SAMPLE as possible. Because the patient cannot provide information, your sources will be her friends and the teacher. Patients with altered mental status can have a wide variety of problems, and SAMPLE will be one of the keys to providing successful treatment.

3. What are some potential differential diagnoses?

Although your rapid trauma survey did not reveal life-threatening injuries, you cannot rule out a head injury as the cause of Julie's altered mental status. Based on the information you have at this point, other differential diagnoses include overdose, hypoglycaemia, and infection.

4. Which interventions should you consider at this point, if any?

By now, you should have delegated the role of cervical-spine immobilisation. The patient is already receiving supplemental oxygen. While you perform a detailed physical assessment, you can ask your colleague to obtain a glucose level and apply the cardiac monitor. Until you obtain more information, no further interventions are needed.

5. Given the current situation, should you consider treating the patient on the scene, or continuing treatment on the way to hospital?

In this case, it is best to package the patient and continue treatment on the way to the hospital. If the patient's condition continues to deteriorate, the optimal place for treatment to be given would be the A&E department.

6. How should your patient management progress?

Maintenance of the ABCs should take priority. Now that you have ruled out trauma as a potential MOI, the patient no longer requires cervical-spine immobilisation. Depending on your department's guideline, you might have to contact the receiving hospital for orders. Remember to bring the medication bottle to hospital. Also, keep a watchful eye on the cardiac monitor for the development of ventricular rhythms associated with the drug's toxicity.

7. Can the information you provide to the hospital staff during your radio report contribute to a negative patient outcome?

Absolutely! Not providing the proper information to the hospital staff can lead to mistreatment of your patient. In this case, not making the A&E department staff aware of the ingestion of amitriptyline, including the dose and number of pills taken, might delay lifesaving treatment or lead to the administration of incorrect treatment that produces unwanted complications, including death. You are the eyes and ears of the doctor—it is your responsibility to paint an accurate picture that enables the doctor to make proper treatment decisions.

8. Are there any potential complications that can arise during transport relative to the patient's condition?

Tricyclic anti-depressants are extremely toxic medications. Life-threatening events potentially include the development of ventricular arrhythmias, convulsions, and pulmonary oedema. Sound knowledge of the effects of tricyclic anti-depressants and good assessment skills are paramount to the delivery of effective patient care.

Prep Kit

Ready for Review

- Toxicological emergencies usually fall under one of two general headings: intentional and unintentional.
- Given the variety of illicit drugs coupled with the continued growth of licit drugs, even the most well-read and experienced paramedic may find it difficult to stay current with the myriad drugs sold in the streets today. For this reason, the NPIS may be an indispensable aid.
- The four primary methods whereby a toxin commonly enters the body are ingestion, inhalation, injection, and absorption.
- Although the sheer number of substances of abuse may seem daunting, the good news is that many drugs, on entering the body, produce similar signs and symptoms.
- Human beings have a long history of abusing drugs and alcohol. With the passing of time, the physiological and societal effects of alcohol abuse have become well known and thoroughly documented. Unfortunately, the area of medicine dealing with drugs of abuse is challenging because of uncertainty about the prevalence of the problem and the continual evolution of the substances themselves.
- Alcohol is the most widely abused drug in the United Kingdom.
- Generally, patients with toxicological emergencies are considered medical patients, although toxicological emergencies may lead to trauma, too.
- From a management perspective, ALS care builds on the basics:
  - Ensure the scene is safe for access and egress.
  - Maintain the airway.
  - Ensure that breathing is adequate.
  - Ensure that circulation isn't compromised (by hypoperfusion or arrhythmia).
  - Administer high-concentration supplemental oxygen.
  - Establish an IV.
  - Be prepared to manage shock, coma, convulsions, and arrhythmias.
  - Transport the patient as soon as possible. Place the patient in the recovery position if there is any risk of vomiting to reduce the risk of aspiration.

Vital Vocabulary

alcoholism A state of physical and psychological addiction to ethyl alcohol.

amphetamines A class of drugs that increase alertness and excitation (that is, stimulants); includes methamphetamine (crank or ice), methylenedioxyamphetamine (MDA, Adam), and methylenedioxymethamphetamine (MDMA, Eve, ecstasy).

antagonist Something that counteracts the action of something else; in relation to drugs, a drug that is an antagonist has an affinity for a cell receptor and, by binding to it, the cell is prevented from responding.

barbiturates Potent sedative-hypnotics historically used as sleep aids, anti-anxiety drugs, and as part of the regime for convulsion control.

benzodiazepines The family of sedative-hypnotics most commonly used to treat anxiety, convulsions, and alcohol withdrawal.

caladium A common houseplant that contains caladium oxalate crystals; ingestion leads to nausea, vomiting, and diarrhoea.

carbamates A more recent development than organophosphates, they are derivatives of carbamic acid. They are mainly used to control insect pests in agriculture and horticulture. As with organophosphates, they inhibit the action of acetylcholine at the nerve synapses.

castor bean A seed that contains the poison ricin; causes a variety of toxic effects: burning of the mouth and throat; nausea, vomiting, diarrhoea, and severe stomach pains; prostration; failing vision and kidney failure, which is the usual cause of death.

caustics Chemicals that are acids or alkalis; cause direct chemical injury to the tissues they contact.

delirium tremens (DTs) A severe withdrawal syndrome seen in people with alcoholism who are deprived of ethyl alcohol; characterised by restlessness, fever, sweating, disorientation, agitation, and convulsions; can be fatal if untreated.

dieffenbachia A common houseplant that resembles "elephant ears"; ingestion leads to burns of the mouth and tongue and, possibly, paralysis of the vocal cords and nausea and vomiting; in severe cases, may be oedema of the tongue and larynx, leading to airway compromise.

drug Substance that has some therapeutic effect (such as reducing inflammation, fighting bacteria, or producing euphoria) when given in the appropriate circumstances and in the appropriate dose.

drug abuse Any use of drugs that causes physical, psychological, economic, legal, or social harm to the user or others affected by the user's behaviour.

drug addiction A chronic disorder characterised by the compulsive use of a substance that results in physical, psychological, or social harm to the user who continues to use the substance despite the harm.

foxglove A plant that contains cardiac glycosides used in making digitalis; ingestion of leaves causes nausea, vomiting, diarrhoea, abdominal cramps, hyperkalaemia, and a variety of arrhythmias.

habituation The situation in which there is a physical tolerance and psychological dependence on a drug or drugs.

hallucinogen An agent that produces false perceptions in any one of the five senses.

hydrocarbons Compounds made up principally of hydrogen and carbon atom mostly obtained from the distillation of petroleum.

illicit In relation to drugs, illegal drugs such as marijuana, cocaine, and LSD.

laburnum A common tree with vibrant yellow flowers and pea-shaped seed pods. Ingestion leads to intense vomiting, convulsions, drowsiness, and coma.

lantana A perennial flowering shrub with clusters of red berries that can lead to serious and even fatal poisoning; Also known as red sage or wild sage; ingestion causes stomach upsets, muscle weakness, shock, and, sometimes, death.

licit In relation to drugs, legalised drugs such as coffee, alcohol, and tobacco.

lithium The cornerstone drug for the treatment of bipolar disorder.

marijuana The dried leaves and flower buds of the *Cannabis sativa* plant that are smoked to achieve a high.

methamphetamine A highly addictive drug in the amphetamine family.

monoamine oxidase inhibitors (MAOIs) Psychiatric medication used primarily to treat atypical depression by increasing noradrenaline and serotonin levels in the central nervous system.

narcotic The generic term for opiates and opioids, drugs that act as a CNS depressant and produce insensibility or stupor.

opiate Various alkaloids derived from the opium or poppy plant.

opioid A synthetic narcotic not derived from opium.

organophosphates A class of chemical found in many insecticides used in agriculture and in the home.

physical dependence A physiological state of adaptation to a drug, usually characterised by tolerance to the drug's effects and a withdrawal syndrome if use of the drug is stopped, especially abruptly.

poison A substance whose chemical action could damage structures or impair function when introduced into the body.

potentiation Enhancement of the effect of one drug by another drug.

psychological dependence The emotional state of craving a drug to maintain a feeling of well-being.

salicylates Aspirin-like drugs.

sedative-hypnotic A drug used to reduce anxiety, calm agitated patients, and help produce drowsiness and sleep (CNS depressants).

selective serotonin reuptake inhibitors (SSRIs) A class of antidepressants that inhibit the reuptake of serotonin.

serotonin syndrome An idiosyncratic complication that occurs with anti-depressant therapy in which patients have lower extremity muscle rigidity, confusion or disorientation, and/or agitation.

synergism The action of two substances such as drugs, in which the *total effects are greater than the sum of the independent effects* of the two substances.

theophylline A naturally occurring alkaloid found in a variety of plants (such as tea leaves).

tolerance Physiological adaptation to the effects of a drug such that increasingly larger doses of the drug are required to achieve the same effect.

toxicological emergencies Medical emergencies caused by toxic agents such as poison.

toxidrome The syndrome-like symptoms of a poisonous agent.

tricyclic anti-depressants (TCAs) A group of drugs used to treat severe depression and manage pain; minimal dosing errors can cause toxic results.

withdrawal syndrome A predictable set of signs and symptoms, usually involving altered central nervous system activity, that occurs after the abrupt cessation of a drug or after rapidly decreasing the usual dosage of a drug.

▬ Points to Ponder

You and your colleague are called to a house near a college campus. When you arrive in front of the house, you notice a large number of college-age people gathered around someone lying supine on the front lawn. A police officer arrives on the scene at the same time you do. You approach the patient and find a female who looks to be in her late teens or early 20s. You hear snoring respirations and notice that the patient is covered in vomit. As your colleague is rolling the patient to her side and clearing her airway, you ask some of the bystanders what happened. They back away, saying, "We were just having a party, and she wasn't feeling good so we brought her outside". Your colleague reports that the patient is breathing and responds to deep painful stimuli but does not have a gag reflex.

What is your first treatment priority? Can you immediately assume that the signs and symptoms you are seeing are caused by alcohol ingestion? What other assessment points should you consider?

Issues: Assessing a Potential Alcohol Overdose, Obtaining Information From Bystanders.

Assessment in Action

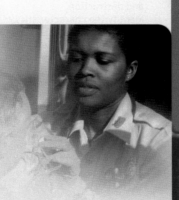

You and your colleague have arrived on the scene of a reported diabetic emergency. When you arrive at the patient's side, you see a 50-year-old man who seems to be unconscious on the floor. The patient's wife states that her husband had been at work all day. When he arrived at home, he stated he had a very bad headache and then collapsed to the floor. The wife confirms that the patient has type 1 diabetes.

As you and your colleague begin your assessment, you notice that he is drooling severely, is perspiring, and has been incontinent. You direct your colleague to obtain a blood glucose level, which comes back as 10 mmol/l. You were assuming that this call was for a diabetic emergency, but now that does not seem to be the case. As you return to your assessment, the patient vomits a large amount, which has a distinct chemical smell. You suction the patient aggressively and complete airway management measures. When you ask the wife what the patient may have been around at work, she says that her husband works at a landscaping business.

1. **What are the two types of toxicological emergencies?**
   A. Licit and illicit
   B. Prescribed and GSL
   C. Intentional and unintentional
   D. Drug or poison

2. **The patient in this scenario may be experiencing signs and symptoms of which toxidrome?**
   A. Stimulant
   B. Narcotic
   C. Sedative-hypnotic
   D. Cholinergic

3. **You determine through further questioning that the patient was using some kind of chemical at work, but the wife does not know what it was. What is your primary concern at this point in your assessment?**
   A. Determine what your colleagues and bystanders have potentially been exposed to.
   B. Move the patient quickly to your ambulance and transport immediately.
   C. Obtain IV access and administer naloxone per guidelines.
   D. Determine the potential for the patient to become violent.

4. **A patient with signs and symptoms of SLUDGE may have been exposed to:**
   A. carbon monoxide.
   B. organophosphates.
   C. barbiturates.
   D. chlorine.

5. **Organophosphates exert their toxic effects on which body system?**
   A. Integumentary
   B. Cardiac
   C. Nervous
   D. Endocrine

6. **The approach to a patient with organophosphate poisoning should start with:**
   A. decontamination and removal of contaminated items.
   B. administering atropine 2.0 mg IV push immediately.
   C. contacting the police to prevent violence.
   D. obtaining an oxygen saturation level on your patient.

Challenging Question

7. **Given that your colleagues and the patient's wife have potentially been contaminated through contact with the patient's clothing and vomit, which component becomes the most important part of decontamination—the patient or everyone else in the room?**

34 Haematological Emergencies

Objectives

Cognitive

- Identify the anatomy of the haematopoietic system.
- Describe volume and volume-control related to the haematopoietic system.
- Identify and describe the blood-forming organs.
- Describe normal red blood cell (RBC) production, function, and destruction.
- Explain the significance of the haematocrit with respect to red cell size and number.
- Explain the correlation of the RBC count, haematocrit, and haemoglobin values.
- Define anaemia.
- Describe normal white blood cell (WBC) production, function, and destruction.
- Identify the characteristics of the inflammatory process.
- Identify the difference between cellular and humoral immunity.
- Identify alterations in immunological response.
- Describe the number, normal function, types, and life span of leucocytes.
- List the leucocyte disorders.
- Describe platelets with respect to normal function, life span, and numbers.
- Describe the components of the haemostatic mechanism.
- Describe the function of coagulation factors, platelets, and blood vessels necessary for normal coagulation.
- Describe the intrinsic and extrinsic clotting systems with respect to identification of factor deficiencies in each stage.

- Identify blood groups.
- Describe how acquired factor deficiencies may occur.
- Define fibrinolysis.
- Identify the components of physical assessment as they relate to the haematological system.
- Describe the pathology and clinical manifestations and prognosis associated with:
  - Anaemia
  - Leukaemia
  - Lymphomas
  - Polycythaemia
  - Disseminated intravascular coagulopathy
  - Haemophilia
  - Sickle cell disease
  - Multiple myeloma
- Integrate pathophysiological principles into the assessment of a patient with a haematological disease.

Affective

- Value the sense of urgency for initial assessment and interventions for patients with a haematological crisis.

Psychomotor

- Perform an assessment of the patient with a haematological disorder.

Introduction

Most ambulance services rarely respond to haematological emergencies. Haematological disorders can be complex, difficult to assess, and challenging to treat in the prehospital setting. Although you may be able to provide only limited interventions, your actions may not only offer support, but actually save the patient's life. As a paramedic, you should have a basic understanding of the haematopoietic system (the blood components and the organs involved in their development and production) and haematological disorders, and you should know how to respond to these kinds of emergencies appropriately.

Anatomy and Physiology

Blood and Plasma

Blood is "the fluid of life": Without it, we would not be able to live. Blood performs the following functions:

- **Respiratory function.** Transports oxygen from the lungs to the tissues and carbon dioxide from the tissues to the lungs
- **Nutritional function.** Carries nutrients (glucose, proteins, and fats) from the digestive tract to cells throughout the body
- **Excretory function.** Transports the waste products of metabolism from the cells where they are produced to the excretory organs
- **Regulatory function.** Transports hormones to their target organs and transmits excess internal heat to the surface of the body to be dissipated
- **Defensive function.** Carries defensive cells and antibodies, which protect the body against foreign organisms

Blood is made up of two main components: plasma and formed elements (cells). Plasma is essentially 92% water and 6% to 7% proteins; the remainder consists of a variety of other elements (including electrolytes, clotting factors, glucose). Plasma accounts for 55% of the total blood volume. It has a specific gravity of around 1.03. Specific gravity is a substance's weight compared with that of an equal volume of water. Water has a specific gravity of 1.0, so anything with a specific gravity greater than 1.0 is "heavier" than water and anything with a specific gravity less than 1.0 is "lighter".

The formed elements account for 45% of the total blood volume. These elements include red blood cells (RBCs) or erythrocytes, white blood cells (WBCs) or leucocytes, and platelets or thrombocytes Figure 34-1 ▾ . Most of these elements (99%) are RBCs.

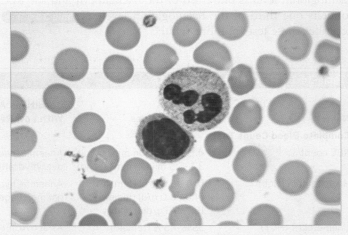

Figure 34-1 The components of blood include RBCs, WBCs, platelets, and plasma.

You are the Paramedic Part 1

It is early evening, and you have just been dispatched to 30 Lyons Road for a 35-year-old man complaining of shortness of breath and severe abdominal pain. You and your colleague respond immediately and arrive on scene within 8 minutes.

You are greeted at the front door by a concerned family member. The woman points to the bedroom and says, "He's in there! He's having another attack!" When you enter the bedroom, you see a man of African origin sitting on the edge of the bed holding his stomach.

Initial Assessment	Recording Time: 0 Minutes
Appearance	Eyes open with pained expression
Level of consciousness	A (Alert to person, place, and day)
Airway	Patent
Breathing	Laboured and shallow
Circulation	Perspiring

1. What, if anything, about his appearance gives you cause for concern?
2. What information do you already have at your disposal?

RBC production occurs within stem cells; this production is stimulated by a protein secreted by the kidneys in response to circulatory need. RBCs may take as long as 5 days to mature and have an average life of about 4 months. Their specific gravity is approximately 1.09. Within the RBCs, iron-rich haemoglobin is responsible for carrying oxygen to the tissues. Oxygen attached to haemoglobin gives blood its characteristic red colour, although many other factors can change the colour of blood.

Three laboratory tests are commonly performed on blood: RBC count, haemoglobin level, and haematocrit. The RBC count measures the number of RBCs in a sample of blood. The haemoglobin level identifies the percentage of haemoglobin found within the RBCs. The haematocrit gives the overall percentage of RBCs in the blood. The patient's blood is considered balanced (even if the numbers are too high or low) if the haemoglobin level is one third of the haematocrit and the RBC count is one third of the haemoglobin level. **Table 34-1 ▾** describes these tests in more detail.

WBCs, which are larger than RBCs, provide the body with immunity against "foreign invaders". They are derived from the stem cells, or cells that develop into other types of cells in the body. Several types of WBCs exist, each of which performs a specific task in relation to maintaining the immune system.

At the Scene

Platelets form the initial plug following vascular injury. The clotting proteins then toughen and complete the blood clot.

Platelets are the smallest of the formed elements and are responsible for the clotting of the blood. (The coagulation process or haemostasis is described in more detail in Chapter 6.) Approximately two thirds of the platelets circulate throughout the blood; the rest are stored in the spleen. Platelets are also derived from stem cells. They have an average life span of up to 11 days.

Table 34-1	RBC and WBC Tests		
Name	**Normal Values**	**Conditions Associated With Low Readings**	**Conditions Associated With High Readings**
Complete Blood Count Test			
RBC count	4.5–6.0 million mm³ (adult) 3.3–5.5 million mm³ (child)	Anaemia, haemorrhage, certain leukaemias, overyhydration, chronic infections	Polycythaemia, cardiovascular disease, haemoconcentration, dehydration
Haemoglobin (Hgb)	12.0–16.0 g/dl (female) 14.0–18.0 g/dl (male) 10.7–17.1 g/dl (child)	Anaemia, hyperthyroidism, liver disease, haemorrhage, haemolytic reactions	COPD, CHF, polycythaemia, high altitude sickness
Haematocrit (HCT)	35%–45% (female) 40%–50% (male) 32%–55% (child)	As above, including leukaemia, lupus, endocarditis, rheumatic fever, nutritional disorders	Polycythaemia and usually anything that produces severe dehydration
WBC Count and Differential			
WBC count	5,000–10,000/mm³ (adult) 4,500–15,500/mm³ (child) 9,400–34,000/mm³ (infant)	Viral infections, bone marrow diseases or disorders, leukaemia, radiation, late-stage AIDS	Viral and bacterial infections, haemorrhage, traumatic tissue injuries, leukaemia, cigarette smoking
Neutrophils (segmented and unsegmented)	50%–60%* 2,500–8,000/mm³	Leukaemia, infections, rheumatoid arthritis, vitamin B$_{12}$ deficiency, enlarged spleen	Bacterial infections, tissue breakdown, haemolytic reactions, tumours, MI, surgical stress, and cancer
Basophils (also known as MAST cells)	0.5%–1%* 25–100/mm³	Allergic reactions, hyperthyroidism, MI, bleeding ulcers, stress	Certain leukaemias, inflammations, allergy, polycythaemia, haemolytic anaemia
Eosinophils	1%–4%* 50–500/mm³	Mononucleosis, CHF, Cushing's disease	Addison's disease, tumours, skin infections, allergies
Lymphocytes	20%–40%* 1,000–4,000/mm³	Hodgkin's disease, burns, trauma, lupus, Cushing's disease, immunodeficiency states	Numerous bacterial and viral infections, hepatitis, leukaemia, toxoplasmosis, Graves' disease
Monocytes	2%–6%* 100–700/mm³	Steroid use, infections, rheumatoid arthritis, HIV	Numerous bacterial and parasitic infections, recovery of acute infections, TB, haematological disorders
Thrombocytes (platelets)	150,000–400,000/mm³	Thrombocytopenia, certain cancers, certain leukaemias, sickle cell disease, systemic lupus erythematosus	Pulmonary embolism, polycythaemia, acute haemorrhage, metastatic cancer, surgical stress

COPD indicates chronic obstructive pulmonary disease; CHF, congestive heart failure; MI, myocardial infarction; and TB, tuberculosis.
*Percentage of the total WBC count.
Example: If the WBC is 5,000, neutrophils should account for 2,500 to 3,000 of this count.

At the Scene

To check whether you might have a low RBC count, look at the palm of your hand and note the creases. Now outstretch your palm and look at those creases. If they are white, your haematocrit (or RBC count) may be low! This test works only on normal-temperature caucasian skin.

Blood-Forming Organs and RBC Production

Although many parts and organs of the human body can alter or affect the haematological system, the major players are the bone marrow, liver, and spleen Figure 34-2 ▾.

The bone marrow is the primary site for cell production within the human body. Bone marrow may be found in most of the long bones plus the pelvis, skull, and vertebrae.

The liver produces the clotting factors found in the blood. It filters the blood, removing toxins, and is essential to normal metabolism and homeostasis. As old RBCs enter the liver, they are broken down into bile. The liver is a highly vascular organ that also stores some blood within itself.

The spleen is also quite vascular. It is involved with the filtering and breakdown of erythrocytes, assists with the production of lymphocytes, and has an important role in providing homeostasis and infection control. If the spleen, which stores about one third of the platelets, has to be removed, the platelets return to the blood.

At the Scene

"Clot busters" (fibrinolytic therapy given in cases of acute myocardial infarction and stroke) activate the body's fibrinolytic system, resulting in clot decomposition (also known as lysis). Such therapy must be monitored closely in patients with haematological disorders because the effect, if exaggerated, may cause excess bleeding.

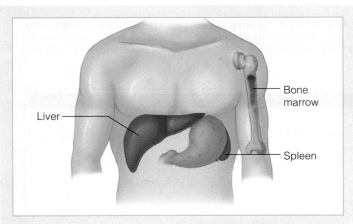

Figure 34-2 The bone marrow, liver, and spleen are the main components of the body related to the blood system.

Inflammatory Response

At birth, all of the body's cells and blood contain antigens—substances within the body that will react with lymphocytes and antibodies within the immune system. Typically, the body keeps these antigens in memory and, when exposed to something for which it already has antibodies, will not initiate a reaction (see Chapter 6). However, when the body is exposed to something it cannot identify in its base antigens, it produces antibodies to counteract the foreign or unidentified antigen. This reaction can also occur in patients with an autoimmune disorder. For unknown reasons, some people develop reactions to their own antigens.

The Immune System

The primary component of the immune system is the WBCs. Like other blood cells, WBCs are produced in the bone marrow. A small number of WBCs are always circulating in the bloodstream, but a larger reserve is ready to spring into action whenever infectious-type material is detected in the blood. Specific laboratory values relating to WBCs and measurement of essential subcomponents—namely, neutrophils, lymphocytes, basophils, and eosinophils—can provide valuable information about the status of the immune system (see Table 34-1).

The baseline WBC count is measured when the body is in a normal state (during times of no known infection or inflammation). The normal range is 5,000 to 10,000 cells/mm^3. Women tend to have higher baseline WBC counts, especially during childbearing years, owing to changes that occur during menstrual periods.

At the Scene

The life cycle of a WBC begins when the bone marrow releases a type of cell called granulocytes, which remain in the circulation for 6 to 12 hours. If the cells travel to tissues, they live for a few more days. Otherwise, WBCs are recycled by the reticuloendothelial system, as are RBCs.

Blood Classifications

To ensure compatibility and prevent medical problems during blood component replacement, blood type classifications have been developed. In the ABO system, the RBC classification types are "O", "A", "B", and "AB"; they indicate which antigens are found in the plasma membrane Table 34-2 ▸.

Blood contains a secondary antigen, known as the Rh antigen (the name signifies that the antigen was first found in the Rhesus monkey). In the United Kingdom, 84% of the population have this antigen. Thus, if an individual has the blood type A-positive (A+), the blood contains the Rh antigen.

Some patients may be receiving or have previously received a blood transfusion. It is important to determine a patient's blood type and the type of blood received. When a

Blood Type	ABO Antigens	ABO Antibodies	Acceptable Blood Donor Types
A	A	Anti-B	A, O
B	B	Anti-A	B, O
AB	A, B	None	A, B, AB, O
O	None	Anti-A Anti-B	O

Table 34-2 Blood Types

Documentation and Communication

Many anti-inflammatory drugs (aspirin, ibuprofen) and some herbals (ginkgo, garlic, ginger, ginseng, feverfew) decrease platelet aggregation. Although this effect may be beneficial (such as in myocardial infarction or stroke prevention), these drugs may also increase the tendency to bleed. Always ask patients about medications, including general sales list and herbal medications!

patient receives blood or plasma that matches his or her classification (A+ into A+) or the universal donor blood type (O), problems rarely arise. However, if a patient receives a blood type that is different than his or her own—for example, a patient with type A receives type B—a transfusion reaction will occur. Also, if a patient with A– blood receives an A+ transfusion, a transfusion reaction could occur, but this is rare. Blood reactions are similar to an anaphylactic reaction—they occur rapidly and can cause severe circulatory collapse and even death. When a patient receives a blood transfusion, it is important to monitor the patient very closely for the first 30 to 60 minutes because transfusion reactions typically begin within this timeframe.

Homeostasis and the Homeostatic Mechanism

The body must work within a close balance, referred to as homeostasis. Put simply, "what goes in" must balance with "what comes out". For example, if you consume 2,500 ml of water, your body must remove 2,500 ml of fluid to maintain balance. The reverse is true as well: If you are working in the hot sun and sweat 2,000 ml, you must replenish that fluid or you will soon feel the effects of dehydration. Many systems and organs are part of the homeostatic mechanism. For more information, go to Chapters 6 and 8.

Epidemiology

Anaemia

Anaemia is defined as a haemoglobin or erythrocyte level that is lower than normal Figure 34-3 ▸. Usually it is associated with some type of underlying disease process. Anaemia may also result from acute or chronic blood loss or a decrease in production or increase in destruction of erythrocytes. Finally, anaemia may be an outcome of a preexisting haemolytic disorder—a disorder related to the breakdown of RBCs.

Iron Deficiency Anaemia

Iron deficiency anaemia, the most common type of anaemia, affects 50 of 1,000 men, 140 of 1,000 women, and 470 of 1,000 children between 1 and 2 years of age. Typical causes include gastrointestinal blood loss, menstrual bleeding (the most common cause in UK women, particularly in the lower socioeconomic groups), and blood loss due to frequent donations or diagnostic tests for patients hospitalised for

You are the Paramedic Part 2

When you introduce yourself, the patient tells you his name and that he has sickle cell anaemia. He reports that he has had similar episodes in the past and is afraid he is having another "flare-up". The patient looks frightened and tells you his grandfather died of sickle cell anaemia at a relatively young age. You apply oxygen at 15 l/min via nonrebreathing mask. Your assessment reveals the following:

Vital Signs	Recording Time: 5 Minutes
Level of consciousness	Alert, with a Glasgow Coma Scale score of 15
Skin	Perspiring and feverish with pale mucous membranes
Pulse	Radial pulse, 112 beats/min, weak and regular
Blood pressure	108/46 mm Hg
Respirations	28 breaths/min and shallow
SpO_2	92% while breathing room air

3. What complications are common with sickle cell anaemia?
4. What are your treatment priorities given your understanding of patients with sickle cell anaemia?

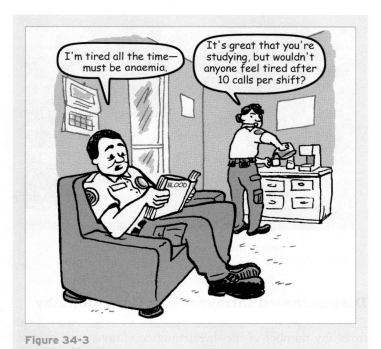

Figure 34-3

Leukaemia

Leukaemia is a disease that develops in the lymphoid system. In this type of cancer, blood cells—particularly WBCs—develop abnormally and/or excessively. Leukaemia can cause anaemia, thrombocytopenia (decrease in platelets), and leucopenia (decrease in WBCs); conversely, it has been noted to produce an extremely high WBC count (leucocytosis). Patients with leukaemia experience frequent bleeding, bruising, infections, and fever **Figure 34-4 ▶**.

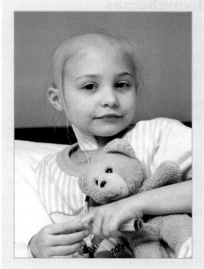

Figure 34-4 People with leukaemia may have frequent bleeding, bruising, infections, and fever.

long periods. In children, it is usually related to premature birth or low birth weight.

Haematological Disorders

These disorders can be hereditary. They include diseases caused by genetic problems within the RBC, such as sickle cell disease and thalassaemia. In these disorders, when the RBCs are first developing their membranes, they may become rigid and deformed. The RBCs may then become lodged in small blood vessels, leading to a thrombosis (blood clot). In many haematological disorders, the defective RBCs migrate to the spleen, where they are destroyed. These disorders may also result from a deficiency of an enzyme known as glucose-6-phosphate dehydrogenase; this enzyme helps protect cells during infections. When levels of this enzyme are low, cells can become damaged. Although glucose-6-phosphate dehydrogenase deficiency is most commonly seen in people of African origin, it can arise in individuals of any race.

The most common type of acquired anaemia develops when the flow of RBCs is disrupted owing to problems with blood vessel linings (aneurysms, weaknesses) or blood clots. In autoimmune disorders, RBCs are destroyed by the body's own antibodies, which erroneously think that the normal blood cells are foreign. RBCs can also be destroyed by microorganisms in the blood.

Anaemia can have serious consequences for people who travel to high-altitude areas. The combination of the lower number of RBCs and reduced oxygen levels in the atmosphere can lead to serious conditions that a healthy individual would not experience, such as hypoxia, difficulty breathing, and chest pain.

Renal failure will produce anaemia in a person because the kidneys will not be producing enough erythropoietin for red blood cell production.

Leukaemia can be classified as acute or chronic. In most situations, but especially in chronic cases, the disease tends to develop more frequently in older populations (65 years or older). In acute leukaemia, bone marrow is replaced with abnormal lymphoblasts. In chronic leukaemia, abnormal mature lymphoid cells accumulate in the bone marrow, lymph nodes, spleen, and peripheral blood. This form of leukaemia is typically found by chance during routine blood tests; suspicions are raised when the tests reveal a high lymphocyte count.

Survival of leukaemia depends on factors such as the stage at which the disease is detected, the patient's underlying medical condition, and the response to treatment. Acute and chronic leukaemia are treated with chemotherapy and radiotherapy. After receiving treatment, most patients will go into remission, especially when their conditions are identified early. Indeed, approximately 80% of children will be cured when their leukaemia is diagnosed and treated early. Owing to the higher occurrence of genetic abnormalities and leukaemic lymphoblasts as a result of the ageing process, the adult cure rate is, at best, 30% to 40%.

At the Scene

When abnormalities of the blood cells are suspected, note the following:
1. Anaemia commonly results in complaints of fatigue, lethargy, and dyspnoea.
2. Low WBC counts (leucopenia) often lead to infection and fever.
3. Low platelet counts (thrombocytopenia) often cause cutaneous bleeding (including petechiae) and bleeding from mucous membranes (nosebleeds, rectal bleeding).

Lymphomas

Lymphomas are a group of malignant diseases that arise within the lymphoid system. They are classified in two categories: non-Hodgkin's lymphoma (accounting for the majority of cases) and Hodgkin's lymphoma.

Non-Hodgkin's lymphoma can occur at any age in any person and can be hereditary. Furthermore, these types of cancer may be characterised based on the progression of the disease: indolent, aggressive, or highly aggressive. With very slow (indolent) progression, the disease may never leave the lymphoid system. In the highly aggressive form, the disease may affect multiple organs in a relatively short period, usually within several months. How well a patient responds to treatment depends on how early the disease is recognised and classified.

Hodgkin's lymphoma is a painless progressive enlargement of the lymphoid glands, most commonly affecting the spleen and the lymph nodes. A highly rare form of lymphoma, it is suspected to have some hereditary components. The incidence of Hodgkin's lymphoma has two peaks: one between 15 and 35 years of age and a second peak after age 55 to 60 years. The disease is twice as common in men as in women. Patients may not show any symptoms for many years, with the disease being discovered only after patients complain of night sweats, chills, persistent coughs, and swelling of various lymph nodes (usually in the neck first). They may also note loss of appetite for an unknown reason, significant weight loss, generalised itching, fatigue, and/or bone pain. With aggressive treatment, symptoms may disappear for long periods; 60% to 90% of patients may actually be cured.

Polycythaemia

Polycythaemia is characterised by an overabundance or overproduction of RBCs. The increased RBC production can be caused by a rare disorder originating in a single stem cell or an existing disease such as congestive heart failure or hypertension. It can also arise in individuals who live in high-altitude areas for long periods. The disease essentially causes hyperviscosity of the circulatory system.

The overabundance of the blood products associated with polycythaemia may lead to many other signs and symptoms, such as strokes, transient ischaemic attacks, headaches, and abdominal pain (usually associated with an enlarged spleen). This disease is often found accidentally when blood cell counts are performed after a patient complains of frequent episodes of the previously mentioned signs and symptoms. Cases of polycythaemia are more frequently found in middle-aged adults (50 years and older).

Clinical treatment usually includes phlebotomy to try to maintain haematocrit levels at less than 45% in men and less than 42% in women. Other treatments have included cancer-type therapy intended to slow the production of new RBCs within the bone marrow. Survival is less than 18 months when the disease goes untreated but can be as long as 15 years for treated patients.

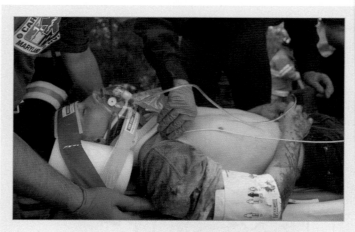

Figure 34-5 Severe trauma and extended hypotension can result in DIC.

Disseminated Intravascular Coagulopathy

Disseminated intravascular coagulopathy (DIC) may result from any number of life-threatening conditions such as massive injury and hypotension due to trauma **Figure 34-5 ▲**. Sepsis and obstetric complications also may cause DIC.

The condition progresses in two stages. First, free thrombin and fibrin deposits in the blood increase, and platelets begin to aggregate. In this stage of the condition, owing to excessive bleeding, massive blood loss, or tissue injury, the coagulation system and fibrinolytic system become overwhelmed. The fibrinolytic system is activated, which causes a breakdown of the fibrin clots, a process known as defibrination. In the second stage of the condition, uncontrolled haemorrhage results from the severe reduction in clotting factors.

DIC can be chronic or acute and is most likely to be encountered by ambulance staff as the result of trauma/nontrauma. The clinical progression of DIC will depend upon the intensity of the stimulus and the health of the patient's liver, bone marrow, and endothelium, prior to any illness or trauma. The mortality of DIC is quite high, especially in acute cases; some studies have shown it to be 75%. The primary causes of death relate to uncontrolled bleeding, hypotension, and shock.

Haemophilia

Haemophilia is a bleeding disorder in which clotting does not occur or occurs insufficiently (von Willebrand disease). It is usually associated with an X-linked recessive inheritance pattern, albeit one that is poorly understood. The disease is classified into two primary types: type A, which is due to low levels of factor VIII (antihaemophilic globulin and antihaemophilic factor), and type B, which is associated with a deficiency of factor IX (plasma thromboplastin component, also known as the Christmas factor). This disease is primarily found in the male population. The levels of factors VIII and IX determine the severity of the disease.

Both type A and type B have the same signs and symptoms. Acute and chronic bleeding can occur at any time and may or may not be life-threatening. Any injury or illness that can cause bleeding should not be taken lightly in a person with haemophilia. Spontaneous intracranial bleeding is common in haemophilia and is a major cause of death. Patients with significant acute bleeding episodes require hospitalisation for transfusion and often require infusion of factors VIII and IX. If a patient has just had or needs surgery, these factors should be at 100% at the beginning of the procedure and should be maintained to a level up to 50% for several weeks thereafter.

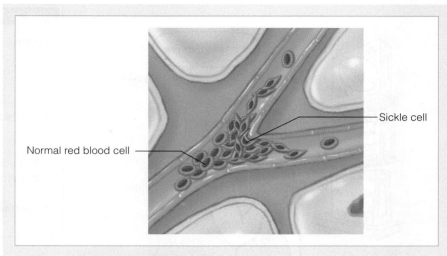

Figure 34-6 Normal RBCs and sickle cells.

At the Scene

Very often patients who have specialist diseases/disorders will know a lot more than you about their care. Work in collaboration with the patient to effect a care package.

Sickle Cell Disease

Sickle cell disease is—by far—the leading inherited blood disorder. Although it primarily affects African, Puerto Rican, and European populations, it can occur in anyone. In the United Kingdom, it is estimated that there are over 6,000 adults and children with sickle cell disease. The numbers are much greater in Africa, where in Nigeria alone it is estimated that 45,000 to 90,000 babies are born with the disease each year. Also, 30% of all newborns in Africa will carry the sickle cell trait, which means they can pass the disease on to future generations, ensuring its continuation. Mortality at younger ages is common, with the average life expectancy being 45 years in men and women. In general, women tend to live slightly longer than men with this disease.

Sickle cell disease starts with a gene defect of the adult-type haemoglobin (HbA). This mutation can be inherited from both parents (HbSS) or one parent (HbS). When the gene is inherited from both parents, there is a high probability the patient will be prone to sickle cells (that is, the person actually has the disease) or the sickle cell trait (the person is a carrier of the mutation). The defective RBCs are misshapen; affected cells have an oblong shape instead of a smooth, round shape 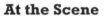. This shape makes the RBC a poor oxygen carrier, which means a patient with this disease is highly susceptible to hypoxia. The odd shape may also cause RBCs to lodge in small blood vessels (thrombotic crisis) or in the spleen, causing the organ to swell and rupture, which can lead to death. Sickle cell disease may also lead to aplastic crises, in which RBC production temporarily stops, or to haemolytic crises, in which the RBCs break down quickly.

In acute crises, patients may have significant pain, which will require aggressive pain management. They may experience frequent infections, which can lead to sepsis and death. Patients may often have signs of mild dehydration and many other complaints.

Multiple Myeloma

In multiple myeloma, abnormal plasma cells infiltrate the bone marrow. These neoplastic (tumour) cells essentially become malignant, allowing tumours to form inside the bones. Neoplastic cells may also accelerate protein development within the bloodstream, leading to organ failure (primarily the kidneys) and eventually death. This disease rarely occurs early in life—most patients are aged above 40 years. Men tend to have this disease more frequently than women.

The mere presence of these malignant cells does not mean a patient has a terminal condition, but patients may be at risk for the development of such a condition. As the disease progresses further and tumours grow or become more numerous, patients may have weakness in the bones, resulting in spontaneous fractures. In advanced cases of myeloma, chemotherapy and other anticancer type treatment may be given but may not cure the disease. Morbidity and mortality primarily depend on the extent of the disease in the patient and any underlying medical conditions.

General Assessment and Management

Assessment of a patient suspected of having a haematological disorder should be no different from assessment of any other patient, albeit with a few additional items to consider and questions to ask. During your initial assessment, note any signs and symptoms that may be immediately life-threatening. When

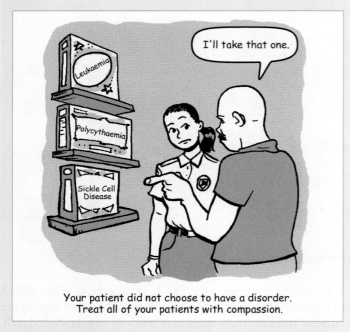

I'll take that one.

Leukaemia

Polycythaemia

Sickle Cell Disease

Your patient did not choose to have a disorder. Treat all of your patients with compassion.

Figure 34-7

Table 34-3	Common Findings With Blood Disorders
System	**Common Findings**
Skin	Uncontrolled bleeding, unexplained or chronic bruising, itching, pallor or jaundice (yellow appearance usually indicates liver problems)
Gastrointestinal	Epistaxis (nose bleed), bleeding or infected gums, ulcers, melaena (blood in the stool), and liver failure (causes jaundice)
Skeletal	Chronic joint or bone pain or rigidity
Cardiovascular	Dyspnoea, tachycardia, chest pain, haemoptysis (coughing up blood)
Genitourinary	Haematuria, menorrhagia, chronic or recurring infections

performing the focused history and physical examination, it is extremely important to understand the chief complaint; to do so, you may need to be very inquisitive about the patient's history and SAMPLE history. Also, be very supportive of the patients and their families—some patients with a blood disorder may not be willing to disclose the condition because they may feel that they will be treated differently (Figure 34-7 ▲).

During the focused history and physical examination, look for changes in level of consciousness and symptoms such as vertigo, feelings of fatigue, or syncopal episodes. Does the patient have any complaints of dyspnoea, chest pain, changes in heart rate and rhythm, or coughing up of blood? Has the patient experienced visual disturbances, muscle pain, or stiffness? Skin changes such as colour changes, burning, or itching? Bleeding problems from the nose, gums, and ulcers? Any history of liver problems or pain for unknown reasons? Problems with the genitourinary system?

When treating a patient with a known or suspected blood disorder, you will need to perform a physical examination. In such cases, it will be extremely important to have a basic understanding of some of the common findings in blood disorders (Table 34-3 ▶).

General management for any patient with problems related to a blood disorder should include the following elements:

- **Oxygen.** The amount needed and how it is given (that is, bag-mask ventilation, nonrebreathing mask) depends on the severity of the patient's condition and respiratory status.
- **Fluids.** Initiate intravenous (IV) fluid replacement as indicated for the specific disorder or chief complaint.
- **Electrocardiogram (ECG).** Monitor and treat symptomatic disturbances as necessary.

- **Transport.** Transport to the closest, most appropriate hospital.
- **Pharmacology.** Pain management is often necessary, especially in the case of a sickle-cell crisis.
- **Psychological support.** Be supportive and communicate with the patient.

Assessment and Management of Anaemia

Your basic assessment should be the same for all patients, although you may want to ask some specific questions when anaemia is suspected. Most commonly, patients with anaemia will complain of feeling worn down, having no energy, or feeling as if they have overexerted themselves. Patients may also complain that they "can't catch their breath". Owing to the reduction of haemoglobin, some may develop anginal-type chest pain related to the reduction in oxygen availability to the heart muscle. Also common in anaemic patients are leucopenia (reduction in WBCs) and thrombocytopenia (reduction in platelets); both conditions can induce more frequent infections, fevers, cutaneous bleeding, and frequent nosebleeds.

In cases of anaemia, check and monitor the airway and the patient's breathing closely, administering high-flow oxygen when necessary. Check vital signs frequently. In cases of chest pain, apply a cardiac monitor and watch the rhythm closely. A 12-lead ECG may also be warranted to make sure the chest pain is not related to a new-onset myocardial infarction. Blood pressure management may also be needed, along with fluid replacement therapy. Monitor patients closely during fluid replacement—IV fluids do not contain RBCs or blood components, so they may induce unwanted or unexpected bleeding. Do not be surprised if you have to control significant nosebleeds in any patient with anaemia.

Allow the patient to rest in a comfortable position and transport him or her to the closest, most appropriate hospital. In most cases, a gentle, easy transport is appropriate. However, if the patient experiences an abrupt change in the level of consciousness, hypotension develops, or other significant perfusion inadequacies arise, consider rapid transport.

Assessment and Management of Leukaemia

How patients with leukaemia present depends on the stage of the leukaemia and the patient's current treatment. Patients typically complain of fatigue, headaches, or dyspnoea or have signs of neurological defects. During the detailed physical examination, fever, bone pain, and perspiration may be evident. Patients may complain of feeling full, soreness in the mid part of the chest, and unexplained bleeding. You should monitor all basic vital signs (blood pressure, pulse, respirations, and temperature) and the cardiac monitor. Do not be surprised if the vital signs indicate shock because the common signs of hypotension and tachycardia are often present.

Management includes providing airway support and oxygen therapy as appropriate. IV fluid therapy and analgesics for comfort may be needed as well. Patients typically need constant positive support because many have a negative outlook toward their condition. The patient's relatives may be quite concerned, especially when the patient is in the advanced stages of the disease; be supportive to them as well. In some cases, you may be called because the patient's condition has deteriorated and the family is uncertain about what to do. In such a scenario, your assessment may indicate normal findings for the patient. The patient or family may change their minds about transport or may have never truly wanted transport but rather professional insight and support. Discuss this situation with ambulance control, on-call clinical advice, the patient's general practitioner, or other named health professional as appropriate. Document all findings before leaving, and have a refusal and/or release form signed.

Few calls for patients with leukaemia require extreme measures or rapid transport, but be alert to rapid changes in the patient's condition. If you transport, be aware that the patient could go into arrest. Make sure you find out the patient's and family's wishes about what to do in this situation.

Assessment and Management of Lymphomas

Generally speaking, lymphomas require specialised levels of treatment involving some form of chemotherapy or radiation therapy. How well a patient responds to these treatments depends on the stage of disease and its classification. As a rule, lymphomas respond well to chemotherapy; in fact, aggressive lymphomas respond better than indolent ones. Even if an indolent lymphoma is not cured with chemotherapy, many patients may survive as long as 10 years.

When assessing patients with lymphoma, ask specific questions such as "What type of lymphoma (cancer) do you have"? and "What type of treatment are you receiving"? As you perform your assessment, you will usually note pallor. The airway will usually be patent and breathing adequate, although sometimes you may note some congestion in the lower lung fields. The patient may complain of being first hot and then cold or even both in different areas of the body. Signs of inadequate perfusion are common, including low blood pressure accompanied by an elevated heart rate. Abnormal ECG rhythms may also be evident.

Patients with lymphoma may be in constant extreme pain; therefore, if pain management is needed and available, it may

You are the Paramedic Part 3

As your colleague obtains IV access, applies 12 litres of oxygen by nonrebreathing mask, and readies the patient for transport, you perform a quick examination. When you ask the patient to point to the area of pain, he puts his hand over his left upper quadrant and says that he has vomited a few times this evening. He also mentions that he has had chills and feels like he cannot catch his breath. You note the presence of dullness when percussing the lowest intercostal space in the anterior axillary line on the left side. On gentle palpation and observation of the patient's face, you note that he has some tenderness in his left upper quadrant, and you can feel a portion of the spleen.

Your partner inserts an 18-gauge IV cannula in the left antecubital vein and begins to administer a 250 ml bolus of normal saline.

Reassessment	Recording Time: 10 Minutes
Level of consciousness	Alert, with a Glasgow Coma Scale score of 15
Skin	Perspiring and feverish with pale mucous membranes
Pulse	Radial pulse, 116 beats/min, weak and regular
Blood pressure	108/44 mm Hg
Respirations	20 breaths/min and shallow
SpO_2	95%
Blood glucose level	4.3 mmol/l
ECG	Sinus tachycardia without ectopics

5. What, if anything, is abnormal about your physical assessment findings?
6. Given your assessment, what do you think are potential sources of the patient's complaints?

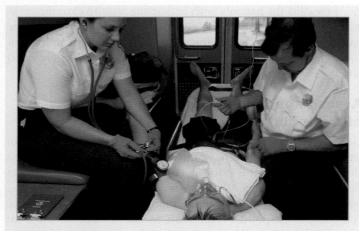

Figure 34-8 Patients with lymphoma who are in extreme pain should receive fluid therapy, oxygen, and analgesics.

have to be aggressive. Treat inadequate perfusion with fluid therapy, and provide supplemental oxygen Figure 34-8 ▲ . If necessary, treat abnormal heart rhythms. If the patient's condition does not improve or even deteriorates following these measures, initiate rapid transport to the closest hospital. As with leukaemia, you may be called to offer support but no transport. Be supportive, discuss your findings with ambulance control, on-call clinical advice, the patient's general practitioner, or other named health professional as appropriate. Explain the options to the patient and family, and allow them to make a decision.

Assessment and Management of Polycythaemia

Owing to the nature of polycythaemia and its plethora of symptoms, your assessment findings may vary widely. Altered levels of consciousness may be evident due to stroke or transient ischaemic attack-like events or hypoxia secondary to poor circulation from lesions within the circulatory system. Respiratory distress is common, as are changes in peripheral pulses, heart rate, and skin colour. Tachycardia is the most common change in heart rhythm. Patients also tend to have purplish skin with red hands and feet.

As you assess the patient, note the extent and duration of dyspnoea. Has the patient experienced uncontrolled itching (pruritus) or noted changes in skin temperature? Make sure to obtain a thorough medical history in cases of known or suspected polycythaemia.

Prehospital care largely consists of supportive care and transporting the patient to an appropriate hospital. Administer oxygen as needed. Establish IV access for possible pharmacological interventions for pain or heart rate control as appropriate. Be supportive to the patient and family.

Assessment and Management of DIC

As you assess and care for critically injured or ill patients, keep in mind the issues that may lead to DIC. Your goal is to identify signs and symptoms commonly associated with DIC or progression toward it. In cases involving severe trauma, patients may have episodes of respiratory difficulty, signs of shock, and skin changes, ranging from cold and clammy to pallor to small black-and-blue marks (purpura) on the chest and abdomen.

It is important to identify the cause underlying the patient's presenting condition and establish treatment early, while not delaying transport to an appropriate hospital. Maintain an airway, administer supplemental oxygen, and treat the patient for shock (keep the patient warm, control bleeding, administer IV fluids for hypotension) as per local protocol. Pharmacological interventions may entail pain management and treatment for abnormal heart rhythms, although treatment for altered heart rhythms should come last. Patients who have DIC due to severe trauma have a poor survival rate; they and family members need strong support. Be optimistic but honest with patients and family, and don't give false impressions regarding survival.

At the Scene

Patients with DIC have a failure of multiple organs (kidneys, lungs, heart) at once, accompanied by bleeding from IV sites, bleeding into joints, and, possibly, intracranial haemorrhage.

Assessment and Management of Haemophilia

When taking the patient's history, you may discover previous or current haemophilia conditions. In addition to taking care of the ABCs, be alert for signs of acute blood loss (pallor, weak pulse, and hypotension). Note any bleeding of unknown origin, such as nosebleeds, bloody sputum, and blood in the urine or stool (melaena). Owing to blood loss, patients may exhibit signs of hypoxia due to the reduction in oxygen-carrying capacity; as a consequence, any patient who complains of respiratory problems should receive high-flow oxygen.

Note ECG findings, and treat symptomatic arrhythmias as appropriate. IV fluid therapy may be necessary in cases of unstable hypotension, but understand that the patient actually needs a transfusion or plasma. Some patients will have significant pain, so analgesics may be appropriate. Although you may be called to treat someone with bleeding of unknown cause only to find that the bleeding stopped before you arrive on scene, you should suggest that the patient get immediate hospital or medical follow-up.

Assessment and Management of Sickle Cell Disease

Do not take a call for a person having a sickle cell crisis lightly. Patients are often in life-threatening situations, characterised by shortness of breath and signs of pneumonia. Their skin will show signs of inadequate perfusion, accompanied by hypotension. They may show signs of jaundice and yellowing in the eye (icteric sclera). High levels of oxygen are recommended to prevent further destruction of the RBCs due to hypoxia. Patients may complain of multiple system involvement, including chest, abdominal, and arthritic-type pain, although some may report only fatigue or achiness along with fever.

Besides providing oxygen therapy and rapid transport to an appropriate hospital, you may need to give IV fluid therapy to counter the patient's dehydration. Remember that patients may have lived with the disease for a long time and, thus, may have a very high pain threshold. As a consequence, they often require a higher level of analgesia.

At the Scene

Sickle cell disease may mimic appendicitis or opiate withdrawal.

Assessment and Management of Multiple Myeloma

Findings during your assessment and management of multiple myeloma depend on the patient's stage of disease. Early-stage complaints may be as simple as fatigue or mild pain. Later-stage disease may be evidenced by unexplained haemorrhage and significant weight loss, frequent bone fractures, and an increase of pain in any number of locations.

Management is similar to that for other blood disorders: IV fluid therapy, pain management, and supportive care. Do not assume that the patient is ready to or is going to die; he or she may just be having a complication of the myeloma. On receiving definitive care at an appropriate hospital, the patient's condition may improve.

You are the Paramedic Part 4

You gently transport the patient to the nearest hospital and continue to monitor his condition en route. Although he reports that his feeling of shortness of breath has decreased, he continues to have abnormal skin signs. When you give your report to the A&E department nurse, she indicates that she is familiar with this patient because he has had periodic exacerbations of sickle cell anaemia. One such incident required multiple blood transfusions secondary to an aplastic crisis.

Reassessment	Recording Time: 20 Minutes
Level of consciousness	Alert, with a Glasgow Coma Scale score of 15
Skin	Perspiring and warm with improved colour of mucous membranes
Pulse	Radial pulse, 98 beats/min, weak and regular
Blood pressure	116/50 mm Hg
Respirations	20 breaths/min
SpO$_2$	98%
Temperature	38ºC
ECG	Sinus rhythm without ectopics

7. Should this patient receive analgesics? Why or why not?
8. Would this call change if the patient had the same or similar signs and symptoms in the presence of trauma?

You are the Paramedic Summary

1. What, if anything, about his appearance gives you cause for concern?

The patient is showing signs of hypoperfusion. He is sweaty, his breathing is laboured, and his facial expression and body position suggest that he is experiencing moderate to severe abdominal pain.

2. What information do you already have at your disposal?

The patient has a medical history that has significantly affected him in the past and could be related to his chief complaint. It is important to absorb all possible information provided by the patient. Information from family, friends, and bystanders may also be helpful.

3. What complications are common with sickle cell anaemia?

Patients struggle with oxygenation and tissue perfusion. They are at high risk for hypoxia owing to the decreased ability for the misshapen red blood cells (RBC) to carry oxygen. They are also at risk for blood clots. They may experience cessation of RBC production and/or RBC breakdown.

4. What are your treatment priorities given your understanding of patients with sickle cell anaemia?

Recognise the potential seriousness of the patient's condition by conducting an appropriate physical examination and history taking, administer high-flow oxygen and IV fluids (as needed), and provide prompt transport to the nearest appropriate facility.

5. What, if anything, is abnormal about your physical assessment findings?

Physical findings point to splenic enlargement or splenomegaly. The spleen can become enlarged for many reasons, including viral, bacterial, and parasitic infections; cancer; and haemolytic anaemias. Because patients with sickle cell anaemia are at greater risk for splenic sequestration (enlargement of the spleen as a result of the trapping of RBCs), if enlargement of the spleen is noted, the patient must be transported quickly and the receiving facility notified immediately.

6. Given your assessment, what do you think are potential source of the patient's complaints?

His abdominal pain could be the result of splenic crisis or his enlarged spleen could be the result of an infection (especially in the presence of fever). No matter what its underlying cause, the patient's condition should be treated as very serious with prompt transport and frequent reassessments for changes in the patient's condition.

7. Should this patient receive analgesics? Why or why not?

Pain management is an essential part of patient care. When dealing with abdominal pain in the prehospital setting, some doctors may not want you to administer medications such as morphine because it can mask the source of pain. In these situations, make every attempt to consult with the receiving hospital before administration of analgesics. If it has been determined that analgesics are inappropriate, make every attempt to address the patient's pain through body position and gentle handling and transport.

8. Would this call change if the patient had the same or similar signs and symptoms in the presence of trauma?

An enlarged spleen with the added history of trauma can equate to a fatal patient outcome. What makes this case even more serious is the RBCs' decreased ability to provide oxygen to the patient's tissues and organs. Bleeding, especially at the volume seen in splenic rupture, is an especially life-threatening situation for a patient with sickle cell anaemia.

Prep Kit

Ready for Review

- Most ambulance services rarely respond to haematological emergencies.
- Blood performs respiratory, nutritional, excretory, regulatory, and defensive functions.
- Blood disorders include anaemia, iron deficiency anaemia, haematological disorders, leukaemias, lymphomas, polycythaemia, DIC, haemophilia, sickle cell disease, and multiple myeloma.
- During the initial assessment of a patient with a haematological disorder, note any signs and symptoms that may be immediately life threatening.
- During the focused history and physical examination, look for changes in level of consciousness such as vertigo, feelings of fatigue, or syncopal episodes.
- General management for any patient with problems related to a blood disorder should include the following elements: oxygen, fluids, ECG, transport, pharmacology, and psychological support.

Vital Vocabulary

ABO system The antigen classification given to blood.

anaemia A lower than normal haemoglobin or erythrocyte level.

antibodies Molecules in the body that react against foreign antigens in the body.

antigens Substances (usually protein) identified as foreign to the body.

autoimmune disorders Disorders in which the body identifies its own antigen as a foreign body and activates the inflammatory system.

clotting factors Substances in the blood that are necessary for clotting; also called coagulation factors.

coagulation Clotting.

disseminated intravascular coagulopathy (DIC) A life-threatening condition commonly found in severe trauma.

erythrocytes Red blood cells.

fibrin A white, insoluble protein formed in the clotting process.

fibrinolytic system The mechanism by which fibrin undergoes dissolution owing to the action of enzymes; clots are destroyed.

haematocrit The percentage of RBCs in total blood volume.

haematopoietic system The system that includes all blood components and the organs involved in their development and production.

haemoglobin The iron-rich protein in the blood that carries oxygen.

haemolytic disorder A disorder relating to the breakdown of RBCs.

haemophilia A bleeding disorder that is primarily hereditary, in which clotting does not occur or occurs insufficiently.

homeostasis The maintenance of constant balance in the body.

homeostatic mechanism The mechanism involving many parts of the body that maintain homeostasis.

iron deficiency anaemia The most common type of anaemia in which iron stores are low or lacking and the serum iron concentration is low.

leucocytes White blood cells.

leucopenia Reduction in the number of WBCs.

leukaemia Cancer or malignancy of the blood-forming organs, particularly affecting the WBCs that develop abnormally and/or excessively at the expense of normal blood cells.

lymphoblasts Lymphocytes transformed because of stimulation by an antigen.

lymphoid system The system primarily made up of the bone marrow, lymph nodes, and spleen that participates in formation of lymphocytes and immune responses.

lymphomas Malignant diseases that arise within the lymphoid system; includes non-Hodgkin's and Hodgkin's lymphomas.

melaena Blood in the stool.

multiple myeloma A disease in which an abnormal plasma cell infiltrates the bone marrow with a cancerous (neoplastic) cell, causing tumours to form inside the bones.

neoplastic cells Another term for cancerous cells.

petechiae Tiny purple or red spots that appear on the skin due to bleeding within the skin or under mucous membranes.

phlebotomy Making an incision into a vein to remove blood.

plasma A component of blood, made of 92% water, 6% to 7% proteins, and electrolytes, clotting factors, and glucose; this makes up 55% of the total blood volume.

polycythaemia An overabundance or production of RBCs, WBCs, and platelets.

pruritus Unspecified itching.

reticuloendothelial system The system in the body that is primarily used to defend against infection.

sickle cell disease A disease that causes the RBCs to be misshapen, resulting in poor oxygen-carrying capability and potentially resulting in lodging of the RBCs in blood vessels or the spleen.

specific gravity The weight of a substance compared with water.

stem cells Cells that can develop into other types of cells in the body.

thalassaemia A type of anaemia in which not enough haemoglobin is produced, or the haemoglobin is defective.

thrombin An enzyme that causes the conversion of fibrinogen to fibrin, which binds to the platelet plugs, forming the final mature blood clot.

thrombocytes Platelets.

thrombocytopenia Reduction in the number of platelets.

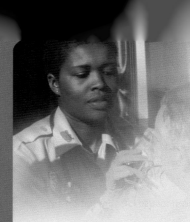

Assessment in Action

You are dispatched for a "sick person". When you arrive on scene, you find a 32-year-old woman lying supine on her sofa. She called 999 because she has not been feeling right for about 1 week and just can't move today. During your assessment, you note that she is very pale; her skin is warm and dry. Her vital signs seem to be within normal limits. The patient says that she is tired all the time and has lost approximately 9 kg during the past 3 to 4 weeks. She denies any chance of pregnancy but reports that her menstrual cycles have been heavier. She denies any medical history of disease and tells you that she takes a daily vitamin and an iron supplement.

You place the patient on high-flow oxygen and as a precaution, place a cannula in the dorsum of her left hand. En route, you manage to find out from her that she previously has been admitted with anaemia.

1. **What is anaemia?**
   A. Reduction below the normal levels of RBCs, as shown by a decreased haemoglobin or haematocrit level
   B. A malignant tumour of blood-forming tissue
   C. Overproduction of RBCs and platelets
   D. A malignant tumour of lymphatic tissues

2. **What is the name of the body system that produces blood cells?**
   A. Circulatory system
   B. Respiratory system
   C. Haematopoietic system
   D. Hepatic system

3. **What are the blood-forming organs in an adult?**
   A. The liver and spleen
   B. Bone marrow
   C. Myocardium
   D. Lungs

4. **What is the normal life cycle of an RBC?**
   A. 1 month
   B. 3 months
   C. 4 months
   D. 1 year

5. **Haematocrit (Hct) is:**
   A. an iron-rich compound responsible for carrying oxygen to the tissues.
   B. a measure of RBCs per unit of blood volume.
   C. the pulse oximetry reading.
   D. the number of leucocytes per unit of blood volume.

6. **Haemoglobin (Hb) is:**
   A. an iron-rich compound responsible for carrying oxygen to the tissues.
   B. a measure of RBCs per unit of blood volume.
   C. the pulse oximetry reading.
   D. the number of leucocytes per unit of blood volume.

7. **Cells that can develop into other types of cells in the body are:**
   A. stem cells.
   B. erythrocytes.
   C. fibrin.
   D. plasma.

8. **_____ are the smallest of the formed elements and are responsible for the clotting of the blood.**
   A. Leucocytes
   B. Erythrocytes
   C. Platelets
   D. Stem cells

9. **Blood transports oxygen from the lungs to the tissues and carbon dioxide from the tissues to the lungs. This is the_____ function.**
   A. respiratory
   B. nutritional
   C. excretory
   D. regulatory

10. **Blood carries glucose, proteins, and fats from the digestive tract to cells through the body. This is the_____ function.**
    A. respiratory
    B. nutritional
    C. excretory
    D. regulatory

11. **Blood transports the waste products of metabolism from the cells where they are produced to excretory organs. This is the _____ function.**
    A. respiratory
    B. nutritional
    C. excretory
    D. regulatory

12. **Blood brings hormones to their target organs and transmits excess internal heat to the surface of the body to be dissipated. This is the _____ function.**
    A. respiratory
    B. defensive
    C. excretory
    D. regulatory

13. **Blood carries defensive cells and antibodies that protect the body against foreign organisms. This is the _____ function.**
    A. respiratory
    B. defensive
    C. excretory
    D. regulatory

Challenging Question

You are dispatched to the local shopping centre for someone who has fallen. On arrival, you find a 42-year-old man sitting at the base of the steps. According to witnesses, he tripped up the steps, lost his balance, and then fell down four steps. He is alert to his name but is confused about what happened. The patient complains of pain to his left axillary area and his left knee. During your assessment, you find him to be tachycardic, tachypnoeic, and grossly perspiring. His blood pressure is 70/30 mm Hg, pulse rate is 118 beats/min, and respiratory rate is 30 breaths/min. While you and your colleague are providing the patient with full cervical-spine precautions, you note a bruise on his left flank area. You provide the patient with 100% supplemental oxygen via a nonrebreathing mask and take him to the ambulance for transport to the A&E department.

During your focused examination, you note a medical ID tag that reads "Haemophilia A". You initiate IV fluid therapy and provide a fluid bolus. The patient is transported to the hospital without any further incident. You give a report to the A&E department nurse and doctor. You overhear the doctor order "factor VIII" from the pharmacy.

14. **What is your primary care in the prehospital environment for a patient with haemophilia?**

15. **What would your primary care be for any patient with a haematopoietic problem?**

Points to Ponder

You respond to a private house, where you find a 28-year-old African-Caribbean woman lying in bed. She complains of pain in her chest with associated shortness of breath. You note swelling of her hands and feet. The patient says that she has had the flu for the past 2 days and has vomited at least four times. She has also had a low-grade fever and generalised body aches. Your physical examination reveals nothing truly remarkable. The patient has a history of high blood pressure and sickle cell disease.

What is happening with this patient physiologically? What, if any, treatment should you administer?

Issues: Understand the Urgency for Assessment and Intervention in Patients With Haematological Crises.

35 Environmental Emergencies

Objectives

Cognitive

- Define "environmental emergency".
- Describe the incidence, morbidity and mortality associated with environmental emergencies.
- Identify risk factors most predisposing to environmental emergencies.
- Identify environmental factors that may cause illness or exacerbate a pre-existing illness.
- Identify environmental factors that may complicate treatment or transport decisions.
- List the principle types of environmental illnesses.
- Define "homeostasis" and relate the concept to environmental influences.
- Identify normal, critically high, and critically low body temperatures.
- Describe several methods of temperature monitoring.
- Identify the components of the body's thermoregulatory mechanism.
- Describe the general process of thermal regulation, including substances used and wastes generated.
- Describe the body's compensatory process for over heating.
- Describe the body's compensatory process for excess heat loss.
- List the common forms of heat and cold disorders.
- List the common predisposing factors associated with heat and cold disorders.
- List the common preventative measures associated with heat and cold disorders.
- Integrate the pathophysiological principles and complicating factors common to environmental emergencies and discuss differentiating features between emergent and urgent presentations.
- Define heat illness.
- Describe the pathophysiology of heat illness.
- Identify signs and symptoms of heat illness.
- List the predisposing factors for heat illness.
- List measures to prevent heat illness.
- Discuss the symptomatic variations presented in progressive heat disorders.
- Relate symptomatic findings to the commonly used terms: heat cramps, heat exhaustion, and heatstroke.
- Correlate the abnormal findings in assessment with their clinical significance in the patient with heat illness.
- Describe the contribution of dehydration to the development of heat disorders.

- Describe the differences between classical and exertional heatstroke.
- Define fever and discuss its pathophysiological mechanism.
- Identify the fundamental thermoregulatory difference between fever and heatstroke.
- Discuss how one may differentiate between fever and heatstroke.
- Discuss the role of fluid therapy in the treatment of heat disorders.
- Differentiate among the various treatments and interventions in the management of heat disorders.
- Integrate the pathophysiological principles and the assessment findings to formulate an initial diagnosis and implement a treatment plan for the patient who has dehydration, heat exhaustion, or heatstroke.
- Define hypothermia.
- Describe the pathophysiology of hypothermia.
- List predisposing factors for hypothermia.
- List measures to prevent hypothermia.
- Identify differences between mild and severe hypothermia.
- Describe differences between chronic and acute hypothermia.
- List signs and symptoms of hypothermia.
- Correlate abnormal findings in assessment with their clinical significance in the patient with hypothermia.
- Discuss the impact of severe hypothermia on standard BCLS and ACLS algorithms and transport considerations.
- Integrate pathophysiological principles and the assessment findings to formulate an initial diagnosis and implement a treatment plan for the patient who has either mild or severe hypothermia.
- Define frostbite.
- Define superficial frostbite (frostnip).
- Differentiate between superficial frostbite and deep frostbite.
- List predisposing factors for frostbite.
- List measures to prevent frostbite.
- Correlate abnormal findings in assessment with their clinical significance in the patient with frostbite.
- Differentiate among the various treatments and interventions in the management of frostbite.
- Integrate pathophysiological principles and the assessment findings to formulate an initial diagnosis and implement a treatment plan for the patient with superficial or deep frostbite.
- Define drowning.
- Describe the pathophysiology of drowning.
- List signs and symptoms of drowning.
- Describe the lack of significance of fresh versus saltwater immersion, as it relates to drowning.

- Discuss the incidence of "wet" versus "dry" drownings and the differences in their management.
- Discuss the complications and protective role of hypothermia in the context of drowning.
- Correlate the abnormal findings in assessment with the clinical significance in the patient with drowning.
- Differentiate among the various treatments and interventions in the management of drowning.
- Integrate pathophysiological principles and assessment findings to formulate an initial diagnosis and implement a treatment plan for the drowning patient.
- Integrate the pathophysiological principles of the patient affected by an environmental emergency.
- Differentiate between environmental emergencies based on assessment findings.

- Correlate abnormal findings in the assessment with their clinical significance in the patient affected by an environmental emergency.
- Develop a patient management plan based on the initial diagnosis of the patient affected by an environmental emergency.

Affective

None

Psychomotor

None

Introduction

Environmental emergencies are medical conditions caused or worsened by the weather, terrain, or unique atmospheric conditions such as high altitude or underwater. Most ambulance service personnel would recognise the obvious problem of a child who has fallen into an icy lake. The challenge lies in recognising patients with environmental emergencies in the unusual settings of endurance sports events or at mass gatherings, and even acutely confused older patients (Figure 35-1 ▾).

Unique to environmental emergencies are the conditions that directly cause harm or complicate treatment and transport considerations. Wind, rain, snow, temperature extremes, and humidity may all affect the body's ability to adapt to its environment. Unprepared hill walkers can experience cold illnesses during summer rainstorms as easily as overdressed snow sports enthusiasts can die of heat illnesses during strenuous outings. The locations of these outings can also have a huge impact on the ability to know about, respond to, and rescue people in remote settings (Figure 35-2 ▾).

Certain generic risk factors predispose people to environmental emergencies. In addition, very young and old people have unique disadvantages when it comes to thermoregulation. Conditions such as diabetes, cardiac disease (for example, coronary artery disease, congestive heart failure), restrictive lung disease, thyroid disease, and psychiatric illnesses can alter

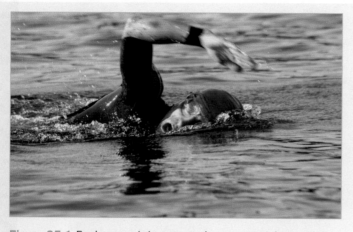

Figure 35-1 Environmental emergencies can occur in a variety of settings, including endurance sports events.

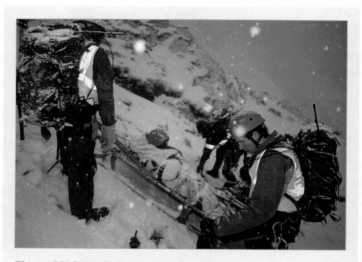

Figure 35-2 Medical attention may be needed in some extreme environments.

You are the Paramedic Part 1

You and your colleague are called to the public library because of a man "acting strangely". You notice that the spring day has turned much cooler as you respond and begin to consider why someone would be acting strangely at the library.

When you arrive, you run through the downpour and wind to the entrance. You recognise one of the police officers. She tells you, "I think he's just drunk", and notes that she arrested the man a month ago after a pub disturbance. After you confirm that the police officer has checked the man for weapons, you ask the bystander who has given up his coat to the patient if he knows what is going on. He reports that the patient was standing outside trying to remove his shirt and trousers. The patient told him that he was "too hot".

Initial Assessment	Recording Time: 0 Minutes
Appearance	Eyes open, no obvious distress
Level of consciousness	V (Responsive to verbal stimuli); slurs words
Airway	Open; odour of alcohol on breath
Breathing	Adequate rate and tidal volume
Circulation	Radial pulse present; cold hands

1. What are three things that could medically harm this man in the next hour?
2. Do you believe the scene to be adequately secured?
3. Where do you believe is the best place to assess the patient properly?

the body's ability to compensate for environmental extremes. Finally, the patient's overall health and fitness status and ability to acclimatise (that is, adjust to the new environment) can mean the difference between life and death.

This chapter first describes the techniques that the healthy body uses to respond to changes in temperature. It then assesses factors that can interfere with the body's ability to shed or gain heat, thereby increasing a person's risk of experiencing an environmental emergency. Next, it examines the pathophysiology, recognition, and treatment of environmental illnesses. Finally, the chapter considers preventive measures for environmental illnesses.

Homeostasis and Body Temperature

Homeostasis refers to body processes that balance the supply and demand of the body's needs. Ensuring the balance between heat production and heat excretion (thermoregulation) is the job of thermosensitive neurons in the anterior hypothalamus. Like a car thermostat, the hypothalamus—the "master thermostat" in the brain—operates according to the principle of negative feedback control: A rise in core body temperature elicits responses that increase heat loss and shut off normal heat production pathways (thermogenesis); a fall in core body temperature prompts heat production and conservation and turns off normal heat-liberating pathways (thermolysis) **Figure 35-3 ▾** .

At the Scene

Do not become a victim yourself. Dress for the weather.

The human body stubbornly defends a constant core temperature of approximately 37°C that represents a balance between the heat produced or absorbed by the body and the heat eliminated to the outside. At this temperature, the metabolic reactions of the body proceed at their optimal level. Temperatures in the core (the brain and thoracoabdominal organs) remain relatively constant. The temperature of the periphery (the skin) can fluctuate a great deal, so this part of the body has a major role in thermoregulation. The lowest body temperature at which human survival of accidental hypothermia has been reported is 9°C. More generally, hypothermia is defined as a body temperature starting at 35°C and heat stroke at 40°C.

In the prehospital setting, the oral temperature is commonly used and is a suitable measurement for general medical conditions such as suspected pneumonia. It can vary dramatically from the core temperature if the patient has been mouth breathing or drinking hot or cold liquids. The axillary temperature, taken in the armpit, can be as much as 17°C cooler than the oral temperature. Tactile temperatures taken by parents are remarkably accurate but only in terms of knowing whether a child has a fever, not in determining the actual temperature. In environmental situations, the most accurate means of determining core temperatures is to use a rectal thermometer capable of measuring extremes of temperatures **Figure 35-4 ▶** . Tympanic temperatures, which are taken with a device that measures the heat reflected off the eardrum, also provide accurate core measurements.

Thermoregulatory Mechanisms

The body's main thermoregulatory centre is located in specialised tissue found in the hypothalamus. The thermogenic (heat-generating) tissues in the hypothalamus are mediated by the sympathetic nervous system; the thermolytic (heat-liberating) tissues are mediated by the parasympathetic nervous system. The hypothalamus receives signals from peripheral receptors (located primarily in the skin and muscles) and central receptors (triggered by changes in blood temperature; located in the core).

At rest, the body produces heat chiefly by the metabolism of nutrients (carbohydrates, fats, and rarely proteins), with the subsequent liberation of primarily water and carbon dioxide. Liver and skeletal muscles are the major contributors to the basal metabolic rate (BMR), the heat energy produced at rest from normal body metabolic

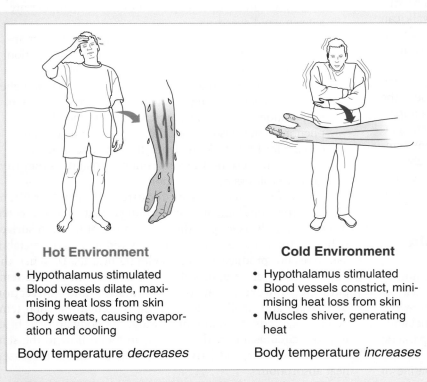

Hot Environment

- Hypothalamus stimulated
- Blood vessels dilate, maximising heat loss from skin
- Body sweats, causing evaporation and cooling

Body temperature *decreases*

Cold Environment

- Hypothalamus stimulated
- Blood vessels constrict, minimising heat loss from skin
- Muscles shiver, generating heat

Body temperature *increases*

Figure 35-3 Like a car thermostat, the hypothalamus notes a rise or fall in core body temperature and elicits responses to regulate it.

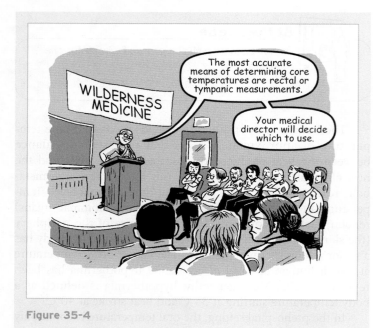

Figure 35-4

reactions. The BMR can be thought of as the minimal caloric energy requirement to sit on the couch all day! The BMR of the average 70-kg adult is in the range of 60 to 70 kilocalories per hour. Many factors affect this rate, including age, sex, stress, and hormones. The most important factor, however, is body surface area. As the ratio of body surface area to body volume increases, heat loss to the environment increases. Thus, when two people have the same weight, the shorter person will have a higher BMR.

Exertion also affects the metabolic rate. A brisk walk can produce heat totaling 300 kcal/h, for example. The recommended daily caloric intake is 2,000 to 2,500 kcal (a food "calorie" is actually a kilocalorie).

Some of the heat generated by metabolism and glycogen breakdown for muscular work is used to warm the body; the excess is excreted, ordinarily by taking advantage of the temperature gradient between the body and the outside environment. If the environmental temperature is higher than the body temperature, there is a third potential source of body heat: absorption of heat from the outside. Standing in bright sunshine on a hot, breezeless day, for example, can add up to 150 kcal/h to the internal heat load.

Physiological Responses to Heat and Cold
Thermolysis

The body reacts to its daily production of heat energy and to hot environmental conditions in much the same way—thermolysis, the release of stored heat and energy from the body. An increase in core temperature causes the hypothalamus to send signals via efferent pathways in the parasympathetic nervous system, causing vasodilatation and sweating.

Because of cutaneous vasodilation, the effective volume of the vascular system is increased (when the diameter of a tube, such as an artery, is increased, its volume increases); the heart must increase its output to compensate for this effect. Heart

rate and stroke volume increase, but the work of the heart is markedly increased. If vasodilation increases dramatically, the person may have a complete loss of vasomotor control (that is, the ability of the arteries to constrict in response to sympathetic stimulation). In that case, blood pools in the periphery, and the patient could experience neurogenic shock.

When warmed blood from the core and overheated muscles heads for the peripherally dilated cutaneous vessels, it may be cooled in four major ways (in addition to behavioural changes, such as slowing down or seeking shade):

- **Radiation**, the transfer of heat via electromagnetic waves, accounts for more than 65% of heat loss in a cooler setting. Heat loss through the head is especially notable. If the ambient temperature is high (20°C or greater), body heat will be gained.
- **Conduction** is the transfer of heat from a hotter object to a cooler object by direct physical contact. Air is a poor conductor of heat (only 2% of body heat is lost to it), whereas the ground is a good conductor. Water is the best conductor. A person who falls into a cold lake will lose heat 25 times faster than a dry person exposed to air of the same temperature. Clothing soaked with rain, snow, or perspiration can be just as dangerous.
- **Convection** refers to the loss of heat that takes place when moving air picks up heat and carries it away. A person instinctively uses this principle when blowing on hot food to cool it. Likewise, air moving across the body surface can pick up heat and carry it away. The faster the air is moving, the faster it can remove heat from the body. The windchill factor measures the chilling effect of a given temperature at a given wind speed.
- **Evaporation**, the conversion of a liquid to a gas, liberates 1 kcal per 1.7 ml of sweat. Sweating and heat dissipation by evaporation normally account for about 30% of cooling. Evaporation is the main mode of cooling in higher temperatures until a high humidity level slows the rate of evaporation. It has a minor role via respiration. This phenomenon is also behind the evaporative method of cooling for heat stroke patients. In cold conditions, wet clothes can cause heat loss by conduction and, as they dry, further heat loss by evaporation.

These four mechanisms require a thermal gradient between the body and its surroundings; that is, the mechanisms work only as long as the temperature of the skin surface is higher than that of the outside environment (and metabolism does not produce an overwhelming heat load). When the outside temperature approaches or exceeds skin surface temperature, however, heat loss by radiation and convection diminishes and finally ceases. When the environmental temperature exceeds the skin temperature, the body absorbs heat. In those circumstances, the increase in blood flow to the skin becomes counterproductive because it promotes increased heat absorption.

The only way the body can dissipate heat when the ambient temperature approaches body temperature is by the evaporation of sweat, up to a point. A healthy adult can sweat a maximum of about 1 l/h but cannot maintain that rate for more than a few hours at a time. Furthermore, for effective evaporation of sweat, the ambient air must be relatively unsaturated with water. As the relative humidity increases, the rate of evaporation decreases; effective sweat evaporation ceases when the relative humidity reaches about 75%.

Thermogenesis

In a cold environment, the skin serves as the body's thermostat. If your skin is cold, your body will shiver even if your core body temperature is not lowered. Thermogenesis, the production of heat and energy for the body, is the main method of dealing with cold stressors. In addition to normal heat production from the BMR and physical exertion, the sympathetic nervous system can increase muscle tone and initiate shivering in the short-term and increase thyroid levels in the long-term. The hypothalamus also stimulates peripheral vasoconstriction, thereby shunting blood to the core. Sweating decreases. The thicker the outer shell, the better the insulation. All other factors being equal, heavier people are more effectively insulated from the cold. This conservation of heat for the sake of the core continues until the body's ability to generate heat becomes overwhelmed, resulting in hypothermia.

▌Heat Illness

Heat illness is an increase in core body temperature (CBT) due to inadequate thermolysis. The fundamental problem is the inability to get rid of the heat buildup in the body, often because of hot and humid conditions. A person's general state of health, clothing, mobility, age, preexisting illnesses, and certain medications ⬤ Table 35-1 ▸ can add to the problem. When the thermoregulatory system is taxed beyond its limits or fails for any reason, the core body temperature soars, sometimes rising from normal to about 41°C in less than 15 minutes. That is the situation in heat stroke, for example.

Risk Factors for Heat Illness

Certain factors increase a person's risk for ill effects from any given heat stress; the factors are summarised in ⬤ Table 35-2 ▾ . Older people are at particular risk because they do not adjust as well to the heat: They perspire less; they acclimatise more slowly; they feel thirst less readily in response to dehydration; and decreased mobility may make getting a glass of water difficult. Older people are also more likely to have chronic conditions, such as diabetes and cardiovascular disease, that interfere with normal heat excretion. In addition, they are more likely to be taking medications that disrupt the body's mechanisms for dissipating heat. For example, diuretics taken for hypertension may result in an older person being dangerously close to dehydration and electrolyte disturbances and interfere with the peripheral vasodilation necessary for heat transfer. Beta blockers can lessen a tachycardic response to heat stress, as can normal age-related

Table 35-1	Medications Contributing to Heat Illness
■ Alcohol ■ Alpha agonists ■ Amphetamines ■ Anticholinergic medications (atropine sulphate, scopolamine, benzatropine mesylate, belladonna, and synthetic alkaloids) ■ Antihistamines ■ Antiparkinsonian agents ■ Antipsychotics (such as haloperidol) ■ Beta blockers ■ Calcium channel blockers ■ Cocaine ■ Diuretics (furosemide, hydrochlorothiazide, bumetanide) ■ Heroin	■ Laxatives ■ Lithium ■ Lysergic acid diethylamide (LSD) ■ Monoamine oxidase inhibitors ■ Phencyclidine hydrochloride ■ Phenothiazines (prochlorperazine, chlorpromazine, promethazine) ■ Sympathomimetic medicines (amphetamines, adrenaline, ephedrine, cocaine, noradrenaline) ■ Thyroid agonists (levothyroxine) ■ Tricyclic antidepressants (amitriptyline, imipramine, nortriptyline, protriptyline)

Table 35-2	Factors That Predispose to Heat Illness	
Factors That Increase Internal Heat Production		**Factors That Interfere With Heat Dissipation**
■ Physical exertion ■ Response to infection (fever) ■ Hyperthyroidism ■ Agitated and tremulous states (Parkinson, psychosis, mania, drug withdrawal—opiate and alcohol) ■ Drug overdoses (such as sympathomimetics, cocaine, caffeine, lysergic acid diethylamide, phencyclidine hydrochloride, methamphetamine, ecstasy)		■ High ambient temperature ■ High humidity ■ Obesity (insulation effect, less efficient dissipation) ■ Impaired vasodilatation ■ Diabetes ■ Alcoholism ■ Drugs: diuretics, tranquilisers, beta blockers, antihistamines, phenothiazines ■ Impaired ability to sweat (cystic fibrosis, skin diseases, healed burns) ■ Heavy or tight clothing
Factors That Increase Heat Absorption		**Factors That Impair the Body's Response to Heat Stress**
■ Confined, unventilated, hot living quarters ■ Working in hot conditions (bakeries, steel works, construction sites) ■ Being in parked motor vehicles in summer		■ Dehydration ■ Prior heat stroke ■ Hypokalaemia ■ Cardiovascular disease ■ Previous stroke or other central nervous system lesion

Table 35-3	Comparing Conditions Resulting From Heat Stress		
Variable	**Heat Cramps**	**Heat Exhaustion**	**Heat Stroke**
Pathophysiology	Sodium and water loss	Sodium and water loss, hypovolaemia	Failure of heat-regulating mechanisms
Mental status	Normal	Normal or mild confusion	Altered, delirium, convulsions
Temperature	May be mildly elevated	Usually mildly elevated	> 40.5°C
Skin	Cool, moist	Pale, cool, moist	Dry, hot, but sweating may persist, especially with exertional heat stroke
Muscle cramping	Severe	May or may not be present	Absent

decreased maximum heart rates. Acclimitasation can decrease the likelihood of heat illness, but it takes days of progressive exertion in a hot environment to be effective.

Among the young and healthy, people most vulnerable to heat stress include infants and young children exposed to a hot environment. Children, compared with adults, have proportionately higher metabolic heat production, have a CBT that rises faster during dehydration, and do not dissipate heat as well owing to their smaller organ and vascular systems. Athletes and military recruits engaging in heavy exertion in hot conditions are also at increased risk.

The following subsections discuss the major types of heat illness Table 35-3 ▲ .

Heat Cramps

Heat cramps are acute and involuntary muscle pains, usually in the lower extremities, the abdomen, or both, that occur because of profuse sweating and subsequent sodium losses in sweat. Three factors contribute to heat cramps: salt depletion, dehydration, and muscle fatigue. Heat cramps most often afflict people in good physical condition—for example, athletes, military personnel, and physical labourers. In fact, British coal miners would add salt to their beer to prevent cramps. A recent study of football players showed a twofold increase in sweat sodium losses in athletes prone to heat cramps. Usually a person exerting himself or herself in a hot environment will become thirsty and increase the intake of fluids. But if the person is sweating heavily, he or she is losing fluids and salt through the skin. If the person drinks plain water, he or she will not replace sweat sodium losses Figure 35-5 ▶ . Hence, the rehabilitation sector at a fire should have watered-down sports drinks available instead of just water.

Heat cramps usually start suddenly during strenuous and/or prolonged physical activity. They may be mild, characterised by only slight abdominal cramping and tingling in the extremities. More often, however, they present with severe, incapacitating pain in the extremities and abdomen. The patient may become hypotensive and nauseated but remains alert. The pulse is generally rapid, the skin pale and moist, and the temperature normal.

Treatment of heat cramps aims to eliminate the exposure and restore lost salt and water to the body:

■ Move the patient to a cool environment. Have the patient lie down if he or she feels faint.

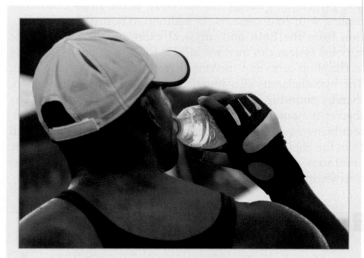

Figure 35-5 If you drink plain water, you will not replace the sweat salt losses.

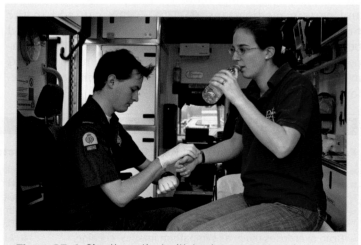

Figure 35-6 Give the patient with heat cramps one or two glasses of rehydration fluids and/or sports drinks if he or she is not nauseated.

■ If the patient is not nauseated, give one or two glasses of rehydration fluids and/or sports drinks containing glucose Figure 35-6 ▲ . Instruct the patient to drink the solution slowly. Have the patient munch on salty crisps.

Salt tablets can irritate the stomach lining and may precipitate or worsen nausea.

- If the patient is too nauseated to take liquids by mouth, establish an intravenous (IV) line and infuse normal saline.
- Do not massage the cramping muscles. That tactic may actually aggravate the pain.
- As the patient's salt balance is restored, the symptoms will abate and the patient may want to resume activity. In the prehospital setting, this decision is best made with caution.

Heat Syncope

Heat syncope is an orthostatic syncopal, or near-syncopal, episode that typically occurs in nonacclimated people who may be under heat stress. It can occur with prolonged standing, as in mass outdoor gatherings, or when standing suddenly from a sitting or lying position. Peripheral vasodilatation, possibly exacerbated by some degree of dehydration, is thought to be the cause. Treatment involves placing the patient in a supine position and replacing fluid deficits. If the patient does not recover quickly in the supine position, suspect heat exhaustion or heat stroke.

Heat Exhaustion

Heat exhaustion is a clinical syndrome thought to represent a milder form of heat illness on a continuum leading to heat stroke. Its hallmarks are volume depletion and heat stress. Classically, two forms are described: water-depleted and sodium-depleted. Water-depleted heat exhaustion occurs primarily in older persons owing to immobility, medications that contribute to dehydration, and decreased thirst sensitivity and in active younger workers or athletes who do not adequately replace fluids in a hot environment. Sodium-depleted heat exhaustion may take hours or days to develop and results from huge sodium losses from sweating but replacing only free water, not sodium.

A concept closely related to sodium-depleted heat exhaustion is exertional hyponatraemia. Studies carried out by the US from the Boston Marathon, the Grand Canyon National Park, and the military point to a common thread: prolonged exertion in a hot environment coupled with excessive hypotonic fluid intake. This phenomenon leads to nausea, vomiting, weight gain, and, in severe cases, mental status changes, cerebral oedema, and convulsions. The practical concern is older, debilitated patients and patients who participate in extreme endurance sports events such as marathons and endurance trainings.

Symptoms of heat exhaustion may include headache, fatigue, dizziness, nausea, vomiting, and, sometimes, abdominal cramping. The patient is usually sweating profusely, and the skin is pale and clammy. He or she may be slightly disorientated. The temperature may be normal or slightly elevated (< 40°C). Tachycardia is present, although this response may be blunted if the patient is taking a beta blocker. Respirations are fast and shallow. Tachypnoea may

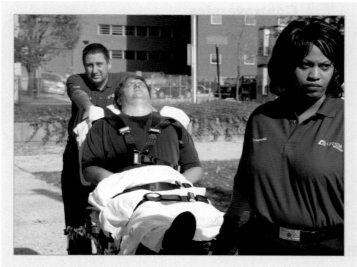

Figure 35-7 Remove the patient from the heat.

produce symptoms of hyperventilation: carpopedal spasm, perioral numbness, and a low end-tidal carbon dioxide level. Blood pressure may be decreased due to peripheral pooling of blood or volume depletion; if not decreased at rest, blood pressure will almost certainly drop when the patient tries to sit or stand from a recumbent position (orthostatic hypotension). If the patient reports brown urine, suspect rhabdomyolysis (the destruction of muscle tissue leading to a release of potassium and myoglobin).

Heat exhaustion is sometimes mistaken for "summer flu", and the condition may be misdiagnosed. If untreated, heat exhaustion may progress to heat stroke. The treatment of heat exhaustion is aimed at removing the patient from exposure to heat and repairing the fluid and electrolyte balance:

- Move the patient to a cool environment Figure 35-7 ▲; remove excess clothing, and place supine with legs elevated.
- If the patient's temperature is elevated, sponge, spray, or drip the patient with tepid water and fan gently to make him or her more comfortable—but don't overdo it. Heroic measures to lower body temperature rapidly are unnecessary, and chilling the patient can cause shivering and thermogenesis.
- Consider specially designed cooling chairs for hand and forearm immersion in cold water for rehabilitation at fire scenes, mass gatherings, and endurance sports.
- Oral hydration with sports drinks may be appropriate. If nausea and vomiting are present, start a normal saline IV and draw blood for electrolyte analysis. Use the heart rate and blood pressure to guide the fluid amounts administered.
- If exertional hyponatraemia is suspected, do not give fluids by mouth. Instead, draw blood for checking the blood sodium level and administer IV normal saline.

- Monitor cardiac rhythm, vital signs, temperature, and end-tidal carbon dioxide.
- If you cannot determine whether the patient has heat exhaustion or heat stroke, treat for heat stroke.

Heat Stroke

Of all heat illnesses, heat stroke is the least common but the most deadly. It is caused by a severe disturbance in the body's thermoregulation and is a profound emergency, with mortality rates as high as 10% in treated patients and 30% to 80% in untreated patients. Experts typically rely on two findings to make this diagnosis: core temperature more than 40°C and altered mental status.

Two heat stroke syndromes are distinguished: classic and exertional Table 35-4 ▾ . Classic heat stroke (passive heat stroke), which usually occurs during heat waves, is most likely to strike very old, very young, or bedridden people. Patients with chronic illnesses, such as diabetes or heart disease, are particularly susceptible, as are people with alcoholism and patients taking certain medications (diuretics, sedatives, anticholinergics). In this syndrome, high environmental temperatures initially elicit thermolysis, but the CBT eventually soars, and the typical signs and symptoms of heat stroke appear.

Exertional heat stroke is typically an illness of young and fit people exercising in hot and humid conditions. When the ambient temperature approaches body temperature, radiation and convection are no longer effective means of shedding excess heat. If the relative humidity rises above 75%, evaporative cooling becomes ineffective. A person who continues exercising in such conditions will continue generating heat without any means of excreting that heat. Heat will then build up within the body, causing the CBT to elevate dramatically.

The Clinical Picture of Heat Stroke

Both types of heat stroke present with similar signs and symptoms, which may or may not be recognised as the consequence of heat exposure. Patients almost certainly won't be able to give a coherent history because they will be confused, delirious, or comatose. Often the very earliest signs of heat stroke are changes in behaviour—irritability, combativeness, signs the patient is hallucinating—which may mislead bystanders and ambulance personnel into thinking the patient is having a behavioural or substance-related emergency. Older patients with heat stroke may present with signs resembling those of a suspected stroke. Other central nervous system disturbances—including tremours, convulsions, constricted pupils, and decerebrate or decorticate posturing—may also be prominent features of heat stroke.

At the Scene

Suspect heat stroke and check a core temperature in any person behaving strangely in a hot environment.

The diagnostic vital sign is, of course, a markedly elevated temperature, usually greater than 40°C. Signs of a hyperdynamic state are usually present: tachycardia, hyperventilation with an end-tidal carbon dioxide of less than 20 mm Hg, and lowered peripheral vascular resistance from efforts of the body to cool itself with vasodilatation. Heat stroke is characterised by some degree of dehydration, which worsens the problem by decreasing the body's ability to get the hotter core blood to the periphery for thermolysis. Blood pressure can be normal or decreased depending on the level of dehydration. The skin can be dry, red, and hot in classic heat stroke or pale and sweaty in exertional heat stroke.

The diagnosis of heat stroke is easy to miss. It may develop rapidly in a patient whose heat exhaustion was mistaken for the flu, or it may present as coma of unknown origin. Unless you keep the possibility of heat stroke constantly in mind during the hot months of the year and routinely take the temperature as part of the vital signs, you may waste precious time searching for some other cause of the patient's symptoms.

Fever and Conditions That Mimic Heat Stroke

New paramedics may face a perplexing challenge: Why is this care home patient's temperature elevated? Is it heat stroke, a febrile illness, or sepsis? Neurological changes can be present in either case. The history, however, may suggest infectious causes. For example, a change in the urine colour in a catheter bag, a recent complaint of cough and dyspnoea, an obvious

Table 35-4	Classic Versus Exertional Heat Stroke	
Characteristic	**Classic Heat Stroke**	**Exertional Heat Stroke**
Age	Older	Younger
General health	Chronic diseases, schizophrenia	Healthy person
Medications	Beta blockers, diuretics, anticholinergics	Often none, consider stimulant abuse
Activity	Very little to bedridden	Strenuous
Sweating	Absent	Present
Skin	Hot, red, dry	Moist, pale
Blood glucose level	Normal	Hypoglycaemic
Rhabdomyolysis	Rare	Common
Acute renal failure	Rare	Common

skin infection, or complaints of a fever, rash, photophobia, and stiff neck may point to meningitis. An intermittent shaking chill also favours infectious causes of increased temperature.

A fever can signal that the body is fighting an infection by inhibiting reproduction of harmful toxins. Pyrogens (proteins secreted by infective organisms and the body's immune system) act on the hypothalamus by increasing the thermal set point, which results in a fever. The body then uses its thermoregulatory tools to maintain the new temperature setting. The patient with a reset temperature may adapt to this change by wearing more clothes, and sometimes the body creates more heat via shivering. Although aspirin and nonsteroidal anti-inflammatory drugs can lower a fever (by blocking prostaglandins), they are dangerous in treating heat illnesses.

Anticholinergic poisoning presents with an elevated temperature; dry, red skin; mental status changes; and tachycardia. Anticholinergic poisonings usually cause dilated pupils, whereas patients with heat stroke usually have constricted pupils.

Two rare syndromes must also be considered. Neuroleptic malignant syndrome (NMS) is caused by antipsychotic and some antiemetic medications and presents with hyperthermia, muscular rigidity, altered mental status, and a hyperdynamic state. Malignant hyperthermia can occur as a result of common anaesthesia medications (notably suxamethonium) and presents similarly to NMS. Researchers are exploring a common genetic contributor to malignant hyperthermia and heat stroke.

Treatment of Heat Stroke

If you are unsure about what exactly is causing the elevated temperature, the prudent step is to treat for heat stroke given the deadly consequences of missing it. Your medical director may also help with treatment plans.

Treatment of heat stroke aims at removing the patient from the environment and promoting rapid cooling. Two main methods are used for rapid cooling: ice water body immersion and evaporative cooling by spraying tepid water over the patient accompanied by the use of fans to promote convection. Placing cold packs on the neck, groin, and axillae can augment the evaporative method. Research has shown that ice water immersion is probably the more effective means of rapid cooling but has obvious limitations in the back of an ambulance, including the need for ice. Conscious patients do not tolerate this measure well, and patients with altered mental status can be challenging to manage in an ice bath. You must also monitor CBT to avoid over cooling, resulting in shivering and even hypothermia.

- Evaluate the ABCs, administer supplemental oxygen, and be prepared to intubate.
- Move the patient to a cool environment, and strip the patient to underclothing. Monitor the rectal temperature every 10 minutes. Cooling efforts should continue until the rectal temperature has fallen below about 39°C.
- Cool as rapidly as possible by the most expeditious means available.
  - Spray the patient with tepid water while fanning constantly to promote rapid evaporation. Ideally, your ambulances will have effective air conditioning in the rear compartment. Apply cold packs to the patient's neck, groin, and axillae to aid in cooling from evaporative techniques.
  - Consider ice water immersion in cases of prolonged transport or delayed evacuation. Cooling with ice water–soaked blankets and fanning is nearly as effective as immersion. Pay close attention to airway status; watch for convulsions and CBT to avoid overcooling.
- Start an IV line, give normal saline, and check the blood glucose level. Be careful with fluids—pulmonary oedema is a known complication of heat stroke. Remember that cooling promotes peripheral vasoconstriction that can raise the blood pressure.
- Monitor cardiac rhythm, and remember that rhabdomyolysis can occur with resultant hyperkalaemia.
- Be prepared to treat convulsions with common anticonvulsive medicines (lorazepam, midazolam, or diazepam).

A few measures are *not* helpful: Covering the patient with wet sheets may impede heat loss by evaporation. Dantrolene, a medication once thought to aid in lowering the temperature, has not been shown to be effective. Last, massaging muscles to combat cutaneous vasoconstriction from cooling too much is not beneficial.

Prevention of Heat Illness

The following measures can help protect you, your colleagues, and the communities you serve from heat illness:

- Paramedics working in hot climates should have appropriate summer uniforms.
- If you are on standby, park the ambulance in the shade and make sure the air conditioning works.
- Increase your daily intake of fluid. Do not rely on thirst to gauge your need. Try to drink something every hour during very hot weather, aiming for urination every 2 hours. Dark urine is concentrated, indicating that the body is dehydrated. Avoid beverages with a high sugar content and those that promote diuresis (such as caffeinated or alcoholic drinks).
- Install or carry a portable fan in the ambulance to improve convection, supplement the air conditioning, and treat patients with heat illness.
- Carry a portable cooler or—if you are lucky enough—an onboard refrigerator for hot weather. Fill the cooler about half full with crushed ice, and stock it with sports drinks or other salt-containing drinks for patients and the ambulance crew.
- Review Figure 35-8 ▶ outlining the relationship of heat and humidity to heat stress.
- Conduct community-based programmes aimed at high-risk populations—for example, care home risk assessments.

Be alert for early symptoms of heat illness, such as headache, nausea, cramps, and dizziness. If you experience any of those symptoms, get out of the hot environment immediately and get medical attention.

Heat Index

Temperature (°C)

Relative Humidity (%)	27	28	29	30	31	32	33	34	36	37	38	39	40	41	43	47
40	27	27	28	29	31	33	34	36	38	41	43	46	48	51	54	58
45	27	28	29	31	32	34	36	38	40	43	46	48	51	54	58	
50	27	28	29	31	33	35	37	39	42	45	48	51	55	58		
55	27	29	30	32	34	36	38	41	44	47	51	54	58			
60	28	29	31	33	35	38	41	43	47	51	54	58				
65	28	29	32	34	37	39	42	46	49	53	58					
70	28	30	32	35	38	41	44	48	52	57						
75	29	31	33	36	39	43	47	51	56							
80	29	32	34	38	41	45	49	54								
85	29	32	36	39	43	47	52	57								
90	30	33	37	41	45	50	55									
95	30	34	38	42	47	53										
100	31	35	39	44	49	56										

Likelihood of heat disorders with prolonged exposure or strenuous activity:

☐ Caution   ☐ Extreme caution   ☐ Danger   ☐ Extreme danger

Figure 35-8 Likelihood of heat disorders.
Adapted from: US National Weather Service. Available at: http://www.nws.noaa.gov/om/heat/index.shtml. Accessed May 2006.

Local Cold Injury

Most injuries from the cold are localised to the extremities or exposed parts of the body, such as the tips of the ears, nose, upper cheek, and tips of the fingers or toes Figure 35-9 ▶. Local freezing injuries fall under the general heading of frost-bite. Frostbite is an ischaemic injury that is classified as superficial or deep depending on whether tissue loss occurs.

A very mild form of frostbite, sometimes called frostnip, comes on slowly and generally is not painful, so the victim tends to be unaware of its occurrence. This problem is easily treated by placing a warm hand firmly over the chilled nose or ear or, when the fingers are frost-nipped, by placing the fingers into the armpit. The return of warmth to a frost-nipped area is usually signaled by some redness and tingling. Windmilling involves rapidly making a large circle with your hand, starting with your hand next to your side, raising it backward and up until you are reaching straight up, and moving it rapidly down frontward. This technique forces blood into the cold hand.

Deeper degrees of frostbite involve freezing of tissues and can occur only in ambient temperatures well below the freezing point. Cells are composed chiefly of water, so when they are subjected to low enough temperatures, the water within them turns into ice crystals, which can damage or destroy the cells. This problem is further complicated by increased viscosity accompanied by "sludging", poor flow, capillary leakage, and resultant thrombus and ischaemic injury.

Risk Factors for Frostbite

Several factors predispose a person to frostbite:
- Going out on a cold, windy day without earmuffs, mittens, a scarf, or a hat.

You are the Paramedic Part 2

You ask the patient what is going on as you assist him to the ambulance. His gait is unsteady. Your colleague obtains an initial set of vital signs. The patient takes a moment and tells you that he had been drinking earlier and got caught in the rain. You notice that the coat he is wearing is dry. When you ask him if it is his coat, the patient says "no". Your colleague informs you that the coat belongs to the bystander who initially helped him and that his identification says he is 44 years old.

As you begin to undress the patient, you notice that his clothes are wet and his appearance is unkempt. The patient states that his head hurts. He says "no" when asked about dizziness, visual disturbances, chest pain, and trouble breathing. He says that his stomach "always hurts", and that he has trouble with his pancreas but can offer no more clarification on his pain or history. There is no nausea, vomiting, diarrhoea, or unusually coloured stools. The patient states he has been drinking most of the afternoon but does not know where he is or what day it is. He denies any psychiatric history.

Vital Signs	Recording Time: 5 Minutes
Skin	Pink, cool, and dry
Pulse	112 beats/min; irregular and weak
Blood pressure	108/60 mm Hg
Respirations	24 breaths/min
SpO$_2$	Not reading

4. Does the additional information narrow the diagnostic possibilities?
5. What interventions might benefit the patient?
6. Why is the pulse oximetry not working?

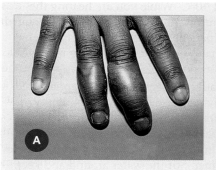 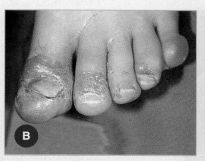 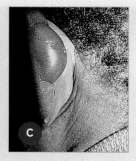

Figure 35-9 The extremities (**A** and **B**) and the ears (**C**) are particularly susceptible to frostbite.

- Impeding the circulation to the extremities:
  - Wearing tight gloves and shoes and too many socks.
  - Lacing boots very tightly and remaining in a cramped position for a while.
  - Wearing plastic boots that won't expand. Preferably, boots should be lined with felt, which will expand when wet.
  - Smoking, which constricts arteries.
  - Drinking, which helps peripherally dilate blood vessels, helping the person to get colder.
- Going out in the cold when tired, dehydrated, or hungry.
- Coming in direct contact with cold objects.
- Not staying hydrated, which would otherwise promote increased blood flow.
- Allowing oneself to become thoroughly chilled. Generalised hypothermia is the most effective way to sustain local cold injury.

To avoid getting frostbite, avoid all of the preceding behaviours! Note the windchill, and always cover your face when you are outside for a long time (such as when skiing). Keep your feet dry and warm, and come in often to warm up. This precaution is especially important for children.

Superficial Frostbite

The most common symptom of frostbite is an altered sensation: numbness, tingling, or burning. The skin typically appears white and waxy and has been compared with frozen halibut **Figure 35-10 ▶** . Because it is frozen, the skin is firm to palpation, but the underlying tissues remain soft. Once thawing occurs, the injured area turns cyanotic, and the patient experiences a hot, stinging sensation. Capillary leakage produces oedema in the frostbitten area, and blebs develop within a few hours after thawing. Dull or throbbing pain may persist for days or weeks after the injury.

The prehospital treatment of superficial frostbite differs significantly from that of deep frostbite, so it is very important to distinguish between the two. Usually it is difficult to determine the depth of the injury when you first see it—even a shallow frostbite injury can appear to be frozen solid. If the tissues beneath the skin are soft when you press down on the skin surface, the frostbite is probably superficial. If not, or if there is

any doubt, treat the injury as deep frostbite.

Mild cold injuries are generally managed by a combination of dressing, rest, food, and limiting exposure to the cold. Once you have determined that the patient has superficial frostbite only, proceed as follows:

- *Remove the patient from the cold.* Take the patient indoors or into a heated ambulance so the body can stop retaining warm blood in the core and instead send some warm blood to the periphery, where it is urgently needed.
- *Rewarm the injured part with body heat.* If an ear, nose, or foot is frostbitten, apply firm, steady pressure against the area with a warm hand. If a hand is frostbitten, have the patient insert the hand into the armpit and hold it there without moving. Do not try to rewarm a frostbitten part with radiant or dry heat.
- *Do not rub or massage the frostbitten area;* massage will cause further damage to injured tissues.
- *Cover blisters with a dry, sterile dressing,* and protect the area from further injury.
- *Transport the patient to the hospital* with the injured area elevated and protected from the cold.

Deep Frostbite

Deep frostbite usually involves the hands or the feet. A frozen extremity looks white, yellow-white, or mottled blue-white, and it is hard, cold, and without sensation. The major tissue damage occurs not from the freezing of the tissues, but rather when the tissues thaw out, particularly if thawing occurs gradually. When tissues thaw slowly, partial refreezing of melted water may

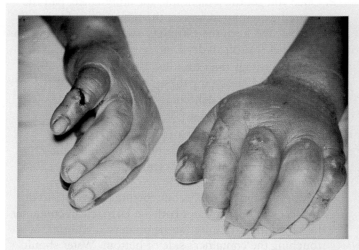

Figure 35-10 Frostbitten parts are hard and usually waxy to the touch.

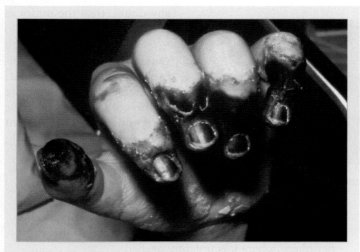

Figure 35-11 Gangrene can occur when tissue is frozen and chemical changes occur in the cells.

occur. Because these new ice crystals tend to be much larger than those formed during the original freeze, they cause even greater tissue damage. As thawing occurs, the injured area turns purple and becomes excruciatingly painful. Gangrene (permanent cell death) may set in within a few days, requiring amputation of all or part of the injured limb **Figure 35-11 ▲** .

The prehospital treatment of deep frostbite depends on two factors: (1) whether the injured extremity has been partially or completely thawed before you arrive and (2) how far the patient is from the hospital.

- If the extremity is still frozen when you find the patient, leave it frozen until the patient reaches the hospital; rapid rewarming is extremely difficult to carry out properly in the prehospital environment. If you are within about an hour's drive of a hospital:
  1. Leave the frozen extremity frozen. As long as the limb is not thawed, the patient may even walk on it if necessary.
  2. Once you get the patient into the ambulance, pad the injured extremity to protect the tissues from further trauma, and keep the extremity away from the heater or any other sources of dry heat.
  3. Do not massage the extremity. The cells are full of ice crystals, and massaging the extremity will cause the ice crystals to lacerate delicate tissues.
  4. Transport without delay.
- If the extremity is already partially thawed or if the evacuation or transport will be delayed, contact the A&E consultant to discuss rewarming in the prehospital environment.
  1. Rewarm the injured extremity before transport. To do so, you will need a water bath—a large, clean container in which the extremity can be immersed without touching the container's side or bottom. Water should be heated in a second container and then stirred into the water bath until the temperature of the bath is

between 35°C and 40°C. While you are heating the water, administer intravenous analgesia such as fentanyl or morphine. The patient will experience very severe pain as the limb thaws out, and you want to mitigate that pain as much as possible.

  2. When the water bath has reached the appropriate temperature, gently immerse the injured extremity. Keep a thermometer in the water. When the water temperature falls below 38°C, temporarily remove the injured extremity from the bath while you add more hot water to the container. Stir the water around and keep adding more hot water until the bath is again in the appropriate temperature range; then reimmerse the injured extremity.

    The rewarming procedure typically takes 10 to 30 minutes. It is complete when the frozen area is warm to the touch and is deep red or bluish (and remains red when you remove the limb from the water bath). While rewarming is in progress, the patient should be kept warm, preferably indoors, with insulated clothing and blankets. Do not permit the patient to smoke, because nicotine causes vasoconstriction and, therefore, interferes with blood flow to the injured area.

  3. Once rewarming is complete, dry the extremity and apply sterile dressings very gently. Use sterile gauze to separate frostbitten fingers and toes.

At the Scene

Do not attempt rewarming in the prehospital environment if there is any possibility of refreezing or if the patient must walk on the frostbitten foot.

Trench Foot

Trench foot involves a process similar to frostbite but can occur at temperatures as high as 15°C. It is caused by prolonged exposure to cool, wet conditions. The mechanism of injury can be explained by conduction: Wet feet lose heat 25 times faster than dry feet. Vasoconstriction and an ischaemic cascade similar to that seen with frostbite then set in. Prevention—keeping the feet dry and warm—is the best treatment.

▌Hypothermia

Hypothermia is defined as a decrease in CBT generally starting at 35°C owing to inadequate thermogenesis and/or excess environmental cold stress. Any temperature below the body's temperature can result in hypothermia. For example, an older person with alcoholism who has had a stroke and is now living alone can become hypothermic in a 15°C home. An unprepared hill walker caught in a summer wind and rainstorm is another classic example, as is a person who becomes submerged in icy water **Figure 35-12 ▶** .

The body regulates cold stress by increasing thermogenesis, decreasing thermolysis, and pursuing adaptive behavioural changes. **Table 35-5 ▾** summarises the factors contributing to thermoregulation and hypothermia.

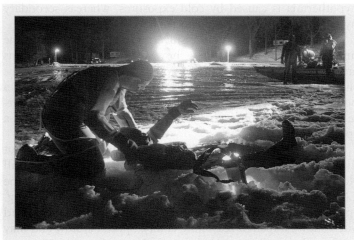

Figure 35-12 Patients who have been submerged in cold water are at high risk for hypothermia.

Table 35-5	Factors Contributing to Thermoregulation and Hypothermia	
If thermogenic factors plus heat retention factors are less than cold factors, then hypothermia results.		
Thermogenic Factors	**Heat Retention Factors**	**Cold Factors**
Muscular exertion	Vasoconstriction	Radiation • Temperature • Surface areas
Shivering (↑ BMR 2–5 times)	Body surface area	Convection • Windchill
Energy stores	Adipose tissue	Conduction • Wetness

Risk Factors for Hypothermia

People at risk for hypothermia have increased thermolysis, decreased thermogenesis, impaired thermoregulation, or other contributing factors. Many issues can lead to the development of a hypothermic condition, including cold temperatures, fatigue, improper gear for adverse conditions, wetness, dehydration, malnutrition, and the length of exposure and intensity of weather conditions **Table 35-6 ▾**.

Alcohol is by far the most common cause of heat loss in urban settings. It predisposes the patient to hypothermia by impairing shivering thermogenesis (decreased thermogenesis) and by promoting cutaneous vasodilatation (increased thermolysis), which hinders the body's attempts to create an insulating shell around its warm core. Liver disease, which leads to inadequate glycogen stores, and the subnormal nutritional status of most people with alcoholism further impair metabolic heat generation. Finally, alcohol impairs judgement, which often leads to inappropriate behaviour in cold conditions. Impaired thermoregulation can also occur with therapeutic or overdoses of sedative medications, tricyclic antidepressants, and phenothiazines, primarily by interfering with central nervous system (CNS)-mediated vasoconstriction.

Older people often cannot generate heat effectively because of reduced muscle mass and a diminished shivering response. Atrophy of subcutaneous fat also reduces elderly patients' insulation against heat loss. Medications commonly prescribed to older people may interfere with vasoconstriction as well. Hypothyroidism and malnutrition may further contribute to an older person's vulnerability (decreased thermogenesis).

Special Considerations

Older people on fixed budgets should be checked on during cold spells. Infants and toddlers, who have a large head-to-body surface area, should always have their heads covered during the winter.

Table 35-6	Factors That Predispose to Cold Illness		
Factors That Increase Heat Loss	**Factors That Impair Thermoregulatory Mechanisms**	**Factors That Decrease Heat Production**	**Miscellaneous Causes**
■ Cold water drowning ■ Wet clothes ■ Windchill ■ Impaired judgement from drugs or alcohol ■ Vasodilatation from: – Alcohol – Acute spinal cord injury ■ Diabetic peripheral neuropathies	■ Dehydration ■ Parkinson's disease or dementias ■ Multiple sclerosis ■ Anorexia nervosa ■ Central nervous system bleeding or ischaemic cerebrovascular accident ■ Multi-system trauma ■ Drugs interfering with vasoconstriction: – Alcohol – Benzodiazepines – Phenothiazines – Tricyclic antidepressants	■ Hypothyroidism ■ Age extremes ■ Hypoglycaemia ■ Malnutrition ■ Inability to shiver and immobility	■ Sepsis ■ Meningitis ■ Overzealous heat stroke treatment

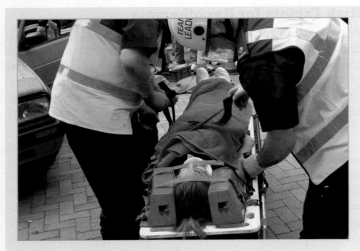

Figure 35-13 Trauma patients need to be moved to the longboard or stretcher with a blanket on it as soon as is safe and medically appropriate.

At the Scene

Simply covering a patient hit by a car and lying in the street is not good enough; body heat continues to be conducted away into the cold pavement. Remove the patient from the street onto a blanket or rescue quickly.

The most important of the other factors contributing to hypothermia is trauma. Hypotension and hypovolaemia can interfere with normal thermoregulation. Patients with CNS trauma or shock will not be able to mount a shivering response owing to the nature of their injuries. Last, hypothermia in trauma patients can lead to serious coagulation problems. If you are wearing protective gear in the cold, make sure your ambulance is warm, ask the patient if he or she is cold, and do what you can to conserve the patient's body heat **Figure 35-13 ▲**.

The Clinical Picture of Hypothermia

Watch for "umbles"—stumbles, mumbles, fumbles, and grumbles. These behaviours are good indicators of how the cold affects the cerebral and cognitive functioning of patients in the early stages of hypothermia.

The clinical definition of mild hypothermia is a CBT greater than 32.2°C. Below this CBT, the condition is considered moderate hypothermia when between 30°C to 32°C and severe hypothermia when below 30°C. In the early stage of hypothermia, the CBT is more than 35°C, but the patient shows obvious signs and symptoms of hypothermia. Luckily, the body may compensate for this condition through thermogenesis until the patient finds a way to increase heat production or the glycogen energy stored in muscles and liver is exhausted.

Hypothermia may also be classified according to the time to onset. Acute occurs rapidly (as in cold water drownings), subacute during a short time (as in exposure to cold conditions during a short time), and chronic that may occur over days (for example, an urban homeless person or a poorly heated home with an elderly resident). In yet another classification, primary hypothermia is caused by cold exposures, whereas secondary hypothermia is due to problems such as severe sepsis.

In mild hypothermia, the shivering is in full force and the umbles are noticeable. Often, however, the initial symptoms are vague. Older people may simply have a more flat affect, be slightly more confused, or develop symptoms suggestive of a possible stroke, including dysarthria and ataxia. No strong correlation has been observed between signs or symptoms and a specific CBT.

The net effect of hypothermia is to slow things down, but different body systems react in different ways. The overall slowdown of function is most dramatically apparent in the CNS, where just about everything slows—thinking, feeling, speaking. A hypothermic patient is typically apathetic and often shows impaired reasoning ability. Speech is slow and may be slurred; coordination is impaired; the gait is ataxic. This picture may closely resemble that associated with stroke, head injury, or alcohol intoxication, which probably explains why so many cases of hypothermia are initially misdiagnosed.

In the cardiovascular system, hypothermia induces several changes. Initially, as peripheral vasoconstriction shunts blood to the body core, the body's volume receptors interpret the increased flow as an increase in volume. They therefore stimulate the kidneys to start producing more urine (cold diuresis). At the same time, cooling of the tissues induces a flow of water from the intravascular to the extravascular spaces. The net effects are to increase the viscosity of the blood, thereby impairing circulation, and to produce a state of hypovolaemia. Meanwhile, the heart is suffering from the drop in body temperature. Cold initially speeds up the heart, then slows the rate and disrupts the electric conduction system. At a CBT of approximately 30°C, the body experiences cardiac arrhythmias, including atrial fibrillation. A unique Osborn wave may be observed if shivering does not obscure the tracing **Figure 35-14 ▼**. Of special concern is ventricular fibrillation (VF), to which a hypothermic heart becomes susceptible at a CBT around 28°C. Once the heart fibrillates, repeated defibrillation is not recommended until the CBT is greater than 30°C.

Initially, the respiratory rate speeds up, but later it slows, leading to a decrease in minute volume. Tracheobronchial secretions increase, and

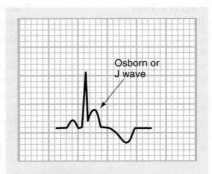

Figure 35-14 Osborn or J wave.

bronchospasm may occur. At 32.2°C, hypoventilation is profound, protective airway reflexes decline, and oxygen consumption decreases by about half.

The muscular system also slows down in response to cold. Although the initial muscular reaction to cold is shivering, that reaction is a mixed blessing. It generates heat, but it also makes skilled movements more difficult. Shivering, in any case, ceases when the CBT falls below 32.7°C. Thereafter, cold muscles become progressively weaker and stiffer, impairing the exposed person's ability to save himself or herself.

Finally, cold affects the body's metabolism. Shivering can deplete the body of glucose, leading to hypoglycaemia. Meanwhile, insulin levels fall, making further glucose metabolism impossible, so the body switches to the metabolism of fat. The liver's metabolism of drugs is also affected by the cold. Because medications are metabolised more slowly than normal, the effects of those drugs last much longer.

At the Scene

If a patient in a road traffic collision is shivering, this is not a good sign. If you need heavy clothing, remember that the patient will also be cold.

Treatment of Hypothermia

This section first discusses general care and then explains how to manage cardiac arrest in a hypothermic patient. General care is aimed at preserving further heat loss and rewarming. The victim should be stripped of wet clothes and insulated from further heat loss.

Breathing Patients With a Pulse
Mild Hypothermia Cases: 32°C to 35°C
The treatment is passive rewarming, which involves removing wet clothing, drying the patient's skin, moving the patient into a warmed ambulance, and using warm blankets or "space" blankets to prevent further conductive heat loss. Depending on the patient's location and the relative ease of transport, you may have to promote heat generation by feeding the patient, giving warm fluids (not caffeine or alcohol), and getting the person to move about.

Moderate Hypothermia Cases: 30°C to 32°C
The treatment is passive rewarming and active external rewarming of the truncal areas. This approach involves the use of several means to directly warm the patient's skin, including heating blankets or radiant heat from hot packs in the groin, neck, and axillae; forced hot air; and warmed IV fluids. Fluids at temperatures from 39°C to 41°C may be infused. It is prudent to administer a 500-ml bolus (unless otherwise contraindicated) to counter the hypovolaemia commonly encountered in hypothermia. Commercial warming devices that use special blankets and a heated fan unit can warm patients up faster than warm blankets. Carefully moni-

tor the patient for haemodynamic changes and direct thermal tissue injury because active external rewarming measures can cause "afterdrop". Afterdrop, the continued lowering of CBT even after the patient is removed from the cold, is more common in chronic hypothermia and hypothermia complicated by frostbitten extremities. Nevertheless, evidence from the United States suggests that forced air rewarming can be effective for some patients, even patients with severe hypothermia.

Severe Hypothermia Cases: Less Than 30°C
The active internal rewarming sequence used to treat severe hypothermia is accomplished in-hospital using the following modalities: warm IV fluids; warm, humid oxygen; peritoneal lavage (potassium chloride–free fluid); extracorporeal rewarming; and oesophageal rewarming tubes. Rewarming should continue until the CBT is greater than 35°C, spontaneous circulation returns, or resuscitative efforts cease.

Patients With No Pulse or Not Breathing
You may need to "look, listen, and feel" for a good 60 seconds to determine whether breathing and a pulse are present and, perhaps, use a portable Doppler device. Patients in cardiac arrest require high-quality CPR (push hard and fast, and allow full chest recoil) and a single shock if in VF/VT. Resume CPR immediately. Establish IV access. Infuse warm normal saline. Attempt to insert an advanced airway, and ventilate with warm, humid oxygen.

Cases of Hypothermia Less Than 30°C
Continue CPR, attempt a single defibrillation for VF/VT, establish IV access, withhold IV medications, and transport to the hospital.

Cases of Hypothermia Greater Than 30°C
Continue CPR, and administer IV medications as indicated by the electrocardiographic rhythm, but space them at longer than standard intervals. Repeat defibrillation for VF/VT as the core temperature rises. Transport the patient to hospital to provide active internal rewarming.

Withholding and Cessation of Resuscitative Efforts

Patients with obvious lethal traumatic injuries or those so frozen as to block the airway or chest compression efforts generally are dead. If submersion preceded the arrest, successful resuscitation is unlikely, with the possible exception of immersion in icy waters. Trauma and alcohol and drug overdoses could have led to hypothermia in the first place and can hamper resuscitation efforts. Try to factor these conditions into your treatment decisions. For example, a heroin user who was found outdoors and quickly recovers after naloxone administration should have a temperature check and should not be left at the scene.

Some believe that patients who appear dead after prolonged exposure to cold temperatures are not dead until "warm and dead". The effects of hypothermia may essentially protect

Controversies

There is a widespread belief that rough handling of a hypothermic heart may cause VF. Although people in severe hypothermia are prone to a VF arrest, it has not been clearly demonstrated that intubation or roughly handling the patient causes VF. In fact, in the US Danzl's multicentre hypothermia survey showed no case of VF in 117 hypothermic patients who were intubated. Do not let your concern for possible VF prevent you from inserting an advanced airway or moving the patient.

the brain and organs if hypothermia develops quickly, a fact that is being used to successfully treat some cardiac arrest patients. Sometimes it may be impossible to know which came first—a cardiac arrest and then hypothermia or vice versa. In those situations, it is prudent to attempt resuscitation.

Drowning or Submersion

There are about 700 deaths per year by drowning or submersion in the UK, and many more times that number of near drownings. A high percentage of these deaths involve children.

The first task in understanding drowning is to define this condition. At one point, 33 different definitions existed. In 2002, the first World Congress on Drowning developed the definition now in use: Drowning is the process of experiencing respiratory impairment from submersion/immersion in liquid. The "Utstein style" guidelines were then modified for drowning, and the term "drowning" was abandoned.

People may live or die based on what happens when a liquid-air interface occurs at the airway's entrance. Consequently, the drowning continuum progresses from breath holding, to laryngospasm, to the accumulation of carbon dioxide and the inability to oxygenate the lungs, to subsequent respiratory and cardiac arrest from multiple-organ failure due to tissue hypoxia. The victim can be resuscitated at any point along this continuum.

Table 35-7 ▾ lists the risk factors for drowning. Note that toddlers typically drown in baths, school-age children in pools, and teenagers in lakes or rivers.

Pathophysiology of Drowning and Submersion

Drowning generally follows a predictable sequence starting when the victim cannot keep his or her face out of the liquid medium:

- The length of breath holding depends on the victim's state of health and fitness, his or her level of panic, and the water temperature.

Table 35-7	Risk Factors for Drowning and Submersion

- Male sex
- Younger than 20 years (even higher for < 5 years)
- Pre-existing conditions, such as convulsion disorders
- Alcohol use
- Ineffective safety barriers (gates, locks, or use of a solar panel on a pool)
- Hyperventilation (may lead to shallow water blackout syndrome)

You are the Paramedic Part 3

After getting the patient out of his wet clothes, you begin your examination. He is barely shivering. He has trouble following your commands but does not seem to have any focal weakness. His pupils are equal, round, and reactive to light. His voice is slurred, but his facial muscles are symmetric and intact. The spine is nontender; the lungs are clear; and there is moderate epigastric tenderness to palpation. You find no evidence of trauma.

You insert an 18-gauge IV cannula, draw a blood sample, and check the patient's glucose level. It is 8.9 mmol/l. Your partner has hung a bag of warm normal saline. The temperature is 32°C. You begin to remove the patient's clothes and place hot packs in the groin, axillae, and neck. You wrap the IV fluid warmer around the bag of the nonrebreathing mask and wrap the oxygen tubing in a hot pack.

Reassessment	Recording Time: 15 Minutes
Skin	Getting pinker, cold, dry
Pulse	108 beats/min; regular and strong
Blood pressure	110/64 mm Hg
Respirations	24 breaths/min
S_PO_2	100% on nonrebreathing mask at 15 l/min supplemental oxygen; good waveform

7. What information is important to convey to the accident and emergency (A&E) department staff when you call?
8. What effect does alcohol have on hypothermia?
9. Why did the patient remove his clothing if he was hypothermic?

- As the victim goes under and water enters the mouth and nose, coughing and gasping ensue, and the victim swallows considerable amounts of water. Note that while some theoretical differences distinguish saltwater and freshwater drownings, this information is neither clinically significant nor useful in resuscitating a patient. In fact, 11 ml of water per kilogram of body weight is required to produce significant blood problems, and 22 ml/kg is needed to create electrolyte problems. Both types of water can lead to pulmonary injuries.

- A very small amount of water is aspirated into the posterior pharynx and perhaps the trachea, setting off spasms of the laryngeal muscles (laryngospasm) that effectively seal off and protect the airway—at least temporarily—from further aspiration.

- Laryngospasm leads to asphyxia—that is, a combination of hypoxaemia and hypercarbia—and the patient may lose consciousness. Hypoxaemia stimulates the body to shift from aerobic to anaerobic metabolism, with the ensuing production of lactate and development of metabolic acidosis. If the patient dies during this phase of laryngospasm, as occurs in 10% to 15% of drowning cases, it is essentially a death from suffocation, because the lungs are still dry ("dry drowning").

- At a certain point, which varies from person to person, water begins to enter the lungs. That event may occur because the hypercarbic and hypoxic drives stimulate inhalation or, if the patient has lost consciousness, because progressive asphyxia causes the laryngeal muscles to relax. In either case, the net effect is to permit water to gain access to the lungs ("wet drowning"). Its entry triggers an increase in peripheral airway resistance along with constriction of pulmonary vessels, all of which decrease the compliance of the lungs. In other words, the lungs become stiff.

- The decompensation stage of drowning occurs next. The victim gasps for air, inhaling yet more water, which mixes with air and chemicals in the lungs to form froth. Apnoea recurs, and the victim loses consciousness (if he or she has not already done so). The process of hypoxic brain damage begins, and cardiac arrest occurs.

Response to Drowning and Submersion Incidents

In general terms, the resuscitation of a victim of a submersion is the same as that for any other patient in respiratory or cardiac arrest, albeit with a few new logistic problems.

First, of course, you must reach the victim. People who have specialised training and experience in water rescue are best able to accomplish this task Figure 35-15 ▶.

When you reach the victim, the steps of treatment follow the usual sequence of ABCs. The first priority is establishing the airway. Cervical spine precautions should then be taken if necessary.

Assist ventilation as soon as possible, even before the patient is removed from the water. Do not perform manual thrusts (Heimlich manoeuvre) to remove water from the lungs because they may displace water from the stomach into the lungs. For adults, use chest compressions.

Start supplementary oxygen at the same time that you quickly determine whether a pulse is present. If there is no pulse, begin high-quality CPR. You may need to suction. One Australian study of drowning victims noted that 66% of patients receiving rescue breathing and 86% getting compressions vomited; one of your primary goals will be to prevent vomiting. In any event, protect the airway from aspiration during vomiting. Advanced airway placement may be appropriate if BLS airway interventions fail.

During normal, spontaneous breathing, the pressure in the airways at the end of exhalation is effectively zero. As a result, some alveoli normally collapse during the expiratory phase of the respiratory cycle. When there is widespread atelectasis and shunt—as in drowning—it is desirable to maintain some positive pressure at the end of exhalation to keep alveoli open and to drive any fluid that may have accumulated in the alveoli back into the interstitium or capillaries. The technique called positive end-expiratory pressure (PEEP) focuses on maintaining some degree of positive pressure at the end of the expiratory phase of respiration. In the prehospital environment, PEEP is indicated for intubated patients who must be transported over long distances to hospital after submersion or who have other conditions that produce significant shunt. Several commercial devices are designed to allow PEEP via an endotracheal tube. In addition, portable ventilators usually have a PEEP setting.

If a pulse is absent, implement advanced life support measures similar to those used in any other case of cardiopulmonary arrest: establish IV access, administer adrenaline, perform cardiac monitoring, and ensure electric conversion of VF.

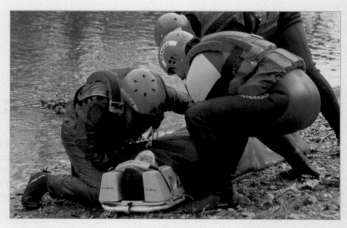

Figure 35-15 Rescuers must wear proper personal protective equipment, including a personal flotation device, when performing a water rescue.

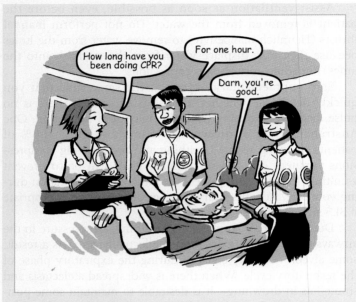

Figure 35-16

Table 35-8 | Management of Drowning and Submersion

- Rescuers trained and practised in doing so should perform the water rescue.
- Ensure basic life support measures are being carried out with an emphasis on airway and oxygenation.
- Anticipate vomiting.
- Administer supplemental oxygen and intubate if needed.
- Establish IV access.
- Measure core temperature, and prevent or treat hypothermia.
- Give a beta-2 adrenergic by metered-dose inhaler or nebuliser for wheezing.
- Monitor end-tidal carbon dioxide and pulse oximetry.
- Insert a nasogastric tube in intubated patients.
- Transport every submersion patient to hospital, including patients who seem to recover at the scene.

Patients rescued from submersion are prone to bronchospasm from the irritation to their airways. If you hear wheezes, administer a beta-2 adrenergic drug, such as salbutamol by nebuliser, as you would for a patient having an acute asthmatic attack.

Do not give up on the victim of submersion, especially if the patient is a child and the incident occurred in icy water **Figure 35-16 ▲** . Successful resuscitations with complete neurological recovery have been reported even in cases in which the victim had been submerged for more than an hour in icy water. Remember to consider the effects of hypothermia on a drowning patient, including measuring a core temperature and using the hypothermia algorithm. Studies indicate that the length of submersion and the response to prehospital resuscitation are major predictors of outcome. In other words, if patients are awake on hospital arrival, they will do better.

Table 35-8 ▲ summarises the management of drowning and submersion.

Postresuscitation Complications

Adult respiratory distress syndrome, chemical or bacterial pneumonitis, and renal failure are common complications that can occur hours to days after a submersion. These factors highlight the importance of an A&E department evaluation of submersion victims. Their symptoms may be subtle (slight cough, mild tachypnoea), or they may be asymptomatic.

You are the Paramedic Part 4

As you roll the patient into the A&E department, a member of the nursing staff comments that she saw him during her last shift. You politely convince her that despite his history, the patient is in moderate hypothermia and may have acute pancreatitis. She is appreciative of the blood draw and the care you've given. You assist the staff as they place the patient on a commercial hot-air warming blanket. When you follow up later, you learn that the patient was eventually rewarmed but was admitted for pancreatitis and observation.

You are the Paramedic Summary

1. What are three things that could medically harm this man in the next hour?

Alcohol abuse has many potential deadly consequences. You should always consider intracranial problems (intracranial bleeding from alcohol-related falls or ischaemic stroke), hypoglycaemia, and hypothermia.

2. Do you believe the scene to be adequately secured?

The presence of the police, the alcohol consumption, the patient's male sex, and the history of mental illness all predict violence toward ambulance personnel. Verify with the police that the patient has been properly searched. If you are uncertain, use your physical examination as a weapons sweep. You must conduct a risk assessment on all potentially violent patients you will be with in the back of the ambulance.

3. Where do you believe is the best place to assess the patient properly?

At this point, you do not have enough information to formulate a proper plan. Preserving the patient's dignity and getting the patient into the back of a warm ambulance are key concerns. Standing outside with the public looking on is not conducive to conducting a hands-on examination.

4. Does the additional information narrow the diagnostic possibilities?

This patient complains of a headache and abdominal pain. A patient with alcoholism with a headache may have something as dangerous as chronic subdural bleeding or as simple as an alcohol-related headache. The abdominal pain suggests acute or chronic pancreatitis, but also oesophageal problems. The fact the patient is wet, is confused, and has been out in the rain and wind suggests hypothermia.

5. What interventions might benefit the patient?

A check of the blood glucose level, core temperature, and a rhythm strip are all indicated at this point. The initiation of IV access must be weighed against relative ease, length of transport, and your guidelines.

6. Why is the pulse oximetry not working?

Hypothermia. Numerous factors can affect the functioning of the pulse oximetry unit. You must analyze the waveform to know if it is truly malfunctioning or if the patient's condition is causing the inability to obtain a reading.

7. What information is important to convey to the accident and emergency department staff when you call?

Your suspicions of hypothermia and pancreatitis, the basics of how the patient was found, and his core temperature should be enough information to alert the staff to a sick patient.

8. What effect does alcohol have on hypothermia?

Alcohol promotes vasodilatation, sending more blood to the skin and promoting further heat loss. It also impairs shivering mechanisms, judgement, and decision making.

9. Why did the patient remove his clothing if he was hypothermic?

Normally constricted blood vessels beneath the skin can dilate on reaching a certain core temperature, causing the patient to suddenly feel warm. It can be a sign of mental impairment from hypothermia.

Prep Kit

Ready for Review

- Environmental emergencies are medical conditions caused or worsened by the weather, terrain, or unique atmospheric conditions such as high altitude or being underwater.
- Risk factors that predispose people to environmental emergencies include being very young, being elderly, being in a poor state of health, and taking certain medications.
- Thermoregulation is the body's ability to ensure a balance between heat production and elimination. The hypothalamus is the organ involved in regulating this balance. The skin also has a major role.
- The body produces heat through metabolism. The basal metabolic rate (BMR) is the heat energy produced at rest from normal metabolic reactions. Metabolism can be increased through exertion, which also creates body heat. Absorption of heat from the environment can also occur.
- Thermolysis is the release of heat and energy from the body. Thermogenesis is the production of heat and energy for the body.
- The body has four main means of cooling itself: radiation—transfer of heat to the environment; conduction—transfer of heat to a cooler object through direct contact; convection—loss of heat to air moving across the skin; and evaporation—conversion of liquid to a gas (sweating).
- Heat illness is the increase in core body temperature due to inadequate thermolysis; the body cannot get rid of a heat buildup.
- Heat cramps are acute, involuntary muscle pains in the abdomen or lower extremities resulting from profuse sweating and sodium loss. The patient's pulse is usually rapid, the skin pale and moist, and the temperature normal. Treatment includes moving the patient to a cool environment, providing a salt-containing solution if the patient is not nauseated, or administering IV normal saline.
- Heat syncope can occur when an overheated patient suddenly changes position. Treatment includes placing the patient supine and replacing fluids.
- Heat exhaustion can result from dehydration and heat stress. Symptoms include headache, fatigue, dizziness, nausea, vomiting, and abdominal cramping. Skin is usually pale and clammy, and heart rate and respirations are rapid. Treatment consists of removing the patient from heat and providing fluids through sports drinks or an IV line.
- Heat stroke is defined as a core temperature above 40°C and altered mental status. Signs include changes in behaviour, nervous system disturbances (such as tremours), elevated temperature, tachycardia, hyperventilation, and skin that is dry and red or pale and sweaty. Treatment is to remove the patient from the heat, perform cooling measures, administer normal saline, and monitor the cardiac rhythm.
- Fever can mimic heat stroke. Take a thorough history, and treat for heat stroke if in doubt.
- To prevent heat illness, dress appropriately, stay hydrated, and stay in the shade or air conditioning. Community-based programmes aimed at high-risk populations can provide valuable education.
- Frostbite is local freezing of a body part; it is classified as superficial or deep. Frostnip is a very mild form of frostbite.

- Superficial frostbite is characterised by numbness, tingling, or burning. The skin is white, waxy, and firm to palpation. When thawed, the skin turns cyanotic and the patient feels a hot, stinging sensation. Treatment is getting the patient out of the cold; rewarming the injured part with body heat; covering with a warm, sterile dressing; and transporting the patient.
- In deep frostbite, the injured body part looks white, yellow-white, or mottled blue-white and is hard, cold, and without sensation. Major tissue damage can occur when the part thaws. Gangrene (permanent cell death) can result in the need for amputation. Treatment includes leaving the part frozen if it is found frozen, or rewarming the part if it is partially thawed.
- Trench foot is similar to frostbite but results from prolonged exposure to cool, wet conditions. Prevention is the best treatment.
- Hypothermia is a decrease in core body temperature. It can be mild, moderate, or severe.
- Mild hypothermia is a core body temperature between 32°C to 35°C. The patient shivers and may be confused, have slurred speech, or have impaired coordination. Treatment is passive rewarming such as removing wet clothing or drying the patient's skin and possibly providing warm fluids.
- Moderate hypothermia is a core body temperature in the range of 30°C to 32°C. Treatment is passive rewarming, active external rewarming of truncal areas, administering warmed IV fluids, and potentially using special rewarming devices.
- Severe hypothermia is a core body temperature less than 30°C. Treatment is active internal rewarming, such as administering warm IV fluids, and in-hospital measures.
- Hypothermic patients who are not breathing or who do not have a pulse need resuscitation. Patients in cardiac arrest require high-quality CPR and possibly a single shock depending on the heart rhythm. Attempt to insert an advanced airway; deliver ventilation with warm, humidified oxygen; and provide IV fluids.
- Hypothermic patients with obvious lethal traumatic injuries or patients who are so frozen as to block the airway or chest compression efforts generally are dead. If the patient appears dead after prolonged exposure, hypothermia may protect the brain and organs. Resuscitation can be attempted in cases of cardiac arrest and hypothermia.
- Drowning or submersion is the process of experiencing respiratory impairment from submersion or immersion in liquid. Drowning progresses from breath holding, to laryngospasm, to respiratory and cardiac arrest.
- Caring for a submersion patient starts with reaching the patient, a task that should be undertaken by specially trained rescuers. Treatment includes caring for the ABCs and taking cervical spine precautions. Positive end-expiratory pressure may be used to keep the alveoli open and drive fluid out. A nasogastric tube may be inserted to decompress the stomach if the patient is intubated. Submersion patients may develop bronchospasm and may require administration of a beta-2 adrenergic drug.
- Shallow water blackout occurs when a person hyperventilates just before diving underwater and passes out before resurfacing. Treatment is the same as for any other submersion.

◼ Vital Vocabulary

afterdrop Continued fall in core temperature after a victim of hypothermia has been removed from a cold environment, due at least in part to the return of cold blood from the body surface to the body core.

ataxia Inability to coordinate the muscles properly; often used to describe a staggering gait.

basal metabolic rate (BMR) The heat energy produced at rest from normal body metabolic reactions, determined mostly by the liver and skeletal muscles.

classic heat stroke Also called passive heat stroke, this is a serious heat illness that usually occurs during heat waves and is most likely to strike very old, very young, or bedridden people.

cold diuresis Secretion of large amounts of urine in response to cold exposure and the consequent shunting of blood volume to the body core.

conduction Transfer of heat to a solid object or a liquid by direct contact.

convection Mechanism by which body heat is picked up and carried away by moving air currents.

core body temperature (CBT) The temperature in the part of the body comprising the heart, lungs, brain, and abdominal viscera.

deep frostbite A type of frostbite in which the affected part looks white, yellow-white, or mottled blue-white and is hard, cold, and without sensation.

drowning The process of experiencing respiratory impairment from submersion or immersion in liquid.

environmental emergencies Medical conditions caused or exacerbated by the weather, terrain, or unique atmospheric conditions such as high altitude or underwater.

evaporation The conversion of a liquid to a gas.

exertional heat stroke A serious type of heat stroke usually affecting young and fit people exercising in hot and humid conditions.

exertional hyponatraemia A condition due to prolonged exertion in hot environments coupled with excessive hypotonic fluid intake that leads to nausea, vomiting, and, in severe cases, mental status changes and convulsions.

frostbite Localised damage to tissues resulting from prolonged exposure to extreme cold.

frostnip Early frostbite, characterised by numbness and pallor without significant tissue damage.

gangrene Permanent cell death.

heat cramps Acute and involuntary muscle pains, usually in the lower extremities, the abdomen, or both, that occur because of profuse sweating and subsequent sodium losses in sweat.

heat exhaustion A clinical syndrome characterised by volume depletion and heat stress that is thought to be a milder form of heat illness and on a continuum leading to heat stroke.

heat illness The increase in core body temperature due to inadequate thermolysis.

heat stroke The least common and most deadly heat illness, caused by a severe disturbance in thermoregulation, usually characterised by a core temperature of more than 40°C and altered mental status.

heat syncope An orthostatic or near-syncopal episode that typically occurs in nonacclimated individuals who may be under heat stress.

homeostasis Body processes that balance the supply and demand of the body's needs.

hyperthermia Unusually elevated body temperature.

hypothalamus Portion of the brain that regulates a multitude of body functions, including core temperature.

hypothermia Condition in which the core body temperature is significantly below normal.

laryngospasm Severe constriction of the larynx in response to allergy, noxious stimuli, or illness.

malignant hyperthermia A condition that can result from common anaesthesia medications (notably suxamethonium) and present with hyperthermia, muscular rigidity, altered mental status, and a hyperdynamic state.

neuroleptic malignant syndrome (NMS) A condition caused by antipsychotic and even common antiemetic medications that presents with hyperthermia, muscular rigidity, altered mental status, and a hyperdynamic state.

orthostatic hypotension A fall in blood pressure that occurs when moving from a recumbent to a sitting or standing position.

superficial frostbite A type of frostbite characterised by altered sensation (numbness, tingling, or burning) and white, waxy skin that is firm to palpation, but the underlying tissues remain soft.

thermogenesis The production of heat in the body.

thermolysis The liberation of heat from the body.

thermoregulation The process by which the body compensates for environmental extremes, for example, balancing between heat production and heat excretion.

trench foot A process similar to frostbite but caused by prolonged exposure to cool, wet conditions.

windchill factor The factor that takes into account the temperature and wind velocity in calculating the effect of a given ambient temperature on living organisms.

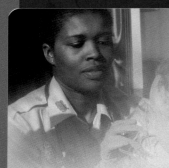

Assessment in Action

You are dispatched to older people's housing complex for an unconscious person. When you arrive on scene and enter the apartment, you find the patient lying on floor. This is the fourth day of a heat wave and the patient did not have her air conditioning unit on. The patient's heart rate is 120 beats/min; the respiratory rate is 36 breaths/min.

1. **What do you suspect is wrong with this patient?**
   A. Heat exhaustion
   B. Heat cramps
   C. Heat stroke
   D. Frostbite

2. **What are the two types of heat stroke?**
   A. Classic heat stroke and exertional heat stroke
   B. Thermolysis and thermoregulation
   C. Orthostatic hypotension and classic hypotension
   D. Classic heat stroke and orthostatic hypotension

3. **A clinical syndrome thought to represent a milder form of heat illness and on a continuum leading to heat stroke is:**
   A. heat cramps.
   B. classic heat stroke.
   C. hyponatraemia.
   D. heat exhaustion.

4. **A condition closely related to sodium-depleted heat exhaustion is:**
   A. classic heat stroke.
   B. exertional heat stroke.
   C. exertional hyponatraemia.
   D. heat exhaustion.

5. **Medical conditions caused or worsened by the weather, terrain, or unique atmospheric conditions such as high altitude or underwater are called:**
   A. hypothermia.
   B. hyperthermia.
   C. weather-related emergencies.
   D. environmental emergencies.

6. **Which of the following terms refers to the body processes that balance the supply and demand of the body's needs?**
   A. Homeostasis
   B. Thermoregulation
   C. Hypothalamus
   D. Body temperature

7. **The body's reaction to its daily production of heat energy and to hot environmental conditions is:**
   A. thermogenesis.
   B. thermolysis.
   C. hypothermia.
   D. hyperthermia.

8. **When warmed blood from the core and overheated muscles heads for the peripherally dilated cutaneous vessels, the four major means of cooling it are:**
   A. thermogenesis, thermolysis, hypothermia, and hyperthermia.
   B. radiation, conduction, convection, and evaporation.
   C. hypothermia, radiation, conduction, and hyperthermia.
   D. conduction, convection, evaporation, and thermogenesis.

Challenging Questions

You are treating a severely hypothermic middle-aged male who is in cardiac arrest. The man was found in a moorland area after being lost for 12 hours. The ambient temperature is −2.2°C. CPR is in progress and the patient has been successfully intubated. The A&E consultant requests over the phone that you attempt defibrillation one time if indicated, withhold all cardiac medications, and rapidly transport the patient to the closest appropriate facility.

9. **What affect would repeated defibrillation attempts have on this patient?**

10. **Why should medication therapy be withheld in cardiac arrest patients with severe hypothermia?**

■ Points to Ponder

You are dispatched for a man who has fallen outside. When you arrive, you find a man lying on the ground responsive to painful stimuli only. It is the middle of winter and is very cold. The patient is wearing only a light jacket and regular clothes. You immediately put the patient in the ambulance and begin assessing the patient. You turn the heat up in the back of the ambulance. The patient is extremely cold to the touch. His heart rate is 50 beats/min; blood pressure is 100/60 mm Hg; and

the respiratory rate is 12 breaths/min. You are unable to obtain a pulse oximetry reading.

What are your main concerns for this patient?

Issues: Understanding the Pathophysiology of Environmental Emergencies. Understanding the Treatment Modalities for Hypothermia. Understanding How Young and Old People Are at Risk for Hypothermia.

36

Infectious and Communicable Diseases

Objectives

Cognitive

- Review the specific anatomy and physiology pertinent to infectious and communicable diseases.
- Define specific terminology identified with infectious/communicable diseases.
- Discuss public health principles relevant to infectious/communicable disease.
- Identify public health agencies involved in the prevention and management of disease outbreaks.
- List and describe the steps of an infectious process.
- Discuss the risks associated with infection.
- List and describe the stages of infectious diseases.
- List and describe infectious agents, including bacteria, viruses, fungi, protozoans, and helminths (worms).
- Describe host defence mechanisms against infection.
- Describe characteristics of the immune system, including the categories of white blood cells, the reticuloendothelial system (RES), and the complement system.
- Describe the processes of the immune system defences, to include humoral and cell-mediated immunity.
- In specific diseases, identify and discuss the issues of personal isolation.
- Describe and discuss the rationale for the various types of PPE.
- Discuss what constitutes a significant exposure to an infectious agent.
- Describe the assessment of a patient suspected of, or identified as having, an infectious/communicable disease.
- Discuss the proper disposal of contaminated supplies (sharps, gauze sponges, tourniquets, etc.).
- Discuss disinfection of patient care equipment, and areas in which care of the patient occurred.
- Discuss the following relative to HIV—causative agent, body systems affected and potential secondary complications, modes of transmission, the seroconversion rate after direct significant exposure, susceptibility and resistance, signs and symptoms, specific patient management and personal protective measures, and immunisation.
- Discuss hepatitis A, including the causative agent, body systems affected and potential secondary complications, routes of transmission, susceptibility and resistance, signs and symptoms, patient management and protective measures, and immunisation.
- Discuss hepatitis B (serum hepatitis), including the causative agent, the organ affected and potential secondary complications, routes of transmission, signs and symptoms, patient management and protective measures, and immunisation.
- Discuss the susceptibility and resistance to hepatitis B.
- Discuss hepatitis C, including the causative agent, the organ affected, routes of transmission, susceptibility and resistance, signs and symptoms, patient management and protective measures, and immunisation and control measures.
- Discuss hepatitis D (hepatitis delta virus), including the causative agent, the organ affected, routes of transmission, susceptibility and resistance, signs and symptoms, patient management and protective measures, and immunisation and control measures.
- Discuss hepatitis E, including the causative agent, the organ affected, routes of transmission, susceptibility and resistance, signs and symptoms, patient management and protective measures, and immunisation and control measures.
- Discuss tuberculosis, including the causative agent, body systems affected and secondary complications, routes of transmission, susceptibility and resistance, signs and symptoms, patient management and protective measures, and immunisation and control measures.
- Discuss meningococcal meningitis (spinal meningitis), including causative organisms, tissues affected, modes of transmission, susceptibility and resistance, signs and symptoms, patient management and protective measures, and immunisation and control measures.
- Discuss other infectious agents known to cause meningitis including streptococcus pneumonia, haemophilus influenza type b, and other varieties of viruses.
- Discuss pneumonia, including causative organisms, body systems affected, routes of transmission, susceptibility and resistance, signs and symptoms, patient management and protective measures, and immunisation.
- Discuss tetanus, including the causative organism, the body system affected, modes of transmission, susceptibility and resistance, signs and symptoms, patient management and protective measures, and immunisation.
- Discuss rabies and hantavirus as they apply to regional environmental exposures, including the causative organisms, the body systems affected, routes of transmission, susceptibility and resistance, signs and symptoms, patient management and protective measures, and immunisation and control measures.
- Identify paediatric viral diseases.
- Discuss chickenpox, including the causative organism, the body system affected, mode of transmission, susceptibility and resistance, signs and symptoms, patient management and protective measures, and immunisation and control measures.
- Discuss mumps, including the causative organism, the body organs and systems affected, mode of transmission, susceptibility and resistance, signs and symptoms, patient management and protective measures, and immunisation.
- Discuss rubella (German measles), including the causative agent, the body tissues and systems affected, modes of transmission, susceptibility and resistance, signs and symptoms, patient management and protective measures, and immunisation.
- Discuss measles (rubeola, hard measles), including the causative organism, the body tissues, organs, and systems affected, mode of transmission, susceptibility and resistance, signs and symptoms, patient management and protective measures, and immunisation.

- Discuss the importance of immunisation, and those diseases, especially in the paediatric population, which warrant widespread immunisation (MMR).
- Discuss pertussis (whooping cough), including the causative organism, the body organs affected, mode of transmission, susceptibility and resistance, signs and symptoms, patient management and protective measures, and immunisation.
- Discuss influenza, including causative organisms, the body system affected, mode of transmission, susceptibility and resistance, signs and symptoms, patient management and protective measures, and immunisation.
- Discuss mononucleosis, including the causative organisms, the body regions, organs, and systems affected, modes of transmission, susceptibility and resistance, signs and symptoms, patient management and protective measures, and immunisation.
- Discuss herpes simplex type 1, including the causative organism, the body regions and system affected, modes of transmission, susceptibility and resistance, signs and symptoms, patient management and protective measures, and immunisation.
- Discuss the characteristics of, and organisms associated with, febrile and afebrile respiratory disease, to include bronchiolitis, bronchitis, laryngitis, croup, epiglottitis, and the common cold.
- Discuss syphilis, including the causative organism, the body regions, organs, and systems affected, modes of transmission, susceptibility and resistance, stages of signs and symptoms, patient management and protective measures, and immunisation.
- Discuss gonorrhoea, including the causative organism, the body organs and associated structures affected, mode of transmission, susceptibility and resistance, signs and symptoms, patient management and protective measures, and immunisation.
- Discuss chlamydia, including the causative organism, the body regions, organs, and systems affected, modes of transmission, susceptibility and resistance, signs and symptoms, patient management and protective measures, and immunisation.
- Discuss herpes simplex 2 (genital herpes), including the causative organism, the body regions, tissues, and structures affected, mode of transmission, susceptibility and resistance, signs and symptoms, patient management and protective measures, and immunisation.
- Discuss scabies, including the aetiologic agent, the body organs affected, modes of transmission, susceptibility and resistance, signs and symptoms, patient management and protective measures, and immunisation.
- Discuss lice, including the infesting agents, the body regions affected, modes of transmission and host factors, susceptibility and resistance, signs and symptoms, patient management and protective measures, and prevention.

- Describe Lyme disease, including the causative organism, the body organs and systems affected, mode of transmission, susceptibility and resistance, phases of signs and symptoms, patient management and control measures, and immunisation.
- Discuss gastroenteritis, including the causative organisms, the body system affected, modes of transmission, susceptibility and resistance, signs and symptoms, patient management and protective measures, and immunisation.
- Discuss the local guideline for reporting and documenting an infectious/communicable disease exposure.
- Articulate the pathophysiological principles of an infectious process given a case study of a patient with an infectious/communicable disease.
- Articulate the prehospital assessment and management, to include safety considerations, of a patient presenting with signs and symptoms suggestive of an infectious/communicable disease.

Affective

- Advocate compliance with standards and guidelines by role modelling adherence to universal precautions and body substance isolation (BSI).
- Value the importance of immunisation, especially in children and populations at risk.
- Value the safe management of a patient with an infectious/communicable disease.
- Advocate respect for the feelings of patients, family, and others at the scene of an infectious/communicable disease.
- Advocate empathy for a patient with an infectious/communicable disease.
- Value the importance of infectious/communicable disease control.
- Consistently demonstrate the use of body substance isolation.

Psychomotor

- Demonstrate the ability to comply with body substance isolation guidelines.
- Perform an assessment of a patient with an infectious/communicable disease.
- Effectively and safely manage a patient with an infectious/communicable disease, including airway and ventilation care, support of circulation, pharmacological intervention, transport considerations, psychological support/communication strategies, and other considerations as mandated by local guideline.

Introduction

In 1913, Randolph Borne said "We can become as much slaves to precaution as we can to fear". This statement is particularly relevant to NHS ambulance care in the streets today, because many care providers are fearful when caring for patients who have or are suspected to have a communicable disease. A paramedic who does not understand how communicable diseases are transmitted and how to take sensible precautions will be hesitant in caring for some patients, no matter what the cause of their illness. This chapter examines the ways in which communicable diseases are transmitted from one person to another. The communicable diseases that paramedics are most likely to encounter in the course of their work are examined, as well as those illnesses that create the greatest anxiety among health care personnel and the public at large. Finally, the chapter reviews the measures that a paramedic can take to protect against communicable disease.

Agencies Responsible for Protecting the Public Health

A number of government agencies are responsible for protecting the health of the general public. Agencies at the national level include the Health Protection Agency (HPA), the National Institute for Clinical Excellence (NICE), the Health and Safety Executive (HSE), the Department for Environment, Food, and Rural Affairs (DEFRA), and the Department of Health (DoH), which have precise rules and regulations designed to protect the employees of public and private organisations. This chapter refers to several regulations, governed by the HSE and the DoH. Data on the numbers of patients infected as well as research and guidance for health care providers and the general public are available from the Department of Health and the Health Protection Agency.

Disease prevention and public health protection are managed at both local and national levels, and whilst paramedics might not feel they are directly responsible for water quality, food hygiene, and immunisation programmes, it is clearly beneficial for ambulance trusts to know their local public health officials and to work with them. When potential threats to a community's health exist—such as anthrax, SARS, and bird flu—a close working relationship between ambulance trusts and public health agencies is essential.

Host Defence Mechanisms

The human body provides "built-in protection" from pathogenic organisms with several defences that protect you against infection.

Skin, which covers the entire exterior of the body, offers a primary protective barrier blocking pathogens' ability to enter through the intact surface. The normal secretions of the skin also provide an antibacterial property that protects against pathogen entry. This is why antibacterial handwashing solutions should not be used; these solutions kill off large amounts of bacteria and viruses on the skin, including normal flora.

Mucous membranes offer another protective barrier. For example, the eyes produce tears that dilute and remove foreign substances. The mucous membranes that line the urinary, respiratory, and gastrointestinal (GI) tract also trap and remove organisms. Cells that line the respiratory tract secrete lysozymes that destroy bacteria, while macrophages trap and destroy bacteria; thus these mucous membranes serve as the first line of defence against airborne and droplet-transmitted diseases. Goblet cells lining the GI tract produce highly acidic and alkaline secretions, which form barriers that prevent penetration by bacteria and some viruses.

You are the Paramedic Part 1

You are dispatched to a house for an older woman who is "not feeling well". You are greeted by a family member who identifies herself as the 999 caller. She tells you that she found her 70-year-old grandmother lying on the floor of the toilet complaining of "feeling sick and hurting all over". She thinks that her grandmother has been on the floor since sometime yesterday.

You are unable to bring all of your bags and equipment into the toilet because of the cramped space, and your patient is wedged behind the toilet door. Before entering, you peek around the door to perform a quick initial assessment. After you squeeze through the doorway, you must close the door to gain complete access to the patient's face and head.

Initial Assessment	Recording Time: 0 Minutes
Appearance	Fetal position, appears tired
Level of consciousness	A (Alert to person, place and day)
Airway	Patent, occasional cough
Breathing	Rapid and shallow
Circulation	Flushed face, sweaty skin, rapid pulse

1. Given your initial findings, what do you know about the patient's overall condition?
2. What are your immediate concerns?

The immune system contains proteins that kill viruses. Immune response ignites the production of antibodies that are directed against a specific invading organism. Both B cells and T cells work together to fight infection.

The Cycle of Infection

Infection involves a chain of events through which the communicable disease spreads. In some cases, solving the puzzle of why a particular individual or group of individuals developed a specific disease may be as simple as retracing steps to find the source of exposure. In other cases, the puzzle is more difficult to solve, with infectious disease experts taking years to find a pattern in the spread of a disease and then plan a strategy to break the chain of the infection. The study of infectious diseases takes into consideration population demographics that can affect the spread of a disease, such as age distributions; genetic factors; income levels; ethnic groups; workplaces and schools; geographical boundaries; and the expansion, decline, or movement of the disease.

Here's a classic tale that illustrates how easily disease may spread. In a local hospital paediatric ward, a visitor brought a bag of sweets for a child. Because of the "no food" rule, his attentive nurse placed the sweets at the nurses' station. Another nurse had emptied a bedpan of stool from a child admitted for hepatitis A infection, but was in such a rush that she forgot to wash her hands. She then noticed the bag of sweets, poked a few selections, and finally found one she wanted to eat. The sweets, being out in a public place, were consumed throughout the morning. Subsequently, another nurse came down with hepatitis A, a disease that is typically spread by the oral–faecal route. Obviously, the chain of infection in this scenario could have been broken by handwashing and following a few simple rules.

Transmission of Communicable Diseases

By the very nature of their work, health care providers come in contact with sick people; a certain proportion of those sick people have contagious diseases. Communicable diseases can be transmitted from one person to another under certain conditions **Figure 36-1 ▶**.

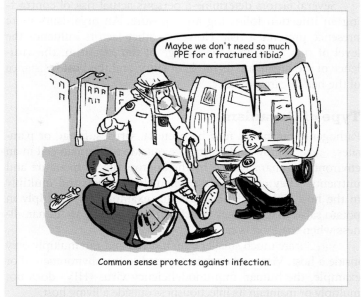

Common sense protects against infection.

Figure 36-1

To understand the principles of prevention, you must first understand how diseases are spread. Communicable diseases are caused by microorganisms—usually bacteria or viruses, but sometimes fungi and parasites. They spread from person to person by several specific mechanisms:

- **Direct contact** with the infected person—that is, by touching. Direct contact may be as brief as touching one patient after caring for another patient or as intimate as sexual intercourse. Most cases of the common cold are thought to be transmitted through casual direct contact. Venereal diseases, such as syphilis and gonorrhoea, are transmitted principally by sexual contact, and are therefore referred to as sexually transmitted infections (STIs).
- **Indirect contact**—for example, touching a bloody stretcher railing with an open cut or sore on your hand. Objects that harbour micro-organisms and can transmit them to others are called fomites. Towels used by a patient are a good illustration of fomites that could transmit the infection.
- **Inhalation** of infected droplets, such as those released into the surroundings when a person with pulmonary tuberculosis (TB) coughs or sneezes.
- **Puncture by a contaminated needle** or other sharp instrument. Punctures may occur if a health care provider is not using needlesafe or needleless devices.
- **Transfusion** of contaminated blood products. Screening tests for bloodborne disease have vastly reduced the risks of contracting illnesses from contaminated blood. However, donated blood is not 100% safe from bloodborne pathogens.
- **Vectorborne.** A vector is a vehicle that transmits infection from a reservoir to a host. For example, a mosquito infected with West Nile virus that bites a susceptible person may transmit the disease.

Several factors determine a person's actual risk of contracting an infection following an exposure. An organism's mere presence presents a risk. However, other factors influence the level of risk, including the dosage of the organism, the virulence of the organism, its mode of entry, and the host resistance of the health care provider.

Type of Organism

Pathogenic organisms may be bacteria, viruses, fungi, or parasites. Bacteria grow and reproduce outside the human cell in an environment characterised by the appropriate temperature and nutrients. They cause disease when they invade and multiply in the host. Salmonella bacteria, for example, can multiply in potato salad that has been unrefrigerated, leading to human illness when the food is eaten.

Viruses are much smaller than bacteria and can multiply only inside a host. Viruses die when exposed to the environment. For example, the human immunodeficiency virus (HIV) does not multiply or maintain its infectiousness outside a living host.

Fungi are similar to bacteria in that they can grow rapidly in the presence of nutrients and organic material. Most fungal infections are acquired from contact with decaying organic matter or from airborne spores in the environment (eg, moulds).

Parasites live in or on another living creature. They take advantage of their host by feeding off its cells and tissues. Scabies and lice are examples. Parasites include both protozoans—single-celled, usually microscopic, eukaryotic organisms (eg, amoebas, ciliates, flagellates, and sporozoans)—and helminths (commonly called worms), which are invertebrates with long, flexible, rounded or flattened bodies.

Dosage of the Organism

A certain number of organisms must be present for infection to occur. For example, the laboratory report on a urine specimen sent for culture may note "greater than 100,000 colonies of bacteria per millilitre of urine" or "infection is not present".

Virulence of the Organism

Virulence is the ability of an organism to invade and create disease in a host. It also encompasses the organism's ability to survive outside the living host. For example, HIV does not pose a risk outside the human body because it dies upon exposure to light and air.

Mode of Entry

If the organism does not enter the body by the correct route, infection cannot occur. Thus if you suspect a patient has a respiratory communicable disease and you mask the patient, you can't inhale the droplets.

Host Resistance

The healthier you are, the less susceptible you are to infection. Your ability to fight off infection is called host resistance. Your immune system will protect you from acquiring disease even though all of the other risk factors may be present. Wellness programmes and vaccine/immunisation programmes serve to boost host resistance.

At the Scene

Exposure does not mean infection.

Once a susceptible person has been exposed to an organism, it takes time for the organism to multiply within the body and produce symptoms. That time period—between exposure to the organism and the first symptoms of illness—is called the incubation period. For example, it usually takes 12 to 26 days from a susceptible person's exposure to the mumps virus until the patient begins to feel feverish and unwell. The incubation period for the influenza virus is much shorter—usually 24 to 72 hours.

Most communicable diseases are contagious only during a portion of the illness. A person may be sick with chickenpox for 2 to 3 weeks, but is capable of transmitting the virus to another individual for only about 1 week—from 1 day before the vesicles appear on the skin to about 6 days after. The period during which a person can transmit the illness to someone else is called the communicable period.

Just as exposure and infection are different concepts, we also need to distinguish between contamination and infection. An object that has organisms on or in it is contaminated. This term applies to water, food, dressing materials, linens, sharps, equipment, and even the ambulance. A person is not infected, however, unless the organisms actually produce an illness. With some diseases, such as hepatitis B or C viral infection, a person may have the disease and not be aware of it; there are no signs or symptoms, and the person is not ill. However, such carriers can pass the disease on to others through their blood or through sexual contact.

In the context of communicable disease, a reservoir is a place where organisms may live and multiply. In institutional settings, for example, air-conditioning systems and showerheads have been identified as reservoirs for the bacterium that causes Legionnaires' disease. Obviously, health care personnel have a responsibility not only to protect themselves from contracting communicable diseases, but also to ensure that they and their equipment do not transmit illness to others.

Precautions for the Health Care Provider

Although the risk of contracting a communicable disease is real, it should not be exaggerated and certainly should not be a source of fear and stress. Fear comes from lack of proper education and training, and there is no reason a paramedic should not be properly educated about disease issues.

At the Scene

Infection control works for the patient and the health care provider.

Designated Infection Control Manager

The HSE requires that each ambulance trust has a designated Infection Control Manager (ICM) or similar. This individual is charged with ensuring that proper post-exposure medical treatment and counselling is provided to the exposed employee/volunteer. Post-exposure medical treatment is offered to prevent the exposed health care provider from contracting the disease to which he or she was exposed. Treatment should be offered within 24 to 48 hours following an exposure, with the actual time frame being based on the diagnosis; exposure to bacterial meningitis, for example, would require treatment within 24 hours. The ICM tracks and follows the correct time frames, serves as a liaison between the exposed employee and the medical facility, ensures that confidentiality is maintained, and makes sure that documentation adheres to guidelines. This is essential to ensure the human rights of the employee are met.

The communication network for exposure reporting varies across ambulance trusts. However each trust will have a documented procedure for managing exposure that complies with Health and Safety Legislation.

Health Protection Agency

The HPA Centre for Infections (CfI) carries out a broad spectrum of work relating to prevention of infectious disease. The remit of the centre includes infectious disease surveillance, collecting and monitoring national disease statistics, providing specialist and reference microbiology and microbial epidemiology, co-ordinating the investigation and cause of national and uncommon outbreaks, helping advise government on the risks posed by various infections, and responding to international health alerts.

Universal Precautions

The term universal precautions is used to describe infection control practices that reduce the opportunity for an exposure to occur in the daily care of patients. It replaces the older terms Category 1 and 11. Universal precautions are measures which must be adopted routinely in dealing with all patients. For example, if a patient has oral herpes lesions and you are suctioning without a glove and have an open cut or sore, your finger could become infected with herpes. These precautions apply to all body substances except sweat.

You are the Paramedic Part 2

Because of the problem with access, you decide to utilise the carry chair to move the patient to your trolley in the next room. During transfer you notice that the patient is quite warm and coughs occasionally. When you ask about her flu-like symptoms, she says she has had chills and a dry cough for a few days.

Vital Signs	Recording Time: 7 Minutes
Level of consciousness	A (Alert to person, place, and day)
Skin	Flushed, warm, and sweaty
Pulse	110 beats/min, weak radial pulse
Blood pressure	118/72 mm Hg
Respirations	36 breaths/min, shallow
S$_P$O$_2$	90% on room air

3. Think of a few potential illnesses that could cause these signs and symptoms.
4. Of those, which are the most serious and why?

Table 36-1	Recommended Immunisations/ Vaccinations for Health Care Providers

- Chickenpox
- Tetanus
- Diphtheria
- Poliomyelitis
- BCG (Tuberculosis)
- Hepatitis B
- MMR (Measles, mumps, rubella)

Adapted from the Department of Health and the Health Protection Agency.

DoH-Recommended Immunisations and Vaccinations

Keeping current with recommended vaccines and immunisations boosts host resistance and the immune response. The DoH guidelines are detailed in the Green Book (revised 2006). The recommended immunisations for health care providers are listed in (Table 36-1 ▲).

Personal Protective Equipment

Personal protective equipment (PPE) serves as a secondary protective barrier beyond what your body provides. The selection and use of PPE depends on the task and procedure at hand. Your trust's Infection Control Policy should contain a listing of its risk procedures and the recommended use of PPE. The DoH has also developed guidelines for PPE (Table 36-2 ▼).

Handwashing is your major protective measure. The current standard for handwashing is the use of antimicrobial, alcohol-based foams or gels (Figure 36-2 ▶).

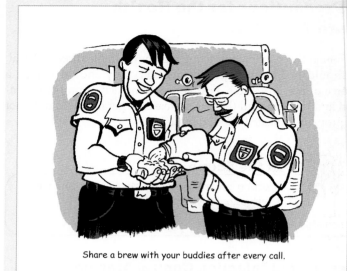

Share a brew with your buddies after every call.

Figure 36-2

Use of antibacterial products is not recommended. The friction used in antimicrobial alcohol-based foams and gels to make them evaporate removes surface organisms and kills viruses, but leaves the normal flora intact.

Notes from Nancy

Wash your hands after every call.

Table 36-2	Recommended Personal Protective Equipment for Prevention of Transmission of HIV and Hepatitis B Virus in the Prehospital Setting			
Task or Activity	**Disposable Gloves**	**Apron**	**Mask**	**Protective Eyewear**
Bleeding control with spurting blood	Yes	Yes	Yes	Yes
Bleeding control with minimal bleeding	Yes	No	No	No
Emergency childbirth	Yes	Yes	Yes, if splashing is likely	Yes, if splashing is likely
Blood drawing	Recommended for health care providers	No	No	No
Starting an intravenous line	Yes	No	No	No
Endotracheal intubation, laryngeal mask airway use	Yes	No	No, unless splashing is likely*	No, unless splashing is likely*
Oral/nasal suctioning, manually cleaning airway	Yes	No	No, unless splashing is likely*	No, unless splashing is likely*
Handling and cleaning instruments with microbial contamination	Yes	No, unless soiling is likely	No	No
Measuring blood pressure	No	No	No	No
Measuring temperature	No	No	No	No
Giving an injection	Recommended for health care providers	No	No	No

*Splashing is often likely, so use PPE accordingly.

Adapted from the Department of Health and the Health Protection Agency.

Rubella occurs most commonly during the winter and spring and is highly communicable to susceptible individuals. Transmission occurs by direct contact with the nasopharyngeal secretions of an infected person—either by droplet spread or by touching the patient or articles freshly contaminated with the patient's secretions. The incubation period is 14 to 23 days. The communicable period starts about a week before the rash appears and continues until 4 days after the rash becomes evident.

As with measles, the only certain protection against rubella is immunity. All paramedics should be immunised against rubella before starting their employment. No special measures are needed to disinfect the ambulance after carrying a patient known to have rubella. Prevention measures include masking the patient with a surgical mask. Post-exposure treatment includes a vaccine if you are not immune. Practise universal precautions and routine cleaning after transport of a rubella patient.

Mumps

Mumps is a viral disease that occurs most commonly in winter and spring. Signs and symptoms in children include fever plus swelling and tenderness of one of the salivary glands, usually the parotid. Mumps in males past the age of puberty may have a very painful complication; inflammation of the testicles occurs in up to 25% of cases, but this does not result in sterility. Thus while rubella is a matter of particular concern for female paramedics, mumps should worry any male paramedic who did not have the illness or receive immunisation against it as a child. All paramedics should be immunised against mumps before starting employment if they are not already immune.

Transmission of mumps occurs by droplet spread or direct contact with the saliva of an infected person. The incubation period is 12 to 26 days. The communicable period lasts 9 days after the salivary glands swell up. As a precaution, place a surgical mask on the mumps patient. Wear gloves when in contact with drainage, and carry out routine cleaning following patient transport. Post-exposure treatment with a vaccine is not recommended. Work restriction will apply.

Chickenpox

Chickenpox, also known as varicella, is a highly contagious viral disease that produces a slight fever, photosensitivity, and a vesicular rash that gradually crusts over, leaving a series of scabs **Figure 36-8 ▸** . The rash comes in crops, moving from the covered areas of the body to uncovered areas. The same virus can lead to herpes zoster ("shingles") in adults. Herpes zoster arises when the chickenpox virus takes up residence in the ganglion of a nerve. When the individual later becomes stressed (physically or emotionally), lesions may appear along the affected nerve pathway. Herpes zoster can be extremely painful.

Transmission of varicella virus occurs by direct contact or droplet spread of respiratory secretions from patients with chickenpox. Contact with the vesicular fluid of patients with either chickenpox or herpes zoster, and probably contact with articles recently contaminated by that fluid, can also transmit the virus. The incubation period for chickenpox is 10 to 21 days. The communicable period starts 1 to 2 days before the appearance of the rash and lasts about 5 days after the first vesicles become apparent.

Having chickenpox as a child usually provides lifelong immunity against infection. When transporting a patient suspected of having chickenpox, place a surgical mask on the patient. Wear gloves when in contact with discharges or drainage from lesions. Post-exposure treatment includes a vaccine if not immune. If the exposed person is pregnant or immunocompromised, varicella zoster immunoglobulin should be offered.

Pertussis

Pertussis (whooping cough) is a bacterial infection. It has an insidious onset and is characterised by an irritating cough that becomes paroxysmal in about 1 to 2 weeks; this cough may last for 1 to 2 months. In recent years, the incidence of this disease has been increasing in adolescents and young adults. Some cases have occurred in previously vaccinated people who have diminished immunity.

Transmission takes place through direct contact with discharges from mucous membranes and/or airborne droplets. The incubation period is 7 to 14 days. This disease is highly communicable in its early stages before the cough becomes paroxysmal, and then becomes negligible in about 3 weeks. Prevention includes placing a surgical mask on the patient. If coughing makes this placement difficult, try a nonrebreathing mask. Post-exposure care may include antibiotic treatment. Good handwashing and routine cleaning of the vehicle are the only special measures required after transporting a patient with pertussis. All paramedics should be assessed for vaccination with DPT (diphtheria, pertussis, tetanus).

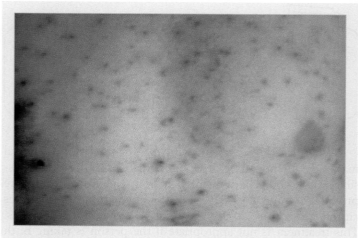

Figure 36-8 The distinctive rash produced by chickenpox.

Other Common or Serious Communicable Diseases

Meningitis

Meningitis is an inflammation of the membranes that cover the brain and spinal cord, called the meninges. Two types of meningitis are distinguished: bacterial and viral. The bacterial form is communicable, and the viral form is not. Meningitis is not transmitted through the air, but rather is a droplet-transmitted disease. The most common bacterial organisms implicated in meningitis are *Neisseria meningitidis, Streptococcus pneumoniae, Haemophilus influenzae,* group B *Streptococcus,* and *Listeria monocytogenes.*

The type of meningitis most often involved in epidemic outbreaks is meningococcal meningitis, which is caused by *N meningitidis.* Sporadic cases of meningococcal meningitis occur most frequently during winter and spring, but epidemic outbreaks can occur at any time, especially where young people live together under crowded conditions, such as in college dorms or military barracks. The classic signs and symptoms of meningitis are the same for both the viral and bacterial forms: sudden-onset fever, severe headache, neck stiffness, photosensitivity, and a pink rash that becomes purple in colour. The patient almost always experiences changes in mental status, ranging from apathy to delirium. Projectile vomiting is common. Diagnosis is made by Gram's stain.

Transmission occurs following direct contact with the nasopharyngeal secretions of an infected person (mouth-to-mouth, suctioning/intubation with spraying of secretions). The incubation period for meningococcal meningitis lasts between 2 and 10 days. The communicable period is variable, as it lasts as long as meningococcal bacteria are present in the patient's nasal and oral secretions. The microorganisms generally disappear from the patient's upper respiratory tract within 24 hours after antibiotic treatment begins.

At the Scene

Meningococcal bacteria are unable to survive outside of the respiratory tract. Therefore, risk of contamination is minimal, except when exposed to large droplets or secretions. All paramedics should in confirmed cases, seek medical advice.

When treating a patient with meningitis, place a surgical mask or nonrebreathing mask on the patient. If this is not possible, mask yourself. Transmission from patient to health care provider is rare. Post-exposure treatment typically includes ciprofloxacin (one dose given orally) or rifampin for 2 days. This treatment is not appropriate if the person is taking birth control pills, and it should not be offered to pregnant personnel. Meningitis vaccine is not recommended for any health care provider group; it is recommended for college students enter-

ing dormitory living for the first time, military recruits, and all secondary school pupils.

Tuberculosis

Tuberculosis (TB) was once widespread in the United Kingdom, but no longer, with an incidence of 161.16 cases per 100,000 population in 2005. This disease remains an important cause of disability and death in much of the developing world, however.

TB is *not* a highly communicable disease. Three types of TB exist: typical, which is communicable, and atypical and extrapulmonary (TB of the bone, kidney, lymph glands, and so on), which are not communicable.

TB infection means that the individual has tested positive for exposure to TB but does not have, and may never develop, active disease. People with TB infection do not pose a risk to others. *TB disease* means that the individual has active TB disease verified by laboratory testing and a positive chest X-ray.

During the 1990s multidrug–resistant TB emerged as a threat in the USA and worldwide. Although it was initially an untreatable disease, therapies for it are now available. Multidrug-resistant TB occurs in immunocompromised people who have not complied with their full course of treatment, but its incidence is quite low. In the UK, 1.1% of all isolates are multidrug-resistant and there is no suggestion of an increase in this type of TB in the UK.

Signs and symptoms of TB include a persistent cough for more than 3 weeks plus one of more of the following: night sweats, headache, weight loss, haemoptysis, or chest pain. Transmission occurs by airborne droplets from a person with active untreated disease. In general, that type of spread occurs among people who have continued, intimate exposure to the infected individual (primarily those living in the same household). For the paramedic, such intense exposure is likely to occur only when mouth-to-mouth ventilation is given to a patient with active untreated TB. Thanks to new medications, 10% of people are no longer communicable after 2 days of treatment.

At the Scene

Notify your ICM if you believe you may have been exposed to TB. The hospital is required to notify the ICM if a patient you have transported may have TB.

The incubation period for TB is 4 to 12 weeks. The disease is communicable only when an active lesion develops in the lungs and droplets are expelled into the air by coughing. Ten percent of patients are no longer communicable after 2 days of treatment. After 14 days of treatment virtually all patients are no longer communicable.

Early infection with TB can be detected either by a tuberculin skin test or by the QFT-TB Gold blood test. All health care providers, including paramedics, may have had a tuberculin test at the beginning of employment and periodically based on the TB risk assessment for the trust. If a known positive history is present on employment, then a questionnaire must be completed. A chest X-ray is indicated only for a first positive test.

As a preventive measure, place a surgical mask on the suspected TB patient. If prevention was not taken, report the incident to your ICM. Given that the incubation period for TB is 4 to 12 weeks, the paramedic who suspects he or she has been exposed to TB should assess the need for baseline testing and then be retested in 8 to 10 weeks. If the test has become positive at that time, the individual will have a chest X-ray to rule out infection and usually will be offered a 6- to 9-month course of antibiotic therapy. Because these drugs are toxic to the liver, the individual should not consume alcohol while on the drugs and liver function tests should be done monthly.

Notes from Nancy

TB is *not* a highly communicable disease.

No special measures are required after transporting a patient suspected of having active TB. The vehicle should be cleaned as usual.

Pneumonia

Pneumonia is the fifth leading cause of death in the UK, with 1 to 3 cases per 1,000 population affected in this way. The cause of pneumonia may be bacteria, viruses, fungi, or other organisms. More than 50 types of pneumonia have been identified, ranging from mild to life-threatening. Individuals who are most susceptible to pneumonia are older adults, heavy smokers or alcoholics, individuals with chronic illnesses, and immunocompromised individuals. Worldwide, pneumonia is a leading cause of death in paediatric patients, particularly infants. Although antibiotics have been very successful in treating the most common forms of bacterial pneumonia, some antibiotic-resistant strains pose a very serious therapeutic challenge.

Other Respiratory Conditions

A number of "other respiratory conditions" may (or may not) be associated with a fever and may (or may not) be infectious. These conditions run the gamut from basic annoyance to potentially life-threatening conditions.

Bronchiolitis is an infection of the lungs and airways that usually occurs in children 3 to 6 months of age. The child starts with a runny nose and slight fever. After 2 to 3 days, the child is wheezing and coughing with tachypnoea and tachycardia. The cause is usually viral (eg, respiratory syncytial virus, parainfluenza, influenza). Transmission of bronchiolitis generally occurs by inhaling droplets of infected mucus or respiratory secretions.

Bronchitis arises when the inner walls of the bronchioles become infected and inflamed. Symptoms include soreness in the chest and throat, congestion, wheezing, dyspnoea, and a slight fever. This condition is caused by the same virus that produces the common cold and gastric reflux disease, as well as by common pollutants and smoking or secondhand smoke. "Chronic" bronchitis patients cough most days for spans of 3 months or more a year, for two or more consecutive years. Chronic bronchitis is discussed further in Chapter 26.

Laryngitis is an inflammation of the voice box due to overuse, irritation, or infection. Its cause is usually viral but can be bacterial. Symptoms include hoarseness, weak voice, sore throat, dry throat, and cough.

Croup is the inflammation of the larynx and airway just below it. It primarily affects children 5 years old or younger. Croup comes on strongest in the nightime and may last 3 to 7 days. Symptoms include a loud, harsh, barking cough; fever; noisy inhalations; hoarse voice; and mild to moderate dyspnoea. This infection is caused by a virus, similar to the common cold, as well as by other viruses (eg, parainfluenza, respiratory syncytial virus, measles, adenovirus). It is spread by respiratory secretions or droplets from coughing, sneezing, and breathing.

Epiglottitis is a life-threatening condition that causes the epiglottis and supraglottic tissue to swell. The pus-filled flap of tissue then partially or completely occludes the glottic opening. Although this disease can affect any age group, it is most prevalent in 2- to 7-year-olds. Its incidence has fallen sharply since 1985, when administration of the Hib vaccine to 2-month-old infants became routine. Symptoms include difficulty breathing and swallowing with stridor and drooling. Patients are very anxious, are cyanotic, and have a muffled voice and fever. Epiglottitis is caused by the *Haemophilus influenzae* type b (Hib) bacteria and is contagious by the droplet route via coughing and sneezing.

The common cold is an infection of the upper respiratory system characterised by a runny nose, sore throat, cough, congestion, and watery eyes. Any one of 200 viruses can cause the cold, so symptoms may vary. Patients do not have a fever. Colds are very common in preschoolers but can occur in patients of all ages. Colds usually last about a week and are spread by droplets, coughing, hand-to-hand contact, and shared utensils.

Respiratory Syncytial Virus

Respiratory syncytial virus (RSV) is the leading cause of lower respiratory tract infections in infants, older people, and immunocompromised individuals. This virus spreads in the hospital environment as well as in the community. In the community setting, outbreaks generally occur in late autumn, winter, and early spring.

Signs and symptoms include those of upper respiratory infection—sneezing, runny nose, nasal congestion, cough, and fever. The disease progression moves to the lower respiratory tract, leading to pneumonia, bronchiolitis, and tracheobronchitis. Hypoxaemia and apnoea are often seen in infants and are usually the leading cause for the child's hospitalisation.

Transmission may occur in two ways: (1) by direct contact with large droplets that do not extend more than 1 m, or (2) by indirect contact with contaminated hands or contaminated items. Research has shown that RSV can survive on hands for less than 1 hour; however, the virus has been shown to survive on other surfaces for as long as 30 hours. The infection's incubation period ranges from 2 to 8 days.

Prevention of RSV transmission relies on proper use of PPE. Gloves should be worn when caring for the RSV-infected patient, and their removal must be followed by good handwashing. The use of alcohol-based foams or gels is acceptable. Post-transport cleaning of the vehicle is important, but special cleaning solutions are not required.

Post-exposure treatment consists of supportive care. If you have been exposed, your ICM will follow your health status. Health care providers who develop RSV infection should be placed on work restrictions—in particular, they should not care for immunocompromised patients.

Mononucleosis

Mononucleosis is caused by the Epstein-Barr virus, a herpes virus. This virus is also suspected of causing a related disease, chronic fatigue syndrome. The virus grows in the epithelium of the oropharynx and sheds into saliva—hence the name "kissing disease" for mononucleosis.

Transmission occurs via direct contact with the saliva of an infected person. Some cases have also been linked to contaminated blood transfusions. The incubation period is 4 to 6 weeks following exposure, with a prolonged communicable period. Pharyngeal excretions may persist for a year or more after infection. Signs and symptoms include sore throat, fever, secretions from the pharynx, and swollen lymph glands, with or without malaise, anorexia, headache, muscle pain, and an enlarged liver and spleen.

Prevention involves the use of gloves and good handwashing techniques when in direct contact with patient oral secretions. No special cleaning solutions are required following patient transport.

Influenza

Influenza (flu) viruses cause acute respiratory illnesses generally presenting as winter epidemics. Influenza activity varies from year to year, but it can become a significant cause of death in susceptible individuals. Infection rates are high in children, but the most deaths occur in the over-65 age group, especially in patients with medical conditions such as chronic pulmonary or heart disease.

At the Scene

A paramedic with a cold or flu can be extremely hazardous to a patient who is immunocompromised.

For this droplet-transmitted disease, transmission occurs from person to person by coughing and sneezing. The incubation period is about 1 to 4 days following exposure. The communicable period in adults lasts from the day before symptoms begin until about 5 days after the onset of the illness. Signs and symptoms include systemic fever, shaking chills, headache, muscle pain, malaise, and loss of appetite. Respiratory symptoms include dry cough, hoarseness, and nasal discharge. The duration of illness is about 3 to 4 days, and complications may include viral or bacterial pneumonia.

Prevention involves placing a surgical mask or nonrebreathing mask on the patient. The key preventive measure, however, is an annual flu shot. Each year, a new vaccine is developed based on the anticipated strains for that year. The injectable form of the vaccine does not contain live virus, so you cannot get the disease from the flu shot. An alternative to the injectable form is the nasal spray, which contains live attenuated virus. This is an option for people younger than age 49. If you do not receive a vaccine and have an exposure, antiviral drugs may be offered within 48 hours to reduce the severity of the flu should you contract it.

Sexually Transmitted Infections

As the name implies, sexually transmitted infections (STIs) are usually acquired by sexual contact. While the term STI ordinarily conjures up diagnoses such as gonorrhoea or syphilis, in fact the range of diseases that are transmitted sexually is very wide and includes such conditions as herpes, hepatitis, and HIV infection. Hepatitis and HIV/AIDS are considered separately in this chapter. This section reviews the features of gonorrhoea, syphilis, scabies, and genital herpes infections.

Gonorrhoea

Gonorrhoea is an infection caused by the gonococcal bacteria, *Neisseria gonorrhoeae*. In 2005, more than 19,000 cases of gonorrhoea were reported. Transmission occurs sexually, by contact with the pus-containing fluid from mucous membranes of infected people. The incubation period is usually 2 to 7 days but may be longer. This infection is communicable for months if not treated. If treated, the individual is noncommunicable within hours.

Signs and symptoms of gonorrhoea differ between males and females. Males usually see a pus-containing discharge from the urethra and often experience pain on urination (dysuria) starting a few days after the exposure. In females, the initial inflammation of the urethra or cervix may be so mild that it passes unnoticed, and the illness may progress until it presents as pelvic inflammatory disease, with signs and symptoms of an acute abdomen. Depending on the patient's sexual practices, gonorrhoeal infection may also involve the anus and throat.

The risk of acquiring any STI through a route other than sexual contact is remote. Prevention includes glove use if touching drainage from the genital area and thorough handwashing.

Syphilis

Syphilis is an acute and chronic disease caused by the spiral-shaped bacteria *Treponema pallidum*. It may sound like a disease that died out in the 19th century but it is still with us. In 2000, there were 333 diagnosed cases of syphilis in the UK. The groups with the highest incidence rates are young people aged 20 to 35 years. High numbers of cases are also reported in urban areas.

Transmission occurs by direct contact with the infectious fluids of the primary lesion(s). The bacteria can be transmitted across the placenta from an infected mother to her fetus and by sexual contact. In some cases, transmission has occurred via blood transfusion. The incubation period is 10 days to 3 months; the communicable period has a variable length. If treated with penicillin, the individual is considered noncommunicable within 24 to 48 hours.

The initial infection with syphilis produces an ulcerative lesion, called a chancre, of the skin or mucous membrane at the site of infection Figure 36-9 ▶ . Chancres are most likely to occur in the genital region. "Secondary infection" is the term used to describe the presence of skin rash, patchy hair loss, and swollen lymph glands. Complications of syphilis can include cardiac, ophthalmic, auditory, and central nervous system complications, as well as lesions of the tissues and bone.

Prevention measures include use of gloves and good handwashing techniques. No special cleaning precautions are required.

Genital Herpes

Genital herpes is a chronic, recurrent illness produced by infection with the herpes simplex virus. The herpes simplex virus is further classified into two types: type 1 is generally transmitted via contact with oral secretions, and type 2 is spread through sexual contact. Genital herpes is characterised by vesicular lesions Figure 36-10 ▶ . In women, the vesicles occur initially on the cervix; during recurrent infections, vesicles may also appear around the vulva, legs, and buttocks. In men, lesions commonly occur on the penis, as well as around the anus, depending on sexual practices. Lesions may also be present on the mouth as the result of oral sex.

Transmission usually occurs through sexual contact, but infants may become infected if delivered through the birth canal of a woman with active disease. The incubation period is 2 to 12 days. Secretion of the virus in saliva has been noted to persist for up to 7 weeks following the appearance of a lesion. Genital lesions are infectious for 4 to 7 days.

This disease is elusive; it can suddenly become reactivated, often repeatedly, over many years. Outbreaks are often stress-related. This disease can be treated with acyclovir, valaciclovir, or famciclovir for 7 to 10 days to reduce outbreaks. There is no

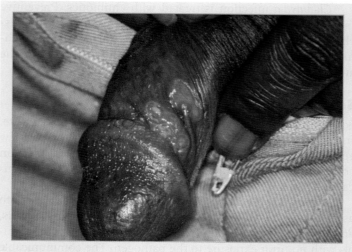

Figure 36-9 A chancre is a sign of syphilis.

cure, however. Preventive measures include the use of gloves when touching drainage from lesions and good handwashing techniques. No special cleaning precautions are necessary.

Chlamydia

Chlamydia infections have the highest incidence of all STIs. In 2005, 109,958 cases were reported to the HPA; the growth in this number is believed to be due to the availability of more sensitive screening tests and the trend

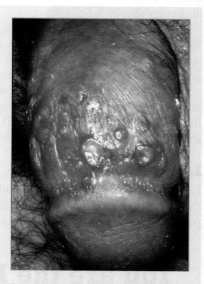

Figure 36-10 Genital herpes.

toward routine screening. In most women, this infection initially remains asymptomatic. However, many women who are infected with *Chlamydia trachomatis* go on to develop pelvic inflammatory disease. In men, infection may lead to epididymitis, prostatitis, proctitis, and proctocolitis.

Transmission occurs through sexual contact. Perinatal infections may result in premature rupture of membranes, premature birth, or stillbirth. The incubation period is believed to be 7 to 14 days or longer. The communicable period is unknown. Signs and symptoms include inflammation of the urethra, epididymis, cervix, and fallopian tubes when the infection is acquired through sexual transmission. Urethral discharge may appear grey or white in colour. The amount of discharge is variable.

Chlamydia infection is treated with antibiotics. Preventive measures include wearing gloves when in contact with discharge from the genital area and using good handwashing techniques. There are no special cleaning requirements for the ambulance or linens.

Scabies

Scabies is caused by infection with *Sarcoptes scabiei*, a parasite. Incidence of this disease has been increasing over the past few years in both the United Kingdom and Europe. This infection commonly affects families, children, sexual partners, chronically ill patients, and people in communal living.

Transmission occurs via direct skin-to-skin contact, such as through wrestling, sexual contact, undergarments, towels, and linens. The incubation period is 2 to 6 weeks for individuals with no prior exposure to the pathogen. The communicable period lasts until the mites and eggs are destroyed by treatment. Signs and symptoms include nocturnal itching and the presence of a rash involving the hands, flexor aspects of the wrists, axillary folds, ankles, toes, genital area, buttocks, and abdomen **Figure 36-11 ▶** .

Prevention consists of wearing gloves and practising good handwashing techniques. Vehicle linens require only routine washing in hot water, with routine cleaning of the vehicle after patient transport. Lindane is a topical treatment for scabies, but no treatment cream or lotion should be applied on a routine basis because of reports of lindane toxicity. In case of documented exposure, treatment will be undertaken and work restrictions from patient care may be ordered.

Lice

Lice are small insects that live in hair and feed on blood through the skin. There are three types of lice: head lice, body lice, and pubic lice. All types of lice are acquired through direct contact with an infested person. Head and body lice can also be acquired from objects such as hats, combs, or clothes infested with lice. Lice eggs look like small white or tan dots on the skin. The eggs hatch after about one week, and then the new lice mature in one to two weeks. Head lice can be found in the hair, as well as in other hairy areas of the head such as eyebrows, eyelashes, moustaches, and beards. Body lice is usually found in the seams of clothing, and can transfer certain diseases. Signs and symptoms of lice include itching and irritation, and possibly sores.

When discussing lice as an STI, the focus is on pubic or crab lice. *Phthirus pubis* is a parasite that is usually greyish in colour. Lice are common in individuals with poor hygiene, communal lifestyles, and multiple sexual partners.

Transmission of pubic lice occurs through intimate physical or sexual contact. The incubation period lasts approximately 8 to

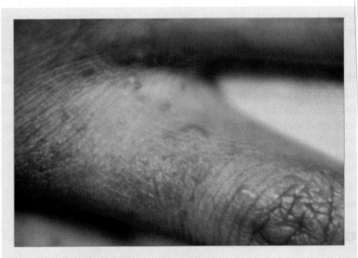

Figure 36-11 Rash produced by scabies.

You are the Paramedic Part 4

When you arrive at the accident and emergency (A&E) department, you are met by the staff as you open your ambulance doors. They are wearing full PPE, including gloves, aprons, goggles, and FFP3 masks. The hospital staff informs you (due to other recent admissions from this same nursing care facility) that they suspect your patient is likely to have SARS and will have to be placed in isolation.

Reassessment	Recording Time: 25 Minutes
Skin	Flushed, warm, and sweaty
Pulse	108 beats/min, weak radial pulse
Blood pressure	116/56 mm Hg
Respirations	36 breaths/min, shallow
S_PO_2	94%
ECG	Sinus tachycardia (no ectopy)

7. After the transfer of care, what steps must be taken with regard to exposure?
8. Will this alter your immediate lifestyle or work habits? If so, how?
9. What are some other considerations with respect to this patient's family?

10 days after the eggs hatch. The communicable period ends when all lice and eggs are destroyed by treatment. Signs and symptoms include slight to severe itching and visual nits clinging to the pubic, perianal, or perineal hair. Pubic lice can also infest eyelashes, eyebrows, axilla, scalp, and other body hairs.

Preventive measures include wearing gloves and practising good handwashing techniques. Routine cleaning of the vehicle after transport is sufficient. In case of documented exposure, permethrin cream treatment may be prescribed and restrictions from patient care may be indicated until the paramedic is free of lice.

Bloodborne Diseases

Viral Hepatitis

Viral hepatitis is an inflammation of the liver produced by a virus. Five distinct forms of viral hepatitis exist (A, B, C, D, and E) that are produced by different viruses and vary somewhat in their means of transmission. All five types present with the same signs and symptoms, so the type causing illness is ultimately determined by blood testing. Hepatitis A and hepatitis E will be discussed as enteric (intestinal) diseases in this chapter, because they are not bloodborne infections.

Hepatitis B Virus Infection

Hepatitis type B virus (HBV), also known as serum hepatitis, cases have greatly diminished in the UK population due to vaccine programmes geared toward health care providers and all children and young adults. In the UK the prevalence of chronic hepatitis B infection is 0.3% with approximately 350 million people affected chronically worldwide. Transmission is through sexual contact, blood transfusion, or puncture of the skin with contaminated needles. Occasionally other objects, such as shared razors, tattoo needles, or acupuncture needles, have been implicated in transmission. Type B hepatitis is particularly common in intravenous drug users who share needles. Health care providers, especially those involved in surgery, dentistry, and emergency medicine, were deemed to carry a particularly high risk of contracting hepatitis through accidental needlestick injuries until vaccination programmes began. Since then, the incidence rate for occupationally acquired HBV infection has fallen by 95%.

Limited data suggest that this virus can survive outside the body in the presence of dried blood for as long as 7 days. The incubation period for HBV varies widely—from 45 to 200 days. The communicable period starts weeks before the first symptoms appear and may persist for years in chronic carriers. It is estimated that 2% to 10% of all HBV-infected individuals will become chronic carriers. Approximately 3% to 5% of infected patients will eventually develop cirrhosis of the liver or liver cancer.

Signs and symptoms of HBV infection include loss of appetite, nausea, vomiting, general fatigue and malaise, low-grade fever, vague abdominal discomfort, and sometimes aching in the joints. The very smell of food may provoke nausea, and smokers often notice a sudden distaste for cigarettes. Signs and symptoms may subside at this point for 50% to 60% of infected patients, which explains why many infected individuals never know that they have acquired the disease. For those who progress into the second phase of the disease, the urine begins to turn dark, and then a day or two later, the patient develops jaundice, a yellowing of the skin, and scleral icterus, a yellowing of the eyes Figure 36-12 ▼ . Type B hepatitis usually lasts several weeks, although complete recovery may take 3 to 4 months.

Prevention of HBV transmission focuses on using gloves when handling blood, OPIM, or materials containing "gross visible" blood. Good handwashing technique is essential. Paramedics should be immunised against HBV when first employed. Vaccination, which is both safe and effective, protects only against HBV but offers that protection for life; it protects indirectly against hepatitis D infection because one must be infected with type B to acquire type D. If you are allergic to yeast or mercury, notify the vaccine administrator and arrangements will be made to obtain the proper vaccine to meet your needs. Vaccine is administered in a three-dose

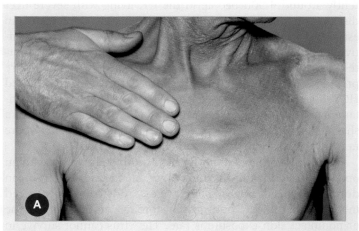
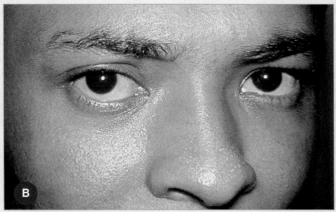

Figure 36-12 Signs of HBV infection. **A.** Jaundice. **B.** Scleral icterus.

Table 36-4	Vaccine Series for Hepatitis B

- Initial dose
- Second dose: 4 weeks from first dose
- Third dose: 6 months from first dose
- Titre: 1 to 2 months after completion of the three-dose series

series Table 36-4 ▲ . After the series is completed, you should have a blood test (titre) performed 1 to 2 months later to ensure that you responded to the vaccine.

Practise routine universal precautions. If you are exposed, notify your ICM. The ICM will verify the source patient's test results. If you have a positive titre on file, no follow-up treatment is needed. If you do not have a titre report on file and the patient is positive for HBV infection, a titre will be ordered on you. Treatment will depend on the results of that titre report. If you have not been vaccinated and the patient is positive for HBV, you will be offered hepatitis B immune globulin and the vaccine series. The risk of infection is 6% to 30% only if you were not vaccinated and did not report the exposure event.

Hepatitis C Virus Infection

The hepatitis C virus (HCV) is the most common chronic bloodborne infection. The HPA estimates that there are currently around 4,500 people in the UK living with severe liver disease as a result of having a chronic hepatitis C infection. An estimated 1% to 4% of health care providers are antibody-positive for HCV. However, this disease is not efficiently transmitted through occupational exposure, and no health care provider group is at increased risk for occupationally acquired HCV infection. Instead, occupational risk is related to a contaminated deep needlestick with visible blood on the sharp, a sharp that has been in the patient's vein or artery, a hollow-bore needle, and a source patient with a high viral load.

Transmission may occur by blood-to-blood contact with an open area of the skin, sexual contact, blood transfusion, organ donation, unsafe medical practices, and from an infected mother to her infant. Transmission through mucous membrane or nonintact skin exposure is rare. The virus cannot survive in the environment long enough to pose a risk for any means of transmission except via bloodborne contact.

Approximately 75% to 80% of HCV-infected individuals progress to long-term chronic infection. The incubation period ranges from 2 to 24 weeks (average is 6 to 7 weeks). Signs and symptoms are the same as those for hepatitis B, and diagnosis is established by testing for HCV antibody. Some 75% of infected people remain unaware that they acquired the infection because they do not develop phase 2 signs and symptoms.

To prevent HCV transmission, use gloves when in direct contact with blood or OPIM, and use needlesafe or needleless devices. No special cleaning requirements apply—just perform routine cleaning of the vehicle and equipment.

If you have sustained an exposure, testing will begin with the source patient providing there is informed consent. If the source is HCV-positive, you will have a baseline HCV antibody test and liver function test. You should have an HCV-RNA test 4 to 6 weeks following the exposure event. If it is negative, you did not acquire HCV from the exposure. If it is positive, you will begin treatment. There is no vaccine to protect against HCV infection, nor can any medication offer post-exposure prevention against infection, however, treatment is available, which is highly successful in preventing chronic infection.

Hepatitis D Virus Infection

Hepatitis type D, also called delta hepatitis, requires the host to be infected with hepatitis B for hepatitis D virus (HDV) infection to occur. For this reason, HDV is considered a parasite for HBV. Hepatitis D is mainly seen in Central Africa, the Middle East and South America, low rates of infection are present in most of Europe, the USA, and Australia. The highest incidence is noted in IV drug users. Transmission is generally by percutaneous exposure, as HDV is not effectively transmitted through sexual contact. Perinatal transmission is rare.

The incubation period for HDV infection ranges from 30 to 180 days. Blood is considered to be infectious during all phases of the illness. Signs and symptoms are the same as those associated with hepatitis B.

To protect against HDV transmission, use gloves when in contact with blood or OPIM, use needlesafe or needleless devices, and perform routine cleaning of the vehicle following patient transport. Remember that you should not go through the pockets of known IV drug users who are found unconscious, as you may get cut with a contaminated sharp. If a documented exposure occurs, testing begins with the source patient in accordance with testing laws. If the source is positive for HDV and you are protected against HBV, no further treatment is indicated.

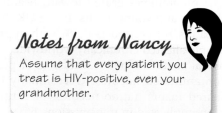

Notes from Nancy

Assume that every patient you treat is HIV-positive, even your grandmother.

Human Immunodeficiency Virus Infection

Human immunodeficiency virus (HIV) type 1 was first identified in the late 1970s. Today, an estimated 60 million people worldwide are infected with this virus. There are an estimated 63,500 HIV-infected adults alive in the UK, a third of whom have not yet had their infections diagnosed. Because of the stigma surrounding the disease, many cases remain undiagnosed.

Although HIV is primarily a sexually transmitted disease, it is also bloodborne and can be transmitted from mother to infant in the birthing process. In 1998 the proportion of pregnant women with HIV in the UK whose diagnosis was known before delivery was very low. This meant that the opportunity for reducing mother-to-child transmission of the virus was being missed. Since that time, enormous strides have been made in improving the uptake of testing in antenatal clinics, achieving the DoH target of 80% uptake by the end of 2002 and since surpassing it. HIV is also transmitted through blood transfusions, albeit at a very low rate since the initiation of testing for the presence of P24 (a protein present from the beginning of the HIV life cycle) in donated blood. With P24 testing, the virus can now be detected 1 to 6 days after infection.

HIV is not transmitted through casual or even household contact. Even among individuals who routinely share eating utensils, toothbrushes, and razors with HIV-infected patients, there is no evidence of an increased rate of HIV infection. This disease is not airborne or droplet transmitted.

The HIV pathogen envelops infected cells and attacks the immune system and other body organs. The immune system is then unable to assist in protecting the infected individual from other diseases. It takes about 7 days for the virus to envelop a cell, and this process may occur 4 to 6 weeks after the exposure event. The communicable period is unknown, but is believed to span from the onset of infection possibly throughout life.

Signs and symptoms may include acute febrile illness, malaise, swollen lymph glands, headache, and possibly rash. Following initial infection, most individuals present with enlargement of the lymph nodes and appear healthy. However, the number of T-helper lymphocytes (CD4 cells) gradually declines. T-helper cells are essential components of the immune system that mediate both cellular and humoral immunity. Seroconversion occurs, meaning that antibodies can be detected in the blood; this usually occurs within the first three months. People who are <u>seropositive</u> for HIV are placed on anti-retroviral drug treatment.

Prevention focuses on the use of gloves when in direct contact with patient blood or OPIM, the use of needlesafe or needleless devices, good handwashing technique, and routine cleaning of the vehicle after transport. Post-exposure medical follow-up is covered in the AIDS section that follows.

The risk for acquiring HIV infection is sharps-related. There have been five cases of occupationally acquired HIV infection in health care workers in the UK. A high-risk exposure to HIV includes *all* of the following: a deep stick with a large-gauge hollow-bore needle, the device has visible blood on it, the patient is HIV-positive with a high viral load, and the device had been in the patient's vein or artery. Following this type of exposure, the risk of transmission is 0.3% for mucous membrane exposure to the eye and 0.09% for nonintact skin.

Acquired Immunodeficiency Syndrome

<u>Acquired immunodeficiency syndrome (AIDS)</u> is the end-stage disease process caused by HIV. The patient with AIDS is extremely vulnerable to numerous bacterial, viral, and fungal infections that would not affect a person with an intact immune system. These *opportunistic infections* include pneumonia in infants or people with compromised immune systems, loss of vision due to cytomegalovirus, reddish/purple skin lesions, atypical TB, and cryptococcal meningitis.

The incubation period of AIDS spans the time between documented infection (ie, becoming HIV-positive) and development of the end-stage disease; it is determined by the CD4 cell count and the presence of opportunistic infections. The communicable period is presumed to last as long as the patient is seropositive, *even before clinically apparent AIDS develops.* Surveys of patients presenting to A&E departments have shown that around 6% of seriously ill or injured patients are HIV-positive.

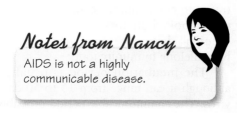

Notes from Nancy

AIDS is not a highly communicable disease.

Prevention involves following universal precautions. Use gloves when in contact with blood or OPIM, use needlesafe or needleless devices, and perform routine cleaning of the vehicle and equipment. There is no need to restrict pregnant care providers from contact with known HIV/AIDS patients.

If an actual exposure occurs, the source patient will be tested, ideally using the rapid HIV testing method. Its results are accurate and are available in less than 1 hour. If the test is negative, then no further testing is indicated for the paramedic. If the source is positive, then blood is sent for assessment of viral load and the paramedic may be offered anti-retroviral drugs for a period of 4 weeks; the criteria for use of these drugs are published by the DoH.

Anti-retroviral drugs are toxic, so careful and complete counselling should be provided to the exposed health care provider. The DoH recommends that a doctor knowledgeable in the use of these drugs be consulted.

At the Scene

Body fluids that do not transmit bloodborne disease: tears, sweat, urine, stool, vomitus, nasal secretions, and sputum.

Enteric (Intestinal) Diseases

Gastroenteritis

<u>Gastroenteritis</u>, also known as the stomach flu, comprises many types of infections and irritations of the gastrointestinal tract. Patients experience symptoms such as nausea and vomiting, fever, abdominal cramps, and diarrhoea. In healthy individuals, gastroenteritis is usually not serious. In children, elderly people, and patients with chronic illness, severe complications such as dehydration may develop.

Hepatitis A Virus Infection

<u>Hepatitis A</u> was a common childhood infection in the early 20th century but now in the 21st century it is an unusual infection in the UK. Transmission is by the faecal–oral route—that is, by ingestion of food or water that has been contaminated by infected faeces. Epidemic outbreaks can usually be

traced to contaminated drinking water, milk, sliced meats, and undercooked shellfish. Hepatitis A is often described as a "benign" disease because once you acquire the disease you have lifelong immunity to it.

The incubation period is usually about 2 to 4 weeks, although it can range from 15 to 50 days after ingestion of the virus. The communicable period probably starts toward the end of the incubation period and continues for a few days after the patient becomes jaundiced. Signs and symptoms in phase 1 include fatigue, loss of appetite, fever, nausea, and abdominal pain; smokers will lose their interest in smoking. In phase 2, patients have jaundice, dark-coloured urine, and whitish stools.

Prevention includes use of gloves and good handwashing technique if in contact with patient stool. No special cleaning of the vehicle is needed. Hepatitis A vaccine is recommended for Emergency Management Agency response team members who may work outside the United Kingdom, but not for any other health care provider groups.

Hepatitis E Virus Infection

Hepatitis E virus (HEV) infection is also referred to as enterically transmitted non-A, non-B hepatitis (ET-NANB). It accounts for an estimated 50% of hepatitis cases in developing countries. Transmission occurs via the faecal–oral route by ingestion of contaminated water. In developing countries, there is a strong association between HEV and floods, poor sanitation, and primitive hygiene. Rare cases of transmission via transfusion have been documented, and sexual transmission is on record.

This disease is not chronic. Its incubation period is about 15 to 64 days. The communicable period is believed to be the same as for hepatitis A. Signs and symptoms are the same as for other forms of hepatitis. Prevention includes the use of gloves when in contact with stool, good handwashing technique, and cleaning contaminated equipment.

Clostridium difficile

Clostridium difficile (otherwise referred to as *C difficile*) was first recognised to cause antibiotic-associated diarrhoea and colitis in the late 1970s. Actual prevalence has historically been difficult as laboratories have only been required to report cases to the HPA voluntarily. Since January 2004, *C difficile* has been part of the mandatory surveillance programme for healthcare associated infections; the number of reports increased from less than 1,000 in the early 1990s to well over 50,000 in the mid 2000s. Some of this was due to improved diagnostic tests and improved reporting by laboratories, but there has clearly been a very significant increase in the number of cases. *C difficile* is a major cause of antibiotic-associated diarrhoea and colitis, and mostly affects elderly patients with other underlying diseases.

C difficilee is a bacterium from the same family that causes tetanus, botulism, and gas gangrene; *Clostridium*. It is an anaerobic bacterium and is usually found in the large intestine, where there is very little oxygen. Although a harmful bacteria, it can be found in low numbers in less than 5% of the healthy adult population. The "host" person can tolerate this as the bacteria is kept in check by the normal, "good" bacterial population of the intestine. However, when this good population is killed off through the use of broad spectrum antibiotics (usually in elderly patients), *C difficile* is able to become established and produces toxins that damage the cells lining the intestine. This results in symptoms ranging from mild diarrhoea to ulcerative colitis and, at worst, perforation of the intestine leading to peritonitis. It can be fatal.

Spread of the disease is based on cross infection from another patient, either through direct patient to patient contact, via health care staff, or via contaminated surroundings. The diarrhoea of a contaminated person contains large amounts of spores that are able to survive for long periods of time and can be picked up and passed on.

█ Vectorborne Diseases

West Nile Virus

West Nile virus (WNV) is a relatively new disease in Europe. The virus was first discovered in Uganda in the 1930s; its first identified appearance in the Western Hemisphere was in New York City in 1999. The risk of contracting WNV in Europe is considered very low but several cases have been reported in Portugal and Southern France.

Transmission is via bite from a mosquito carrying the virus (only about 1% of mosquitoes carry WNV). This infection is not transmitted from person to person, so there is no period of communicability. WNV has been transmitted via donated blood and organs, as well as during haemodialysis; two cases have involved needlestick injuries in laboratory workers working with this virus. The incubation period is from 3 to 14 days following the bite.

In the majority of cases, this disease is mild and uneventful. Indeed, 80% of people who acquire WNV infection remain unaware that they have it. The 20% of people who are symptomatic exhibit fever, headache, body rash, and swollen lymph glands. Mild symptoms appear in older people and immunocompromised people. In healthy individuals, the immune system fights off the disease. About 1 in 150 symptomatic individuals will go on to develop severe signs and symptoms, which include encephalitis, meningitis that can lead to neurological complications, and death.

Use needlesafe devices systems to avoid a contaminated sharps injury when WNV infection is suspected. If you sustain a contaminated sharps injury involving a patient with WNV, notify your ICM. There is no recommended medical follow-up treatment. No special cleaning of the vehicle is needed or recommended.

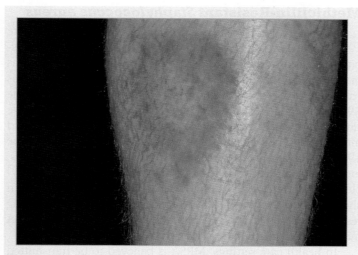

Figure 36-13 The bull's-eye rash of Lyme disease is most common in the area of the groin, thigh, or axilla.

Lyme Disease

Lyme disease is caused by a bacterium transmitted via a tick bite. Lyme disease is rare in the UK. The disease is usually found in people who have visited areas where ticks are present such as the New Forest, the Highlands, and Exmoor.

Lyme disease primarily affects the skin, heart, joints, and nervous system. Some patients remain asymptomatic. This disease occurs more often in children younger than age 10 years and in middle-aged adults. Lyme disease is not transmitted from person to person. Its incubation period ranges from 3 to 32 days.

Lyme disease is usually divided into three stages: early localised, early disseminated, and late manifestations. The early stage is characterised by a round, red skin lesion. This bull's-eye rash (so called because it extends outward with a ring in the centre) is most common in the area of the groin, thigh, or axilla **Figure 36-13 ▲**. If present, it is warm to the touch, and may blister or scab. In the early disseminated stage, secondary lesions may develop within days and the patient may complain of flu-like symptoms—fever, chills, headache, malaise, and muscle pain. Nonproductive cough, testicular swelling, sore throat, enlarged spleen, and enlarged lymph nodes may be present. Neurologic involvement may occur in 15% to 20% of untreated patients within 2 to 8 weeks; cardiac involvement may occur in 10% of untreated patients. In the third phase of the illness, arthritis occurs in about 60% of untreated patients, beginning days to years after the initial infection. Intermittent joint pain affects about 50% of patients, and lasts from days to months. Chronic neurological symptoms are uncommon. Memory impairment, depressed mood, and severe fatigue are the most common symptoms of Lyme disease.

Prevention includes wearing long sleeves and trousers when in tick-infested areas, plus use of insecticides that contain carbaril, diazinon, chlorpyrifos, or cyfluthrin. If you sustain a tick bite, use proper technique for removing ticks. Post-exposure treatment with antibiotics is not warranted or recommended.

Zoonotic (Animal-borne) Diseases

Hantavirus

Hantavirus, also known as haemorrhagic fever with renal syndrome, is associated with the deer mouse, white-footed mouse, and cotton rat. It has also been found in rats in urban areas. This disease was first identified in Korea in the early 1950s and in the Southwestern United States in 1993. Hantavirus infection is rare in the UK; in the whole of 2005 there were no reported cases at all.

Hantavirus is found in the urine, faeces, and saliva of chronically infected rodents. Transmission occurs via direct contact with rodent waste matter, often through aerosol inhalation. The incubation period usually lasts 12 to 16 days following exposure but has been noted to range from 5 to 42 days. This disease is not transmitted from person to person, so there is no period of communicability. Signs and symptoms begin with the sudden onset of fever, which lasts 3 to 8 days. It is accompanied by headache, abdominal pain, loss of appetite, and vomiting.

Prevention focuses on universal precautions. Routine cleaning of the vehicle is all that is indicated.

Rabies

Rabies (hydrophobia) is found worldwide and accounts for about 300,000 deaths each year in developing countries. In the UK the last human death from indigenous classical rabies occurred in 1902, and the last case of indigenous terrestrial animal rabies was in 1922. Most cases of rabies in the UK now occur in quarantined animals, or in people infected abroad. The vaccination of domestic animals and the development of vaccine and rabies immunoglobulin have greatly reduced the number of deaths in humans who contract rabies. However, as many as 39,000 people still receive post-exposure prophylaxis annually worldwide.

Transmission is primarily related to the direct bite of an infected animal. The virus is shed in the saliva of the infected animal from the time it becomes infected. Other routes of transmission include contamination of mucous membranes (eyes, mouth) and one case suspected to be related to a cornea organ transplant. In general, however, nonbite exposures to rabies—scratches, abrasions, open wounds, or mucous membranes contaminated with saliva or other potentially infectious material from a rabid animal—are rare. There are no documented cases of human-to-human transmission of rabies.

The incubation period is usually 2 to 8 weeks, but varies depending on the severity of the bite and the location of the wound. Signs and symptoms in human infection are generally nonspecific: fever, chills, sore throat, malaise, headache, and weakness. Paraesthesia (skin sensation with no apparent cause) may develop at or near the site of exposure. Following these initial signs, the neurological phase of the disease begins—hyperactivity, convulsions, bizarre behaviour, and hydrophobia. Patients also have fear of the sight of water or while drinking it as a result of severe spasms of the throat and masseter (chewing) muscles. As the disease progresses, patients may develop paralysis and deterioration of mental status leading to coma. Although rabies is generally viewed as a fatal disease, several cases of survival have been reported recently.

For prevention, follow universal precautions for patient care and cleaning of the vehicle. If you are bitten by a suspect animal, you will be offered human rabies vaccine if deemed appropriate.

Tetanus

Tetanus is a vaccine-preventable disease for which there is a national immunisation programme in the UK. Tetanus is a notifiable disease by law and should be reported on suspicion of the diagnosis to the proper officer, normally the local consultant in communicable disease control (CCDC).

Transmission occurs when tetanus spores enter the body by either of two means: (1) a puncture wound contaminated with animal faeces, street dust, or soil, or (2) contaminated street drugs. Tetanus is not transmitted from person to person. Occasionally, cases have occurred postoperatively or following seemingly minor injuries.

The incubation period is usually about 14 days from the exposure but has been documented to be as short as 3 days. The cases that have short incubation periods tend to feature a higher level of contamination. Signs and symptoms begin at the site of the wound, followed by painful muscle contractions in the neck and trunk muscles. The key sign that suggests tetanus is abdominal rigidity, although this rigidity may be confined to the location of the injury.

Prevention involves the use of gloves when handling any patient wounds and drainage. No special cleaning routines are necessary after transport of a patient with tetanus.

Antibiotic-Resistant Organisms

The overuse and misuse of antibiotics has led some pathogens to develop resistance to the antibiotic drugs commonly prescribed to eradicate them. As a consequence, both pharmacies and the DoH now restrict the use of many antibiotics. There has also been an attempt to educate the population regarding the risks associated with the overuse of antibiotics.

Methicillin-Resistant *Staphylococcus aureus*

Staphylococcus aureus became resistant to penicillin in the late 1950s. Today almost 90% of community (CA-MRSA) and hospital isolates are resistant to penicillin. The drug methicillin was made available in the early 1960s to treat infections with this pathogen. MRSA strains were first seen in many countries in the 1960s but new strains appeared in the 1980s, which have caused outbreaks of infection in hospitals throughout the world including the UK. Further new strains also emerged during the 1990s. MRSA strains are also resistant to some other antibiotics, including cephalosporins, erythromycins, clindamycin, tetracyclines, and aminoglycosides. Although vancomycin has been shown to effectively treat MRSA, some mild strains are showing resistance to this drug as well. Other drugs used to treat MRSA include quinupristin/dalfopristin, linezolid, and daptomycin.

In health care settings, MRSA is believed to be transmitted from patient to patient via unwashed hands of health care providers. Studies have shown that 50% to 90% of health care providers carry MRSA in their nares; the pathogen can subsequently be transferred to skin and other areas of the body through a break in the skin. Surfaces contaminated with MRSA do not seem to be important in transmission. Factors that increase the risk for developing MRSA include antibiotic therapy, prolonged hospital stays, a stay in intensive care or a burn unit, and exposure to an infected patient. Many patients who contract MRSA live in long-term care facilities.

Patients with MSRA may be either colonised with this organism or infected. The incubation period appears to be between 5 to 45 days. The communicable period varies, as patients who have active infection may carry MRSA for months. MRSA results in soft-tissue infections. Its signs and symptoms may involve localised skin abscesses and cellulites, empyemas, and endocarditis. Sepsis is found in older patients with S aureus infections. After bloodstream infection with this organism, secondary infections such as osteomyelitis and septic arthritis may develop at other body sites.

To prevent MRSA transmission, use universal precautions (gloves and good handwashing technique) when in contact with patient wounds and nonintact skin. If you are in direct contact with wound drainage but your skin is intact, no exposure will occur. If you have a true exposure, no post-exposure treatment is recommended. The incident must still be documented, however.

Vancomycin-Resistant Enterococci

Enterococcus is a common, normal organism of the GI tract, urinary tract, and genitourinary tract. More than 450 species of enterococci exist, many of which are resistant to antimicrobial agents. These organisms grow under both reduced and oxygenated conditions. When they become resistant to the main drug used for treating enterococcal infection, vancomycin, the patient is said to have vancomycin-resistant enterococci (VRE). VRE is primarily a hospital-acquired (nosocomial) infection.

Patients identified with VRE outside the hospital setting typically reside in nursing homes or visit haemodialysis centres.

VRE may be found in urinary tract infections and bloodstream infections; it has also been identified in manure, uncooked chicken, and individuals who work at farms or processing plants. The infectious organisms can live on surfaces for long periods of time, so transmission may occur by direct contact with contaminated surfaces or equipment. A person can be either colonised or infected with VRE, but only infected patients can transmit this organism. Thus transmission may occur when you have direct contact with wound drainage and an open cut or sore allows entry of the organism. This illness can be treated with a new synthetic antibiotic, linezolid.

Prevention relies on the use of universal precautions, gloves, and good handwashing technique when in contact with wound drainage. An apron is necessary only if your uniform may come in contact with wound drainage. Post-transport cleaning of all areas that came in contact with the patient is important, but no special cleaning solution is required. If you sustain direct contact with an open wound and VRE body fluids, notify your ICM and complete an exposure report. No post-exposure medical treatment is indicated.

New and Emerging Diseases

In the past, a disease would jump from animals to humans every 20 to 30 years. Today, this transmission is occurring much more frequently. Recent examples include HIV infection, monkeypox, SARS, and avian flu. The latter two are discussed here.

Severe Acute Respiratory Syndrome

Severe acute respiratory syndrome (SARS) is a new disease that arose from the merger of two viruses, one from mammals and one from birds. The source of this virus has been identified as bats found in Hong Kong. SARS was first reported in Asia in February 2003. Within a few months, the disease had spread from Asia to Canada, South America, and Europe. By early 2003, the World Health Organisation (WHO) reported a total of 8,098 cases worldwide and 774 deaths. In the United Kingdom, the HPA reported eight confirmed cases (all mild) and no deaths; all of the UK cases involved people who had travelled to areas where SARS cases had previously been reported. The latest cases of SARS were reported in April 2004 in China and resulted from a laboratory accident. In the United Kingdom, no health care providers have contracted SARS. The exact current figures are dynamic as most "suspected" cases turn out to be other illnesses.

Transmission is by close personal contact—that is, living with and caring for a person with the disease or having direct contact with respiratory secretions or body fluids of

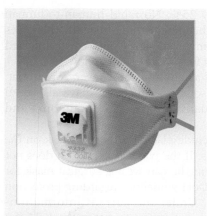

Figure 36-14 Wear an FFP3 respirator that has been properly fit-tested to protect yourself from SARS.

an infected person (eg, kissing or hugging, talking within 1 m, sharing eating utensils). The incubation period is about 10 days from the date of exposure; the communicable period has not been well defined. Signs and symptoms include a fever of greater than 38°C, head-ache, overall feeling of discomfort, and body aches. SARS resembles any general flu-like illness; however, after 2 to 7 days a dry cough appears, and patients with severe illness progress to pneumonia and may need respiratory support.

Care for a person suspected of having SARS begins with an assessment and taking of a travel history. Place a surgical mask on a patient who presents with signs and symptoms of SARS in order to contain secretions. Interim DoH guidelines indicate that the paramedic should wear an FFP3 respirator that has been properly fit-tested Figure 36-14 ▲ . Under the current reporting system, medical facilities are required to notify the ICM if a patient transported is later diagnosed with SARS. If an unprotected exposure occurs, notify the ICM and complete an exposure report form. If a true exposure occurred, a 10-day quarantine may be recommended. This time off will be covered by workers' compensation. The exposed paramedic will be asked to take a temperature check at least daily.

Avian Flu

Avian (bird) flu is caused by a virus that occurs naturally in the bird population. This virus is carried in the intestinal tract of wild birds and does not usually cause illness. However, in domestic bird populations (eg, chickens, ducks, and turkeys), it is very contagious. Birds acquire the illness from contact with contaminated excretions or surfaces that are contaminated with excretions. If an infected bird is used for food and is cooked, it does not pose a risk to those who eat it.

The first cases of avian flu in humans were reported in Hong Kong in 1997; 18 people became infected and 6 died in this outbreak. In the cases that have occurred since then, the

At the Scene

Travel history should be a routine part of patient assessment.

death rate is approximately 25%. No rapid human-to-human cases of this disease has been reported. Instead, the cases occurring in humans have involved close contact with infected birds. The transmission risk for humans is quite low.

Signs and symptoms of avian flu include fever, sore throat, cough, and muscle aches; some eye infections have also been noted. Illness may eventually progress to pneumonia and severe respiratory distress.

Preventive measures include placing a surgical mask on the patient to contain secretions. If the patient's condition does not permit this action, the paramedic can wear a surgical mask for protection. Follow current DoH guidelines regarding protection for health care providers. Under the current information-sharing system, the hospital is required to notify the ICM if a patient transported is later diagnosed with avian flu. If an exposure is documented, then an antiviral drug may be offered within 48 hours of exposure. Antiviral drugs do not prevent the flu, but rather reduce the severity of the illness. It is also important to get an annual flu shot to ensure protection from type A viruses. Some concern exists that someone infected with a regular type A flu virus may become co-infected with avian flu, allowing the two to merge and form a new virus.

Notes from Nancy

Don't drive a four-wheeled fomite. Clean and air the ambulance after every call.

At the Scene

The lead agency for responding to potential pandemic diseases is the Health Protection Agency. The Centre for Infections is part of this Agency.

Ambulance Cleaning and Disinfection

The paramedic has an obligation to protect patients from nosocomial infections (infections acquired from a health care setting—in this instance, an ambulance). One way to protect patients is by complying with work restriction guidelines: Reporting for work when you have a sore throat or the flu is *not* in the best interests of your patients or your colleagues.

Another way to protect patients from nosocomial infections is to keep the ambulance interior and its equipment clean and disinfected. When cleaning equipment, select cleaning solutions to fit the equipment category:

- **Critical equipment:** items that come in contact with mucous membranes; laryngoscope blades, endotracheal tubes, etc. These items are single use and disposable.
- **Semicritical equipment:** items that come in direct contact with intact skin; stethoscopes, blood pressure cuffs, splints. Clean with solutions that have a label claiming to kill HBV. Bleach and water at 1:100 dilution fits this requirement.
- **Noncritical equipment:** cleaning surfaces, floors, ambulance seats, work surfaces. Hospital-grade cleaner or bleach and water mixture is effective for this equipment.

General cleaning routines need to be listed in the trust's Infection Control Policy. A basic rule of thumb is to do the following after *every* call:

1. Strip used linens from the stretcher immediately after use, and place them in a plastic bag or in the designated receptacle in the A&E department.
2. In an appropriate receptacle, discard all disposable equipment used for care of the patient that meets your trust's definition of medical waste. Most items will be considered clinical waste.
3. Wash contaminated areas with soap and water. For disinfection to be effective, cleaning must be done first.
4. Clean the stretcher with germicidal/virucidal solution or bleach and water at 1:100 dilution.
5. If any spillage or other contamination occurred in the ambulance, clean it up with the same germicidal/virucidal or bleach/water solution.
6. Create a timetable for routine full cleaning for the vehicle, as required by the Infection Control Policy. Name the brands of solution to be used.
7. Have a written policy/procedure for cleaning each piece of equipment. Refer to the manufacturer's recommendations as a guide.

You are the Paramedic Summary

1. Given your initial findings, what do you know about the patient's overall condition?

Her flushed, sweaty skin points to the possibility of fever and infection. Depending on her health history, she may or may not be able to compensate for the vasodilation and the resultant increased myocardial workload and oxygen consumption.

2. What are your immediate concerns?

Before moving this patient, you must determine that no trauma has occurred. Also note the length of time that this patient has been on the floor and whether any loss of consciousness occurred.

3. Think of a few potential illnesses that could cause these signs and symptoms.

Viral, bacterial, fungi, and other parasitic infections can result in pneumonia, bronchitis, and influenza, to name just a few.

4. Of those, which are the most serious and why?

Communicable, contagious, or infectious diseases not only place your patient at risk but all those individuals around the patient, including friends, family, health care providers, and the general public.

5. Why is it important to periodically reconsider your differential diagnosis throughout the call?

You must remain mentally flexible and periodically rethink your list of possible causes related to the patient's signs and symptoms. Failure to do so can result in a pigeon-holing of your differentials and can cause you to make errors in patient care. Critical thinking skills are the key to delivering good medicine.

6. Given your updated differential, what would be considered "high-risk" procedures for this patient?

Any airway manoeuvres, procedures, or treatment that could potentially spread the disease and/or place the health care provider at elevated risk for exposure would be considered "high risk". Examples include endotracheal intubation, laryngeal mask airway, CPAP, BiPAP, bag-valve-mask ventilations (without appropriate filtration), and use of nebuliser treatments.

7. After the transfer of care, what steps must be taken with regard to exposure?

Immediately notify your trust's ICM and complete an exposure report form. During this call, which included close patient contact in an enclosed space as well as carrying the patient to the trolley, you have received a true exposure. Your ICM and clinical director will be likely to remove you from duty and place you on a 10-day quarantine. Because your partner did not receive the same level of exposure, he or she may or may not be removed from active duty.

8. Will this alter your immediate lifestyle or work habits? If so, how?

Yes—a 10-day quarantine means that you will not be going to work on an ambulance and potentially coming in contact with sick patients (for your sake and theirs).

9. What are some other considerations with respect to this patient's family?

The granddaughter and any other family members will need to be notified and watched for signs and symptoms of SARS. Due to family stressors and mortality rates associated with SARS in older people, they may also need some form of mental health counselling.

Prep Kit

Ready for Review

- Government agencies such as the HPA and the DoH bear the responsibility for protection of the public health, prevention of epidemics, and management of outbreaks.
- The human body offers several defences to protect against infection, such as skin, the mucous membranes, and the immune system.
- Infection involves a typical chain of events through which the communicable disease spreads.
- Communicable diseases can be transmitted from one person to another under certain conditions.
- Precautions against communicable diseases include the infection control manager, the Department of Health, universal precautions, immunisations and vaccinations, personal protective equipment, post-exposure medical follow up, and an infection control policy.
- The overuse and misuse of antibiotics has led some pathogens to develop resistance to the antibiotic drugs commonly prescribed to eradicate them.
- New and emerging diseases of concern include SARS and avian flu.
- Clean and disinfect the ambulance and your equipment to protect patients from infection.

Vital Vocabulary

acquired immunodeficiency syndrome (AIDS) The end-stage disease process caused by the human immunodeficiency virus (HIV). A person with this is extremely vulnerable to numerous bacterial, viral, and fungal infections that would not affect a person with an intact immune system.

avian (bird) flu A disease caused by a virus that occurs naturally in the bird population. Signs and symptoms include fever, sore throat, cough, and muscle aches.

bacteria Small organisms that can grow and reproduce outside the human cell in the presence of the temperature and nutrients, and cause disease by invading and multiplying in the tissues of the host.

bloodborne pathogens Pathogenic microorganisms that are present in human blood and can cause disease in humans. These pathogens include, but are not limited to, hepatitis B virus (HBV) and human immunodeficiency virus (HIV).

carrier An individual who harbours an infectious agent and, although not personally ill, can transmit the infection to another person.

chancre The primary hard lesion or ulcer of syphilis that occurs at the entry site of the infection.

chickenpox A very contagious disease caused by varicella zoster virus, which is part of the herpes virus family, occurring most often in the winter and early spring.

Chlamydia A sexually transmitted disease that has the highest incidence. Signs and symptoms include inflammation of the urethra, epididymis, cervix, fallopian tubes, and discharge from the urethra.

communicable disease A disease that can be transmitted from one person to another under certain conditions.

communicable period The period during which an infected person is capable of transmitting illness to someone else.

contaminated The presence or the reasonably anticipated presence of blood or other potentially infectious materials on an item or surface.

enterococcus A common, normal organism of the GI tract, urinary tract, and genitourinary tract, and which may become resistant to vancomycin.

fomite An inanimate object contaminated with microorganisms that serves as a means of transmitting an illness.

fungus (plural: fungi) A small organism that can grow rapidly in the presence of nutrients and organic material, and can cause infection related to contact with decaying organic matter or from airborne spores in the environment such as moulds.

gastroenteritis A term that comprises many types of infections and irritations of the gastrointestinal tract; symptoms include nausea and vomiting, fever, abdominal cramps, and diarrhoea.

gonorrhoea A sexually transmitted disease which results in infection caused by the gonococcal bacteria, *Neisseria gonorrhoea*. Signs and symptoms include pus-containing discharge from the urethra and painful urination in males, and signs and symptoms of an acute abdomen in females.

hantavirus Also known as haemorrhagic fever with renal syndrome, this is a type of virus found in wild rodents, which can also cause disease in humans, characterised by fever, headache, abdominal pain, loss of appetite, and vomiting.

helminths Invertebrates with long, flexible, rounded, or flattened bodies, commonly called worms; a type of parasite.

hepatitis A An inflammation from a virus that causes mild fatigue, loss of appetite, fever, nausea, abdominal pain, and eventually, jaundice, dark-coloured urine, and whitish stools.

host resistance One's ability to fight off infection.

human immunodeficiency virus (HIV) The virus that causes AIDS (acquired immunodeficiency syndrome), which kills or damages the cells in the body's immune system so that the body is unable to fight infections and certain cancers.

icterus Jaundice; the yellow appearance of the skin and other tissues caused by an accumulation of bile pigments.

incubation period The time period between exposure to an organism and the first symptoms of illness, during which the organism multiplies within the body and starts to produce symptoms.

infection The abnormal invasion of a host or host tissue by organisms such as bacteria, viruses, or parasites, with or without signs or symptoms of disease.

Infection Control Manager (ICM) An individual trained to ensure that proper post-exposure medical treatment and counselling is provided to an exposed employee or volunteer.

influenza The flu, a respiratory infection caused by a variety of viruses. It differs from the common cold in that the flu involves a fever, headache, and extreme exhaustion.

jaundice The presence of excessive bile pigments in the bloodstream that give the skin, mucous membranes, and eyes a distinct yellow colour; jaundice is often associated with liver disease.

lice Tiny, wingless, parasitic insects that feed on the patient's blood. This infestation is easily spread through close personal contact. Several types exist: head, body, and pubic.

Lyme disease A tick-borne disease which primarily affects the skin, heart, joints, and nervous system, and characterised by a round, red lesion or bull's-eye rash.

measles An infectious viral disease that occurs most often in late winter and spring. It begins with a fever followed by a cough, running nose, and pink eye. Then a rash spreads from the face and neck down the back and trunk.

meningitis An inflammation of the meningeal coverings of the brain and spinal cord; it is usually caused by a virus or bacterium.

meningococcal meningitis An infection of the fluid of a person's spinal cord and the fluid that surrounds the brain. Sometimes referred to as spinal meningitis, it is caused by bacteria or virus. The viral type is less severe than the bacterial; the bacterial type can result in brain damage, hearing loss, learning disability, or death.

mononucleosis Infectious mononucleosis or mono (glandular fever), caused by the Epstein-Barr virus, is often called the kissing disease. It is also spread by coughing or sneezing.

mumps A viral infection that primarily affects the parotid glands, which are one of the three pairs of salivary glands, causing swelling in front of the ears.

nosocomial infection An infection acquired from a health care setting.

OPIM An acronym that stands for other potentially infectious materials. These include CSF, pericardial fluid, synovial fluid, pleural fluid, amniotic fluid, peritoneal fluid, and any fluid containing gross visible blood.

parasite Any living organism in or on any other living creature; takes advantage of the host by feeding off cells and tissues.

pertussis An acute infectious disease characterised by a catarrhal stage, followed by a paroxysmal cough that ends in a whooping inspiration. Also called whooping cough.

pneumonia An inflammation of the lungs caused by bacteria, viruses, fungi, or other organisms.

protozoans Single-celled, usually microscopic, eukaryotic organisms such as amoebas, ciliates, flagellates, and sporozoans; a type of parasite.

rabies A fatal infection of the central nervous system caused by a bite from an animal that has been infected with the rabies virus.

reservoir In the context of communicable disease, a place where organisms may live and multiply.

respiratory syncytial virus (RSV) A labile paramyxovirus that produces its characteristic fusion of human cells in a tissue culture known as the syncytial effect. Two subtypes, A and B, have been identified. RSV can affect both the upper and lower respiratory tracts but is more prevalent with the lower, causing pneumonias and bronchiolitis.

rubella A viral disease similar to measles, best known by the distinctive red rash on the skin. It is not nearly as infectious or severe as measles.

scabies An infestation of the skin with the mite *Sarcoptes scabei*. It spreads rapidly when there is skin-to-skin contact.

seropositive Having a positive blood test for an infectious agent, such as HIV or hepatitis B or C virus.

serum hepatitis The hepatitis type B virus (HBV), which is transmitted through sexual contact, blood transfusion, or puncture of the skin with contaminated needles, and whose signs and symptoms include loss of appetite, nausea, vomiting, general fatigue and malaise, low-grade fever, vague abdominal discomfort, and sometimes aching in the joints. Eventually, jaundice will occur.

severe acute respiratory syndrome (SARS) Potentially life-threatening viral infection that usually starts with flu-like symptoms.

sexually transmitted infections (STIs) A group of diseases usually acquired by sexual contact, and which include gonorrhoea, syphilis, chlamydia, scabies, pubic lice, herpes, hepatitis, and HIV infection.

source individual Any individual, living or dead, whose blood or other potentially infectious materials may be a source of occupational exposure to the member/volunteer. Examples include, but are not limited to, hospital and clinic patients; clients in institutions for the developmentally disabled; trauma victims; clients of drug and alcohol treatment facilities; residents of hospices and nursing homes; human remains; and individuals who donate or sell blood or blood components.

Staphylococcus aureus A strain of bacteria that became resistant to the drug methicillin, creating a new strain called methicillin-resistant *staphylococcus aureus;* symptoms include infection and possibly localised skin abscesses and cellulites, empyemas, and endocarditis.

syphilis A sexually transmitted disease caused by the spiral-shaped bacteria *Treponema pallidum* and whose signs and symptoms include an ulcerative lesion or chancre of the skin or mucous membrane at the site of infection, commonly in the genital region.

tetanus A disease caused by spores that enter the body through a puncture wound contaminated with animal faeces, street dust, or soil, or which can enter through contaminated street drugs, and whose signs and symptoms include pain at the wound site and painful muscle contractions in the neck and trunk muscles.

tuberculin skin test A test to determine if a person has ever been infected with tuberculosis.

tuberculosis (TB) An infection which can progress to a disease characterised by a persistent cough for 2 to 3 weeks plus night sweats, headache, weight loss, haemoptysis, or chest pain.

universal precautions The term used to describe the infection control practices that will reduce the opportunity for exposure of providers in the daily care of patients.

vesicle A tiny fluid-filled sac; a small blister.

viral hepatitis An inflammation of the liver produced by one of five distinct forms a virus—A, B, C, D, and E. The five types differ in transmission but present with the same signs and symptoms.

virulence The ability of an organism to invade and create disease in a host. Also refers to the ability of an organism to survive outside the living host.

virus A small organism that can only multiply inside a host, such as a human, and cause disease.

West Nile virus (WNV) A type of virus that is transmitted by mosquitos, and which usually only causes mild disease in humans, but can cause encephalitis, meningitis, or death. Symptoms, if exhibited, include fever, headache, body rash, and swollen lymph glands.

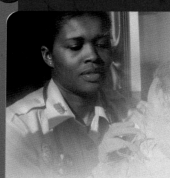

Assessment in Action

A call goes out for a patient complaining of fever, rash, and weakness. The location given is the local university. When the paramedics arrive, they are taken to a dorm room where a student is lying on the sofa. Patient assessment reveals a pinkish-coloured rash, rapid onset of a headache and stiff neck; also, the patient does not want to be in bright light.

During transport to the local hospital, the patient vomits. The next day, a rumour circulates that the student was diagnosed with bacterial meningitis. The hospital contacts the ICM, who then contacts the paramedics who were on the call.

1. **What is meningitis?**
   A. Inflammation of the lining of the myocardium
   B. Inflammation of the meninges, the membranes that cover the brain and spinal cord
   C. Inflammation of the pleura
   D. Inflammation of the endocrine system

2. **What is the transmission mode for meningitis?**
   A. Vectorborne
   B. Direct contact with the nasopharyngeal secretions of an infected person
   C. Indirect contact
   D. Inhalation of infected droplets

3. **How is the diagnosis of meningitis made?**
   A. Gram's stain
   B. Standard blood work
   C. Chest X-rays
   D. Arterial blood gas analysis

4. **What is the incubation period of meningitis?**
   A. 12 to 24 hours
   B. 8 to 36 hours
   C. 2 to 10 days
   D. 10 to 21 days

5. **Which type of meningitis is communicable?**
   A. Viral
   B. Bacterial

6. **Communicable diseases are caused by microorganisms. How many means of transmission are there?**
   A. 3
   B. 6
   C. 8
   D. 4

7. **What are bacteria?**
   A. Small organisms that can grow and reproduce outside the human cell in the presence of the right temperature and nutrients
   B. Small organisms that multiply inside a host; they die when exposed to the environment
   C. Organisms that grow rapidly in the presence of nutrients and organic material
   D. Small living organisms in or on any living creature

8. **Who does the post-exposure medical management begin with?**
   A. Employee
   B. Source individual
   C. Family members
   D. ICM

9. **The liaison who handles notification between the hospital and an exposed responder is the:**
   A. clinical director.
   B. ICM.
   C. paramedic supervisor.
   D. ambulance control

10. **In an approach to infection control, which of the following is based on the assumption that all blood and body fluids are potentially infectious?**
    A. PPE
    B. Handwashing
    C. Biohazard labeling
    D. Universal precautions

Challenging Question

It's 02:00 and you are dispatched to a house for a man who doesn't feel well. When you arrive on the scene, the patient tells you he has been coughing for approximately 2 weeks. During that time he has had a headache, unexplained weight loss, and night sweats. On the way to hospital, the patient begins to cough uncontrollably, including in your face.

11. **What are some communicable diseases this patient may possibly have, and how can you prevent becoming exposed to them?**

■ Points to Ponder

You are sent to the home of a 42-year-old man complaining of right-sided chest pain. During your assessment you find the patient to be in supraventricular tachycardia at a rate of 220 beats/min, with blood pressure of 100/70 mm Hg and a respiratory rate of 22 breaths/min. He is pale in colour and slightly perspiring. Before starting an IV, your partner practises the appropriate universal precautions. You are helping your partner clean up when you suddenly feel a sharp prick in the palm of your hand. You have just received a needlestick from the used cannula. Your palm has small specks of blood coming from it. When you arrive at hospital, the patient informs you that he has hepatitis C virus and is currently under treatment for this disease.

What should you do now? Could you have prevented this exposure?

Issues: Safe Management of a Patient With an Infectious and Communicable Disease, Compliance With Universal Precautions, Managing an Exposure.

37 Behavioural Emergencies

Objectives

Cognitive

- Define behaviour and distinguish between normal and abnormal behaviour.
- Define behavioural emergency.
- Discuss the prevalence of behaviour and psychiatric disorders.
- Discuss the factors that may alter the behaviour or emotional status of an ill or injured individual.
- Describe the medicolegal considerations for management of emotionally disturbed patients.
- Discuss the pathophysiology of behavioural and psychiatric disorders.
- Describe the overt behaviours associated with behavioural and psychiatric disorders.
- Define the following terms:
  - Affect
  - Anger
  - Anxiety
  - Confusion
  - Depression
  - Fear
  - Mental status
  - Open-ended question
  - Posture
- Describe the verbal techniques useful in managing the emotionally disturbed patient.
- List the reasons for taking appropriate measures to ensure the safety of the patient, paramedic, and others.
- Describe the circumstances when relatives, bystanders, and others should be removed from the scene.
- Describe the techniques that facilitate the systematic gathering of information from a disturbed patient.
- List situations in which the paramedic is expected to transport a patient forcibly and against his will.
- Identify techniques for physical assessment in a patient with behavioural problems.
- Describe methods of restraint that may be necessary in managing an emotionally disturbed patient.
- List the risk factors for suicide.
- List the behaviours that may be seen indicating that a patient may be at risk for suicide.
- Integrate the pathophysiological principles with the assessment of the patient with behavioural and psychiatric disorders.
- Differentiate between the various behavioural and psychiatric disorders based on the assessment and history.
- Formulate an initial diagnosis based on the assessment findings.
- Develop a patient management plan based on the initial diagnosis.

Affective

- Advocate for empathetic and respectful treatment for individuals experiencing behavioural emergencies.

Psychomotor

- Demonstrate safe techniques for managing and restraining a violent patient.

Introduction

Problems related to abnormal behaviour are commonly the result of "mental problems", implying that they originate in some ephemeral place called the mind, as opposed to "real" medical problems, which originate in the solid, tangible structures of the body. In reality, the mind and the body are not separate entities; they are inseparable parts of a whole human being. When a person becomes ill with any disease, that illness will inevitably affect the individual's behaviour—often making him or her anxious or depressed. Similarly, changes in mental state influence the body's

Notes from Nancy

Abnormal behaviour may be due to many conditions other than mental illness.

physical health. A depressed person, for example, may lose appetite or become more susceptible to bodily disease. Thus, whenever we examine a patient, it is important to view the patient as a whole person and try to understand both the physical and the mental factors that contribute to the patient's distress **Figure 37-1 ▶** .

For specific details on the Mental Health Act 1983 and the Mental Capacity Act 2005, please refer to the current JRCALC National Clinical Guidelines.

What Is a Behavioural Emergency?

The concept of behaviour has been widely debated over the years. Most experts define it as the way people act or perform—for example, how they react to a situation. Behaviour includes all the things people do and the reasons why they do those things. Who defines when the behaviour becomes abnormal

is also a source of debate, as is who defines what is normal—society in general, a particular community or social group, a parent, a boss, a friend, or even a stranger. Abnormal behaviour in and of itself may not be a medical problem and is hardly cause for alarm. The real questions are "When does abnormal behaviour require medical intervention"? and "When does it require an ambulance response"? Almost all disordered behaviour represents the individual's effort to adapt to some stress, whether internal or external. In most cases the disruptive behaviour is a temporary action, abating when the individual has managed to mobilise his or her psychological defence mechanisms.

Behavioural emergencies are situations in which the patient's presenting problem is some disorder of mood, thought, or behaviour that interferes with his or her activities of daily living (ADLs); ADLs are normal, everyday activities such as getting dressed and taking out the rubbish. When a

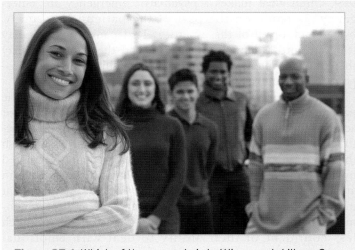

Figure 37-1 Which of these people is battling mental illness?

You are the Paramedic Part 1

You are dispatched to 49 Midway Drive for a 37-year-old man who is "acting crazy". The ambulance dispatcher informs you that police officers have been sent as well. You pull-up around the corner from the scene and wait for an update from the police. A few minutes later, they notify you that the scene is safe and one man is in custody.

You arrive to find a man in his late 30s lying on the ground with his hands cuffed behind his back. He is yelling about seeing flashing green and yellow lights from the sky. After you introduce yourself, he tells you that his name is Matt.

Initial Assessment	Recording Time: 0 Minutes
Appearance	Sweaty, anxious
Level of consciousness	A (Alert to person, place, and day)
Airway	Patent
Breathing	Fast and deep
Circulation	Fast, slightly irregular pulse

1. What are some medical conditions that can give the appearance of "acting crazy"?
2. What are some considerations to discuss with your crewmate while you parked away from the scene?

person becomes so depressed that he or she cannot get up in the morning, shower, and make breakfast, or when someone has delusions or hallucinations that prohibit them from holding down a job, a behavioural emergency exists.

A psychiatric emergency exists when the abnormal behaviour threatens an individual's health and safety or the health and safety of another. The most extreme examples are situations in which a person becomes suicidal, homicidal, or has a psychotic episode. In a psychotic episode, a person often experiences delusions (false beliefs) or hallucinations (false perceptions) that result in loss of contact with reality. For example, a patient who has taken illegal drugs may experience an alteration of reality—a "bad trip". Psychotic episodes can have very dangerous consequences because the individual's behaviour becomes violent, usually from exaggerated fear or paranoia.

No matter what definition of a psychiatric emergency a textbook may furnish, the *operative* definition of a behavioural or psychiatric emergency is provided by the person who dials 999. Often what makes a psychiatric emergency an "emergency" is panic on the part of the patient, the family, bystanders, or all of these parties. That panic, in turn, may translate into a demand for action, and the paramedic may therefore face intense pressure to do something (such as transport the patient to an accident and emergency department).

Paradoxically, it is precisely in this situation—when the patient is behaving strangely and bystanders are clamouring for action—that the paramedic usually feels least *able* to do something. Most paramedics would rather deal with a train crash than with the tangle of confused and frayed feelings presented by a psychiatric emergency. Most people prefer to operate in areas in which they feel competent. For paramedics, that means dealing with problems like broken legs, cardiac arrhythmias, or narcotic overdoses. Ambulance personnel feel much less confident of their ability to deal with emotional disturbances—especially since most paramedic training programmes don't delve into such matters. Furthermore, paramedics tend to be action-orientated people. They like to see tangible results of what they do—a hypoglycaemic patient coming around after an injection of glucagon, a clinically dead patient restored to life by CPR and defibrillation. What tangible rewards can there be in escorting a confused, hallucinating patient to the hospital, let alone in dealing with a belligerent and violent patient who is screaming obscenities?

In fact, prehospital intervention *is* possible and often critical in behavioural emergencies. Paramedics can make a huge difference in the life of a disturbed patient, and the skills for doing so can be learned just like any other skill. Indeed, the skills for dealing with abnormal behaviour may ultimately be much more important to the paramedic's work than skills such as endotracheal intubation. After all, how many calls require placing an advanced airway? Many more calls require the paramedic to deal with people who are angry, depressed, agitated, panicky, or out of control. Clearly, it's worthwhile learning an organised and systematic approach to emergencies that involve abnormal behaviour.

Causes of Abnormal Behaviour

Anyone who has seen a paranoid, belligerent diabetic transformed into a paragon of courtesy and charm by the mere addition of 10 to 30 g of glucose to the bloodstream knows that not everyone who acts crazy *is* crazy. Similarly, no one would diagnose mental illness in a person who was stunned and mute after the unanticipated death of a husband or wife. Abnormal behaviour typically results from a complex interaction of biological or organic causes, developmental factors, psychological stressors, emotional stimuli, and sociocultural influences. Those causes can be classified into three broad categories: (1) biological or organic causes, (2) psychosocial causes, and (3) sociocultural causes.

Biological or Organic Causes of Abnormal Behaviour

Many patients presenting with psychiatric symptoms are actually suffering from a physical illness or are under the influence of a substance that interferes with normal cerebral function. Such patients are generally classified as having organic brain syndrome. Diabetes, convulsion disorders, severe infections, metabolic disorders, head injury, stroke, alcohol, tumours in the brain, and drugs may all cause derangements in behaviour. When faced with abnormal behaviour, always look for situational and organic causes, as they're the ones you'll be best able to treat in an acute emergency.

The conditions and substances that can produce psychiatric symptoms are summarised in [Table 37-1 ▶]. Probably the most common offenders are alcohol and drugs. Besides intoxication with alcohol or drugs, other common forms of organic brain syndrome include delirium and dementia. Delirium is characterised by a global impairment of cognitive function that comes on quite rapidly and may fluctuate in severity over the course of a day. Delirium is almost always a disturbance in mental status. Dementia is a more chronic process that produces severe deficits in memory, abstract thinking, and judgement.

Psychosocial Causes of Abnormal Behaviour

Normal individuals may develop abnormal reactions to stressful psychosocial events (eg, childhood trauma) or developmental influences (eg, parents who deprived them of love, caring, support, and encouragement). When a person's basic needs are threatened, that individual faces a crisis. A person in crisis has two alternatives for dealing with this threat: (1) cope with it, finding ways to alter the situation or his or her perception of it so that it is no longer so stressful, or (2) attempt to alleviate the discomfort by escaping from the stress. Escape may take many forms, including alcohol, drugs, psychiatric symptoms, and even suicide.

Sociocultural Causes of Abnormal Behaviour

Chapter 2 considered the responses of patients, their families, bystanders, and rescue personnel to the stresses of emergencies and the various ways that people react to death and dying.

Table 37-1	Selected Disease States That May Produce Psychotic Symptoms	
Disease State	**Psychotic Symptoms**	
Toxic and deficiency states	Drug-induced psychoses, especially from: • Digitalis • Steroids • Disulfiram • Amphetamines • LSD, PCP, and other psychedelics Nutrition disorders: • Alcohol abuse • Vitamin deficiencies Poisoning with bromide or other heavy metals Kidney failure Liver failure	
Infections	Syphilis Parasites Viral encephalitis (eg, after measles) Brain abscess UTI Chest infections (particularly ones in the elderly)	
Neurological disease	Convulsion disorders (especially temporal lobe convulsions) Primary and metastatic tumours of the brain Dementia Cerebrovascular accident Closed head injury	
Cardiovascular disorders	Low cardiac output (eg, in heart failure)	
Endocrine disorders	Thyroid hyperfunction (thyrotoxicosis) Adrenal hyperfunction (Cushing's syndrome)	
Metabolic disorders	Electrolyte imbalances (eg, after severe diarrhoea) Hypoglycaemia Diabetic ketoacidosis	

Humans are social animals; we prefer to live in groups. Not surprisingly, then, social and cultural factors directly affect biology, behaviour, and responses to the stress of emergencies. For example, the effects of assault, rape, and racial attacks or the death of a loved one may produce significant changes in an individual's behaviour.

Psychopathology

Many factors contribute to disturbances of behaviour. Some of these influences are easily identified and treated, while others may never be clearly understood. The causes, signs, symptoms, and management of abnormal behaviour can be grouped into several common areas of psychopathology:

- Anxiety disorders
- Mood disorders and suicide
- Personality disorders
- Somatoform (a disorder involving excessive concern with one's physical health and appearance) and dissociative disorders
- Eating, impulse control, and substance-related disorders
- Schizophrenia and other psychotic disorders
- Hostile and violent patients

The remainder of this chapter focuses on these areas of psychopathology. Before considering those categories in detail, however, you need to learn about assessing a patient with a behavioural emergency.

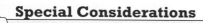

Special Considerations

The American Psychiatric Association (APA) is a scientific and professional organisation whose goals are to promote quality care, education, and research in mental health.

The APA publishes the *Diagnostic and Statistical Manual of Mental Disorders, Fourth Edition, Text Revision (DSM IV TR)*, a comprehensive reference manual focusing on mental health disorders, including symptomatic and diagnostic information. In the UK this role is undertaken by the Royal College of Psychiatrists and a number of charities supporting patients, relatives, carers, and health care providers.

Psychiatric Signs and Symptoms

When an organ begins functioning abnormally, the human body mobilises various defences to correct the abnormality. The patient experiences those corrective measures as symptoms, and the paramedic observes their effects as signs. Physical symptoms and signs reflect the body's attempts to maintain its balance in the face of physical stress.

Psychiatric signs and symptoms serve the same function for the mind. They reveal the personality trying to maintain the optimal internal balance in the face of a stressor. Like the symptoms and signs of physical illness, psychiatric symptoms and signs can be grouped according to the "systems" they affect. Here, however, the focus is on systems of psychological (rather than physiological) functioning. The psychological functions involved are consciousness, motor activity, speech, thought, affect, memory, orientation, and perception. Psychiatric signs and symptoms are categorised by disorder in **Table 37-2 ▸**.

Disorders of Consciousness

Consciousness refers to the degree to which a person is aware of and attentive to the external world. Disorders of consciousness such as delirium, stupor, and coma usually indicate an organic basis for the patient's disorder. Other disorders of consciousness, however, are seen in psychiatric patients. Inattention in patients means that it is difficult to gain their attention; with distractibility, their attention is easily diverted; and confusion refers to impaired understanding of their surroundings.

Table 37-2	Classification of Psychiatric Signs and Symptoms
Disorder	**Psychiatric Signs and Symptoms**
Disorders of consciousness	Distractibility and inattention Confusion Delirium Stupor and coma
Disorders of motor activity	Restlessness Stereotyped movements Compulsions Retarded movements
Disorders of speech	Retarded speech Acceleration or pressure 　of speech Neologisms (words the patient 　invents) Echolalia (the patient echoes 　words he or she hears) Mutism
Disorders of thinking	Disordered thought progression: 　• Flight of ideas 　• Retardation of thought 　• Perseveration 　• Circumstantial thinking Disordered thought content: 　• Delusions 　• Obsessions 　• Phobias
Disorders of mood and affect	Anxiety Euphoria Depression Inappropriate affect Flat affect
Disorders of memory	Amnesia Confabulation
Disorders of orientation	Disorientated to person, place, 　and time
Disorders of perception	Illusions Hallucinations
Disorders of intelligence	Mental retardation

Disorders of Motor Activity

Motor activity in a disturbed patient may be increased, decreased, or bizarre in some way. Restlessness refers to the situation in which a patient cannot sit still; when restlessness occurs in association with extreme anxiety, it's called agitation. At the other end of the spectrum, a very depressed or psychotic patient may exhibit exceptionally slow or retarded movements. In some cases, the patient appears to have little or no control over motor activity. Stereotyped activity involves a repetition of movements that don't seem to serve any useful purpose—for instance, a patient's repetitive touching of the elbow, nose, and forehead in succession. Compulsions are repetitive actions that are carried out to relieve the anxiety of obsessive thoughts.

Disorders of Speech

Like motor activity, speech may be abnormally fast or abnormally slow. Retardation of speech is seen in severely depressed patients, whereas manic patients often show accelerated speech and pressure of speech (ie, words pour out like water escaping under pressure). The words the patient uses may themselves be strange or unusual. Neologisms are words that the patient invents. In echolalia, the patient echoes the words of the examiner. When the patient doesn't speak at all, the condition is called mutism.

Disorders of Thinking

Thinking is the highest of the mental functions, requiring integration of knowledge, perception, and memory. Thinking may be disordered in its progression or in its content.

The *progression* of thought, like motor activity and speech, may be speeded up or slowed down. Flight of ideas, which occurs in some manic conditions, refers to accelerated thinking in which the mind skips so rapidly from one idea to another that the listener finds it difficult to grasp the connection between them. At the other end of the spectrum, depressed patients may experience retardation of thought, in which it seems to take a very long time to get from one thought to the next. In circumstantial thinking, the patient includes many irrelevant details in his or her account of things. Perseveration refers to repetition of the same idea over and over again.

The *content* of thought may also be abnormal in a patient with psychiatric problems. The patient may, for example, express delusions—fixed beliefs that are not shared by others of the same culture or background and that the patient is not willing to change by reasonable explanation. With delusions of persecution, the individual believes that others are plotting against him or her. With delusions of grandeur, the patient believes he or she is someone of great importance. Other delusions that suggest psychoses include thought broadcasting (the belief that others can hear one's thoughts) and thought control (the belief that outside forces are controlling one's thoughts).

Obsessions are thoughts that will not go away, despite attempts to forget them. Usually the person with an obsession knows that the idea is unreasonable, but can't stop thinking about it. Patients may, for example, have an obsessional belief that the gas stove hasn't been turned off, so they'll return again and again to the kitchen to make sure. Each time they do so, their anxiety will be relieved for a short time, but then they must go back and check yet again. Phobias are obsessive, irrational fears of specific things or situations, such as fear of heights, fear of open places, fear of confined places, or fear of certain animals ◀ Figure 37-2 ▶.

Disorders of Mood and Affect

Mood refers to a person's sustained and pervasive emotional state; affect is the outward expression of a person's mood. A person's mood may be described as *depressed, euphoric,* or *anxious.* Affect is described as *appropriate* or *inappropriate.* A

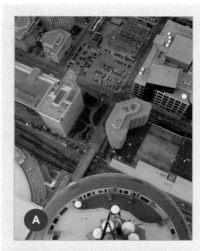

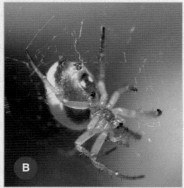

Figure 37-2 Phobias are irrational fears of specific things, such as fear of heights (**A**) or fear of certain animals (**B**).

patient who puts on a waxy smile as he tells you of a parent's death would be considered to be showing inappropriate affect—that is, the emotion expressed is out of synch with the situation. Affect is characterised as labile when it shifts rapidly, as in the patient who is laughing one moment and crying the next. With a flat affect, the patient does not seem to feel much of anything at all.

Disorders of Memory

The most profound disorder of memory is amnesia, the loss of memory. Memory is a complex process consisting of four separate functions: registration, the ability to add new items to the cerebral data bank; retention, the ability to store those items in an accessible place in the mind;

recall, the ability to retrieve a specific piece of stored information on demand; and recognition, the ability to identify information that one has encountered before. Amnesia may reflect the disruption of one or several of those functions. In delirium, for example, a person may be unable to register events properly and thus can't recall what happened while he or she was delirious. When painful memories are repressed, recall is impaired.

Sometimes patients with severe memory deficits from organic brain disease will invent experiences to "paper over" the gaps in memory; this behaviour is called confabulation.

Disorders of Orientation

Orientation refers to a person's sense of who one is (person), where one is (place), and at what day of the week one finds himself or herself (day). A person who is confused about those particulars is said to be disorientated. Disorientation is most common in organic brain syndromes.

Disorders of Perception

Perception refers to the way a person processes the data supplied by the five senses. Two disorders of perception are illusions and hallucinations. An illusion is a misinterpretation of sensory stimuli—for example, mistaking a piece of rope for a snake or a cat's meowing for a human voice. A hallucination is a perception that has no basis in reality and occurs without any external stimuli. Hallucinations may involve any of the five senses—a person may hear, see, feel, taste, or smell something that isn't there. Auditory hallucinations (eg, hearing voices) are the most common. Hallucinations involving other senses (eg, the frightening visual hallucinations in delirium tremens) suggest an organic cause.

You are the Paramedic Part 2

After a few minutes, you are able to calm the patient. When you ask why he's upset, he tells you that he came home from work to find the neighbour's dog barking. He tells you that the barking changed into understandable words. The dog said that it would tell his boss that he was stealing at work. Your patient also tells you that things have been stressful at work with many cutbacks and layoffs, and he's afraid he might lose his job if his boss thought he was stealing. After you display concern for his well being, Matt agrees to let you "check him over".

Vital Signs	Recording Time: 5 Minutes
Skin	Sweaty, flushed, and warm
Pulse	100 to 120 beats/min (dependent upon emotional state)
Blood pressure	146/90 mm Hg
Respirations	24 to 42 breaths/min (dependent upon emotional state)
SpO2	99% ambient air

3. What are the medical implications when police control the scene of a violent patient?

4. Is it wise to agree with or validate a patient's hallucinations?

Disorders of Intelligence

Intelligence refers to a person's intellectual ability. A person's intelligence is not necessarily a function of his or her education. For example, a person with a disorder of intelligence may have been born with mental retardation or may have suffered from a disease that makes it more difficult to process, remember, and communicate information.

At the Scene

Many people have mental disorders, and many individuals who don't currently have such a disorder may develop one at some point in their lives. It's no cause for shame. With so many stressors in today's society, it's quite understandable.

■ Assessment of the Patient With a Behavioural Emergency

Assessment of the patient with a behavioural emergency differs in at least two ways from the methods of patient assessment studied so far. In assessing the patient with trauma or acute illness, you use a variety of diagnostic instruments to measure vital functions and detect abnormalities—a stethoscope to evaluate breath sounds, a sphygmomanometer to measure the blood pressure, and so forth. In assessing the disturbed patient, *you* are the diagnostic instrument. You must use your thinking processes to evaluate someone else's thinking processes, your perceptions to test the validity of someone else's perceptions, your feelings to measure someone else's feelings. That takes practice, because most ambulance personnel are not accustomed to using their feelings in this way. For example, if someone makes you feel very angry, your reaction is apt to be "That guy infuriates me. I'd like to knock his teeth in". In conducting the psychiatric examination, however, a more useful paradigm is "That guy infuriates me, so it is quite likely he's paranoid, because paranoid patients often elicit anger in others".

A second way in which the assessment of a patient with a behavioural emergency differs from that of a patient with a nonmental medical problem is that the assessment is part of the treatment. As soon as you speak to the patient, your voice and manner will influence his or her condition, for better or worse. The very process of listening to the patient describe the issue at hand can also mitigate the problem.

Scene Assessment

The patient's overall condition and the nature of his or her psychiatric problem will determine how much of the assessment you are able to perform. A disturbed patient may prefer not to be touched, and you must respect that wish unless there's a compelling medical reason for doing otherwise (eg, profuse bleeding from slashed wrists or a decreased level of consciousness from an overdose). At the very least, you should be able to assess the patient's general appearance—for example, the patient's dress, cleanliness, and grooming, all of which provide clues to the way the patient perceives himself or herself. Pay attention to the patient's posture. Does the patient appear frustrated, angry, sobbing, or catatonic (lacking expression or movement, or appearing rigid)? Observe the scene carefully for weapons, remembering that almost anything—a chair, a lamp, or a book—can be used as a weapon. If you have any questions about your ability to manage the situation safely, call for assistance.

Initial Assessment

Identify yourself clearly. Tell the patient who you are and what you are trying to do. If the patient is confused or delusional, you may have to explain who you are at frequent intervals. Do so without arguing, in an emotionally neutral tone of voice. ("No, Mr. Jones, I'm not from MI5. I'm a paramedic with the ambulance service, and I'm here to help you".)

Attend first to priority problems—airway, breathing, or circulatory concerns. In most patients with behavioural emergencies, the problem will be more psychiatric than physiological in presentation. However, your assessment must look for signs and symptoms of abnormal functioning as well as abnormal behaviour.

Be prepared to spend time with the disturbed patient. Don't be in a hurry; rather, convey the message that you have the time and concern to learn what's bothering the patient. Assess the patient wherever the emergency occurs. Don't rush off immediately to the hospital, because the hospital is likely to be a strange, intimidating place for the patient; your haste to get there may reinforce the patient's belief that something is terribly wrong. Let the patient recover his or her bearings in familiar surroundings when medically possible.

Patients who are seriously disturbed should be seen by a doctor and evaluated for possible hospitalisation. Many of these patients will agree to their transport to the hospital. Others may not want your help and try to prevent you from taking them to a hospital. Because this kind of transport deprives the patient of his or her civil liberties, it must never be undertaken lightly. Even an experienced psychiatrist may find it difficult to define what kind of behaviour justifies removing a person from society or what constitutes "dangerous behaviour".

As a general rule, a conscious adult must consent to be taken to hospital. If the patient withholds this consent, he or she may be taken against his or her will only under an appropriate section of the Mental Health Act 1983, which will require the presence of a police officer and/or appropriate doctor and approved social worker to be present. The same applies to the use of forcible restraint. Where such measures are deemed necessary, police officers should be summoned. In addition, every ambulance service should have clearly defined guidelines, drawn up with legal advice, for dealing with patients who require involuntary commitment. Be familiar with these guidelines and the Mental Health Act 1983, and seek advice from your ambulance service if in doubt.

Focused History and Physical Examination

Begin your focused history and physical examination for individuals who are behaving abnormally by obtaining both their past medical history and their history of present illness. To gather the necessary information, talk with the patient and use your interviewing skills. Set some ground rules for your interview. Let the patient know what you expect, and what he or she may expect of you. ("It's okay to cry or even scream, but we aren't going to let you hurt yourself or anyone else".) Allow the patient to tell the story in his or her own way. Don't attempt to direct the conversation, but allow the patient to vent his or her feelings.

Interviewing Techniques

When evaluating a trauma patient, you can generally obtain enough information to provide appropriate initial treatment just from the physical examination, even if the patient is unconscious and can't give a history. When evaluating a patient with a behavioural emergency, by contrast, virtually all of the diagnostic information (and much of the therapeutic benefit) must come from talking with the patient. Skill in interviewing a disturbed person, therefore, is central to dealing with psychiatric emergencies. Here are some guidelines:

- *Begin the interview with an open-ended question*. An open-ended question doesn't provide possible answers for the patient, but rather allows the patient to select the answer. For example, say "It's clear you've been feeling bad. Tell me something about the kind of troubles you've been having". (The only circumstance in which you should begin with more direct questioning is when it is essential to obtain specific information in a hurry, such as "What kind of pills did you take? How many"?)
- *Let the patient talk* and tell the story in his or her own way, even if it takes a little more time. Letting patients talk allows them to gain some control over themselves and their situation. At the same time, it enables *you* to assess the patient's speech, affect, and thought processes.
- *Listen, and show that you're listening*. Your facial expression, posture, eye contact, an occasional nod—all of these things can convey to the patient that you're paying close attention to what he or she is saying **Figure 37-3 ▶**.
- *Don't be afraid of silences*, even though they may seem intolerably long. Maintain an attentive and relaxed attitude until the patient takes up the story again. It's especially important to be silent when the patient stops speaking because of overwhelming emotion. Avoid the temptation to jump into the silence with a hasty "There, there", to forestall the patient's expressions of emotion, such as crying. The expression of feelings is often therapeutic in itself—that's why people speak of having "a good cry"— and patients are often able to express themselves more easily after intense emotion has been released.

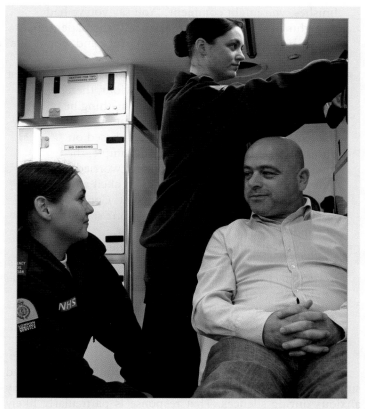

Figure 37-3 Making eye contact with a patient can provide useful clues about his or her emotional state—but don't stare at the patient.

Furthermore, your silence gives patients a chance to get control of themselves in their own way.

- *Acknowledge and label the patient's feelings*. The disturbed patient may feel overwhelmed by intense and chaotic feelings. Identifying those feelings and giving them a name (eg, "You seem very angry") can help the patient gain control over them.
- *Don't argue*. If the patient misperceives reality, make note of the misperceptions, but don't try to talk the patient out of them. When a misperception is very frightening or distressing to the patient, you might try just once to provide a simple and factual statement, in a neutral tone of voice ("Yes, that does look a lot like a snake, but actually it's just a shadow"). But don't get into a dispute on the nature of reality.
- Facilitation is a technique of encouraging the patient to communicate by using gestures or noncommittal words, such as a nod of the head or a phrase like "Go on", "I see", or "What happened after that"? You can also use facilitation to return the patient to a topic on which you'd like some elaboration. For example, a patient may have made a passing reference to suicidal thoughts and then moved on to another subject. When the patient

finishes, you might comment, "You say you've had thoughts of suicide"? This remark tells the patient that you've been paying attention to the story and would like to learn more.

■ Confrontation refers to pointing out something of interest in the patient's conversation or behaviour, thereby directing the patient's attention to something he or she may have been unaware of. Confrontations describe how the patient appears to the interviewer based on observations, *not* judgements. For example, the interviewer might remark, "You seem worried" or "You look very sad". Such comments often elicit a freer expression of feelings from the patient. Confrontations must be carefully phrased, so they won't sound nagging or condescending.

■ When the patient finishes giving the initial account of the problem, you will have to *ask questions*. Keep the questions as nondirective as possible. Avoid asking questions that can be answered with a yes or no ("Are you very angry"?) or asking leading questions ("Do you think that your husband is a part of the problem"?). *How* and *what* questions are preferred ("How did you feel when that happened"?).

Some patients find it difficult to deal with the unstructured situation of nondirective questioning and may become very anxious during silences. That response is particularly likely among adolescents, severely depressed patients, and confused or disorganised patients. When your open-ended questions meet with uncomprehending silence, try another approach and perform a more structured interview.

The Mental Status Examination

The mental status examination (MSE) is a key part of your focused physical examination of a patient who is experiencing an acute psychiatric problem. To conduct the MSE, you must check each of the "systems" of mental function in an orderly way. A useful mnemonic for the elements of the MSE is COASTMAP, also discussed in Chapter 14 (**Figure 37-4 ▶**):

■ **Consciousness.** Determine the patient's level of consciousness (alert, confused, responds to pain, unresponsive). Note the patient's ability to *pay attention* to a discussion and *concentrate*. Is the patient easily distracted, or can he or she focus on the events at hand?

■ **Orientation.** Ask what the year or month is. Ask the patient to state where he or she is at the moment—the country, county, town, or specific location. If the patient is not sure, have the patient make a best guess.

■ **Activity.** Examine the patient's behaviour. Is the patient restless and agitated, pacing up and down? Experiencing tremors? Sitting very still, scarcely moving at all? Making any strange or repetitive movements (scanning of the environment, odd or repetitive gestures)?

■ **Speech.** Identify the form, rather than the content of the patient's speech. Note the rate, volume, flow, articulation, and intonation of speech. Is it too fast or too slow? Too

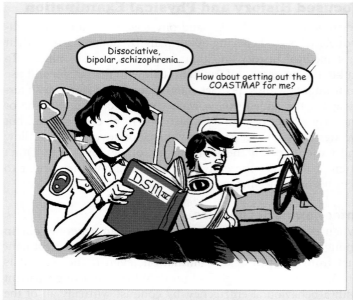

Figure 37-4

loud or too soft? Is the speech garbled or slurred (dysarthria)? Is the patient stuttering or mumbling? Using any strange words?

■ **Thought.** Listen to the patient's story. What's on his or her mind? Is the patient making sense? Is there anything unusual about his or her reasoning? Is the patient expressing apparently false ideas (delusions), such as a belief that MI5 is after him/her? Is the patient experiencing any false sensory impressions (hallucinations), such as hearing voices? Is he/she experiencing a flight of ideas?

■ **Memory.** Form an impression of the patient's memory—recent, remote, and immediate. If memory loss is present, determine whether it is constant or variable. Some patients may create memories to take the place of things they can't recall (confabulation).

■ **Affect and mood.** The patient's mood may be objectively noted via body language. Is the mood euphoric or sad? Is it labile? Does the affect—the expression of inner feelings—seem appropriate to the situation or is it animated, angry, flat, or withdrawn?

■ **Perception.** Detecting disorders of perception may be difficult, because patients often hesitate to answer direct questions about hallucinations or illusions. Sometimes it is helpful to ask the patient, "Do you ever hear things that other people can't hear"?

You can conduct nearly all of the MSE just by watching and listening (and knowing what to watch and listen *for!*). Only the assessment of memory, orientation, and perhaps perception requires you to ask some direct questions. Practise being an observer. Get into the habit of *noticing* how other people talk, move, and express their feelings.

Documentation and Communication

The mental status examination (MSE) contains many new terms that most health care and mental health professionals use to describe behaviour. Using the same terms will help you avoid ambiguous meanings and communicate a clear description of the behaviour.

At the Scene

The physical assessment of a patient with an acute injury or illness relies on the evaluation of specific criteria. The psychological assessment (MSE) of a patient with an acute behavioural emergency also has specific criteria. Most of the information in the MSE is gathered in the initial assessment and the focused history and physical examination.

Patients with psychiatric problems may be taking any of several types of psychotropic drugs—that is, drugs that affect mood, thought, or behaviour. During your assessment, you should determine which medications have been prescribed for your patient, and whether he or she is actually taking them. Psychotropic drugs are among the most widely prescribed medications in the United Kingdom. Most of these medications target the autonomic nervous system by either inhibiting or enhancing the sympathetic or parasympathetic nervous systems. The paramedic will have a thorough understanding of these two systems as well as knowledge of how the drugs in the paramedic's kit may potentially interact with these types of medications.

Many acute problems arise when patients fail to take their medications. Acute symptoms can be relieved by transporting the patient to hospital safely and quickly. In hospital, crisis workers may assist patients in getting their medications to prevent recurring episodes.

The Rest of the Focused History and Physical Examination

While much of your focused history and physical examination involves interviewing the patient about psychiatric history and performing the MSE, you must also look for signs of an organic cause of the patient's behaviour:

- Measure the **vital signs** for fever or indications of increased intracranial pressure.
- Examine the **skin** temperature and moisture. Scars may indicate deliberate self-injury in borderline personality disorders.
- Inspect the **head** for evidence of major trauma.

- Check the **pupils** for size, equality, and reaction to light. Pupillary abnormalities may indicate a toxic ingestion or an intracranial process as the source of the patient's behaviour.
- Note any unusual **odours on the patient's breath** such as poisons, alcohol, or ketones from diabetic ketoacidosis.
- In examining the **extremities**, check for needle tracks, tremors, and unilateral weakness or loss of sensation.

Detailed Physical Examination and Ongoing Assessment

Unless a significant traumatic problem exists, a detailed physical examination may be conducted to provide helpful information. Based on your transport time and the patient's mental status, the detailed physical examination may be deferred. However, during transport, when the ongoing assessment is routinely done, is a good time to assess more details of your patient's mental status.

Often patients with abnormal behaviour may have settled down physically, but their minds may still be in a state of flux; this could lead to very impulsive behaviour. Monitor patients vigilantly for sudden changes in thought or behaviour, particularly as you near the hospital. If patients don't want help, they may try to jump from the ambulance or hurt themselves. Medical and traumatic conditions may cause a deterioration in a condition identified earlier in the assessment.

General Principles

The following guidelines apply to the care of *any* patient with a psychiatric problem:

- *Be as calm and direct as possible.* Disturbed patients are often frightened of losing self-control. Your behaviour should indicate that you have confidence in the patient's ability to maintain control. Indeed, one of the main purposes of the interview is to help the patient re-establish some self-mastery. If you show anxiety or panic, you merely affirm the patient's conviction that the situation is overwhelming.
- *Exclude disruptive people from the interview.* In most cases, you should interview the patient alone, while relatives and bystanders wait in another room (your partner can interview them). Some patients, however, will become anxious if separated from an important person—a parent, or perhaps a friend. If another person has a calming effect on the patient, ask that person to remain present.
- *Sit down* to interview the patient, preferably at a 45° angle from the individual so you don't encroach on the patient's "personal space" **Figure 37-5 ▶**.
- *Maintain a nonjudgemental attitude.* Accept the patient's right to have his or her own feelings about things, and don't blame, judge, or criticise him or her for those feelings.
- *Provide honest reassurance.* Give supportive, truthful information—for example, "Many people experience periods of hopelessness like you're having, but today there

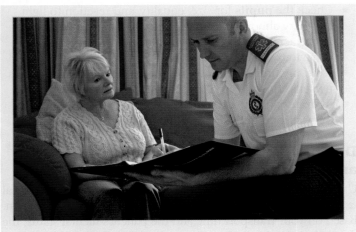

Figure 37-5 When interviewing the patient, sit at a 45° angle to avoid encroaching on personal space.

are effective treatments for those feelings". Avoid excessive reassurance, however, such as "Everything's going to be all right". Such statements will merely convince the patient that you don't understand how bad things are.

- After the patient has finished telling his or her story and you have concluded your assessment, *develop a definite plan of action*. This step gives the patient the feeling that something is being done to help, which in turn relieves anxiety. Furthermore, people in crisis need direction. Don't confront the patient with an array of decisions (eg, "Do you want to go to the hospital, or would you rather stay at home and call your doctor tomorrow"?); rather, state what you think is the best course of action ("I think it's important for you to go to hospital. There are doctors there who can help you"). Once the plan is determined and you have

begun to carry it out, allow the patient to make choices and thereby exercise some control over the situation. You might ask the patient, for example, whether he or she prefers to be carried on a stretcher or to walk to the ambulance on his or her own. These small decisions may seem minor, but they allow the patient to attain a measure of self-respect.

- *Encourage some motor activity*. Moving about often helps ease anxiety. If you are taking the patient to the hospital, have the patient gather up the things he or she wants to bring along. Let the patients do as much for themselves as possible, to reinforce the feeling that you expect them to improve.
- *Stay with the patient at all times*. Once you have responded to the emergency, the patient's safety becomes your responsibility. If the patient politely excuses himself or herself, locks the bathroom door, and swallows the contents of a bottle of sleeping pills, you'll have a lot of explaining to do—at least to your own conscience.
- *Bring all of the patient's medications to the hospital*. If the patient is receiving treatment for psychiatric problems, knowing which medications have been prescribed can help the doctors at the hospital identify the condition for which the patient has been treated.
- *Never assume that it's impossible to talk with any patient until you've tried*. Even if the patient sits silently and appears unaware of your presence, assume that he or she can hear and understand everything you say.

General Management

General management of the patient with a psychiatric problem follows the approach stressed throughout this text. After ensuring that the scene is safe, which may require assistance

You are the Paramedic Part 3

Matt explains that he's been struggling with his finances and may lose his house. His wife divorced him last year after she said he was a lazy husband. He says, "I still love her and wish I knew how to win her back, but it's been difficult to think clearly for the last couple of years". He starts to cry and whispers to you, "I wish I was dead". Given his behaviour and statements, you suggest that he come with you to hospital to be evaluated. He hesitantly agrees.

Reassessment	Recording Time: 10 Minutes
Skin	Warm, pink, and sweaty
Pulse	100 beats/min, regular
Blood pressure	140/88 mm Hg
Respirations	24 breaths/min
SpO2	100% on ambient air
Blood glucose	5 mmol/l

5. How important is police involvement if the patient apparently becomes agreeable?
6. What are the risk factors for suicide, and do they apply in this situation?
7. Would you talk with Matt about his comment or wait and let the hospital staff explore these issues?

from police officers, focus on any life-threatening conditions discovered in the initial assessment. If immediate life threats are not present, perform a focused history and physical examination to uncover any medical abnormalities that should be considered. If the erratic behaviour might possibly be caused by a medical disorder (eg, hypoglycaemia, overdose, or hypoxia), treat the individual for the medical disorder before presuming that the patient's behaviour is due to an emotional or psychiatric cause. These measures may include oxygen therapy, testing of the blood glucose level, and administration of glucose, as well as general interventions for hypothermia or shock management.

Disorganisation and disorientation are *not* diagnoses, but rather ways in which various conditions such as schizophrenia or organic brain syndromes (eg, head injury, drug ingestion, and metabolic disorders) may present themselves. These presentations account for a large number of ambulance calls, particularly those involving older people. While the paramedic doesn't need to make a specific diagnosis in such cases, he or she does need to know how these patients should be managed in the prehospital environment.

Disorganised patients are characterised by uncontrolled and disconnected thought. They are usually incoherent or rambling in their speech, although they may be orientated to person and place. Often such patients are found wandering aimlessly down the centre of the street, dressed peculiarly, uttering meaningless words and sentences. A thorough examination of such a patient is rarely possible, and the principal objective is to transport the patient to the hospital in a nontraumatic fashion.

The disorganised patient needs structure. The paramedic should explain in very plain language what's being done and what the patient's role will be. Directions should be simple, consistent, and firm. It may be useless to try to take a detailed history; a name and address may be all that can be obtained. Explain to such patients that they need to be seen by a doctor, and that you'll take them to the hospital to get help.

In managing the disorientated patient, the key is to *keep orienting the patient* to time, place, and the people in the environment. Tell the patient who you are, and explain what you're doing. You may have to identify yourself several times en route. Reassure the patient, and point out landmarks that will help the patient orientate himself/herself.

Specific Conditions

Anxiety Disorders

Anxiety disorders are mental disorders in which the dominant moods are fear and apprehension. Everyone experiences anxiety occasionally, and a certain amount of anxiety helps people adapt constructively to stress. Patients with anxiety disorders, by contrast, experience persistent, incapacitating anxiety in the absence of external threat. Almost one fifth of adults will experience some form of anxiety disorder in any given year. Several types of anxiety disorders are likely to elicit a call for an ambu-

lance or affect the delivery of prehospital care, including generalised anxiety disorder, phobias, and panic disorder.

Generalised Anxiety Disorder

Although some anxiety in everyday activity is normal, when a person worries about everything for no particular reason, or if that worrying is unproductive and the individual can't decide what to do about an upcoming situation, the person may be suffering from generalised anxiety disorder (GAD). To make a diagnosis of GAD, symptoms (anxiety and worry) must be present more days than not for a period of at least 6 months and the worry must be difficult to turn off or control. GAD is one of the most common anxiety disorders. Patients suffering from GAD are often treated with both pharmacological agents and counselling. The acute symptoms of anxiety and worry can become overwhelming in GAD, however, prompting a family member or colleague to call for an ambulance.

When dealing with a patient with GAD, identify yourself in a calm, confident manner. Listen attentively to the patient and talk with the individual generally about his or her feelings.

Phobias

Phobic disorders involve an unreasonable fear, apprehension, or dread of a specific situation or thing. The patient with a simple phobia focuses all his or her anxieties onto one class of objects (eg, mice, spiders, dogs) or situations (eg, high places, darkness, flying). Almost one tenth of adults have social phobias, or fear of everyday social situations such as fear of going to parties, meeting new people, speaking, eating in public, etc. When confronted with the feared object or situation, the phobic person experiences intolerable anxiety and all of the autonomic symptoms that anxiety brings. The patient usually recognises that the fear is unreasonable but is unable to do anything about it.

In managing a phobic patient, explain each step of treatment in detail before you carry it out Figure 37-6 ▾. "First we'll give you oxygen to help you breathe. Then we're going to move you onto this chair, so that we can carry you downstairs".

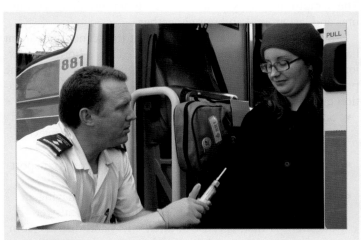

Figure 37-6 With a phobic patient, explain each step of treatment in detail before carrying it out.

Table 37-3	Signs and Symptoms of a Panic Attack
■ Shortness of breath or a sensation of being smothered ■ Palpitations or tachycardia ■ Sweating ■ Nausea or abdominal distress ■ Flushes or chills ■ Fear of dying ■ Feelings of unreality or of being detached from oneself	■ Dizziness or feeling faint ■ Trembling ■ Feeling of choking ■ Paraesthesias ■ Chest pain or discomfort ■ Fear of going crazy

Source: Adapted from American Psychiatric Association, *Diagnostic and Statistical Manual of Mental Disorders, Fourth Edition, Text Revision.* Washington, DC: APA, 2000.

Panic Disorder

Panic disorder is characterised by sudden, usually unexpected, and overwhelming feelings of fear and dread, accompanied by a variety of other symptoms produced by a massive activation of the autonomic nervous system. Women are two thirds more likely to be affected by this condition than are men, and the disorder tends to run in families. The attacks usually begin when the patient is in her 20s. Most affected individuals can identify a stressful event that preceded their first attack, such as an illness or loss of a loved one. Thereafter, the attacks may come "out of the blue", without any apparent precipitating stress. If allowed to continue, panic attacks may cause severe restrictions in the patient's lifestyle. The individual becomes afraid to go to work, to go shopping, or to leave the house at all, out of fear that an attack will occur away from home. The fear of going into public places is called agoraphobia (literally, "fear of the marketplace").

The classic signs and symptoms of panic disorder are summarised in   Table 37-3 ▲ . A large percentage of the signs and symptoms—such as palpitations and sweating—are a consequence of autonomic nervous system discharge, while others (chest discomfort, paresthesias) may reflect hyperventilation. The symptoms usually peak in intensity within about 10 minutes and last around an hour altogether.

By the time the paramedics arrive at the scene, the patient having a panic attack may be surrounded by a horde of anxious and excited people, who will themselves contribute to the problem. Accordingly, you'll need to take control of the situation quickly:

- *Separate the patient from panicky bystanders.* If you can find a calm friend or member of the patient's family, however, having this person present may be helpful.
- *Provide as calm an environment* as possible as you transport the patient to the hospital.
- *Be tolerant of the patient's disability.* The patient having an anxiety attack may not be able to cooperate or answer questions at first, because of intense fear and distress. Your manner must convey that everything is under control.

- *Reassure the patient that he or she is safe.* The word "safe" can be a magic pill that will often de-escalate symptoms to a more manageable level. "We're going to take you down these stairs on this chair. It's going to be okay; we'll go slowly and be very careful to keep you safe while we move you".
- *Give the patient's symptoms a name.* Once you have checked the vital signs and the electrocardiogram (ECG) monitor, you should be in a position to reassure the patient that he or she is not in immediate danger of dying. "I know that your symptoms are very distressing, but they're not a life-threatening condition".
- *Encourage the patient to do things for himself or herself* to the extent that he or she is able, to help regain a sense of being in control.

Panic attacks may mimic a range of physical disorders in their presentation. Conversely, symptoms of anxiety may be the presenting complaint in medical conditions such as cardiac arrhythmias, withdrawal states, anaphylaxis, hyperthyroidism, and certain tumours. For that reason, any patient experiencing a panic attack—especially a first panic attack—should be fully evaluated in hospital. Hyperventilating patients should probably not be treated with the "paper bag therapy". Patients whose anxiety results from an unsuspected pulmonary embolism or cardiac problem may suffer serious complications and even die from the hypoxaemia induced by this treatment. Hyperventilation is best managed by coaching patients to slow their breathing until they regain control.

Post-traumatic Stress Disorder

The number of traumatic events occurring in the general population has increased in both frequency and intensity in recent years. Post-traumatic stress disorder (PTSD) is a severe form of anxiety that stems from a traumatic experience; it is characterised by the patient reliving the stress and nightmares of the original situation. Causes can be as general as combat military service and terrorist attacks or as personal as a road traffic collision or sexual assault   Figure 37-7 ▼ .

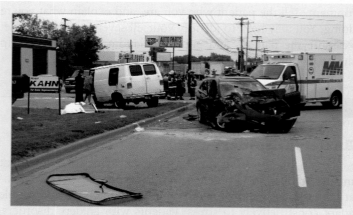

Figure 37-7 Post-traumatic stress disorder can be caused by a traumatic event such as a car crash with a fatality.

Table 37-4 Medications for Anxiety

Class	Generic Name	Trade Name
Antidepressants		
Selective serotonin reuptake inhibitors	Citalopram	Cipramil
	Escitalopram	Cipralex
	Fluoxetine	Prozac
	Fluvoxamine	Faverin
	Paroxetine	Seroxat
	Sertraline	Lustral
Monoamine oxidase inhibitors	Phenelzine	Nardil
Serotonin-noradrenaline reuptake inhibitors	Venlafaxine	Efexor
Anxiolytics		
Benzodiazepines	Alprazolam	Xanax
	Chlordiazepoxide	Librium
	Clonazepam	Rivotril
	Diazepam	Valium
	Lorazepam	Ativan
Nonbenzodiazepines	Buspirone	Buspar
Other Classes		
Antihistamines	Hydroxyzine	Atarax Ucerax
Beta blockers	Propranolol	Inderal
Anti-convulsants	Carbamazepine	Tegretol
	Gabapentin	Neurontin
	Valproic acid	Depakote

One symptom commonly associated with PTSD is flashbacks—sudden memories in which the victim relives the event. Sleep disturbances, including nightmares, and depression or survivor guilt are other signs and symptoms of PTSD. Treatment in the prehospital setting is intended to protect the patient, support the individual in a positive way, and transfer the individual to a medical facility for a more thorough evaluation.

Medications for Anxiety

Several classes of medications are effective in the treatment of anxiety disorders, including many antidepressants **Table 37-4 ▲**. In the past, drugs that exert a tranquilising or sedative effect, thereby reducing anxiety, were the most commonly prescribed (and overprescribed) psychotropic agents. Today, much safer drugs such as the selective serotonin reuptake inhibitors are more frequently prescribed.

Benzodiazepines serve such functions—as antianxiety agents, muscle relaxants, anticonvulsants, and sedatives. Unfortunately, they are often the source of overdoses. Some prehospital providers may use these drugs for chemical restraint, reduction of pain or rapid sequence induction; paramedics can only administer benzodiazepines to treat prolonged convulsions. Beware of the signs and symptoms of potential overdose: severe hypotension, bradycardia, slurred speech, altered mental status, and impaired coordination. Management of a benzodiazepine overdose includes airway management and IV fluids for hypotension.

Mood Disorders

Mood disorders, formally known as affective disorders, are among the most prevalent psychiatric disorders. As much as 10% of the UK population will experience a mood disorder, such as a major depression or a manic-depressive illness, at some point in their lives. Although feelings such as depression and joy are universal, mood disorders differ from normal bouts of sadness or happiness. In mood disorders, the changes in affect are accompanied by other symptoms, and the net effect is to cause a major disturbance in the person's ability to function. Patients who experience either depression or mania suffer from a unipolar mood disorder; that is, their mood remains at only one pole of the depression-mania continuum. Patients who alternate between mania and depression (both poles of the continuum) have bipolar mood disorder. The majority of patients with a unipolar mood disorder are depressed. Unipolar mania is relatively rare.

Depression and Suicidal Behaviour

Depression is the leading cause of disability in people between 15 and 44 years of age. It affects women more frequently than men and may occur at any age (the mean age of onset is 32 years). The depressed patient is often readily identified by a sad expression, bouts of crying, and listless or apathetic behaviour. He or she expresses feelings of worthlessness, guilt, and pessimism. These patients may want to be left alone, asserting that no one understands or cares and that their problems are hopeless.

Depression may occur in episodes with a sudden onset and limited duration; this is common in major depressive disorder, in which the patient feels substantial suffering and pain that interfere with social or occupational functioning. In other cases, the onset of depression may be insidious and chronic in nature. When a person experiences signs and symptoms of depression for the majority of days for at least two years, he or she may be suffering from a chronic form of depression known as dysthymic disorder. The signs and symptoms of dysthymic disorder cause social and occupational distress but rarely require hospitalisation unless the individual becomes suicidal.

The diagnostic features of depression are most easily remembered by the mnemonic GAS PIPES:

- **Guilt** and self-reproach are characteristic features of depression. One way to try to get at the patient's guilt feelings is to ask a question such as "Are you down on yourself"? or "Do you ever feel as if you're worthless"?
- **Appetite** is abnormal in depression. Usually it is *decreased,* but a minority of depressed patients may report increased appetite.

- **Sleep disturbance** usually takes the form of insomnia. The typical depressed patient will report that he or she awakens at 3:00 or 4:00 in the morning and can't get back to sleep again.
- **Paying attention.** The depressed patient has difficulty paying attention; that is, the ability to concentrate is impaired, sometimes severely. Ask the patient, "When you're reading a book or a newspaper, can you get all the way through what you're reading, or does your mind start to wander after a couple of minutes"?
- **Interest.** The depressed patient loses interest in things that were once important. He or she can no longer summon enthusiasm for work or hobbies. You might ask the patient, "Are you a [local team name] fan"? If the answer is yes, ask, "How are they doing this season"? The depressed patient will tell you, "Well, I haven't really been following them lately".
- **Psychomotor abnormalities** in the depressed patient can take the form of either retardation or agitation. Although many depressed patients seem to do everything in slow motion, a significant percentage show agitated behaviour, such as pacing, wringing their hands, or picking at themselves.
- **Energy.** Depressed people have no energy. They are tired all the time and don't feel like doing anything.
- **Suicide.** Most worrying is that depressed people tend to have pervasive and recurrent thoughts of suicide.

Medications for Depression

Antidepressants are prescribed to combat the symptoms of depressive illness ◖ **Table 37-5 ▸** ◗. They are classified into three categories:

- *Tricyclic antidepressants (TCAs) and related drugs,* like the neuroleptics, produce atropine-like side effects and may cause orthostatic hypotension.
- *Monoamine oxidase (MAO) inhibitors* are usually prescribed when TCAs are not effective. Their most notable side effect is *hypertensive crisis,* which may occur in patients taking MAO inhibitors if they receive certain other drugs (eg, sympathomimetics, narcotics) or if they eat certain foods (eg, cheese, yogurt, sour cream, beer, wine, chopped liver).
- *Other agents* include the very widely prescribed fluoxetine (Prozac).

Suicidal Ideation

Suicide is any willful act designed to end one's own life. It is the third leading cause of death among 15- to 25-year-olds and the fourth leading cause of death in the 25- to 44-year age group. For people aged 45 to 64 years, suicide rates are the eighth leading cause of death. Suicide is more common

Notes from Nancy

Evaluate the suicide risk in every depressed patient.

among men, especially those who are white and single, widowed, or divorced. The risk of suicide is also high among depressed patients, one sixth of whom will succeed in taking their own lives. Alcoholism is another important risk factor. Notably, more than half of all successful suicides have made a previous attempt, and three fourths have given a clear warning of their intent to kill themselves. The risk factors for suicide are summarised in ◖ **Table 37-6 ▾** ◗.

Suicide attempts typically occur when a person feels that close emotional attachments are endangered or when the person has lost someone or something important in his or her life. The suicidal person may also have feelings characteristic of depression—feelings of worthlessness, lack of self-esteem, and a sense of being unable to manage his or her life.

Evaluation of Suicide Risk

The assessment of *every* depressed patient must include an evaluation of the suicide risk. Many paramedics are reluctant to ask a patient directly about suicidal thoughts, because they fear that

Table 37-5	Medications for Depression	
Class	**Generic Name**	**Trade Name**
Tricyclic antidepressants and related drugs	Amitriptyline	Contained in Triptafen
	Doxepin	Sinequan
	Nortriptyline	Allegron
	Trimipramine	Surmontil
MAO inhibitors	Isocarboxazid	Marplan
	Phenelzine	Nardil
Serotonin reuptake inhibitors	Fluoxetine	Prozac
	Citalopram	Cipramil
Others	Trazodone	Molipaxin
	Clomipramine	Anafranil
	Dosulepin	Prothiaden
	Lofepramine	Gamanil

Table 37-6	Risk Factors for Suicide
- Depression, or sudden improvement in depression - Male sex, age > 55 - Age < 19 - Single, widowed, or divorced - Alcohol or other drug abuse - Recent loss of spouse or significant relationship - Chronic, debilitating illness	- Schizophrenia - Expresses suicidal thoughts and concrete plans for carrying them out - White - Social isolation - Previous suicide attempt(s) - Financial setback or job loss - Family history of suicide

they might "put ideas into the patient's head" **Figure 37-8** ▼. The paramedic should realise, however, that suicide is not such an original idea that a depressed patient will not have thought of it. Most depressed patients, in fact, are relieved when the topic is brought up, as this discussion gives them "permission" to talk about their suicidal ideas. Often it is easier for both the paramedic and the patient to broach the subject in a stepwise fashion. You might start by asking, "Have you ever thought that life wasn't worth living"? From there, you may proceed by degrees. "Did you ever feel that you would be better off dead? Have you ever thought of harming yourself? Do you feel that way now? Do you have a plan of how you would go about it?

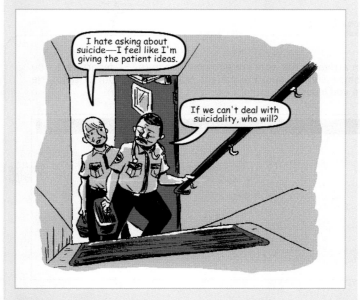

Figure 37-8

Do you have the things you need to carry out the plan? Has anyone in your family ever committed suicide? Have you ever tried to kill yourself before"? Patients who have made previous attempts; who have fashioned detailed, concrete plans for suicide; or who have a history of suicide among close relatives are at higher risk and must be evaluated at the hospital.

Many patients make last-minute efforts to communicate their suicidal intentions. When an individual phones to threaten suicide, someone should stay on the line until the ambulance crew has reached the scene. On arrival, quickly survey the area for

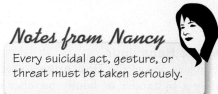

Notes from Nancy

Every suicidal act, gesture, or threat must be taken seriously.

any implements that the patient might use to injure himself or herself and discreetly remove those items. Make certain that you account for your own safety. Talk with the patient, and encourage him or her to discuss feelings. Ask the same questions mentioned earlier regarding the patient's suicidal ideas and plans.

Management of the Patient at Risk of Suicide

Whenever you find a patient to be severely depressed or you have another reason to suspect that a patient is at risk of suicide, follow these guidelines:

- Don't leave the patient alone. The patient's well-being is your responsibility until transferred to the care of another medical professional.
- Bring any implements of potential self-destruction you may have found at the scene (pill bottles, weapons) to the hospital.
- Acknowledge the patient's feelings. Don't argue with the wish to die, but provide honest reassurance. ("It's not unusual for a person to feel like you do after losing someone close to them. Sometimes it helps to talk about it".)
- If the patient refuses transport, try to involve persons close to him or her in eliciting cooperation. If resistance persists, it may be necessary to obtain police assistance.

When a person has *attempted* suicide, medical treatment has priority. The patient who has taken an overdose of sedative or depressant drugs must be managed for possible respiratory depression or circulatory collapse; the patient who has slashed his or her wrists must be treated to control bleeding and restore circulating volume. Nonetheless, if the patient is conscious, try to establish communication and ask the patient to talk about the situation.

A person who attempts suicide is in enormous distress. Among the most important skills that any health care provider can acquire is the ability to see beyond another person's behaviour to the underlying distress. When called to treat a person who has attempted suicide, it's worthwhile to say to the person, and to remind yourself, "You must have been very unhappy to do something like this. It's time to get some help or to talk to someone".

Table 37-7	Medications for Mania
Generic Name	**Trade Name**
Lithium carbonate	Camcolit, Lithonate, Liskonum, Priadel
Lithium citrate	Li-Liquid, Priadel
Carbamazepine	Tegretol
Valproic acid	Depakote

Manic Behaviour

Mania is one of the most striking psychiatric conditions. Typically a bystander or family member calls for an ambulance, because the patient is unlikely to believe there's anything wrong. On the contrary, the manic patient is more apt to report being "on top of the world—never felt better in my life". Individuals experiencing mania typically have abnormally exaggerated happiness, joy, or euphoria with hyperactivity and insomnia.

Medications for Mania

Drug therapy for bipolar (manic-depressive) disorder usually requires multiple medications (Table 37-7 ▲). Antianxiety drugs may help reduce agitation or anxiety, while antipsychotic drugs may help reduce psychomotor activity and delusions or hallucinations. Antidepressants may help reduce depression. While these agents may be used for a limited period of time, mood stabilisers are considered lifetime therapy for bipolar patients. Lithium carbonate and valproic acid (Depakote) are commonly used as first-line therapy. Unfortunately, some patients taking lithium preparations develop symptoms of toxicity, including nausea and vomiting, dysarthria, tremors, and lethargy. Lithium toxicity may lead to brain damage if not treated, so patients showing signs of toxicity require medical attention. Antiepileptic medications such as valproic acid (Depakote) or carbamazepine (Tegretol) are frequently used for lithium nonresponders, who account for 20% to 40% of bipolar patients.

The Mental Status Examination in the Manic Patient

In manic patients, the MSE is likely to reveal the following findings:

- **Consciousness**—awake and alert, but easily distracted. The patient may complain of an inability to concentrate.
- **Orientation to time and place**—commonly disturbed in manic patients.
- **Activity**—markedly hyperactive. Almost all manic patients report a significantly decreased need for sleep, and they may go for days without sleeping.
- **Speech**—pressured and rapid. The patient is also very talkative.
- **Thought**—flight of ideas and delusions of grandeur. Patients may report that their thoughts are racing; their monologues may skip rapidly from one topic to another (tangential thinking). Their ideas are often grandiose, such as unrealistic plans to embark on a large business venture or to run for high public office. Patients may also believe that they have special powers or they are famous and wealthy.
- **Memory**—usually intact in manics, but may be distorted by underlying delusions.

You are the Paramedic Part 4

You contact the hospital and notify them of your patient's status. Upon arrival at the accident and emergency (A&E) department, you are met by a nurse and a security guard. They are very calm and compassionate, and the patient readily trusts both of them. He remains calm throughout your stay there, even falling asleep just before you leave for another call.

Reassessment	Recording Time: 20 Minutes
Skin	Warm, pink, and slightly moist
Pulse	90 beats/min, regular
Blood pressure	140/88 mm Hg
Respirations	20 breaths/min
S_PO_2	100% ambient air
Temperature	37°C
Pupils	4 mm/PEARRL
Blood glucose	5 mmol/l
ECG	Sinus rhythm

8. How can your professionalism and general demeanour affect patient care in scenarios such as these?

9. What would you tell the hospital in your pre-alert call to help personnel there prepare for the patient?

- **Affect**—an apparently elated affect (the hallmark of mania). The patient seems to be on a "high", and is unusually and infectiously cheerful. The good cheer may be quite brittle, however, and the person may quickly become irritable, sarcastic, and hostile with very little provocation.
- **Perception**—may be disturbed. A person having an acute manic episode may show psychotic symptoms such as hallucinations.

Management of the Manic Patient

Individuals experiencing acute manic episodes have a high probability of getting themselves into trouble of one sort or another—for example, going on wild spending sprees, making foolish business investments, driving recklessly, committing sexual indiscretions, or picking fights. Generally it is when someone has got themselves into some sort of trouble, or when his or her behaviour has become intolerably disruptive, that an ambulance is summoned.

Because manic patients are unlikely to consider themselves ill, they may not agree that they need treatment. In dealing with the manic patient, be calm, firm, and patient; don't argue or get into a power struggle. Minimise external stimulation. Talk to the patient in a quiet place, away from other people. (Meanwhile, have your partner obtain the history separately from relatives or bystanders.) When it's time to transport, don't use sirens.

If the patient refuses transport, request a doctor and, if necessary, police assistance.

Personality Disorders

Personality disorders are "enduring patterns of perceiving, relating to and thinking about the environment and one's self that are exhibited in a wide range of social and personal contexts" and are "inflexible and maladaptive, and cause significant functional impairment or subjective distress". Common definitions of "personality" include the ways a person behaves or thinks. How people think or behave in the world and with others may be suspicious, outgoing, fearful, or overly dramatic. When these ways of relating to others become dysfunctional or cause distress to other people, that person is considered to have a personality disorder. Usually the person with the personality disorder doesn't feel any subjective distress but such distress may be acutely felt by others. The *Diagnostic and Statistical Manual of Mental Disorders, Fourth Edition, Text Revision (DSM IV TR)*, classifies personality disorders into three categories: odd or eccentric disorders; dramatic, emotional or erratic disorders; and anxious or fearful disorders.

True personality disorders are rare in the general population. When a person does have a personality disorder, another psychiatric illness is likely to be present at the same time. Such patients tend to do poorly during treatment. For example, individuals who are depressed in addition to having a personality disorder usually have more difficulty managing the depression.

Ambulance crews will have difficulty influencing personality disorders over the long term because of their limited interaction with patients. Nevertheless, they need to understand these abnormal behaviours to be aware of how they should react in the current situation. A patient with an antisocial personality will not think twice about hurting you if agitated. One with a histrionic personality may be demanding and dictate the level of care. Be calm and professional in your interactions with patients exhibiting these traits.

Somatoform Disorders

People who are overly concerned with their physical health and appearance may have a somatoform disorder if their preoccupation dominates their life. A hypochondriac provides the classic example of a somatoform disorder. In hypochondriasis, patients have a great deal of anxiety or fear that they may have a serious disease. They are so convinced that they're ill that even a doctor can't convince them otherwise. Although the problem in hypochondriasis is anxiety, the individual is preoccupied with other supposed symptoms. With somatisation disorder, individuals also have multiple complaints, but are more concerned with the symptoms than with their meaning. In conversion disorders, a physical problem (eg, paralysis, blindness, or convulsions) has no identifiable pathophysiology, but results from malingering or faking a physical disorder.

Similar to conversion disorder and malingering are factitious disorders, in which the symptoms the patient is experiencing are under voluntary control but there is no obvious reason for producing the symptoms except to assume the "sick role" and receive extra attention. This type of behaviour has also been referred to as Munchausen syndrome. When a parent (typically a mother) intentionally makes a child sick to garner attention and pity, it is referred to as factitious disorder by proxy or Munchausen syndrome by proxy. This is an atypical form of child abuse.

Dissociative Disorders

People who have mild feelings of being detached from themselves, as if they were dreaming, are said to be having a dissociative experience. When this dissociation becomes so intense that they lose their identity and assume new ones or are unable to function because they have lost their memory or sense of reality, a dissociative disorder may be present. Somatoform and dissociative disorders have been linked historically and share many common traits. Management of these patients centres on careful observation to prevent injury and management of symptomatic signs and symptoms based on local guidelines. Because treatment to correct the disorder is difficult and often unsuccessful, it should be carried out in the safety and security of a hospital. Talk with the patient about what is happening so you have detailed information to report to the hospital staff.

A stressful event, exhaustion, or physical or mental pressures—usually extreme in nature—may cause a feeling of dreaming or slow motion. These alterations in perceptions of reality are often referred to as dissociative experiences; they can be either mild and readily explained or extraordinarily frightening. Two types of experiences are distinguished—depersonalisation and derealisation. As a paramedic, you may have responded to a horrible road traffic collision where a patient described the event as "dreamlike" or "as if time had stopped". In such a case of depersonalisation, the patient loses his or her own sense of reality. In derealisation, objects seem to change size or shape; people may seem dead or behave like robots. In their most severe forms, dissociative disorders result in abnormal functioning, amnesia, a trance, or even a new identity (formerly known as multiple personality disorder).

Eating, Impulse Control, and Substance-Related Disorders

Disorders of personal control, motivation, and substance use generally evolve over a relatively long period of time. Because of the chronic nature of these problems, ambulance crews will typically be called when an acute exacerbation of the underlying problem occurs—for example, when a bulimic patient experiences electrolyte imbalances that produce a sudden onset of weakness, dizziness, cardiac or respiratory complaints, or convulsions, or when an alcoholic suffers respiratory depression from binge drinking. Emergency management of these patients typically focuses on treating symptomatic complaints and the presenting signs and symptoms.

Eating Disorders

Eating disorders have been around for many decades, although their incidence began to increase rapidly in the 1950s and 1960s. Today, eating disorders are widespread in the developed world and are emerging as a problem in developing countries. Some countries are experiencing a fourfold increase in eating disorders. Individuals most likely to be affected by these disorders are young females of upper-middle-class or upper-class socioeconomic status who live in socially competitive surroundings.

There are two major types of eating disorders: bulimia nervosa and anorexia nervosa. In both forms, individuals may experience severe electrolyte imbalances leading to cardiac problems, convulsions, and renal failure as well as less severe erosion of dental enamel and salivary gland enlargement. Anxiety, depression, and substance abuse disorders are noted in as many as two thirds of those diagnosed with eating disorders.

Bulimia nervosa is characterised by consumption of large amounts of food, typically more junk food than fruits and vegetables; many individuals with this disorder describe their eating as "out of control". Most patients compensate for the binge eating by using purging techniques such as vomiting, laxatives, diuretics, or excessive exercise. Individuals with bulimia are humiliated by both their problem and their lack of control.

People with anorexia differ from those with bulimia in one important characteristic—they are successful at losing weight. Unfortunately, they are so effective at losing weight that they jeopardise their health and even their lives. They may even binge, albeit on smaller quantities of food. These individuals diet by exerting extraordinary control over their eating. The typical anorexic has decreased body weight based on age and height, demonstrates an intense fear of obesity even though the person is underweight, and experiences amenorrhoea (the absence of menstruation).

Impulse Control Disorders

Individuals who have impulse control disorders lack the ability to resist a temptation or can't avoid acting on a drive. Examples of impulse control disorders include intermittent explosive disorder (acting on aggressive impulses involving the destruction of property), kleptomania (acting on the urge to steal things), pyromania (acting on the urge to set fires), and pathological gambling.

Of course, not every arsonist is a pyromaniac, nor is everyone who steals a kleptomaniac. Impulse control disorders are typically associated with other disorders, such as depression, antisocial or borderline personality disorders, and Alzheimer's disease. Treatment relies on cognitive and behavioural interventions to identify underlying triggers and influences. This group of disorders is rare; only 4% of arsonists are diagnosed with pyromania, for example.

Substance-Related Disorders

Substance-related disorders include psychological disorders associated with the use of alcohol, cigarettes, illicit drugs, and other substances that change the way a person feels, behaves, or thinks. These disorders have been known for thousands of years and now cost thousands of lives and millions of pounds annually. It was not until 1980; however, that substance-related disorders were recognised as a complex biological and psychological problem rather than a sign of moral weakness.

Substance-related disorders are regarded on four levels. In substance use, a person may use moderate amounts of a substance without seriously affecting ADLs (eg, a social drinker). Substance intoxication describes use that results in impaired thinking and motor function (eg, a drunk driver). Substance abuse occurs when the use of a substance disrupts ADLs (eg, a person has difficulty with work, school, or relationships). Substance dependence describes an addiction to a substance. The person is physiologically dependent and requires increasingly larger amounts to produce the same effect. An addict may display "drug-seeking behaviours" such as the repeated use of the substance or taking desperate measures to ingest more of the substance (stealing money, standing out in the cold for a smoke).

Determining the most effective treatment for substance-related disorders requires an integrative approach of examining the social, biological, cultural, cognitive, and psychological dimensions of the problem. As a paramedic, it will be difficult to explore these areas during a short transport to the hospital, particularly given that much of your time will be devoted to ensuring the safety of your crew and the patient's ABCs. Understanding the complex nature of substance-related disorders is the first step in providing professional, competent, and compassionate care to the homeless drug addict as well as the substance-dependent businessperson.

Psychosis

Psychosis is a state of delusion in which the individual is out of touch with reality. Affected people are tuned into their own internal reality of ideas and feelings, which they mistake for the reality of the external world. To the person experiencing a psychotic episode, the line differentiating reality from fantasy is blurred—not distinct, as it is in those without psychoses. That internal reality may make patients belligerent and angry toward others. Alternatively, they may become mute and withdrawn as they give all their attention to the voices and feelings within. Psychoses or psychotic episodes occur for many reasons; the use of mind-altering substances is one of the most common causes, and that experience may be limited to the duration of the substance within the body. Other causes include intense stress, delusional disorders, and, more commonly, schizophrenia. Some psychotic episodes last for brief periods; others last a lifetime.

Schizophrenia

Schizophrenia is a complex disorder that is neither easily defined nor readily treated, yet has a dramatic effect on society. One in 100 people will be affected by schizophrenia in their lifetimes. An estimated 0.2% to 1.5% of the world's population has schizophrenia. The typical onset occurs during early adulthood, with dysfunctional symptoms becoming more prominent over time. Some individuals diagnosed with schizophrenia display signs during early childhood; their disease may be associated with brain damage suffered early in life. Other influences thought to contribute to this disorder include genetics, neurobiological influences, and psychological and social influences.

Individuals with schizophrenia may experience positive, negative, or disorganised symptoms. Positive symptoms include delusions and hallucinations. Negative symptoms (a lack of normal behaviour) include apathy, mutism, a flat affect, and a lack of interest in pleasure. Disorganised symptoms include erratic speech, emotional responses, and motor behaviour.

Schizophrenia can be divided into several subclasses. The paranoid type is characterised by delusions or hallucinations usually centred on a specific theme, while cognitive functions remain intact. Individuals with the disorganised type of schizophrenia usually display the wrong emotion for a particular situation and are often self-absorbed. Patients with the catatonic type display odd motor activity, such as strange expressions in their face or remaining rigid, while the undifferentiated type features behaviours that don't fit neatly into another category.

Medications for Psychosis

Antipsychotic drugs are separated into two groups: atypical antipsychotic (AAP) agents and typical (traditional) antipsychotic agents (also known as neuroleptics). Both classes are prescribed to control psychotic symptoms, no matter what their cause. Antipsychotic medications are listed in **Table 37-8**.

Table 37-8	Antipsychotic Medications	
Type	**Generic Name**	**Trade Name**
Atypical antipsychotic (AAP) agents	Clozapine	Clozaril
	Olanzapine	Zyprexa
	Quetiapine	Seroquel
	Risperidone	Risperidal
	Ziprasidone	Geodon
	Aripiprazole	Abilify
Traditional antipsychotics	Chlorpromazine	Thorazine
	Chlorprothixene	Taractan
	Fluphenazine	Modicate, Moditen
	Haloperidol	Haldol
	Loxapine	Loxitane
	Mesoridazine	Serentil
	Molindone	Moban
	Perphenazine	Fentazin
	Thiothixene	Navane
	Trifluoperazine	Stelazine

Patients taking typical antipsychotic agents may occasionally experience an acute dystonic reaction, in which the individual develops muscle spasms of the neck, face, and back within a few days of starting treatment with the drug. An acute dystonic reaction can be rapidly corrected by giving diphenhydramine, 25 to 50 mg IV, but the muscle spasms are apt to recur after the diphenhydramine wears off. Neuroleptics also have atropine-like effects (anticholinergic effects), so patients taking antipsychotic medications may suffer the side effects associated with atropine use, such as dry mouth, blurred vision, urinary retention, and cardiac arrhythmias.

The AAP agents are often used as first-line therapy because they not only relieve symptoms such as delusions and hallucinations but also enhance the quality of life for schizophrenics by improving the affective symptoms of anxiety and depression and decreasing suicidal tendencies. However, the AAP medications may cause metabolic side effects such as glucose deregulation, hypercholesterolaemia, and hypertension.

The Mental Status Examination of the Psychotic Patient

The most characteristic feature of psychosis is a profound thought disorder, often accompanied by disturbances in mood and perception. The following list outlines disturbances of mood and perception.

- **Consciousness.** The psychotic is awake and alert, but may be easily distracted, especially if paying attention to hallucinations. If the level of consciousness is fluctuating, suspect an organic brain syndrome.

- **Orientation.** Disturbances in orientation are more common in organic disorders than in psychoses, but the severely psychotic patient may be disorientated as to time and place.
- **Activity.** Activity is most commonly accelerated, with agitation and hyperactivity, but can be retarded. Bizarre, stereotyped movements are common.
- **Speech.** Speech may be pressured or sound strange because of unusual words that the patient has invented (neologisms).
- **Thought.** Thought is disturbed in progression and content and may show any of the following disorders:
  - Flight of ideas, the headlong plunge from one thought to another.
  - Loosening of associations, in which the logical connection between one idea and the next becomes obscure, at least to the listener. In extreme cases, the patient's speech may be entirely incomprehensible.
  - Delusions, especially of persecution.
  - Thought broadcasting (the belief that thoughts are broadcast aloud and can be heard by others).
  - Thought insertion (the belief that thoughts are being thrust into his or her mind by another person) and thought withdrawal (the belief that thoughts are being removed).
- **Memory.** Memory can be relatively or entirely intact in psychosis. It may be difficult to obtain the cooperation of the patient for formal memory testing.
- **Affect and mood.** Mood is likely to be disturbed in psychosis. The disturbance may take the form of euphoria, sadness, or wide swings in mood; affect may reflect those inner states or be flat.
- **Perception.** Auditory hallucinations are common in psychosis. Patients hear voices commenting on their behaviour or telling them what to do. Suspect that patients are hearing such voices when they seem to be attending a conversation other than yours or talking to themselves.

Management of the Patient With Psychotic Symptoms

Dealing with a psychotic patient is difficult. The usual methods of reasoning with a patient are unlikely to be effective, because the psychotic person has his or her own rules of logic that may be quite different from those that govern nonpsychotic thinking. Furthermore, the paramedic is likely to feel uncomfortable in the presence of a psychotic person. Those uncomfortable feelings are one of your built-in diagnostic instruments. They

Notes from Nancy

Warning! The patient who hears voices commanding him to hurt himself or others must be considered dangerous.

are elicited by the fear, suspicion, and hostility that the patient is broadcasting through body language. Use your uncomfortable feelings to help make a tentative diagnosis of a psychotic problem. Then proceed as follows:

- *Assess the situation for danger* to yourself or others.
- *Identify yourself clearly*, and explain your mission. ("I'm Stan Elson. I'm a paramedic with the ambulance service, and this is my colleague, Steve O'Donnel. We've come to see if we can help. Can you tell us about your problem"?)
- *Be calm, direct, and straightforward.* Your calmness and confidence can do a great deal toward calming the patient.
- *Maintain an emotional distance.* Don't touch the patient, and don't be overly friendly or effusively reassuring. Convey an attitude of emotional neutrality.
- *Don't argue.* Don't challenge patients regarding the reality of their beliefs or the validity of their perceptions. Don't go along with their delusions simply to humour them, but don't make an issue of the delusions either. Talk about real things.
- *Explain your expectations of the patient.* ("We're not going to let you hurt anyone with that cricket bat. . . .")
- *Explain each step of management.* ("Let's walk downstairs to the ambulance".)
- *Involve people the patient trusts*, such as family or friends, in managing the patient and gaining cooperation.

Special Considerations

Paediatric Behavioural Problems

Behavioural disorders are estimated to affect as many as one in five children and adolescents, with two thirds of those having a mental health problem not receiving proper treatment. When not treated properly, such a problem is very likely to persist into adulthood. Given that suicide is the third leading cause of death in adolescents and the seventh leading cause of death in school-aged children, more attention has been given to mood disorders, anxiety, and other behavioural problems in this population. Children are also more likely to have coexisting problems (eg, attention deficit hyperactivity disorder, conduct disorder, and oppositional defiant disorder) along with the more traditional mental health disorders.

Mental health problems in children are difficult to diagnose because the lines between normal and abnormal behaviour are less clear in this population. Diagnosis and treatment may be difficult when trying to distinguish between organic, genetic, and environmental causes. Cultural and ethnic factors also blur the line between normal and abnormal coping mechanisms. The mental status assessment of the child is similar to that of an adult, but takes the child's developmental level into consideration. Abnormal findings in the developmental and MSE are often related to adjustment disorders and stress rather than to the more serious disorders. Your assessment must

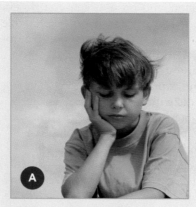

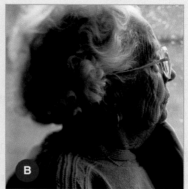

Figure 37-9 Children as well as older adults are affected by behavioural problems.

include an assessment of suicide risk in any child Figure 37-9 ◄.

Behavioural Problems in Older People

As people age, they are exposed to new experiences and alterations to routines that may have become well established over the course of many years. Some of these experiences may result in physical and psychological changes in the older adult. For example, dementia, a gradual loss of mental capabilities, may result from Alzheimer's disease, chronic alcohol abuse, after effects of multiple strokes, or nutritional deficiencies. The loss of loved ones or family moving away may cause loneliness. Financial worries, dissatisfaction with living arrangements, or doubts about the significance of one's life accomplishments may become a significant concern as well. These issues often produce psychological distress and physical pain, which may manifest as abnormal behaviour. Anxiety disorders, substance abuse disorders (particularly alcohol abuse), and mood disorders such as depression and even suicide are common among older people.

An elderly person is less likely to be accurately diagnosed with a mental illness than a similarly affected younger person. All too often, anxiety and depression are incorrectly considered a normal part of ageing. Ageism is discrimination against older people because of their age. To avoid engaging in ageism and to provide proper care for the older population, particularly those with mental health issues, you must first take stock of your own attitudes toward older people and the mentally ill. With this awareness, you will be able to perform a complete physical and psychosocial assessment without bias, and will understand the complex issues surrounding the care of older people.

■ Hostile and Violent Patients

Few situations are as difficult for the paramedic as dealing with a hostile, angry patient. It takes a great deal of maturity and a lot of experience to understand that <u>anger</u> may be a response to illness and aggressive behaviour may be the patient's way of dealing with feelings of helplessness. Sometimes the patient seems to be implying, "There's something very wrong with me, and you're not doing everything possible to help". The temptation is to respond with anger, but doing so rarely serves any useful purpose. Most angry patients can be calmed by a trained person who conveys an impression of confidence that the patient will behave well. It may be helpful to ask the patient directly about his or her anger. "Can you explain why you're so angry with me"? Giving the patient a chance to talk about these feelings often enables the patient to gain mastery over those feelings.

A patient who is violent or threatening violence poses one of the most difficult management problems for ambulance crews. Most ambulance technicians and paramedics see themselves as caregivers, not as "heavies", and often find themselves unprepared—both psychologically and tactically—to deal with hostile or violent behaviour. Furthermore, the encounter with a violent patient carries the constant risk that someone may get hurt—the patient, a bystander, the paramedics, or all of them. The best way to ensure that no one is harmed is to take preventive action—that is, to assess the potential for violence in *every* call and to take steps to prevent violence from happening.

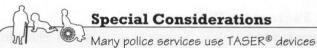

Special Considerations

Many police services use TASER® devices Figure 37-10 ► to immobilise people who are behaving in a violent or aggressive manner. TASER® devices were designed as an alternative to more violent immobilisation methods. There is some controversy in the use of these weapons in the in-custody death phenomenon. There is data supporting the assertion that these weapons are temporally, but not causally, related to these deaths in custody. More studies are being done. Ambulance crews need to be aware that many of the patients subjected to a TASER® exposure are at high risk for medical problems due to the underlying condition which is affecting their behaviour. It is important for paramedics to identify these underlying conditions and to ensure appropriate medical care. Conditions to be vigilant for include: drug overdose syndromes, excited delirium, acute psychiatric decompensation, hypoglycaemia, heat stroke, hepatic encephalopathy, convulsion disorders, dementia, and encephalitis. Police officers are not routinely trained to recognise these conditions, and will rely on ambulance personnel to make appropriate decisions at the scene.

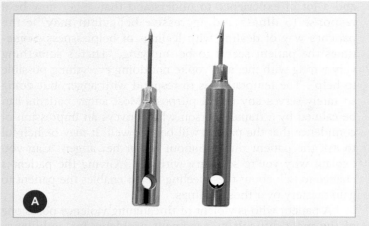
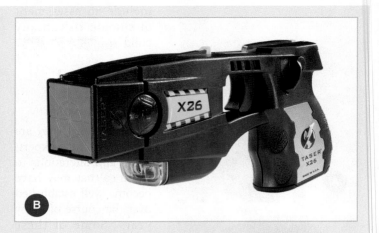

Figure 37-10 A. TASER® probes. **B.** TASER® Electronic Control Device.

Identifying Situations With the Potential for Violence

Preventive action starts with being psychologically prepared for a possible violent encounter and keeping that possibility somewhere in the back of your mind in your response to *every* call. Don't rely too heavily on the information you get from your dispatcher—the "elderly woman with a possible stroke" may have a disgruntled son with a shotgun! Being psychologically prepared for violence does *not* mean becoming paranoid or treating every patient with distrust. It *does* mean developing a "nose for danger", also known as "survival awareness".

Risk Factors for Violence

Scenarios in which violence is more likely to occur include any situation where alcohol or illicit drugs are being consumed (eg, public house, night club, party), crowd incidents, and incidents in which violence has already occurred (eg, shooting, stabbing, domestic disturbances). People who are more likely to be violent include those who are intoxicated with alcohol or drugs (especially PCP, LSD, amphetamines, and cocaine), experiencing withdrawal from alcohol or drugs, psychotic (especially manic and paranoid types), or delirious from any cause (eg, hypoglycaemia, sepsis).

The most important clues to the patient's potential for violence are found in the individual's behaviour and body language. Look for these warning signals:

- **Posture**—the patient who sits tensely at the edge of the chair or grips at the armrest.
- **Speech**—loud, critical, threatening, full of profanity.
- **Motor activity**—unable to sit still; pacing back and forth or in circles; easily startled.
- **Other body language**—clenched fists, avoidance of eye contact, turning away when spoken to.

- **Your own feelings**—your own "gut" response to the patient. If your instinct tells you that you're in danger, pay attention!

Management of the Violent Patient

Once you have concluded, for *any* reason, that there is a potential for violence in a situation, take the following steps.

Assess the whole situation. Are factors in the surroundings contributing to the escalation of violence (eg, friends who are egging the patient on)? Can those factors be removed? Does evidence suggest drug use, alcohol use, head injury, or diabetes? Can anyone present give you some background information? (Did the patient's behaviour come on gradually or suddenly? Does he or she have a history of violent behaviour? Are there any known medical problems, such as diabetes?)

Observe your surroundings. Make sure you have an escape route. Place yourself between the patient and the door, but don't move behind an agitated patient. Don't turn your back on the patient—not even for a moment. Note any furniture or other potential barriers. Scan the area for anything that could be used as a weapon (eg, heavy or sharp objects) if the level of violence escalates. If a violent patient is armed with a weapon, don't try to deal with the situation yourself; back off and notify the police. Make sure that others at the scene are not endangered while you await the arrival of the police.

Maintain a safe distance. Moving too close to a potentially violent patient is likely to increase his or her anxiety level. Maintain a safety zone of two arm lengths; if the patient is backing away from you, it's a sign that you're too close. Let the patient find a comfortable distance. Don't position yourself directly face-to-face with the patient but rather slightly to the side at a 45° angle, with your escape route unobstructed.

Try verbal restraints first. Anger and aggressive behaviour are often responses to illness or to feelings of helplessness. Just

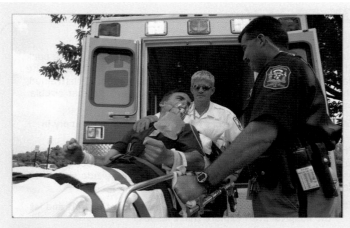

Figure 37-11 You may use physical restraints only to protect yourself or others or to prevent a patient from causing injury to himself or herself.

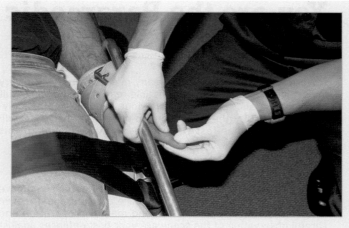

Figure 37-12 If the patient is restrained, frequently assess circulation distal to the restraints.

talking to the angry person in a calm, sympathetic way may defuse some of the anger.

- Take a moment to concentrate your own thoughts so that you can convey an impression of calmness and self-control to the patient.
- Identify yourselves as medical personnel who are there to try to help. Keep your voice low—that forces the patient to stop what he or she is doing to focus on what you are saying.
- Acknowledge the patient's behaviour, and restate your willingness to help. ("You look very upset. How can we help you"?).
- Encourage the patient to talk about what is bothering him or her. *Listen* to what is said, and *show* that you are listening by paraphrasing the words back to the patient. ("I think I understand. Are you saying that . . ."?)
- Ask the patient specifically if he or she might lose control or is carrying any sort of weapon.
- Define your expectations of the patient's behaviour. Acknowledge his or her potential to do harm ("You could really hurt someone with that crowbar . . ."), but assure the patient that losing control won't be permitted.
- If "verbal de-escalation" isn't working, back off and get help. ("Look, I've been trying to talk to you for the past 15 minutes and we're just going in circles. I'm going to leave you alone for a few minutes and see if you can get hold of yourself. When I come back, we'll try talking again, but if that still doesn't work, I'm going to have some people with me to keep you from hurting anyone".)

When verbal restraint fails, the use of physical restraint should be considered Figure 37-11 ▲ . Unless in immediate danger from the patient, restraint should be applied by police officers or other members of staff with appropriate training in these techniques (eg, care home staff from centres for patients with

mental illness). The majority of staff in the ambulance service are trained in diffusion techniques, awareness of the signs of impending violence, and break-away techniques.

Check the patient's peripheral circulation every few minutes to make sure the restraints aren't too tight Figure 37-12 ▲ . Check the radial pulses in the arms and the dorsalis pedis pulses in the feet.

Document everything in the patient's chart—the reasons for using restraints (be specific, giving examples of the patient's behaviour and the indications of the violence potential); the number of people used to subdue the patient; the restraining devices used; the status of the peripheral circulation after restraints were applied; and who travelled in the ambulance. Make sure you attempt to carry out normal baseline checks if at all possible.

Controversies

Physical restraint is not without complications and hazards. One alternative is to use chemical restraints, although this can only be used if a medical practitioner with the necessary skills is present. Until recently, benzodiazepines, droperidol, and haloperidol were the only medications available for chemical restraint in the prehospital arena. Droperidol is associated with prolonged QT syndromes and is therefore no longer used. Benzodiazepines and haloperidol carry their own risks. Newer atypical antipsychotic (AAP) agents, such as the injectable ziprasidone (Geodon), hold promise for preventing injuries to patients and providers.

You are the Paramedic Summary

1. What are some medical conditions that can give the appearance of "acting crazy"?

Abnormal behaviour may have many medical causes. It is very important to look at all of the possible reasons that could result in combative and aggressive behaviour. Hypoxia and hypoglycaemia are two of the most common underlying medical conditions that can manifest themselves in ways similar to this patient's behaviour.

2. What are some considerations to discuss with your crewmate while you are parked away from the scene?

Every situation has a potential for danger. Situations you have been asked to attend in which the police are on scene are even more likely to have problems. Good mental preparation and careful observation of the scene are your best defences against harm. Follow the lead of the police, but realise that even they are caught off guard at times.

3. What are the medical implications when police control the scene of a violent patient?

When the police are present, they control the scene. Ambulance staff should follow their direction on when and how to approach. Police officers are not responsible for medical care. The most important rule is for everyone to work together to ensure the safety of the responders and safeguard the best interest of the patient.

4. Is it wise to agree with or validate a patient's hallucinations?

If the patient asks you what a dog is saying, truthfully and neutrally answer that you don't hear it. This response does not deny the patient's own experience, but does inform the patient that others are not having the same experience.

5. How important is police involvement if the patient apparently becomes agreeable?

A patient's attitude and general demeanour can change in a flash. You must always consider this potential for change, especially if you will be providing patient care while alone in the back of the ambulance. Ask for escorts, including an officer in the back, if you feel it's appropriate. When the patient is restrained, check the extremities every five minutes to ensure that circulation and neurological function are not compromised.

6. What are the risk factors for suicide, and do they apply in this situation?

This man is in danger of losing his job, he has an altered perception of reality, he is recently divorced, and he is under the influence of drugs. He has several risk factors for suicide even if he doesn't express the intent.

7. Would you talk with Matt about his comment or wait and let the hospital staff explore these issues?

Every statement regarding suicide must be taken seriously, even if it's made impulsively or casually. You must determine the patient's seriousness by asking whether he or she has plans or has made preparations. The patient's responses may affect your immediate safety.

8. How can your professionalism and general demeanour affect patient care in scenarios such as these?

Talking with the patient is therapeutic. Take the time to build trust and rapport. Let the patient tell the story in his or her own way. Listen. Don't argue or dispute the nature of reality.

9. What would you tell the hospital in your pre-alert call to help personnel there prepare for the patient?

Hospital personnel need to know the basics of the patient's thinking and state of mind. They also need to know if and why the patient is restrained. If a patient is out of control, the hospital may want additional security or chemical restraints immediately available. Don't bring behavioural emergency patients into the accident and emergency department unannounced.

Prep Kit

■ Ready for Review

- Behaviour includes the things we do—how we act or react to situations.
- Behaviour may be abnormal as defined by society, your boss, a parent, or friend. Abnormal behaviour by itself may not be an emergency.
- In a behavioural emergency, the individual's presenting problem is a disorder of thought, mood, or behaviour that interferes with the activities of daily living.
- The behavioural emergency becomes a psychiatric emergency when the patient becomes suicidal, homicidal, or acutely psychotic.
- Abnormal behaviour can stem from a situational crisis, organic problems, or psychiatric causes.
- When assessing psychiatric problems, you collect information about the person's state of mind and thinking. Your actions and attitude often provide some of the therapy sought by the patient. Be prepared to spend some time with the patient as you assess his or her thinking.
- Dissociative disorders are characterised by depersonalisation (stepping out of one's current experience) and derealisation (an altered perception of objects or people in an experience). In the most severe form of dissociative disorders, multiple personalities may emerge.
- The mind generates specific signs and symptoms when it is not functioning well. Paramedics must sharpen their assessment skills to properly identify how the patient is functioning mentally. The COASTMAP mnemonic can be used to remember various disorders of behaviour.
- In anxiety disorders, the dominant mood is fear and apprehension. Fear can turn into a phobia when it becomes unreasonable. Anxiety, when sudden and overwhelming, may become a panic disorder. Anxiety, phobias, and panic disorder may complicate your efforts to treat a person.
- Mood disorders are the most common psychiatric disorders. In mania, the patient often feels great to the point of exaggeration, with hyperactivity, insomnia, and grandiose ideas. Feelings of depression can be accompanied by guilt, apathy, and sleep disturbances. Depression may become so severe that the person may attempt suicide.
- Suicide and attempted suicide are problems affecting all age groups and people of all socioeconomic status. Men are often more successful at suicide because they use more lethal means, although women make more attempts. Every suicidal gesture must be assessed and taken very seriously. Don't be afraid to talk with patients about their suicidal thoughts.
- Personality disorders are exaggerations in how people think about or perceive their environment and surroundings. They are classified into three categories: odd or eccentric behaviours; dramatic, emotional, or erratic behaviours; and anxious or fearful behaviours.
- In somatoform disorders, such as factitious disorders and hypochondriasis, patients are overly concerned with their physical health or appearance to the point that this concern dominates their lives.
- Eating disorders, such as anorexia nervosa and bulimia nervosa, are disorders of personal control related to eating. They can result in acute and chronic problems.
- Impulse control disorders include impulsive gambling, kleptomania, and pyromania. They reflect the inability to resist temptation.
- Substance-related disorders are associated with the use of alcohol and drugs. A variety of social, biological, cultural, and physiological dimensions define substance-related disorders.

- Psychosis is a state of delusion in which individuals are out of touch with reality. Causes include psychiatric problems (eg, schizophrenia), drug-induced psychotic states, and intense stress.
- Individuals with schizophrenia may display positive symptoms (hallucinations and delusions), negative symptoms (apathy and a flat affect), or disorganised symptoms (erratic speech or motor function). Dealing with psychotic patients is difficult because their behaviour may be dangerous.
- Disorganisation and disorientation describe how conditions may present themselves. Disorganised patients have uncontrolled and disconnected thoughts. They need structure, explanations, and directions. Disorientated patients may not know where they are, what day it is, or even who they are. These patients need continuous orienting.
- Dealing with hostile, combative, and violent patients can be emotionally and physically demanding for emergency responders. Be cautious when approaching these individuals and evaluating situations where violent or potentially violent patients may be. Know the specific risk factors and signs of hostile situations.
- Combative patients may need to be restrained. In such cases, the police should be requested to attend the scene to assist by providing this skill. Remember, you are an advocate for the patient at all times.

■ Vital Vocabulary

activities of daily living (ADLs) Normal everyday activities such as getting dressed, brushing teeth, taking out the rubbish, etc.

acute dystonic reaction A syndrome that may occur in patients taking typical antipsychotic agents. The patient develops muscle spasms of the neck, face, and back within a few days of starting treatment with the drug.

affect The outward expression of a person's mood.

agitation Extreme restlessness and anxiety.

agoraphobia Literally, "fear of the marketplace"; fear of entering a public place from which escape may be impeded.

amnesia Loss of memory.

anger A strong, negative emotion that may be a response to illness, and which could result in aggressive behaviour on the part of the patient.

anorexia nervosa An eating disorder in which a person diets by exerting extraordinary control over his or her eating, and loses weight to the point of jeopardising his or her health and life.

antipsychotic drugs Medications used to control psychosis.

anxiety disorder A mental disorder in which the dominant mood is fear and apprehension.

atropine-like effects Results of some antipsychotic medications that include side effects similar to atropine, resulting in dry mouth, blurred vision, urinary retention, and cardiac arrhythmias.

behaviour The way people act or perform, for example how they react/respond to a situation.

behavioural emergencies An emergency in which the patient's presenting problem is some disorder of mood, thought, or behaviour that interferes with their activities of daily living (ADLs).

bipolar mood disorder A disorder in which a person alternates between mania and depression.

borderline personality disorder A disorder characterised by disordered images of self, impulsive and unpredictable behaviour, marked shifts in mood, and instability in relationships with others.

bulimia nervosa An eating disorder characterised by consumption of large amounts of food, and for which the patient then sometimes compensates by using purging techniques.

catatonic Lacking expression or movement, or appearing rigid.

catatonic type A type of schizophrenia in which the person displays odd motor activity, such as strange facial expression or rigidity.

circumstantial thinking Situation in which a patient includes many irrelevant details in his or her account of things.

compulsion A repetitive action carried out to relieve the anxiety of obsessive thoughts.

confabulation The invention of experiences to cover gaps in memory, seen in patients with certain organic brain syndromes.

confrontation Interviewing technique in which the interviewer points out to the patient something of interest in his/her conversation or behaviour.

confusion An impaired understanding of one's surroundings.

delirium An acute confessional state characterised by global impairment of thinking, perception, judgement, and memory.

delusion A fixed belief that is not shared by others of a person's culture or background and that can't be changed by reasonable argument; a false belief.

delusions of grandeur A state in which a person believes oneself to be someone of great importance.

delusions of persecution A state in which a person believes that others are plotting against him or her.

dementia Chronic deterioration of mental function.

depersonalisation A type of dissociative disorder in which a person loses his or her sense of reality, and may experience events as being "dream-like".

depression A persistent mood of sadness, despair, and discouragement; may be a symptom of many different mental and physical disorders, or it may be a disorder on its own.

derealisation A symptom of a dissociative disorder in which objects seem to change size or shape; people may seem dead or behave like robots when viewed during a moment of acute stress.

disorganisation A condition in which a person is characterised by uncontrolled and disconnected thought, is usually incoherent or rambling in speech, and may or may not be orientated to person and place.

disorganised symptoms Refers to erratic speech, emotional responses, and motor behaviour.

disorganised type A type of schizophrenia in which the person usually displays the wrong emotion for a particular situation, often self-absorbed.

disorientation Confusion regarding a person's sense of who one is (person), where one is (place), and at what point in time one finds oneself (time).

dissociation Feelings of being detached from yourself, as if you were dreaming.

distractibility The patient's attention is easily diverted.

echolalia Meaningless echoing of the interviewer's words by the patient.

facilitation An interviewing technique in which the interviewer uses noncommittal words and gestures to encourage the patient to proceed.

fear Also sometimes referred to as a phobia, this is an anxious feeling, usually about specific things or situations.

flat Used to describe behaviour in which the patient doesn't seem to feel much of anything at all.

flight of ideas Accelerated thinking in which the mind skips very rapidly from one thought to the next.

generalised anxiety disorder (GAD) A disorder in which a person worries about everything for no particular reason, or their worrying is unproductive and they can't decide what to do about an upcoming situation.

hallucination A sense perception not founded on objective reality; a false perception.

illusion A misinterpretation of sensory stimuli.

impulse control disorders A condition in which an individual lacks the ability to resist a temptation or can't stop acting on a drive.

inattention Used to describe patients with whom it is difficult to gain their attention or focus.

labile Used to describe a rapid shift in mood.

loosening of associations A situation in which the logical connection between one idea and the next becomes obscure, at least to the listener.

mania A mental disorder characterised by abnormally exaggerated happiness, joy, or euphoria with hyperactivity, insomnia, and grandiose ideas.

manic-depressive illness A bipolar disorder in which mood fluctuates between depression and mania. The alterations in mood are usually episodic and recurrent.

mental status examination (MSE) A way of measuring the "mental vital signs" in a disturbed patient. The mnemonic COASTMAP can be used to conduct this examination, assessing consciousness, orientation, activity, speech, thought, memory, affect and mood, and perception.

mood A person's sustained and pervasive emotional state.

mood disorder A group of disorders in which the disturbance of mood is accompanied by full or partial manic or depressive syndrome.

mutism The absence of speech.

negative symptoms Evidence of a disease or condition, noted by lack of normal circumstances, rather than the presence of new physical evidence or a physical change; with regard to schizophrenia, refers to a lack of normal behaviour, and apathy, mutism, a flat affect, and a lack of interest in pleasure.

neologism An invented word that has meaning only to its inventor.

obsession A persistent idea that a person cannot dismiss from his or her thoughts.

organic brain syndrome Temporary or permanent dysfunction of the brain, caused by a disturbance in the physical or physiological functioning of brain tissue.

orientation A person's sense of who one is (person), where one is (place), and at what day of the week one finds oneself (day).

paranoid type A type of schizophrenia in which the person experiences delusions or hallucinations usually centered around a specific theme, where their cognitive functions remain intact.

perception The way a person processes the data supplied by the five senses.

perseveration Repeating the same idea over and over again.

personality disorder The term used to describe a condition a person has when he or she behaves or thinks in a way that is dysfunctional or causes distress to other people.

phobia An abnormal and persistent dread of a specific object or situation.

positive symptoms Evidence of or physical change due to a disease or condition, which can be physically noted by the patient or health care provider; with regard to schizophrenia, refers to delusions and hallucinations.

post-traumatic stress disorder (PTSD) A severe form of anxiety that stems from a traumatic experience. PTSD is characterised by the reliving of the stress and nightmares of the original situation.

posture The position of one's body.

pressure of speech Speech in which words seem to tumble out under immense emotional pressure.

psychiatric emergency An emergency in which abnormal behaviour threatens an individual's health and safety or the health and safety of another person, for example when a person becomes suicidal, homicidal, or has a psychotic episode.

psychosis A mental disorder characterised by loss of contact with reality.

psychotropic drugs Drugs that affect mood, thought, or behaviour.

recall The ability to retrieve a specific piece of stored information on demand.

recognition The ability to identify information that one has encountered before.

registration The ability to add new items to the cerebral data bank.

restlessness A situation in which the patient can't sit still.

retardation of thought The patient seems to take a very long time to get from one thought to the next.

retention The ability to store items in an accessible place in the mind.

simple phobia A fear that is focused on one class of objects (eg, mice, spiders, dogs) or situations (eg, high places, darkness, flying).

somatoform disorder A condition in which a person is overly concerned with physical health and appearance to the point that it dominates his or her life; an example is hypochondria.

stereotyped activity Repetitive movements that don't appear to serve any purpose.

substance abuse Use of a substance that disrupts activities of daily living.

substance dependence Use of a substance that results in addiction and physiological dependence on the substance.

substance intoxication Use of a substance that results in impaired thinking and motor function.

substance use Use of moderate amounts of a substance without seriously affecting activities of daily living.

suicide Any willful act designed to bring an end to one's own life.

tangential thinking Leaving the current topic midconversation to talk about something else, inhibiting interpersonal communication.

thought broadcasting The belief that others can hear one's thoughts.

thought control The belief that outside forces are controlling one's thoughts.

thought insertion The belief that thoughts are being thrust into one's mind by another person.

thought withdrawal The belief that thoughts are being removed from one's mind.

undifferentiated type Schizophrenia that does not fit neatly into another category.

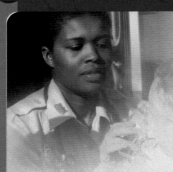

Assessment in Action

Ambulance control requests that you respond with the police service to "check the welfare" of an older woman. They received a call from the woman's niece, who lives in another part of the country. She said her aunt called and told her that her house was being robbed by an "invisible man". This behaviour is not normal for her.

On your arrival, the police service has to use force to gain access to the flat. You find the patient squatting in the corner. She is belligerent and screaming obscenities to the "invisible robber". You spend some time trying to speak with her, but she isn't cooperative. It is time to transport the patient to hospital, but she refuses to go.

1. **This patient is likely to be having a(n) _____ type of behavioural emergency.**
   A. organic
   B. situational
   C. psychiatric
   D. depressive

2. **What type of psychiatric disorder could this be considered?**
   A. Mood disorder
   B. Eating disorder
   C. Somatoform disorder
   D. Schizophrenic/psychotic disorder

3. **Which of the following statements regarding open-ended questions is not true?**
   A. They can lead patients to give a specific answer.
   B. They give patients an opportunity to express themselves.
   C. They encourage better patient responses.
   D. They are less likely to provoke unwanted answers.

4. **Classifications of psychiatric signs and symptoms include:**
   A. disorders of consciousness.
   B. disorders of motor activity.
   C. disorders of speech.
   D. all of the above.

5. **Delusions of persecution fall under which classification?**
   A. Disorders of thinking
   B. Disorders of orientation
   C. Disorders of perception
   D. Disorders of memory

6. **Disorder of perception refers to a:**
   A. person's sense of who one is, where one is, and what time it is.
   B. person's ability to process the data supplied by the five senses.
   C. person's intellectual ability.
   D. person's sustained and pervasive emotional state.

7. **The patient in the above scenario is having which of the following?**
   A. A hallucination
   B. An illusion
   C. Acute depression
   D. Organic symptoms

8. **When examining a patient's mental status, use the mnemonic:**
   A. SAMPLE.
   B. AMPLE.
   C. MSE.
   D. COASTMAP.

9. **Psychosis is defined as a(n):**
   A. state of delusion and describes individuals who are out of touch with reality.
   B. complex disorder that is neither easily defined nor easily treated, and that dramatically affects today's society.
   C. inability to resist a temptation.
   D. eating disorder.

10. **The best way to deal with a patient having hallucinations is to:**
    A. use physical restraints.
    B. use the talk-down method.
    C. administer antipsychotic medications.
    D. scream at the patient.

Challenging Question

You are sent to a private house for a 96-year-old woman. The patient's daughter found her sitting in a chair, not responding as she would normally. Her daughter initially thought she might have awakened her mother, and her mother was just "a little slow". After approximately 30 minutes, she called 999. Upon your arrival, you find the patient to be resting comfortably in her chair. She is alert and responsive to her name and address only. She doesn't remember her daughter's name, nor does she know what month or year it is. Her daughter states that she has had a stroke in the past and has a history of high blood pressure. The patient denies any complaints, has no chest pain, and no shortness of breath. During your assessment you find no neurological deficits, and the patient has equal hand grips, negative facial droop, and negative slurred speech. Her blood glucose level is 6.2 mmol/l. She doesn't remember getting out of bed this morning and doesn't remember going to her chair. She continuously asks you who you are and why you're there.

11. **As the paramedic, what is your differential diagnosis?**

Points to Ponder

Toward the end of your shift, you are sent to a private house for a 24-year-old man having chest pain. When you arrive on scene, you find the young man lying on the ground, complaining of reproducible chest pain and trembling. He appears to be hyperventilating. He does not answer questions, but does follow commands. His vital signs are all within normal limits, except he's breathing approximately 30 times per minute. As you attempt to speak to the patient, his father keeps interrupting, wanting to know whether his son is having a heart attack. The father is upset that you're not transporting right away. While you're attempting to take control of the scene, his sister tells you that the patient was on the phone with his girlfriend and she was breaking up with him. He became very agitated, and then began to breathe "very fast". She called 999. The patient has a history of anxiety/panic attacks, but this episode was different from previous ones.

What are some possibilities for what could be happening with this patient? How can you calm this patient down?

Issues: Empathy for Patients With Behavioural Emergencies, Respectful Approach to Patients and Family Members.

38 Gynaecological Emergencies

Objectives

Cognitive

- Review the anatomic structures and physiology of the female reproductive system.
- Identify the normal events of the menstrual cycle.
- Describe how to assess a patient with a gynaecological complaint.
- Explain how to recognise a gynaecological emergency.
- Describe the general care of any patient experiencing a gynaecological emergency.
- Describe the pathophysiology, assessment, and management of specific gynaecological emergencies.

Affective

- Value the importance of maintaining a patient's modesty and privacy while still being able to obtain necessary information.
- Defend the need to provide care for a patient of sexual assault, while still preventing destruction of crime scene information.
- Serve as a role model for other ambulance clinicians when discussing or caring for patients with gynaecological emergencies.

Psychomotor

- Demonstrate how to assess a patient with a gynaecological complaint.
- Demonstrate how to provide care for a patient with:
  - Excessive vaginal bleeding
  - Abdominal pain
  - Sexual assault

Introduction

The *Merriam-Webster Dictionary* defines gynaecology as "a branch of medicine that deals with the diseases and routine physical care of the reproductive system of women" and obstetrics as "a branch of medical science that deals with birth and with its antecedents and sequels". Although the medical specialities of obstetrics and gynaecology are separate fields of study, the two are so inextricably entwined—as these definitions make clear—that it is virtually impossible to write about one without referencing the other.

Before the 20th century, both fields of study were relegated to the realm of "subjects not discussed in polite society". Despite the work of pioneering doctors dating back as far as 98 AD, most of the knowledge of these two sciences was held by midwives, who jealously guarded the "secrets" of women with almost religious fervour.

One of the earliest medical texts covering obstetrics and gynaecology was written by Soranus (98 AD), a Greco-Roman doctor. His obstetric textbook, which was used until the 1600s, described podalic version (delivery of the infant feet first), the obstetric chair, and instructions for the newborn: "boiled water and honey for the child for the first two days, then on to the mother's breast". Unfortunately for women, the enlightened science of the Romans did not survive their empire. In 1522, a German doctor named Wert masqueraded as a woman to sneak a peek at the mysteries of the birthing room. He was unmasked and burned at the stake for his intellectual curiosity.

Three other doctors of the 1500s fared better than the hapless Dr Wert. Ambrose Pare was a surgeon-barber who apprenticed at the famous Paris Hotel Dieu, the first midwife school in Paris, and was one of the first doctors to record dilating the cervix to induce labour. Thomas Raynalde penned *The Birth of Mankynde* in 1544, which described caesarean section. In 1554, Jacob Rueff published *De Conceptu Generationis Hominis,* which described the whole process of pregnancy.

Despite the advances of these forward-thinking minds, childbirth and female medical conditions remained in the realm of superstition and folk medicine until well into the 1900s. The women's suffrage movement (1848–1920) and the women's liberation movement of the 1960s not only catalysed progress in equal rights, but also made strides in the scientific study of women's unique medical problems.

The physiological, emotional, and mental processes experienced by the two sexes are widely disparate, despite sharing many similarities. The physiological, chemical, hormonal, and even mental differences between men and women are beyond the scope of this book. The most obvious difference between the two sexes, however, is that women are uniquely designed to conceive and give birth.

This chapter first discusses the female anatomy, then outlines issues that are unique to female patients, including problems that may be encountered in the emergency setting. We next consider the gynaecological causes of abdominal pain in women and look in detail at life-threatening conditions. We also briefly examine vaginal bleeding, both traumatic and organic, and discuss how it should be managed in the prehospital environment. Finally, we consider the principles of managing a woman who has been the victim of sexual assault.

Female Anatomy

The female external genitalia, collectively called the vulva, are the structures seen from the outside of the body **Figure 38-1 ▶**. The mons pubis is a rounded pad of fatty (adipose) tissue that overlies the symphysis pubis, located anterior to the urethral and vaginal openings. The mons pubis is not an organ, but rather a "landmark". Coarse, dark hair normally

You are the Paramedic Part 1

You are dispatched to the home of a 40-year-old woman with abdominal pain and vaginal bleeding. You arrive to find an apparently healthy middle-aged woman, Lara Adams, lying on her side on the bed with her knees drawn up.

The patient tells you that she has been experiencing spotting for 10 to 15 minutes and is now having abdominal pain and cramping. She is 6 weeks pregnant, and this is her first pregnancy. She immediately phoned her general practitioner when the spotting started and was heading out the door to his surgery when the pain began.

Initial Assessment	Recording Time: 0 Minutes
Appearance	Anxious and tearful
Level of consciousness	A (Alert to person, place, and day)
Airway	Patent; patient is talking
Breathing	Rapid with adequate tidal volume
Circulation	Strong, slightly fast radial pulse

1. Based on your general impression and initial assessment, how would you categorise this patient?
2. What interventions would you choose to initiate at this point?

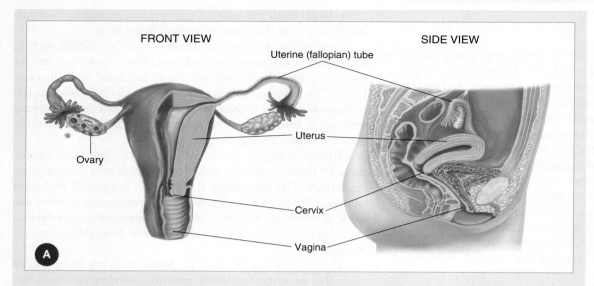

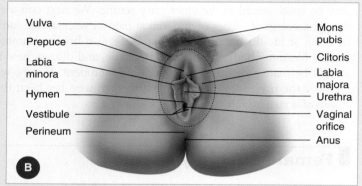

Figure 38-1 The anatomy of the female reproductive system. **A.** Front and side views. **B.** External genitalia.

The vagina, or lower portion of the birth canal, serves as a passage for menstrual flow and as the receptacle of the penis during sexual intercourse. Just inside the lower vagina are two tiny openings that lead to the Bartholin glands. These glands secrete mucus that acts as a lubricant during intercourse. Bacterial infection, particularly gonorrhoea, may cause these openings to become abscessed and cystic.

Before first intercourse, the vaginal orifice is protected by the hymen. This membrane forms a border around the vaginal orifice, partially enclosing it. The hymen may be ruptured before first intercourse by trauma or by such mundane events as horse riding, gymnastics, or other sports. Pain and vaginal bleeding will generally be present in such an event; because this usually occurs in young women, it may be of concern to the patient and her parents. In some cases, the hymen may completely cover the vaginal orifice, a condition called imperforate hymen. If it remains undetected until puberty, this condition will block the flow of first menses, resulting in relatively acute pain, with severe constipation and low back pain among the presenting symptoms. Such a condition may lead to endometriosis or cause other secondary painful effects as well. Imperforate hymen can also be caused by childhood sexual abuse, in which the imperforation results from scarring from digital or penile penetration.

About 2.5 cm below the vaginal opening is the anal opening, which allows for the passage of faeces and bowel gases. The area of skin between the vagina and the anus is called the clinical perineum.

appears over the mons in early puberty, becoming sparser later in life with the advent of menopause. The labia majora and labia minora, described as "lips", surround and protect the vaginal opening together with the more anterior opening of the urethra. The labia majora are covered with pubic hair, but the labia minora are devoid of it. The area between the vaginal opening and the anus is called the perineum. The clitoris is located at the anterior junction of the labia minora, just below a layer of skin called the prepuce. The clitoris is a small, cylindrical mass of erectile tissue and nerves that is homologous to the glans penis of the male. Like the male penis, the clitoris becomes enlarged with blood flow on tactile stimulation, and it has an important role in the sexual excitement of the female.

Between the labia minora is a cleft referred to as the vestibule. Located within the vestibule is the urethral opening (orifice), the vaginal opening (orifice), and the hymen. The urethra, which leads to the bladder, allows for passage of urine. The length of the urethra in females averages approximately 3.8 cm. This short length is one reason why women are more prone than men to urinary tract infections and bladder infections.

Menstruation

Of the many emergencies that paramedics are called on to treat, one of the most common calls is bleeding. For gynaecological emergencies, that would translate into bleeding from the vagina, also called bleeding "PV". However, before we embark on the

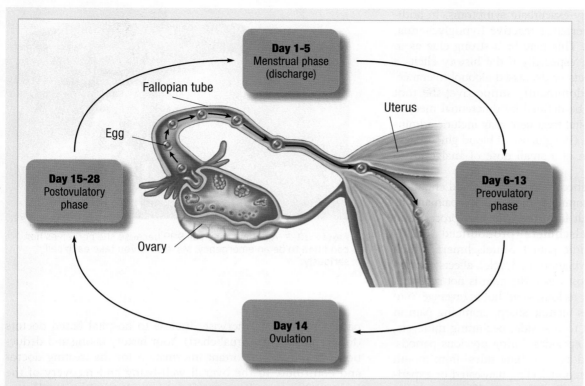

Figure 38-2 The menstrual cycle, based on an average 28-day cycle. The length of the cycle and number of days in each phase vary from woman to woman, but generally fall within a range of 24 to 35 days.

The onset of first menses, when a female reaches childbearing age, is called menarche. Depending on genetics, socioeconomic factors, and individual health, this event may take place anywhere between the ages of 10 and 16 years. The last menses, when a woman has reached the end of childbearing age, is called menopause. The advent of menopause typically begins between the ages of 40 and 50, with menstrual cycles becoming less frequent. This last phase of a woman's entire birth cycle, including the period of life that follows it, is called the climacteric.

Owing to gradually decreasing production of oestrogen and other hormones during the climacteric, a woman may experience a range of symptoms due to hormonal imbalance. These symptoms may be as benign as copious perspiration, hair loss, and hot flushes (sometimes accompanied by tachycardia) or as ominous as the symptoms seen often in the emergency setting such as severe muscle aches and pains, headache, dyspnoea, vertigo, digestive problems, and emotional instability. Postmenopausal women no longer have to deal with the discomfort and irritation of monthly menses, but the decreased hormone production makes them more susceptible to atherosclerosis, osteoporosis, and coronary heart disease. Diminished oestrogen may also result in atrophy of genitourinary organs, resulting in vaginal dryness and discomfort. Atrophy of the bladder and urethral mucosa can result in urinary frequency, nocturia, and incontinence.

Menstruation is predominantly related to the discussion of obstetrics, but is also a necessary component of the gynaecological examination. Disorders of the menstrual cycle may be seen in the prehospital setting, actually putting the call for emergency service in motion. Some of these disorders are classified in the following paragraphs.

Premenstrual syndrome (PMS) (also called premenstrual tension) is a cluster of all or some of the troubling symptoms mentioned in the discussion of the menstrual cycle. It normally occurs 7 to 14 days before the onset of the menstrual flow, then generally subsides once the flow begins. Premenstrual syndrome affects about one third of all premenopausal women, particularly in the 30- to 40-year-old group, and may be significantly debilitating. Stress, diet, alcohol consumption, and use of prescription

emergency treatment of vaginal bleeding, we must first consider what is "normal" vaginal bleeding.

One way in which women are uniquely different from men is the physiological phenomenon of menstruation. Also called the menses, period, or menstrual cycle, menstruation is the cyclic and periodic vaginal discharge of 25 to 65 ml of blood, epithelial cells, mucus, and tissue. The duration of the cycle differs from woman to woman, ranging from an average of 24 days to 35 days. Unless told otherwise by the patient, assume the average cycle to be 28 days. Three phases make up the entire menstrual cycle: the menstrual phase (the first phase), the preovulatory phase, and the postovulatory phase. Based on a 28-day cycle, the menstrual (discharge) phase lasts about 5 days. The preovulatory phase lasts from about day 6 to 13, and the postovulatory phase lasts from day 15 to 28 **Figure 38-2 ▲**.

During the menstrual cycle, a woman experiences several systemic changes as her hormonal levels ebb and flow. She may experience a weight gain of several pounds due to extracellular oedema (fluid retention) that tends to localise in the abdomen, fingers, and ankles; muscle sensitivity due to the extracellular oedema (hypertonicity); vascular alterations that increase her susceptibility to bruising; breast pain and tenderness resulting from swelling; mild to severe headache, including "menstrual migraine" (a vascular headache resulting from the hormonal "dump"); severe cramping; and emotional changes, such as agitation, irritability, depression, anger, and moodiness.

or non-prescription drugs may exacerbate symptoms. In addition, some women may experience reactive hypoglycaemia, resulting in increased fatigue. This may be a strong clue as to what is troubling the patient, especially if the history elicits a recent intense craving for sweets or decreased alcohol tolerance. Prehospital treatment is predominantly supportive; the root cause of the symptoms must be defined by differential medical diagnosis. Supportive prehospital treatment may include administration of oral or intravenous (IV) glucose, if blood glucose levels indicate, or administration of a small dose of analgesics to reduce patient anxiety.

Some women may experience abdominal pain and cramping in the 2 weeks before the beginning of menses. This pain and its accompanying symptoms result from the ovulatory process and are collectively called mittelschmerz (pronounced "MITT-ul-shmurz"; German for "middle pain"). Mittelschmerz, which may start at any time during ovulation (midcycle), affects approximately 20% of women. In most cases, the pain is not severe; it may last only a few minutes or as long as 48 hours (average, 6 to 8 hours). Signs and symptoms include sharp, cramping pain in the lower abdomen, localised to one side, beginning midcycle, with a history of similar pain episodes during previous periods. The pain may also be reported as "switching sides" from month to month. Some women also report feeling nauseated or experiencing minor blood spotting. The condition itself is not serious, and the pain can often be relieved by general-sales-list analgesics. Any persistent pain or any abnormal symptoms are cause for concern and should be evaluated by a doctor.

Dysmenorrhoea is painful menses. It is classified into two categories: primary and secondary. Primary dysmenorrhoea occurs with the advent of the menstrual flow and normally lasts for the first 1 to 2 days with gradual relief. Severe cramping may precede the period, with pain originating in the area of the symphysis pubis and radiating downward to the vulva and outward to the thighs. Nausea, vomiting, and diarrhoea may accompany the pain. Primary dysmenorrhoea accounts for about 80% of patients presenting with painful menses and accompanies a "regular" period. Secondary dysmenorrhoea is pain that is present before, during, and after the menstrual flow. It is generally organic in nature (not hormonal) and may signal an underlying illness or dysfunction. As with premenstrual syndrome, prehospital treatment is largely supportive.

At this point, you may be asking why this information is important and whether anyone would actually call the ambulance service for "menstrual" problems. In fact, people call the ambulance service for virtually anything. If the situation is an emergency to the patient, professionally, it should be an emergency to you as well. Generally, for menstrual-related conditions, paramedics are called because (1) the symptoms are new for the patient, (2) the symptoms are worse than in the past, or (3) the patient innately "feels" that something is wrong Figure 38-3 ▶ . You are in the unique position of being one of the few remaining medical specialities that make "house calls". As a consequence, you are able to examine the patient's living conditions, estimate domestic tensions (if evident), and obtain information that a

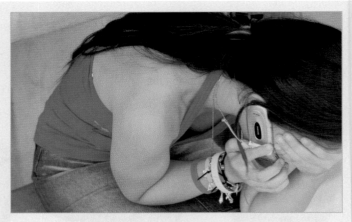

Figure 38-3 A patient may call 999 because she perceives her condition to be an emergency. Make sure you take each call seriously.

patient might not otherwise disclose to hospital based doctors (for example, a menstrual chart). Your history taking and deduction can provide important information for the treating doctor and contribute to the overall well-being and recovery of the patient. Of course, for you to ascertain what is "abnormal", you must know what is "normal".

Amenorrhoea is the absence or cessation of menses. This condition may be caused by a number of factors, but *the most common cause is pregnancy.* Exercise-induced amenorrhoea is common in female athletes, particularly those who participate in physically intense sports. Amenorrhoea can also be caused by emotional problems or extreme stress. In an adolescent or young adult, the condition may have its origination in anorexia nervosa; in this case, it is a symptom of the patient's malnutrition and emotional state.

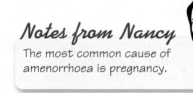

Notes from Nancy

The most common cause of amenorrhoea is pregnancy.

Vaginal bleeding is one of the most frequent reasons for women to consult a gynaecologist. The assessment and management of a patient with this chief complaint depend largely on whether there is a mechanism of injury. Vaginal bleeding, when not in the course of regular menstruation, is always an abnormal finding. The cause may be as benign as emotional stress or as serious as pelvic, cervical, or uterine cancer. Likewise, a disturbance in the normal menstrual cycle is cause for concern. If the flow of blood lasts several days longer than normal or is excessive, the condition is called menorrhagia. If the blood flow occurs more often than a 24-day interval, it is termed epimenorrhoea (usually caused by physical or emotional stress). Blood flow or intermittent spotting of blood occurring irregularly but frequently is termed metrorrhagia.

Documentation and Communication

Your attempts to obtain accurate, truthful information from the patient may be hindered by the presence of family members, loved ones, or bystanders. Removing nonessential personnel from the area will increase the likelihood that you obtain accurate information.

Metrorrhagia is of greatest concern to paramedics because its causes range from hormonal imbalance to malignancies to spontaneous abortion (miscarriage). Endometritis, inflammation of the endometrium, often associated with a bacterial infection, may be another cause of vaginal bleeding.

Pathophysiology

Causes of gynaecological emergencies range from disease to ectopic pregnancy to trauma.

Endometritis

Endometritis is an inflammation or irritation of the endometrium (uterine lining), most commonly caused by infection. Sexually transmitted infections (STIs) are a frequent culprit (gonorrhoea and chlamydia, predominantly), but endometritis may also occur after gynaecological surgery, abortion (elective, miscarriage, or therapeutic), or use of an intrauterine device (IUD). Symptoms may include malaise, fever (high- or low-grade), constipation or uncomfortable bowel movements, vaginal bleeding or discharge (or both), abdominal distension, and lower abdominal or pelvic pain.

Abdominal auscultation may reveal decreased bowel sounds, and pain may be elicited by palpation of the abdomen. Left untreated, endometritis may lead to septic shock or cause spontaneous abortion in a pregnant patient.

Endometriosis

Endometriosis affects approximately 1 in 10 women of childbearing age. This condition can be extremely painful, or there may be no symptoms. It results when endometrial tissue grows outside the uterus, generally on the surface of abdominal and pelvic organs. Organs of the pelvic cavity are the most common locations for the ectopic growths, but endometrial tissue can occasionally be found in the lungs or other parts of the body. This condition is one of the leading causes of infertility in women, with 30% to 40% of affected women unable to conceive. Many women do not even realise they have endometriosis until they encounter difficulties trying to get pregnant.

In women who experience symptoms, the most common complaint is pain, generally localised in the lower back, pelvic, and abdominal regions, that may be chronic. Other symptoms include painful coitus (during and after), gastrointestinal pain, dysuria and painful bowel movements during the menstrual cycle, fatigue (perhaps leading to misdiagnosis as chronic fatigue syndrome), extremely painful and escalating menstrual cramping, and very heavy menstrual periods. Patients may also experience bleeding between periods or report premenstrual spotting.

Pelvic Inflammatory Disease

Approximately 1 in 50 sexually active women in the UK develop pelvic inflammatory disease (PID) each year. One fourth of the women will require hospitalisation. PID is one of the most common causes of women presenting to

You are the Paramedic Part 2

You administer oxygen to the patient, obtain vital signs, establish intravenous access, and apply the cardiac monitor and note a normal sinus rhythm. As you continue your assessment, she says, "Please just take me to hospital. Please". You can tell that she is very frightened. You assist her to the ambulance, where she finds her original position of comfort.

Vital Signs	Recording Time: 5 Minutes
Level of consciousness	Alert, with a Glasgow Coma Scale score of 15
Skin	Warm, pink, and dry
Pulse	90 beats/min and regular
Blood pressure	110/68 mm Hg
Respirations	30 breaths/min
SpO2	100% with supplemental oxygen at 10 l/min via nonrebreathing mask

3. What other information would you like to know?

4. What issues do you foresee that will likely impact patient care?

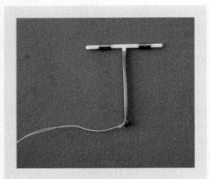

Figure 38-4 The IUD contraceptive device can increase a woman's risk of developing PID and ectopic pregnancy and may cause pain and bleeding.

emergency care services with a chief complaint of abdominal pain. One of every four women who contract PID will have severe abdominal pain or experience sterility or childbirth complications. Many women may have PID for years but do not realise it until they learn they are infertile.

PID is an infection of the female upper organs of reproduction— specifically, the uterus, ovaries, and fallopian tubes. Disease-causing organisms enter the vagina, generally by the process of sexual activity, and migrate through the opening of the cervix and into the uterine cavity, where they invade the mucosa. The infection may then expand to the fallopian tubes (producing scarring that can lead to life-threatening ectopic pregnancy or sterility), eventually involving the ovaries (leading to the development of a life-threatening tubo-ovarian abscess) and the peritoneal cavity. Although PID itself is seldom a threat to life, its ultimate consequences can be lethal.

Risk factors for PID include the use of an IUD as a contraceptive device Figure 38-4 ▲ , frequent sexual activity with multiple partners, and a history of previous PID. The disease is most prevalent in women aged between 15–24 and statistically decreases after age 30 years (the typical monogamy and marriage years).

Gardnerella Vaginitis

The *Gardnerella* bacterium normally resides in the genital area in women. It can cause an infection called Gardnerella vaginitis if the bacteria become too numerous. Young, sexually active women are the most likely to be affected, but it can develop in any female—adult or child. This infection can also occur in the urethra of males. It can be associated with PID, and recent use of antibiotics can increase the risk of contracting the infection. Gardnerella vaginitis can cause complications in pregnant women.

Gardnerella vaginitis is often confused with a yeast infection. Signs and symptoms include a "fishy" vaginal odour, itching, irritation, and a smooth, thin, sticky, white or grey discharge. Patients often describe their symptoms as being worse after intercourse or menstruation. Patients, although they are not in acute distress, should be seen by a doctor, who will most likely treat the condition with antibiotics.

Interstitial Cystitis

The prevalence of interstitial cystitis/painful bladder syndrome (IC/PBS) in the United Kingdom is approximately 18 cases per 100,000 women. Although the condition affects men and women, 90% of diagnosed cases are in women. IC/PBS is a chronic bladder condition with an unknown cause; it results in an inflamed or irritated bladder wall. In severe cases, the irritation can lead to the formation of ulcers in the bladder and bleeding into the bladder lining. The bladder may become internally scarred and stiff, resulting in markedly reduced bladder capacity. Symptoms vary but may mimic the symptoms associated with urinary tract infections and sexually transmitted diseases: pressure or tenderness in the bladder and surrounding pelvic region, pain that ranges from mild discomfort to severe, and urinary frequency or urgency. Some patients report urinating as many as 60 times per day. Painful coitus is not uncommon, and many women report that their symptoms become worse during their menstrual cycle.

There is currently no cure for IC/PBS (antibiotics are ineffective), so patients are generally treated so as to provide symptomatic relief. Some doctors may prescribe antihistamines or antidepressants, whereas others give ibuprofen, aspirin, or even opiates for severe cases.

Ectopic Pregnancy

The word *ectopic* means "located away from a normal position". In ectopic pregnancy, a fertilised egg is implanted somewhere besides the uterus Figure 38-5 ▶ . In 97% of cases, the egg is fertilised inside one of the fallopian tubes and has been blocked from passing into the uterus, generally by an obstruction, such as PID-related tubal scarring or as a result of tubal surgery (ligation or reverse ligation). The other 3% of ectopic pregnancies occur in the abdomen, within the cervix, or on an ovary. Ectopic pregnancy is the leading cause of maternal death in the first trimester. Approximately 1 in 100 pregnancies are ectopic in the UK and the condition occurs indiscriminately in any sexually active woman. In cases where a previous ectopic pregnancy has presented, there is a 1 in 10 chance that a future pregnancy will also be ectopic. Although PID is the most common cause of ectopic pregnancy, other causes include pelvic surgery, smoking, IUD use (IUDs do not cause ectopic pregnancy but, by blocking uterine pregnancy, may cause fertilisation to occur higher up), fibroids, tumours or cysts in the tubes, fallopian endometriosis, hormonal imbalance, and fertility treatments.

With a tubal pregnancy, the fertilised egg implants in the fallopian tube, then begins to grow and produce hormones in the same way a normally implanted egg does, taking nourishment from the maternal blood supply. Owing to the production of hormones, the woman begins to experience the early physiological changes of pregnancy. Her period stops, her breasts become enlarged and tender, and the uterine environment changes just as it would with a normal pregnancy. The fallopian tube, lacking the expansive muscle capacity of the uterus, has little stretching ability, so the developing embryo will soon run out of growing room. When this occurs, the tube is likely to rupture, causing massive intra-abdominal haemorrhage and shock.

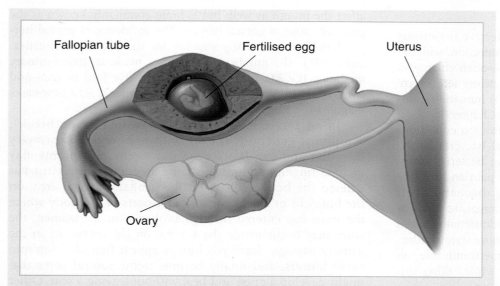

Fallopian tube   Fertilised egg   Uterus

Ovary

Figure 38-5 In an ectopic pregnancy, a fertilised egg implants somewhere other than the uterus. Here it is implanted in one of the fallopian tubes.

Ruptured Ovarian Cyst and Tubo-ovarian Abscess

Ruptured ovarian cysts and tubo-ovarian abscesses present with similar findings to ectopic pregnancy, so their prehospital management is identical to that for ectopic pregnancy.

An ovarian cyst is essentially a fluid-filled sac that forms on or within an ovary. Of the many types of cysts, the most common is the *functional cyst,* which generally develops during the menstrual cycle. During the cycle, the ovaries form tiny sacs (cysts) to hold the eggs. Once an egg matures, the sac breaks open and releases the egg, which then begins its journey through the fallopian tube for fertilisation; the sac itself dissolves. If the sac fails to break open, however, the egg may continue to mature and form a *follicular cyst.* Under normal circumstances, this type of cyst spontaneously disappears within a 1- to 3-month period. A *corpus luteum cyst* develops if the sac seals itself after release of the egg. Fluid then accumulates inside the cyst, and the cyst continues to grow. These cysts usually resolve spontaneously but may grow up to 10 cm. At this size, they can twist the ovary, causing bleeding and pain. Fertility drugs can increase the chances of corpus luteum cysts developing.

If the cycle of forming sacs is repeated excessively and the eggs do not release, *polycystic ovaries* may develop. This hormonal reproductive disorder is characterised by lack of progesterone and high levels of androgens (male hormone). It can have a negative impact on normal insulin production, leading to diabetes (especially gestational). It can also initiate heart and blood vessel problems, such as hypertension, and produce pelvic pain and irregular menstrual cycles.

Dermoid cysts lead to growths of formational tissue, such as teeth and hair, and may become very large and painful. Endometriomas form in women who have endometriosis, when uterine tissue attaches to the ovaries and begins to grow. Pain from this type of cyst usually manifests during menstruation or sexual intercourse. Cystadenomas are formed from cells on the outer surface of the ovary. These cysts are usually filled with a sticky gel substance or other fluid. They can become large and cause pain. A haemorrhagic cyst forms when a blood vessel bursts in the cyst wall and the blood fills the sac. Occasionally, these cysts will rupture and spill blood into the abdominal cavity, resulting in great pain.

Tubo-ovarian abscess is encountered secondary to a primary infectious agent—typically, the ones that cause PID. The most common underlying cause is gonorrhoea. Diverticulitis and appendicitis have also been found to be compounding factors. In this condition, the fallopian tubes or ovaries become blocked by an infectious mass, which grows and forms an abscess.

Toxic Shock Syndrome

Toxic shock syndrome (TSS) is a form of septic shock. The disease made headlines in the 1980s, when it was identified as a syndrome affecting women who used tampons. A connection was made between the use of super-absorbency tampons and a risk of contracting the disease, but the panic that ensued was out of proportion to the actual threat. The disease has been identified as having *Streptococcus pyogenes* (group A strep) or *Staphylococcus aureus* as the causative agent. TSS affects men and women, and it can involve several of the body's systems, including the hepatic, cardiovascular, central nervous, and renal systems. It can result when minor infections of the lungs, sinuses, skin lesions, or the vagina progress to actual TSS, which can be fatal. Menstruating women appear particularly prone to developing TSS—hence, the original association between the syndrome and tampon use. Initial symptoms include syncope, myalgia, diarrhoea, vomiting, headache, fever, and sore throat. Other symptoms may include diverse petechiae, light rash, and scleral injection (bloodshot eyes). As the disease progresses, signs of systemic shock will begin to appear. Disseminated intravascular coagulation, severe hypotension, adult respiratory distress syndrome, and arrhythmias may develop, and the patient may show signs of kidney and liver failure.

Rapid transport is indicated in cases of TSS. Provide high-flow supplemental oxygen, IV therapy, and cardiac monitoring. Little more can be done for a patient with TSS in the prehospital environment because aggressive antibiotic therapy and possible surgical intervention are required.

Sexually Transmitted Infections

As mentioned earlier, PID results from infective organisms crossing the cervix. It is typically a secondary infection, with the primary infection being sexually transmitted—often chlamydia or gonorrhoea. Sexually transmitted infections (STIs) are reviewed briefly here, with the exception of the human immunodeficiency virus (HIV), which is discussed in Chapter 36.

Bacterial vaginosis is one of the most common conditions to afflict women. In this infection, normal bacteria in the vagina are replaced by an overgrowth of other bacterial forms. Symptoms may include itching, burning, or pain and may be accompanied by a "fishy", foul-smelling discharge. Left untreated, bacterial vaginosis can lead to premature birth or low birthweight in the case of pregnancy. Additionally, it can make the patient increasingly susceptible to more serious infections and result in PID. It is treated with metronidazole, an antibiotic. If the patient consumes alcohol while taking this therapy, severe nausea and vomiting may develop.

Chancroid is caused by infection with the bacterium *Haemophilus ducreyi*. This highly contagious yet curable disease causes painful sores (ulcers), usually of the genitals. Swollen, painful lymph glands or inguinal buboes in the groin area may be present as well. Women may be asymptomatic and, thus, unaware they have the disease. Chancroid is known to facilitate the transmission of HIV.

Chlamydia is caused by the bacterium *Chlamydia trachomatis*. It is the most common sexually transmitted bacterial infection in the UK and is most prevalent in women under 20. Although symptoms of chlamydia are usually mild or absent, some women may have symptoms including lower abdominal pain, low back pain, nausea, fever, pain during intercourse, to bleeding between menstrual periods. Chlamydial infection of the cervix can spread to the rectum, leading to rectal pain, discharge, or bleeding. Left untreated, the infection can progress to PID. In rare cases, chlamydia causes arthritis that may be accompanied by skin lesions and inflammation of the eye and urethra (Reiter syndrome).

Cytomegalovirus (CMV) is a member of the herpes virus family. This very common viral infection has no known cure, and the virus can remain dormant in the body for years. An estimated 50% of pregnant women in the UK have antibodies to CMV. In its active stages, CMV may produce symptoms including prolonged high fever, chills, headache, malaise, extreme fatigue, and an enlarged spleen. People with an increased risk for developing active infection and more serious complications (such as fever, pneumonia, liver infection, and anaemia) include people with immune disorders, people receiving chemotherapy, and pregnant women. Newborns who acquire CMV are susceptible to lung problems, blood problems, liver problems, swollen glands, rash, and poor weight gain.

Genital herpes is an infection of the genitals, buttocks, or anal area caused by herpes simplex virus, type I or type II. Type I, which is the most common form, infects the mouth and lips, causing cold sores or "fever" blisters; it may also produce sores on the genitals. Type II, the more serious infection, can affect the mouth as well, but is more commonly known as the primary cause of genital herpes. The incidence of genital herpes has been increasing steadily for the last three decades. Since 1971, the number of diagnoses made at genito-urinary medicine (GUM) clinics has increased five-fold in men and twenty-fold in women. In 2003, there were 17,932 new cases diagnosed in England, Wales and Scotland.

In an active herpes infection (called an outbreak), symptoms generally appear within 2 weeks of primary infection and can last for several weeks. Symptoms may include tingling or sores near the area where the virus has entered the body, such as on the genital or rectal area, on the buttocks or thighs, or on other parts of the body where the virus has entered through broken skin. In women, the sores may occur inside the vagina, on the cervix, or in the urinary passage. Small red bumps appear first, develop into small blisters, and finally become itchy, painful sores that might develop a crust and heal without leaving a scar. Other symptoms that may accompany the first outbreak, and possibly subsequent outbreaks, include fever, muscle aches and pains, headache, dysuria, vaginal discharge, and swollen glands in the groin area.

Gonorrhoea is caused by *Neisseria gonorrhoeae*, a bacterium that can grow and multiply rapidly in the warm, moist areas of the reproductive tract, including the cervix, uterus, and fallopian tubes in women and in the urethra in women and men. The bacterium can also grow in the mouth, throat, eyes, and anus. Symptoms, which are generally more severe in men than in women, appear approximately 2 to 10 days after exposure. Women may be infected with gonorrhoea for months but experience virtually no symptoms until the infection has spread to other parts of the reproductive system. When symptoms do appear in women, they generally manifest as dysuria (painful urination), with associated burning or itching, a yellowish or bloody vaginal discharge, usually with a foul odour, and occult blood associated with vaginal intercourse. More severe infections may present with cramping and abdominal pain, nausea and vomiting, and bleeding between periods; these symptoms indicate that the infection has progressed to PID. Rectal infections generally present with anal discharge and itching, plus occasional painful bowel movements with faecal blood spotting. Infection of the throat (for which oral sex is the introducing factor) is called gonococcal pharyngitis. Its symptoms are usually mild, consisting of painful or difficult swallowing, sore throat, swollen lymph glands, and fever. Headache and nasal congestion may also be present. If the infection is not treated, the bacterium may enter the bloodstream and spread to other parts of the body, including the brain—a condition known as disseminated gonococcaemia.

Genital warts (also called condylomata acuminata and venereal warts) are caused by the human papilloma virus (HPV). Of the more than 100 types of HPV that have been identified (most are harmless), about 30 types are spread through sexual contact. HPV is the second most common STI in the UK, with over 81,137 new cases being diagnosed in 2005. Some infected people have no symptoms. In others, multiple growths develop in the genital areas—that is, the vagina, vulva, cervix, or rectum, or the penis and scrotum in men. HPV has been identified as a contributing factor in cervical, vulvar, and anal cancers. In pregnant women, warts may develop that become large enough to impede urination or obstruct the birth canal. If the virus is passed to the foetus, the child may develop *laryngeal papillomatosis* (throat warts that block the airway), a potentially life-threatening condition.

Syphilis is caused by the bacterium *Treponema pallidum*. Because many of its signs and symptoms mimic other diseases, syphilis is sometimes called the "great imitator" by clinicians. The disease manifests in three stages: primary, secondary, and late. Approximately 400 new cases of syphilis are reported each year in the UK, which represents a substantial increase in its diagnoses of over 2,000% since 1996. Transmission occurs through direct contact with open sores, which may arise anywhere on the body, but tend to appear on the genitals, anus, rectum, lips, or mouth. A person with syphilis may remain asymptomatic for years, not realising that his or her sores are manifestations of a disease.

The primary stage of syphilis is usually marked by the appearance of a single sore (a chancre), although in some people, multiple sores develop. The chancre is usually painless and is small, firm, and round. It usually goes away after 3 to 6 weeks, at which point the disease has progressed to the second stage.

The secondary stage of syphilis is characterised by the development of mucous membrane lesions and a skin rash. The characteristic rash may manifest on the palms of the hands and the bottoms of the feet as rough, red or reddish brown spots. Alternatively, it may be barely discernible or resemble rashes from other diseases. The rash generally does not itch. Symptoms of secondary syphilis may include fever, swollen lymph glands, sore throat, patchy hair loss, headaches, weight loss, muscle aches, and fatigue. Like the chancre of the primary stage, these symptoms will resolve without treatment. Left untreated, the secondary stage invariably leads to late-stage syphilis.

In the late stage, syphilis has no signs or symptoms, but internal damage is accumulating. Syphilis attacks the brain, nerves, eyes, heart, blood vessels, liver, bones, and joints, although the damage may not become evident for years. Paralysis, numbness, dementia, gradual blindness, and difficulty coordinating muscle movements are possible physical manifestations and may be serious enough to cause death. Pregnant women with syphilis may have stillborn babies, babies who are born blind, developmentally delayed babies, or babies who die shortly after birth.

Trichomoniasis is caused by a single-celled protozoan parasite, *Trichomonas vaginalis*. This parasite is transmitted through sexual contact, with the vagina being the most common site of infection. The infected person may be asymptomatic or may experience signs and symptoms including a frothy, yellow-green vaginal discharge with a strong odour. The infection may also cause irritation and itching of the female genital area, discomfort during intercourse, dysuria, and lower abdominal pain. When present, symptoms usually appear in women within 5 to 28 days of exposure to *Trichomonas vaginalis*. Left untreated, the

infection can lead to low birthweight or premature birth in pregnant women and to increased susceptibility to HIV infection. The number of cases of trichomoniasis diagnosed in the UK each year is fairly constant with a total of 6,435 presentations detected in 2003. (This consisted of 6,152 cases in women and 283 cases in men, which is probably explained by the infection being generally asymptomatic in men).

Vaginal yeast infections are typically caused by the *Candida albicans* fungus. Yeasts are tiny organisms that normally live in small numbers inside the vagina and on the skin. The normal acidic environment of the vagina helps keep yeast from growing. If the vagina becomes less acidic, however, the yeast population may increase dramatically and result in infection. Conditions that may alter the acidic balance of the vagina include the use of oral contraceptives, menstruation, pregnancy, diabetes, and some antibiotics. Moisture and irritation of the vagina also seem to encourage yeast growth. Stress from lack of sleep, illness, or poor diet are other contributing factors. Women with immunosuppressive diseases such as HIV infection or diabetes are also at increased risk. More than half of all women will experience at least one infection during their lifetime. Symptoms include itching, burning, soreness in the vagina and around the vulva, and vulvar swelling. Some women may report a thick, white vaginal discharge ("cottage cheese" appearance), pain during sexual intercourse, and burning on urination.

Patient Assessment

Obtaining an accurate and detailed patient assessment is of utmost importance when dealing with gynaecological issues. You may not be able to make a specific diagnosis in the prehospital environment, but a thorough detailed examination and patient history will help determine just how sick the patient is and whether lifesaving measures should be initiated. This is especially true when dealing with abdominal pain.

Women have many of the same conditions that cause abdominal pain in men—for example, renal colic, ulcers, gastroenteritis, cholecystitis, diverticulitis, pancreatitis, appendicitis, mesenteric ischaemia, and dissecting aneurysm. In addition, there are numerous gynaecological causes of abdominal pain. An old medical maxim states, "Anyone who neglects to consider a gynaecological cause in a woman of childbearing age who complains of abdominal pain will miss the diagnosis at least 50% of the time". Missing the diagnosis may be fatal for the patient.

Scene Assessment

Every emergency call—including calls involving gynaecological emergencies—begins with a thorough scene assessment. Is the scene safe? Will you need assistance? Is it a medical call, a trauma call, or both? How many patients do you have? What is the mechanism of injury or nature of illness? Have you taken adequate universal precautions to guard against contamination with body fluids? Gynaecological emergencies can be very messy, sometimes involving large amounts of blood and body fluids contaminated with communicable diseases.

Where is the patient found? If she is at home, what is the condition of the house? Is it clean, filthy, or neglected? Do you see evidence of a fight? Are alcohol, tobacco products, or drug paraphernalia present? Are there pictures of loved ones or, conversely, a noticeable absence of pictures? Does the patient live alone or with other people? All information you obtain will contribute to your assessment of the patient's overall health and the safety of the scene. In case of a crime scene, you may also be required to testify in court regarding the conditions on your arrival.

Initial Assessment

What is the overall presentation of the patient? Are there any obvious threats to life? Is she conscious? Does she have obvious breathing difficulty or evidence of injury? Does she appear pale, cyanotic, red, or grey? Is she alert and oriented or confused? Is she calm or not? What is her emotional state? What is her physical appearance—well kept or unkempt? Do you find the patient sitting up, lying down, prone, supine, in the fetal position, in the tripod position, in the bath, or on all fours? (The last position is common for patients in severe pain from renal colic).

Once you have answered these basic questions and treated any immediate threats to airway, breathing, or circulation, you can proceed with the focused physical examination, rapid medical assessment, or rapid trauma assessment as the situation dictates. Conduct rapid medical or trauma assessment if the patient is not responsive or has a significant mechanism of injury but threats to life are not immediately obvious. In the focused history and physical examination, pay special attention to gynaecological and reproductive history in addition to the usual criteria.

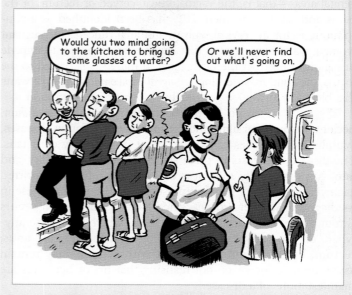

Figure 38-6

Try to protect the patient's modesty at all times during your history and physical examination. Gynaecological emergencies can be highly embarrassing for the patient, and many women may be extremely uncomfortable about discussing their sexual history in front of strangers or even close family members **Figure 38-6 ▲**. A teenage or adolescent girl may want to keep her sexual history from her parents, and few women are comfortable with having their genitals exposed to a crowd of family, neighbours, paramedics, or police officers. Limit the crowd to personnel

You are the Paramedic Part 3

You continue to ask questions about Mrs. Adams' pain and pregnancy using the LORDS TRACHEA mnemonic (see the "Focused History Physical Examination" section of this chapter). You obtain her orthostatic vital signs and perform a focused physical examination. No changes in positional vital signs are noted, and you find no signs of shock or trauma. You believe that Mrs Adams is in stable condition but requires immediate clinical evaluation in hospital. En route to hospital, you advise the accident and emergency (A&E) personnel of the patient's signs, symptoms, and other pertinent information regarding your assessment and interventions.

Vital Signs	Recording Time: 15 Minutes
Level of consciousness	Alert, with a Glasgow Coma Scale score of 15
Skin	Warm, pink, and dry
Pulse	86 beats/min and regular
Blood pressure	110/66 mm Hg
Respirations	24 breaths/min
SpO_2	100% with supplemental oxygen at 10 l/min via nonrebreathing mask

5. Given the information you have so far, will this patient require aggressive prehospital care?
6. What are the three true life-threatening gynaecological emergencies?
7. Does your differential diagnosis include any of these conditions?

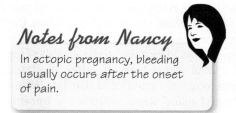

typically diffuse and is spread over both quadrants of the lower abdomen. It may be described as "achy", and the patient may volunteer that the pain is made worse by walking or by sexual intercourse. The latter revelation usually indicates cervical involvement in the infective process. Pain localised to the right upper quadrant is indicative of infection that has spread to the abdominal cavity. Associated symptoms may include vaginal discharge, fever and chills, and pain or burning on urination (dysuria).

Any woman with PID who feels sick enough to call for an ambulance probably has a severe infection and is likely to present pyrexic and look unwell. Physical examination findings may be sparse or may include the entire textbook profile. Be alert for signs of peritoneal irritation (that is, the patient winces on palpation of the abdomen or every time the ambulance hits a bump). Be very gentle should you decide to palpate this patient's abdomen as part of the examination.

PID cannot be treated in the prehospital environment by ambulance clinicians because it generally requires administration of an appropriate antibiotic for 10 to 14 days. The best you can do is obtain a thorough history, make the patient as comfortable as possible, and transport with as gentle a ride as can be managed.

At the Scene

The ambulance does not carry the appropriate supplies and equipment for a definitive diagnosis in the prehospital environment. Look for threats to life, treat for shock, and transport in a position of comfort.

Ectopic Pregnancy

Nearly all women with ectopic pregnancy will present with a chief complaint of abdominal pain. This pain will generally be localised to one side of the abdomen and, in the early stages, will be described as crampy and intermittent. As the pregnancy progresses, the embryo will abort or the tube will rupture. Either event will produce severe abdominal pain, localised to one side. By the time the ambulance service is involved, the patient is likely to be in constant pain, which will be diffused throughout the abdomen. Diffuse pain is especially likely if there is significant haemoperitoneum (blood in the abdominal cavity). Referred pain to the shoulder is ominous because it indicates massive haemoperitoneum. Vaginal bleeding is another sign of ectopic pregnancy, occurring in approximately 50–80% of women. This bleeding will usually occur *after* onset of pain in ectopic pregnancy, in contrast with spontaneous abortion, in which bleeding usually *precedes* pain.

In the history, you need to establish the intervals between the manifestations of the various symptoms. Part of the blood

volume in ectopic pregnancy originates in the shedding of the uterine lining as the embryo is displaced from its site of implantation and the production of hormones ceases. Vaginal bleeding may itself be light, so it is not a good indicator of internal blood loss. Look for a positive Cullen's sign or Grey Turner's sign and for signs of shock and abdominal distension and tenderness to help gauge internal bleeding. Signs of shock will generally be a pulse greater than 100 beats/min; systolic blood pressure less than 90 mm Hg, cold, moist skin; fatigue with associated restlessness and anxiety.

The classic triad for diagnosing ectopic pregnancy is amenorrhoea (75–90% of women), vaginal bleeding, and abdominal pain. A history of ectopic pregnancy, IUD use, and a history of PID also significantly raise the index of suspicion. *Always treat for shock in any woman presenting with abdominal pain and vaginal bleeding, regardless of whether shock symptoms are actually present* Figure 38-9 ▾ . Follow these steps in the management of a patient with a suspected ectopic pregnancy:

- Ensure an adequate airway, and administer high-concentration supplemental oxygen.
- Keep the patient left laterally recumbent, even if unconscious and intubated.
- Insert at least one large-bore IV cannula and administer a crystalloid solution (normal saline or Hartmann's); be prepared to run it wide open if signs of shock develop.
- Give nothing by mouth, including water.
- Anticipate vomiting. Have a vomit bowl and suction close at hand.
- Keep the patient warm.
- Monitor the patient's ECG.
- Transport.
- Pre-alert the receiving hospital of the patient's suspected diagnosis, her condition, and your estimated time of arrival.
- Use caution administering strong analgesia.
- Recheck vital signs frequently during transport.

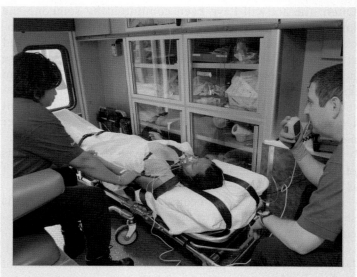

Figure 38-9 Always treat for shock in any woman with abdominal pain and vaginal bleeding.

Ruptured Ovarian Cyst and Tubo-ovarian Abscess

A patient with an ovarian cyst may complain of dull, achy pain in the lower back and thighs, abdominal pain or pressure, nausea and vomiting, breast tenderness, abnormal bleeding and painful menstruation, and painful intercourse. A patient with a tubo-ovarian abscess may present with severe abdominal pain, guarding and rebound tenderness, nausea and vomiting, abdominal distension, and fever. If the abscess ruptures, infectious matter can spread throughout the entire body. The prehospital management of ruptured ovarian cyst and tubo-ovarian abscess are the same as for ectopic pregnancy.

Sexual Assault

Sexual assault is a horrific crime that is as old as humankind. It can take many forms, but the most common is rape. Among the crimes that humans commit against their fellow humans, rape ranks as one of the most perverse and devastating. The Sexual Offences Act (2003) took full effect in April 2004 and altered the way offences were measured and recorded. At the time a Home Office study suggested there was an estimated 190,000 incidents of serious sexual assault of which an estimated 80,000 females were the victim of rape or attempted rape.

Paramedics called on to treat a victim of sexual assault, indecent assault, or actual or alleged rape face many complex issues, ranging from obvious medical ones to serious psychological and legal issues. In particular, you may be the first person the victim has contact with after the encounter, and how the situation is managed from first contact throughout treatment and transport may have lasting effects for the patient and you. Professionalism, tact, kindness, and sensitivity are of paramount importance.

A rape victim has just had a major traumatic experience. Often, the act will have been committed by someone she knew and trusted. The last thing she wants to do is give a concise, detailed report of what she has just experienced, and attempting to elicit such information will be likely to cause her to "shut down". Whenever possible, a female rape victim should be given the option of being treated by a female paramedic because the patient may be experiencing ambivalent feelings toward men in general; these feelings will hinder assessment and the patient's well-being.

The job of paramedics is to deal with the medical aspects of the case and to act as the patient advocate. In this capacity, it is important for you to focus on several key issues.

The first issue is the medical treatment of the patient. Is she physically injured? Are any life-threatening injuries present? Does the patient complain of any pain?

The second issue is your psychological care of the patient. Do not cross-examine her or attempt to elicit information for the benefit of the police. Do not pass judgement on the patient, and protect her from the judgement of others on the scene. It

does not matter how the patient is dressed, what her local reputation is, where she was, or what she was doing when the assault occurred. The concept of a woman "deserving" to be raped is just as ludicrous as you "deserving" to be assaulted for wearing the colours of a rival sports team. A crime has been committed, and you need to remain mindful of that fact. Many women report feeling "raped again" when subjected to interrogation, criticism, or scepticism.

Last, remember that you are at a crime scene and expect police involvement early in the situation. In many cases the ambulance service may be called by the police. Police officers are trained in basic first aid skills, but their primary function is to investigate criminal activity and not to manage patient care. Your job is to treat the medical aspects of the incident, but you still have a responsibility to *preserve* evidence. If the victim of an assault does not have a life-threatening injury and would like to press charges against the assailant, the police may isolate the patient for forensic purposes and take the patient to a rape suite at the police station rather than to the A&E department at hospital. Do not cut through any clothing or throw away anything from the scene. Place bloodstained articles in separate paper (not plastic) bags. Obtain evidence bags from the police if necessary. Paper bags allow wet items to dry naturally, whereas plastic allows mould to grow and may destroy biological evidence.

It may also be necessary to gently persuade the patient to *not* clean herself up. This will be a natural desire on the part of the patient, stemming from the desire to "wash away" the humiliation and embarrassment of the assault. Valuable evidence can be destroyed in this process. The patient also needs to be discouraged from urinating, changing clothes, opening her bowels, or rinsing out her mouth. She will need to be photographed by police personnel and the photographic record needs to be as accurate as possible. If the patient cannot be discouraged from taking these actions, respect her feelings. Remember, some patients may refuse transport altogether, and they have the right to do so. Do not simply accept this refusal and leave. Instead, try to persuade the patient to allow you to call a friend or relative who can stay with her or, better still, with whom she can stay. Getting the patient away from the scene keeps her from having to constantly relive the experience by being subjected to the environment where the assault occurred. Many communities also have rape crisis centres, which offer confidential victim support and counselling services. Such professional guidance will aid the explanation and necessity of evidence preservation and can support the victim through the immediate crisis phase, the subsequent legal proceedings (if she decides to prosecute) and beyond.

Notes from Nancy

Find out if the woman has been injured. Do not ask questions about the incident itself.

chancroid A highly contagious STI caused by the bacteria *Haemophilus ducreyi*, which causes painful sores (ulcers), usually of the genitals.

chlamydia An STI caused by the bacterium *Chlamydia trachomatis*.

climacteric End phase of a woman's life menstrual cycle.

clitoris A small, cylindrical mass of erectile tissue and nerves located at the anterior junction of the labia minora, homologous to the glans penis of the male.

contraceptive device A device used to prevent pregnancy.

cystadenomas Fluid-filled cysts that form on the outer ovarian surface.

cytomegalovirus (CMV) A herpes virus that can produce the symptoms of prolonged high fever, chills, headache, malaise, extreme fatigue, and an enlarged spleen.

dermoid cysts Ovarian cysts containing formational tissue, such as hair and teeth.

dysmenorrhoea Painful menstruation.

ecstasy A drug officially named methylenedioxymethamphetamine (MDMA) that is sometimes used to facilitate date rape; a methamphetamine derivative with hallucinogenic properties; street names include E, XTC, disco biscuit, rhubarb and custard, smarties, Rolex, and dolphins.

ectopic pregnancy A pregnancy in which the egg implants somewhere other than the uterine endometrium.

endometriomas Ovarian cysts formed from endometrial tissue.

endometriosis A condition in which endometrial tissue grows outside the uterus.

endometritis An inflammation of the endometrium that often is associated with a bacterial infection.

endometrium The inner mucous membrane of the uterus.

epimenorrhoea Menstrual blood flow that occurs more often than a 24-day interval.

gamma-hydroxybutyrate (GHB) A drug used to facilitate date rape; is colourless and odourless with a salty taste disguised when mixed with a drink; street names include liquid E, grievous bodily harm, easy lay, G, scoop, liquid X, soap, and salty water.

Gardnerella vaginitis An infection caused by a bacterium that normally resides in the genital area in women but that can cause infection if the bacteria become too numerous; signs and symptoms include a vaginal odour that may be fishy, itching, irritation, and, possibly, a smooth, thin, sticky, white or grey discharge.

genital herpes An infection of the genitals, buttocks, or anal area caused by herpes simplex virus (HSV), which may cause sores of the genitals, mouth, or lips.

genital warts Warts caused by the human papilloma virus (HPV), an STI; also called condylomata acuminata or venereal warts.

gonorrhoea An STI caused by *Neisseria gonorrhoeae*.

gravid Pregnant; the number of times a woman has been pregnant is indicated by gravida, for example, gravida 3 indicates three pregnancies.

haemoperitoneum Blood in the peritoneal cavity.

haemorrhagic cyst A blood-filled sac that forms when a blood vessel bursts in a cyst wall and the blood fills the sac.

hymen A membrane that protects the vaginal orifice before first intercourse.

imperforate hymen A situation in which the hymen completely covers the vaginal orifice.

ketamine hydrochloride A powerful general anaesthetic drug used to facilitate date rape as it depresses the nervous system and causes a temporary loss of body sensation. Its application is beneficial in both human and veterinary operations; street names include special K, vitamin K, K, super K, and green.

labia majora Outer fleshy "lips" covered with pubic hair that protect the vagina.

labia minora Inner fleshy "lips" devoid of pubic hair that protect the vagina.

menarche The beginning phase of a woman's life cycle of menstruation.

menopause The ending phase of a woman's life cycle of menstruation.

menorrhagia Menstrual blood flow that lasts several days longer than it should or flow that is abnormally excessive.

menstrual cycle The entire monthly cycle of menstruation from start to finish.

menstruation Monthly flow of blood.

metrorrhagia Irregular but frequent vaginal bleeding.

mons pubis This is a rounded pad of fatty tissue that overlies the symphysis pubis and is anterior to the urethral and vaginal openings.

parietal pain Pain caused by inflammation of the parietal peritoneum that is generally described as steady, aching, and aggravated by movement.

parity Number of live births a woman has had.

perineum The area between the vaginal opening and the anus.

pelvic inflammatory disease (PID) An infection of the female upper organs of reproduction, specifically the uterus, ovaries, and fallopian tubes.

premenstrual syndrome (PMS) A cluster of all or some of the troubling symptoms that occur during a woman's menstrual phase that can include fluid retention, breast pain and tenderness, headache, severe cramping, and emotional changes, including agitation, irritability, depression, and anger.

prepuce In the anatomy of the female genitalia, a layer of skin directly above the clitoris.

rape Is any act of non-consensual intercourse by a man with a person; the victim can be either male or female. Intercourse can be vaginal, anal or oral. According to the Sexual Offences Act (2003) a person consents if he or she agrees by choice, and has the freedom and capacity to make that choice. The law does not require the victim to have resisted physically.

referred pain Pain that seems to radiate or travel as it becomes more intense.

Rohypnol A benzodiazepine used to facilitate date rape and that can create memory loss; street names include roofies, roof, R2, and rocha.

ruptured ovarian cyst A fluid-filled sac within the ovary that bursts from internal pressure.

sexual assault An attack against a person that is sexual in nature, the most common of which is rape.

syphilis An STI caused by the bacterium *Treponema pallidum*, which manifests in three stages—primary, secondary, and late—and is transmitted through direct contact with open sores.

toxic shock syndrome (TSS) A form of septic shock caused by *Streptococcus pyogenes* (group A strep) or *Staphylococcus aureus*; initial symptoms include syncope, myalgia, diarrhoea, vomiting, headache, fever, and sore throat.

trichomoniasis A parasitic infection.

tubo-ovarian abscess An infectious mass growing within the ovaries and fallopian tubes.

vagina The lower portion of the birth canal, which also serves as a passage for menstrual flow and as the receptacle of the penis during sexual intercourse.

vaginal bleeding Bleeding from the vagina.

vaginal yeast infection An infection caused by the fungus, *Candida albicans*, in which fungi over populate the vagina.

vestibule A cleft between the labia minora, where the urethral opening (orifice), the vaginal opening (orifice), and the hymen are located.

visceral pain Pain caused by some dysfunction of the hollow abdominal organs and is generally poorly localised and diffuse.

vulva The female external genitalia.

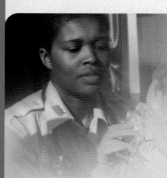

Assessment in Action

You are dispatched to an office building for a patient complaining of abdominal pain. When you arrive on scene, you are led to the 21-year-old woman who is bent over at the waist complaining of severe pain in her pelvic region. She states her pain began last night while she was watching TV and states that it's becoming unbearable. Her vital signs are a respiratory rate of 24 breaths/min, blood pressure of 130/74 mm Hg, a heart rate of 120 beats/min, sinus tachycardia on the ECG monitor, and a pulse oximetry reading of 100% while breathing room air. She tells you that she is currently menstruating so there is no chance she is pregnant. Her bleeding is normal. She takes birth control pills.

1. **How long does the normal menstrual cycle last?**
   A. Generally 14 days and occurs at regular intervals from puberty to menopause
   B. Generally 21 days and occurs at regular intervals from puberty to menopause
   C. Generally 28 days and occurs at regular intervals from puberty to menopause
   D. Generally 35 days and occurs at regular intervals from puberty to menopause

2. **When should you ask about sexual activity?**
   A. Whenever you have a patient who might be pregnant
   B. In all patients with abdominal pain
   C. In all adult women but not children
   D. In all women except older women

3. **Some potential causes of this patient's pain include all the following, EXCEPT:**
   A. ectopic pregnancy.
   B. pelvic inflammatory disease.
   C. ruptured ovarian cyst.
   D. none of the above.

4. **An infection in the female reproductive system and surrounding organs that can lead to sepsis and infertility is called:**
   A. ruptured ovarian cyst.
   B. endometriosis.
   C. pelvic inflammatory disease.
   D. spontaneous abortion.

5. **The inflammation of PID frequently follows the onset of menstrual bleeding by:**
   A. 1 to 3 days.
   B. 4 to 6 days.
   C. 7 to 10 days.
   D. 14 to 21 days.

6. **A ruptured ovarian cyst may mimic all of the following, EXCEPT:**
   A. appendicitis.
   B. cholecystitis.
   C. ectopic pregnancy.
   D. salpingitis.

7. **Ectopic pregnancy usually presents with:**
   A. missed periods, watery periods, nausea, vomiting, or frequent urination.
   B. the Kehr sign, breast tenderness, nausea, vomiting, and shortness of breath.
   C. chest pain, low blood glucose level, and frequent urination.
   D. elevated white blood cell count, low S_PO_2, and hyperglycaemia.

8. **Gynaecological emergencies are classified into which of the following three groups?**
   A. Nontraumatic, traumatic, and sexual assault
   B. Normal, traumatic, and sexual assault
   C. Self-inflicted, nontraumatic, and sexual assault
   D. Sexual assault, nontraumatic, and hereditary

9. **What is mittelschmerz?**
   A. Lower abdominal pain experienced by some women at the time of ovulation
   B. Upper abdominal pain experienced by some women at the time of ovulation
   C. The absence of pain during menstruation
   D. Painful menses but also may be associated with headache, syncope, backache, and leg pain

10. **Endometritis is inflammation of the:**
    A. uterine lining.
    B. ovaries.
    C. fallopian tubes.
    D. endometrial wall.

11. **What are the complications of vaginal bleeding?**
    A. Uncontrolled vaginal bleeding can lead to hypovolaemic shock and death.
    B. Uncontrolled vaginal bleeding can lead to hypertension.
    C. Uncontrolled vaginal bleeding can lead to endometriosis.
    D. Uncontrolled vaginal bleeding can lead to cystitis.

Challenging Question

12. **What is the treatment for a ruptured ectopic pregnancy?**

Points to Ponder

You are dispatched to the local university campus for an assault. When you arrive on scene, you are met by university staff and informed of an alleged assault on a 19-year-old female student. When you begin your assessment, you note that the patient is in a fetal position and appears to be in a catatonic state. She is not speaking and stares at the wall. The patient does not make any eye contact with you when you call her name. You note that she has bruises on her face and her wrists and is wrapped in a blanket.

How can you interview this patient in a way that will produce the information you need without further upsetting her?

Issues: Protecting a Patient's Modesty and Privacy, Obtaining Necessary Information in a Sensitive Way, Providing Appropriate Care for a Victim of a Sexual Assault.

39 Obstetric Emergencies

Objectives

Cognitive

- Review the anatomical structures and physiology of the reproductive system.
- Identify the normal events of pregnancy.
- Describe how to assess an obstetric patient.
- Identify the stages of labour and the paramedic's role in each stage.
- Differentiate between normal and abnormal delivery.
- Identify and describe complications associated with pregnancy and delivery.
- Identify predelivery emergencies.
- State indications of an imminent delivery.
- Explain the use of the contents of a maternity pack.
- Differentiate between the management of a patient with predelivery emergencies from a normal delivery.
- State the steps in the predelivery preparation of the mother.
- Establish the relationship between universal precautions and childbirth.
- State the steps to assist in the delivery of a newborn.
- Describe how to care for the newborn.
- Describe how and when to cut the umbilical cord.
- Discuss the steps in the delivery of the placenta.
- Describe the management of the mother post-delivery.
- Summarise neonatal resuscitation procedures.
- Describe the procedures for handling abnormal deliveries.
- Describe the procedures for handling complications of pregnancy.
- Describe the procedures for handling maternal complications of labour.
- Describe special considerations when meconium is present in amniotic fluid or during delivery.
- Describe special considerations of a premature baby.

Affective

- Advocate the need for treating two patients (mother and baby).
- Value the importance of maintaining a patient's modesty and privacy during assessment and management.
- Serve as a role model for other ambulance clinicians when discussing or performing the steps of childbirth.

Psychomotor

- Demonstrate how to assess an obstetric patient.
- Demonstrate how to provide care for a patient with:
  - Excessive vaginal bleeding
  - Abdominal pain
  - Hypertensive crisis
- Demonstrate how to prepare the obstetric patient for delivery.
- Demonstrate how to assist in the normal cephalic delivery of the fetus.
- Demonstrate how to deliver the placenta.
- Demonstrate how to provide post-delivery care of the mother.
- Demonstrate how to assist with abnormal deliveries.
- Demonstrate how to care for the mother with delivery complications.

Introduction

In Chapter 38, we discussed gynaecology and medical emergencies unique to the female. This chapter goes a step further by discussing obstetric emergencies.

When you are responding to an obstetric incident, keep several key issues in mind. Firstly, pregnancy itself is not a disease that needs treatment; it is the natural continuation of the human species. Women have been having children without the benefit of accident and emergency (A&E) departments, painkillers, and enhanced 999 since time began. For the most part, childbirth is a happy event for all involved. Emotions may run high, however, ranging from delirious exuberance to panicked distress. You need to be the eye in the centre of the emotional storm, bringing professional calm and control to the scene. Secondly, the number of patients increases to a minimum of two—the expectant mother and the baby—or perhaps even more if more than one baby is expected.

While childbirth and pregnancy are both naturally occurring states, they are not without potential complications, including maternal death and fetal death. With the advent of modern medicine, maternal and infant mortality rates have been significantly reduced, and close medical monitoring usually discovers problems long before childbirth. In developing nations, however, mortality remains high. Contributing factors include malnutrition, disease, lack of education, and lack of adequate medical care.

Anatomy of the Female Reproductive System

The female reproductive organs include the external organs that constitute the pudendum: mammary glands (breasts), vagina, uterus (womb), and ovaries and fallopian tubes. The ovaries are the starting point for reproduction. These paired glands are found next to the uterus, one ovary on either side. They are about the size and shape of an unshelled almond and are homologous to the testes in the male (ie, they are essentially the female gonads). The ovaries are positioned in the upper pelvic cavity but typically descend to the brim of the pelvis during the third month of fetal development.

Each ovary contains about 200,000 follicles, and each follicle contains an oocyte (egg). The human female is born with all the eggs she will ever release (approximately 400,000). Each month, during the menstrual cycle, about 20 of these follicles begin the process of maturation, but only a single follicle ultimately matures and releases an ovum; the other follicles die in a process called atresia. (Chapter 38 covers the menstrual cycle.)

The maturation of an oocyte occurs when the follicular cells respond to follicle-stimulating hormone (FSH) released by the anterior pituitary gland, which is first stimulated by the release of gonadotrophin-releasing factor (GnRF) from the hypothalamus. As the preovulatory phase of the menstrual cycle progresses, the anterior pituitary gland releases luteinising hormone (LH), which stimulates the process of ovulation—that is, the release of the egg (or at this point, the ovum). LH continues to be excreted throughout the ovarian cycle and subsequent pregnancy, should it occur, stimulating the ovarian cells to produce the hormones relaxin, progesterone, and various oestrogens.

What is left of the follicle after the egg has been released becomes the corpus luteum, which in turn secretes another female hormone, progesterone. Under the influence of progesterone, the secretory phase (the second phase of the menstrual cycle) takes place. The glands of the endometrium increase in size and secrete the materials on which the fertilised egg will implant and grow. There it will develop into an embryo and then a fetus Figure 39-1 ▶ . If the ovum is *not* fertilised, however, it dies and degenerates 36 to 48 hours after being released. The corpus luteum also degenerates about 10 days later, and the endometrium then breaks down and is shed as menstrual flow on about the 28th day of the cycle (ie, about 14 days after ovulation).

You are the Paramedic Part 1

You are sent to a house for a woman in labour. Upon arriving at the scene, you are escorted to the patient by her husband, who is clearly excited. He tells you that his wife's waters broke about 3 hours ago, and that she is now having contractions. You find the patient lying on her left side on her bed. She is having regular contractions every 3 minutes—each lasting approximately 45 seconds. You perform an initial assessment.

Initial Assessment	Recording Time: 0 Minutes
Appearance	Conscious; holding her lower back; panting
Level of consciousness	A (Alert to person, place, and day)
Airway	Patent
Breathing	Increased respirations; adequate depth
Circulation	Radial pulses, rapid and strong; skin, pink and moist

1. What specific questions should you ask this patient?

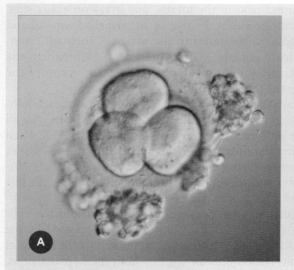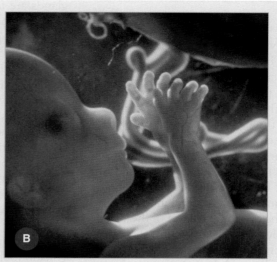

Figure 39-1 A. Embryo. **B.** Fetus.

mucous membrane composed of two layers, the stratum basalis and the stratum functionalis. The stratum functionalis, the layer innermost to the uterine cavity, is shed during menstruation. The stratum basalis is permanent and produces a new stratum functionalis following the period. As the follicle starts developing and pumping out oestrogen, the endometrium is stimulated to increase its thickness in preparation for the reception and future growth of a fertilised egg (proliferative phase).

The ova passes from the ovaries to the uterus through the fallopian tubes, or oviducts. These paired structures measure about 10 cm long. Each tube extends out laterally from the uterus, terminating just short of an ovary. The proximal end of each fallopian tube is very thick and narrow and connects to the uterus itself. Each fallopian tube comprises three layers of tissue: the internal mucosa, the muscularis, and the serosa. The serosa—the outer layer—consists of a serous membrane that protects the tubes. The muscularis—the middle layer—is made of smooth muscle; contractions of this layer help move the ovum through the tube and into the uterus. The internal mucosa—innermost layer—contains secretory cells and ciliated columnar cells, which also move the ovum along and may play a part in providing nutrition to the ovum. In summary, when an ovary releases an egg, the ciliary action of the fimbriae sweeps the egg into the infundibulum, and the actions of the internal mucosa and the muscularis provide the ovum with a short tube ride to the uterus. If the egg collides with a sperm cell somewhere along the length of the ampulla, it may become fertilised. Fertilisation can occur at any time within about a 24-hour window following ovulation.

The uterus is a muscular, inverted pear-shaped organ that lies between the urinary bladder and the rectum. The dome-shaped top of the uterus is called the fundus. Below the dome, the uterus begins to taper and narrow, forming the body. The narrowest portion of the uterus, called the cervix, opens into the vagina; the junction of the two is called the external os. The interior of the body of the uterus is the uterine cavity, and the interior of the cervix is the cervical canal.

The uterus is where the fertilised ovum will implant, where the fetus will develop, and where the act of labour takes place. It consists of three layers of tissue: the perimetrium (outer protective layer), the myometrium (middle layer), and the endometrium (inner lining). The myometrium is composed of three layers of muscle fibres; the contractions of these muscles help expel the fetus during childbirth. The endometrium is a

The vagina is a highly muscular, tubular organ lined with mucous membranes. It serves as a receptacle for the male penis during sexual intercourse, and allows for the exit of the menstrual flow. The interior of the vagina is acidic owing to the breakdown of glycogen (found in large amounts in the vaginal mucosa), which creates a low-pH environment that inhibits bacterial growth. This acidity, while beneficial, is injurious to sperm cells. Semen is alkaline in nature and likewise has antibacterial properties. The alkalinity of seminal fluid neutralises the acidity of the vagina, allowing the sperm cells to survive and fertilise the ovum.

The vagina is the lower portion of the birth canal and can stretch widely to accommodate the delivery of a fetus. If the vagina is unable to stretch far enough, then the tissues in and around the perineum may tear, causing much pain and bleeding. In such cases, the attending doctor may make an incision in the perineal skin called an episiotomy. In the prehospital setting, you are limited to providing gentle pressure against the infant's head to prevent an explosive birth and give the tissues time to expand.

The mammary glands (breasts) are modified sweat glands that are mainly composed of adipose tissue. Their primary purpose is lactation, or milk secretion, to provide nourishment to the newborn. Milk is carried to the surface of each breast through lactiferous ducts that terminate in a nipple. The nipple of the breast is surrounded by a darker pigmented area called the areola. Breast enlargement, tenderness, and milk excretion are all signs that a woman is probably pregnant. Unilateral enlargement, discoloured or foul fluid excretion, or pain and tenderness in the breasts may indicate a more serious underlying condition.

Conception and Gestation

Once the egg has been fertilised and implanted in the endometrium of the uterus, both the egg and the pregnant woman begin to undergo major physiological, hormonal, and chemical changes. The egg, upon entering the uterus, begins absorbing uterine fluid through the cell membrane. As the fluid fills the interior of the egg, cell division increases rapidly, and the cells multiply on the outside of the egg surface, forming layers that will eventually generate the fetal membrane, placenta, and embryo. The egg, now called a blastocyst, will migrate to the endometrial wall and become implanted there approximately 1 week after conception. Upon implantation, the egg will adhere to the endometrium, and enzymatic activity from the egg will dissolve endometrial tissue and provide nourishment for its development. Occasionally, the mechanism of implantation may result in vaginal bleeding that is spotty and painless, but of concern to the patient who does not yet realise her condition.

The implantation and subsequent actions of the blastocyst trigger the development of placental tissues, whose formation stimulates the release of human chorionic gonadotrophin hormone, which in turn sends signals to the corpus luteum that pregnancy has begun. The corpus luteum then begins to produce hormones designed to support the pregnancy until the placenta has developed. By the second week after conception, the blastocyst has evolved into an embryonic disc, and the amniotic sac and placenta are starting to differentiate into their specialised duties. The developing placenta produces projections that tap into the external tissue layer (extra-embryonic ectodermal) tissue of the blastocyst, where spaces called lacunae have been formed. These spaces are filled with maternal blood, and the connection allows both the embryo to draw on the maternal circulation for oxygenation and nutrition and embryonic waste products to be shunted safely away. This connection serves as the beginning of the umbilical cord.

In the third week after conception, the egg, now officially the *embryo,* is ready to begin the process of forming specialised body systems. The rudiments of the central nervous system, cardiovascular system, spine, and portions of the skeletal anatomy begin to appear. At the end of this week, an S-shaped tubular heart begins to beat, and blood cells produced in the yolk sac begin to circulate. The pregnant woman, by this point, may notice that she has missed her period and begin to suspect that she is pregnant.

At around the 14th day after ovulation, the placenta begins to develop. Essentially an enlarged endocrine gland, the placenta carries out a number of crucial functions during pregnancy. The placenta serves as an early liver, taking care of the synthesis of glycogen and cholesterol, metabolises fatty acid, and produces antibodies that protect the fetus. It also provides the following:

- **Respiratory gas exchange.** The placenta functions as the fetal lungs, enabling the fetus to exchange its carbon dioxide-laden blood for oxygen-rich blood.
- **Transport of nutrients** from maternal to fetal circulation.
- **Excretion of wastes,** some of which pass into the maternal circulation and others of which are excreted into the amniotic fluid.

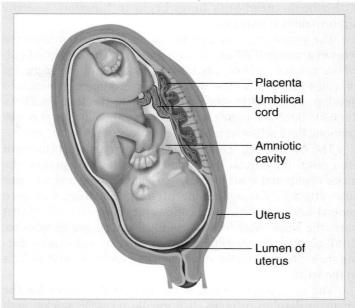

Figure 39-2 The umbilical cord and other structures of the pregnant uterus.

- **Transfer of heat** from mother to fetus.
- **Hormone production.** The placenta produces chorionic gonadotrophin, a hormone that maintains the pregnancy and stimulates changes in the mother's breasts, vagina, and cervix that prepare her for delivery and motherhood.
- **Formation of a barrier** against harmful substances in the mother's circulation, such as chemicals or microorganisms. When the placenta blocks a drug from reaching the fetal bloodstream, we say that the drug "does not cross the placenta". The placenta is not able to exclude every harmful substance, so you need to be very careful about which drugs are administered to women during pregnancy. The umbilical cord connects the placenta to the fetus via the fetal umbilicus (navel) Figure 39-2 ▲ . The cord is grey, easily compressed, soft, and pliant though structurally tough. The interior of the cord contains a mucoid material (Wharton's jelly—it keeps the umbilical cord from becoming knotted) and a supportive framework of loose connective tissue. The umbilical cord also contains two arteries and one vein. Occasionally, a child will be born with only a single umbilical artery (SUA). SUA may be genetically normal in some children, but may also indicate a congenital abnormality, such as heart or kidney malformations.

Fetal circulation differs from that of the mother. The umbilical *vein* carries oxygenated blood from the placenta to the fetus, while the umbilical *arteries* carry arteriovenous blood to the placenta. Since the fetus obtains its oxygen via the placenta, the fetal circulation bypasses the lungs until birth. A duct connects the umbilical vein and the inferior vena cava, another duct connects the pulmonary artery and the aorta, and an opening separates the right and left atria of the fetal heart.

At birth, the newborn's lungs begin to function, and the arteriovenous shunts close.

The amniotic sac is a membranous bag that encloses the fetus in a watery fluid called amniotic fluid. The amniotic fluid, whose volume reaches about 1 litre by the end of pregnancy, provides the fetus with a weightless environment in which to develop. In the latter stages of pregnancy, the fetus swallows amniotic fluid and passes wastes out into the fluid. In this way amniotic fluid assists in fetal excretory function.

The 4th through the 8th weeks of embryonic development are critical for normal development. During this period, the major organs and other body systems are forming and are most susceptible to damage. Some prescription drugs and even general-sales-list (GSL) medications may have side effects that harm the fetus. Women who use illicit drugs, smoke tobacco, drink alcohol, or are exposed to other toxic substances during their pregnancy also run the risk of creating birth defects in the fetus.

The gestational period is the time that it takes for the infant to develop in utero. It normally takes 38 weeks, with significant developmental progress occurring each week. The time of pregnancy is calculated from the first day of the pregnant woman's last menstrual period. As the placental tissues normally start sending hormonal signals to the corpus luteum to start changing the internal environment in the second week after conception, this dating method adds 2 weeks to the entire calculation, leading to 40 total weeks of pregnancy from conception to birth (antenatal period).

Physiological Maternal Changes During Pregnancy

When a woman conceives, carries a baby to term, and then gives birth, several physiological changes occur within her body. Many of these changes can alter the normal response to trauma or exacerbate or create medical conditions that can threaten the health of both the woman and baby. In particular, hormonal changes precipitate physiological changes, and the rapidly changing internal environment puts stress on the woman. Metabolic demands increase during pregnancy, and the enlarging uterus with its significant vascularity creates mechanical changes as well.

The most significant physiological changes occur in the uterus. Before a woman's first pregnancy, the uterus measures about 7 cm long by 5 cm wide and is approximately 3 cm thick. After pregnancy has stretched the uterus, it will rarely return to its previous dimensions. In the nonpregnant patient, the uterus weighs only about 2 g and has a fluid capacity of about 10 ml. By the end of pregnancy, the uterus may weigh as much as 1 kg and have a capacity of about 5,000 ml.

The measurement of the fundus of the uterus (the top portion, opposite the cervix) can indicate possible developmental problems. The fundus is measured in centimetres by running a

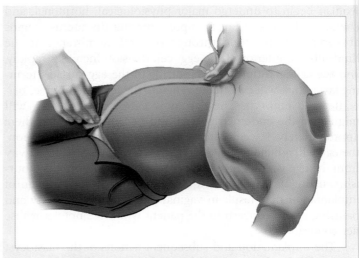

Figure 39-3 Measuring the fundus.

measuring tape vertically from the top of the pubic bone to the top of the fundus **Figure 39-3 ▲**. The length in centimetres roughly corresponds to length of gestation. For example, if the patient is 32 weeks' pregnant, the measurement would be 32 cm. If the length is longer or shorter than expected, it could indicate uterine growth problems or breech position (if shorter) or the possibility of twins (if longer).

The circulatory system of a woman is impacted by pregnancy in several ways. The average woman has about 4 to 5 litres of blood available as total circulating volume. Blood volume in the pregnant female increases gradually throughout gestation, such that there may be as much as a 40% to 50% overall increase at term. The level of increase depends on such factors as patient size, number of times gravid (total pregnancies, but not necessarily carried to term) and para (pregnancies carried to more than 28 weeks' gestation, regardless of whether delivered dead or alive), and number of fetuses she is carrying. This increase in blood volume is necessary for meeting the metabolic needs of the developing fetus, to perfuse maternal organs adequately—especially the uterus and kidneys—and for helping compensate for blood loss during delivery. At term, the uterus normally contains 15% to 16% of the mother's total circulating blood volume. During vaginal delivery, a woman may lose as much as 500 ml of blood (1,000 ml in case of caesarean section). The uterus, as it contracts, tends to shunt blood back into maternal circulation (autotransfusion), thereby preserving maternal circulatory haemostasis.

As blood volume increases, so does the number of red blood cells (RBCs), which increase by as much as 33% over the normal count. The increase in RBCs heightens the pregnant woman's need for iron, which is why most women have to take antenatal vitamins. If the woman does not take iron supplements, the fetus will rob maternal stores for its needs, resulting in anaemia for the woman—and often leading to preterm labour and spontaneous abortion. Women who live in socioeconomically deprived areas and lack access to antenatal health care are the most likely to experience pregnancy-related anaemia.

A woman's white blood cell (WBC) count also increases during pregnancy, with an average of 4,300 to 4,500 ml before pregnancy to as high as 12,000 ml or more in the third trimester of pregnancy. Clotting factors are similarly increased, while fibrinolytic factors are depressed. These issues are important considerations if the paramedic has to deal with obstetric haemorrhage or thromboembolic disease.

As blood volume increases, so does the size of the pregnant woman's heart, by an average of 10% to 15% from prepregnancy levels, with a collateral capacity increase of 70 to 80 ml. Cardiac output increases to about 40% more than before pregnancy, reaching its maximum capacity at about 22 weeks' gestation and then maintaining this level until term. As the uterus enlarges and the diaphragm becomes elevated, internal maternal organs begin to shift to make room. The myocardium is displaced upward and to the left with a slight rotation in its long axis, which causes the apex of the heart to shift laterally (remember this point when auscultating the S_3 and S_4 heart sounds). In addition, the intensity of the "lub-dub" S_1 heart sound increases, while the S_2 heart sound generally remains normal. Increased cardiac output can also cause a benign systolic flow murmur, which results from hypertrophy of the heart and dilation across the tricuspid valve.

A pregnant woman's heart rate gradually increases during pregnancy, by an average of 15 to 20 beats/min by term. ECG changes that can occur during pregnancy include ectopic beats and supraventricular tachycardia, which is often considered normal. Other changes include a slight left axis deviation and lead III changes such as low-voltage QRS, T-wave inversion or flattening, or even occasional Q waves.

As gestation increases, a woman's sensitivity to body positioning increases as well. Resting or lying supine can cause the uterus to impinge upon the inferior vena cava, thereby decreasing venous return to the heart. Pressure by the fetus on the common iliac vein creates this problem as well. Over time, if pressure is not relieved, cardiac output is decreased, blood pressure drops, and lower extremity oedema will result. In about the 12th week of gestation, systolic pressure may drop slightly, but diastolic pressure usually declines by 5 to 10 mm Hg. Diastolic pressure usually returns to normal prepregnancy levels at about 36 weeks' gestation.

The pressures exerted upon the circulatory system and the increased blood volume combine to produce venous distension of about 150% of prepregnancy levels. Blood return to the heart is reduced as the venous ends of the capillaries become dilated. Pregnant women who are bedridden or who spend a great deal of time lying down are in particular danger of experiencing deep venous thrombosis, which can lead to pulmonary embolism. The slow return also causes delayed absorption of subcutaneously or intramuscularly injected medications.

When a gravid patient goes into labour, the position she is in stresses the cardiovascular system as well. In the United Kingdom, the standard position is the lithotomy position, in

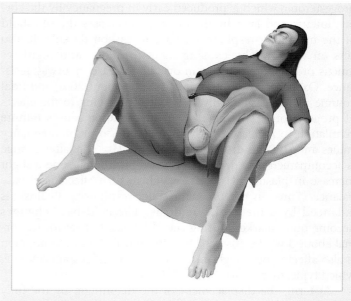

Figure 39-4 Lithotomy position.

which the woman is supine (on her back) with her knees spread apart, or her feet in stirrups **Figure 39-4 ▲**. Most ambulance cots don't have stirrup attachments, so let's assume that birth will occur in the supine or semi-recumbent position. In the supine position, maternal cardiac output can increase as much as 25% from uterine contractions, with pulse pressure increasing by about the same percentage. Impingement of the uterus on the inferior vena cava may cause the heart rate to decrease about 15%, in turn causing stroke volume to increase as much as 30%. Intra-abdominal pressure combined with the intensity of uterine contractions then causes central venous pressures to rise. Blood volume also increases during contractions to about 300 to 500 ml.

The workload of the heart increases significantly during both gestation and labour. For a healthy woman, this presents no undue complications. For a woman with heart disease or other forms of cardiac compromise, however, the increased work can result in ventricular failure or pulmonary oedema, culminating in congestive heart failure. The pain and pressures of labour can further stress the heart, resulting in cardiac arrest.

During pregnancy, the respiratory system undergoes stresses as well. The uterus pushes the diaphragm up toward the abdominal cavity, resulting in about a 4-cm displacement of the diaphragm. To compensate for this change, the rib margins flare outward, increasing the lower thoracic diameter by about 2 cm and the total thoracic circumference by as much as 6 cm. This flaring allows the respiratory system to maintain intrathoracic volume. The abdominal muscles tend to lose their tone during pregnancy, which allows respiration to be more diaphragmatic.

As maternal oxygen demand increases, the respiratory physiology changes to accommodate this need. The hormone progesterone, which is produced early in pregnancy by the corpus luteum and later by the placenta, decreases the threshold of the medullary respiratory centre to carbon dioxide. It also acts on the bronchi, causing them to dilate, and regulates mucus production, causing an overall decrease in airway resistance. Oxygen consumption increases by about 20%, and tidal volume increases gradually to about 40% owing to the effects of progesterone. The increase in tidal volume causes minute ventilation to increase by as much as 50% over prepregnancy values and pCO_2 to drop by about 5 mm Hg. The latter change is accompanied by a decrease in blood bicarbonate and a slight increase in plasma pH levels, which in turn affects acid-base balance. Thus, in the pregnant state, respiratory alkalosis is balanced by a metabolic acidosis. The acid-base changes become quite marked during actual labour, but return to normal about 3 weeks postpartum (after birth). Minute ventilation is also affected by a slight increase in maternal respiratory rate, which typically rises to about 10 l/min.

At term, the displacement of the diaphragm by the fully enlarged uterus causes a decrease in expiratory reserve volume, functional residual capacity, and residual volume. Tidal volume and inspiratory reserve volume increase, causing the inspiratory capacity to increase. Structural changes within the respiratory mucous membrane result in increased vascularity and oedema. For these reasons, you should avoid nasal intubation in pregnant patients and (if necessary) choose the next smaller size ET tube for oral intubation, to avoid creating additional complications from trauma to the respiratory tract. Oestrogen also affects the nasal tract, leading the respiratory membrane to become friable, and making epistaxis a potential emergency condition with the pregnant patient.

As the pregnancy progresses, the maternal metabolism undergoes phenomenal changes—most obviously, weight gain and alterations in physical structure. Weight gain is partly due to increased blood volume and increases in intracellular and extracellular fluid (3 kg), uterine growth (1.5 kg), placental growth (1 kg), fetal growth (3 kg), and increased breast tissue (1 to 1.5 kg). Some weight gain is also attributable to increased proteins and fat deposits, with the average weight gain in pregnancy being 12.3 kg.

The hormone relaxin, which is released during pregnancy, causes collagenous tissues to soften and produces a generalised relaxing of the ligamentous system, especially along the spine; this effect contributes to the characteristic lordosis of latter pregnancy and the increased flexion of the neck, both of which help the pregnant patient compensate for balance. Animal studies have shown that relaxin also appears to enhance mammary gland enlargement, soften the cervix, and increase pelvic joint motility.

Pregnancy increases the demand for carbohydrates, which seems to be based on fetal demand for glucose. Because the insulin molecule is too large to pass through the placental barrier, several fetoplacental and maternal hormones are utilised to compensate for the increased carbohydrate requirement. Women who are predisposed to a diabetic state may become chemical diabetics during pregnancy, but return to a normal carbohydrate metabolism postpartum. During pregnancy, the pancreas secretes insulin in greater amounts and at a faster pace, while cellular sensitivity to insulin declines. The increased production of insulin is the result of increased levels of free cortisol and progesterone. Oestrogen has the effect of blunting the action of insulin, whereas progesterone decreases the utilisation of insulin by the cells. Human chorionic somatomammotropin (hCS) is released to help stimulate lypolysis; it also acts on glucose to increase peripheral utilisation. The net effect is to make glucose available to the fetus from increased energy production from fat. In a healthy woman, these systems work a very fine balancing act to maintain homeostasis. In obese women or women who have been diagnosed with or are predisposed to diabetes, this balance is much harder to achieve. In such cases, gestational diabetes or eclampsia is a possibility.

You are the Paramedic Part 2

The patient tells you that this is her second pregnancy. She has a healthy 5-year-old boy, and did not have any complications with his pregnancy. She further tells you that she feels as though she needs to move her bowels. The closest appropriate hospital is approximately 25 miles away. As you perform a physical examination on the patient, your partner obtains her baseline observations.

Vital Signs	Recording Time: 5 Minutes
Level of consciousness	A (Alert to person, place, and day)
Respirations	26 breaths/min; adequate depth
Pulse	110 beats/min; strong and regular at the radial artery
Skin	Pink, warm, and moist
Blood pressure	104/64 mm Hg
SpO_2	98% on room air

2. On the basis of what the patient has told you, what do you expect to find during your physical examination?

3. Is there adequate time to transport this patient to hospital, or should you prepare for imminent delivery?

Gestational diabetes mellitus (GDM) is the inability to process carbohydrates during the pregnancy. Increased maternal insulin production results in increased placental production of human placental lactogen, which leads to an imbalance between the supply of the mother's insulin and glucose production. The patient may be asymptomatic or may exhibit the same signs observed in patients with diabetes mellitus, polyuria, polydipsia, and polyphagia. Treatment consists of diet control and oral hypoglycaemic medications. As GDM may occur early in the pregnancy, it is recommended that patients undergo a fasting glucose test as part of routine antenatal testing.

Medical Conditions That Can Be Detrimentally Affected by Pregnancy

Several medical conditions may adversely affect the health of both the woman and the developing fetus. Pregnancy has the tendency to aggravate preexisting medical conditions and give rise to new ones. Pregnancy is also associated with some unique conditions, such as placentitis, a viral or bacterial infection of the placental surface. Only the most common pregnancy-related complications are discussed here.

Heart Disease

Heart disease is of major concern when dealing with a pregnant patient. When you are obtaining the patient's medical history, find out the nature and treatment of any heart conditions. Which cardiac medications has the patient been taking? Has she previously been diagnosed with arrhythmias or heart murmurs? Has she had a history of rheumatic fever, or was she born with a congenital heart defect? Such heart defects may be benign under normal conditions, but the added stresses of pregnancy could create major problems. Has the patient experienced any episodes of dizziness, lightheadedness, or syncopal episodes with the pregnancy? Such episodes can be indicative of arrhythmias that can become critical during the stresses of labour.

Hypertension

A major cause of mortality and morbidity in the pregnant woman is hypertension. Blood pressure is generally lower during the gestational period than at prepregnancy levels, but women who are hypertensive or borderline hypertensive may have their hypertension exacerbated by pregnancy.

Chronic hypertension is a blood pressure that is equal to or greater than 140/90 mm Hg, which exists prior to pregnancy, occurs before the 20th week of pregnancy, or continues to persist postpartum. Diastolic pressures higher than 110 mm Hg place the patient in an increased risk category for stroke and other cardiovascular dangers.

Gestational hypertension develops after the 20th week of pregnancy in women with previously normal blood pressures and resolves spontaneously in the postpartum period. It is more commonly experienced by women who are obese or glucose intolerant. Gestational hypertension may be an early sign of preeclampsia but, if no other signs or symptoms manifest, it is generally benign.

Preeclampsia (also called toxaemia of pregnancy) is the most serious of the hypertensive disorders. It occurs in about 8% of all pregnancies and, along with the other hypertensive disorders, accounts for about 15% of direct maternal deaths annually in the United Kingdom. Women younger than 20 years who are experiencing their first pregnancy are at highest risk, followed by women with advanced maternal age, histories of multiple pregnancies, and risk factors of chronic hypertension, renal disease, and diabetes. Race also tends to play a factor, with black women being most susceptible. The disorder manifests after the 20th week of pregnancy, with the onset of a triad of symptoms: oedema, usually of the face, ankles, and hands; gradual onset of hypertension; and protein in the urine. Other symptoms include severe headache, nausea and vomiting, agitation, rapid weight gain, and visual disturbances. Preeclampsia can lead to chronic hypertension, which can retard growth and development of the fetus, impair liver and renal function, cause pulmonary oedema, or progress to life-threatening tonic-clonic convulsions, a state called eclampsia. Other risk factors that may accompany preeclampsia include liver or renal failure, cerebral haemorrhage, placental abruption, and HELLP syndrome (Haemolysis, Elevated Liver enzymes, Low Platelets), the presence of which necessitates immediate delivery of the fetus to save the woman's life. A systolic pressure exceeding 160 to 180 mm Hg and a diastolic pressure exceeding 105 mm Hg, in the presence of these other risk factors, may require administration of emergency hypertensive medications, such as labetalol or hydralazine; however, these are not currently given under normal UK prehospital guidelines. Preeclampsia normally resolves with delivery, but can manifest postpartum.

Diabetes

Diabetes may be markedly affected by pregnancy. As the hormones of pregnancy alter the insulin-regulating mechanisms, diabetics may experience wildly fluctuating blood glucose levels, manifested as hyperglycaemic or hypoglycaemic episodes. Unfortunately, oral hypoglycaemic agents can cross the placental barrier and affect the fetus, so people with insulin-dependent diabetes may have to adjust their daily dosing during pregnancy.

Respiratory Disorders

One of the most common complaints of pregnant patients is breathlessness or general dyspnoea, which is often precipitated by hormone-related anatomical changes to the respiratory system and is generally only of minor concern and discomfort to the patient. In the pregnant patient, it is important to distinguish between this kind of *physiological* dyspnoea and *pathological* dyspnoea. In the latter case, careful evaluation of the patient, identification of signs and symptoms, or a medical history may reveal an underlying condition that is being aggravated by the pregnancy.

Asthma is one of the most common conditions that can complicate pregnancy. It can either be aggravated as a preexisting illness or occur for the first time during pregnancy, triggered by the effects of stress or respiratory irritants on an already-sensitised respiratory system. Acute asthma attacks render the fetus and woman vulnerable to progressive hypoxia. Maternal complications of an asthma attack may include premature labour, preeclampsia, respiratory failure, vaginal haemorrhage, or eclampsia. Fetal complications may include premature birth, low birth weight, growth retardation, and quite possibly fetal death.

Tuberculosis is not directly aggravated by pregnancy, but the effects of the disease on the respiratory tree can overtax the respiratory system burdened by pregnancy. Women with tuberculosis are more prone to experience premature delivery as well as spontaneous abortion. Endometritis and placentitis with tuberculosis as the causative agent are also potential complications.

Cystic fibrosis (CF) is a hereditary disease that affects the whole body. It results from an autosomal-recessive mutation that impairs the genes responsible for creating sweat, mucus, and digestive juices. CF is basically an exocrine system disorder, whose mechanism causes intense scarring of targeted organs. The lungs are particularly susceptible, with the result that patients experience frequent lung infections. There is no cure for the disease, and it often proves fatal before a person reaches 40 years of age. CF does not appear to affect pregnancy directly, or vice versa, although women with CF have a greater chance of diabetes developing. The primary effects of CF on pregnancy appear to be collateral, with pregnancy exacerbating other disease processes that CF has affected. Reduced pulmonary function in a patient with CF may also lead to complications in pregnancy.

Pneumonia is a major indirect cause of maternal death in the United Kingdom. This illness of the respiratory system and lungs results in alveolar inflammation and oedema. Pneumonia can be caused by fungal, viral, or bacterial infection; parasitical infestation; or traumatic or chemical insult to the lungs (eg, aspiration of vomitus). Alcohol abuse is another factor. Pneumonia can be especially virulent during pregnancy, due to the mother's already depressed immune system. In conjunction with disorders such as CF, it can have a significant impact on maternal mortality and morbidity. Low birth weight and premature labour are common complications, with preterm delivery occurring in as many as 43% of cases and before 36 weeks' gestation.

Renal Disorders

As pregnancy progresses, a woman's kidneys increase in length by up to 2 cm, and her ureters get longer, wider, and more curved. Although these changes increase the capacity of the ureters, they can also lead to urinary stasis, resulting in urinary tract infections. These infections can be mild, but they may also progress to states that result in low fetal birth weight and retarded fetal development, premature labour, or even intrauterine fetal death.

Pressure on the bladder as the uterus enlarges can also result in increased urinary frequency. The renal plasma flow rate increases by as much as 25% to 50%, and the glomerular filtration rate increases by about 50%. Patients with preexisting renal disease are likely to experience compounding of associated problems, and those without a diagnosis of renal disease may experience renal malfunctions or failure due to hypertensive disorders or conditions such as hyperemesis gravidarum.

Haemoglobinopathies

About 13,000 people in the UK have inherited (genetic) haemoglobin disorders. These disorders affect persons of a variety of ethnic and racial backgrounds, but are most prominent in Black Caribbean, Black African, and Black British communities. Haemoglobin, the protein in RBCs responsible for oxygen transport, changes structurally as a result of genetic mutation, which in turn creates syndromes in the affected person. The two most clinically significant haemoglobinopathies are sickle cell anaemia (SSA) and thalassaemia.

In sickle cell disease, under certain physiological conditions the mutation causes the RBCs to become malformed, assuming a sickle shape. This cell alteration inhibits the RBCs from passing smoothly through the small capillaries, which in turn can block blood flow. Complications arising from this blockage include severe acute pain, strokes, and target organ damage, especially the spleen and liver. Because these individuals are anaemic, they are prone to infectious states, particularly pneumonia, which is a common cause of death of those with SSA. SSA affects an estimated 12,500 people with an estimated 240,000 carriers in the United Kingdom.

Pregnant patients with SSA are prone to pain crises, convulsion disorders, and thrombosis. Anaemia can also significantly affect fetal growth and mortality. Episodes of SSA can mimic several other conditions (eg, chest pain, abdominal pain) and can cause conditions such as kidney failure and congestive heart failure. Treatment for pregnant patients follows the same modality as for nonpregnant patients. Pain management in the field is controversial, and should be determined by local guidelines.

Genetic mutations in the thalassaemias result in a decrease in the amount of normal haemoglobin. Thalassaemias are more common in peoples of Mediterranean descent as well as in African and Middle Eastern populations. The severity of the condition depends on the severity of mutation. In pregnant women with severe cases, the anaemia causes such a high level of oxygen deprivation that the fetus cannot survive, and a massive fluid accumulation can manifest in the fetus (hydrops fetalis) resulting in neonatal death. The most severe form of thalassaemia, called Cooley's anaemia, greatly increases an infant's susceptibility to infection and causes growth retardation and skeletal malformations.

Isoimmunisation (Rh Disease)

Rh factor is a protein found on the RBCs of most people. When this factor is absent, the person is said to be Rh negative. When a woman who is Rh negative becomes pregnant by a man who has the Rh factor (Rh positive) and the fetus inherits this factor, the fetal blood can pass into the mother's circulation and produce maternal antibody (isoimmunisation) to the factor.

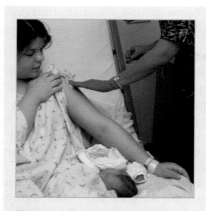

Figure 39-5 An Rh-negative woman who becomes pregnant by an Rh-positive man should receive an injection of anti-D immunoglobulin, which prevents the woman's body from attacking subsequent Rh-positive pregnancies.

Rh disease is normally not a problem in first pregnancies, but in subsequent pregnancies the antibody will aggressively cross the placental barrier to attack the fetal RBCs, which the mother's body identifies as foreign proteins Figure 39-5 ◄ . This attack can result in death for the fetus or cause haemolytic disease (erythroblastosis fetalis) in a newborn. Newborns with haemolytic disease may present with jaundice, anaemia, and hepatomegaly.

Group B Streptococci Perinatal Infections

Group B streptococcus (GBS) is the leading cause of life-threatening infections in newborns, yet remains one of conditions for which pregnant women are not routinely screened. This infection is caused by *Streptococcus agalactiae,* bacteria that live in the genitourinary and gastrointestinal tracts of healthy individuals, generally without causing any ill effects. In pregnancy, the bacteria can proliferate, resulting in urinary tract infection, infection of the uterus, and stillbirth. If the infection is passed on to the newborn, it can cause respiratory problems, pneumonia, septic shock, and meningitis. Infant illness generally manifests within the first 7 days after birth, but can occur several months later.

Perinatal Viral and Parasitic Infections

Viral and parasitic infections in pregnancy can cause significant problems for the pregnant woman and child. Infections early in pregnancy can affect the formation of the organ systems of the fetus; infections later in pregnancy can result in neurological impairments, growth disturbances, and heart and respiratory effusions. The most commonly encountered infections include varicella zoster virus, human parvovirus B19 (fifth disease), toxoplasmosis, and cytomegalovirus.

Epilepsy

Most women with epilepsy have normal pregnancies. In women who take medication to control convulsions, however, the altered haemodynamics of pregnancy can affect medication levels, possibly resulting in convulsions. Nearly one third of epileptic women will experience an increase in convulsions, regardless of medication alterations. Generalised tonic-clonic convulsions have been known to cause miscarriages, and the onset of labour can trigger convulsions in some women, which will ultimately result in fetal distress. Women with epilepsy also tend to have an increased risk of vaginal bleeding, both during and after pregnancy.

Convulsions

When a convulsion occurs in pregnancy, two patients are involved—the pregnant woman and the fetus. Convulsions can be caused by hypertension, toxaemia, preeclampsia, or a preexisting convulsion disorder. Treatment for a pregnant patient is especially difficult because diazepam—the drug commonly used to treat convulsions—can cross the placental barrier, causing fetal distress. In pregnant patients, magnesium sulphate is the recommended treatment, especially in the patient with eclampsia. In addition, high-flow supplemental oxygen is needed for both patients to counteract the hypoxia that occurs in convulsions. Potential complications in such cases may include abruptio placenta, haemorrhage, disseminated intravascular coagulation, and death.

Thyroid Disorders

The thyroid is a butterfly shaped endocrine gland that is located in the neck, directly in front of the trachea. It is responsible for production of several hormones, including thyroxine (T_4) and triiodothyronine (T_3). These hormones regulate the metabolic rate and affect the functions and growth of other organ systems. Calcitonin, which controls calcium blood levels, is also produced in the thyroid. Thyroid disorders affect about 2% of pregnant women and, if left untreated, can lead to complications for both patients. Some pregnant women have pre-existing thyroid conditions, while others experience thyroid problems during or after pregnancy, secondary to metabolic alterations.

When the thyroid produces too much thyroid hormone, hyperthyroidism results. Symptoms of hyperthyroidism in pregnancy include fatigue, forgetfulness, constipation, bradycardia, feeling cold, and muscle and joint aches. One of the serious complications of hyperthyroidism is preeclampsia.

When the thyroid produces too little thyroid hormone, the condition is called hypothyroidism. Symptoms of hypothyroidism include nervousness and irritability, tachycardia, and feeling warm. Hypothyroidism can cause long-term neurological or developmental deficits in the fetus, and may result in mental retardation.

Cholestasis

Cholestasis is a disease of the liver that occurs only during pregnancy. Hormones affect the gallbladder by slowing down or blocking the normal bile flow from the liver. Bile, which aids the process of digestion by breaking down fats, is produced in the liver and stored in the gallbladder. When its normal flow is altered, bile acids build up in the liver, then spill out into the bloodstream. The most common symptom of this condition is profuse, painful itching, particularly of the hands and feet. Patients may also complain of fatigue or depression, nausea, and right upper quadrant pain. They may also notice colour changes in waste elimination—dark urine and light grey or yellow stools. Women who are carrying multiple fetuses are at a higher risk for the development of cholestasis, as are women who have a family history of cholestasis or who have had previous liver damage.

Cholestasis is relatively benign and transitory for the pregnant woman, but can have serious effects on the fetus. Because the fetus relies on the woman's liver to remove bile acids from the blood, any impediment to this process puts stress on the developing fetal liver. Preterm birth and stillbirth are potential complications of untreated cholestasis.

Complications of Pregnancy

Most pregnancies proceed uneventfully, but paramedics are likely to be summoned when they do not.

Cephalopelvic Disproportion

In cephalopelvic disproportion, the head of the fetus is larger than the pelvis. Cephalopelvimetry (an X-ray measurement) may be performed to acquire the dimensions of the fetal head. In most cases, a caesarean section will be required to prevent maternal and fetal distress. You should ask the patient about this complication before you attempt delivery in the field. Cephalopelvic disproportion may cause massive haemorrhage, along with other postpartum complications.

Abortion

Abortion is defined as expulsion of the fetus, from any cause, before the 20th week of gestation (some sources consider any loss of the pregnancy up to the 28th week of gestation to be an abortion). Most abortions occur during the first trimester, before the placenta is fully mature.

Spontaneous Versus Induced Abortion

Abortions can be broadly classified as spontaneous or induced. A spontaneous abortion (miscarriage) occurs naturally, affecting about 1 of every 5 pregnancies. Causes may include acute or chronic illness in the pregnant woman, maternal exposure to toxic substances (illicit drugs), abnormalities in the fetus, or abnormal detachment of the placenta. In many cases, the cause of a spontaneous abortion cannot be found.

An induced abortion is brought about intentionally. When you are taking a medical history that includes an abortive history, you must be dispassionate and professional regardless of your personal convictions. You may encounter a patient who is experiencing complications following an induced abortion, such as vaginal bleeding or sepsis from having parts of the fetus in utero. You may also encounter a patient who has "self-medicated" in an attempt to induce an abortion and is experiencing toxic effects of the herbal remedy as well as a threatened or progressing abortion. Herbal preparations work by making the uterus and bloodstream too toxic for the fetus to survive, which in turn may be too toxic for the woman to survive.

Stages of Abortion

Sooner or later, you are likely to find yourself attempting to manage an abortion that is occurring spontaneously. The specific management of such a case depends to some extent on the stage of the abortion when the patient presents for treatment. All pregnant patients presenting with vaginal bleeding or abdominal pain should be transported and evaluated at a definitive care facility.

A threatened abortion is an abortion that is attempting to take place. It is generally characterised by vaginal bleeding during

You are the Paramedic Part 3

Your visual examination of the patient's vaginal area reveals crowning of the baby's head. After ensuring that you and your colleague are wearing the appropriate PPE, you open the sterile maternity pack, position the patient properly, and prepare for imminent delivery. You ask the patient's husband to sit next to his wife's head.

Reassessment	Recording Time: 10 Minutes
Level of consciousness	A (Alert to person, place, and day)
Respirations	28 breaths/min; adequate depth
Pulse	118 beats/min; strong and regular
Skin	Pink, warm, and moist
Blood pressure	Not obtained; you and your partner are preparing to deliver the baby
SpO₂	98% on room air

As the baby's head delivers, you note the presence of a nuchal cord. You instruct the patient to stop pushing so you can correct the situation. Your colleague applies oxygen to the patient via nonrebreathing mask.

4. What is a nuchal cord? How should you manage this situation?

the first half of pregnancy—usually in the first trimester. The patient may present with abdominal discomfort or complain of menstrual cramps. Severe pain is rarely a presenting complaint, as uterine contractions are not rhythmic. The cervix remains closed. A threatened abortion can progress to an incomplete abortion, or it may subside, allowing the pregnancy to go to term. The treatment for a threatened abortion is usually complete bed rest, often in a hospital environment, so that the woman's condition can be monitored. Your role in this case is usually transport and emotional support.

An inevitable abortion is a spontaneous abortion that cannot be prevented. The patient will generally present with severe abdominal pain caused by strong uterine contractions. Vaginal bleeding, often massive, will be present, as well as cervical dilation, as the uterus is preparing to expel the products of conception. When you are treating a patient who is experiencing a spontaneous abortion, your goals are to maintain blood pressure and prevent hypovolaemia. Treatment consists of establishing an IV line of normal saline to maintain blood pressure, 100% supplemental oxygen via nonrebreathing mask at 15 l/min, acquiring an ECG, and providing emotional support with rapid transport. Be alert for signs of shock.

An incomplete abortion occurs when part of the products of conception are expelled but some remain in the uterus. (For example, the fetus is expelled but the placenta remains, or only part of the fetus is expelled.) As the cervix has dilated to expel the fetus, vaginal bleeding will be present, which may be slight or profuse, but will be continuous. Be alert for signs and symptoms of shock, and start an IV line of normal saline. If products of conception are protruding from the vagina, you will find that gentle removal of protruding tissues may prevent or relieve signs of shock. You will most often encounter this situation when you find the patient on the toilet, having attempted a bowel movement, with the fetus in the toilet still attached to the umbilical cord hanging from the vagina. The fetus should be gently collected, and emotional support provided to the patient. Fundal massage may be beneficial in stimulating the placenta to deliver. All products of conception need to be collected and presented to the receiving hospital. Do not deter the patient from viewing the fetus if she wishes, but be prepared for a strong emotional reaction. A complete abortion has occurred when all the products of conception have been expelled.

In a missed abortion, the fetus dies during the first 20 weeks of gestation but remains in utero. There is no field management of a missed abortion other than transport and emotional support. Management at the hospital will consist of a dilation and curettage (D&C), in which the cervix will be manually dilated and the endometrial lining scraped and suctioned. You should suspect a missed abortion when the patient presents with a history of threatened abortion. The typical history will be a cessation of vaginal bleeding followed by a gradual diminishing of the signs of pregnancy, such as uterine and breast enlargement. The mother may also report having had a brownish vaginal discharge, possibly accompanied by a rank smell. On examination, the uterus may feel like a hard mass in the abdomen, and fetal

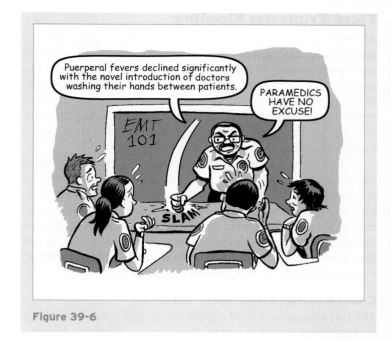

Figure 39-6

heart sounds cannot be heard. Missed abortion is generally caused by anembryonic gestation (blighted ovum), maternal disease, uterine anomalies, embryonic anomalies, placental abnormalities, or fetal chromosomal abnormalities. It almost always occurs because of a problem with the fetus, but occasionally a healthy fetus can be expelled by a diseased or damaged uterus. A missed abortion generally precedes a spontaneous abortion.

Septic abortion was once the leading cause of maternal death worldwide. In medical literature, a common complication of childbirth was puerperal fever, which was caused by a streptococcal infection of the genital tract. The incidence of puerperal fever declined significantly in the early 20th century when doctors began routinely washing their hands between patients Figure 39-6 ▲ . Septic abortion occurs when the uterus becomes infected—often by common vaginal bacterial flora—following any type of abortion. The patient will generally give a history of fever and bad-smelling vaginal discharge, usually starting within a few hours after abortion. Physical examination will generally reveal fever and abdominal tenderness. In severe cases, the infection will have progressed to septicaemia, resulting in septic shock. For this life-threatening emergency, prehospital management consists of starting an IV line of normal saline, administering 100% supplemental oxygen via nonrebreathing mask, ECG monitoring, and rapid transport. The fluid administration rate should maintain the patient's blood pressure at an acceptable level.

Notes from Nancy

Any vaginal bleeding during the third trimester of pregnancy must be regarded as a dire medical emergency until proved otherwise.

Third-Trimester Bleeding

Abortion accounts for the majority of vaginal bleeding that results in an emergency call. Any detachment of the ovum or embryo from the uterine wall will result in bleeding. The patient may complain of light or heavy bleeding, normally accompanied by cramping abdominal pain. She may also report the passage of tissue or clots. Vaginal bleeding is a serious sign at any stage of pregnancy, but the complications of bleeding increase as the gestation time lengthens.

Third-trimester bleeding presents the greatest danger of haemorrhage, which becomes more acute as the woman approaches term. A complicating factor of third-trimester bleeding is the large volume of blood present within the pregnant woman's body and the compensatory mechanisms that are functioning as a result of pregnancy. A pregnant woman can lose a full 40% of her circulating volume before significant signs and symptoms of hypovolaemia become apparent.

Causes of Third-Trimester Bleeding

The three major causes of significant antepartum haemorrhage (haemorrhage before delivery) are abruptio placenta, placenta praevia, and uterine rupture.

Abruptio placenta refers to a premature separation of a normally implanted placenta from the wall of the uterus **Figure 39-7 ▾**. It most commonly occurs during the last trimester of pregnancy, but can take place in the second trimester as well. Abruptio placenta affects about 1 of every 100 pregnancies that go to term. Maternal hypertension is the most common cause of abruption (44%), followed by trauma (eg, road traffic collisions), assault, falls, and infection. Drug abuse, alcohol use, and smoking are also contributing factors. Incidence is greater among multiparous women and those who have previously experienced abruptio placenta.

The patient with abruptio placenta will usually report vaginal bleeding, with bright red blood, although in some cases the blood does not emerge through the cervix and the bleeding may remain concealed within the endometrium. In any case, the woman will experience the sudden onset of severe abdominal pain, and she may report that she no longer feels the baby moving inside her. Physical examination may reveal signs of shock, often out of proportion to the apparent volume of blood loss. The abdomen will be tender and the uterus rigid to palpation. Fetal heart sounds are often absent because the fetus, being partly or completely cut off from its blood supply, is likely to die. Other complications include severe haemorrhaging. If the haemorrhaging cannot be controlled after delivery, a hysterectomy may be necessary.

In placenta praevia, the placenta is implanted low in the uterus and, as it grows, it partially or fully obscures the cervical canal **Figure 39-8 ▾**. This condition is the leading cause of vaginal bleeding in the second and third trimesters of pregnancy, with the majority of problems occurring near term, as the cervix begins to dilate in preparation for delivery. Maternal age and multiparity are risk factors, with women older than 30 years being three times as likely to experience the condition as will women in their 20s. Placenta praevia occurs in about 5 of every 1,000 births, with a maternal mortality rate of 0.03%. Complications include disseminated intravascular coagulation, haemorrhage, and low fetal birth weight.

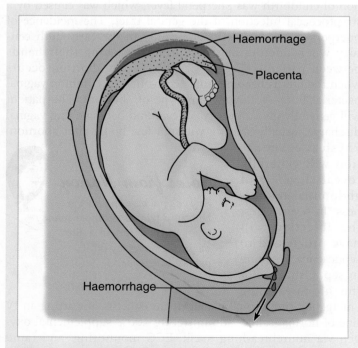

Figure 39-7 In abruptio placenta, the placenta separates prematurely from the wall of the uterus.

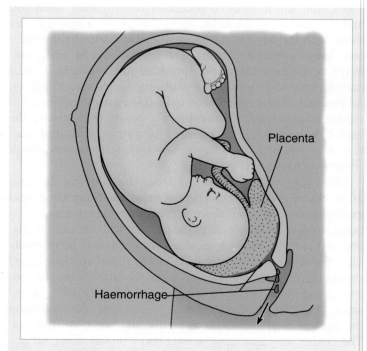

Figure 39-8 In placenta praevia, the placenta develops over and covers the cervix.

The chief complaint of a woman with placenta praevia is usually painless vaginal bleeding, with the loss of bright red blood. Because the blood supply to the fetus is not immediately jeopardised, fetal movements continue and fetal heart sounds remain audible. On gentle palpation, the uterus is soft and nontender. (Do *not* try to palpate the abdomen deeply in any woman with third-trimester bleeding; if she does have placenta praevia, deep palpation may induce heavy bleeding.)

If the uterus ruptures, it will happen during labour. Patients at greatest risk are women who have had many children and those with a scar on the uterus (eg, from a previous caesarean section). Typically, you will be called for a "possible obstetric emergency", and find a woman in active labour complaining of weakness, dizziness, and thirst. She may tell you that initially, she had very strong and painful contractions, but then the contractions slackened off. Physical examination will reveal signs of shock—sweating, tachycardia, and falling blood pressure. Significant vaginal bleeding may or may not be obvious.

Assessment and Management of Third-Trimester Bleeding

Assessment of third-trimester bleeding is much the same as assessment of vaginal bleeding. When the patient presents with the chief complaint of vaginal bleeding, try to determine as much as possible about the nature of the bleeding. When did it start? What activity was the woman engaged in at the onset? Was she active or at rest? How much blood has been lost? (Use the blood loss chart in Chapter 38 to quantify this amount.) Is the patient experiencing abdominal pain? What is the nature of the pain? Sharp? Cramping? Dull? Achy? Use OPQRST to elaborate on the chief complaint of labour pain. Rate its severity on a scale of 1 to 10. During the physical examination, identify any changes in orthostatic vital signs. Orthostatic changes indicate a significant blood loss, which may be contrary to the physical evidence of bleeding, which may be slight. Look for a positive Grey Turner's sign or Cullen's sign, which can help correlate the presence of internal bleeding.

You do not need to identify the underlying cause of the third-trimester bleeding to treat it. Regardless of the source of haemorrhaging, prehospital management is the same as follows:

1. Keep the woman recumbent, lying on her left side.
2. Administer 100% supplemental oxygen via nonrebreathing mask at 15 l/min.
3. Rapid transport to an appropriate hospital, notifying the facility of the patient's condition en route.
4. Start an IV line of normal saline with a large-bore IV cannula. Infuse at a rate necessary to maintain blood pressure. An additional IV line may be indicated.
5. Establish an ECG and obtain baseline vital signs. Do not attempt to examine the woman internally or pack the vagina with trauma pads.
6. Use loosely placed trauma pads over the vagina in an effort to stop the flow of blood.

Disorders of Pregnancy States

Hyperemesis Gravidarum

Hyperemesis gravidarum is a condition of persistent nausea and vomiting during pregnancy. Nearly all women experience the infamous—but normal—"morning sickness", especially during the first trimester of pregnancy. Hyperemesis gravidarum is a much more serious condition, with about 1% of pregnant women being affected. Prolonged vomiting leads to dehydration and malnutrition, which have negative effects on the woman and fetus. The exact cause of the condition is unknown, but suspects include increased hormone levels—especially oestrogen and human chorionic gonadotropin (hCG)—stress, and changes to the gastrointestinal system. Hyperemesis gravidarum is most common in first-time pregnancies, with multiple gestations, and in women who are obese. This condition may also present in conjunction with molar pregnancy (discussed below) and HELLP syndrome. Symptoms include severe and persistent vomiting, in excess of three or four times daily. Vomiting is usually projectile and generally consists of bile and possibly blood. Severe nausea, pallor, and possibly jaundice may also be seen.

Prehospital treatment of hyperemesis gravidarum includes the following steps:

1. Provide 100% supplemental oxygen via nonrebreathing mask.
2. Start an IV line of normal saline and administer the first 250 ml of fluid, if clinically indicated.
3. Check blood glucose level.
4. Check orthostatic vital signs, and obtain an ECG.
5. Transport. Severe cases will ultimately require hospitalisation.

Molar Pregnancy

Molar pregnancies (hydatidiform mole) arise when a malfunction of the egg or sperm creates a problem at the fertilisation stage, resulting in an abnormal placenta. A complete mole occurs when an empty egg is fertilised, which triggers the normal progression of pregnancy, but there is no fetus present. A partial mole occurs when two sperm fertilise the same egg; instead of twins, a malfunction occurs resulting in an abnormal placenta and a fetus with an abnormal chromosome count.

In cases involving molar pregnancies, you are most likely to be responding to a call for vaginal spotting or bleeding (usually dark brown) or excessive nausea and vomiting. Preeclampsia is also a potential complication. Molar pregnancies are particularly frightening and heartbreaking as well, as the woman truly believes she is having a normal pregnancy. Antenatal screenings tend to find most instances of molar pregnancy, and a D&C is scheduled early on.

Pseudopregnancy

Pseudocyesis ("psychogenic" pregnancy) is a false pregnancy that develops all the typical signs and symptoms of true pregnancy, including weight gain, menstrual cessation, tender breasts, enlarged uterus, and even labour pains. Its exact cause is unknown, but it is presumed to be caused by the emotional desire to be pregnant. There is little for you to do for these cases except provide emotional support.

Ectopic Pregnancy

Ectopic pregnancy is a severe disorder of pregnancy with potentially life-threatening consequences. In an ectopic pregnancy, a fertilised ovum becomes implanted somewhere other than in the uterus, usually in one of the fallopian tubes. All the normal signs and symptoms of pregnancy are usually present. The patient is in severe pain, possibly in hypovolaemic shock. It is important for you to be understanding, empathetic, and, above all, supportive and patient.

Notes from Nancy

A pregnant woman may lose a lot of blood before she shows signs of shock. Don't wait for signs and symptoms. Suspect shock from the mechanisms of injury.

Pregnancy and Drugs

When a pregnant woman is a drug addict, the illicit drugs she uses pass through the placenta barrier and enter into the fetal circulation. The fetus may then develop birth defects (see Chapter 44) and also becomes an addict. When you are delivering the baby of a woman with a history of drug abuse, be aware that the baby may have signs of withdrawal after it is born—for example, respiratory depression, bradycardia, tachycardia, convulsions, and cardiac arrest. Treatment should revolve around cardiorespiratory support.

■ General Assessment of the Pregnant Patient

Some Definitions

When you are talking about the characteristics of labour and delivery in women with different obstetric histories, special terminology is used. Gravidity refers to a uterus that contains a fetus, whatever the outcome (ie, abortion, stillbirth, or live birth). Parity refers to delivery of a infant after the 28th week of gestation, irrespective of whether the infant was born alive or dead. We classify a woman, then, according to the number of times her uterus has been occupied (gravidity) and the number of times she has carried a fetus more than 28 weeks (parity).

- **Primigravida**—a woman who is pregnant for the first time.
- **Primipara** ("primip")—a woman who has had only one delivery.
- **Multigravida**—a woman who has had two or more pregnancies, irrespective of the outcome.
- **Multipara** ("multip")—a woman who has had two or more deliveries. A woman who has had more than five deliveries is referred to as a "grand multipara".

- **Nullipara**—a woman who has never delivered.

For example, a woman who has had four pregnancies but carried only one of them to term—the three others ended in miscarriage—would be classified as gravida 4, para 1. The medical shorthand annotation would be G4P1. You could also write the preceding case history as G4A3P1, showing abortive history.

Scene Assessment and Initial Assessment

Proper physical assessment and medical history are an important part in treating the obstetric patient. Perform a scene assessment as with any other call. Likewise, the initial assessment should be the same as with any patient.

> **At the Scene**
>
> Blood pressure is an unreliable indicator of perfusion in any patient, but it is even less reliable in the pregnant patient because a greater volume of blood can be lost before hypotension develops.

Focused History and Physical Examination

Determine the patient's chief complaint, elaborate on this chief complaint using the OPQRST, and obtain the SAMPLE history. Specifically, you want to know if the patient is pregnant, how many times she has been pregnant (gravida), and how many times she has had a live birth (para). The first question can generally be bypassed if the patiently is obviously pregnant. Asking a woman who is near term if she is pregnant (the unspoken implication is that she is just fat) is not a good way to develop trust or gain a friend—but, if in doubt, ask. The number of times pregnant may also need to be clarified, as many women do not count abortions or miscarriages as pregnancies, and tend to think only of actual deliveries. Also ask about the length of gestation and her estimated due date or date of confinement.

Ask the patient whether she has experienced complications with any of her pregnancies, or whether she has had any obstetric or gynaecological complications. Has she ever had a caesarean section? If so, is the current baby planned for caesarean delivery or does the patient intend to have a vaginal birth after caesarean (VBAC)? Complications of VBAC can include uterine rupture. Is the patient currently under a doctor's care? Has she been taking antenatal vitamins? When was her last visit to her doctor? Has her doctor indicated any concerns about this pregnancy?

Has the patient had a recent ultrasound? What were the findings? Did the ultrasound reveal more than one fetus or any abnormal presentations? Is the patient taking any current medications? Any GSL drugs, recreational drugs, or herbals? Does the patient have any allergies? (This subject should have been covered in the SAMPLE history, but ask again now.)

What is your general impression of the patient's overall health? Has she been smoking, consuming alcohol, or used any illicit drugs during the pregnancy? If yes, how recently? Is the patient currently experiencing pain? If yes, what is the quality and duration? Where is it located and does it radiate? Was the onset gradual or sudden? When did the pain start, and does anything relieve it? Has the patient experienced this type of pain before? When? Is the pain occurring regularly? Is it sporadic or constant?

Has the patient noticed any vaginal bleeding or spotting? If so, what was the amount of bleeding? How long did the bleeding last? What colour was the blood? What was the patient doing prior to the bleeding? Did she use sanitary pads to stop the bleeding? How many pads? Did the bleeding stop? Has the patient passed any clots or tissue? If so, try to obtain samples to give to the A&E department. Has the patient experienced any other type of vaginal discharge? What was the amount, colour, and duration of that discharge? Was any identifiable or disagreeable odour associated with the discharge?

If the patient is in active labour, have her waters broken? Does she need to move her bowels or push? If she answers yes to these last questions, delivery may be imminent.

Focused Physical Examination

Your physical examination should be based on the patient's chief complaint. Just because a woman is pregnant, you should not rule out the possibility of asthma, heart attack, or allergic reactions, for example. No matter what the chief complaint, the detailed physical examination should also include fetal heart sounds and heart rate. By feeling the abdomen, you can roughly palpate the fetal position. Pay close attention to the vital signs of both patients—the woman and the fetus. If the patient tells you she has abdominal pain, ask her to describe the pain; this information will help determine whether she is having contractions.

Inspect the vaginal area for crowning or vaginal bleeding or discharge. Crowning indicates that you will need to deliver the baby on scene. If there is no crowning, ask the mother

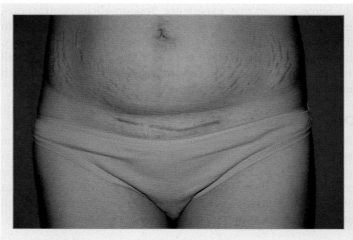

Figure 39-9 A scar from a caesarean section.

> ### At the Scene
>
> If you note a scar above a woman's pubic hair line **Figure 39-9 ▲**, it may mean she has delivered once before by caesarean. Ask whether she knows of any reason why she would not be able to deliver vaginally, and report her response. Women who have previously delivered by caesarean section are not necessarily precluded from having a normal, vaginal delivery.

how far apart the contractions are, and then time them. Ask the patient if her waters have broken, and, if so, how long ago. First-time mothers (gravida 1) typically take more time to deliver, whereas multigravida and multipara mothers can deliver very quickly.

If you see bleeding or discharge, ascertain when it started and check the abdomen for tenderness and rigidity. Normal abdomens are not rigid during pregnancy. Assessment of the serial vital signs will tell you if the woman or fetus is in distress.

You are the Paramedic Part 4

After successfully managing the nuchal cord, you immediately deliver the rest of the body. The infant is blue, but begins breathing spontaneously within a few seconds. The mother remains haemodynamically stable. Next, you pat the infant dry, and wrap the baby in warm blankets. Finally, you place the infant in the correct position and continue to monitor the infant's overall condition.

Newborn Assessment	Recording Time: 14 Minutes
Respirations	Rapid and irregular; adequate tidal volume
Pulse rate	130 beats/min; strong and regular
Colour	Central and peripheral cyanosis

5. What three parameters should be used to determine the need for newborn resuscitation?
6. Is additional treatment required for this infant other than maintaining airway patency and providing thermal management?

Some women may experience Braxton-Hicks contractions, or intermittent uterine contractions that may occur every 10 to 20 minutes. Usually seen in the third month of the pregnancy, this condition is also known as false labour. It is prudent to call the patient's midwife to ensure a full assessment of both mother and fetus will be performed.

Ongoing Assessment

Ongoing examination should include an assessment of the woman's serial vital signs and the fetal heart rate and heart tones. Also, time the contractions and perform a head-to-toe examination of the woman (if you have not already done so) to avoid missing other possible injuries and complications. Check any interventions and transport to a delivery suite.

Trauma During Pregnancy

Trauma is a serious complicating factor in pregnancy, partly because of the many physiological changes that occur during pregnancy, but mostly because of the involvement of two patients—the woman and her fetus. Both patients are particularly vulnerable to trauma because of the unique features of pregnancy.

Although not the most prolific cause of maternal death in the UK, traumatic injury continues to have a marked effect on pregnant women each year, with 6% to 8% of pregnant women experiencing some type of trauma during the pregnancy, usually in the last trimester. The major causes of injury to pregnant women are road traffic collisions, falls, and domestic abuse. Road traffic trauma accounts for 60% to 67% of trauma in pregnancy, but accounts for only 21% of maternal deaths.

At the Scene

Throughout pregnancy, seatbelts should be used with *both* the lap belt and the shoulder harness in place. The lap belt portion should be placed under the abdomen and over the iliac crests and the pubic symphysis. The shoulder harness should be positioned between the breasts.

Vulnerability of the Pregnant Woman to Trauma

In general, abdominal trauma occurs from the same mechanisms in pregnant women as in nonpregnant women. However, because the likelihood of domestic abuse increases greatly during a woman's pregnancy, prehospital personnel should be suspicious for evidence of this crime.

The anatomical changes during pregnancy have important implications for trauma. As the woman approaches term, her abdominal contents are compressed into the upper abdomen.

The diaphragm is elevated by about 4 cm, so there is a higher incidence of abdominal injuries in association with chest trauma. Meanwhile, because the peritoneum is maximally stretched, significant abdominal trauma may occur without peritoneal signs.

In the first trimester of pregnancy, the uterus is well protected in the woman's bony pelvis and is rarely damaged from abdominal trauma. In the second and third trimesters of pregnancy, the uterus grows out from the pelvis and extends into the abdomen, making it more vulnerable to blunt and penetrating trauma. In road traffic collisions, for example, the use of a lap belt increases the likelihood of uterine damage because the lap belt compresses the uterus. Shoulder restraints, by contrast, decrease the chance of uterine injury. In penetrating injuries, the large uterus protects the other organs from injury. Because the uterus shields the other organs, pregnant women with penetrating wounds can have excellent outcomes, although the fetus is often injured by the trauma. In addition to abdominal tenderness, the examination of an injured pregnant woman may reveal an abnormal fetal position, an easily palpated fetus, inability to palpate the top of the uterus, or vaginal bleeding.

As early as the second trimester of pregnancy, the bladder is displaced upward (superior) and forward (anterior) so that it lies outside the pelvic cavity. It is therefore at increased risk of injury, particularly from a deceleration injury caused by a lap seatbelt. Should you encounter a restrained pregnant patient in a road traffic collision, make a note of belt placement. If the patient is found with the belt placed over the abdomen or on top of the uterine dome, this positioning should dramatically increase your index of suspicion for internal injuries to the woman and fetus. The uterus also becomes more vulnerable to injury as it increases in size, and deceleration forces, such as those produced by vehicular trauma, may bring about abruptio placenta or uterine rupture.

As noted earlier, pregnancy is accompanied by a significant increase in vascular volume. Normal vascular volume increases by nearly 50% during the first 6 months of pregnancy as a result of the pregnant woman having to perfuse her own circulation and that of the fetus. To meet this demand, normal cardiac output increases by about 40% as a result of the increasing pulse rate and stroke volume. The resting pulse rate increases by 15 to 20 beats/min over the rate in a nonpregnant patient, so the resting pulse may be as high as 100 beats/min by the end of the second trimester of pregnancy. This physiological change makes it much more difficult to interpret tachycardia. Furthermore, because of the pregnant woman's vastly expanded blood volume, other signs of hypovolaemia, such as a falling blood pressure, may not be evident until she has lost as much as 40% of her blood volume. Therefore you need to be aggressive in managing a pregnant woman with a mechanism of injury (MOI) that indicates shock.

A relative redistribution of blood volume also occurs during pregnancy, with blood flow to the pelvic region increasing tenfold. If a pregnant woman sustains a pelvic fracture, her chances of bleeding to death are therefore significantly higher than those of a nonpregnant woman. A good deal of blood volume can be lost before signs and symptoms of shock develop because other mechanisms are compensating for the loss.

Regarding respiration, the pregnant woman has a higher basal metabolism and therefore an increased need for oxygen. At the same time, she has more carbon dioxide to eliminate—hers and that produced by fetal metabolism. She responds by increasing her tidal volume and, therefore, her minute volume. If she should need artificial ventilation, you will have to administer supplemental oxygen at a higher minute volume than usual.

During pregnancy, digestion slows and bowel motility decreases, resulting in the stomach staying full longer. With the gravid uterus placing pressure on the stomach, the chances of aspiration are dramatically increased.

Vulnerability of the Fetus to Trauma

The muscular wall of the uterus acts as a cushion for the fetus against the direct effects of blunt trauma, but fetal injury can occur as a result of rapid deceleration of circulation or may be secondary to impaired fetal circulation. The most common cause of fetal death from trauma is maternal death, but a woman will often survive an incident that proves fatal for the fetus. Blunt trauma resulting in abruptio placenta, for instance, provides a good statistical outcome for the mother but often results in the death of the fetus.

Notes from Nancy
A fetal heart rate lower than 120 per minute means fetal distress.

If the pregnant woman has sustained trauma and is bleeding massively, the maternal circulation will shunt blood away from fetal circulation to maintain maternal homeostasis—maternal circulation takes precedence over the requirements of the fetus. Therefore, any injury that involves significant maternal bleeding will threaten the life of the fetus. By the time the woman shows clinical signs of shock, fetal circulation will be so compromised that you can expect a fetal mortality of 70% to 80%.

The best indication of the status of the fetus after trauma is the fetal heart rate. A normal fetal heart rate is between 120 and 160 beats/min. A rate slower than 120 beats/min

Notes from Nancy
Every pregnant woman who has been in a collision must be evaluated at hospital, even if her own injuries appear trivial.

means fetal distress and signals a dire emergency. To measure the fetal heart rate, listen with the bell of the stethoscope over the pregnant woman's abdomen. You may have to move the stethoscope around the abdomen until you can hear the fetal heart sounds. Palpate the woman's pulse at the same time as you count the fetal heart rate. If the fetal heart rate is identical to the maternal pulse, you are probably listening to an echo of the maternal heartbeat and not the fetal heart, so change the position of your stethoscope and try again. It takes a lot of practice to hear fetal heart tones and requires quiet surroundings. Some modern ambulances may be equipped with Doppler stethoscopes, which make assessment of fetal heart sounds much easier.

Treatment of the Pregnant Trauma Patient

Although trauma in a pregnant woman involves at least *two* patients, we can treat only one of them directly: the woman. In general, what is good for the woman will be good for the fetus. For example, any effort to improve maternal perfusion will have a collateral effect of improving fetal circulation. Potential damage to the fetus cannot be assessed adequately in the field, however, only presumed or suspected. While a decreased fetal heart rate signals an emergency situation, a normal fetal heart rate does not guarantee that all is well. Even minor deceleration forces can cause significant injury to the fetus.

In general, the prehospital management of pregnant women with abdominal trauma is the same as for nonpregnant patients. Airway, breathing, and circulation remain the highest priorities. However, because the large uterus can compress the vena cava (decreasing right atrial preload), a pregnant woman should be transported to the hospital on her left side unless a spinal injury is suspected **Figure 39-10 ▾**. If you must transport a patient in the supine position, elevate her right hip about 15 cm to minimise the pressure of the

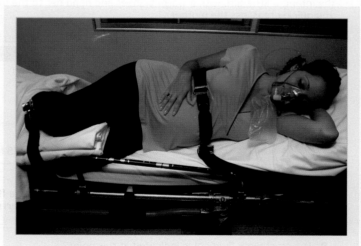

Figure 39-10 Whenever possible, transport a pregnant patient lying on her left side to allow for sufficient circulation through the vena cava.

vena cava. Be aware that because of the physiological changes that occur in a woman's body during pregnancy, the fetus may lack appropriate circulation even if the woman's vital signs appear normal. In other words, the fetus may be in shock before signs appear in the mother, so initiate early, aggressive fluid resuscitation.

Field treatment of a pregnant trauma patient is as follows:

1. *Ensure an adequate airway.* Regurgitation and aspiration are much more likely in a pregnant woman than in a patient who is not pregnant, so if the patient is unconscious, provide early endotracheal intubation to isolate the airway. Provide cricoid pressure until the airway is secured.

2. *Administer oxygen.* A pregnant woman's oxygen needs are 10% to 20% higher than normal, so provide 100% supplemental oxygen via nonrebreathing mask if the patient is conscious.

3. *Assist ventilations as needed, and provide a higher minute volume than usual.* Because the uterus of a pregnant woman presses up against the diaphragm, she will be more difficult to ventilate. Once the patient is intubated, therefore, you may want to use a positive-pressure ventilator periodically to ensure visible chest rise (representing an adequate tidal volume).

4. *Control external bleeding promptly.* Splint any fractures.

5. *Start one or two IV lines of normal saline.* Use large-bore cannulas and macro drip sets. Administer a bolus if signs

and symptoms of haemodynamic compromise are present, with the goal of maintaining blood pressure. Remember that a larger volume of fluid is necessary for the pregnant patient.

6. *Notify the receiving hospital* of the patient's status and your estimated time of arrival.

7. *Transport* the woman in the lateral recumbent position. If she is on a longboard, tilt the longboard 30° to the left by wedging pillows beneath it. This will cause the uterus to shift, taking the weight off the inferior vena cava and improving venous return to the heart.

If cardiac arrest occurs, provide CPR and ALS as you would for a nonpregnant patient.

If resuscitation efforts are not effective within 5 minutes, an emergency caesarean section must be performed to save the woman and possibly the baby. Immediate evacuation of the uterine contents provides the most favourable resuscitation scenario for the woman. If a caesarean is done within 5 minutes of maternal death, the fetus at term has a 70% chance of survival. Paramedic caesarean section guidelines are not commonplace and remain highly controversial; therefore, your patient requires rapid transport and prior notification to the closest A&E department. Even if the woman is *obviously* dead (eg, in case of decapitation), good CPR and ventilatory support may keep the fetus viable until a caesarean section can be performed.

You are the Paramedic Part 5

The infant's trunk is pink following the administration of blow-by oxygen; however, the infant's hands and feet remain somewhat cyanotic. The infant is breathing adequately and has a heart rate of 130 beats/min. After clamping and cutting the umbilical cord, you wrap the infant, a little girl, with a warm blanket and hand her to the mother. As your colleague retrieves the stretcher from the ambulance, you quickly reassess the mother.

Reassessment	Recording Time: 21 Minutes
Level of consciousness	A (Alert to person, place, and day)
Respirations	24 breaths/min; adequate depth
Pulse	104 beats/min; strong and regular
Skin	Pink, warm, and moist
Blood pressure	100/60 mm Hg
SpO$_2$	99% on nonrebreathing mask of 15 l/min oxygen

During transport, you initiate an IV of normal saline and set the flow rate to keep the vein open. You reexamine the mother and note a moderate amount of vaginal bleeding. Your estimated time of arrival at hospital is 20 minutes.

7. How will you treat this patient's postpartum bleeding?

8. Is a crystalloid fluid bolus indicated at this point?

Following your interventions, the patient's bleeding has subsided. The placenta delivers shortly before you arrive at hospital. The mother and baby remain stable.

Assisting Delivery

With the woman prepared as described, take up a position just distal to her buttocks (on her right side if you are right-handed and on her left side if you are left-handed) and follow these steps.

1. Control the delivery. When crowning occurs, place *gentle* pressure on the baby's head with the palm of your gloved hand to prevent the head from delivering too quickly and tearing the perinium.

2. As the baby's head begins to emerge from the vagina, it will start to turn. Support the head as it turns. Do *not* attempt to pull the baby from the vagina! If the membranes cover the head after it emerges, tear the amniotic sac with your fingers or forceps to permit escape of amniotic fluid and enable the baby to breathe.

3. Slip your middle finger alongside the baby's head to check for a nuchal cord. In such a case, the umbilical cord becomes wrapped around part of the infant's body, generally the neck and as a single loop. In most cases, a nuchal cord is not a significant problem, but as the fetus descends during labour, cord compression may occur, causing the fetal heart rate to slow and resulting in fetal distress.

4. If you find a nuchal cord, try to slip it gently over the baby's shoulder and head. Should this manoeuvre fail, and if the cord is wrapped tightly around the neck, place umbilical clamps 5 cm apart and cut the cord between the clamps.

5. Gently guide the baby's head downward to allow delivery of the upper shoulder **Figure 39-16 ▸**. Do not pull on the baby to facilitate the delivery.

6. Gently guide the head upward to allow delivery of the upper shoulder **Figure 39-17 ▸**.

7. Once the shoulders are delivered, the baby's trunk and legs will follow rapidly **Figure 39-18 ▸**. Be prepared to grasp and support the infant as it emerges, keeping in mind an important fact: *Newborn babies are wet and slippery.*

8. Once the baby is delivered, lay the baby along your arm with one arm and shoulder between your fingers and the head held dependent to aid drainage.

9. Wipe any blood or mucus from the baby's nose and mouth with a sterile gauze. Use an appropriate suction device (eg, bulb syringe) to suction the baby's mouth and nostrils, if needed. Be sure to squeeze the bulb *before* inserting the tip, and only *then* place the tip in the baby's mouth or nostril and release the bulb slowly. Withdraw the bulb, expel its contents into a waste container, and repeat suctioning as needed.

10. Dry the baby with towels (wet babies lose heat faster than dry ones) and wrap with a dry blanket.

11. Record the time of birth for your patient clinical record.

Notes from Nancy
Babies are slippery!

In a normal delivery, the baby will usually be breathing on his or her own, if not shrieking, by the time you finish suctioning the airway.

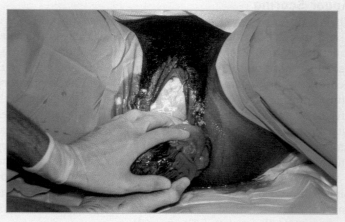

Figure 39-16 Gently guide the baby's head downward to allow delivery of the upper shoulder.

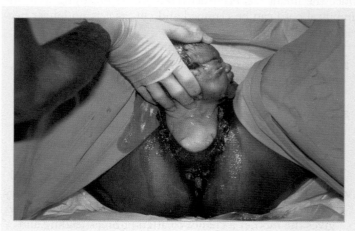

Figure 39-17 Gently guide the head upward to allow delivery of the upper shoulder.

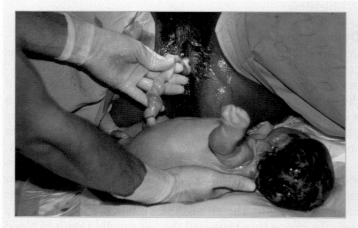

Figure 39-18 Once the shoulders are delivered, the baby's trunk and legs will follow rapidly.

Babies are usually born blue, but with a few good howls they should turn a nice pink, although their extremities may remain dusky.

Apgar Scoring

The Apgar scoring system (devised by Virginia Apgar, MD) is a useful means of evaluating the adequacy of a newborn's vital functions immediately after birth; such information will prove useful to those who take over the care of the baby after your delivery. In this system, five parameters—heart rate, respiratory effort, muscle tone, reflex irritability, and colour—are each given a score from 0 to 2 both 60 seconds and then 5 minutes after birth. The majority of infants are vigorous and have a total score of 7 to 10; they cough or cry within seconds of delivery and require no further resuscitation. Infants with a score in the 4 to 6 range are moderately depressed; they may be pale or blue 1 minute after delivery, with poorly sustained respirations and flaccid muscle tone. Such infants will require some form of resuscitation (discussed in Chapter 40).

Cutting the Umbilical Cord

Once the infant has been delivered and is breathing well, the umbilical cord can be clamped and cut, as it is no longer necessary for the infant's survival.

1. Handle the umbilical cord with care.
2. Tie or clamp the cord about 20 cm from the infant's navel, with two ties (or clamps) placed 5 cm apart. Cut the cord between the two ties or clamps.
3. Examine the cut ends of the cord to be certain there is no bleeding. If the cut end attached to the infant is bleeding, tie or clamp the cord *proximal* to the previous clamp, and examine it again (do *not* remove the first clamp). There should not be any oozing from the infant's end of the cord.
4. Once the cord is clamped and cut, wrap the baby in a dry blanket and place him or her at the mother's breast. This gives the mother a chance to attempt breastfeeding and allows for bonding between the mother and child. The suckling reflex also triggers the uterus to contract, which will speed the delivery of the placenta and reduce bleeding.

Delivery and Management of the Placenta

With the delivery of the baby, the second stage of labour is complete, and the third stage—delivery of the placenta—begins. The placenta is usually delivered within 20 minutes of the baby's arrival. Your job is to make stimulating conversation with the mother and bystanders as you wait patiently for the placenta to begin to separate spontaneously. Do not attempt to speed delivery of the placenta by pulling on the umbilical cord.

The first sign that the placenta is separating from the uterine wall is usually the patient's complaint that her contractions are starting again. The uterus rises in the abdomen and feels hard to palpation. The end of the umbilical cord protruding from the vagina lengthens, and there is usually a gush of blood from the vagina. When these signs occur:

1. Instruct the patient to bear down to expel the placenta.
2. As she does so, hold the placenta with both hands and gently twist it so that the membranes will peel completely off the uterine wall.

3. Gently massage the abdomen over the uterus to aid in its contraction.
4. If your local guidelines says to do so, administer oxytocin. Before you start oxytocin, make absolutely sure the woman isn't delivering a second baby!

Once you have the placenta in your hand, examine it for completeness. One side (fetal side) should be grey, shiny, and smooth; the other side (maternal side) should be dark maroon with a rough texture Figure 39-19 ▶. There may also be a white fringe around the placenta, which is the remnant of the amniotic sac. Pallor of the maternal surface of the placenta may indicate haemorrhage or fetal anaemia. Blood clots adhering to the surface suggest abruption. Try to determine whether the placenta is malformed in any way or if pieces are obviously missing; retained pieces of placenta will cause persistent bleeding. Place the placenta in one of the plastic bags from the maternity pack, and transport it with you to the hospital for examination by the pathology lab.

Examine the perineum for lacerations and apply pressure to any bleeding tears. Clean up and place a sanitary pad over the mother's vaginal opening, lower her legs, and prepare for transport. If the placenta has not delivered after 15 minutes, transport the patient anyway. Transport the patient in the supine recumbent position, with pads and draping in place, maintaining universal precautions.

Some women may ask if they can keep the placenta. This is standard practice in some parts of the world, where consumption of the placenta is considered a means for the mother to regain her strength quickly. Women from some cultures may want to keep the placenta to bury it and plant a tree over the spot, so that the tree and the child grow together. You need to respect such requests. If the patient refuses transport to the hospital, try to follow local guidelines and law as to who should receive the placenta.

Abnormal Deliveries

Most deliveries are normal. The baby arrives headfirst, followed shortly by the placenta; the mother and paramedics come through the event like champions. Occasionally, however, complications arise. To deal with obstetric complications successfully, the paramedic must know when to anticipate them, how to recognise them when they

> **Notes from Nancy**
>
> Never pull on the umbilical cord to try to hasten delivery of the placenta.

> **Notes from Nancy**
>
> Any baby who is not coming headfirst must be delivered at the hospital.

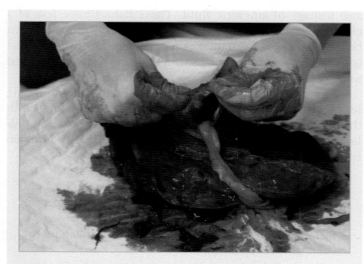

Figure 39-19 A whole placenta.

do occur, and what action to take to ensure that everyone makes it through the event successfully.

Breech Presentations

Most term babies enter the world headfirst (vertex presentation). The baby's head serves to open a path through the cervix for the narrower shoulders and hips. In a breech presentation,

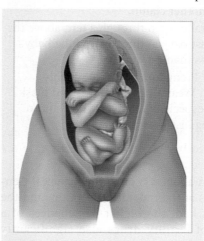

Figure 39-20 In a breech presentation, the buttocks are delivered first. These deliveries are usually slow, so you will often have time to transport the mother to the hospital.

however, another part of the body leads the way, usually the buttocks (the word *breech* means "buttocks") Figure 39-20 ◂ , but sometimes one of the feet comes first. Breech presentations occur in 4% of all deliveries and are more common with premature births.

The best place for a breech presentation to be delivered is in the hospital. Of course, sometimes you won't realise that you are dealing with a breech until the mother is crowning and you notice that the presenting part does not have any hair but rather has a suspicious indentation down the middle. By the time you have made that astute observation, it's usually too late to get the woman to the hospital.

If you have determined that the buttocks are the presenting part and that delivery is imminent, proceed as follows:

- Position the woman with her buttocks at the edge of the bed or stretcher and her legs flexed.

- Allow the buttocks and trunk of the baby to deliver spontaneously. *Do not pull on the baby.*
- Once the baby's legs are clear, support the baby's body on the palm of your hand and volar surface of your arm.
- Lower the baby slightly so that it very nearly hangs by its own weight downward; that will help the head pass through the pelvic outlet. You can tell when the head is in the vaginal canal because you'll be able to see the baby's hairline at the nape of his or her neck just below the woman's symphysis pubis.
- When you can see the baby's hairline, grasp the baby by the ankles and lift him or her upward in the direction of the woman's abdomen. The head should then deliver without difficulty.
- If the baby's head does not deliver within 3 minutes, the child is in danger of suffocation, and immediate action is indicated. Suffocation may occur when the baby's umbilical cord is compressed by his or her head against the birth canal, which cuts off the baby's supply of oxygenated blood from the placenta, and the face is pressed against the vaginal wall, which prevents the baby from breathing on his or her own. Place your gloved hand in the vagina, with your palm toward the baby's face. Form a V with your fingers on either side of the baby's nose, and push the vaginal wall away from the baby's face, thus establishing an airway, until the head is delivered.
- Remember: *This is a delivery, not an extrication.* Do not attempt to forcibly pull the baby out or allow an explosive delivery. If the head does not deliver within 3 minutes of establishing the airway, provide rapid transport to the hospital, with the mother's buttocks elevated on pillows. Try to maintain the baby's airway throughout transport. En route, pre-alert the hospital so that it can have the appropriate personnel on hand when the mother arrives.

Other Abnormal Presentations

There are a variety of other abnormal ways in which the baby may present for delivery, most of them fortunately quite rare. In a footling breech, one or both feet will dangle down through the vaginal opening Figure 39-21 ▸ . In a transverse presentation (transverse lie), the fetus lies crosswise in the uterus and may wave at the paramedic with one hand protruding through the vagina. Even the baby who is coming headfirst may extend the

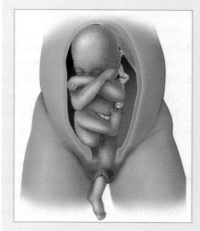

Figure 39-21 In very rare instances, an infant's limb—usually a single arm or leg—presents first. This is a serious situation, and you must provide prompt transport for hospital delivery.

neck and present with the face or brow instead of the top of the head (vertex). With all of those abnormal presentations, the most important point is *not to attempt delivery in the prehospital environment*. Nearly all of these abnormal presentations will require delivery by caesarean section, so prehospital management is to provide rapid transport.

Prolapsed Umbilical Cord

With a <u>prolapsed umbilical cord,</u> the cord emerges from the uterus ahead of the baby (Figure 39-22 ▾). With each uterine contraction, the cord is then compressed between the presenting part and the bony pelvis, shutting off the baby's supply of oxygenated blood from the placenta. Fetal asphyxia may ensue if circulation through the cord is not rapidly reestablished and maintained until delivery. Cord prolapse occurs in 3% of deliveries and is more likely when the presenting part does not completely fill the pelvic brim, such as in abnormal presentations or with small babies (premature births, multiple births).

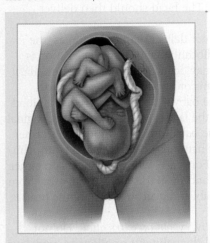

Figure 39-22 A prolapsed umbilical cord, another rare situation, is very dangerous and must be cared for at the hospital.

Treatment of cord prolapse is clearly urgent. Take the following steps:

1. Position the woman supine with her hips elevated as much as possible on pillows.
2. Administer 100% supplemental oxygen via nonrebreathing mask.
3. Instruct the woman to pant with each contraction, which will prevent her from bearing down.
4. With two fingers of a gloved hand, gently push the baby (not the cord) back up into the vagina until the presenting part no longer presses on the cord
5. While you maintain pressure on the presenting part, have your colleague cover the exposed portion of the cord with dressings moistened in normal saline.
6. Somehow, you must try to maintain that position, with a gloved hand pushing the presenting part away from the cord, throughout *urgent transport* to the hospital.

Premature and Small Infants

Preterm labour occurs late in the second trimester or early in the third trimester of pregnancy. The pregnant woman will start to experience contractions; she also may have spotting and leakage of amniotic fluid. These babies have less of a chance of survival and more birth defects if they are born before 37 weeks of gestation. The treatment for this condition is to prevent labour from occurring, thereby allowing the fetus to more fully develop and have a better chance of survival.

Any baby born before 37 weeks' gestation *or* weighing less than 2.5 kg needs special care. Chapter 40 discusses the care of neonates in more detail. For our purposes here, follow these guidelines when dealing with small, red, wrinkled babies:

1. Keep the baby warm. Babies lose heat by the same mechanisms that adults do—radiation, convection, conduction, and evaporation. But babies—and especially "premies"—have less natural insulation and a larger surface area in relation to mass, so they are much more vulnerable to rapid heat loss.
    - Dry the baby thoroughly as soon as possible after birth.
    - Cover the baby with a dry blanket.
    - Place the baby on the mother's chest, and cover both with another blanket.
2. Keep the ambulance interior nice and warm. If it's comfortable for you, it's too cold for the premie.
3. Maintain the baby's airway. Use a bulb syringe to keep the baby's nose and mouth clear of fluid, if present.
4. Prevent bleeding from the umbilical cord; a very small baby cannot afford to lose even a little bit of blood. If the cord is oozing, apply another clamp.
5. Administer supplemental oxygen through a tent above the infant's head; do *not* blast oxygen directly into the baby's eyes. Use low flow—less than 4 l/min.
6. Prevent contamination. Premature babies are highly susceptible to infection. Wear a surgical gown and mask, and keep bystanders—especially relatives who want to "give the new baby a big kiss"—at a distance.

Multiple Births

Multiple gestations occur in about 3% of all pregnancies. Generally, the older a woman is at the time of conception, and the more pregnancies she has had, the higher her chances of a multiple birth. The use of fertility drugs also significantly increases a woman's odds of being pregnant with more than one child, including quadruplets and quintuplets.

The incidence of multiple births in the United Kingdom has risen significantly in recent years, so the odds of a paramedic having to assist in the delivery of multiple births is not necessarily a remote one. This is one of the reasons the maternity pack has more than you can use with a single birth, and why there should always be a spare maternity pack on the vehicle. As a rule, the delivery of multiple births does not pose any special problems, except that you have to do a few things twice (or three times!). There is a greater chance of encountering breech presentations in such births. Because the babies are usually smaller, however, delivery is easier than in a single breech birth.

Prep Kit

■ Ready for Review

- The ovaries are the starting point for reproduction. During the menstrual cycle, one follicle releases an ovum. If the ovum becomes fertilised, it develops into an embryo, and then into a fetus.
- The fallopian tubes are the structures that transport the ovum from the ovary to the uterus (a muscular, inverted pear-shaped organ). Once an egg is fertilised, it implants in the endometrium (the inner lining of the uterus).
- The fetus is enclosed in the amniotic sac, which contains amniotic fluid, allowing the fetus to develop in a weightless environment.
- The gestational period (the time that it takes for the infant to develop in utero) normally lasts 38 weeks.
- In the first trimester of pregnancy, the placenta, umbilical cord, specialised body systems, and limbs form. In the second trimester of pregnancy, the fetus gains weight and body systems become more specialised. In the last trimester of pregnancy, the fetus primarily puts on weight.
- Pregnancy is considered at term by week 37. Babies born before 37 weeks of gestation are considered premature.
- Physiological changes during pregnancy can alter a woman's normal response to trauma or exacerbate or create medical conditions that can threaten the health of woman and fetus.
- Conditions that can be exacerbated by pregnancy include heart disease, hypertension, diabetes, respiratory disorders, renal disorders, haemoglobin disorders, epilepsy, and thyroid disorders.
- Preeclampsia is the most serious hypertensive disorder, manifesting after the 20th week of pregnancy. Symptoms include oedema, gradual onset of hypertension, protein in the urine, severe headache, nausea and vomiting, agitation, rapid weight gain, and visual disturbances.
- Cholestasis is a liver disease that occurs only during pregnancy. In this condition, the flow of bile is altered, causing acid buildup. The acid eventually spills into the bloodstream, causing profuse and painful itching.
- Abortion is expulsion of the fetus, from any cause, before the 20th week of gestation.
- An incomplete abortion occurs when only some of the products of conception are expelled. In such cases, be alert for signs and symptoms of shock.
- The three major causes of significant antepartum haemorrhage are abruptio placenta, placenta praevia, and uterine rupture.
- Assessment of third-trimester bleeding is much the same as the assessment of other vaginal bleeding. Keep the woman lying on her left side, administer supplemental oxygen, provide rapid transport, provide IV fluids and ECG monitoring, and place sanitary pads over the vagina.
- Ectopic pregnancy occurs when a fertilised ovum has implanted somewhere other than the uterus, usually in one of the fallopian tubes. The patient will be in severe pain and possibly hypovolaemic shock.
- In assessing a patient with an obstetric emergency, identify the length of gestation, estimated due date, any complications with this pregnancy or others, and the presence of any vaginal bleeding.
- The major causes of injury to pregnant women are road traffic collisions, falls, domestic abuse, and penetrating injuries such as gunshot wounds. Treatment of trauma in a pregnant woman is the same as treatment of a nonpregnant woman, except that the pregnant patient should be transported on her left side unless spinal injury is suspected.
- Labour may begin with a release of a mucus plug (sometimes with blood) from the vagina.
- The first stage of labour begins with the onset of contractions—crampy abdominal pains that may radiate into the lower back. The amniotic sac may also rupture.
- The second stage of labour begins when the baby's head enters the birth canal. The woman's contractions become more intense and more frequent. When the baby's head becomes visible at the vaginal opening (crowning), delivery is imminent.
- The third stage of labour occurs when the placenta is expelled.
- In assessing a pregnant patient, determine whether there is time to take her to hospital.
- If delivery is imminent, prepare a private clean area as quickly as possible. Behave in a calm and reassuring way. Control the delivery. Clear the baby's airway.
- Never pull on the umbilical cord to deliver the placenta. Gently massage the abdomen to aid in delivery of the placenta. Once the placenta is delivered, examine it for completeness.
- A baby born before 37 weeks' gestation or weighing less than 2.5 kg is premature. Keep a premie warm, maintain the airway, prevent umbilical cord bleeding, administer supplemental oxygen, and prevent contamination.
- Complications of labour include postpartum haemorrhage. In such cases, massage the abdomen, infuse normal saline, and transport urgently.
- Meconium is the baby's first stool. A yellow or greenish black tint to the amniotic fluid indicates the presence of meconium.
- Pulmonary embolism can cause maternal death during childbirth or postpartum. Suspect this complication if the patient experiences sudden dyspnoea, tachycardia, atrial fibrillation, or postpartum hypotension.
- Pharmacology during pregnancy may include magnesium sulphate for eclampsia; calcium chloride to reverse respiratory depression following magnesium sulphate administration; salbutamol for asthma and as a uterine relaxant and occasionally for cord prolapse; diazepam for treating anxiety, diphenhydramine for treating hyperemesis gravidarum, and oxytocin for treatment of postpartum haemorrhage.

■ Vital Vocabulary

abortion Expulsion of the fetus, from any cause, before the 20th week of gestation.

abruptio placenta A premature separation of the placenta from the wall of the uterus.

amniotic fluid A watery fluid that provides the fetus with a weightless environment in which to develop.

amniotic sac The fluid-filled, baglike membrane in which the fetus develops.

antenatal The state of the pregnant woman before birth.

antepartum Before delivery.

Apgar scoring system A scoring system for assessing the status of a newborn that assigns a number value to each of five areas of assessment.

atresia The process by which an oocyte dies.

blastocyst The term for an oocyte once it has been fertilised and multiplies into cells.

body In the context of the uterus, the portion below the fundus that begins to taper and narrow.

breech presentation A delivery in which the buttocks come out first.

cervical canal The interior of the cervix.

cervix The narrowest portion of the uterus that opens into the vagina.

cholestasis A common liver disease that occurs only during pregnancy, in which the flow of bile is altered resulting in acids being released into the bloodstream, causing profuse and painful itching.

chronic hypertension A blood pressure that is equal to or greater than 140/90 mm Hg, which exists prior to pregnancy, occurs before the 20th week of pregnancy, or continues to persist postpartum.

complete abortion Expulsion of all products of conception from the uterus.

corpus luteum The remains of a follicle after an oocyte has been released, and which secretes progesterone.

crowning The appearance of the infant's head at the vaginal opening during labour.

ectopic pregnancy An egg that attaches outside the uterus, typically in a fallopian tube.

embryo The fetus in the earliest stages after fertilisation.

endometrium The innermost layer of tissue in the uterus.

episiotomy An incision in the perineal skin made to prevent tearing during childbirth.

external os The junction where the uterus opens into the vagina.

fallopian tubes The vehicles of transportation of the ova from the ovaries to the uterus; also called oviducts.

fetus The developing, unborn infant inside the uterus.

first stage of labour The stage of labour that begins with the onset of regular labour pains, crampy abdominal pains, during which the uterus contracts and the cervix effaces.

follicle-stimulating hormone (FSH) A hormone produced by the anterior pituitary gland which is important in the menstrual cycle.

footling breech A delivery in which one or both feet dangle through the vaginal opening.

fundus The dome-shaped top of the uterus.

gestational diabetes Diabetes that develops during pregnancy in women who did not have diabetes before pregnancy.

gestational hypertension High blood pressure that develops after the 20th week of pregnancy, in women with previously normal blood pressures, and resolves spontaneously in the postpartum period.

gestational period The time that it takes for the infant to develop in utero, normally 38 weeks.

GnRF A chemical released by the hypothalamus that stimulates the release of follicle-stimulating hormone.

gravid The number of all pregnancies a woman has had, including those not necessarily carried to term.

gravidity A term used to refer to a uterus that contains a pregnancy, whatever the outcome.

Group B streptococcus (GBS) A bacterium that lives in the genitourinary and gastrointestinal tracts of normal healthy individuals, but which can cause life-threatening infections in newborn babies.

human chorionic gonadotropin hormone A hormone that sends signals to the corpus luteum that pregnancy has initiated.

hyperemesis gravidarum A condition of persistent nausea and vomiting during pregnancy.

incomplete abortion Expulsion of the fetus which results in some products of conception remaining in the uterus.

induced abortion Intentional expulsion of the fetus.

inevitable abortion A spontaneous abortion that cannot be prevented.

internal mucosa The inner layer of tissue in the fallopian tubes.

labour The mechanism by which the baby and the placenta are expelled from the uterus.

luteinising hormone (LH) A hormone released by the anterior pituitary gland that stimulates the process of ovulation.

meconium A dark green material in the amniotic fluid that can indicate disease in the newborn; the meconium can be aspirated into the infant's lungs during delivery; the baby's first bowel movement.

missed abortion A situation in which a fetus has died during the first 20 weeks of gestation, but has remained in utero.

molar pregnancy Pregnancy in which there is a problem at the fertilisation stage, with a malfunction of the egg or sperm that results in an abnormal placenta and a fetus with an abnormal chromosome count, or which results in an empty egg.

multigravida A woman who has had two or more pregnancies, irrespective of the outcome.

multipara A woman who has had two or more deliveries.

muscularis The middle layer of tissue in the fallopian tubes.

myometrium The middle layer of tissue in the uterus.

nullipara A woman who has never delivered.

oocyte An egg produced from the female ovary.

ovulation A process in which an ovum is released from a follicle.

ovum A mature oocyte.

para The number of pregnancies a woman has carried to more than 28 weeks, regardless of whether the fetus was delivered dead or alive.

parity Number of live births a woman has had.

perimetrium The outer protective layer of tissue in the uterus.

placenta The tissue attached to the uterine wall that nourishes the fetus through the umbilical cord.

placenta praevia A condition in which the placenta develops over and covers the cervix.

postpartum After birth.

preeclampsia A condition of late pregnancy that involves gradual onset of hypertension, headache, visual changes, and swelling of the hands and feet; also called pregnancy-induced hypertension or toxaemia of pregnancy.

primigravida A woman who is pregnant for the first time.

primipara A woman who has had one delivery only.

progesterone A hormone that influences the second phase of the menstrual cycle, when the oocyte is either fertilised or dies.

prolapsed umbilical cord A situation in which the umbilical cord comes out of the vagina before the infant.

pseudocyesis A false pregnancy that develops all the typical signs and symptoms of true pregnancy, but in which no actual pregnancy exists.

Rh factor A protein found on the red blood cells of most people; when a woman without this protein is impregnated by a man with this protein, the woman's body can create antibodies against the protein and attack future pregnancies.

second stage of labour The stage of labour in which the baby's head enters the birth canal, during which contractions become more intense and more frequent.

secretory phase The second phase of the menstrual cycle.

septic abortion A life-threatening emergency in which the uterus becomes infected following any type of abortion.

serosa The outermost layer of tissue in the fallopian tubes.

spontaneous abortion Expulsion of the fetus that occurs naturally; also called miscarriage.

stratum basalis A permanent mucous membrane that makes up part of the outer endometrium.

stratum functionalis An inner mucous membrane that makes up part of the endometrium, and which is renewed following menstruation.

supine hypotensive syndrome Low blood pressure resulting from compression of the inferior vena cava by the weight of the pregnant uterus when the mother is supine.

third stage of labour The stage of labour in which the placenta is expelled.

threatened abortion Expulsion of the fetus that is attempting to take place but has not occurred yet; usually occurs in the first trimester.

transverse presentation A delivery in which the fetus lies crosswise in the uterus; one hand may protrude through the vagina.

umbilical cord The conduit connecting mother to infant via the placenta; contains two arteries and one vein.

uterine cavity The interior of the body of the uterus.

uterine inversion A potentially fatal complication of childbirth in which the placenta fails to detach properly and results in the uterus turning inside-out.

uterus A muscular inverted pear-shaped organ, that lies situated between the urinary bladder and the rectum.

vagina A tubular organ lined with mucous membranes, which is the lower portion of the birth canal.

Assessment in Action

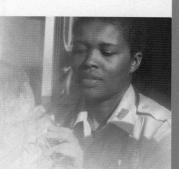

You are called to the street corner for a person who fell. When you arrive, you see an obviously pregnant woman who has fallen and sprained her ankle. As you are assessing the patient's ankle, you note that both of her ankles are swollen. You obtain a set of vital signs that include a pulse rate of 110 beats/min; blood pressure, 150/92 mm Hg; respiratory rate, 20 breaths/min; and a pulse oximetry reading of 100% on room air. When you took the patient's pulse rate, you noticed that her hands and wrists appeared swollen as well. You prepare her for transport to hospital and while you are driving to hospital, the patient begins to complain of abdominal cramping. The woman's eye's roll back and she has a full-body convulsion.

1. **This patient's medical condition is probably related to:**
   A. preeclampsia.
   B. eclampsia.
   C. abruptio placenta.
   D. spontaneous abortion.

2. **Treatment of the above patient includes all of the following, EXCEPT:**
   A. splinting of the ankle.
   B. placing the patient in the recovery position on a stretcher.
   C. administering IV normal saline and oxygen.
   D. placing the patient in the right lateral recumbent position on a stretcher.

3. **The criteria for the diagnosis of preeclampsia includes all of the following, EXCEPT:**
   A. hypertension.
   B. proteinuria.
   C. excessive weight gain with oedema.
   D. hypotension.

4. **Which medications should you be prepared to administer?**
   A. Magnesium sulphate and diazepam
   B. Morphine and diazepam
   C. Magnesium sulphate and morphine
   D. Adrenaline and atropine

5. **When does ectopic pregnancy occur?**
   A. When a fertilised ovum implants in the uterine cavity
   B. When a fertilised ovum implants anywhere other than the uterine cavity
   C. Usually later in pregnancy
   D. When a patient becomes hypertensive

6. **The absence of abdominal pain is associated with:**
   A. spontaneous abortion.
   B. placenta praevia.
   C. uterine rupture.
   D. abruptio placentae.

7. **How many stages of labour are there?**
   A. 3
   B. 5
   C. 4
   D. 6

8. **The period during which intrauterine fetal development takes place is known as:**
   A. gestation.
   B. para.
   C. uterine contractions.
   D. gravida.

9. **Pregnant patients are described by their gravid and parous states. What is the correct terminology?**
   A. Gravida and parachute
   B. Gravida and para
   C. Live and aborted
   D. Para and gravitation

10. **Uterine rupture refers to:**
   A. painless, bright red bleeding without uterine contraction.
   B. localised uterine tenderness.
   C. absent fetal heart tones.
   D. spontaneous or traumatic rupture of the uterine wall.

Challenging Question

11. **What special considerations will you need to take into account for this trauma patient?**

▬ Points to Ponder

You respond to an obstetric emergency. On arrival you find a 23-year-old woman in the final trimester of pregnancy. She is seated in the living room on a chair. She is sobbing uncontrollably. You notice that she is sitting on a towel that has blood on it. Her chief complaint is a sudden onset of vaginal bleeding that has been occurring for 20 minutes. You ask if she is in pain, and she replies "a little".

You ask if she has ever been pregnant, and she replies "once before, and I began haemorrhaging 2 weeks before delivery. I delivered a stillborn baby". She sobs.

How will you address this patient's emotions?

Issues: Dealing With Personal Tragedy, Determining a Pregnant Woman's History, Empathetic Response, Implementing a Treatment Plan.

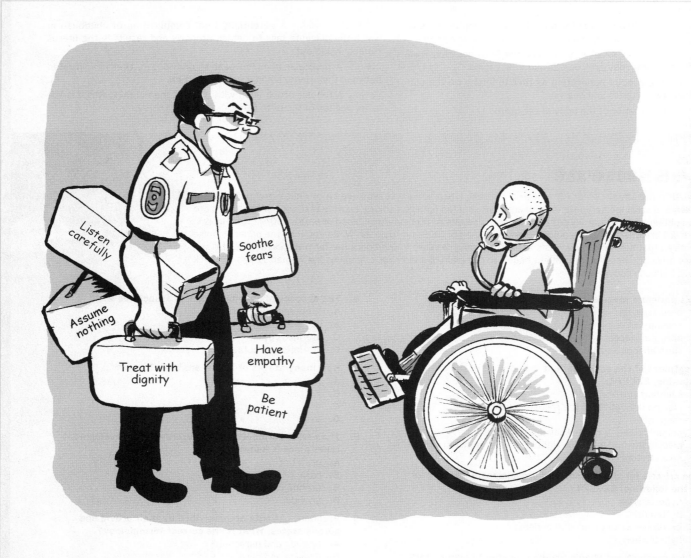

> Special problems . . . require special approaches".

—Nancy L. Caroline, MD

Special Patient Groups

Section Editor: Mark Woolcock

6

Section

40 Neonatology

Objectives

Cognitive

- Define the term newborn.
- Define the term neonate.
- Identify important antepartum factors that can affect childbirth.
- Identify important intrapartum factors that can term the newborn high risk.
- Identify the factors that lead to premature birth and low birth weight newborns.
- Distinguish between primary and secondary apnoea.
- Discuss pulmonary perfusion and asphyxia.
- Identify the primary signs utilised for evaluating a newborn during resuscitation.
- Formulate an appropriate treatment plan for providing initial care to a newborn.
- Determine when ventilatory assistance is appropriate for a newborn.
- Prepare appropriate ventilation equipment, adjuncts, and technique for a newborn.
- Determine when chest compressions are appropriate for a newborn.
- Discuss appropriate chest compression techniques for a newborn.
- Assess patient improvement due to chest compressions and ventilations.
- Determine when endotracheal intubation is appropriate for a newborn.
- Discuss appropriate endotracheal intubation techniques for a newborn.
- Assess patient improvement due to endotracheal intubation.
- Identify complications related to endotracheal intubation for a newborn.
- Determine when vascular access is indicated for a newborn.
- Discuss the routes of medication administration for a newborn.
- Determine when blow-by oxygen delivery is appropriate for a newborn.
- Discuss appropriate blow-by oxygen delivery devices and technique for a newborn.
- Assess patient improvement due to assisted ventilations.
- Determine when an orogastric tube should be inserted during positive-pressure ventilation.
- Discuss the signs of hypovolaemia in a newborn.
- Discuss the initial steps in resuscitation of a newborn.
- Assess patient improvement due to blow-by oxygen delivery.
- Discuss the effects maternal narcotic usage has on the newborn.
- Determine the appropriate treatment for the newborn with narcotic depression.
- Discuss appropriate transport guidelines for a newborn.
- Determine appropriate receiving facilities for low- and high-risk newborns.
- Describe the epidemiology, including the incidence, morbidity/mortality, risk factors, and prevention strategies for meconium aspiration.
- Discuss the pathophysiology of meconium aspiration.
- Discuss the assessment findings associated with meconium aspiration.

- Discuss the treatment/management plan for meconium aspiration.
- Describe the epidemiology, including the incidence, morbidity/mortality, risk factors, and prevention strategies for apnoea in the neonate.
- Discuss the pathophysiology of apnoea in the neonate.
- Discuss the assessment findings associated with apnoea in the neonate.
- Discuss the treatment/management plan for apnoea in the neonate.
- Describe the epidemiology, pathophysiology, assessment findings, and treatment/management plan for diaphragmatic hernia.
- Describe the epidemiology, including the incidence, morbidity/mortality, and risk factors for bradycardia in the neonate.
- Discuss the pathophysiology of bradycardia in the neonate.
- Discuss the assessment findings associated with bradycardia in the neonate.
- Discuss the treatment/management plan for bradycardia in the neonate.
- Describe the epidemiology, including the incidence, morbidity/mortality, and risk factors for premature infants.
- Discuss the pathophysiology of premature infants.
- Discuss the assessment findings associated with premature infants.
- Discuss the treatment/management plan for premature infants.
- Describe the epidemiology, including the incidence, morbidity/mortality, and risk factors for respiratory distress/cyanosis in the neonate.
- Discuss the pathophysiology of respiratory distress/cyanosis in the neonate.
- Discuss the assessment findings associated with respiratory distress/cyanosis in the neonate.
- Discuss the treatment/management plan for respiratory distress/cyanosis in the neonate.
- Describe the epidemiology, including the incidence, morbidity/mortality, and risk factors for convulsions in the neonate.
- Discuss the pathophysiology of convulsions in the neonate.
- Discuss the assessment findings associated with convulsions in the neonate.
- Discuss the treatment/management plan for convulsions in the neonate.
- Describe the epidemiology, including the incidence, morbidity/mortality, and risk factors for fever in the neonate.
- Discuss the pathophysiology of fever in the neonate.
- Discuss the assessment findings associated with fever in the neonate.
- Discuss the treatment/management plan for fever in the neonate.
- Describe the epidemiology, including the incidence, morbidity/mortality, and risk factors for hypothermia in the neonate.
- Discuss the pathophysiology of hypothermia in the neonate.
- Discuss the assessment findings associated with hypothermia in the neonate.

- Discuss the treatment/management plan for hypothermia in the neonate.
- Describe the epidemiology, including the incidence, morbidity/mortality, and risk factors for hypoglycaemia in the neonate.
- Discuss the pathophysiology of hypoglycaemia in the neonate.
- Discuss the assessment findings associated with hypoglycaemia in the neonate.
- Discuss the treatment/management plan for hypoglycaemia in the neonate.
- Describe the epidemiology, including the incidence, morbidity/mortality, and risk factors for vomiting in the neonate.
- Discuss the pathophysiology of vomiting in the neonate.
- Discuss the assessment findings associated with vomiting in the neonate.
- Discuss the treatment/management plan for vomiting in the neonate.
- Describe the epidemiology, including the incidence, morbidity/mortality, and risk factors for diarrhoea in the neonate.
- Discuss the pathophysiology of diarrhoea in the neonate.
- Discuss the assessment findings associated with diarrhoea in the neonate.
- Discuss the treatment/management plan for diarrhoea in the neonate.
- Describe the epidemiology, including the incidence, morbidity/mortality, and risk factors for common birth injuries in the neonate.
- Discuss the pathophysiology of common birth injuries in the neonate.
- Discuss the assessment findings associated with common birth injuries in the neonate.
- Discuss the treatment/management plan for common birth injuries in the neonate.
- Describe the epidemiology, including the incidence, morbidity/mortality, and risk factors for cardiac arrest in the neonate.
- Discuss the pathophysiology of cardiac arrest in the neonate.
- Discuss the assessment findings associated with cardiac arrest in the neonate.
- Discuss the treatment/management plan for cardiac arrest in the neonate.

- Discuss the pathophysiology of post arrest management of the neonate.
- Discuss the assessment findings associated with post arrest situations in the neonate.
- Discuss the treatment/management plan to stabilise the post arrest neonate.

Affective

- Demonstrate and advocate appropriate interaction with a newborn/neonate that conveys respect for their position in life.
- Recognise the emotional impact of newborn/neonate injuries/illnesses on parents/guardians.
- Recognise and appreciate the physical and emotional difficulties associated with separation of the parent/guardian and a newborn/neonate.
- Listen to the concerns expressed by parents/guardians.
- Attend to the need for reassurance, empathy, and compassion for the parent/guardian.

Psychomotor

- Demonstrate preparation of a newborn resuscitation area.
- Demonstrate appropriate assessment technique for examining a newborn.
- Demonstrate appropriate assisted ventilations for a newborn.
- Demonstrate appropriate endotracheal intubation technique for a newborn.
- Demonstrate appropriate meconium aspiration suctioning technique for a newborn.
- Demonstrate appropriate insertion of an orogastric tube.
- Demonstrate needle chest decompression for a newborn or neonate.
- Demonstrate appropriate chest compression and ventilation technique for a newborn.
- Demonstrate appropriate techniques to improve or eliminate endotracheal intubation complications.
- Demonstrate vascular access cannulation techniques for a newborn.
- Demonstrate the initial steps in resuscitation of a newborn.
- Demonstrate blow-by oxygen delivery for a newborn.

Introduction

The care of a newborn or neonate must be tailored to meet the unique needs of this population. A <u>newborn</u> refers to an infant within the first few hours after birth; a <u>neonate</u> refers to an infant within the first month after birth. A healthy neonate is completely dependent on others for nourishment, warmth, and protection from the environment. Most parents recognise this need and instinctively wish to fulfil the role of nurturer and parent. When a newborn needs special support that necessitates intervention by trained paramedics, the parents may feel isolated and inadequate. It is important for you to support the needs of both the newborn and the parents by allowing them to be physically close as much as possible, explaining what is being done, and providing details of the plan for transport to the next level of care.

This chapter reviews the physiological changes that occur in a newborn during birth, the care that should be provided during and immediately after birth, and the special needs of premature births or those complicated by other factors. It also reviews the steps involved in neonatal resuscitation and outlines the process of transporting an infant to hospital or between hospitals.

General Pathophysiology and Assessment

Additional skilled care intervention is needed for approximately 6% of newborn deliveries, with the rate of complications increasing as the newborn's birth weight and gestational age decrease. In the United Kingdom, approximately 80% of the babies born each year weighing less than 1.5 kg require

Table 40-1	Antepartum (Before Birth) Risk Factors
<ul><li>Multiple gestation</li><li>Pregnant woman's age < 16 y or > 35 y</li><li>< 35 weeks' gestation</li><li>Post-term (> 42 weeks') gestation</li><li>Toxaemia, hypertension, diabetes</li><li><u>Polyhydramnios</u> (excessive amount of amniotic fluid)</li><li>Premature rupture of the membrane and fetal malformation</li></ul>	<ul><li>Inadequate antenatal care</li><li>History of perinatal morbidity or mortality</li><li>Use of drugs/medications</li><li>Fetal anaemia</li><li><u>Oligohydramnios</u> (decreased volume of amniotic fluid during a pregnancy)</li></ul>

Table 40-2	Intrapartum (During Birth) Risk Factors
<ul><li>Premature labour</li><li>Rupture of membranes > 24 hours before delivery</li><li>Abnormal presentation</li><li><u>Prolapsed cord</u></li><li>Chorioamnionitis</li></ul>	<ul><li>Meconium-stained <u>amniotic fluid</u></li><li>Use of narcotics within 4 hours of delivery</li><li>Prolonged labour or precipitous delivery</li><li>Bleeding</li><li><u>Placenta previa</u></li></ul>

resuscitation. **Table 40-1 ▲** and **Table 40-2 ▲** outline risk factors for complications before and during birth. Because both short- and long-term outcomes in newborns have been linked to initial stabilisation efforts, it is imperative that you anticipate problems with newborns, are knowledgeable about how to deal with them, have the appropriate resuscitation equipment readily available, and carefully consider the newborn's definitive transport destination.

You are the Paramedic Part 1

You are called to the home of a 24-year-old woman who is 39 weeks' pregnant. She was alone when her waters ruptured. She is experiencing regular contractions that are 3 minutes apart and was afraid to drive to hospital, so she called 999. When you and your colleague arrive, you find your patient sitting on the sofa. After you introduce yourselves, the patient tells you that she has already called her husband, who said he will meet her at hospital. According to the patient, her waters broke around 15 minutes ago and the fluid was clear.

Initial Assessment	Recording Time: 0 Minutes
Appearance	Obviously pregnant; very nervous and in pain
Level of consciousness	A (Alert to person, place, and day)
Airway	Patent
Breathing	Respirations, increased; adequate tidal volume
Circulation	Radial pulses, increased rate and regular; no gross bleeding

1. Why is it important to determine the colour of the amniotic fluid?
2. What are some reliable indicators of imminent delivery?
3. What specific questions should you ask that will allow you to anticipate the need for resuscitation of the newborn?

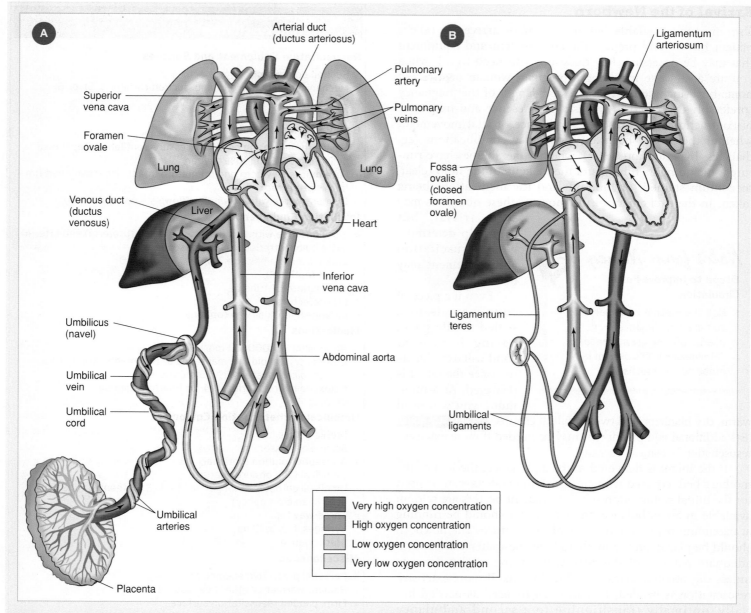

Figure 40-1 Fetal circulation. **A.** Oxygenated blood from the placenta reaches the fetus through the umbilical vein. Blood returns to the placenta via two umbilical arteries. Right-to-left shunts occur at the foramen ovale and the ductus arteriosus. **B.** Fetal circulation following transition.

Transition From Fetus to Newborn

In utero (ie, in the pregnant woman's womb), a fetus receives its oxygen from the placenta **Figure 40-1 ▲**. The fetal lung is collapsed and filled with fluid, and most of the fetal blood flow is diverted away from the lungs. As the baby is delivered, a rapid series of events needs to occur to enable the baby to breathe; this process is called fetal transition. During fetal transition, the newborn's lungs need to expand with air within seconds. As the baby's lungs become filled with air, the pulmonary pressure drops and blood begins to flow to the lungs, picking up oxygen. Anything that delays this decline in pulmonary pressure can lead to delayed transition, hypoxia, brain damage, and, ultimately, death **Table 40-3 ▶**.

Table 40-3	Causes of Delayed Transition in Newborns
■ Hypoxia	■ Hypothermia
■ Meconium or blood aspiration	■ Pneumonia
■ Acidosis	■ Hypotension

An infant delivered at less than 37 completed weeks of gestation is considered preterm; an infant born at 38 to 42 weeks of gestation is described as term; and an infant born at more than 42 weeks of gestation is described as post-term (or post-dates). These gestational lengths change if there is more than one fetus in the uterus.

Arrival of the Newborn

Use any time available before the infant arrives to take a patient history and prepare the environment and equipment that may be necessary. Key questions you need to ask when you are at a scene involving a pregnant woman or a recent home birth include the mother's age; length of the pregnancy (preferably expressed in weeks); the presence and frequency of contractions; the presence or absence of fetal movement; whether there have been any pregnancy complications (eg, diabetes, hypertension, fever); whether membranes have ruptured, including its timing and the makeup of the fluid (clear, meconium stained, or bloody); and the medications being taken. In the excitement of the moment these questions may seem trivial, but they help determine what resuscitation and equipment may be needed.

Even if a piece of equipment is in a sealed sterile pack, having it near at hand will expedite its use once the infant is delivered. At a minimum, you will need warm, dry blankets, and two umbilical clamps. **Table 40-4 ▶** lists additional equipment that may be needed if more extensive resuscitation becomes necessary.

If the infant is delivered in the ambulance, the foot of the mother's bed, covered with clean, warm blankets, can be used for the initial stabilisation steps. As radiant heaters are seldom available in an ambulance, the rear heater should be running at maximum before the delivery of the neonate. The newborn should be placed on the mother's bare chest after you confirm adequate patency of the airway, breathing, and pulse rate unless the situation does not allow for this. If more extensive resuscitation is needed, this area can be used as needed initially, optimally transitioning to a second ambulance equipped with a neonatal transport incubator to allow maintenance of a thermoneutral environment and observation of the newborn's colour and tone.

If the umbilical cord comes out ahead of the baby (which is more common with polyhydramnios, a condition characterised by extra amniotic fluid), the blood supply through the umbilical cord may be cut off. In this case, relieving pressure on the cord (by gently moving the presenting part of the body off the cord and pushing the cord back) can be lifesaving.

Notes from Nancy

Steps to Improve Fetal Circulation

- Roll the mother onto her side, to take the weight of her uterus off the great vessels.
- Administer 100% oxygen by mask to the mother.

Special Considerations

A delay in clamping the umbilical cord and keeping the infant below the placenta may allow blood to flow into the infant, which can in turn lead to polycythaemia (an abnormally high red blood cell count).

Table 40-4	**Preparation of Area for Newborn Resuscitation***

Resuscitation Equipment and Supplies

- Suction equipment
- Mechanical suction and tubing, suction catheters, 5F or 6F
- 8F feeding tube and 20-ml syringe
- Meconium aspirator

Bag-Valve-Mask Equipment

- Device for delivering positive-pressure ventilation, capable of delivering 90% to 100% oxygen
- Face masks, newborn and premature infant size (cushioned-rim masks preferred)
- Oxygen source with flowmeter (flow rate up to 10 l/min)

Intubation Equipment

- Laryngoscope with straight blades, size 0 (preterm) and 1 (term)
- Extra bulb, batteries for laryngoscope
- Endotracheal tubes size 2.5, 3.0, 3.5, and 4.0
- Stylet (optional)
- Appropriate ET tube tie
- CO_2 detectors
- Laryngeal mask airway (optional)

Medications

- Adrenaline 1:10,000 (0.1 mg/ml)
- Isotonic crystalloid (normal saline or Hartmann's solution)
- Sodium bicarbonate, 4.2% (5 mEq/10 ml)
- Naloxone hydrochloride, 0.4- or 1-mg/ml ampoule
- Glucose 10%

Umbilical Catheterisation Equipment

- Sterile gloves
- Scalpel or scissors
- Antiseptic solution (optional)
- Umbilical tape or cord ligature
- Umbilical catheters, 3.5F, 5F (a sterile 3.5F feeding tube can be used in an emergency)
- Three-way tap
- Syringes, 1, 2, 5, 10 ml
- Sterile gauze

Miscellaneous

- Personal protective equipment
- Radiant warmer or other heat source
- Firm, padded resuscitation surface
- Clock with second hand, timer optional
- 2 x towels
- Stethoscope, neonatal or paediatric preferred
- Oropharyngeal airway (0, 00, and 000 sizes)

*Reproduced from *Newborn Life Support—Resuscitation at Birth*, 2nd edition. © European Resuscitation Council.

After the infant is delivered, keep the baby at the level of the mother, with the head slightly lower than the body, while you clamp the umbilical cord in two places (5 cm and 10 cm from the baby) and then cut between the clamps. Where this is normal practice in a managed delivery (use of oxytocin to deliver the third stage) it can be appropriate just to clamp once and cut the maternal side in a physiological delivery of the third stage.

Your initial rapid assessment of the newborn may be done simultaneously with any treatment interventions. Note the time of delivery, and monitor the ABCs. In particular, assess respiratory rate, respiratory effort, pulse rate, colour, and tone.

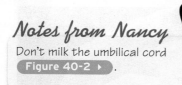

Notes from Nancy

Don't milk the umbilical cord Figure 40-2 ▶.

Nearly 90% of newborns are vigorous term babies. To ensure thermoregulation in a healthy newborn, put the baby directly on the mother's chest after birth, drying, and then covering with a dry towel. Position the baby to ensure a patent airway, clear the airway of secretions as needed, and assess the baby's colour. All newborns are cyanotic immediately after birth. If the newborn remains vigorous and quickly becomes pink, ongoing observation and continued thermoregulation with direct skin-to-skin contact with the mother should be maintained while on the way to the maternity hospital. Bonding with the mother should be encouraged in a newborn.

Need for Resuscitation

Not all deliveries go so smoothly. Approximately 10% of newborns need additional assistance and 1% need major resuscitation to survive. If a problem arises, it is important to follow the clearly defined algorithm developed by the Resuscitation Council (UK) to optimise the outcome. In this algorithm, interventions, assessment, and determination of need to progress to the next level of resuscitation are delineated in 30-second intervals.

Notes from Nancy

Do not suction deep into the oropharynx. Do not suction for more than 10 seconds at a time.

The initial steps following delivery (drying, warming, stimulating) are carried out for 30 seconds. If the newborn has not responded, further interventions are indicated. Assess the newborn's respiratory rate, respiratory effort, heart rate, tone, and colour. Count the respiratory rate and pulse rate. The heart rate can be determined either by auscultation or by feeling the base of the umbilical cord at the baby's abdomen, as the umbilical artery should still have pulsatile flow. However, palpation of the umbilical pulse can be difficult unless it is practised regularly Figure 40-3 ▶. Many newborns become centrally pink but have blue hands and feet (acrocyanosis). If the baby maintains central cyanosis of the trunk or mucous membranes, but has good respiratory rate and depth and an adequate circulation, provide supplemental free-flow oxygen. Keep the baby on the mother's chest unless you need to manage the airway.

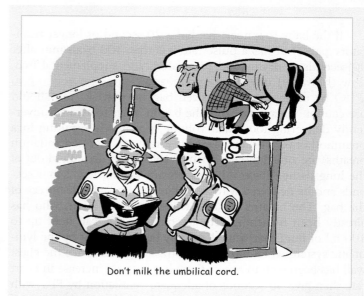

Don't milk the umbilical cord.

Figure 40-2

You are the Paramedic Part 2

Your patient tells you that this is her third pregnancy and that her first two pregnancies resulted in normal deliveries. At her last doctor's appointment, her obstetrician told her that he did not anticipate any problems and that the baby was in a head-down position in the uterus (fully engaged).

Your colleague obtains baseline vital signs as you perform a visual examination of the patient's vaginal area and put on appropriate personal protective equipment. Your examination reveals crowning of the baby's head. You immediately position the patient appropriately and open the maternity pack.

Vital Signs	Recording Time: 3 Minutes
Skin	Pink, warm, and moist
Pulse	110 beats/min, strong and regular
Blood pressure	106/60 mm Hg
Respirations	24 breaths/min; adequate tidal volume
S_PO_2	98% on room air

4. What equipment and supplies should be available in case the infant requires resuscitation?

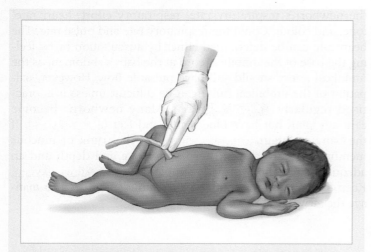

Figure 40-3 Feel for a pulse at the base of the umbilical cord.

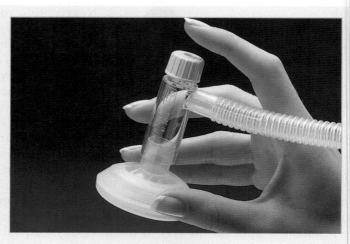

Figure 40-4 Free-flow oxygen device.

If the baby is apnoeic (ie, has a 20-second or longer respiratory pause) or has a pulse rate less than 100 beats/min after 90 seconds of drying and stimulation and supplemental free-flow (blow-by) oxygen, begin positive-pressure ventilation (PPV) by using a newborn sized bag-valve-mask. You should use caution when squeezing the bag in order to avoid inadvertently delivering too much volume, potentially resulting in a pneumothorax. The first five breaths given (termed inflation breaths) are aimed to help open alveoli and to drive fluid out of the lung tissue. These inflation breaths should last 2 to 3 seconds and be delivered with a constant and sustained squeeze of the bag. The breaths are not necessary in an infant who has already been breathing. The neonate's airway can hold up to 100 ml of fluid that will adequately be reabsorbed by the lymphatic system when inflation breaths are given. Once the chest wall has been seen to rise or there has been an increase in heart rate then give 30 seconds of adequate ventilation by PPV with free flow supplemental oxygen via a bag-valve-mask device. If the infant's pulse rate is less than 60 beats/min, begin chest compressions. Effective chest compressions should result in palpable pulses.

Fewer than 1% of deliveries involve bradycardia that requires treatment with chest compressions. The most common aetiology for bradycardia in a neonate is hypoxia, which is readily reversed by effective PPV. Profound hypoxia or shock is also the cause of cardiac arrest, which is almost always a secondary event in these small patients. Another less common aetiology—but one that requires prompt intervention—is tension pneumothorax. If ventilation and chest compressions do not improve the bradycardia, administer adrenaline via IV or IO line. Endotracheal (ET) drug delivery has poor absorption and can increase the difficulty in providing good ventilations in the neonate. For these reasons drug delivery via the ET tube should be considered a last resort intervention. Even infants who have been resuscitated for 20 minutes can have positive long-term outcomes. Newborns are very resilient, and most respond readily to interventions.

Specific Intervention and Resuscitation Steps

Drying and Stimulation

After ensuring the patency of the airway, dry and stimulate the infant (in the absence of meconium-stained fluid or thick vernix). Flick the soles of the baby's feet and gently rub the baby's back. Avoid rubbing too roughly or slapping the baby, since these actions may lead to traumatic injury.

Free-Flow Oxygen

If an infant is cyanotic or pale, but has adequate respiratory effort, provide supplemental oxygen. Given that 5 g/100 ml of deoxygenated haemoglobin is needed before clinical cyanosis becomes apparent, a severely anaemic hypoxic infant will be pale, but not cyanotic. Warm and humidify the oxygen (if this is available) where it will be provided for more than a few minutes. If PPV is not indicated (ie, the pulse rate is greater than 100 beats/min and the infant has adequate respiratory effort), oxygen can initially be delivered through an oxygen mask or via oxygen tubing within a hand that is cupped and held close to the infant's nose and mouth **Figure 40-4 ▲**. The oxygen flow rate should be set at 5 l/min. Do not blow oxygen directly into or onto the newborn's eyes.

Oral Airways

Oral airways are rarely used for neonates, but they can be lifesaving if airway obstruction leads to respiratory failure. Bilateral choanal atresia (bony or membranous obstruction of the back of the nose preventing air flow) can be rapidly fatal, but usually responds to placement of an oral airway (or a gloved finger until an adequate oral airway is located). The Pierre Robin sequence is a series of developmental anomalies including a small chin and posteriorly positioned tongue that frequently lead to airway obstruction. Positioning the patient prone (chest down) may relieve the obstruction. If not, insert an appropriately measured oral or nasal airway. As with infants and small children, use a tongue blade to depress the tongue and insert the oral airway without rotating it. Remember that the optimal position for a neonate's head is in a *neutral position;* you will need to place a towel or similar under the baby's shoulders to ensure this position is maintained.

Bag-Valve-Mask Ventilation

Bag-valve-mask ventilation is indicated when an infant is apnoeic, has inadequate respiratory effort, or has a pulse rate less than 100 beats/min (bradycardia) after you clear the airway of secretions, relieve obstruction from the tongue, and dry and stimulate the infant. Signs of respiratory distress that suggest a need for bag-valve-mask ventilation include periodic breathing, intercostal recessions (sucking in between the ribs), nasal flaring, and grunting on expiration. Respiratory distress occurs in approximately 8 of every 1,000 live births and accounts for approximately 15% of neonatal deaths. Table 40-5 ▼ summarises the most common conditions leading to respiratory distress.

Three devices may be used to deliver bag-valve-mask ventilation to a neonate. First, you may use a self-inflating bag with an oxygen reservoir (an oxygen source is not necessary to provide PPV but is necessary to provide supplemental oxygen). Second, you may use a flow-inflating bag, though it needs a gas source to provide PPV; this technique is therefore more common in the operating theatre. Third, you may apply a T-piece resuscitator (mostly found in neonatal intensive care units and on most resuscitaires).

In the prehospital environment, you will most likely use a self-inflating bag for bag-valve-mask ventilation. If available, always use the infant size (240 ml). Given that the breath size (tidal volume) of a neonate is only 5 to 8 ml/kg, only one tenth of the bag's volume will be used for each breath—which explains why a larger bag can easily create problems. If a neonatal bag is not available and the infant is in severe respiratory distress, has apnoea, or has bradycardia, you can use a bag designed for adults or older children (750 ml or greater volume) as long as you keep the delivered breath size appropriately small and monitor chest rise to avoid excessive volumes of delivered breaths.

When you are administering bag-valve-mask ventilation with supplemental oxygen, the face mask needs to provide an

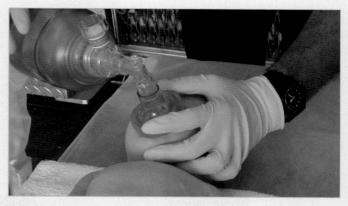

Figure 40-5 Bag-valve-mask ventilation of the newborn. Hold the mask securely to the face with your thumb and index finger. Apply countertraction under the bony part of the chin with your middle finger.

airtight seal, fitting over the newborn's mouth and nose, and extending down to the chin but not over the eyes Figure 40-5 ▲. The newborn needs to have a patent airway, cleared of secretions, with his or her neck in a neutral position. The first five breaths after birth may frequently require higher pressures (perhaps 30 cm H_2O or even higher) because the lungs are not yet expanded and are still full of fluid. To deliver these initial breaths, you may need to manually (cover with your finger) disable the spring-loaded pop-off valve (it is usually set by the manufacturer at 30 to 40 cm H_2O). Subsequent breaths should be delivered with sufficient pressure to result in visible but not excessive chest rise.

In a newborn, the correct timing for ventilation is 40 to 60 breaths/min. In the excitement of the moment, with your adrenaline surging, it is easy to inadvertently deliver breaths at a much higher rate, which can lead to hypocapnia, air trapping, or pneumothorax. To help with the timing, count "breath–two–three, breath–two–three" as you ventilate: Give a breath on "breath", and release on "two–three". Continue PPV as long as the pulse rate remains less than 100 beats/min or respiratory effort is ineffective. If prolonged PPV is needed, hook the system to a pressure manometer to aid in monitoring and minimising excessive pressures where available (target peak inspiratory pressure less than 25 cm H_2O in full-term newborns, less in preterm infants).

The most common reasons for ineffective bag-valve-mask ventilation are inadequate seal of the mask on the face and incorrect head position. Other causes such as mucous plug, pneumothorax, or equipment malfunction need to be considered as well.

Notes from Nancy

Indications for Artificial Ventilation of the Newborn

- Apnoea
- Pulse rate less than 100 beats/min
- Persisting central cyanosis despite breathing supplemental oxygen

Table 40-5	Common Causes of Respiratory Distress
■ Lung or heart disease	■ Persistent pulmonary hypertension
■ Central nervous system disorders	■ Mucous/vernix obstruction of nasal passages
■ Pneumothorax	■ Choanal atresia
■ Meconium aspiration	■ Amniotic fluid aspiration
■ Lung immaturity	■ Pneumonia
■ Shock and sepsis	■ Metabolic acidosis
■ Diaphragmatic hernia	

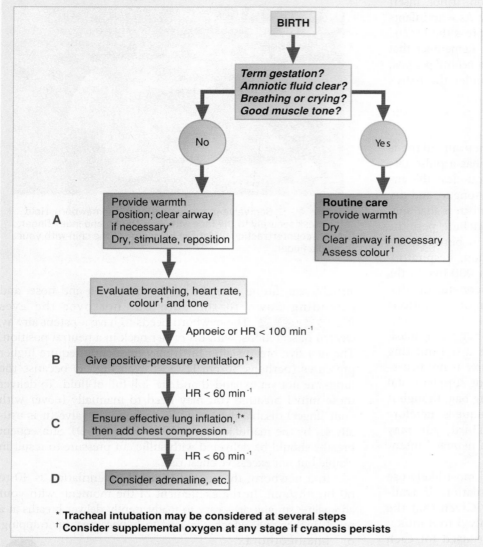

Figure 40-6 Newborn life support algorithm.

Adapted from *2005 Resuscitation Guidelines* with permission from Resuscitation Council (UK).

Intubation

Bag-valve-mask ventilation provides successful resuscitation of most newborns. Intubation, however, may be necessary if the newborn requires resuscitation beyond simple interventions (Figure 40-6 ▲). Intubation is indicated in the following situations:

- Meconium-stained fluid is present and the infant is not vigorous (ie, poor muscle tone, bradycardia, inadequate

Controversies

Resuscitation with supplemental oxygen is the norm in the United Kingdom and is currently recommended by the Resuscitation Council (UK); however, a growing body of evidence suggests that resuscitation with room air is a safe alternative. Bag-valve-mask ventilation can be initiated with room air while an oxygen source is being secured.

ventilation), a condition for which tracheal suctioning is indicated.

- Congenital diaphragmatic hernia (a congenital defect in which abdominal organs herniate through an opening in the diaphragm into the chest cavity) is suspected and respiratory support is indicated.
- The infant does not respond to bag-valve-mask ventilation and chest compressions, necessitating endotracheal administration of adrenaline (ie, no IO site or umbilical cannula can be established).
- Prolonged PPV is needed.

Before you begin ventilation, make sure that you have the following equipment available:

- Suction equipment (10F tubing, with 5F to 8F being available, suction set to 100 cm H_2O or its lightest setting)
- Laryngoscope (check the light to ensure that the bulb is bright and screwed in tightly)
- Blades—straight: No. 1 for full-term infants, No. 0 for preterm infants
- Shoulder towel
- Adhesive tape, to tape the endotracheal tube
- Endotracheal tube: 2.5 to 4.0 mm (2.5 mm if the newborn is delivered before 28 weeks of gestation, 3.0 mm if delivered before 28 to 34 weeks of gestation, 3.5 mm if delivered before 34 to 38 weeks of gestation, and 4.0 mm if delivered after 38 weeks of gestation)

Some paramedics use a stylet to provide rigidity to the ET tube. In such a case, you must secure the stylet (bending it over at the top of the ET tube so it can't advance) and make sure that it does not extend beyond the ET tube, or tracheal perforation may occur.

Intubation of the neonate is discussed in the following steps and shown in (Skill Drill 40-1 ▶):

1. Be sure the newborn is preoxygenated by bag-valve-mask ventilation with high-flow supplemental oxygen prior to making an intubation attempt (Step 1).
2. Suction the oropharynx if necessary to remove any excess secretions (Step 2). This is a vagal stimulus, so pay close attention to pulse rate. Bag-valve-mask ventilation may be needed if the newborn develops bradycardia at this point.
3. Place the laryngoscope blade in the oropharynx and then visualise the vocal cords (Step 3). Avoid applying torque to the blade, as it increases the risk of trauma. Place the ET

Skill Drill 40-1: Intubation of a Neonate

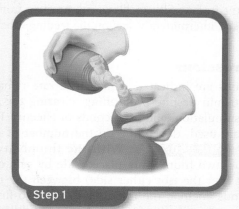

Step 1

Preoxygenate the infant by bag-valve-mask ventilation with 100% supplemental oxygen.

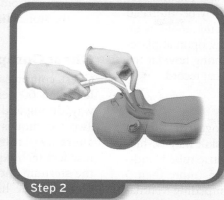

Step 2

Suction the oropharynx. Provide bag-valve-mask ventilation if bradycardia results.

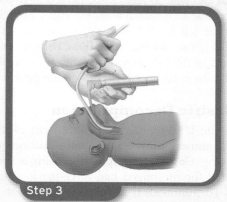

Step 3

Place the laryngoscope blade in the oropharynx. Visualise the vocal cords. Place the ET tube between the vocal cords until the black line on the ET tube is at the level of the cords.

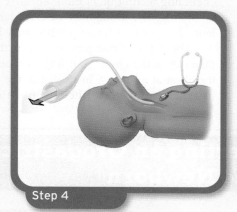

Step 4

Confirm placement. Observe chest rise, auscultate laterally and high on the chest, note the absence of significant air sounds over the stomach, and note mist in the ET tube.

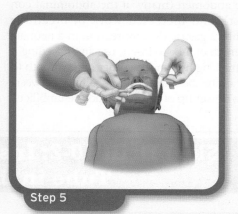

Step 5

Tape the ET tube in place. Monitor the newborn closely for complications.

tube between the vocal cords until the black line on the tube is at the level of the cords. For full-term babies, the ET tube is usually advanced until it is at 9 cm at the lip. A premature baby may need to have the ET tube advanced to only 6½ to 7 cm at the lip. Limit the intubation attempt to 20 seconds, and initiate bag-valve-mask ventilation if it is unsuccessful or if significant bradycardia develops.

4. Confirm placement (Step 4) by observing chest rise when applying positive pressure through the ET tube, auscultating laterally and high on the chest, noting the absence of significant air sounds over the stomach, noting mist in the ET tube (seen when the patient exhales through the tube from condensation of humidified air leaving the lungs), and observing for clinical improvement.

5. Tape the ET tube in place on the face to minimise the risk of the tube dislodging (Step 5). Monitor the infant closely for complications such as tube dislodgement, tube occlusion by mucous plug or meconium, or pneumothorax.

Notes from Nancy

Indications for Endotracheal Intubation of the Newborn

- Inability to ventilate effectively by bag-valve-mask device
- Necessity to perform tracheal suctioning, especially if meconium is present and infant depressed at birth
- When prolonged ventilation will be necessary

Complications of ET tube placement include oropharyngeal or tracheal perforation, oesophageal intubation with subsequent persistent hypoxia, and intubation of either bronchus intubation that can lead to atelectasis, persistent hypoxia, and pneumothorax (due to neonatal anatomy either bronchus may be intubated as the left bronchus is not yet at the same acute angle as an adult). You can minimise these risks by ensuring optimal placement of the laryngoscope blade and carefully noting how far the ET tube is advanced. Record on the patient clinical record.

Gastric Decompression

In the UK, prehospital placement of an orogastric tube is uncommon; however, in some situations this skill may be life-saving. Gastric decompression using an orogastric tube is indicated for prolonged bag-valve-mask ventilation (more than 5 to 10 minutes), if abdominal distension is impeding ventilation, or in the presence of diaphragmatic hernia. Many diaphragmatic hernias are diagnosed antenatally by routine ultrasound; they are suspected clinically if there are decreased breath sounds (90% of diaphragmatic hernias are on the left), a scaphoid or concave abdomen (many of the abdominal contents are in the chest), and increased work of breathing. `Skill Drill 40-2 ▾` shows gastric decompression in a neonate.

1. To determine the length of tube to insert, use an 8F feeding tube and measure the length from the corner of the mouth to the bottom of the earlobe then to a position halfway between the xiphoid process (lower tip of sternum) and the umbilicus.

2. Insert the tube through the mouth (Step 1).
3. Attach a 20-ml syringe and suction the stomach contents (Step 2). Tape the tube to the baby's cheek. Remove the syringe from the feeding tube to allow venting of air from the stomach, and intermittently suction the feeding tube.

Chest Compressions

Chest compressions are indicated if the pulse rate remains less than 60 beats/min despite positioning, clearing the airway, drying and stimulation, and 30 seconds of effective PPV. Two techniques are used, depending on the number of rescuers available (Figure 40-7 ▸). With the thumb (two-rescuer) technique, two thumbs are placed side by side over the sternum (not over the ribs either side) between the nipples, and the hands encircle the torso. With the two-finger (one-rescuer) technique, the tips of the index and middle fingers are placed over the sternum between the nipples and the sternum is compressed between the fingers at a rate of three compressions to one ventilation. Evidence has shown that the encircling technique is more effective; however, in a prehospital setting, the availability of extra hands is not always prevalent, thus the two-finger method may be the only option.

The depth of compression is one third of the anteroposterior diameter of the chest. Your fingers should remain in contact with the chest at all times. In neonates, the chest compressions occur in synchrony with artificial ventilation, which you continue

Skill Drill 40-2: Inserting an Orogastric Tube in the Newborn

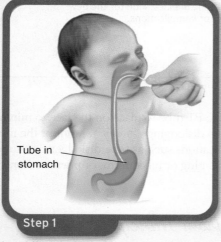

Tube in stomach

Step 1

Insert the tube to the appropriate depth. Leave the nose open to allow for ventilations.

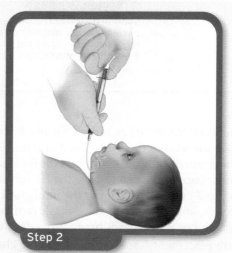

Step 2

Remove the gastric contents with a 20-ml syringe. Remove the syringe and leave the tip of the tube open to allow air to vent from the stomach. Tape the tube to the newborn's cheek.

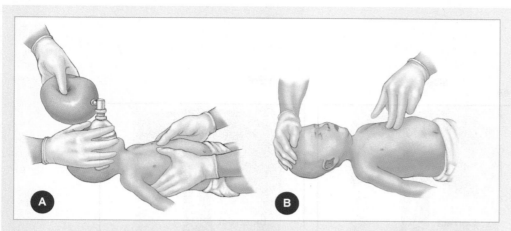

Figure 40-7 Chest compressions in the newborn. **A.** When there are two rescuers, use your thumbs side by side, placed just below an imaginary line drawn between the two nipples. **B.** When working alone, or when the baby is large, use two fingers to depress the sternum.

during chest compressions. The person delivering the chest compression counts out loud, "One and two and three and breath and. . . ." Downward strokes of chest compressions should be delivered while saying, "One and two and three". Release of the strokes should occur while saying "and". The person ventilating delivers a breath during the sequence "breath and". This results in 90 compressions and 30 breaths/min. Pulse rate is assessed at 30-second intervals, and chest compressions stop when the pulse rate is greater than 60 beats/min. Liver laceration and rib fractures are some possible risks of delivering chest compressions. Refer to Appendix A for coverage of infant/neonate CPR.

Venous Access

Emergency access becomes necessary when fluid administration is needed to support circulation, when resuscitation medications (eg, adrenaline, sodium bicarbonate) must be administered IV, and when therapeutic drugs (eg, IV glucose, antibiotics) must be given IV. Establishing peripheral access in an infant can prove difficult, however.

The umbilical vein can be cannulated using an umbilical vein line in a newborn and can be used up to 7 days after birth.

1. Clean the cord with alcohol or another antiseptic. Place a sterile tie firmly, but not too tightly, around the base of the cord to control bleeding. Place a sterile drape over the site. Although the line must be placed quickly in an emergency situation, maintain sterile technique as much as possible.

2. Prefill a sterile 3.5F to 5F umbilical vein line cannula (a comparable-size sterile feeding tube can be used in an emergency) with normal saline using a 5-ml syringe.

3. Cut the cord with a scalpel below the clamp placed on the cord at birth about 1 to 2 cm from the skin (between the clamp and the cord tie).

4. The umbilical vein is a large, thin-walled vessel usually found at the 12 o'clock position, as compared to the two thick-walled umbilical arteries usually found at 4 and 8 o'clock (Figure 40-8 ▶). Insert the cannula into this

vein for a distance of 2 to 4 cm (less in preterm infants) until blood can be aspirated. If the cannula is advanced into the liver, the infusion of hypertonic solutions may lead to irreversible damage (Figure 40-9 ▶). If the cannula is advanced into the heart, arrhythmias may develop.

5. Flush the cannula with 1 ml of normal saline and tape it in place.

Pharmacological Interventions

Medications are rarely needed in neonatal resuscitation, as most infants can be resuscitated with ventilatory support. Medications in neonates are based on weight, so you may need to estimate the infant's weight for dosing. A full-term infant usually weighs 3 to 4 kg;

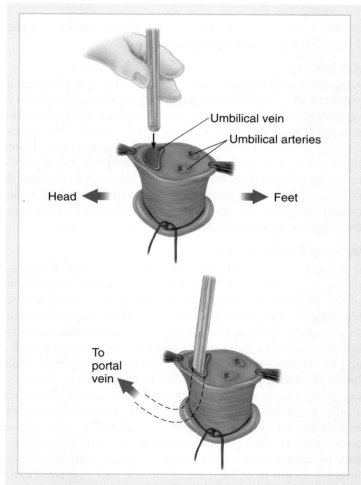

Figure 40-8 Location of the umbilical vein.

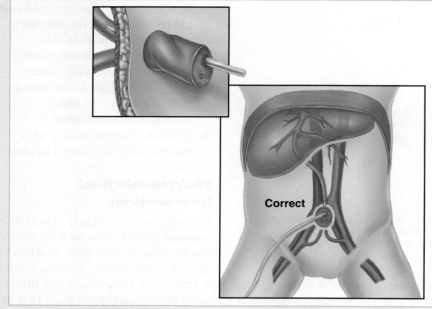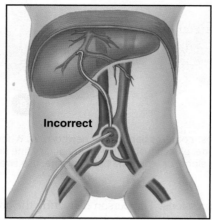

Figure 40-9 Umbilical vein cannulation.

an infant born at 28 weeks of gestation, on average, weighs 1 kg and is approximately 37.5 cm long.

Adrenaline

Administration of adrenaline is indicated when the infant has a pulse rate of less than 60 beats/min after 30 seconds of effective ventilation and 30 seconds of chest compressions. The recommended concentration for newborns is 1:10,000. The recommended dose is 0.1 to 0.3 ml/kg of 1:10,000 adrenaline IV or IO, equal to 0.01 to 0.03 mg/kg, administered rapidly, followed by a 0.5 to 1 ml normal saline flush to clear the line. If IV/IO access is not yet established, the use of the tracheal route (which was previously advocated) is now thought to be ineffective whilst using standard doses.

Volume Replacement

If the infant has significant intravascular volume depletion owing to conditions such as placental abruption (separation of the placenta from the uterus, which leads to excessive bleeding) or septic shock, fluid resuscitation may be needed. In a newborn, place a low umbilical vein line as outlined earlier. In a newborn more than a few days old, place a peripheral IV or intraosseus (IO) line. Placement of an intraosseus line is discussed in Chapter 8. While the technique for placing an IO line is similar to that used with older children or adults, a smaller needle should be used in neonates to avoid exiting the far side of the bone. A fluid bolus in an infant consists of 10 ml/kg of normal saline IV. Multiple boluses may be administered if the patient remains clinically hypovolaemic. Signs of hypovolaemia include pallor, delayed capillary refill, and weak pulses despite a good pulse rate or high-quality chest compressions.

▌Specific Conditions

Acidosis

If bradycardia persists after adequate ventilation, chest compressions, and volume expansion, and you suspect metabolic acidosis, sodium bicarbonate may be indicated. Although this is seldom used in the UK in the prehospital situation, a dose of 1–2 mmol/kg (2–4 ml/kg of 4.2%) can be given. This is an attempt to correct the intracardiac, not the systemic, acidosis. If this is effective an increase in heart rate is usually seen within a few minutes. Sodium bicarbonate must never be given ET and rapid administration should be avoided, especially in premature infants. On some occasions, sodium bicarbonate may be given before adrenaline as some evidence shows that adrenaline is less effective in an acidotic environment.

Respiratory Suppression Secondary to Narcotics

In the case of a drug-addicted mother, administration of naloxone to the newborn to reverse the narcotic effect may precipitate convulsions that can potentially cause death, so this intervention is no longer recommended as a first line drug in resuscitation. In the case of respiratory suppression from chronic narcotics in the prehospital environment, provide ventilatory support and transport immediately. If respiratory depression is from the mother being treated acutely with narcotics, and there is no chronic narcotic exposure, naloxone, 0.1 mg/kg, may be administered to the newborn via the IV/IM route to reverse the narcotic effect.

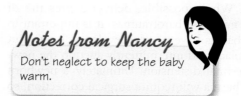

Pneumothorax Evacuation

If an infant has signs of a significant pneumothorax— severe respiratory distress unresponsive to PPV with unilateral decreased breath sounds and (if the pneumothorax is on the right) shift of heart sounds—a needle evacuation of the pneumothorax may be necessary.

At the Scene

While positive-pressure ventilation and chest compressions can be performed in a moving emergency vehicle, you should pull the vehicle over to the side of the road while placing and securing an advanced airway.

Apnoea

Apnoea is common in infants delivered before 32 weeks of gestation, but is rarely seen in the first 24 hours after delivery, even in premature infants. If prolonged (more than 20 seconds), it can lead to hypoxaemia and bradycardia. Risk factors for apnoea include prematurity, infection, prolonged or difficult labour and delivery, drug exposure, gastroesophageal reflux, central nervous system abnormalities including convulsions, and metabolic disorders.

The pathophysiology of apnoea depends on the underlying aetiology. Apnoea of prematurity is due to an underdeveloped central nervous system. Gastroesophageal reflux can trigger a vagal response, leading to apnoea. Drug-induced apnoea frequently results from direct central nervous system depression. Regardless of the cause, a newborn with apnoea needs respiratory support to minimise hypoxic brain damage and other organ damage.

Assessment of an apnoeic infant includes a careful history to elicit possible aetiologic risk factors and a physical examination that focuses on neurological signs and symptoms or signs of infection. At birth it is important to differentiate between primary apnoea and secondary apnoea (also called *terminal apnoea*). If the newborn has experienced a relatively short period of hypoxia, he or she will have a period of rapid breathing, followed by apnoea and bradycardia. At this point, drying and stimulation may suffice to cause a resumption of breathing and improvement in pulse rate. If hypoxia continues during primary apnoea, the infant will gasp and enter secondary apnoea. At this point, stimulation alone will not restart the baby's breathing. Instead, PPV by bag-valve-mask device is required.

Meconium-Stained Amniotic Fluid

Meconium-stained amniotic fluid, which is present in 10% to 15% of deliveries, carries a high risk of morbidity. Passage of meconium may occur either before or during delivery. It is more common in post-term infants and in those who are small for their gestational age (weigh less than the 10th percentile for their age). Infants do not normally pass stool before birth, but if they do and then inhale the meconium-stained amniotic fluid either in utero or at delivery, their airways may become plugged. The passage of meconium in utero indicates that the baby has been gasping and has passed through primary apnoea; this is a sign that the baby has sustained an hypoxic event in utero. It is this event that has most likely led to the passage of the meconium and its subsequent inhalation. This, in turn, can lead to atelectasis, persistent pulmonary hypertension (delayed transition from fetal to neonatal circulation), pneumonitis, or pneumothorax, which may require needle aspiration.

When a newborn is delivered through meconium-stained amniotic fluid, determine whether the fluid is thin and green stained versus thick and particulate. Assess the newborn's activity level. If the baby is crying and vigorous, employ standard interventions. If the baby is depressed, do not dry or stimulate him or her. It is imperative to inspect the airway

You are the Paramedic Part 3

A little girl is delivered to you. There is no evidence of meconium on the infant's face. You dry the infant, place her in a supine position with her head in the neutral position, and perform an assessment.

Newborn Assessment	Recording Time: 9 Minutes
Respiratory effort	Rapid and irregular; strong cry
Pulse rate	130 beats/min, regular
Colour	Cyanosis to the trunk and extremities

5. What treatment is indicated for this infant?
6. When is positive-pressure ventilation indicated for the newborn?

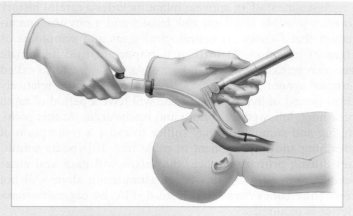

Figure 40-10 Meconium aspiration.

under direct vision. Perform a laryngoscopy and suction where appropriate. If the child remains unresponsive, intubate the trachea and suction through the end of the ET tube. Be sure to cover the hole of the meconium aspirator with your finger while you are suctioning **Figure 40-10 ▲**. Once all large particles of meconium have been removed, continue with normal resuscitative measures. As ever, although an airway and breathing problem is being addressed, it is worth considering the effect that a laryngoscope may have on instigating vagal stimulus and thus creating a circulation problem as well.

After tracheal suctioning, drying and stimulation are often enough to establish adequate breathing and pulse rate; in many cases, however, oxygen and PPV are needed. If intubation for direct tracheal suctioning is unsuccessful and the newborn has significant bradycardia, continue with standard resuscitation guidelines, recognising that the newborn will be at high risk of aspiration from meconium or from thick vernix, both of which can be lethal to the infant. If the newborn has prolonged hypoxia after significantly delayed resuscitation, the outcome is likely to be poor. When transporting such an infant with respiratory symptoms, contact a unit with the facilities and skills in managing high-risk newborns. To help support the family, explain what is being done for the newborn but do not discuss "chance of survival".

Diaphragmatic Hernia

Diaphragmatic hernia—that is, an abnormal opening in the diaphragm, most commonly on the left side—has an incidence of 1 in 2,200 live births. This diagnosis is often made on antenatal ultrasound before the baby's birth. The diagnosis is suspected clinically in a newborn with respiratory distress, heart sounds shifted to the right, decreased breath sounds on the left (which can also be signs of a pneumothorax), and scaphoid abdomen (ie, the abdomen, rather than being round, is sunken due to the abdominal contents being in the chest cavity). Mortality may be as high as 50% for this condition.

If a newborn has a diaphragmatic hernia, bag-valve-mask ventilation will introduce air that distends the intestines in the chest cavity, further compromising the newborn's ability to ventilate. If PPV is needed in such a newborn, place an ET tube and deliver a peak ventilatory pressure sufficient to allow for the chest to rise. Where possible, deliver a pressure of 25 cm H_2O or less to minimise barotraumas. It is important to remember that these babies have poorly developed lungs. Put an orogastric tube in place and intermittently suction the newborn to minimise intestinal distension. Ultimately, a newborn with a diaphragmatic hernia will require surgical correction, so transport him or her to a facility with a neonatal intensive care unit and a paediatric surgical team.

Additional Conditions

Additional conditions that you may encounter and your treatment response include the following:

- **Choanal atresia.** Place an oral airway.
- **Pierre Robin sequence.** Position the infant prone to maintain the airway. Use an oral or nasal airway if needed.
- **Cleft lip and/or palate.** Airway resuscitation is not needed, but you may need to apply some cricoid pressure if intubation becomes necessary. Consider delivering PPV via bag-valve-mask device. You may need to use a little extra positive pressure in the case of a cleft palate. Owing to the risk of aspiration and regurgitation, do not feed the newborn with a cleft lip and palate in the prehospital environment.
- **Exposed abdominal contents.** A developmental defect may lead to intestines appearing outside the abdomen. In this situation, while providing standard resuscitation, place the newborn from the waist down into a sterile, clear plastic bag to keep the bowel clean and minimise heat/fluid loss. Monitor the colour of the intestines (pink is good, blue/black is bad) and, if necessary, reposition the newborn, and if necessary the intestines, so that the intestines remain pink and he or she cannot turn and cut off the blood supply.

Premature and Low Birth Weight Infants

Infants delivered before 37 completed weeks of gestation are considered premature **Figure 40-11 ▶**. Infants born weighing less than 2.5 kg are considered low birth weight. The most common aetiology for low birth weight is prematurity. A number of factors can predispose a woman to deliver prematurely, including genetic factors, infection, cervical incompetence (early opening of cervix), abruption (blood under the placenta), multiple gestations (eg, twins, triplets), previous delivery of a premature infant, drug use, and trauma. Other factors that may contribute to low birth weight include chronic maternal hypertension, smoking, placental anomalies, and chromosomal abnormalities. If an infant is delivered prior to 24 weeks of gestation or weighs less than 500 g and is born outside of a centre that is equipped to manage such deliveries, the baby is unlikely to survive. The degree of immaturity can be estimated by physical characteristics such as skin appearance (more thin and translucent in more premature infants). If you observe signs of life, it is advisable to attempt resuscitation until the newborn can be transported to an appropriate facility.

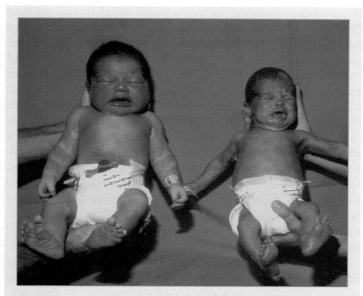

Figure 40-11 Premature infants (right) are smaller and thinner than full-term infants (left).

Morbidity and mortality in this population are, in large part, related to the degree of prematurity. Most infants delivered after 28 weeks of gestation who receive needed cardiovascular support after birth survive and do well over the long term. Infants delivered at 24 weeks of gestation have a high morbidity and mortality. Approximately one third die and one third experience significant long-term problems—typically respiratory issues, related to the need for long-term ventilation and oxygen treatment, and neurological issues, related to bleeding into the brain.

If an infant is delivered prematurely in the prehospital environment, providing cardiorespiratory support and a thermoneutral environment will optimise his or her survival and long-term outcome. Premature infants are at higher risk for respiratory distress owing to surfactant deficiency. Their thermoregulation can be improved with careful environmental control by use of warm blankets, plastic wrap, and in very preterm babies, the use of a plastic bag up to their head. If this latter method is used, the child should not be dried but placed immediately into the bag and the bag left uncovered and placed under a radiant heater. This will not be available in ambulances in the UK. The lungs of a premature infant are weak, so use only the minimum pressure necessary to move the chest when you are providing PPV. Brain injury can result from hypoxaemia, rapid changes in blood pressure, or hyperosmolarity leading to intraventricular haemorrhage. Premature infants are also at risk of retinopathy of prematurity (abnormal vascular development of the retina), which may be worsened by long-term oxygen exposure over several hours. Because hypoxia causes irreparable brain damage, however, do not withhold oxygen from a cyanotic premature infant.

Convulsions in the Neonate

Convulsions are the most distinctive sign of neurological disease in the newborn. A convulsion is defined clinically as a paroxysmal alteration in neurological function (ie, behavioural and/or autonomic function). Convulsions are more common in premature infants. The incidence in this population can be as high as 57.5 per 1,000 infants who weigh less than 1.5 kg at birth, compared with 2.8 per 1,000 infants who weigh between 2.5 kg and 4 kg at birth. In the prehospital environment, convulsions are identified by direct observation; in the hospital, an electroencephalogram is used to confirm the diagnosis of convulsions.

Newborns may exhibit normal motor activity that can sometimes be mistaken for convulsions. These myoclonic, dysconjugate eye movements or sucking movements are often seen when the newborn is drowsy or asleep. In addition, jitteriness is often confused with a convulsion (**Table 40-6 ▼**). Jitteriness is characteristically a disorder of the newborn and is rarely seen at a later age. Jitteriness is most commonly seen with hypoxic ischaemic encephalopathy, hypocalcaemia, hypoglycaemia, and drug withdrawal.

Convulsions, by contrast, represent a relative medical emergency. They are usually related to a significant underlying abnormality—one that often requires specific therapy. Convulsions may also interfere with cardiopulmonary function, feeding, and metabolic function. Finally, prolonged convulsions may even cause brain injury.

Types of Convulsions

Four major types of convulsions are distinguished as follows:

- **Subtle convulsion.** A convulsion characterised by eye deviation, blinking, sucking, and pedalling movements of the legs and apnoea.
- **Tonic convulsion.** A convulsion characterised by tonic extension of the limbs. Less commonly, flexion of the arms and extension of the legs may also occur. This type of convulsion is more common in premature infants, especially in those with intraventricular haemorrhage.
- **Focal clonic convulsion.** A convulsion characterised by clonic localised jerking. This type of convulsion can occur in both full-term and premature infants.

Table 40-6	Jitteriness Versus Convulsions in the Newborn	
Characteristic	**Jitteriness**	**Convulsions**
Ocular phenomenon (deviation or fixation of the eyes)	Not seen	Commonly associated
Stimulus sensitive (may be triggered by a stimulus)	Yes	No
Dominant movement	Tremor	Clonic jerking
Application of gentle pressure to limb	Stops jitteriness	Does not stop convulsions
Autonomic phenomenon	Not associated	Common association

Table 40-7	Causes of Neonatal Convulsions
■ Hypoxic ischaemic encephalopathy ■ Intracranial infections (meningitis) ■ Hypoglycaemia ■ Other metabolic disturbances ■ Epileptic syndromes	■ Intracranial haemorrhage ■ Development defects ■ Hypocalcaemia

■ **Myoclonic convulsion.** A convulsion characterised by flexion jerks of the upper or lower extremities. This type of convulsion may occur singly or in a series of repetitive jerks.

When describing convulsions, *multifocal* refers to clinical activity that involves more than one site, is asynchronous, and is usually migratory. *Generalised* refers to activity that is bilateral, synchronous, and nonmigratory.

Causes of Convulsions

Table 40-7 ▲ lists the most common (and important) causes of neonatal convulsions. The time of onset for hypoxic ischaemic encephalopathy, hypoglycaemia, and other metabolic disturbances is up to 3 days after delivery. With all other causes listed in Table 40-7, convulsions may begin 3 days or longer after birth.

Hypoxic ischaemic encephalopathy, usually secondary to perinatal asphyxia (lack of oxygen to tissues) is the single most common cause of convulsions in both term and preterm infants. Convulsions characteristically occur in the first 24 hours and usually become severe. Metabolic abnormalities include disturbances in the levels of glucose, calcium, magnesium, or electrolytes. Other metabolic disturbances include abnormalities of amino acids, organic acids, blood ammonia, and certain toxins.

Hypoglycaemia is most frequently seen in infants who are small for their gestational age, those who are large for their gestational age, and those whose mothers were diabetic during pregnancy. Neurological symptoms consist of jitteriness, stupor, hypotonia (floppy), apnoea, poor feeding, and convulsions.

Hypocalcaemia has two major peaks of incidence. The first peak occurs at 2 to 3 days after delivery and is most commonly seen in low birth weight infants and in infants of diabetic mothers. Late-onset hypocalcaemia is rare in the United Kingdom but may be seen in infants who consume cow's milk or synthetic formulas high in phosphorous.

Other metabolic disturbances are uncommon in neonates, although hyponatraemia, hyperammonaemia, other amino acid and organic acid abnormalities, or convulsions from drug withdrawal (eg, narcotic analgesics, sedative hypnotics, tricyclic antidepressants, cocaine, or alcohol) may be seen.

Assessment and Management of Convulsions

Evaluation of a newborn with convulsions must include a quick evaluation of antenatal and birth history and a careful physical examination. You may observe a quiet, often hypotonic infant. The newborn may be lethargic or apnoeic.

Hypoglycaemia must be recognised quickly and treated promptly. In these cases, blood glucose measurement and administration of glucose may be lifesaving in the prehospital environment. Obtain the newborn's baseline vital signs and oxygen saturation readings and provide additional oxygen, assisted ventilation, blood pressure evaluation, and IV access as necessary. A 10% glucose solution may be given as an IV bolus (2.5 ml/kg) if the newborn's blood glucose level is less than 2.6 mmol/l, with a recheck of the blood glucose level in about 30 minutes. All newborns have a drop in blood glucose levels in the first few hours of birth. These levels may drop as low as 1–2 mmol/l. In adults these levels may cause severe physiological derangement but not so in the newborn as they begin to burn alternative forms of energy. Newborns can be found to be ketogenic in the first 72 hours after birth until feeding becomes established.

Giving anticonvulsant medication such as diazepam or diazemuls (benzodiazepine)—the drugs most commonly used in such cases—requires care in administration, as they may interfere with respiratory and cardiac function.

Monitor the newborn's respiratory status and saturations carefully. Maintain the newborn's normal body temperature and keep the family informed about what you are doing for their infant as transport gets under way.

Thermoregulation

Thermoregulation is the body's ability to balance heat production and heat loss so as to maintain normal body temperature. This ability is very limited in the newborn. The average normal temperature of a newborn is 37.5°C. For the neonate, the thermoneutral temperature range is 36.6 to 37.2°C.

Nonshivering thermogenesis, the production of heat by metabolism, is the primary source of heat production in the neonate. Brown fat (deposited in the fetus after 28 weeks of gestation, and principally stored around the scapula, kidneys, adrenal glands, neck, and axilla) is a thermogenic tissue unique to the newborn.

Heat loss occurs when heat is lost to the environment, through any of the following four mechanisms. In evaporation, heat is lost when water evaporates from the skin and respiratory tract. In convection, heat is lost to cooler surrounding air; the extent of heat loss depends on the air temperature and air movement. In conduction, heat is lost to cooler solid objects in direct contact with the body. In radiation, heat is lost to cooler surrounding objects not in direct contact with the body.

Fever

Fever is defined as a rectal temperature greater than 38°C. Oral and axillary temperatures are, respectively, 0.6°C and 1.1°C lower than the rectal temperature on average.

A newborn's temperature regulation system is relatively immature, so fever may not always be a presenting feature with infection or illness. In fact, neonates may become hypothermic with infection. No matter what the presenting symptoms are, it is important to identify newborns with serious bacterial infection (eg, bacteraemia, urinary tract infection, meningitis, bacterial gastroenteritis, and pneumonia) or serious viral infection (eg, herpes simplex) for which treatment is available. Approximately 13% of infants younger than 28 days with a temperature of more than 38.1°C will have a serious bacterial infection.

Fever may also be caused by overheating. Babies can easily become too hot when dressed in many layers of clothing, over-bundled in a heated car, or placed in direct sunlight, even through a window, or near heating vents at home. Fever related to dehydration is an important consideration in breastfeeding babies, especially in the first week after birth. These infants have often lost more than 10% of their weight and may have a history of difficulty in initiating breastfeeding.

Newborns have limited ability to control their temperature. They do not sweat when they are hot, to allow cooling, and they do not shiver to raise their temperature, when they are cold. Term infants may produce sweat over their brow but not the rest of their body. Premature infants do not produce sweat. Moreover, many newborns with serious life-threatening infections may actually see their core temperature drop; these infants are at a higher risk for hypoglycaemia and metabolic acidosis. A careful examination will reveal irritability, <u>somnolence</u>, and decreased feeding. The infant may feel warm to touch. Some infants with fever, however, may be initially asymptomatic.

When fever is suspected, observe the newborn for the presence of rashes, especially petechiae or pinpoint pink or red skin lesions **Figure 40-12 ▸**. Obtain a careful history regarding general activity, feeding, voiding, and stooling. Obtain the newborn's vital signs and ensure adequate oxygenation and ventilation, providing free-flow supplemental oxygen if necessary. Perform chest compressions, if indicated. Administration of antipyretic agents such as paracetamol or ibuprofen is controversial in the prehospital setting; do not give ibuprofen to an infant. To cool the newborn, remove additional layers of clothing and improve ventilation in the environment. Rapid cooling is to be avoided.

Hypothermia

Hypothermia is a drop in body temperature to less than 35°C. Hypothermia in the newborn occurs in all climates, but is more common during the winter months. It has been linked to impaired growth and may make the newborn vulnerable to infections. Moderate hypothermia is associated with an

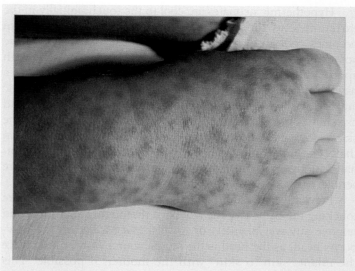

Figure 40-12 A newborn with a fever may also have petechiae or pinpoint pink or red skin lesions.

increased risk of death in low birth weight infants. Sick or low birth weight infants admitted to hospital with hypothermia are more likely to die than those admitted with normal temperature. Infants may die of cold exposure at temperatures adults find comfortable. **Table 40-8 ▾** lists risk factors for hypothermia.

Newborn infants have increased surface area-to-volume ratio, making the newborn extremely sensitive to environmental conditions, especially when wet after delivery. An increase in metabolic function in an attempt to overcome the heat loss can cause hypoglycaemia, metabolic acidosis, <u>pulmonary hypertension</u>, and hypoxaemia. Every hypothermic newborn should also be investigated for infection.

Table 40-8	Risk Factors for Hypothermia

- All neonates in the first 8 to 12 hours after birth
- Home delivery
- Prolonged resuscitation
- <u>Small for gestational age</u> infant
- Infant with central nervous system problems
- Prematurity
- Sepsis
- Inadequate measures to keep the infant warm during transport

You are the Paramedic Part 4

After delivery of blow-by oxygen, the baby's trunk is now pink; her hands and feet, however, remain cyanotic. You take appropriate actions to keep her warm. Further assessment reveals that her respirations are rapid and her pulse rate is 120 beats/min. She resists your attempts to straighten her hips and knees and moves her foot away when you snap your finger against it.

7. Does this child require resuscitation?

8. Is it safe to clamp and cut the umbilical cord?

Hypothermic neonates are cool to the touch, initially in the extremities; as their temperature drops, however, the skin becomes cool all over. The infant may also be pale and have acrocyanosis. The hypothermic newborn may present with apnoea, bradycardia, cyanosis, irritability, and a weak cry. As a newborn's temperature drops, he or she may become lethargic and sluggish. In severely hypothermic babies, the face and extremities may appear bright red. Sclerema—hardening of the skin associated with reddening and oedema—may be seen on the back, limbs, or all over the body. Thermal shock, disseminated intravascular coagulopathy, and death may occur in more serious cases.

Preventive measures include warming your hands before touching the baby. Dry the newborn thoroughly after birth and remove any wet blankets or towels. Place a hat on the newborn's head, as the head is the largest source of heat loss. Place the infant "skin to skin" with the mother, if possible. This serves two purposes: The mother keeps the baby warm, and mother and baby can more readily bond. Ensure adequate oxygenation and ventilation, and perform chest compressions if necessary. If the infant is hypoglycaemic, you may administer 10% glucose. Warm IV fluids can assist in rewarming the newborn. The critically ill newborn, once stabilised, should be placed in a prewarmed incubator or, if none is available, covered with warm blankets and kept on mother's chest.

At home, skin-to-skin contact is the best method to rewarm a baby with mild hypothermia. Ideally, the room should be warm (24°C to 26.5°C), and the baby should be covered with a warm blanket and wear a prewarmed cap. Continue the rewarming process until the baby's temperature reaches the normal range or his or her feet are no longer cold. Do not use hot water bottles—they may cause burns because blood circulation is poor in the cold skin of babies.

Recent studies in neonates with hypoxic-ischaemic injury indicate improved outcomes when the infant is provided mild therapeutic hypothermia within 6 hours of birth. This approach is not recommended in the prehospital environment, although it is prudent to prevent hyperthermia. Maintain the infant at the lower margin of normal temperature (axillary temperature no higher than 36.5°C).

Hypoglycaemia

In full-term or preterm infants, hypoglycaemia is a blood glucose level of less than 2.6 mmol/l. This condition represents an imbalance between glucose supply and utilisation. Glucose levels may be low due to inadequate intake or storage or increased utilisation of glucose. Most infants remain asymptomatic until the glucose falls below 1.1 mmol/l for a significant period of time. Because the brain relies on glucose as its primary fuel, hypoglycaemia may result in convulsions and severe, permanent brain damage. **Table 40-9 ▶** lists risk factors for hypoglycaemia in the newborn.

The fetus receives glucose from the mother and deposits glycogen in the liver, lung, heart, and skeletal muscle in utero. The infant then begins to utilise those glycogen stores to meet glucose needs after birth; most full-term infants will have sufficient glycogen stores to meet their glucose needs for 8 to 12 hours. Disorders related to decreased glycogen stores (small for gestational age, prematurity, postmaturity) or to increased utilisation of glucose (infant of a diabetic mother, large for gestational age, hypoxia, hypothermia, sepsis) place the infant at increased risk for hypoglycaemia. Metabolic adaptations to maintain normal glucose levels are regulated by counter regulatory hormones such as glucagon, adrenaline, cortisol, and growth hormone. Frequently, stressed infants will become hypoglycaemic.

Symptoms of hypoglycaemia may include cyanosis, apnoea, irritability, poor sucking or feeding, and hypothermia. These symptoms may also be associated with lethargy, tremors, twitching or convulsions, and coma. They may also have tachycardia, tachypnoea, or vomiting.

Check the blood glucose level in all sick newborns (by heel stick) and evaluate the newborn's vital signs. After you establish good oxygenation, ventilation, and circulation (ABCs), manage the hypoglycaemia. The administration of a 10% glucose solution as a bolus at 2.5 ml/kg via IV access should be considered if the newborn's blood glucose level is less than 2.6 mmol/l. This intervention may be followed by an IV infusion of 10% glucose based on the infant's gestational age (60 ml/kg/d for a full-term infant; adjust upward based on the recommendations

Table 40-9	Risk Factors for Hypoglycaemia in the Newborn
Risk Factor	**Specific Indicators**
Disorders of fetal growth and maturity	Small for gestational age
	Smaller of discordant twins (weight difference > 25%)
	Large for gestational age
	Low birth weight infant (birth weight < 2,500 g)
Prematurity	Less than 37 weeks of gestation or less than 2.5 kg
Disorders of maternal glucose regulation	Insulin-dependent diabetic mother
	Gestational diabetic mother
	Morbid obesity in mother
Neonatal conditions with disturbed oxidative metabolism	Perinatal distress
	Hypoxaemia due to cardiac or lung disease
	Shock, hypoperfusion, sepsis, cold stress
Severe anaemia	Pallor (in the absence of hypovolaemia)
Congenital anomalies and genetic disorders	Visible anatomical deformities/abnormalities

of the referring hospital for premature infants). As always, maintain normal body temperature—hypothermia places additional stress on glucose demand.

Vomiting

Vomiting is very common in newborns. Approximately 85% of infants vomit during the first week of life, and another 10% have vomited by 6 weeks of age. Vomiting ranges from "spitting up" to severe, bloody or bilious, projectile vomiting. Most episodes of vomiting are benign and do not result in weight loss, dehydration, or other ill effects. Bilious and/or bloody emesis (vomiting) indicates a pathologic condition that needs medical attention. Persistent vomiting is a warning sign and can cause excessive loss of fluid, dehydration, and changes in electrolyte levels (ie, sodium, potassium, and glucose).

Vomiting mucus, occasionally blood streaked, in the first few hours of life is not uncommon. Persistent vomiting in the first 24 hours of life suggests obstruction in the upper digestive tract or increased intracranial pressure. Vomitus containing dark blood is often a sign of a life-threatening illness; it indicates bleeding in the gut. Sometimes, vomitus may be accompanied by bloody or tarry stool, another worrying sign. Aspiration of vomitus can cause respiratory insufficiencies or obstruction of the airway.

Causes of Vomiting

A newborn's presenting symptoms may give a clue to the site of obstruction or other problem that is causing the vomiting. One possible cause is oesophageal atresia (narrowing) with or without tracheo-oesophageal fistula. Its incidence is 1 case per 3,000 to 4,500 births. Infants are seen with excessive frothing soon after birth and may choke when attempting to feed, because the swallowed milk is returned promptly. This condition can also lead to an acute gastric perforation when the infant cries or strains and the air from the fistula enters the stomach; this problem is often lethal.

Another possible cause of vomiting, pathogenic gastro-oesophageal reflux (GOR), is common in infants, with a reported prevalence of 2% to 10%. GOR is most commonly seen in infancy, with its incidence peaking in the 1- to 4-month age group. The infant may vomit either immediately or a few hours after a feeding. The vomiting may not be forceful. In uncomplicated GOR, the vomitus is not bile stained or bloody. GOR in infants and young children can present as typical or atypical crying and/or irritability, apnoea and/or bradycardia, poor appetite, apparent life-threatening event, vomiting, wheezing, stridor, weight loss or poor growth (failure to thrive), hoarseness, and/or laryngitis.

In infantile hypertrophic pyloric stenosis (IHPS), marked hypertrophy and hyperplasia of the two (circular and longitudinal) muscular layers of the pylorus occur. As a consequence, the pylorus becomes thickened and obstructs the end of the stomach. The incidence of IHPS is 2 to 4 cases per 1,000 live births, with a male-to-female predominance of 4:1; 30% of patients with IHPS are first-born males. The usual age of presentation is approximately 3 weeks of life (range, 1 to 18 weeks). In IHPS, the stomach muscles contract forcibly to overcome the obstruction. Affected infants usually present with projectile vomiting, dehydration, malnutrition, and electrolyte changes. The vomitus in this case is not bile stained, but it can be brown or coffee coloured due to blood, resulting from gastritis or to a Mallory Weiss tear at the gastro-oesophageal junction.

Malrotation is a congenital anomaly of rotation of the midgut. In this condition, the small bowel is found predominantly on the right side of the abdomen; the caecum is found in the epigastrium–right hypochondrium. In cases of malrotation, the vomitus is bile stained and may be feculent (like faeces/stool) if the obstruction is distal in the intestines. Malrotation is estimated to occur in 1 of every 500 live births. Approximately 40% of patients are diagnosed within the first week of life; 75% are diagnosed by 1 year of age; and the remaining 25% are diagnosed later in life. With symptomatic malrotation, 75% to 90% of cases occur in infants younger than 1 year, 50% to 64% of cases occur in infants younger than 1 month, and 25% to 40% of cases occur in the first week of life. During the first week of life, the ratio of male-to-female presentation is 2:1. Since the advent of corrective surgical procedures, the morbidity and mortality have decreased significantly. Early mortality rate ranged from 23% to 33%, with most deaths resulting from bowel dysfunction and malnutrition.

Another cause of vomiting, meconium plug, is seen in Hirschsprung disease, wherein the last segment of colon fails to relax and causes mechanical obstruction. (This condition is due to the distal bowel not receiving a nerve supply.) The infant usually has a history of not passing meconium in the first 24 hours of life.

Vomiting may also happen in conjunction with asphyxia, meningitis (infection of the layers covering the brain and spine), and hydrocephalus (large head size is a clue). It is often sudden, unexpected, and forceful in such cases, and it may be accompanied by persistent irritability. Meningitis and hydrocephalus may also be associated with increased intracranial pressure (ICP).

Use of drugs during pregnancy can lead to several withdrawal symptoms in infants, including vomiting. The drugs that most commonly cause vomiting in newborns are barbiturates.

Assessment and Management of Vomiting

On physical examination, you may note a distended stomach that has been caused by vomiting. Suspect an infection if the newborn has a fever or a history of contact with sick people.

Initial management steps for a newborn with vomiting start with the ABCs. Maintain a patent airway, while staying aware that a vomiting infant can aspirate the vomitus and compromise the airway. Keep the infant's face turned to one side to prevent further aspiration. Suction or clear the vomitus from the airway with the help of a suction catheter. Ensure adequate oxygenation, providing either free-flow supplemental oxygen or bag-valve-mask ventilation as necessary. Bradycardia may be caused by vagal stimulus and is usually transient; it may resolve with stimulation and free-flow oxygen.

Antiemetics should not be administered in the prehospital environment. The infant may be dehydrated, however, and need fluid resuscitation. Dry mucous membranes, tachycardia, or a sunken fontanelle are clues that the patient needs hydration. Normal saline (10–20 ml/kg) may be required in that case.

On transport, place the newborn on his or her side, identify a facility capable of managing a high-risk infant, and explain what is being done for the infant to the family.

Diarrhoea

A normal number of stools per day for an infant is five to six, especially if the infant is breastfeeding, when infants often stool after every feeding. Diarrhoea is an excessive loss of electrolytes and fluid in the stool. In the United Kingdom, infants younger than 3 years have 1 to 2 episodes of diarrhoea each year. The prevalence is higher in infants attending daycare centres. Nine percent of all hospitalisations of children younger than 5 years of age are for diarrhoea.

The most common cause of acute diarrhoea in children is viral infection (especially rotavirus infection during the winter months). Less frequently encountered causes include poisoning due to insecticides, organophosphates, and carbamates. Diarrhoea related to these agents is accompanied by profuse sweating, lacrimation, hypersalivation, and abdominal cramps, or more serious conditions such as intussusception, malrotation, increased ICP, and metabolic acidosis. Other causes of diarrhoea include gastroenteritis, lactose intolerance, neonatal abstinence syndrome, thyrotoxicosis, and cystic fibrosis.

Severe cases of diarrhoea can cause dehydration and subsequent electrolyte imbalance. Combinations of physical signs—such as ill general appearance, poor vital signs, capillary refill of greater than 2 seconds, dry mucous membranes, absent tears, weight loss, and low urine output—are good objective predictors of the degree of dehydration.

Assessment and Management of Diarrhoea

Assessment includes estimating the number and volume of loose stools, urinary output, and degree of dehydration based on skin turgor, mucous membranes, presence of sunken eyes, and other signs. Patient management, as always, begins with the ABCs. The newborn's airway and ventilation may be compromised if he or she is severely dehydrated and is sluggish, so ensure adequate oxygenation and ventilation. Perform chest compressions in addition to PPV in a newborn if the pulse rate is less than 60 beats/min.

Fluid therapy may be indicated when a newborn has diarrhoea. Normal saline (10 ml/kg) may be needed immediately to fluid resuscitate the infant.

Common Birth Injuries in the Newborn

Birth trauma includes both avoidable and unavoidable injuries to the infant resulting from mechanical forces (ie, compression, traction) during the delivery process. Such trauma is estimated to occur in 2 to 7 of every 1,000 live births. Most birth injuries are self-limiting and have a favourable outcome. Nearly half are potentially avoidable with recognition and anticipation of obstetric risk factors.

Birth injuries account for 2% to 3% of all infant deaths, with 5 to 8 of every 100,000 newborns dying of birth trauma and 25 of every 100,000 newborns dying of anoxic injury. Separating the effects of a hypoxic ischaemic insult from the effects of a traumatic birth injury may prove difficult.

A difficult birth or injury to the baby can occur because of the infant's size or position during labour and delivery. Conditions associated with a difficult birth include primigravida (first pregnancy), prolonged labour, cephalopelvic disproportion (the size and shape of the maternal pelvis are not adequate for the vaginal delivery of the infant), prolonged or rapid labour, abnormal presentation (eg, breech), large size (birth weight exceeding 4 kg), prematurity, or low birth weight.

Birth trauma includes a variety of injuries. For example, abrasions, lacerations, bruises, and subcutaneous fat necrosis can occur with deliveries that involve instruments (eg, a vacuum or forceps). Moulding of the head and overriding parietal bones are part of the normal process of labour, but occasionally excessive moulding may be seen.

Caput succedaneum is swelling of the soft tissue of the baby's scalp as it presses against the dilating cervix. This type of cranial injury is very common. The swelling usually disappears in the first day or two after birth.

A cephalhaematoma is an area of bleeding between the parietal bone and its covering periosteum. It often appears several hours after birth as a raised lump on the newborn's head, is limited by the boundaries of the bone, and may take 2 weeks to 3 months to resolve. If the bleeding is severe, jaundice may be seen as the red blood cells break down. Babies born by instrumental vaginal delivery are more likely to have a cephalhaematoma.

Linear fractures are occasionally seen with difficult births (spontaneous vaginal deliveries or deliveries using instruments).

Brachial plexus injuries typically occur in large babies and have an incidence of 0.5 to 2.0 cases per 1,000 live births. The most common brachial plexus injury is Erb palsy (involvement of C5, C6). Klumpke paralysis (C7–C8, T1) is rare and results in the weakness of the intrinsic muscles of the hand.

Although branches of the facial nerve may be injured in forceps delivery, most facial nerve palsy is unrelated to trauma. Physical findings include asymmetric facies with crying (lack of movement on the affected side makes the face appear to be "pulled" to the opposite side). Full resolution of cranial nerve injuries may take several weeks.

Diaphragmatic paralysis may occur as an isolated finding when the cervical roots supplying the phrenic nerve are injured or in association with brachial plexus injury. The newborn may experience respiratory distress with hypoxaemia, hypercapnoea, and acidosis. Approximately 80% of the lesions are on the right side, and 10% are bilateral.

Laryngeal nerve injury appears to result from an intrauterine posture in which the head is rotated and flexed laterally. The infant presents with stridor or a hoarse cry. Bilateral injury may be associated with severe respiratory distress needing respiratory support. The paralysis often resolves in 4 to 6 weeks, but may occasionally take as long as 6 to 12 months to clear up.

Spinal cord injury may result from excessive traction (in a breech delivery) or rotation and torsion (in a vertex delivery). The clinical presentation is stillbirth or rapid neonatal death with failure to establish an adequate airway.

The clavicle is the most frequently fractured bone in the newborn; such a bone injury is most often an unpredictable, unavoidable complication of normal birth. Risk factors may include large size, mid-forceps delivery, and shoulder dystocia (ie, the baby's shoulders get stuck in the birth canal). The infant may present with pseudoparalysis as he or she tries not to move the affected extremity to minimise pain. Examination will show crepitus and palpable bony irregularity.

Loss of spontaneous arm or leg movement is an early sign of long bone fracture. The femur and humerus are the most commonly affected long bones. The fractures are treated by splinting. Look for signs of radial nerve injury with a humerus fracture. Intra-abdominal injury is uncommon and may be overlooked as a cause of death in a newborn. Haemorrhage is the most serious complication, and the liver is the organ most commonly injured. The bleeding may be catastrophic or insidious, and the patient presents with circulatory collapse. Consider intra-abdominal bleeding in every infant presenting with shock, or unexplained pallor, plus abdominal distension.

Family and Transport Considerations

Once the infant is stabilised as much as possible in the prehospital environment, transport the patient to the nearest facility that can provide the next level of care. This facility will not necessarily be a tertiary hospital. A nearby community hospital, if it is located much closer, may be able to perform additional stabilisation procedures for a very ill baby, such as placement of a chest tube for a clinically significant pneumothorax. Ideally, someone will contact this facility to discuss the situation and obtain advice regarding care and disposition. Throughout the process, ongoing communication with the family regarding what is being done for the infant and what care is planned will help allay fears. Do not be specific about survival statistics. Many factors play into mortality and morbidity, and you don't want to be misleading. If family members have questions you can't answer, be straightforward. Tell them that you don't have a definite answer, but you will help put them in touch with the people who do (ie, the centre to which the infant is being transferred) **Figure 40-13 ▸** .

During transport, ongoing observation and frequent reassessment will ensure timely intervention should the newborn's status change. Attention to thermoregulation, respiratory effort, patency of airway, skin colour, and pulse rate is vital. If the infant is being transferred between facilities after the initial stabilisation, continue to provide close observation and assessment of these factors to facilitate initiation of interventions should the infant's condition change.

You are the Paramedic Part 5

You prepare both the infant and mother for transport, load them into the ambulance, and begin the journey to a hospital located 20 miles away. En route, the mother experiences mild vaginal bleeding, which you control with fundal massage. As the infant is nursing, you establish an IV of normal saline on the mother and administer supplemental oxygen. After delivery of the placenta, you reassess the mother.

Reassessment	Recording Time: 19 Minutes
Skin	Pink, warm, and moist
Pulse	84 beats/min, strong and regular
Blood pressure	104/58 mm Hg
Respirations	20 breaths/min; adequate tidal volume
SpO₂	99% on oxygen

When you arrive at the delivery suite, you are met by a neonatologist and a doctor. Both the mother and baby are haemodynamically stable and are admitted to hospital.

9. When are chest compressions indicated for the newborn?
10. When is adrenaline indicated during newborn resuscitation?

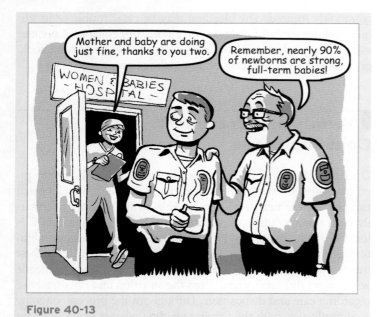

Figure 40-13

The development of new and more sophisticated techniques for the care of newborn infants, especially premature infants, together with round-the-clock care by expert medical personnel, has significantly reduced the mortality among high-risk newborns in hospitals where such capabilities are available. Because the average community hospital cannot provide the specially trained doctors and nurses or the expensive equipment needed for such care, it sometimes becomes necessary to transfer the critically ill infant to a regional centre, where the infant may benefit from highly skilled personnel and sophisticated equipment. In the well-organised regional referral system, transport of a high-risk newborn proceeds through the following several steps:

1. A doctor at the referring hospital initiates a request for transport. A doctor in the regional centre decides if the intensive care nursery can accommodate the patient and gives the referring doctor advice on management of the infant until the transport team arrives.

2. A mode of transportation is chosen—ground transportation, helicopter, or fixed-wing aircraft, depending on the distance, availability of services, and weather conditions.

3. The transport team is mobilised, and equipment is assembled. The ideal team consists of a nurse with special training in neonatal intensive care, a neonatologist, and a paramedic who has spent a period of training and education in a neonatal intensive care unit. The equipment is highly specialised, requiring appropriately designed ventilation and oxygenation units and an incubator meeting stringent criteria.

4. On arriving at the referring hospital, the transport team continues to stabilise the infant before embarking on transport. Conditions such as hypoxaemia, acidosis, hypoglycaemia, and hypovolaemia must be treated before leaving the referring hospital.

5. While stabilising the infant, the team collects information and materials including a copy of the mother's and infant's charts and any X-rays taken of the infant.

You are the Paramedic Summary

1. Why is it important to determine the colour of the amniotic fluid?

A crucial part of your predelivery evaluation is to determine the colour of the amniotic fluid. Normally, it should be clear. Amniotic fluid that is brown or contains thick, particulate meconium—the baby's first bowel movement—indicates that the newborn may have aspirated the meconium. In such a case, the newborn may be severely hypoxic and may require aggressive resuscitation.

2. What are some reliable indicators of imminent delivery?

When determining whether you have time to transport the mother to hospital or must prepare for imminent delivery, there are some key questions to ask and some key observations to make. Regular contractions that are less than 5 minutes apart—even if the amniotic sac has not ruptured—should be considered a sign of impending delivery. If the woman says that she feels the urge to move her bowels, the baby is pressing on her rectum and is in the birth canal. Clearly, crowning of the baby's head indicates that delivery is in progress. Perhaps one of the most reliable indicators of impending delivery is when the mother states that she is going to have her baby "now"! If she tells you this, believe her—even if it is her first baby.

3. What specific questions should you ask that will allow you to anticipate the need for resuscitation of the newborn?

Although it's impossible to predict all of the complications that might potentially occur following delivery, a thorough maternal assessment—if time permits—will enable you to identify risk factors that should increase your suspicion for a distressed newborn who will require resuscitation. Establishing how far along a woman is into her pregnancy is a key consideration. If a fetus is less than 37 weeks of gestation—in which case the woman would be in premature labour—the risk for a distressed newborn increases. You should also ask if the patient is carrying more than one baby. Of course, if she has had regular antenatal care—which typically includes an ultrasound—she will know the answer. Inquire about the use of drugs (legal and illegal), alcohol, or cigarettes during the mother's pregnancy; these factors clearly increase the risk of newborn distress. Finally, ask about her medical history, focusing specifically on conditions that can complicate pregnancy (ie, pregnancy-induced hypertension [preeclampsia] or gestational diabetes).

4. What equipment and supplies should be available in case the infant requires resuscitation?

Although approximately 90% of babies are born normal and require little more than drying, warming, and suctioning, you should be adequately prepared in the event that the infant requires more aggressive resuscitative measures. In addition to the sterile maternity pack, you should have a neonatal-size bag-valve-mask device, equipment and supplies required to perform tracheal suctioning of meconium (ie, newborn-size ET tubes, meconium aspirator, suction, laryngoscope and blades), and adrenaline (1:10,000 only) for refractory cardiopulmonary depression. Consider carrying this equipment and supplies in a special newborn resuscitation kit, which should be checked daily, along with the other equipment and supplies on the ambulance.

5. What treatment is indicated for this infant?

Although the infant is breathing adequately and has a pulse rate greater than 100 beats/min, the presence of central cyanosis indicates the need for free-flow supplemental oxygen. It can be delivered using an oxygen mask or oxygen tubing held near the baby's nose and mouth. Set the oxygen flow rate at 5 l/min and observe the infant for improving colour. Avoid blowing oxygen directly into the baby's eyes, as it may dry out the mucosa.

6. When is positive-pressure ventilation indicated for the newborn?

PPV is indicated in the newborn if the infant is apnoeic or has gasping respirations, if the infant's pulse rate is less than 100 beats/min, or if central cyanosis persists despite the delivery of free-flow supplemental oxygen. The proper ventilation rate for the newborn is 30 to 40 breaths/min.

7. Does the child require further resuscitation?

From these observations no further resuscitation actions are required at this time. However, the child and mother should be carefully monitored for any change whilst being transported.

8. Is it safe to clamp and cut the umbilical cord?

The umbilical cord should not be clamped and cut until the baby is breathing adequately on its own and the cord has stopped pulsating. If neither of these has occurred, do not clamp and cut the cord. Instead, keep the baby at the level of the perineum, wrap the cord with sterile, moist dressings, and transport immediately with continued resuscitation en route to hospital. The infant in this case has adequate breathing and a pulse rate greater than 100 beats/min; therefore, it is haemodynamically stable, and it is safe to clamp and cut the umbilical cord.

9. When are chest compressions indicated for the newborn?

Chest compressions are rarely needed during newborn resuscitation. However, if there is no pulse or if the pulse rate falls below 60 beats/min despite *adequate* oxygenation and ventilation, begin chest compressions immediately. In the newborn, chest compressions are delivered using the two-finger technique (one rescuer) or the two-thumb encircling-hands technique (two rescuers). Compress the chest one third to one half the anteroposterior depth of the chest at a rate of 120 interventions/min (90 compressions/30 ventilations). After 30 seconds of chest compressions, reassess the infant.

10. When is adrenaline indicated during newborn resuscitation?

As with chest compressions, medication therapy is rarely needed during newborn resuscitation. However, if the pulse is absent *or* less than 60 beats/min despite 30 seconds of *adequate* oxygenation and ventilation *plus* an additional 30 seconds of chest compressions (1 minute total), you should administer adrenaline. The proper newborn dose for adrenaline is 0.1 to 0.3 ml/kg of a 1:10,000 solution via rapid administration. *Never use adrenaline 1:1,000 during newborn resuscitation; it is too concentrated and may result in a spontaneous intracranial haemorrhage!* Adrenaline can be administered via a peripheral IV line or through the umbilical vein (if you are able to cannulate the umbilical vein). If adrenaline is administered via the ET tube, consider giving a higher dose—0.3 to 1 ml/kg.

Prep Kit

Ready for Review

- The care of a newborn or neonate must be tailored to meet the unique needs of this population.
- Additional skilled care intervention is needed for approximately 6% of newborn deliveries, with the rate of complications increasing as birth weight and gestational age decrease.
- In the United Kingdom, approximately 80% of babies born each year weighing less than 1.5 kg require resuscitation.
- Both short- and long-term outcomes have been linked to initial stabilisation efforts.
- Your initial rapid assessment of the infant may be done simultaneously with any treatment interventions.
- Nearly 90% of newborns are vigorous full-term babies.
- Not all deliveries go smoothly. Approximately 10% of newborns need additional assistance and 1% need resuscitation to survive.
- Infants born before 37 weeks of gestation are considered premature.
- Convulsions are the most distinctive sign of neurological disease in the newborn.
- Thermoregulation is very limited in the newborn, so the paramedic must take an active role in keeping the newborn's body temperature in the normal range.
- In full-term or preterm neonates, hypoglycaemia is a blood glucose level of less than 2 mmol/l.
- Vomiting is common in infants.
- For an infant who is breastfeeding, five to six stools per day is normal.
- Birth trauma includes both avoidable and unavoidable injuries to the infant resulting from mechanical forces during the delivery process. A difficult birth or injury to the baby can occur because of the infant's size or position during labour or delivery.
- Once the infant is stabilised as much as possible in the prehospital environment, he or she needs to be transported to the nearest facility that can provide the next level of care.

Vital Vocabulary

acrocyanosis A decrease in the amount of oxygen delivered to the extremities. The hands and feet turn blue because of narrowing (constriction) of small arterioles (tiny arteries) toward the end of the arms and legs.

amniotic fluid A clear, slightly yellowish liquid that surrounds the unborn baby (fetus) during pregnancy; contained in the amniotic sac.

apnoea Respiratory pause greater than or equal to 20 seconds.

asphyxia Condition of severely deficient supply of oxygen to the body leading to end organ damage.

bradycardia A pulse rate of less than 100 beats/min in the newborn.

central cyanosis Bluish colouration of the skin due to the presence of deoxygenated haemoglobin in blood vessels near the skin surface.

choanal atresia A narrowing or blockage of the nasal airway by membranous or bony tissue; a congenital condition, meaning it is present at birth.

cleft lip An abnormal defect or fissure in the upper lip that failed to close during development. It is often associated with cleft palate.

cleft palate A fissure or hole in the palate (roof of the mouth) that forms a communicating pathway between the mouth and nasal cavities.

convulsion A paroxysmal alteration in neurological function, ie, behavioural and/or autonomic function.

diaphragmatic hernia Passage of loops of bowel with or without other abdominal organs, through the diaphragm muscle; occurs as the bowel from the abdomen "herniates" upward through the diaphragm into the chest (thoracic) cavity.

Erb palsy Lack of movement at the shoulder due to nerve injury resulting from the stretching of the cervical nerve roots (C5 and C6 most commonly) during delivery of the baby's head during birth. The effect is usually transient, but can be permanent

free-flow oxygen Oxygen administered via oxygen tube and a cupped hand on patient's face.

gestation Period of time from conception to birth. For humans, the full period is normally 9 months (or 40 weeks).

grunting Noises heard when a baby is having difficulty breathing; short inarticulate guttural sounds as effort is expended.

hypoglycaemia A deficiency of glucose in the blood caused by too much insulin or too little glucose; in the newborn it is a level less than 2 mmol/l, and in older neonates it is a level less than 3 mmol/l.

hypotonia Low or poor muscle tone (floppy).

hypovolaemia An abnormal decrease in blood volume or, strictly speaking, an abnormal decrease in the volume of blood plasma.

hypoxic ischaemic encephalopathy Damage to cells in the central nervous system (the brain and spinal cord) from inadequate oxygen.

intercostal recessions Skin sucking in between the ribs, seen when a patient creates increased negative intrathoracic pressure to breathe.

intussusception An event where one part of the intestine folds into another part of the intestines lead to a blockage.

Klumpke paralysis An injury of childbirth affecting the spinal nerves C7, C8, and T1 of the brachial plexus. It can be contrasted to Erb palsy, which affects C5 and C6.

malrotation A congenital anomaly of rotation of the midgut, the small bowel is found predominantly on the right side of the abdomen.

meconium A dark green faecal material that accumulates in the fetal intestines and is discharged around the time of birth.

nasal flaring Intermittent outward movements of the nostrils with each inspiration; indicates an increase in the work needed to breathe.

neonate Infant during the first month after birth.

newborn Infant within the first few hours after birth.

oligohydramnios Decreased volume of amniotic fluid during a pregnancy; a risk factor associated with abnormalities of the urinary tract, postmaturity (birth after a prolonged pregnancy), and intrauterine growth retardation.

persistent pulmonary hypertension Delayed transition from fetal to neonatal circulation.

Pierre Robin sequence A condition present at birth marked by a very small lower jaw (micrognathia). The tongue tends to fall back and downward (glossoptosis), and there is a cleft soft palate.

placenta previa Abnormal location of the placenta in the lower part of the uterus, near or over the cervix.

polycythaemia Abnormally high red blood cell count.

polyhydramnios An excessive amount of amniotic fluid. May cause preterm labour.

positive-pressure ventilation (PPV) Method for assisting ventilation (bag-valve-mask or intubated) with high-flow air or supplemental oxygen.

post-term Any pregnancy that lasts more than 42 weeks.

premature Underdeveloped; the condition of an infant born too soon. Refers to infants delivered before 37 weeks from the first day of the last menstrual period.

preterm Used to describe an infant delivered at less than 37 completed weeks.

primary apnoea Apnoea caused by oxygen deprivation; usually corrected with stimulation, such as drying or slapping the newborn's feet. Primary apnoea is typically preceded by an initial period of rapid breathing.

primigravida First pregnancy.

prolapsed cord When the umbilical cord presents itself outside of the uterus while the fetus is still inside; an obstetric emergency during pregnancy or labour that acutely endangers the life of the baby; can happen when the water breaks and with the gush of water the cord comes along.

pulmonary hypertension Elevated blood pressure in the pulmonary arteries from constriction; causes problems with the blood flow in the lungs, and makes the heart work harder.

retinopathy of prematurity A disease of the eye that affects prematurely born babies, thought to be caused by disorganised growth of retinal blood vessels resulting in scarring and retinal detachment; can lead to blindness in serious cases.

secondary apnoea When asphyxia continues after primary apnoea, infant responds with a period of gasping respirations, falling pulse rate and falling blood pressure.

small for gestational age An infant whose size and weight are considerably less than the average for babies of the same age.

somnolence Sleepiness.

surfactant A substance formed in the lungs that helps keep the small air sacs or alveoli from collapsing and sticking together; a low level in a premature baby contributes to respiratory distress syndrome.

term Used to describe an infant delivered at 38 to 42 weeks of gestation.

umbilical vein Blood vessel in umbilical cord used to administer emergency medications.

vernix A white, cheesy substance that covers the fetus' skin in utero and at birth.

Assessment in Action

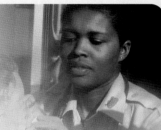

A 21-year-old woman who is 41 weeks' pregnant felt a few contractions and had the urge to go the toilet. Her membranes ruptured (her "water broke") during this process, and she noticed it looked like "pea soup". She remembered from her antenatal visits that this wasn't a good sign and called 999. You arrive at the scene and find the infant's head presenting at the perineum.

1. **What does the "pea soup" appearance of the amniotic fluid indicate?**
   A. Dehydration of the newborn
   B. Meconium staining
   C. Cardiac arrest of the newborn
   D. Normal delivery

2. **How are delivery and resuscitation of a meconium-stained infant different from other full-term deliveries?**
   A. Higher rate of morbidity
   B. Lower rate of morbidity
   C. Higher rate of breech presentation
   D. Lower rate of breech presentation

3. **What is the most essential piece of equipment you need to prepare for this delivery?**
   A. Items to warm and dry the newborn
   B. Pulse oximeter
   C. Cardiac monitor
   D. ET tube and meconium aspirator

4. **What is the primary use of the ET tube once you have it placed in the meconium-stained newborn?**
   A. It supplies positive-pressure ventilation.
   B. It serves as a suction device.
   C. It holds the airway open.
   D. It provides standard ventilation.

Challenging Question

5. **What measures will you take to care for the mother of this child?**

■ Points to Ponder

For the infant born through meconium-stained amniotic fluid discussed previously, the infant is depressed and you intubated and suctioned the trachea using a meconium aspirator while providing free-flow oxygen. You've dried and stimulated the newborn without causing injury. It is almost 2 minutes past delivery. The infant's pulse rate is 85 beats/min.

What is the next step in managing the airway—PPV or intubation?

Issues: Infant Airway Intubation, Neonatal Resuscitation.

41 Paediatrics

Objectives

Cognitive

- Discuss the paramedic's role in the reduction of infant and childhood morbidity and mortality from acute illness and injury.
- Identify methods/mechanisms that prevent injuries to infants and children.
- Identify key growth and developmental characteristics of infants and children and their implications.
- Identify key anatomical and physiological characteristics of infants and their implications.
- Describe techniques for successful assessment of infants and children.
- Describe techniques for successful treatment of infants and children.
- Identify the common responses of families to acute illness and injury of an infant or child.
- Describe techniques for successful interaction with families of acutely ill or injured infants and children.
- Outline differences in adult and childhood anatomy and physiology.
- Identify "normal" age group related vital signs.
- Discuss the appropriate equipment utilised to obtain paediatric vital signs.
- Determine appropriate airway adjuncts for infants and children.
- Discuss complications of improper utilisation of airway adjuncts with infants and children.
- Discuss appropriate ventilation devices for infants and children.
- Discuss complications of improper utilisation of ventilation devices with infants and children.
- Discuss appropriate endotracheal intubation equipment for infants and children.
- Identify complications of improper endotracheal intubation procedures for infants and children.
- List the indications and methods for gastric decompression for infants and children.
- Define respiratory distress.
- Define respiratory failure.
- Define respiratory arrest.
- Differentiate between upper airway obstruction and lower airway disease.
- Describe the general approach to the treatment of children with respiratory distress, failure, or arrest from upper airway obstruction or lower airway disease.
- Discuss the common causes of hypoperfusion in infants and children.
- Evaluate the severity of hypoperfusion in infants and children.
- Identify the major classifications of paediatric cardiac rhythms.
- Discuss the primary aetiologies of cardiopulmonary arrest in infants and children.
- Discuss age appropriate vascular access sites for infants and children.
- Discuss the appropriate equipment for vascular access in infants and children.
- Identify complications of vascular access for infants and children.
- Describe the primary aetiologies of altered level of consciousness in infants and children.
- Identify common lethal mechanisms of injury in infants and children.
- Discuss anatomical features of children that predispose or protect them from certain injuries.
- Describe aspects of infant and children airway management that are affected by potential cervical spine injury.
- Identify infant and child trauma patients who require spinal immobilisation.
- Discuss fluid management and shock treatment for infant and child trauma patients.
- Determine when pain management and sedation are appropriate for infants and children.
- Define child abuse.
- Define child neglect.
- Define sudden unexpected death in infancy (SUDI).
- Discuss the parent/caregiver responses to the death of an infant or child.
- Define children with special health care needs.
- Define technology assisted children.
- Discuss basic cardiac life support (CPR) guidelines for infants and children.
- Identify appropriate parameters for performing infant and child CPR.
- Integrate advanced life support skills with basic cardiac life support for infants and children.
- Discuss the indications, dosage, route of administration and special considerations for medication administration in infants and children.
- Discuss appropriate transport guidelines for infants and children.
- Discuss appropriate receiving facilities for low and high risk infants and children.
- Describe the epidemiology, including the incidence, morbidity/mortality, risk factors and prevention strategies for respiratory distress/failure in infants and children.
- Discuss the pathophysiology of respiratory distress/failure in infants and children.
- Discuss the assessment findings associated with respiratory distress/failure in infants and children.
- Discuss the management/treatment plan for respiratory distress/failure in infants and children.
- Describe the epidemiology, including the incidence, morbidity/mortality, risk factors and prevention strategies for hypoperfusion in infants and children.
- Discuss the pathophysiology of hypoperfusion in infants and children.
- Discuss the assessment findings associated with hypoperfusion in infants and children.
- Discuss the management/treatment plan for hypoperfusion in infants and children.
- Describe the epidemiology, including the incidence, morbidity/mortality, risk factors and prevention strategies for cardiac arrhythmias in infants and children.

- Discuss the pathophysiology of cardiac arrhythmias in infants and children.
- Discuss the assessment findings associated with cardiac arrhythmias in infants and children.
- Discuss the management/treatment plan for cardiac arrhythmias in infants and children.
- Describe the epidemiology, including the incidence, morbidity/mortality, risk factors and prevention strategies for neurological emergencies in infants and children.
- Discuss the pathophysiology of neurological emergencies in infants and children.
- Discuss the assessment findings associated with neurological emergencies in infants and children.
- Discuss the management/treatment plan for neurological emergencies in infants and children.
- Describe the epidemiology, including the incidence, morbidity/mortality, risk factors and prevention strategies for trauma in infants and children.
- Discuss the pathophysiology of trauma in infants and children.
- Discuss the assessment findings associated with trauma in infants and children.
- Discuss the management/treatment plan for trauma in infants and children.
- Describe the epidemiology, including the incidence, morbidity/mortality, risk factors and prevention strategies for abuse and neglect in infants and children.
- Discuss the pathophysiology of abuse and neglect in infants and children.
- Discuss the assessment findings associated with abuse and neglect in infants and children.
- Discuss the management/treatment plan for abuse and neglect in infants and children.
- Describe the epidemiology, including the incidence, morbidity/mortality, risk factors and prevention strategies for SUDI in infants and children.
- Describe the epidemiology, including the incidence, morbidity/mortality, risk factors and prevention strategies for children with special health care needs including technology assisted children.
- Discuss the pathophysiology of children with special health care needs including technology assisted children.
- Discuss the assessment findings of children with special health care needs including technology assisted children.
- Discuss the management/treatment plan for children with special health care needs including technology assisted children.
- Describe the epidemiology, including the incidence, morbidity/mortality, risk factors and prevention strategies for SUDI in infants and children.
- Discuss the pathophysiology of SUDI in infants and children.
- Discuss the assessment findings associated with SUDI in infants and children.
- Discuss the management/treatment plan for SUDI in infants and children.

Affective

- Demonstrate and advocate appropriate interactions with the infant/child that conveys an understanding of their developmental stage.
- Recognise the emotional dependence of the infant/child to their parent/guardian.
- Recognise the emotional impact of the infant/child injuries and illnesses on the parent/guardian.

- Recognise and appreciate the physical and emotional difficulties associated with separation of the parent/guardian of a child with special needs.
- Demonstrate the ability to provide reassurance, empathy and compassion for the parent/guardian.

Psychomotor

- Demonstrate the appropriate approach for treating infants and children.
- Demonstrate appropriate intervention techniques with families of acutely ill or injured infants and children.
- Demonstrate the appropriate assessment for different developmental age groups.
- Demonstrate an appropriate technique for measuring paediatric vital signs.
- Demonstrate the use of a length-based resuscitation device for determining equipment sizes, drug doses or other pertinent information for a paediatric patient.
- Demonstrate the appropriate approach for treating infants and children with respiratory distress, failure, and arrest.
- Demonstrate proper technique for administering blow-by oxygen to infants and children.
- Demonstrate the proper utilisation of a paediatric nonrebreather oxygen mask.
- Demonstrate proper technique for suctioning of infants and children.
- Demonstrate appropriate use of airway adjuncts with infants and children.
- Demonstrate appropriate use of ventilation devices for infants and children.
- Demonstrate endotracheal intubation procedures in infants and children.
- Demonstrate appropriate treatment/management of intubation complications of infants and children.
- Demonstrate appropriate needle cricothyroidotomy in infants and children.
- Demonstrate proper placement of a gastric tube in infants and children.
- Demonstrate an appropriate technique for insertion of peripheral intravenous cannulas for infants and children.
- Demonstrate an appropriate technique for administration of intramuscular, inhalation, subcutaneous, rectal, endotracheal and oral medication for infants and children.
- Demonstrate an appropriate technique for insertion of an intraosseous line for infants and children.
- Demonstrate appropriate interventions for infants and children with a partially obstructed airway.
- Demonstrate age appropriate basic airway clearing manoeuvres for infants and children with a completely obstructed airway.
- Demonstrate proper technique for direct laryngoscopy and foreign body retrieval in infants and children with a completely obstructed airway.
- Demonstrate appropriate airway and breathing control manoeuvres for infant and child trauma patients.
- Demonstrate appropriate treatment of infants and children requiring advanced airway and breathing control.
- Demonstrate appropriate immobilisation techniques for infant and child trauma patients.
- Demonstrate appropriate treatment of infants and children with head injuries.
- Demonstrate appropriate treatment of infants and children with chest injuries.

- Demonstrate appropriate treatment of infants and children with abdominal injuries.
- Demonstrate appropriate treatment of infants and children with extremity injuries.
- Demonstrate appropriate treatment of infants and children with burns.

- Demonstrate appropriate parent/carer interviewing techniques for infant and child death situations.
- Demonstrate proper infant CPR.
- Demonstrate proper child CPR.
- Demonstrate proper techniques for performing infant and child defibrillation and synchronised cardioversion.

Introduction

Children differ anatomically, physiologically, and emotionally from adults. In addition, the types of illnesses and injuries they sustain and their responses to them vary across the paediatric age span. For these reasons, you must tailor your approach to accommodate the developmental and social issues unique to paediatrics. Some children may be afraid of the ambulance crew. Depending on the age of the child, he or she may not be able to tell you what is wrong. Also, each paediatric call involves one or more parents or carers who may be stressed or frightened themselves.

This chapter addresses some of the special considerations that will enhance your effectiveness in caring for an ill or injured child. It begins by discussing the approach to paediatric patients, with an eye toward their developmental level and the anatomical or physiological differences unique to the age group. This information is used to outline an approach to paediatric assessment, review specific paediatric emergencies, and address their prehospital management. Finally, the chapter details the skills needed to care efficiently and effectively for paediatric patients, regardless of the diagnosis.

Approach to Paediatric Patients

Sick or injured children present unique challenges in evaluation and management. Their perceptions of their illness or injury, their world, and you differ from the perceptions of adults. Depending on their age, they may not be able to report what is bothering them. Fear or pain may make children difficult to assess as well. In addition, you will have to work with

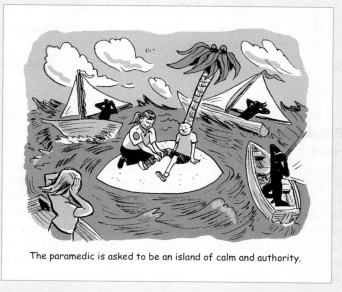

The paramedic is asked to be an island of calm and authority.

Figure 41-1

concerned parents who may themselves be acting irrationally. In the midst of this challenge, you are expected to be an island of calm and authority, carrying out your job systematically, carefully, and confidently Figure 41-1 ▲.

The manner in which you approach a sick or injured child will depend on the child's age and developmental level. Childhood extends from the neonatal period, just after birth, until aged 18 years. An enormous amount of physical and psychological development occurs in these 18 years. A child's anatomy, physiology, and psychosocial development will all influence your assessment and treatment.

You are the Paramedic Part 1

You and your colleague are on station when you receive a call to a child who has fallen from a second floor window. When you arrive, you are flagged down by a frantic mother who points towards her 2-year-old son. You see a toddler lying face up on the pavement approximately 1 metre from the block of flats. Mum tells you that she has turned her son over but did not move him any further.

The toddler is lying motionless. His eyes are open, but he does not focus on you or his mother as she stands crying beside him. You observe an adequate respiratory rate with good bilateral chest expansion. The boy appears pale and has cool, dry skin.

Initial Assessment	Recording Time: 0 Minutes
Appearance	Pale toddler, lying motionless, making no eye contact
Level of consciousness	V (Responsive to verbal stimuli)
Airway	Open
Breathing	Adequate rate and volume; no recession or audible sounds
Circulation	Weak radial pulses with pale, cool, dry skin

1. What assessment tool will you use to form your general impression of your patient?
2. What can you do to assist the panicked mother?

Paediatric Anatomy and Physiology

Head

You may have seen an infant or young child and noted the size of the child's head: Little children have very big heads. In fact, an infant's head is already two thirds the size it will be in adulthood. The large head means more surface area for heat loss. It also means more mass relative to the rest of the body—an important factor in the incidence of head injuries in young patients, who tend to lead with the head in a fall. During the school-age years, the head and body become more proportional.

Neck and Airway

Children have short, stubby necks, which can make it difficult to feel a carotid pulse or see jugular veins. Not surprisingly, the airway of a young child is also much smaller than an adult airway. That smaller diameter makes the airway more prone to obstruction, either by foreign body inhalation, inflammation with infection, or the child's disproportionately large tongue. During the first few months of life, infants are obligate nose breathers, and nasal obstruction with mucus can result in significant respiratory distress. Their epiglottis is quite floppy and U-shaped, which can make it difficult to visualise the cords during intubation. Finally, the narrowest part of a young child's airway occurs at the level of the cricoid cartilage, rather than at the vocal cords as in adults; this issue should influence your choice of endotracheal (ET) tubes.

Chest and Lungs

A child's chest wall is quite thin, with less musculature and less subcutaneous fat than in an adult. The thin chest wall makes it easy to hear heart and lungs sounds but also means that sounds are readily transmitted throughout the chest. Sounds originating from the nose or throat can be heard quite clearly on auscultation, for example. The rib cage is more compliant, making recession easy to see. Use of the diaphragm as a muscle of respiration is pronounced in infants, leading to belly breathing at baseline.

Heart

Circulation in the fetus is much different from that in the newborn, and large right-sided forces on the electrocardiogram (ECG) are normal in young infants. During the first year of life, the ECG axis and voltages shift to reflect left ventricular dominance. Cardiac output is rate-dependent in infants and young children. They have relatively poor ability to increase stroke volume, which is reflected in their normal heart rates (higher in newborns than in older children and adults) and in rate response to physiological stress and hypovolaemia.

Abdomen

The appearance of abdominal distension in a healthy infant is due to two factors: the weak abdominal wall muscles and the size of the solid organs. The liver extends below the ribcage in infants, making it more vulnerable to injury. As the child grows, the liver becomes more proportionate and is better protected by the bony ribcage.

Musculoskeletal System

Reaching adult height requires active bone growth. The growth plates (ossification centres) of a child's bones are made of cartilage, are relatively weak, and are easily fractured. As a consequence, the bones of growing children are weaker than their ligaments, making fractures more common than sprains. Bones finish growing at differing times, but most growth plates will be closed by late adolescence.

Brain and Nervous System

The brain and nervous system continue to develop once the baby is born. As the brain matures, the infant's responses to the environment, outside stimuli, and even pain become more organised and purposeful. The speed of brain development can be appreciated by comparing the abilities and interactions of a 4-day-old baby, whose repertoire is limited to eating, sleeping, and defecating, with those of a 4-month-old, who smiles socially, rolls over, and plays with a rattle, and with those of a 12-month-old, who walks, is beginning to talk, and expresses preferences for individuals and activities.

Developmental Stages

Neonate and Infant

The first month of life is called the neonatal period, whereas infancy refers to the first 12 months of life. A lot of development occurs in this interval. Neonates don't do very much, other than eat, sleep, and cry. During the first months of life, a baby will have longer awake periods and interact more with the environment. Infants between 2 and 6 months of age are more active and social and can recognise their parents. By 4 months of age, infants are able to hold their heads up. Infants between 6 and 12 months of age babble, can sit unsupported, reach for objects, and are becoming more mobile—crawling and even walking. At 9 months of age, most infants develop stranger anxiety, with a strong preference for their parents.

Because infants cannot communicate their feelings or needs verbally, it is especially important to respect a parent's perception that "something is wrong". Nonspecific concerns about a young infant's behaviour, feeding, or sleep pattern may be tip-offs to a serious underlying illness or injury.

Consider the best location for performing your initial assessment. Although separating a 2-week-old from a parent will not cause distress, an older infant in stable condition will be calmest in a parent's arms. Make sure that your hands and stethoscope are warm—a startled, crying infant will be difficult to examine. Be opportunistic with your examination. If the child is quiet, listen to the heart and lungs first, perhaps listening over the clothes before you expose the chest and disturb the infant. If a young infant starts crying, letting the baby suck on a dummy or gloved finger may quiet the child enough to allow you to complete your assessment. Jingling keys or shining a penlight may distract an older infant for long enough for you to finish an examination.

Toddler

The toddler period includes the ages from 1 to 3 years. It includes the "terrible twos", a behavioural manifestation of the child's struggle between continued dependence on parents for food, shelter, and love and his or her emerging drive for independence. Children in this age group are not capable of reasoning, and they have a poorly developed sense of cause and effect. Language development is occurring rapidly, as is the ability to explore the world by crawling, walking, running, and climbing. Many toddlers will begin to have associations—possibly negative—with health care providers.

Your assessment of a toddler begins with observation of the child's interactions with the parent, vocalisations, and mobility, measured through the Paediatric Assessment Triangle (PAT), which is described in detail later. Examine a toddler in stable condition on the parent's lap. Get down to the child's level, sitting or squatting for the examination. You may need to be creative to get a good examination on a toddler with stranger anxiety: Use a parent to lift the shirt so that you can count respiratory rate, or have the parent press on the abdomen to see if that appears painful. Use play and distraction techniques whenever possible—listening to the doll's chest first may buy you a few minutes of cooperation. Offer toddlers limited choices when possible because they like to be in control. If you ask yes or no questions, the answer is likely to be "No"! Consider saving the more upsetting parts of the examination, such as palpating a tender abdomen or examining an injured extremity, for last. Be flexible in your approach—some toddlers will not let you complete an orderly head-to-toe examination.

Preschool-Age Child

During the preschool years (3 to 5 years), the child is becoming much more verbal and interactive. He or she can understand directions and be engaged with an activity or set of goals.

At the Scene

Keep infants and young children close to their parents during your assessment to help them feel safe and to improve your ability to perform the assessment.

Generally, a preschooler will be able to tell you what hurts and may have a story to share about the illness or injury. Preschoolers will understand as you explain what you are going to do, but choose your words carefully because preschoolers are very literal. Saying "I'm going take your pulse" may lead preschoolers to believe that you are taking something from them and wonder if you plan to give it back! Speak to them in very plain language about what you are going to do and provide lots of reassurance—this is the stage of monsters under the bed and many other fears.

As you perform your assessment, take advantage of the child's curiosity and desire to cooperate. If the patient is in medically stable condition, offer to take turns with the child in listening to the heart and lungs. Let the preschooler play with or hold equipment that is safe. To help give the child some sense of control, offer simple choices. Avoid yes or no questions. Set limits on behaviour if the child acts out. For the most part, you should be able to talk a preschooler through an orderly head-to-toe examination.

School-Age Child

As a child enters the school-age period (5 to 12 years), he or she becomes much more analytic and capable of abstract thought. At this age, the child can understand cause and effect. School-age children will have their own stories to tell about the illness or injury and may have their own ideas about the care to be given. By 8 years, the child's anatomy and physiology are similar to those of adults.

Ask the child about the history leading to calling 999 and let the child describe the symptoms, rather than focusing on the parent. Explain what you plan to do in simple language, and answer the child's questions. Give the child appropriate choices and control whenever possible, and provide ongoing reassurance and encouragement.

Adolescent

The adolescent years, from 13 to 18 years, can be difficult. Adolescents are struggling with issues of independence, body image, sexuality, and peer pressure. Friends are key support figures, and this is a time of experimentation and risk-taking behaviours.

With respect to CPR and foreign body airway obstruction procedures, once secondary sexual characteristics have developed (breasts or facial/axillary hair), the child should be treated as an adult. During the assessment, you must address the patient. Failure to do so can result in the adolescent feeling left out of his or her own care, which can alienate the patient, making it difficult to get an accurate assessment or give appropriate treatment. Encourage the patient's questions and involvement. Also, provide accurate information—a teen may become alienated and uncooperative if you are suspected of being misleading. When you perform the physical examination, respect the patient's privacy. If the adolescent's friends are present, he or she may want them to remain during the assessment. Let the patient have as much control over the situation as appropriate.

Parents of Ill or Injured Children

The majority of children you will treat will come with at least one parent or carer. Thus, in many paediatric calls, you will be dealing with more than one patient—even if only the child is ill or injured. Serious illness or injury to a child is one of the most stressful situations parents can face. Some may react to this stress by becoming angry—at the fact that their child is sick, at the person or situation that caused the injury, or at you simply because they need someone to blame! Other parents will be frightened or guilty about the circumstances that led to the illness or injury. Establishing rapport with parents is vital, however, because they will be a source of important information and assistance. Children look to their parents when they are frightened and often mimic their response, so helping calm a parent may also help the patient cope.

Approach stressed parents in a calm, quiet, and professional manner. Enlist their help in caring for the child. Along the way, explain what you are doing and provide honest reassurance and support. Above all, don't blame the parent for what has happened. Finally, transport at least one parent or carer with the child.

If the parent is extremely emotional, provide support, but remember that your first priority is the child. Don't let a distraught or aggressive parent interfere with your care. If necessary, enlist the help of other family members or the police.

Paediatric Assessment

Just as your general approach to a paediatric patient differs somewhat from your approach to an adult patient, so, too, will your assessment. In particular, you may need to adapt your assessment skills.

General Impression Using the Paediatric Assessment Triangle

After ensuring scene safety, the first step in an initial assessment of any patient begins with your general assessment of how the patient looks (the "sick–not sick" classification). An assessment tool called the <u>Paediatric Assessment Triangle (PAT)</u> **Figure 41-2 ▶** has been developed to help ambulance clinicians form a "from-the-doorway" general impression of paediatric patients. Paramedics with experience in treating ill and injured children intuitively use some version of the PAT to make the important distinction between sick and not-sick patients. The PAT standardises this approach by including three elements—the child's appearance, work of breathing, and circulation—that collectively paint an accurate clinical picture of the patient's cardiopulmonary status and level of consciousness. It applies a rapid, hands-off systematic approach to observing an ill or injured child and helps answer three questions:

- Is this patient sick or not sick?

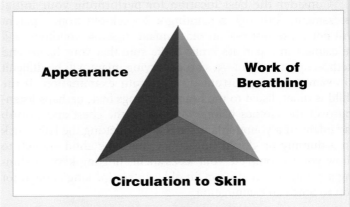

Figure 41-2 The Paediatric Assessment Triangle.

At the Scene

Use the PAT to help with your hands-off, from-the-doorway general impression of paediatric patients.

- What is the most likely physiological abnormality?
- Does this child require emergency treatment?

Appearance

The first element of the PAT is the child's appearance. In many cases, this is the most important factor in determining the severity of illness, the need for treatment, and the response to therapy. Appearance reflects the adequacy of ventilation, oxygenation, brain perfusion, body homeostasis, and central nervous system (CNS) function. The TICLS (tickles) mnemonic highlights the most important features of a child's appearance: Tone, Interactiveness, Consolability, Look or gaze, and Speech or cry **Table 41-1 ▶**.

To assess appearance, observe the child from a distance, allowing the child to interact with the parent or carer as he or she chooses. Walk through the characteristics of the TICLS mnemonic while observing the child from the doorway. Delay touching the patient until you have developed your general impression because the child may become agitated by your touch. Unless a child is unconscious or critically ill, take your time in assessing his or her general appearance by observation before you begin the hands-on assessment and take vital signs. **Figure 41-3 ▶** and **Figure 41-4 ▶** demonstrate examples of an infant with a normal appearance and one with an appearance that worries you.

An abnormal appearance may result from numerous underlying physiological abnormalities. A child may show evidence of inadequate oxygenation or ventilation, as in respiratory emergencies; inadequate brain perfusion, as from cardiovascular emergencies; systemic abnormalities or metabolic derangements,

Table 41-1	Characteristics of Appearance: The TICLS Mnemonic
Characteristic	**Features to Look For**
Tone	Is the child moving or resisting examination vigorously? Does the child have good muscle tone? Or is the child limp, listless, or flaccid?
Interactiveness	How alert is the child? How readily does a person, object, or sound distract the child or draw the child's attention? Will the child reach for, grasp, and play with a toy or examination instrument, like a penlight torch or tongue blade? Or is the child uninterested in playing or interacting with the parent or ambulance clinician?
Consolability	Can the child be consoled or comforted by the parent or by the ambulance clinician? Or is the child's crying or agitation unrelieved by gentle reassurance?
Look or gaze	Does the child fix his or her gaze on a face, or is there a "nobody home", glassy-eyed stare?
Speech or cry	Is the child's cry strong and spontaneous or weak or high-pitched? Is the content of speech age-appropriate or confused or garbled?

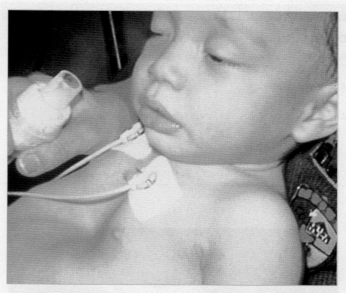

Figure 41-4 A child with an abnormal appearance. A limp child unable to maintain eye contact may be critically ill or injured.

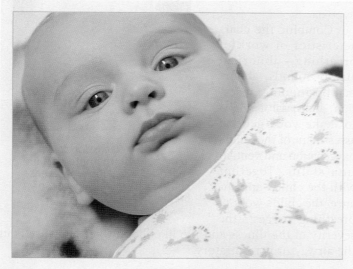

Figure 41-3 A child with a normal appearance. An infant or child who is not very sick will make good eye contact.

such as with poisoning, infection, or hypoglycaemia; or acute or chronic brain injury. In any event, a child with a grossly abnormal appearance is seriously ill and requires immediate life-support interventions and transport. The remainder of the PAT—work of breathing and circulation—plus the initial assessment may help identify the cause of the abnormal appearance and determine the severity of a child's illness and the need for treatment and transport to hospital.

Work of Breathing

A child's work of breathing is often a better assessment of his or her oxygenation and ventilation status than the auscultation or respiratory rate. The work of breathing reflects the child's attempt to compensate for abnormalities in oxygenation and ventilation and, therefore, it is a proxy for effectiveness of gas exchange. The hands-off assessment of work of breathing includes listening for abnormal airway sounds and looking for signs of increased breathing effort Table 41-2 ▶ .

Some abnormal airway sounds can be heard without a stethoscope and can indicate the likely physiology and anatomical location of the breathing problem. For example, snoring, muffled or hoarse voice, or stridor can indicate obstruction at the level of the oropharynx, glottis or supraglottic structures, or glottis or subglottic structures, respectively. Such an upper airway obstruction may result from croup, bacterial upper airway infections, or bleeding or oedema.

Lower airway obstruction is suggested by abnormal grunting or wheezing. Grunting is a form of auto-PEEP (positive end-expiratory pressure), a way to distend the lower respiratory air sacs or alveoli to promote maximum gas exchange. Grunting involves exhaling against a partially closed glottis. This short, low-pitched sound is best heard at the end of exhalation and is often mistaken for whimpering. Grunting suggests moderate to severe hypoxia and is seen with lower airway conditions such as pneumonia and pulmonary oedema. It reflects poor gas exchange because of fluid in the lower airways and air sacs. Wheezing is a musical tone caused by air being forced through

Table 41-2	Characteristics of Work of Breathing
Characteristic	**Features to Look For**
Abnormal airway sounds	Snoring, muffled or hoarse speech, stridor, grunting or wheezing
Abnormal posturing	Sniffing position, tripod position, refusing to lie down
Recession	Supraclavicular, intercostal, subcostal, or substernal recession of the chest wall; head bobbing in infants
Flaring	Flaring of the nares on inspiration

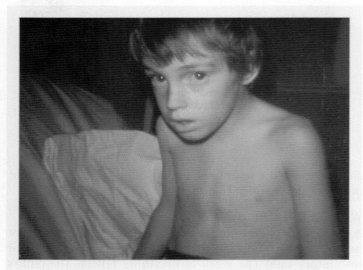

Figure 41-5 A child in a sniffing position is trying to align the airway to increase patency and improve airflow.

constricted or partially blocked small airways. It often occurs during exhalation only but can occur during inspiration and expiration during severe asthma attacks. Although this sound is often heard only by auscultation, severe obstruction may result in wheezing that is audible even without a stethoscope.

Abnormal positioning and recession are physical signs of increased work of breathing that can easily be assessed without touching the patient. A child who is in the sniffing position is trying to align the axes of the airways to improve patency and increase air flow Figure 41-5 ▲ ; such a position often reflects a severe upper airway obstruction. The child who refuses to lie down or who leans forward on outstretched arms (tripoding) is creating the optimal mechanical advantage to use accessory muscles of respiration Figure 41-6 ▶ .

Recession represents the recruitment of accessory muscles of respiration to provide more "muscle power" to move air into the lungs in the face of airway or lung disease or injury. To observe recession optimally, expose the child's chest. Recession is a more useful measure of work of breathing in children than in adults because a child's chest wall is less muscular, so the inward excursion of skin and soft

tissue between the ribs is more apparent. Recession may be evident in the supraclavicular area (above the clavicle), the intercostal area (between the ribs), the subcostal area (below the rib line), or the substernal area (under the sternum) Figure 41-7 ▶ . Another form of recession that is seen only in infants is head bobbing, the use of neck muscles to help breathing during severe hypoxia. The infant extends the neck as he or she inhales, then allows the head to fall forward during exhalation. Nasal flaring is the exaggerated opening of the nostrils during laboured inspiration and indicates moderate to severe hypoxia.

Combine the characteristics of work of breathing—abnormal airway sounds, abnormal positioning, recession, and nasal flaring—to make your general assessment of the child's oxygenation and ventilation status. Together with the child's appearance, the child's work of breathing suggests the severity of the illness and the likelihood that the cause is in the airway or is respiratory.

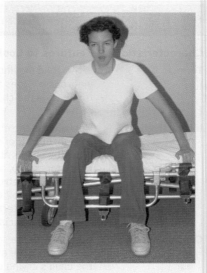

Figure 41-6 A child in a tripod position is maximising his or her accessory muscles of respiration.

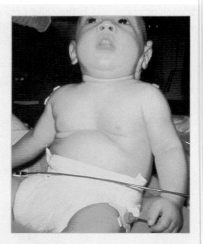

Figure 41-7 Recession can occur in the suprasternal, intercostal, subcostal, and substernal areas and indicate increased work of breathing.

Circulation

The goal of rapid circulatory assessment is to determine the adequacy of cardiac output and core perfusion. When cardiac output diminishes, the body responds by shunting circulation from nonessential areas (eg, skin) toward vital organs. Therefore, circulation to the skin reflects the overall status of core circulation. The three characteristics considered when assessing the circulation are pallor, mottling, and cyanosis Table 41-3 ▶ .

Pallor may be the initial sign of poor circulation or even the only visual sign in a child with compensated shock. It indicates

Table 41-3	Characteristics of Circulation to Skin
Characteristic	**Features to Look For**
Pallor	White or pale skin or mucous membranes from inadequate blood flow
Mottling	Patchy skin discolouration due to vasoconstriction or vasodilation
Cyanosis	Bluish discolouration of skin and mucous membranes

At the Scene

Note the line of demarcation of any mottling or pallor on the child's limbs during your initial assessment. An increase in mottling or pallor with movement toward the core of the body indicates a worsening "shell to core" shunt from peripheral vasoconstriction.

reflex peripheral vasoconstriction that is shunting blood toward the core. Pallor may also indicate anaemia or hypoxia.

Mottling reflects vasomotor instability in the capillary beds demonstrated by patchy areas of vasoconstriction and vasodilation. It may also be a child's physiological response to a cold environment.

Cyanosis, a bluish discolouration of the skin and mucous membranes, is the most extreme visual indicator of poor perfusion or poor oxygenation. Acrocyanosis, blue hands or feet in an infant younger than 2 months, is distinct from cyanosis; it is a normal finding when a young infant is cold. True cyanosis is seen in the skin and mucous membranes and is a late finding of respiratory failure or shock.

After assessing the child's appearance and work of breathing, visually scan the child's skin and mucous membranes looking for pallor, mottling, and cyanosis. You can then combine the three pieces of the PAT to estimate the severity of illness and the likely underlying pathological cause. For example, a child with an abnormal appearance with poor circulation may be in shock from a cardiovascular cause.

Initial Assessment

After using the PAT to form a general impression of the patient, you will need to complete the rest of the initial assessment—that is, you must assess the child's mental status and ABCs and prioritise the care and need for transport. Threats to the ABCs are managed as they are found, providing a prioritised sequence of life-support interventions to reverse critical physiological abnormalities. The steps are the same as with adults, albeit with differences related to the child's anatomy, physiology, and signs of distress.

Early in your assessment of a young child, you will need to estimate the child's weight, because much of your care will depend on the child's size. Ask the parent how much the child

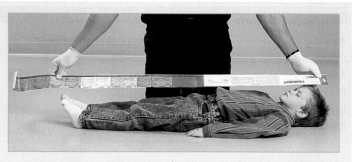

Figure 41-8 Use of a length-based resuscitation tape is one way to estimate a child's weight and identify the correct size for paediatric equipment and medication doses.

weighs or make your own estimate, using a tool such as a length-based resuscitation tape **Figure 41-8**.

1. Measure the child's length, from head to heel, with the tape (with the red portion at the head).
2. Note the weight in kilograms that corresponds to the child's measured length at the heel.
3. If the child is longer than the tape, use adult equipment and medication doses.
4. From the tape, identify appropriate equipment sizes.
5. From the tape, identify appropriate medication doses.

Airway

The PAT may suggest the presence of an airway obstruction based on abnormal airway sounds and increased work of breathing. As with adults, determine if the airway is open and the patient has adequate chest rise with breathing. Check for mucus, blood, or a foreign body in the mouth or airway. If there is potential obstruction from the tongue or soft tissues, position the airway and suction as necessary. Determine whether the airway is open and patent, partially obstructed, or totally obstructed. Do not keep the suction tip or catheter in the back of a child's throat too long because young patients are extremely sensitive to vagal stimuli and the heart rate may plummet.

Breathing

The breathing component of the initial assessment involves calculating the respiratory rate, auscultating breath sounds, and checking pulse oximetry for oxygen saturation. Verify the respiratory rate per minute by counting the number of chest rises over 60 seconds. Healthy infants may show periodic breathing, or variable respiratory rates with short periods of apnoea (< 20 s). As a consequence, counting for only 10 to 15 seconds may give a falsely low respiratory rate. Interpreting the respiratory rate requires knowing the normal values for the child's age **Table 41-4** and putting the respiratory rate in context with the rest of the PAT and initial assessment. Rapid respiratory rates may simply reflect high fever, anxiety, pain, or excitement. Normal rates, by contrast, may occur in a child who has been breathing rapidly with increased work of breathing and is becoming fatigued. Serial assessment of respiratory rates may

Table 41-4	Normal Respiratory Rate by Age
Age	**Respiratory Rate (breaths/min)**
Infant	25–50
Toddler	20–30
Preschool-age child	20–25
School-age child	15–20
Adolescent	12–16

Table 41-5	Normal Pulse Rates for Age
Age	**Pulse Rate (beats/min)**
Infant	100–160
Toddler	90–150
Preschool-age child	80–140
School-age child	70–120
Adolescent	60–100

At the Scene

Consider pulse oximetry readings in terms of the environmental context and the physiological status of the child. Peripheral vasoconstriction from hypothermia or poor perfusion may alter these readings. Always correlate the pulse oximetry waveform with the patient's pulse rate and ECG reading.

be especially useful because the trend may be more accurate than any single value.

Auscultate the breath sounds with a stethoscope over the midaxillary line to hear abnormal lung sounds during inhalation and exhalation. Listen for extra breath sounds such as inspiratory crackles, wheezes, or rhonchi; rhonchi often indicate harsh breath sounds or sounds that may be transmitted from the upper airways. If you cannot determine whether the sounds are being generated in the lungs or the upper airway, hold the stethoscope over the nose or trachea and listen. Also, listen to the breath sounds for adequacy of air movement. Diminished breath sounds may signal severe respiratory distress. Auscultation over the trachea may also help distinguish stridor from other sounds.

Check the pulse oximetry reading to determine the oxygen saturation while the child breathes ambient air. You can place the pulse oximetry probe on a young child's finger just as you would with an adult. In infants or young children who try to remove the probe, it may be helpful to place the probe on a toe, possibly with a sock covering it. A pulse oximetry reading of greater than 95% saturation while breathing room air indicates good oxygenation.

As with the respiratory rate, evaluate the pulse oximetry reading in the context of the PAT and remainder of the initial assessment. A child with a normal pulse oximetry reading, for example, may be expending increasing amounts of energy and increasing the work of breathing to maintain his or her oxygen saturation. The PAT and initial assessment would identify the respiratory distress and point to the need for immediate intervention despite the normal oxygen saturation.

Circulation

The information obtained from the PAT about circulation to the skin directs the next step of the initial assessment. Integrate this assessment of circulation with the pulse rate and quality,

skin CTC (colour, temperature, and condition plus capillary refill time), and blood pressure to obtain an overall assessment of the child's circulatory status.

Obtain the child's pulse rate by listening to the heart or feeling the pulse for 60 seconds. As with respiratory rates in paediatric patients, it is important to know normal pulse rates based on age (Table 41-5 ▲). Interpret the pulse rate within the context of the overall history, PAT, and initial assessment. Tachycardia may indicate early hypoxia or shock or a less serious condition such as fever, anxiety, pain, or excitement.

Feel for the pulse to ascertain the rate and quality of pulsations. If you cannot find a peripheral (distal) pulse (that is, radial or brachial), feel for a central pulse (that is, femoral or carotid). Check the femoral pulse in infants and young children and the carotid pulse in older children and adolescents. As with adults, if there is no pulse, start CPR.

After checking the pulse rate, do a hands-on evaluation of skin CTC. Check whether the hands and feet are warm or cool to the touch. Check capillary refill time on the sternum or the forehead of the child. A normal refill time is less than 2 seconds. These two pieces of information need to be placed in context with the PAT and remainder of initial assessment because cool extremities and delayed capillary refill are commonly seen in a child in a cool environment.

The last step in the circulation assessment is to measure the blood pressure. It may be difficult to obtain an accurate measurement in a young child or infant because of a lack of cooperation and need for proper cuff size. Nevertheless, you should attempt to measure the blood pressure on the upper arm or thigh, making sure the cuff has a width two thirds the length of the upper arm or thigh. One formula for determining the lower limit of acceptable blood pressure in children ages 1 to 10 years is this: minimal systolic blood pressure = 80 + (2 × age in years).

At the Scene

Blood pressure is just one component of the overall assessment of paediatric patients. Determination of physiological stability should be based on all data collected from the PAT, physical examination, and initial vital signs. Remember that compensated shock can exist in the face of adequate blood pressure.

Table 41-6	Normal Blood Pressure for Age
Age	Minimal Systolic Blood Pressure (mm Hg)
Infant	>70
Toddler	>80
Preschool-age child	>80
School-age child	>80
Adolescent	>90

Table 41-7	AVPU Scale		
Category	Stimulus	Response Type	Reaction
Alert	Normal environment	Appropriate	Normal interactiveness for age
Verbal	Simple command or sound stimulus	Appropriate	Responds to name
		Inappropriate	Nonspecific or confused
Painful	Pain	Appropriate	Withdraws from pain
		Inappropriate	Makes sound or moves without purpose or localisation of pain
		Pathological	Posturing
Unresponsive			No perceptible response to any stimulus

At the Scene

For children 1 to 10 years, calculate the lower limit of acceptable blood pressure for age with the following formula:

Minimal systolic blood pressure = 80 + (2 × age in years)

For example, a 2-year-old toddler should have a minimal systolic blood pressure of 84; a lower rate indicates decompensated shock. (Table 41-6 ▲ shows normal minimal systolic blood pressure values for different ages.) Given the technical difficulty of trying to measure a blood pressure, make one attempt in the prehospital environment; if unsuccessful, move on to the rest of the assessment.

Mental Status

Your general impression of the patient should provide the first clues about the child's neurological status. As you begin the initial assessment, use the AVPU scale Table 41-7 ▲ to evaluate the cerebral cortex. The AVPU scale is a conventional way of assessing any patient's level of consciousness (LOC) or mental status. It categorises motor response based on simple response to stimuli, classifying the patient as alert, responsive to verbal stimuli, responsive to painful stimuli, or unresponsive.

After evaluating the patient's response with the AVPU scale, assess the pupillary response to a beam of light to assess brain stem response. Next, evaluate motor activity, looking for symmetric movement of the extremities, convulsions, posturing, or flaccidity. Combine this information with the PAT results to determine the child's neurological status.

Exposure Considerations

Proper exposure of the child is necessary to complete the initial assessment. During the PAT, the child will have been at least partially undressed to assess the work of breathing and circulation. It is also important to evaluate the child from head to toe and to look at the child's back during the initial assessment. Be careful to avoid heat loss, especially in infants, by covering the child up as soon as possible. Keep the temperature in the ambulance high, and use blankets when necessary.

Assessment of Pain

Numerous studies have found that children are much less likely than adults to receive effective pain medications. Inadequate treatment of pain has many adverse effects on the child and family. Pain causes morbidity and misery for the child and parents, and it interferes with your ability accurately to assess physiological abnormalities. Children who do not receive appropriate analgesia may be more likely to have exaggerated pain responses to subsequent painful procedures. Also, post-traumatic stress may be more common among children who experience pain during an illness or injury.

Assessment of pain must consider developmental age. The ability to identify pain improves with the age of the child. In infants and preverbal children, it may be difficult to distinguish crying and agitation due to hypoxia, hunger, or pain. Further assessment and discussion with parents about their perceptions of the child's pain are essential to identify pain in this age group. For verbal children, pain scales using pictures of facial expressions, such as the Wong-Baker FACES scale, may prove helpful Figure 41-9 ▶ .

Remaining calm and providing quiet, professional reassurance to parents and child is critical for managing paediatric pain and anxiety. A calm parent will help keep the child calm and more at ease. Distraction techniques with toys or stories may prove helpful in reducing pain, as may visual imagery techniques and music. Sucrose dummies may reduce pain in neonates. Pharmacological methods for reducing pain—such as paracetamol, opiates, benzodiazepines, and Entonox—are available to paramedics in a number of ambulance services. The benefit of such analgesic or anxiolytic medication must be weighed against the risks of its administration (respiratory depression, bradycardia, hypoxaemia, and hypotension are potential side effects of sedatives), including the potential route of administration. Medications that are given intravenously are

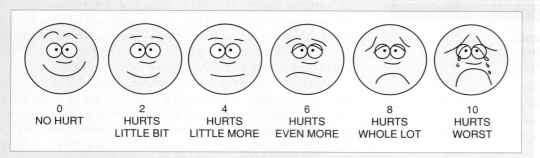

| 0 NO HURT | 2 HURTS LITTLE BIT | 4 HURTS LITTLE MORE | 6 HURTS EVEN MORE | 8 HURTS WHOLE LOT | 10 HURTS WORST |

Figure 41-9 Pictures such as the Wong-Baker FACES Pain Rating Scale allow for self-assessment of pain in young children.

From Hockenberry MJ, Wilson D, Wikelstein ML: *Wong's Essentials of Paediatric Nursing*, ed. 7, St. Louis, 2005, p. 1259. Used with permission. Copyright, Mosby.

Special Considerations

Consider pain to be a vital sign in paediatric patients. Assess and reassess pain along with the other vital signs. Treat pain accordingly.

often most effective at reducing pain, but they require establishing intravenous (IV) access, which itself is a painful procedure.

Today, assessment of pain is recognised as part of vital sign assessment, and management of paediatric pain and anxiety should be a routine part of prehospital care. This effort requires a thorough understanding of nonpharmacological techniques, drugs, potential drug contraindications and complications, and management of the complications.

Transport Decision

After completing the initial assessment and beginning resuscitation when necessary, you must make a crucial decision: whether to transport the child to the accident and emergency (A&E) department immediately or continue the additional assessment and treatment on scene. Immediate transport is imperative if the emergency call is for trauma and the child has a serious mechanism of injury (MOI), a physiological abnormality, or a potentially significant anatomical abnormality or if the scene is unsafe. In these cases, stabilise the spine, manage the airway and breathing, stop external bleeding, and begin transport. Attempt vascular access on the way to the A&E department. If the emergency call is for an illness, the decision to stay or go is less clear-cut and depends on the following factors: expected benefits of treatment, ambulance service guidelines, comfort level, and transport time.

Additional Assessment

Focused History and Physical Examination

The focused history and physical examination, which is performed on medical and trauma patients, has four objectives:

- To obtain a complete description of the chief complaint (for example, OPQRST and SAMPLE)
- To determine the MOI or nature of an illness

You are the Paramedic Part 2

You use the PAT to form a general impression of the patient. Based on his abnormal appearance and circulation, you determine that the child is sick and requires rapid treatment. The combination of your knowledge that children are more prone to head injuries than adults because of the larger size and weight of their heads compared with rest of their bodies, the MOI, and your general impression of the patient leads you to suspect that the child may have a closed head injury.

You immediately assign one of the fire fighters the task of maintaining manual cervical spine immobilisation. You ask your partner to apply 100% supplemental oxygen via nonrebreathing mask as you expose the child to complete a rapid trauma assessment. This examination reveals a mildly distended abdomen and an obviously deformed right thigh. You ask your colleague to issue a pre-alert, citing the combination of your physical assessment findings and the MOI.

Vital Signs	Recording Time: 5 Minutes
Skin	Pale, cool, and dry
Pulse	170 beats/min, regular; weak distally but strong centrally
Blood pressure	86/48 mm Hg
Respirations	40 breaths/min; unlaboured, clear breath sounds
SpO_2	99% on nonrebreathing mask at 12 l/min of oxygen
Capillary refill	2–3 seconds

3. What do you need to carefully monitor the patient for?
4. Which interventions should you consider at this point, if any?

Table 41-8	**Paediatric SAMPLE Components**
Component	**Explanation**
Signs and symptoms	Onset and nature of symptoms of pain or fever
	Age-appropriate signs of distress
Allergies	Known drug reactions or other allergies
Medications	Exact names and doses of ongoing drugs (including general-sales-list, prescribed, herbal, and recreational drugs)
	Timing and amount of last dose
	Time and dose of analgesics or antipyretics
Past medical history	Previous illnesses or injuries
	Immunisations
	History of pregnancy, labour, delivery (infants and toddlers)
Last oral intake	Timing of the child's last food or drink, including bottle or breastfeeding
Events leading to illness or injury	Key events leading to the current incident
	Fever history

- To perform a rapid trauma or medical assessment or a focused or vectored physical examination of a specific body part or body system
- To obtain baseline vital signs

If the child seems to be in physiologically unstable condition based on the initial assessment, you may decide to begin transport immediately and conduct the focused history and physical examination in the ambulance. If the child is in stable condition and the scene is safe, perform the focused history and physical examination on the scene, before transport. The detailed physical examination is conducted en route to the hospital for trauma patients with a significant MOI. It can be done on the scene if you are waiting for the ambulance to arrive or if patient removal is delayed because of entrapment. As opposed to the initial assessment, which addresses immediately life-threatening pathological problems, the focused history and physical examination narrows the focus to assessing the body part or body system specifically involved, obtaining a complete set of baseline vital signs, elaborating on the chief complaint (ie, OPQRST), and obtaining a patient history (ie, SAMPLE).

To obtain the focused history, use the SAMPLE mnemonic **Table 41-8 ▲**. Tailor the physical examination to the child's age and developmental stage. In trauma patients, after the detailed physical examination is complete, reconsider the need for immediate transport.

Ongoing Assessment

The elements in the ongoing assessment include the PAT, reassessment of patient priority, vital signs (every 5 minutes if unstable condition and every 15 minutes if stable), assessment of the effectiveness of interventions (eg, medications adminis-

Documentation and Communication

Perform frequent reassessment of serial vital signs, and record them on your documentation form. By recording each set of vital signs, you can visualise trends and transfer important information to the accepting doctors.

tered, splints applied, bleeding controlled), and reassessment of the focused examination areas. Perform this kind of ongoing assessment on all patients to observe their response to treatment, to guide ongoing treatments, and to track the progression of identified pathological and anatomical problems. New problems may also be identified on reassessment. The elements in the ongoing assessment also guide the choice of an appropriate transport destination and your radio or telephone communications with hospital staff.

Respiratory Emergencies

Respiratory problems are among the most common medical emergencies that you will frequently encounter in children. Paediatric patients with a respiratory chief complaint will span the spectrum from mildly ill to near death. In paediatrics, respiratory failure and arrest precede the majority of cardiopulmonary arrests; by contrast, a primary cardiac event is the usual cause of sudden death in adults. Early identification and intervention can stop the progression from respiratory distress to cardiopulmonary failure and help to avert much paediatric morbidity and mortality.

General Assessment and Management

When faced with a respiratory emergency, the first step is to determine the severity of the disease: Is the patient in respiratory distress, respiratory failure, or respiratory arrest?

Respiratory distress entails increased work of breathing to maintain oxygenation and/or ventilation; that is, it is a compensated state in which increased work of breathing results in adequate pulmonary gas exchange. The hallmarks of respiratory distress—which is classified as mild, moderate, or severe—are recession (suprasternal, intercostal, subcostal), abdominal breathing, nasal flaring, and grunting.

A patient in respiratory failure can no longer compensate for the underlying pathological or anatomical problem by increased work of breathing, so hypoxia and/or carbon dioxide retention occur. Signs of respiratory failure may include decreased or absent recession owing to fatigue of the chest wall muscles, altered mental status owing to inadequate oxygenation and ventilation of the brain, and an abnormally low respiratory rate **Table 41-9 ▶**. Respiratory failure is a decompensated state, requiring urgent intervention to ensure adequate oxygenation and ventilation and prevent respiratory arrest. Do not be afraid to assist ventilations at this point if you judge the tidal volume or respiratory effort to be inadequate.

Table 41-9	Signs of Impending Respiratory Failure
Assess	**Sign**
Mental status	Agitation, restlessness, confusion, lethargy (VPU of AVPU)
Skin colour	Cyanosis, pallor
Respiratory rate	Tachypnoea → bradypnoea → apnoea
Respiratory effort	Severe recession, nasal flaring, grunting, paradoxical abdominal motion, tripod positioning
Auscultation	Stridor, wheezing, rales, or diminished air movement
Blood oxygen saturation	< 90% with supplemental oxygen
Pulse rate	Tachycardia, bradycardia, or cardiac arrest

At the Scene

Initiate aggressive airway management and ventilatory support with a bag-valve-mask device and supplemental oxygen as soon as possible for a child with respiratory failure.

Table 41-10	Key Questions in Respiratory Emergencies
Component	**Key Questions**
Signs and symptoms	Shortness of breath? Hoarseness? Stridor? Wheezing? Cough? Chest pain? Choking? Rash/Hives? Cyanosis?
Allergies	Known drug or food allergies; smoke exposure
Medications	Names and doses of ongoing medications; recent use of corticosteroids
Past medical history	History of asthma, chronic lung disease, heart problems, prematurity; prior hospitalisations and intubation for breathing problems; history of choking or anaphylaxis; immunisations
Last oral intake	Timing of last food, including bottle or breastfeeding
Events leading to illness or injury	Fever history or recent illness; history of injury to chest; history of choking on food or object

Respiratory arrest implies that the patient is not breathing spontaneously. Administer immediate bag-valve-mask ventilation with supplemental oxygen to prevent progression to cardiopulmonary arrest. Resuscitation of a child from respiratory arrest is often successful, whereas resuscitation of a child in cardiopulmonary arrest usually fails.

By combining the three components of the PAT, you can determine the severity of disease before you even touch the patient. The child's appearance will give you clues about the adequacy of CNS oxygenation and ventilation. If a child with trouble breathing is sleepy, assume the child is hypoxic. Assess the work of breathing by noting the patient's position of comfort, presence or absence of recession, and grunting or flaring. A patient who prefers to sit upright, in the sniffing position, or to use his or her arms for support is trying to optimise breathing mechanics. Deep recession heralds the use of accessory muscles of respiration to move air. Assessment of circulation for the presence of pallor or cyanosis will give further information on the adequacy of oxygenation.

After forming a general impression using the PAT, move on to the hands-on initial assessment. For respiratory emergencies, focus on the child's airway and breathing. Assess the airway by listening for stridor in awake patients or checking for obstruction in sluggish patients. Assess breathing by determining the child's respiratory rate, listening to the lungs for adequacy of air entry and abnormal breath sounds, and checking pulse oximetry readings. A rate that is too low may be more worrisome than a rate that is too high for the child's age. The presence of abnormal breath sounds may identify the anatomical or pathological abnormality and suggest a likely diagnosis.

For example, symmetric, diffuse wheezing implies bronchospasm and possibly asthma, whereas diffuse rhonchi, rales, and wheezing in an infant or toddler are typical signs of lower airway inflammation associated with bronchiolitis. The presence of stridor in the context of clear lung fields is consistent with upper airway obstruction, often due to croup. Poor air entry with decreased breath sounds is an ominous sign that must be addressed immediately. Determine oxygen saturation by assessing pulse oximetry via a finger or toe or, in a small infant, around the foot.

Your determination of whether the patient is in respiratory distress, respiratory failure, or respiratory arrest will drive your next steps, by indicating the urgency for treatment and transport. You can obtain the SAMPLE history at the scene or during transport, depending on the patient's stability. ◖ Table 41-10 ▲ lists key questions to ask during a respiratory emergency.

Most paediatric patients with a primary respiratory complaint will have respiratory distress and require only generic treatment. Allow the child to assume a position of comfort, and provide supplemental oxygen. The choice of oxygen delivery method will depend on the severity of illness and the child's developmental level. Young children may become agitated by a nasal cannula or face mask. Because crying and thrashing increase metabolic demands and oxygen consumption, you must weigh the benefits of this therapy against the potential cost. Allowing a caregiver to deliver blow-by oxygen to a calm toddler may be your best choice, if the child does not show signs of respiratory failure.

As a child becomes fatigued, respiratory distress may progress to respiratory failure. As part of your ongoing assessment, electronically monitor the patient's pulse rate, respiratory

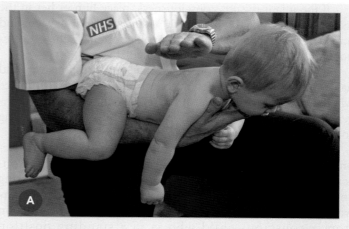

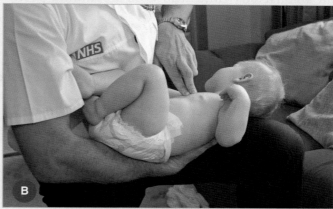

Figure 41-10 Perform back slaps and chest thrusts to clear a foreign body airway obstruction in an infant. **A.** Hold the infant face down with the body resting on your forearm. Support the jaw and face with your hand, and keep the head lower than the rest of the body. Give the infant five back slaps between the shoulder blades, using the heel of your hand. **B.** Give the infant five quick chest thrusts, using two fingers placed on the lower half of the sternum.

Special Considerations

Respiratory distress, respiratory failure, and respiratory arrest exist along a continuum. Intervene early to prevent progression to respiratory arrest in paediatric patients.

rate, and oxygen saturation. A significant change or trend in any of these variables requires prompt patient reassessment. You should also perform frequent reassessment to evaluate the effects of your treatment.

Upper Airway Emergencies

Foreign Body Aspiration or Obstruction

Infants and toddlers explore their environment by putting everything and anything into their mouths, resulting in a high risk of foreign body aspiration. Any small object or food item has the potential to obstruct a young child's narrow trachea. Peanuts, sweets, grapes, balloons, and small toys or pieces of toys are frequent offenders. Swallowed foreign bodies can also cause respiratory distress in infants and young children because a rigid oesophageal foreign body can compress the relative pliable trachea. In addition, the tongue, owing to its large size relative to the upper airway, frequently causes mild upper airway obstruction in a child with a decreased LOC and diminished muscle tone.

Suspect foreign body aspiration when you encounter signs of mild or severe airway obstruction on the PAT or initial assessment. An awake patient with stridor, increased work of breathing, and good colour on the PAT has mild upper airway obstruction. Auscultation may reveal fair to good air entry, and the presence of unilateral wheezing may tip you off to a foreign body lodged in a mainstem bronchus. In contrast, a patient with severe airway obstruction is likely to be cyanotic and unconscious when you arrive, owing to profound hypoxia. If the child has spontaneous respiratory effort, you will hear poor air entry, but you may *not* hear stridor owing to minimal air flow through the trachea. A typical SAMPLE history for foreign body aspiration reveals a previously healthy child with sudden onset of coughing, choking, or gagging while eating or playing.

Initial management of mild airway obstruction involves allowing the patient to assume a position of comfort, providing supplemental oxygen as tolerated, and transporting the child to an appropriate hospital. Avoid agitating the child because this stimulus could worsen the situation. Continuous monitoring and frequent reassessments are needed to ensure that the problem does not progress to severe airway obstruction.

In severe airway obstruction, the initial management steps are different for conscious and unconscious patients. For an infant who is responsive and conscious (Figure 41-10 ▶):

1. Hold the infant face down, with the body resting on your forearm. Support the infant's head and face with your hand, and keep the head lower than the rest of the body.

2. Deliver five back slaps between the shoulder blades using the heel of your hand.

3. Place your free hand behind the infant's head and back, and bring the infant upright on your thigh, sandwiching the infant's body between your two hands and arms. The infant's head should remain below the level of the body.

4. Give five quick chest thrusts in the same location and manner as for chest compressions, using two fingers placed on the lower half of the sternum. For larger infants, or if you have small hands, you can place the infant in your lap and turn the infant's whole body as a unit between back slaps and chest thrusts.

5. Check the airway. If you can see the foreign body now, remove it. If not, repeat the cycle as often as necessary. Do not stick your fingers in the child's mouth to remove an object unless you can actually visualise the object.

6. If the infant becomes unresponsive or apnoeic, open the airway, give 5 breaths and commence CPR.

If the infant regains consciousness, place him or her in the recovery position, administer 100% supplemental oxygen, and transport immediately. If you are unable to relieve the obstruction after several attempts, begin immediate transport.

If you have reason to believe that an unresponsive child has a foreign body obstruction, check the upper airway to see whether an object is visible. If so, try to remove it using a finger sweep motion. Never perform blind finger sweeps; doing so may push the object further into the airway.

Abdominal thrusts (alternating with back slaps) are recommended to relieve a severe airway obstruction in a conscious child. They increase the pressure in the chest, creating an artificial cough that may force a foreign body from the airway. Follow these steps to remove a foreign body obstruction from a conscious child who is in a standing position **Figure 41-11 ▾** :

1. Give five back slaps, striking the child firmly between the shoulder blades.
2. Give the child rapid, distinct abdominal thrusts in an upward direction. Be careful to avoid applying force to the lower ribcage or sternum.
3. Give five back slaps, repeating the above sequence until the child expels the foreign object or becomes unresponsive.
4. If the child becomes unresponsive, place him or her supine on a firm, flat surface and inspect the airway using the head tilt–chin lift. If you can see the foreign body, try to remove it. Do not perform blind finger sweeps.
5. Attempt rescue breathing. If the first attempt fails, reposition the head and try again.
6. If the airway remains obstructed, begin CPR with chest compressions at the 15:2 compression/ventilation ratio and prepare for immediate transport.

If you manage to clear the airway obstruction in an unresponsive child (older than 1 year), but he or she remains apnoeic and pulseless, begin CPR and attach the automated external defibrillator (AED) as soon as possible, using appropriately sized AED pads. If you are unable to relieve the obstruction after several attempts, transport immediately.

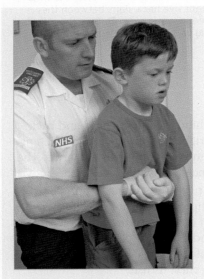

Figure 41-11 To relieve a foreign body obstruction in a responsive child who is standing, kneel behind the child, wrap your arms around his or her body, and place your fist just above the umbilicus and well below the xiphoid process.

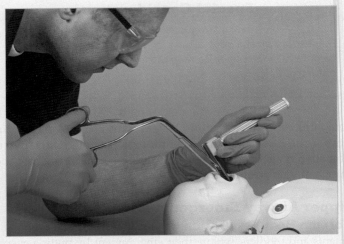

Figure 41-12 Using Magill forceps and direct laryngoscopy to remove foreign body airway obstruction.

If the BLS procedures do not dislodge the obstruction and severe airway obstruction remains, advanced airway procedures may be required. If the obstruction is more proximal, direct laryngoscopy with removal of the foreign body with Magill forceps may be successful **Figure 41-12 ▴** :

1. Hold the laryngoscope handle with your left hand.
2. Uncompensate the mouth by exerting thumb pressure on the chin.
3. Insert a paediatric straight blade into the mouth, and lift the tongue with the blade.
4. Exert gentle traction upward along the axis of the laryngoscope handle at a 45° angle, and advance the blade. Do not use the teeth or gums for leverage.
5. Watch the tip until the foreign body is visible. Do not go past the vocal cords.
6. Use suction to improve visibility if secretions are present.
7. Insert the Magill forceps into the mouth with the tips closed.
8. Grasp the foreign object and remove while looking directly at it.
9. Look at the airway to ensure that it is clear of debris. Remove the laryngoscope blade.

If you manage to remove the object, recheck the patient's breathing and circulation. Begin rescue breathing and CPR as needed and arrange for immediate transport. If direct laryngoscopy does not reveal the foreign body, use bag-valve-mask ventilation. If bag-valve-mask ventilation does not provide adequate ventilatory support, attempt to insert an advanced airway (such as ET tube or laryngeal mask airway). Immediate transport to an appropriate hospital is required.

Anaphylaxis

Anaphylaxis is a potentially life-threatening allergic reaction, triggered by exposure to an antigen (foreign protein). Food—especially nuts, shellfish, eggs, and milk—and bee stings are among the most common causes, although anaphylaxis to

curve. In some cases, bending the tube into the shape of a hockey stick is beneficial.

Preparing for and Performing Endotracheal Intubation

Paediatric patients should be preoxygenated (but not hyperventilated) with a bag-valve-mask device and 100% supplemental oxygen for at least 30 seconds before you attempt intubation using the "squeeze, release, release" technique. Adequate preoxygenation cannot be overemphasised because respiratory failure or arrest is the most common cause of cardiopulmonary arrest in the paediatric population. During this time, you must also ensure that the child's head is in the proper position—the neutral position for patients with suspected spinal trauma or the sniffing position for patients without trauma. Insert an airway adjunct if one is needed to ensure adequate ventilation. Apply cricoid pressure once positive-pressure ventilation is initiated,

and maintain it until the ET tube is correctly placed, verified, and secured.

Because stimulation of the parasympathetic nervous system and bradycardia can occur during intubation, you should apply a cardiac monitor if one is available. Use a pulse oximeter before, during, and after the intubation attempt to monitor the patient's pulse rate and oxygen saturation.

To perform endotracheal intubation in an infant or a child, follow the steps listed in **Skill Drill 41-4 ▾**:

1. Take universal precautions (gloves and face mask) **Step 1**.
2. Check, prepare, and assemble your equipment **Step 2**.
3. Manually open the patient's airway, and insert an adjunct if needed **Step 3**.

Skill Drill 41-4: Performing Paediatric Endotracheal Intubation

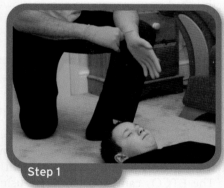

Step 1

Take universal precautions (gloves and face mask).

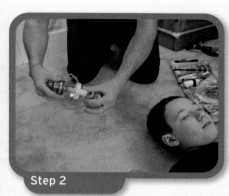

Step 2

Check, prepare, and assemble your equipment.

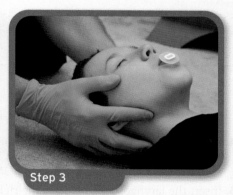

Step 3

Manually open the patient's airway and insert an adjunct if needed.

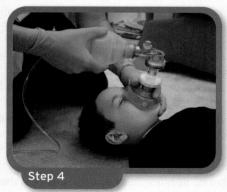

Step 4

Preoxygenate the child with a bag-valve-mask device and 100% oxygen for at least 30 seconds.

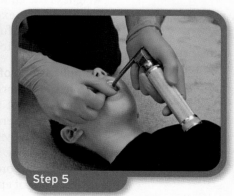

Step 5

Insert the laryngoscope blade in the right side of the mouth, and sweep the tongue to the left. Lift the tongue with firm, gentle pressure. Avoid using the teeth or gums as a fulcrum.

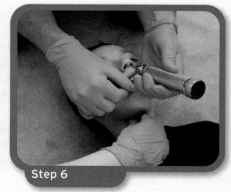

Step 6

Identify the vocal cords. Pay particular attention to the length of the tube that has been chosen. If the cords are not visible, instruct your partner to apply cricoid pressure.

Skill Drill 41-4: Performing Paediatric Endotracheal Intubation (*continued*)

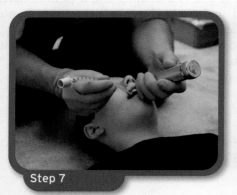

Step 7

Introduce the ET tube in the right corner of the patient's mouth.
   Pass the ET tube through the vocal cords to approximately 2 to 3 cm below the vocal cords. Inflate the cuff if you are using a cuffed tube.
   Attach an ETCO$_2$ detector.

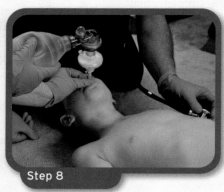

Step 8

Attach the bag-valve-mask device, ventilate, and auscultate for equal breath sounds.

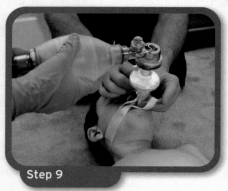

Step 9

Secure the ET tube. Reconfirm tube placement.

4. Preoxygenate the child with a bag-valve-mask device and 100% supplemental oxygen for at least 30 seconds (Step 4).

5. Insert the laryngoscope blade in the right side of the mouth, and sweep the tongue to the left. Lift the tongue with firm, gentle pressure. Avoid using the teeth or gums as a fulcrum (Step 5).

6. Identify the vocal cords. If they are not visible, instruct your partner to apply cricoid pressure (Step 6).

7. Introduce the ET tube in the right corner of the patient's mouth (Step 7). Pass the ET tube through the vocal cords to approximately 2 to 3 cm below the vocal cords. Inflate the cuff if you are using a cuffed tube. Attach an end-tidal carbon dioxide (ETCO$_2$) detector.

8. Attach the bag-valve-mask device, ventilate, and auscultate for equal breath sounds over each lateral chest wall high in the axillae. Ensure absence of breath sounds over the abdomen (Step 8).

9. Secure the ET tube, noting the placement of the distance marker at the patient's teeth or gums, and reconfirm tube placement (Step 9).

Although tape may be applied in several ways to secure ET tubes, no single method is failsafe. One person should always hold the tube in place while another secures the device.

A critical step in endotracheal intubation is confirmation of correct placement of the tube. Watch the ET tube pass through the vocal cords, listen for breath sounds, and document the presence of ETCO$_2$. The ETCO$_2$ can be detected by using a colourimetric monitor or can be measured by capnometry. The colourimetric devices, which should be selected based on the weight of the child, are very accurate, even in infants and small children. The exception is in cardiac arrest, a situation in which poor perfusion may result in levels of exhaled carbon dioxide too low to be detected by these devices.

Complications of Endotracheal Intubation

Frequent monitoring of proper tube placement, especially during any move of the patient (such as from the ground to the stretcher) is essential. The following clinical findings indicate immediate removal of the ET tube:

- No chest rise with ventilation
- Absence of breath sounds during auscultation
- Presence of epigastric gurgling sounds or vomitus in the ET tube
- Failure to confirm proper tube position with detection devices

In a patient with spontaneous circulation, lack of a colour on a colourimetric device indicates oesophageal intubation. In such a case, the ET tube should be removed, bag-valve-mask

Table 41-11	DOPE: Troubleshooting the ET Tube	
Problem	**Assessment**	**Intervention**
Dislodgement		
Oesophageal intubation	No ETCO$_2$ reading or colour change Oxygen saturation < 90% Bradycardia Lack of chest rise with ventilation Auscultation of bubbling over stomach	Extubate Bag-valve-mask ventilation Reintubate
Mainstem bronchus intubation	Asymmetric chest rise Asymmetric breath sounds	Pull tube back until breath sounds and chest rise are symmetric
Accidental extubation	Same as oesophageal intubation Poor or absent air movement on auscultation	Bag-valve-mask ventilation Reintubate
Obstruction		
Tube blocked with blood, secretions, or kink	Decreased chest rise Decreased breath sounds bilaterally Oxygen saturation < 90% Increased resistance to bagging	Suction Extubate Bag-valve-mask ventilation Reintubate
Pneumothorax		
Tension pneumothorax, spontaneous or induced	Asymmetric chest rise Asymmetric breath sounds Shock Oxygen saturation < 90% Jugular venous distension* Tracheal deviation*	Needle thoracostomy
Equipment		
Big air leak around tube Activated pop-off valve on resuscitator Oxygen tubing disconnected Oxygen tank empty		Check equipment "patient to cylinder"

*Not easily accessed or frequently seen in young children.

ventilation resumed for 2 minutes, and endotracheal intubation reattempted, preferably with a new tube.

If an intubated patient experiences a sudden decline in respiratory status, use the DOPE mnemonic (Dislodgement, Obstruction, Pneumothorax, Equipment) to identify the potential problem, and institute an appropriate intervention Table 41-11 ▲ .

Orogastric and Nasogastric Tube Insertion

During positive-pressure ventilation, it is common to inflate the stomach, as well as the lungs, with air. Gastric distension slows downward movement of the diaphragm and decreases tidal volume, making ventilation more difficult and necessitating higher inspiratory pressures. It also increases the risk that the patient will vomit and aspirate stomach contents into the lungs. Placement of a nasogastric (NG) tube or an orogastric (OG) tube decompresses the stomach and makes assisted ventilation easier.

At the Scene

Calculate the endotracheal tube size for a child between 1 and 10 years as follows:

(Age ÷ 4) + 4 = Internal diameter (in mm)
(Age ÷ 2) + 12 = Length (in cm)

Documentation and Communication

Vital signs, especially pulse rate and oxygen saturation, should be recorded before and after each intubation attempt. Record the size of the ET tube and the depth of insertion as measured at the patient's lip.

Gastric decompression with an NG or OG tube is contraindicated in unresponsive children with a poor or absent gag reflex and an unsecured airway. Instead, you should perform endotracheal intubation first to decrease the risk of vomiting and aspiration.

Special Considerations

A single intubation attempt should be limited to 20 seconds. If the attempt is not successful after 20 seconds, resume bag-valve-mask ventilation and preoxygenate the child for the next attempt.

Preparation of Equipment

To perform NG or OG tube insertion, you will need an appropriately sized NG or OG tube; a 30- to 60-ml syringe with a funnel-tipped adapter for manual removal of stomach contents through the tube; mechanical suction; adhesive tape; and a water-soluble lubricant. To prepare the patient and the equipment for NG or OG tube placement:

1. Select the proper size of tube. Use a length-based resuscitation tape to determine the proper size, or use a tube size twice the ET tube size that the child would need. For example, a child who needs a 5.0-mm ET tube requires a 10F OG or NG tube.

2. Measure the tube on the patient. The length of the tube should be the same as the distance from the lips or tip of the nose (depending on whether the OG or NG route is used) to the earlobe *plus* the distance from the earlobe to the xiphoid process **Figure 41-19** ▶ .

3. Mark this length on the tube with a piece of tape. When the tip of the tube is in the stomach, the tape should be at the lips or nostril.

4. Place the patient in a supine position.

5. Assess the gag reflex. If the patient is unresponsive and has a poor or absent gag reflex, perform endotracheal intubation before gastric tube placement.

6. In a trauma patient, maintain in-line stabilisation of the cervical spine if a neck injury is possible. Choose the OG route of insertion if the patient has a severe head or midfacial injury.

7. Lubricate the end of the tube.

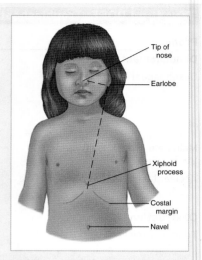

Figure 41-19 Technique for measuring the distance to insert an NG or OG tube.

You are the Paramedic Part 3

As you prepare to immobilise the patient for transport, he begins to vomit. You, your colleague, and the fire fighter maintaining manual cervical spine stabilisation log roll the child using a coordinated movement directed by you. You suction what appear to be chunks of pizza from the child's mouth and back of his throat. After suctioning, the child's oxygen saturation falls to 90%, his respiratory rate decreases to 16 breaths/min, and work of breathing increases. Your partner immediately begins bag-valve-mask ventilation using 100% oxygen, while you quickly measure the child using a length-based resuscitation tape and gather the appropriate intubation equipment.

The child is successfully intubated with a 4.5 uncuffed ET tube using in-line cervical spine stabilisation for potential cervical spine injury. You confirm ET tube placement by direct visualisation of the vocal cords, bilateral breath sounds, and a positive colour change on the colourimetric ETCO$_2$ detector. You then secure the ET tube at the 13-cm mark at the child's lip. Your partner continues to provide bag-valve-mask ventilation at a rate of 20 breaths/min with 100% supplemental oxygen while you reassess the patient.

Reassessment	Recording Time: 10 Minutes
Skin	Pale, cool, and dry
Pulse	190 beats/min, regular; weak distally but strong centrally
ECG	Narrow complex tachycardia
Blood pressure	78/46 mm Hg
Respirations	20 breaths/min via bag-valve-mask ventilation
S$_P$O$_2$	97% on bag-valve-mask ventilation at 100% oxygen
Pupils	Equal and reactive to light
Capillary refill	4 seconds

5. Is this child in shock? If so, is it compensated or decompensated?

6. How should your patient management progress?

OG Tube Insertion

Follow these steps to insert an OG tube in an infant or child:

1. Insert the tube over the tongue, using a tongue blade if necessary to facilitate insertion.
2. Advance the tube into the hypopharynx, then insert it rapidly into the stomach.
3. If the child begins coughing or choking or has a change in voice, immediately remove the tube; it may be in the trachea.

NG Tube Insertion

Follow these steps to insert an NG tube in an infant or child:

1. Insert the tube gently through the nostril, directing the tube straight back. Do not angle the tube superiorly.
2. If the tube does not pass easily, try the opposite nostril or a smaller tube. Never force the tube.
3. If NG passage is unsuccessful, use the OG approach.

Assessing Placement of OG and NG Tubes

Follow these steps to confirm successful placement of an NG or OG tube:

1. Check tube placement by aspirating stomach contents. Use a syringe with an appropriate adapter to quickly instill 10 to 20 ml of air through the tube while auscultating over the left upper quadrant. If you hear a rush of air (or gurgling) over the stomach, the placement is correct.
2. If correct placement cannot be confirmed, remove the tube.
3. Secure the tube to the bridge of the nose or to the cheek, using adhesive tape.
4. Aspirate air from the stomach, using a 30- to 60-ml cannula-tipped syringe, or connect the tube to mechanical suction at a low, continuous suction of 20 to 40 mm Hg or to the intermittent setting.

Complications of OG or NG Tube Insertion

As with endotracheal intubation, you must be aware of the potential complications associated with the placement of an NG or OG tube—namely, placement of the tube into the trachea, resulting in hypoxia; vomiting and aspiration of stomach contents; airway bleeding or obstruction; and passage of the tube into the cranium. The last complication can occur if you insert an NG tube into a patient with severe head or midfacial trauma because the tube may be passed through the fracture and into the brain.

▌Cardiovascular Emergencies

Cardiovascular emergencies are relatively rare in children. When such problems arise, they are often related to volume or infection rather than a primary cardiac cause, unless the child has congenital heart disease. Through the PAT and initial assessment, you can quickly identify a cardiovascular emergency, understand the likely cause, and institute potentially lifesaving treatment.

General Assessment and Management

As with all paediatric emergencies, when called to a scene for a suspected cardiac complaint, begin the hands-off assessment by using the PAT and then move on to the initial assessment using the ABCs. The child's appearance gives an overview of perfusion, oxygenation, ventilation, and neurological status. For a suspected cardiovascular problem, an abnormal appearance may indicate inadequate brain perfusion and the need for rapid intervention. Tachypnoea, without recession or abnormal airway sounds, is common in an infant or child with a primary cardiac problem; it is a mechanism for blowing off carbon dioxide to compensate for metabolic acidosis related to poor perfusion. In contrast, when cardiac compromise progresses to congestive heart failure, pulmonary oedema leads to increased work of breathing and a fast respiratory rate. The presence of pallor, cyanosis, or mottling may tip you off to this problem.

For suspected cardiovascular compromise, start with airway and breathing, and provide supportive care as needed. Ensure adequate oxygenation and ventilation, and then assess the circulation by checking heart rate, pulse quality, skin CTC, and blood pressure when possible. Combine information from the PAT and initial assessment to make an initial decision about the likely underlying cause, the patient's priority, and the need for immediate treatment or transport.

If you determine that the patient's condition is stable enough for you to continue the assessment on site, continue with the SAMPLE history and the focused physical examination. (Table 41-12 ▶ reviews key elements of a cardiovascular SAMPLE history.) Repeat the PAT and ABCs after each intervention, and monitor trends over time.

Shock

Shock is defined as inadequate delivery of oxygen and nutrients to tissues to meet metabolic demand. The types of shock that you may encounter are the same in adults and children: hypovolaemic, distributive, and cardiogenic.

Besides determining the cause of shock, you must quickly determine whether the child is in a compensated or decompensated state. In compensated shock, although the child has critical abnormalities of perfusion, his or her body is (for the moment) able to mount a physiological response to maintain adequate perfusion to vital organs by shunting blood from the periphery, increasing the heart rate, and increasing the vascular tone. A child in compensated shock will have a normal appearance, tachycardia, and signs of decreased peripheral perfusion, such as cool extremities with prolonged capillary refill. Timely intervention is needed to prevent a child in compensated shock from decompensating.

Decompensated shock is a state of inadequate perfusion in which the body's own mechanisms to improve perfusion are no longer sufficient to maintain a normal blood pressure. By definition, a child in decompensated shock will be hypotensive for age (Table 41-13 ▶ . In addition to being profoundly tachycardic and showing signs of poor peripheral perfusion, a child in decompensated shock may have an altered appearance,

Table 41-12	SAMPLE Components for a Child With Cardiovascular Problems
Components	**Features**
Signs and symptoms	Presence of vomiting or diarrhoea Number of episodes of vomiting or diarrhoea Vomiting blood or bile; blood in stool External haemorrhage Presence or absence of fever Rash Respiratory distress or shortness of breath
Allergies	Known allergies History of anaphylaxis
Medications	Exact names and dosages of ongoing medications Use of laxative or anti-diarrhoeal medications Long-term diuretic therapy Potential exposure to other medications or drugs Timing and dosages of analgesics or antipyretics
Past medical problems	History of heart problems History of prematurity Prior hospitalisations for cardiovascular problems
Last oral intake	Timing of the child's last food or drink, including bottle or breastfeeding
Events leading to injury or illness	Travel Trauma Fever history Symptoms in family members Potential toxic exposure

Table 41-13	Lower Limits of Normal Systolic Blood Pressure by Age
Age	**Minimal Systolic Blood Pressure**
Infant (1 month to 1 year)	> 70 mm Hg
1-year-old child	> 80 mm Hg
Child (1–10 years)	80 + (2 × age in years)
Child or adolescent > 10 years	> 90 mm Hg

reflecting inadequate perfusion of the brain. Because children typically have strong cardiovascular systems, they are able to compensate for inadequate perfusion by increasing heart rate and peripheral vascular resistance more efficiently than adults. Hypotension is, therefore, a late and ominous sign in an infant or a young child, and urgent intervention is needed to prevent cardiac arrest.

Initial management involves allowing the child to assume a position of comfort and starting supplemental oxygen. After completing the initial assessment, make a transport decision based on the severity of the problem. Start resuscitation on scene for any child who shows signs of decompensated shock. While rapid transport is imperative, the risk of deterioration to cardiac arrest is too high to permit a "load-and-go" approach.

Hypovolaemic Shock

Hypovolaemia is the most common cause of shock in infants and young children, with loss of volume occurring due to illness or trauma. Because of their small blood volume (80 ml/kg body weight), a combination of excessive fluid losses and poor intake in an infant or a young child with gastroenteritis ("stomach flu") can result in shock relatively quickly. The same vulnerability exists with haemorrhage from trauma.

A patient with hypovolaemic shock will often appear listless or lethargic and may have a compensatory tachypnoea. The child may appear pale, mottled, or cyanotic. In medical shock, further assessment may identify signs of dehydration such as sunken eyes, dry mucous membranes, poor skin turgor, or delayed capillary refill with cool extremities. In an injured child, the site of bleeding may be identified on the initial assessment or detailed physical examination.

Allow the child to remain in a position of comfort, administer supplemental oxygen, and keep the child warm. Apply direct pressure to stop any external bleeding. Volume replacement is the mainstay of treatment for hypovolaemic shock, whether medical or traumatic in origin.

If the child is in compensated shock, you can attempt to establish IV en route to the hospital. As with all procedures, gather all the equipment necessary before beginning this step. Cannulas—preferably an over-the-needle cannula—are available in paediatric sizes of 20, 22, and 24 gauge. A butterfly needle is a temporary alternative if an over-the-needle cannula is unavailable; this stainless steel needle stays in the vein, predisposing it to infiltration.

Many of the sites used for IV access in adults are the same for children. The most commonly used sites are the dorsum of the hand and the antecubital fossa. In children, veins in the foot may also be used Figure 41-20 ▶ . Scalp veins and the external jugular veins are used less commonly.

The procedure for establishing IV access is as follows:
1. Select the vein that you will use.
2. Secure the appropriate limb to minimise movement during the procedure.
3. Apply a tourniquet proximal to the selected site.
4. Clean the site with alcohol.
5. Insert the cannula through the skin with the bevel facing upward. Be sure to enter the skin at a shallow angle parallel to the vein.
6. Advance the cannula until you see blood return into the hub.
7. Continue to gently advance the cannula over the needle into the vein until the hub of the cannula is flush with the skin.
8. Completely remove the needle and attach IV tubing.
9. Flush the cannula with saline. Note if the line is easily flushed or if there is resistance. Resistance may mean that the cannula tip is located outside of the lumen. Carefully

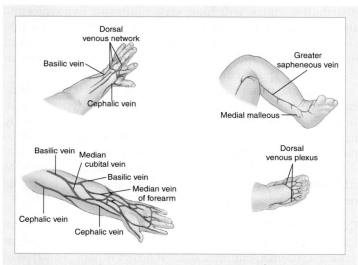

Figure 41-20 Sites for IV access in infants and children include the hands, antecubital fossa, saphenous veins at the ankle, and feet.

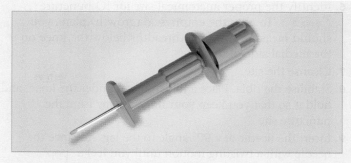

Figure 41-21 Standard paediatric IO needle.

look at the surrounding skin for infiltration of fluids. If the line is infiltrated, remove it.

10. Secure the cannula with a clear plastic dressing. Wrap the IV tubing with extra gauze to prevent the child from pulling out the IV cannula.

Once IV access is established, fluid resuscitation should begin with isotonic fluids *only,* such as normal saline or lactated Ringer's. In medical emergencies, the initial fluid challenge should be calculated accurately at 20 ml/kg of isotonic fluid, and then reassess the patient's condition. In emergencies that are traumatic in origin, the fluid challenge should still be drawn up as 20 ml/kg but must be administered in 5 ml/kg boluses; titrated against haemodynamic response. The use of warm IV fluids (when possible) can counteract the effects of systemic hypothermia from environmental exposure, blood loss, or open wounds. Multiple fluid boluses may be necessary during transport.

Volume resuscitation should be addressed separately from treatment of hypoglycaemia. In a child with shock due to medical illness, perform a blood glucose check; treat with glucose (10% dextrose) only for a documented low blood glucose level, and certainly only after any circulatory compromise has been stabilised. Hypoglycaemia is unlikely in shock due to acute injury.

Notes from Nancy

Be alert for signs of shock or respiratory insufficiency in any child who has sustained blunt chest trauma.

If a child is in decompensated shock with hypotension, begin initial fluid resuscitation at the scene. Make one attempt at IV access. If it is unsuccessful, begin IO infusion. When an IO needle

is placed correctly, it will rest in the medullary canal, the space within the bone that contains bone marrow. An IO infusion is contraindicated if a secure IV line is available or if a fracture (or possible fracture) exists in the same bone in which you plan to insert the IO needle. Anything that can be administered IV can be administered through an IO line (such as isotonic fluids, medications).

The IO needles are usually double needles, consisting of a solid-bore needle inside a sharpened hollow needle **Figure 41-21 ▲**. This double needle is pushed into the bone (usually the proximal tibia) with a screwing, twisting action. Once the needle pops through the bone, the solid needle is removed, leaving the hollow steel needle in place. Standard IV tubing is attached to this hub.

The IO lines require full and careful immobilisation because they rest at a 90° angle to the bone and are easily dislodged. Stabilise the IO needle, thereby ensuring adequate flow, in the same manner that you would any impaled object. As with any invasive procedure, several complications may be associated with IO infusion: compartment syndrome, failed infusion, growth plate injury, bone inflammation caused by infection (osteomyelitis), skin infection, and bony fracture. Proper technique will help to minimise these complications.

Follow the steps in **Skill Drill 41-5 ▶** to establish an IO infusion in paediatric patients:

1. Check the IV fluid for proper fluid, clarity, and expiry date. Look for any discolouration or particles floating in the fluid. If any are found, discard and choose another bag of fluid.

2. Select the appropriate equipment, including an IO needle, syringe, saline, and extension set **Step 1**. A three-way tap should also be used to facilitate easier fluid administration.

3. Select the proper administration set. Connect the administration set to the bag. Prepare the administration set. Fill the drip chamber, and flush the tubing. Make sure no air bubbles remain in the tubing.

4. Prepare the syringe, extension tubing, and three-way tap **Step 2**.

5. Take universal precautions. This must be done before the IO puncture.

6. Identify the proper anatomical site for IO puncture (Step 3). To miss the epiphyseal (growth) plate, you should measure two fingerbreadths below the knee on the medial side of the leg.

7. Cleanse the site.

8. Stabilise the tibia. Place a folded towel under the knee, and hold it so that you keep your fingers away from the puncture site.

9. Insert the needle at a 90° angle to the leg. Advance the needle with a twisting motion until you feel a "pop" (Step 4). Unscrew the cap, and remove the stylet from the needle (Step 5).

10. Attach the syringe and extension set to the IO needle. Pull back on the syringe to aspirate blood and particles of bone marrow to ensure placement and use sample for blood glucose measurement. If you are not able to aspirate marrow but the IO flushes easily with no signs of infiltration (swelling around insertion site), then continue to flush. Consider using the aspirated marrow for a blood glucose test.

11. Slowly inject saline to ensure proper placement of the needle. Watch for infiltration, and stop the infusion immediately if any is noted.

12. It is possible to fracture the bone during insertion of the IO. If this happens, you should remove the IO needle and switch to the other leg.

13. Connect the administration set, and adjust the flow rate. Fluid does not flow well through an IO needle, and boluses are given under pressure by administering the fluid using a syringe and a three-way tap (Step 6).

14. Secure the needle with tape, and support it with a bulky dressing. Be careful not to tape around the entire circumference of the leg, which could impair circulation and create compartment syndrome.

15. Dispose of the needle in the proper container (Step 7).

As with IV administration, give 20-ml/kg boluses of isotonic fluid via IO infusion to treat hypovolaemia of a medical origin or 5ml/kg when trauma is the cause of the hypovolaemia, reassessing after each bolus and repeating as needed based on physiological response. As much as 60 ml/kg may be needed during transport to improve the child's blood pressure, pulse rate, mental status, and peripheral perfusion. Rapidly transport the patient to an appropriate hospital.

Distributive Shock

In distributive shock, decreased vascular tone develops, resulting in vasodilation and third spacing of fluids due to increased vascular permeability (leakage of plasma out of the blood vessels and into the surrounding tissues). This results in a drop in effective blood volume and functional hypovolaemia. Distributive shock may be due to sepsis, anaphylaxis, and spinal cord injury; sepsis accounts for the bulk of paediatric cases.

Early in distributive shock, the child may have warm, flushed skin and bounding pulses as a result of peripheral vasodilation. In contrast, the symptoms and signs of *late* distributive shock will look very similar to hypovolaemic shock on initial assessment. Fever is a key finding in septic shock, whereas urticarial rash and wheezing may be noted in anaphylaxis, and neurological deficits are apparent in shock due to spinal cord injury.

Front-line treatment of distributive shock is volume resuscitation because the child is in a state of relative hypovolaemia. In a child with apparent sepsis who remains persistently hypotensive despite a total of 60 ml/kg of isotonic fluid, vasopressor support to improve vascular tone may be considered.

Anaphylactic shock should be treated immediately with IM adrenaline and in accordance with local guidelines. It may be necessary to repeat doses to stabilise the child.

Cardiogenic Shock

Cardiogenic shock is the result of pump failure: Intravascular volume is normal, but myocardial function is poor. This type of shock is uncommon in the paediatric population but may be present in children with underlying congenital heart disease, myocarditis, or rhythm disturbances. It is important to recognise cardiogenic shock by the child's history or from the initial assessment because the treatment for this type of shock is very different from that for hypovolaemic or distributive shock.

A child in cardiogenic shock will appear listless or lethargic (like children in hypovolaemic or distributive shock) but is likely to show signs of increased work of breathing owing to congestive heart failure and pulmonary oedema. Circulation will be impaired, and skin will look pale, mottled, or cyanotic. Your initial assessment may reveal an abnormal heart rate or rhythm or a murmur or gallop. The child's skin may feel clammy, and you may feel an enlarged liver. The parent may describe the infant sweating with feeding and, in many cases, will recount a history of congenital heart disease.

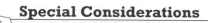

Special Considerations

Shock in children is commonly due to hypovolaemia. Fluid resuscitation with isotonic fluid is the mainstay of treatment.

If you suspect cardiogenic shock, allow the child to remain in a position of comfort (often sitting upright), administer supplemental oxygen, and transport. The transport destination is a critical decision because the ultimate management requires paediatric critical care capability. Supplemental oxygen may not increase the SpO_2 in children with particular types of congenital heart disease, and parents will often alert you to this fact. Consider establishing IV access en route to the receiving hospital. Unless you are sure of the diagnosis of cardiogenic shock (the child has a history of congenital heart disease, is afebrile, and has no history of volume loss), err on the side of fluid resuscitation. If you suspect cardiac dysfunction, administer a single isotonic

Skill Drill 41-5: Paediatric IO Infusion

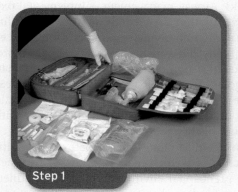

Step 1

Check selected IV fluid for proper fluid, clarity, and expiry date.

Select the appropriate equipment, including an IO needle, syringe, saline, and extension.

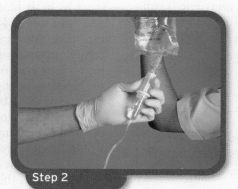

Step 2

Select the proper administration set. Connect the administration set to the bag. Prepare the administration set. Prepare the syringe and three-way tap.

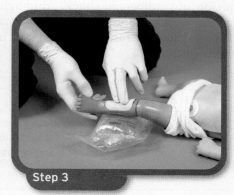

Step 3

Take universal precautions.

Identify the proper anatomical site for IO puncture.

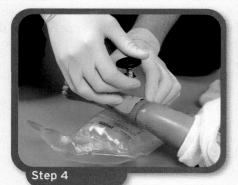

Step 4

Cleanse the site appropriately.

Stabilise the tibia.

Insert the needle at the proper angle.

Advance the needle with a twisting motion until a "pop" is felt.

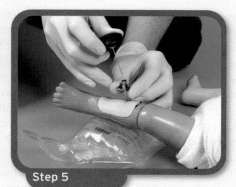

Step 5

Unscrew the cap, and remove the stylet from the needle.

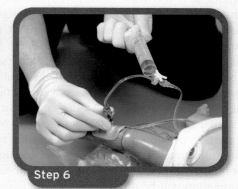

Step 6

Attach the syringe and three-way tap to the IO needle.

Pull back on the syringe to aspirate blood and particles of bone marrow to ensure placement and use sample for blood glucose measurement.

Slowly inject saline to assure proper placement of the needle.

Watch for infiltration, and stop the infusion immediately if noted.

Connect the administration set.

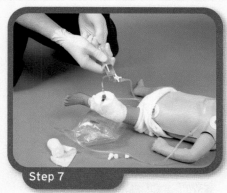

Step 7

Secure the needle with tape, and support it with a bulky dressing.

Dispose of the needle in the proper container.

fluid bolus slowly, and monitor carefully to assess its effect. Increased work of breathing, a drop in oxygen saturation, or worsening perfusion after a fluid bolus will confirm your suspicion of cardiogenic shock. Although inotropic agents may be needed to improve cardiac contractility and improve perfusion, they are rarely administered in the prehospital environment.

> ### At the Scene
> A child with decompensated shock from hypovolaemia needs fluid resuscitation. Do not waste time with multiple IV insertion attempts. Insert an IO needle, and begin fluid therapy.

Arrhythmias

Rhythm disturbances can be classified based on whether the heart beat is too slow (bradyarrhythmias), too fast (tachyarrhythmias), or absent (pulseless). The signs and symptoms associated with a rhythm disturbance are often nonspecific—for example, the patient or parent may report fatigue, irritability, vomiting, chest or abdominal pain, palpitations, and shortness of breath. If you suspect a rhythm disturbance, quickly move through the PAT and initial assessment, supporting the airway and breathing as necessary. An ECG or rhythm strip will help to identify the underlying rhythm and suggest which specific management steps should be initiated. Address reversible causes of arrhythmias such as hypoxaemia. The decision to stay on scene to obtain additional history and perform a focused physical examination will be dictated by the child's overall physiological status.

Bradyarrhythmias

Bradyarrhythmias in children most often occur secondary to hypoxia, rather than as a result of a primary cardiac problem (such as heart block). Airway management, supplemental oxygen, and assisted ventilation as needed are always first-line treatment. Also, treat any underlying respiratory problem. Less common causes of bradycardia include congenital or acquired heart block and toxic ingestion of beta blockers, calcium channel blockers, or digoxin. Elevated ICP can also cause bradycardia and should be considered in children with ventricular shunts, a history of head injury, or suspected child abuse without a consistent injury history.

Initiate electronic cardiac monitoring as part of your initial assessment. If the child is asymptomatic, no further treatment is indicated in the prehospital environment. Healthy, athletic adolescents may have bradycardia as an incidental finding and should be transported to a hospital for further evaluation.

If the child's pulse rate is lower than 60 beats per minute despite oxygenation and ventilation and perfusion is poor, begin chest compressions and attempt IV or IO access. For chest compressions to be effective, the patient should be placed on a firm, flat surface with the head at the same level as the body. If you need to carry an infant while providing CPR, your forearm and hand can serve as the flat surface.

Follow the steps in **Skill Drill 41-6 ▾** to perform infant chest compressions:

1. Place the infant on a firm surface, using one hand to keep the head in an open airway position. You can also use a pad or wedge under the shoulders and upper body to keep the head from tilting forward.
2. Follow the lines of the ribcage until they meet at the xiphisternum; place two fingers in the middle of the sternum, one fingerbreadth above this point **Step 1**.

Skill Drill 41-6: Performing Infant Chest Compressions

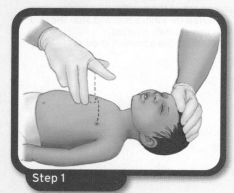

Step 1
Position the infant on a firm surface while maintaining the airway. Place two fingers in the middle of the sternum, one fingerbreadth above the xiphisternum.

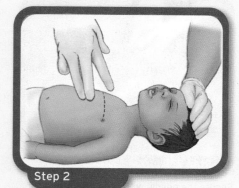

Step 2
Using two fingers, compress the chest by approximately one third of its depth at a rate of 100 compressions/min. Allow the sternum to return briefly to its normal position between compressions.

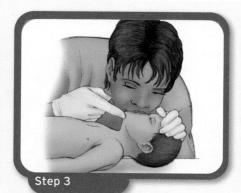

Step 3
Coordinate rapid compression and ventilation in a 15:2 ratio.

3. Using two fingers, compress the chest by approximately one third of its depth at a rate of 100 compressions/min. Allow the chest to recoil. Minimise interruptions in chest compressions.

4. After each compression, allow the sternum to return briefly to its normal position. Allow equal time for compression and relaxation of the chest. Avoid jerky movements of your compressing fingers (Step 2).

5. Coordinate rapid compression and ventilation in a 15:2 ratio, making sure the infant's chest rises with each ventilation. You will find this easier to do if you use your free hand to keep the head in the open airway position. If the chest does not rise or rises only a little, use a chin lift to open the airway. If you are finding the transition difficult between compressions and ventilations, you may consider using a 30:2 ratio.

6. It is not recommended to stop BLS for breathing or pulse checks until ALS intervention is available (Step 3).

Skill Drill 41-7 ▸ shows the steps for performing chest compressions in children between 1 year and puberty (approximately 12 years):

1. Place the child on a firm surface, and use one hand to maintain the head tilt–chin lift (Step 1).

2. Place the heel of your hand over the middle of the sternum (between the nipples). Avoid compression over the lower tip of the sternum, which is called the xiphoid process (Step 2).

3. Compress the chest about one third its total depth (100 compressions/min) and allow full chest recoil. Minimise interruptions in chest compressions. Compression and relaxation should be about the same duration. Use smooth movements, and hold your fingers off the child's ribs.

4. Coordinate rapid compression and ventilation in a 15:2 ratio, making sure that you see a visible chest rise with each ventilation (Step 3).

5. Continue with BLS until an AED arrives or the child shows signs of recovery.

6. If the child resumes effective breathing, place him or her in the recovery position (Step 4).

Quickly transport the patient to an appropriate hospital, while performing ongoing reassessments. If the child still has symptomatic bradycardia, medications are indicated. Adrenaline is the initial medication of choice; the dose should be repeated every 3 to 5 minutes as needed for symptomatic bradycardia. If you identify heart block, give atropine as the second medication. If the child continues to have symptomatic bradycardia, cardiac pacing may be indicated. If the child's rhythm deteriorates, switch to the appropriate treatment algorithm.

Tachyarrhythmias

Sinus tachycardia, a pulse rate higher than normal for age, is common in children. Although it may be a sign of serious underlying illness or injury, it may also be due to fever, pain, or

Skill Drill 41-7: Performing Chest Compressions on a Child

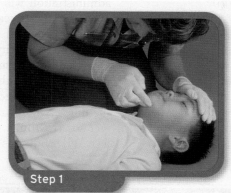

Step 1
Place the child on a firm surface, and use one hand to maintain the head tilt-chin lift.

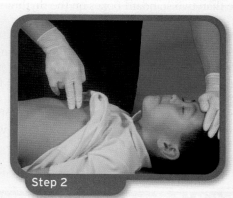

Step 2
Place the heel of your hand over the middle of the sternum (between the nipples); avoid compression of the xiphoid process.

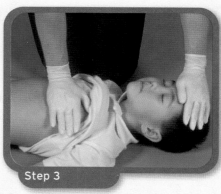

Step 3
Coordinate compression with ventilation in a 15:2 ratio, pausing for ventilation.

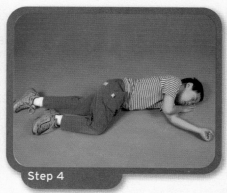

Step 4
If the child resumes effective breathing, place him or her in the recovery position.

At the Scene

The preferred agent for paediatric bradycardia is adrenaline unless the bradycardia is suspected to be from increased vagal tone.

anxiety. Interpret the presence of tachycardia in the context of the remainder of the PAT and initial assessment. For example, if a child appears well but has a fever, sinus tachycardia is likely and treatment with antipyretics is all that is necessary. If a tachycardic child has a history of copious vomiting or diarrhoea, fluid resuscitation is the appropriate treatment.

If a tachycardic child appears ill and has poor perfusion with no history of fever, trauma, or excessive volume loss, continue your assessment for a primary cardiac cause while initiating resuscitation. Your assessment should include determination of pulse rate along with interpretation of an ECG or rhythm strip.

Tachyarrhythmias are subdivided into two types based on the width of the QRS complex. A narrow complex tachycardia exists when the QRS complex is 0.08 second or less (less than two standard boxes on the rhythm strip); a wide complex tachycardia exists when the QRS complex is greater than 0.08 second (more than two standard boxes on the rhythm strip).

Narrow Complex Tachycardia

Although sinus tachycardia is the most common arrhythmia in children, supraventricular tachycardia (SVT) is the most frequent tachyarrhythmia requiring anti-arrhythmic treatment. Table 41-14 ▾ compares sinus tachycardia, reentry SVT, and ventricular tachycardia (VT). You may identify sinus tachycardia based on the presence or absence of P waves, pulse rate, and history of preceding illness or injury. Its treatment is

geared toward the underlying cause and may include oxygen, fluids, splinting, and analgesia.

SVT, which involves abnormal conduction pathways, can be identified by a narrow QRS complex, absence of P waves, and an unvarying pulse rate of more than 220 beats/min in an infant or more than 180 beats/min in a child. The child may have a history of SVT or exhibit nonspecific signs and symptoms, including irritability, vomiting, and chest or abdominal pain. Parents of young infants may report poor feeding for several days. The treatment of SVT depends on the patient's perfusion and overall stability. If the child is in stable condition, consider attempting vagal manoeuvres before obtaining IV access: Have an older child hold his or her breath, blow into a straw with the end crimped over, or bear down as if having a bowel movement; in a younger child, place an examination glove filled with ice firmly over the midface, being careful not to obstruct the nose and mouth. Attempt these techniques only once, while continually monitoring the child's rhythm.

If the child has adequate perfusion and vagal manoeuvres do not succeed in converting SVT to a sinus rhythm, they will require adenosine, which is outside many local guidelines. Adenosine has a short half-life and must be injected quickly into a vein near the heart, usually an antecubital vein. Its administration will be followed by a brief run of bradycardia, ventricular tachycardia, ventricular fibrillation, or asystole, which will convert spontaneously to sinus rhythm. Persistence of any of these rhythms is rare, but be prepared to switch arrhythmia algorithms if necessary.

For a child with SVT who has poor perfusion, synchronised cardioversion is recommended. Synchronised cardioversion is the timed administration of electrical energy to the heart to correct an arrhythmia. If the child is generating a regular but ineffective rhythm, it is important to time the jolt of electricity with

Table 41-14	Features of Sinus Tachycardia, SVT, and VT					
	History	Pulse Rate	Respiratory Rate	QRS Interval	Assessment	Treatment
Sinus tachycardia	Fever Volume loss Hypoxia Pain Increased activity or exercise	< 220 beats/min (infant) < 180 beats/min (child)	Variable	Narrow: < 0.08 s	Hypovolaemia Hypoxia Painful injury	Fluids Oxygen Splinting Analgesia or sedation
Supraventricular tachycardia	Congenital heart disease Known SVT Nonspecific symptoms (such as poor feeding, fussiness)	> 220 beats/min (infants) > 180 beats/min (child)	Constant	Narrow: < 0.08 s	CHF* may be present	Vagal manoeuvres (ice to face) Adenosine Synchronised electrical cardioversion
Ventricular tachycardia	Serious systemic illness	> 150 beats/min	Variable	Wide: > 0.08 s	CHF may be present	Synchronised electrical cardioversion Amiodarone Procainamide

*CHF indicates congestive heart failure.

the appropriate phase of the electrical activity (corresponds with the R wave on an ECG). A burst of electricity to the myocardium during the relative refractory period (the downward slope of the T wave) can precipitate ventricular fibrillation (VF)—a potentially lethal effect. Follow the same steps with synchronised cardioversion as with defibrillation, except that you must press the "sync" button on the defibrillator to alert the machine to time the electrical jolt. The dose of the initial synchronised cardioversion attempt is 0.5 to 1.0 joules per kilogram of body weight (J/kg). If the first dose is unsuccessful, a repeated dose of 2 J/kg can be given. In the hospital setting, sedation is provided before cardioversion, but its administration must not delay the procedure in a child in unstable condition.

An alternative approach to treating the child in SVT with poor perfusion is to give a dose of IV adenosine if vascular access is readily available. Do not delay synchronised cardioversion if vascular access is not already established, however. If the child remains in SVT and is in unstable condition or shock or is unconscious, you may give additional anti-arrhythmic medications in conjunction with cardiology consultation.

Wide Complex Tachycardia

A child with a wide QRS complex tachycardia with a palpable pulse is probably in VT, a rare, but potentially life-threatening rhythm in children. Its presence may reflect underlying cardiac pathology. SVT may sometimes manifest as a wide complex rhythm, and distinguishing between the two can be challenging.

If a child with suspected VT is in haemodynamically stable condition and IV access is available, consider giving anti-arrhythmic medication. Amiodarone is the drug of choice for VT with a pulse. If a child with VT is in unstable condition or shock or is unconscious, the treatment is synchronised cardioversion. Prior sedation is ideal, but do not delay cardioversion for this reason. The same dose of synchronised cardioversion is used for SVT and VT.

Special Considerations

The most common cause of tachycardia in an infant or a young child is sinus tachycardia from fever, dehydration, or pain.

If a child with a tachyarrhythmia is or becomes pulseless, begin CPR and follow the pulseless arrest treatment guidelines. Prepare to immediately transport any child with an arrhythmia to an appropriate receiving hospital. Copies of rhythm strips or ECG tracings will be helpful to hospital personnel for diagnostic and therapeutic purposes.

Pulseless Arrest

Cardiopulmonary arrest exists when the child is unresponsive, apnoeic, and pulseless. In children, this type of arrhythmia is usually a secondary event—that is, the end result of profound hypoxaemia and acidosis owing to respiratory failure. Asystole is the most common arrest rhythm. Pulseless electrical activity

Table 41-15	Paediatric Defibrillation Paddle Size
Age/Weight	**Paddle Size**
Older than 12 mo or > 10 kg	8-cm (adult) paddles
Up to 12 mo or < 10 kg	4.5-cm (paediatric) paddles

(PEA), VT, and VF are seen with lower frequency in children than in adults. The survival rate for children with asystolic arrest in the prehospital setting is poor, and few survivors have good neurological outcomes. The survival rate for children with VF arrest is slightly better and, as in adults, depends on early defibrillation.

When confronted with a paediatric patient in cardiopulmonary arrest, the most important consideration is to provide high-quality BLS skills. Support the airway and breathing, and begin chest compressions. Attempt IV or IO access. Attach a monitor or defibrillator to determine the underlying cardiac rhythm. If it is asystole or PEA, defibrillation is not indicated, and additional treatment is limited to adrenaline or a single dose of vasopressin. After administering the medication, perform five cycles of CPR (approximately 2 minutes) before rechecking the rhythm and assessing for the presence of a pulse. If asystole or PEA persists, continue with CPR and adrenaline. High-dose adrenaline is not routinely recommended. Consider the four "Hs" and he four "Ts" as the potential causes—for example, Hypoxia, Hypothermia, or Hypovolaemia (refer to Appendix A).

Defibrillation is performed before administration of medication in the treatment of VF or pulseless VT. Follow these steps to perform manual defibrillation in an infant or a child:

1. Confirm unresponsiveness, pulselessness, and apnoea.
2. Begin CPR if a defibrillator is not immediately available.
3. Select the proper paddle size `Table 41-15 ▲` .
4. Apply conductive gel to the child's chest. Place one paddle on the anterior chest wall to the right of the sternum, inferior to the clavicle; place the other paddle on the left midclavicular line at the level of the xiphoid process `Figure 41-22 ▶` . Apply firm pressure to the paddles. For children who are younger than 12 months or who weigh less than 10 kg, you may use anterior-posterior paddle placement `Figure 41-23 ▶` .

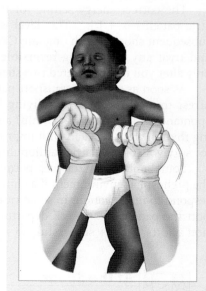

Figure 41-22 Site for defibrillation paddles on anterior chest wall in small infants.

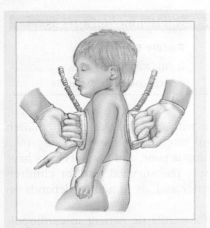

Figure 41-23 Site for defibrillation paddles placed in anterior-posterior position for larger infants and children.

5. Assess the cardiac rhythm to confirm the presence of VF or pulseless VT.

6. Select the appropriate energy setting, and charge the defibrillator.

7. Verbally and visually ensure that no one is in contact with the patient; stop CPR if it is in progress.

8. Deliver the shock at the appropriate energy setting.

9. Give 5 cycles of CPR (approximately 2 minutes).

10. Reassess the rhythm.

11. If a shockable rhythm persists, give an additional shock at the same energy, and immediately resume CPR.

12. Insert an advanced airway, establish IV access, and begin medication therapy if indicated. Repeat the defibrillation after 5 cycles of CPR (approximately 2 minutes) if refractory VF or pulseless VT persists.

Many ambulance services use pregelled defibrillator pads instead of gel. If your system uses defibrillator pads, place them in the same location as you would when using an AED. When applying the pads, ensure that there are no air pockets in the pad-skin interface because they may result in skin burns and decreased defibrillation effectiveness.

The correct energy setting for the defibrillation of paediatric patients is 4 J/kg. This level is used for initial and any subsequent shocks. With ongoing CPR, remember to search for and treat any underlying reversible causes. Give adrenaline only after you have delivered two shocks.

As soon as possible, transport patients in cardiopulmonary arrest to an appropriate receiving hospital. Early return of spontaneous circulation (< 5 min) and VF or VT as a presenting rhythm are associated with improved neurological outcome for survivors of paediatric cardiopulmonary arrest.

Some ambulance services permit recognition of death in the prehospital environment if a child in cardiac arrest does not respond to resuscitation. In some cases, you may elect to transport the patient to an A&E department, even when resuscitation efforts are not successful, so as to provide bereavement support to the family. A child's death is a devastating event for the family and the ambulance service crew, and this may be one of your most difficult calls.

■ Medical Emergencies

Approximately one third of all prehospital calls for paediatric patients are trauma-related; two thirds are medical. Medical calls may include respiratory complaints (as previously discussed in this chapter), fever, convulsions, and altered LOC.

Fever

Fever is a common paediatric complaint but often not a true medical emergency. A symptom of an underlying infectious or inflammatory process, fever can have multiple causes. Most paediatric fevers are caused by viral infections, which are often mild and self-limiting. In other cases, fever is a symptom of a more serious bacterial infection.

Your general impression and initial assessment will help you determine the severity of illness. Remember that young children with a fever can look quite ill—even if they only have a "bug"—because increased body temperature causes increased metabolism, tachycardia, and tachypnoea. Record temperature as part of the vital signs, but recognise that the height of the fever does not reflect the severity of the illness. If the patient is a young infant, a rectal temperature is most accurate, but recognition that fever is present is more important than the exact temperature. As you move through the initial assessment, look for signs of respiratory distress, shock, convulsions, stiff neck, petechial or purpuric rash, or a bulging fontanelle in an infant. These signs may tip you off to the presence of pneumonia, sepsis, or meningitis, all of which can be life threatening and require prompt transport to an appropriate hospital.

Very young infants (younger than 2 months) should always be considered at risk for serious infection. Young infants have few ways of interacting with the world, and a fever (defined as body temperature > 38°C) may be the only sign of a potentially life-threatening illness. Regardless of how well a child in this age group looks, he or she should be assessed and transported quickly to a hospital for a full sepsis screening, including blood, urine, and cerebrospinal fluid (CSF) analysis.

The focused history and physical examination will help to determine the underlying cause of the fever and the severity of illness. Perform this assessment on scene if the child is in stable condition or en route to the hospital if the child appears seriously ill. Ask about the presence of vomiting, diarrhoea, poor feeding, headache, neck pain or stiffness, and rash. A history of infectious exposure may provide clues to the likely cause of the child's current illness. The focused medical history may also identify a child at high risk for serious

At the Scene

Keep a laminated copy of the paediatric algorithms with you at all times for your reference during a cardiovascular emergency.

Notes from Nancy

The majority of emergencies requiring CPR in children are preventable.

bacterial illness. For example, sickle cell disease, human immunodeficiency virus infection, and childhood cancers may all lead to an immunocompromised state.

A child with a fever may require little intervention in the prehospital environment. Simply support the ABCs as needed. Although fever by itself is not dangerous, temperature control will make the child with a minor acute illness look and feel better. Consider treating with paracetamol or ibuprofen, but avoid aspirin in children. Use of aspirin in children has been linked with a rare illness, Reye's syndrome, which can result in cerebral oedema and liver failure. Other cooling measures should be limited to undressing the child. Transport the patient to an appropriate hospital with ongoing reassessment for clinical deterioration.

Meningitis

Meningitis entails inflammation or infection of the meninges, the covering of the brain and spinal cord. It is usually caused by a viral or bacterial infection. Although children may look and feel quite ill, viral meningitis is rarely a life-threatening infection. By contrast, bacterial meningitis is potentially fatal. Children with bacterial meningitis can progress rapidly from mildly ill-appearing to coma and even death. In the early stages of illness, it is difficult to tell which type of infection is present, so take the safe route: Always proceed as if the child may have bacterial meningitis.

The symptoms of meningitis vary depending on the age of the child and the agent causing the infection. In general, the younger the child, the more vague the symptoms. A newborn with early bacterial meningitis may have fever as the only symptom. Young infants will often have fever and perhaps localising signs such as lethargy, irritability, poor feeding, and a bulging fontanelle. Young children rarely show typical "meningeal signs" such as nuchal rigidity (neck stiffness with movement of the neck) until they are a bit older. Verbal children will often complain of headaches and neck pain. An altered LOC and convulsions are ominous symptoms at any age.

The most common way in which neonates contract meningitis-causing bacteria is during the birthing process: The bacteria that are a normal part of the mother's vaginal tract—*Escherichia coli,* group B *Streptococcus,* and *Listeria monocytogenes*—can produce serious infections in newborns. Older infants and young children are at risk for contracting viral meningitis from enteroviruses, which are widespread during the summer and autumn. Bacterial meningitis in this age group most often involves *Streptococcus pneumoniae* (also known as pneumococcus) and *Neisseria meningitidis* (also known as meningococcus), although pneumococcus infection is becoming less frequent as more young children are vaccinated against this bacterium.

Meningitis from *H influenzae* is rare because a vaccine against this pathogen was introduced several years ago.

Neisseria meningitidis may also cause sepsis (an overwhelming bacterial infection in the bloodstream). Meningococcal meningitis with sepsis is typically characterised by a petechial (small, pinpoint red spots) or purpuric (larger purple or black spots) rash in addition to the other symptoms of meningitis **Figure 41-24** .

Infection control is an important part of managing a child who may have meningitis. Meningococcus, in particular, is quite contagious. Protect yourself and others from contracting this illness by being vigilant about using standard and respiratory precautions. Wear a gown, gloves, and a mask if meningitis is a possibility.

Children with meningococcal sepsis and meningitis get very sick, very fast, so move quickly through your assessment. Form your general impression, and perform the initial assessment as usual, while recognising that the initial presentation of a child with meningitis can be highly variable. Look for fever, altered mental status, bulging fontanelle, photophobia, nuchal rigidity, irritability, petechiae, purpura, and signs of shock. Perform a glucose check because hypoglycaemia may result from the hypermetabolic state. Helpful components of a SAMPLE history are shown in **Table 41-16** .

For children in physiologically unstable condition, treat with benzylpenicillin given by slow IV administration (IM can be used if IV access is difficult). For a child less than 1 year, the dose is 300 mg; for a child between 1 and 9 years, 600 mg; and for over 9 years, 1.2 g. Following administration of benzylpenicillin, the child may experience hypotension due to toxin release into the bloodstream, thus fluid replacement is advocated at 20 ml/kg. After providing lifesaving interventions, transport quickly, ideally to a hospital with a paediatric intensive care unit. En route, perform frequent reassessments—one of the hallmarks of this disease is rapid deterioration. Monitor vital signs and changes in physical examination findings closely to anticipate a child's needs and continue with therapeutic treatment as indicated by local guidelines.

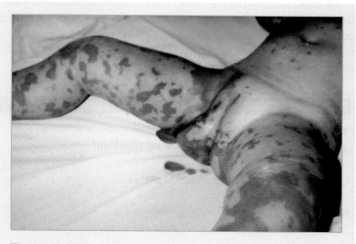

Figure 41-24 Purpura in a child with meningococcal sepsis.

Table 41-16	Paediatric SAMPLE History for Suspected Meningitis
Component	**Explanation**
Signs and symptoms	Onset and duration of illness, including "cold symptoms" (runny nose, cough) Onset and duration of fever Rash? Headache? Neck pain? Photophobia? Irritability?
Allergies	Known drug reactions or other allergies
Medications	Exact names and doses of ongoing drugs Timing and amount of last dose Time and dose of analgesics and antipyretics
Past medical history	Previous illnesses or injuries Immunisations Perinatal history for young infants
Last oral intake	Timing of the child's last food or drink, including bottle or breastfeeding
Events leading to illness or injury	Any known exposures to children with illnesses and what kind of illnesses

Table 41-17	AEIOU-TIPPS: Possible Causes of Altered LOC and Mental Status
A	Alcohol
E	Epilepsy, endocrine, electrolytes
I	Insulin
O	Opiates and other drugs
U	Uraemia
T	Trauma, temperature
I	Infection
P	Psychogenic
P	Poison
S	Shock, stroke, space-occupying lesion, subarachnoid haemorrhage

Altered LOC and Mental Status

An altered LOC or mental status is an abnormal neurological state in which a child is less alert and interactive with the environment than normal. **Table 41-17 ▶** uses the mnemonic AEIOU-TIPPS to highlight some common causes of altered LOC. Without a good history, it may be difficult to determine the underlying cause, and you may find yourself simply identifying and treating worrying symptoms.

Run through the PAT and ABCs quickly to determine possible points of intervention. Pay special attention to possible disability and glucose issues. Use the AVPU scale (Alert, responsive to Voice, responsive to Pain, Unresponsive) to identify the level of disability. In addition, check the patient's glucose level because hypoglycaemia (defined as a plasma glucose level of < 4 mmol/l in infants and children) is easily treatable.

The focused history and physical examination, whether performed at the scene or en route to hospital, may also provide clues about the underlying cause. For example, a child with a history of epilepsy may be in a postictal state after an unwitnessed convulsion; a child with diabetes may be hypoglycaemic or in diabetic ketoacidosis. A history of toxic ingestion, recent illness, or injury may also reveal the cause of the altered mental status.

Regardless of the cause, the initial management of altered mental status is the same. Support the ABCs by carefully assessing the patient's airway and breathing. Provide assisted ventilation or airway support as needed. If the child is hypoglycaemic, give an infusion of glucose (5ml/kg of 10% dextrose). Always recheck the blood glucose level after giving IV glucose. The goal is to maintain a *normal* glucose level: Hyperglycaemia is associated with worse neurological outcomes in patients with cerebral isschaemia. For children with altered mental status and signs or symptoms suggestive of an opiate toxidrome **Table 41-18 ▼**, consider giving naloxone. All patients with altered mental status should be transported expeditiously to the nearest or most appropriate hospital.

Convulsions

Convulsions result from abnormal electrical discharges in the brain. Although many types of convulsions exist, generalised convulsions manifest as abnormal motor activity and an altered LOC. Some children are predisposed to convulsions because of underlying brain abnormalities, whereas others experience

At the Scene

Always check the glucose level for a patient with altered mental status.

Table 41-18	Common Toxidromes	
Toxidrome	**Agent**	**Signs and Symptoms**
Anticholinergic	Antihistamines, cyclic anti-depressants	"Hot as a hare, red as a beet (hot, dry skin; hyperthermia), blind as a bat (dilated pupils), mad as a hatter (delirium, hallucinations)"
Cholinergic	Organophosphates	DUMBELS: Diarrhoea/diaphoresis, Urination, Miosis, Bradycardia/bronchoconstriction, Emesis, Lacrimation, Salivation
Narcotic	Morphine, methadone	Bradycardia, hypoventilation, miosis, hypotension
Sympathomimetic	Cocaine, amphetamines	Tachycardia, hypertension, hyperthermia, mydriasis (dilated pupils), diaphoresis (sweating)

convulsions as a result of trauma, metabolic disturbances, ingestion, or infection. Convulsions associated with fever (febrile convulsions) are unique to young children.

The physical manifestation of a convulsion will depend on the area of the brain firing the electrical discharges and the age of the child. Infants have immature brains, so convulsions in this age group may be subtle. Repetitive movements such as lip smacking, chewing, and "bicycling" suggest convulsion activity. Apnoea and cyanosis can also be signs of underlying convulsion activity.

The prognosis following a convulsion is closely linked to the underlying cause. For example, a child with a febrile convulsion will not have brain damage as a consequence of the event, whereas a child who has a convulsion as a complication of a head injury or meningitis may have long-term neurological abnormalities. All types of convulsions (but especially first-time convulsions) are frightening to parents, and they often result in a 999 call.

Types of Convulsions

The classification system for convulsions is the same for children and adults (see Chapter 28 for an in-depth discussion of convulsions). Briefly, convulsions that involve the entire brain are considered generalised convulsions, whereas those that involve only one part of the brain are called partial convulsions. The most common type of convulsions are generalised tonic-clonic convulsions (grand mal), which involve jerking of both arms and/or legs. Absence convulsions (petit mal) are generalised convulsions that involve brief loss of attention without abnormal body movements. Partial convulsions can be further subclassified into simple partial convulsions, which involve focal motor jerking without loss of consciousness, and complex partial convulsions, which feature focal motor jerking with loss of consciousness.

Febrile Convulsions

Febrile convulsions occur in about 2% to 5% of young children. To make this diagnosis, the child must be between 6 months and 6 years old, have a fever, and have no identifiable precipitating cause (such as head injury, ingestion, or meningitis). Most febrile convulsions occur in children between the ages of 6 months and 3 years. The strongest predictor for having a febrile convulsion is a history of this diagnosis in a first-line relative.

Simple febrile convulsions are brief, generalised tonic-clonic convulsions (lasting < 15 minutes) that occur in a child without underlying neurological abnormalities. Complex febrile convulsions are longer (lasting > 15 minutes), are focal, or occur in a child with baseline developmental or neurological abnormality. They may also be associated with serious illness.

Special Considerations

Febrile convulsions are unique to children. Reassure the parents of a child with a simple febrile convulsion that the child has an excellent prognosis.

The majority of your calls for fever and convulsions will involve simple febrile convulsions. The postictal phase after a brief convulsion tends to be short, so the child will often be waking up or back to baseline by the time you arrive at the scene. Depending on your trust's policy, a well-appearing child who has a history consistent with a simple febrile convulsion may be transported by ambulance service or by parents but will often benefit from assessment at an A&E department.

The prognosis for children with simple febrile convulsions is excellent. Although one third of children who have one simple febrile convulsion will have another such convulsion, their prognosis does not change. There is no relationship between simple febrile convulsions and brain damage or future developmental or learning disabilities, and children with this diagnosis have only a slightly increased risk for subsequent development of epilepsy.

Assessment of Convulsions

The general impression and initial assessment of a child with a history of convulsions should give special attention to compromised oxygenation and ventilation and signs of ongoing convulsion activity. Convulsions place a child at risk for respiratory distress or failure because of airway obstruction (often from the tongue), aspiration, or depressed respiratory drive. Given the typical ambulance service response time, any child who is still having a convulsion when you arrive is likely to have been having convulsion activity for at least 10 minutes beforehand, and should be considered to be in status epilepticus; initiate treatment to stop the convulsion in such cases. Status epilepticus has historically been defined as any convulsion lasting more than 30 minutes or two or more convulsions without return to neurological baseline between convulsions. In recent years, however, neurologists have begun urging treatment for any convulsion lasting more than 5 minutes. As part of your SAMPLE history, ask about prior convulsions; anti-convulsant medications; recent illness, injury, or suspected ingestion; duration of the convulsion activity; and the character of the convulsion.

Treatment of Convulsions

Treatment at the scene will be limited to supportive care if the convulsion has stopped by your arrival, but status epilepticus requires more extensive intervention. For a child with ongoing convulsion activity, uncompensate the airway using the chin-lift or jaw-thrust manoeuvre. Very proximal airway obstruction is common during a convulsion or postictal state because the tongue and jaw fall backward owing to the decreased muscle tone associated with altered mental status. If the airway is not maintainable with positioning, consider inserting a nasopharyngeal airway. Suction for secretions or vomitus, and consider the recovery position in case of ongoing vomiting. Do not attempt to intubate during an active convulsion because endotracheal intubation in this setting is associated with serious complications and is rarely successful. You are better off using BLS airway management, stopping the convulsion, and then considering the child's need for ALS airway support.

Provide high-flow supplemental oxygen to the patient, and start bag-valve-mask ventilation as indicated for hypoventilation.

Assess the child for IV sites. Measure the blood glucose level, and treat any hypoglycaemia.

Consider your options for anti-convulsant administration. Insertion of an IV line can be difficult in a child having a convulsion, and alternative routes for medication delivery may be needed. The goal of medical therapy is to stop the convulsion while minimising anti-convulsant side effects.

First-line anti-convulsant treatment consists of a benzodiazepine—lorazepam, diazepam, or midazolam. All benzodiazepines can cause respiratory depression, so monitor oxygenation and ventilation carefully, especially when you give repeated doses or combinations of anti-convulsants. Lorazepam is an excellent choice for convulsion management because of its rapid onset, lower risk of respiratory depression, and relatively long half-life. Its usefulness in the prehospital environment is limited because it must be refrigerated. Diazepam is frequently used in the prehospital setting, given by the IV or rectal route. The advantages of rectal administration include ease of access and a lower rate of respiratory depression, although onset of action is longer (approximately 5 minutes). The half-life of diazepam is relatively short, however, and breakthrough convulsions may occur with longer transport times. Midazolam may be administered by the IV, IM, buccal, and intranasal routes. Although it has excellent anti-convulsant effects, it has the shortest duration of action of the three benzodiazepines mentioned. Be prepared to repeat dosing for recurrent convulsions.

If the convulsions do not stop after two or three doses of a benzodiazepine, a second-line agent is necessary; however, this will usually occur in the hospital environment. Phenobarbital is the second-line agent of choice for neonates. Phenobarbital, phenytoin, and fosphenytoin are acceptable second-line agents for infants and children outside of the neonatal age group. Phe-nobarbital has sedative effects and causes respiratory depression, so be vigilant if you give it after a benzodiazepine. Although phenytoin has the advantage of not compromising the respiratory system or causing sedation, it is difficult to administer and can cause hypotension and bradycardia. Fosphenytoin, a drug that is metabolised to phenytoin, allows for more rapid infusion with fewer side effects; it may be administered by the IV route. Paraldehyde can also be used as a second-line drug; given via the PR route it causes little respiratory depression.

Any child with a history suggestive of convulsions requires A&E evaluation to look for the cause. Although treatment at the scene is appropriate for a child in status epilepticus, detailed assessment should be performed during transport. Monitor cardiorespiratory status in any postictal child, and reassess frequently for recurrent convulsion activity.

■ Toxicology Emergencies

Toxic exposures account for a significant number of paediatric emergencies. Every year around 40,000 children attend A&E departments following accidental poisoning. By far the largest group is the under 5 and the normal route for poisoning is ingestion.

Toxic exposures can take the form of ingestion, inhalation, injection, or application of a substance (see Chapter 33 for more on specific exposures). A toddler or preschool-age child is most likely to have an unintentional exposure, the result of developmentally normal exploration. In this age group, ingestion tends to involve small quantities of a single cleaning product, cosmetic, or plant or a few pills. In contrast, toxic exposures in adolescents are typically the result of recreational drug use or suicide

You are the Paramedic Part 4

Based on the patient's vital signs and condition, you determine that he is in compensated shock. You insert a 20-gauge peripheral IV cannula into one antecubital fossa, and initiate a normal saline bolus. When you used the length-based resuscitation tape earlier, you estimated the child's weight to be approximately 12 kg, so you plan to administer a total of 60 ml (5 ml/kg). While the fluid is being delivered, you and your crew apply a cervical collar, secure the child to a paediatric longboard, and pad the natural hollows with a blanket. You then load the patient in the ambulance, making sure to keep him warm, and contact the receiving hospital.

Reassessment	Recording Time: 18 Minutes
Skin	Pale, cool, and dry
Pulse	165 beats/min, regular; weak distal pulses but strong central pulses
ECG	Narrow complex tachycardia
Blood pressure	84/56 mm Hg
Respirations	20 breaths/min via bag-valve-mask ventilation
SpO_2	98% on bag-valve-mask ventilation with high-flow supplemental oxygen
Pupils	Equal and reactive to light

7. What do you think is the cause for shock in this patient?

8. What criteria were used to determine that this patient was a "trauma alert"?

attempts and often involve multiple agents. Although intentional exposures among adolescents lead to greater morbidity and mortality, in small children the toxic effects of some medications are such that "one pill can kill".

Assessment

The evaluation of a child who has experienced a potentially toxic exposure follows the standard assessment sequence. Take a focused history to identify the agents to which the child was exposed, the quantity, and the route and time of exposure. Findings of physical assessment will vary widely based on these factors. Make special note of vital signs, pupillary changes, skin temperature and moisture, and any unusual odours. Putting together these pieces of the puzzle may allow you to identify a toxidrome—a pattern of symptoms and signs typical of a particular poisoning.

When performing the initial assessment, attend to airway, breathing, and circulatory support as indicated. A glucose check is an important test because ingestion of some common substances can lead to hypoglycaemia—namely, ethanol and other alcohols, insulin, oral hypoglycaemic agents, and beta blockers. Treat hypoglycaemia as part of your resuscitation.

If the child is in stable condition without physiological abnormalities and without a serious toxic exposure, stay on scene to obtain additional history and perform an expanded physical examination. See Table 41-19 ▶ for the SAMPLE history for a paediatric patient with a potential toxic exposure. During the expanded physical examination, look for toxidromes by assessing the patient's mental status, pupillary changes, skin CTC, gastrointestinal activity (bowel sounds, emesis, or diarrhoea), and abnormal odours. Perform frequent reassessments because the child's condition may change.

At the Scene

Have the UK National Poisons Information Service number (0870 600 6266) handy for suspected poisonings.

Children with potentially life-threatening toxic exposures may be asymptomatic on your arrival, and the dose of drug in an accidental toddler ingestion may be high. Always attempt to collect any pill containers or bottles and transport them with the patient to the hospital to assist the A&E staff in making treatment decisions.

Management

The management of any potential toxic exposure begins with supportive care and attention to the ABCs. Other management options include reducing the absorption of the substance by decontamination, enhancing elimination of the substance, and/or providing an antidote. Give special attention to the risks of environmental exposures for the ambulance service crew, who may also require decontamination measures.

Table 41-19	The Paediatric SAMPLE for Toxic Exposures	
Components	**Features**	
Signs and symptoms	Time of suspected exposure Behaviour changes in child Emesis and content of vomit	
Allergies	Known drug reactions or other allergies	
Medications	Identity of suspected toxin Amount of toxin exposure (count pills or measure volume) Pill or chemical containers on scene Exact names and doses of prescribed medications	
Past medical problems	Previous illnesses or injuries	
Last oral intake	Timing of the child's last food or drink Type and time of home treatment (such as ipecacuanha mixture [Ipecac])	
Events leading to injury or illness	Key events leading to the exposure Type of exposure (inhaled, injected, ingested, or absorbed through the skin) Poison Centre contact	

Decontamination

If the substance has been applied to the skin, reducing absorption involves removal of all clothing and a thorough washing of the skin. With ocular exposure, immediately wash out the eyes. For ingested toxins, options to reduce gastric absorption include dilution, syrup of ipecac, gastric lavage, and activated charcoal.

Depending on the substance ingested, it may be useful to dilute the substance by getting the child to drink a glass of milk or water. This decision should be made in conjunction with an A&E consultant or NPIS. If the child has any airway or breathing concerns, do not to allow the child to drink.

Ipecac does not remove significant amounts of ingested toxins and can cause prolonged emesis. It should not be used in the prehospital management of paediatric toxic ingestion.

The most common method currently used for gastrointestinal decontamination in the A&E setting is the administration of activated charcoal. Activated charcoal adsorbs many ingested toxins in the gut, making less drug available for systemic absorption. If it is administered within the first hour after exposure; however, some common toxins do not bind to charcoal—for example, heavy metals, alcohols, hydrocarbons, acids, and alkalis. Activated charcoal is messy to administer and is rarely readily accepted by paediatric patients. For these reasons, as well as the risk of severe chemical pneumonia if a child with altered mental status or vomiting aspirates the charcoal, this treatment may be best given in the hospital setting.

Enhanced Elimination

Cathartics such as sorbitol are sometimes combined with activated charcoal. They work by speeding up elimination. In general, cathartics are not recommended for young children because they have been known to cause significant diarrhoea with serious—sometimes life-threatening—electrolyte abnormalities. Hospital providers have additional options for enhancing elimination, such as whole bowel irrigation, urinary alkalinisation for salicylate overdoses, dialysis, and haemoperfusion.

Antidotes

Antidotes can be lifesaving but are available for only a few poisonings. They work by reversing or blocking the effects of the ingested toxin. **Table 41-20** lists some of the more commonly available antidotes; indications for their use are the same for young children as for adults. The dose depends on the weight of the child.

> **Notes from Nancy**
>
> Any child with unexplained tachypnoea should be suspected of having salicylate poisoning.

Sudden Unexpected Death in Infancy

Sudden unexpected death in infancy (SUDI), formerly known as cot death and also known as sudden infant death syndrome (SIDS), is the sudden and unexpected death of an infant younger than 1 year for whom a thorough postmortem examination fails to demonstrate an adequate cause of death. Whatever the cause, the sudden death of an apparently healthy baby is devastating to families and to the ambulance service crew that responds to the call. Risk factors associated with SUDI include male sex; prematurity; low birth weight; young maternal age; sleeping in the prone position; sleeping with soft, bulky blankets or soft objects; sleeping on soft surfaces; and exposure to tobacco smoke.

Congenital abnormalities has replaced SUDI as the leading cause of death in infants aged 1 month to 1 year. With a peak of incidence between 2 and 4 months, the Office for National Statistics stated that there were 183 recorded cases in 2003, compared to 396 in 1995; the trend continues down each year.

Table 41-20	Common Antidotes
Poison	**Antidote**
Carbon monoxide	Oxygen
Organophosphate	Atropine/pralidoxime
Tricyclic anti-depressants	Bicarbonate
Opiates	Naloxone
Beta blockers	Glucagon
Calcium channel blockers	Calcium
Benzodiazepine	Flumazenil

Assessment and Management

The typical scenario for an SUDI call is that of a healthy infant who was put down for a nap and later found dead in bed. On arrival of ambulance service, the baby will be lifeless and, depending on discovery time, may have rigor mortis and dependent lividity (pooling of blood on the underside of the body). The presence of frothy or blood-tinged fluid in the mouth or nose or on the bedding is typical of SUDI. Be alert for clues to other potential causes of death, such as trauma, suffocation, or maltreatment.

Your decision to start resuscitative efforts, or to stop CPR that was started by first responders or family members, can be difficult in cases of suspected SUDI. Your actions will be guided by local guidelines on declaring death in the prehospital environment and by your assessment of the patient and the needs of the family. Although a victim of SUDI cannot be resuscitated, failure to initiate care may not be acceptable to the shocked family. Likewise, A&E care will not change the outcome for the infant, but hospital-based social services for the family may be an important resource. Where death has been recognised at scene, it is necessary to notify the police. This is obviously a distressing time and the notion of calling the police is often difficult to understand by the parents. You may also be required to contact other support mechanisms such as neighbours, other family members, or even members of the clergy.

Despite the emotionally charged atmosphere, doing a thorough scene assessment and obtaining the pertinent history is important. A history of recent illnesses, chronic conditions, medications, or trauma may decrease the likelihood of SUDI as the cause of death.

Death of a Child

Whatever you suspect as the cause of death, be compassionate and non-judgemental in dealing with parents. Find out the infant's name, and use it. Don't hesitate to tell the family how sorry you are. Families in this situation will often look to you for answers. Even when there is nothing to do medically, you can make a big impact by providing emotional support and care to the surviving family members.

Apparent Life-Threatening Event

An apparent life-threatening event (ALTE) is an episode during which an infant becomes pale or cyanotic; chokes, gags, or has an apnoeic spell; or loses muscle tone. These changes are sufficiently dramatic for the parent to become frightened, and even may think that the baby is dying. ALTEs frequently prompt 999 calls. Their causes may include benign diagnoses, such as a brief episode of laryngospasm during feedings or gastro-oesophageal reflux, and serious diagnoses, such as sepsis, congenital heart disease, and convulsions.

ALTEs were once thought of as existing along a spectrum with SUDI; hence they were called near-miss or aborted SUDI. More recent evidence demonstrates that although both events occur in early infancy, the two are not related.

It is common to find a distraught parent and a well-appearing baby on arrival at the scene of an ALTE call. Provide life support if the infant shows signs of cardiorespiratory compromise or altered mental status, and transport all infants with a history of an ALTE to an appropriate hospital for evaluation. This is a challenging age group to assess, and overtriage is the safest path.

Child Abuse and Neglect

Sadly, child abuse is prevalent in our society. The NSPCC reports that around 33,000 children are on a Child Protection Register. Every week, one child is killed by their parent or carer in England and Wales. Chapter 43 covers the subject in more depth and provides statistical breakdowns.

Child abuse or maltreatment comes in many forms: physical abuse, sexual abuse, emotional abuse, and child neglect. Physical abuse involves the infliction of injury to a child. Sexual abuse occurs when an adult engages in sexual activity with a child; it can range from inappropriate touching to intercourse. Emotional abuse and child neglect are often difficult to identify and may go unreported.

Keep the possibility of child abuse and neglect in mind when you are called to assist with an injured child. The information you gather from the initial scene assessment and interviews may prove invaluable. If you suspect child abuse, you should act on your suspicions because child abuse involves a pattern of behaviour. A child who is abused once is likely to be abused again—and next time, it may be more serious or even fatal.

Risk Factors for Abuse

No child asks to be abused, but certain risk factors make abuse more likely. Younger children are more often abused than older children, perhaps a function of their helplessness and limited ability to communicate their needs. Children who require a lot of extra attention, such as children with disabilities, chronic illnesses, or other developmental problems, are also more likely to be abused.

Child abuse occurs across all socioeconomic levels, although it is more prevalent in lower-socioeconomic families. Divorce, financial problems, and illness can contribute to the overall stress level of parents, placing them at higher risk to abuse their children. Drug and alcohol abuse can also interfere with a parent's ability to parent, and both are associated with higher rates of abusive behaviour. Domestic violence in the home places a child at a much higher risk for child abuse.

Table 41-21	CHILD ABUSE Mnemonic for Suspicion of Child Abuse
C	Consistency of the injury with the child's developmental age
H	History inconsistent with injury
I	Inappropriate parental concerns
L	Lack of supervision
D	Delay in seeking care
A	Affect (of the parent or parent and the child in relation to the parent)
B	Bruises of varying ages
U	Unusual injury patterns
S	Suspicious circumstances
E	Environmental clues

Suspecting Abuse

When you are called to the home of an injured child and suspect abuse or neglect, trust your instincts. Use your scene assessment, focused history, and physical examination to gather additional information. Look for "red flags" that could suggest child maltreatment (summarised in the mnemonic CHILD ABUSE; Table 41-21 ▲):

- A history inconsistent with the type of injury sustained—for example, a child who fell from a tree but whose bruises are only on the buttocks
- An account of the injury that is inconsistent with the developmental abilities of the child—for example, a 2-month-old child rolling off a bed
- An old injury that went unreported
- Inappropriate actions or language from the parent

Assessment and Management
Scene Assessment

To recognise abuse, you first have to suspect it. Once you begin to question whether abuse or neglect is involved, it becomes important to document what you see very carefully. Although it may be difficult to remain impartial when child abuse or neglect is suspected, it is an important part of professionalism. Record what you see and hear, but do not editorialise. Be detailed in your incident report about the child's environment, noting the condition of the home and the interactions among the parents, the child, and the ambulance service crew. Record verbatim any comments that concern you.

Documentation and Communication

If you suspect child abuse, take extra care with your documentation. Record conversations verbatim (in quotes) and document on your patient clinical record what you see and hear.

Do not approach the parent with your concerns, but make sure that you pass them on to staff at the receiving hospital. In the UK, ambulance service providers are required to report any incidences where child abuse is suspected.

General and Initial Assessments

Although child abuse can generate a big emotional response from the ambulance service crew, remember that your primary focus should be on trauma assessment and management and on ensuring the safety of the child. Base your general impression on the PAT, which may range from normal in a child with minor inflicted injuries to grossly abnormal in a child with severe internal or CNS injuries. In shaken baby syndrome you may encounter a child with a very abnormal appearance but no external signs of injury. In such a case, the child receives a severe brain injury when a parent violently shakes the infant, often when the child is crying inconsolably. Given that few parents will admit to having hurt the child, be alert for a history that is inconsistent with the clinical picture.

Give special attention to the child's skin while looking for bruises, especially of different ages or in concerning locations. Active toddlers often have bruises on their shins from falls and active playing but rarely on their backs or buttocks. Bruises in identifiable patterns such as belt buckles, looped cords, or straight lines are rarely incurred accidentally. Figure 41-25 ▾ and Figure 41-26 ▸ are examples of bruises that are suggestive of abuse.

Use the CHILD ABUSE mnemonic when you obtain additional history. Ask yourself, "Does the parent's explanation make sense? Could this child produce this bruise or injury through his or her normal activities"?

Mimics of Abuse

It can be difficult to distinguish some normal skin findings from inflicted injuries. For example, Mongolian spots Figure 41-27 ▸ can mimic bruises. These birthmarks are generally found on the lower back and buttocks of children of Asian or African-American descent; they may be mistaken for bruises because of their unique bluish colouring.

Certain cultural customs also produce skin markings that can mimic child abuse. Coining and cupping Figure 41-28 ▸ and Figure 41-29 ▸ are traditional Asian healing practices, often used in the treatment of fever. Although the skin markings can be impressive, the practice is not harmful and does not necessarily represent abuse.

■ Trauma

Paediatric trauma is the leading cause of death among children older than 1 year. Motor vehicle collisions cause the most deaths in this age group, followed by falls and submersions. Among adolescents, murder and suicide are major causes of death.

Children's age-related anatomy and physiology make their injury patterns and responses to trauma different from those seen in adults. In addition, a child's developmental stage will affect his or her response to injury. For a young child, being strapped to a longboard may be as traumatic as the injury leading to the ambulance service call!

Anatomical and Physiological Differences

Head

Recall that infants and young children have heads that are large relative to the rest of their bodies. The head also

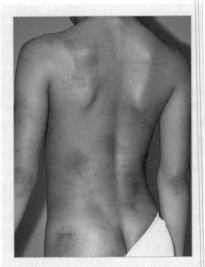

Figure 41-26 Bruises from child abuse. Multiple bruises or injuries that are in different stages of healing are concerns for abuse.

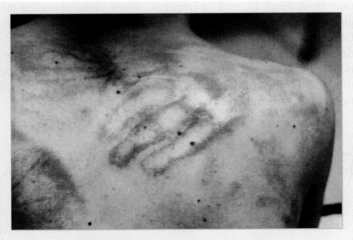

Figure 41-25 Bruises from child abuse. Look for bruises that look like finger or hand marks.

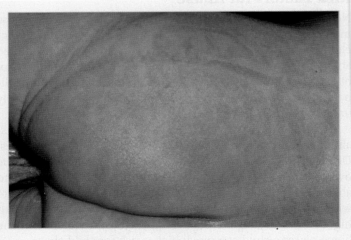

Figure 41-27 A Mongolian spot is a birthmark that can mimic a bruise. It may be on the back, buttocks, or extremities.

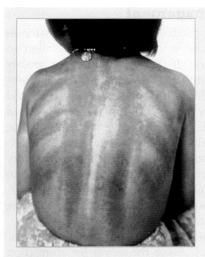

Figure 41-28 Coining, the practice of rubbing hot coins on the back as a treatment of medical illnesses, can leave impressive markings that can mimic child abuse.

has a larger mass compared with adults. The head's larger size and weight make it more prone to injury. A young child falling from a height, for example, is more likely to fall on his or her head. Traumatic brain injury is the leading cause of death and significant disability in paediatric trauma patients.

Spinal Column

The vertebral column continues to develop along with the child. When the child is younger, the cervical spine fulcrum (or bending point) is higher because the head is heavier. As the child grows, the fulcrum descends to "adult level", around C5 through C7. An infant who sustains blunt head trauma involving acceleration-deceleration forces is at high risk for a fatal, high cervical spinal injury. By comparison, a school-age child who experiences the same injury will be likely to sustain a lower cervical spinal injury and be paralysed.

Fortunately, vertebral fractures and spinal cord injuries in young children are uncommon. Spinal ligaments are more lax in children than in adults, leading to increased mobility and the phenomenon of cord injury in the absence of identifiable vertebral bony fracture or dislocation.

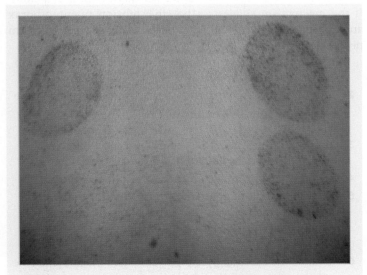

Figure 41-29 Round, flat, red circles on a child's back may be from the practice of cupping—placing warm cups on the skin to draw out illness from the body.

Thoracic and lumbar spinal injuries are also encountered relatively infrequently until a child is pursuing adult activities, such as driving and diving. Nevertheless, these injuries are seen in children in association with specific mechanisms—for example, seatbelt-associated lumbar spine injuries (often associated with abdominal injury) and compression fracture due to axial loading in a fall. When confronted with a significant MOI, the safest course is to assume that the child has a bony injury and transport with spinal immobilisation precautions.

It is often difficult to coax a young child to remain immobilised in a longboard apparatus. In this case, a vacuum mattress may be more comforting, particularly if lined with a familiar smelling blanket or mum's jumper, etc. As a last resort, your overall objective is to immobilise the spine, and this may only be achieved through a parent holding the child and you packing supporting blankets, etc. around both parent and child; however, if the child is still, the spinal column is still.

Chest

Chest trauma is the third leading cause of serious injury in paediatric trauma. A child's chest wall is more pliable and flexible than that of an adult. As a result, children have fewer rib fractures and flail chest events, but injuries to the thoracic organs may be more severe because the pliable ribcage is more easily compressed during blunt trauma. As a consequence, children are more vulnerable than adults to pulmonary contusions, pericardial tamponade, and diaphragmatic rupture. Be sure to look for signs of these injuries in a child with suspected chest trauma, but note that the signs of pneumothorax or haemothorax in children are often subtle. You may not see signs such as neck vein distension, and it may be difficult to determine tracheal deviation.

Abdomen and Pelvis

Abdominal injuries are the second leading cause of serious trauma in children (after head injuries). In paediatric patients, the intra-abdominal organs are relatively large, making them vulnerable to blunt trauma. For example, the abdomen in an infant or toddler often seems protuberant because of the large liver. The liver and the spleen extend below the ribcage in young children and, therefore, do not have as much bony protection as they do in an adult. These organs have a rich blood supply, so injuries to them can result in large blood losses. The kidneys are also more vulnerable to injury in children because they are more mobile and less well supported than in adults. Finally, the duodenum and pancreas are likely to be damaged in handlebar injuries.

Pelvic fractures are relatively rare in young children and are generally seen only with high-energy MOIs. The risk for pelvic fracture increases in adolescence, when the skeleton and MOIs become more like those of adults.

Extremities

The bones of young children continue growing until well into adolescence, resulting in a higher rate of fractures than in adults. This susceptibility to fractures is a function of bone density and the presence of cartilaginous growth plates.

Growth plate fractures can be seen with low-energy MOIs, and they may not evidence the degree of tenderness, swelling, and bruising usually associated with a broken bone. Because a young child's ligaments are sturdier than the long bones, sprains are relatively uncommon, and joint dislocations without associated fractures are not often encountered.

Injury Patterns

Blunt trauma is the MOI in more than 90% of paediatric injury cases. Because they have less muscle and fat mass than adults, children have less protection against the forces transmitted in blunt trauma.

Falls are common in paediatric patients, and the injuries sustained will reflect the anatomy of the child and the height of the fall. For example, a 6-year-old playing on the swings is most likely to sustain an upper extremity fracture when falling onto an outstretched arm. Internal or head injuries would be uncommon with this mechanism. Conversely, an infant, with a big head and no protective reflexes, who pitches out of a backpack or shopping trolley is likely to sustain a skull fracture and could have an intracranial haemorrhage. Falls from a standing position usually result in isolated long bone injuries, whereas high-energy falls (such as from a window, ejection from a motor vehicle, car-versus-pedestrian collision) may result in multiple trauma.

Injuries from bicycle handlebars typically produce compression injuries to the intra-abdominal organs. Duodenal haematomas and/or pancreatic injuries are common with this MOI, as are upper extremity injuries. You must also consider a head injury if the patient went over the handlebars, especially if not wearing a helmet.

Motor vehicle collisions can result in a variety of injury patterns depending on whether the child was properly restrained and where the child was seated in the car. For unrestrained passengers, assume multiple trauma. Restrained passengers may sustain chest and abdominal injuries associated with seatbelt use. If you see chest or abdominal bruising in a seatbelt pattern, have a high suspicion for spinal fractures. Air bags pose a particular threat for head and neck injuries in young children.

A child who is the victim of a car-versus-pedestrian collision is likely to sustain multi-system trauma. Depending on the child's height and the height of the vehicle's bumper, a child may receive chest, abdominal, and lower extremity injuries at impact. Head and neck injuries may result from the fall when the child is thrown.

Special Considerations

Always consider multiple trauma in paediatric patients. Consider head or abdominal injuries, even if they are not readily apparent.

Assessment and Management

The first steps in managing paediatric trauma are the same as for medical emergencies. Use your hands-off assessment to establish a general impression. If the PAT findings are grossly abnormal, quickly move to initial assessment and management to prevent death or disability. Abnormal appearance should make you think immediately of a head injury. With an isolated closed head injury, the child's breathing and circulation may be normal. Of course, abnormal appearance may also reflect inadequate oxygenation of the brain owing to shock or respiratory failure. Abnormalities in work of breathing will tip you off to chest or airway injury and abnormal circulation to a haemorrhage problem. If multi-system injuries are present, all three sides of the PAT may be abnormal.

Begin the initial assessment, initiating life support interventions as you identify problems. Assess the airway for obstruction with teeth, blood, vomit, or oedema. Provide suction as required. For cervical spinal injury, uncompensate the airway using the jaw-thrust manoeuvre. If the child cannot maintain the airway, consider placement of an oropharyngeal airway. If you attempt endotracheal intubation, maintain cervical spinal precautions. Establishment of an emergency surgical airway in a child is fraught with complications, and the failure rate is high; for these reasons, tracheotomy should be reserved for the most expert surgeons in a controlled setting. The chances of needing to perform a needle cricothyroidotomy in a child are remote. In younger children, identification of the cricothyroid membrane is difficult. Appropriate needle cricothyroidotomy is described in Chapter 11.

Breathing assessment includes evaluation for symmetric chest rise and equal breath sounds. Provide 100% supplemental oxygen, give bag-valve-mask ventilation as needed.

Pneumothorax is not common in paediatric blunt chest injury, but it may be present with penetrating trauma of the chest or upper abdomen. Remember that you are less likely to see jugular venous distension and tracheal deviation in a child. If the mechanism suggests a possible tension pneumothorax and the patient is in significant respiratory distress, perform needle decompression **Skill Drill 41-8 ▶** :

1. Assess the patient to ensure that the presentation is due to a tension pneumothorax.
2. Prepare and assemble the necessary equipment: large-bore IV cannula, preferably 14 to 16 gauge, alcohol wipes and IV dressing.
3. Locate the appropriate site. Find the second intercostal space in the midclavicular line on the affected side.
4. Cleanse the appropriate area using aseptic technique.
5. Insert the needle at a 90° angle, just superior to the third rib (nerves, arteries, and veins run along the inferior borders of each rib), and listen for the release of air (Step 1).
6. Advance the cannula over the needle, and place the needle in the sharps container.
7. Secure the cannula in place the same way you would secure an impaled object.

8. Monitor the patient closely for recurrence of the tension pneumothorax.

Any trauma patient should be considered to be at risk for developing shock from visible external bleeding or internal bleeding. Assess the child's circulation by checking the heart rate and quality, capillary refill, skin temperature, and blood pressure. In paediatric patients, the only sign of compensated shock might be an elevated heart rate—children have a remarkable capacity for peripheral vasoconstriction and can maintain their blood pressure despite significant blood loss. If the MOI is concerning and the child is tachycardic, assume the presence of compensated shock and initiate volume resuscitation with 5 ml/kg of isotonic fluid. Ideally, you will insert a peripheral IV line, but an IO line may be best in a child with haemorrhagic shock who is unconscious. Control external bleeding as you would in any trauma patient. Once the ABCs are stabilised, continue your assessment of disability with the AVPU scale. Your assessment of appearance in the PAT will already have identified an altered LOC. Check the child's pupils and motor function. Place a cervical collar, and immobilise the child on a longboard as indicated.

If increased ICP is a concern, keep the head midline to facilitate jugular venous return to the heart. If the patient is not in shock, elevate the backboard or head of the stretcher to 30°. Perform shock resuscitation with IV fluids—brain hypoperfusion will make matters worse. If the child has acute signs of herniation such as a "blown" pupil or the Cushing's triad (elevated blood pressure, bradycardia, abnormal respiratory pattern), consider mild hyperventilation guided to an ETCO$_2$ of 32 to 35 mm Hg and giving mannitol if your guidelines allow.

The last piece of the initial assessment will be "exposure"—that is, a head-to-toe examination to identify all injuries. Log roll the child, and examine the back and buttocks. Once you have completed this examination, cover the child in blankets. Don't forget to cover the head, especially in infants and young children, and avoid drafts from heating or air-conditioning units. Children have a relatively large skin surface area–body mass ratio, increasing their risk for heat loss and hypothermia. Consider the use of warm IV fluids, warm oxygen, and a warm patient transport environment and keeping the patient covered. Also be sure to remove any wet clothing that could conduct heat away from the patient.

Treat any fractures—open or closed—as you would in an adult. Check out your equipment ahead of time to ensure that you have splints appropriate for smaller children.

Transport Considerations

After initial assessment and stabilisation, you are faced with the transport decision. Some traumas are load-and-go situations because of the severity of injuries and the patient's unstable condition. Examples include trauma involving an ominous MOI regardless of how the patient looks on scene, a child with an unstable or compromised airway, a child in shock, a child with difficulty breathing, and a child with a severe neurological disability. For these patients, perform lifesaving procedures on

Skill Drill 41-8: Decompression of a Tension Pneumothorax

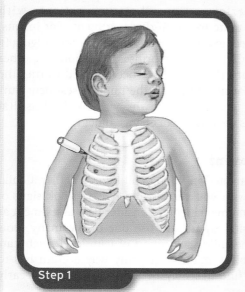

Step 1
Locate the appropriate site. Find the second intercostal space in the midclavicular line on the affected side.

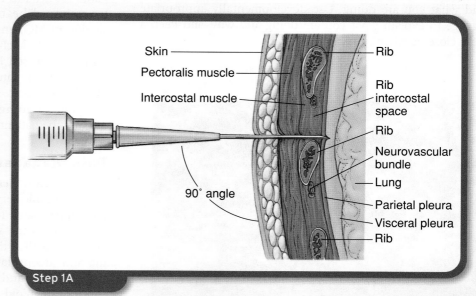

Step 1A
Cleanse the appropriate area using aseptic technique. Insert the needle at a 90° angle and listen for the release of air.

Skin — Rib
Pectoralis muscle — Rib
Intercostal muscle — Rib intercostal space
Rib
Neurovascular bundle
90° angle — Lung
Parietal pleura
Visceral pleura
Rib

scene or en route, and quickly transfer them to an appropriate trauma centre according to local trauma triage guidelines.

All trauma victims for whom spinal injury is suspected require appropriate spinal stabilisation. The indications are the same for children and adults. You may have difficulty finding an appropriately sized cervical collar for infants or very young children. Do not attempt to place a collar that is too big on a small child—use towel rolls and tape to immobilise the head. Apply the tape across the temples and forehead, but ensure that the chin strap/tape allows the child to breathe adequately. As not all services carry paediatric immobilisation devices, it is recommended that an adult longboard is utilised. Remember to pad under the shoulders of smaller children and infants to counter their larger occiput, maintaining neutral alignment Figure 41-30 ▾ .

Immobilise a child with the following steps Skill Drill 41-9 ▸ :

1. Maintain a small child's head in a neutral position by placing a towel under the a small child's shoulders Step 1 .
2. Place an appropriately sized cervical collar on the patient Step 2 .
3. Carefully log roll the child onto the immobilisation device Step 3 .
4. Secure the patient's torso to the immobilisation device first Step 4 .
5. Secure the child's head to the immobilisation device Step 5 .
6. Complete immobilisation by ensuring that the child is strapped in properly Step 6 .

Secure the child firmly onto the longboard but leave room for adequate chest expansion. Being immobilised is a frightening experience, especially for a young child who cannot understand what you are doing. Use developmentally appropriate language to explain what you are doing and why, and keep a parent close by when possible.

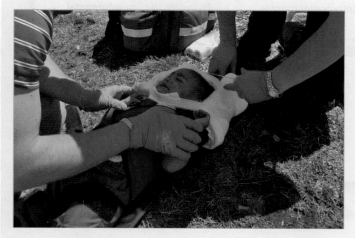

Figure 41-30 Cervical spinal stabilisation with towels and tape for a young infant.

Follow the steps in Skill Drill 41-10 ▸ to immobilise an infant:

1. Carefully stabilise the infant's head in a neutral position and lay the seat down into a reclined position on a hard surface Step 1 .
2. Position a paediatric board or other similar device between the patient and the surface on which the infant is resting Step 2 .
3. Carefully slide the infant into position on the board Step 3 .
4. Make sure the infant's head is in a neutral position by placing a towel under the infant's shoulders Step 4 .
5. Secure the torso first, and place padding to fill any voids Step 5 .
6. Secure the infant's head to the backboard Step 6 .

Consideration should also be given to securing an infant in a vacuum-style mattress, as these often provide high levels of immobilisation and are tolerated more. The identification of the nearest appropriate hospital depends on local guidelines and the capabilities of local hospitals. In some areas of the country, you may be directed to take the patient directly to a paediatric trauma centre or to arrange for air transport to a paediatric trauma centre. In other areas of the country, children are evaluated primarily at local hospitals and then transferred on to a paediatric trauma centre.

Expanded History and Examination

If the patient is in stable condition and does not meet the load-and-go criteria, obtain additional history as outlined in Table 41-22 ▸ and perform a more thorough physical examination. A head-to-toe, back-to-front detailed physical examination should be performed on all trauma patients with significant MOI en route to the A&E department. For infants, this will include checking the anterior fontanelle for bulging (a sign of increased ICP). Look for bruises, abrasions, or other subtle signs of injury that may have been missed during the initial assessment. Be sure to revisit the initial assessment during your ongoing assessment on the way to the hospital because the patient's condition can change quickly.

Pain Management

Pain is often undertreated in young children. Whether a child can communicate with you verbally, do not overlook signs of pain in paediatric trauma patients. Consider pain assessment as important as the vital signs, and use one of the many tools available to elicit the child's self-report of pain level. Tachycardia and inconsolability may be the only way a child has to express pain, and findings may be similar to those of early shock or plain old fear.

Pain treatment includes use of a calm, reassuring voice, distraction techniques, and, when appropriate, medications. Commonly used pain medications include morphine. Patients who are intubated should receive pain medication and sedation

Skill Drill 41-9: Immobilising a Child

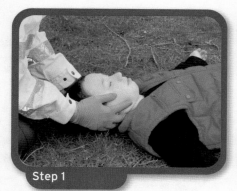

Step 1

Use a towel under the shoulders of a small child to maintain the head in a neutral position.

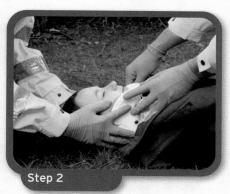

Step 2

Apply an appropriately sized cervical collar.

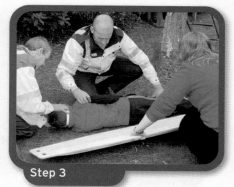

Step 3

Log roll the child onto the immobilisation device.

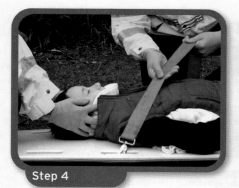

Step 4

Secure the torso first.

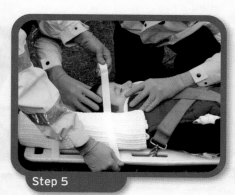

Step 5

Secure the head last.

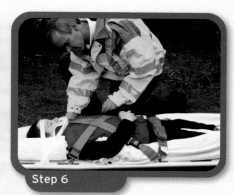

Step 6

Ensure that the child is strapped in properly.

Table 41-22	SAMPLE History in Paediatric Trauma
Component	**Explanation**
Signs and symptoms	Time of event Nature of symptoms or pain Age-appropriate signs of distress
Allergies	Known drug reactions or other allergies
Medications	Timing and last dose of long-term medications Timing and dose of analgesics or antipyretics
Past medical history	Prior surgeries Immunisations, especially last tetanus
Last oral intake	Time of child's last food and drink, including bottle or breastfeeding
Events leading to the injury	Key events leading to the current incident MOI Hazards at the scene

(such as diazepam and midazolam) if they are in haemodynamically stable condition.

You must weigh the risks and benefits when deciding to administer these medications. Children who are in shock and haemodynamically unstable condition are not good candidates for opiates or sedatives; these medications may worsen their already precarious status. All children receiving such medications should be carefully monitored in terms of their pulse rate, respiratory rate, pulse oximetry, and blood pressure.

Burns

The initial assessment and management of paediatric burn victims is similar to that of adults, with a few key differences. The larger skin surface–body mass ratio of children makes them more susceptible to heat and fluid loss. Worrying patterns of injury or suspicious circumstances should also raise concerns of child abuse.

Skill Drill 41-10: Immobilising an Infant

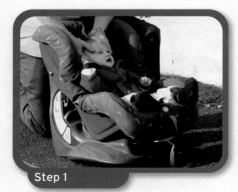

Step 1

Stabilise the head in a neutral position.

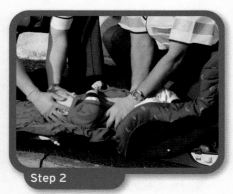

Step 2

Place an immobilisation device between the infant and the surface on which he or she is resting.

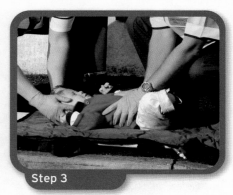

Step 3

Slide the infant onto the board.

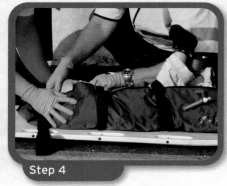

Step 4

Ensure the neutral head position. Secure the torso first; pad any voids.

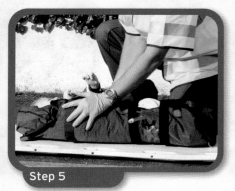

Step 5

Secure the head.

Assessment

The assessment of scene safety is an important element in a call to someone who has been burnt. Check for ongoing dangers such as fire, chemicals, or other hazardous materials. Your from-the-doorway assessment may identify signs of smoke inhalation, such as abnormal airway sounds and respiratory distress, or soot around the nose. Quickly move the patient and crew to a well-ventilated area.

An estimation of the percentage of body surface area burned may affect your decision to start fluid resuscitation in the prehospital environment and influence the transport destination. For adolescents, use the same rule of nines that you use for adult burn victims. For younger children, this rule of nines is modified to account for a child's disproportionately larger head size. For infants, the head and trunk each account for 18% of body surface area, the arms each count as 9%, and the legs each count as 14%. The size of a child's palm (not including fingers) represents about 1% total body surface area. You can also use this rule of palm to assess the extent of the burn **Figure 41-31 ▶** .

Burns suggestive of abuse include those in which the mechanism or pattern observed does not match the history or the child's developmental capabilities. For example, a child who cannot stand independently is unlikely to pull a hot cup of coffee off a table. Splash burns—as from tipping over a pot of boiling water—should have an irregular configuration because the hot liquid runs down the child's body. Be suspicious if a burn has clear demarcation lines or is on the buttocks.

Management

Initial management begins with removal of burning clothing and support of the ABCs. If you observe signs of smoke inhalation, consider early intubation. Make sure that you have a range of tubes available because airway oedema and sloughing may mandate use of a smaller tube than originally estimated.

All burn victims should be provided 100% supplemental oxygen, regardless of the presence or absence of signs of respiratory distress. Smoke inhalation may cause bronchospasm resulting in wheezing and mild respiratory distress. Consider using a bronchodilator such as salbutamol.

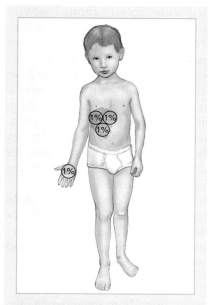

Figure 41-31 Using the child's palm to estimate burned body surface area.

Cannulate the child and initiate fluid resuscitation during transport for patients with large burns (25% of burned body surface area). Depending on age, give up to 20 ml/kg of isotonic fluid, and reassess the need for additional boluses—as large burns can lead to huge fluid shifts.

Clean burned areas minimally to avoid hypothermia, and cover them with clean, dry cloth. Avoid putting lotions or ointments on burned skin because they can trap heat and bacteria. It is important to keep the patient warm whilst simultaneously cooling the burn—*cool the burn not the patient.*

Analgesia is a critical part of the early management of burns; these injuries can be incredibly painful. Assess and treat pain and anxiety as discussed previously. Carefully monitor any child given narcotics for signs of respiratory or haemodynamic compromise.

Once the patient's condition is stabilised, begin transport to an appropriate hospital. Larger burns, full-thickness burns, and burns involving the face and neck are best treated at a regional burn centre, if there is one, otherwise go to the nearest A&E department.

At the Scene

Use the rule of palm to estimate the percentage of body surface area burned in a young child or infant: A child's palm is equal to 1% of body surface area.

Children With Special Health Care Needs

Children with special health care needs include those with physical, developmental, and learning disabilities. The disabilities have a broad range of causes, including premature birth, traumatic brain injury, congenital anatomical anomalies, and acquired illnesses. Advances in technology and drugs have enabled an increasing number of children with disabilities to receive care in the community, leading to a corresponding increase in the number of ambulance service calls for this medically complex population.

Technology-Assisted Children

Technology-assisted children constitute a subset of children with special health care needs that may require your assistance. It is important to familiarise yourself with the various types of medical technology that you may encounter and have to troubleshoot.

Tracheostomy Tubes and Artificial Ventilators

Tracheostomy is surgical procedure, involving creation of a stoma—in this case, a permanent connection between the skin of the throat and trachea—through which a tracheostomy tube can be placed for long-term ventilatory needs Figure 41-32 ▶ . A child might need a tracheostomy for a variety of reasons, including long-term ventilator support for chronic lung disease, inability to protect the airway because of neurological impairment, and a congenital airway anomaly leading to airway obstruction. Parents have been trained in the use and care of their child's tracheostomy and are a source of valuable information. In general, they will have a spare tracheostomy tube available.

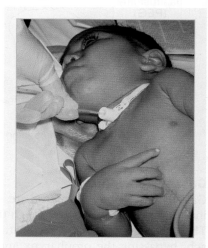

Figure 41-32 A tracheostomy is a surgical opening in the neck into the trachea, creating an artificial airway.

A child with a tracheostomy tube may breathe spontaneously with room air, if the function of the tube is simply to bypass mechanical upper airway obstruction. Alternatively, the child may be dependent on a home ventilator and supplemental oxygen if he or she has severe lung disease or problems with respiratory drive.

Although a tracheostomy tube is intended to provide a secure, permanent airway, problems can arise, as with any mechanical device. The most common problem is obstruction of the tracheostomy tube with secretions, resulting in respiratory distress or respiratory failure. Displacement of the tube is another potential problem. If you are faced with a child with a tracheostomy tube and respiratory distress, start by assessing tube position and suctioning the tube. If the child is using a home ventilator, disconnect the circuit and provide bag-valve-mask ventilation. If these measures fail to lead to improvement or if the child is cyanotic or in severe distress, you may need to remove and replace the tracheostomy tube, preferably using a tube of the same diameter and length. Confirmation of tube position is done in the same manner as for an ET tube.

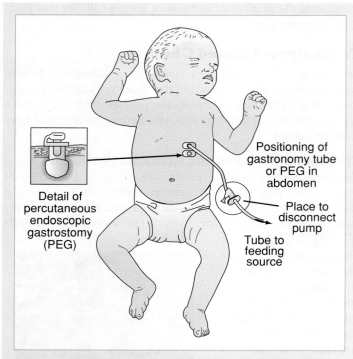

Figure 41-33 A G-tube is an opening through the skin directly into the stomach.

Gastrostomy Tubes

Gastrostomy tubes (G-tubes) are surgically placed directly into the patient's stomach through the skin **Figure 41-33 ▲**. They provide nutrition or medications directly into the stomach, bypassing the oropharynx and oesophagus. Some children are unable to take food or medication by mouth and depend on a G-tube for all of their nutrition; for other patients, the tube is used to supplement intake and ensure adequate nutrition.

Problems such as obstruction, dislodgement, or leakage of a G-tube are not uncommon but rarely represent an emergency. Most such calls can be managed by supportive care and transport. Urgent A&E evaluation is needed if a G-tube has been pulled out because the opening on the abdominal wall tends to constrict quickly, making replacement difficult.

Central Venous Cannulas

A central venous cannula may be inserted when a child needs long-term IV access for medications or nutrition. Such a device is placed surgically or by interventional radiologists into large central veins, such as the subclavian. Completely implanted central lines, with a port or reservoir accessible under the skin, may be left in place for months to years. For example, they are commonly placed in children with cancer who are undergoing long courses of chemotherapy. Partially implanted central lines have tubing external to the skin.

Complications associated with central venous cannulas include infections, obstruction, and dislodged or broken cannulas. Children with an infection of the central line may have redness, swelling, tenderness, or pus at the skin site of insertion; they may also have systemic signs of infection (such as fever) or signs of septic shock. Central line obstruction may be a medical emergency, depending on what is infusing through the line. If the child is not in urgent need of the infusion, simply assess the patient and transport to a hospital. Dislodged or broken cannulas may result in leakage of fluid or blood. In such a case, use sterile technique to clamp off the broken line to minimise risk of infection or air embolus.

On rare occasions, you will be confronted with a child who has a functioning central line but requires emergency IV access for prehospital treatment. Because these permanent lines carry a high risk for infection, look for peripheral access and avoid using the central line whenever possible.

CSF Shunts

Hydrocephalus is a condition resulting from impaired circulation and absorption of CSF, leading to increased size of the ventricles (fluid-filled spaces in the brain) and increased ICP. Hydrocephalus may be congenital or acquired; it is most commonly seen in children born with brain malformations as a complication of prematurity or following surgery for a brain tumour. Cerebrospinal fluid shunts are inserted to drain excessive fluid from the brain, thereby normalising ICP **Figure 41-34 ▶**. A neurosurgeon places the tube and connects it to a one-way, pressure-sensitive valve that runs from the enlarged ventricle subcutaneously into the abdominal peritoneal space. When pressure builds up in the ventricle, the one-way valve uncompensates, and CSF drains into the peritoneum, where it is reabsorbed.

A CSF shunt obstruction occurs when the drainage of fluid from the brain through the shunt tubing becomes blocked— perhaps due to a break in the tubing, problems with the valve, or buildup of debris in the tubing. Without adequate fluid drainage, the CSF fluid continues to accumulate, resulting in hydrocephalus. A child with a shunt obstruction will show signs of increased ICP, which may range from subtle changes in behaviour to impending brain herniation. Typical symptoms include headache, fatigue, vomiting, and even coma. Late signs include the Cushing's triad (hypertension, bradycardia, respiratory compromise).

A CSF shunt infection results from bacterial contamination during the surgery to place the shunt or from bacteria in the blood adhering to and infecting the hardware. Infections are encountered most frequently within months of shunt surgery. Children with shunt infections are generally very sick and have fever and signs of shunt obstruction.

Shunt obstructions and shunt infections are true medical emergencies. The patient should be transported to appropriate

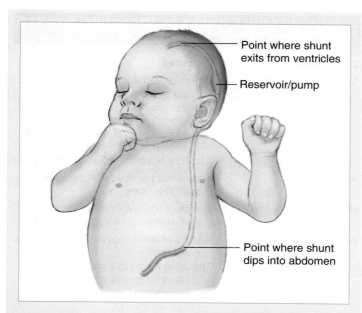

Point where shunt exits from ventricles

Reservoir/pump

Point where shunt dips into abdomen

Figure 41-34 A CSF shunt directs CSF away from the ventricles in the brain to the abdomen to relieve pressure.

treatment facilities where neurosurgical evaluation is available. The child's condition can deteriorate rapidly, so maintain continuous cardiopulmonary monitoring during transport.

Assessment and Management

Follow the standard paediatric assessment sequence when approaching children with special health care needs. Ask questions of the carer or parent to establish the child's baseline level of neurological function and baseline physiological status. Meet every child at his or her unique developmental level. An otherwise healthy 10-year-old with a perinatal brain injury may have the developmental skills of a toddler. Conversely, a 6-year-old with severe cardiopulmonary compromise may be ventilator-dependent and have oxygen saturation in the 80s but be cognitively intact.

Your treatment goal is to restore a child to his or her own physiological baseline, which will require collaboration with parents to determine what is normal for the child and management strategies that have been successful in the past.

Special Considerations

Parents will be key resources when managing a child with special health care needs. Draw on their expertise to assist you in assessing and managing the child.

Transport

Most children with special health care needs will have a medical home—that is, a hospital or clinic where they receive their care. Transporting to a hospital where the clinical team is familiar with the patient's history and needs will streamline their care. If this is not possible, take along any medical records available to assist the team at the receiving hospital to sort out the potentially complex issues faced by the patient. Take any assistive devices as well, including home ventilators and feeding pumps. Most important, take the parent or parent of the child! Children with special health care needs rely on their parents for much—if not all—of their care-taking needs, so it can be emotionally difficult for the child to be separated from the parent.

Paediatric Mental Health

During your time as a paramedic, you will undoubtedly encounter children with behavioural and psychiatric problems. The call may be for out-of-control behaviour or for a suicide attempt. Unfortunately, ambulance service calls for behavioural emergencies are increasing, reflecting in part the limited community resources available for children with mental health problems. A recent study of one A&E department found that 5% of all paediatric A&E visits were for mental health concerns.

Safety

When you are called to a home for a behavioural or psychiatric emergency, safety should be your first priority. Assess the scene for your own safety and for the safety of your patient. If weapons are involved or you cannot determine the degree of risk, call for police backup.

Approach the child calmly, letting him or her know you are there to help. Address the patient directly when obtaining the history, and explain clearly what you are doing and why. Some children may make a run for it, so carefully plan where you position yourselves.

The laws regarding restraining patients in the UK are quite clear. Unless the patient will do harm to themselves or another, you must not restrain any patient. In circumstances where you believe the child will not wait to be assessed or treated, it is prudent to call the police.

Assessment and Management

The PAT will give you a general impression of the child's mental status and cardiovascular stability. A child who has attempted suicide by ingestion may have life-threatening medical complications that trump his or her psychiatric concerns.

In the absence of acute medical issues, the bulk of your assessment will be based on observation and history. In cases involving a very agitated child, your hands-on examination may be limited. **Table 41-23 ▶** lists specific SAMPLE questions for behavioural emergencies. As always, treat any existing medical problems or injuries by using standard guidelines.

▋Promoting Prevention

Emergency care for children involves a team approach by health care professionals in the community and in the hospital. Paramedics are a critical part of the community responsible for caring for sick and injured children, but their role in prevention is not always highlighted, even though this is an area where they can have a greater public health impact than possible by running a code or controlling an airway. To be an effective child safety advocate, you must be knowledgeable about local and national prevention programmes, such as those conducted through the NSPCC or RoSPA.

Prevention of Injuries

Most injuries are not accidents, but rather are predictable and preventable events. Knowledge of injury patterns helps target potential areas for intervention and prevention. For example,

Table 41-23	SAMPLE History for Behavioural Problems in Children
Component	**Features**
Signs and symptoms	Out-of-control behaviour? Suicidal or homicidal thoughts or actions? Harm to self, others, or pets? Recent change in behaviour? Recent change in medication? Auditory or visual hallucinations?
Allergies	Known food or drug allergies and their reactions
Medications	List of all patient's medications and vitamins, prescribed and GSL
Past medical history	History of any behaviour or psychiatric problems? Therapist or psychiatrist contact information? Prior psychiatric or behavioural hospitalisations? Any medical illnesses?
Last oral intake	Timing and identification of last food and drink
Events leading to behavioural problems	Ongoing or new stressors? Argument or fight with boyfriend, girlfriend, or family members?

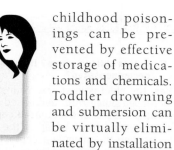

Notes from Nancy

In the seriously injured child, all organ systems must be assumed to be injured until proved otherwise.

childhood poisonings can be prevented by effective storage of medications and chemicals. Toddler drowning and submersion can be virtually eliminated by installation of four-sided pool fencing. The risk of serious injury from a bike crash is lessened by use of a helmet. The morbidity and mortality from road traffic collisions is dramatically decreased by the appropriate use of child restraint devices.

As you care for children, you may be frustrated by the illnesses and injuries that you encounter, especially when they are preventable. Take this frustration as a call to action. Get involved in your community. Participate in existing prevention programmes or start your own programme. Numerous types of paediatric injury can be targeted Table 41-24 ▶ ; choose something that interests you, and take a leadership role.

Table 41-24	Examples of Common Injuries and Possible Prevention Strategies
Injury	**Preventive Measures**
Vehicle trauma	Infant and child restraint seats Seatbelts and air bags Pedestrian safety programmes Motorcycle helmets
Cycling	Bicycle helmets Bicycle paths separate from vehicle traffic
Recreation	Appropriate safety padding and apparel Cyclist, skateboard, and skater safety programmes Soft, energy-absorbent playground surfaces
Drowning and submersion	Four-sided locked pool enclosures Pool alarms Immediate adult supervision Caretaker CPR training Swimming lessons Pool and beach safety instruction Personal flotation devices
Poisoning and household injuries	Proper storage of chemicals and medications Child safety packaging
Burns	Proper maintenance and monitoring of electrical appliances and cords Fire and smoke detectors Proper placement of cookware on stove top
Other	Discouragement of infant walker use Gated stairways Babysitter first-aid training Child care worker first-aid training

You are the Paramedic Summary

1. What assessment tool will you use to form your general impression of your patient?

The PAT provides emergency care providers with a quick hands-off approach to patient assessment. It can provide you with information about your patient in less than 30 seconds and without touching the patient. The three sides of the PAT—appearance, breathing, and circulation—will aid you in determining whether the child is sick or not sick. The PAT will also assist you in figuring out the physiological status of your patient: Is he or she in respiratory distress or failure; in shock; or experiencing a neurological problem?

2. What can you do to assist the panicked mother?

If you are a parent, you can probably relate to the fear and panic the mother is experiencing. Your best approach is to let the mother know everything that you are doing as you are doing it. Reassure her that you are doing everything possible to take care of her child, but be careful not to offer false hope by saying "Everything will be okay". Above all, remain calm and in charge of the scene. The mother needs to see that you are confident and secure with what you are doing. If possible, ask the mother to help care for the child and allow her to accompany her child to the hospital.

3. What do you need to carefully monitor your patient for?

Although the patient seems to be in stable condition at this time, he can begin to decompensate at any time without warning. The physical examination revealed a potential head injury, abdominal injury with bleeding, and a fractured femur. Any of these injuries can cause rapid deterioration of the patient's condition. Be alert for further changes in mental status, decline in respiratory status, and signs of shock.

4. Which interventions should you consider at this point, if any?

You have delegated the role of cervical spine immobilisation, and the patient is receiving supplemental oxygen. At this time, you can consider establishing IV access, applying a cardiac monitor, applying a cervical collar, and immobilising the child on a longboard.

5. Is this child in shock? If so, is it compensated or decompensated?

Yes, the child is in shock. Your patient assessment reveals an increased pulse rate, decreased respiratory status, decreased blood pressure, and increased capillary refill. Currently, he is in compensated shock based on the blood pressure, which remains lower than the minimal acceptable blood pressure. The formula for calculating minimal acceptable blood pressure for children younger than 10 years is 80 + (2 × age in years); this patient is 2 years old, so the minimal acceptable blood pressure would be 84 mm Hg.

6. How should your patient management progress?

Once the airway has been secured, you should focus on correcting the problems with circulation. Establish vascular access so you can administer fluids. Time is of the essence, meaning you should not spend a great deal of time trying to secure peripheral IV access. If you experience difficulty trying to find a vein, obtain vascular access using an IO needle. After securing vascular access, administer a fluid bolus at 5 ml/kg.

7. What do you think is the cause for shock in this patient?

This child has two potential causes for shock: abdominal injury with bleeding and a fractured femur. Both injuries could lead to a significant blood loss. Head injury will cause the blood pressure to increase as the pressure within the skull rises.

8. What criteria were used to determine that this patient was a "trauma alert"?

A trauma alert was called for this patient owing to the MOI, potential for a closed head injury, possible abdominal bleeding, and a femoral fracture.

Prep Kit

Ready for Review

- Children differ anatomically, physiologically, and emotionally from adults.
- Sick or injured children present unique challenges in evaluation and management. Their perceptions of their illness or injury, their world, and of paramedics differ from the perceptions of adults.
- The majority of children you treat will come with at least one parent or carer. Thus, in many paediatric calls, you will be dealing with more than one patient—even if only the child is ill or injured.
- Serious illness or injury to a child is one of the most stressful situations parents can face.
- An assessment tool called the Paediatric Assessment Triangle (PAT) has been developed to help ambulance service providers form a from-the-doorway general impression of paediatric patients.
- Respiratory problems are among the medical emergencies that you will most frequently encounter in children. Paediatric patients with a respiratory chief complaint will span the spectrum from mildly ill to near death.
- In paediatrics, respiratory failure and arrest precede the majority of cardiopulmonary arrests; by contrast, a primary cardiac event is the usual cause of sudden death in adults.
- Cardiovascular emergencies are relatively rare in children. When such problems arise, they are often related to volume or infection rather than to a primary cardiac cause, unless the child has congenital heart disease.
- Through the PAT and initial assessment, you can quickly identify a cardiovascular emergency, understand the likely pathological cause, and institute potentially lifesaving treatment.
- Paediatric medical calls may include respiratory complaints, fever, convulsions, and altered LOC.
- Toxic exposures account for a significant number of paediatric emergencies.
- The sudden death of an apparently healthy baby is devastating to families and the ambulance service crew that responds to the call.
- An apparent life-threatening event (ALTE) is an episode during which an infant becomes pale or cyanotic; chokes, gags, or has an apnoeic spell; or loses muscle tone.
- Child abuse or maltreatment comes in many forms: physical abuse, sexual abuse, emotional abuse, child neglect.
- Paediatric trauma is the leading cause of death among children older than 1 year.
  - Motor vehicle collisions cause the most deaths in this age group, followed by falls and submersions.
  - Among adolescents, murder and suicide are major causes of death.
- The initial assessment and management of paediatric burn victims is similar to that of adults, with a few key differences.
  - The larger skin surface–body mass ratio of children makes them more susceptible to heat and fluid loss.
  - Worrying patterns of injury or suspicious circumstances should raise concerns of child abuse.
- Children with special health care needs include children with physical, developmental, and learning disabilities.
  - These disabilities have a broad range of causes, including premature birth, traumatic brain injury, congenital anatomical anomalies, and acquired illnesses.
  - Advances in technology and drugs have enabled an increasing number of children with disabilities to receive care in the community, leading to a corresponding increase in the number of ambulance service calls for this medically complex population.
- During your time as a paramedic, you will undoubtedly encounter children with behavioural and psychiatric problems.
  - The call may be for out-of-control behaviour or for a suicide attempt.
  - Ambulance service calls for behavioural emergencies are increasing, reflecting in part the limited community resources available for children with mental health problems.

Vital Vocabulary

absence convulsions The type of convulsions characterised by a brief lapse of attention in which the patient may stare and not respond; formerly known as petit mal convulsions.

acrocyanosis Cyanosis of the extremities.

apparent life-threatening event (ALTE) An unexpected sudden episode of colour change, tone change, or apnoea that required mouth-to-mouth resuscitation or vigorous stimulation.

blow-by technique A method of delivering oxygen by holding a face mask or similar device near an infant's or a child's face; used when a nonrebreathing mask is not tolerated.

bronchiolitis A condition seen in children younger than 2 years, characterised by dyspnoea and wheezing.

central venous cannula A cannula inserted into the vena cava to permit intermittent or continuous monitoring of central venous pressure and to facilitate obtaining blood samples for chemical analysis.

cerebrospinal fluid shunts Tubes that drain fluid manufactured in the ventricles of the brain from the subarachnoid space to another part of the body outside of the brain, such as the peritoneum; lowers pressure in the brain.

complex febrile convulsions An unusual form of convulsions that occurs in association with a rapid increase in body temperature.

complex partial convulsions Convulsions characterised by alteration of consciousness with or without complex focal motor activity.

cricoid pressure The application of posterior pressure to the cricoid cartilage; minimises gastric distension and the risk of vomiting and aspiration during ventilation; also referred to as the Sellick manoeuvre.

croup A childhood viral disease characterised by oedema of the upper airways with barking cough, difficult breathing, and stridor.

cyanosis Slightly bluish, greyish, slatelike, or dark purple discolouration of the skin due to hypoxia.

epiglottitis Inflammation of the epiglottis.

generalised convulsions The convulsions characterised by manifestations that indicate involvement of both cerebral hemispheres.

grunting A short, low-pitched sound at the end of exhalation, present in children with moderate to severe hypoxia; reflects poor gas exchange because of fluid in the lower airways and air sacs.

head bobbing A sign of increased work of breathing in which the head lifts and tilts back during inspiration, then moves forward during expiration.

hydrocephalus The increased accumulation of cerebrospinal fluid within the ventricles of the brain.

meningitis Inflammation of the membranes of the spinal cord or brain.

Mongolian spots Blue-grey areas of discolouration of the skin caused by abnormal pigment, not by trauma or bruising.

mottling A condition of abnormal skin circulation, caused by vasoconstriction or inadequate circulation.

nasal flaring The flaring out of the nostrils, indicating increased work of breathing and hypoxia.

neonatal period The first month of life.

nuchal rigidity A stiff or painful neck; commonly associated with meningitis.

ossification centres Areas where cartilage is transformed through calcification into a new area of bone.

osteomyelitis Inflammation of the bone due to infection; a potential complication of intraosseous infusion.

pallor Lack of colour; paleness.

Paediatric Assessment Triangle (PAT) An assessment tool that allows rapid formation of a general impression of the type and level of illness or injury in an infant or child without touching him or her; consists of assessing appearance, work of breathing, and circulation to the skin.

petechial Characterised by small purplish, nonblanching spots on the skin.

purpuric Pertaining to bruising of the skin.

respiratory arrest The absence of respirations with detectable cardiac activity.

respiratory distress A clinical state characterised by increased respiratory rate, effort, and work of breathing.

respiratory failure A clinical state of inadequate oxygenation, ventilation, or both.

respiratory syncytial virus (RSV) A virus that commonly causes bronchiolitis; usually results in lifelong immunity following exposure.

recession Physical drawing in of the chest wall between the ribs that occurs with increased work of breathing.

rhonchi Rattling respiratory sounds; also called crackles.

sepsis A pathological state, usually in a febrile patient, resulting from the presence of invading microorganisms or their poisonous products in the bloodstream.

shaken baby syndrome A syndrome seen in abused infants and children; the patient has been subjected to violent, whiplash-type shaking injuries inflicted by the abusing individual that may cause coma, convulsions, and increased intracranial pressure due to tearing of the cerebral veins with consequent bleeding into the brain.

simple febrile convulsions A brief, self-limited, generalised convulsion in a previously healthy child between the ages of 6 months and 6 years that is associated with the onset of or sudden increase in fever.

simple partial convulsions Focal convulsions that involve a motor or sensory abnormality in a patient who remains conscious.

sinus tachycardia Rapid heart rate in a child with normal conduction.

sniffing position An upright position in which the patient's head and chin are thrust slightly forward to keep the airway open; appears to be sniffing.

status epilepticus A state of continuous convulsions or multiple convulsions without a return to consciousness for 30 minutes.

stoma A small opening, especially an artificially created opening, such as that made by tracheostomy.

stridor A harsh sound during inspiration, high-pitched due to partial upper airway obstruction.

subglottic space The narrowest part of the paediatric airway.

sudden unexpected death in infancy (SUDI) The abrupt and unexplained death of an apparently healthy child younger than 1 year.

supraventricular tachycardia (SVT) An abnormal heart rhythm with a rapid, narrow QRS complex.

synchronised cardioversion The timed delivery of energy into the myocardium to correct rapid, regular cardiac rhythms in patients who are in unstable condition.

tonic-clonic convulsions Convulsions that feature rhythmic back-and-forth motion of an extremity and body stiffness.

tripoding An abnormal position to keep the airway open; involves leaning forward onto two arms stretched forward.

vasoconstriction A decrease in the calibre of blood vessels.

ventilation-perfusion mismatch A pathological state in which the oxygen entering the lungs is not mixing properly with the blood circulating through the lungs.

wheezing The production of whistling sounds during expiration such as occurs in asthma and bronchiolitis.

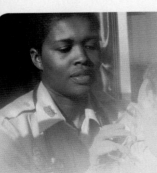

Assessment in Action

You arrive on the scene of a 6-year-old girl having difficulty breathing. Your assessment reveals that she is breathing about 40 times per minute. Her chest muscles seem to be tight and sunken between her ribs. She appears to be working very hard to breathe, and you hear grunting sounds, but the patient's skin colour and mental state seem within normal limits.

1. **Which phase of physiological response is this patient in?**
    A. Respiratory distress
    B. Respiratory failure
    C. Respiratory arrest
    D. Cardiac arrest

2. **A child who appears to be sleepy or drowsy in addition to having difficulty breathing is called:**
    A. obtuse.
    B. obstructed.
    C. sluggish.
    D. compromised.

3. **A child who uses chest muscles to help breathe is said to be using:**
   A. excessive muscles.
   B. accessory muscles.
   C. retractive muscles.
   D. tripod muscles.

4. **Which phase of physiological response represents the point at which the patient will decompensate?**
   A. Respiratory distress
   B. Respiratory failure
   C. Respiratory arrest
   D. Cardiac arrest

5. **What is the best way to manage a paediatric patient in respiratory arrest?**
   A. Face mask with oxygen at 15 l/min
   B. Bag-valve-mask ventilation with oxygen at 15 l/min
   C. ET tube with bag-valve-mask ventilation
   D. Chest compressions, ET tube with bag-valve-mask ventilation

Challenging Question

6. **Why are paediatric patients more likely to have respiratory arrest before cardiac arrest?**

Points to Ponder

You have been dispatched to a paediatric patient who has a low oxygen saturation level. During your response, you wonder how this call came in for a specific problem like "low oxygen saturation level", so you ask your ambulance control to find out more about the call. The ambulance control reports that the call came from the child's mother. When you arrive at the scene, you find a child lying on a bed. The patient is connected to a number of tubes, and you notice a tracheostomy tube in place. The mother states that his saturation level is lower than normal and she is concerned that one of the drains is not working. When you look around the room, you realise that you are not familiar with any of the equipment present.

What is the best way to proceed with your assessment and treatment of this child?

Issues: Technology-Assisted Children, Work of Breathing, Airway Obstruction.

42 Older People

Objectives

Cognitive

- Discuss population demographics demonstrating the rise in elderly population in the UK.
- Discuss society's view of ageing and the social, financial, and ethical issues facing the elderly.
- Assess the various living environments of elderly patients.
- Describe the local resources available to assist the elderly and create strategies to refer at risk patients to appropriate community services.
- Discuss issues facing society concerning the elderly.
- Discuss common emotional and psychological reactions to ageing to include causes and manifestations.
- Apply the pathophysiology of multi-system failure to the assessment and management of medical conditions in the elderly patient.
- Discuss the problems with mobility in the elderly and develop strategies to prevent falls.
- Discuss the implications of problems with sensation to communication and patient assessment.
- Discuss the problems with continence and elimination and develop communication strategies to provide psychological support.
- Discuss factors that may complicate the assessment of the elderly patient.
- Describe principles that should be employed when assessing and communicating with the elderly.
- Compare the assessment of a young patient with that of an elderly patient.
- Discuss common complaints of elderly patients.
- Compare the pharmacokinetics of an elderly patient to that of a young adult.
- Discuss the impact of polypharmacy and medication non-compliance on patient assessment and management.
- Discuss drug distribution, metabolism, and excretion in the elderly patient.
- Discuss medication issues of the elderly including polypharmacy, dosing errors and increased drug sensitivity.
- Discuss the use and effects of commonly prescribed drugs for the elderly patient.
- Discuss the normal and abnormal changes with age of the pulmonary system.
- Describe the epidemiology of pulmonary diseases in the elderly, including incidence, morbidity/mortality, risk factors, and prevention strategies for patients with pneumonia, chronic obstructive pulmonary diseases and pulmonary embolism.
- Compare and contrast the pathophysiology of pulmonary diseases in the elderly with that of a younger adult, including pneumonia, chronic obstructive pulmonary diseases, and pulmonary embolism.
- Discuss the assessment of the elderly patient with pulmonary complaints, including pneumonia, chronic obstructive pulmonary diseases, and pulmonary embolism.
- Identify the need for intervention and transport of the elderly patient with pulmonary complaints.
- Develop a treatment and management plan of the elderly patient with pulmonary complaints, including pneumonia, chronic obstructive pulmonary diseases, and pulmonary embolism.
- Discuss the normal and abnormal cardiovascular system changes with age.
- Describe the epidemiology for cardiovascular diseases in the elderly, including incidence, morbidity/mortality, risk factors, and prevention strategies for patients with myocardial infarction, heart failure, arrhythmias, aneurysm, and hypertension.
- Compare and contrast the pathophysiology of cardiovascular diseases in the elderly with that of a younger adult, including myocardial infarction, heart failure, arrhythmias, aneurysm, and hypertension.
- Discuss the assessment of the elderly patient with complaints related to the cardiovascular system, including myocardial infarction, heart failure, arrhythmias, aneurysm, and hypertension.
- Identify the need for intervention and transport of the elderly patient with cardiovascular complaints.
- Develop a treatment and management plan for the elderly patient with cardiovascular complaints, including myocardial infarction, heart failure, arrhythmias, aneurysm, and hypertension.
- Discuss the normal and abnormal changes with age of the nervous system.
- Describe the epidemiology for nervous system diseases in the elderly, including incidence, morbidity/mortality, risk factors, and prevention strategies for patients with cerebrovascular disease, delirium, dementia, Alzheimer's disease, and Parkinson's disease.
- Compare and contrast the pathophysiology of nervous system diseases in the elderly with that of a younger adult, including cerebrovascular disease, delirium, dementia, Alzheimer's disease, and Parkinson's disease.
- Discuss the assessment of the elderly patient with complaints related to the nervous system, including cerebrovascular disease, delirium, dementia, Alzheimer's disease, and Parkinson's disease.
- Identify the need for intervention and transport of the patient with complaints related to the nervous system.
- Develop a treatment and management plan of the elderly patient with complaints related to the nervous system, including cerebrovascular disease, delirium, dementia, Alzheimer's disease, and Parkinson's disease.
- Discuss the normal and abnormal changes of the endocrine system with age.

- Describe the epidemiology for endocrine diseases in the elderly, including incidence, morbidity/mortality, risk factors, and prevention strategies for patients with diabetes and thyroid diseases.
- Compare and contrast the pathophysiology of diabetes and thyroid diseases in the elderly with that of a younger adult.
- Discuss the assessment of the elderly patient with complaints related to the endocrine system, including diabetes and thyroid diseases.
- Identify the need for intervention and transport of the patient with endocrine problems.
- Develop a treatment and management plan of the elderly patient with endocrine problems, including diabetes and thyroid diseases.
- Discuss the normal and abnormal changes of the gastrointestinal system with age.
- Discuss the assessment of the elderly patient with complaints related to the gastrointestinal system.
- Identify the need for intervention and transport of the patient with gastrointestinal complaints.
- Develop and execute a treatment and management plan of the elderly patient with gastrointestinal problems.
- Discuss the assessment and management of an elderly patient with GI haemorrhage and bowel obstruction.
- Compare and contrast the pathophysiology of GI haemorrhage and bowel obstruction in the elderly with that of a young adult.
- Discuss the normal and abnormal changes with age related to toxicology.
- Discuss the assessment of the elderly patient with complaints related to toxicology.
- Identify the need for intervention and transport of the patient with toxicological problems.
- Develop and execute a treatment and management plan of the elderly patient with toxicological problems.
- Describe the epidemiology in the elderly, including the incidence, morbidity/mortality, risk factors, and prevention strategies, for patients with drug toxicity.
- Compare and contrast the pathophysiology of drug toxicity in the elderly with that of a younger adult.
- Discuss the assessment findings common in elderly patients with drug toxicity.
- Discuss the management/considerations when treating an elderly patient with drug toxicity.
- Describe the epidemiology for drug and alcohol abuse in the elderly, including incidence, morbidity/mortality, risk factors, and prevention strategies.
- Compare and contrast the pathophysiology of drug and alcohol abuse in the elderly with that of a younger adult.
- Discuss the assessment findings common in elderly patients with drug and alcohol abuse.
- Discuss the management/considerations when treating an elderly patient with drug and alcohol abuse.
- Discuss the normal and abnormal changes of thermoregulation with age.
- Discuss the assessment of the elderly patient with complaints related to thermoregulation.
- Identify the need for intervention and transport of the patient with environmental considerations.
- Develop and execute a treatment and management plan for the elderly patient with environmental considerations.
- Compare and contrast the pathophysiology of hypothermia and hyperthermia in the elderly with that of a younger adult.

- Discuss the assessment findings and management plan for elderly patients with hypothermia and hyperthermia.
- Discuss the normal and abnormal psychiatric changes of age.
- Describe the epidemiology of depression and suicide in the elderly, including incidence, morbidity/mortality, risk factors, and prevention strategies.
- Compare and contrast the psychiatry of depression and suicide in the elderly with that of a younger adult.
- Discuss the assessment of the elderly patient with psychiatric complaints, including depression and suicide.
- Identify the need for intervention and transport of the elderly psychiatric patient.
- Develop a treatment and management plan of the elderly psychiatric patient, including depression and suicide.
- Discuss the normal and abnormal changes of the integumentary system with age.
- Describe the epidemiology for pressure ulcers in the elderly, including incidence, morbidity/mortality, risk factors, and prevention strategies.
- Compare and contrast the pathophysiology of pressure ulcers in the elderly with that of a younger adult.
- Discuss the assessment of the elderly patient with complaints related to the integumentary system, including pressure ulcers.
- Identify the need for intervention and transport of the patient with complaints related to the integumentary system.
- Develop a treatment and management plan of the elderly patient with complaints related to the integumentary system, including pressure ulcers.
- Discuss the normal and abnormal changes of the musculoskeletal system with age.
- Describe the epidemiology for osteoarthritis and osteoporosis, including incidence, morbidity/mortality, risk factors, and prevention strategies.
- Compare and contrast the pathophysiology of osteoarthritis and osteoporosis with that of a younger adult.
- Discuss the assessment of the elderly patient with complaints related to the musculoskeletal system, including osteoarthritis and osteoporosis.
- Identify the need for intervention and transport of the patient with musculoskeletal complaints.
- Develop a treatment and management plan of the elderly patient with musculoskeletal complaints, including osteoarthritis and osteoporosis.
- Describe the epidemiology for trauma in the elderly, including incidence, morbidity/mortality, risk factors, and prevention strategies for patients with orthopaedic injuries, burns, and head injuries.
- Compare and contrast the pathophysiology of trauma in the elderly with that of a younger adult, including orthopaedic injuries, burns, and head injuries.
- Discuss the assessment findings common in elderly patients with traumatic injuries, including orthopaedic injuries, burns, and head injuries.
- Discuss the management/considerations when treating an elderly patient with traumatic injuries, including orthopaedic injuries, burns, and head injuries.
- Identify the need for intervention and transport of the elderly patient with trauma.

Affective

- Demonstrate and advocate appropriate interactions with the elderly that conveys respect for their position in life.
- Recognise the emotional need for independence in the elderly while simultaneously attending to their apparent acute dependence.
- Recognise and appreciate the many impediments to physical and emotional well being in the elderly.

- Recognise and appreciate the physical and emotional difficulties associated with being a carer of an impaired elderly person, particularly the patient with Alzheimer's disease.

Psychomotor

- Demonstrate the ability to assess an older patient.
- Demonstrate the ability to adjust their assessment to an older patient.

Introduction

Approximately one fifth of the UK population is over 60 years of age. Between 1995 and 2025 the number of people over 80 will increase by almost 50% and the number over 90 will double.

Older people constitute an ever-increasing proportion of patients in the health care system, particularly the emergency care sector. The NHS spent around £10 million, about 40% of its budget, on patients over 65 in 1998–99. This means almost two thirds of its general and acute hospital beds are committed to patients over 65. This population also has more contacts with doctors than those under 65 years of age.

The old-age dependency ratio depicts the dependency individuals place upon society as they age. It is defined as the number of older people for every 100 adults (potential carers) between the ages of 18 and 64. In 1990, there were 20 older people for every 100 "carers". By 2025, it is projected that there will be 32 older people for every 100 "carers". The supply of carers is not keeping pace with the growth of the older population. The need for carers is going to increase, and society is going to have difficulty keeping up with the demand for services as the population continues to age. As the older population grows, ambulance clinicians will be required to offer services that are cost effective and efficient. Costs associated with providing care and facility issues will make finance a continuing concern.

Most of your older patients will not reside in nursing homes. Although nursing home admissions are increasing owing to the larger number of older people in the United Kingdom, a countertrend is for elderly people to maintain independent lives. Many older adults continue to live at home with support from a spouse or family member and a visiting nurse; others live in a more dependent care environment such as a warden-assisted or sheltered accommodation.

Determining how and where older adults will spend their retirement years is a difficult and complex process involving numerous social and economic issues such as the person's marital status, financial resources, religious beliefs, ethnicity, sex, and general health. Because such decisions may place a burden on family members, their wishes must be considered by health care providers. When making these decisions, older adults and their families can seek advice from medical social workers, professional care managers, discharge planners at health care facilities, and a large number of private and public resources. The range of services available includes delivered meals, personal care, housekeeping, adult day care, transportation, carer support, respite care, and crisis response systems, including ambulance services and lifelines Figure 42-1 ▶ .

Psychosocial factors may influence successful ageing. For example, at retirement, a person may no longer feel useful or productive in society and may experience diminished self-esteem. Age also brings bereavement—sadness over the loss of friends and loved ones. Notably, the likelihood of death increases during the year following the death of one's spouse. As friends and family members die, elderly persons tend to experience increasing loneliness and isolation—factors shown to have negative effects on health.

Finally, the health problems of older people are quantitatively and qualitatively different from the problems of younger people. One cannot simply transfer the principles of caring for

You are the Paramedic Part 1

You are working with Mike, a newly qualified paramedic who has joined your station. Your focus for the day has been on older people emergencies because your ambulance service provides service to six care homes and sheltered housing accommodations. As luck would have it, you are dispatched to one of the smaller community care homes for a sick person.

Upon arrival you are escorted to the day room where the residents spend most of their time. A nurse sitting next to a patient seated in a wheelchair by the window waves you over. She introduces you to Mrs Howard, a frail-looking 86-year-old widow. The nurse explains that Mrs Howard has been running a low-grade fever since the previous evening and is "not acting like her normal self". The doctor has requested that she be transferred to hospital to be evaluated. When asked how she is feeling, Mrs Howard slowly turns her head away from the window toward you and replies "not well".

Initial Assessment	Recording Time: 0 Minutes
Appearance	Frail, weak, elderly woman
Level of consciousness	A (Alert to person, place, and day)
Airway	Open and clear
Breathing	Adequate chest rise and volume
Circulation	Strong, rapid radial pulse, slightly irregular

1. Why is it important to review common medical problems of elderly people?
2. Which organ systems are greatly affected by age-related changes?

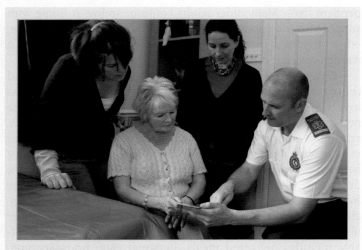

Figure 42-1 Emergency care professionals should be familiar with available resources.

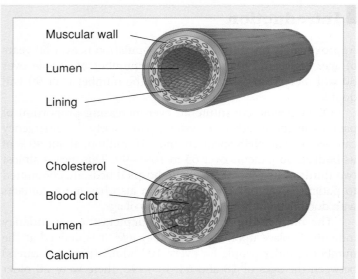

Figure 42-3 Atherosclerosis, the buildup of fatty plaque on arterial walls.

the younger population without modification. The special problems of older people require special approaches.

Anatomy and Physiology

Human growth and development peaks in the late 20s and early 30s, at which point the ageing process sets in. Ageing is a *linear* process; that is, the rate at which we lose functions does not increase with age. A 35-year-old is ageing just as fast as an 85-year-old, but the older person exhibits the cumulative results of a longer process. Of course, the ageing process can vary dramatically from one person to another. Most of us can report having seen 60-year-olds who look frail and elderly and 80-year-olds who run marathons **Figure 42-2 ◂** .

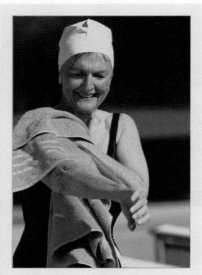

Figure 42-2 Many older people, especially those who have hobbies and activities, are healthy and outgoing.

The ageing process is inevitably accompanied by changes in physiological function, such as a decline in the function of the liver and kidneys. All tissues in the body undergo ageing, albeit not at the same rate. The decrease in the functional capacity of various organ systems is normal but can affect the way in which a patient responds to illness.

It can also affect the way health professionals respond to a patient's illness. For example, a health care provider who is unaware of the normal changes of ageing may mistake the changes for signs of illness and be tempted to give treatment when none is necessary. At the other end of the spectrum, there is a widespread—and unfortunate—tendency to attribute genuine disease symptoms to "just getting old" and to neglect their treatment.

Changes in the Cardiovascular System

A variety of changes occur in the cardiovascular system as a person grows older, with their net effect being to decrease the efficiency of this system. Specifically, the heart hypertrophies (enlarges) with age, probably in response to the chronically increased afterload imposed by stiffened blood vessels. Bigger is not better, however. Over time, cardiac output declines, mostly as a result of a decreasing stroke volume. Arteriosclerosis—the stiffening of vessel walls—contributes to systolic hypertension in many older patients, which places an extra burden on the heart. This phenomenon may be a consequence of disease states such as diabetes, atherosclerosis **Figure 42-3 ▴** , and renal compromise, and it is associated with an increased risk of cardiovascular disease, dementia, and death. Compliance of vascular walls depends on the production of collagen and elastin, proteins that are the primary components of muscle and connective tissue. An increase in pressure (normal hypertension seen in ageing) leads to overproduction of abnormal collagen and decreased quantities of elastin, both of which contribute to vascular stiffening. The result is a widening pulse pressure, decreased coronary artery perfusion, and changes in cardiac ejection efficiency.

At the same time, the electric conduction system of the heart deteriorates over time. For example, the number of pacemaker cells in the sinoatrial node decreases dramatically as a person ages. In many cases, the changes in the conduction system lead to bradycardia, which can in turn contribute to the decline in cardiac output.

Some changes in cardiovascular performance are probably not a direct consequence of ageing, but rather reflect the deconditioning effect of a sedentary lifestyle. Whether because of other disabilities (such as arthritis) or for psychological reasons, many people tend to limit physical activity as they grow older. The bodybuilder's slogan, "Use it or lose it", applies just as much to the cardiac muscle as to the biceps.

Changes in the Respiratory System

A person's respiratory capacity also undergoes significant reductions with age, largely due to decreases in the elasticity of the lungs and in the size and strength of the respiratory muscles. In addition, calcification of costochondral cartilage tends to make the chest wall stiffer. As a result of these changes, the vital capacity (the amount of air that can be exhaled following a maximal inhalation) decreases, and the residual volume (the amount of air left in the lungs at the end of a maximal exhalation) increases. Thus, although the total amount of air in the lungs does not change with age, the proportion of that air usefully used in gas exchange progressively declines. Air flow, which depends largely on airway size and resistance, also deteriorates somewhat with age.

Meanwhile, changes in the distribution of blood flow within the lungs result in declining pO_2. At age 30, the pO_2 of a healthy person breathing ambient air is usually around 90 mm Hg; at 80 years, the pO_2 under the same conditions is around 75 mm Hg ($pO_2 = 100 - age/3$). Furthermore, the respiratory drive becomes dulled as a person ages because of decreased sensitivity to changes in arterial blood gases or decreased central nervous system (CNS) response to such changes. As a consequence, elderly people have a slower reaction to hypoxaemia and hypercarbia.

Musculoskeletal changes, such as kyphosis (outward curvature of the thoracic spine; also called hunchback), may also affect pulmonary function by limiting lung volume and maximal inspiratory pressure. In addition, the lung's defence mechanisms become less effective as a natural consequence of ageing. The cough and gag reflexes decrease with age, increasing the risk of aspiration. Furthermore, the ciliary mechanisms that normally help remove bronchial secretions are markedly slowed.

Changes in the Renal System

Age brings changes in the kidneys as well. The kidneys are responsible for maintaining the body's fluid and electrolyte balance and have important roles in maintaining the body's long-term acid-base balance and eliminating drugs from the body. In a young adult, the kidneys weigh 250 to 270 g; in a healthy 70-year-old, they weigh 180 to 200 g. This decline in weight results from a loss of functioning nephron units, which translates into a smaller effective filtering surface. At the same time, renal blood flow decreases by as much as 50% as a person ages.

Although the kidneys of an elderly person may be capable of dealing with day-to-day demands, they may not be able to meet unusual challenges, such as those imposed by illness. For that reason, acute illness in elderly patients is often accompanied by derangements in fluid and electrolyte balance. Ageing kidneys, for example, respond sluggishly to sodium deficiency. An elderly patient may lose a great deal of sodium before the

You are the Paramedic Part 2

You begin a physical examination while your partner obtains a set of vital signs. The nurse caring for your patient is new to the care home and is not very familiar with her. She is able to tell you that your patient has a history of atrial fibrillation, congestive heart failure, diabetes, and hypertension. She is currently prescribed digoxin, pioglitazone, enalapri, ezetimibe, and simvastatin.

While you are speaking with the nurse, another patient approaches you and sets her hand on your patient's shoulder. She introduces herself as Mrs Jessup, a good friend of Mrs Howard. She tells you that it is normal for them to go for a walk every night after dinner; however, they have not walked for the past couple of evenings because Mrs Howard has been feeling weak. She also volunteers that Mrs Howard has not been eating much the past few days. Mrs Howard brushes off her friend's concerns. You are able to ascertain from Mrs Howard that the last meal she had was a bowl of soup yesterday at lunch.

Vital Signs	Recording Time: 5 Minutes
Level of consciousness	Alert
Pulse	110 beats/min, strong and irregular
Blood pressure	168/94 mm Hg
Respirations	22 breaths/min, regular
Skin	Hot, pink, and dry
SpO_2	93% on room air

3. Why might obtaining an accurate medical history and history of the present illness be challenging when interviewing an elderly patient?

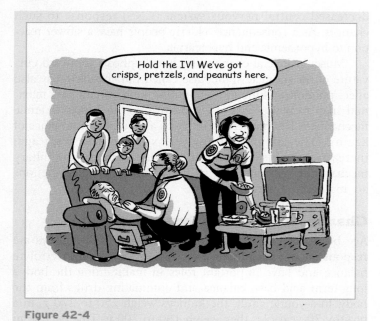

Figure 42-4

kidneys halt urinary sodium excretion, a problem that is exacerbated by the markedly decreased thirst mechanism in elderly people. The net result may be a rapid development of severe dehydration.

Conversely, elderly patients are at considerable risk of overhydration if they are exposed to large sodium loads (such as from intravenous [IV] saline solutions or heavily salted foods) **Figure 42-4 ▲**. Because of its lower glomerular filtration rate, the ageing kidney is less able than its younger counterpart to excrete a large sodium load, making the patient vulnerable to acute volume overload.

The same factors that reduce an older person's ability to handle sodium also affect the body's ability to handle potassium. Thus, elderly patients are prone to hyperkalaemia, which can reach serious—even lethal—levels if the patient becomes acidotic or if the potassium load is increased from any source.

Bowel and bladder continence require anatomically correct gastrointestinal (GI) and genitourinary tracts, functioning and intact sphincters, and properly working cognitive and physical functions. Urinary incontinence (involuntary loss of urine) can have significant social and emotional impact, but relatively few people admit to the problem and even fewer seek treatment. Incontinence is not a normal part of ageing and can lead to skin irritation, skin breakdown, and urinary tract infections. As people age, the capacity of the bladder decreases. As a consequence, an older person may find it difficult to postpone voiding or may have involuntary bladder contractions. Two major types of incontinence are distinguished: stress and urge. Stress incontinence occurs during activities such as coughing, laughing, sneezing, lifting, and exercise. Urge incontinence is triggered by hot or cold fluids, running water, and even thinking about going to the toilet. Treatment of incontinence consists of medications, physical therapy, and, possibly, surgery.

The opposite of incontinence is urinary retention or difficulty urinating. Patients may have difficulty voiding or absence of voiding as a result of many medical causes. In men, enlargement of the prostate can place pressure on the urethra, making voiding difficult. Bladder and urinary tract infections can also cause inflammation. In severe cases of urinary retention, patients may have acute or chronic renal failure.

Changes in the Digestive System

The process of digestion begins in the mouth, which is also where ageing-related changes in the digestive system may first be noted. A decrease in the number of taste buds and changes in olfactory receptors may diminish an older person's senses of taste and smell, which may in turn interfere with the enjoyment of food. The consequent decrease in appetite may lead to malnutrition. Other changes in the mouth include a reduction in the volume of saliva, with a resulting dryness of the mouth. Dental loss is *not* a normal result of the ageing process, but rather the result of disease of the teeth and gums; nevertheless, dental loss is widespread in the elderly population and contributes to nutritional and digestive problems.

Like oral secretions, gastric secretions are reduced as a person ages—although enough acid is still present to produce ulcers under certain conditions. Changes in gastric motility also occur, which may lead to slower gastric emptying—a factor of some importance when assessing the risk of aspiration.

Function of the small and large bowel changes little as a consequence of ageing, although the incidence of certain diseases involving the bowel (such as diverticulosis) increases as a person grows older.

In the liver, there are changes in hepatic enzyme systems, with some systems declining in activity and others increasing. Notably, the activity of the enzyme systems concerned with the detoxification of drugs *declines* as a person ages.

Changes in the Musculoskeletal System

Ageing brings a widespread decrease in bone mass in men and women, but especially among postmenopausal women. Bones become more brittle and tend to break more easily. Narrowing of the intervertebral discs and compression fractures of the vertebrae contribute to a decrease in height as a person ages, along with changes in posture. Joints lose their flexibility and may be further immobilised by arthritic changes. In fact, more than half of all elderly people have some form of arthritis. Muscle mass decreases throughout the body, with an accompanying decrease in muscle strength. From your perspective, the

At the Scene

Growing old does not naturally or normally include confusion, dementia, delirium, depression, falls, weakness, syncope, and other conditions related to disease processes.

changes in the musculoskeletal system most often translate into fractures incurred as the result of falls.

Changes in the Nervous System

Ageing produces changes in the nervous system that are reflected in the neurological examination. Changes in thinking (cognitive) speed, memory, and postural stability are the most common normal findings in older people. Studies have documented age-associated declines in mental function, especially slower central processing of sensory stimuli and language, and longer retrieval times for short- and long-term memory. Collectively, these changes affect performance on the mental status portion of the neurological examination, with common findings including slow responses to questioning or requests to repeat a question.

The brain decreases in terms of weight (5% to 10%) and volume as a person ages. The functional significance of these changes is not clear, however. The human brain has an enormous reserve capacity, and having a smaller and lighter brain does not interfere with the mental capabilities of productive elderly people.

Undeniably, though, the performance of most of the sense organs suffers with increasing age. The senses of taste and smell become diminished as a person ages.

Visual changes may begin as early as 40 years, so that as many as 50% of patients older than 65 years have vision problems. Causes of visual impairment in elderly people may include diabetic retinopathy and age-related macular degeneration.

The two most common causes of visual disturbances in elderly people, however, are cataracts and glaucoma. Cataracts are a result of hardening of the lenses over time. The lenses eventually become opaque, which prevents light and images from being transmitted to the rear of the eye. Patients with cataracts may complain of blurred vision, double vision, spots, and/or ghost images. Surgical repair may be required to gain vision. By contrast, glaucoma is caused by an increase in intraocular pressure severe enough to damage the optic nerve, potentially resulting in permanent loss of peripheral and central vision. Treatment of glaucoma consists of oral medications and eye drops.

Decreases in visual acuity are common in older people, even without disease processes such as cataracts. Night vision becomes impaired, as does the ability to adjust to rapid changes in lighting conditions, depth perception, and perception of colour. Changes in a patient's vision can affect independence, ability to read, and ability to drive a vehicle.

The possibility of hearing loss increases with age. A common cause of hearing impairment in older patients is presbycusis, a progressive hearing loss, particularly in the high frequencies, along with lessened ability to discriminate between a particular sound and background noise. Patients who lose the ability to interpret most speech experience a decreased ability to communicate, which may lead to isolation and depression.

Another hearing-related impairment noted in the elderly population is Meniere disease (prevalence, 2 people per 1,000 population). Onset of symptoms usually occurs in early middle age, with symptoms presenting in cycles that last several months at a time. The typical symptoms include vertigo (a sudden loss of normal balance or equilibrium), hearing loss, tinnitus, and pressure in the ear.

For many older people, physiological changes make it difficult to produce speech that is loud enough, clear, and well spaced. Weakness, paralysis, poor hearing, or brain damage can damage the delicate functions that make these abilities possible.

Sense of body position (proprioception) also becomes impaired with age. Proprioception enables us to maintain postural stability by using a variety of receptors in the joints and information provided by the eyes. As these mechanisms fail with age, people become less steady on their feet, and the tendency to fall increases markedly.

Changes in the Integumentary System

Wrinkling and loss of resiliency of the skin are the most visible signs of ageing. Wrinkling occurs because the skin becomes thinner, drier, less elastic, and more fragile. Subcutaneous fat becomes thinner, resulting in a loosened outer cover for the body. Elastin (the substance that makes the skin pliable) and collagen (the substance that makes the skin strong) decrease with age. Thinner skin tears much more easily, and the loss of elasticity allows for more bleeding before tamponade occurs.

As a person ages, the sebaceous glands produce less oil, making dryer skin. Sweat gland activity also decreases, hindering the ability to sweat and to regulate heat. Hair follicles produce thinner hair or may stop producing hair. Follicles produce less melanin (the pigment that gives hair colour), making the hair colour revert to grey or white.

The blood vessels that supply the skin also are affected by atherosclerosis and provide less oxygenated blood at the cellular level. As a consequence of the skin's lower metabolism, epidermal cells develop more slowly and do not replace outgoing cells as quickly as with younger skin. Elderly patients, therefore, are at higher risk for secondary infection after the skin breaks, for skin tumours, and for fungal or viral infections of the skin.

Homeostatic and Other Changes

Homeostasis is the process by which the body maintains a constant internal environment. Many homeostatic mechanisms work on a feedback principle, much like the thermostat in a house—that is, a change in the internal environment feeds back to the control system to induce a corrective response. For example, when the body temperature starts to rise, temperature sensors are activated, which in turn activate compensatory responses: Cutaneous blood vessels dilate, and

Special Considerations

With patients who have some degree of hearing loss, don't shout! Lean closer and speak into the patient's ear using a somewhat low pitch. Remember that patients with limited vision are not necessarily hard of hearing.

excess heat is transferred from the body to the environment. Similarly, when the concentration of glucose in the blood rises, the pancreas is stimulated to secrete insulin, which leads to uptake of glucose by cells and reduction of the blood glucose level back toward normal.

Across the board, ageing is accompanied by a progressive loss of these homeostatic capabilities. For that reason, a specific illness or injury in elderly people is more likely to result in generalised deterioration. For example, the thirst mechanism, which ordinarily protects a person from dehydration, becomes depressed in elderly patients. Likewise, temperature-regulating mechanisms tend to become disordered, which makes elderly patients much more vulnerable to environmental stresses such as heat exhaustion and accidental hypothermia after relatively minor exposures. A defect in temperature regulation also may account for the absence of a febrile response to illness in many elderly people. Infections that would ordinarily produce high fever, such as pneumococcal pneumonia, may produce only a low-grade or no fever in elderly people.

Notes from Nancy

A specific illness or injury in the elderly is more likely to result in generalised deterioration.

The regulatory system that manages the blood glucose level similarly becomes impaired with increasing age, such that an elevated blood glucose level occurs quite commonly in older patients. Ordinarily, moderate hyperglycaemia does no harm, but overly aggressive treatment of this problem may produce damaging hypoglycaemia.

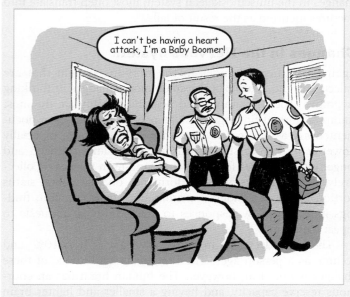

Figure 42-5

Pathophysiology

Cardiovascular System

Diseases of the heart remain the leading cause of death among older adults in the United Kingdom, and coronary artery disease (CAD) is the number one culprit. Heart attack is the major cause of morbidity and mortality in people older than 65 years, and its potential for mortality increases significantly after a person reaches 70 years **Figure 42-5 ▶**.

Myocardial infarction (MI) is the death of part of the heart muscle due to the blockage of one of the coronary arteries. Although chest pain is a common presentation for acute myocardial infarction in older patients, it may be decreased in intensity or atypical. In fact, it may even be absent, with the patient complaining primarily of dyspnoea or fatigue. Major risk factors for MI include tobacco use, hypertension, diabetes, obesity, psychosocial factors, physical activity, and alcohol consumption. Preventive strategies include measures to prevent the first MI, avoidance of recurring MIs, and lifestyle changes. Lifestyle changes include the cessation of tobacco use, eating a healthy diet, good control of blood glucose (in diabetics), exercise, weight control, and control of hypertension. A general practitioner may also order aspirin to help reduce the risk of heart attack.

People 65 years and older are a high-risk group for heart failure. In fact, this problem is the most common reason for hospitalisation in the older population. Heart failure is on the rise in this cohort for two paradoxical reasons: better care of the diseases that might otherwise result in failure (such as CAD and hypertension), which enables patients to live long enough to develop heart failure, and more effective management of heart failure once it develops. Risk factors include sex, ethnicity, family history and genetics, long-term alcohol abuse, and multiple medical conditions—CAD, emphysema, hyperthyroidism, thiamine (vitamin B) deficiency, and human immunodeficiency virus infection, among others. As with MI, prevention is aimed at lifestyle changes: cessation of tobacco use, eating a healthy diet, good control of blood glucose (in diabetics), exercise, weight control, and control of hypertension.

Rhythm disturbances (arrhythmias) of the heart occur when the electrical system controlling the heartbeat experiences an interruption or malfunction. These irregularities cause heartbeats that are too fast, too slow, irregular, or absent. Many people experience an occasional or harmless arrhythmia, which they may describe as a skipping, fluttering, or fast heartbeat. Arrhythmias in older people are generally a result of age-related changes in the heart, existing cardiac disease, adverse drug effects, or a combination of these factors.

Cardiac arrhythmias are classified by the part of the heart from which they originate. Unlike tachyarrhythmias or bradyarrhythmias, which speed up or slow down the heart, premature beats signify no change in speed but rather alter the regularity of the heartbeat. In contrast, atrial fibrillation (coming from the atria), which is the most common arrhythmia among elderly people, increases the risk of stroke and heart failure. The fibrillating atria allow stasis of the blood, thereby encouraging clot formation and increasing the chances that a clot fragment might travel to the brain and cause a stroke. Most of the blood in the atria enters the ventricles when the valves open, with about 20% being forced in by contraction of the atria. The ageing heart may function adequately when preload provided by the atria ends up in the ventricles; however, when that 20% remains in the atria, new signs or symptoms of heart failure may develop or stable heart failure may decompensate.

Bradycardias are also more common in elderly people. The ageing conduction system may produce sinus abnormalities such as sick sinus syndrome. CAD may produce high-degree blocks, whereas medications such as beta blockers or calcium channel blockers can slow the heart too much.

The human heart beats 2.5 thousand million times and moves 200 million litres of blood in an average lifetime. Not surprisingly, this workload affects the cardiovascular system throughout the entire body over the lifespan. For example, the incidence of aneurysm increases with age. An aneurysm is a weakness in any artery that produces a balloon defect, weakening the arterial wall. This weakness may be congenital (present at birth) or acquired. In the latter case, hypertension, atherosclerotic disease, and obesity are contributing factors to development of such a defect. For example, blood pressure greater than 160/95 mm Hg doubles the mortality risk in men and can lead to kidney loss and blindness by damaging the blood vessels that supply the kidney and eyes. Life-threatening aneurysms can develop in the brain, chest, or abdomen. A new headache or a change in chronic headache patterns, for example, may signal early cerebral bleeding from an aneurysm; all too often, the first manifestation is a sudden and devastating stroke. Preventive measures—proper diet, exercise, smoking cessation, and cholesterol control—aim to control the risk factors associated with hypertension and atherosclerotic diseases.

Aortic dissection occurs when the inside wall of the artery becomes torn and allows blood to collect between the arterial wall layers. It may occur with trauma or sustained hypertension. Dissection weakens the arterial wall, making it prone to rupture. A thoracic dissection, for example, can produce chest pain that is difficult to differentiate from cardiac ischaemia. Therefore, it is helpful to take blood pressure readings in both arms in all patients with chest pain. A systolic blood pressure difference of 15 mm Hg or higher suggests a thoracic dissection.

More than half of all older persons are hypertensive. The majority have isolated systolic hypertension resulting from a loss of arterial elasticity. Controlling systolic and/or diastolic hypertension in elderly people helps prevent strokes and MIs. Hypertensive emergencies in older people require a controlled decline in blood pressure that often cannot be achieved in the field.

Stroke is a significant cause of death and disability in elderly people. More than 80% of all stroke deaths occur in persons older than 65 years, and stroke is the leading cause of long-term disability at any age. Strokes, which are mainly caused by atherosclerosis, affect 130,000 people in the UK every year. The risk of stroke doubles each decade after 35 years, mirroring the increase in risk factors such as hypertension and atrial fibrillation. Hypertension is the primary risk for stroke, but age, family history, smoking, diabetes, high cholesterol, and heart disease also contribute. Prevention is aimed at reduction of risk factors, improving diet and exercise, and lowering cholesterol.

Transient ischaemic attacks (also called TIAs and ministrokes) entail a temporary disturbance of blood supply to the brain that results in a sudden, temporary decrease in brain function. The symptoms are the same as those for a stroke but generally last less than 24 hours; they are warning signs of a future stroke.

Respiratory System

Although tobacco abuse seems to be decreasing among elderly people, chronic lower respiratory disease, influenza, and pneumonia remain in the top five causes of deaths in the elderly. In fact, one of the most common causes of death in older patients is infection with *Pneumococcus* bacteria.

Pneumonia involves an inflammation of the lung, secondary to infection by bacteria, viruses, or other organisms. Although it can affect people at any age, this disease has its biggest impact on very young and elderly people, typically during the colder seasons (winter and early spring). People considered at risk include elderly people; people with underlying health problems such as chronic obstructive pulmonary disease (COPD), diabetes mellitus, and vascular diseases; and any person with a depressed immune system because of acquired immunodeficiency syndrome, cancer therapy, or organ transplantation. Treatment is primarily supportive, consisting of bed rest, fluids, oxygen therapy via nasal cannula or mask to relieve dyspnoea, analgesics to reduce fever, and antibiotics. Preventive measures include a vaccine given once and boosters after 3 to 5 years.

COPD includes chronic asthma, chronic bronchitis, and emphysema, all of which are characterised by the presence of bronchial obstruction and airway inflammation. Distinguishing these diseases can be difficult, so the problem may not be diagnosed or treated correctly. COPD affects approximately 10% of the older population, mostly owing to tobacco use. Its effects reflect the age-related loss of elastic tissue in the lungs (*senile emphysema*) and a decreased ability to defend against infection. These factors may increase the baseline disability of COPD and predispose older patients for an increased risk of acute exacerbation, often caused by infection.

Measures that are known to reduce potential exacerbations of COPD include immunisation for influenza and pneumococcal pneumonia. Long-term oxygen therapy has proven helpful in hypoxaemic patients. In addition, pulmonary rehabilitation may improve functional status and the quality of life for some patients.

Approximately 1 in 20 elderly people has a history of asthma or is affected by it. Onset can occur in old age with presenting symptoms of shortness of breath (especially with effort), chronic or nocturnal cough, and wheezing.

A pulmonary embolus arises when a blood vessel supplying the lung becomes blocked by a clot. Any obstruction in blood flow to the lung can result in irreversible damage or infarction. An embolus is often released from a vein in a lower extremity, the pelvis, or the abdomen but could also result from a damaged heart. The risk of pulmonary embolus increases with age because of increasing immobility. Older patients may also be bedridden after recent surgery (such as abdominal procedures). Finally, elderly patients have an increased incidence of diseases associated with a higher risk of pulmonary embolus, such as cancer, heart attack, cardiac arrhythmias, and clotting disorders.

Prevention of thromboembolism is based on the patient's risk level—high, moderate, or low. Surgical patients are in the highest-risk category for potential emboli, and prophylaxis is recommended, including warfarin and/or heparin and compression stockings.

Endocrine System

Diabetes arises when the body cannot oxidise complex carbohydrates (sugars) due to impaired pancreatic activity—namely, production of insulin. Insulin moves carbohydrates out of the bloodstream, through the cellular walls, and into the cells to be metabolised. With diabetes, more glucose is present in the blood than the body can handle. Elderly patients with diabetes are at increased risk for hypoglycaemia for several reasons: medications, inadequate or irregular dietary intake, inability to recognise the warning signs due to cognitive problems, and/or blunted warning signs. Delirium may be the only indication of hypoglycaemia in an elderly patient.

About 1,400,000 people in the UK are known to have diabetes. About 80% of these people have type 2 diabetes. The average age for developing type 2 diabetes is 52 years. About 10 in 100 people over age 65 have type 2 diabetes. The most common risk factor for this disease is having more than one chronic disease, and many elderly people with diabetes also have hypertension, heart disease, and stroke. Other risk factors for diabetes include a family history of diabetes, genetics, age, diet, obesity, and a sedentary lifestyle. Symptoms of an elevated blood glucose level (that is, hyperglycaemia) include fatigue, poor wound healing, blurred vision, and frequent infections. Other symptoms of diabetes include the three Ps: Polyuria, Polydipsia, and Polyphagia. Prevention of type 2 diabetes is aimed at changes in lifestyle that include dietary restrictions, exercise, and controlling obesity.

Older diabetics whose blood glucose levels tend to be high are more prone to hyperosmolar hyperglycaemic nonketotic (HHNK) coma than diabetic ketoacidosis. The most frequent cause for HHNK coma is infection. Presentation is likely to be acute confusion with dehydration, although signs of dehydration may be altered in elderly patients (**Table 42-1** ▶). Prehospital treatment remains the same as for younger patients, albeit with a cautious approach to fluid resuscitation.

Thyroid abnormalities also increase with ageing. Many older patients remain asymptomatic, and the disease is diagnosed only when a routine blood test reveals a thyroid prob-

Table 42-1	Signs of Dehydration in Elderly People

- Dry tongue
- Longitudinal furrows in the tongue
- Dry mucous membranes
- Weak upper body musculature
- Confusion
- Difficulty in speech
- Sunken eyes

lem. With hypothyroidism, for example, the signs and symptoms may match those seen with normal ageing: cold intolerance, constipation, dry skin, weakness, and so on. For acute-onset hyperthyroidism (*thyrotoxicosis*), the presentation can be blunted; although tachycardia is generally present, older patients may experience less tremor, anxiety, or hyperactive reflexes than their younger counterparts. Atrial fibrillation is more likely to be induced by an overactive thyroid gland in a older patient. A smaller percentage of elderly hyperthyroid patients present with symptoms opposite those expected: weakness, lethargy, and depression.

Gastrointestinal System

Constipation is a frequent and significant problem in elderly people. Although it can cause acute abdominal pain, it should not be the initial suspect when a patient experiences such discomfort. Instead, causes with high mortality, such as bleeding from an acute abdominal aneurysm or dead bowel from mesenteric ischaemia, should be investigated first. Many elderly people have diverticulosis (small outward pouches in the colon wall) and are at risk for diverticulitis and/or perforation. Appendicitis can be difficult to diagnose in older people, which probably accounts for the high perforation rate (50%) seen with this condition. The incidence of peptic ulcer disease is also increased among the older population, probably because of their relatively high use of nonsteroidal anti-inflammatory drugs (NSAIDs) for pain management.

Large bowel obstructions in elderly people are likely to be caused by cancer, impacted stool, or sigmoid volvulus. In addition, small bowel obstruction secondary to gallstones increases significantly with age. One third to one half of all elderly people have cholelithiasis (gallstones), although most remain asymptomatic for life. With one or more episodes of cholecystitis (inflammation of the gallbladder), the gallbladder adheres to the small bowel and, over time, creates an opening or fistula. The stone(s) drop into the bowel and produce the obstruction. Such a *gallstone ileus* may account for as many as 25% of small bowel obstructions in elderly patients. The large and small intestines are at risk for obstruction from adhesions due to previous surgery or infection or when a segment of bowel is forced into a fascial defect (hernia) in the abdominal wall.

Older patients are more likely than younger ones to have stomach or duodenal ulcers (peptic ulcer disease). The main risk factors for peptic ulcers are regular use of NSAIDs and infection with *Helicobacter pylori* (an ulcer-associated bacteria of the stomach), both of which are more common in older patients. Other medications have also been implicated in ulcer formation. The main symptom of peptic ulcer disease is dyspepsia (gnawing, burning pain in the upper abdomen), which usually improves immediately after eating but returns several hours later. Other causes of dyspepsia include acid reflux, gastritis, and gastric cancer.

Musculoskeletal System

Changes in physical abilities can affect older adults' confidence in their mobility. The muscle system atrophies and weakens with age. Muscle fibres become smaller and fewer, motor neurons decline in number, and strength declines. The ligaments and cartilage of the joints lose their elasticity. Cartilage also goes through degenerative changes with ageing, contributing to arthritis.

The stooped posture of older people comes from atrophy of the supporting structures of the body. Two of every three older patients will show some degree of kyphosis (also called humpback, hunchback, and Pott curvature). Lost height in older adults generally results from compression in the spinal column, first in the discs and then from the process of osteoporosis in the vertebral bodies.

Osteoporosis, a condition that affects men and women, is characterised by a decrease in bone mass leading to reduction in bone strength and greater susceptibility to fracture. The extent of bone loss that a person undergoes is influenced by numerous factors, including genetics, smoking, level of activity, diet, alcohol consumption, hormonal factors, and body weight. The most rapid loss of bone occurs in women during the years following menopause, and many postmenopausal women use hormone replacement therapy as a means to reduce the loss of bone. Calcium and vitamin D supplementation is another treatment for the condition, and many other medications are available to improve bone strength. Older people should remain active and perform low-impact exercises to maintain bone and muscle strength.

Osteoarthritis is a progressive disease of the joints that destroys cartilage, promotes the formation of bone spurs in joints, and leads to joint stiffness. This type of arthritis is thought to result from "wear and tear" and, in some cases, from repetitive trauma to the joints. It affects 35% to 45% of the population older than 65 years. Typically, osteoarthritis affects several joints of the body, most commonly those in the hands, knees, hips, and spine. Patients complain of pain and stiffness that gets worse with exertion. The end result is often substantial disability and disfigurement. Patients are typically treated with anti-inflammatory medications and physiotherapy to improve the range of motion.

Nervous System

Normal age-related cognitive changes have two major features: (1) They are relatively isolated (that is, they are not associated with multiple abnormal neurological findings that suggest specific disease states), and (2) the onset and progression of these findings are "in time" with the person's ageing process (that is, the findings are not sudden or extreme, and they do not extend to other abnormalities).

Delirium (also known as acute brain syndrome or acute confusional state) is a symptom, not a disease. A reflection of an underlying disturbance to a person's well-being (usually a treatable physical or mental illness), this temporary, usually reversible condition results in rapid changes in brain function. In elderly people, delirium often replaces or confounds the typical presentation caused by a medical problem, an adverse medication effect, or drug withdrawal. Disorders that cause delirium may also include poisons, electrolyte imbalances, nutritional deficiencies, and infections such as urinary tract infections and pneumonia. Onset of confusion or disorientation is abrupt (occurring during hours to days) but generally resolves with treatment of the underlying problem. The confusion and disorientation fluctuate with time, and hallucinations may occur. The patient experiences a rapid alteration between mental states, such as lethargy and agitation, serious attention disruption, disorganised thinking, and changes in perception and sensation.

Unlike delirium, dementia is a disease that produces irreversible brain failure. Disorders that cause dementia include conditions that impair vascular and neurological structures within the brain, such as infections, strokes, head injuries, poor nutrition, and medications. The two most common degenerative types of dementia in older people are Alzheimer's disease (one of the fastest-growing health care problems) and multi-infarct or vascular dementia, both of which cause structural damage to the brain. An estimated 6% to 10% of elderly people will eventually have dementia, although this percentage increases with advancing age. Dementia may be diagnosed when two or more brain functions are impaired. These cognitive and psychomotor functions consist of language, memory, visual perception, emotional behaviour and/or personality, and cognitive skills. Other risk factors that may predispose a patient to dementia include lower level of education, female sex, and Afro-Caribbean ethnicity. Although most cases of dementia cannot be prevented, some experts suggest that low-fat diets and exercise may help ward off vascular dementia.

Experts have not identified a single cause for Alzheimer's disease, but most believe it is not a normal part of the ageing process. Although age is a significant risk factor for this disease (Alzheimer's disease typically affects patients older than 60 years), but age alone is not the cause. This progressive disease cannot be cured or reversed by any known treatment or intervention. Symptoms are subtle at onset. Over time, patients lose their ability to think, reason clearly, solve problems, and concentrate; they may present with altered behaviour that includes paranoia, delusions, and social inappropriateness. In the later stages of Alzheimer's disease, patients cannot take care of themselves and may lose the ability to speak. People with severe Alzheimer's disease become completely debilitated and totally dependent on others.

Patients with Parkinson's disease—another age-related neurological disorder—have two or more of the following symptoms: resting tremor of an extremity, slowness of movement (bradykinesia), rigidity or stiffness of the extremities or trunk, and poor balance. Parkinson's disease is caused by degeneration of the substantia nigra, an area of the brain that controls voluntary movement by producing the neurotransmitter dopamine. Cells use dopamine to transmit impulses, so a loss of dopamine results in the loss of muscle function. Parkinson's disease can affect one or both sides of the body and produces a wide range of functional loss.

The incidence of convulsions (including status epilepticus) is also increased in elderly people, partly because of the increase in risk factors such as stroke, dementia, primary or metastatic brain tumours, and acute metabolic disorders (such as hyperglycaemia, hyponatraemia, alcohol withdrawal). Prehospital treatment for convulsions is the same for younger and older patients.

Toxicology

As the number of uses for medications increases, there is a proportional increase in the likelihood of adverse drug reactions and interactions. Elderly people are particularly prone to adverse reactions, even when they take drugs at doses that would be safe in younger people. This increased incidence of adverse drug reactions among elderly people seems to reflect changes in drug metabolism because of diminished hepatic function; in drug elimination because of diminished renal function; in body composition, including increased body fat and decreased body water, altering the distribution of drugs through the various body compartments; and in the responsiveness to drugs that affect the CNS. A change in any one of these processes can lead to toxic effects in elderly people.

Other body changes may affect medication use by older patients in a more general way. As vision declines with age, reading small print becomes more difficult. Night vision becomes less acute, so reading labels in dim light can lead to errors. Short-term memory loss may lead to forgetfulness about whether medications have been taken. An inability to distinguish flavours may cause patients to take multiple doses of medications before they detect problems.

Elderly people consume more than 25% of all prescribed and general-sales-list drugs sold in the United Kingdom. Community-dwelling older persons take an average of three to five medications per day. Nursing home patients take an average of six to seven routinely scheduled medications daily (polymedicine) and two to three additional medications on an as-needed basis. This kind of polypharmacy may be therapeutic when multiple drugs are needed to manage different medical problems, but it may prove harmful when these medications interact. Elderly patients are particularly prone to having multiple chronic diseases, which may lead to a vicious circle: The presence of multiple disease states leads to the use of multiple medications, which increases the likelihood of adverse reactions, which in turn leads to treatment with more

medications. In turn, a person's chance of ending up in hospital because of an adverse reaction to a medication increases with the number of drugs taken. Ultimately, the best dosage of a drug for an elderly patient is the lowest dosage that will achieve a therapeutic effect.

Medication noncompliance in older patients is also associated with negative effects on health. Many patients—not just older patients—do not follow instructions or advice on the use of their medications. Because elderly people use more medications than the rest of the population, noncompliance issues are more likely. Noncompliance issues include failure to pick up a prescription (for example, the patient isn't able to get to the local pharmacy or doesn't see the benefits of it), improper administration of medication (for example, the patient decreases the dosage to make the prescription last longer), discontinuation of medication (for example, the patient feels better and decides not to take the medication), and taking inappropriate medications (for example, the patient had medication left over from a previous prescription or shares the medicine with family members or friends).

Older patients are predisposed to medicine-related reactions owing to the previously mentioned age-related physiological changes that occur in body systems and body composition. For example, an increase in the proportion of adipose tissue can prolong the half-life of a drug. In particular, medications that affect the CNS are the most common source of adverse or unexpected reactions, and barbiturates and benzodiazepines are the drugs most often associated with toxic effects. A reduction in the nervous system response—especially the decrease in parasympathetic activity typically seen with the ageing process—increases the risk that adverse anticholinergic effects will occur. Reduced beta-adrenergic receptor sensitivity (which is responsible for bronchodilation) makes most bronchodilator medications less effective. The use of diuretics and anti-hypertensive medications by older patients can cause hypotension and orthostatic changes due to reduced cardiac output and a decrease in total body water. Finally, decreased glucose tolerance may cause medications such as diuretics and corticosteroids to have hyperglycaemic effects.

> **Notes from Nancy**
> The best dosage of a drug for an elderly patient is the lowest dosage that will achieve a therapeutic effect.

Drug and Alcohol Abuse

Alcohol is the preferred substance of abuse among older people, in whom its use is on the rise. A much smaller but increasing segment of the older population uses illegal drugs. Most users are men, and more than half carry their addiction into old age. About one third develop an abuse problem after reaching 65 years, often in response to a life-changing event such as the loss of a spouse, declining health, or low self-esteem.

The prevalence of alcohol and drug misuse among older people is also attributable to the multiplicity of medications that are prescribed for them and their heightened vulnerability to abuse owing to the effects of ageing. Decreased body mass and total body water means higher concentrations of blood alcohol; at the same time, the combination of digestive, renal, and hepatic system changes means slower elimination of alcohol from the body.

As the older population continues to grow and experiences even more chronic disabilities, the likelihood of substance abuse–related problems in this group will increase. Recognising substance abuse in older people can be difficult. If they have engaged in this behaviour for a long time, it may be well hidden from—or even accepted by—family members and friends. Because substance abuse can complicate your prehospital assessment and treatment, it is important to ask about this issue.

Psychiatric Conditions

Depression is not part of normal ageing, but rather a medical disease that occurs in about 6% of the population older than 65 years. The good news is that it is treatable with medication and therapy. The bad news is that if depression goes unrecognised or untreated, it is associated with a higher suicide rate in the elderly population than in any other age group. Depression in elderly patients can mimic the effects of many other medical problems (such as dementia). Risk factors for depression in older people include a history of depression, chronic disease, and loss (function, independence, or significant others). This condition may be difficult to recognise in older people because many don't want to complain about feeling sad, worthless, or unwanted.

Disturbingly, the majority of elder suicides occur in people who have recently been diagnosed with depression. In addition, the majority of suicide victims have seen their general practioner within the month before the event. Unlike younger people, older patients typically do not make suicidal gestures or attempt to get help. Instead, the rate of completed suicide is disproportionately high in the older population. Many older patients see no other way out when they have a terminal illness or debilitating cardiac or neurological condition (such as severe heart disease or stroke).

Injury in Elderly People
Environmental Injury

Internal temperature regulation is slowed in elderly people and gets slower with increasing age. The body's ability to recognise fluctuations in temperature becomes delayed owing to a slowed endocrine system. Heat gain or loss in response to environmental changes is delayed by atherosclerotic vessels, slowed circulation, and decreased sweat production in the skin. In addition, thermoregulation can be adversely affected by chronic disease, medications, and alcohol use, all of which are more frequent in elderly people.

Not surprisingly, about half of all deaths of hypothermia occur in elderly people, and most *indoor* hypothermia deaths involve elderly patients. Although living where harsh winters occur is a risk factor, hypothermia can develop at temperatures above freezing when an older person is exposed for a prolonged period.

The death rates from hyperthermia are more than doubled in elderly people compared with younger persons; people older than 85 years are at highest risk.

Trauma in Elderly People

Trauma is one of the top 10 causes of death among elderly people. The mortality rate for trauma in patients older than 65 years is 55 per 100,000, versus 50 per 100,000 for all other age groups. Deaths from injury in people older than 65 years account for one fourth of all trauma deaths in the United Kingdom, and injury is the seventh leading cause of death in the older population.

Several factors place an elderly person at higher risk of trauma than a younger person—namely, slower reflexes, visual and hearing deficits, equilibrium disorders, and an overall reduction in agility. In particular, changes in the body's homeostatic compensatory mechanisms combined with the effects of ageing on body systems and any preexisting conditions usually add up to less-than-favourable outcomes in trauma situations. Compensation in trauma is successful when increased heart rate, increased respiration, and adequate vasoconstriction make up for trauma-related deficits. Reduced cardiac reserve, decreased respiratory function, impaired renal activity, and ineffective vasoconstriction, by contrast, may lead to unsuccessful recovery from traumatic situations. Furthermore, an elderly person is more likely to sustain serious injury in case of trauma because stiffened blood vessels and fragile tissues tear more readily, and brittle, demineralised bone is more vulnerable to fracture.

At the Scene

Compensatory mechanism changes + ageing systems + preexisting conditions = bad outcomes.

Most older trauma cases involve falls or road traffic collisions. The incidence of falls, for example, increases with increasing age. Although most falls do *not* produce serious injury, elderly people account for 75% of all fall-related deaths. This increased mortality in elderly patients is directly related to the patient's age, preexisting disease processes, and complications related to the trauma. Falls are associated with a higher incidence of anxiety and depression, a loss of confidence, and postfall syndrome. With this syndrome, older patients develop a lack of confidence and anxiety about potential falls. Ultimately, they may become immobile, risk incontinence, and develop pneumonia or pressure ulcers from lack of movement.

Table 42-2	Causes of Falls in Elderly People
Cause	**Clues to Suggest This Cause**
Extrinsic (mechanical)	Obvious environmental hazard at the scene, such as poor lighting, scatter rugs, uneven pavement, ice or other slippery surface
Intrinsic drop attacks	Sudden fall; patient found on the ground somewhat confused, often temporarily paralysed and unable to get up; no premonitory symptoms
Postural hypotension	Fall when getting up from a recumbent or sitting position (Check medications the patient is taking, and ask about occult blood loss, such as presence of black stools. Measure blood pressure in recumbent and sitting positions.)
Dizziness or syncope	Marked bradycardia or tachyarrhythmias
Stroke	Other characteristic signs of stroke, such as hemiparesis, hemiplegia, or dysphasia
Fracture	Patient felt something snap before falling.

Falls among elderly people are evenly divided between those resulting from extrinsic (external) causes, such as tripping on a loose rug or slipping on ice, and those resulting from intrinsic (internal) causes, such as a dizzy spell or a syncopal attack (Table 42-2 ▲). The risk of falls increases in people with preexisting gait abnormalities (such as from neurological or musculoskeletal impairment) and cognitive impairment. Older patients with osteoporosis have lower-density bones, so even a sudden, awkward turn may fracture a bone. When treating a patient who has fallen, you need to take a careful history. Although the patient often attributes the fall to an accidental cause ("I must have tripped over the rug"), meticulous questioning often reveals a period of dizziness or palpitations just before the fall, suggesting a different cause. Home safety assessments by emergency care—during a routine visit or as part of an outreach programme—may reduce the incidence of falls.

After falls, road traffic collisions are the second leading cause of accidental death among elderly people. Of licensed drivers, 10% are elderly people. They account for 10% of all traffic deaths, 11% of all vehicle occupant deaths, and 16% of all pedestrian deaths. Impaired vision, errors in judgement, and underlying medical conditions contribute to the higher risk. Impairments in vision and hearing, along with diminished agility, also contribute to pedestrian deaths involving elderly people.

Types of Injuries Commonly Seen in Elderly People

Changes associated with normal ageing and with diseases of ageing make elderly people particularly vulnerable to certain types of injuries. In particular, head trauma or injury is a serious problem. The increased fragility of cerebral blood vessels, enlargement of the subdural space, and a decrease in the supportive tissue of the meninges all contribute to make an elderly person more vulnerable than a younger person to intracranial bleeding, particularly subdural haematoma. In many cases, the haematoma develops slowly, during days or weeks. By the time the patient becomes symptomatic, the person or his or her carers may not remember the incident, or the family members or carers may feel guilty about their own negligence in the incident. As a result, it may be difficult to obtain an accurate history of the initial trauma. The most important early symptom of a subdural haematoma is headache, which may be worse at night. Sometimes the headache occurs on the same side of the head as the blood clot. With increasing intracranial pressure, the state of consciousness becomes depressed, and the patient becomes increasingly drowsy.

Elderly people are also more vulnerable than their younger counterparts to cervical spinal cord injury and cord compression, even after apparently minor trauma. Degenerative changes in the cervical spine (cervical spondylosis) cause arthritic "spurs" and narrowing of the vertebral canal; the nerve roots exiting from the cervical spine gradually become compressed, and pressure on the spinal cord increases. Any injury to the cervical spine, therefore, is much more likely to injure the already compromised spinal cord. Even a sudden movement of the neck may result in spinal cord injury.

Injuries to the chest in elderly people are much more likely to produce rib fracture and flail chest, owing to the brittleness of the ribs and overall stiffening of the chest wall as the costochondral cartilage becomes calcified. Abdominal trauma often produces liver injury, perhaps because the liver is less protected by abdominal musculature.

Orthopaedic injuries are a common result of falls in older patients, with hip fractures the most common acute orthopaedic injury, followed, in severity and frequency, by fractures of the femur, pelvis, tibia, and upper extremities. Hip fracture may also occur without trauma, simply because of vigorous contracture of the hip musculature. The most important risk factor for hip fracture is osteoporosis: Approximately half of older women and one of eight older men will have an osteoporosis-related fracture (hip or other). The cost to the NHS each year due to osteoporosis is £1.5 thousand million. Annually it accounts for 60,000 hip fractures and 50,000 wrist fractures, and results in the occupancy of 20% of all orthopaedic beds in hospitals.

Burns are a significant risk of morbidity and mortality in elderly people because of physiological and pathophysiological changes. The risk of mortality is increased when preexisting medical conditions exist, defence mechanisms to protect against infection are weakened, and fluid replacement is complicated by renal compromise. In the assessment of a burn patient, prehospital providers need to monitor the patient's hydration status by assessing current vital signs, mucous membranes, and urine output, which is typically 50 to 60 ml/h or 1 to 2 ml/kg/h.

Assessment of Older Patients

Although illness is common among elderly people, it is *not* an inevitable part of ageing. Complaints of elderly people cannot be ascribed simply to "getting old". Ageing is a continuous

there signs of violence, such as broken glassware, that might provide clues to elder abuse? Are the patient's living conditions adequately heated or cooled? Is the patient living alone? Does the patient have pets? (If so, you should make arrangements for someone, such as a neighbour, to assume their care until the patient returns.) Record these observations on the patient record form to enable social service personnel to make appropriate arrangements for follow-up care.

Measure the patient's vital signs carefully. Postural changes in blood pressure vary among elderly people, but changes increase with increasing frailty and heighten the person's risk for falls. Marked postural changes in blood pressure and pulse may indicate hypovolaemia or overmedication. As you measure the vital signs, bear in mind that normal blood pressure for a young person may represent significant hypotension in an elderly patient. If possible, determine the patient's baseline blood pressure. When obtaining a patient's blood pressure, be aware of the possibility of significant hypertension and orthostatic changes. Consider taking vital signs in both arms and checking pulses proximally and distally in all extremities. This process will allow you to gather information and observe for signs of dependent oedema, dehydration, and the patient's circulatory status without raising his or her anxiety level.

Pay attention to the respiratory rate. Tachypnoea can be a very sensitive indicator of acute illness in elderly people—especially pulmonary infection—even when patients show few, if any, other signs. When assessing the patient's respirations, listen to lung sounds in all fields, noting adventitious sounds that might aid in development of a treatment plan. You can also use the stethoscope to listen for carotid bruits; note jugular vein distension.

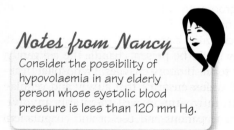

Notes from Nancy

Consider the possibility of hypovolaemia in any elderly person whose systolic blood pressure is less than 120 mm Hg.

Detailed Physical Examination

Conduct the detailed physical examination as you would for any other patient. When examining the mouth, make a note of any upper or lower dentures. In the chest examination, keep in mind that elderly people may have pulmonary crackles without apparent pathology—so don't lunge for the GTN and furosemide at the first crackle you hear in the chest. Similarly, oedema in the legs may be the result of chronic venous insufficiency and not right-sided heart failure.

Assessment and Management of Medical Complaints in Elderly People

Cardiovascular Complaints

Prehospital treatment for chest pain remains essentially unchanged in elderly patients, albeit with extra cautions because of the increased potential for medication side effects.

At the Scene

If the patient is hypotensive and is wearing a GTN patch, remove it. The patient's complaint could be caused by too much or too little of this medication.

As in all prehospital emergencies, health care providers must prioritise the patient's airway, breathing, and circulatory status. GTN and morphine may produce more hypotension or respiratory compromise than in younger patients or may react adversely with long-term medications. Aspirin may increase bleeding in a patient who is already taking anti-coagulants. For patients 75 years or older with ST-segment elevation infarcts, angioplasty offers a better outcome than thrombolysis.

The presentation of heart failure in an older person can be confused by symptoms and signs symbolic of old age and shared by a number of chronic diseases—for example, dyspnoea on exertion, easy fatigability (especially with left-sided heart failure), confusion, crackles on lung examination, orthopnoea, dry cough progressing to productive cough, and dependent peripheral oedema in right-sided heart failure. Acute exacerbations of heart failure are often related to poor diet, medication noncompliance, onset of arrhythmias such as atrial fibrillation, or acute myocardial ischaemia.

Prehospital treatment is unchanged from that of younger patients, although greater consideration is given to becoming familiar with the patient's medications and their implications for your proposed treatment. For example, the patient taking long-term furosemide may not respond to the usual dose of the same drug that you administer as an acute therapy. Additional treatments by prehospital providers (specifically those not bound by JRCALC guidelines) should include close monitoring of fluids and avoidance of excessive fluid overload, use of beta blockers in patients with systolic dysfunction (low ejection fraction), use of digoxin in patients with atrial fibrillation or atrial flutter, and, possibly, use of anti-coagulation therapy in patients with atrial arrhythmias to prevent thromboembolism.

Nonperfusing rhythms receive the same treatment as given to younger adults. Survival depends on the prearrest health of the patient and the usual factors: early recognition, prompt and effective CPR, and early defibrillation.

Thoracic aneurysms generally remain asymptomatic until they become large or rupture. Early symptoms may be related to compression by the aneurysm, such as difficulty swallowing or hoarseness from laryngeal nerve pressure. Abdominal aortic aneurysms present typically with abdominal pain or possibly only with back pain. Asymptomatic thoracic and abdominal aneurysms that do not exceed a certain size and are not expanding are generally treated without surgery but are reassessed on a regular timetable. In an older patient with back pain, examine the chest and abdomen carefully. The treatment of abdominal emergencies is surgical, so early recognition, assessment, stabilisation, and rapid transport to an appropriate medical facility are essential.

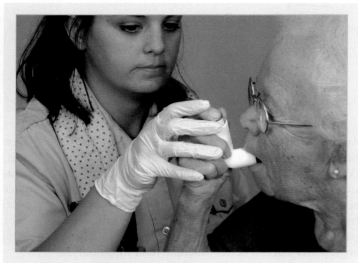

Figure 42-6 A patient having an asthma attack may have a bronchodilator medication in a metered-dose inhaler. Older patients often do not use an inhaler correctly, so you may need to help with its use if your guidelines allow it.

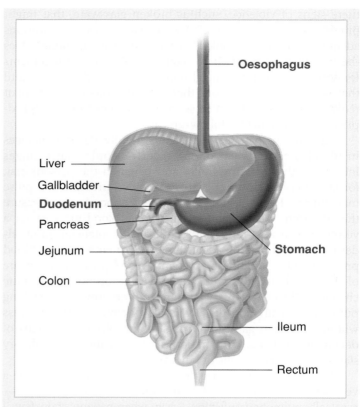

Figure 42-7 Upper GI bleeding occurs in the stomach, oesophagus, and duodenum.

The usual treatments for systolic hypertension usually prove safe and effective in older patients. In case of rapid onset of symptomatic systolic hypertension, treatment aims to reduce the systolic pressure with anti-hypertensive therapy, which can minimise cardiovascular and cerebrovascular morbidity and mortality.

Respiratory Complaints

An older patient with pneumonia often does not have the classic presentation of chills, fever, and productive cough. Instead, these symptoms are often supplanted by acute confusion (delirium), normal temperature, and a minimal to absent cough. Prehospital treatment is supportive and includes oxygen and IV access as indicated. At the receiving facility, providers will determine whether antibiotics or admission is appropriate.

Asthma clinical practice guidelines are the same for younger and older patients Figure 42-6 ▲ . On rare occasions, adrenaline may be indicated for a life-threatening asthma exacerbation.

In a patient of any age, treatment goals for COPD are to reduce the symptoms and complications. Along with shortness of breath, presenting symptoms may include fatigue and a decreased activity level. Treatment consists of immediate assessment and correction of respiratory difficulties with the application of supplemental oxygen. The patient may also receive bronchodilators to decrease the shortness of breath, inhaled or oral steroids to decrease inflammation, and antibiotics to treat infection.

Many pulmonary emboli are silent or present with tachypnoea alone—that is, the classic triad of dyspnoea, chest pain, and haemoptysis is often altered or absent. If you suspect a pulmonary embolus, check for swelling, erythema, and warmth or tenderness of the lower leg; all of these are signs of a deep venous

thrombosis, which is a common cause of pulmonary embolus. If deep venous thrombosis might be present, handle the leg gently and monitor the patient for respiratory changes. Prehospital treatment is largely supportive after ensuring that airway and ventilation are adequate. Future treatment will inevitably involve prehospital lysing of the thrombus and use of anti-coagulation therapies after a risk assessment is performed, with these measures being followed by rapid transport to a coronary care unit.

GI Complaints

Many causes are possible for gastric complaints. Constipation and its accompanying abdominal pain, for example, are some of the more common complaints of older patients. In your assessment of a gastric emergency, ask the patient about food and fluid intake, history of abdominal complaints, current bowel and bladder habits, and medications and supplements before proceeding with a physical examination. Symptoms are often vague and manifest only as diffuse abdominal pain with no particular point of origin. Abdominal and gastric complaints often require surgical treatment, so early recognition and rapid transport for definitive hospital care are the best practice.

Upper GI haemorrhage occurs when there is bleeding from the oesophagus, stomach, or duodenum Figure 42-7 ▲ . When severe, this condition is a true medical emergency that must be recognised and assessed quickly. Not only are older people more prone to upper GI bleeding, they are also at a greater risk of complications, the need for urgent surgery, and death.

It is not possible to determine the cause of upper GI bleeding without an endoscopic examination (inspection of the inside of a hollow organ or body cavity) of the oesophagus, stomach, and duodenum. However, the history can offer clues to the cause. Regular use of NSAIDs or alcohol may result in bleeding from irritation of the lining of the stomach or from ulcers (a hollowing out or disintegration of tissue) in the stomach or duodenum. Forceful vomiting can cause tears in the oesophagus that may bleed. Cirrhosis of the liver from long-term alcohol use or chronic infectious hepatitis may cause enlargement of the veins (varices) in the oesophagus. These varices can rupture and result in massive bleeding. Stomach cancer or oesophageal cancer can also produce upper GI bleeding. Recent weight loss or difficulty swallowing would raise the suspicion of cancer as the source of bleeding.

On arrival at the scene, even more important than knowing the cause of bleeding is being able to assess its severity. Slower bleeding is characterised by emesis with coffee-grounds appearance. With minor bleeding, the heart rate and systolic blood pressure are normal. Brisk bleeding presents with haematemesis (vomiting red blood) or melaena (black, tarlike stools). It is important to note that melaena, not pain, is the most common presenting symptom of GI bleeding. Prehospital treatment is supportive, including adequate pain control.

Lower GI haemorrhage primarily describes bleeding from the colon and rectum Figure 42-8 ▸ and should never simply be attributed to haemorrhoids. Colon polyps and colon cancer are also possible causes, among others. Minor lower GI bleeding is characterised by small amounts of red blood covering formed brown stools or scant amounts of red blood noticed on the toilet paper. Severe lower GI bleeding is characterised by passing significant amounts of red blood or maroon-coloured stools.

Assessment should begin with identifying risk factors such as a history of previous lower GI bleeding, symptoms or signs suggestive of colon cancer, recent constipation or diarrhoea, and use of medications such as blood thinners. Treat for shock. Severe lower GI bleeding requires immediate transport to the nearest emergency department.

Neurological and Endocrine Complaints

Effective prehospital acute stroke care includes early recognition, discovery of stroke-mimics such as hypoglycaemia or hypoxia, and timely transport to the most appropriate hospital. Use a stroke assessment tool as appropriate, taking the patient's history into account when assessing the components of the scale. An older person with severe arthritis may not move as well on one side, or damage from a previous stroke may make his or her speech difficult to assess. Always ask family members or carers for information that may help you identify deviations from the patient's normal pattern of behaviour or activity. Assess for new weakness, fatigue, syncope,

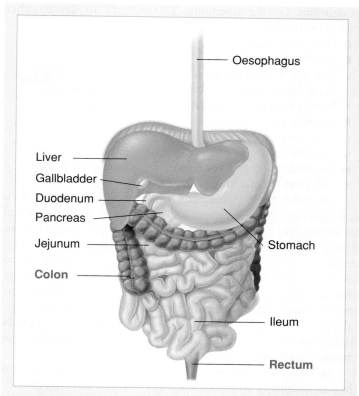

Figure 42-8 Lower GI bleeding takes place primarily in the colon and rectum.

Documentation and Communication

A stroke is a traumatic and emotional event for the patient, and a sensitive and compassionate approach is essential. Even though patients may not be able to communicate with you, they can often understand. Communicate with them as you would any other patient—in a calm and reassuring manner.

and near syncope and for changes in these symptoms and in mood and sleep patterns.

Dementia signs and symptoms take months to years to become apparent and may include short-term memory loss or shortened attention span, jargon dysphasia (talking nonsense), hallucinations, confusion, disorientation, difficulty in learning and retaining new information, and personality changes such as social withdrawal or inappropriate behaviour. Dementia is not synonymous with delirium, however, and a patient with dementia can also have delirium. In delirium, assess for recent changes in the patient's level of consciousness or orientation. Specifically, look for an acute onset of anxiety, an inability to think logically or maintain attention, and an inability to focus. Also assess for changes in vital signs, temperature (indicating infection), glucose level, and medications—all frequent causes of delirium. Use the mnemonic "DELIRIUMS" to identify other causes of delirium:

D Drugs or toxins

E Emotional (psychiatric)

L Low pO_2 (carbon monoxide poisoning, COPD, congestive heart failure, acute myocardial infarction, pneumonia)

I Infection (pneumonia, urinary tract infection, sepsis)

R Retention of stool or urine

I Ictal (convulsions)

U Undernutrition or underhydration

M Metabolism (thyroid or endocrine, electrolytes, kidneys)

S Subdural haematoma

Altered mental status is a symptom, not a disease. As a consequence, the assessment and subsequent management of its numerous causes is complicated. Always consider head injury (medical or traumatic), heart rhythm disturbances, dementia, medications, fluid balance changes (such as blood loss), respiratory disorders (such as hypoxia), endocrine changes (such as blood glucose level fluctuations), hyperthermia or hypothermia, and infection. Most important, prehospital providers need to consider neurological causes (such as Alzheimer's disease and Parkinson's disease) and endocrine changes (such as diabetes).

In Alzheimer's disease, symptoms may present as confusion (lack of familiarity with surroundings), changes in personality or judgement, and extreme difficulty with daily activities, such as feeding, bathing, and bowel and bladder control. Parkinson's disease may present as dyskinesia (involuntary movements or tremors affecting one or both sides of the body), dementia, depression, autonomic dysfunction (bladder and GI problems), and postural instability (loss of reflexes or inability to "right oneself").

Many endocrine changes may have occurred earlier in life and been diagnosed before intervention by prehospital providers became necessary. Older patients may have diseases such as Grave's disease (hyperthyroidism), Addison's disease (hypoadrenalism), Cushing's syndrome (hyperadrenalism), osteoporosis, or diabetes. In the assessment of older patients with diagnosed diabetes, look for signs of dehydration or hyperglycaemia (the three Ps: Polyuria, Polydipsia, and Polyphagia). New-onset diabetes in older patients is often a mild progression that produces no symptoms.

> **Notes from Nancy**
> Delirium in the elderly is always a sign of physical illness or drug intoxication and is always an emergency.

Toxicologic Complaints

The most common therapeutic error in cases of reported poison exposure is "inadvertently took/given medication twice" or "double dosing". In essence, medications are poisons with beneficial side effects. This definition emphasises the need for obtaining a careful history and collecting and transporting all medications with the patient.

As mentioned earlier, many elderly people take a variety of drugs. Patients may also take general-sales-list medications or medications prescribed for a family member or friend.

Another factor contributing to the toxic effects of drugs in elderly people is ageing-related alterations in pharmacokinetics (that is, the absorption, distribution, metabolism, and excretion of drugs). Pharmacokinetics may also be influenced by diet, smoking, alcohol consumption, and use of other drugs. Drugs such as digoxin that depend on the liver and kidney for metabolism and excretion are particularly likely to accumulate to toxic levels in older patients. With most drugs, we know little about the optimal dosage for elderly people because nearly all clinical trials to establish the safe dosages of drugs are performed in young populations. For the most part, dosages for elderly people need to be *reduced* compared with those for younger patients ("Start low, go slow").

Although almost any drug can produce toxic effects in an older person, certain drugs and classes of drugs are implicated more often than others; **Table 42-4 ▶** lists the "dirty dozen". Typically toxic effects present with psychiatric symptoms (such as hallucinations, paranoia, delusions, agitation, and psychosis) and cognitive impairment (such as delirium, confusion, disorientation, amnesia, stupor, and coma) **Figure 42-9 ▼**.

> **Notes from Nancy**
> Bring all of the patient's medications—prescription and non-prescription—to the hospital.

Sepsis

Infections in older persons can be severe and dangerous. Sepsis is the disease state that results from the presence of microorganisms or their toxic products in the bloodstream. This is a serious

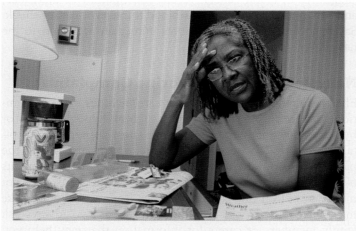

Figure 42-9 The toxic effects of drugs may initially manifest in the form of confusion.

Table 42-4 Drugs Most Likely to Cause Toxic Reactions in Elderly People	
Medication	**Symptoms**
Anti-inflammatory agents (NSAIDs, steroids)	Drowsiness, dizziness, confusion, anxiety, bradypnoea, tachypnoea, GI bleeding
Antibiotics	GI signs, altered mental status, convulsions, coma
Anticholinergics and antihistamines	Urination difficulty, constipation, drowsiness, restlessness, irritability, hypertension
Anti-coagulants (warfarin)	Bruising, epistaxis, haematuria, abdominal pain, vomiting, faecal blood
Anti-arrhythmics (amiodarone, lignocaine)	Restlessness, hypotension, bradycardia, tachycardia, palpitations, angina
Anti-depressants (tricyclics, long-acting selective serotonin reuptake inhibitors)	Confusion, delirium, disorientation, memory impairment
Anti-hypertensives (diuretics, alpha blockers, beta blockers; angiotensin-converting enzyme inhibitors)	Hypotension, palpitations, angina, fluid retention, headache
Antipsychotics (phenothiazines, atypicals)	Drowsiness, tachycardia, dizziness, restlessness
Digoxin	Headache, fatigue, malaise, drowsiness, depression
Insulin and oral antidiabetic medications	Hypoglycaemia presenting as confusion
Opiates	Delirium, respiratory depression, apnoea, involuntary muscle movements
Sedative-hypnotics (benzodiazepines, barbiturates)	Incoordination, dizziness, disturbances in cognitive function

problem that every ambulance clinicians should know how to recognise and treat. Think of sepsis whenever you see a hot, flushed patient who is also tachycardic and tachypnoeic. Other signs of sepsis include an oral temperature greater than 38°C or less than 36°C, a respiratory rate of more than 20 breaths/min or $_pCO_2$ less than 32 mm Hg, and pulse rate of greater than 90 beats/min. Sepsis can be caused by bacteria, fungi, and viruses.

Skin Complaints

Herpes zoster (shingles) is caused by the reactivation of varicella virus on nerve roots. This condition is more common in the older population. Most people with herpes zoster are in good health, but people with cancer or immunosuppression are at higher risk. This condition affects any nerve in the body, but the thoracic nerves and the ophthalmic division of the trigeminal nerve are most common. The disease usually starts with pain in the affected area. Subsequently, a cluster of tiny blisters (vesicles) erupts on reddened skin in the same area. The rash is typically unilateral; it rarely crosses the midline.

One of the most common complications of herpes zoster is pain, or postherpetic neuralgia. During the acute phase of the infection, the person may have severe pain and require narcotic pain relievers. Antiviral medications such as aciclovir and famciclovir can be used, preferably within 48 hours of the activation of the disease. These medications decrease healing time, new lesion formation, and pain.

Cellulitis is an acute inflammation in the skin caused by a bacterial infection Figure 42-10 ▶ . This condition usually affects the lower extremities. Symptoms include fever, chills, and general malaise. Cellulitis can cause warmth, swelling, redness, tenderness, and enlarged nodes in the affected area. Blood tests may show elevation of the white blood cell count and the presence of bacteria. Treatments include antibiotic therapy, ensuring adequate fluid intake, and local dressings if there is an open sore.

Psychological Complaints

Depression can be a normal, short-term reaction to a particular event. When sadness, restlessness, fatigue, and hopelessness persist for weeks, however, it becomes a larger concern. Depression in the elderly population is a major health problem with an incidence growing in tandem with the progressive ageing of the population. This trend can be attributed to increases in polypathology, psychosocial stress, and ageing-related changes in the brain that collectively lead to greater cognitive impairment, increased medical illness, dependency on health care services, and more suicide attempts Figure 42-11 ▶ . Depression may also occur when a patient takes a variety of medications; such polypharmacy is more likely when the person has multiple medical conditions that result in more vulnerability to toxic effects.

When dealing with psychological emergencies with older patients, health care providers need to determine whether the situation is a true behavioural emergency or a behavioural crisis. A behavioural emergency implies a significant risk of

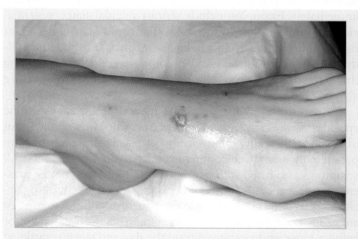

Figure 42-10 Cellulitis is a diffuse, acute inflammation in the skin caused by bacterial infection.

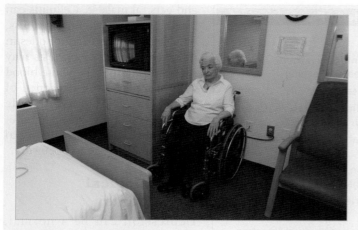

Figure 42-11 Isolation and chronic medical problems are among the factors that contribute to depression in older adults.

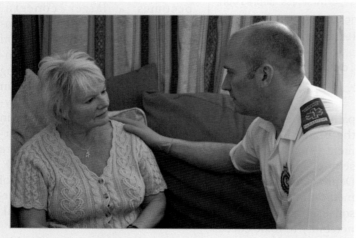

Figure 42-12 A patient in a behavioural crisis may be searching for alternative methods of coping.

serious harm to self or others unless intervention is undertaken immediately. Examples include serious suicidal states, potential violence, and impaired judgement that could leave a person at risk of injury or death. In a behavioural crisis, the patient's ability to cope is insufficient and becomes overwhelmed, sending the patient in search of alternative methods of coping **Figure 42-12 ▲** .

When dealing with a patient's mental illness or psychotic episodes, always remember that a person who is psychotic is out of touch with reality. Many forms of psychotic behaviour are possible, including schizophrenic and paranoid behaviours. All symptoms associated with psychotic conditions may not be present when a patient is having an episode, however. Clues to psychotic behaviour might include the patient becoming excited or angry for no apparent reason, engaging in antisocial activity or being a loner, and sleeping during the day and staying awake at night. Information about changes in the patient's normal routine may be obtained from family members, friends, or carers.

Management of Medical Emergencies in Elderly People

The assessment and management of medical emergencies in older patients can be complex. If you are well prepared to deal with these complex situations, you will not feel quite so overwhelmed and helpless.

In every emergency, you should first complete a scene assessment to confirm the scene safety, determine the nature of the call, identify the number of potential patients, and ascertain the need for additional resources. Next, you should perform an initial assessment, which consists of several quick, yet complex observations. First, formulate a general impression based on the patient's mental status and the status of his or her airway, breathing, and circulatory systems. Then, determine transport priorities.

With the exception of patients who require immediate interventions to maintain a patent airway, adequate and supportive breathing, or circulatory status, most prehospital care is supportive and focuses on pain relief and palliative interventions. Additional steps in the patient treatment plan will depend on the patient's specific medical emergency and chief complaint.

Table 42-5 ▶ reviews common medical complications encountered with older patients and their management strategies.

Assessment and Management of Trauma in Elderly Patients

Begin the assessment by looking at the mechanism of injury. Falls account for the largest number of injuries in elderly people, followed by injuries related to road traffic (including passenger and pedestrian trauma) and then burns and other injuries. Always look for signs or symptoms that the patient may have experienced a medical problem before the trauma. A syncopal event while driving, for example, may result in a collision.

The initial management of an injured elderly patient follows the basic ABC pattern of trauma care with some special concerns.

While securing the airway, check for dentures. If they are intact and in place, leave them where they are; if the dentures are broken or loose in the mouth, remove them and place them in a safe container. Aggressive suctioning of blood or secretions is required because of the older patient's lessened airway and gag reflexes **Figure 42-13 ▶** .

When assessing breathing, check for rib fracture. If assisted ventilation is required, use a bag-valve-mask gently, exerting just enough pressure to inflate the lungs so as to lessen the chance of creating a pneumothorax. Administer supplemental oxygen early to assist the body in compensating for early states of trauma.

Table 42-5	Common Medical Complications in Elderly People and Their Management
Medical Complication	**Management**
Incontinence	Some cases are managed surgically. Other considerations include absorptive devices for faecal and urinary incontinence, placement of catheters, and awareness of the patient's self-esteem and social issues.
COPD	Nebuliser treatment with a bronchial dilator could include ipratropium or salbutamol.
Pulmonary emboli	Lysing the thrombus and anti-coagulation therapies are indicated, although not prehospitally at present. Once all risk factors for bleeding have been reviewed, anti-coagulants such as heparin or enoxaparin can be considered.
Heart failure	Heart failure that produces signs and symptoms of pulmonary oedema can be managed with sublingual GTN and IV furosemide. Some providers can also consider a vasoactive medication such as dopamine for patients with haemodynamically unstable hypotension.
Arrhythmias	Unless a patient is in unstable condition, arrhythmias are handled with supportive care only. Unstable arrhythmias are treated following current CPR and electrocardiographic guidelines.
Aneurysm	Treatment is handled surgically, and prehospital interventions focus on supportive care.
Hypertension	Hypertensive emergencies require a controlled decline in blood pressure, which is not often feasible in prehospital care.
Cerebrovascular disease	Prehospital management targets recognition, resuscitation, and rapid transfer to the A&E or preferably a specialist stroke unit.
Delirium, dementia, Alzheimer's disease, Parkinson's disease	Recognise and treat the underlying cause, and provide supportive interventions. Provide supportive care.
Diabetes	In hypoglycaemia, treatments address the decrease in the blood glucose level with IM or IV injections when not contraindicated. In hyperglycaemia, some providers can initiate treatment that aims to eliminate additional glucose by using fluid boluses for patients with adequate renal function.
GI problems	Few treatments using medications for GI problems are possible in the prehospital environment, other than anti-emetics. For nausea and vomiting, consider metoclopramide.
Drug toxic effects	• Lignocaine. CNS depression may occur, so be alert for respiratory changes. No antidote is used in prehospital care to reverse its effects. • Beta blockers. Provide supportive care; definitive care may involve activated charcoal, the use of atropine, adrenaline, and glucagon in symptomatic patients. • Anti-hypertensives. Provide supportive care. No antidote is used in prehospital care to reverse the drugs' effects. • Diuretics. Provide supportive care. Consider treatments aimed at restoring volume depletion and electrolyte imbalance. No antidote is used in prehospital care to reverse the drugs' effects. • Digitalis. Provide supportive care. Consider fluid replacement. Definitive care may consider vasoactive medications such as dopamine and activated charcoal. • Psychotropics. Provide supportive care. Consider aggressive fluid replacement if appropriate. • Anti-depressants. Provide supportive care. Give fluid therapy for hypotension.
Alcohol abuse	Provide supportive care. Later care includes identification of abuse potential and referral to an appropriate treatment facility.
Behavioural disorders	Use psychological support and communication strategies.
Depression, suicide	Provide supportive care. Later care includes identification of the potential condition and referral to an appropriate treatment facility.

When evaluating circulation, remember that what is a normal blood pressure in a younger person may mean hypotension in an older person. If possible, try to determine the patient's normal baseline blood pressure and circulatory status.

The initial assessment of disability (neurological status) should include an evaluation of the pupils and the level of consciousness, according to the AVPU scale. Finally, be sure to expose the entire injured area, even if it means peeling away many layers of clothing.

Once the initial assessment is complete, try to obtain a complete history of the trauma event from the patient and from anyone who may have witnessed the event Figure 42-14 ▶. If the patient fell, from what height? Did the patient have any symptoms beforehand, such as dizziness? If the patient was

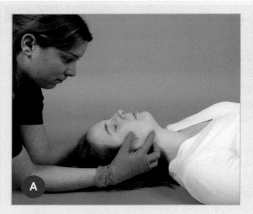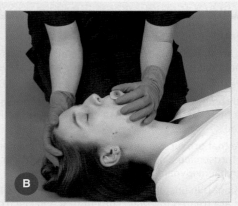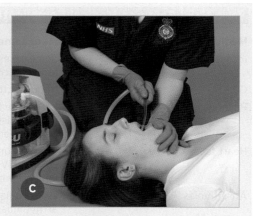

Figure 42-13 The airway should initially be addressed using simple techniques, such as (**A**) the modified jaw-thrust, (**B**) placement of an oropharyngeal or nasopharyngeal airway, and (**C**) suctioning.

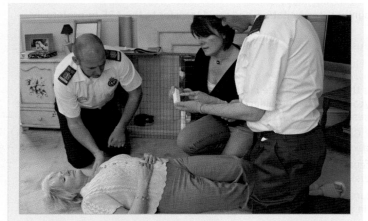

Figure 42-14 History is especially important in older patients who have lost consciousness.

struck by a car, how fast was the car moving? If the patient was the driver of a car involved in a collision, did he or she feel dizzy or black out before the crash? Did the patient have chest pain? Did witnesses notice the car moving erratically before it crashed?

Obtain a complete list of all medications the patient takes regularly. Inquire in particular about beta blockers, anti-hypertensives, and medications for diabetes because they may affect the patient's response to resuscitation measures and to anaesthesia.

Conduct the focused physical examination as usual, staying particularly alert for signs of injuries to the head, cervical spine, ribs, abdomen, and long bones. Pain from fractures or peripheral injury may be difficult to assess if the patient has decreased pain perception.

You are the Paramedic Part 4

You place your patient on a stretcher in a semi-recumbent position and move her to the ambulance. While en route to hospital, she begins to complain of a being "a little breathless". A reassessment reveals no changes in her status. Your colleague suggests administering a nebuliser treatment with salbutamol. You agree, and the patient receives a nebuliser treatment with 5 mg of salbutamol. A pre-alert is given en route to the accident and emergency (A&E) department.

As you arrive at the A&E department your patient says that she is breathing easier and thanks you for being so caring. She is observed in the A&E department for a few hours, and right lower lobe pneumonia is diagnosed by chest X-ray. She is admitted to hospital for treatment with IV antibiotics and is discharged to the care home on the fifth day.

Reassessment	Recording Time: 20 Minutes
Skin	Pink, hot, and dry
Pulse	113 beats/min, strong and irregular
Blood pressure	158/96 mm Hg
Respirations	22 breaths/min regular
S_PO_2	95% with supplemental oxygen at 12 l/min by mask
ECG	Atrial fibrillation

6. Does pneumonia present in the same way in elderly people as in younger people?

7. How is pneumonia managed in the prehospital setting?

Additional treatment will depend on the patient's specific injuries, although there are a few general principles to keep in mind:

- Insert an IV cannula and give an isotonic solution, but use caution. It is very easy to overload an elderly person with sodium, and you must balance that with the need to maintain adequate perfusion pressure. Use small boluses, and reassess the patient frequently, especially for signs of pulmonary oedema.
- Monitor cardiac rhythm throughout care of the patient, and be alert for changes. Previous or continuing cardiac disease predisposes a person to ECG changes.
- Take steps to preserve temperature in elderly trauma patients. Regulation of temperature is slowed in elderly people, and the blood in cold patients does not clot as well.
- Frail elderly patients may not do very well with a traction splint for a femoral fracture. If possible, place the patient on a well-padded longboard and pad him or her well with pillows secured firmly in place.
- Immobilise the cervical spine before transporting the patient. Pad the longboard generously, because the skin of an older person may be damaged by the direct trauma of the pressure and the decrease in blood flow. Target areas where the bone is near the surface, from top to bottom: occiput, scapula, spinous processes, elbows, sacrum, and heels. A pressure ulcer can develop in as little as 45 minutes and can complicate the original injury.

Elder Abuse

One category of older person trauma that deserves special mention is elder abuse—that is, any form of mistreatment that results in harm or loss to an older person. Five types of abuse are distinguished: physical, sexual, emotional, neglect, and financial. The first four are similar to the forms found in child abuse. Financial abuse involves improper use of an older person's funds, property, or assets. The average victim of elder abuse is 80 years old, is female, and has multiple chronic conditions. These conditions make patients unable to function on their own, leaving them dependent on others for at least part of their care. The abuser is almost always known to the abused and is often a family member (such as adult children or a spouse).

One clue to elder abuse is unexplained injuries that do not fit the stated cause. Assessment of elder abuse must include not only the physical examination, but also the environmental and social clues. Look at the patient's overall hygiene, and review how he or she interacts with family members or carers. Take adequate time to listen patiently to any concerns expressed by

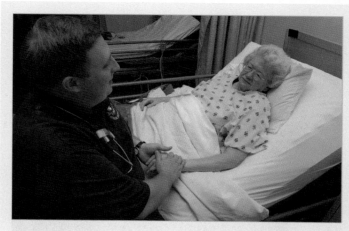

Figure 42-15 Take time to listen patiently to older patients.

older patients about their care (or lack of it) **Figure 42-15 ▲**. If the patient's condition is stable but the situation is unsafe, see if the patient will agree to let you take him or her to hospital. If the patient refuses transport, see if he or she will accept help from social services. If the situation is immediately unsafe, notify the police and remain with the patient only if the scene remains safe to do so.

The UK has widespread guidelines on elder abuse. Nevertheless, only one of five cases of elder abuse is ever reported. The way elder abuse is defined varies considerably, so it is advisable to become familiar with the legislation that applies to your own area. However, regardless of the legislation, if you have any reason to suspect elder abuse in a given case of injury—for example, if you found evidence of gross patient neglect in the patient's residence—carefully document your observations and report your findings and suspicions to the receiving hospital. For more information on this topic, see Chapter 43.

End-of-Life Care

You will inevitably be involved with end-of-life care for many patients. Of course, "do not attempt resuscitation" (DNAR) does *not* mean "do not respond to the needs of a terminal patient". There is much you can do, beginning with demonstrating a caring and concerned attitude and approach. Many of your visits may be "no transport" decisions, but they prove no less valuable to the patient than more aggressive measures. Many communities have a local hospice, an organisation that provides terminal care for patients and support for their families. If one exists in your community, consider how you or your service might collaborate on providing quality care for a person at the end of life **Figure 42-16 ▶**.

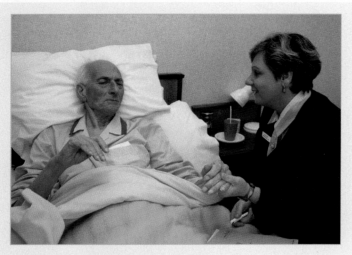

Figure 42-16 Hospice care allows people with terminal illnesses to receive palliative care in their own homes.

You are the Paramedic Summary

1. Why is it important to review common medical problems of elderly people?

Well, like it or not, we are not getting any younger. Approximately one fifth of the UK population is over 60 years of age. Between 1995 and 2025 the number of people over 80 could increase by almost 50% and the number over 90 will double. As we age, our bodies undergo numerous physical changes that affect the way we respond to illness and disease. Keeping up-to-date with medical problems of elderly people is just as important as staying current on other kinds of emergencies.

2. Which organ systems are greatly affected by age-related changes?

Although the ageing process affects all body systems, the organ systems most relevant to older patients are the respiratory, cardiovascular, renal, nervous, and musculoskeletal.

3. Why might obtaining an accurate medical history and history of the present illness be challenging when interviewing an elderly patient?

The elderly patient can present with numerous challenges that might make patient assessment tricky. These include having more than one chronic illness, not feeling pain the same way a younger person might, difficulty distinguishing acute from chronic problems, fear of being hospitalised, and fear of losing control over their ability to care for themselves. It is important to be patient and look for subtle clues when assessing an older person.

4. What are some specific respiratory illnesses commonly seen in elderly people?

Respiratory illnesses commonly seen in elderly people include bacterial pneumonia, COPD, and pulmonary embolism.

5. What are the risk factors for pneumonia in elderly people? Are any present here?

Residing in an institutional environment, chronic illness, and a compromised immune system are all risk factors for contracting pneumonia. In our case, Mrs Howard resides in a care home and has diabetes, which increases her chances of getting pneumonia.

6. Does pneumonia present in the same way in elderly people as it does in younger people?

If you are expecting to find a patient presenting with fever, productive cough, chest discomfort, and chest congestion, keep looking! The clinical presentation of pneumonia in elderly people will fool you. Rather than presenting with the "classic clinical picture" described above, an elderly person with pneumonia might present with altered mental status, cough, fever, shortness of breath, tachycardia, and tachypnoea.

7. How is pneumonia managed in the prehospital setting?

Prehospital management of pneumonia is aimed at supportive care. Ensuring an adequate airway and oxygenation and a little tender loving care will go a long way for most of your patients. Definitive treatment for pneumonia is the administration of antibiotics.

Prep Kit

Ready for Review

- Elderly people constitute an ever-increasing proportion of patients presenting to the health care system, particularly to the emergency care sector.
- The health problems of older people are quantitatively and qualitatively different from those of younger people. The special problems of older people require special approaches.
- The ageing process is accompanied by changes in physiological function. The decrease in the functional capacity of various organ systems can affect the way in which the patient responds to illness.
- A variety of changes occur in the cardiovascular system as a person ages. The heart hypertrophies (enlarges), arteriosclerosis (the stiffening of vessel walls) develops, and the electric conduction system of the heart deteriorates.
- A person's respiratory capacity also undergoes significant reductions with age due to decreases in the elasticity of the lungs and in the size and strength of the respiratory muscles, calcification of costochrondral cartilage in the chest wall, and musculoskeletal changes.
- Older patients may experience renal system changes. Although the kidneys of an elderly person may be capable of dealing with day-to-day demands, they may not be able to meet unusual challenges, such as those imposed by illness. Therefore, acute illness in elderly patients is often accompanied by derangements in fluid and electrolyte balance.
- Changes in the endocrine system may lead to diabetes and thyroid abnormalities in older patients.
- Ageing brings a widespread decrease in bone mass in men and women, but especially among postmenopausal women. Bones become more brittle and tend to break more easily.
- Changes in the nervous system lead to a decrease in the performance of sense organs, as evidenced by visual changes (glaucoma and cataracts are common) and hearing loss.
- Diseases of the heart remain the leading cause of death among older adults in the United Kingdom. Heart attack is the major cause of morbidity and mortality in people older than 65 years, and its potential for mortality increases significantly after 70 years.
- Stroke is a significant cause of death and disability in elderly people. More than 80% of all stroke deaths occur in persons older than 65 years, and stroke is the leading cause of long-term disability at any age.
- Chronic lower respiratory disease, influenza, and pneumonia remain in the top five causes for elderly deaths.
- An older patient with diabetes is at increased risk for hypoglycaemia for several reasons: medications, inadequate or irregular dietary intake, inability to recognise the warning signs due to cognitive problems, and/or blunted warning signs. Delirium may be the only indication of hypoglycaemia in an elderly patient.
- Older diabetics whose blood glucose levels tend to be high are prone to hyperosmolar hyperglycaemic nonketotic (HHNK) coma. The most frequent cause for HHNK is infection. Presentation is likely to be acute confusion with dehydration.
- Gastrointestinal problems in elderly people include peptic ulcer disease, small bowel obstruction due to gallstones, and stomach or duodenal ulcers (peptic ulcer disease).
- Osteoporosis is characterised by a decrease in bone mass leading to reduction in bone strength and greater susceptibility to fracture. Osteoarthritis is a progressive disease process of the joints that destroys cartilage, promotes the formation of bone spurs in joints, and leads to joint stiffness.

- In elderly people, delirium often replaces or confounds the typical presentation caused by a medical problem, an adverse medication effect, or drug withdrawal. Disorders that cause delirium may also include poisons, electrolyte imbalances, nutritional deficiencies, and infections such as urinary tract infections and pneumonia.
- Unlike delirium, dementia is a disease that produces irreversible brain failure. Disorders that cause dementia include conditions that impair vascular and neurological structures within the brain, such as infections, stroke, head injuries, poor nutrition, and medications.
- The two most common degenerative types of dementia in older people are Alzheimer's disease and multi-infarct or vascular dementia, both of which cause structural damage to the brain.
- Elderly people are particularly prone to adverse drug reactions because of changes in the following: drug metabolism because of diminished hepatic function; drug elimination because of diminished renal function; body composition, including increased body fat and decreased body water, altering the distribution of drugs through the various body compartments; and the responsiveness to drugs of the central nervous system.
- Alcohol is the preferred substance of abuse among older persons, in whom its use is on the rise. A much smaller but increasing segment of the older population uses illicit drugs.
- Depression in elderly patients can mimic the effects of many other medical problems (such as dementia). Risk factors for depression in an older person include a history of depression, chronic disease, and loss (function, independence, or significant others).
- Several factors place an elderly person at higher risk of trauma than a younger person: slower reflexes, visual and hearing deficits, equilibrium disorders, and an overall reduction in agility.
- Most elderly trauma cases involve falls or road traffic collisions. Falls among elderly people are evenly divided between those resulting from extrinsic (external) causes, such as tripping on a loose rug or slipping on ice, and those resulting from intrinsic (internal) causes, such as a dizzy spell or a syncopal attack.
- Knowing what is and what is not part of the ageing process constitutes the first challenge in assessing elderly patients. A second challenge is that signs and symptoms of disease may be altered from their presentation in younger patients as a consequence of ageing.
- When a patient's chief complaint seems trivial, it may be necessary to go through a review of systems to confirm that you are not missing important pieces of information. If any of the screening questions yields a positive answer, follow up with further questions.
- The physical examination of older patients can be difficult. Poor cooperation and easy fatigability may require that you keep manipulations of the patient to a minimum. You may have to peel many layers of clothing off elderly patients to perform an adequate examination.
- Infections in older people can be severe and dangerous. Consider sepsis whenever you see a hot, flushed patient who is also tachycardic and tachypnoeic.
- Elder abuse is any form of mistreatment that results in harm or loss to an older person. Five types of abuse are distinguished: physical, sexual, emotional, neglect, and financial.

Vital Vocabulary

bereavement Sadness from loss; grieving.

delirium An acute confusional state characterised by global impairment of thinking, perception, judgement, and memory.

dementia A chronic deterioration of mental functions.

homeostasis A tendency to constancy or stability in the body's internal milieu.

hospice An organisation that provides end-of-life care to patients with terminal illnesses and their families.

osteoporosis A decrease in bone mass and density.

polypharmacy The use of multiple medications.

presbycusis Progressive hearing loss, particularly in the high frequencies, along with lessened ability to discriminate between a particular sound and background noise.

proprioception The ability to perceive the position and movement of one's body or limbs.

review of systems A systematic survey of the patient's symptoms according to the major organ systems.

sepsis A disease state that results from the presence of microorganisms or their toxic products in the bloodstream.

spondylosis Immobility and consolidation of a vertebral joint.

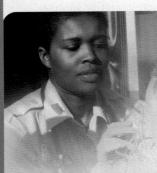

Assessment in Action

You are dispatched to a house for a fall. When you arrive on scene, you find an elderly man lying on his back. A large pool of blood is around his head. The patient is conscious, alert, and orientated to person, place, and day. He denies experiencing any loss of consciousness. He states that he was trying to get around the corner and tripped over his feet. His wife tells you that he has neuropathy to both his lower legs, bilateral knee replacements, and a hip replacement. He also has a history of blood clots and hypertension. His medications include lisinopril and warfarin. He has a large laceration to the back of his head. His vital signs are stable.

1. **A common change seen in the cardiovascular system of the elderly patient is:**
   A. neuropathy.
   B. hypertrophy.
   C. increased inotropy.
   D. increased automaticity.

2. **Changes in thinking, speed, memory, and postural stability are effects of the:**
   A. cardiovascular system.
   B. nervous system.
   C. pulmonary system.
   D. renal system.

3. **What is homeostasis?**
   A. Maintaining the constancy of the external environment
   B. An acute confusional state
   C. A decrease in bone mass and density
   D. Maintaining the constancy of the internal environment

4. **What is osteoarthritis?**
   A. A progressive disease process of the joints resulting in the destruction of cartilage
   B. A condition that affects only women and is characterised by a decrease in bone mass
   C. Atrophy of the supporting structures of the body
   D. A condition in which muscle fibres are smaller and fewer in numbers

5. **For what reasons are elderly persons particularly prone to adverse drug reactions?**
   A. Changes in drug metabolism because of diminished hepatic function
   B. Changes in drug elimination because of diminished renal function
   C. Changes in body composition, increased body fat, and decreased body water
   D. Changes in responsiveness to drugs that affect the central nervous system
   E. All of the above

6. **The underlying causes of falls among the elderly are classified as being:**
   A. extrinsic and intrinsic.
   B. medical illness and trauma.
   C. extrinsic and external.
   D. intrinsic and internal.

7. **In the elderly, _____ are MOST common after a fall.**
   A. extradural haematomas
   B. subdural haematomas
   C. intracerebral aneurysms
   D. ruptured cerebral arteries

Challenging Question

8. **Why do many older patients present atypically when they experience and injury or illness that causes shock?**

Points to Ponder

It's 07:00 hrs and your shift has just begun. You are dispatched to sheltered housing accommodations across town for an 86-year-old woman with chest pain. You recognise the address and flat as one that you have been to on several occasions. When you arrive, the patient's condition appears stable, but she has chest pain on palpation, inspiration, and movement. Her vital signs are as follows: pulse rate, 58 beats/min with sinus bradycardia on the cardiac monitor; blood pressure, 110/72 mm Hg; respiratory rate, 16 breaths/min; and pulse oximetry, 95% on room air. The patient tells you that this pain began after she received a phone call from her daughter, who was supposed to come and visit her and is now unable to do so.

Does this patient need to be transported immediately? How will you manage this patient?

Issues: Being an Advocate for the Elderly, Recognising the Need for Independence in the Elderly.

43 Protection of Vulnerable Adults and Children

Objectives

Cognitive

- Discuss the incidence of abuse and assault.
- Describe the categories of abuse.
- Discuss examples of spouse abuse.
- Discuss examples of elder abuse.
- Discuss examples of child abuse.
- Discuss examples of sexual assault.
- Describe the characteristics associated with the profile of the typical abuser of a spouse.
- Describe the characteristics associated with the profile of the typical abuser of the elder.
- Describe the characteristics associated with the profile of the typical abuser of children.
- Describe the characteristics associated with the profile of the typical assailant of sexual assault.
- Identify the profile of the "at-risk" spouse.
- Identify the profile of the "at-risk" elder.
- Identify the profile of the "at-risk" child.
- Discuss the assessment and management of the abused patient.
- Discuss the legal aspects associated with abuse situations.
- Identify community resources that are able to assist victims of abuse and assault.
- Discuss the documentation associated with abused and assaulted patients.

Affective

- Demonstrate sensitivity to the abused patient.
- Value the behaviour of the abused patient.
- Attend to the emotional state of the abused patient.
- Recognise the value of non-verbal communication with the abused patient.
- Attend to the needs for reassurance, empathy, and compassion with the abused patient.
- Listen to the concerns expressed by the abused patient.
- Listen and value the concerns expressed by the sexually assaulted patient.

Psychomotor

- Demonstrate the ability to assess a spouse, elder, or child abused patient.
- Demonstrate the ability to assess a sexually assaulted patient.

Introduction

Abuse, neglect, and assault are, unfortunately, all too common in the United Kingdom ◀ Table 43-1 ▾ . Because these issues are frequently encountered reasons for calls to the ambulance service, it is important for you to recognise the signs and symptoms. You must know not only how to recognise and differentiate among abuse, neglect, and assault, but also how to protect yourself from injury while maintaining optimal care for the patient. Victims who survive abuse or neglect often have permanent disabilities, mental and physical. Although prevention strategies have improved in recent years, paramedics may be on the front lines for getting help to victims of abuse ◀ Figure 43-1 ▶ .

Table 43-1	Incidence of Child Abuse
Type of Abuse	**Percentage**
Neglect	43
Emotional abuse	21
Physical abuse	16
Sexual abuse	8
Mixed abuse	11

Source: Referrals, assessments and children and young people on child protection registers, England — Year ending 31 March 2006. Available at: http://www.dfes.gov.uk/rsgateway/DB/SFR/s000692/SFR45-2006.pdf Accessed 26 November 2006.

Child Abuse

Child abuse includes any improper or excessive action that injures or otherwise harms a child or infant, including physical abuse, sexual abuse, neglect, and emotional abuse. Many survivors are negatively affected by such abuse for the rest of their

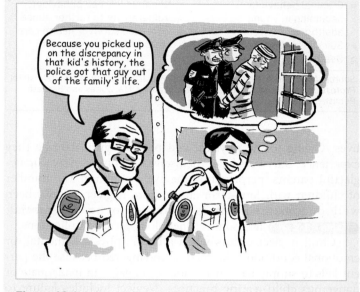

Figure 43-1

You are the Paramedic Part 1

You respond to a call for a "child who fell". On arrival, you find an unconscious 5-month-old boy. The mother had just come home from work; her boyfriend had been watching the baby. The boyfriend states that the baby "fell off the sofa" approximately 30 cm from the carpeted floor. The child is comatose and has ataxic breathing.

The boyfriend appears nervous. He tries to answer all questions asked of the mother and to control the scene. In the same flat, you find a 7-year-old girl with wheezing in all fields. The mother states that the child has a puffer, but it is empty and the mother has no prescription to obtain a refill. Five other children are in the cramped flat, all under age 10 years. The one-bedroom flat is clean but very small, and children must sleep on a bare mattress in the living room. The mother sleeps in the bedroom with the baby (in the same bed).

Initial Assessment	Recording Time: 0 Minutes	
	5-month-old patient	**7-year-old patient**
Appearance	Comatose	Agitated, pensive
Level of consciousness	U (Unresponsive)	A (Alert to person, place, and day)
Airway	Mildly obstructed	Mildly obstructed
Breathing	22 breaths/min, irregular	> 40 breaths/min, shallow
Circulation	78 beats/min; irregular	> 140 beats/min; regular
Skin	Acrocyanotic	Flushed

1. What are your first priorities after assessing scene safety?
2. What should raise your index of suspicion?
3. What is the 5-month-old patient's transport and treatment status, in your judgement?

Table 43-2	Potential Complications of Maltreatment

- Low self-esteem and underachievement
- Abnormal growth and development
- Poor school performance
- Social withdrawal
- Substance abuse
- Criminal behaviour beginning in young adulthood
- Suicidal tendencies
- Death
- Psychological disorders or psychiatric symptoms
- Permanent physical or neurological damage
- Teen promiscuity and pregnancy
- Eating disorders
- Negative learned behaviour
- Vulnerability to further abuse
- Increased survivor health care costs to family and society

Source: American Academy of Pediatrics. *Pediatric Education for Prehospital Professionals*, 2nd ed. Table 12-1, p.244. Sudbury, MA: Jones and Bartlett Publishers, Inc.

Table 43-3	Risk Factors for Child Abuse

Parent or Carer
- Parental history of abuse as a child
- Substance abuse by parents
- Insufficient or inaccurate parental knowledge about child development

Family
- Disorganised and disruptive family structure
- Marital or partner discord
- Financial or outside stressors present
- Inappropriate or dysfunctional parent–child interaction

Child
- Disability of the child
- Attention deficits or difficult temperament of child

Environment
- Home life affected by poverty or unemployment
- Isolation of parents; lack of social support
- Violent, crime-filled community

Source: Child Welfare Information Gateway. Available at: http://www.childwelfare.gov/pubs/usermanuals/foundation/foundatione.cfm. Accessed 24 July 2006.

lives. Owing to the physical and psychological damage they experience, survivors may themselves become abusive or neglectful parents, perpetuating the cycle of abuse. The number of children with long-term effects from neglect has not been well documented but is believed to be substantial. **Table 43-2 ▲** lists some of these long-term complications.

Child neglect occurs when a child's physical, mental, or emotional condition is harmed or endangered because the parent fails to supply basic necessities or engages in inadequate or dangerous child-rearing practices. Neglect includes failure to provide adequate food, clothing, or shelter; the parent's misuse of drugs or alcohol; failure to provide support or affection necessary to the child's psychological and social development; or child abandonment. Children who are neglected are often dirty or too thin or appear developmentally delayed because of a lack of stimulation.

As a paramedic, you will often be called to scenes because of a reported injury to a child. Many abused children have permanent or life-threatening injuries, and some die. If suspected child abuse is not reported, the child is likely to be victimised repeatedly. Therefore, you must be aware of the signs of child abuse and neglect, and mindful of your responsibility to report suspected abuse to the police or social services. When in doubt as to whether abuse or neglect is involved, it is always better to err on the side of caution to protect the victim.

Profile of an At-Risk Child

Child abuse and neglect occurs in all communities and among all socioeconomic groups. Younger children are at higher risk for fatal abuse and neglect than are older children. On average one child is killed by their parent or carer every week in England and Wales, with babies under the age of one being at a four times greater risk to die of a violent assault than the average person in England and Wales. Although no geographic, ethnic, or economic setting is free of child abuse or neglect, children from low-income or single-parent families have more *reported* occurrences of abuse and neglect than children from higher-income families. **Table 43-3 ▶** lists other factors that put a child at risk of abuse.

At the Scene

It is a good idea to establish a "code" between you and your colleague indicating that they should discreetly call for police. This signal can be as simple as "Could you go to the ambulance and get the extra set of latex-free gloves"? This way, you will not aggravate or "tip off" the abuser to your request for police, further riling the abuser.

When assessing a potential child abuse case, be attuned to suspicious behavioural traits. A child who does not become agitated when a parent leaves the room or who does not look to a parent for reassurance may be abused. Children who are abused may also cry excessively or not at all, may be wary of physical contact, or may appear apprehensive.

People Who Abuse Children

Child maltreatment can be done by any person who has care, custody, or control of the child, including parents, step-parents, foster parents, babysitters, and relatives. Abusive parents frequently receive little enjoyment from parenting and are more isolated from the community than are nonabusive parents. They have unrealistic expectations of their child and try to control the child through negative and authoritarian means. Abusive parents are often afraid of, or emotionally unable to ask for help from, sources of support in their community. Most were themselves abused or neglected as children. Many view themselves as victims in life generally or in the parent–child relationship in particular. They feel that they have lost control of their children and their own lives. When their children behave in a manner

Table 43-4	"Red Flag" Behaviours

- Apathy
- Bizarre or strange conduct
- Little or no concern about the child
- Overreaction to child misbehaviour
- Not forthcoming with events surrounding injury
- Intoxication
- Overreaction to child's condition

Source: American Academy of Pediatrics. *Pediatric Education for Prehospital Professionals*, 2nd ed. Table 12-7, p. 250. Sudbury, MA: Jones and Bartlett Publishers, Inc.

that parents perceive as disrespectful, they lash out in an effort to establish control. Abusive parents may prefer to discipline using other means but are pushed to violence by stress.

Characteristics shared by parents of maltreated children include drug use, poor self-concept, immaturity, lack of parenting knowledge, and lack of interpersonal skills. Table 43-4 ▲ lists additional "red flag" behaviours.

Assessment and Management of Child Abuse

One of the most important indicators of possible abuse is repeated calls to the same home or family for a child injury or medical problem. Nevertheless, the best indicator by far is the physical examination of the child, conducted with a keen ear for inconsistencies in the history. The physical examination must take into consideration the mental and emotional age of the child. Examining the child from toe to head may work best on toddlers and preschoolers, whereas an infant may be best examined in a parent's arms. Preadolescents and teenagers have modesty and body awareness concerns, which should be respected.

If possible, do the examination with another colleague. This approach will verify your findings and help prevent false accusations of impropriety. Also, make certain that you are very objective on your documentation. Do not include opinions or draw nonmedical conclusions; list only the objective information, and stick to the facts.

When assessing for possible child abuse, you may find the CHILD ABUSE mnemonic helpful:

C   *Consistency* of the injury with the child's developmental age
H   *History* inconsistent with injury
I   *Inappropriate* parental concerns
L   *Lack* of supervision
D   *Delay* in seeking care
A   *Affect*
B   *Bruises* of varying ages
U   *Unusual* injury patterns
S   *Suspicious* circumstances
E   *Environmental* clues

Soft-tissue injuries are the most common findings in the physical examination of an abused child. Multiple bruises in various stages of healing are another red flag Figure 43-2 ▶. Be alert for bruises on areas of the body where they would not be expected, such as the buttocks Figure 43-3 ▶, back, face, and upper legs. Bites and burns may also be noted. Stocking/glove burns and doughnut burns occur when a child is immersed in hot water Figure 43-4 ▶.

Fractures can result from falls, twisting, or jerking injuries. Multiple fractures or fractures in various stages of healing are indicators of abuse, as are "self-healing" fractures. Head injuries are the most deadly for children; even if not fatal, they can easily produce permanent disability. Look for scalp wounds, signs and symptoms of haematoma, and concussion Figure 43-5 ▶.

You are the Paramedic Part 2

You decide to call the police to the scene, owing to the injuries and current history of the 5-month-old patient. The boyfriend becomes visibly agitated when he hears you on the radio. "What do we need the police for? Just take care of the kid", he states. After making sure you have a visible escape route, you continue caring for the child and tell the man, "It's just routine". You then ask the mother for the medical history of the child, hoping to deflect the man's attention. At this time, the 5-month-old boy is having difficulty in breathing, his extremities are becoming cyanotic, and he does not respond to external stimuli. The 7-year-old girl with asthma is in moderate distress as your partner sets up the nebuliser with the paediatric dose of salbutamol.

Vital Signs	Recording Time: 5 Minutes	
	5-month-old patient	7-year-old patient
Skin	Cool and dry, cyanotic extremities	Warm, wet
Pulse	62 beats/min	120 beats/min
Blood pressure	Unobtainable	96/50 mm Hg
Respirations	20 breaths/min; irregular	32 breaths/min
SpO_2	89% on room air	97% on room air

4. Do you think you will have to ventilate the 5-month-old boy? Why or why not?
5. Do you think you will have to ventilate the 7-year-old girl? Why or why not?

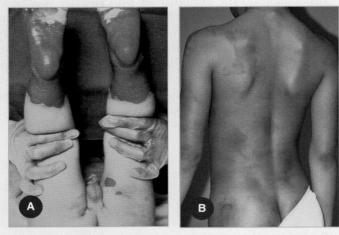

Figure 43-2 Signs of child abuse. **A.** Scald. **B.** Multiple injuries at different stages of healing.

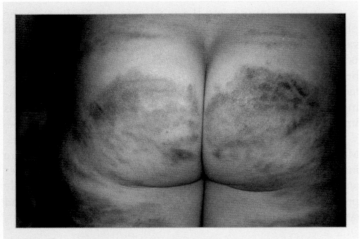

Figure 43-3 Bruises on the buttocks are usually inflicted injuries.

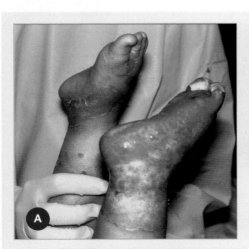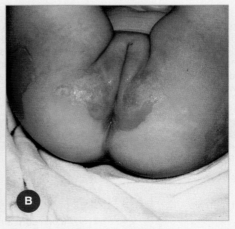

Figure 43-4 A. Stocking/glove burns of the feet or hands in an infant or a toddler are almost always inflicted injuries. **B.** A doughnut burn occurs when a child is held in a hot bath and the area in contact with the cooler porcelain is spared.

Although abdominal injuries are rare in child abuse cases, they are usually serious. Remember, small children have thin and underdeveloped abdominal muscles. Note the colour and rigidity of the abdomen and tenderness to palpation. Injuries to the abdomen may result in injuries to the intestines or rupture of the liver.

Sometimes, normal physical findings may suggest an inflicted injury. Other benign skin findings can also suggest abuse, although the lesions are actually produced by cultural rituals intended to treat illness. Some medical or folk remedies may be foreign to you or inconsistent with your training. For example, cupping (**Figure 43-6 ▶**) and coin rubbing (**Figure 43-7 ▶**) are alarming to most paramedics, but a reasonable explanation of the practice, which is common in some Asian cultures, should allay your suspicions.

It is important to observe the scene, including the household dynamics, as you care for the patient. In the "You are the Paramedic" scenario in this chapter, the paramedics discovered two patients; be aware that more than one victim may be encountered. It is important to keep the scene as safe and calm as possible while still providing life support for any critical and moderately distressed patients.

In a case involving child abuse or neglect, the patient clinical records, with objective observations, will be very important to the police and social services. Paramedics have a duty to report cases of child abuse or neglect. Don't assume that someone else has already called or that the accident and emergency (A&E) department will call! It is better to have more than one person call the hotline for the same case than to see the case "fall through the cracks". Most communities also have parenting classes available through county social services.

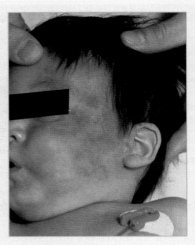

Figure 43-5 The face is a common target for physical abuse.

Elder Abuse

The incidence of older patient abuse and neglect is growing in the United Kingdom. The ageing of the population and the strains placed on carers and the nursing home systems contribute to this

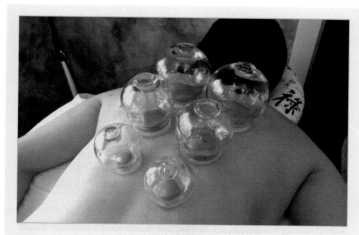

Figure 43-6 Cupping is the cultural practice of placing warm cups on the skin to pull out illness from the body. The red, flat, rounded skin lesions are often more intensely red at the borders.

Table 43-5	Profile of Abused Older Patients

- Women
- People older than 75 years
- People with one or more chronic physical or mental impairments placing them in a care-dependent position
- People who live with their abusers
- Socially isolated people
- People who exhibit problematic behaviour (such as incontinence or shouting)

Table 43-6	Profile of a Person Who Abuses Elders

- Lives with the victim
- Has drug or alcohol dependency problems
- Is older than 50 years
- Depends on the victim for financial support
- Has poor impulse control
- Is ill prepared or reluctant to provide care
- Has a history of domestic violence

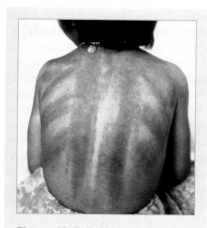

Figure 43-7 Rubbing hot coins, often on the back, produces rounded and oblong red, patchy, flat skin lesions.

problem. You must use sound judgement and learn to develop good observational skills. Because older patients present very differently from children and younger adults, you must be especially attuned to the possibility of abuse in this population. Consider the following scenario:

You respond to a call for a collapse. On arrival, you find an 86-year-old man lying on his side in the living room, bleeding from the mouth and nose. He appears confused, and you cannot understand what he is trying to say. His 56-year-old daughter states that her father tripped and fell. His vital signs are as follows: pulse, 68 beats/min; respirations, 14 breaths/min; and blood pressure, 100/68 mm Hg. The patient's skin is warm and wet. You see a walking aid in the kitchen approximately 8 m away. The daughter states that the patient doesn't really need it, stating, "He just uses it to get sympathy". The daughter is very upset that the police have just pulled up. Your colleague tells you that she has been to this home several times before for falls, that the patient has Alzheimer's disease, and that the daughter seems to lose patience with him, sometimes refusing to cooperate with the ambulance service. The daughter then states, "Would you people hurry up and get him out of here? He's getting blood all over the rug".

In this scenario, the elderly patient clearly needs assistance, but his daughter also seems to be overwhelmed. This situation is not unusual: Because people are living longer than ever before, their children (often baby boomers) must assume responsibility for their care. The stress on these carers is real—physical, emotional, and financial burdens can wear them down. Ambulance clinicians should be familiar with local resources to assist carers and patients. This assistance can be as simple as a visiting nurse or a community care agency to take the patient to his or her doctor's appointments.

As with child abuse, elder abuse involves a direct action causing harm to the victim. Abuse of older patients includes sexual abuse, psychological or emotional abuse, neglect, and abandonment. Neglect can be active or passive. Active neglect refers to the deliberate withholding of companionship, medicine, food, exercise, or assistance with mobility; passive neglect occurs when an older person is ignored, left alone, isolated, or forgotten. Abandonment is the desertion of an older person by a person who has physical custody of the older person or by a person who has assumed responsibility for providing care. **Table 43-5 ▲** lists the characteristics of older abused patients. In domestic abuse cases, the abusers are quite often the children of the abused person **Table 43-6 ▲**.

Factors Contributing to Elder Abuse

Although paramedics are concerned with treating and managing the results of abuse and neglect, an understanding of why these problems occur can be beneficial. In some cases, the violence may be a learned response. Children who were abused may ultimately be in a position to abuse their elderly parents. The stress of caring for an older person may push some carers into abuse or neglect. Factors such as a diminishing social network, frailty, and medical illness also put older people at risk for maltreatment. Older people are at an increased risk for abuse in nursing facilities that have a history of providing inadequate care, are understaffed, and provide poor training for their employees.

Signs of Elder Abuse

The signs and symptoms of elder abuse and neglect can be subtle and, in the emergency setting, can often be overlooked. Evaluate each situation involving an older person with a critical eye toward potential abuse and neglect.

Be on the lookout for a fearful patient with unexplained bruises or sores that have not been tended to. Of course, the patient may naturally be fearful of the whole emergency situation, and there may well be a reasonable explanation for the marks on the body. Be alert for a situation in which you find an unkempt, dirty patient while the carer is clean. Generally speaking, a solicitous carer will keep the patient and the patient's surroundings tidy. Watch for a patient who allows the carer to answer all of your questions, while appearing mentally competent to do so; this person may look to the carer for approval when you ask the patient a direct question. If a patient tells you that items are being taken or money confiscated, such a complaint may be an indication of paranoia or a symptom of dementia—but it could very well be true. Don't investigate these claims; simply document them thoroughly. Be wary if a patient states that he or she is not allowed to socialise with peers and is kept in isolation.

Generally speaking, abused elders do not seek help. This reluctance may be due to fear of being institutionalised, fear of getting the abuser into "trouble", polypharmacy, confusion, or brain disorders such as Alzheimer's disease. In such cases, the physical examination, history, and observation of scene surroundings and patient interaction with parents are of paramount concern. The physical examination and history should address the following issues:

- Is the patient capable of answering your questions in an appropriate way?
- Is the patient fearful?
- Does the patient look clean?
- Are the pill bottles marked appropriately and consistent with purchase dates and use?
- Does the patient have bruises or sores?
- Is the patient's current history consistent with the report given by the carer?

Objectively record your observations on the patient clinical record (PCR), avoiding drawing conclusions and giving opinions. Social Services could use these observations as an indicator of whether assistance is required.

As far as the scene goes, ask these questions (Figure 43-8 ▶):

- Is the home tidy, and are the surroundings orderly?
- Is there food in the refrigerator?
- What is the heating situation, and is it appropriate to the weather?
- Does the patient use a walking or wheelchair device?

For patients who reside in nursing homes, signs of abuse include undocumented decubitus ulcers, tied-off catheters, and dangerous use of restraints. Some nursing home residents who are victims of abuse may not have a way to report the abuse, may not know how to report the abuse, may not be physically able to report it, or may fear retaliation for reporting it. Others may be victims of abuse by visiting family members.

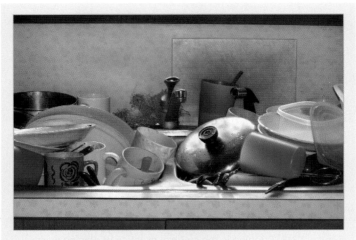

Figure 43-8 The patient's environment can provide clues to abuse or neglect.

Although the ageing of the population has placed increased demands on the system, institutional carers have a legal obligation to meet accepted standards of care. The provision of social services is governed by primary and secondary legislation (ie, Acts of Parliament and Rules and Regulations) together with government guidance which must be followed by local authorities. The NHS and Community Care Act 1990 Section 47(1) imposes a duty on local authorities to carry out an assessment of need for community care services with people who appear to them to need such services and then, having regard to that assessment, decide whether those needs call for the provision by them of services. If the patient is institutionalised in a nursing or residential home or receiving care by a domiciliary care agency and abuse or neglect is suspected, you will need to notify social services and the Regional Office of the Commission for Social Care Inspection (CSCI) who are responsible for overseeing the facility. In circumstances where there is an immediate risk, cases should be referred directly to the police.

Domestic Abuse

Violence within the family has a long history. In ancient Rome, for example, husbands had the legal right to administer physical punishment to their wives within their own homes and in public. Today, ambulance services are frequently called for assault and battery situations in the home. The statistics on intimate-partner abuse are sobering: Millions of women are abused by an intimate partner each year.

Calls of this nature challenge the skills of ambulance clinicians. Scene safety is a paramount concern, and preservation of evidence is a necessity. Consider the following scenario:

You are called for a "woman bleeding". When you arrive, a man opens the door and tells you that his wife fell down the stairs. You find a 42-year-old woman crying and bleeding from her mouth. She has obvious contusions and abrasions on her face. Vital signs are a pulse of 124 beats/min, respirations of 28 breaths/min, and blood pressure of 132/84 mm Hg. The patient is alert and orientated to

At the Scene

If you and your colleague can safely get the patient and the person suspected of abuse away from each other, by all means do so. This separation will help make the scene safer; it also gives you a chance to compare current histories.

person, place, and day; her skin is warm and dry. Her husband tries to answer all of the questions you pose to her. The stairwell is carpeted and has only seven risers, but there is no blood on the stairs. Two children, ages 6 and 12, are crying in an adjacent bedroom. The father tells them to stay in the bedroom. Police have not been dispatched to this call yet.

Is there significance to the husband dominating the patient interview? Should the crying children raise any red flags? The children's concern and the husband's control of the scene could be perfectly normal behaviour. You must look at all the pieces of the puzzle. Document what you have observed, not what you think.

As a paramedic, you must be able to recognise the scope of domestic abuse and understand its various forms:

- **Physical abuse**—hitting, kicking, pushing, shoving, choking, beating
- **Emotional abuse**—making negative comments, calling names, playing mind games
- **Economic abuse**—trying to keep a person from getting a job and gaining his or her own economic independence
- **Sexual abuse**—making a person perform sexual activities against his or her will

Even though the awareness of domestic abuse has been raised in recent years, dealing with these cases in the prehospital environment presents a challenge to ambulance clinicians. Battered patients may not give accurate details about their injuries, and they may avoid seeking help. Indeed, victims typically report their abuse only as a last resort, for many reasons—for example, embarrassment, financial considerations, and low self-esteem. Often, they believe the behaviour will change, as is promised so frequently by the abuser. Sometimes the victim believes that he or she is the reason for the abuse and somehow deserved it (also called the Stockholm syndrome).

Profile of an Abused Spouse

Physical injuries from abuse include broken bones, cuts, head injuries, bruises, burns, scars from old injuries, and internal injuries. An abused spouse may have feelings of anxiety, distress, or hopelessness and may show signs of depression, make suicide attempts, or engage in substance abuse.

Although in the overwhelming majority of cases the victim is a woman, men also are abused. Men who are battered may be too humiliated to report the incident as it happened but still feel the same emotions as their female counterparts: guilt, loss of control, and shame. Because society tends to be less empathetic toward abused men and because fewer resources exist for them, the situation can be all the more difficult.

Same-sex relationships can be as fraught with peril as heterosexual unions. A common misconception is that participants in same-sex relationships are "on an equal playing field", so that the abuse cannot be as serious as that found in heterosexual relationships. In reality, concerns about "coming out" may prevent these victims from seeking help. You must be aware of and sensitive to their concerns.

Battered patients may appear fearful, apprehensive, or nonverbal. They may avoid eye contact, and their answers may be incorrect or inconsistent. Be alert for verbal clues such as "It was my fault—I really shouldn't push him" or "He's a good person—it's just that when he drinks . . ." In the UK the police operate

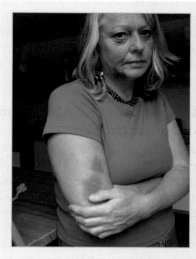

Figure 43-9 Injuries associated with intimate-partner abuse.

a low tolerance towards domestic violence and where there are signs of physical abuse or in situations where acts of verbal abuse are witnessed by the police, arrests will be made at scene of one or all parties involved **Figure 43-9 ▲** .

People Who Abuse Their Partners

People who commit domestic abuse may be paranoid, overly sensitive, obsessive, or threatening. They often abuse alcohol or drugs and have access to weapons. **Table 43-7 ▾** lists other characteristics of abusers.

People who abuse partners or spouses may use intimidation and threats to maintain their control over the person. They may throw objects in a rage or threaten regarding what he or she will do if the spouse leaves or reports the abusive behaviour. An abusive spouse may also use isolation as a means to dominate the partner, not allowing the spouse to visit friends or talk openly with others, and may feel that he or she is providing discipline or is justified in these actions. Many times, an abusive person is immediately remorseful and promises never

Table 43-7	**Characteristics of a Person Who Abuses a Partner**

- Was abused as a child
- Becomes more violent with each ensuing attack
- Usually comes from a family of abusers
- Very low self-esteem
- Remorseful after the attack; promises it will never happen again (but it does)
- May direct violence at children, especially children from a partner's previous relationship(s)

to let the problem happen again. Historically, this is rarely true; the abuse usually continues and becomes even more violent.

Never forget that domestic violence calls can be dangerous. You may be dealing with a potentially violent person, and emotions on the scene will be highly charged. If the person appears to be hostile or violent, remove all unnecessary people (such as family, friends, and bystanders) from the scene. It is imperative that you put your safety and the safety of your colleague first. If there is any doubt about scene safety, call for police assistance (see Chapter 51).

Assessment and Management of Domestic Abuse

Identifying a battered patient can be difficult because the victim may be protective of the attacker, frightened, or honestly unable to recall details. Patients may avoid eye contact or be otherwise evasive about their injuries. Listen for verbal clues regarding the incident, such as "We've been having some problems". On approach to the patient, use direct questioning to ascertain whether the domestic problems led to the physical harm. Try to empathise and reassure the patient; this caring attitude alone may instil confidence. Be as objective and nonjudgemental as possible. Listen attentively, and be supportive. Give the patient a sense of control as much as possible. You may be the last or only chance a victim has to escape this situation, so encourage the patient to consider where he or she can go or whom he or she can call for help.

In cases involving domestic abuse, the PCR is more than just documentation of the transfer of care; it is a permanent record of treatment and disposition. More important, from a legal viewpoint, it represents hard evidence for the prosecution and the defence. Your statements and assessments must be objective, nonjudgemental, exact (when quoting a statement from the scene), and as neat as possible. If you make an error and want to change it, draw a line through the error and initial the lined-out statement. Usually, before testifying in court, you are allowed to review your PCR, but remember that your testimony may come many years and many patients later.

Intimate-partner abuse is not simply a "family issue"; it is a crime to beat another person, regardless of the relationship. The presence of police personnel may be helpful in these cases. If the patient refuses to be transported, consider leaving information on domestic abuse support services, which the patient may reference later. Learn what services are available in your area.

■ Sexual Assault

Sexual assault is another call that the ambulance service receives all too often. Although most victims are women, men and children may also be attacked sexually. There are no typical characteristics of sexual offenders and unfortunately, they are very difficult to detect. Often, you can do little beyond providing compassion and transportation to the A&E. On some occasions, patients may have multiple-system trauma and need treatment for shock. Your actions will go a long way toward providing relief. From arrival on scene to possible judicial system involvement, your professionalism is the key to proper care.

Consider the following scenario:

> You are sent to an "assist police" call. On arrival at the scene, you find a 20-year-old woman covered in a blanket and bleeding from several abrasions on her face. The police officer pulls you aside and states that the patient may have been assaulted in the alleyway on her way home from night class. Vital signs include a pulse of 134 beats/min, respirations of 32 breaths/min and irregular, and blood pressure of 122/80 mm Hg. The patient is alert and orientated to person, place, and day; her skin is warm and wet. She is very quiet, appears confused, and tells you she doesn't remember what happened. She wants to go home and shower.

The victim of sexual assault is often found in a state of denial or disbelief. Likewise, the desire to shower is common. The patient should be encouraged to go to hospital, where evidence can be collected and where access to professional services is more readily available.

Sexual assault and rape are crimes of power, force, and violence. Essentially, sexual assault refers to any unwanted sexual contact and rape is described as an act of non-consensual sexual intercourse (ie, vaginal, anal, or oral penetration) by a man with another person; victims can be either male or female (Sexual Offences Act, 2003). When the victim is underage, it is called statutory rape. Rape is a serious offence, and you have a

You are the Paramedic Part 3

Vital Signs	Recording Time: 10 Minutes	
	5-month-old patient	7-year-old patient
Skin	Good colour; cool and dry	Warm, wet
Pulse	98 beats/min	110 beats/min
Blood pressure	60/P	96/50 mm Hg
Respirations	Ventilated	Nebuliser treatment; normal breaths/min
SpO$_2$	98%	100%

6. What further treatment do you need for the 5-month-old boy? How can you check for level of consciousness at this point?

7. Is the small-volume nebuliser treatment working for the 7-year-old girl? Does this patient need to go to the hospital? Why or why not?

At the Scene

It is usually preferable to have a same-gender paramedic assist with the victim of sexual abuse. If you have this capability and there is no unreasonable time lag for that type of response, you should consider this option as an enhancement to the treatment process.

responsibility to preserve the crime scene in addition to treating the patient (see Chapter 51).

Treatment and Documentation

A victim of sexual assault may be hysterical, embarrassed, and/or frightened. You must be vigilant, but above all, you must be professional and compassionate. If you do not observe life-threatening signs and symptoms on arrival, avoid any aggressive treatment behaviour. Leave evidence as untouched as possible, and encourage the patient to leave the same clothes on as were worn at the time of the assault, and not to throw away or destroy any clothing. Encourage the patient not to bathe, shower, urinate, or defecate, if possible. If oral penetration has occurred, advise the patient not to eat, drink, brush the teeth, or use mouthwash until he or she has been examined.

Treat all other injuries according to appropriate procedures and guidelines for your service. Observe universal precautions. Take the patient's history, perform a limited physical examination, and provide treatment as quickly, quietly, and calmly as possible. Take care to shield the patient from onlookers. Help the patient regain a sense of control by posing open-ended questions and allowing him or her to make decisions.

The patient may refuse assistance or transport, often because he or she wants to maintain privacy and avoid public exposure. Adult patients have the right to decline care. In these cases, you should follow your service's refusal of treatment procedure without being judgemental or condescending. It is also important to advise patients to seek further medical attention as they may require post exposure prophylaxis and/or contraceptive advice. Your compassion is the best tool to win the patient's confidence to get further help.

Because you may need to appear in court as much as 2 or 3 years later, you should document the patient's history, assessment, treatment, and response to treatment in detail. Record only the objective facts. Subjective statements made by those on the scene or the patient should be in quotes on the PCR. Thoroughly document all patient statements pertaining to the crime, as well as statements, names, addresses, and contact information of any witnesses.

Like a battered partner, a victim of sexual abuse must be treated and protected by the ambulance service and police. Conscientious paramedics will make a huge difference in the recovery of patients through their professional conduct.

Child Victims

In most cases of child sexual abuse, the person who abused the child is an adult who knows the child and may be living under the same roof. Children of any age and either sex can be victims of sexual abuse. Although most victims of rape are older than 10 years, younger children may also be victims.

Child sexual abuse usually does not occur as a single incident. It does not always involve violence and physical force, and it commonly leaves no visible signs. The power of authority or the parent–child bond may be used to victimise the child instead of force or violence. The child may be manipulated into thinking that the acts are acceptable and normal behaviour. The child may also be made to feel deeply ashamed and powerless or even be kept silent by threats. The insidious nature of this abuse makes it difficult to detect unless the child discloses the information to a confidant or a prehospital professional.

Your assessment of a child who has been sexually abused should be limited to determining the type of dressing any injuries require. Sometimes, a sexually abused child is also beaten. In such cases, you should treat bruises and fractures as well. Do not examine the genitalia of a young child unless you see evidence of bleeding or an injury to this region that must be treated. In some cases, the child may present with behavioural or physical problems, such as hostility or restlessness.

You are the Paramedic Summary

1. What are your first priorities after assessing scene safety?

Your first priority in the scenario should be to open the airway of the 5-month-old boy. Your next priority is to call for a second paramedic unit to help care for the 7-year-old girl.

2. What should raise your index of suspicion?

Your index of suspicion should be raised by the nervousness of the boyfriend and his attempts to control the scene.

3. What is the 5-month-old patient's transport and treatment status, in your judgement?

The 5-month-old boy should be considered to be in unstable condition, and treatment and transport should occur as rapidly as possible after airway manoeuvring.

4. Do you think that you will have to ventilate the 5-month-old boy? Why or why not?

You will have to ventilate this patient on the scene because you can control his airway better than the boy can himself.

5. Do you think you will have to ventilate the 7-year-old girl? Why or why not?

This patient does not have to be ventilated at this point; give the salbutamol and/or ipratropium bromide treatment a chance to work before you take this step.

6. What further treatment do you need for the 5-month-old boy? How can you check for level of consciousness at this point?

This patient needs to be evaluated for brain damage due to the "fall" or to hypoxia. At this point, it is a good idea to check for painful stimuli and watch the boy's reaction, if any. A pinch of the foot may provide a response.

7. Is the nebuliser treatment working for the 7-year-old girl? Does this patient need to go to hospital? Why or why not?

The nebuliser seems to be working for the 7-year-old girl; however, she should still be transported to hospital. There the patient can be interviewed by professionals and, at the very least, receive another prescription for her metered-dose inhaler.

Prep Kit

Ready for Review

- Abuse, neglect, and assault occur at all levels of society. Because maltreatment and assault are common reasons for calls to the ambulance service, you must recognise the signs and symptoms of these problems.

- Child abuse includes any improper or excessive action that injures or otherwise harms a child or infant, including physical abuse, sexual abuse, neglect, and emotional abuse. Many survivors are negatively affected for the rest of their lives.

- Social services and the police have statutory authority and responsibility to investigate allegations or suspicions about child abuse. The ambulance service must refer all such concerns to social services. In circumstances where the child is considered to be in immediate risk, cases should be referred directly to the police.

- Watch for the telltale signs of abused children and people who abuse children.

- Abuse and neglect of elderly people are on the rise. Because elderly patients present very differently from the way child and adult patients do, you must be especially attuned to the possibility of abuse in the elderly population.

- Elder abuse can be domestic or institutional. Adult children are often the ones who abuse their elderly parents.

- Social services exist for carers and victims alike.

- Domestic abuse happens in heterosexual and homosexual relationships.

- Victims of sexual abuse may not be inclined to report the crime.

Vital Vocabulary

abuse Any form of maltreatment that results in harm or loss. Maltreatment may be physical, sexual, psychological, or financial/material.

active neglect The refusal or failure to fulfil an obligation; a conscious or intentional attempt to inflict physical or emotional stress. Examples include abandonment and denial of food or health-related services.

assault Unlawfully placing a person in fear of immediate bodily harm.

battery Unlawfully touching a person; this includes providing emergency care without consent.

coin rubbing A cultural ritual intended to treat an illness by rubbing hot coins, often on the back, which produces rounded and oblong red, patchy, flat skin lesions.

cupping The cultural practice of placing warm cups on the skin to pull out illness from the body. The red, flat, rounded skin lesions are often more intensely red at the borders.

neglect Refusal or failure on the part of the carer to provide life necessities, such as food, water, clothing, shelter, personal hygiene, medicine, comfort, and personal safety.

passive neglect An unintentional refusal or failure to fulfil an obligation, which results in physical or emotional distress. Examples include forgetting or isolating the person.

polypharmacy Simultaneous use of many medications.

rape Sexual intercourse inflicted forcibly on another person, against that person's will.

sexual assault An attack against a person that is sexual in nature, the most common of which is rape.

Social Services Organisation that is responsible for the well-being, protection and care of children, elderly and disabled people and for the promotion of that well-being and protection through the use of direct services as well as their co-ordination of, and liaison with, voluntary agencies, private companies and other public authorities.

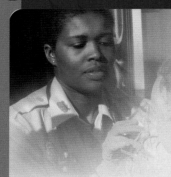

Assessment in Action

You have responded to a report of a female patient in her 40s with a possible fractured arm. As you enter the home, you notice it is immaculately clean. Your patient is sitting on a sofa holding her left forearm, which is bruised and appears to be very tender. You ask the woman what happened, and she says that she fell on a wet floor that she had just finished mopping. As you begin your assessment, you notice a man has walked into the room. He tells you that his wife is very clumsy and "runs into everything". He states that he is sure it is not as bad as she is making it sound. As the husband is speaking, you notice the patient looks down at the floor and will not make eye contact with you.

1. **What is your primary concern in this situation?**
   A. Gathering more information about the patient
   B. Your safety
   C. Splinting the patient's arm
   D. Questioning the husband further

2. **When you begin your assessment of the patient, you notice some bruising on her right arm. When you ask the patient how that happened, she states that she must have obtained the bruising when she fell today. How can you tell if bruising is new or old?**
   A. The bruise is larger if it is a new injury.
   B. The bruise is smaller if it is a new injury.
   C. The bruise will be a different colour or appearance.
   D. The bruise will be the same colour or appearance.

3. **As you ask the patient further about her medical history, she states that she is very clumsy and has broken that arm before. When you ask her when this occurred and what hospital treated her injuries, she states she cannot remember. The husband states that the injury was years ago and it does not matter in this case. What action should you take at this point?**
   A. If it is safe to do so, interview the husband away from the wife.
   B. Immediately remove the patient to the safety of your ambulance.
   C. Ask the patient if there are any children in the home.
   D. You and your colleague should leave the scene and call the police.

4. **When you and your colleague come back together, you find that the history of events does not match between husband and wife. You choose to splint the patient's arm and transport her to hospital of her choice. When you advise her of your intentions, she states that she does not want to go to hospital. What is your next course of action?**
   A. Have the patient sign a refusal, and leave the scene.
   B. Have your colleague go outside and contact the police.
   C. Have a neighbour come over to take the patient to hospital.
   D. Contact your supervisor.

5. **After police personnel arrive, you are able to treat and transport the patient to hospital of her choice. Once inside your ambulance, what is a recommended way to obtain more information on how the injury occurred?**
   A. Have a police officer ride in with you and the patient.
   B. Do not ask direct questions because they will upset the patient.
   C. Ask direct questions about the potential that the injury was caused by abuse.
   D. Wait until you arrive at hospital, and let the doctor obtain the information.

Challenging Question

6. **You and your colleague begin to write your patient clinical record concerning this call. What should you be aware of during your documentation?**

Points to Ponder

You and your colleague are called to a local preschool for an ill child. When you arrive at the school office, you find a 5-year-old Asian child who appears to have a common cold. You notice the child is coughing and is tugging at his ears. The head teacher pulls you aside and says that she suspects child abuse. When you ask why, she directs the child to come into her office and asks him to raise up his shirt. You notice large, red marks extending from the shoulders to the lumbar region of the child's back. You ask the child what happened to make these marks and the child states, "my grandmother is trying to make me better". The head teacher insists that the police be contacted to arrest the grandmother.

What is your opinion?

Issues: Abuse, Cultural Differences, Child Abuse, Physical Abuse.

Patients With Special Needs

Objectives

Cognitive

- Describe the various aetiologies and types of hearing impairments.
- Recognise the patient with a hearing impairment.
- Anticipate accommodations that may be needed in order to properly manage the patient with a hearing impairment.
- Describe the various aetiologies of visual impairments.
- Recognise the patient with a visual impairment.
- Anticipate accommodations that may be needed in order to properly manage the patient with a visual impairment.
- Describe the various aetiologies and types of speech impairments.
- Recognise the patient with speech impairment.
- Anticipate accommodations that may be needed in order to properly manage the patient with speech impairment.
- Describe the various aetiologies of obesity.
- Anticipate accommodations that may be needed in order to properly manage the patient with obesity.
- Describe paraplegia/quadriplegia.
- Anticipate accommodations that may be needed in order to properly manage the patient with paraplegia/quadriplegia.
- Define mental illness.
- Describe the various aetiologies of mental illness.
- Recognise the presenting signs of various mental illnesses.
- Anticipate accommodations that may be needed in order to properly manage the patient with a mental illness.
- Define the term "developmentally disabled".
- Recognise the patient with a developmental disability.
- Anticipate accommodations that may be needed in order to properly manage the patient with a developmental disability.
- Describe Down's syndrome.
- Recognise the patient with Down's syndrome.
- Anticipate accommodations that may be needed in order to properly manage the patient with Down's syndrome.
- Describe the various aetiologies of emotional impairment.
- Recognise the patient with an emotional impairment.
- Anticipate accommodations that may be needed in order to properly manage the patient with an emotional impairment.
- Define emotional/mental impairment (EMI).
- Recognise the patient with an emotional or mental impairment.
- Anticipate accommodations that may be needed in order to properly manage patients with an emotional or mental impairment.
- Describe the following diseases/illnesses:
  - Arthritis
  - Cancer
  - Cerebral palsy
  - Cystic fibrosis
  - Multiple sclerosis
  - Muscular dystrophy
  - Myasthenia gravis
  - Spina bifida
  - Patients with a previous head injury
- Identify the possible presenting sign(s) for the following diseases/illnesses:
  - Arthritis
  - Cancer
  - Cerebral palsy
  - Cystic fibrosis
  - Multiple sclerosis
  - Muscular dystrophy
  - Myasthenia gravis
  - Spina bifida
  - Patients with a previous head injury
- Anticipate accommodations that may be needed in order to properly manage the following patients:
  - Arthritis
  - Cancer
  - Cerebral palsy
  - Cystic fibrosis
  - Multiple sclerosis
  - Muscular dystrophy
  - Myasthenia gravis
  - Spina bifida
  - Patients with a previous head injury
- Define cultural diversity.
- Recognise cultural diversity in patients.
- Anticipate accommodations that may be needed in order to manage a patient whilst being sensitive to culture.
- Identify a patient who is terminally ill.
- Anticipate accommodations that may be needed in order to properly manage a patient who is terminally ill.
- Identify a patient with a communicable disease.
- Recognise the presenting signs of a patient with a communicable disease.
- Anticipate accommodations that may be needed in order to properly manage a patient with a communicable disease.

Affective

None

Psychomotor

None

Introduction

Throughout the ages, humans have learned to adapt to the challenges they encounter. In the prehospital environment, you will encounter patients who face a variety of special challenges. Some conditions or anomalies are congenital; others have developed during the patient's lifetime or occurred as the result of a sudden event (eg, the transection of the spinal cord during a diving accident). Whatever the source of the challenge, these patients will require you to adapt your assessment and management to accommodate their needs.

Although you can still use the standard assessment plan with these patients, sometimes it may be necessary to adapt to meet a patient's unique needs. Can the patient see you? Can the patient hear you? Can the patient normally move all extremities? You will need to formulate a plan to care for these patients in a short amount of time. Be willing to incorporate "the experts" (ie, the patient, family members, or carers) as essential team members. Learn to solve problems as part of a group, and remember your ultimate goal: to give the patient the best care possible, in the most efficient way, and still accommodate for his or her individual needs. Your confidence and caring attitude will promote trust between you, your patient, and the other members of your team.

Physical Challenges

Humans use all five senses to gather information, but we often take that sensory feedback for granted. Imagine what it would be like to go bowling while blindfolded. You hear the pins dropping—but did you knock down a couple of pins, get a strike, or just leave a seven–ten split? Imagine how frustrating it might be to see that you need to tie your shoe but to be unable to do so because an injury resulted in the loss of motor function in your hand.

Hearing Impairments

Hearing challenges are generally classified into two types: conductive and sensorineural deafness. Conductive deafness often a curable condition caused by an injury to the eardrum, an infection, or simply a buildup of earwax in the external auditory canal. Sensorineural deafness, which is permanent, may be caused by a lesion of, or damage of the inner ear, or the eighth cranial nerve. This type of hearing impairment may be congenital or secondary to a birth injury, but it may also have occurred over time from disease, medication complications, viral infections, or tumours. People may also lose their hearing due to ageing (*presbycusis*) or from prolonged exposure to loud noise.

Hearing impairment may range from a slight hearing loss to total deafness. Some patients may have difficulty with pitch, volume, and speaking distinctly. Some have learned to speak even though they have never heard speech. Others may have heard speech and learned to talk, but have since lost some or all of their hearing, leading them to speak too loudly. Parkinson's disease or other disease processes may cause the patient to slur words, speak very slowly, or speak in a monotone voice.

At the Scene

Consider the excess use of sirens and protect your hearing . . . before it's too late.

You are the Paramedic Part 1

You and your colleague are dispatched to a local park for a child in respiratory distress. When you arrive at the entrance you are guided by member of the public to a pavilion, where you find a group of active 8-year-olds enjoying a school picnic. As you get closer to the pavilion, you notice that all the children in this group have Down's syndrome.

Seated on one of the picnic benches is a girl in obvious respiratory distress. You observe that she is in a tripod position and is using accessory muscles to breathe. As you get closer, you hear audible expiratory wheezes. Her teacher is next to her trying to provide reassurance.

Initial Assessment	Recording Time: 0 Minutes
Appearance	Anxious; child seated in a tripod position
Level of consciousness	A (Alert to person, place, and day)
Airway	Open
Breathing	Tachypnoea with accessory muscle use; audible wheeze
Circulation	Strong radial pulse, elevated rate

1. What is Down's syndrome?
2. What are the characteristic physical features of Down's syndrome?

Interaction With a Hearing-Impaired Patient

Clues that a person could be hearing impaired include the presence of hearing aids, poor pronunciation of words, or failure to respond to your presence or questions. While communicating, face the patient so that he or she can see your mouth; don't exaggerate your lip movements or look away. Position yourself approximately 50 cm directly in front of the patient. Most people who are hearing impaired have learned to use body language, such as hand gestures and lipreading. Because hearing-impaired patients typically have more difficulty hearing higher-frequency sounds, if the patient seems to have difficulty hearing you, don't just speak louder—try lowering the pitch of your voice.

Ask the patient, "How would you like to communicate with me"? British Sign Language (BSL) may be his or her preferred method of communication **Figure 44-1**. An interpreter, family member, or friend may prove to be a valuable team member. If an interpreter is not readily available, call your receiving hospital early on to request one. Ideally, an interpreter will arrive before you begin your assessment. Other patients may prefer written communication or communication of concepts or procedures with gestures or pictures. Simply asking a team member to retrieve the patient's hearing aid may help a great deal.

Here are some helpful hints for working with patients with hearing impairments:

- Speak slowly and distinctly into a less impaired ear, or position yourself on that side.
- Change speakers. Given that 80% of hearing loss is related to inability to hear high-pitched sounds, look for a team

At the Scene

Some hearing-impaired patients' ears are overly sensitive to very loud noises close to their ears. Remember to use a normal level of voice when speaking to them.

At the Scene

When caring for a hearing-impaired patient, one easy solution is to place the ear pieces of your stethoscope into the patient's ears while you speak into the bell of the stethoscope.

member with a low-pitched voice if you think this may be the issue.

- Provide paper and pencil so that you may write your questions and the patient may write his or her responses.
- Only one person should ask interview questions, to avoid confusing the patient.
- Try the "reverse stethoscope" technique: put the earpieces of your stethoscope in the patient's ear and speak softly into the bell of the stethoscope. This will amplify your voice.

At the Scene

Many patients with borderline hearing impairments may not be aware of the extent of their problem. The distracting and noisy prehospital environment may worsen the situation. If a patient frequently asks you to repeat things, suspect a hearing impairment.

Hearing Aids

A hearing aid is essentially a device that makes sound louder. Hearing aids cannot restore hearing to normal, but they do improve hearing and listening ability. Several types of hearing aids are available **Figure 44-2**:

- *In-the-canal* and *completely in-the-canal*. These hearing aids are contained in a tiny case that fits partly or completely into the ear canal.
- *In-the-ear*. All parts are contained in a shell that fits in the outer part of the ear.

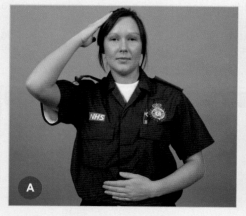
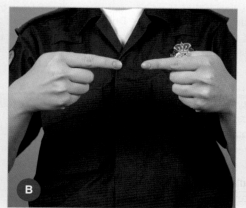
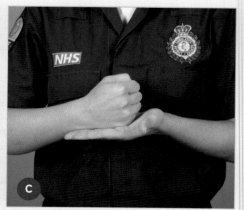

Figure 44-1 Consider learning the BSL signs for common terms related to illness and injury. **A.** Sick. **B.** Hurt. **C.** Help.

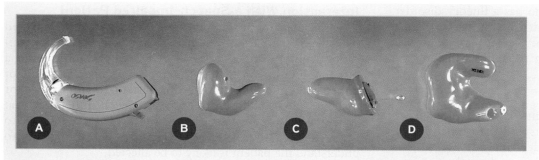

Figure 44-2 Different types of hearing aids. **A.** Behind-the-ear type. **B.** Conventional body type. **C.** In-the-canal type. **D.** In-the-ear type.

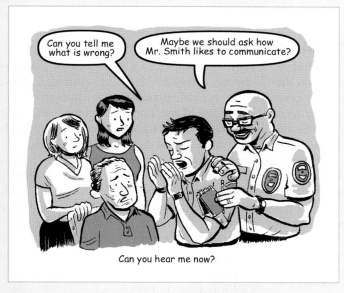

Figure 44-3

- *Behind-the-ear.* All parts are contained in a plastic case that rests behind the ear. The NHS typically uses digital BTE (behind-the-ear) hearing aids.
- *Conventional body type.* This older style is generally used by people with profound hearing loss.

Implantable hearing aids are also an option for patients with less profound hearing loss.

To insert a hearing aid, follow the natural shape of the ear. The device needs to fit snugly without forcing. If you hear a whistling sound, the hearing aid may not be in far enough to create a seal, or the volume may be too loud. Try repositioning the hearing aid, or remove it and turn down the volume. If you can't insert the hearing aid after two attempts, put it in the box, take it with you, and document the transport and transfer of hearing aids to hospital personnel. Never try to clean hearing aids, and never get them wet.

If a patient's hearing aid is not working, try troubleshooting the problem. First, make sure the hearing aid is turned on **Figure 44-3 ▲** . Try a fresh battery, and check the tubing to make sure it isn't twisted or bent. Check the switch to make sure it's set on M (microphone), not T (telecoil). For a body aid, try a spare cord, as the old one may be broken or shorted. Finally, check the ear mould to make sure it isn't plugged with wax.

Speech Impairments

For most people, the spoken word is the primary mechanism for communicating thoughts and ideas. For some, speech may be delayed by psychological or psychosocial factors. For others, it may be altered by injury, illness, or hearing impairment.

Articulation Disorders

Articulation disorders cause the majority of speech difficulties. Dysarthria—the inability to make speech sounds correctly—results from a lack of muscle control and coordination of the larynx, tongue, mouth, and lips. Speech can be slurred, indistinct, slow, or nasal. Commonly, articulation disorders result from damage to nerve pathways passing from the brain to muscles in the larynx, mouth, or lips; delayed development from hearing problems; or slow maturation of the nervous system due to brain damage or motor disability. Articulation disorders affect both children and adults.

Language Disorders

Stroke, traumatic head/brain injury, brain tumour, delayed development, hearing loss, lack of stimulation, or emotional disturbance may cause damage to the language centre of the brain and lead to dysphasia. Dysphasia is the partial loss of the ability to communicate in speech, writing, or signs (aphasia refers to the total loss). It can range from being very mild to making communication with the patient almost impossible. Dysphasia is usually categorised as expressive or receptive. Those with expressive dysphasia can often mentally formulate sentences but cannot then express these in normal speech; this usually causes a high degree of frustration for that individual, so make sure you put them at ease. Receptive dysphasia refers to an individual who is able to articulate words normally but is unable to process what is being said to them.

When communicating with a dysphasic patient, remember to talk to the patient as an adult, not as a child. Use focused questions rather than open-ended questions, and minimise background noise.

Fluency Disorders

In fluency disorders, the person's speech pattern is broken, interrupted, or repetitious. An example of this type of disorder is stuttering. Stuttering may be noticed only when the person attempts certain words or sounds, and it may become worse when the individual is under stress. Stuttering is normal for young children and will usually disappear gradually over time. The specific causes of stuttering are unknown.

When dealing with a person who has a fluency disorder, patience is the key. Impatience with or interruption of a patient who stutters may frustrate the patient more and cause the stuttering to get worse, making receiving a history and assessment difficult.

Voice Production Disorders

Voice production disorders refer to the way the voice sounds and may be slightly easier to understand than other speech impairments. Signs of these disorders include hoarseness, harshness, inappropriate pitch, or abnormal nasal resonance. Causes include the closure of vocal cords, hormonal or psychiatric disturbance, or severe hearing loss.

Hypernasality may be a complication of a cleft palate, a deformity in which the two sides of the palate fail to fuse in the midline during in-utero development (**Figure 44-4** ◄), or it may accompany enlarged adenoids.

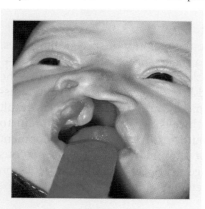

Figure 44-4 Cleft palate.

Inflammation of the larynx is called laryngitis. Laryngitis is a common occurrence in cases involving overuse of the voice, throat infections, heavy smoking, smoke inhalation, allergic reaction, or exposure to fumes. The cause of the laryngitis may provide clues about the patient's reason for calling for your services and the severity of the situation.

Chronic laryngitis may point to long-term exposure to laryngeal irritants, which may cause polyps to develop in the larynx. Occurring more commonly in men, progressive hoarseness is usually the chief complaint in such cases. Long-term exposure to toxins such as chemicals, smoking, or weakened vocal cords from continuous strain are other risk factors.

The most ominous cause of chronic laryngitis is carcinoma of the larynx. A laryngectomy—either partial or total removal of the larynx—may be performed to battle the cancer. In the case of a total laryngectomy, the patient would have *aphonia,* an inability to produce normal speech sounds. The patient would receive a tracheostomy, and might communicate by burping sounds or by using an electronic or mechanical device.

At the Scene

As with all barriers to communication, remember to document whenever you enlist the help of an interpreter or a person who signs. Also remember that conclusions reached based on the information from interpreters may not be valid.

Interaction With a Speech-Impaired Patient

When establishing communication, ask the speech-impaired patient how he or she would be most comfortable communicating with you. Allow an appropriate amount of time for a response and listen carefully to establish an understanding, or enlist someone who knows the patient to interpret. For instance, small children often have speech difficulties that spontaneously resolve, but may be difficult for a stranger to understand. If the patient prefers to speak, your ability to understand the patient is likely to be affected.

When working with a patient with a voice production disorder, offer a pencil and paper or listen carefully if the patient prefers to speak. Repeat what the patient said to allow for correction or further clarification. Avoid speaking for the patient or finishing sentences for him or her. And above all, have patience!

Visual Impairments

Visual impairments may result from a multitude of causes—congenital defect, disease, injury, infection (eg, cytomegalovirus), or degeneration of the eyeball, optic nerve, or nerve pathway (eg, with ageing). The degree of visual impairment may range from partial to total. Some patients lose peripheral or central vision; others can distinguish light from dark or discern general shapes.

Visual impairments may be difficult to recognise. During your scene assessment, look for signs that indicate the person is visually impaired, such as the presence of spectacles, a white stick, or a guide dog. Make yourself known when you enter the room; introduce yourself and others in the room, or have others introduce themselves so that the patient can identify their placement and voice. In addition, retrieve any visual aids to make the interaction more comfortable for your patient (**Figure 44-5** ▼).

A visually impaired person may feel vulnerable, especially during the chaos of an accident scene. He or she may have learned to use other senses such as hearing, touch, and smell to compensate for the loss of sight, and the sounds and smells of an accident may be disorienting. Remember to tell

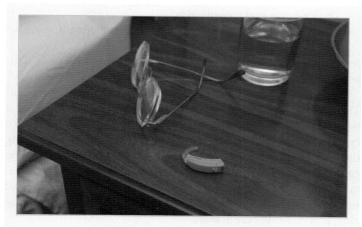

Figure 44-5 If a patient normally uses spectacles or a hearing aid, try to ensure he or she is using them. This may reduce the patient's disorientation and stress, and will probably improve your communication with the patient during assessment.

the patient what is happening, identify noises, and describe the situation and surroundings, especially if you need to move the patient.

At the Scene

Remember that guide dogs are "working dogs". Don't play with the animal or distract it unless the patient gives permission to do so.

To ambulate safely, the patient may use a stick or Zimmer frame. Even if the individual will be carried out on your trolley, don't forget to take the patient's stick or zimmer frame. Unless the patient is critical, the guide dog can remain in the room and will provide reassurance for the patient and prevent delays in transport. Take the dog with you in the ambulance.

An ambulatory patient may be led by a light touch on the arm or elbow. You may also allow the patient to rest his or her hand on your shoulder, as this may enhance the patient's sense of balance and security while moving. You may also ask the patient which method he or she prefers to use while travelling to the ambulance. Patients should be gently guided but never pushed. Obstacles need to be communicated in advance. Statements such as "You're approaching the stairs", and instructions about how many stairs to expect, will allow the patient to anticipate and navigate the obstacles safely. They will also appreciate your consideration and concern.

Paralysis

Paralysis is the inability to move one or more body parts. It may be caused by cerebrovascular events (CVE), trauma, or birth defects, among other things. Paralysis does not always entail a loss of sensation, however. In some cases, the patient will have normal sensation or hyperaesthesia (increased sensitivity), which may cause the individual to interpret touch as pain in the affected area. Paralysis of one side of the face may cause subsequent communication challenges as well.

Special Considerations

- Hemiplegia. Paralysis of one side of the body, possibly from CVE or head injury
- Paraplegia. Paralysis of the lower part of the body, possibly from thoracic or lumbar spinal injury or spina bifida
- Quadriplegia. Paralysis of all four extremities and the trunk, possibly from a cervical spine injury; also called tetraplegia.

Paralysed patients may have diaphragmatic involvement requiring the use of a ventilator. They may also rely on specialised equipment such as halo traction, Foley catheters, tracheostomies, colostomies, or feeding tubes. Each spinal cord procedure requires its own equipment and may have its own complications (see Chapter 45).

Dysphagia, which can be caused by partial paralysis of the pharynx or oesophagus, is the inability to swallow. Patients with dysphagia may choke or aspirate food and drink very easily, leading to the need for emergency airway interventions.

If patients have lost some or all of the sensation in the affected limbs, they cannot tell you when you are hurting them. Always take great care when lifting or moving a paralysed patient. Because paralysed limbs lack muscle tone, provide intravenous access and medication administration on the nonaffected side whenever possible. Check intravenous sites frequently for infiltration, especially after medication administration.

Special Considerations

Moving the patient without dislodging or compromising his or her extra equipment takes planning and coordination. You may need to recruit more team members so that you can efficiently move the patient without causing further complication. Strategically placed padding or pillows may also keep the patient more comfortable during transport.

Obesity

Obesity is the result of a serious imbalance between food eaten and calories used. The solution to the obesity problem may sound relatively simple—re-establish the balance and cure the problem. Unfortunately, obesity can be a much more complex situation. Causes of obesity are not fully understood. This problem may be attributed to low basal metabolic rate or genetic predisposition.

Obesity is defined and classified in many different ways; however, one of the most scientific ways is to calculate an individual's body mass index (BMI). This is weight in kilograms divided by the square of height in metres. In the UK, people with a body mass index between 25 and 30 are categorised as overweight, and those with an index above 30 are categorised as obese. Severe obesity affects almost one quarter of British adults. These individuals are often ridiculed publicly and sometimes are victims of discrimination. Mobility and the patients' general quality of life are often negatively affected by being overweight, and the extra weight can cause a myriad of health problems.

Interaction With an Obese Patient

Obese patients may be embarrassed by their condition or fearful of ridicule as a result of past experiences. Some of those negative interactions may have occurred at the hands of an insensitive health care professional. As with any patient, work hard to put these individuals at ease early. Establish the patient's presenting complaint and then communicate your plan to help. Many severely obese patients have a complex and extensive past medical history, so mastering the art of conducting a patient interview will serve you well in your interactions with these individuals.

If transport is necessary, plan early for extra help and don't be afraid to call for more help if necessary. In particular, send a member of your team to find the easiest and safest exit. Remember, everyone's safety is at stake! You don't want to risk dropping the patient or injuring a team member by trying to lift too much weight. Moves, no matter how simple they may seem, become far more complex with an oversized patient.

Interaction With a Morbidly Obese Patient

Morbidly obese patients may overcome mobility difficulties by pulling, rocking, or rolling into a position. The constant strain on their body's structures may leave them with chronic joint injuries or osteoarthritis.

Some morbidly obese patients suffer from a condition called obesity hypoventilation syndrome, also known as Pickwickian syndrome. Patients with Pickwickian syndrome are usually *extremely* obese. They experience hypoxaemia (deficient oxygenation of the blood), hypercapnia (excess carbon dioxide in the blood), and polycythaemia (overabundance or overproduction of red blood cells). Physical findings may include headache, apnoea (especially during sleep), sleepiness, red face, muscle twitching, and signs of right-sided heart failure. Some of these symptoms may necessitate emergency intervention in the prehospital environment.

Weight reduction is the ultimate remedy for Pickwickian syndrome. Some patients may be on a carefully monitored diet; others may benefit from surgical intervention, such as gastric by-pass surgery. Surgery carries a high risk of complications, however, and not all patients are suitable candidates.

When you are moving a morbidly obese patient, follow these helpful tips:

- Treat the patient with dignity and respect.
- Ask your patient how best to move him or her before attempting to do so.

At the Scene

When transporting an obese patient, be sure to alert the receiving hospital in advance if special accommodations, equipment, or other resources may be needed.

- Avoid trying to lift the patient by only one limb, which would risk injury to overtaxed joints.
- Co-ordinate and communicate all moves to all team members *prior* to starting.
- If the move becomes uncontrolled at any point, stop, reposition, and resume.
- Look for pinch or pressure points from equipment, as they could cause a deep vein thrombosis.
- Very large patients may have difficulty breathing if you lay them flat. Keep this possibility in mind when you position these individuals.
- Many manufacturers now make specialised equipment for morbidly obese patients, and some areas have specially equipped ambulances for such patients. Become familiar with the resources available in your area.
- Plan egress routes to accommodate for a large patient, equipment, *and* the lifting crew members. Remember: Do no harm!
- Notify the receiving hospital early to allow special arrangements to be made prior to your arrival to accommodate the patient's needs.

You are the Paramedic Part 2

You kneel down in front of the young girl, introduce yourself, and ask her name. She tells you that her name is Allison. You note that she has to take a breath after every two words. She tells you that she is having a hard time "catching her breath", points to her emblem, and starts to cry. You hold her hand and reassure her that you are going to help her feel better very soon. While you are doing this you look at a medical identification emblem on her right wrist, which reveals that Allison has asthma and is allergic to penicillin. You ask the teacher if she can provide any additional information. She relates that Allison was playing rounders with her classmates when she sat down on the grass and didn't get up. One of the helpers went over to Allison and found her to be having a hard time breathing. She was brought over to the pavilion and someone called 999. Allison normally has an inhaler of salbutamol but it was accidentally left at the school. She has no other medical history or drug allergies. She has the emotional and developmental skills of a 4-year-old. A call was placed to her mother who authorised treatment, and she will meet you at the hospital.

Vital Signs	Recording Time: 5 Minutes
Level of consciousness	Alert
Skin	Pale, warm, and dry
Pulse	126 beats/min, regular
Blood pressure	106/72 mm Hg
Respirations	36 breaths/min, laboured
SpO₂	89% on ambient air

3. What medical conditions are commonly seen in patients with Down's syndrome?
4. Why is it important to be physically at the patient's level to speak with her?

Mental Challenges

Mental Illness

Mental illness is a generic term for a variety of illnesses that result in perceptive, cognitive, emotional, or memory dysfunction. These conditions include bipolar disorder, depression, schizophrenia, and drug or alcohol abuse. See Chapter 37 for more detail.

Learning Disabilities

Learning disability or difficulty is insufficient development of the brain resulting in the inability to learn and socially adapt at the usual rate. It may be caused by genetic factors, congenital infections, complications at birth, malnutrition, or environmental factors. Prenatal drug or alcohol use may also cause disability, as in fetal alcohol syndrome. Postnatal causes may include traumatic brain injury or poisoning (eg, with lead or other toxins).

Although IQ testing can identify the extent of the person's ability to learn and reason, just speaking to the patient and family members will give you a good idea of how well the patient can understand you and interact. A person with a slight impairment may appear slow to understand or have a limited vocabulary. Such an individual may act in an immature manner in comparison to peers. Because the individual may also have difficulty adjusting to change or a break in routine, an emergency call that generates a roomful of strangers can be overwhelming. The patient may become more difficult to interact with as his or her anxiety level increases. A severely disabled person may not have the ability to care for himself or herself, communicate, understand, or respond to the surroundings.

Treatment of these patients should be based on the complaint unless the illness is related to the learning disability. Patients with learning disabilities are prone to the same disease processes as any other patients, including diabetes, cardiac events, and respiratory difficulties. Transport should be accomplished without causing any more stress than necessary. In most cases, supportive care is all that is needed.

Down's Syndrome

Down's syndrome is characterised by a genetic chromosomal defect that can occur during fetal development, resulting in mild to severe learning difficulties (Figure 44-6 ▶). The normal human somatic cell contains 23 chromosomes. Down's syndrome, which is also known as Trisomy 21, usually occurs when chromosome 21 fails to separate, so that the ovum contains 24 chromosomes. When the ovum is fertilised by a normal sperm with 23 chromosomes, a triplication ("Trisomy") of chromosome 21 occurs.

Increased maternal age (more than 35 years old) and a family history of Down's syndrome are known risk factors for this condition. A variety of abnormal physical features may be associated with Down's syndrome: a round head with a flat occiput; an enlarged, protruding tongue; slanted, wide-set eyes

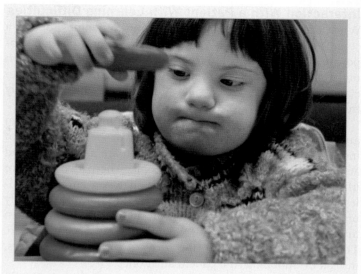

Figure 44-6 A child with Down's syndrome.

and folded skin on either side of the nose, covering the inner corners of the eye; short, wide hands; a small face and features; congenital heart defects; thyroid problems; and hearing and vision problems. Patients do not usually have all of these symptoms, but will have a combination of them to such a degree that the diagnosis is usually made rapidly at birth.

Patients with Down's syndrome are at increased risk for medical complications, including those that affect the cardiovascular, sensory, endocrine, orthopaedic, dental, gastrointestinal, neurological development, and haematological systems. As many as 40% may suffer from heart conditions, hearing, and vision problems. In particular, two thirds of children born with Down's syndrome have congenital heart disease (eg, endocardial cushion defects, or ventricular or atrial septal defects). Emergency treatment should therefore include airway management, supplemental oxygen, and IV access. In patients with heart failure, administer diuretics with judicious fluid resuscitation only if necessary.

Because people with Down's syndrome often have large tongues and small oral and nasal cavities, intubation of these patients may be difficult. These individuals may also have malocclusions and other dental anomalies (eg, abnormal contact of the upper and lower teeth). The enlarged tongue and dental anomalies can lead to speech abnormalities as well. In an emergency situation, if airway management is necessary, mask ventilation and intubation can be challenging. In the case of airway obstruction, a simple jaw-thrust manoeuvre may be all that is needed to clear the airway. In an unconscious patient, either the jaw-thrust manoeuvre or a nasopharyngeal airway may be necessary.

Many people with Down's syndrome have epilepsy. Most of the convulsions are of the tonic-clonic type. Management is the same as with other patients with convulsions.

Interaction With a Patient With Learning Difficulties

When caring for a patient with learning difficulties, obtain a complete history, treat the presenting illness, and provide supportive care. It is normal to feel somewhat uncomfortable when initiating contact with a patient with learning difficulties, especially if you've encountered such situations infrequently. Simply treating the patient as you would anyone else is the best plan.

Approach the patient with learning difficulties in a calm and friendly manner, watching him or her for signs of increased anxiety or fear. Remember, you are a "stranger" and are approaching with a group of people. The patient may not understand your uniform or realise that you and your colleague are there to help. It may be helpful to hold back slightly until you can establish a rapport with the patient. You can then introduce your colleague and explain what you are going to do. This method will slowly bring forward the other providers, instead of "mobbing" the patient all at once.

You might interact with a patient as follows: "Hello Mr Pemberton. My name is John Brown". (Shake Mr Pemberton's hand if he will allow it.) "We're here to help you. Your sister called us. She says you're not feeling well today, and we're here to help you feel better. My friend Tim is going to take your blood pressure. Do you remember having that done before"? (Allow Mr Pemberton to see and touch the blood pressure cuff as Tim moves forward. Move slowly but deliberately, explaining beforehand what you are going to do, just like you would with any other patient. Watch carefully for signs of fear or reluctance from the patient.)

Do your best to soothe the patient's anxiety and/or discomfort as you work through your assessment and treatment. By initially establishing trust and communication, you'll have more success executing your treatment plan, even if you eventually need to do something painful such as starting an IV.

Emotional/Mental Impairment

In the Victorian era, an emotional stress condition associated with chronic fatigue, anxiety, depression, sleep disturbances, headache, and sexual dysfunction might be lumped into the category known as *neurasthenia*—in modern terms, a "nervous breakdown". Today, doctors diagnose specific disorders such as anxiety, depression, obsessive compulsion, or mania.

Mental illness can occur in people with mental or emotional disability just as it can in anyone else. (The care of mentally ill patients is discussed in depth in Chapter 37.) In the broader sense, a person's mental status can influence his or her physical well-being, and vice versa. Emotionally or mentally impaired individuals may be difficult to assess due to the body's normal stress response, which may alter their respiratory rate, heart rate, or perception of physical illness. Gathering a detailed history will be useful in the assessment and development of a treatment plan for these patients. Calmly ascertain the chief complaint and treat the patient accordingly, with care and understanding.

One of the key components of effective communication—with any type of patient—is to be a good listener. Always "listen" carefully to your patient—not just the words spoken, but also heeding the patient's tone, facial expressions, and body language. Watch for signs of aggression, clenched fists, or aggressive agitated movements or speech; they may be your only warning of an impending dangerous confrontation. Implementing active listening skills by repeating what you heard will reassure the patient that you understand and are there to help. Although mentally ill patients may present an

You are the Paramedic Part 3

Your colleague prepares a nebuliser containing 5.0 mg of salbutamol and 500 mcg of ipratropium whilst you obtain a peak expiratory flow measurement; after the third attempt it registers at around 50% of what the teacher states is her normal figure. You continue your assessment, taking care to let your patient know everything that you are doing. Examination reveals significant diminished air movement bilaterally with faint expiratory wheezes.

You ask your colleague to place her on the cardiac monitor. You assist the patient onto the stretcher and into the ambulance to continue your treatment prior to leaving for the hospital.

In the back of the ambulance you give the patient a teddy bear and tell her how brave she is. She responds with a weak smile. A 20-gauge IV is started in the left dorsum and 100 mg of hydrocortisone is given slowly. As the ambulance departs, you refill the nebuliser with another 5.0 mg of salbutamol.

Reassessment	Recording Time: 12 Minutes
Skin	Pale, warm, and dry
Pulse	138 beats/min, regular
Blood pressure	110/72 mm Hg
Respirations	28 breaths/min, laboured
SpO_2	92% on nebuliser treatment driven by oxygen at 10 l/min
ECG	Sinus tachycardia
Pupils	Reactive to light

5. What anatomical features of Down's syndrome can make airway management challenging?

assessment challenge, they are still patients and are prone to the same illnesses and disease processes as anyone else. Consequently, treatment and transport of such patients should focus on the chief complaint and supportive care.

When treating patients with emotional/mental impairment, take care in establishing communication with the patient and/or the parent. Establish a baseline for the patient's emotional/mental ability so that you will be able to identify any changes. Speak in a calm voice, even if the patient does not have the ability to understand, and explain what you're going to do before doing it.

Pathological Challenges

Pathological challenges require special consideration when you formulate your treatment plan. Pathologies you may encounter during your career may include arthritis, cancer, cerebral palsy, cystic fibrosis, multiple sclerosis, muscular dystrophy, previous head injury, spina bifida, and myasthenia gravis. Many of these patients will be well versed in the progression, treatment, and unique nuances of their current health status.

Cancer

Simply stated, cancer is the uncontrolled overgrowth of tissue cells. If this growth is left unchecked, these cells can spread, damage body systems and may ultimately lead to death. More than 200 different kinds of cancer are believed to exist; the type is determined by where the cancer originates. (Cancer is discussed in greater detail in Chapters 6 and 45.)

Numerous types of treatment regimes are available for cancer—surgery, medications, radiation, and chemotherapy, to name a few. Cancer treatment may follow a single pathway, or be orchestrated into a complex combination of therapies and medications. Surgical removal has long been one of the primary methods of controlling or terminating cancer's progression; it is often used in tandem with other therapies.

Arthritis

Arthritis is a joint inflammation that causes pain, swelling, stiffness, and decreased range of motion, all of which leave patients more vulnerable to falls. Many types of arthritis are distinguished, with symptoms ranging from mild to debilitating. For example, osteoarthritis is a degenerative joint disease associated with ageing Figure 44-7 ▸ . It initially targets the distal finger joints, base of the thumb, cervical and lumbar spine, hips, and knees. The pain of osteoarthritis usually grows throughout the day, with stiffness increasing following prolonged rest. In contrast, rheumatoid arthritis is an autoimmune disorder that causes inflammation and destruction of the joints and connective tissues. Some patients may experience periods of remission while others may have rapid progression of the disease.

Be sure to ask the patient with arthritis about his or her current medications before administering additional ones. Take

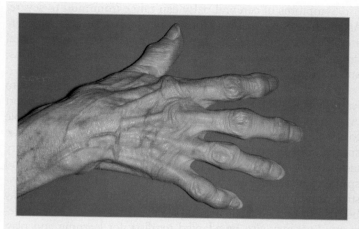

Figure 44-7 Osteoarthritis may cause substantial disfigurement.

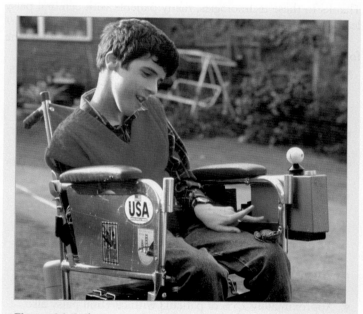

Figure 44-8 A person with cerebral palsy.

special care when moving such a patient so as to incur the least amount of discomfort. Make sure the patient is as comfortable as possible and remember to use equipment that fits the patient properly.

Cerebral Palsy

Cerebral palsy is a nonprogressive, bilateral neuromuscular disorder in which voluntary muscles are poorly controlled. It results from developmental brain defects in utero (eg, cerebral hypoxia, maternal infection, or kernicterus), brain trauma at birth or in early childhood, or postpartum infections (eg, encephalitis or meningitis.) Patients often have spastic movements of their limbs and display poor posture Figure 44-8 ▲ , which impairs their ability to move in a controlled manner.

Symptoms of cerebral palsy can range from mild to severe. As children grow, these symptoms may either become exaggerated or stay the same. Related complications include visual impairments, hearing and language difficulties, convulsions, and learning difficulties.

Some children with severe cases of cerebral palsy are able to learn to walk with assistive devices, whereas others need support even to sit and cannot stand, walk, or speak. If the patient is able to speak, grimacing and uncontrolled movement may make speech difficult and hard to understand. To cope with ordinary tasks, many patients use computerised household controls and speaking aids. Electric wheelchairs may be controlled with a joystick or mouth control. Specially shaped chairs and pillows may be custom-built to facilitate the patient's comfort and ease movement. Toys may also be adapted to allow for learning and play. In addition, computers may be specially configured to aid the patient with speech simulation and provide the ability to perform household tasks, such as temperature control and lighting. Thanks to these technologies, many patients with cerebral palsy lead near-normal lives and live independently.

When caring for a patient with cerebral palsy, note the following:

- Do not assume that patients with cerebral palsy are always mentally impaired. Although 75% of patients have some mental impairment, many people with cerebral palsy have a normal IQ or only slight mental impairment.
- Patients' limbs are often underdeveloped and are prone to injury (eg, from a fall from a wheelchair).
- Patients who have the ability to walk may have an ataxic or unsteady gait and are prone to falls.
- If the patient has a specially made pillow or chair (paediatric patients), the patient may prefer to use it during transport. Remember to pad the patient to ensure his or her comfort, and never force a patient's extremities into any position.
- Whenever possible, take Zimmer frames or wheelchairs along during transport.
- Approximately 25% of patients with cerebral palsy also have convulsions. Be prepared to care for the patient if a convulsion occurs, and keep suction available.

Cystic Fibrosis

Cystic fibrosis (mucoviscidosis) is a chronic dysfunction of the endocrine system that targets multiple body systems, but primarily the respiratory and digestive systems. This inherited disease affects approximately 7,500 people in the United Kingdom. Although it is found in all races and ethnic groups, it most commonly occurs in Caucasian individuals of Northern European descent. The disease is a life limiting illness and the average ife expectancy is 31 years.

Cystic fibrosis is caused by a defective gene, which makes it difficult for chloride to move through cells. This causes unusually high sodium loss (resulting in salty skin) and abnormally thick mucus secretions. The secretions in the lungs cause breathing difficulties and provide an ideal growing medium for bacteria, leaving the patient highly susceptible to infection. Ultimately, the lung damage from the condition leads to lung disease, which is the primary cause of death in affected individuals.

Respiratory difficulties associated with cystic fibrosis include tachypnoea, productive cough, shortness of breath, barrel chest, clubbed fingers, and cyanosis. The thick mucus may also collect in the intestines. Malnutrition and poor growth rate are not uncommon symptoms, as are intestinal blockages. Doctors strive to reduce the progression of the disease with physiotherapy, exercise, vitamin supplements, and medications. Some patients may also benefit from a lung transplant.

Care of these patients should primarily focus on treating the individual's chief complaint. Keep a keen eye out for respiratory insufficiency, signs of a respiratory infection, intestinal blockage, or cardiac arrhythmias (as a result of the electrolyte imbalance). Suctioning, high-flow supplemental oxygen, and breathing therapies may also be required during transport.

Multiple Sclerosis

Multiple sclerosis is a chronic disease of the central nervous system characterised by destruction of the myelin and nerve axons within the brain and spinal cord. It has no known cause, but is an autoimmune disorder or in some cases is genetically inherited. This disease strikes women in their 20s to 40s two to three times more often than men. Approximately 85,000 people in the United Kingdom have multiple sclerosis, some with serious handicaps.

Myelin is a fatty covering that shields the axons; axons are responsible for electrical conduction from neurons to muscles, leading to muscle response and communication from the body to the brain. Multiple sclerosis causes areas of myelin in random places to become inflamed, detach from the axon, and ultimately self-destruct. The area of destruction becomes scarred over—hence the name multiple (*many*) sclerosis (*to harden*) **Figure 44-9 ▸** .

Two types of multiple sclerosis are distinguished: relapsing/remitting and progressive. The relapsing/remitting form, which affects 90% of patients, presents with bouts of worsening symptoms. Signs and symptoms of multiple sclerosis can be divided into those associated with the brain and those associated with the spinal cord **Table 44-1 ▸** and include numbness or tingling in parts of the body, unexplained weakness, dizziness, fatigue, double or blurry vision, and visual impairment. Periods of relapse leave the patient feeling marked improvement, with stiffness and weakness lingering for some. The other 10% of patients have the progressive form, in which symptoms get progressively worse with no periods of improvement or relief. Half of all people who have the relapsing/remitting form of the disease will develop the progressive form within 15 years if they remain untreated.

There is no cure for multiple sclerosis, although many treatments can significantly reduce the frequency of attacks and lessen symptoms when they occur. As with other illnesses, your treatment may be limited to supportive care. You may also be called to the patient's side due to tertiary complications

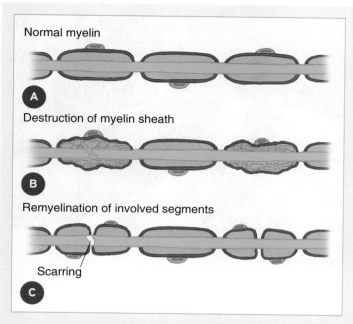

Figure 44-9 Progression of multiple sclerosis. **A.** Normal myelin. **B.** Destruction of myelin sheath. **C.** Scarring.

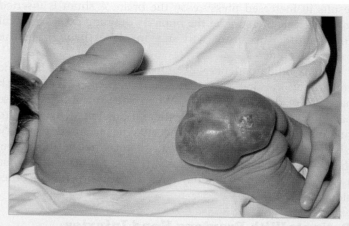

Figure 44-10 Spina bifida is characterised by exposure of part of the spinal cord.

Table 44-1	Signs and Symptoms of Multiple Sclerosis
Brain-Related	**Spinal Cord-Related**
■ Slurred speech	■ Stiffness
■ Confusion	■ Muscle spasms
■ Forgetfulness	■ Bowel and bladder problems
■ Pain	■ Sexual dysfunction
■ Depression	■ Paralysis
	■ Numbness
	■ Muscle weakness

of multiple sclerosis, such as a fall. Because of the disease process, the patient may lack sensation in some areas, so the physical examination may be difficult. A detailed medical history will help elucidate the diagnosis.

As with paralysed patients, you must take special care when lifting and moving patients with multiple sclerosis. When these individuals are in crisis, they may not be able to walk even with their mobility devices.

Muscular Dystrophy

Muscular dystrophy is an inherited muscular disease that causes degeneration of the muscle fibres. In many cases, the destroyed fibres are replaced by fat or connective tissue. The result is a gradual weakening of muscles, slowing of motor development, and loss of muscle contractility. More than 30 types of muscular dystrophy have been identified. Some strike in early childhood and progress rapidly. Others don't strike until the late teens into the forties and progress much more slowly. Duchenne muscular dystrophy, the most common type, chiefly affects boys (1 of every 3,500 male births).

Muscular dystrophy may not be apparent in infancy, but appears as the child grows, presenting as muscle weakness during childhood or early adulthood. Parents or doctors may notice a delay in the normal developmental landmarks such as sitting, walking, or climbing stairs. The wasting of skeletal muscles ultimately leads to increasing disability and deformity. Kyphoscoliosis—an outward hump of the upper spine accompanied by curvature of the lower spine—may compromise pulmonary function. Cardiac involvement may also be present in as many as 95% of patients. Unfortunately, only 25% of those affected live to age 21 years, with pulmonary or cardiac complications usually being the cause of death.

Spina Bifida

Spina bifida is the most common permanently disabling birth defect. In this disorder, during the first month of pregnancy, the fetus's spinal column does not close properly or completely and vertebrae do not develop, leaving a portion of the spinal cord exposed Figure 44-10 ▲. Regularly taking the B vitamin folic acid prior to becoming pregnant reduces the risk of spinal defects. Other maternal risk factors for spina bifida include previous neural tube defect pregnancy (increases risk by 20%), diabetes, medically diagnosed obesity, some anticonvulsion medications, exposure to increased temperature in early pregnancy (ie, hot baths or hot tubs, infection resulting in fever), Caucasian or Hispanic ethnicity, and lower socioeconomic status.

Symptoms of spina bifida may include partial or full paralysis (usually of the lower extremities), bladder or bowel control difficulties, learning disabilities, and latex allergy. In addition, as many as 70% to 90% of individuals with the most severe form of spina bifida also have hydrocephalus. In hydrocephalus, an increase in the amount of cerebral spinal fluid results in increased pressure on the brain. A shunt is inserted to relieve this pressure on the brain by draining excess cerebral spinal fluid; the shunt will stay in place throughout the patient's lifetime.

Spina bifida patients will probably benefit from the same considerations that you offer when treating a patient with paralysis or difficulty moving. When you are caring for these patients, ask how best to move them if possible. Remember to rule out a fall or other event that may have caused an injury. Check carefully for injuries, as patients may not be able to feel them—or the pain of an infiltrated IV, for that matter. Also, be aware that these patients may have urinary catheters or other aids in place.

Patients With Previous Head Injuries

Patients who previously experienced head injuries may be difficult to assess and treat. Brain-injured patients may face a complex array of challenges related to their injury. In such cases, gathering a complete medical history from the patient, family, and friends will assist you in the formation of a treatment plan. (Treatment will be primarily supportive care.) Your interaction with the patient will need to be tailored to his or her specific abilities. Take the time to speak with the patient and the family to establish what is normal for the patient—for example, whether the patient has cognitive, sensory, communication, motor, behavioural, or psychological deficits.

When you are caring for a patient with a previous head injury, talk to him or her in a calm and soothing tone, and watch the patient closely for signs of anxiety or aggression. In some cases, the patient may need to be specially positioned to ensure the safety of both you and the patient. Do not expect such an individual to walk to the ambulance or trolley. As always, treat the patient with respect, use his or her name, explain procedures, and reassure the patient throughout your care.

Myasthenia Gravis

Myasthenia gravis is an abnormal condition characterised by chronic weakness of muscles, especially in the face and throat. It is the result of a defect in the conduction of nerve impulses at the nerve junction, caused by a lack of acetylcholine. In myasthenia gravis, antibodies keep acetylcholine from reaching the muscles by blocking or damaging the receptor sites. This interruption in communication results in sudden bouts of muscle weakness, usually during activity, although the condition improves with rest.

The first symptoms usually present as weakness in eye or eyelid movement. Myasthenia gravis may also affect facial muscle control, changing the person's facial expression. In many cases, the disease is noticed initially as a sudden difficulty swallowing or chewing, or as slurred speech. Other symptoms may include blurry vision, weakness or difficulty moving the neck, shortness of breath, and weakness or difficulty moving limbs. Myasthenia gravis may be difficult to diagnose because these symptoms can be attributed to many illnesses and disease processes.

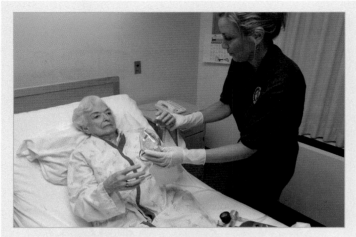

Figure 44-11 You will sometimes encounter patients with a terminal illness.

A crisis may occur if the patient's respiratory muscles are damaged by infection, stress, or side effects of medications. These muscles could become so weak that the patient suffers an acute onset of respiratory failure. In such a case, you need to intervene immediately with airway management and ventilatory support.

■ Terminally Ill Patients

Unfortunately, some illnesses currently cannot be cured. As health care providers, you will be called upon to assist a patient who is facing imminent death, or terminal illness **Figure 44-11 ▲** . Signs of impending death include decreased intake of food and drink, confusion, withdrawal, irregular breathing patterns, bradycardia, or tachycardia.

Although the goal of end-of-life care is to provide patients with a meaningful, dignified, and comfortable death, there is a surprising lack of data describing what patients and their families believe constitutes a "good death". While some patients with terminal illness choose to have the most aggressive care possible, others have a goal of comfort rather than cure or prolonging of life. In general, seriously ill patients identify pain and symptom management, preparation for death, and achieving a sense of completion as important factors in a good death.

If you are called to a scene in which death is imminent, the actions you take will have a lasting impact on the family. This is a time when compassion, understanding, and sensitivity are most needed. The family may be having a difficult time coping with the situation, and they may act with anger and hostility. Treat everyone with compassion and understanding. Your colleague may be able to separate individuals and speak

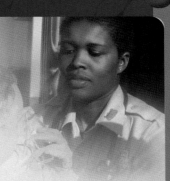

Assessment in Action

You are dispatched to a house for a 32-year-old patient with shortness of breath. When you arrive on scene, you find a male patient supine in his bed. You noticed medical and patient moving equipment whilst walking to the patient. You are told by his family that he had a spinal cord injury a year ago and is paralysed from the neck down. They inform you that the patient is prone to pneumonia and they believe he has it now. His blood pressure is 140/70 mm Hg; pulse rate, 120 beats/min; respiratory rate, 26 breaths/min; pulse oximetry reading on room air, 95%; and the ECG shows sinus tachycardia.

1. _____ is paralysis of all four extremities and the trunk, possibly from a cervical spine injury.
   A. Hemiplegia
   B. Paraplegia
   C. Quadriplegia
   D. Hyperaesthesia

2. True or false? Paralysed patients always have diaphragmatic involvement.
   A. True
   B. False

3. A paralysed patient may have normal sensation or:
   A. hyperaesthesia.
   B. hypoaesthesia.
   C. diaphragmatic involvement.
   D. hemiparesis.

4. _____ is paralysis of one side of the body.
   A. Hemiplegia
   B. Hyperaesthesia
   C. Hemiparesis
   D. Paraplegia

5. _____ is defined as a nonprogressive bilateral neuromuscular disorder in which voluntary muscles are poorly controlled.
   A. Arthritis
   B. Osteoarthritis
   C. Cerebral palsy
   D. Cystic fibrosis

6. _____ is a chronic dysfunction of the endocrine system that affects multiple body systems.
   A. Arthritis
   B. Cerebral palsy
   C. Pleurisy
   D. Cystic fibrosis

7. _____ is a chronic disease of the central nervous system in which destruction of the myelin and nerve axons occur within several regions of the brain and spinal cord.
   A. Cerebral palsy
   B. Multiple sclerosis
   C. Cystic fibrosis
   D. Arthritis

Challenging Questions

You are dispatched to a house for an unresponsive patient. When you arrive on scene, you are greeted by the patient's daughter, who tells you she believes her mother is dead, or is dying. After speaking to the daughter, you find out the patient is home with end-stage liver cancer. The patient is taking agonal respirations at a rate of 2 to 4 breaths/min. She has weak, slow pulses and an unpalpable blood pressure.

8. What should you do for this patient?

9. What should you do for the family?

Points to Ponder

You and your crewmate are dispatched to a local residential home for a convulsion. You are familiar with this facility, as it is known as the home of severely impaired individuals. When you arrive, you find a female patient who appears postictal. The patient is normally nonverbal, and her body is severely contracted. She has a history of severe learning difficulties, convulsions, diabetes, and CVE. The patient's vital signs are as follows: blood pressure, 180/90 mm Hg; respiratory rate,

24 breaths/min; pulse rate, 110 beats/min; pulse oximetry reading on room air, 96%; and the ECG shows sinus tachycardia.

How do you assess her mental status?

Issues: Understanding the Challenges of Caring for Patients With Special Needs

www.Paramedic.EMSzone.com/UK/

45 Chronic Care Patient Interventions

Objectives

Cognitive

- Compare and contrast the primary objectives of the paramedic and the home care professional.
- Identify the importance of home health care medicine as related to the ALS level of care.
- Differentiate between the role of ambulance clinician and the role of the carer.
- Compare and contrast the primary objectives of acute care, home care, and hospice care.
- Summarise the types of home health care available in your area and the services provided.
- Discuss the aspects of home care that result in enhanced quality of care for a given patient.
- Discuss the aspects of home care that have a potential to become a detriment to the quality of care for a given patient.
- List complications commonly seen in the home care patients which result in their hospitalisation.
- Compare the cost, mortality, and quality of care for a given patient in the hospital versus the home care setting.
- Discuss the significance of palliative care programmes as related to a patient in a home health care setting.
- Define hospice care, comfort care, and DNAR as they relate to local practice, law, and policy.
- List the stages of the grief process and relate them to an individual in hospice care.
- List pathologies and complications typical to home care patients.
- Given a home care scenario, predict complications requiring ALS intervention.
- Given a series of home care scenarios, determine which patients should receive follow-up home care and which should be transported to an emergency care facility.
- Describe airway maintenance devices typically found in the home care environment.
- Describe devices that provide or enhance alveolar ventilation in the home care setting.
- List modes of artificial ventilation and an out-of-hospital situation where each might be employed.
- List vascular access devices found in the home care setting.
- Recognise standard central venous access devices utilised in home health care.
- Describe the basic universal characteristics of central venous cannulas.
- Describe the basic universal characteristics of implantable injection devices.
- List devices found in the home care setting that are used to empty, irrigate or deliver nutrition or medication to the GI/GU tract.
- Describe complications of assessing each of the airway, vascular access, and GI/GU devices described above.
- Given a series of scenarios, demonstrate the appropriate ALS interventions.
- Given a series of scenarios, demonstrate interaction and support with the family members/support persons for a patient who has died.
- Describe common complications with central venous access and implantable drug administration ports in the out-of-hospital setting.
- Describe the indications and contraindications for urinary cannula insertion in an out-of-hospital setting.
- Identify the proper anatomy for placement of urinary cannulas in males or females.
- Identify failure of GI/GU devices found in the home care setting.
- Identify failure of ventilatory devices found in the home care setting.
- Identify failure of vascular access devices found in the home care setting.
- Identify failure of drains.
- Differentiate between home care and acute care as preferable situations for a given patient scenario.
- Discuss the relationship between local home care treatment guidelines/SOPs and local ambulance service guidelines/SOPs.
- Discuss differences in individual's ability to accept and cope with their own impending death.
- Discuss the rights of the terminally ill.

Affective

- Value the role of the home care professional and understand their role in patient care along the life-span continuum.
- Value the patient's desire to remain in the home setting.
- Value the patient's desire to accept or deny hospice care.
- Value the uses of long term venous access in the home health setting, including but not limited to:
  - Chemotherapy
  - Home pain management
  - Nutrition therapy
  - Congestive heart therapy
  - Antibiotic therapy

Psychomotor

- Observe for an infected or otherwise complicated venous access point.
- Demonstrate proper tracheostomy care.
- Demonstrate the insertion of a new inner cannula and/or the use of an endotracheal tube to temporarily maintain an airway in a tracheostomy patient.
- Demonstrate proper technique for drawing blood from a central venous line.
- Demonstrate the method of accessing vascular access devices found in the home health care setting.

Introduction

Breakthrough technologies, newer drugs, and research have combined to increase the average life expectancy. Thanks to these advances, people who might have died from injuries or illnesses 50 years ago may now continue to lead satisfying and productive lives. Many of these individuals, however, require physical support and care of chronic illnesses—care that may take place in the home setting. As a result of this trend, paramedics are being called upon more frequently to interact with chronic care providers and patients who are receiving home care **Table 45-1 ▾**.

Quality patient care is the ultimate goal for providers, but the aims for specific patient populations are often quite different. In the acute care setting (hospital), objectives include stabilisation, diagnosis, and treatment. In the prehospital setting, emergency care has historically been associated with these objectives.

In rehabilitation care, the objective is to restore a person with disabilities to his or her maximum potential in several areas: physical, social, spiritual, psychological, and vocational.

Formerly, this kind of healing, exercise, and development of skills took place in hospitals. In recent years, however, rehabilitation programmes have shifted from the hospital to specialised rehabilitation centres and expanded home health care programmes. Rehabilitation centres are designed to promote healing and the gradual return of the patient to the community.

In patients who are unable to return to their homes, the long-term care objectives include maintenance of a safe, stimulating environment for the patient. Although prehospital providers often equate long-term care with nursing homes for the elderly, facilities also exist for children and patients with specific health care needs. Some long-term care facilities offer custodial care; others provide life enhancement. Clearly, long-term care covers a broad range of services.

The philosophy of hospice care began in England in the 1960s. This multidisciplinary approach sought to improve the quality of a person's end-of-life experience through pain and symptom management. Because many patients felt more comfortable in their own homes, surrounded by familiar people and objects, and living on their own timetable, ensuring this comfort was the primary part of the palliative plan of care.

Originally, patients resided in *hospices* (from the same Latin root as *hospitality*) to receive end-of-life care that included pain management without cure management. Over time, hospice care grew to include home and in-hospital care designed to support the dying patient and his or her

Table 45-1	Home Care Patients in the United Kingdom, 1992 and 2000				
Year	Number of Persons Receiving Home Care	> 65 Years Old	< 65 Years Old	Female	Male
1992	1,232,200	23.1%	76.9%	66.8%	33.2%
2000	1,355,290	29.5%	70.5%	64.8%	35.2%

Source: www.cdc.gov/nchs/fastats/homehealthcare.htm (retrieved August 1, 2006).

You are the Paramedic Part 1

You and your partner are dispatched to a private home for a severe headache. As your partner approaches the address, you both make mention of the wheelchair access ramp leading up to the side entrance. The door is opened by a young woman as you make your way up the walkway. She leads you into the home, explaining that her 36-year-old husband, Michael, has been experiencing a severe headache for the past 2 hours and has not experienced any relief from his normal medication.

You enter the living room and find the patient sitting in a wheelchair. He is awake, alert, and in obvious distress. You observe that he has a tracheostomy tube in place although he is not receiving supplemental oxygen. His wife tells you that he is able to breathe on his own during the day without additional oxygen, but needs a ventilator for support at night. He does not require any other special equipment or treatment.

Initial Assessment	Recording Time: 0 Minutes
Appearance	Seated upright in an electric wheelchair, face wet with sweat, grimacing
Level of consciousness	A (Alert to person, place, and day)
Airway	Open and clear
Breathing	Adequate chest rise and volume
Circulation	Slow, strong radial pulse

1. Does treating a patient with chronic health problems affect the way you deliver emergency care?
2. What types of patients are likely to benefit from home care?

Special Considerations

Chronic conditions necessitating home care occur across all ages. Different conditions are more prevalent in certain age groups. In addition, the age of the person affects his or her response to the chronic condition.

In childhood, chronic conditions may impede the attainment of normal developmental milestones and affect trust and autonomy. In adolescence, body image and peer acceptance become primary concerns, and normal teenage rebellion may interfere with treatment plans. The development of intimate relationships and achievement of vocational goals may be impaired when chronic illness strikes in early adulthood. Chronic illness in middle age may hinder professional or career growth, resulting in early retirement and the need to use retirement income for medical expenses. Spouses of older patients may become the primary carer even though they are experiencing a similar decline in health.

family during the terminal illness and afterwards through the bereavement process. Patients admitted to hospice care have an incurable or terminal illness, which requires symptomatic control of their condition to the end of life with support for carers and relatives beyond that point.

Home care used to be the norm for terminally ill patients because few patients could afford private hospital care and, therefore, were cared for at home. To assist some families with care of the sick, certain religious groups provided home health care, while public health nurses and visiting nurse societies provided education to home health care providers on cleanliness and prevention of disease in addition to care. Over the years, visiting nursing has evolved into a multidisciplinary specialty. Today, home health care providers are usually referred by a general practitioner and associated with a hospital or primary care trust.

Previously, patients receiving home health care often relied on accident and emergency (A&E) department visits for management of acute incidents even when the incident could be managed at home. As a paramedic, your role in the care of these patients has expanded as more advanced technology emerges in support of specialist health care providers such as Acute Care in the Home Practitioners and Macmillan Nurses.

Home health care has become an increasingly attractive alternative both to patients, who often want to maintain control over their health care decision making, and to the Department of Health, which wants to control acute care costs.

Because the Department of Health pays for the majority of home services that are reimbursed, it regulates home health care agencies to ensure they meet certain quality standards. In addition, each public programme has its own method of determining reimbursement (ie, through reimbursement guidelines and financial ceilings).

Costs for similar home care services vary substantially. Nevertheless, studies show that home-based health care costs less than institutional health care, gives more satisfaction to those who receive it because they can remain in familiar surroundings, and often results in fewer and shorter hospital stays.

Measurement of the quality of health care is difficult in any setting but is particularly complex when care is delivered in the home. Consumers of home health care are vulnerable, are frequently too sick to advocate for themselves, and may lack advocates. Paramedics have a unique opportunity to listen to these patients and their families, observe the home care situation, and assist in securing additional resources or reporting to protective agencies. In addition, you can offer guidance for in-home injury prevention as you observe the patient at home.

The Role of the Paramedic in Injury Prevention in the Home Care Setting

The role of the paramedic is ideal for identifying and preventing illness and injury in the home care setting. You may be able to help identify causes of illness or injury, or prevention of either, in the future. For example, you may be called to the home of a patient who has fallen while trying to walk to the toilet unassisted. As you arrive, you observe that the patient has tripped over a bath rug which caught under her mobility device. Your teachable moment comes in assisting the patient and family to recognise the need to remove scatter rugs and other hazards that might add to the cause of falls. Injuries include unintentional injuries, such as those caused by road traffic collisions, drowning, falls, and fires, and intentional injuries, such as suicide and violence.

An injury is defined by the US Centers for Disease Control (CDC) as "unintentional or intentional damage to the body resulting from acute exposure to thermal, mechanical, electrical or chemical energy, or from the absence of such essentials as heat or oxygen". Injuries and illness may be preventable by changing the environment or individual behaviour. One useful framework for injury prevention is the Haddon matrix.

The Haddon matrix, developed by Dr. William Haddon, who was the first administrator of what is now the US National Highway Traffic Safety Administration, can be a useful tool for identifying injury prevention opportunities. According to the Haddon matrix framework, injuries occur in a certain time sequence: the pre-event phase, the event phase, and the post-event phase. Each event has a host (the person who is involved in the injury) and the equipment that is involved in the injury. There are also different environmental situations in which an injury might occur. Prevention can be focused in any "cell" of the matrix. For example, teaching the patient and family about the hazards of having scatter rugs is an intervention that addresses the host/pre-event cell; removing the rugs may address the pre-event/equipment cell.

Assessment of the Chronic Care Patient

Scene Assessment

Scene safety follows the same guidelines as for any call. Pets that live in homes with chronically ill individuals may be agitated because the household has changed from a living quarters to a care facility—full of strange noises, new faces, and smells. Remember, however, that you are entering someone's home, not a health care facility. Carer stress, exhaustion, and pressure may cause some family members to react negatively to your presence or rely on you to help relieve stress Figure 45-1 ▾. The house may have been renovated to accommodate large equipment that may make entrances unsafe (eg, ramps intended to accommodate a wheelchair).

In addition to the usual scene assessment, perform a quick assessment of the supporting equipment. How can it be moved safely? Are backup batteries for the equipment available? Is the equipment compatible with the ambulance electrical system? Will the equipment fit?

When you assess the patient's environment, note whether nutritional support is adequate; basic needs such as a reliable, safe heat source, good ventilation, electricity, and available water are important.

Body Substance Isolation

BSI or universal precautions in the home care scenario are the same as in any setting. Keep contaminated supplies and equipment together and off the floor and furniture. Bring two disposable bags for supplies: Contaminated but disposable supplies can go in one bag, while contaminated but reusable

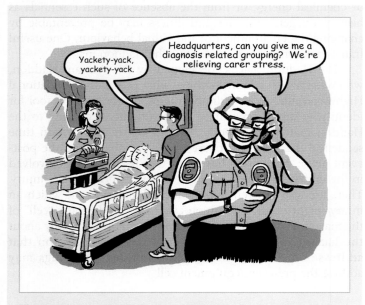

Figure 45-1

supplies go in the other. Follow your ambulance service trust's plan for cleaning supplies and returning them to use.

The most effective means of preventing transmission of microorganisms is handwashing. Use a waterless gel with at least 60% alcohol content before applying your gloves and after removing them. Use a mask, goggles, and apron if you will be exposed to respiratory secretions or if your patient is immunosuppressed and should be protected from the provider. Most chronically ill patients have had multiple exposures to latex, so avoid wearing latex gloves when caring for these patients. This consideration is especially critical in the paediatric population, particularly for children with spina bifida.

Basic principles of infection control should be applied to the home care setting. The US Centers for Disease Control and Prevention suggests a focus on infection control strategies in home care that target reducing infections related to home infusion therapy, urinary tract care, respiratory care, wound care, and enteral therapy. As a paramedic you should adhere to standard and droplet precautions for home care patients to protect your health as well as the health of others you will come in contact with.

Initial Assessment

To conduct the initial assessment of patients with chronic illness, first gather a general impression. Does the patient appear to be on the point of death? If so, do not try to troubleshoot any home care devices. Instead, remove the patient as quickly as possible from the equipment and transfer him or her to your ambulance equipment. Apply portable oxygen while you assess the situation, but troubleshoot any malfunctioning devices later if you cannot fix the malfunction or failure.

Assess the patient's airway. Many patients receiving home care have artificial or altered airways such as tracheostomies or laryngectomies. Your evaluation of patients receiving home oxygen or support ventilation are no different than for any other patient. Assess the work of breathing. Look for accessory muscle use, posture, grunting, or pursed lip breathing to keep the alveoli uncompensated. Listen to the patient's breath sounds and compare them on a side-to-side basis. Finally, assess pulse oximetry.

Assess the patient's level of consciousness (LOC) or mental status. In the chronic care patient, a common alteration in LOC is dementia. Document the patient's behaviour, including accusations, but remain non-judgemental toward carers. Another possible change in LOC is delirium, an often acute, reversible

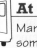

At the Scene

Many factors vary the results of pulse oximetry, some of which are patient age, gender, and peripheral circulation. Compare your results to the usual patient results and intervene based on your overall assessment.

change in behaviour that may be caused by glucose or electrolyte imbalances, nutritional deficiencies, hypothermia, or hyperthermia.

Focused History and Physical Examination

In a trauma patient, stabilise the patient's cervical spine, perform a rapid physical examination, provide comfort, and assess for other injuries. In a medical patient, gather a SAMPLE history, perform an assessment of the chief complaint, and take the patient's vital signs before you develop the plan of care. Once you have obtained the history, you may complete a physical examination. Treatment is based on both history and examination.

Medication Interactions in Home Care

Each patient may react differently to a particular medication. You are expected to treat any possible medication interactions by maintaining the patient's airway, breathing, and circulation.

Untoward reactions to medication interactions may be accidental. Observe the scene for signs of unsafe medication administration practices (eg, Does the patient understand his or her dosing requirements? Could similar-sounding medications cause confusion?), inadequate lighting, or problematic equipment (eg, faulty infusion pumps or failing electrical supply). Not all medications are meant to be crushed, yet some patients or carers may crush tablets before placing them in a gastric tube. Crushed extended-release medications may enter the patient's bloodstream too rapidly, causing an accidental overdose. Be suspicious for potential, accidental, or deliberate overdosing by the patient or carer. Report any suspicion of abuse to the proper social services or the primary care trust.

Using the Home Health History

Carers may range from professional to friends, family, or members of voluntary or church groups. Informal caregiving networks often keep few records about the patient's care. In contrast, when home care is more formal—for example, occurring through hospitals or community care agencies—providers may be required to keep detailed records similar to those in hospitals or nursing homes. In particular, medical insurance agencies expect detailed records to support a claim. The Department of Health promotes the access of information sharing and permits paramedic access to such confidential records for the treatment and transport of the patient.

Compliance Issues

Calls to patients receiving home care sometimes result from inoperative or damaged equipment such as IVs, tubes, artificial airways, and ventilators. Always consider that a call to a chronically ill patient may result from equipment failure rather than a worsening of the patient's condition. In such a case, care should be directed toward maintaining the patient on ambulance equipment while the patient's own equipment is repaired or the patient can be transferred to new equipment. Inability to easily or expeditiously repair or replace the equipment will often result in a transfer to hospital.

Special Considerations

Culture plays a significant role in determining what the patient and family consider adequate care. Assess the adequacy of care by speaking with the patient and family—not by making assumptions about what would be adequate in your own home. Learn the customs and cultural needs of people in your area.

Assessing Dementia

When you are assessing a patient with dementia (or any patient, for that matter), ask two critical questions: What is the patient's usual baseline functioning? How does function today vary from baseline? Once you have identified a change from baseline behaviour, either from carers or from a health record, determine whether a reversible condition needs to be treated—for example, hypoglycaemia, hypoxia, or hypothermia.

If no reversible conditions can be diagnosed, transport the patient to the A&E department for further evaluation. Dementia

Documentation and Communication

Paramedics are often frustrated because they expect a certain level of reporting, including written transfer paperwork from a patient's carer. Respectfully ask the carer about his or her involvement with the patient. Treat this provider in the same manner as you would a close family member if he or she is unable to answer all of your questions. Whenever possible, explain the rationale for your treatment plan. Remember—you have been called because the home care treatment is not working or the situation has changed. In addition, explain that once you arrive on the scene, the law requires you to assume responsibility of the patient since you are now the primary care provider.

At the Scene

Use the mnemonic AEIOU-TIPS to determine possible causes of altered mental status:

A Alcohol or acidosis
E Epilepsy, environment, electricity
I Insulin
O Overdose
U Uraemia
T Trauma
I Infection
P Poisoning or psychosis
S Convulsion, stroke, or shock

alone does not render a patient incompetent. In this country, patients cannot be transported against their will unless they are a hazard to themselves or others. Call ambulance control or the patient's general practitioner if the patient is unwilling to be transported. Document all assessments and interventions on your patient clinical record (PCR).

Detailed Physical Examination

The detailed physical examination assesses a specific region or body system in the case of trauma with significant MOI. Most calls to the chronic care home will be medical in nature. A systematic approach to the clinical examination may clue you into the mechanism or cause of the illness. The level of detail required for a physical examination in the home care setting is similar to any other physical examination encountered in paramedic practice. The need for a comprehensive examination depends on the acuity of the patient and the risk factors for further injury or illness. Do bear in mind that carers will often resist calling for help until the patient is quite unwell. So be mindful of the presenting complaint and its history leading up to the request for your help.

Ongoing Assessment

If you are unable to resolve the patient's problem, plan to transport the patient to the appropriate facility or treat at home as per clinical guidelines. Streamline the patient's equipment by removing components that will not be used during transport (eg, a humidification device for a home ventilator). Document your care on the PCR or hand-over report.

If the patient's own equipment will be used during transport, be sure to have battery backup for electrical devices in case of ambulance mechanical difficulties. Home care equip-

ment is either purchased or loaned, and the patient may be financially liable if it is lost or damaged. Be sure that all equipment is clearly labelled with the patient's name and contact information **Figure 45-2 ▾**. Document which pieces of equipment were transported as well as the name of the person assuming responsibility for the patient and equipment at the receiving facility.

Should the patient's problem resolve before transport, follow your guidelines for referring the patient to his or her own general practitioner or hospital doctor.

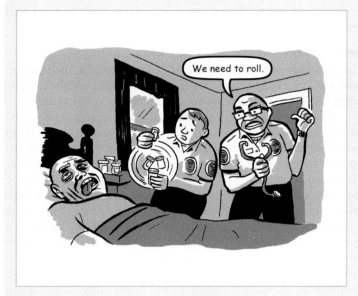

Figure 45-2

You are the Paramedic Part 2

You begin your assessment while your partner takes a set of vital signs. The patient was involved in a road traffic collision 6 months ago, resulting in a ruptured spleen, multiple rib fractures, a fractured left arm, and a C4 fracture of the neck. The spinal fracture and resulting spinal cord injury left your patient a quadriplegic. He is able to move using an electronic wheelchair. His wife was taught to straight catheterise her husband every 6 to 8 hours and assist with a bowel regime. She is also skilled in providing tracheostomy care and setting up the ventilator at night. A home health nurse visits five times a week to provide additional assistance. He is prescribed 15 mg of baclofen three times a day to help with muscle spasms and cramping and paracetamol as needed for pain or fever.

The patient tells you that his headache began approximately 2 hours earlier while watching a football game on television. He had taken the paracetamol as prescribed with no relief. The pain has gradually got worse and is now a 10 on a scale of 1 to 10. He describes the pain as a relentless pounding that does not radiate. He does admit to having blurred vision. At this time he denies having experienced nausea, vomiting, chest pain, or shortness of breath.

Vital Signs	Recording Time: 5 Minutes
Level of consciousness	Alert
Pulse	56 beats/min, regular
Blood pressure	194/100 mm Hg
Respirations	16 breaths/min, regular
Skin	Flushed, warm, and perspiring about the face; cool, pale, and clammy elsewhere
SpO2	99% on room air

3. What type of equipment might you encounter with patients receiving home health care?

At the Scene

Transporting equipment not designed to be used during a transport may increase the risk of injury to patients and ambulance service professionals.

Types of Patients Who Receive Home Health Care

Chronically ill patients are cared for at home by a wide range of carers who may include family members, unlicensed carers, licensed nonprofessional carers, licensed professionals, or a combination of these. Many family members who care for chronically ill patients are medically knowledgeable and are often the paramedic's best source of information and care guidelines.

In addition to frail or chronically ill elderly patients in the home care setting, you may encounter individuals, for example, who have recently had a hospital stay, surgery, or a high-risk pregnancy, or a newborn with medical complications. Chronic illness or permanent injury may also necessitate home care **Table 45-2 ▾**. Many of these patients experience similar physical problems regardless of the initial cause.

Table 45-2	Chronic Illnesses and Injuries Encountered in the Home Care Setting
Type of Disease, Injury, or Abnormality	**General Long-Term Problem**
Neuromuscular disease	Hypoventilation
Guillain-Barré syndrome	Decreased cough mechanism
Muscular dystrophy	Inability to maintain airway
Amyotrophic lateral sclerosis Multiple sclerosis Polio/postpolio syndrome Spinal cord injury Sleep apnoea	Immobility: deep vein thrombosis, pulmonary embolus, pressure ulcers

Musculoskeletal abnormalities:
  Scoliosis or lordosis
  Pectus excavatum
  Pectus carinatum
  Pickwickian syndrome
	Hypoventilation

Pulmonary abnormalities:
  Bronchopulmonary dysplasia
  Chronic obstructive pulmonary disease
  Cystic fibrosis
	Decreased oxygen diffusion, infection

Cardiac abnormalities: Advanced-stage congestive heart failure	Decreased oxygen diffusion

Patients With Abnormal Airway Conditions

Patients with respiratory compromise generally are unable to ventilate themselves adequately. In chronic obstructive pulmonary disease (COPD), loss of alveolar surface area or damage to the bronchial lining reduces the volume of air delivered to the alveoli and increases the work of breathing. Cystic fibrosis increases the amount of mucous present in the airway, limiting air flow and reducing diffusion across the pulmonary capillary membrane. Bronchopulmonary dysplasia results from early oxygen administration to (usually premature) newborns and causes permanent changes in the cells of the respiratory tract. Musculoskeletal changes such as scoliosis and chest wall abnormalities make it difficult to expand the chest adequately. Excess weight over the chest (Pickwickian syndrome) or sleep apnoea may leave the patient hypoventilated during sleep. In isolated cases, ventilation would normally be adequate but the patient is experiencing an increased metabolic demand from fever or infection.

Home Oxygen-Delivery Systems

With any type of respiratory abnormality, the home care treatment plan is designed to supplement the patient's respiratory effort. Any stressor such as infection, exposure to an allergen, or psychological upset can increase the severity of signs and symptoms and render the current respiratory support inadequate.

The simplest home oxygen systems involve a nasal cannula and oxygen in various delivery systems, ranging from small portable cylinders to large oxygen-enrichment systems **Figure 45-3 ▸**. The patient usually receives oxygen from a supplier after being contracted by the patient's general practitioner. Patients who are anxious breathe faster, use more of the oxygen, and may run out prior to delivery; you may be called when a person's oxygen demand

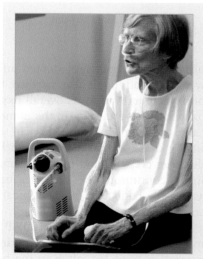

Figure 45-3 Home oxygen systems involve a nasal cannula and oxygen.

exceeds the current supply. If your assessment reveals that the patient needs to have more stored oxygen available, call the general practitioner's surgery or the out of hours service. Meanwhile, use your cylinders to keep the patient calm and prevent decompensation. Be sure the cylinders are stored safely and within reach of the patient or carer.

Some patients use oxygen concentrators, which are large electrical devices that concentrate the oxygen in ambient air and eliminate other gases. Such a system eliminates frequent delivery of oxygen cylinders, is less expensive, and is easy to maintain. Its large size means that the device is not portable, however, and many concentrators are noisy and give off heat. Patients should have backup oxygen cylinders available in the event of electrical failure.

A liquid oxygen system **Figure 45-4** may also be used. With this system, more gas can be kept in a smaller container, making it an attractive option for active patients. Oxygen cannot be stored as a liquid for long as it will evaporate.

To decrease the work of breathing by keeping the air passages and alveoli uncompensated during the expiratory phase, patients may use continuous positive airway pressure (CPAP) **Figure 45-5**. By keeping the airway pressure slightly higher than atmospheric pressure, CPAP keeps alveoli and airway passages stented and open, and decreases the work of breathing. It also increases the driving (diffusing) force of oxygen and improves overall oxygenation if a supplemental oxygen line is attached. In the home care setting, CPAP is typically used for sleep apnoea. The device consists of a tight-fitting mask or nasal prongs with a thick pillow of air to decrease pressure and prevent damage to the nose and upper lip. A continuous pressure measured in centimetres of H_2O assists the patient in taking a breath and makes it difficult to completely exhale.

Bilevel airway pressure (BiPAP) exerts a different level of inspiratory pressure versus expiratory pressure. This type of support is used less often in the home care setting and does not ventilate the patient.

A ventilator, also called a respirator, mechanically delivers air to the lungs. Home ventilators are smaller than most

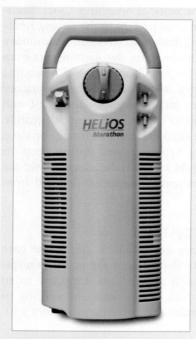

Figure 45-4 Liquid oxygen system.

At the Scene

Both CPAP and BiPAP can be administered in the home by nasal or face mask without endotracheal intubation. This technique is referred to as "noninvasive ventilation".

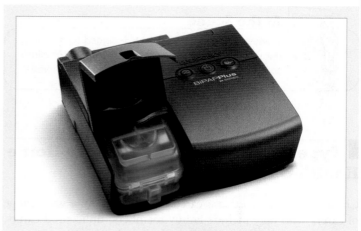

Figure 45-5 Continuous positive airway pressure machine.

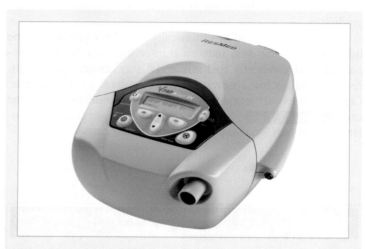

Figure 45-6 Home ventilator.

microwave ovens, use regular household electricity, and may include a battery backup **Figure 45-6**. It is important for you to become familiar with the types of units available to transport your patient effectively, or assist with an equipment malfunction.

Ventilators may be set to deliver a certain volume of gas to the lungs. For example, the machine setting may specify the tidal volume (volume of air breathed in and out during a normal breath) to be delivered. This target tidal volume is based on patient-specific factors, such as resistance to flow or lung compliance (elasticity), and general practitioner preference. Other ventilators are designed to deliver a certain pressure. Volume ventilators and pressure ventilators are used most often with an invasive airway, endotracheal intubation, or tracheostomy (discussed later in this section).

Normal breathing relies on increasing the size of the chest so that intrapulmonary and intrapleural pressures fall and air

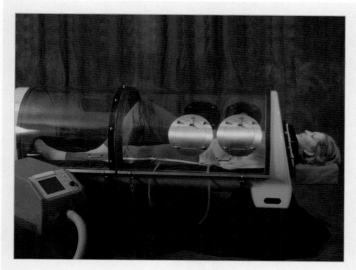

Figure 45-7 Negative-pressure ventilator.

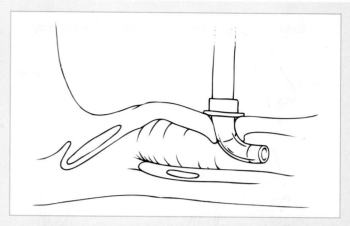

Figure 45-8 A tracheostomy is a planned surgical procedure in which an opening is placed in the trachea below the cricoid ring.

 At the Scene

Monitor the patient's blood pressure and pulse if you are going to begin positive-pressure ventilation after a period of normal breathing.

 At the Scene

If a tracheostomy becomes plugged, the patient may be ventilated by deflating the cuff, covering the nose and mouth with a mask, and using the bag-valve-mask device. If you are unable to ventilate the patient through the tracheostomy, plug the tracheostomy stoma and attempt to ventilate the patient in the traditional manner with a bag-valve-mask device.

rushes in (negative-pressure ventilation). Most mechanical ventilators rely on positive-pressure ventilation—that is, air is pushed into the lungs. (You may be most familiar with positive-pressure ventilation when you are using the bag-valve-mask device.) This type of ventilation alters the haemodynamics of the body by decreasing venous return to the heart; the thoracic pump pulls blood back to the heart when the pressure within the chest is less than atmospheric pressure. During positive-pressure ventilation, the pump is not as effective and cardiac output can drop.

Negative-pressure ventilators mimic the body's normal method of breathing. These devices—which may be called ponchos, turtleshells, or belts Figure 45-7 ▲ —enlarge the chest, dropping intrapulmonary pressure below the atmospheric pressure and allowing air to rush in. Negative-pressure ventilators do not need an invasive airway and do not alter haemodynamics. They depend on a patent airway.

Invasive Airways

Improvements in artificial ventilation have transformed many homes into satellite intensive care units. As a consequence, paramedics may encounter patients who are ventilated through a tracheostomy, a surgical airway in which an opening is placed in the trachea below the cricoid ring Figure 45-8 ▶ . A tracheostomy may become necessary when prolonged use of an endotracheal (ET) tube might predispose the patient to tra-

cheal necrosis, tracheo-oesophageal fistula, ventilator-acquired pneumonia, or oral damage. (ET tubes and intubation are covered in depth in Chapter 11.)

A laryngectomy is a surgical procedure in which the larynx is removed, usually because of cancer. The trachea is then curved anteriorly and sewn to tissues of the neck. The opening that is created in the neck is called a stoma. A patient with a laryngectomy cannot be manually bagged through the nose and mouth, and you must be careful not to introduce liquids into the stoma. Most of these patients use a stoma cover to act as a filter and prevent mucus from being coughed onto others. A patient with a laryngectomy cannot produce normal speech and must learn to swallow and regurgitate air from the stomach or use an assistive device Figure 45-9 ▶ .

Tracheostomy tube designs vary, so ask the carer about the tube prior to beginning care. General types of tracheostomy

 At the Scene

If you are transporting a child with a tracheostomy in a standard car seat, avoid using seats with a tray or shield. The tray or shield could come into contact with the tracheostomy and injure the child or block the airway.

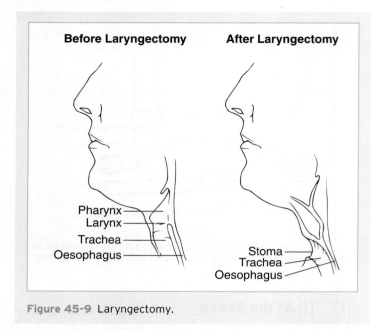

Before Laryngectomy **After Laryngectomy**

Pharynx
Larynx
Trachea
Oesophagus

Stoma
Trachea
Oesophagus

Figure 45-9 Laryngectomy.

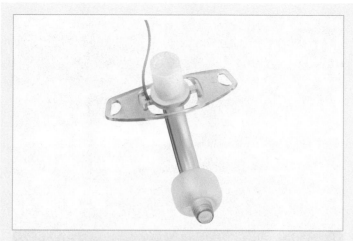

Figure 45-10 Tracheostomy tube.

tubes include a one-piece metal tube that can be plugged for speech. Such tubes are usually placed in patients weeks to months after the tracheostomy surgery when the opening has healed well.

Airway Management

It is important to assess for airway patency in all patients, but it is especially important in patients with artificial airways. The basic airway techniques of opening, repositioning, and clearing (especially suctioning) the airway are the most critical steps in improving airway clearance and patency, thereby improving oxygenation and ventilation.

Assess the flow of oxygen and ensure that there is sufficient oxygen in the system. If you are uncertain about the oxygen flow, transfer the patient to the transport oxygen source. If a patient is on a ventilator when you arrive, assess the patient's chest for synchronous movement with the ventilator. If you have any doubt about ventilator function, do not be afraid to remove the patient from the ventilator and use manual positive-pressure ventilation. Avoid adjusting home ventilator settings unless you have specific credentials to work with the particular device. Soliciting the help of the patient, family, and carers can assist in assessment and troubleshooting of equipment.

Occasionally an artificial airway will need to be exchanged or replaced. Tracheostomy tubes are easily removed (Figure 45-10 ▶). Untie the tracheostomy strings or device used to secure the tube, and gently slide the tube out on exhalation. When replacing this tube, have the patient take a deep breath and gently follow the contour of the tube during inhalation.

One-piece plastic tubes come either with or without cuffs. When you are working with plastic tubes, suction the patient orally with a blue-tip catheter. Deflate the cuff and remove it

At the Scene

For infants and small children, the tracheostomy tube is usually a single-cannula plastic tube and is generally not cuffed (even if mechanical ventilation is required).

during exhalation. To replace the tracheostomy, insert an obturator (guide) into it, gently guide the tube in on inhalation, remove the obturator, and add air to the cuff.

Two-piece tracheostomies have an outer cannula that is guided into place by the obturator. When the obturator is removed, insert the inner cannula and turn the standard connector until it clicks or locks into place. Add air to the cuff, and apply the holder to secure the device around the neck. Never let go of the tube until it is secured.

On rare occasions, the paramedic will need to replace a tracheostomy with an ET tube. The easiest method is to remove the tracheostomy tube and gently guide a slightly smaller ET tube into place. (The size of the tracheostomy tube appears on its neck piece.) The ET tube will extend out from the neck, so take care to stabilise the tube. Confirm chest rise with ventilation, as it is possible—especially with new tracheostomies—to misplace the tube within the neck but outside of the trachea.

If the tracheostomy has inadvertently closed, you may intubate the patient orally or nasally. Place an occlusive dressing over the tracheostomy site to prevent air loss and observe the patient carefully for adequate chest rise.

To suction and clean a tracheostomy, follow the steps given here and in (**Skill Drill 45-1** ▶):

1. Wash your hands and apply a mask, goggles, and clean nitrile gloves. Suctioning a home care patient is a clean procedure, not a sterile one.

2. Open supplies may be used. For cost reasons, home care patients often reuse their suction catheters. If the catheters

Skill Drill 45-1: Cleaning a Tracheostomy

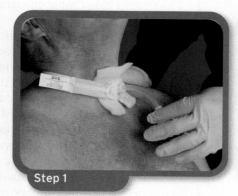

Step 1

Remove the inner cannula and place the device to soak in the cleansing solution.

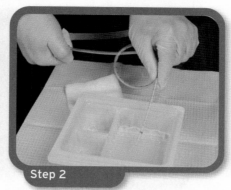

Step 2

Attach the cannula to negative pressure. Check the suction and clear the cannula by drawing up a small amount of saline.

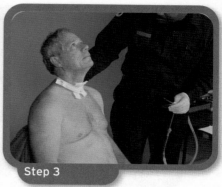

Step 3

Ask the patient to take a deep breath or pre-oxygenate him or her using the ventilator.

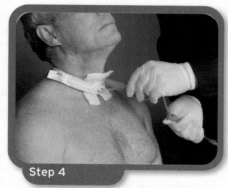

Step 4

Insert the cannula into the trachea without suction. Apply intermittent suction while removing the cannula. Repeat as necessary.

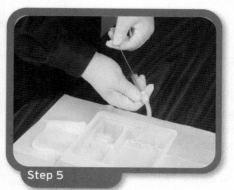

Step 5

Clean the inner cannula with the tracheostomy brush, rinse, and replace and lock into place.

do not have visible contamination and have been stored in a clean manner, they are acceptable for use.

3. Remove the inner cannula. Check with your patient's carer, if available, and place the device to soak in the appropriate recommended solution. Placing the cannula in plain water is acceptable in short-term situations. With one-piece tracheostomy tubes, this step is unnecessary. If the patient is dependent on a ventilator, have a replacement cannula immediately available (Step 1).

4. Attach the cannula to negative pressure. Check the suction and clear the cannula by drawing up a small amount of saline (Step 2).

5. Ask the patient to take a deep breath or preoxygenate him or her (Step 3).

6. Insert the cannula into the trachea without suction. Apply intermittent suction while removing the cannula. Repeat as necessary. Keep the patient well oxygenated during the procedure (Step 4).

7. Clean the inner cannula with the tracheostomy brush, rinse, and replace and lock into place. Omit this step for a one-piece tracheostomy (Step 5).

8. Remove your gloves and wash your hands.

9. Document the procedure and assessment on your PCR.

In asthmatic patients, peak flow readings are usually obtained immediately before and after treatment for bronchospasm. A peak flow meter measures the rate of air being expired in litres per minute and gives the provider an indication about the condition of the larger airways. To take a peak flow reading, follow the steps in **Skill Drill 45-2 ▶**:

1. Help the patient into a position of comfort, either sitting upright or standing upright, if safe to do so.

2. Place the indicator at the base of the numbered scale (Step 1).

3. Ask the patient to take a deep breath through the mouth.

4. Ask the patient to put the meter in the mouth and close his or her lips around the end.

Skill Drill 45-2: Obtaining a Peak Flow Reading

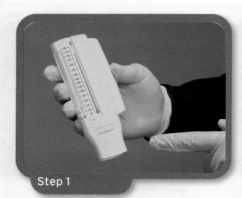

Step 1

Help the patient into a position of comfort. Place the indicator at the base of the numbered scale. Describe to the patient what you would like them to do.

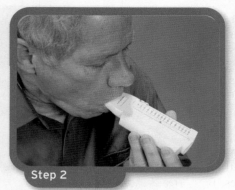

Step 2

Ask the patient to take a deep breath through the mouth and put the meter in the mouth. Patient blows out as hard as possible through the device for approximately 1 second. If possible, repeat two more times to obtain an average result.

5. Ask the patient to blow out as hard as possible through the device for approximately 1 second (Step 2).

6. If time and conditions permit, ask the patient to repeat steps 2 to 5 two more times to obtain an average result. Allow rest periods.

7. Document the results on the PCR.

8. Assist in cleaning the device and storing it correctly, and dispose of cardboard tube.

Patients With Acute Cardiovascular Disease and Vascular Access

Patients who have chronic cardiovascular disease are often cared for in the home setting. Many patients have cardiac insufficiency or heart failure, an inability of the heart to keep up with the demands placed on it and failure of the heart to pump blood efficiently. The heart is then unable to provide adequate blood flow to other organs. The signs and symptoms of heart failure depend on which side of the heart is failing and include dyspnoea, cardiac asthma, pooling of blood (stasis) systemically or in the liver's circulation, oedema, cyanosis, and hypertrophy (enlargement) of the heart. There are many causes of congestive heart failure: coronary artery disease, leading to heart attacks and heart muscle weakness; primary heart muscle weakness from viral infections or toxins such as prolonged alcohol exposure; heart valve disease causing heart muscle weakness due to too much leaking of blood; heart muscle stiffness from a blocked valve; and hypertension. Treatment is aimed at improving the pumping function of the heart. Some patients may have an implantable pacemaker that delivers synchronised electrical stimulation to three chambers of the heart, enabling the heart to pump blood more efficiently throughout the body.

Cardiomyopathy, a condition in which the heart muscle does not work at the optimal level, can be caused by many disease processes. Primary cardiomyopathy cannot be traced to a single cause. Hypertension, coronary artery disease, and viral infections might combine to decrease the ability of the muscle to eject blood. Secondary cardiomyopathy can be traced to a single cause, usually one that affects other body organs at the same time. All types of cardiomyopathy result in inadequate cardiac output, limiting the patient's activity. Many treatments require long-term venous access devices.

The heart never ejects 100% of the blood in the left ventricle during a heartbeat, but an ejection fraction greater than 55% is considered adequate. An ejection fraction less than 55% may limit the patient's activity level and indicates the presence of cardiomyopathy. An ejection fraction less than 20% can significantly alter a patient's lifestyle. In a home care patient, a change in the previous level of activity is a red flag that the heart may be temporarily or permanently deteriorated.

Vascular Access

A central venous cannula—a venous access device with the tip of the cannula in the vena cava—is used for many types of home care patients, including those receiving chemotherapy, long-term antibiotic or pain management, high-concentration glucose solutions, and haemodialysis. In contrast, a midline cannula is located in a large vessel but not the vena cava (Table 45-3 ▸).

Because the devices are used intermittently, they must be flushed to keep them open. In the past, low-concentration heparin has been the flush of choice. However, research has shown that low platelet counts develop in some patients following long-term use of heparin even at low concentrations, a condition known as heparin-induced thrombocytopenia. Flushing the device with saline eliminates the possibility of heparin-induced thrombocytopenia but means the patency of the device must be assessed frequently. Patients who are chronically ill or fragile may have devices that allow medications and fluids to be infused or body fluids to be removed and monitored. These devices place the patient at increased risk for cardiovascular complications including anticoagulation, embolus formation, stasis, air embolus, and obstructed or malfunctioning devices.

Table 45-3	Venous Access Devices	
Type	**Use**	**Prehospital Precautions**
Midline cannulas	Short-term fluids, analgesia, antibiotics	Moderate-length cannula, not good for rapid fluid resuscitation
Peripherally inserted central cannula	Long-term fluids, analgesia, chemotherapy, antibiotic therapy	Long cannula; not good for fluid resuscitation; may require online medical direction for use
Central lines, tunnelled implanted	Long-term fluids, analgesia, chemotherapy, antibiotic therapy, multiple blood draws	Have a non-cutting/crush clamp available, as not all have a clamp; may require online medical direction for use
Implanted infusion device	Long-term fluids, analgesia, chemotherapy, antibiotic therapy	Use a non-cutting or non-bevelled needle for access; may require online medical direction for use

Cannula dysfunction occurs frequently in patients receiving home infusions. Cannula-associated thrombosis can be life threatening and limit future vascular sites. Both of these complications can be minimised and treated when the paramedic is aware of preventative measures.

If a device does not seem to be working properly, ensure that it is not used for medications or any other purpose. If the patient has a gastric tube (which places him or her at increased risk for aspiration of stomach contents), position the patient in a semi-recumbent or upright position if tolerated. Inspect and secure all external devices prior to moving the patient, especially when preparing for transport—it takes relatively little tension to inadvertently displace a tube, line, or device.

There are several things that a paramedic can do to reduce or prevent complications of vascular access devices: check the devices carefully before any treatment; keep device area clean; check that the correct medication and dose or nutrition are being infused into the device; use the device site only for what it was designed for (eg, dialysis cannulas should only be used for dialysis treatment); avoid placing a blood pressure cuff on an arm that has an device port; and check pulses carefully in the device area.

Occasionally, it will be necessary to access a device for assessment, to draw blood, or to infuse medications. Proper technique is important. Patients and their carers will be your best resource in performing these functions. In addition, check with your ambulance training officer regarding accessing a venous access device when there is a need for resuscitation and you are unable to obtain any other vascular access.

Drawing Blood From a Central Venous Cannula

Central venous cannulas (CVCs) offer easy access to the venous system but may present resistance to rapid fluid infusion due to their length. Because they enter the central circulation in the chest, negative pressure may draw in air (air embolus) or provide entry to microorganisms. To draw blood from a CVC, follow the steps illustrated in **Skill Drill 45-3 ▶** :

1. Wash your hands and apply a mask, goggles, and nitrile gloves.
2. Draw the flush solution (usually normal saline but may be a heparin solution) into a syringe (Step 1).
3. Set up the supplies, including the port access kit.

4. Swab the port with an appropriate cleansing solution (eg, Betadine) *or* clamp the cannula and remove the cap (Step 2).
5. Attach an empty syringe or Vacutainer adapter to the hub or port (Step 3).
6. Release the clamp (if clamped), and aspirate 5 ml of blood (Step 4).
7. Reclamp the cannula if necessary and discard the aspirated blood (Step 5).

8. Attach a new syringe or adapter (Step 6).
9. Obtain the blood samples (Step 7).
10. Reclamp the cannula if necessary and attach the syringe with the flush solution (Step 8).
11. Release the clamp and flush the line (Step 9).
12. Reclamp and recap the line (Step 10).
13. Identify the vials of blood by writing the date and time drawn and the paramedic's name on the side of the tube, and prepare them for transport by securing them in a leak-proof protected container. Transport tubes to the patient's general practitioner, hospital personnel, or usual lab. Do not shake blood collection tubes, as this may cause the blood to haemolyse.
14. Document the procedure and assessment on the PCR.
15. Dispose of contaminated equipment.

Accessing an Implantable Venous Access Device

Usually phlebotomy is carried out in the home by community nurses. However, paramedics may be called on to conduct this procedure. Most haematology laboratories insist on three separate means of patient identification on the form and two on the sample, except for transfusion, when it must be three on each. This is in addition to the date and time of the sample and the name of the clinician who carried out the procedure. To access an implantable venous access device, follow the steps in **Skill Drill 45-4 ▶** :

1. Wash your hands and apply a mask, goggles, and nitrile gloves.
2. Open supplies including the port access kit.
3. Palpate the skin over the device (Step 1).
4. Cleanse the skin over the device using a cleansing solution (Step 2).

Skill Drill 45-3: Drawing Blood From a Central Venous Cannula

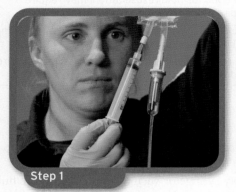

Step 1

Draw the flush solution into a syringe.

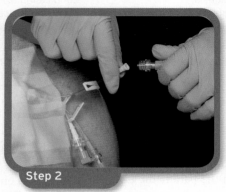

Step 2

Swab the port with an appropriate cleansing solution *or* clamp the cannula and remove the cap.

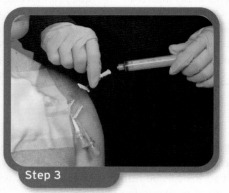

Step 3

Attach an empty syringe or Vacutainer adapter to the hub or port.

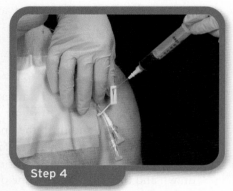

Step 4

Release the clamp (if clamped), and aspirate 5 ml of blood.

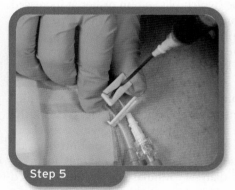

Step 5

Reclamp if necessary and discard the aspirated blood per your exposure control plan.

5. Prime the needle tubing and needle with saline. Use a special access needle called unbevelled or non-cutting to avoid slicing the silicone reservoir wall (Step 3).

6. While stabilising the device, insert the needle at a 90° angle to the skin until the needle tip reaches the back of the device (Step 4).

7. Aspirate 5 ml of blood (Step 5).

8. Discard the aspirate and obtain blood samples if necessary (Step 6).

9. Flush the line with normal saline (Step 7).

10. Administer medications or fluids as directed (Step 8).

11. Flush the device (Step 9).

12. Secure the needle with a sterile dressing *or* remove by pulling straight out of the device (Step 10).

13. Apply a dressing to the skin over the device if the needle was removed.

14. Identify the samples of blood by writing the date and time drawn and the patient's and paramedic's information on the side of the tube, and protect them for transport by securing them in a leak-proof protected container. Transport tubes to the patient's general practitioner, hospital personnel, or usual lab. Do not shake blood collection tubes, as this may cause the blood to haemolyse.

15. Document the procedure and assessment on the PCR.

16. Dispose of contaminated equipment.

Anticoagulant therapy is common in home care patients, so you should consider covert bleeding as a likely cause of hypovolaemic shock in such individuals. A sudden onset of chest pain, shortness of breath, and decreased cardiac output during or immediately after opening an implanted or tunnelled port may be indicators of an air embolus. Turn the patient on his or her left side to keep the embolus sequestered in the right atrium, so that air can be absorbed a little at a time, and transport the patient in that position.

Management of Vascular Access Devices

Vascular access devices relieve anxiety and the pain of frequent insertion attempts for patients. At the same time, they

Skill Drill 45-3: Drawing Blood From a Central Venous Cannula (*continued*)

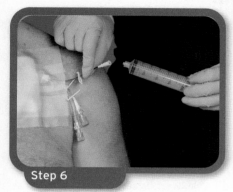

Step 6

Attach a new syringe or adapter.

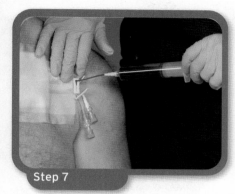

Step 7

Obtain the blood samples.

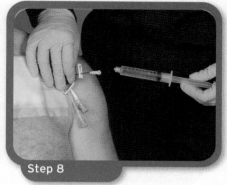

Step 8

Reclamp if necessary and attach the syringe with the flush solution.

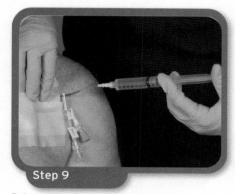

Step 9

Release the clamp and flush the line.

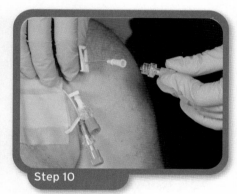

Step 10

Reclamp and recap the line.

create potential complications. Common complications resulting from vascular access, assessment findings, and emergency interventions are shown in **Table 45-4 ▶**. If a device complication is suspected, the paramedic should not attempt to access the device. A device complication requires additional medical intervention. While not all patients will need to be transported immediately to a hospital, contact should be established and a plan made with the patient's usual health care professional. Serious complications require immediate transport of the patient to an acute care facility for further evaluation and treatment.

Patients With Gastrointestinal/Genitourinary Access

A gastric tube may be placed when the patient cannot ingest fluids, food, or medications by mouth. Tubes may be inserted through the nose or mouth into the stomach (using nasogastric or orogastric tubes). Alternatively, endoscopy procedures may be undertaken to guide the surgical entrance of the tube into the stomach, such as a percutaneous endoscopic gastric

tube or placement of a percutaneous endoscopic jejunum tube into the jejunum. The patient must have adequate stomach function to support use of a gastric tube. If there has been

Table 45-4	Serious Complications Associated With Vascular Access Devices
Complication	**Assessment Findings**
Occlusion	Cannot aspirate blood; infusion doesn't run
Cannula thrombosis	Swelling of arm, neck, or shoulder; pain
Sepsis	Fever, chills, malaise
Cannula migration	Change in length of exposed cannula
Cannula breakage	Leaking or bleeding from cannula
Embolism (air)	Chest pain, shortness of breath, tachycardia, hypotension, decreased level of consciousness
Embolism (PICC/midline cannula)	Inadvertent removal with distal portion of cannula missing

Skill Drill 45-4: Accessing an Implantable Venous Access Device

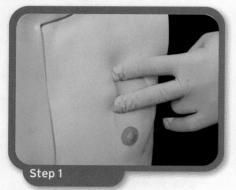

Step 1

Palpate the skin over the device.

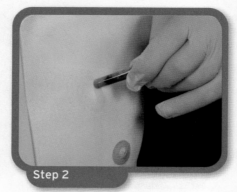

Step 2

Cleanse the skin over the device.

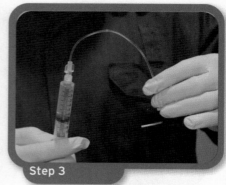

Step 3

Prime the needle tubing and needle with saline.

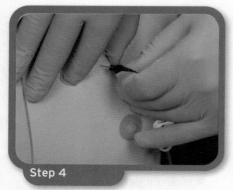

Step 4

While stabilising the device, insert the needle at a 90° angle to the skin until the needle tip reaches the back of the device.

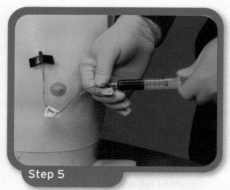

Step 5

Aspirate 5 ml of blood.

damage to the stomach, the tube may be placed into the jejunum of the small intestine.

Patients who have gastric tubes in place may still be at increased risk for aspiration. To minimise the risk of regurgitation and aspiration, the patient should be upright, at least to 30° when medications or nutrition are being infused. They should ideally be kept upright for 30 to 60 minutes after feeding. To prevent further complications such as cramping, nausea, vomiting, and diarrhoea, liquids should be infused slowly. Some home care patients with gastric tubes may have their liquids delivered by an infusion pump. Occasionally a gastric tube may become nonfunctional when noncommercial foods are infused through it. This practice is highly discouraged by nutrition experts. Gastric tubes should be flushed, usually with cooled, boiled water, before and after medications or nutritional fluids.

Any abdominal surgery places the patient at risk for development of adhesions. Adhesions are scar tissue that may con-

nect one loop of bowel to another or encircle a segment of bowel, constricting it and resulting in a bowel obstruction. A large-bowel obstruction (ie, obstruction in the colon) usually results from a growth within the bowel rather than adhesions. A small-bowel obstruction occurs when the small intestine becomes blocked. Improperly dissolved medications, food supplements, or the actions of certain types of medications can all lead to bowel obstruction.

Chronically ill patients who receive care at home are especially vulnerable to difficulties with normal elimination, especially normal urinary function. Such patients may require a long-term indwelling urinary catheter. Conversely, patients with neurological damage may require intermittent urinary catheterisation or placement of an indwelling catheter. The bladder is normally sterile, so introduction of any device can introduce bacteria. Unless the patient is immunocompromised, however, there is low risk that clean (rather than sterile) catheterisation will cause an infection **Figure 45-11 ▸**.

Skill Drill 45-4: Accessing an Implantable Venous Access Device (continued)

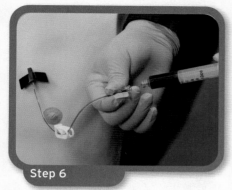

Step 6

Discard the aspirate and obtain blood samples if necessary.

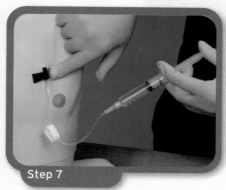

Step 7

Flush the line with normal saline.

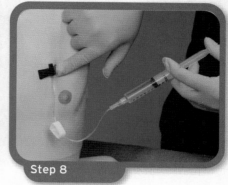

Step 8

Administer medications or fluids as directed.

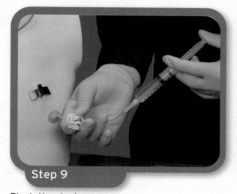

Step 9

Flush the device.

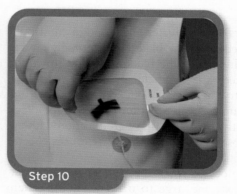

Step 10

Secure the needle with a sterile dressing.

You are the Paramedic Part 3

You perform a physical examination and find that the patient's abdomen is distended and firm upon palpation. No other significant findings are observed. Unsure of what to make of your clinical findings and the patient's clinical presentation, you decide to contact the patient's GP for guidance.

The patient's GP advises you to catheterise the patient in an attempt to relieve any pressure caused by a full bladder and to transport for further evaluation and management of the blood pressure. While you explain the doctor's recommendation for treatment and transport, the patient's wife goes to get the catheterisation kit. The patient informs you that he and his wife have discussed resuscitation measures in the event that they are required and that they wish to have everything attempted.

Reassessment	Recording Time: 12 Minutes
Skin	Flushed, warm, and perspiring about the face; cool, pale, and clammy elsewhere
Pulse	52 beats/min, regular
Blood pressure	208/120 mm Hg
Respirations	16 breaths/min, regular
SpO_2	98% on room air
ECG	Sinus bradycardia with no ectopy
Pupils	PEARRL

4. Why did the doctor recommended catheterising the patient's bladder prior to transport?

5. Why is it important that the patient's wishes for a full resuscitation be known?

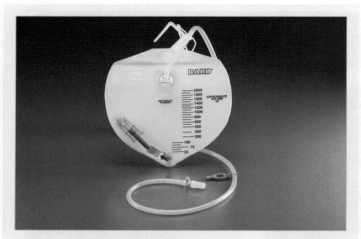

Figure 45-11 Urinary drainage bag.

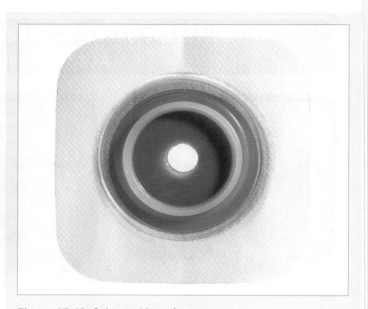

Figure 45-12 Ostomy skin wafer.

© 2007 E.R. Squibb & Sons, LLC. Reprinted with permission.

Indwelling catheters have a greater likelihood of contributing to urinary tract infections. The bladder is normally closed to the outside by a sphincter at the bladder-urethra junction. Indwelling catheters keep the sphincter open and provide a continuous route of entry for bacteria. Due to the short urethra in the female, women are at greater risk for urinary tract infections than men. Given the ongoing risk of an infection with an indwelling catheter, urosepsis is one of the likely causes of septic shock in such patients.

The urge to urinate occurs when the bladder fills to about 150 ml of fluid. An extreme urge to urinate occurs when approximately 400 ml of fluid fills the bladder. In susceptible individuals (eg, those with a disruption in the spinal cord), a full bladder can lead to dangerously high blood pressure, which places the patient at risk for stroke.

Patients with small-bowel disease may need large portions of the small intestine removed (ileostomy). A stoma is constructed that connects the small intestine to the outside of the abdomen where the patient attaches a collection bag. The intestinal waste from an ileostomy is irritating to skin, as it contains some of the digestive juices. The bag must be emptied frequently.

At the Scene

Signs of potential failure of a gastrointestinal or genitourinary device in the home care setting include abdominal pain or distension, decreased or absent bowel sounds, bladder distension, dysuria, and changes in urinary output or colour.

A colostomy is a surgical opening in the large intestine that is brought to the surface of the abdomen to drain solid waste **Figure 45-12 ▲**. The drainage varies from loose (if the colostomy is along the ascending colon) to soft (if the colostomy is along the transverse or descending colon). A temporary colostomy allows the bowel to rest and heal, and is intended to be reversed at a later date. In a permanent colostomy, stool is always diverted to the stoma.

Occasionally, the ureters will be brought to the surface to a stoma, and urine will then drain directly into an appliance. Such an ureterostomy differs from a suprapubic catheter in that the catheter is surgically placed into the bladder. In the latter case, the ureters remain intact and continue to drain the kidneys into the urinary bladder.

Signs and symptoms of a large-bowel obstruction include changes in stool (may be very watery), abdominal distension, and localised pain. Signs and symptoms of a small-bowel obstruction include diffuse pain, nausea, and vomiting (often containing faecal material). Bowel sounds may vary from hypoactive to high pitched and frequent.

A bladder overfilled with urine may appear as abdominal distension. If the bladder is distended, its upper margin can usually be palpated. In abdominal distension, no upper margin will be evident. Urine production depends on factors such as fluid intake, fluid losses other than urine, and the condition of the kidneys. Urine is normally clear yellow and sterile with a slight odour. A strong ammonia smell indicates a urinary tract infection.

Skill Drill 45-5: Catheterising an Adult Male Patient

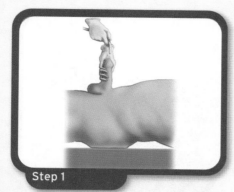

Step 1

Hold the penis at a 90° angle to the body and insert the catheter.

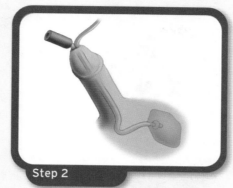

Step 2

Insert the catheter until the Y between the drainage port and the balloon port is at the tip of the penis. For a straight catheter, insert approximately 2 to 3 cm more.

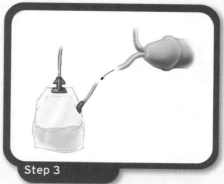

Step 3

Allow urine to drain.

At the Scene

When you are assessing bowel sounds, listen for 1 minute over each abdominal quadrant. Have a quiet atmosphere and auscultate *before* you palpate the abdomen.

Inserting a Catheter

Patients who are not able to void (urinate) on their own may need to be catheterised. Catheters may remain in place (ie, indwelling catheters such as Foley catheters) or may be used intermittently (straight catheters). While the principles for catheterisation remain the same for either gender, anatomy differences change the process.

To catheterise adult male patients, follow these steps **Skill Drill 45-5 ▲**:

1. Help position the patient supine with legs slightly spread apart. Maintain privacy as much as possible.
2. Wash your hands and apply a mask, goggles, and clean nitrile gloves.
3. Conduct the procedure using aseptic techniques throughout. Double gloving will avoid any delay when going from the "dirty" to the "clean" or aseptic side of the procedure. Open supplies including the urinary catheter and placement kit. Place necessary supplies onto a clean area within reach. If you are inserting an indwelling catheter, connect a syringe filled with saline to the balloon port. Also connect the indwelling catheter to the drainage system. There are no connecting ports for either a balloon or a drainage bag on a straight catheter.
4. If possible wash the penis with soap and water (or have the patient do so if he is able). Make sure that the foreskin has been retracted. Clean the external meatus with sterile normal saline solution.
5. Coat the end of the catheter with a water-soluble gel. An anaesthetic gel is preferred for patients with sensation in the penile area. Allow time for the anaesthetic to become effective.
6. Hold the penis at a 90° angle to the body and insert the catheter **Step 1**.
7. When urine is evident in the tubing, insert the catheter until the Y between the drainage port and the balloon port is at the tip of the penis. For a straight catheter, insert approximately 2 to 3 cm more **Step 2**.
8. Inflate the balloon with sterile water for injection and gently pull back on the catheter until you feel resistance, which indicates that the balloon is snug against the neck of the bladder. This step is unnecessary for a straight catheter.
9. Allow urine to drain. Note the amount and colour **Step 3**.
10. To remove a catheter, remove the saline in the balloon port and pull back gently until the catheter is free of the tip of the penis. *Never* remove an indwelling catheter without using a syringe to remove the saline from the balloon, as it may damage the urinary sphincter. For a straight catheter, simply pull back gently to remove the catheter. Dispose according to local clinical waste procedures.

Skill Drill 45-6: Catheterising an Adult Female Patient

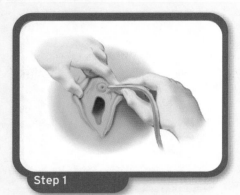

Step 1

Locate the urinary meatus anterior to the vagina and insert the catheter.

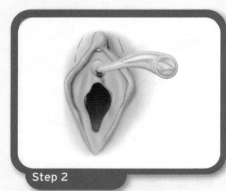

Step 2

When urine is evident in the tubing, insert the catheter another 2 to 8 cm.

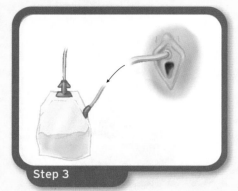

Step 3

Allow urine to drain.

11. Remove your gloves and wash your hands, following universal precautions.

12. If the catheter is to remain in place, secure it to the patient's leg according to the home care instructions.

13. Document the procedure and assessment on the PCR.

To catheterise an adult female patient, follow these steps **Skill Drill 45-6 ▲** :

1. Help position the patient supine with legs spread apart or side lying with the top knee flexed. Maintain privacy as much as possible.

2. Wash your hands and apply clean nitrile gloves.

3. Open supplies including the urinary catheter and placement kit. Place necessary supplies onto a clean area within reach. If you are inserting an indwelling catheter, connect a syringe filled with saline to the balloon port. Also connect the indwelling catheter to the drainage system. There are no connecting ports for either a balloon or a drainage bag on a straight catheter.

4. Wash the postnatal area with soap and water (or have the patient do so if she is able). First cleanse the outer area of the perineum, and then spread the labia minora and thoroughly wash the mucosa surrounding the vagina and the urinary meatus. Dry with a clean towel. Clean the urinary meatus with sterile normal saline solution.

5. Coat the end of the catheter with a water-soluble gel. An anaesthetic gel is preferred for patients with sensation in the postnatal area. Allow time for the anaesthetic to become effective.

6. Locate the urinary meatus anterior to the vagina and insert the catheter **Step 1** .

7. When urine is evident in the tubing, insert the catheter another 2 to 8 cm **Step 2** .

8. Inflate the balloon with sterile water for injection and gently pull back on the catheter until you feel resistance,

which indicates that the balloon is positioned against the neck of the bladder. This step is unnecessary for a straight catheter.

9. Allow urine to drain. Note the amount and colour **Step 3** .

10. To remove a catheter, remove the saline in the balloon port and pull back gently until the catheter is free of the tip of the meatus. Never remove an indwelling catheter without using a syringe to remove the saline from the balloon, as it may damage the urinary sphincter. For a straight catheter, simply pull back gently to remove the catheter. Dispose according to local clinical waste procedures.

11. Remove your gloves and wash your hands.

12. If the catheter is to remain in place, secure it to the patient's leg or abdomen according to the patient's needs.

13. Document the procedure and assessment on the PCR.

Replacing an Ostomy Device

To replace an ostomy device, follow the steps in **Skill Drill 45-7 ▶** :

1. Help position the patient in a comfortable area in which to change the appliance and easily dispose of the contaminated articles.

2. Wash your hands and apply a mask, goggles, and clean nitrile gloves.

3. Open supplies. Ostomy equipment includes a skin barrier called a wafer and one of several styles of drainage bags. Some bags can be opened along the bottom and emptied at regular intervals; others are sealed around a system similar to a urine drainage bag.

4. Empty/remove the current appliance and dispose of it appropriately **Step 1** .

5. Wash the area around the stoma with soap and water. Cleanse the stoma with water only, being careful not to rub or irritate the area **Step 2** .

6. Place a clean gauze pad over the stoma to prevent contamination of the clean skin with stool or urine (Step 3).

7. Cut the wafer to the correct size using the patient's measurement or tracing. Home care patients usually have the stoma already sized or have a tracing to cut a hole in the wafer large enough for the stoma but keeping exposed skin to a minimum (Step 4).

8. Attach the appliance to the wafer. Be sure the distal end is open (Step 5).

9. Remove the gauze (Step 6).

10. Remove the paper backing from the wafer (Step 7).

11. Apply the appliance with the stoma centred in the wafer cutout (Step 8).

12. Remove your gloves and wash your hands.

13. Document the procedure and assessment on the PCR.

 At the Scene

Be careful not to cut the ostomy appliance when using trauma shears to cut away clothing. The drainage can contaminate wounds and damage intact skin.

Patients With Wounds and Acute Infections

Wounds associated with trauma or surgery result in a break in the skin. These wounds, which may be either intentional (as with surgery) or unintentional (as during trauma), then undergo healing—that is, regeneration of living tissue.

Factors that affect wound healing include nutritional status, activity level, medications (including use of nicotine, anti-inflammatory drugs, heparin, and chemotherapy), chronic illness or immobility, diabetes, and the presence (or absence) of infection.

Immunosuppressed patients—such as early transplant recipients or individuals with human immunodeficiency virus infection—are at greater risk for acquiring infections, including wound infections. Immunocompromised patients have alterations in their immunity that increase both the risk for infection and the ability to combat infection, especially respiratory infections. Fever is often the only symptom of infection in the immunocompromised patient and always requires further investigation. Special care should be taken for protection of these patients.

Drainage from a wound (called exudate) consists of fluid and cells. Serous exudate is a clear, watery drainage. Purulent exudate is pus, which consists of white blood cells, liquefied dead tissue, and bacteria. The colour of the exudate often provides a clue about the types of bacteria present. Sanguinous exudate is bloody; fresh, oxygenated blood is light red, while older blood is darker red.

Patients with vascular access devices are at increased risk for infections. Observe the device area for signs of infection, especially a hot to touch, reddened area that may indicate an abscess at the site. Practise good hand hygiene and site care when working with these devices.

Immobile patients with chronic illnesses are at high risk for skin breakdown, leaving them susceptible to infection. Perform a careful assessment of your patient's skin. Assess a surgical or treated wound by noting the following:

- **Appearance.** Healing appears as a pink to reddened area.
- **Size.** Measure the wound. Note any changes in size as described by the patient or carer.
- **Drainage.** Observe the colour, consistency, odour, and number of gauze pads soaked in a timeframe to help measure the amount of drainage.
- **Swelling.** This can occur throughout the body (generalised) or in a specific area (localised). Generalised swelling or oedema is a common sign in severely ill patients.
- **Pain.** Using a pain score, ask your patient to rate his or her level of pain; ask the patient or a family member for any observations of changes in level of pain. Many patients who are chronically ill may not be able to communicate their pain using a traditional 1 to 10 pain score, so be prepared to use a nonverbal scoring tool.
- **Drains or tubes.** Check the amount of drainage.
- **Temperature.** Warm to hot skin indicates a possible infection. Temperature regulation in many chronically ill or fragile patients is poor, however, so patients who have infections may not always feel warm to the touch or have a fever. Ask the patient or carer what is considered a normal temperature and what is different, if anything, today.

A wound with minor redness, slight warmth to the touch, and swelling may indicate a superficial infection. A painful reddened area that may have cracks or serous drainage, sometimes with red streaks extending from the area, may indicate that the patient has cellulitis. Patients with a fever and chills with an area that is hot to the touch, has purulent exudate, and is the source of pain may have a more serious infection. Cellulitis is usually treated with antibiotics, rest and elevation of the affected area, and warm compresses. Cellulitis may be more severe and require hospitalisation in patients who have venous stasis, diabetes, or who are immunocompromised. If left untreated, wound infections in chronically ill patients may lead to sepsis—a serious systemic infection.

An important complication of wound healing is separation of the edges of the wound, called dehiscence. If the amount of drainage from a wound increases, especially 4 to 5 days after injury, dehiscence is likely.

 At the Scene

Methicillin-resistant *Staphylococcus aureus* (MRSA) is a serious problem in the community, especially among chronically ill patients. MRSA can colonise the skin and body of an individual without causing sickness and, in this way, unknowingly be passed on to other individuals.

Skill Drill 45-7: Replacing an Ostomy Device

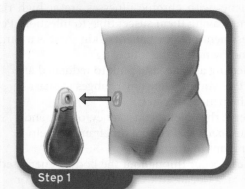

Step 1

Empty/remove the current appliance and dispose of it appropriately.

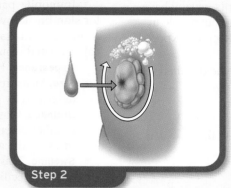

Step 2

Wash the area around the stoma with soap and water. Cleanse the stoma with water.

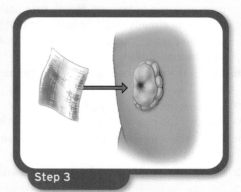

Step 3

Place a clean gauze pad over the stoma.

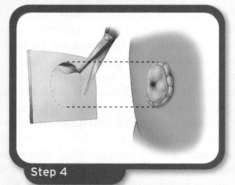

Step 4

Cut the wafer to the correct size using the patient's measurement or tracing.

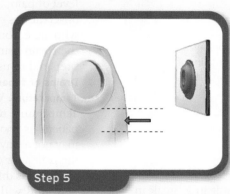

Step 5

Attach the appliance to the wafer.

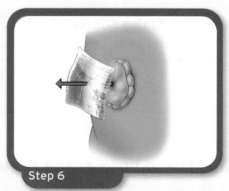

Step 6

Remove the gauze.

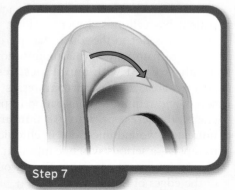

Step 7

Remove the paper backing from the wafer.

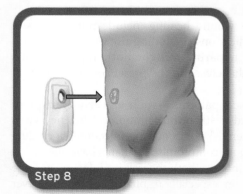

Step 8

Apply the appliance with the stoma centred in the wafer cutout.

Some wounds may be left open and unsutured to promote healing from within. In other cases, sutures or staples are used to hold the edges of a wound together; most are removed 5 to 10 days after repair. In contrast, stay sutures and retention sutures hold both skin and underlying fat or muscle together and may be left in place for 14 to 21 days.

Drains may also be sutured into place to allow liquids to escape and decrease tension on the sutures or staples. Drains are usually flat pieces of tubing that remain open on both ends. One end is placed deep within the wound; the other end lies on the skin, draining onto gauze dressing. Closed wound drainage systems rely on a tubing drain plus some type of negative pressure (suction). This kind of system prevents the entry of microorganisms into the drain and thus into the wound.

Wound Care

After exposing a wound for assessment, you should redress it to prevent further contamination. Encourage the patient to lie still while the wound is redressed. Apply a sterile dressing and secure it to the area prior to transport. This dressing should cover the surface of the wound and the surrounding area and should not be either too tight or too loose. You may need to apply a bulky dressing to a wound to help protect it during transfer and transport.

Always reassess the patient's pain level and tolerance to the dressing following the procedure. Patients with limited mobility may be uncomfortable during movement with a dressing in place. Providing reassurance, direction, and comfort to the patient and carers during these procedures will enhance their sense of control and comfort. Provide pain relief as required.

Maternal/Child Health Risks

Each year in the United Kingdom there are approximately 4 million births. More than a half million infants were born preterm in 2004, and infants were also more likely to be born low birth weight (< 2,500 g). In addition, the percentage of preterm births (infants born at less than 37 weeks of gestation) has increased slightly. Caesarean deliveries are also at an all-time high. Women may deliver at home, or may spend anything from a few hours to several days in a health care setting, typically a hospital maternity unit. Each of these factors contributes to the increased need for home care for women and infants in the postpartum period.

Complications in the postpartum period include postpartum bleeding, depression, sepsis, pulmonary embolus, and infant septicaemia. Postpartum bleeding or haemorrhage is the leading cause of maternal death. This occurs in as many as 10 out of 100 births. When you are obtaining the mother's history, asking her about postpartum bleeding in a previous pregnancy is important as a significant risk factor.

Pulmonary embolus is another complication that may occur in the postpartum period. The risk of pulmonary embolus is increased in both pregnancy and in the postpartum period. The incidence of thromboembolic disease in pregnancy has been reported to range from 1 case in 200 deliveries to 1 case in 1,400 deliveries and is caused by venous stasis, decreasing fibrinolytic activity, and increased procoagulant factors.

Depression that occurs during pregnancy or within a year after delivery is called perinatal or postnatal depression. During pregnancy the amount of oestrogen and progesterone increases greatly. In the first 24 hours after childbirth, the amount of hormones rapidly drops back down to their normal prepregnancy levels. After pregnancy, similar hormonal changes may trigger symptoms of depression. The number of women affected with depression during this time is unknown, but some researchers suggest that depression is one of the most common complications during and after pregnancy. It is often not recognised or treated because normal changes during pregnancy such as fatigue, insomnia, strong emotional reactions, and changes in body weight may occur during pregnancy and after pregnancy. These same symptoms may also be signs of depression. The key to treatment is early recognition and referral.

Infants have immature physiology that can result in an inability to regulate temperature, adapt to respiratory problems, or respond to infection because of poorly functioning

You are the Paramedic Part 4

The patient's wife was able to catheterise her husband while he sat upright in his wheelchair. The catheter drained 800 ml of urine. An IV line was established in the right antecubital with an 18-gauge needle. During transport you note that the swelling in the patient's abdomen has almost resolved and it is now soft upon palpation. He states that his headache is almost relieved and that he no longer has blurred vision.

Upon arrival to the A&E department, the patient's symptoms have almost resolved. He is monitored in the emergency room and discharged after a short period of observation, with a diagnosis of autonomic hyperreflexia syndrome.

Reassessment	Recording Time: 18 Minutes
Skin	Pale, warm, and dry
Pulse	80 beats/min
Blood pressure	144/82 mm Hg
Respirations	16 breaths/min, unlaboured
S_PO_2	99% on room air
ECG	Sinus rhythm without ectopy

6. What is the pathophysiology of autonomic hyperreflexia syndrome?

7. What are signs and symptoms of autonomic hyperreflexia syndrome?

immune systems. All of these factors have an impact on sepsis, which is one of the most common causes of infant death.

In 2002, infant death from sepsis was 7 per 1,000 live births. Some pregnancy complications that can increase the risk of sepsis for a newborn include maternal bleeding, maternal fever, infection in the uterus, and premature rupture of membranes. Sepsis in newborns produces few symptoms and is difficult to determine. Frequently, these babies suddenly don't seem to be feeling well or "just don't look right" to those who care for them. Listen to the carer: any baby who has a change in mental status should be transported immediately for further evaluation and treatment.

Less than 1% of births occur unexpectedly at home. Once the baby has delivered, either before or on your arrival, a newborn examination should be conducted. Most newborns are healthy and need little treatment. Make sure the midwife, if not present, has been contacted. Transport decisions should be based on local guidelines and family requests. Discuss child safety restraint issues of newborns before you encounter an emergency delivery in the home. The five steps to follow in the approach to assessing a newborn are the same in any setting:

- Dry and warm the baby.
- Clear the airway.
- Assess breathing.
- Assess pulse rate.
- Assess colour.

A depressed newborn does not respond to drying, warming, and clearing the airway. These babies require resuscitation.

Paediatric Apnoea

Premature newborns or those with congenital heart, lung, or neurological problems often require home care, including an apnoea monitor. Healthy infants may experience periods of apnoea, especially during sleep. If the apnoea is prolonged, is frequent, or occurs with a drop in pulse rate or a change in skin colour or muscle tone, it is not normal. Home monitoring of apnoea may be indicated when an infant:

- Has unresolved apnoea of prematurity at the time of hospital discharge.
- Has severe gastroesophageal reflux.
- Has a history of an apparent life-threatening event.
- Is the sibling of a baby who had sudden unexplained death in infancy.

Carers are taught to stimulate the infant if the low pulse rate or apnoea alarm sounds; you may be called if stimulation doesn't work. Be prepared to provide positive-pressure ventilation and remember that newborns—especially premature

At the Scene

False alarms are common with apnoea monitors and may be caused by movement, loose lead wires, or improperly placed electrodes. When in doubt, follow your local ambulance service guidelines and have the family contact the manufacturer of the device.

babies—have difficulty in controlling their body temperatures. Keep the infant warm, including covering the infant's head.

Hospice/Comfort Care

Patients in hospice care can experience pain and discomfort from tumour growth, treatment modalities (eg, radiation and chemotherapy), immobility, inflammation, or infection. Treatment of hospice patients is based on the type and severity of pain. Patients initially receive around-the-clock anti-inflammatory medications, often coupled with antianxiety or antiemetic agents. When this regime no longer manages the pain, the patient may receive a mild opioid/opiate. A strong opioid/opiate may be added later, along with antianxiety and antiemetic medications.

Pain may also be managed by mechanical or electrical means. Transcutaneous electrical nerve stimulators (TENS) relieve pain by competing for nerve transmission pathways with the painful stimulus. Less pain stimulation reaches the brain, so the patient feels less pain. In addition, simple comfort measures are important in providing pain reduction and comfort to the patient. Turning, positioning, and supporting body parts with blanket rolls or pillows can increase comfort. Maintaining a comfortable room temperature helps. Hands-on or energy-based therapies such as massage may be used.

Some health care providers are concerned that hospice patients may overdose on pain medications. This problem, however, is not as frequent as patients being undermedicated. If you suspect that a hospice patient has received too much medication, you should begin the assessment and treatment as for any other patient. Opioids/opiates affect the respiratory drive centre, so pay close attention and care to breathing adequacy. Although naloxone can reverse the effects of opioids/opiates, the goal in these cases is to enable the patient to breathe sufficiently on his or her own. Complete reversal of the effects of the opioid/opiate will return the patient to intractable pain, initiation of the sympathetic response, and a sudden increase in blood pressure and pulse rate.

Progressive Dementia

Dementia is a progressive brain disorder with an insidious onset in which cognitive activities are lost first, followed by physical abilities. Causes of dementia may include Alzheimer's disease, Pick's disease, Parkinson's disease, and stroke. Some nutritional disorders, such as Wernicke disease or Korsakoff psychosis, can also cause dementia.

Concerns regarding patients with dementia include injuries resulting from loss of judgement and insight, confusion when using medications, and becoming lost when leaving home or a familiar environment. Carers may also be at risk if the patient experiences paranoia. Early dementia can be managed in the home setting, but advanced dementia generally requires nursing home care.

Chronic Pain Management

Pain is a subjective term. *Nociception* is a term that more accurately describes the transmission of stimuli over specific nerve pathways. All nociceptors (ie, pain receptors) begin as free nerve endings and end in the dorsal (ascending) roots of the spinal cord. Some respond to mechanical damage, some to thermal damage, and some to chemical damage. The skin, joints, and musculature are well supplied with pain receptors, whereas the visceral organs have a limited number of pain receptors and the brain has no pain receptors. There are two major types of nociceptors: alpha (fast) fibres, which transmit a sharp, localised type of pain usually associated with an injury, and C (slow) fibres, which transmit a slow pain (often described as burning, throbbing, or aching) typically associated with long-term conditions.

Acute pain occurs immediately after an injury or surgery. Chronic pain occurs long after relief of the initiating cause is achieved; it may also be defined as pain lasting for 6 months or longer. Some research indicates that failure to treat acute pain adequately may lead to chronic pain.

The body perceives pain as a stressor. In response, it activates the sympathetic nervous system, leading to elevated blood pressure, tachycardia, and tachypnoea. Energy stores are needed to maintain this sympathetic response, even though they could be better used for healing. Effective management of pain reduces energy consumption and allows for rest and healing.

Home Chemotherapy

Chemotherapy refers to the introduction of either single cytotoxic drugs or combinations of cytotoxic drugs into the body for the purpose of interrupting or eradicating malignant cellular growth. The many side effects of these treatments include alopecia (hair loss), anorexia, fatigue, leucopenia (decreased numbers of leucocytes), thrombocytopenia (decreased numbers of platelets), anaemia, and increased risk of infections. During radiation therapy, painful blisters may develop at the treatment site.

Patients receiving chemotherapy routinely take multiple medications. Some of these drugs are given to battle the disease process, while others are intended to manage the symptoms of the side effects of chemotherapy. Analgesic medication patches and antiemetics are commonly prescribed. In addition, peripheral access devices may be surgically placed to aid in the delivery of these medications. Use of these devices to deliver medication requires specialised training. Follow your local guideline or direction from a GP when using these devices.

Patients with cancer often have seriously depressed immune systems, owing to either the treatment regime or the disease process. To safeguard patients from infection, wash your hands before and after contact and wear a mask. Reverse isolation, in which the patient wears a mask, is also suggested.

Transplant Recipients

Organ transplants are considered for the treatment of a failing organ or organs. The paramedic must remember that a patient who has recently undergone a transplant is at risk of infection and take steps to protect the patient—for example, by using reverse isolation, in which the patient wears a mask.

You should encourage transplant patients and carers to bring all medications and any other information to hospital with them if transport is indicated.

Psychosocial Support

Adaptation and adjustment to a chronic illness do not occur all at once. Stages of adaptation and adjustment are varied and individual, and an unexpected event can trigger readjustment needs in a patient thought to have adjusted to his or her condition. When faced with such an illness, individuals are likely to proceed through a sense of loss or mourning that is similar to that experienced by survivors of a loved one's death Table 45-5 ▾ . The goal of adjustment is acceptance of the

At the Scene

Prehospital providers often find it most difficult to work with patients who are in the acceptance stage of the dying process because the patient appears to have given up. In chronic illness or during injury adjustment, this stage may be the easiest. Allow the patient to do as much as possible for himself or herself. Talk with the patient or carer so that you are aware of what the patient expects from your treatment.

Table 45-5	Stages of Adjustment to Chronic Illness	
Stages	**Behaviours**	**Paramedic Response**
Denial	Refusal to follow plan	Treat result of refusal; stay non-judgemental/non-argumentative; educate/reinforce plan
Anger	Verbal or physical abuse	Anger is an acceptable emotion, abuse is not; set limits; retreat if the scene is unsafe; call for assistance; provide care when the scene becomes safe; document
Bargaining	Refusal to follow plan as part of bargain	Restate options; incorporate the bargain as possible
Withdrawal with depression	Profound sadness, reduction in interaction and eye contact, listlessness	Provide reassurance
Acceptance	Adaptive behaviours	Be supportive

At the Scene

A terminally ill patient has the following rights:
1. The right to know the truth
2. The right to confidentiality and privacy
3. The right to consent to treatment
4. The right to choose the place to die
5. The right to determine the disposition of his or her body

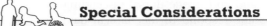

Special Considerations

Paramedics must often assume the role of health educators. At the appropriate time during a call, encourage the carer to prepare a list including the following items:

- Telephone list of all family and friends who should be notified of a change in the patient's condition
- Current medications, ventilator settings, tracheostomy tube type and care, tube feeding type and amount, ostomy type and appliance

condition and construction of a realistic life plan incorporating the new strengths and limitations.

Patients receiving home care are encouraged to make end-of-life decisions early in their care, if they haven't already. A durable power of attorney (DPOA; also called a health care proxy) allows a patient to appoint someone to make health care decisions in the event that he or she becomes incapacitated. The decisions covered by a DPOA include discontinuation of life support in the event of a terminal illness or injury, discontinuation and removal of life-sustaining equipment in the event of an irreversible coma, and termination of artificial nutrition and hydration. For more information, see Chapter 4.

Do not attempt resuscitation (DNAR) and do not intubate forms are general practitioners' orders to withhold life-sustaining treatment in the event of cardiac or respiratory arrest. These orders do *not* mean that no treatment should be given. That is, patients should receive pain medication, supplemental oxygen therapy, nutrition, and hydration as needed based on assessment.

You are the Paramedic Summary

1. Does treating a patient with chronic health problems affect the way you deliver emergency care?

The emergency care given to a patient with a chronic illness is no different from the care given to a person who is acutely ill. What may change is the method of delivery. For example, medications may be administered through an indwelling cannula such a peripheral inserted central catheter (PICC) line or oxygen therapy may be delivered via a tracheostomy tube.

2. What groups of patients are likely to benefit from home care?

Quite a few groups of patients benefit from home health care. As technology advances, the number of illnesses that can be treated at home is on the rise. For example, you might treat patients with spinal cord injuries, chronic neuromuscular disorders such as multiple sclerosis, respiratory illnesses such as cystic fibrosis, and patients with advanced heart failure. One important thing to remember is that there is no age limit to those receiving home health care, as diseases have no age barriers.

3. What type of equipment might you encounter with patients receiving home health care?

Just as the types of disease processes you will encounter are wide and varied, so is the type of equipment you might encounter. Common examples of equipment used in the home setting include tracheostomy tubes, ventilators, CPAP machines, urinary catheters, gastrostomy tubes, and indwelling IV cannulas. A good rule of thumb to follow is: if you are unfamiliar with the equipment do not use it! Carers are excellent resources for you to use. Ask for help in understanding how a specific piece of equipment works. When you are in doubt how to use a piece of equipment, call the patient's GP for guidance.

4. Why did the doctor recommended catheterising the patient's bladder prior to transport?

Spinal cord injuries can make the body work in strange ways! In some spinal cord injury patients, the pressure of a full bladder can trigger a significant rise in blood pressure. If the pressure is not relieved, the hypertension can lead to further damage or death.

5. Why is it important that the patient's wishes for a full resuscitation be known?

Knowing a person's wishes regarding resuscitation is important because the person may have a completely different view of life with a chronic illness or injury. Your patient has had time to adjust to living as a quadriplegic and may view his life as meaningful and fulfilling in a new way. You must abide by your patient's wishes and not try to impose your impressions of how a person's life must be on the patient. Remember, what you may consider as a handicap may be considered a blessing to someone who is living with the condition.

6. What is the pathophysiology of autonomic hyperreflexia syndrome?

Autonomic hyperreflexia syndrome (also called autonomic dysreflexia) is seen in patients with a spinal cord injury above the T6 level. It results from a stimulus being introduced to areas of the body below the spinal cord. Common stimuli are the pressure caused by a distended bladder or rectum. The stimulus travels up the spinal cord until it becomes blocked, preventing it from reaching the brain. As a result, the sympathetic nerve receptors below the injury site cause a rise in blood pressure. This increase in pressure is then detected by the baroreceptors, which stimulate the parasympathetic nervous system in an attempt to lower the blood pressure. Since the signals cannot travel below the injury, the blood pressure remains elevated while the pulse rate decreases. If the blood pressure remains elevated it can become life-threatening.

7. What are signs and symptoms of autonomic hyperreflexia syndrome?

The signs and symptoms include paroxysmal hypertension (systolic pressure can reach as high as 300 mm Hg), pounding headache, blurred vision, sweating above the level of injury, increased nasal congestion, nausea, bradycardia, and a distended rectum or bladder.

Prep Kit

■ Ready for Review

- Breakthrough technologies, newer drugs, and research have combined to increase the average life expectancy. People who might have died of injuries or illnesses 50 years ago may now continue to lead satisfying and productive lives.
- Many of these patients require physical support and care of chronic illnesses—care that may take place in the home setting.
- In rehabilitation care, the focus is on restoration of a person with disabilities to his or her maximum potential along several fronts: physical, social, spiritual, psychological, and vocational areas.
- Chronically ill patients are cared for at home by a wide range of carers, who may include family members, unlicensed carers, licensed nonprofessional carers, licensed professionals, or a combination of these.
- Consumers of home health care are vulnerable, are frequently too sick to advocate for themselves, and may lack advocates. Paramedics have a unique opportunity to assist in securing additional resources, reporting to protective agencies, and offering guidance for in-home injury prevention.
- Many family members who care for chronically ill patients are medically sophisticated and are often the paramedic's best source of information and care guidelines.
- In the home care setting, you may encounter patients who are chronically ill or permanently injured, as well as those who have recently had a hospital stay, surgery, or a high-risk pregnancy. You may also encounter newborns with medical complications. Many of these patients experience similar physical problems regardless of the initial cause.
- Assessment of the chronic care patient follows the standard guidelines. Ask the carers how the patient's condition differs today.
- It is important to assess for airway patency in all patients, but especially in patients with artificial airways.
- Patients with respiratory compromise have the inability to adequately ventilate themselves. The home care treatment plan is designed to supplement the patient's loss of respiratory effort. Any stressor can tip the balance, increase the severity of signs and symptoms, and render the current respiratory support inadequate.
- Ventilators mechanically deliver air to the lungs. Home ventilators are smaller than most microwave ovens, use regular household electricity, and may include a battery backup.
- Patients who have chronic cardiovascular disease are often cared for in the home setting. Many patients have cardiac insufficiency or heart failure, an inability of the heart to keep up with the demands placed on it and failure of the heart to pump blood efficiently.
- Central venous cannulas are used for many types of home care patients, including those receiving chemotherapy, long-term antibiotic therapy or pain management, high-concentration glucose solutions, and haemodialysis.
- A gastric tube may be placed when a patient cannot ingest fluids, food, or medications by mouth.
- Chronically ill patients and patients with neurological damage may require a long-term indwelling urinary catheter or intermittent urinary catheterisation.
- A wound with minor redness, slight warmth to the touch, and swelling may indicate a superficial infection. A painful reddened area with cracks, serous drainage, or red streaks extending from the area may indicate that the patient has cellulitis. Cellulitis may be more severe and require hospitalisation in patients who have venous stasis, diabetes, or who are immunocompromised.
- Complications in the postpartum period that you may see in the prehospital environment include postpartum bleeding, depression, sepsis, pulmonary embolus, and infant septicaemia. You may also be called to assist with paediatric apnoea monitors.
- Patients in hospice care can experience pain and discomfort from tumour growth, treatment modalities (eg, radiation and chemotherapy), immobility, inflammation, or infection. Treatment of hospice patients is based on the type and severity of pain.
- Patients receiving home care are encouraged to make end-of-life decisions early in their care. A durable power of attorney allows a patient to appoint someone to make health care decisions in the event that he or she becomes incapacitated.

■ Vital Vocabulary

chemotherapy The introduction of either single cytotoxic drugs or combinations of cytotoxic drugs into the body for the purpose of interrupting or eradicating malignant cellular growth.

chronic obstructive pulmonary disease (COPD) Illnesses that cause obstructive problems in the lower airways, including chronic bronchitis, emphysema, and sometimes asthma.

colostomy Establishment of an opening between the colon and the surface of the body for the purpose of providing drainage of the bowel.

dehiscence Separation of the edges of a wound.

dementia Chronic deterioration of mental functions.

Do Not Intubate Written documentation by a general practitioner giving permission to medical personnel not to attempt intubation.

Do Not Attempt Resuscitation (DNAR) Written documentation by a general practitioner giving permission to medical personnel not to attempt resuscitation in the event of cardiac arrest.

ejection fraction The fraction of the end-diastolic volume that is ejected with each ventricle beat; it is the stroke volume divided by end-diastolic volume and is expressed as a percentage.

ileostomy Surgical procedure to remove large portions of the small intestine.

laryngectomy A surgical procedure in which the larynx is removed.

negative-pressure ventilation Drawing of air into the lungs; airflow from a region of higher pressure (outside the body) to a region of lower pressure (the lungs); occurs during normal (unassisted breathing).

oxygen concentrators Large, electrical devices that concentrate the oxygen in ambient air and eliminate other gases

positive-pressure ventilation Forcing of air into the lungs.

purulent exudates Discharge that contains pus.

serous exudates Discharge that contains serum, a thin watery substance.

tidal volume Amount of air inhaled or exhaled during normal, quiet breathing; the volume of one breath.

tracheostomy Surgical opening into the trachea.

ureterostomy The formation of an opening to allow the passage of urine.

Assessment in Action

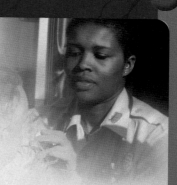

You are dispatched to the home of a 68-year-old man for an altered mental status. When you arrive on scene, you are greeted by his daughter, who tells you that the patient is an insulin-dependent diabetic whose blood sugar is 34. He is also a paraplegic from a traumatic accident 5 years before. His daughter tells you that the night before her father was experiencing upper body pain, which is typical, but it seemed to be worse yesterday. You administer glucagon and oral carbohydrates. The patient becomes alert and orientated and refuses transport to hospital. His only remaining complaint is his increased pain.

1. **Pain can be classified as _____ and _____.**
   A. Acute, surgical
   B. Chronic, traumatic
   C. Acute, chronic
   D. Subjective, stimuli

2. **Chronic pain is defined as:**
   A. pain lasting up to 3 months.
   B. pain lasting longer than 6 months.
   C. pain lasting only 2 months.
   D. pain lasting less than 3 months.

3. **The _____ nervous system is activated in the face of pain.**
   A. sympathetic
   B. parasympathetic
   C. cholinergic
   D. anticholinergic

4. **_____ is the more accurate term describing transmission of stimuli over specific nerve pathways.**
   A. Nociception
   B. Parasympathetic
   C. Sympathetic
   D. Receptor

5. **Management of pain _____, which allows for rest and healing.**
   A. increases energy consumption
   B. reduces energy consumption
   C. does nothing
   D. maintains the sympathetic response

6. **Ambulance clinicians must assume:**
   A. the patient is well cared for.
   B. the patient is being abused.
   C. the role of the legal guardian.
   D. the role of health educators.

7. **True or false? Conduct the initial assessment of the patient with chronic illness in the same way as for any other patient.**
   A. False
   B. True

Challenging Question

You are dispatched to the private home of an 84-year-old man. When you arrive, the family greets you and tells you that the patient called 999 complaining of chest pain, but the patient has Alzheimer's disease. The family does not believe the patient has any complaints, and they do not want him transported to hospital.

8. **What course of action should you take?**

Points to Ponder

You and your partner are dispatched to the home of a 72-year-old woman with a complaint of respiratory distress. When you arrive on scene, you are greeted by the patient's home health care provider. She tells you that the patient has terminal cancer. For the last 2 days, the patient has experienced an increase in shortness of breath. Her respiratory rate is 32 breaths/min; blood pressure, 100/60 mm Hg; pulse oximetry on supplemental oxygen, 94%; and pulse rate, 110 beats/min, sinus tachycardia on the monitor. The patient has breast cancer with metastasis to the lungs. Her family is in the process of placing the patient into hospice care, but the paperwork has not been completed yet.

Given the history of lung cancer and immunosuppression, what condition do you suspect? Should you transport the patient?

Issues: The Role of the Home Health Care Professional, Dealing With Family and Friends as Home Health Care Providers.

www.Paramedic.EMSzone.com/UK/

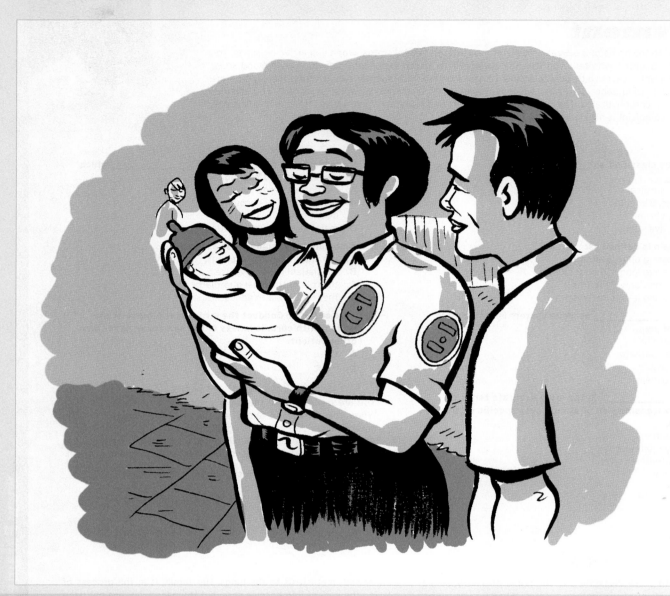

" It's not the ones you lose, but the ones you save by being there just when they needed you. We provide countless numbers of sons and daughters, husbands and wives, fathers and mothers with the precious gift of more time".

—Garry Briese

Operations

7

Section

Section Editors: David G. Jones and Tim Jones

46 Ambulance Operations

Objectives

Cognitive

- Identify current government policy, legislation, and performance standards that influence ambulance design, deployment, equipment requirements, and staffing.
- Discuss the importance of completing an ambulance vehicle daily inspection (VDI) and checklist.
- Discuss the factors to be considered when determining ambulance dispatch points within communities.
- Describe the advantages and disadvantages of air ambulance transport.
- Identify the conditions/situations in which specialised support, including air ambulances, may be beneficial.

Affective

- Reflect on personal practices relative to ambulance operations which may affect the safety of your colleagues, the patient, and bystanders.
- Serve as a role model for others relative to the operation of ambulances.
- Value the need to serve as the patient advocate to ensure appropriate patient care at all times.

Psychomotor

- Demonstrate safe use of a variety of patient manual handling aids to care safely for a patient in various settings, including how to place a patient in, and remove a patient from, an ambulance.

Introduction

Driving an emergency vehicle is an enormous responsibility. Not only do you have to be aware of the safety of yourself and colleagues, you are also responsible for the safety of patients and carers as well as the safe passage of other road users. This responsibility is not optional; it goes with the job, the uniform and the vehicle. The public will look to you to set exemplary standards: an ambulance is a conspicuous vehicle and the manner in which it is driven will not go unnoticed. Whether driving an ambulance routinely or undertaking an emergency journey, you are expected to abide by all aspects of the law and the Highway Code. Whilst you are not entitled to break the law, there are certain exemptions that can be claimed to facilitate an emergency response. Activating the lights and sirens does not guarantee that you will be seen, heard, or understood by other road users. Using blues and twos does not give you the automatic right of way, but can improve the progress you make, however they are also associated with an increase in risk. Do not use them lightly. Do not abuse the privilege, and never be fooled into thinking that they will prevent accidents or collisions.

History of Ground Ambulances

Over the years, much has changed in the way that patients are transported to emergency care facilities. During the French Revolutionary Wars (1790s), Dr. Dominique-Jean Larrey conceived the idea of a mobile transport system for casualties. The first vehicles used for this purpose were horse-drawn wagons called flying ambulances and were part of an ambulance corps. This corps consisted of a doctor, a quartermaster, a non-commissioned officer, a drummer boy to carry bandages, and 24 infantrymen to protect them. Even with such a large entourage they were able to remove victims from the battlefield within 15 minutes (**Figure 46-1 ▶**).

The first recognisable ambulances in the United Kingdom are likely to have been "pest coaches" as referred to by Samuel Pepys in his diary of August 3, 1665. This transport of the sick was initially provided for the benefit of the "well" populations. Those poor souls suffering signs of plague were removed from their neighbourhoods in an attempt to halt its rapid spread. For years transport for the sick was generally haphazard and often inappropriate. However there were instances of recognis-

able beneficence; for instance in 1767, records for Staffordshire Royal Infirmary detail a "sprung carriage for the conveyance of the sick or maimed—from any distance". Fever hospitals and asylums sporadically provided transport in the form of sedan chairs and later a chaise or litter. It is the city of Liverpool that is generally acknowledged as one of the pioneers of organised horse drawn transport for the sick and injured. Across the UK, each city, town, and borough developed its own ambulance systems, often initiated with police constables conveying injured people from public places.

The 999 telephone number was introduced in the late 1930s but it was not until the Second World War that "prehospital care" rather than the simple transport of casualties became a real consideration. Traditionally, the art of medicine was delivered by general practitioners (GPs) within their own communities. At the scene of a road traffic collision the prime consideration would be to transport the casualty to skilled help rather than get the help to the patient. First aid became an integral skill for many and with the knowledge gained in theatres of war—from Napoleonic times through to Korea and Vietnam, it became more generally accepted that certain key interventions should be undertaken without delay and would subsequently reduce mortality. "Stretcher bearers" and ambulance "drivers" progressed by acquiring enhanced training; police constables, first aiders, and civil defence corps slowly gave way to the professional ambulance services of today, staffed by highly skilled, well trained and educated dispatchers, emergency medical technicians, and paramedics.

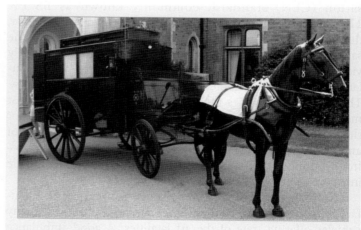

Figure 46-1 Horse-drawn ambulance carriage.

You are the Paramedic Part 1

You and your colleague have been dispatched to the scene of a road traffic collision on the nearby dual carriageway. Ambulance control advises you that they have received several calls regarding the accident, with the potential for multiple casualties. It is approaching 15.30 hrs and you realise that the schools have turned out, it is raining heavily and the roads are already congested.

1. What are some of the potential hazards you may encounter en route to the scene?
2. What dangers must be considered when approaching the scene with regard to parking and personnel protection?

Ambulance Equipment

Along with the acquisition of new skills, ambulance staff were required to be familiar with increasing amounts of equipment. From resuscitators and oxygen regulators, airway adjuncts and splints, trolley cots, and stretchers the equipment lists grew and included in some services "surgeon's tools" such as scalpels and amputation saws. An influential parliamentary review in the mid 1960s, known as the Millar Report, recommended not only standardisation of equipment for ambulance services but more importantly rigorous standards for training. Since then, advances in technology and medical sciences means procedures and treatments once confined to hospital premises are now commonplace "in the street". Today's ambulance will have numerous pieces of equipment on board and ambulance crews need to be able to use a full range of diagnostic and monitoring equipment. They also need an underpinning knowledge of how to interpret their findings.

Although ambulance designs vary depending on the base chassis and local needs, they are now all recognisable as sharing a common goal, that of providing a safe, prompt, and clinically effective environment for patient care. These days many ambulance service vehicles are not equipped to convey patients but are still used by ambulance technicians and paramedics as fast or rapid response vehicles.

Basic layout and capabilities for ambulances have been recommended across Europe by the Comité Européen de Normalisation (CEN) standard, commonly known as BS EN 1789:2000—Medical Vehicles and their Equipment. However, due to the importance of the requirements for ensuring the safety of both patients and ambulance staff, it has been widely viewed as a standard specification requirement for new ambulances and therefore adopted within most of the health industry. The standard "specifies the requirements for the design, test methods, performance, and equipping of road ambulances for the transport of sick or injured persons". Various levels of ambulance fitment are covered depending on intended use—from routine transports (types A_1 and A_2) through to mobile intensive care front line specifications (type C).

Collaborative design of ambulances between users, manufacturers, academics, and patients has now produced many vehicles offering state of the art facilities. A good ambulance design should allow you to treat your patient safely. Equipment should be easily accessible but safely stowed. Surfaces should be of the type that are easily cleaned and have no sharp edges, and ergonomic considerations should influence the placement and detail of the layout and design. Ambulances should be highly conspicuous even in the poorest visibility, provide a level of comfort for the patient, and a suitable safe and clean working environment for you and your colleagues.

Checking the Ambulance

Getting ready to respond to a call is an essential part of patient care. At the beginning of each shift, you must check the ambulance to ensure the proper equipment is available and in good working order. Every time supplies and equipment are used, they should be properly cleaned or replaced and returned to service for the next call. Some ambulance trusts now assist crews with the provision of "make ready" services where specialised staff check, restock, and deep-clean vehicles on a regular basis, sometimes after each shift or every 24 hours. It may be considered more efficient for you to be starting a shift on a pre-checked vehicle rather than being delayed sourcing supplies. It should never be forgotten however that the roadworthiness of an ambulance is still the responsibility of the person driving the vehicle. The legal requirements are the same as for driving other vehicles and you must ensure that you comply fully—there are no exemptions because of emergency or "blue-light" status. Visual inspection of the vehicle for any defects or damage should be a daily routine, as should checking fluid levels in the engine compartment and serviceability of lights, windscreen washers, horn or sirens, etc. Ambulance crews will still want to reassure themselves that their ambulance is ready for the first call, equipment is in place, monitors powered and calibrated, medications secure and in date, documentation to hand, and personal issue protective equipment ready for wearing. Whatever systems are in place within your area, it is vital that the vehicle daily inspection (VDI) process is followed and documented.

Ambulance Compartments

All compartments in the ambulance should be checked regularly, both inside and out. Most ambulances carry the larger immobilisation and splinting equipment in the outside compartments for easy access when speed may be an important factor in patient care `Figure 46-2 ▶`. Medications and temperature-sensitive equipment are generally stored in the patient compartment area. The following list specifies some examples of the detail contained in CEN recommendations for essential equipment that should be found on front line emergency ambulances:

- Main stretcher/undercarriage EN 1865
- Pick up stretcher EN 1865
- Vacuum mattress EN 1865
- Device for conveying a seated patient EN 1865
- Carrying sheet or transfer mattress EN 1865
- Longboard complete with head immobiliser and securing straps EN 1865
- Traction device
- Immobilisation set for fractures
- Immobilisation devices for cervical and upper spine
- Cervical collar-set

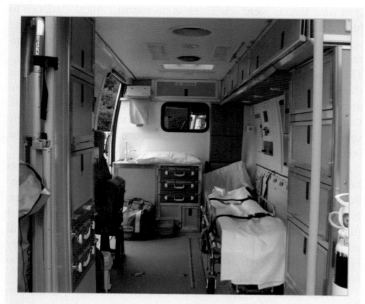

Figure 46-2 Equipment found in an ambulance.

- Extrication devices or short longboard
- Stationary oxygen—minimum 2,000 l; Portable oxygen— minimum 400 l; Resuscitators with oxygen inlet and masks and airways for all ages and oxygen reservoir
- Mouth-to-mask ventilator with oxygen inlet
- Non-manual suction device with a minimum pressure of −65 kPa with a minimum capacity of 1 litre
- Manual BP monitor, cuff size 10 cm to 66 cm
- Automatic BP monitor, cuff size 10 cm to 66 cm
- Oximeter EN 1865
- Stethoscope
- Thermometer
- Device for blood glucose determination

Documentation and Communication

The mechanical aspects of emergency work, such as driving and moving patients, can have an impact on your safety and the safety of others. Your service should have specific procedures for daily inspections and documenting vehicle movements throughout the shift. Following these procedures protects you physically, and documenting your compliance is an important legal protection. Procedures should call for dating and signing of the check sheets. Store these sheets in conjunction with your services policy, so they can be referenced later if needed.

Ambulance Staffing and Development

During the 1990s and since the turn of the millennium, the provision of a wide range of health care services have come under review. How and when patients access care and the role of ambulance services in England has come under scrutiny, with particular focus on which health care needs ambulance trusts can, and should, provide for. Various government papers have discussed National Health Service urgent, emergency, and out-of-hours care. The most influential for ambulance services has been "Taking Healthcare to the Patient, Transforming NHS Ambulance Services" published by the Department of Health in June 2005. Setting the direction for future developments, the main recommendations of this document are for an improvement in the provision of clinical advice to callers (hear and treat); a greater range of mobile health care providers (see and treat); an enhanced range of primary care, diagnostic, and health promotion services, as well as continued excellence in providing emergency care.

It is likely that these proposed changes in service provision will see some fundamental changes in how ambulance services are delivered in the future. It is also likely that there will need to be a significant reduction in double-staffed stretcher ambulances in favour of an increase in mobile single responders responsible for initial assessment, face-to-face triage, and the onward referral of patients. It should be remembered that ambulance services are only a part of NHS health care provision and do not function in isolation. It will ultimately be up to the public, politicians, and health commissioners (who buy in services) what level of care will be provided, where, and by whom.

The implementation of these recommendations has required a significant change in ambulance service structure and staffing. As of July 2006, ambulance trusts in England have merged to form 13 regional ambulance trusts from the previous 31 county based services. Services in Wales, Scotland, Northern Ireland, and the Channel Islands are not directly affected by the review.

It is recognised that the traditional model of transporting the majority of patients seen by ambulance crews to an accident and emergency (A&E) department does not meet the needs of many patients who activate the 999 system. It is becoming increasingly accepted that ambulance staff can deal with the patient's needs safely and effectively and can arrange safe and appropriate referral of patients onto a variety of care pathways other than routine admission to A&E. This may occur as the result of telephone advice to callers (supported by clinical decision making software) or a face-to-face assessment of the patient's true clinical need. Options of care may include simple surgical procedures provided at home such as primary wound closure, administration of primary care medicines using patient group directions (PGDs), or referral to an integrated primary care service such as community nurses or general practitioners. If you are to undertake such management and referrals safely, you will need to undertake thorough holistic assessments of patients' needs.

Although demand for ambulance services has been increasing year on year, many callers do not need the attendance of a paramedic-crewed ambulance with all its life saving skills and equipment. Increasingly patients access the emergency services with complex health and social needs and recent figures relating to ambulance calls suggest that only 15% of demand is for patients with possibly life-threatening conditions. It is quite likely that an increased range of responses will become available to ambulance services and the challenge will be to meet correctly the needs of those contacting the service.

Call Taking

Identifying emergency callers with life-threatening conditions and responding quickly with the right resource will always be the prime objective for any ambulance service. This process starts in the control centre where specialist staff triage calls to prioritise and identify the most appropriate response. This process of triage is driven by clinical algorithms that elicit priority symptoms from callers who often have no medical knowledge and, in some cases, no knowledge of the patient. As soon as key information is obtained resources can be activated to attend. Increasingly initial responses may differ from the traditional double-crewed ambulances and can involve skilled solo responders travelling by methods most suited to the environment, such as motorcycles, cars or even bicycles.

Without the support of technology, getting the right resource to the right patient in the right time would rely a lot on good fortune. Modern computer-aided dispatch (CAD) and automated vehicle location systems (AVLS) allow the pinpointing of resources which are linked to mapping systems. This enables real-time identification of resources and their status and the near instant transfer of information to data terminals or in-vehicle computer screens. If resources are pre-located in known areas of high demand, fast response times are far more likely.

Performance Measurements

Since the mid 1970s, ambulance services have been reporting on prompt performance rather than on clinical outcome. Traditionally all 999 calls were deemed an emergency and were responded to on a "first come first served" basis. More recently, requirements were stipulated to attend 75% of life-threatening calls within 8 minutes and 95% of calls in 14 minutes (urban) and within 19 minutes (rural). Following the NHS executive's commissioned "Review of Ambulance Performance Standards" in July 1996, services were strongly encouraged to prioritise 999 calls according to the clinical needs of the patients. Two commercial systems were available to assist in this task, criteria based dispatch (CBD) and advanced medical priority dispatch systems (later known as AMPDS). Having identified the priority of clinical need, it was then for the most serious or life threatened that strin-

gent time targets were set. There is no robust clinical evidence to justify 8 minutes as a target time for life-threatened patients. The origins are found within the science that predicts that, after 8 minutes of oxygen starvation, the brain can suffer irreversible damage. This was why the benchmark came into being. It is slightly ironic that an ambulance trust's *performance* has been measured on an arrival time and not the clinical care delivered following arrival. Current performance of UK ambulance services is monitored by various bodies. Latest figures for England can be accessed from the NHS via "The Information Centre" at the NHS web site.

It is only in the last decade that increased attention has been given to clinical audit and outcome measures for the prehospital phase of a patient's journey through the NHS. Some National Service Frameworks (NSFs) acknowledge the part played by ambulance staff in treating patients prior to hospital admission. Performance measures within the NSF for Coronary Heart Disease (March 2000) first cited the "call to door" time as well as "door to needle" time for thrombolytic therapy.

With good progress being made in developing common electronic systems for recording clinical patient details, much more emphasis is likely to be given to the benefits of the care delivered, rather than how quickly something was done.

When comparing ambulance trusts it may be useful to understand some of the key factors that are analysed in an effective, cost-efficient service as summarised below.

- **Response times.** High-performance systems typically use a fractile response time standard in which a significant fraction (usually 75% or 90%) of all responses must be achieved in an established time—for example, 8 minutes or less.
- **Clock start.** When the time keeping clock starts; currently when the chief complaint and address details are established, often 60 to 90 seconds after the call is connected. From April 2008, the "clock start" is taken from when the 999 call is connected to the control room.
- **Clock stop/on scene.** When help arrives at the patient or the location given (for instance, at the entrance to a block of flats). It should be noted that it is not necessary for an "ambulance" to arrive on scene, but the arrival of help or a responder that will have been dispatched by the ambulance service, but who should be suitably trained and equipped with a defibrillator.
- **Productivity.** The ambulance trust measures how many patient transports per hour each ambulance accomplishes (known as "unit-hour utilisation").
- **Unit costs.** Determined by the cost to respond to each call as well as the actual number of hours the units were actively operating, these costs include the crew members' salaries plus the operational cost of vehicles and equipment (fuel, routine maintenance, and repairs).

Some other factors to be taken into account might include geographical area and population served, demand patterns, budget and financial balance, clinical governance (which includes risk, complaints, patient satisfaction, clinical audit, effectiveness, clinical key performance indicators, and staff training and development).

System Status Management

System Status Management (SSM) is a concept that was developed by Jack Stout in 1983. The goals of SSM are to maximise efficiency and reduce response time. SSM uses historical data to determine ambulance service demands and then tries to take fluctuations in demand into consideration when organising service. For example, an increased demand for service may be noted during certain hours of the day or in certain geographical locations. These demands are termed peak loads. In an urban area, the demand for an ambulance service may be higher during the daytime but lower during the night. SSM attempts strategic deployment of ambulance resources in order to minimise response times. The strategic deployment of an ambulance to a location, known as listening watch or standby, can take advantage of developments in satellite vehicle location and GPS technologies.

Another component of SSM is peak demand staffing. Shift schedules are designed to provide a sufficient number of ambulances during peak load hours. For example, more ambulances might be staffed between 12:00 and 18:00 than between midnight and 06:00. One potentially negative aspect of SSM is the toll that it can take on personnel who have less time to get out of the vehicle and relax in the ambulance station between calls. To mitigate this, some services invest in standby points for ambulances that provide a parking bay for the vehicle and rest/refreshment facilities for crews. One service is reputed to have found it cost effective to rent a motel room to allow crews a comfortable, if brief, place of rest between calls.

Locating Ambulance Stations

The goals for establishing ambulance stations are to maximise efficiency and to minimise response times. In most urban and suburban areas, the distance factor may not be as important as the demand patterns and call volume. In a rural setting, both availability of first responders and distance may be equally important. Also, an area may have special features that create increased ambulance demand, for example major transport hubs, a high density of residential homes for the elderly or perhaps a particular area of social deprivation and poverty; all of which are factors known to increase demand for ambulance services. Although traditionally many communities have had their own ambulance stations, demand patterns can make these stations, with their associated overheads, difficult to justify. Consideration now is given to deploying resources into an area for cover and then returning to a more central ambulance depot for shift change-over, re-supply, and other support functions.

The Paramedic as an Emergency Health Care Professional

Since 2003 the term *paramedic* has been a registered title and can only be used by those who meet the standards of proficiency stipulated by the UK Health Professions Council. All staff, irrespective of grade or qualification, working on an ambulance have a responsibility to conduct themselves as professionals. Even in times of severe stress or fatigue, you should act as an advocate for the patient. You should always seek to deliver high-quality care without regard to time of day, the location of the call, or the appearance or conduct of the patient. Always remember that you represent your service, and your profession to the public, to your colleagues, and most importantly, to your patients and their families in their time of need.

> **Notes from Nancy**
>
> Even when you are attending a late job and in times of severe stress or fatigue, you should always act as an advocate for the patient.

▮ Emergency Vehicle Operation

All the advances made in prehospital care mean nothing if you never arrive. Driving an emergency vehicle requires you to be aware of *all* dangers on the roadway, including some that are not factors when you drive your private vehicle Figure 46-3 ▸ . Knowing where to look for these dangers is your responsibility whenever you get behind the wheel of an ambulance. Part of the ambulance service basic training requirement is to acquire advanced driving skills appropriate to the role you undertake. It is part of your continuing responsibility to refresh those skills, and to exercise caution at all times.

Use of Escorts

It is typically *not* a good idea to follow another emergency vehicle, such as a police car, through traffic as an escort. Many drivers will see only the first set of lights and sirens and assume that the way is clear once that vehicle has passed. If you are following another emergency vehicle, leave enough space between the vehicles so that other drivers (and you) have enough time to react and safely stop should someone pull in front of you unexpectedly.

You are the Paramedic Part 2

En route to the call you have received updated information that an ambulance and officer are on scene and report that there are four paediatric casualties, one of whom is still trapped in the wreckage.

3. How will knowing that there are multiple patients, including children, affect your driving?

4. Where should the ambulance be positioned at the scene of a road traffic collision if you are the *first* to arrive?

5. Where should the ambulance be positioned at the scene of a road traffic collision if you are *not* the first to arrive?

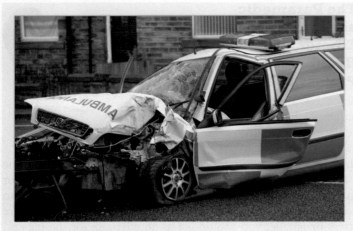

Figure 46-3 Always take care when driving.

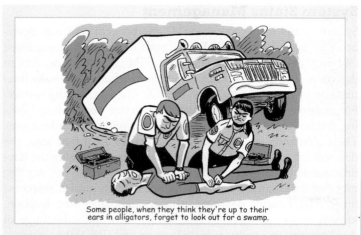

Some people, when they think they're up to their ears in alligators, forget to look out for a swamp.

Figure 46-4 Some people can't see the woods for the trees.

Another potential danger can occur when family members wish to follow closely behind you on the way to hospital. Both the ambulance and other drivers may have difficulty seeing the vehicles that are following. If you need to stop suddenly, there may be no time to react and the vehicle could collide with the ambulance. It is very important to advise family members before you leave the scene that they do not need to drive closely behind you and they must obey normal driving rules and regulations.

Use of Lights and Sirens

Despite improvements in the sophistication of 999 answering systems and in the accuracy of telephone triage protocols, most emergency ambulance crews are required to use their lights and sirens most of the time when responding to calls. In contrast, the decision to use lights and sirens when transporting patients to the hospital calls for judgements primarily based on the patient's clinical needs. The decision should not be taken lightly and is a balance of risk. There can be no set rules, as variables such as distance, travelling times, and traffic conditions will all impact on your decision to use lights and sirens when moving to hospital. Local guidelines usually require the ambulance control to be informed even if a hospital pre-alert is not required, even then, you must proceed with due regard for everyone's safety.

Driving to the Scene

The type of call can sometimes affect how an inexperienced driver might respond. When you hear that the call involves children, a cardiac arrest or a severe trauma, you may want to drive with less caution, feeling that speed is more important than safety. Nothing will speed up a driver's adrenaline more than hearing that the call involves a baby or a colleague. As a professional, you must not let the nature of the call affect your judgement—always drive with caution.

Parking at an Emergency Scene

Safety at an accident scene is paramount, but can be neglected while your concerns are for others. If you are first on scene at a road traffic collision, park the ambulance beyond the crash site to allow easy egress onto the hospital. Only block the road when necessary and, if possible, allow entry for other emergency vehicles. If other emergency services are on site providing protection, try to park for ease of access and loading, while leaving yourself a clear exit.

Sometimes the general public complains about the way a stationary ambulance inconveniences other drivers. It may be difficult to understand why people object to blocked roads when you are working diligently to save people's lives. However, sometimes the ambulance *is* parked in such a way that it impedes traffic flow unnecessarily. If you need to park an ambulance in such a way that it blocks a traffic lane for safety reasons, do it; see Chapter 51 for more information. At the same time, however, maintain concern for others who are not involved in the incident. For example, if you are parking at a block of flats, be aware that other people may need to leave while you are inside and try not to block parked vehicles.

Always wear highly visible protective clothing when you get out of the vehicle on roads or are working in any public areas, whatever the time of day or night. Reflective vests/ Hi Viz tabards are lightweight and have the added benefit of increasing visibility during the day as well as at night **Figure 46-4 ▲** .

Reversing the Emergency Vehicle

Most ambulance services have an established policy about vehicle reversing. Reversing a vehicle is the most common source of vehicle damage and often results in costly repairs. If possible, avoid situations in which the ambulance will have to be backed up; good forward vision and anticipation are essential at all times. Although some ambulances are fitted with reversing cameras, distance warning beepers, and reversing alarms, these alone do not make the manoeuvre safe. If you must reverse the ambulance, follow these rules:

- Use a lookout to guide you **Figure 46-5 ▶** .
- Try to complete reversing manoeuvres before loading a patient

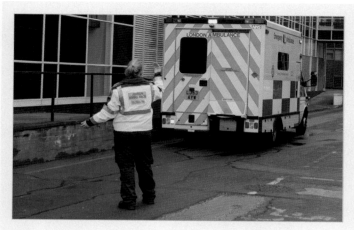

Figure 46-5 Always use a lookout when reversing the ambulance.

- Consider reversing into a cul-de-sac rather than out of one.
- Agree directions with the lookout *before* you place the vehicle in reverse. You may be attempting to back to the left while your lookout is trying to direct you to the right.
- Keep your lookout in view at all times. If you lose sight of the lookout, stop until he or she is back in your line of vision.
- Never allow anyone to stand between a reversing vehicle and a stationary object
- Agree on hand signals with your lookout before moving. Some people have different ideas of which gesture means "stop".
- Keep your window rolled down when in motion. This may allow you to hear instructions and people warning you of unseen dangers.

- Do a walk-around before getting behind the wheel and look up as well as down. Overhanging objects, tree branches/canopies, etc. and objects in the ground, such as a low wall, may not be visible once you start reversing.
- Use audible warning devices whenever the ambulance is reversing.

Loading and Unloading the Patient

When you are loading or unloading the ambulance, care must be taken to ensure that the patient is moved safely and considerately. Many patients will be loaded into the ambulance while on a stretcher or carry chair; this can be most disconcerting and possibly frightening for the patient. Take time to reassure your patient and explain how they will be moved into the ambulance *before* you move them. Some patients may be allowed to enter the patient compartment with little assistance from the crew, if it is safe to do so, but they should always be supervised. Always secure the patient, and make him or her comfortable, either on a stretcher or in a seat, with appropriate safety restraints.

If the patient is to be accompanied, ensure any escort is safely seated and using the fitted seatbelts. When police presence is required, as when transporting a prisoner, the officer may need to ride in close proximity to the patient. In all cases, the escorts should be secured using the fitted belts/restraint devices, if at all possible.

You must ensure that you are fully familiar with all patient handling equipment available within your service. It is vital that you fully understand the capabilities, capacity, loads, safety features and functions of carry chairs, trolley cots, stretchers, slides, lifts, hoists, or wheelchairs. It is not acceptable to be stuck trying to release a stretcher from the ambulance while your colleague is performing CPR. Make sure you are completely familiar with your equipment before you are required to use it.

You are the Paramedic Part 3

On scene, you are greeted by the ambulance officer who directs you to the trapped casualty. He tells you that the 7-year-old child has a severe head injury and has mobilised the air ambulance to transport the child once the child is freed from the wreckage.

Initial Assessment	Recording Time: 0 minutes
Appearance	Pale and limp
Level of consciousness	P (Responds to painful stimuli)
Airway	Manually maintained by a fire fighter
Breathing	Shallow, irregular
Circulation	Slow, full pulse

6. What information should you provide for the HEMS team?
7. What safety considerations are necessary when approaching any helicopter?

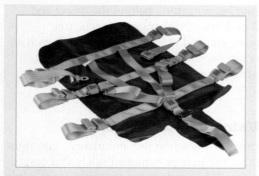

Figure 46-6 Paediatric stretcher securing device.

Use of Safety Restraints

Standard operating procedures should make it obligatory for everyone in the ambulance to use seatbelts, not just the patient. Familiarise yourself with all safety restraints in use within your vehicle and service before you need to use them. Children should not be transported on the stretcher unless properly restrained. It is not advisable to use adult seatbelts for children. Many paediatric transport devices are available, and they should be used when appropriate Figure 46-6 ▲ . Of course, when you are driving the ambulance you should always use a seatbelt.

Air Ambulances or Helicopter Emergency Medical Services (HEMS)

Air ambulance operations in the UK have been prevalent since 1987 when the first air ambulance was introduced in Cornwall. Ever since, they have increased in numbers and now serve as a major part of ambulance service responses across the whole of the United Kingdom. In the UK there are three main types or models of helicopter ambulance systems:

- The first is the "ambulance resource" system where suitably trained paramedics are flown to the scene, the patient assessed and stabilised, and then flown to the most appropriate hospital. These paramedics will attend a whole variety of ill or injured patients in support of ground ambulances and are particularly beneficial in accessing difficult terrain and remote areas Figure 46-7 ▶ .
- The second helicopter system is staffed by a senior doctor with appropriate trauma care experience assisted by an extended trained paramedic. This airborne crew is only dispatched to patients suffering severe or multi-system trauma. The interventions that can be instigated on scene by the crew and the prompt removal of the casualty to a specialised treatment centre can greatly assist the land-based ambulance resources
- Thirdly, rather than a dedicated air ambulance, some services are supported by a shared response where a paramedic is on duty with a police helicopter crew. This obviously has funding benefits, and patient care duties and transport will usually take precedence over police work.

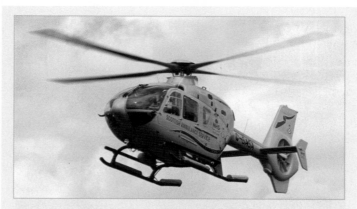

Figure 46-7 Rotary-wing ambulance.

Separate to HEMS operations, all ambulance services can have access to search and rescue (SAR) helicopters under military command. These aircraft are usually used for undertaking mountain rescue or coastguard type duties, but they can also be requested for various humanitarian "civilian" journeys.

Fixed-wing ambulance aircraft are also used around the country, and the Scottish ambulance service is probably the most experienced user. You should be familiar with your local protocols for interacting with any aircraft operations, whether scheduled transports and repatriations from overseas or HEMS trauma care, your knowledge and skills will contribute to the teamwork essential for patient care.

Air medical transport—especially the use of helicopters—has done much to speed up the transfer of patients from the trauma scene to definitive care and in bringing specialist skills to the patient. With the movement of many medical resources to specialist centres, it can be a long journey by land to the nearest burns unit, neurology, or trauma centre. For time-critical patients, helicopter journeys can have enormous benefits. This mode of transport however presents certain risks, and is not appropriate in all circumstances. Some patients, such as those in the advanced stages of pregnancy, will not benefit from the confined space in most helicopters, or an aggressive, unsedated patient could present undue risk inside the aircraft. After sunset and at other times of poor visibility HEMS activities are generally grounded as it is essential for the pilot to be able to see clearly where it is safe to land. Although advice on preparing a landing site will be available to emergency crews, the decision on where to land will always rest with the pilot. Your skills can be better used ensuring that patients are cared for and protected from any downdraft caused by HEMS operations.

Use of an air ambulance may also be warranted if the patient has a spinal injury and the terrain over which the patient must be carried is very rough. Even though the patient is immobilised, ground transport in a vehicle that is bouncing on the road could cause further injuries. The paramedic on scene is the best judge of the patient's clinical condition and possible transport needs.

After the helicopter has landed, *no one* should approach the helicopter until signalled to do so by the pilot. If possible, all rotors should be stopped before you approach the aircraft. If the aircraft continues to operate in a "hot" mode (with rotor blades active), the tail rotor is the most dangerous part of the aircraft and should be avoided at all times. Always approach helicopter from the front and keep the pilot in view at all times. Follow the air crew's instructions.

Table 46-1 ▾ summarises the advantages of using an air ambulance.

Table 46-2 ▾ summarises the disadvantages of using an air ambulance.

Table 46-2	Disadvantages of Using an Air Ambulance
■ Weather/environment restrictions/hours of operation
■ Altitude limitations with certain chest injuries
■ May be slower for short transports
■ Aircraft cabin size, usually only suitable for one stabilised casualty
■ Terrain
■ Cost
■ Patient's condition

Table 46-1	Advantages of Using an Air Ambulance
■ Specialised skills or equipment is needed
■ Rapid transport is possible
■ Quick over longer distances
■ Prompt access to specialist treatment centres
■ Can provide access to patients in remote areas
■ Helicopter hospital helipads are available

You are the Paramedic Part 4

The patient is freed by the fire service and immobilised on a longboard. The HEMS doctor performs rapid sequence induction in order to ventilate the patient. Once packaged, the patient is loaded onto the helicopter which then transports the child to the nearest trauma hospital for care.

Reassessment	Recording Time: 15 Minutes
Level of consciousness	U (Unresponsive) with a Glasgow Coma Scale score of 3 prior to sedation
Skin	Pale, dry
Pulse	55 beats/min, regular
Blood pressure	170/96 mm Hg
Respirations	Ventilated, 20 breaths/min
SpO_2	100%
Pupils	Unequal, left pupil larger than right
Blood glucose	4.7 mmol/l

8. What advantages does the utilisation of HEMS offer the patient in this incident?

You are the Paramedic Summary

1. What are some of the potential hazards you may encounter en route to the scene?

- Whenever an ambulance is en route to an emergency call, you must approach every road junction and hazard cautiously and be prepared to change your driving plans accordingly.
- In multiple vehicle responses, always approach every junction with extra caution and with the thought that you could be meeting another emergency vehicle at that exact point (police or fire).
- Remember that the average road user can react in a number of ways once they realise that you are coming up behind them. They may:
  - Brake suddenly
  - Change lanes
  - Not give way
- Developing your hazard awareness skills will enable you to anticipate potential problems.
- When the roads are wet (or in other adverse conditions) remember the effect on vehicle braking distances. Also in heavy rain, other road users such as pedestrians and cyclists may be distracted and less observant.
- At the start and end of the school day there is a significant increase in associated hazards for all road users. Not only numerous young people using roads, crossings, bus stops, and pavements, but parents are stopping, starting, and manoeuvring vehicles.

2. What dangers must be considered when approaching the scene with regard to parking and personnel protection?

Always approach the scene cautiously and with the thought that you could be meeting other emergency vehicles and personnel or dazed and confused patients/bystanders at the scene. If the scene has already been secured, park beyond the incident to prevent your ambulance from being exposed to the traffic. You may also receive arrival instructions if you are not the first on scene. The arrival instructions may specify where the police would like you to park your ambulance and to whom you should report. All ambulance personnel should ensure that the appropriate PPE is donned before approaching the scene of any accident.

3. How will knowing that there are multiple patients, including children, affect your driving?

It should not affect your driving at all. Your professional driving technique will ensure you drive within your limits and with due regard for the safety of other road users. There is a state of mind know as "red mist"; where the driver of the emergency vehicle becomes too focused on the incident and casualties (especially if the injured are children) and the desire to reach the scene quickly overrides normal driving safety margins. Drivers should learn to recognise this common trait and ensure their driving allows them to reach the scene as quickly and as safely as possible.

4. Where should the ambulance be positioned at the scene of a road traffic collision if you are the *first* to arrive?

If you are the first to arrive at the scene of any incident, take time to perform a scene assessment for potential hazards to you, your crew, and the patients. Headlights may need to be turned off to avoid dazzling vehicles approaching from the opposite carriageway. In the case of fire or any escaping hazardous liquids, it may be necessary to park at least 50 m from the wreckage, upwind and uphill (if possible).

5. Where should the ambulance be positioned at the scene of a road traffic collision if you are *not* the first to arrive?

If the scene has already been secured, park beyond the incident to prevent your ambulance from being exposed to the traffic. Follow directions from the police or ambulance officers if they are on scene. Try to ensure you can leave the scene safely and are not likely to be blocked by other emergency vehicles.

6. What information should you provide for the HEMS team?

To assist with early triage decisions a concise medical report is helpful. Include a description of the mechanism of injury (ejected onto the bonnet, thrown 5 m from motorbike, etc) the patient's gender, approximate age and vital signs following an ABC and AVPU format: "25-year-old male motorcyclist impact into car approx 40 mph; airway clear, breathing laboured, respiratory rate 30, poorly perfused, pulse 140, BP not yet known, responding only to pain, possible head, spinal, and abdominal injury".

7. What safety considerations are necessary when approaching any helicopter?

- Never approach the aircraft unless instructed to by the pilot.
- The general rule is that you should not approach a helicopter when the rotor blades are turning, unless instructed to do so by the pilot. If you are instructed to approach while the rotors are turning, approach from the front and keep eye contact with the pilot.
- When the rotors are turning do not go anywhere near the tail area of the aircraft
- If the aircraft is on a slope always try to approach from the downhill angle.
- Be aware of the wash from rotors, it can throw up dirt, debris, and light objects that are not properly secured. If you are wearing a helmet, ensure it is securely fastened.

8. What advantages does the utilisation of HEMS offer the patient in this incident?

In this case, the activation of HEMS facilitated the availability of a prehospital clinician with the skills and competency to secure the child's airway by means of drug-induced intubation. Although not all HEMS operations are in a position to offer such advanced treatment, they can all facilitate rapid removal of patients to a specialist facility appropriate to a patient's clinical needs—in this case, a hospital with a paediatric neurological specialty.

Prep Kit

Ready for Review

- Check the ambulance at the beginning of every shift to ensure that all equipment is available and in good working order.
- Any specific exemption from traffic laws does not negate your responsibility to proceed with due regard to other road users.
- Other blue-light escorts should not be used due to the danger to other motorists not seeing both the ambulance and the escort.
- Lights and sirens should be used when required on responding to emergencies but used considerately and to serve a purpose.
- Avoid reversing the vehicle if possible. If it is necessary, use a lookout to assist in the procedure. Make sure everyone is clear on where the vehicle is to be placed and that hand signals used are agreed upon.
- All drivers and passengers should use safety restraints while a vehicle is in motion.
- Air transport should be considered whenever time is of the essence and for the best patient outcome.

Vital Vocabulary

fractile response time A fraction (not average) of all emergency responses for the purpose of setting standards in response times.

listening watch The placement of an ambulance at a specific geographic location in order to cover larger areas of territory and reduce response times. Also called standby.

peak load A time of day or day of week in which the call volume is at its highest.

strategic deployment Nominating listening watch and standby locations for ambulances to enhance the geographical coverage of emergency resources to attend 999 calls.

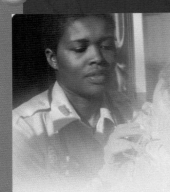

Assessment in Action

At the end of your shift you are dispatched to the scene of a vehicle that has crashed into a tree. When you arrive, you are approached by a fire fighter who tells you that the patient "is in there and well trapped" and there will be a delay in accessing the patient due to extrication. You see that there is heavy damage to the driver's side of the vehicle. The A post is crushed to the ground and the steering wheel and dashboard are crushing the patient in the vehicle. The patient appears unresponsive and copious amounts of blood are coming from his head. You notice a compound fracture of his left femur with extensive bleeding. You and your colleague decide to request an air ambulance due to the patient's condition and extended extrication time. After 15 minutes of extrication, you are able to free the patient from the vehicle. You secure the patient properly to a longboard and transfer him to the ambulance. While en route to the air ambulance landing zone, you intubate him and start two large-bore IVs. When you arrive at the air ambulance landing zone, the air ambulance has just landed.

1. **What was the advantage to using the air ambulance for this patient?**
   A. Reduced transport time; it helped the patient receive definitive treatment quickly.
   B. It was the end of your shift and you and your colleague will be able to leave on time.
   C. You didn't have to deal with an unstable patient for the next 20 minutes driving the patient to the hospital.
   D. The fire service and other personnel wanted to practise their skills of having an air ambulance land.

2. **While intubating this patient, you need to suction blood out of the airway. You were unable to find your suction unit. At the beginning of every shift you should:**
   A. check the ambulance to ensure the proper equipment is both available and in good working order.
   B. make sure that there is enough fuel and then go and get coffee.
   C. document what the previous crew has to say about supplies and equipment.
   D. start your personal work that needs to get done before anything else.

3. **Which of the following safety measures should be used when approaching the air ambulance to load the patient?**
   A. Approach the air ambulance as soon as it lands.
   B. At least eight people should help load the air ambulance.
   C. The air ambulance should be approached from the front.
   D. The air ambulance should be approached from the rear.

4. **During the vehicle daily inspection (VDI), it is important to check the following to ensure the road worthiness of your ambulance.**
   A. Tyre tread pressure and wheel nut security
   B. Oil and water control levels

   C. Integrity of all normal and emergency warning lights
   D. All of the above

5. **Air ambulance transportation is not suitable for the following groups of patients:**
   A. Serious trauma patients from road traffic collisions
   B. Patients who are over 1 hour away from care and require rapid intervention
   C. Patients with suspected spinal injuries
   D. Patients who are in the late stage of pregnancy and birth is imminent

6. **Paramedics who meet all the Standards stipulated by the _____ are eligible to register and thus entitled to legally practise in the UK.**
   A. BPA (British Paramedic Association)
   B. ASA (Ambulance Service Association)
   C. HPC (Health Profession Council)
   D. RCUK (Resuscitation Council UK)

Challenging Questions

7. **Ambulance response times in rural areas are expected to be similar to urban areas. Is it more beneficial to have more rapid response cars to achieve the response time or double the ambulances to transport the patients to hospital?**

8. **What is the best way of measuring the efficacy of the ambulance service—reviewing response time or patient outcomes?**

▇ Points to Ponder

You are sent to a shopping centre for a patient who is convulsing. You are responding with lights and sirens. The quickest route is via a ring road that skirts the busy town centre; however, the road still has many roundabouts and traffic lights along its course.

On approaching a set of traffic lights, you realise that the green light changes to amber, and then red. As you pass the now stationary line of traffic and enter the junction, you notice a car, on the right, start to drive forward (it is, obviously, their right of way). You think they see you because they slow down, but as you continue, you realise they have not in fact seen you and a collision is unavoidable.

What actions should you take subsequent to the collision?

Issues: Assessing Personal Safety Practices While Operating Your Emergency Vehicle, Knowledge of Legal Exemptions to the Road Traffic Act, Notifying Ambulance Control and Other Appropriate Agencies, Exchange of Driver Documentations and Details With Those Involved.

47 Incident Command

Objectives

Cognitive

- Explain the need for the incident command system (ICS) in managing emergency medical services incidents.
- Define the term major incident.
- Define the term disaster management.
- Describe essential elements of the situation report when arriving at a potential major incident.
- Describe the role of the paramedics and ambulance services in planning for major incidents and disasters.
- Define the following types of incidents and how they affect medical management:
  - Uncompensated incident
  - Compensated incident
- Describe the functional components of the incident command system in terms of the following:
  - Command
  - Communications
  - Equipment
  - Tactical operations
  - Strategic (Gold) command
  - Delegated key roles
- Differentiate between singular and unified command and when each is most applicable.
- Describe the principal role of the ambulance commander (AC).
- Describe the need for transfer of command and procedures for transferring it.
- Differentiate between command procedures used at small, medium, and large scale incidents.
- Explain the local/regional threshold for establishing command and implementation of the incident command system including the threshold for major incident declaration.
- List and describe the key responsibilities associated to the following designated tasks within the ICS:
  - Command
  - Safety
  - Communications
  - Assessment
  - Triage
  - Treatment
  - Transport
  - Logistics
  - Rest area
  - Parking
  - Extrication/rescue
  - Disposition of deceased (body holding area)
- Describe the rationale for identifying specific personnel to these roles.
- Describe the role of the medical commander (MC) at major incidents.
- Define triage and describe the principles of triage.
- Given colour coded labels and numerical priorities, assign the following terms to each:
  - Immediate
  - Urgent
  - Delayed
  - Expectant
- Define triage Sieve and triage Sort.
- Describe when triage Sieve and triage Sort techniques should be implemented.
- Describe the need for and techniques used in tracking patients during major incidents.
- Describe techniques used to allocate patients to hospitals and track them.
- Describe modifications of telecommunications procedures during major incidents.
- List and describe the essential equipment to provide logistical support to major incident operations to include:
  - Airway, respiratory, and haemorrhage control
  - Burn management
  - Patient packaging/ immobilisation
- List the physical and psychological signs of critical incident stress.
- Describe the role of critical incident stress management during or immediately after a major incident.
- Describe the role of the following exercises in preparation for major incidents:
  - Simulated exercises
  - Table top exercises

Affective

- Understand the rationale for initiating incident command even at a relatively small incident, such as a road traffic collision.
- Explain the rationale for having efficient and effective communications as part of an incident command system.
- Explain why common problems encountered at a major incident can have an adverse effect on an entire incident.
- Explain the organisational benefits for having a major incident plan and for using the incident command system.

Psychomotor

- Demonstrate the use of local/regional triage labelling system used for triage Sieve and triage Sort.
- Given a simulated major incident:
  - Establish unified or singular command
  - Conduct a scene assessment
  - Determine scene objectives
  - Formulate an incident plan
  - Request appropriate resources
  - Determine need to initiate ICS and allocate specific management roles within the system's structure
  - Coordinate communications
  - Coordinate with outside agencies

- Demonstrate effective initial scene assessment and constant reappraisal by providing effective situation reports.
- Given a table top major incident exercise, fulfill the role of triage officer.
- Given a table top major incident exercise, fulfill the role of casualty clearing officer.
- Given a table top major incident exercise, fulfill the role of ambulance loading officer.

Introduction

The most challenging situations you can be called to are disasters and major incidents. These incidents can be overwhelming because you will find a large number of patients and a lack of specialised equipment and/or adequate help. When you respond to an event with a large number of patients, you must use a systematic approach to manage the incident most efficiently. By learning to use the principles of an incident command system (ICS), you will be able to do the greatest good for the greatest number. As a paramedic you will typically be required to work in one of the Bronze Command roles at the incident site. To promote more efficient coordination of emergency incidents at a large scale incident the Integrated Emergency Management System (IEMS) was developed. To reduce on-scene problems and to increase your efficiency, you should attend training and have a solid understanding of the basics of IEMS. As a practitioner, it is your responsibility to be familiar with both local and national major incident guidelines and plans.

Disasters

Disasters overwhelm ambulance service and community resources because critical infrastructure has been damaged or destroyed Figure 47-1 . Critical infrastructure includes the electrical power grid, communication systems, fuel for vehicles, water, sewage removal, food, hospitals, and transportation systems. Disaster management requires planners to take a broad look at anticipation, assessment, prevention, preparation, response, and recovery management.

Major Incidents

The Department of Health (2005) defines a major incident as "any occurrence that presents serious threat to the health of the community, disruption to the service, or causes (or is likely to cause) such numbers of casualties as to require special arrangements to be implemented by hospitals, ambulance trusts, or primary care organisations Figure 47-2 . Indeed, a road traffic collision with several critical patients may constitute a major incident for a town with a single ambulance resource, so the principal management system can be effectively used in a relatively routine incident.

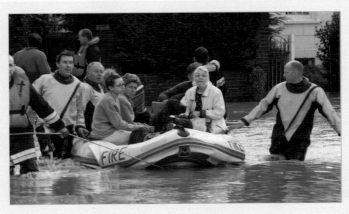

Figure 47-1 Disasters can overwhelm ambulance service resources and can damage critical infrastructure.

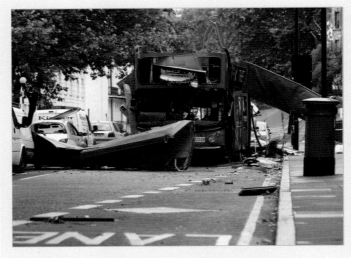

Figure 47-2 Major incidents can be large, such as the attack on the London Underground, or can be much smaller in scope.

Your response to major incidents will differ depending on a number of factors, such as the area of land covered by the incident and the location and how spread out your patients are. You should be able to recognise a major incident as an uncompensated incident or a compensated incident. An uncompensated incident is where the incident creates a demand that cannot be met from local resources. A compensated incident is where the incident, although large, can be met from local resources.

You are the Paramedic Part 1

You have been sent to the scene of a commercial plane crash. You are the first ambulance crew to arrive. There is no fire or other hazard noted initially. From inside the ambulance, you see approximately 30 to 40 victims walking or lying about the scene. As you arrive, 10 to 15 people approach your ambulance with cuts, bruises, and abrasions.

1. What is your plan of action?
2. Why is an incident command system (ICS) needed for handling major incidents?
3. What is an "uncompensated" incident? What is a "compensated" incident?

At the Scene

Simulated and table top major incident exercises are an effective way for emergency services to learn their individual roles at a major incident and the collaborative strategies, tactical, and operational processes facilitated through the integrated emergency management system (IEMS).

In addition you should be able to recognise whether the incident is simple, where the local infrastructure (eg, electricity supplies, water supplies, roads, hospitals, and so on) is intact, or whether the incident is compound, where local infrastructure has been destroyed, leading to long-term recovery management.

Organisations may establish different standards for what constitutes a major incident or for when to declare a major incident, but experience is helpful when determining the severity of an incident and the capacity to effectively manage the expected demand. Emergency services that have regular exposure to major incidents will gain valuable experience and will be better prepared to respond to them. You can make significant contributions to the effectiveness of your practice at such an event by participating in major incident exercises (simulated and table top), in collaboration with other emergency services and responding agencies.

Preparing for the Major Incident: The Incident Command System

It is important for you to be familiar with the terminology and concepts of a structured incident command system (ICS), such as the principles of Major Incident Medical Management and Support (MIMMS). As you know, communication is the building block of good patient care. Common terminology and the use of "clear text" communications (plain English as opposed to radio jargon) help responders from emergency services to work efficiently together.

Using the ICS gives you a modular organisational structure that is built on the size and complexity of the incident. The goal of a structured response to a major incident is to make the best use of your resources to manage the environment around the incident and to treat patients during an emergency. Make certain to follow your local standard operating procedures for establishing an ICS. This system is designed to control duplication of effort and freelancing, in which individual ambulances or different organisations make independent and often inefficient decisions about the next appropriate action. It is essential that any individual assigned a management role in a major incident is not assigned more than he or she can deal with. In the event that you find that you have more tasks or people than you can deal with, delegate tasks to other practitioners.

One of the organising principles of the ICS is limiting the span of control of any one individual, keeping the supervisor/worker ratio at one supervisor for three to seven workers. A supervisor who finds that his or her effective span of control is exceeded—that is, has more than seven people reporting to him or her—needs to divide tasks and delegate supervision of some tasks to another person.

Organisational divisions may include the medical commander (MC) and ambulance commander at the silver level, and ambulance and medical staff at the bronze level **Figure 47-3 ▾**.

The individuals who will participate in the many tasks in a major incident or a disaster should use a common major incident plan. You should find out from your service if one exists, who is in charge, how it is activated, and what your expected role will be.

ICS Roles and Responsibilities

There are many roles defined in the ICS, with gold, silver, and bronze being the levels of command. Gold is strategic, silver is tactical, and bronze is operational. It is important for you to understand the specific duties of each and how they work in coordinating the response. Command functions at scene include the ambulance commander (AC), forward incident officer, safety officer, primary triage officer, casualty clearing officer, loading officer, and parking officer. These roles are often used with "bronze" prefixes, for example Bronze Forward, Bronze Parking, Bronze Safety, etc. This helps to highlight their operational, rather than tactical, role.

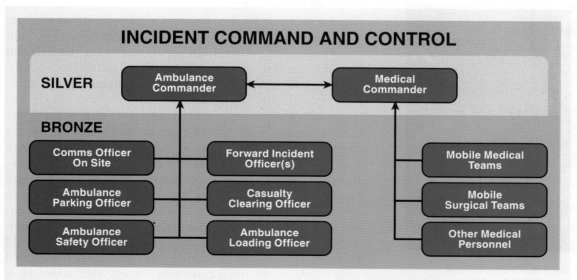

Figure 47-3 Incident command and control. Not all positions will be filled in every incident. However, the ambulance commander is ultimately responsible for all activity. Subordinates may be appointed to assist in managing the incident.

Command

The <u>ambulance commander (AC)</u> is the person on scene in charge of the overall medical activity at the incident. The AC will assess the incident, establish the tactical objectives and priorities, and develop a plan to manage the incident **Figure 47-4 ▾** . The number of command duties (public relations, safety, and liaison) the AC takes on often varies by the size of the incident. Small incidents often mean the AC will do it all. In an incident of medium size or complexity, the AC may delegate some functions but retain others. For example, at a road traffic collision with multiple patients, the AC may designate a safety officer or assign a public relations (PR) officer to manage the media, but maintain responsibility for the other command functions. In a complex situation, the AC may appoint team members to all of the command roles.

Large major incidents, such as a hazardous materials incident, require a multiagency or inter-regional response and need to use an <u>Integrated Emergency Response</u>. Plans are usually drawn up and revised at the Regional Resilience Forum, where representatives from various organisations, including emergency services, local organisations, and transport networks collaborate. In this case, plans are drawn up in advance by all cooperating agencies that assume a shared responsibility for decision making and cooperation. The response plan should designate the lead and support agencies in several kinds of major incidents. (The CCBRN/hazardous materials team will take the lead in a chemical leak, for example. However, a medical lead might be required in a serious road traffic collision). Ultimately, the police retain the overall lead during the response phase of a major incident, only delegating authority where there is a specific requirement for expert opinion. Trusts bordering each other should practise with each other to ensure that an Integrated Emergency Response will function well and that communication among the people involved is well established before a real incident occurs.

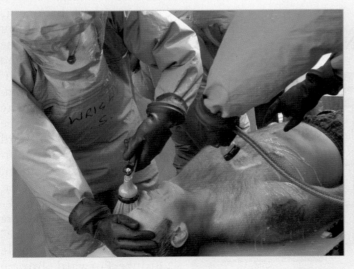

Figure 47-4 The person in command at a major incident oversees the incident and develops a plan for response.

A <u>single command system</u> is one in which one person is in charge. Ideally, it is used for short duration, limited incidents that require the services of a single agency.

Your AC should be on or near the scene, where he or she can easily communicate with all emergency services operating at the scene. It is important that you know who the AC is, where the command post is located, and how to communicate with your supervisor. If the incident is very large, you will be reporting to a supervisor working under the AC. (Remember the rule of span of control? The number of people who can be effectively supervised is between three and seven.) To make the AC easily identifiable, some type of garment can be worn, such as a green/white chequered tabard inscribed with the words *Ambulance Commander*. If the command post is set up in a vehicle, it should be well marked, and you should know its location. Most UK ambulance services will provide a command and communication vehicle for use in such circumstances. These vehicles will liaise with vehicles from other emergency services to form the Joint Emergency Services Control Centre (JESCC) where the respective organisations' silver commanders will collocate.

This communication is particularly important if a <u>transfer of command</u> takes place. Because a major incident can be ever-changing and ever-increasing in scope, an AC may turn over command of the medical management to someone with more experience in a critical area. This change, or transfer of command, must take place in an orderly manner and, if possible, face to face. In extreme situations, it could be done by phone or radio. Your service should have procedures in the major incident plan that govern the transfer of command. Make certain to follow these procedures. When an incident draws to a close, there should be a <u>termination of command</u>. Your service should have <u>demobilisation</u> procedures to implement as the situation declines or comes to an end.

Communications

Communications is the one area of response that receives criticism in every incident debrief. Communication to and from the scene to the control room must be maintained and logged. Communications between the AC and the bronze officers working at the scene must be maintained and logged. Sometimes this is delegated to a support officer who writes down all communication between Silver and others. The mobile control vehicle will provide hand held radios for communication at the site for both the ambulance service and other delegated medical staff who attend the scene. Although numerous communication systems can be used ranging from mobile phones, landlines, hand signals, pagers, and runners, they all negate the requirement to have a central point of contact; and potentially command of the incident can be placed in jeopardy. Use of such methods should therefore be utilised with caution, and links must be retained with the AC to ensure a consistent management approach is maintained.

Table 47-1	MI Equipment and Supplies*
Airway control	PPE (gloves, face shield, European standard EN149: 2001 FFP3 respirator) Oral airways, nasal airways Suction units (manual units) Rigid tip Yankeur and flexible suction catheters LMA, ET tubes Laryngoscope and blades Tube check, tube restraint, tape, syringes, stylet End-tidal CO_2 device
Breathing	Pocket mask and one-way valve Bag-valve-mask device(s) (adult and child), spare masks Oxygen delivery devices (nonrebreathing mask, cannula, extension tubing) Oxygen cylinder, regulator Occlusive dressings Large-bore IV cannula for thoracic decompression
Circulation	Dressings, bandages, tape Sphygmomanometer, stethoscope Burn dressings, burn sheets, sterile water for irrigation One-handed tourniquets 1,000 mL bags of normal saline, IV giving sets, cannulas
Disability	Adjustable rigid collars (one size fits all) Head immobilsers, wide tape, longboard straps Torches, spare batteries
Exposure	Space blanket to cover patients Scissors
Logistic/Command	Major incident vests (triage, treatment, transport, parking, commander) Pads of paper, pencils, pens, markers Triage labels or kits used by your ambulance service Assessment cards

Equipment Officer

The bronze equipment officer has responsibility for facilities, food and water, fuel, lighting, and medical equipment and supplies for patients and ambulance personnel. Local standard operating procedures will list the medical equipment needed for the incident, depending on the type of incident. **Table 47-1 ◄** lists common major incident equipment and supplies. Logistics personnel are designated to source food, shelter, and health care for you and the other ambulance personnel at the scene of a major incident **Figure 47-5 ▼**. In a large incident, it is often necessary for many people to handle logistics, even though only one person will report to the AC.

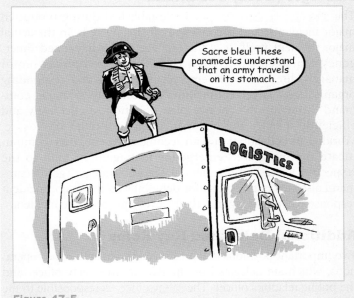

Figure 47-5

You are the Paramedic Part 2

As more ambulances arrive on scene, you take on the role of the forward incident officer. The first patient you see is walking towards you.

Initial Assessment: Patient 1	Recording Time: 5 minutes
Appearance	Pale, cool, dry skin
Level of consciousness	Well orientated; pupils equal and reactive
Airway	Open
Breathing	12 breaths/min, deep, regular, and by mouth
Circulation	Pulse rapid, full, and regular

4. How should you triage this patient?
5. What is the difference between single and unified command?
6. What is "span of control"?

Forward Incident Officer

The AC is in command of all ambulance and medical personnel at the scene of a major incident. At large major incidents, the AC takes a holistic and tactical role, which necessitates delegation of some specific operational roles to facilitate this. A significant appointment in this instance is that of a forward incident officer. The forward (bronze) incident officer is responsible to the AC for the management of ambulance resources and acts as the ACs eyes and ears at the site of the incident, supervising people working at the scene and directing rescue efforts in close liaison with the AC. Bronze officers often have experience in management within the ambulance service, although this appointment should be made based on competence and experience and not purely on a hierarchal position.

Strategic (Gold) Command

The strategic (gold) command is established during protracted major incidents, and is convened off-site, away from the actual major incident itself. It is the top tier of the Integrated Emergency Management System (IEMS) and comprises senior managers/directors of all emergency services and responding organisations' silver commanders. Ultimately, strategic command formulates a cohesive plan of action to effectively and efficiently manage the major incident to a point of closure. Working in collaboration with technical experts, they communicate the integrated emergency management plan to the respective silver commanders at scene. Strategic (gold) command also sets out a course for demobilising the major incident response when moving into the recovery phase of the incident.

Additional Delegated Key Roles

Two important positions that are crucial to the ambulance operations, which are delegated by the AC, are the safety officer and the public relations officer. The safety officer is responsible to the AC and monitors the scene for conditions or operations that may present a hazard to ambulance clinicians, medical personnel, and patients. The safety officer may need to work with environmental health and hazardous materials specialists. The importance of the safety officer cannot be underestimated—he or she has the authority to stop an emergency operation whenever a rescuer is in danger. A safety officer should ideally remove hazards to paramedics and patients before the hazards cause injury.

The public relations (PR) officer provides the media and the public with clear and understandable information. A wise PR officer positions his or her base station at a safe distance from the incident to minimise distractions. Also, the PR officer must keep the media updated whilst the police attempt to restrict them from becoming part of the incident. The designated PR officer may work in collaboration with fellow PR officers from responding agencies at the joint information centre (JIC); in which case the police are likely to take the lead in all PR announcements. It is normal for the JIC to agree on casualty numbers before releasing the information to the press. In some circumstances, the JIC may be responsible for disseminating a message designed to help a situation, prevent panic, and provide evacuation directions.

The Integrated Emergency Management System (IEMS)

The Civil Contingencies Act was implemented in 2004. This Act was designed to provide a framework under which responders to an incident shared information and worked together, using the Integrated Emergency Management System. Major incidents require the involvement and coordination of multiple jurisdictions, functional agencies, and emergency service disciplines. IEMS provides a consistent nationwide template to enable government, as well as private-sector and nongovernmental organisations, to work together effectively and efficiently. IEMS is used to prepare for, prevent, respond to, and recover from domestic incidents, regardless of cause, size, or complexity, including acts of catastrophic terrorism.

Two important underlying principles of IEMS are flexibility and standardisation. The organisational structure must be flexible enough to be rapidly adapted for use in any situation. IEMS provides standardisation in terminology, resource classification, personnel training, certification, and more. Another important feature of IEMS is the concept of operational integration in which agencies of different types or from different jurisdictions can communicate with each other.

The ICS, which is the focus of this chapter, is one component of IEMS. The major IEMS components are:

- **Command and management.** The IEMS standardises incident management for all hazards and across all levels of government. The IEMS standard incident command structures are based on three key constructs: ICS, integrated emergency management, and public relations.
- **Preparedness.** IEMS establishes measures for all responders to incorporate into their systems in preparation to respond to all incidents at any time.
- **Resource management.** IEMS sets up mechanisms to describe, audit, track, and dispatch resources before, during, and after an incident. IEMS also defines standard procedures to recover equipment used during the incident.
- **Communications and information management.** Effective communications and information management and sharing are critical aspects of domestic incident management. IEMS communications and information systems enable the essential functions needed to provide interoperability.
- **Supporting technologies.** IEMS promotes national standards and operational integration for supporting technologies to provide structure for the science and technology used in incident management.
- **Ongoing management and maintenance.** The UK Government has the ability to open up a Cabinet Operations Briefing Room (COBRa), which will establish a multijurisdictional, multidisciplinary IEMS Intelligence Centre. This centre will provide strategic direction for and oversight of IEMS, supporting routine maintenance and continuous improvement of the system in the long term. Similar establishments exist in Scotland (Scottish Executive Emergency Room [SEER]) and in Wales.

Ambulance Service Response Within the Major Incident Plan

Preparedness

Preparedness involves the decisions made and basic planning done before an incident occurs. Some parts of every country are prone to natural disasters, such as hurricanes, floods, earthquakes, or landslides. Therefore, preparedness in a given area would involve decisions and planning about the most likely natural disasters for the area, among other disasters.

Your ambulance service should have written major incident plans that you are regularly trained to carry out. A copy of the major incident plan should be kept on every ambulance station. Ambulance service facilities should have major incident supplies for at least a 72-hour period of self-sufficiency. Your ambulance service should have mutual aid agreements with surrounding organisations so that requests for help can be accelerated in an emergency. All groups with mutual aid agreements should practise using the plans frequently. Organisations should share a list of resources with each other so they will know early on what they can access. Also, your local ambulance service should develop an assistance programme for the families of ambulance service personnel. If ambulance service personnel have concerns about their families during a major incident, their effectiveness could be diminished. Regional Resilience Forums are vital in assisting with this process and creating a good dialogue with other health care practitioners and other emergency services.

Situation Report (Sit Rep)

You remember that assessing the scene starts with ambulance control. If control information indicates a possible unsafe scene, you should stay away from the scene or get only close enough to make an assessment without putting yourself in harm's way. When you arrive first on the scene of a major incident, you will make an initial assessment and some preliminary decisions.

The situation report (sit rep) has seven questions, which will allow you to report what you see accurately and will assist you in requesting assistance. They can be remembered by the mnemonic METHANE: Major incident standby/declared, stating your call sign, Exact location of incident, Type of incident, Hazards at scene, Access and egress routes from the scene, Number of patients involved, Emergency services at scene or required.

The sit rep can be a constantly changing as new information is obtained, and should be updated when this occurs.

M The initial call for a *major incident* is made and ensures that the call sign of the attending vehicle is logged by ambulance control.

E Confirmation of the *exact location* of the incident is a must for all other attending ambulances, police, and fire staff. The use of a six-figure map reference will, if available, reduce the opportunity for error.

T The *type of incident* will be important for the control to ensure that the correct assistance is provided at the scene. In addition the fire service will need to know the type of incident in order to ensure the correct PDA (predetermined attendance to the incident).

H Identification of the actual or potential *hazards* will become part of the dynamic risk assessment of the first crew on scene. Ensuring that the correct assistance is requested to scene. It will also ensure that the 1-2-3 of safety (self, scene, survivors) is followed.

A *Access and egress.* The initial sitrep will concentrate on the most appropriate route of entry to the incident for supporting staff and vehicles, to avoid traffic congestion or partially blocked routes.

N The *number of casualties* that can be seen or that you believe may be involved. The initial number will change as a more careful examination of the scene can be carried out. An initial over estimation of casualties is better than an under estimation.

E A report of the *emergency services* which are already at the scene or a request for those services which need to be on scene. This should also include specialist services and other relevant organisations required on scene.

Conversely, the mnemonic CHALET (Casualties, Hazards, Access, Location, Emergency services, Type of incident) serves a similar purpose to that of METHANE when constructing a situation report. However, it is not as robust or systematic in its presentation of information.

Establishing Command

Once you have performed a comprehensive situation report; it is crucial to follow three simple steps; *establish command, notify all other emergency services at scene,* and *identify the additional resources required and request them.* A command system ensures that resources are effectively and efficiently coordinated. Command must be established early, preferably by the first arriving, most experienced ambulance clinician who will initially assume the role of AC. Other organisations will identify a service lead in a similar fashion, which will include a police commander, fire commander, and local government officials.

 At the Scene

Participating in a simulated major incident can help the paramedic better understand how command is established, the scene is assessed, how scene objectives are determined, how an incident plan is created, how resources are requested, when ICS needs to expand, how communication is coordinated, and how the ambulance service works with other agencies during a large emergency.

Incident Control

One emergency service at the scene of a major incident will take principal responsibility, which in the UK will normally be the police. The controlling organisation should be seen as a facilitator for the other emergency services, ensuring close communication and collaborative work. A fundamental element of incident control is the protection of the scene. This is established through the creation of an outer and inner cordon to restrict and monitor movement of personnel, vehicles, and equipment within the scene. The outer cordon surrounds the entire incident and can encompass an area with a radius of several miles. Where possible the outer cordon is a physical barrier consisting of road blocks, traffic cones, police line tape, portable metal fencing, and authorised personnel preventing entry. Conversely, the inner cordon does not always have such clear demarcation unless there is a hazardous material at the scene. Indeed, in a hazardous material incident the inner cordon boundary forms the entry point to the cold zone. Although the police will retain control of the entire incident as the principal emergency service, they may initially surrender their control within the inner cordon to the fire service depending on the nature of hazards at the scene.

Communications

Communications is often the key problem at a major incident. The infrastructure can be damaged or communications capabilities can be overwhelmed, as happened on the 7th of July. If possible, use face-to-face communications to limit radio traffic. Some organisations responding to a major incident might not know how to use a radio, however if they are being used, for this reason avoid using jargon or code words. Most communications problems should be worked out before a major incident happens by designating channels strictly for command during an incident. Whatever form of communications equipment is used, it is imperative that it is reliable, durable, field-tested, and that there are backups in place if the primary communications system does not work. It is very important that you include a "Plan B" in case of a communications failure, such as the utilisation of the Emergency Reserve Channel (ERC).

▌Ambulance Service Responsibilities

The ambulance service branch of the ICS renders the AC accountable for all medical activity at the scene. Where medical activity is high, the AC will appoint a forward incident officer to supervise the primary roles—triage, treatment, and transport **Figure 47-6 ▸**. On arrival at scene, ambulance personnel should initially report to the parking officer who will ensure they receive a briefing before entering the inner cordon. Generally, one member of the crew will remain with the vehicles at the ambulance parking area, while the second crew member presents to the AC for deployment within the scene. **Figure 47-7 ▸** and **Figure 47-8 ▸** show diagrams of components within the ICS.

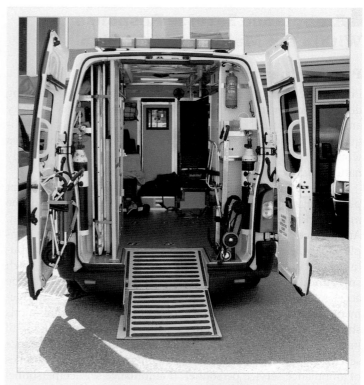

Figure 47-6 This mobile emergency room is staffed by paramedics and doctors who are able to provide advanced life support to multiple patients simultaneously on the scene of a major incident.

Triage Unit

The primary triage officer is ultimately in charge of counting and prioritising patients using the triage Sieve. During large incidents, a number of triage personnel may be needed. The primary duty of the triage officer is to ensure that every patient receives initial assessment of his or her condition. Paramedics doing triage will help move patients to the appropriate treatment sector. One of the most difficult parts of being a triage officer is that you must not begin treatment until all patients are triaged, or you will compromise your triage efforts.

Casualty Clearing Officer

The casualty clearing officer will locate and set up the casualty clearing station with a tier for each priority of patient. Casualty clearing officers ensure that triage Sort of patients is performed and that adequate patient care is given as resources allow. Casualty clearing officers also have a responsibility to assist with moving patients to the transportation area. The casualty clearing officer liaises with the medical team to request sufficient quantities of supplies, including bandages, burn supplies, airway and respiratory supplies, and patient packaging equipment.

Ambulance Loading Officer

The ambulance loading officer coordinates the transportation and distribution of patients to appropriate receiving hospitals. Transportation requires coordination with AC to help ensure

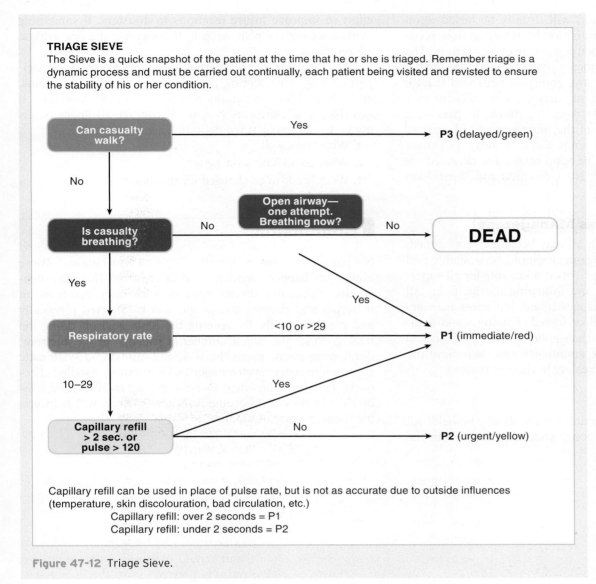

TRIAGE SIEVE

The Sieve is a quick snapshot of the patient at the time that he or she is triaged. Remember triage is a dynamic process and must be carried out continually, each patient being visited and revisted to ensure the stability of his or her condition.

Can casualty walk? — Yes → **P3** (delayed/green)

No ↓

Is casualty breathing? — No → Open airway— one attempt. Breathing now? — No → **DEAD**

Yes ↓   Yes ↘

Respiratory rate — <10 or >29 → **P1** (immediate/red)

10–29 ↓   Yes ↗

Capillary refill > 2 sec. or pulse > 120 — No → **P2** (urgent/yellow)

Capillary refill can be used in place of pulse rate, but is not as accurate due to outside influences (temperature, skin discolouration, bad circulation, etc.)
        Capillary refill: over 2 seconds = P1
        Capillary refill: under 2 seconds = P2

Figure 47-12 Triage Sieve.

Paediatric triage Sieve is usually undertaken using a paediatric triage tape. This has been developed to quickly show the appropriate respiratory and haemodynamic states for the child using the child's height as its discriminator. If a tape is not available, use the adult parameters to triage the child. Although this will overestimate the child's actual state, it is safer to be cautious at this stage, before a more accurate assessment is carried out using the triage Sort at the casualty clearing station.

Triage Sort

When patients arrive in the casualty clearing station they are re-triaged using the triage Sort. This reassessment measures physiological parameters to gauge a more accurate indication of the patient's clinical condition. The triage Sort consists of a weighted score being awarded following an assessment of the patients Triage Revised Trauma Score (TRTS), which measures the patient's respiratory rate, systolic blood pressure, and Glasgow Coma Scale score. A TRTS of 12 is categorised as delayed (green), a TRTS of 11 is categorised as urgent (yellow) and a TRTS of 1–10 is categorised as immediate (red). Where the use of the expectant category has been authorised by the medical commander, a TRTS of 1–3 constitutes this category with a TRTS of 0 identifying the dead.

Triage Special Considerations

There are a few special situations in triage. Patients who are hysterical and disruptive to rescue efforts may need to be made an immediate priority and transported out of the major incident site, even if they are not seriously injured. Panic breeds panic, and this type of behaviour could have a detrimental impact on other patients and on the emergency services personnel.

Emergency services personnel who become sick or injured during the rescue effort should be handled as an immediate priority and be transported off the site as soon as possible to avoid negative impact to the morale of remaining teams.

Hazardous materials incidents force the hazardous materials team to identify patients as contaminated or decontaminated before the regular triage process. Contamination by chemicals or biological weapons in a treatment area, a hospital, or trauma centre could obstruct all systems and organisations coping with the major incident. Bear in mind that some incidents may require multiple triage areas or teams because the victims are located far apart.

Transportation of Patients

All patients triaged as Immediate (red) or Urgent (yellow) should preferably be transported by ambulance (including air ambulance where available and appropriate). In extremely large situations, a bus may transport the walking wounded. If a bus is used for minimal priority patients, it is strongly suggested that they be transported to a hospital some distance from the major incident site to avoid overwhelming the local area hospital resources.

Priority for transportation will usually be based upon triage category. However, prioritisation for transport from scene to hospital must be based upon a number of key factors. The loading officer will use the patient's triage category, the type of transport available, and the availability of beds and theatre space at hospitals. Some patients may require specialist care not available at the closest facilities (eg, burns or paediatric surgery) and therefore some of the more severely ill patients may be sent to destinations some distance away. For these patients, air ambulances may be appropriate. The deceased are handled or transported under strict direction and supervision of the police.

Critical Incident Stress Management

Responders at a disaster or an MI may become overwhelmed. Critical incident stress management should be available and spoken about to all personnel. This is a key role for all supervising officers, both during and following the incident. All responders are encouraged to participate, but stress management should not be imposed or forced. Forcing stress management can do more harm than good to the psychological well-being of rescuers. Some ambulance clinicians have the ability and resilience for self-healing in these situations.

After-Action Reviews

After any incident, an after-action review should be held. All agencies involved in the response should participate in the effort to improve future reactions to disasters. If something worked well in the plan, keep it. If something did not work at all, remove it or fix it.

No response is ever perfect, but it is up to all participants to keep perfecting their training, equipment, plans, and skills. All observations should be noted, in writing if possible, to allow future review. Discourage all finger pointing by use of a structured debrief. This identifies:

1. What went well
2. What could have gone better
3. What needs to be changed for the future.

Conclusion

No paramedic ever wants the "Big One" to happen. These events can happen anywhere and at anytime. They can overwhelm ambulance service systems with huge demands on materials and people, and people can be affected physically and psychologically. By keeping the basic goal of "doing the most good for the largest number of patients" in the forefront, developing plans, using the ICS, and applying a systematic approach to triage, even a major incident can be handled effectively. Practise plans often or on everyday smaller scale incidents, and they will become instinctive, which will help you use them in larger incidents.

You are the Paramedic Summary

1. What is your plan of action?

After assuming command of the incident and making sure that you and your colleagues safety is ensured, you would pass a situation report back to ambulance control (METHANE or CHALET). You would then be able to triage Sieve the walking wounded by labelling them green, and designating an area for them to be placed.

2. Why is an incident command system (ICS) needed for handling major incidents?

Any incident that involves multiple vehicles responding to an incident requires management of the resources and personnel for a timely and efficient operation. When multiple agencies are involved, it is even more urgent that a system be in place to manage the incident and coordinate the response, facilitating easy communication between agencies. Paramedics are trained to manage a single patient with multiple priorities. This is practised on a daily basis. When a situation arises in which multiple patients must be managed and multiple ambulances are responding (not a daily practice), there must be an ICS that is simple and well understood by all emergency services personnel. Each service needs to have an ICS that has been practised and is understood by all staff in each of the agencies that may be asked to respond to any major incident.

3. What is a "compensated" incident? What is an "uncompensated" incident?

A compensated incident is one where casualties can be effectively managed by mobilising additional resources to cope with the increase in workload for the health service, the demand is less than the capacity. An uncompensated incident is where demand for health care exceeds the capacity despite the mobilisation of additional resources, examples can be seen in mass casualty disasters such as earthquakes.

4. How should you triage this patient?

Delayed (Green).

5. What is the difference between single and unified command?

Single command usually only works well when there is one emergency service agency responsible for the entire operation and no need for other disciplines to be involved. A unified command structure is more common and a key component of an ICS. This means that all involved agencies contribute to the command process by determining the overall goals and objectives, joint planning for tactical activities, and maximising the use of all assigned resources at the incident.

6. What is "span of control"?

Another key component of an ICS is the span of control. A manageable span of control is the number of officers that one supervising officer can manage effectively. The desired range is from three to seven. It can be very easy to lose track of workers at an incident if they are not assigned to small groups.

7. How should you triage this patient?

Immediate (Red).

8. Why is there an essential need for common terminology in an ICS?

Because there may be crews from many different services, it is easier to use simple sector titles indicating the function they serve (eg, commander, parking, primary triage, treatment, loading, safety). A major incident is not the time to begin figuring out another agency's "code system". Plain English works best in these situations. It is much easier for responding vehicles to report to the IC instead of trying to remember that the paramedic supervisor on Vehicle 881 is the person commanding the incident response at the scene.

9. How should you triage this patient?

Immediate (Red).

10. What is the value of triage labels?

Triage labels can be very useful tools. The hardest part is getting crews to start using them! Typically, there are a few different types of triage labels commercially available for services to purchase. The key thing to remember is that any system will work, as long as everyone follows it; it has been known for coloured tags to be attached to patients in some instances to allow their triage state to be recognised. One very useful aspect to triage labels is that they help to eliminate the need to reassess the same patient over and over again. Once the patient is labelled, it is clear that an ambulance clinician has assessed them at least once.

Prep Kit

Ready for Review

- Major incident management requires planners to take a broad look at preparedness, planning, training, response, and after-action review.
- A major incident is any occurrence that presents serious threat to the health of the community, disruption to the service, or causes (or is likely to cause) such numbers or types of casualties as to require special arrangements to be implemented by hospitals, ambulance trusts, or primary care organisations.
- Using the incident command system (ICS) gives you a modular organisational structure that is built on the size and complexity of the incident.
- Major incidents require the involvement and coordination of multiple jurisdictions, functional agencies, and emergency response disciplines. The Integrated Emergency Management System (IEMS) is used to prepare for, prevent, respond to, and recover from domestic incidents, regardless of cause, size, or complexity, including acts of terrorism.
- Your ambulance service should have written major incident plans that you are regularly trained to carry out.
- At incidents that have a significant medical demand, the ambulance commander should appoint bronze officers who will supervise triage, treatment, and transport of injured patients.
- The goal of triage is to do the greatest good for the greatest number. This means that the triage assessment is brief and patient condition categories are basic.

Vital Vocabulary

ambulance commander (AC) The overall leader (silver) of ambulance operations, and accountable for all medical activity at the scene.

ambulance loading officer Delegated role from the ambulance commander, the person who coordinates transportation and distribution of patients to appropriate receiving hospitals.

ambulance parking officer Delegated role from the ambulance commander, the person who locates an area to store equipment and personnel and tracks ambulance arrival and deployment from the parking area.

body holding area An area near to but separate from the casualty clearing area where the deceased can be stored prior to their removal from the scene. This area is usually guarded by a police officer and should be shielded as far as practicable from public view.

bronze equipment officer Delegated role from the ambulance commander, the position that helps procure and stockpile equipment and supplies during an incident.

casualty clearing officer Delegated role from the ambulance commander, the person responsible for locating, setting up, and supervising casualty clearing station.

compensated An incident, although large, which can be met from local resources.

compound incident An incident where local infrastructure has been destroyed, leading to long term recovery management (see critical infrastructure).

critical infrastructure The external foundation in communities made up of structures and services critical in the day-to-day living activities of humans: energy sources, fuel, water, sewage removal, food, hospitals, and transportation systems.

demobilisation The process of "standing-down" from the emergency response of the major incident and implementing the recovery phase.

disaster management A planned, coordinated response to a disaster that involves cooperation of multiple agencies and enables effective triage and provision of care according to triage decisions.

disasters Widespread events that disrupt community resources and functions, in turn threatening public safety, lives, and property.

forward incident officer Delegated role from the ambulance commander, the person who supervises the people working at the scene of a complex incident.

freelancing When individual units or different organisations make independent and often inefficient decisions about the next appropriate action.

incident command system (ICS) A system implemented to manage disasters and major incidents in which senior managers and directors of an emergency service direct their respective incident commander at the scene.

Integrated Emergency Response A command system used in larger incidents in which there is a multiagency response or multiple jurisdictions are involved.

joint information centre (JIC) An area designated by the incident commander, or a designee, in which public relations officers from multiple agencies disseminate information about the incident.

major incident Any occurrence that presents serious threat to the health of the community, disruption to the service, or causes (or is likely to cause) such numbers or types of casualties as to require special arrangements to be implemented by hospitals, ambulance trusts, or primary care organisations.

medical commander (MC) A specific part of the ICS, which requires a doctor to operate in a managerial and not treatment role, alongside the AC.

primary triage officer The person in charge of prioritising patients, whose primary duty is to ensure that every patient receives initial triage.

public relations (PR) officer Delegated role from the ambulance commander, the person who keeps the public informed and relates any information to the press.

safety officer Delegated role from the ambulance commander, the person who gives the "go ahead" to a plan or who may stop an operation when rescuer safety is an issue.

simple incident Incident where local infrastructure (i.e., electricity supplies, water supplies, roads, hospitals, and so forth) is intact.

single command system A command system in which one person is in charge, generally used with small incidents that involve only one responding agency.

span of control The subordinate positions under the commander's direction to which the workload is distributed; the supervisor/worker ratio.

strategic (Gold) command Established during protracted major incidents, and is convened off-site, away from the actual major incident itself. It is the top tier of the Integrated Emergency Management System and comprises senior managers/directors of all emergency services and responding organisations.

termination of command The end of the incident command structure when an incident draws to a close.

transfer of command When an incident commander turns over command to someone with more experience in a critical area.

triage To categorise patients based on the severity of their conditions and prioritise them for care accordingly.

triage Sieve The initial categorisation of patients at the site where they are found using three parameters: mobility, respiratory rate, and circulatory status. This is sometimes referred to as primary triage.

triage Sort The categorisation of patients using three parameters: respiratory rate, systolic blood pressure, and Glasgow Coma Scale score. This is carried out in the casualty clearing station and is sometimes referred to as secondary triage.

uncompensated Where the incident creates a demand that cannot be met from local resources.

Assessment in Action

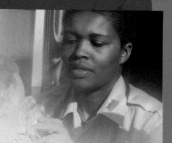

You are sent to a road traffic collision involving a single-decker bus on a dual carriageway. You are the first ambulance on scene. When you leave your vehicle, you immediately begin your initial scene assessment. There are several walking wounded, and you are informed that the bus was full, was cut up by another vehicle, and swerved to the left. It travelled down an embankment, rolled over, and landed on its wheels. There are no other vehicles involved, but many people are leaving their vehicles to try to help.

1. **As the first paramedic arriving at the scene, your first priority should be to:**
   A. start treating the injured.
   B. assume control of the scene.
   C. prepare a casualty clearing station.
   D. start triaging patients.

2. **The first situation report to your control is very important and should include all of the following, EXCEPT:**
   A. location of the casualty clearing station.
   B. exact location of the incident.
   C. type of incident.
   D. approximate number of patients involved.

3. **A major incident is defined for health agencies as:**
   A. the greatest challenge facing an ambulance service practitioner because the resources are severely limited initially.
   B. an event that is relatively simple to manage without compromise to day-to-day activities.
   C. an event in which the number of patients exceeds the number of patient care providers or the resources available to responders.
   D. the result of a natural or man-made disaster, subcategorised as uncompensated or compensated.

4. **Regardless of the cause of this major incident, how would this scenario be subcategorised?**
   A. Compensated incident
   B. Uncompensated incident
   C. Open-ended incident
   D. Man-made disaster

5. **What are the two types of incident command systems?**
   A. Single command and unified command systems
   B. Span of control and consolidated action systems
   C. Unified command and dual command systems
   D. Single command and multiple command systems

6. **What is span of control?**
   A. Individual units or different organisations making independent and often inefficient decisions about the next appropriate action
   B. The establishing of objectives and priorities by the person overseeing the incident
   C. The positions under a commander's direction to which the workload is distributed; the supervisor/worker ratio
   D. Assistance in procuring and stockpiling equipment

7. **The ambulance commander should remain in continuous contact with the:**
   A. fire commander.
   B. medical commander.
   C. police commander.
   D. WRVS.

8. **There are several positions that fall under the responsibility of the ambulance commander. They are the:**
   A. safety officer.
   B. forward incident officer.
   C. loading officer
   D. all of the above.

Challenging Question

You arrive to work your night shift. You learn that the day crew has been at a factory fire all afternoon. Your supervisor asks you to relieve your colleagues who are still at scene. You arrive at the incident and are asked to take over the primary triage officer role. The off-going triage officer informs you that they have already triaged 22 patients and that they are expecting another 15 to 20 patients. You've never done this before and are a little nervous. After taking in a few deep breaths, you begin your role.

9. **What is your role?**

Points to Ponder

You are sent to your local sixth form college at 13:15 because of the smell of smoke. When you arrive, the local fire brigade is on scene assessing the situation. The canteen staff left something burning on the stove, and it caught fire. There are approximately 10 to 15 students who were in the canteen and are experiencing possible smoke inhalation symptoms.

What should you do first? Who should you contact?

Issues: Initiating Incident Command at Smaller Events, Knowing Your Trust's Standard Operating Procedures for a Major Incident, Understanding Why Common Problems of a Major Incident Can Have an Adverse Effect on an Entire Incident.

48 Terrorism

Objectives

Cognitive

- Define terrorism.
- List the different terrorist agenda categories.
- Describe the five threat levels used by the Home Office to notify responders and the public of the potential for a terrorist attack:
  - Critical—an attack is expected imminently.
  - Severe—an attack is highly likely.
  - Substantial—an attack is a strong possibility.
  - Moderate—an attack is possible but not likely.
  - Low—an attack is unlikely.
- On the basis of Home Office threat levels, discuss what actions paramedics should take during the course of their work to heighten their ability to respond to and survive a terrorist attack.
- Recognise the hallmarks of a terrorist event.
- List potential terrorist targets and their vulnerability.
- Discuss these key principles to assuring responder safety at the scene of a terrorist event:
  - Establishing scene safety
  - Approaching the scene
  - Protective measures
  - Establishing a safety zone
  - Ongoing reevaluation of scene safety
  - Awareness of secondary devices
- Discuss the following critical actions that the paramedic must perform to operate on the scene following a terrorist attack:
  - Notification
  - Establish command
  - Patient management

- Describe and list the five weapons of mass destruction (WMD).
- Describe historical events dealing with terrorism.
- List conventional/chemical/biological/radiological/nuclear agents that may be used by a terrorist.
- Describe the routes of exposure for chemical agents.
- Describe the routes of exposure for biological agents.
- Describe the routes of exposure for nuclear/radiological dispersal devices (RDD).
- Discuss the clinical manifestations of exposure to the various WMD agents.
- Describe the treatment to be rendered to a victim of a conventional/chemical/biological/radiological/nuclear attack.

Affective

- Discuss the 21st century terrorist's trend towards mass violence and indiscriminate death.
- Explain the rationale behind not entering the WMD scene or being unable to treat contaminated patients, and the possible impact on the paramedic.

Psychomotor

- Demonstrate the patient assessment skills to assist the patient involved in a conventional/chemical/biological/radiological/nuclear agent.
- Given a scenario of a terrorist event, establish scene safety and begin patient management.

Introduction

As a result of the increase in terrorist activity, it is possible that you may respond to a terrorist event during your career. Throughout the world, international terrorists as well as domestic groups have increased their targeting of civilian populations with acts of terror. The question is not will terrorists strike again, but rather when and where they will strike. The paramedic must be mentally and physically prepared for the possibility of a terrorist event.

The use of weapons of mass destruction (WMD), or weapons of major incident (WMI), further complicates the management of the terrorist incident and places the paramedic in greater danger. Although it is difficult to anticipate and plan a response to many terrorist events, there are several key principles that apply to every response. This chapter describes how you can prepare to respond to these events by discussing types of terrorist events, personnel safety, and patient management. You will learn the signs, symptoms, and treatment of patients who have been exposed to a conventional, chemical, biological, radiological, or nuclear attack. At the end of this chapter, you will be able to answer the following key questions:

- What are your initial actions?
- Who should you notify, and what should you tell them?
- What type of additional resources might you require?
- How should you proceed to address the needs of the victims?

- How do you ensure your own and your colleague's safety, as well as the safety of the victims?
- What is the clinical presentation of a patient exposed to a WMD?
- How are WMD patients to be assessed and treated?
- How do you avoid becoming contaminated or cross-contaminated with a WMD agent?

What Is Terrorism?

No one is quite sure who the first terrorist was, but terrorist forces have been at work since early civilisations. The British Terrorism Act 2000 defines terrorism so as to include not only violent offences against people and physical damage to property, but also acts, "designed seriously to interfere with or seriously to disrupt an electronic system". However this, and any of the other acts covered by the definition, would also need to be (a) designed to influence the government or to intimidate the public or a section of the public, and (b) be done for the purpose of advancing a political, religious, or ideological cause **Figure 48-1 ▶** . Today, terrorists pose a threat to countries and cultures everywhere. International terrorism has brought a new fear into the lives of many British citizens.

Modern-day terrorism is common in the Middle East, where terrorist groups have frequently attacked civilian populations. In Colombia, political terrorist groups target oil resources as a means to instill fear.

You are the Paramedic Part 1

You and your colleague are dispatched to the Mountjoy shopping centre for a patient having a convulsion. While en route ambulance control informs you that they have received numerous 999 calls from within the shopping centre. Callers are stating that a large number of people are vomiting and having convulsions. Many appear to be unconscious.

Additional information received from ambulance control states that security is reporting a high-pitched whistling sound, much like a gas leak. The Special Operations Response Team (SORT), has been dispatched and has an estimated time of arrival (ETA) of 4 minutes. All vehicles are given the order to not enter until the SORT personnel have evaluated the scene.

On arrival in the primary car park, you note that your supervisor is on the scene and has donned the "Ambulance Commander" vest. Your supervisor, as well as numerous other responders from police, fire, and security, meets you at the front entrance. Your ambulance is assigned to report to the casualty clearing station that has been set up in a restaurant across the street. As part of the Sieve triage system, the "walking wounded" who have already exited the building were told to go to the restaurant to be medically evaluated. There are a number of higher priority patients who are being evaluated or are yet to be assessed pending authorisation that the site is actually safe to enter, but they are clearly not your responsibility at this time. You are assigned a female patient in her 30s who is pacing around and appears to be crying.

Initial Assessment	Recording Time: 0 Minutes
Appearance	Female in her 30s who is pacing around and appears to be crying
Level of consciousness	A (Alert to person, place, and day)
Airway	Open and clear
Breathing	Rapid and shallow
Circulation	Weak, slow radial pulse

1. What is your first priority on arrival in this situation?
2. What does the ambulance control information indicate as far as the need for additional resources?

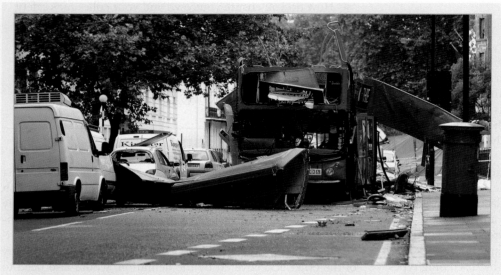

Figure 48-1 The attack on the transport system in London killed 52 innocent people.

Terrorist organisations are generally categorised. Only a small percentage of groups, such as the following, actually turn towards terrorism as a means to achieve their goals:

1. **Violent religious groups/doomsday cults.** These include groups such as Aum Shinrikyo, who carried out chemical and biological attacks in Tokyo between 1994 and 1995. Some of these groups may participate in apocalyptic violence.

2. **Extremist political groups.** They may include violent separatist groups and those who seek political, religious, economic, and social freedom.

3. **Technology terrorists.** Those who attack a population's technological infrastructure as a means to draw attention to their cause, such as cyberterrorists.

4. **Single-issue groups.** These include animal rights groups, anarchists, racists, or even ecoterrorists who threaten or use violence as a means to protect the environment.

Most terrorist attacks require the coordination of multiple terrorists or "actors" working together. Nineteen hijackers worked together to commit the worst act of terrorism in US history on 11th September, 2001. At least four terrorists worked together to commit the London Underground bombings on 7th July, 2005. However, in a few instances there has been a single terrorist who struck with devastating results.

▌Weapons of Mass Destruction

What Are Weapons of Mass Destruction?

A weapon of mass destruction (WMD), or weapon of major incident (WMI), is any agent designed to bring about mass death, casualties, and/or massive damage to property and infrastructure (bridges, tunnels, airports, and seaports). These instruments of death and destruction include conventional, chemical, biological, radiological, and nuclear weapons. To date, the preferred WMD for terrorists have been explosive devices. Terrorist groups have favoured tactics that use lorry bombs or car or pedestrian suicide bombers. Many previous terrorist attempts to use either chemical or biological weapons to their full capacity have been unsuccessful. Nonetheless, as a paramedic you should understand the destructive potential of these weapons.

As discussed earlier, the motives and tactics of the 21st century terrorist groups have begun to change. As with the doomsday cults, many terrorist groups participate in large-scale, indiscriminate killing. This doctrine of total carnage would make the use of WMDs highly desirable. WMDs are easy to obtain or create and are specifically geared toward killing large numbers of people. Had the proper techniques been used during the 1995 attack on the Tokyo underground, there would have been tens of thousands of casualties. With the fall of the former Soviet Union, the technology and expertise to produce WMDs may be available to terrorist groups with sufficient funding. Moreover, the technical recipes for making nuclear, biological, and chemical (NBC) weapons and explosive devices can be found readily on the Internet; in fact, they have even been published on terrorist group websites.

There are five categories of terrorist incidents that first responder agencies may confront in the prehospital environment. They are easily remembered with the mnemonic CCBRN:

C	Conventional (incendiary, explosives)
C	Chemical
B	Biological
R	Radiological
N	Nuclear

Conventional—Explosives/Incendiary Weapons

Explosives are the most likely method to be used by terrorists **Figure 48-2 ▶**. Incendiary weapons involve agents and chemicals used to start fires. Incendiary agents, such as acetone, can be combined with chemicals to produce explosives capable of massive destruction. Ranging from suicide bombings on public buses to lorries loaded with explosives set to go off in underground parking garages of government buildings, these explosions can be very destructive. Explosives are substances that fit into one of the following two categories:

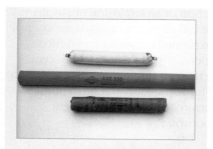

Figure 48-2 Every year, tons of explosives are stolen, some by potential terrorists.

- A substance or article, including a device designed to function by explosion
- A substance or article, including a device, which by chemical reaction within itself can function in a similar manner even if not designated to function by explosion, unless the substance or article is other wise classified.

Chemical Terrorism/Warfare

Chemical agents are manmade substances that can have devastating effects on living organisms. They can be produced in liquid, powder, or vapour form depending on the desired route of exposure and dissemination technique. Developed during World War I, these agents have been implicated in thousands of deaths since being introduced on the battlefield, and since then have been used to terrorise civilian populations. These agents consist of the following five categories:

- Vesicants or blister agents (ie, mustard gas and Lewisite)
- Respiratory or choking agents (ie, phosgene or chlorine)
- Nerve agents (ie, sarin, soman, tabun, or V agent)
- Metabolic or blood agents (ie, hydrogen cyanide, cyanogens chloride)
- Irritating agents (ie, mace, chloropicrin, tear gas, capsicum/pepper spray, and dibenzoxazepine)

Biological Terrorism/Warfare

Biological agents are organisms that cause disease or death. They are generally found in nature; for terrorist use, however, they are cultivated, synthesised, and mutated in a laboratory. The weaponisation of biological agents is performed to artificially maximise the target population's exposure to the germ, thereby exposing the greatest number of people and achieving the desired result.

The primary types of biological agents that you may come into contact with during a biological event include:

- Viruses
- Bacteria
- Toxins

Radiological/Nuclear Terrorism

There have been only two publicly known incidents involving the use of a nuclear device. During World War II, Hiroshima and Nagasaki were devastated when they were targeted with nuclear bombs. It has been estimated that a death toll of 214,000 occurred due to the two bombs and their associated effects. The awesome destructive power demonstrated by the attack ended the last stages of the second world war involving Japan, and served as a deterrent to nuclear war.

There are also nations that hold close ties with terrorist groups (known as state-sponsored terrorism) and have obtained some degree of nuclear capability. It is also possible for a terrorist to secure radioactive materials or waste to perpetrate an act of terror. Such materials are far easier for the determined terrorist to acquire and would require less expertise to use. The difficulties in developing a nuclear weapon are well documented. Radioactive materials, however, such as those in

You are the Paramedic Part 2

The SORT personnel are on the scene and have entered the shopping centre. The Ambulance Command reports that they believe a small canister of a nerve gas was released in the sports shop. The actual number of patients still inside the shopping centre who are unconscious or may have had convulsions is approximately eight patients. The SORT personnel, in conjunction with the fire service HazMat team, are rapidly decontaminating patients so they can be removed to the cold zone and receive lifesaving treatment. The Ambulance Commander has already been in contact with the National Poisons Information Service and they have advised that all patients, even those who are alert like your patient, be evaluated for nerve agent symptoms (DUMBELS) and if necessary managed with a nerve agent antidote kit (NAAK). You begin to evaluate your patient further and note she is still crying and has vomited. You start administration of oxygen at 15 litres per minute via nonrebreathing mask.

Vital Signs	Recording Time: 10 Minutes
Level of consciousness	Alert, with a Glasgow Coma Scale score of 15
Skin	Pale, warm and dry
Pulse	Weak radial at 52 beats/min
Respirations	12 breaths/min
SpO$_2$	97% with oxygen at 15 l/min via nonrebreathing mask

3. What precautions can you take to ensure your own safety?
4. What does your index of suspicion tell you about this scene?

Radiological Dispersal Devices (RDDs), also known as "dirty bombs", can cause widespread panic and civil disturbances. More on these devices will be covered later in this chapter.

Paramedic Response to Terrorism

Recognising a Terrorist Event (Indicators)

Most acts of terror are covert, which means that the public safety community generally has no prior knowledge of the time, location, or nature of the attack. This element of surprise makes responding to an event more complex. You must constantly be aware of your surroundings and understand the possible risks for terrorism associated with certain locations, at certain times. It is therefore important that you know the current threat level issued by HM Government through the home office.

This system alerts responders to the potential for an attack, although the specifics of the current threat will not be given. On the basis of the current threat level, the paramedic should take appropriate actions and precautions while continuing to perform daily duties and responding to calls. The system is used to inform the public safety community of the climate of terrorism (derived from intelligence gathering and the amount of terrorist communication) and to heighten the awareness of the potential for a terrorist attack. The system is designed to save lives, including yours. Follow your local guidelines, policies, and procedures.

It is your responsibility to make sure you know the advisory level at the start of your workday. Daily newspapers, television news programmes, and multiple websites all give up-to-date information on the threat level. Many ambulance service organisations are starting to display the advisory system on boards where they can be seen once staff arrive for a shift.

Understanding and being aware of the current threat is only the beginning of responding safely to calls. Once you are on duty, you must be able to make appropriate decisions regarding the potential for a terrorist event. In determining the potential for a terrorist attack, on every call you should observe the following:

- **Type of location.** Is the location a monument, infrastructure, government building, or a specific type of location such as a place of worship? Is there a large gathering? Is there a special event taking place?

At the Scene

A new system has been created by the Home Office to keep the public informed about the level of threat to the UK from terrorism.

- Critical—an attack is expected imminently.
- Severe—an attack is highly likely.
- Substantial—an attack is a strong possibility.
- Moderate—an attack is possible but not likely.
- Low—an attack is unlikely.

- **Type of call.** Is there a report of an explosion or suspicious device nearby? Does the call come into ambulance control as someone having unexplained coughing and difficulty breathing? Are there reports of people fleeing the scene?
- **Number of patients.** Are there multiple patients with similar signs and symptoms? This is probably the single most important clue that a terrorist attack or an incident involving a WMD has occurred.

At the Scene

STEPS 1-2-3
Safety Triggers for Emergency Personnel.
To be used when a cause is unknown.
Step 1—One casualty
Approach using normal procedures.
Step 2—Two casualties
Approach with caution, consider all options, do not discount anything, report on arrival and update control.
Step 3—Three casualties or more
Do not approach the scene. Withdraw—contain—report—isolate yourself and send for specialist help.

- **Victims' statements.** This is probably the second best indication of a terrorist or WMD event. Are the patients fleeing the scene giving statements such as, "Everyone is passing out", "There was a loud explosion", or "There are a lot of people shaking on the ground". If so, something is occurring that you do not want to rush into, even if it turns out not to be a terrorist event.
- **Pre-incident indicators.** Is the terror alert level critical or severe? Has there been a recent increase in violent political activism? Are you aware of any credible threats made against the location, gathering, or occasion?

Response Actions

Once you suspect that a terrorist event has occurred or WMD have been used, there are certain actions to take to ensure that you will be safe and be in the proper position to help the community.

Scene Safety

Ensure that the scene is safe. If you have any doubt that it may not be safe, do not enter. When dealing with a WMD scene, it is safe to assume that you will not be able to enter where the event has occurred—nor do you want to. The best location for standing off is upwind and uphill from the incident. Wait for assistance from those who are trained in assessing and managing WMD scenes Figure 48-3 ▶ . Also remember:

- Failure to park your vehicle at a safe location can place you and your colleague in danger Figure 48-4 ▶ .
- If your vehicle is blocked in by other emergency vehicles or damaged by a secondary device (or event), you will be unable to provide patients with transportation, or escape yourself Figure 48-5 ▶ . Remember not to block others in.

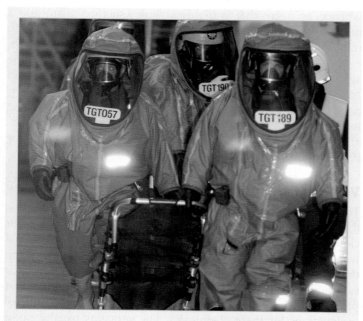

Figure 48-3 Ineffective command and control at a mass-casualty scene could lead to injury or even death of ambulance service personnel.

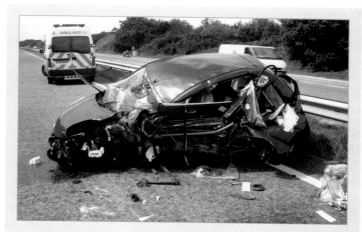

Figure 48-4 Park your vehicle at a safe location and distance.

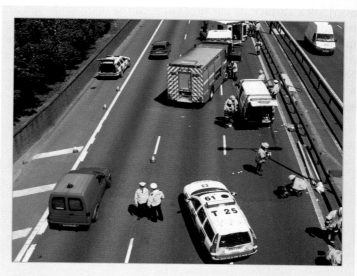

Figure 48-5 Make sure that your vehicle is not blocked in by other emergency vehicles.

Responder Safety (Personnel Protection)

The best form of protection from a WMD agent is preventing yourself from coming into contact with the agent. The greatest threats facing a paramedic in a WMD attack are contamination and cross-contamination. Contamination (primary exposure) with an agent occurs when you have direct contact with the WMD or are exposed to it. Cross-contamination (secondary exposure) occurs when you come into contact with a contaminated person who has not yet been decontaminated.

Notification Procedures

When you suspect a terrorist or WMD event has taken place, notify ambulance control, provided that communication is functioning properly. Vital information needs to be communicated effectively if you are to receive the appropriate assistance (see Chapter 16 for information on effective communication). Inform ambulance control of as much information as possible, including the exact location of the incident and any rendezvous point; the type of incident; the actual and potential hazards involved; the size, shape, and colour of any suspicious containers; and the information displayed on the associated placards. Specify access and egress routes to the scene, estimate the number of casualties involved and any common clinical presentations, as well as detail the emergency services already at scene and those still required.

Fundamentally, trained personnel equipped with the appropriate CCBRN personal protective equipment are the only people skilled to handle a WMD incident. These specialised units, whether SORT, in the case of the ambulance service, or HazMat teams, in relation of the fire service or the military, must be requested as early as possible due to the time required to assemble and dispatch them. Few services have

SORT teams on immediate call and the team may have to travel a long distance to reach the location of the event. It is always better to be safe than sorry; call the team early and the outcome of the call will be more favourable. Keep in mind that there may be more than one type of device or agent present.

Establishing Command

The first arriving paramedic on the scene must begin to sort out the chaos and define his or her responsibilities under the Incident Command System (ICS). As the first person on scene, the paramedic may need to assume initial command by becoming the Ambulance Commander until additional personnel arrive.

At the Scene

Secondary devices may include various types of electronic equipment such as mobile phones or pagers that are detonated when "answered".

Depending on the circumstances, you and other paramedics may function as bronze officers, safety officers, casualty clearing officers or any of the roles commensurate with the major incident command hierarchy. If the ICS is already in place, then you should immediately seek out the Ambulance Silver Commander to receive your assignment. The incident command system and its components are discussed in further detail in Chapter 47.

Secondary Device or Event (Reassessing Scene Safety)

Terrorists have been known to plant additional explosives that are set to explode after the initial bomb. This type of second-ary device is intended primarily to injure responders and to secure media coverage, because the media generally arrives on scene just after the initial response. Do not rely on others to secure your safety. It is every paramedic's responsibility to constantly assess and reassess the scene for safety. It is easy to overlook a suspicious package lying on the floor while you are treating casualties. Stay alert. Something as subtle as a change in the wind direction during a gas attack or an increase in the number of contaminated patients can place you in danger. Never become so involved with the tasks that you are performing that you do not look around and make sure that the scene remains safe.

At the Scene

You are of no help to the public if you become a patient. More importantly, once you become a casualty of the event, you place an additional burden on your fellow responders, who must treat you. Assess the scene and resist the urge to run in and help (do not develop tunnel vision). You may place your life and your colleague in danger. Remember . . . do not become a victim.

Chemical Agents

Chemical agents are liquids or gases that are dispersed to kill or injure. Chemical weapons were first deployed during World War I. During the Cold War, many of these agents were perfected and stockpiled. Whilst many nations have renounced the use of chemical weapons, just as many nations still develop and stockpile them. These agents are deadly and pose a threat if acquired by terrorists.

Chemical weapons have several classifications. The properties or characteristics of an agent can be described as liquid, gas, or solid material. Persistency and volatility are terms used to describe how long the agent will stay on a surface before it evaporates. Persistent or nonvolatile agents can remain on a surface for long periods of time, usually longer than 24 hours. Nonpersistent or volatile agents evaporate relatively fast when left on a surface in the optimal temperature range. An agent that is described as highly persistent (such as VX, a nerve agent) can remain in the environment for weeks to months,

whereas an agent that is highly volatile (such as sarin, also a nerve agent) will turn from liquid to gas (evaporate) within minutes to seconds.

Route of exposure is a term used to describe how the agent most effectively enters the body. Chemical agents can have either a vapour or contact hazard. Agents with a vapour hazard enter the body through the respiratory tract in the form of vapours. Agents with a contact hazard (or skin hazard) give off very little vapour or no vapours and enter the body through the skin.

Vesicants (Blister Agents)

The primary route of exposure of blister agents, or vesicants, is the skin (contact); however, if vesicants are left on the skin or clothing long enough, they produce vapours that can enter the respiratory tract. Vesicants cause burn-like blisters to form on the patient's skin as well as in the respiratory tract. The vesicant agents consist of sulphur mustard (H), Lewisite (L), and phosgene oxime (CX) (the symbols H, L, and CX are military designations for these chemicals). The vesicants usually cause the most damage to damp or moist areas of the body, such as the armpits, groin, and the respiratory tract. Signs of vesicant exposure on the skin include:

- Skin irritation, burning, urticaria, and erythema
- Immediate intense skin pain (with L and CX)
- Formation of large blisters
- Grey discolouration of skin (a sign of permanent damage seen with L and CX)
- Swollen and closed or irritated eyes
- Permanent eye injury (including blindness)

If vapours were inhaled, the patient may experience the following:

- Hoarseness and stridor
- Severe cough
- Haemoptysis (coughing up of blood)
- Severe dyspnoea

Sulphur mustard (agent H) is a brownish, yellowish oily substance that is generally considered very persistent. When released, mustard has the distinct smell of garlic or mustard and is quickly absorbed into the skin and/or mucous membranes. As the agent is absorbed into the skin, it begins an irreversible process of damage to the cells. Absorption through the skin or mucous membranes usually occurs within seconds, and damage to the underlying cells takes place within 1 to 2 minutes.

Mustard is considered a mutagen, which means that it mutates, damages, and changes the structures of cells. Eventually, cellular death will occur. On the surface, the patient will generally not produce any signs or symptoms until 4 to 6 hours after exposure (depending on concentration and amount of exposure) **Figure 48-6** ▶ 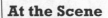.

The patient will experience a progressive urticaria and erythema of the affected area, which will gradually develop into large blisters. These blisters are very similar in shape and appearance to those associated with thermal partial thickness burns. The fluid within the blisters does not contain any of the agent; however,

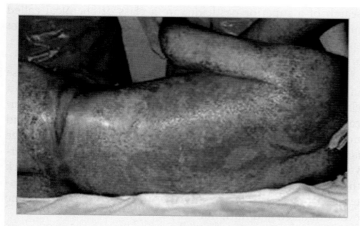

Figure 48-6 Skin damage resulting from exposure to sulphur mustard (agent H).

the skin covering the area is considered to be contaminated until decontamination by trained personnel has been performed.

Mustard also attacks vulnerable cells within the bone marrow and depletes the body's ability to reproduce white blood cells. As with burns, the primary complication associated with vesicant blisters is secondary infection. If the patient does survive the initial direct injury from the agent, the depletion of the white blood cells leaves the patient with a decreased resistance to infections. Although sulphur mustard is regarded as persistent, it does release enough vapours when dispersed to be inhaled. This creates upper and lower airway compromise. The result is damage and swelling of the airways. The airway compromise makes the patient's condition far more serious.

Lewisite (L) and phosgene oxime (CX) produce blister wounds very similar to mustard. They are highly volatile and have a rapid onset of symptoms, as opposed to the delayed onset seen with mustard. These agents produce immediate intense pain and discomfort when contact is made. The patient may have a greyish discolouration at the contaminated site. While tissue damage also occurs with exposure to these agents, they do not cause the secondary cellular injury that is associated with mustard.

Vesicant Agent Treatment

There are no antidotes for mustard or CX exposure. BAL (British Anti-Lewisite) is the antidote for agent L; however, it is not carried by civilian ambulance services. The paramedic must ensure that the patient has been decontaminated before ABCs are initiated. The patient may require prompt airway support if any agent has been inhaled, but this should not occur until after decontamination. Initiate transport and gain IV access as soon as possible. Generally, burn centres are best equipped to handle the wounds and subsequent infections produced by vesicants. Follow your local guidelines when deciding what hospital to transport the patient to.

Pulmonary Agents (Choking Agents)

Pulmonary agents are gases that cause immediate harm to people exposed to them. The primary route of exposure for these agents is through the respiratory tract, which makes them an inhalation or vapour hazard. Once inside the lungs, they damage the lung tissue and fluid leaks into the lungs. Pulmonary oedema develops in the patient, resulting in difficulty breathing due to the ineffectiveness of diffusion through external respiration. These agents produce respiratory-related symptoms such as dyspnoea, tachypnoea, and pulmonary oedema. This class of chemical agents consists of chlorine (CL) and phosgene.

Chlorine (CL) was the first chemical agent ever used in warfare. It has a distinct odour of bleach and creates a green haze when released as a gas. Initially it produces upper airway irritation and a choking sensation. The patient may later experience:

- Shortness of breath
- Chest tightness

You are the Paramedic Part 3

Your patient receives a rapid decontamination and she is now the first patient who is ready to be transported to the nearest hospital. You are notified that the patient has been administered a nerve agent antidote which involved administration of atropine, pralidoxime mesylate, and obidoxime chloride. Your patient, who is a 30-year-old woman who was working in the shopping centre when the incident took place, is still conscious, alert, and orientated. She is complaining of nausea and vomiting. She is experiencing excessive lacrimation and has already urinated twice while in the treatment area. She also has pinpoint pupils and denies any pertinent medical history.

Reassessment	Recording Time: 20 Minutes
Skin	Pale, warm, dry
Pulse	110 beats/min (after atropine) bounding at the radius and regular rate
Blood pressure	150/92 mm Hg
Respirations	12 breaths/min
SpO₂	97% with supplemental oxygen at 15 l/min via nonrebreathing mask
ECG	Sinus tachycardia without ectopics

5. What could your patient's signs and symptoms represent?

6. What are your treatment options for this patient?

- Hoarseness and stridor due to upper airway constriction
- Gasping and coughing

With serious exposures, patients may experience pulmonary oedema, complete airway constriction, and death. The fumes from a mixture of household bleach (CL) and ammonia create an acid gas that produces similar effects. Each year, such mixtures overcome hundreds of people when they try to mix household cleaners.

Phosgene should not be confused with phosgene oxime, a blistering agent, or vesicant. Not only has phosgene been produced for chemical warfare, but it is a product of combustion such as might be produced in a fire at a textile factory or house, or from metalwork or burning Freon (a liquid chemical used in refrigeration). Therefore, you may encounter a patient who was exposed to this gas during the course of a normal call or at a fire scene. Phosgene is a very potent agent that has a delayed onset of symptoms, usually hours. Unlike CL, when phosgene enters the body, it generally does not produce severe irritation, which would possibly cause the patient to leave the area or hold his or her breath. In fact, the odour produced by the chemical is similar to that of freshly mowed grass or hay. The result is that much more of the gas is allowed to enter the body unnoticed. The initial symptoms of a mild exposure may include:

- Nausea
- Chest tightness
- Severe cough
- Dyspnoea upon exertion

The patient with severe exposure may present with dyspnea at rest and excessive pulmonary oedema. The pulmonary oedema that is seen with a severe exposure produces such large amounts of fluid from the lungs that the patient may actually become hypovolaemic and subsequently hypotensive.

Pulmonary Agent Treatment

The best initial treatment for any pulmonary agent is to remove the patient from the contaminated atmosphere. This should be done by trained personnel in the proper PPE. Aggressive management of the ABCs should be initiated, paying particular attention to oxygenation, ventilation, and suctioning if required. Do not allow the patient to be active, as this will worsen the condition much faster. There are no antidotes to counteract the pulmonary agents. Performing the ABCs, gaining IV access, allowing the patient to rest in a position of comfort with the head elevated, and initiating rapid transport are the primary goals for care provided in the prehospital setting. Pharmacological therapy of this patient may include the standard treatment for bronchospasm, pulmonary oedema, potential steroid use (per local clinical guidelines) and positive-pressure ventilation with supplementary oxygen.

Nerve Agents

The nerve agents are among the most deadly chemicals developed. Designed to kill large numbers of people with small quantities, nerve agents can cause cardiac arrest within seconds to minutes of exposure. Nerve agents, discovered while in search of a superior pesticide, are a class of chemical called organophosphates, which are found in household insect sprays, agricultural pesticides, and some industrial chemicals, at far lower strengths than in nerve agents.

There are hundreds of different pesticides available for use in the United Kingdom. Approximately 37 of these belong to a class of insecticides known as organophosphates. The chemicals in this class kill insects by disrupting their brains and nervous systems. Unfortunately, these chemicals or nerve agents (at greater strengths) also can harm the brains and nervous systems of animals and humans. These chemicals block the essential enzyme in the nervous system called cholinesterase from working, causing the body's organs to become overstimulated and burn out.

G agents came from the early nerve agents, the G series, which were developed by German scientists (hence the G) in the period after WWI and into WWII. There are three G series agents, which are all designed with the same basic chemical structure with slight variations to produce different properties. The two variations of these agents are lethality and volatility. The following G agents are listed from low to high, based on lethal properties:

- **Tabun (GA).** Approximately half as lethal as sarin and 36 times more persistent; under the proper conditions it will remain for several days. It also has a fruity smell and an appearance similar to sarin. The components used to manufacture GA are easy to acquire and the agent is easy to manufacture, which make it unique. GA is both a contact and inhalation hazard that can enter the body through skin absorption as well as through the respiratory tract.
- **Sarin (GB).** Highly volatile colourless and odourless liquid. Turns from liquid to gas within seconds to minutes at room temperature. Highly lethal, with an LD_{50} of 1,700 mg/70 kg (about 1 drop, depending on the purity). The LD_{50} is the amount that will kill 50% of people who are exposed to this level. Sarin is primarily a vapour hazard, with the respiratory tract as the main route of entry. This agent is especially dangerous in enclosed environments such as office buildings, shopping centres, or underground trains. When this agent comes into contact with skin, it is quickly absorbed and evaporates. When sarin is on clothing, it has the effect of off-gassing, which means that the vapours are continuously released over a period of time (like perfume). This renders the patient as well as the patient's clothing contaminated.
- **Soman (GD).** Twice as persistent as sarin and five times as lethal. It has a fruity odour as a result of the type of alcohol used in the agent and generally has no colour. This agent is both a contact and inhalation hazard that can enter the body through skin absorption and through the respiratory tract. A unique additive in GD causes it to bind to the cells that it attacks faster than any other agent. This irreversible binding is called ageing, which makes it more difficult to treat patients who have been exposed.

■ **V agent (VX).** Clear oily agent that has no odour and looks like baby oil. V agent was developed by the British after World War II and has similar chemical properties to the G series agents. The difference is that VX is over 100 times more lethal than sarin and is extremely persistent Figure 48-7 . In fact, VX is so persistent that given the proper conditions it will remain relatively unchanged for weeks to months. These properties make VX primarily a contact hazard, because it lets off very little vapour. It is easily absorbed into the skin, and the oily residue that remains on the skin's surface is extremely difficult to decontaminate.

Nerve agents all produce similar symptoms but have varying routes of entry. Nerve agents differ slightly in lethal concentration or dose and also differ in their volatility. Some agents are designed to become a gas quickly (nonpersistent or highly volatile), while others remain liquid for a period of time (persistent or nonvolatile). These agents have been used successfully in warfare and to date represent the only type of chemical agent that has been used successfully in a terrorist act. Once the agent has entered the body through skin contact or through the respiratory system, the patient will begin to exhibit a pattern of predictable symptoms. Like all chemical agents, the severity of the symptoms will depend on the route of exposure and the amount of agent to which the patient was exposed. The resulting symptoms are described below using the military mnemonic SLUDGEM and the medical mnemonic DUMBELS. These two mnemonics are used to describe the symptoms of nerve agent exposure and are shown in Table 48-1 . The medical mnemonic is more useful to you because it lists the more dangerous symptoms associated with exposure to nerve agents, such as bradycardia and bronchorrhoea.

There are only a handful of medical conditions that are associated with the bilateral pinpoint constricted pupils (miosis) seen with nerve agent exposure. Conditions such as a suspected stroke, direct light to both eyes, and a drug overdose all can cause bilateral constricted pupils. You should therefore assess the patient for all of the SLUDGEM/DUMBELS signs and symptoms to determine whether the patient has been exposed to a nerve agent.

Miosis is the most common symptom of nerve agent exposure and can remain for days to weeks. This symptom, along with the others listed in Table 48-1, will help you recognise exposure to a nerve agent early. The convulsions that are

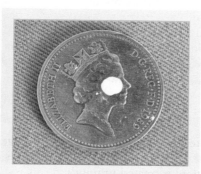

Figure 48-7 VX is the most toxic chemical ever produced. The dot demonstrates the amount needed to achieve the lethal dose.

Table 48-1	Symptoms of People Exposed to Nerve Agents
Military Mnemonic: SLUDGEM	
S	Salivation
L	Lacrimation
U	Urination
D	Defecation
G	GI distress
E	Emesis
M	Miosis
Medical Mnemonic: DUMBELS	
D	Defecation
U	Urination
M	Miosis
B	Bradycardia, Bronchorrhoea
E	Emesis
L	Lacrimation
S	Salivation

associated with nerve agent exposure are unlike those found in patients with a history of convulsion. The patient will continue to have convulsions until death or until treatment is given with a nerve agent antidote kit (NAAK).

Nerve Agent Treatment (NAAK)

Fatalities from severe exposure occur as a result of respiratory complications, which lead to respiratory arrest. Once the patients have been decontaminated, the paramedic should be prepared to treat these patients aggressively, if they are to be saved. You can greatly increase the patient's chances of survival simply by providing airway and ventilatory support. As with all emergencies, managing the ABCs is the best and most important treatment that you can provide. Often patients exposed to these agents will begin convulsing and will not stop. These patients will require administration of nerve agent antidote kits in addition to support of the ABCs.

Fortunately, there is an antidote for nerve agent exposure. The Department of Health recommends that nerve agent antidote kits (NAAK) contain 2 mg atropine, 2 g pralidoxime mesylate, and 250 mg obidoxime chloride. In some regions, paramedics may routinely carry NAAK, conversely paramedics may have to request them to be brought to the scene.

Atropine is used to block the nerve agent's overstimulation of the body. However, because the nerve agent may remain in the body for long periods of time, pralidoxime mesylate and obidoxime chloride is used to decrease the amount of excess acetylcholine being produced. Many of the symptoms described in the DUMBELS mnemonic will be reversed with the use of atropine; however, many doses may need to be administered to see these results. If your service carries a nerve agent antidote, please refer to your local guidelines for dose and usage information.

Table 48-2 ▾ has been provided for quick reference and comparison of the nerve agents.

Industrial Chemicals/Insecticides

As previously mentioned, the basic chemical ingredient in nerve agents is organophosphate. This is a common chemical that is used in lesser concentrations for insecticides. While industrial chemicals are not sufficiently lethal to be effective WMD, they are easy to acquire, inexpensive, and would have similar effects as the nerve agents. Crop-duster planes could be used to disseminate these chemicals. You should be cautious when responding to calls where insecticide equipment is stored and used, such as a farm or supply shop that sells these products. The symptoms and medical management of patients poisoned by organophosphate insecticide are identical to those of the nerve agents.

Metabolic Agents (Cyanides)

Hydrogen cyanide (AC) and cyanogens chloride (CK) are both agents that affect the body's ability to use oxygen. Cyanide is a colourless gas that has an odour similar to almonds. The effects of the cyanides begin on the cellular level and are very rapidly seen at the organ system level. Beside the nerve agents, metabolic agents are the only chemical weapons known to kill within seconds to minutes. Unlike nerve agents, however, these deadly gases are commonly found in many industrial settings. Cyanides are produced in massive quantities globally every year for industrial uses such as gold and silver mining, photography, and plastics processing. They are often present in fires associated with textile or plastic factories. In fact, cyanide is naturally found in the pits or stones of many fruits in very low doses. There is very little difference in the symptoms found between AC and CK. In low doses, these chemicals are associated with dizziness, light-headedness, headache, and vomiting. Higher doses will produce symptoms that include:

- Shortness of breath and gasping respirations
- Tachypnoea
- Flushed skin colour
- Tachycardia
- Altered mental status
- Convulsions
- Coma
- Apnoea
- Cardiac arrest

The symptoms associated with the inhalation of a large amount of cyanide will all appear within several minutes. Death is likely unless the patient is treated promptly.

Cyanide Agent Treatment

Cyanide binds with the body's cells, preventing oxygen from being used. Several medications act as antidotes, but many services do not carry them. Once trained personnel wearing the proper PPE have removed the patient from the source of exposure, even if there is no liquid contamination, all of the patient's clothes must be removed to prevent contamination of the ambulance. Trained and protected personnel must decontaminate any patients who may have been exposed to liquid contamination before a paramedic can initiate treatment. Then you should support the patient's ABCs and gain

At the Scene

On 20th March, 1995, members of a Japanese cult released sarin (GB) in the Tokyo underground. The first arriving medical responders were met with chaos as hundreds and then thousands of people fled the underground system. Many were contaminated and showing signs and systems of nerve agent exposure. In the end more than 5,000 people sought medical care for exposure to sarin, and 12 people died. None of the ambulance service personnel wore protective clothing and most became cross-contaminated. Remember, you can avoid becoming exposed. Don't become a victim yourself!

Table 48-2	Nerve Agents					
Name	Code Name	Odour	Special Features	Onset of Symptoms	Volatility	Route of Exposure
Tabun	GA	Fruity	Easy to manufacture	Immediate	Low	Both contact and vapour hazard
Sarin	GB	None (if pure) or strong	Will off-gas while on victim's clothing	Immediate	High	Primarily respiratory vapour hazard; extremely lethal if skin contact is made
Soman	GD	Fruity	Ages rapidly, making it difficult to treat	Immediate	Moderate	Contact with skin; minimal vapour hazard
V agent	VX	None	Most lethal chemical agent; difficult to decontaminate	Immediate	Very low	Contact with skin; no vapour hazard (unless aerosolised)

At the Scene

Always make sure that your patients have been thoroughly decontaminated by trained personnel before you come into contact with them. Chemical agents are primarily a vapour hazard, and all of the patient's clothing must be removed to prevent cross-contamination. Finally, never perform mouth-to-mouth or mouth-to-mask ventilation on a victim of a chemical agent. Many of the vapours may linger in the patient's airway and cross-contamination may occur.

IV access. Mild effects of cyanide exposure will generally resolve by simply removing the victim from the source of contamination and administering high-flow supplementary oxygen. Severe exposure, however, will require aggressive oxygenation and perhaps ventilation with supplementary oxygen. Always use a bag-valve-mask device or oxygen-powered ventilator device to ventilate a patient exposed to a metabolic agent. The agent can easily be passed on from the patient to the paramedic through mouth-to-mouth or mouth-to-mask ventilations. If no antidote is available, initiate transport immediately.

Table 48-3 ▼ summarises the chemical agents. The odours of the particular chemicals are provided for information purposes only. The sense of smell is a poor tool to use to determine whether there is a chemical agent present. Many people are unable to smell the agents, and the odour could be derived from another source. This information is useful to you if you receive reports from victims claiming to smell bleach or garlic, for example. You should never enter a potentially hazardous area and "sniff" to determine whether a chemical agent is present.

Biological Agents

Biological agents pose many difficult issues when used as a WMD. Biological agents can be almost completely undetectable. Also, most of the diseases caused by these agents will be similar to other minor illnesses commonly seen by paramedics.

Biological agents are grouped as viruses, bacteria, or neurotoxins and may be spread in various ways. Dissemination is the means by which a terrorist will spread the agent—for example, poisoning the water supply or aerosolising the agent into the air or ventilation system of a building. A disease vector is an animal that spreads disease, once infected, to another animal. For example, the plague may be spread by infected rats, smallpox by infected people, and West Nile virus by infected mosquitoes. How easily the disease is able to spread from one human to another human is called communicability. Some diseases, such as those caused by human immunodeficiency virus, are difficult to spread by routine contact. Therefore communicability is considered low. In other instances when communicability is high, such as with smallpox, the person is considered contagious. Typically, your universal precautions are enough to prevent contamination from contagious biological organisms.

Incubation describes the period of time between the person becoming exposed to the agent and when symptoms begin. The incubation period is especially important for the paramedic to understand. Although your patient may not exhibit signs or symptoms, he or she may be contagious.

Paramedics need to be aware of when they should suspect the use of biological agents. If the agent is in the form of a powder, such as in the October 2001 incidents in the United States involving anthrax powder posted in letters, the call must

Table 48-3	Chemical Agents					
Class	**Military Designations**	**Odour**	**Lethality**	**Onset of Symptoms**	**Volatility**	**Primary Route of Exposure**
Nerve agents	Tabun (GA) Sarin (GB) Soman (GD) VX	Fruity or none	Most lethal chemical agents can kill within minutes; effects are reversible with antidotes	Immediate	Moderate (GA, GD) Very high (GB) Low (VX)	Vapour hazard (GB) Both vapour and contact hazard (GA, GD) Contact hazard (VX)
Vesicants	Mustard (H) Lewisite (L) Phosgene oxime (CX)	Garlic (H) Geranium (L)	Causes large blisters to form on victims; may severely damage upper airway if vapours are inhaled; severe intense pain and greyish skin discolouration (L, CX)	Delayed (H) Immediate (L, CX)	Very low (H, L) Moderate (CX)	Primarily contact; with some vapour hazard
Pulmonary agents	Chlorine (CL) Phosgene (CG)	Bleach (CL) Cut grass (CG)	Causes irritation; choking (CL); severe pulmonary oedema (CG)	Immediate (CL) Delayed (CG)	Very high	Vapour hazard
Cyanide agents	Hydrogen cyanide (AC) Cyanogens chloride (CK)	Almonds (AC) Irritating (CK)	Highly lethal chemical gases; can kill within minutes; effects are reversible with antidotes	Immediate	Very high	Vapour hazard

be handled by specialists. Patients who have come into direct contact with the agent need to be decontaminated before any ambulance service contact or treatment is initiated.

Viruses

Viruses are disease causing micro-organisms that require a living host to multiply and survive. A virus is a simple organism and cannot thrive outside of a host (living body). Once in the body, the virus will invade healthy cells and replicate itself to spread through the host. As the virus spreads, so does the disease that it carries. Viruses survive by moving from one host to another by using its transport system-vectors.

Viral agents that may be used during a biological terrorist release pose an extraordinary problem for health care providers, especially those in the ambulance services. Although some viral agents do have vaccines, there is no treatment for a viral infection other than antivirals for some agents. Because of this characteristic, the following viruses have been used as terrorist agents.

Smallpox

Smallpox is a highly contagious disease. All forms of universal precautions must be used to prevent cross-contamination to health care providers. Simply by wearing examination gloves, a filtered respirator, and eye protection, you will greatly reduce your risk of contamination. The last natural case of smallpox in the world was seen in 1977. Before the rash and blisters show, the illness will start with a high fever and body aches and headaches. The patient's temperature is usually in the range of 38°C to 40°C.

An easy, quick way to differentiate the smallpox rash from other skin disorders is to observe the size, shape, and location of the lesions. In smallpox, all the lesions are identical in their development. In other skin disorders, the lesions will be in various stages of healing and development. Smallpox blisters also begin on the face and extremities and eventually move toward the chest and abdomen. The disease is in its most contagious phase when the blisters begin to form **Figure 48-8 ▸**. Unprotected contact with these blisters will promote transmission of the disease. There is a vaccine to prevent smallpox; however, it has been linked to medical complications and in very rare cases death **Table 48-4 ▸**. Vaccination against the disease is part of a national strategy to respond to a terrorist threat. Because the vaccine does have some risk, only first responders have been offered the vaccine. Should an outbreak occur, vaccine would be offered to people at risk.

Viral Haemorrhagic Fevers

Viral haemorrhagic fevers (VHF) consist of a group of diseases that include the Ebola, Rift Valley, and yellow fever viruses, among others. This group of viruses causes the blood in the body to seep out from the tissues and blood vessels

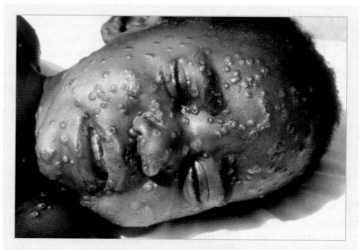

Figure 48-8 In smallpox, all the lesions are identical in their development. In other skin disorders, the lesions will be in various stages of healing and development.

Table 48-4	Characteristics of Smallpox
Dissemination	Aerosolised for warfare or terrorist uses
Communicability	High from infected individuals or items (such as blankets used by infected patients). Person-to-person transmission is possible.
Route of entry	Through inhalation of coughed droplets or direct skin contact with blisters
Signs and symptoms	Severe fever, malaise, body aches, headaches, small blisters on the skin, bleeding of the skin and mucous membranes. Incubation period is 10 to 12 days and the duration of the illness is approximately 4 weeks.
Medical management	Universal precautions. There is no specific treatment for smallpox victims. Patients should be provided with supportive care (ABCs).

Figure 48-9 ▸. Initially, the patient will have flu-like symptoms, progressing to more serious symptoms such as internal and external haemorrhaging. Outbreaks are not uncommon in Africa and South America. Outbreaks in Britain, however, are extremely rare. All universal precautions must be taken when treating these illnesses. Mortality rates can range from 5% to 90%, depending on the strain of virus, the patient's age and health condition, and the availability of a modern health care system **Table 48-5 ▸**.

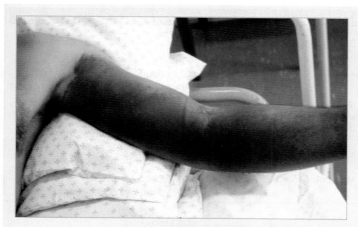

Figure 48-9 Viral haemorrhagic fevers cause the blood vessels and tissues to seep blood. The end result is bruising, haemoptysis, and blood in the patient's stool. Notice the severe discolouration in this patient with Crimean Congo haemorrhagic fever, indicating internal bleeding.

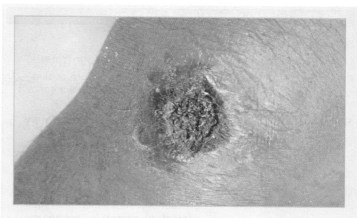

Figure 48-10 Cutaneous anthrax.

Table 48-5	Characteristics of Viral Haemorrhagic Fevers
Dissemination	Direct contact with an infected person's body fluids. It can also be aerosolised for use in an attack.
Communicability	Moderate from person to person or from contaminated items.
Route of entry	Direct contact with an infected person's body fluids.
Signs and symptoms	Sudden onset of fever, weakness, muscle pain, headache, and sore throat. All of these symptoms are followed by vomiting and as the virus runs its course, internal and external bleeding.
Medical management	Universal precautions. There is no specific treatment for viral haemorrhagic fever. Patients should be provided supportive care (ABCs) and treatment for shock and hypotension, if present.

Bacteria

Unlike viruses, bacteria do not require a host to multiply and live. Bacteria are much more complex and larger than viruses and can grow up to 100 times larger than the largest virus. Bacteria contain all the cellular structures of a normal cell and are completely self-sufficient. Most importantly, bacterial infections can be fought with antibiotics.

Most bacterial infections will generally begin with flu-like symptoms, which make it quite difficult to identify whether the cause is a biological attack or a natural epidemic. Biological agents have been developed and used for centuries during times of war.

Inhalation and Cutaneous Anthrax (*Bacillus anthracis*)

Anthrax is a deadly bacteria that lays dormant in a spore (protective shell). When exposed to the optimal temperature and moisture, the germ will be released from the spore. The routes of entry for anthrax are inhalation, cutaneous, or ingestion (from consuming food that contain spores) Figure 48-10 ▲ . Pulmonary anthrax (inhalation) is the most deadly and often presents as a severe cold. Pulmonary anthrax infections are associated with a 90% death rate if untreated. Antibiotics can be used to treat anthrax successfully. There is also a vaccine to prevent anthrax infections Table 48-6 ▶ .

Plague—Bubonic/Pneumonic

Of all the infectious diseases known to humans, none has killed as many as the plague. The 14th century plague that ravaged Asia, the Middle East, and finally Europe (the Black Death) killed an estimated 33 to 42 million people (half the population of Europe). Later on, in the early 19th century, almost 20 million people in India and China perished due to plague. The plague's natural vectors are infected rodents and fleas. When a person is either bitten by an infected flea or comes into contact with an infected rodent (or the urine of the rodent), the person can contract bubonic plague.

Bubonic plague infects the lymphatic system (a passive circulatory system in the body that bathes the tissues in lymph and works with the immune system). When this occurs, the patient's lymph nodes (area of the lymphatic system where infection-fighting cells are housed) become infected and grow. The glands of the nodes will grow large (up to the size of a tennis ball) and round, forming buboes Figure 48-11 ▶ . If left untreated, the infection may spread through the body, leading to sepsis and possibly death. This form of plague is not contagious and is not likely to be seen in a bioterrorist incident.

Table 48-6	Characteristics of Anthrax
Dissemination	Aerosol
Communicability	Only in the cutaneous form (rare)
Route of entry	Through inhalation of spore or skin contact with spore or direct contact with skin wound (cutaneous)
Signs and symptoms	Flu-like symptoms, fever, respiratory distress with tachycardia, shock, pulmonary oedema and respiratory failure after 3 to 5 days of flu-like symptoms
Medical management	Pulmonary/inhalation: universal precautions, supplemental oxygen, ventilatory support for pulmonary oedema or respiratory failure and transport. Cutaneous: universal precautions, apply dry sterile dressing to prevent accidental contact with wound and fluids.

Table 48-7	Characteristics of Plague
Dissemination	Aerosol
Communicability	Bubonic: low, only from contact with fluid in buboe Pneumonic: high, from person to person
Route of entry	Ingestion, inhalation, or cutaneous
Signs and symptoms	Fever, headache, muscle pain and tenderness, pneumonia, shortness of breath, extreme lymph node pain and enlargement (bubonic)
Medical management	Universal precautions, ABCs, provide supplemental oxygen, and transport

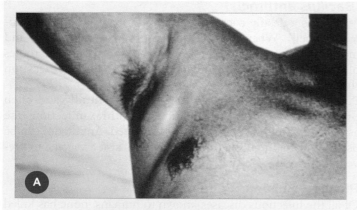

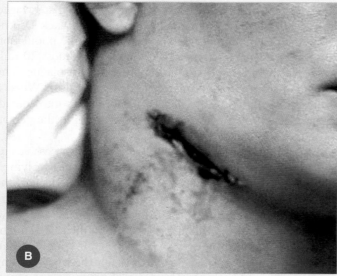

Figure 48-11 A. Plague buboe at lymph node under arm. **B.** Plague buboe at lymph node on neck.

Pneumonic plague is a lung infection, also known as plague pneumonia, that results from inhalation of plague bacteria. This form of the disease is contagious and has a much higher death rate than the bubonic form. This form of plague therefore would be easier to disseminate (aerosolised), has a higher mortality, and is contagious Table 48-7 ▲ .

Neurotoxins

Neurotoxins are the most deadly substances known to humans. The strongest neurotoxin is 15,000 times more lethal than VX and 100,000 times more lethal than sarin. These toxins are produced from plants, marine animals, moulds, and bacteria. The route of entry for these toxins is through ingestion, inhalation from aerosols, or injection. Unlike viruses and bacteria, neurotoxins are not contagious and have a faster onset of symptoms. Although these biological toxins have immense destructive potential, they have not been used successfully as a WMD.

Botulinum Toxin

The most potent neurotoxin is botulinum, which is produced by bacteria. When introduced into the body, this neurotoxin affects the nervous system's ability to function. Voluntary muscle control will diminish as the toxin spreads. Eventually the toxin will cause muscle paralysis that begins at the head and face and travels downward throughout the body. The patient's accessory muscles and diaphragm will become paralysed, and the patient will go into respiratory arrest Table 48-8 ▶ .

Ricin

While not as deadly as botulinum, ricin is still five times more lethal than VX. This toxin is derived from mash that is left from the castor bean Figure 48-12 ▶ . When introduced into the body, ricin causes pulmonary oedema and respiratory and circulatory failure leading to death Table 48-9 ▶ .

The clinical picture depends on the route of exposure. The toxin is quite stable and extremely toxic by many routes of exposure, including inhalation. Perhaps 1 to 3 mg of ricin can kill an adult, and the ingestion of one seed can probably kill a child.

Table 48-8	Characteristics of Botulinum Toxin
Dissemination	Aerosol or food supply sabotage or injection
Communicability	None
Route of entry	Ingestion or gastrointestinal
Signs and symptoms	Dry mouth, intestinal obstruction, urinary retention, constipation, nausea and vomiting, abnormal pupil dilation, blurred vision, double vision, drooping eyelids, difficulty swallowing, difficulty speaking, and respiratory failure due to paralysis
Medical management	ABCs, provide supplemental oxygen and transport. Ventilatory support may be needed due to paralysis of the respiratory muscles. A vaccine is available.

Table 48-9	Characteristics of Ricin
Dissemination	Aerosol or contamination of a food or water supply by sabotage
Communicability	None
Route of entry	Inhalation, ingestion, injection
Signs and symptoms	Inhaled: Cough, difficulty breathing, chest tightness, nausea, muscle aches, pulmonary oedema, and hypoxia Ingested: Nausea and vomiting, internal bleeding, and death Injection: No signs except swelling at the injection site and death
Medical management	ABCs. No treatment or vaccine exists.

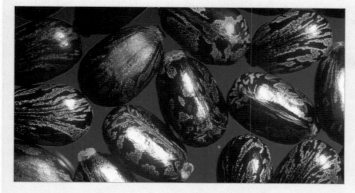

Figure 48-12 These seemingly harmless castor beans contain the key ingredient for ricin, one of the most potent toxins known to humans.

Although all parts of the castor bean are actually poisonous, it is the seeds that are the most toxic. Castor bean ingestion causes a rapid onset of nausea, vomiting, abdominal cramps, and severe diarrhoea, followed by vascular collapse. Death usually occurs on the third day in the absence of appropriate medical intervention.

Ricin is least toxic by the oral route. This is probably a result of poor absorption in the gastrointestinal tract, some digestion in the gut, and, possibly, some expulsion of the agent as caused by the rapid onset of vomiting. Ingestion causes local haemorrhage and necrosis of the liver, spleen, kidney, and gastrointestinal tract. Signs and symptoms appear 4 to 8 hours after exposure.

Signs and symptoms of ricin ingestion are as follows:

- Fever
- Chills
- Headache
- Muscle aches
- Nausea
- Vomiting
- Diarrhoea
- Severe abdominal cramping
- Dehydration
- Gastrointestinal bleeding
- Necrosis of liver, spleen, kidneys, and gastrointestinal tract

Inhalation of ricin causes nonspecific weakness, cough, fever, hypothermia, and hypotension. Symptoms occur about 4 to 8 hours after inhalation, depending on the inhaled dose. The onset of profuse sweating some hours later signifies the termination of the symptoms.

Signs and symptoms of ricin inhalation are as follows:

- Fever
- Chills
- Nausea
- Local irritation of eyes, nose, and throat
- Profuse sweating
- Headache
- Muscle aches
- Nonproductive cough
- Chest pain
- Dyspnoea
- Pulmonary oedema
- Severe lung inflammation
- Cyanosis
- Convulsions
- Respiratory failure

Treatment is supportive and includes both respiratory support and cardiovascular support as needed. Early intubation, ventilation, and positive end expiratory pressure, combined with treatment of pulmonary oedema, are appropriate. Intravenous fluids and electrolyte replacement are useful for treating the dehydration caused by profound vomiting and diarrhoea. **Table 48-10 ▶** summarises the biological agents.

Other Paramedic Roles During a Biological Event

Surveillance of Syndromes

Surveillance of syndromes is the monitoring, usually by public health departments, of patients presenting to accident and emergency departments and alternative care facilities, and the recording of ambulance service call volume and the use of general-sales-list medications. Patients with signs and symptoms that resemble influenza are particularly important. Public health departments monitor for an unusual influx of patients with these symptoms in hopes of catching an outbreak early. The ambulance service role in this surveillance is a small one, yet valuable in the overall tracking of a biological terrorist event or infectious disease outbreak. Quality assurance and ambulance control need to be aware of an unusual number of calls from patients with "unexplainable flu" coming from a particular region or community.

▋ Radiological/Nuclear Devices

What Is Radiation?

Ionising radiation is energy that is emitted in the form of rays, or particles. This energy can be found in radioactive material, such as rocks and metals. Radioactive material is any material that emits radiation. This material is unstable, and attempts to

Table 48-10	Biological Agents			
Disease	Transmission Risk Person to Person	Incubation Period	Duration of Illness	Lethality (approximate case fatality rates)
Inhalation anthrax	No	1 to 6 d	3 to 5 d (usually fatal if untreated)	High
Pneumonic plague	High	2 to 3 d	1 to 6 d (usually fatal)	High unless treated within 12 to 24 h
Smallpox	High	7 to 17 d (average 12 d)	4 wk	High to moderate
Viral haemorrhagic fevers	Moderate	4 to 21 d	Death between 7 to 16 d	High to moderate, depending on type of fever
Botulinum	No	1 to 5 d	Death in 24 to 72 h; lasts months if patient does not die	High without respiratory support
Ricin	No	18 to 24 h	Days; death within 10 to 12 d for ingestion	High

You are the Paramedic Part 4

Your patient has a patent airway. You continue to apply high-flow oxygen via a nonrebreathing mask. Lung sounds are crepitus and moist. Her oxygen saturation is at 97% on 15 l/min of oxygen. Since the patient report that you received from the SORT personnel indicates that a nerve agent antidote kit was used on the patient, you will need to monitor her vital signs closely and watch to see if symptoms develop. You take along another NAAK and send a pre-alert whilst en route to the local accident and emergency (A&E) department.

While en route your patient states that she does not feel right. She is becoming disorientated. She suddenly begins to have a convulsion. You quickly place padding around the patient to keep her from injuring herself. She becomes incontinent, again.

Reassessment	Recording Time: 30 Minutes
Skin	Pale, warm, dry
Pulse	120 beats/min
Blood pressure	148/94 mm Hg
Respirations	12 breaths/min
S_PO_2	97% with supplemental oxygen of 15 l/min via nonrebreathing mask
ECG	Sinus tachycardia with an occasional PVC

7. What does the nerve agent antidote kit include?

8. Is this kit part of your local guideline in dealing with patients exposed to a nerve agent?

9. What is your next step in treatment?

stabilise itself by changing its structure in a natural process called decay. As the substance decays, it gives off radiation until it stabilises. The process of radioactive decay can take from as little as minutes to billions of years; meanwhile, the substance remains radioactive.

The energy that is emitted from a strong radiological source is either alpha, beta, gamma (X-rays), or neutron radiation **Figure 48-13 ▾** . Alpha is the least harmful penetrating type of radiation and cannot travel fast or through most objects. In fact, a sheet of paper or the body's skin easily stops it. Beta radiation is slightly more penetrating than alpha and requires a layer of clothing to stop it. Gamma or X-rays are far faster and stronger than alpha and beta rays. These rays easily penetrate through the human body and require either several inches of lead or concrete to prevent penetration. Neutron energy is the fastest moving and most powerful form of radiation. Neutrons easily penetrate through lead and require several feet of concrete to stop them.

Sources of Radiological Material

There are thousands of radioactive materials found on the earth. These materials are generally used for purposes that benefit humankind, such as medicine, killing germs in food (irradiating), and construction work. Once radiological material has been used for its purpose, the material remaining is called radiological waste. Radiological waste remains radioactive but has no more usefulness. These materials can be found at:

- Hospitals
- Colleges and universities

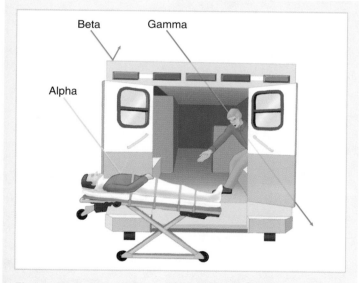

Figure 48-13 Alpha, beta, and gamma radiation.

- Chemical and industrial sites
- Power plants

Not all radioactive material is tightly guarded, and the waste is often not guarded. This makes use of radioactive material and substances appealing to terrorists.

Radiological Dispersal Devices

A radiological dispersal device (RDD) is any container that is designed to disperse radioactive material. This would generally require the use of a bomb, hence the nickname dirty bomb. A dirty bomb would carry the potential to injure victims with not only the radioactive material but also the explosive material used to deliver it. Just the thought of an RDD creates fear in a population, and so the ultimate goal of the terrorist—fear—is accomplished. In reality, however, the destructive capability of a dirty bomb is limited to the explosives that are attached to it. Therefore, if the explosive is sufficient to kill 10 people without radioactive material, it will also kill 10 people with the radioactive material added. There may be long-term injuries and illness associated with the use of an RDD, yet not much more than the bomb by itself would create. In short, the dirty bomb is an ineffective WMD.

Nuclear Energy

Nuclear energy is artificially made by altering (splitting) radioactive atoms. The result is an immense amount of energy that usually takes the form of heat. Nuclear material is used in medicine, weapons, naval vessels, and power plants. Nuclear material gives off all forms of radiation including neutrons (the most deadly type). Like radioactive material, when nuclear material is no longer useful it becomes waste that is still radioactive.

Nuclear Weapons

The destructive energy of a nuclear explosion is unlike any other weapon in the world. That is why nuclear weapons are kept only in secure facilities throughout the world. There are nations that have ties to terrorists and that have actively attempted to build nuclear weapons. However, the ability of these nations to deliver a nuclear weapon, such as a missile or bomb, is as of yet, incomplete. There is also the deterrent of complete mutual annihilation. Therefore, the likelihood of a nuclear attack is extremely remote.

How Radiation Affects the Body

The effects of radiation exposure will vary depending on the amount of radiation that a person receives and the route of entry. Radiation can be introduced into the body by all routes of entry as well as through the body (irradiation). The patient can inhale radioactive dust from nuclear fallout or from a dirty bomb, or have radioactive liquid absorbed into the body through the skin. Once in the body, the radiation source will irradiate the person from within rather than from an external source (such as X-ray equipment). Some common signs of acute radiation sickness are nausea, vomiting, and diarrhoea. Additional injuries will occur with a nuclear blast such as thermal and blast trauma, trauma from flying objects, and eye injuries.

Medical Management

Being exposed to a radiation source does not make a patient contaminated or radioactive. However, when patients have a radioactive source on their body (such as debris from a dirty bomb), they are contaminated and must be initially cared for by the SORT personnel. Once the patient is decontaminated and there is no threat to you, you may begin treatment with the ABCs and treat the patient for any burns or trauma.

Protective Measures

There are no suits or protective gear designed to completely shield from radiation. Those who work in high-risk areas do wear some protection (lead-lined suits); however this equipment is not available to the paramedic.

> **Notes from Nancy**
> Before you enter the hazardous area, remember: Your best allies are time, distance, and shielding.

The best ways to protect yourself from the effects of radiation are to use time, distance, and shielding.

- **Time.** Radiation has a cumulative effect on the body. The less time that you are exposed to the source, the less the effects will be. If you realise that the patient is near a radiation source, leave the area immediately. Personal dosimeters are being carried by many frontline ambulance personnel nowadays to ensure that continual monitoring of exposure is treated as importantly as major exposures.

> **Notes from Nancy**
> The further away you get from a radioactive source the better, but moving even a small distance away reduces exposure a great deal.

- **Distance.** Radiation is limited as to how far it can travel. Depending on the type of radiation, often moving only a few feet is enough to remove you from immediate danger. Alpha radiation cannot travel more than a few inches. You should take this into account when responding to a nuclear or radiological incident and make certain that emergency services personnel are stationed far enough from the incident.

- **Shielding.** As discussed earlier, the path of all radiation can be stopped by a specific object. It will be impossible for you to recognise the type of radiation being emitted, or even from which direction it is coming. Therefore, you should always assume that you are dealing with the strongest form of radiation and use concrete shielding (such as buildings or walls) between yourself and the incident. The importance of shielding cannot be overemphasised. In one atomic test, a car was parked by the side of a house and opposite the direction of the oncoming blast. The house was completely destroyed, yet the car that was directly next to it sustained almost no damage.

You are the Paramedic Summary

1. What is your first priority on arrival in this situation?

Since there are multiple patients and a potential hazard to the rescuers, the first priority is your personal safety and that of your colleagues. That is why it was appropriate to park the vehicles until more information was determined about the cause of the incident.

2. What does the ambulance control information indicate as far as the need for additional resources?

The ambulance control information paints a picture of multiple patients with medical complaints. While it is not uncommon to get multiple patients with traumatic complaints at a typical road traffic collision, we rarely get multiple patients with medical complaints unless there is something they all were exposed to causing the symptoms.

3. What precautions can you take to ensure your own safety?

Make sure you use STEP 1-2-3 to reduce your risk of contamination.

4. What does your index of suspicion tell you about this scene?

The specifics are slowly being identified as the SORT personnel identifies the product that the patients were exposed to. However, the slow pulse rate, vomiting, and tearing lead you in the direction of a nerve agent even before the actual substance is identified.

5. What could your patient's signs and symptoms represent?

As you have learned, patients who have been exposed to a nerve agent are likely to have the symptoms paramedics remember using the mnemonic DUMBELS. That stands for: Defecation, Urination, Miosis, Bradycardia/bronchorrhoea, Emesis, Lacrimation, and Salivation.

6. What are your treatment options for this patient?

In a case of suspected nerve gas exposure implement immediate decontamination of the patients. It is then appropriate to commence treatment of the symptoms with a nerve agent antidote kit. Then transport the patient with ongoing assessment and support of her ABCs.

7. What does the nerve agent antidote kit include?

The Department of Health recommends that nerve agent antidote kits (NAAK) contain 2 mg atropine, 2 g pralidoxime mesylate, and 250 mg obidoxime chloride. In some regions, paramedics may routinely carry NAAK.

8. Is this kit part of your local guideline in dealing with patients exposed to a nerve agent?

If it is not, you should ask your Emergency Planning Officer what the plan is for treating large numbers of patients who have been exposed to a nerve agent.

9. What are your next steps in treatment?

Ongoing assessment, manage the ABCs, and transport the patient. Depending on how fast she comes out of the convulsion and how well she can ventilate, it may be necessary to consider intubation and the need to support or assist her ventilations with a bag-valve-mask device and supplementary oxygen. Consult with A&E to consider the potential need to medicate the patient for (1) nausea and vomiting, (2) pulmonary oedema, and (3) convulsion activity if lengthy.

Prep Kit

Ready for Review

- As a result of the increase in terrorist activity, it is possible that you could witness a terrorist event. You must be mentally and physically prepared for the possibility of a terrorist event.
- The use of weapons of mass destruction or major incident further complicates the management of the terrorist incident. Be aware of your surroundings at all times. The best form of protection from a WMD agent is to avoid contact with the agent.
- A WMD is any agent designed to bring about mass death, casualties, and/or massive damage to property and infrastructure (bridges, tunnels, airports, and seaports). These can be conventional, chemical, biological, radiological, or nuclear weapons.
- Be aware of the current threat level issued by the Home Office. This threat level can be critical, severe, substantial, moderate, or low. On the basis of the current threat level, take appropriate actions and precautions. Be aware of established policies that your organisation may have regarding the current threat level.
- Indicators that may give you clues as to whether the emergency is the result of an attack include the type of location, type of call, number of patients, patients' statements, and preincident indicators.
- If you suspect that a terrorist or WMD event has occurred, ensure that the scene is safe. If you have any doubt that it may not be safe, do not enter. Wait for assistance.
- Notification of the ambulance control is essential. Inform ambulance control of the nature of the event, any additional resources that may be required, the estimated number of patients, and the upwind route of approach or optimal route of approach.
- Establish a parking area, where other vehicles will rendezvous. Be mindful of access and exit routes.
- Terrorists may set secondary devices to explode after the initial bomb, to injure responders and secure media coverage. Constantly assess and reassess the scene for safety.
- Paramedics may be called upon to assist in the delivery of the medications to the public. The paramedic's role may include triage, treatment of seriously ill patients, and patient transport to the hospital.

Vital Vocabulary

alpha Type of energy that is emitted from a strong radiological source; it is the least harmful penetrating type of radiation and cannot travel fast or through most objects.

anthrax A deadly bacteria (*Bacillus anthracis*) that lays dormant in a spore (protective shell); the germ is released from the spore when exposed to the optimal temperature and moisture. The route of entry is inhalation, cutaneous, or gastrointestinal (from consuming food that contains spores).

bacteria Micro-organisms that reproduce by binary fission. These single-cell organisms reproduce rapidly. Some can form spores (encysted variants) when environmental conditions are harsh.

beta Type of energy that is emitted from a strong radiological source; is slightly more penetrating than alpha, and requires a layer of clothing to stop it.

botulinum Produced by bacteria, this is a very potent neurotoxin. When introduced into the body, this neurotoxin affects the nervous system's ability to function and causes muscle paralysis.

buboes Enlarged lymph nodes (up to the size of tennis balls) that were characteristic of people infected with the bubonic plague.

bubonic plague An epidemic that spread throughout Europe in the Middle Ages, causing over 25 million deaths, also called the Black Death, transmitted by infected fleas and characterised by acute malaise, fever, and the formation of tender, enlarged, inflamed lymph nodes that appear as lesions, called buboes.

CCBRN A mnemonic for the five types of terrorist incidents that emergency services may be confronted with in the prehospital environment.

chlorine (CL) The first chemical agent ever used in warfare. It has a distinct odour of bleach, and creates a green haze when released as a gas. Initially it produces upper airway irritation and a choking sensation.

communicability Describes how easily a disease spreads from one human to another human.

contact hazard A hazardous agent that gives off very little or no vapours; the skin is the primary route for this type of chemical to enter the body; also called a skin hazard.

contagious A person infected with a disease that is highly communicable.

covert Act in which the public safety community generally has no prior knowledge of the time, location, or nature of the attack.

cross-contamination Occurs when a person is contaminated by an agent as a result of coming into contact with another contaminated person.

cyanide Agent that affects the body's ability to use oxygen. It is a colourless gas that has an odour similar to almonds. The effects begin on the cellular level and are very rapidly seen at the organ system level.

decay A natural process in which a material that is unstable attempts to stabilise itself by changing its structure.

dirty bomb Name given to a bomb that is used as a radiological dispersal device (RDD).

disease vector An animal that once infected, spreads a disease to another animal.

dissemination The means with which a terrorist will spread a disease, for example, by poisoning of the water supply, or aerosolising the agent into the air or ventilation system of a building.

G agents Early nerve agents that were developed by German scientists in the period after WWI and into WWII. There are three such agents: sarin, soman, and tabun.

gamma (X-rays) Type of energy that is emitted from a strong radiological source that is far faster and stronger than alpha and beta rays. These rays easily penetrate through the human body and require either several inches of lead or concrete to prevent penetration.

incubation Describes the period of time from a person being exposed to a disease to the time when symptoms begin.

international terrorism Terrorism that is carried out by those not of the host's country; also known as cross-border terrorism.

ionising radiation Energy that is emitted in the form of ray or particles.

LD$_{50}$ The amount of an agent or substance that will kill 50% of people who are exposed to this level.

Lewisite (L) A blistering agent that has a rapid onset of symptoms and produces immediate intense pain and discomfort on contact.

lymphatic system A passive circulatory system that transports a plasma-like liquid called lymph, a thin fluid that bathes the tissues of the body.

lymph nodes Area of the lymphatic system where infection-fighting cells are housed.

miosis Bilateral pinpoint constricted pupils.

mutagen Substance that mutates, damages, and changes the structures of DNA in the body's cells.

NAAK A nerve agent antidote kit. According to the Department of Health, a NAAK should contain 2 mg atropine, 2 g pralidoxime mesylate, and 250 mg obidoxime chloride.

nerve agents A class of chemicals called organophosphates; they function by blocking an essential enzyme in the nervous system, which causes the body's organs to become overstimulated and burn out.

neurotoxins Biological agents that are the most deadly substances known to humans; they include botulinum toxin and ricin.

neutron radiation Type of energy that is emitted from a strong radiological source; neutron energy is the fastest moving and most powerful form of radiation. Neutrons easily penetrate through lead, and require several feet of concrete to stop them.

off-gassing The emitting of an agent after exposure, for example from a person's clothes that have been exposed to the agent.

persistency Term used to describe how long a chemical agent will stay on a surface before it evaporates.

phosgene A pulmonary agent that is a product of combustion, such as might be produced in a fire at a textile factory or house, or from metalwork or burning Freon. Phosgene is a very potent agent that has a delayed onset of symptoms, usually hours.

phosgene oxime (CX) A blistering agent that has a rapid onset of symptoms and produces immediate intense pain and discomfort on contact.

pneumonic plague A lung infection, also known as plague pneumonia, that is the result of inhalation of plague bacteria.

radioactive material Any material that emits radiation.

radiological dispersal device (RDD) Any container that is designed to disperse radioactive material.

ricin Neurotoxin derived from mash that is left from pressing oil from the castor bean; causes pulmonary oedema and respiratory and circulatory failure, leading to death.

route of exposure Manner by which a toxic substance enters the body.

sarin (GB) A nerve agent that is one of the G agents; a highly volatile colourless and odourless liquid that turns from liquid to gas within seconds to minutes at room temperature.

secondary device Additional explosives used by terrorists, which are set to explode after the initial bomb.

smallpox A highly contagious disease; it is most contagious when blisters begin to form.

soman (GD) A nerve agent that is one of the G agents; twice as persistent as sarin and five times as lethal; it has a fruity odour as a result of the type of alcohol used in the agent, and is both a contact and inhalation hazard that can enter the body through skin absorption and through the respiratory tract.

state-sponsored terrorism Terrorism that is funded and/or supported by nations that hold close ties with terrorist groups.

sulphur mustard (H) A vesicant; it is a brownish-yellowish oily substance that is generally considered very persistent; has the distinct smell of garlic or mustard and, when released, it is quickly absorbed into the skin and/or mucous membranes and begins an irreversible process of damaging the cells.

surveillance of syndromes The monitoring, usually by public health departments, of patients presenting to accident and emergency departments and alternative care facilities, the recording of ambulance service call volume, and the use of general-sales-list medications.

tabun (GA) A nerve agent that is one of the G agents; is 36 times more persistent than sarin and approximately half as lethal; has a fruity smell and is unique because the components used to manufacture the agent are easy to acquire and the agent is easy to manufacture.

V agent (VX) One of the G agents; it is a clear, oily agent that has no odour and looks like baby oil; over 100 times more lethal than sarin and is extremely persistent.

vapour hazard An agent that enters the body through the respiratory tract.

vesicants Blister agents; the primary route of entry for vesicants is through the skin.

viral haemorrhagic fevers (VHF) A group of diseases that include the Ebola, Rift Valley, and yellow fever viruses among others. This group of viruses causes the blood in the body to seep out from the tissues and blood vessels.

viruses Disease-producing micro-organisms that require a living host to multiply and survive.

volatility Term used to describe how long a chemical agent will stay on a surface before it evaporates.

weapon of major incident (WMI) Any agent designed to bring about mass death, casualties, and/or massive damage to property and infrastructure (bridges, tunnels, airports, and seaports); also known as a weapon of mass destruction (WMD).

weapon of mass destruction (WMD) Any agent designed to bring about mass death, casualties, and/or massive damage to property and infrastructure (bridges, tunnels, airports, and seaports); also known as a weapon of major incident (WMI).

weaponisation The creation of a weapon from a biological agent generally found in nature and that causes disease; the agent is cultivated, synthesised, and/or mutated to maximise the target population's exposure to the germ.

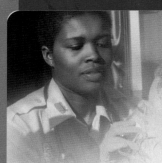

Assessment in Action

Events over the past thirty plus years have shown that terrorists, foreign and domestic, are willing to attack UK interests at home and abroad. Terrorists now have access to a broad array of lethal materials worldwide and can strike a specific target at any given time. Terrorists are no longer limited to conventional weapons.

1. As a paramedic you must be familiar with the nonconventional agents that may be used in a WMD attack. All of the following are nonconventional weapons, EXCEPT:
   A. chemical.
   B. nuclear.
   C. biological.
   D. explosives.

2. A weapon of mass destruction is any agent that will bring about:
   A. major incident.
   B. mass death.
   C. massive damage to infrastructure.
   D. all of the above.

3. Terrorism carried out by individuals or groups who are not from the host country is known as:
   A. domestic terrorism.
   B. doomsday terrorism.
   C. international terrorism.
   D. declaration terrorism.

4. When starting your shift, you see a notice to all crews that the Home Office considers the threat of attack is highly likely. What word would they use to describe this level?
   A. Severe
   B. Low
   C. Moderate
   D. Static

5. Chemical agents are manmade substances that can have devastating effects on living organisms. All of the following are agents that can be used for chemical warfare, EXCEPT:
   A. nerve agents.
   B. pulmonary agents.
   C. bacterial agents.
   D. blood agents.

6. Time, distance, and shielding are the three most important factors in staying safe when dealing with what type of WMD?
   A. Chemical weapon
   B. Radiological weapon
   C. Biological weapon
   D. Bacterial weapon

7. A chemical agent that is described as highly persistent can:
   A. evaporate relatively fast.
   B. remain in the environment for weeks to months.
   C. cause extensive blistering within minutes.
   D. all of the above.

Challenging Questions

You are responding to a railway station where there was a reported small explosion. Ambulance control reports there are now a number of patients complaining of difficulty breathing and nausea. As you walk into the station you observe that two patients are unconscious and convulsing, while numerous others are pleading with you to help them.

8. What type of event do you suspect?

9. What concerns do you have for your safety?

Points to Ponder

You are responding to a WMD incident where a primary explosion has disseminated chemical agents at the County Council offices. You are told by the Ambulance Commander (AC) to park up about two streets from the incident location while they wait for the SORT personnel to evaluate the situation. The parking area is near a park and the AC wants triage to be set up in the park. There are about 40 patients confirmed by the AC. A total of six ambulances within the city are responding.

What are your concerns with both the location of the triage area and the number of ambulances that are responding? What do you want to know about the chemical agent?

Issues: Scene Safety, Parking Location, Ambulance Commander, Need for Decontamination, Secondary Devices.

Objectives

Cognitive

- Define the term rescue.
- Explain the medical and mechanical aspects of rescue situations.
- Explain the role of the paramedic in delivering care at the site of the injury, continuing through the rescue process and to definitive care.
- Describe the phases of a rescue operation.
- Explain the differences in risk between moving water and flat water rescue.
- Explain the effects of immersion hypothermia on the ability to survive sudden immersion and self rescue.
- Explain the phenomenon of the cold protective response in cold water drowning situations.
- Identify the risks associated with low head dams and the rescue complexities they pose.
- Given a picture of moving water, identify and explain the following features and hazards associated with:
  - Hydraulics
  - Strainers
  - Dams/hydroelectric sites
- Explain why water entry techniques are methods of last resort.
- Explain the rescue techniques associated with reach-throw-row-go.
- Explain the self rescue position if unexpectedly immersed in moving water.
- Given a series of pictures identify which would be considered "confined spaces" and potentially oxygen deficient.
- Identify the hazards associated with confined spaces and risks posed to potential rescuers to include:
  - Oxygen deficiency
  - Chemical/toxic exposure/explosion
  - Engulfment
  - Machinery entrapment
  - Electricity
- Identify components necessary to ensure site safety prior to confined space rescue attempts.

- Identify the poisonous gases commonly found in confined spaces to include:
  - Hydrogen sulphide (H_2S)
  - Carbon dioxide (CO_2)
  - Carbon monoxide (CO)
  - Low/high oxygen concentrations (FiO_2)
  - Methane (CH_4)
  - Ammonia (NH_3)
  - Nitrogen dioxide (NO_2)
- Explain the hazard of cave-in during trench rescue operations.
- Describe the effects of traffic flow on the motorway rescue incident.
- List and describe the following techniques to reduce scene risk at motorway incidents:
  - Apparatus placement
  - Headlights and emergency vehicle lighting
  - Cones
  - Reflective and high visibility clothing
- Given a diagram of a passenger car, identify the following structures:
  - A, B, C, D posts
  - Firewall
  - Unibody versus frame designs
- Describe methods for emergency stabilisation.
- Describe the electrical hazards commonly found at motorway incidents (above and below ground).
- Explain techniques to be used in non-technical stretcher carries over rough terrain.
- Develop specific skill in emergency stabilisation of vehicles and access procedures and an awareness of specific extrication strategies.
- Explain assessment procedures and modifications necessary when caring for entrapped patients.
- List the equipment necessary for an "off road" medical pack.
- Explain specific methods of improvisation for assessment, spinal immobilisation, and extremity splinting.

- Explain the indications, contraindications and methods of pain control for entrapped patients.
- Explain the need for and techniques of thermal control for entrapped patients.
- Explain the pathophysiology of "crush" syndrome.
- Develop an understanding of the medical issues involved in providing care for a patient in a rescue environment.
- Develop proficiency in patient packaging and evacuation techniques that pertain to hazardous or rescue environments.

Affective

None

Psychomotor

- Demonstrate in-water spinal immobilisation techniques.
- Demonstrate donning and properly adjusting a personal flotation device (PFD).
- Demonstrate use of a throw bag.

Introduction

"Rescue" means to deliver from danger or imprisonment. As paramedics, we must remove from peril or confinement every patient we encounter. Prehospital providers can't simply push a button and magically transport patients to an accident and emergency department—which means technically that every emergency scene is a rescue situation. Patients are found in every imaginable situation. Imagine you have a patient on the second floor of a three-story building. You find a morbidly obese patient who is lying on the floor of the toilet in the back of the building. Your assessment shows the patient is experiencing a myocardial infarction and acute exacerbation of chronic obstructive pulmonary disease (COPD). The treatment is easy, but the rescue is difficult. You must extricate this patient to your waiting ambulance with a monitor, an IV cannula in his arm, and high-flow oxygen **Figure 49-1 ▶**.

Rescue and removal of patients involves several steps. You must access the patient and then quickly assess him or her for medical/trauma complications to determine which treatments should be started. Treatment must begin at the site, but this is often difficult because of the circumstances surrounding the event. The patient must be released or removed from the entrapment, and medical care must continue throughout the incident. The most difficult process in any rescue is neither the rescue nor the treatment process, but rather the coordination and balance of both.

A technical rescue incident (TRI) is a complex rescue incident involving vehicles, water, trench collapse, confined spaces, or wilderness search and rescue that requires specially trained personnel and special equipment. This chapter

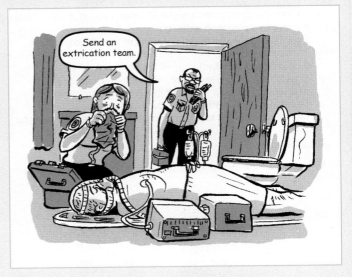

Figure 49-1

describes how to assist specially trained rescue personnel in carrying out the tasks, but it will not make you an expert in the skills that require specialised training.

Training in technical rescue areas is conducted at three levels:

- **Awareness.** This training level is an introduction to the topic, with an emphasis on recognising the hazards, securing the scene, and calling for appropriate assistance. There is no actual use of rescue skills at the awareness level.
- **Operations.** Geared toward working in the "warm zone" of an incident (the area directly around the hazard area), this

You are the Paramedic Part 1

It is a blistering hot summer day in July and your ambulance is sent to a road traffic collision. A lorry has struck a bridge and is now in a ditch, just off the A30. Upon arrival, you and your colleague are stunned as you navigate through what appears to be at least 100 chickens wandering aimlessly across the road. Beyond the chickens, buried in a ditch, is a flatbed lorry turned on its side. Wire mesh cages, feathers, and dead chickens are strewn about. The cab of the lorry has landed on the driver's side with major intrusion into the driver's compartment and you notice the windscreen is "bulls-eyed".

Inside you find a middle-aged man with active bleeding from a forehead laceration. He is screaming that he has severe abdominal pain and cannot move his legs, which are pinned beneath the dashboard. You let him know that help is here and advise him to keep as still as possible and not to move his neck. The scene is safe for you to proceed and you diligently apply in-line immobilisation.

Initial Assessment	Recording Time: 0 Minutes
Appearance	Middle-aged man in obvious pain
Level of consciousness	A (Alert to person, time, and day)
Airway	Open
Breathing	Adequate chest rise and volume
Circulation	Strong, rapid radial pulse

1. What are your initial thoughts about the specialised help you are going to require for this specific incident?
2. Identify the ten steps of a special rescue sequence.

At the Scene

One of the benefits of rescue awareness and operations education is that it helps you avoid rescue situations that you are not trained to handle.

kind of training will allow you to provide direct assistance to those conducting the rescue operation.

- **Technician.** At this level, you are directly involved in the rescue operation itself. Training includes the use of specialised equipment, care of patients during the rescue, and management of the incident and of all personnel at the scene.

Most of the training and education ambulance clinicians receive is aimed at the awareness level, enabling them to identify the hazards and secure the scene to prevent additional people from becoming patients. Your function as a paramedic in rescue operations depends on the type of services you provide and the level of expertise you and your colleagues have attained. All providers must wear proper personal protective equipment (PPE) to allow them to access patients and safely administer treatment that will continue throughout the incident. Once the scene is safe, and the technical aspects of the patient rescue or extrication are understood, patient access and care can begin.

Notes from Nancy

The paramedic's job at the scene of an accident is to take care of the patients.

Types of Rescues

Most ambulance services respond to a variety of special rescue situations Figure 49-2 ▶ , including vehicle, confined space, trench, water, and mountain/fell and cave rescue. It's important for awareness-level responders to have an understanding of these types of rescues. Often, the first emergency vehicle to arrive at a rescue incident is an ambulance with ambulance clinicians who will not be trained in special rescue techniques. The initial actions taken by paramedics may determine the safety of both patients and other emergency service personnel. They may also determine how efficiently the rescue is completed.

At the Scene

Just as in patient care, the first priority in rescue is "rescuer safety".

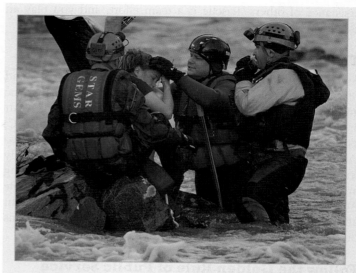

Figure 49-2 Most ambulance services respond to a variety of special rescue situations.

Guidelines for Operations

When assisting rescue team members, the following guidelines will prove useful:

- Be safe.
- Work as a team.
- Think.
- Follow the golden rule of public service.

Be Safe

Rescue situations have many hidden hazards, including oxygen-deficient atmospheres and strong water currents. Knowledge, education, and training are required to recognise the signs that indicate that a hazardous rescue situation exists. Once the hazards are identified, determine what actions are necessary to ensure your own safety as well as the safety of your colleague, the patients, and any bystanders. It requires skill and experience to determine whether a rescue scene is safe to enter, a skilled judgement that could save lives.

At the Scene

All rescue teams should have written safety procedures or standard operating procedures (SOPs) that are familiar to every team member.

Work as a Team

Rescue efforts often require many people to complete a wide variety of tasks. Some personnel may be trained in specific tasks, such as rope/cave rescue or fast-flowing water rescue. However, they can't do their jobs without the support and assistance of others. Rescue is a team effort, and you play an essential role on this team.

Think

As you're working on a rescue situation, you must assess and reassess the scene constantly. You may see something that the ambulance commander (AC) doesn't see. If you think your assigned task may be unsafe, bring it to the attention of the AC, safety officer, or fire officer. Don't try to reorganise the total rescue effort, if it is being directed by people who are highly trained and experienced, but don't ignore what is happening around you either. Observations that you should bring to the AC's attention include changing weather conditions that might affect the rescue scene operations, suspicious packages or items on the scene, and broken equipment.

Follow the Golden Rule of Public Service

When you're involved in carrying out a rescue effort, it's all too easy to concentrate on the technical aspects of the rescue and forget to focus on the scared person who needs your emotional support and encouragement. It's helpful to have emergency personnel stay with the patient whenever possible, keeping the patient updated on which actions will be performed during the rescue process.

Steps of Special Rescue

The role of the paramedic in special rescue operations is often vague and can change as the rescue operation progresses. All

At the Scene

F-A-I-L-U-R-E

The reasons for rescue failures can be referred to by the mnemonic FAILURE:

F Failure to understand the environment, or underestimating it
A Additional medical problems not considered
I Inadequate rescue skills
L Lack of teamwork or experience
U Underestimating the logistics of the incident
R Rescue versus recovery mode not considered
E Equipment not mastered

ambulance clinicians must have some formalised education or training in rescue techniques. This educational process is aimed at preparing them to understand and identify potential hazards and to determine when it's safe or potentially unsafe to access and rescue patients. All prehospital clinicians will be involved with a rescue at some point in their careers, so they must be skilled in specialised patient packaging techniques to allow for a safe extrication and medical care.

Although special rescue situations may take many different forms, all rescuers should follow ten steps to perform these rescues in a safe, effective, and efficient manner:

1. **Preparation**
2. **Response**
3. **Arrival and assessment**
4. **Stabilisation**
5. **Access**

You are the Paramedic Part 2

You are slightly relieved by the sight of a fire appliance arriving on scene, but you know that you require additional resources for extrication and transport. The closest fire rescue tender with extrication capabilities is 30 minutes away, and transport time to the nearest hospital is approximately 45 minutes by land. Your colleague provides a situation report to your ambulance control and asks them to make sure the police are en route and requests assistance from the air ambulance.

You ask assistance from one of the fire fighters to hold the patient's c-spine by leaning through the window on the driver's side of the cab, thus allowing you to commence a more detailed examination. The patient tells you that he was driving down the road when his over-loaded lorry struck the low wall, causing him to veer off into the ditch. The patient denies having any loss of consciousness, headache, dizziness, or visual disturbances. He has a medical history of panic attacks, for which he takes 40 mg of Prozac every day. He has no known drug allergies.

Vital Signs	Recording Time: 5 Minutes
Level of consciousness	Alert
Pulse	122 beats/min, strong and regular
Blood pressure	134/72 mm Hg
Respirations	22 breaths/min
Skin	Pink, warm, and slightly perspiring
SpO₂	95% on normal air

3. Why is it important to maintain good communication with the patient during a special rescue incident?
4. What is the patient at risk of experiencing as a result of being pinned underneath the dashboard from the pelvis down?

6. **Disentanglement**

7. **Removal**

8. **Transport**

9. **Security of the scene and preparation for the next call**

10. **Postincident analysis**

Preparation

You can prepare for responses to emergency rescue incidents by training with fire services and special rescue teams in your area. This educational process will prepare you to respond to a multi-agency call and teach you about the type of rescue equipment other services have access to and the training levels of their personnel. Knowing the terminology used in practice will also make communicating with other rescuers easier and more effective.

Prior to any technical rescue call, your service must consider the following issues:

- Does the service have the personnel and equipment needed to handle a technical rescue incident (TRI) from start to finish? If not, who will they contact?
- What equipment and which personnel will the service send on a technical rescue call?
- Do members of the service know the potential hazard areas in their response area? Have they visited those areas with local representatives?

Response

In the UK, incidents that require specialist rescue techniques will usually be responded to by both the ambulance service and other specialist agencies, such as the Coastguard, Royal National Lifeboat Institution (RNLI), mountain or cave rescue, and of course, the Fire Service.

Arrival and Assessment

Immediately upon arrival, the AC will assume command of the ambulance resources. A rapid and accurate scene assessment is needed to avoid placing rescuers in danger and to determine what additional resources may be needed. Paramedics must assess the extent of injuries and the number of patients; this information will then help to determine how many ambulances and other resources are needed.

Do *not* rush into the incident scene until an assessment of the situation is complete. A paramedic approaching a trench collapse may cause further collapse. A paramedic entering a swiftly flowing river might be knocked off his or her feet straight away and carried downstream. A paramedic climbing into a well to evaluate an unconscious patient may be overcome by an oxygen-deficient atmosphere. There is a clear need to *stop and think about the dangers that may be present.* Don't make yourself part of the problem.

Stabilisation

Once the resources are on the way and the scene is safe to enter, it's time to stabilise the incident. Look around you, identifying and evaluating the hazards at the scene, observing the geographical area, noting the routes of access and egress, observing weather and wind conditions, and considering evacuation problems and transport distances. Establish an outer cordon to keep the public and media out of the working area and maintain a smaller cordon directly around the rescue. The rescue area is the area that surrounds the incident site (eg, collapsed structure, collapsed trench, hazardous spill area). The size of the rescue area is proportional to the hazards that exist.

As part of the stabilisation effort, you should establish three controlled zones:

- **Hot zone.** For fire and rescue teams only. This zone immediately surrounds the dangers of the site (eg, hazardous materials releases) to protect personnel outside the zone.
- **Warm zone.** For properly trained and equipped personnel only. This zone is where personnel and equipment decontamination and hot zone support take place.
- **Cold zone.** For holding vehicles and equipment. This zone contains the command post. The public and the media should be kept clear of the cold zone at all times.

Police or fire cordon tape is often used to demarcate these controlled zones. Of course, someone must ensure that the zones of the emergency scene are enforced. Scene control activities are usually assigned to the police.

During stabilisation, atmospheric monitoring should be started to identify any environments immediately dangerous to life or health (IDLH) for rescuers and patients. After considering the type of incident, you may begin planning how to rescue patients safely. In a trench rescue, for example, the fire service might set up ventilation fans for air flow, set up lights for visibility, and protect the trench from further collapse.

Access

With the scene stabilised, now you must gain access to the patient. How is he or she trapped? In a trench situation, the culprit may be an earth mound. In a rope rescue, scaffolding may have fallen. In a confined space, a hazardous atmosphere may have caused the patient to collapse. To reach a patient who is buried or trapped beneath debris, it is sometimes necessary to dig a tunnel as a means of rescue and escape. Identify the actual reason for the rescue and work toward freeing the patient safely.

Communicate with patients at all times during the rescue to make sure they are not injured further by the rescue operation. Even if they're not injured, they need to be reassured that the team is working as quickly as possible to free them.

Emergency medical care should be initiated as soon as access to the patient is achieved. Technical rescue paramedics are crucial resources at TRIs; not only can these responders start IVs and treat medical conditions, but they also know how to deal with the special equipment being used and the procedures taking place around them. It's vitally important that the actions of ambulance service personnel be effectively coordinated into ongoing operations during rescue incidents. Their main functions are to treat patients and to stand by in case a rescue team member needs medical assistance. As soon as a rescue area is secured and stabilised, ambulance service personnel must be allowed access to the patients for medical assessment and stabilisation. Throughout the course of the rescue operation, which may span many hours, ambulance service personnel must continually monitor and ensure the stability of all patients.

Gaining access to the patient depends on the type of incident. For example, in an incident involving a motor vehicle, its location and position, the damage to the vehicle, and the position of the patient are important considerations. The means of gaining access to the patient must also take into account the nature and severity of the patient's injuries. The chosen means of access may change during the course of the rescue as the nature or severity of the patient's injuries becomes apparent.

Disentanglement

Once precautions have been taken and the reason for entrapment has been identified, the patient needs to be freed as safely as possible. A team member should remain with the patient to direct the rescuers who are performing the disentanglement. In a trench incident, this would include digging either with a shovel or by hand to free the patient.

In a road traffic collision, the vehicle may have to be removed from around the patient rather than trying to remove the patient through the wreckage. Parts of the car—for example, the steering wheel, seats, pedals, and dashboard—may trap the occupants. Disentanglement is the cutting of a vehicle (or machinery) away from trapped or injured patients, using extrication and rescue tools along with various extrication methods.

Removal

Once the patient has been disentangled, efforts shift to removing the patient Figure 49-3 ▸ . In some instances, this may simply amount to having someone assist the patient up a ladder; in other situations, it may require removal with spinal immobilisation due to possible injuries. A wide variety of equipment, including longboards, stretchers, and other immobilisation devices, are used to remove injured patients from trenches, confined spaces, and elevated points.

Preparing the patient for removal involves maintaining continued control of all life-threatening problems, dressing all wounds, and immobilising all suspected fractures and spinal

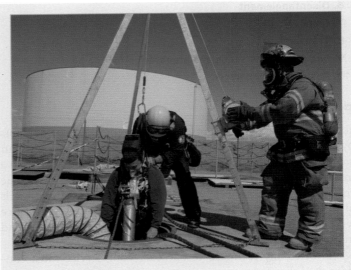

Figure 49-3 Patient removal.

injuries. The use of standard splints in confined areas is difficult and frequently impossible, but stabilisation of the arms to the patient's body and of the legs to each other will often suffice until the patient is positioned on a longboard, which may serve as the ultimate splint for the whole body. The shortboard or Kendrick Extrication Device (KED) is typically used for stabilisation of a sitting patient.

Sometimes a patient must be removed quickly (rapid extrication; covered in Chapter 25) because his or her general condition is deteriorating and time does not permit meticulous splinting and dressing procedures. Quick removal may also occur if hazards are present, such as spilled fuel or other materials that could endanger the patient or rescue personnel. The only time the patient should be moved prior to completion of initial care, assessment, stabilisation, and treatment is when the patient's or emergency services personnel life is in immediate danger.

Packaging is preparing the patient for movement as a unit. It is often accomplished by means of a longboard or similar device. These boards are essential for moving patients with potential or actual spine injuries.

Rough-terrain rescues may require multiple rescuers passing a stretcher over uneven ground, rocks, or fording streams. These operations require at least one person to take each corner of the stretcher or longboard if possible. In extreme cases, a four-person team may have to hand a rescue stretcher around or over obstacles to another team ("leapfrogging"). Rescues in rough terrain often require ingenuity to suspend or pad a stretcher so that the patient is provided with a reasonably comfortable ride. Padding usually consists of foam padding or loosely rolled blankets. This technique is superior to "slinging" the stretcher on straps, which may lead to excessive swaying and bouncing.

Transport

Once the patient has been removed from the hazard area, ambulance service personnel will undertake transport to an appropriate hospital. Depending on the severity of the patient's injuries and the distance to hospital, the type of transport will vary. For example, if a patient is critically injured or if the rescue is taking place some distance from the hospital, or an air ambulance may be more appropriate than a ground ambulance.

In rough-terrain rescues, four-wheel drive, high-clearance vehicles may be required to transport patients on stretchers to an awaiting ambulance. Helicopters are increasingly used for quick evacuation from remote areas, but they have limitations in bad weather conditions and after the hours of darkness.

General Rescue Scene Procedures

As a paramedic, you know that your own safety, as well as the safety of your colleague and the public, is paramount. At a TRI, while you may be tempted to approach the patient or the accident area, it is critically important to slow down and evaluate the situation properly. Consider the potential general hazards and risks of utilities, confined spaces, and environmental conditions, as well as hazards that are IDLH. In confined-space rescue incidents, potential hazards may include deep or isolated spaces, multiple complicating hazards (eg, water or chemicals), failure of essential equipment or service, and environmental conditions (eg, snow or rain).

Approaching the Scene

Beginning with the initial details of the 999 call, you should be compiling facts and impressions about the call. Scene assessment begins with the information gained from the person reporting the incident and then from the bystanders at the scene upon arrival.

The information gathered when an emergency call is received is important to the success of the rescue operation. Information collected should include the following:

- Location of the incident
- Nature of the incident (kinds and number of vehicles)
- Condition and position of patients
- Condition and position of vehicles
- Number of people trapped or injured and types of injuries
- Any specific or special hazard information
- Name of person calling and a number where the person can be reached

As you approach the scene of a TRI, however, you may not always know what kind of scene you are entering. Is it a building site? Do you see piles of earth that would indicate a trench? What actions are the members of the public taking? Are they attempting to rescue trapped people, possibly placing themselves at considerable danger? Identify any life-threatening hazards, and take corrective measures to mitigate them. Determine

whether the situation is a search, rescue, or recovery. If additional resources are needed, they should be ordered by the AC.

A scene assessment should include the initial and ongoing evaluation of the following issues:

- Scope and magnitude of the incident
- Risk and benefit analysis
- Number of known and potential patients
- Hazards
- Access to the scene
- Environmental factors
- Available and necessary resources
- Establishment of a controlled cordon

Utility Hazards

In case of utility hazards, your goal is to control as many of the hazards as possible. Minimise all risks and ensure that all emergency service personnel are using appropriate PPE. Are there any fallen power lines near the scene Figure 49-4 ▾ ? Is equipment or machinery electrically charged so as to present a danger to the patient or the rescuers? The AC should ensure that the proper procedures are taken to shut off the utilities in the rescue area. Remember—utility hazards can be above or below ground, and the rescue situation will dictate which ones need to be addressed first.

At the Scene

Treat all fallen power lines as if they are live until you receive specific clearance from the electricity supplier. Even if the lights are out along the street where the power lines have fallen, never assume that the wires are dead. Be especially alert for fallen power lines after a storm that has blown down trees or tree branches.

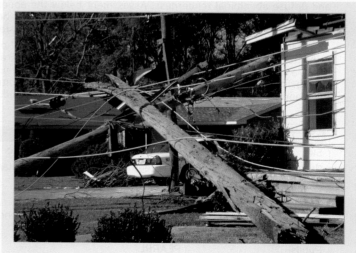

Figure 49-4 Fallen power lines present a hazard.

Utility hazards require the assistance of trained personnel. For electrical hazards, such as fallen power lines, park at least 25 metres away. Watch for falling utility poles; a damaged pole may bring other poles down with it. Don't touch any wires, power lines, or other electrical sources until they have been turned off by a power company representative. It isn't just the wires that are hazardous; any metal that they touch is also live. Metal fences or guardrails may become live along their entire unbroken length. Be careful around running or standing water, as water is an excellent conductor of electricity.

Natural gas and liquefied petroleum gas are nontoxic but are classified as asphyxiates because they displace breathable air. In addition, both are explosive. If a call involves leaking gas, call the gas company immediately.

Scene Security

Has the area been secured to prevent people from entering? Colleagues, family members, and even other rescuers may unwittingly enter an unsafe scene and become patients themselves. The AC should coordinate with police to help secure the scene and control access. In addition, the fire service should implement a strict accountability system to control access to the rescue scene.

Incident Management System

The first arriving officer immediately assumes command and starts using the integrated emergency management system (IEMS). This step is critically important because many TRIs will eventually become very complex and require a large number of assisting units. Without the IEMS in place, it will be difficult—if not impossible—to ensure the rescuers' safety.

Patient Contact

At any rescue scene, you must try to communicate with the patient. Technical rescue situations often last for hours, with the patient being left unmoved and alone for long periods of time. If at all possible, you should attempt to communicate via a radio, mobile phone, or yelling. Reassure the patient that everything is being done to ensure his or her safety.

If you succeed in making contact, it's important to stay in communication with the patient. Ideally, someone should be assigned to talk to the patient, while others focus on making the rescue. Realise that the patient could be sick or injured and is probably frightened. If you are calm, your manner will in turn calm the patient:

- Make and keep eye contact with the patient.
- Tell the truth. Lying destroys trust and confidence. You may not always tell the patient everything, but if the patient asks a specific question, answer truthfully.
- Communicate at a level that the patient can understand.
- Be aware of your own body language.
- Always speak slowly, clearly, and distinctly.
- Use a patient's proper name. Use the patient's surname, preceded by the proper qualifier (ie, Mr or Ms, unless they say that they would like you to use their given name).
- If a patient is hard of hearing, speak clearly and directly at the person, so that he or she can read your lips.

At the Scene

Always assume that oncoming traffic can't see you, and act appropriately.

You are the Paramedic Part 3

Your rapid trauma assessment yields no respiratory compromise, an actively bleeding 10 cm laceration across the patient's forehead, and diffuse abdominal tenderness. Assessment below the abdomen is not possible because the patient is pinned beneath the dashboard from the pelvis down. The patient is anxious about not being able to feel his legs. You do your best to reassure him that additional help is on its way and encourage him to focus on taking slow, deep breaths.

You place the patient on a nonrebreathing mask at 15 l/min of oxygen. Your colleague applies a c-collar and manual c-spine continues to be held by the fire fighter. Bleeding from the forehead laceration is controlled with direct pressure and bandaging. You are able to insert a 16-gauge cannula in the right antecubital fossa and begin a normal saline infusion at a to-keep-vein-open rate. Ambulance control advises that the estimated time of arrival (ETA) for an additional vehicle is approximately 20 minutes and the ETA for the helicopter is approximately 10 minutes. The police are on scene and secure a landing area.

Reassessment	Recording Time: 13 Minutes
Skin	Pink, warm, and slightly perspiring
Pulse	130 breaths/min, strong and regular
Blood pressure	128/70 mm Hg
Respirations	22 breaths/min, regular
SpO_2	98% on 15 l/min of oxygen via nonrebreathing mask
ECG	Sinus tachycardia
Pupils	PEARRL

5. What needs to be monitored on this patient?

- Allow time for the patient to answer or respond to your questions.
- Try to make the patient comfortable and relaxed whenever possible.

Assisting Rescue Crews

If you will be assisting a technical rescue team, training with the team is probably the most important step you can take so that you can work together effectively during a TRI. Training allows you to get a feel for how the team members operate; likewise, they can get an idea of which duties they can trust you with. The more knowledge you have, the more you'll be able to do.

At any TRI, follow the AC's orders. Your ultimate goal is to protect the team and patients. No matter what type of rescue scene you enter, keep these three guidelines in mind:

- Approach the scene cautiously.
- Position apparatus properly.
- Assist specialised team members as necessary.

At the Scene

Most newer cars have driver-side and passenger-side airbags. Some newer vehicles have supplemental airbags in other places as well. Airbags that don't activate during a collision present a danger to rescuers until they're deactivated.

Vehicles

Determine where to locate your emergency vehicle, taking into account the safety of emergency workers, patients, and other motorists. Whenever possible, park emergency vehicles in a manner that will ensure safety and not disrupt traffic any more than necessary. Traffic flow is the largest single hazard associated with any operation that takes place on a motorway. Provide a safe ambulance loading zone. On limited-access motorways, keep vehicles and apparatus not directly involved in the rescue off the motorway. Have parking areas away from the scene. Don't hesitate to request that the road be closed if necessary.

Use large emergency vehicles to provide a barrier against motorists who fail to heed emergency warning lights. Many fire services place appliances at an angle to the accident. This position ensures that the applicance is pushed to the side of an accident in the event that it is struck from behind. You can normally rely on the police to place traffic cones to direct motorists away from the scene.

You need to be visible at an accident scene. Use only essential warning lights, because too many lights tend to distract or confuse other drivers. Consider the use of blue lights at the scene, but ensure that your engine remains running to

avoid a flat battery. Your PPE should be bright to help ensure your visibility during daylight hours. Any PPE that is used at night needs to be equipped with reflective material to increase your visibility in the darkness. PPE must be worn at all road traffic collisions. Before exiting the ambulance at an emergency scene, be alert for any vehicles that might cause you injury. Don't assume that motorists will heed your warning lights. Let the police coordinate traffic control.

Ambulance service providers must be aware of all potential hazards at rescue scenes—both obvious (eg, sharp metal and broken glass) and less obvious or hidden dangers. Power lines may fall from above, and underground electrical feeds may become exposed. Energy-absorbing bumpers can explode when subjected to heat and can spring out when loaded. Airbags or supplemental restraint systems (SRS) can deploy at any time after an accident and must be deactivated even if the power supply to the vehicle has been disconnected. Conventional fuel systems with highly flammable vapours may ignite if they come in contact with hot catalytic converters or heated engine components. New vehicles that use alternative fuel sources (eg, electric or propane-fuelled vehicles) can also pose problems for rescuers. For example, providers must be aware of the electrical power, any storage cells, and high-pressure cylinders used in natural-gas–powered vehicles.

Vehicle-Related Terminology

To reduce confusion and mistakes at extrication scenes, it's important to use standardised terminology when referring to specific parts of vehicles. It may appear obvious, but the front of a vehicle normally travels down the road first. The bonnet is located on the front of the vehicle. The rear of a vehicle is where the boot is usually located.

The right side of the vehicle is on your right as you sit in the vehicle. In the UK, the driver's seat is on the right side of the vehicle. The left side is where the passenger is located. Always refer to left and right as they relate to *the vehicle*—not as they refer to *your* left and right.

Vehicles contain A, B, C, and D posts, which are the vertical supports that hold up the roof and form the upright columns of the occupant cage. The A posts are located closest to the front of the vehicle; they form the sides of the windscreen. In four-door vehicles, the B posts are located between the front and rear doors of a vehicle; in some vehicles, they don't reach all of the way to the roof. In four-door vehicles, the C posts are located behind the rear doors, if present. D posts can be found on larger vehicles such as sport utility vehicles and vans that have a passenger window on the side behind the rear doors. The D post is located behind the rear passenger windows.

The bonnet covers the engine compartment. The bulkhead divides the engine compartment from the passenger compartment. An insulating metal piece known as the firewall protects the passengers in the event of an engine fire. The passenger compartment includes the front and back seats. This

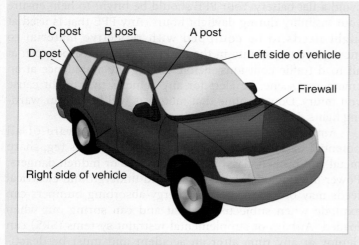

Figure 49-5 The anatomy of a vehicle.

part of a vehicle is sometimes called the occupant cage or occupant compartment **Figure 49-5 ▲** .

There are two common types of vehicle frames: *platform frame* construction and *unibody* construction.

Platform frame construction uses beams to fabricate the load-bearing frame of a vehicle. The engine, transmission, and body components are then attached to this basic platform frame. This type of frame construction is found primarily in lorries and sport utility vehicles; it is rare in smaller passenger cars. Platform frame construction provides a structurally sound base for stabilising the vehicle and an anchor point for attaching cables or extrication tools.

Unibody construction, which is used for most modern cars, combines the vehicle body and the frame into a single component. By folding multiple thicknesses of metal together, a column can be formed that is strong enough to serve as the frame for a lightweight vehicle. Unibody construction allows car manufacturers to produce lighter weight vehicles. When extricating a person from such a vehicle, remember that unibody vehicles don't have the frame rails that are present with platform frame–constructed vehicles.

Vehicle Stabilisation

Unstable objects pose a threat to both rescuers and casualties at the scene. These objects—most often, the damaged vehicles—need to be stabilised before your approach.

Vehicles that end up on their wheels need to be stabilised with chocking in the front and back of the wheels. Chocking is short lengths of robust timber (10 cm × 10 cm) used to stabilise a vehicle. It prevents the vehicle from rolling backward or forward.

After the chocking has been placed, a vehicle can still move because of the give and motion generated by the suspen-

At the Scene

Even vehicles that are positioned upright on all four wheels should be stabilised.

sion system. This motion may occur as rescuers enter the vehicle and the patients are extricated from the vehicle, and it can cause further injuries to the patients of the collision. The suspension system of most vehicles can be stabilised with step blocks, which are stairstep-shaped blocks that are placed under the side of the vehicle.

After a collision, some vehicles will come to rest on their roof or sides. These vehicles are very unstable, and the slightest weight on them can cause them to move.

Gain Access to the Patient
Open the Door

After stabilising the vehicle, the simplest way to access the casualty is to open a door. Try all of the doors first—even if they appear to be badly damaged. It's an embarrassing waste of time and energy to open a jammed door with heavy rescue equipment when another door can be opened easily and without any special equipment.

Attempt to unlock and open the least damaged door first. Make sure the locking mechanism is released. Try the outside and inside handles at the same time if possible.

Notes from Nancy

You don't get extra points for doing things the hard way.

If you have an open door but still need more room, have two rescuers lean against the door and push; most car doors will easily bend open, creating a much wider opening for patient removal.

Break Tempered Glass

If a patient's condition is serious enough to require immediate care and you can't

Notes from Nancy

The easiest way to enter a car is through a door.

enter the vehicle through a door, consider breaking a window. Don't try to break and enter through the windscreen because it's made of laminated windscreen glass, which is difficult to break. The side and rear windows are made of tempered glass, also known as safety glass, and will break easily into small pieces when hit with a sharp, pointed object such as a spring-loaded centre punch **Figure 49-6 ▶** . Because these windows do not pose as great a safety threat, they can be your primary access route.

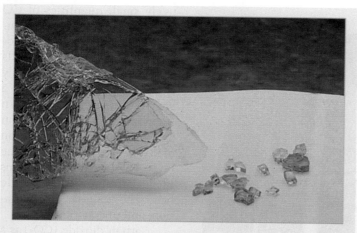

Figure 49-6 The two types of glass in vehicles: laminated glass (left) and tempered glass (right).

At the Scene

Always warn trapped car passengers that you're going to break the glass!

If you must break a window to unlock a door or gain access, try to break one that's far away from the patient. If the patient's condition warrants your immediate entry, however, don't hesitate to break the closest window. Small pieces of tempered glass do not usually pose a danger to people trapped in cars.

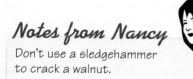

Notes from Nancy

Don't use a sledgehammer to crack a walnut.

During this step of the rescue, all rescuers should be in proper PPE, including safety glasses or goggles. Attempt to lower windows as far as possible before breaking glass, and then select a spring-loaded centre punch. If you're using something other than a spring-loaded centre punch, always aim for a low corner. The window frame will help prevent the tool from sailing into the vehicle and hitting the person inside. Personnel are given a verbal warning "breaking glass", unless a stop/rest call is made. After breaking the window, pull the remaining glass out of the window frame so it doesn't fall onto any passengers or injure any rescuers.

Once you have removed the pieces of glass from the frame, try to unlock the door again. Release the locking mechanism, and then use both the inside and outside door handles at the same time. This action may force a jammed locking mechanism, even in a door that appears to be badly damaged.

Breaking the rear window will sometimes provide an opening large enough to enable a rescuer to reach a patient if there is no other rapid means for gaining access. Using the simple techniques of opening a door or breaking the rear window will enable you to gain access to most patients in vehicle accidents, even those in upside-down vehicles.

Force the Door

If you can't gain access to the vehicle by the methods already described, heavier extrication tools must be used to gain access to the patient. The most common technique is door displacement. The opening and displacement of vehicle doors may be difficult and somewhat unpredictable.

Confined Spaces

A confined space is a location surrounded by a structure that isn't designed for continuous occupancy. Confined spaces have limited openings for entrance and exit. Confined spaces can occur in farm, commercial, and industrial settings. Structures such as grain silos, industrial pits, tanks, and below-ground structures are all considered confined spaces. Car boots are also considered confined spaces. Cisterns, well shafts, and septic tanks are also confined spaces that are found in many residential settings Figure 49-7 ▶ .

Confined spaces present a special hazard because they may have limited ventilation to provide for air circulation and

At the Scene

Airbag Safety

- Steering wheels on most recently manufactured vehicles contain a driver's side airbag, which is a lifesaving safety feature for the occupants of the vehicle.
- If the airbag has deployed during the collision, it does not present a safety hazard for rescuers.
- If not deployed during the collision, an airbag presents a hazard for the passenger of the vehicle and for emergency services personnel. It could potentially deploy if wires are cut or if it becomes activated during the rescue operation.
- If the airbag did not deploy, disconnect the battery and allow the airbag capacitor to discharge. The time required to discharge the capacitor varies from one model of airbag to another.
- Some newer-model vehicles have a switch mounted on or under the dashboard that allows drivers to disconnect or shut off the SRS.
- Don't place a hard object such as a longboard between the patient and an undeployed airbag.
- For your safety, never get in front of an undeployed airbag. You could suffer serious injury if it's unexpectedly activated.
- Some vehicles contain side-mounted airbags or curtains that provide lateral protection for passengers. Check vehicles for the presence of these devices.

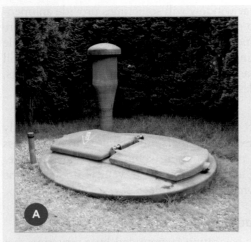
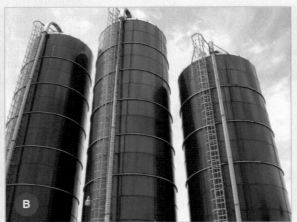

Figure 49-7 Confined spaces **A.** Below ground. **B.** Silo.

At the Scene

Confined spaces such as manholes can be deceiving. They may look habitable but can contain minimal oxygen or deadly invisible toxins.

exchange, which can make them an oxygen-deficient atmosphere, or they may contain poisonous gases. Entering a confined space without testing the atmosphere for safety and without the proper breathing apparatus can result in death. Additionally, there is a risk of fire and explosion in confined spaces because inadequate ventilation may trap flammable mixtures. Grain silos and trenches can suddenly become "quicksand" and lead to engulfment. Machinery may often have confined spaces containing augers or screws that can be hazardous to rescue workers. All rescue personnel must consider the potential for stored electrical energy in any machinery and should never attempt any rescue without being properly trained.

Don't be overwhelmed by the urgency to start treating patients; scene safety must always be considered first. A confined-space call is sometimes dispatched as a heart attack or medical illness call, because the caller assumes the person who entered a confined space and became unresponsive suffered a heart attack or medical illness.

Examples of Oxygen Deficiency/Poisonous Gases in Confined Spaces

Hydrogen sulphide (H_2S) is a colourless, toxic, flammable gas that is released when bacteria break down organic matter in the absence of oxygen. It can be found in swamps, standing water, sewers, natural gas, and in some wells. Hydrogen sulphide is heavier than air and has a very pungent odour at first but deadens the sense of smell very quickly.

Carbon monoxide (CO) is a colourless, odourless, tasteless gas that can't be detected by your normal senses. Inhaling rela-

tively small quantities of CO gas can result in severe poisoning because it binds to haemoglobin in the red blood cells about 240 times more readily than oxygen. Therefore, a small quantity of CO can "monopolise" the haemoglobin and prevent the transportation of oxygen to all parts of the body. The signs and symptoms of CO poisoning include headache, nausea, disorientation, and unconsciousness.

Carbon dioxide (CO_2) is a colourless gas associated with asphyxiation risks. It is actually the end product of a metabolism process in which sugar and fats combine with oxygen. Carbon dioxide is used to make dry ice and is found in fire extinguishers. It produces a sour taste in the mouth and a stinging sensation in the nose and mouth.

Methane (CH_4)—the principal component of natural gas—isn't toxic but will cause burns if ignited. Flammable or explosive mixtures form at much lower concentrations than the concentrations at which asphyxiation risks arise. Methane is used as a fuel from natural gas fields but can also be generated from fermentation of organic matter (eg, manure, waste water, sludge, and municipal solid waste).

Ammonia (NH_3) is a toxic and corrosive chemical with a characteristic pungent odour. Because ammonia is lighter than air, it rises to the upper atmospheric level in confined spaces. It's typically found in rural areas and is used extensively for fertilising agricultural crops.

Nitrogen dioxide (NO_2) is a reddish-brown gas that has a characteristic sharp, biting odour. It is most prominent in air pollution and is considered toxic by inhalation.

Safe Approach

As you approach a confined-space rescue scene, look for a bystander who might have witnessed the emergency. Information gathered prior to the technical rescue team's arrival will save valuable time during the actual rescue. Don't automatically assume that a person in a pit has simply suffered a heart attack; instead, assume that there's an IDLH atmosphere at any confined-space call. An IDLH atmosphere can immediately incapacitate anyone who enters the confined space without a respirator. Toxic gases may be present, or oxygen levels may be

At the Scene

More rescuers die in confined spaces than casualties! Do not enter a confined space without proper breathing apparatus and special training.

insufficient to support life. Inevitably, it will take some time for qualified rescuers to arrive on the scene and prepare for a safe entry into the confined space. The casualty of the original incident may have died before your arrival—don't put your life in danger for a confirmed dead patient.

Assisting Other Rescuers

You and your colleague can prevent a confined-space incident from becoming worse by recognising it, securing the scene, and ensuring that no one enters the space until additional rescue resources arrive. As highly trained personnel arrive, you may provide help by giving these rescuers a situation report.

The first responding rescuers must share whatever information is discovered at the rescue scene with the arriving crew. Anything that may be important to the response should be noted by the first arriving ambulance. Observed conditions should be compared to reported conditions, and continual reassessment should be conducted throughout the incident period. Whether an incident appears to be stable or has changed significantly since the first report will affect the operation strategy for the rescue. An assessment should be quickly completed immediately upon arrival, and this information should be relayed to the specialised rescue team members when they arrive at the scene. Other items of importance that should be included in a situation report are a description of any rescue attempts that have been made, exposures, hazards, extinguishment of fires, the facts and probabilities of the scene, the situation and resources of the fire service, the identity of any hazardous materials present, and a progress evaluation.

Confined-space rescues can be complex and can take a long time to complete. By understanding the hazards of confined spaces, you will be better prepared to assist a specialised team that's dealing with an emergency involving a confined space.

Trenches

Trench rescues may become necessary when earth is removed for placement of a power line or for other construction and the sides of the excavation collapse, trapping a worker **Figure 49-8 ▶** . Entrapments may also occur when children play around a pile of sand or earth that collapses. Unfortunately, many entrapments occur because the required safety precautions were not taken.

Whenever a collapse occurs, you need to understand that the collapsed product is unstable and prone to further collapse. Earth and sand are very heavy, and a person who's partly entrapped can't simply be pulled out. Instead, the patient must be carefully dug out after shoring has stabilised the sides of the excavation.

Vibration or additional weight on top of displaced earth will increase the probability of a secondary collapse. A secondary collapse occurs after the initial collapse; it can be caused by equipment vibration, personnel standing at the edge of the trench, or water eroding away the soil. Safe removal of trapped persons requires a special rescue team that is trained and

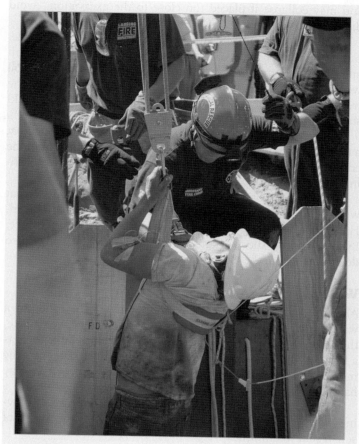

Figure 49-8 Trench rescue.

At the Scene

Most trench collapses occur in trenches less than 4 m deep and 2 m wide. Patients are suddenly covered with heavy soil, resulting in asphyxia. Specially trained rescuers should make safe access only after shoring is in place.

equipped to erect shoring that will protect the rescuers and the entrapped person from secondary collapse.

Safety is of paramount importance when approaching a trench or excavation collapse. Walking close to the edge of a collapse can trigger a secondary collapse. Stay away from the edge of the site, and keep all workers and bystanders away. Vibration from equipment and machinery can cause secondary collapses, so shut off all heavy equipment. Vibrations caused by nearby traffic can also cause collapse, so it may be necessary to stop or divert traffic.

Soil that has been removed from the excavation and placed in a pile is called the spoil pile. This material is very unstable and may collapse if placed too close to the excavation. Avoid disturbing the spoil pile.

Make verbal contact with the trapped person if possible, but do *not* place yourself in danger while doing so. If you approach the trench, do so from the narrow end, where the soil will be more stable. However, it's best *not* to approach the trench unless absolutely necessary; ambulance clinicians should stay out of a trench until it is safe.

Provide reassurance by letting the trapped person know that a trained rescue team is on the way. By removing people from the edges of the excavation, shutting down machinery, and establishing contact with the patient, you start the rescue process.

You can also assess the scene, looking for evidence that would indicate where the trapped workers may be located. Hand tools and hard hats are one indicator of their presence. By questioning the workers, ambulance clinicians may also determine where the patients were last seen.

Water

Almost all ambulance services may potentially be called to a water rescue—whether from a small stream, a large river, a lake, the sea, a reservoir, or a swimming pool. A static source such as a lake may have no current and is considered flat water or slow moving. In contrast, a whitewater stream or flooded river may have a very swift current.

Rescuers may suddenly find themselves immersed in moving water during a water rescue, so they should be aware of self-rescue techniques. A personal flotation device (PFD) is essential. In addition, if suddenly immersed in fast-moving water, rescuers should adopt the self-rescue position. The first step is to roll into a face-up arched position with the lower back higher than the feet to avoid subsurface objects. Keep the feet together and facing in the direction of travel (feet first) with arms to the side. Use the hands for changing direction to avoid objects and for diversion to a safe area. Keep the head down, with the chin tucked in. This position protects the rescuer's head, face, and lower back from striking objects and provides a means for controlling direction.

Cold Water Rescue

Water temperature varies widely by season and by geographical area. Even on warm days, water temperatures can be very low. Water causes heat loss 25 times greater than ambient air temperature. Indeed, any water temperature less than normal body temperature will cause hypothermia; patients who become hypothermic lose the ability to self-rescue. Maintaining body heat is critical because hypothermia becomes an immediate problem that progresses to unconsciousness and death. In

At the Scene

Don't attempt a water rescue unless you are specially trained.

extremely cold water (2°C), a submersion time of 15 to 20 minutes will cause the body to shut down and lead to death.

If you find yourself in cold water, make every effort to keep your face above water, protect your head, and assume the heat-escape-lessening position (HELP) **Figure 49-9 ▾**, which helps keep heat in the core of your body. Immersion casualties should minimise movement and assume the HELP position. In a group, casualties should huddle together to share body warmth.

At the Scene

The colder the water, the faster the loss of heat. Compared with air, water causes a heat loss at a rate 25 times faster. Immersion for 15 to 20 minutes in 2°C water is likely to be fatal.

In water colder than 21°C, immersion casualties may actually benefit from a phenomenon known as the cold protective response. Essentially, when a person is submerged in cold water, heat is conducted from the body to the water. The resulting hypothermia can protect vital organs from the lack of oxygen. In addition, exposure to cold water will occasionally activate certain primitive reflexes, which may preserve body functions for prolonged periods. In one case, a 2½-year-old girl recovered after being submerged in cold water for at least 66 minutes. For this reason, you should continue to provide full resuscitative efforts for a casualty of cold water submersion until the patient recovers or is pronounced dead in hospital (see Chapter 35 for a more detailed discussion of hypothermia).

Whenever a person dives or jumps into very cold water, the diving reflex (also known as the mammalian diving reflex)

At the Scene

The HELP position can decrease heat loss by 60% compared with treading water.

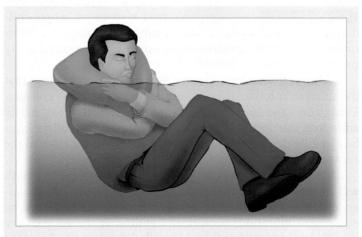
Figure 49-9 The heat-escape-lessening position (HELP).

causes slowing of the heart rate due to submersion in cold water and may cause profound bradycardia. Although loss of consciousness may follow, the person may be able to survive for an extended time under water because of a lowering of the metabolic rate and decreased oxygen demand and consumption associated with hypothermia.

At the Scene

Remember that hypothermic patients are dehydrated due to "cold diuresis", and should be removed from the water in a horizontal position to avoid orthostatic changes.

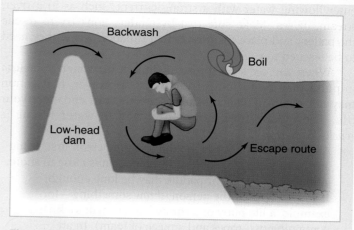

Figure 49-10 Recirculating current at a low-head dam.

Other Water Rescue Situations

In surface water rescues, attending crews must consider hazards such as the dangerous turbulence created by moving water as well as "strainers" (objects in the water such as trees, branches, debris, or wire mesh that can pose a serious risk for rescuers). Dams and hydroelectric sites are also treacherous for even the most skilled rescuers. It's important to remember that the height of a dam does not indicate the degree of hazard to rescuers. Intakes at the base of a dam can act like strainers. Low-head dams are often associated with recirculating currents (sometimes referred to as a "boil") **Figure 49-10**. These currents can trap casualties and unwary rescuers alike, forcing them underwater, away from the dam, and back to the surface again, where the cycle repeats itself. For this reason, low-head dams are often referred to as "drowning machines". Never underestimate the power or intensity of moving water.

Safe Approach

When responding to water incidents, your safety and the safety of other rescuers are your primary concerns. Your standard

At the Scene

The hydraulics of moving water change with variables such as depth, velocity, and obstruction to flow.

equipment is not designed for water rescue activities. When working at a water rescue scene, you should use personal protective equipment designed for water rescue. Whenever you are within 3 metres of the water, you should wear an approved PFD. Shoes that provide solid traction are preferable to boots.

If you are part of the first arriving ambulance's crew, and the endangered people are in a vehicle or holding on to a tree or other solid object, try to communicate with them. Let them know that more help is on the way.

Don't exceed your level of training. If you can't swim, operating around or near water is not recommended. A person who is trained as a lifeguard for still water is not prepared to

You are the Paramedic Part 4

About 5 minutes later, the patient becomes extremely anxious and complains about abdominal pain. A re-assessment of the abdomen shows marked distension and rigidity. The patient is becoming pale and increasingly sweaty. His radial pulses are weakening. Despite your best efforts to be reassuring, the patient's anxiety continues to escalate and he keeps repeating "I'm dying". You reassure the patient that he will soon be freed as you hear the air ambulance landing.

Reassessment	Recording Time: 23 Minutes
Skin	Pale, cool, and perspiring
Pulse	140 beats/min, carotid
Blood pressure	92/68 mm Hg
Respirations	24 breaths/min
SpO2	97% on oxygen at 15 l/min via nonrebreathing mask
ECG	Sinus rhythm

6. Why is it important to be cautious when administering strong opioids to release the patient's pain?

enter flowing water with a strong current, such as in a river, stream, or sea. Make sure that bystanders don't try to rescue the patient and place themselves in a situation where they need to be rescued too.

When you see a person struggling in the water, your first impulse may be to jump in to assist. However, that action may not result in a successful rescue and can endanger your life. The model most commonly used in water rescue is *reach-throw-row-go*:

- Attempt to *reach* out to the threatening person first, using any readily available object. If the person is close to shore, a branch, pole, oar, or paddle may be long enough.
- If you can't reach the person, *throw* something—for example, a life buoy or a throw bag (a small sack containing two ropes and a piece of foam). In an emergency situation, a rescuer opens the bag, pulls out enough rope to grasp firmly, and then throws the bag to the casualty. The casualty should be instructed to grab the rope and not the bag, because the bag may contain more rope that can uncoil.
- If you can't reach the person by throwing something that floats, you may be able to *row* out to the drowning person if a small boat or canoe is available. Do so only if you know how to operate or propel the craft properly. Protect yourself by wearing an approved PFD.

At the Scene

Personal flotation devices (PFDs) that are not worn are not helpful!

Spinal Incidents in Submersion Incidents

Submersion incidents may be complicated by spinal fractures and spinal cord injuries. You must assume that spinal injury exists with the following conditions:

- The submersion has resulted from a diving mishap or fall.
- The patient is unconscious, and no information is available to rule out the possibility of a mechanism causing neck injury.
- The patient is conscious but complains of weakness, paralysis, or numbness in the arms or legs.
- You suspect the possibility of spinal injury despite what witnesses say.

Most spinal injuries in diving incidents affect the cervical spine. When spinal injury is suspected, the neck must be protected from further injury. This means that you will have to stabilise the suspected injury while the patient is still in the water. Follow the steps in **Skill Drill 49-1 ▶**:

1. Turn the patient supine. Two rescuers are usually required to turn the patient safely, although in some cases one rescuer will suffice. Always rotate the entire upper half of the patient's body as a single unit. Twisting only the head, for example, may aggravate any injury to the cervical spine (**Step 1**).
2. Restore the airway and begin ventilation. Immediate ventilation is the primary treatment of all submersion patients as soon as the patient is face up in the water. Use a pocket mask if it is available. Ask the other rescuer to support the head and body as a unit while you open the airway and begin artificial ventilation (**Step 2**).
3. Float a buoyant longboard under the patient as you continue ventilation (**Step 3**).
4. Secure the body and head to the longboard to eliminate motion of the cervical spine. Do not remove the patient from the water until this is done (**Step 4**).
5. Remove the patient from the water, on the longboard (**Step 5**).
6. Cover the patient with a blanket. Give supplemental oxygen if the patient is breathing spontaneously. Begin CPR if there is no respiration. Effective CPR is extremely difficult to perform when the patient is still in the water (**Step 6**).

Search and Rescue

Search and rescue (SAR) is an activity that is conducted by a limited number of services. SAR missions consist of two parts: search (looking for a lost or overdue person) and rescue (removing a patient from a hostile environment).

Several types of situations may result in the initiation of SAR missions. Small children may wander off and be unable to find their way back to a known place. Older adults who are suffering from Alzheimer's disease may fail to remember where they're going and become lost. People who are hiking, walking, or participating in other activities may become lost because they lack the proper training or equipment, because the weather changes unexpectedly, or if they become sick or injured.

Safe Approach

The countryside can include many different environments, such as forests, mountains, cliffs, natural parks, moors, and coastlines. Depending on the terrain and environmental factors, the countryside can be as little as a few minutes from major services. Despite the short access time, the scene could require an extended evacuation. Examples of countryside terrains include cliffs, steep slopes, rivers, streams, valleys, mountainsides, and beaches. Terrain hazards include cliffs, caves, wells, mines, and rock slides.

Skill Drill 49-1: Stabilising a Suspected Spinal Injury in the Water

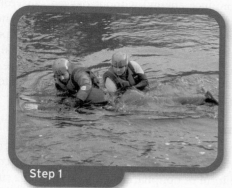

Step 1

Turn the patient to a supine position in the water by rotating the entire upper half of the body as a single unit.

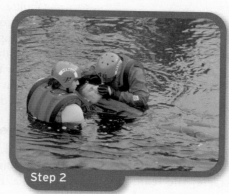

Step 2

As soon as the patient is turned, begin artificial ventilation using the mouth-to-mouth method or a pocket mask.

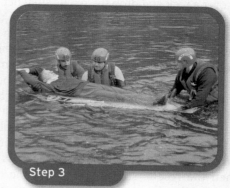

Step 3

Float a buoyant longboard under the patient.

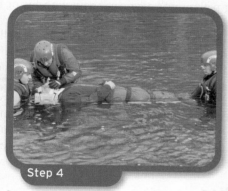

Step 4

Secure the patient to the longboard.

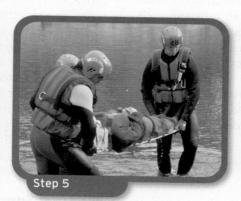

Step 5

Remove the patient from the water.

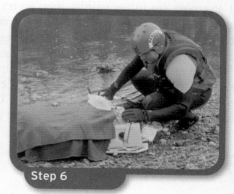

Step 6

Cover the patient with a blanket and apply oxygen if breathing. Begin CPR if breathing is still absent.

When you participate in SAR missions, prepare for the weather conditions by bringing suitable clothing. Make sure that you don't exceed your physical limitations, and don't get into situations that are beyond your ability. Request specialist assistance from mountain, moorland, cliff, cave, coastguard, or marine rescue teams in your area.

Using a Rescue Stretcher

Rescue stretchers facilitate moving patients to a place of safety and can be used in a variety of situations. The manner in which a patient is packaged in a rescue stretcher depends on his or her medical condition, the environment, and the manner in which the patient will be evacuated. Rescue stretchers can be lifted by rope, carried by vehicles, or, most commonly, hand-carried by rescuers. In case of vertical evacuation, pack excess padding around the patient to prevent undue movement. While handling the patient, be sure to communicate and keep him or her apprised of the situation and your progress.

The standard rescue stretcher carry involves a team of six to eight rescuers distributed around the rescue stretcher, three or four to a side. Normally, the person at the front of the left side is in charge and directs the activities of the others. This method has the advantages of being fast, as little teamwork is required, and it usually gives the patient a comfortable ride. Its disadvantages include the fact that this carrying method is very tiring for the rescuers, because it puts constant strain on certain muscles, and ground vision is difficult, especially at night; a rescuer can easily trip over a rock and drop the rescue stretcher.

More than one team will be needed if the rescue stretcher must be carried over a distance further than the team can cover in about 15 to 20 minutes. Team *leapfrogging* is a good method to use on long evacuations, ie, one team takes the rescue stretcher for a given distance while the other team goes ahead to rest and preplan the next stretch. At the handover point, the first team advances to the next point for rest and planning.

When footing is highly unstable, and obstacles prevent the rescue stretcher team from progressing, or falling becomes a possible hazard, the caterpillar or lap pass is a useful option. When the rescue stretcher reaches the obstacle, the team pauses while every extra person lines up on the route ahead of the difficult terrain or obstacles. The rescuers form two lines facing each other about the width of the rescue stretcher apart and alternate (in other words, they aren't all opposite each other). They usually sit down and try to make themselves as stable as possible. When everyone is set, rescuers pass the rescue stretcher down between the two lines. As the rescue stretcher passes a person, he or she gets up and carefully but quickly moves around the line in the direction of travel, and gets set to pass the rescue stretcher again. Done correctly, this technique provides a very stable and secure passage.

Patient Care

Many medical and trauma conditions can and will be assessed during the rescue process. In confined-space rescues, especially with cave-ins and trench rescues, paramedics need to consider the potential for crush injuries—in particular, the possibility of compartment syndrome. When human tissue goes without an adequate supply of oxygen-enriched blood, tissue (cells) continues to metabolise (produce energy) without oxygen (anaerobic metabolism), producing lactic acid as a byproduct. When entrapped or compressed areas of the body are eventually reperfused, these metabolic byproducts are released into the circulation. Treatment with high-flow oxygen therapy and aggressive IV fluid resuscitation can help to reverse the effects of respiratory and metabolic acidosis.

Pain Management

Patients involved in many rescue situations will be experiencing pain from injuries received during the incident. Pain control should take the form of nonpharmacological methods such as splinting to minimise movement, gentle handling, or talking with patients to create a distraction during assessment and movement. Ambulance clinicians must also keep patients warm, as a shivering patient will aggravate pain with his or her every movement.

Pharmacological pain management by paramedics is limited. Careful consideration must be given to early medical advice or assistance if the paramedic feels that the current medications are either inappropriate or insufficient. **Table 49-1 ▶** lists some of the medications that can be considered in the pain management of patients during rescue efforts. Because most analgesics have the potential to induce nausea and vomiting, all medications must be administered slowly and use of antiemetics should be considered.

Medical Supplies

Table 49-2 ▶ lists the basic medical supplies that you should carry in an off-road medical pack.

You are the Paramedic Part 5

The fire service has been on scene for 45 minutes and just finished securing the cab of the lorry. They are now ready to begin the process of removing the dashboard. Ear defenders are provided for both you and the patient to protect your hearing from the hydraulic tools that will be used to remove the dashboard. A blanket is placed over the two of you to prevent injury from debris. The helicopter crew is waiting, ready to assist in extrication and packaging.

Prior to the start of the dashboard removal, you were able to increase the patient's blood pressure to 114/66 mm Hg. Your main concerns are keeping him calm and being prepared for the inevitable decline in his condition once the dashboard is lifted off of his pelvis. As anticipated, once the pressure of the dashboard is relieved from your patient's pelvis, he becomes pale and loses consciousness. One of the helicopter crew is able to palpate a weak carotid pulse. The patient is quickly extricated onto a longboard, secured, and taken to the helicopter. He is immediately intubated, placed on a transport ventilator, and has a second large-bore IV line placed.

Upon arrival at the A&E department, the patient is found to have a shattered pelvis, bilateral femur fractures, and a small subdural haematoma. He is stabilised and subsequently admitted to the trauma intensive care unit for further evaluation and treatment.

Table 49-1 | Medications for Pain Management in Rescue Situations

Medication	Characteristics
Morphine sulphate	Opioid analgesic and central nervous system depressant often used in the treatment of myocardial infarction, kidney stones, and pulmonary oedema. It is contraindicated in patients who are profoundly hypovolaemic or suffering from severe hypotension.
Entonox	This central nervous system depressant with analgesic properties is used for musculoskeletal pain, fractures, and burns. It should not be used in patients who can't follow verbal instructions, those with head injuries, COPD patients, and patients with thoracic injuries or possible pneumothorax. Use caution in environments less than −6°C, which could cause the component gases in Entonox to separate.
Fentanyl citrate	Unrelated to morphine but with similar analgesic effects, it is considered 50 to 100 times more potent than morphine; however, its duration of action is much shorter. It can be used for the management of severe pain, but is contraindicated with severe haemorrhage, shock, or known hypersensitivity.
Nalbuphine	Synthetic analgesic with the same effects as morphine. Nalbuphine has the haemodynamic effects of morphine and is used in patients with moderate to severe pain.

Table 49-2 | Supplies for an Off-Road Medical Pack

- Vinyl or latex gloves
- Face masks
- Hand sanitiser
- Mouth-to-mask resuscitation device
- 1 triangular bandage
- Universal trauma dressings
- 10 cm × 10 cm and 12.5 cm × 22.5 cm sterile dressings
- Roller gauze bandage
- Gauze-adhesive strips
- Occlusive dressing for sealing chest wounds
- Adhesive tape
- Blankets
- Cold packs
- Alcohol wipes
- 50-ml or larger syringe for irrigation of wounds
- 2 glucose or energy gel packets
- Heat packs
- Abdominal dressing
- Survival blankets
- Scissors
- Irrigation fluid or wound cleansing soap
- Goggles
- SAM splint
- Steri-strips
- Cervical collars
- Blood pressure cuff
- Immobilisation straps
- Pocket torch
- Batteries

Patient Packaging

A number of special patient packaging tools are available to help you extricate patients out of their situation and up, down, or out to your ambulance. The Stokes basket, for example, is a rigid framed structure into which the patient is placed and then secured. It comes in two general types. The most common is the wire Stokes basket, which consists of a rigid metal (aluminium, steel, or titanium) frame and ribs with a chicken-wire mesh attached to the frame. The other style is the plastic or fibreglass Stokes basket, which consists of a steel or aluminium frame with a rigid plastic or fibreglass basket. Both types of Stokes baskets are available as one- or two-piece units that can be latched or joined together for easier packing into the rescue scene.

You are the Paramedic Summary

1. What are your initial thoughts about the specialised help you are going to require for this specific incident?

It is quite clear that this patient is trapped, not only in wreckage, but HGV wreckage. The potential equipment needed to release him may not be carried on all "first-away" fire appliances. The length of journey to hospital may necessitate transport by air, thus the earlier the call for air support, the swifter the response.

2. Identify the ten steps of a special rescue sequence.

The ten steps of a special rescue sequence are as follows: (1) preparation, (2) response, (3) arrival and assessment, (4) stabilisation, (5) access, (6) disentanglement, (7) removal, (8) transport, (9) security of the scene and preparation for the next call, and (10) post-incident analysis.

3. Why is it important to maintain good communication with the patient during a special rescue incident?

Patients need to know that you are there and that everything possible is being done to remove them from the situation and provide the necessary care. In our case, communication is easily maintained because you are able to be in the vehicle with the patient. This is not possible in all special rescue incidents. It is not uncommon for the patient or patients to remain alone for several hours while the scene is made safe and access can be made. This is a traumatic time for the patient. A reassuring voice can go a long way to helping keep the patient calm and maintain his or her level of confidence.

4. What is the patient at risk of experiencing as a result of being pinned underneath the dashboard from the pelvis down?

The patient is at risk for experiencing crush syndrome. While his inability to feel his legs may be the result of a spinal cord injury, lack of perfusion can also produce loss of sensation to the areas distal to the source of obstruction, which in this case is the dashboard.

5. What needs to be monitored on this patient?

In a word, SHOCK! Currently he is compensating for the injuries we suspect; at the very minimum you can suspect an abdominal bleed and fractured pelvis. There is no way of knowing how long his body can compensate for the blood loss. Also keep in mind that the dashboard is acting as a tourniquet. You need to anticipate that once the dashboard is removed from the pelvis and blood flow is restored to the lower extremities, the blood pressure is going to change significantly.

6. Why is it important to be cautious when administering strong opioids to release the patient's pain?

It is not hard to imagine that the patient is experiencing a significant amount of pain, but administering drugs such as morphine in large dosages can do a lot more than relieve pain. Although opioids relieve pain they can also mask the presence of injuries, making them difficult to identify or monitor for changes. One of the side effects of opioids is nausea and vomiting. While you can administer an anti-emetic, such as metoclopramide with the opioid, it is not wise to tempt fate with an unprotected airway and risk aspiration. Finally, opioids can decrease the patient's blood pressure. In cases of shock, you need to maintain a perfusing blood pressure as long as possible.

Prep Kit

Ready for Review

- "Rescue" means to deliver from danger or imprisonment.
- The most difficult process in any rescue is neither the rescue or the treatment process, but rather the coordination and balance of both.
- A technical rescue incident (TRI) is a complex rescue incident involving vehicles, water, trench collapse, confined spaces, or wilderness search and rescue that requires specially trained personnel and special equipment.
- Technical rescue training occurs on three levels: awareness, operations, and technician. Most of the training and education ambulance personnel receive is aimed at the awareness level, enabling them to identify the hazards and secure the scene to prevent additional people from becoming patients.
- When assisting rescue team members, the following guidelines will prove useful:
  – Be safe.
  – Work as a team.
  – Think.
  – Follow the golden rule of public service.
- Although special rescue situations may take many different forms, all rescuers should follow ten steps to perform these rescues in a safe, effective, and efficient manner:
  – Preparation
  – Response
  – Arrival and assessment
  – Stabilisation
  – Access
  – Disentanglement
  – Removal
  – Transport
  – Security of the scene and preparation for the next call
  – Postincident analysis
- At a TRI, it is critically important to slow down and properly evaluate the situation. Consider the potential general hazards and risks of utilities, confined spaces, and environmental conditions, as well as hazards that are immediately dangerous to life or health (IDLH).
- The first arriving officer at a rescue scene should immediately assume command and starts using the integrated emergency management system (IEMS). This step is critically important because many TRIs will eventually become very complex and require a large number of assisting units.
- Whenever possible, park emergency vehicles in a manner that will ensure safety and not disrupt traffic any more than necessary. Traffic flow is the largest single hazard associated with any operation that takes place on a motorway.
- A confined space is a location surrounded by a structure that isn't designed for continuous occupancy. Confined spaces have limited openings for entrance and exit.
- Confined spaces present a special hazard because they may have limited ventilation to provide for air circulation and exchange, which can make them an oxygen-deficient atmosphere, or they may contain poisonous gases.
- Trench rescues may become necessary when earth is removed for placement of a utility line or for other construction and the sides of the excavation collapse, trapping a worker.
- Wilderness search and rescue (SAR) missions consist of two parts: search (looking for a lost or overdue person) and rescue (removing a patient from a hostile environment).
- Rescue stretchers facilitate moving patients to a place of safety and can be used in a variety of situations. The manner in which a patient is packaged in a rescue stretcher depends on his or her medical condition, the environment, and the manner in which the patient will be evacuated.

- Pain control in rescue situations should take the form of nonpharmacological methods such as splinting to minimise movement, and gentle handling in association with cautious pharmacological administration.
- A number of special patient packaging tools are available to help extricate patients out of their situation and up, down, or out to the ambulance. The Stokes basket is an example of a packaging tool.

Vital Vocabulary

awareness The first level of rescue training provided to all responders, with an emphasis on recognising the hazards, securing the scene, and calling for appropriate assistance. There is no actual use of rescue skills.

chocking Short lengths of wood that are used to stabilise vehicles.

cold protective response Phenomenon associated with cold water immersion in which reflexes in the body and a lowered metabolic rate help preserve basic body functions.

cold zone A safe area for those agencies involved in the operations; the ambulance commander (AC), command post, emergency services personnel, and other support functions necessary to control the incident should be located in the cold zone.

confined space A space with limited or restricted access that is not meant for continuous occupancy, such as a manhole, well, or tank.

entrapment A situation in which a patient is trapped by debris, soil, or other material and is unable to extricate himself or herself.

hot zone The area immediately surrounding an incident site that is directly dangerous to life or health. All personnel working in the hot zone must wear complete and appropriate protective clothing and equipment. Entry requires approval by the AC or a designated sector officer. Complete backup, rescue, and decontamination teams must be in place before operations begin.

immediately dangerous to life or health (IDLH) An atmospheric concentration of any toxic, corrosive, or asphyxiant substance that poses an immediate threat to life or could cause irreversible or delayed adverse health effects. There are three general IDLH atmospheres: toxic, flammable, and oxygen-deficient.

laminated windscreen glass Type of window glazing that incorporates a sheeting material that stops the glass from breaking into shards.

operations The technical rescue training level required to work in the warm zone of an incident. Training at this level allows responders to provide direct assistance to those conducting the rescue operation and to use certain rescue skills and procedures.

personal flotation device (PFD) Also commonly known as a life jacket, a PFD allows the body to float in water.

search and rescue (SAR) The process of locating and removing a patient from the wilderness.

secondary collapse A collapse that occurs following the primary collapse. This can occur in trench, excavation, and structural collapses.

self-rescue position Position used in fast-flowing water rescue situations. The rescuer rolls into a face-up arched position with the lower back higher than the feet to avoid objects below the surface. The feet should be together and facing in the direction of travel (feet first), with arms at the sides.

shoring A method of supporting a trench wall or building components such as walls, floors, or ceilings using either hydraulic, pneumatic, or wood shoring systems. Shoring is used to prevent collapse.

spoil pile The pile of earth that has been removed from an excavation. The pile may be unstable and prone to collapse.

step blocks Specialised chocking assemblies made out of wood or plastic blocks in a step configuration.

technical rescue incident (TRI) A complex rescue incident involving vehicles or machinery, water or ice, rope techniques, a trench or excavation collapse, confined spaces, a structural collapse, wilderness search and rescue, or hazardous materials, and which requires specially trained personnel and special equipment.

technical rescue team A group of rescuers specially trained in the various disciplines of technical rescue.

technician The training degree that provides a high level of competency in the various disciplines of technical or hazardous materials

rescue for rescuers who will be directly involved in the rescue operation itself.

tempered glass A type of safety glass that is heat-treated so that it will break into small pieces.

warm zone The area located between the hot zone and the cold zone at an incident. Decontamination stations are located in the warm zone.

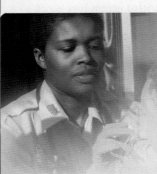

Assessment in Action

You are dispatched to the scene of a road traffic collision. Upon your arrival, you find a single-car collision involving one patient. You immediately notice parts of the vehicle that lie approximately 30 cm away from the vehicle body. You safely and cautiously approach the vehicle, performing your mental scene assessment. The patient is heavily trapped in the driver's seat of the vehicle. The fire service is preparing their jaws of life and other rescue equipment to extricate the patient from the vehicle. You notice the patient is gurgling and unconscious; you ask the ambulance commander approximately how long the extrication will take. They inform you that it will be at least 20 minutes due to the type of entrapment.

1. **At which three levels is training in technical rescue areas conducted?**
   A. Awareness, operations, training
   B. Awareness, technician, basic
   C. Awareness, operations, technician
   D. Awareness, basic level, advanced level

2. **Most of the training and education ambulance personnel receive is aimed at the _____ level.**
   A. basic
   B. operations
   C. technician
   D. awareness

3. **In a road traffic collision, what is the most important thing to remember?**
   A. The vehicle is to be removed from around the patient rather than trying to remove the patient through the wreckage.
   B. The patient is to be removed through the wreckage rather than trying to remove the vehicle from around the patient.
   C. You need to remove the patient immediately without any securing of the vehicle or scene assessment.
   D. Allow the family of the patient to climb into the car and be with the patient to calm him or her.

4. **The fire commander informs you that the vehicle's A post has been crushed onto the patient's upper torso. You understand the A post to be:**
   A. between the front and rear doors of a vehicle.
   B. between the rear doors of the vehicle and the boot.

   C. near the front bumper.
   D. closest to the front of the vehicle—it forms the sides of the windscreen.

5. **You notice that the vehicle remains unstable and could pose a threat to the rescuers. What type of objects can be used to help support this vehicle?**
   A. Chocking or step blocks
   B. Cutting the battery cable
   C. Deflating the tyres
   D. Removing the key from the ignition

6. **The next step after the extrication is completed is to:**
   A. perform patient care.
   B. disentangle the patient.
   C. displace the seat.
   D. remove the windscreen.

Challenging Question

You are sent to the scene of a 25-year-old man who fell into a lake. The patient had been drinking alcohol heavily throughout the course of the day. The water is extremely cold, and the patient begins to panic.

7. **What should you do?**

www.Paramedic.EMSzone.com/UK/

Points to Ponder

Towards the end of your shift, you're sent to a residential area for a construction worker who fell into a hole. When you arrive on scene, you find a 30-year-old man lying in a prone position at the bottom of a hole, which is about 3 m deep and 3 m wide. The fire service is shoring up the hole to allow you access to the patient.

You are told by his foremen that the patient was climbing up a ladder while carrying a bucket; he slipped on the ladder and fell. His foreman tells you that the patient was not responsive initially and stayed that way for approximately 2 minutes. The patient is verbally responsive now, and complains of back and head pain.

What PPE should you don? What is your plan of action?

Issues: Understanding What Your Needs Are at the Scene of a Technical Rescue Incident; Knowing What Information You Should Have at Initial Dispatch, En Route, and Arriving on Scene; Understanding the Importance of Scene Assessment.

Objectives

Cognitive

- Explain the role of the paramedic/ambulance service responder in terms of the following:
  - Incident assessment
  - Assessment of toxicologic risk
  - Appropriate decontamination methods
  - Treatment of semi-decontaminated patients
  - Transportation of semi-decontaminated patients
- Assess a hazardous materials incident and determine the following:
  - Potential hazards to the rescuers, public and environment
  - Potential risk of primary contamination to patients
  - Potential risk of secondary contamination to rescuers
- Identify resources for substance identification, decontamination and treatment information including the following:
  - National Poisons Information Service (NPIS) centre
  - Ambulance control
  - Control of Substances Hazardous to Health (COSHH) and Hazchem data sheets
  - Reference textbooks
  - Computer databases (CHEMDATA)
  - CHEMSAFE
  - Technical specialists
  - Agency for toxic substances and disease registry
- Explain the following terms/concepts:
  - Primary contamination risk
  - Secondary contamination risk
- List and describe the following routes of exposure:
  - Topical
  - Respiratory
  - Gastrointestinal
  - Parenteral
- Explain the following toxicological principles:
  - Acute and delayed toxicity
  - Route of exposure
  - Local versus systemic effects
  - Dose response
  - Synergistic effects
- Explain how the substance and route of contamination alters triage and decontamination methods.
- Explain the limitations of prehospital environment decontamination procedures.
- List and explain the common signs, symptoms, and treatment for the following substances:
  - Corrosives (acids/alkalis)
  - Pulmonary irritants (ammonia/chlorine)
  - Pesticides (carbamates/organophosphates)
  - Chemical asphyxiants (cyanide/carbon monoxide)
  - Hydrocarbon solvents (xylene, methylene chloride)
- Explain the potential risk associated with invasive procedures performed on contaminated patients.
- Given a contaminated patient determine the level of decontamination necessary and:
  - Level of rescuer personal protective equipment (PPE)
  - Decontamination methods
  - Treatment
  - Transportation and patient isolation techniques
- Identify local facilities and resources capable of treating patients exposed to hazardous materials.
- Determine the hazards present to the patient and paramedic given an incident involving hazardous materials.
- Define the following and explain their importance to the risk assessment process:
  - Boiling point
  - Flammable/explosive limits
  - Flash point
  - Ignition temperature
  - Specific gravity
  - Vapour density
  - Vapour pressure
  - Water solubility
  - Alpha radiation
  - Beta radiation
  - Gamma radiation
- Define the toxicological terms and their use in the risk assessment process:
  - Threshold limit value (TLV)
  - Lethal concentration and doses (LD)
  - Parts per million/thousand million (ppm/pptm)
  - Immediately dangerous to life or health (IDLH)
  - Permissible exposure limit (PEL)
  - Threshold limit value, short term exposure limit (TLV-STEL)
  - Threshold limit value, ceiling level (TLV-C)

- Given a specific hazardous material be able to do the following:
  - Research the appropriate information about its physical and chemical characteristics and hazards
  - Suggest the appropriate medical response
  - Determine risk of secondary contamination
- Determine the factors which determine where and when to treat a patient to include:
  - Substance toxicity
  - Patient condition
  - Availability of decontamination
- Explain specific decontamination procedures.
- Explain the four most common decontamination solutions used to include:
  - Water
  - Water and tincture of green soap
  - Isopropyl alcohol
  - Vegetable oil
- Identify the areas of the body difficult to decontaminate to include:
  - Scalp/hair
  - Ears/ear canals/nostrils
  - Axillae
  - Finger nails
  - Navel
  - Groin/buttocks/genitalia
  - Popliteal fossa
  - Web spaces between toes and toe nails
- Explain the requirements of medical monitoring for hazardous material team members both pre- and post-exposure to a hazardous material scene, including:
  - Vital signs
  - Body weight
  - General health
  - Neurological status
  - ECG

- Explain the factors that influence the heat stress on hazardous material team members including:
  - Hydration
  - Physical fitness
  - Ambient temperature
  - Activity
  - Level of PPE
  - Duration of activity
- Explain the documentation necessary for medical monitoring and rehabilitation operations.
  - The substance
  - The toxicity and danger of secondary contamination
  - Appropriate PPE and suit breakthrough time
  - Appropriate level of decontamination
  - Appropriate antidote and medical treatment
  - Transportation method
- Given a simulated hazardous substance, use reference material to determine the appropriate actions.
- Integrate the principles and practices of hazardous materials response in an effective manner to prevent and limit contamination, morbidity, and mortality.

Affective

None

Psychomotor

None

Introduction

One of the inevitable consequences of living in an industrialised world is the proliferation of hazardous materials. The products of our civilisation require the manufacture, transport, storage, use, and disposal of thousands of potentially toxic substances. Each year in the United Kingdom there are many incidents involving hazardous materials that result in injury and death.

This chapter will take a broad look at some of the special considerations involved in responding to incidents that may involve hazardous materials. It is not intended to be a comprehensive coverage of hazardous materials. The general rule for ambulance service personnel responding to industrial, highway, and many other types of incidents is to maintain a high index of suspicion and to stay away from the hazardous materials at the incident.

Paramedics and Hazardous Materials Incidents

Paramedics must be able to identify potential hazardous materials at a scene and determine how to manage the incident during the initial phase if they are the first to arrive at the incident. Early recognition will aid a coordinated and multidisciplinary response including the attendance of specialist hazardous material (HazMat) teams to manage the contaminated areas, in support of National Health Service (NHS) Special Operations Response Teams (SORT) who will assist in the casualty decontamination process. Although these teams will manage the contaminated areas, paramedics must understand how the entire scene should be organised, as well as their specific role of providing emergency care. It is also advantageous to know the principles of personal protective equipment (PPE) used at a hazardous materials scene; how the HazMat team and SORT personnel will decontaminate patients; and what immediate actions should be taken and how exposures should be treated. Sources such as the National Poisons Information Service (NPIS) and ambulance control can assist with such complex clinical management decisions. Paramedics may also be required to monitor the physical effects encountered by the specialist teams deployed at the scene.

Hazardous materials incidents may include:

- A lorry or train crash in which a substance is leaking from a tank or rail container
- A leak, fire, or other emergency at an industrial plant, refinery, or other complex where chemicals or explosives are produced, used, or stored
- A leak or rupture of an underground natural gas pipe
- Deterioration of underground fuel tanks and seepage of oil or petrol into the surrounding ground
- Buildup of methane or other by-products of waste decomposition in sewers or sewage processing plants
- A road traffic collision in which a petrol tank has ruptured

Often, the presence of hazardous materials is easily recognised from warning signs, placards, or labels found in the following locations:

- On buildings or in areas where hazardous materials are produced, used, or stored
- On lorries and railway carriages that carry any hazardous material
- On barrels or boxes that contain hazardous material

You are the Paramedic Part 1

You are responding to a chemical spill at a manufacturing plant. Ambulance control reports that there is one patient who has been removed from the structure by a fire service HazMat team. When you arrive at the scene, you report to the fire commander who advises you that cordons have been established and the patient is just entering from the cold zone from the decontamination corridor. The patient is conscious, well orientated, and answering all questions appropriately, although she is in pain. The fire commander reports that a forklift inside the building collided with some shelving, causing it to fall. The shelving stored several different chemicals and you are handed a number of Hazchem data sheets that were provided by the manufacturing facility.

Among the chemicals you notice a variety of acids (including 70% hydrofluoric, 10% sulphuric, and 20% acetic acid), 50% sodium hydroxide, a solvent, and methylene chloride. The patient was the driver of the forklift. She is a 35-year-old woman who is conscious and experiencing minor pain. Fire personnel on-scene are currently providing supportive high-flow supplemental oxygen at 15 l/min through a nonrebreathing mask.

Initial Assessment	Recording Time: 0 Minutes
Appearance	Entering the "cold zone" by fire personnel on-scene
Level of consciousness	A (Alert to person, place, and day)
Airway	Patent
Breathing	Hyperventilating at a rate of 36 breaths/min
Circulation	Flushed skin

1. What is a hazardous material?
2. What is your role during an incident such as this?
3. How would you manage this patient?

Specialised Team Medical Monitoring Worksheet

Date:_____ Entry Person:_____

Incident #_____ Medical Monitor:_____

Important: Specialised team members shall not be allowed to don PPE if any of the following conditions are present: systolic BP < 100 or > 160, diastolic BP > 100, pulse rate > 120, oral temperature > 37°C, Respirations > 24. Medical monitors must read and be familiar with the "Medical Monitoring Guidelines" before beginning medical evaluations.

Pre-entry Evaluation
Before donning PPE, take and record baseline vital signs.

Time_____ BP_____ Pulse Rate_____ Resp._____ Oral Temp._____°C

Post-entry Evaluation
Immediately after doffing PPE, take vital signs and assess for hyperthermia.

Time_____ BP_____ Pulse Rate_____ Resp._____ Oral Temp._____°C

Re-entry Evaluation
Before redonning PPE, take vital signs and reassess for hyperthermia.
Entry person must remain in rehab for a minimum of 30 minutes between entries.

Time_____ BP_____ Pulse Rate_____ Resp._____ Oral Temp._____°C

Exposure Suspected?
Immediately contact Specialised Team Leader
and see "Exposure Guidelines."

Figure 50-2 Sample rehabilitation log.

You are the Paramedic Summary

1. What is a hazardous material?

There are many different definitions used, but in essence, any substance that causes or may cause adverse effects on the health or safety of employees, the general public, or the environment; any biological agent and other disease-causing agent, or a waste or combination of wastes may be construed as being a hazardous material.

2. What is your role during an incident such as this?

The role of paramedics is to first keep from being exposed or injured. Then a scene assessment is performed to assess for risks of primary or secondary contamination of the patient and the responding staff, determine the need for additional resources, and decide what safety parameters must be immediately established. Depending on the role your Ambulance Trust plays in local hazardous materials response plans and the level of training provided, you may also assess the level of decontamination, treatment, and transportation considerations.

3. How would you manage this patient?

Don the appropriate level PPE for the specific type of substance exposure. Then an initial assessment can be performed. If able to walk, the patient should be instructed to remove all clothing and move to a predetermined decontamination centre. In most Ambulance Trust areas, SORT teams are able to wash and rinse the patient for you.

4. Evaluating the symptoms presented by this patient, what do you expect to be the primary offending chemical?

Hydrofluoric as well as sulphuric acids.

5. You have confirmed your diagnosis. Now how would you treat the patient? What supportive care would you use (include any drugs and dosages)?

- **Hydrofluoric acid.** Once the affected areas are decontaminated, the burned areas should be covered with calcium gluconate gel. If calcium gluconate is not available, Epsom salt (magnesium sulphate), magnesium-containing antacids such as Tums can be used as a topical agent. This will all have to be actioned in line with local guidelines and/or medical advice. In the case of hydrofluoric acid burns, pain is an excellent indicator that the injury is continuing. If pain continues after calcium gluconate gel is applied, then calcium gluconate infiltration is needed.
- **Cardiac symptoms of hypocalcaemia.** Provide continuous monitoring of the ECG, watching for prolongation of the Q-T interval. Muscle contractions or cardiac arrest will need to be treated, ideally by an incident doctor.

6. What information about hazardous materials medical monitoring and rehabilitation operation must be documented?

The type of substance involved, its toxicity, and the danger of secondary contamination must be documented. Additional information to record includes appropriate PPE and suit breakthrough time, appropriate antidotes, medical treatment, and transportation method.

Prep Kit

■ Ready for Review

- Handling hazardous materials emergencies requires specialised extra training and equipment.
- Ambulance clinicians should only enter a hazardous materials scene if they are appropriately trained and have the correct level of PPE necessary.
- The great majority of hazardous materials emergencies are transportation incidents.
- When you are approaching transport incidents, especially those involving commercial vehicles, you should be alert for signs of hazardous materials.
- Signs of hazardous materials include vapour clouds, strange odours, spilled liquids, and multiple victims.
- Hazardous material incidents have hot, warm, and cold zones.
- Sources of information about hazardous materials include placards, transport documents, and COSHH and Hazchem data sheets.
- Primary hazardous materials contamination comes from direct contact with the toxin.
- Secondary contamination is spread by people (patients or ambulance clinicians), clothing, or objects.
- Effects from hazardous materials exposure may be local on the body or systemic.
- Routes of exposure include dermal, respiratory, parenteral, and gastrointestinal.
- Rescue and decontamination of victims is secondary to rescuer and public protection.
- Treatment of hazardous materials victims is usually symptomatic and supportive of the ABCs.
- Invasive procedures should be minimised to avoid the risk of introducing contamination.
- Paramedics may be directed to support a hazardous materials operation with medical monitoring of the HazMat teams or SORT personnel.

■ Vital Vocabulary

absorption A type of decontamination that is done with large pads that the hazardous materials team carry to soak up liquid and remove it from the patient.

asphyxiant Any gas that displaces oxygen from the atmosphere; can be deadly if exposure occurs in a confined space.

carbon monoxide A chemical asphyxiant that results in a cellular respiratory failure; this gas has roughly a 240 times greater affinity for haemoglobin than oxygen, which leads to oxygen becoming inaccessible at cellular level.

chemical asphyxiants Substances that interfere with the utilisation of oxygen at the cellular level.

CHEMSAFE An organisation that provides expert advice and information in the event of chemical incidents. It can be contacted via ambulance control.

cold zone The outermost zone of management at a hazardous materials scene; the area where paramedics typically first encounter the patient.

corrosives A class of chemicals with either high or low Ph levels. Exposure can cause severe soft-tissue damage.

cyanide A chemical asphyxiant used in many industrial processes; exposure can occur from by-products of combustion and fires.

decontamination The process of removing hazardous materials from the body or clothing of victims or rescuers. Includes the methods of dilution, absorption, disposal, and (in rare cases only) neutralisation.

dermal exposure Skin exposure, also known as topical exposure. Some hazardous materials may be absorbed through the skin to produce a systemic effect.

dilution A type of decontamination method that uses copious amounts of water to irrigate the contaminant from the skin or eyes.

disposal A type of decontamination in which as much clothing and equipment as possible is disposed of to reduce the magnitude of the problem.

dose effect The principle that the longer a hazardous material is in contact with the body or the greater the concentration, the greater the effect will probably be.

flash point The temperature at which a vapour can be ignited by a spark.

gastrointestinal exposure Exposure to a hazardous material through intentional or unintentional ingestion of the substance.

hazardous material Any substance that is toxic, poisonous, radioactive, flammable, or explosive and causes injury or death with exposure.

hot zone The central area of a hazardous materials scene and the location of the greatest hazard.

ignition temperature The temperature at which a vapour will burst into sustained burning.

immediately dangerous to life or health (IDLH) A phrase that means the atmospheric concentration of any toxic, corrosive, or asphyxiant substance will pose an immediate threat to life, irreversible or delayed adverse effects, or serious interference for a team member attempting to escape from the dangerous atmosphere; a respirator is mandatory.

lethal dose (LD) Amount of a hazardous substance sure to cause death.

local effect An effect of a hazardous material on the body that is limited to the area of contact.

lower explosive limit (LEL) The concentration of the hazardous material that can burn or explode in the air when it mixes with air.

medical monitoring The process of assessing the health status of specialised team members before and after entry to a hazardous materials incident site.

neutralisation A type of decontamination that uses one chemical to change the hazardous material into two less harmful substances; rarely used by specialised teams.

parenteral exposure Entry of a hazardous material into the bloodstream, either through force of injection or through an open wound.

permissible exposure limit (PEL) The maximum concentration of a chemical that a person may be exposed to under Health and Safety Commission regulations.

ppb Parts per billion; an expression of concentration.

ppm Parts per million; an expression of concentration.

primary contamination An exposure that occurs with direct contact with the hazardous material.

respiratory exposure Exposure of the airways and lungs to a gas or vapour.

secondary contamination Exposure to a hazardous material by contact with a contaminated person or object.

SLUDGE An mnemonic that stands for Salivation, Lacrimation, Urination, Defecation, Gastrointestinal activity, and Emesis, which are the signs and symptoms that can be produced by exposure to organophosphate and carbamate pesticides or other nerve-stimulating agents.

specific gravity The measure that indicates whether or not a hazardous material will sink or float in water.

synergistic effect When two substances interact to produce an overall greater effect than either alone or combined.

systemic effect A physiological effect on the entire body or one of the body's systems.

Transport Emergency Card (TREMCARD) A document that is legally required to be carried by drivers of commercial vehicles that should provide specific information about what is carried on the vehicle.

threshold limit value (TLV) The concentration of a substance that is supposed to be safe for exposure no more than 8 hours per day and 40 hours per week.

threshold limit value ceiling exposure limit (TLV-C) The concentration that a person should never be exposed to.

threshold limit value short-term exposure limit (TLV-STEL) The concentration of a substance that a worker can be exposed to for up to 15 minutes but no more than four times per day with at least an hour between each exposure.

TOXBASE An NHS information source for poisons.

toxicity levels Measures of the risk that a hazardous material poses to the health of an individual who comes into contact with it.

upper explosive limit (UEL) The concentration of a hazardous material at which there is not enough oxygen to support the combustion in air.

vapour density A measure that compares the hazardous material gas to air; toxic gases that are heavier than air will sink, while vapours that are lighter than air will dissipate and travel with the wind.

vapour pressure The pressure exerted by a vapour when the liquid and vapour states of a material are in equilibrium; this measure changes as a material is heated.

warm zone The division of the hazardous materials scene that surrounds the hot zone and is inside the cold zone.

water reactive A property that indicates that a material will undergo a chemical reaction (for example, explosion) when mixed with water.

water soluble A property that indicates that a material can be dissolved in water.

Assessment in Action

You are sent to an overturned tanker on a busy motorway. When you arrive, you notice the truck is leaking something. You're not sure what it is. You immediately call for additional resources.

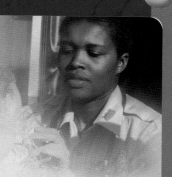

1. **On arrival, you see a placard with white and red stripes. This truck is most likely carrying:**
   A. oxidizers.
   B. flammable liquids.
   C. flammable solids.
   D. explosives.

2. **The standard rule of thumb for hazardous materials scene assessment is:**
   A. if the entire scene cannot be covered by your thumb held out at arm's length, then you are too close.
   B. approach to possible hazardous materials incident should include stopping at a distance away.
   C. the identification of the hazardous material on scene.
   D. preparing the paramedic for the possible health risks.

3. **You should stay _____ from any hazardous material scene.**
   A. uphill and upwind
   B. downhill and downwind
   C. uphill and downwind
   D. upwind and downhill

4. **The measure of health risk that a substance poses to someone who comes into contact with it is called the:**
   A. health hazard.
   B. bill of lading.
   C. toxicity level.
   D. primary contamination.

Challenging Questions

You are sent to a warehouse for three patients who are complaining of nausea, vomiting, diarrhoea, and sweating. When you arrive on scene, you find the patients located outside on a bench. During your assessment, you note that the patients are also hypotensive and have constricted pupils. You begin to ask questions and you find out that this warehouse manufactures pesticides.

5. **What should you immediately suspect?**

6. **What treatment should you provide for these patients?**

Points to Ponder

You are sent to an explosion at a block of flats. While you en route, you see red balls of flames high in the air in the distance. When you arrive, several fire appliances are already on scene. They are keeping you at a parking area until they figure out what happened and if any hazardous materials were involved.

What can you do while waiting for clearance? Once you enter the scene, what precautions should you take?

Issues: Understanding What to Do at a Hazardous Materials Incident.

www.Paramedic.EMSzone.com/UK/

Objectives

Cognitive

- Describe warning signs of potentially violent situations.
- Explain ambulance service considerations for the following types of violent or potentially violent situations:
  - Hostage situations
  - Clandestine drug laboratories
  - Domestic violence
  - Emotionally disturbed people
- Describe police evidence considerations and techniques to assist in evidence preservation.

Affective

None

Psychomotor

None

Introduction

Thousands of times each year, paramedics face potentially violent situations. With any call, you may find yourself in the middle of a physical domestic argument when responding to an injured patient **Figure 51-1 ▼** . As you read the many cautions in this textbook about questionable scenes, remember that ambulance staff in various parts of the world have been severely injured or killed in violent incidents while attempting to reach and treat sick and injured people.

As an educated and effective health care provider, you need to know how to avoid violence when possible and how to protect yourself when violence erupts. Because all emergency services respond to potentially life-threatening situations daily, you should make time for any self-protection course that you can. Sound conflict resolution training will help you identify potentially dangerous situations. Once you recognise a violent situation, you will be able to retreat to a safe location and await the assistance of police. *Your main mission is to return home safely at the end of each shift.*

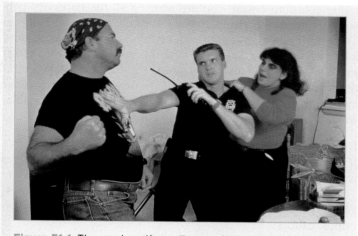

Figure 51-1 The most routine call can quickly turn violent.

Awareness

Some trainee ambulance staff are surprised to hear how serious and widespread attacks against ambulance clinicians have become. Violence is not only an urban event; a call in a rural area can be just as deadly as a call in a large city. In many rural areas, paramedics may arrive at the scene of an emergency long before police. You should never be complacent about the possibility of encountering violence. Problems can occur at every social and economic level and in every size of community.

From the moment you are dispatched to a call, and before you begin patient care, you need to undertake a dynamic risk assessment. Dynamic risk assessments are fluid and flexible, and allow your action plan to change as the situation evolves. If you feel the scene is not safe, contact the police and wait for them to secure the scene. Remember: If you rush in to a scene and are injured by violence, you become a nuisance to your colleagues and fellow emergency services personnel, not a trained care provider.

Body Armour

Body armour does not shield your neck or head, so whatever your level of protection, you will still be vulnerable to injury. Consult with the police to decide if you need protection and at what level. Remember that using sound conflict resolution skills to avoid dangerous situations gives you more protection than body armour. If you are issued with body armour, wear it in all dangerous situations.

Indicators of Violence

Violence can often be predicted, as most experienced ambulance clinicians already know. If you are dispatched to a shooting, stabbing, or attempted suicide, the potential for violence can be obvious. You may not expect aggressive behaviour when you arrive at the scene of an injured person. But if you are met by an agitated family member pacing the room with fists clenched and swearing, your suspicions should be heightened. The potential for such behaviour to escalate to physically violent behaviour

You are the Paramedic Part 1

You and your colleague have just finished your meal break on a warm summer evening. In your community, you respond mainly to cardiac incidents and the occasional road traffic collision. You see very few incidents involving violence, especially domestic violence. In fact, you can't remember responding to a domestic violence incident.

Shortly after your break, you and your colleague are dispatched to a house to care for an injured person. Information about the injury is unavailable. You and your colleague head over to the house.

1. Does the lack of domestic violent incidents in your patch ensure your safety?

2. What measures will you take to stay safe on this call?

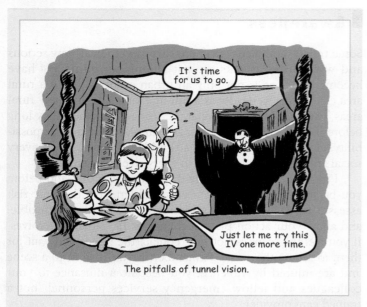

It's time for us to go.

Just let me try this IV one more time.

The pitfalls of tunnel vision.

Figure 51-2

At the Scene

Violence can often be predicted. If your ambulance is dispatched to a shooting, stabbing, or attempted suicide, the potential for violence should be obvious, and you should be very cautious in your approach to the area and scene.

should not be discounted. You must quickly identify potentially dangerous situations and act to remove yourself, your team, and, if possible the patient, to a safe place. You must not become so completely involved with patient care that you fail to see the possibility of physical harm to the patient or other health care providers. Experts call this tunnel vision Figure 51-2 ▲ . Ambulance staff should also realise that sometimes violence is *not* predictable and will be sudden and unexpected. The behaviour of patients and bystanders is not always predictable, particularly if they are intoxicated or have mental health problems. Always have an escape plan when you approach the scene—no matter how safe it initially seems.

Standard Operating Procedures

Some services have developed standard operating procedures (SOPs) for dealing with potentially violent incidents. If your service has an SOP manual, make sure you have read it for direction on handling specific situations.

■ Motorway Incidents

Reality television programmes which show police dashboard cameras mounted in vehicles have provided the public a rare view of the dangers routinely faced by the police when approach-

ing vehicles. You could face similar dangers whenever you walk to the door of a vehicle. Calls to a "man slumped over the steering wheel" or an "unconscious person in a vehicle" can be disastrous for an unsuspecting paramedic. If the occupant of the vehicle has been consuming alcohol or illegal drugs, they are much more likely to become violent.

First Emergency Vehicle at an Unprotected Scene

Incidents on the Hard Shoulder

If the incident is located on the hard shoulder, position your vehicle 50 metres before the incident, parking in a straight line parallel with the carriageway. Point the front wheels towards the nearside verge if there is no physical barrier or obstruction. If you are parked next to a barrier, bridge, or other obstruction, turn the front wheels outward towards the carriageway. This will ensure that if your vehicle is struck, it will be moved either to the left or right of you and the incident.

Turn off forward-facing warning lights and headlights where possible. Use rear-facing blue and/or red lights if fitted, side lights, and hazard lights. Keep the rear doors shut as much as possible to use the reflective markings. As with any road traffic collision, ensure you are wearing all the necessary personal protective equipment prior to alighting the ambulance. This includes a high visibility jacket (done up at the front) and a helmet with eye protection, in addition to standard universal precautions. When walking towards the incident, stay behind the barrier, if possible. If no barrier is present, then stay as far away from the live carriageway as you can. Where possible, watch the approaching traffic.

Incidents in Multiple Lanes

If you are first on scene of an incident on any of the carriageway lanes, your vehicle can be parked in the fend off position. This involves using the vehicle to block one or more lanes. This is extremely hazardous and should be performed with utmost caution.

Your vehicle must be positioned 50 metres before the incident and should use all rear-facing warning lights. The vehicle should be positioned to afford maximum use of rear visual devices and reflective/high visibility markings. If parking to fend off lane one, the vehicle should park at a slight angle, but not intrude into lane two. If it is necessary to fend off lane two, the vehicle should park at an angle to obstruct lanes one and two. Do not intrude into lane three. If it is necessary to fend off lane three, adopt the same principle as for lane one. Do not intrude into lane two. If it is necessary to fend off lanes two and three, adopt the same principle as for lanes one and two. The police will allow ambulance staff to block as many lanes as necessary for their own and the patient's safety.

When parking in the fend off position, ensure the front wheels are turned in a safe direction to reduce the risk of the vehicle being pushed into the incident if it is collided with. Once parked in the fend off position, no one should return to the vehicle unless absolutely necessary.

Retreating From Danger

You will be in situations in which unsafe circumstances dictate your retreat to a safe area. The safest means of retreat is to back away and call for police assistance. If your colleague is injured while approaching a motor vehicle, the best way to ensure help will arrive quickly is to back away and call for assistance yourself. Back away from the danger zone, remain in your vehicle, and provide ambulance control with all the necessary information. This would include:

- The number of aggressors involved
- The number and type of injuries
- The number and type of weapons involved
- The model, colour, and licence plate of the vehicle involved
- The direction of travel if the vehicle leaves the scene before the police arrive
- Confirm your call sign.

In addition, make certain to document in detail why you had to leave the scene. Whilst your safety is paramount, a duty of care is still owed to people who call for help, so you must justify the reasons for not providing this care.

Residential Incidents

Warning Signs

Paramedics may be called to residential areas to assist someone injured in an assault, domestic dispute, shooting, or stabbing. These calls require an obvious level of caution. But many routine calls have the potential for violent outcomes. An attempted suicide may turn into a murder, with you as the victim. The response to an "injured person" may have been an intentional attack by a person who remains on the scene as you arrive.

Your standard procedure for responding to any call involving violence should be to allow the police to arrive and secure the scene before your entry. Securing a scene demands more than the simple presence of a police officer at the scene. Responding paramedics must ensure that the scene is safe before going in to provide patient care.

Approaching a House

Information provided to ambulance control may be limited, and a complete picture of the circumstances at the scene may not be available to paramedics. Keep in mind that all calls have a potential for violence. When arriving at a house, listen for loud, threatening voices. Glance through available windows for signs of a struggle. In addition, look for visible weapons. By obtaining such information, you can make a decision about the relative safety of the scene. Anytime you perceive danger, abort the approach and back away to your vehicle. Call for police assistance, and wait for the officers to arrive.

Entering a House

You should stand to the doorknob side of the door when preparing to knock   Figure 51-3 ▾ . If you stand on the hinged side of the door, any person in the room can observe you by opening the door only slightly, and you would have a limited view of conditions inside the room. Knock on the door and announce: "Ambulance service". Ask whoever answers the door to lead you to the patient. If you do this, you will not only get to the patient quickly, but the person who leads you acts as a shield for you and gives you a few extra moments to react if the situation deteriorates.

When entering any type of structure you should pick a primary exit and a secondary exit. Your primary exit is usually the door that was used to enter the building. A secondary exit might be a rear door or, in an emergency, a window. Whenever you are in a building, try to keep at least one means of escape accessible at all times. If necessary, use of a rendezvous point (RVP) should be considered. If using an RVP, ensure all attending emergency services are aware of its exact location.

As you arrive at the patient's location, scan the room for weapons. If there is a gun or knife,

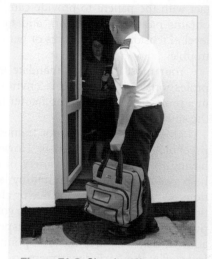

Figure 51-3 Stand on the doorknob side of the entrance when announcing your arrival.

back your way out of the house and call for police assistance. Be aware that objects like ashtrays, scissors, bottles, fireplace pokers, and knitting needles can be used as weapons. Move any potential weapon out of the patient's reach. Sadly, the use of weapons is escalating in the community and personal safety must always remain paramount. Regardless of the patient's age or that of witnesses and bystanders, you must exercise caution as even young people are increasingly carrying illegal guns and knives.

Domestic Violence

Domestic disturbances are among the most dangerous situations faced by police officers and paramedics. For an in-depth discussion on domestic violence, refer to Chapter 43. As a paramedic, you must be aware of the dangers involved and handle these incidents with extreme caution.

If a violent or physical dispute is in progress when you arrive at a house, wait for police assistance before you enter. Tempers may flare while you are treating a patient. Using good communication skills in conjunction with eye contact and appropriate body language can defuse the situation. Your voice is the most effective tool you can use to keep out of trouble in a dispute. Many ambulance staff are able to talk themselves and their colleagues out of trouble; knowing what words to use or not to use in a situation is only part of your goal. You must also be aware of the tone, pace, pitch, and rhythm of your voice. Talk to people with the same respect that you expect from them, in a non-judgemental and non-prejudicial manner. A good paramedic is always respectful because it puts patients at ease and can suppress the anger of a violent person who is not the patient. That person may turn on you, and the situation can quickly deteriorate to a dangerous level if you do not use respectful language and tone.

You may also use a technique known as contact and cover. One aspect of the technique involves a paramedic making contact with the patient to provide care. The second crew member obtains patient information, and more important, gauges the level of tension and warns his or her colleague at the first sign of trouble.

Your most important mandate is to conduct yourself as a professional in a patient-care environment. Your duty is to act in a professional manner, no matter how unpleasant or difficult the situation.

Most paramedics are not trained as marriage counsellors, psychologists, or psychiatrists. However you will find yourself having to intervene for a variety of crises as you are the only help available. You are required by law to report certain conditions such as domestic violence or child abuse to local authorities. As a health care professional, you should be aware of local procedures for reporting the suspected child or vulnerable adult at risk. The first and best point is with nursing and medical staff at the A&E department.

Violence on the Streets

The increase in gang activity and the emergence of clandestine drug laboratories pose unique challenges to paramedics. In addition, you may be responding to an assault or robbery scene before police arrive.

Clandestine Drug Laboratories

Clandestine drug laboratories are a growing problem in the UK. The most popular substance manufactured in clandestine laboratories is methamphetamine, known on the street as crystal meth, speed, and crank. With a small investment of a few hundred pounds, a drug producer, or "cooker", can begin producing methamphetamine Figure 51-4 ▾ .

Everything associated with a clandestine laboratory is hazardous! Because of the highly flammable properties of some chemicals associated with cooking methamphetamine and the toxic nature of others, extreme caution must be exercised when a laboratory is found. Although some methamphetamine "cooking" operations may look like a typical school chemistry laboratory, others are much harder to recognise and may just resemble an untidy kitchen. Large quantities of over-the-counter cold remedies containing ephedrine or pseudoephedrine, litre containers of camping fuel, and sulphuric acid in the form of lye may be the only signs of methamphetamine production. Almost every chemical involved is a hazardous material Figure 51-5 ▸ .

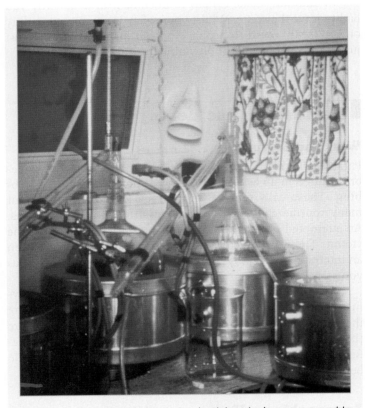

Figure 51-4 Some methamphetamine laboratories may resemble a high school chemistry laboratory. Do not touch anything!

You are the Paramedic Part 2

You arrive at a house. You gather your equipment and prepare to approach the house. While walking toward the house, you can hear a female screaming. A male voice is aggressively swearing over the woman's screaming. Your colleague pauses on the path and looks over at you, eyebrows raised.

3. What information can be obtained as you walk toward the house?

4. What actions should you take in response to the hostilities heard from within the house?

Prep Kit

Ready for Review

- No community, socioeconomic group, race, or religion is immune to violence. The use of sound conflict resolution skills will reduce the potential for you to fall victim to an act of violence while on an emergency call.
- Allow the police to secure the scene of violent incidents before you enter.
- Should violence erupt while you are on scene, retreat to a safe place and summon the police.

Vital Vocabulary

clandestine drug laboratories Locations where illegal drugs such as methamphetamine, lysergic acid diethylamide (LSD), and ectasy are manufactured.

concealment Protection from being seen.

contact and cover Technique that involves one paramedic making contact with the patient to provide care, while the second paramedic obtains patient information, gauges the level of tension, and warns his or her colleague at the first sign of trouble.

cover Obstacles that are difficult or impossible for bullets to penetrate.

physical evidence The evidence that ties a suspect or victim to a crime. It may include body materials, objects, and impressions.

primary exit The main means of escape should violence erupt. This is usually the door you used to enter the building.

secondary exit Any other means of egress, including windows and rear doors.

testimonial evidence The verbal documentation by a witness of the facts of a criminal act.

tunnel vision Dangerous situation when a paramedic becomes so completely involved with patient care that he or she fails to see the possibility of physical harm to the patient or other care providers.

Points to Ponder

You are sent to an assault on a street corner in your town. The police ask you to park approximately two streets away. After approximately 10 minutes, you are notified that the scene is safe. When you approach the patient, you see that he has two stab wounds to his chest. You and your colleague provide spinal precautions and initiate immediate lifesaving care to him. You transport him to the nearest trauma centre.

What would you have done if you arrived at the scene before the police? If the assailant were on the scene, what would you do?

Issues: Potential Exposure to Scene Violence, How to Approach the Scene.

Assessment in Action

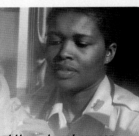

You and your colleague are sent to the M6 for an unconscious patient in a car. You are informed by your control that the scene appears to be safe. The person who called 999 was travelling in the opposite direction and noticed the vehicle pulled over on the hard shoulder of the motorway.

1. **How and where should you approach the vehicle on the shoulder?**
   A. At a minimum of 50 m to the rear and a 20° angle
   B. At a minimum of 50 m in front of the vehicle on a 1° angle
   C. At a minimum of 50 m to the rear of the vehicle and parked in a straight line with wheels facing the nearside
   D. At a minimum of a 30 m to the rear of the vehicle and on a 15° angle

2. **What should you do if the situation turns unsafe?**
   A. Stay and deal with it.
   B. Adapt and overcome.
   C. Retreat from the scene.
   D. Try to talk to the patient.

3. **Information that you need to give to ambulance control if there is an unsafe condition includes all of the following, EXCEPT:**
   A. the number of aggressors involved.
   B. the patient's name and estimated transport time to the hospital.
   C. the number and type of weapons involved, if any.
   D. the model, colour, and licence plate of the vehicle.

4. **True or false? Once on the scene, and there do not appear to be any threats to the ambulance clinicians, you can move on to other things, such as treating the patient.**
   A. True
   B. False

5. **True or false? Only certain calls require a scene assessment for violence hazards.**
   A. True
   B. False

Challenging Question

You are sent to the scene of a paediatric pedestrian struck by a car outside a block of flats. When you arrive on scene, you see a crowd of approximately 100 angry individuals. You find a police officer and you ask her to lead you to the patient. When you arrive at the patient's side, your rapid assessment reveals no life-threatening or serious injuries; you secure the patient, who appears to be stable, and transfer him to the ambulance.

6. **What dangers do large crowds pose to the ambulance clinicians?**

www.Paramedic.EMSzone.com/UK/

Objectives

- Review the purpose of CPR.
- Emphasise the importance of the links in the Chain of Survival to a successful resuscitation.
- List the skill steps of one-rescuer and two-rescuer CPR for the adult, child, and infant patient.
- Discuss the latest guidelines issued by the European Resuscitation Council (December 2005) as they apply to the health care provider.
- Review the management of a cardiac arrest based on analysis of the ECG as either a shockable (VF or VT) or a nonshockable (PEA or asystole) rhythm.
- Review devices that may be useful adjuncts at a resuscitation to increase the probability of increasing the return of spontaneous circulation (ROSC).
- Describe the typical roles of the resuscitation team leader and first ALS trained paramedic on scene.
- Discuss the value of scene choreography at a resuscitation.

Introduction

Paramedics and technicians are frequently dispatched to calls involving a cardiac arrest. An estimated 60% to 70% of all pre-hospital cardiac arrests occur in the home; the remainder occur in public places. Having a bystander who has initiated the proper care at the scene is definitely a plus—indeed, it often means the difference between life or death. Some paramedics might even find it difficult to remember successfully resuscitating a patient from cardiac arrest who did not either have bystander CPR or for whom the arrest was a witnessed event and an AED was immediately available.

This appendix explores planning for the resuscitation, the roles of the subsequent crews to arrive, referred to as the resuscitation team leader/first paramedic on scene, and the resuscitation team, and ways that practice and planning can help increase your resuscitation success. The European Resuscitation Council, in conjunction with the international resuscitation community, revises the guidelines for emergency cardiovascular care and CPR every 5 years. This appendix describes how your organisation can incorporate the latest guidelines into your practice.

Managing Cardiac Arrest

According to the ERC, the "Chain of Survival" includes four essential links: early recognition/early access, early CPR, early defibrillation, and early definitive care Figure A-1 ▸ . Those areas that have made survival of a prehospital cardiac arrest a benchmark for measurable improvements in their health care systems have worked hard on each of these links.

2005 Guidelines: A Reemphasis on Quality CPR

During the past 15 years the emphasis on quality CPR has seemed to slip as providers became more focused on intubation, drug administration, defibrillation, and other aspects of resuscitation and cardiac arrest management. Recent studies have shown that the quality of CPR is poor in both in-hospital and prehospital settings: The depth of compressions is inadequate, the rate of compressions is too slow, almost half the time no compressions are provided, the ventilations are too fast, and the chest is rarely allowed to recoil fully. Studies investigating the value of intubation and resuscitation drugs are inconclusive

You are the Paramedic Part 1

Jim, a 54-year-old man, is playing football on a Saturday afternoon for the local team. He leaves the game to get a drink and starts to feel dizzy as he returns to the pitch. He suddenly drops to his knees and then to the floor. Fortunately, one of his teammates, Tom, took a cardiopulmonary resuscitation (CPR) course about 2 months ago, so he takes charge of the situation. Tom orders a teammate, "Go and call 999 and tell them we have a cardiac arrest". Next, he tells someone else, "Go and find an AED".

About 8 minutes pass as the ambulance, which was located only a few streets away, arrives on the scene.

Upon arrival of your paramedic ambulance, you are led onto the pitch by a teammate. As you approach the patient's side, you do a quick assessment of the scene for safety and potential hazards and then begin an initial assessment. Your general impression indicates a middle-aged, overweight male who is receiving good-quality CPR as judged by the counting you hear and the compressions. A first responder is attaching the electrodes to the AED. These cables can easily be switched to your monitor, but this can wait until after the first shock.

You note the following findings while getting an initial report.

Initial Assessment	Recording Time: 2 Minutes
Appearance	CPR is in progress, patient is not vomiting, and the abdomen is not distended
Level of consciousness	U (Unresponsive)
Airway	Open with a head tilt-chin lift
Breathing	Being ventilated with a bag-valve-mask device

1. Arriving on the scene of an apparent cardiac arrest with bystanders who have initiated care, how should you evaluate the quality of the CPR?

2. Many sports centres and public places have an AED available. How might that have helped in this situation?

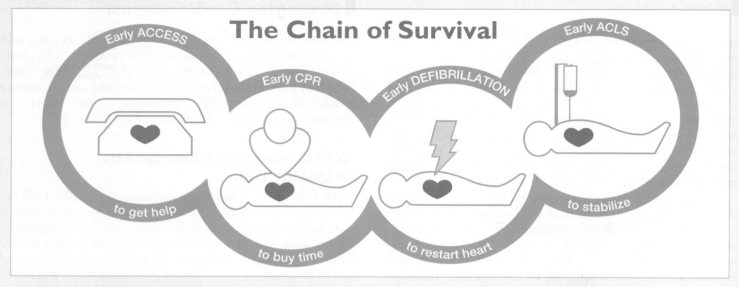

Figure A-1 The four links of the Chain of Survival.

Notes from Nancy

Don't let your CPR skills get rusty. A patient's life may depend on them.

at best, but CPR is clearly important both before and after defibrillation. In addition, immediate CPR can double or triple the rate of survival from ventricular fibrillation (VF) sudden cardiac arrest.

The 2005 resuscitation guidelines reemphasise the importance of providing high-quality CPR (push hard and fast, and allow full chest recoil). In fact, the "resuscitation pyramid" is built on a strong base of high-quality CPR as illustrated in **Figure A-2** ▶. The recognition that a paramedic's best chance of succeeding at resuscitation hinges on continuous, uninterrupted high-quality CPR changes the focus of care.

As you arrive on the scene of the resuscitation/cardiac arrest, you need to clearly understand that the success of the cardiac arrest relies on high-quality compressions and not on an IV, an ET tube, or any drug in your box. Work together with the BLS providers, assist them, complement their efforts, and relieve them as they tire but do not interrupt or disrupt their efforts!

The Steps of CPR

The basic life support steps of CPR for the adult patient follow the algorithm shown in **Figure A-3** ▶. They presume that an AED is not immediately available at the patient's side. Integration of the AED will be discussed later in this appendix.

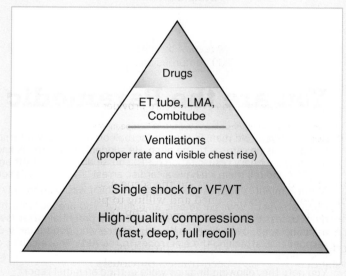

Figure A-2 The resuscitation pyramid. The success of a resuscitation relies on high-quality CPR.

Health care providers (first responders, technicians, and paramedics) who work in the prehospital setting must be trained and prepared to provide either one-rescuer CPR or two-rescuer CPR as available personnel dictate.

In some instances, single-rescuer CPR may have been started before ambulance personnel arrive. To help make CPR easier to learn, remember, and perform, the general public or "lay rescuers" are taught a universal compression–ventilation ratio of 30:2. They are not taught to take a pulse, to perform rescue breathing, or to perform two-rescuer CPR. Paramedics

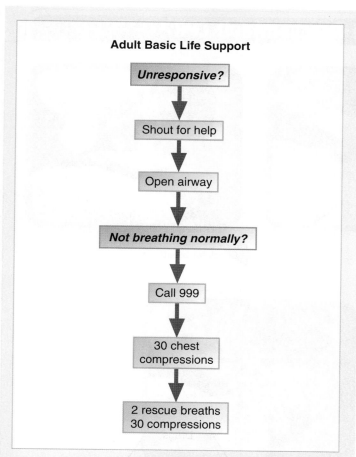

Adult Basic Life Support

Unresponsive?

↓

Shout for help

↓

Open airway

↓

Not breathing normally?

↓

Call 999

↓

30 chest
compressions

↓

2 rescue breaths
30 compressions

Figure A-3 The BLS adult health care provider algorithm.

Reproduced from *Adult Basic Life Support.* © European Resuscitation
Council.

should be thankful to arrive on the scene and find a bystander who is both properly trained and willing to provide CPR. Sadly, studies have shown that bystander CPR is performed in only one third or fewer of witnessed cardiac arrests and that when performed, even by health care providers, it is not done well. Bystanders who have been trained previously in CPR are often reluctant to begin this procedure for the following reasons:

- CPR steps may have been too complicated and included too many steps to remember. The 2005 guidelines made a significant effort to simplify the steps taught to the public.
- Training methods may have been inadequate, and skill retention typically declines very rapidly after a course. This issue is being studied to try to determine which methods of training will produce the greatest skill retention. A video-based watch-and-do method, as opposed to watch-then-do, has been incorporated into many course revisions.
- Some members of the public may be afraid of transmitted diseases and therefore may be reluctant to perform mouth-to-mouth resuscitation. Although the 2005 guidelines strongly emphasise that the risk of transmission of

infection is very low, those who are still concerned are encouraged to use barrier devices. In addition, the technique of compression-only CPR is encouraged for those who are reluctant to do ventilations and for dispatcher-assisted CPR instruction.

Single-Rescuer CPR

Tom immediately began single-rescuer CPR when his teammate Jim dropped suddenly on the football pitch. The steps are shown in **Skill Drill A-1 ▶**.

1. Establish responsiveness. If there is no movement or response to shouting and shaking the adult patient, then the patient is considered "unresponsive" **Step 1**.
   - If you are by yourself, phone 999 (or the emergency number) and make sure the AED is immediately available.
   - If there is a second rescuer, send him or her to call 999 (or the emergency number) and get the AED.
2. Open the airway **Step 2**. Use the head tilt–chin lift method unless trauma to the neck is suspected, in which case the jaw-thrust manoeuvre may be more appropriate.
3. Check for breathing **Step 3**. Look, listen, and feel for up to 10 seconds.
   - If the patient is breathing or resumes effective breathing, place him or her in the recovery position and monitor closely.
4. If the patient is not breathing, start chest compressions **Step 4**. Compressions are delivered in the centre of the chest between the nipples with the heel of the hand and with the second hand on top of the first. Compressions on an adult should be provided at a rate of 100/min, pressing 4 to 5 cm and ensuring full chest recoil after each compression.
5. Ventilate twice (for 1 second each), ensuring visible chest rise. Combine chest compressions with ventilations at a ratio of 30:2 **Step 5**.
   - Continue until either the patient starts breathing or an AED arrives. Once the AED has arrived, attach the pads without interrupting compressions.
6. Do not touch the patient whilst the AED is analysing the patient's rhythm. Follow the voice/visual prompts.

Two-Rescuer CPR

Two-rescuer adult CPR provides the same cycle of 30 compressions to every two breaths as in the single-rescuer technique. Because the work is split between the two rescuers, it is more efficient and there is less interruption in the chest compressions to provide the ventilations. If an advanced airway has been inserted, asynchronous compressions and ventilations are possible. That is, the compressor simply presses hard, fast, and with full chest recoil at the rate of 100/min while the ventilator provides one breath (over 1 second's time, while observing for visible chest rise) every 6 seconds.

Skill Drill A-1: Single-Rescuer Adult CPR

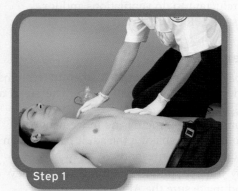

Step 1

Establish responsiveness.

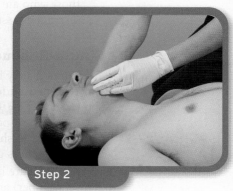

Step 2

Open the airway.

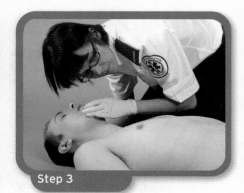

Step 3

Check for breathing.

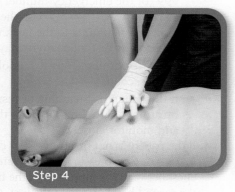

Step 4

If the patient is not breathing, start 30 chest compressions in the centre of the chest at a rate of 100/min and to a depth 4 to 5 cm.

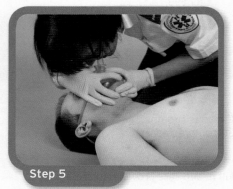

Step 5

Ventilate twice (1 second each) ensuring visible chest rise. Combine chest compressions with ventilations at a ratio of 30:2. Continue until either the patient starts breathing or an AED arrives. Once the AED has arrived, attach the pads without interrupting compressions. Do not touch the patient whilst the AED is analysing the patient's rhythm. Follow the voice/visual prompts.

When you are using the two-rescuer technique, rotate the compressor every 2 minutes. To do so, ask the bystander to continue to assist and kneel on the other side of the patient. Now you can have an "active compressor" and a "waiting compressor" who is ready to take over after the five cycles or 2-minute interval. Studies of rescuer fatigue show that the compressor tires after 2 to 5 minutes and that the quality of compressions will suffer if the compressor is not replaced. The steps in two-rescuer CPR are outlined here and in **Skill Drill A-2 ▶**:

1. Establish responsiveness. Send a helper to phone 999 and get the AED (**Step 1**).
2. Open the airway using the head tilt–chin lift manoeuvre (**Step 2**).
3. Check for breathing for up to 10 seconds (**Step 3**).
4. One rescuer begins 30 compressions—centre of the chest, push hard and fast (rate of 100/min), and allow full chest recoil (**Step 4**). Count out loud.
5. The second rescuer ventilates twice, using a pocket mask or bag-valve-mask. Then the rescuer applies AED pads to

Skill Drill A-2: Two-Rescuer Adult CPR

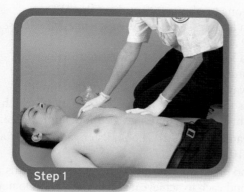

Step 1

Establish responsiveness.

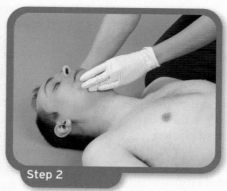

Step 2

Open the airway.

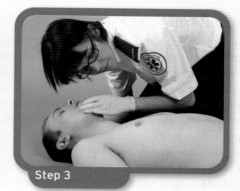

Step 3

Check for breathing.

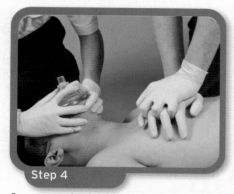

Step 4

One rescuer begins 30 chest compressions in the centre of the chest, counting out loud.

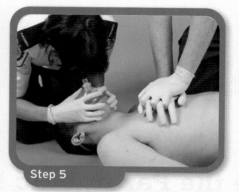

Step 5

The second rescuer ventilates twice using either a pocket face mask or bag-valve-mask. Then the rescuer applies AED pads while waiting. Combine chest compressions with ventilations at a ratio of 30:2. Do not touch the patient whilst the AED is analysing the patient's rhythm. Follow the voice/visual prompts.

the patient while waiting. Combine chest compressions with ventilations at a ratio of 30:2 (Step 5).

6. Do not touch the patient whilst the AED is analysing the patient's rhythm. Follow the voice/visual prompts.

Note: Once an advanced airway has been inserted, the compressions and ventilations are no longer in cycles. Instead, they are asynchronous, with the compressor providing 100/min without pauses for breaths and the ventilator giving 10 breaths/min (every 6 to 8 seconds). The compressor will get tired so be prepared to switch compressors every 2 minutes.

■ Modification in Technique for Children

Definitions

The age-old question asked of paediatricians has been "For the purposes of resuscitation, what age defines a child"? Many paediatricians would simply say, "If the patient looks like a child, then he or she is a child; if the patient looks like an adult, then he or she is an adult". This vagueness is further complicated by the epidemic of childhood obesity. The 2005 guidelines use the following definitions of age groups for the purposes of resuscitation:

- **Neonate**—the first 28 days of life
- **Infant**—between 28 days and 1 year
- **Child**—age 1 year to adolescence (signs of puberty)
- **Adult**—adolescent and older

This appendix concentrates on infant, child, and adult patients. The care of newborn and neonate patients is discussed in Chapter 40.

Child CPR

The technique of CPR has a few slight variations for children, as shown below in italics. **Skill Drill A-3 ▸** shows the steps of one-rescuer child CPR.

1. Establish unresponsiveness. If there is no movement or response to *tapping and asking loudly "Are you okay"?* the child is unresponsive.
   - Send someone to phone 999 and get the AED.
   - If you are a lone rescuer *for a sudden witnessed collapse,* phone 999 and get the AED.
   - If you are a lone rescuer and it was an unwitnessed collapse, proceed to the next step.
2. Open the airway **Step 1**. Use the head tilt–chin lift method unless trauma to the neck is suspected, in which case the jaw-thrust manoeuvre may be more appropriate.
3. Check for breathing **Step 2**. Look, listen, and feel for a maximum of 10 seconds.
   - If there is no breathing, give five *effective* rescue breaths over 1 second each to achieve a visible chest rise. Do not over-ventilate the patient, as it can cause gastric distention and regurgitation. *Use a child-sized bag-valve-mask* device with supplementary oxygen, insert an oropharyngeal airway, and position the second rescuer or ventilator above the supine child's head. Use the "E-C" or "OK" grip to ensure a proper mask seal.
   - If the patient is breathing or resumes effective breathing, place him or her in the recovery position and monitor closely.

You are the Paramedic Part 2

During the first 2 minutes of CPR with Tom and the ambulance crew, a lot of teamwork has been going on. Tom is beginning to tire yet still wants to stay involved, so he becomes the "waiting compressor". Your colleague has pulled out the bag-valve-mask, connected it to supplemental oxygen, and inserted an oropharyngeal airway in the patient; he becomes the ventilator. You place the AED next to Jim and relieve Tom; you now become the compressor.

After approximately 2 minutes (five cycles) of CPR, a brief pause in care allows the responder to analyse Jim's ECG. The AED begins to charge up, displaying a shockable rhythm such as ventricular fibrillation. In the meantime, you administer a few more compressions, and the ventilator removes the bag-valve-mask so oxygen does not flow near the patient. You state loudly, "Stand clear" and proceed to deliver a single shock. The resuscitation team immediately begins the next five cycles of 30 compressions and two ventilations.

Vital Signs	Recording Time: 3 Minutes
Skin	Pale and clammy
Pulse	None palpable at carotid
Blood pressure	None
Respirations	Being ventilated with a bag-valve-mask device

Previously, the duration of time from stopping compressions to analysing to charging and providing the traditional three-shock series would have been almost 2 minutes of no chest compressions. No perfusion of the brain and vital organs occurs when there is no circulation from rescuers compressing the chest properly. Every pause in compressions, even when it lasts for as little as a few seconds, requires the next few compressions to reprime the pump. For this reason, a pause to analyse the rhythm should last no longer than 10 seconds without chest compressions.

When a patient has a shockable rhythm and does respond appropriately to a shock, it often takes a minute or so for return of spontaneous circulation (ROSC). Unless the patient actually wakes up, immediately after the shock the rescuers should begin CPR with chest compressions.

3. What could you do next as the paramedic on the scene?
4. What is the advantage to perfusion and chest compressions from inserting an advanced airway during two-rescuer CPR?

Skill Drill A-3: Single-Rescuer Child CPR

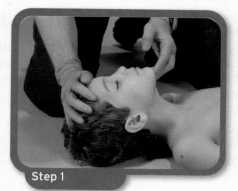

Step 1

Establish unresponsiveness. Open the airway.

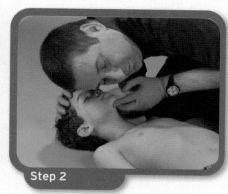

Step 2

Check for breathing (look, listen, and feel). If no breaths, administer five effective breaths.

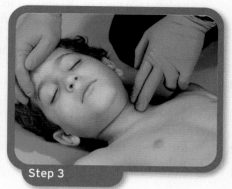

Step 3

Perform a carotid pulse check for 5 seconds (maximum of 10 seconds).

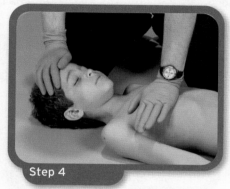

Step 4

Begin 30 compressions—centre of the chest, push hard and fast (rate of 100/min), and allow full chest recoil—using either one or two hands depending on the child's size. Compress one third the depth of the chest.

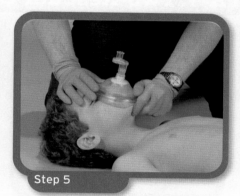

Step 5

Ventilate two times for 1 second each to achieve visible chest rise. Use a child-sized pocket mask with a one-way valve.

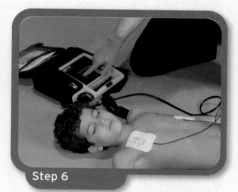

Step 6

Complete five cycles (approximately 2 minutes) and reassess the patient for a maximum of 10 seconds. If the AED has arrived, attach it, using paediatric electrodes if the child is between 1 and 8 years old. Decrease the AED energy level. Analyse the rhythm.

If the rhythm is shockable, administer a single shock and then resume CPR immediately for five cycles. Re-analyse the rhythm.

If the rhythm is not shockable, resume CPR immediately for five cycles.

4. At this point the lay rescuer begins compressions. Health care providers are taught to check for a carotid pulse in the child (as long as they do not exceed 10 seconds) (**Step 3**). Compressions are delivered in the centre of the chest between the nipples with the heel of *either one hand or both hands as in the adult technique.* They should be provided at a rate of 100/min, pressing *one third the depth of the chest* and ensuring full chest recoil after each compression (**Step 4**).

- If a pulse is present, the health care provider gives one rescue breath *every 3 to 5 seconds* (**Step 5**).
- If no pulse is present, the health care provider begins chest compressions. Be prepared to change compressors every 2 minutes.

5. *If not already done, phone 999.*

6. Continue the cycles of 30 compressions (push hard and fast, and allow full chest recoil) and two breaths (1-second duration each to achieve visible chest rise) until the AED or defibrillator arrives. *If there are two rescuers, health care providers are taught to give cycles of 15 compressions to two ventilations.*

7. Check the patient's rhythm once the AED arrives, with the least amount of interruption in chest compressions as possible (**Step 6**). *If the child is between 1 and 8 years old, use paediatric electrodes if available. If the AED has a key or switch to deliver a child shock dose, activate it to decrease the energy level. If no paediatric electrodes are available, use adult pads.*

- If there is a shockable rhythm, administer a single shock. Resume CPR immediately for five cycles (approximately 1 minute), and then re-analyse the rhythm.

- If there is not a shockable rhythm, resume CPR immediately for five cycles (approximately 2 minutes). Some of the public are trained to continue until ALS providers take over or the child starts to move. The health care provider would determine whether the patient has a pulse at this point.

Skill Drill A-4 ▾ shows the steps of two-rescuer child CPR, also summarised here.

1. Establish unresponsiveness, and send a helper to phone 999 and get the AED. If there is no helper, continue with the steps of CPR and then phone and look for an AED at the 1-minute point.
2. Open the airway using the head tilt–chin lift manoeuvre **Step 1**.

3. Check for breathing (look, listen, and feel) **Step 2**. If there is no breathing, administer five effective breaths, each lasting 1 second and achieving visible chest rise.
4. Perform a carotid pulse check (maximum of 10 seconds) **Step 3**.
5. One rescuer begins 15 compressions—centre of the chest, push hard and fast (rate of 100/min), and allow full chest recoil **Step 4**. Count out loud so the second rescuer is prepared to ventilate as you get to "13 and 14 and 15".
6. The second rescuer ventilates two times, each lasting 1 second and achieving visible chest rise **Step 5**. The ventilator should use a child-sized bag-valve-mask device with supplementary oxygen and an OP airway. Position

Skill Drill A-4: Two-Rescuer Child CPR

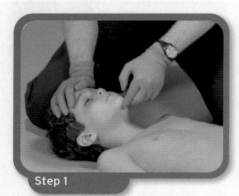

Step 1

Establish unresponsiveness. Open the airway.

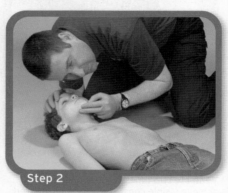

Step 2

Check for breathing (look, listen, and feel). If no breaths, administer five effective breaths.

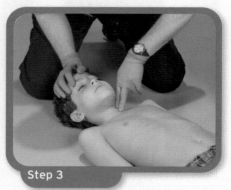

Step 3

Perform a carotid pulse check (maximum of 10 seconds).

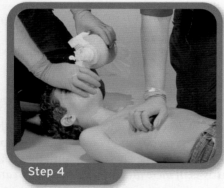

Step 4

One rescuer begins 15 compressions—centre of the chest, push hard and fast (rate of 100/min) and allow full chest recoil.

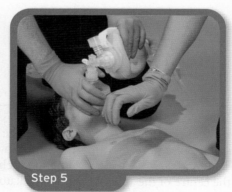

Step 5

The second rescuer ventilates two times for 1 second each to achieve visible chest rise. The ventilator should use a child-sized bag-valve-mask device with supplementary oxygen and an oropharyngeal airway. Position yourself above the head of the supine patient to allow for the proper hand position/mask seal.

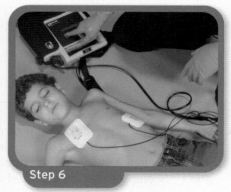

Step 6

Continue uninterrupted BLS until an AED arrives. If an AED has arrived and is attached, analyse the patient's ECG rhythm. Use paediatric electrodes if the child is between 1 and 8 years old. Decrease the AED energy level if not using an alternator.

If the rhythm is shockable, administer a single shock.

If the rhythm is not shockable or immediately following the shock, begin five cycles of 15 compressions to two ventilations.

Introduction

This appendix reviews the standardised approach to patient assessment, which is the format used and reinforced throughout each chapter of this text. Mastery of the standardised approach to patient assessment is a key clinical skill that helps characterise the best paramedics. Only after you have developed a strong foundation in patient assessment and broad clinical experience can you confidently make clinical judgements and adapt the standardised format to meet each patient's immediate needs.

This appendix also covers some of the finer points about assessment, dealing with people, and the importance of working as a team. Many of these strategies are presented throughout the text in the cases and will be used in the clinical skills exercises in your paramedic training programme.

Effective Assessment

The care that you provide is built on a strong base consisting of quality assessment of the patient. For this reason, much of your training programme emphasises assessment, and the scenarios or simulations you participate in during your classroom activities involve constant practice assessing patients. You simply cannot treat a patient properly without taking the time and effort to assess his or her situation. Likewise, you cannot make patient management and treatment interventions without first making a patient assessment.

Paramedics follow a format to gather, evaluate, and synthesise the information. This consistency helps you to make the right patient care management decisions and take the corresponding appropriate actions. Conversely, not doing an effective assessment can have disastrous results for the patient.

Accurate information is critical to your decision making. If a paramedic is too embarrassed to admit he or she could not really hear the patient's blood pressure and makes up data, this can lead to inappropriate decision making, poor patient care, or a lack of confidence in the paramedic's abilities. If you cannot feel, hear, or interpret essential information, such as vital signs, the best course is to immediately say you are having some difficulty obtaining the information and get some help or at least record that it was not found. Perhaps the blood pressure is so low that it is not easy to hear or feel, or perhaps you are just having a bad day. It isn't always important that you make a mistake—it is what you do with your mistakes when they occur that is very important!

You are the Paramedic Part 1

After completing your vehicle daily inspection (VDI) and ensuring that the ambulance is fully stocked, you grab a quick cup of coffee, and book your vehicle on at 07:00 hours precisely. The pager goes off and the MDT screen alerts you to an incoming call. A head-on collision has just occurred outside the Spar shop not far from your station. The police, the fire service, a second ambulance, and a supervisor are all en route because they have received multiple calls on the collision that may involve a fire and entrapment.

The police arrive first and begin to control the flow of traffic. They report that the smoke was from an airbag, not a car fire. They notify ambulance control to continue the response because there are two older patients, one in each vehicle, and it is not clear whether either is trapped. The fire service arrives next, and the incident command system is set up. The senior fire officer reports that there is no fire, but a rescue tender is needed to open the car doors. Both patients are conscious, elderly women. One patient may have her legs trapped; the other is very confused.

Your ambulance arrives next, and you assess the scene as you approach it. The mechanism of injury (MOI) is significant: There is a considerable amount of damage to the front ends of both vehicles, and the rear of the second vehicle has been pushed into a lamp post. There are also some cracks in the windscreen, which may explain the bleeding from the driver's head.

The fire officer fills you in on the details as you quickly don your personal protective gear. The police officer said that one woman is acting as if she is highly intoxicated but he has not yet got a Breathalyser reading on her. The second ambulance and the supervisor are just arriving, so you decide to deal with the confused woman who, according to the police, "May have been the one to cause the collision".

Initial Assessment	Recording Time: 1 Minute
Appearance	A woman in her late 60s. She is bleeding from a head laceration, nervous, scared, and very confused.
Level of consciousness	V (Verbal–knows name, not sure of day or where she is)
Airway	Open and clear
Breathing	Rapid but no obvious life threats at this time
Circulation	She has a weak radial pulse and no life-threatening bleeding.

1. What are some of the potential causes of a head-on collision in which the driver never hit the brakes?
2. What is the significance of the MOI in this collision for your patient?
3. If it is clear that your patient was not wearing a seatbelt, how could this fact change things?

In patient assessment, the history is critically important. Some experts believe that 80% of a medical diagnosis is based solely on the history and not on objective data, such as vital signs, laboratory test results, and ECGs. If you have gained a broad knowledge of diseases and medical conditions through your education, training, reading, and street experience, you will have many profiles with which you can compare the objective and subjective findings of the history. This "pattern recognition" helps you develop a "working differential diagnosis". With excellent history gathering and interviewing skills, you can focus the physical examination and assessment to arrive at the most accurate initial diagnosis and assist accident and emergency (A&E) department staff in arriving at the admission diagnosis.

The Importance of the Physical Examination

The physical examination should be focused on the body system that the chief complaint and history suggest is the source of the problem. **Table B-1 ▼** summarises the types of physical examinations that you have encountered in this text.

You will practise these physical examinations as part of your training programme numerous times until you master them. The examinations will then be incorporated into clinical workshop simulations of patient scenarios to help prepare you for their application in the prehospital environment.

Observational studies show that paramedics who have clearly demonstrated in practical skills testing that they know the steps and sequences of the examinations and know when they are supposed to use them nevertheless overlook the physical examinations or apply them in only a cursory manner at the scene. Ideally, your paramedic instructors and partners will model and instil excellent work habits and a practice ethic so that you will conduct the physical examinations appropriately when your patient's condition warrants their use.

Table B-1	Types of Physical Examinations
Examination	**Description**
Rapid trauma examination/ assessment	Provided for a trauma patient with significant MOI
Rapid physical examination/ assessment	Provided for a medical patient who is not responsive
Detailed physical examination	Provided en route to the A&E for a trauma patient with a significant MOI
Neurological examination	Assesses the cranial nerves, and sensory and motor function in each extremity
Cardiopulmonary (heart/lungs) examination	Includes an assessment of the lung sounds, heart sounds, JVD (jugular venous distension), pedal oedema, and ECG
Obstetric examination	Includes checking for crowning in a woman in labour
Other examinations	For specific patient complaints

Developing an Action Plan

After you obtain subjective information from the patient through your interviewing skills (that is, OPQRST and SAMPLE) and then obtain objective findings by obtaining vital signs and other parametres (such as ECG, SpO_2, $ETCO_2$ blood glucose level, and other clinical findings), the next step is assessment and developing a treatment plan. The more extensive the knowledge base of clinical profiles (that is, typical clinical pictures) you have, the better your chances of making an accurate assessment. Pattern recognition and "gut instinct" based on lots of experience have key roles in this decision process. Once the assessment has been completed, a treatment or action plan must be developed. Some of the treatment will have already begun if the initial assessment revealed life threats based on the patient's mental status or ABCs.

Your action plan for treatment of the patient must consider the priority and severity of the patient's condition, the environmental conditions, and the BLS and ALS treatment guidelines used in your region. Most ambulance services in the UK use the national clinical practice guidelines produced by the Joint Royal Colleges Ambulance Liaison Committee. These guidelines cover the full range of medical, surgical, and trauma conditions typically encountered by the paramedic.

The guidelines are written in a symptom-based assessment format and the topics are typical assessment findings such as abdominal pain, breathlessness, chest pain, headache, mental illness, unconsciousness, etc. Most of the guidance—including asthma, allergic reaction, head trauma, and suspected stroke—involve a combination of assessment findings and presumptive clinical assessments (a "working diagnosis"). You would need to arrive at the right clinical impression to know which guideline to use. In most guidelines, a statement in the preface discusses the issue of clinical judgement. Sometimes it takes this kind of clinical judgement to realise which specific guideline is the best to follow, especially when a patient has multiple presenting problems. Good judgement is developed over time and is based on supervised clinical experience plus common sense.

Factors Affecting the Ability to Assess Patients and Make Decisions

Your attitude can significantly influence your assessment and decision-making abilities. We all have spent a good part of our lives developing attitudes, values, and biases—some helpful and some less than helpful. When you become a paramedic, you must attempt to leave your attitude and your ego at the door! Not everyone keeps their home the way you do, nor does every person look the same, act the same, or have the same values. They just might be different from what you have become accustomed to. Steer clear of assigning "labels" to or stereotyping patients and their families. Referring to patients by derogatory names or slurs is disrespectful and distracting and often leads to a biased and incomplete assessment. Remember, patients call us to provide medical care. Don't try to judge your patients, but rather treat them as you would expect care to be provided to one of your loved ones.

Quality management of the patient depends on an accurate medical assessment, not whether you like the patient. Attempting to prejudge the situation or the patient leads to tunnel vision, as if you have blinkers on and miss everything in the periphery. This behaviour can hamper your information gathering and cause you not to collect enough information for a thorough assessment. It is distracting and leads you to "lock on" to an initial impression too early before you have analysed all the facts. Such an inappropriate gut instinct can cause you to make poor judgements about a patient's medical condition based on past experiences. If you have collected insufficient information to recognise the patterns of injury or a medical condition, you may not be able to make an accurate assessment, or if you do, it will often take longer.

Uncooperative patients can be difficult to assess. When a patient is being difficult, your first reaction may be to pack up and leave. Nevertheless, it is important to remember that this person may be "under the influence"—not necessarily of alcohol or drugs. Many patients who are acting out, belligerent, or restless may be reacting to a medical or traumatic situation such as hypoxia, hypovolaemia, hypoglycaemia, hypothermia, head injury, or concussion. Always rule out medical or traumatic causes for irritability and lack of cooperation before assuming the behaviour is due to intoxication or a behavioural problem.

Sometimes patients have a very distracting injury, such as the fracture shown in **Figure B-1 ▾**. Always follow the plan you have been taught: scene assessment, initial assessment (mental status, ABCs, priority decision), determination of the significance of the MOI, and then appropriate focused history and physical examination. Do not allow a distracting injury to divert your attention from the assessment plan. If necessary, temporarily cover the injury with a towel and continue your assessment! You will ultimately get to it at the proper point in the assessment. You do not want to treat the leg and lose the life because the patient was not breathing adequately.

The number of responders is a factor that definitely needs to be worked into the team's approach to patient assessment and management. Regardless of the various ways in which your local ambulance service responds, once at the scene, the team can consist of two to four or more responders with varying levels of training. How the scene is managed, who the team leader is, and how assessment information is gathered (sequential versus simultaneous) needs to be practised in advance. Patients dislike assessment by committee, in which two or more providers grill the patient at the same time. This practice can be confusing, often no one gets the entire story, and the patient may repeatedly be asked the same questions.

Sometimes the prehospital environment can prove a major distraction to your assessment. If you are prepared for the possibilities, you can consider strategies to deal with them proactively rather than reacting to them. Examples of environmental distracters include crowds, unruly bystanders, potentially violent or dangerous situations, high noise levels, and an excessive number of ambulance clinicians at the scene. If the presence of too many people makes it difficult for you to do your job, politely ask them to wait elsewhere or release the extra service personnel from the scene.

Finally, patient compliance issues may sometimes present obstacles to assessment and management. If the patient has difficulty confiding in you or any of the other rescuers, it can limit the information you have to make accurate decisions. Some patients simply will not tell you their medical history. Be careful not to spark this "problem" by displaying an attitude or body language that says you are disinterested or not really someone the patient can trust. Sensitivity to cultural and ethnic factors is also important and should be included in your training and clinical workshop simulations.

Scene Choreography

The importance of a team leader choreographing the activities of the team at the scene of an emergency cannot be overstated. As described in Appendix A, the resuscitation team leader and resuscitation team members have specific roles that must be constantly practised and carried out correctly to increase the success of prehospital resuscitations. Indeed, the role of the team leader is key to the coordinated effort of the entire team. Achieving this kind of coordination can be challenging when there are too few or too many responders at the scene. Clearly, the team gives its best response when a single leader manages and monitors the team's efforts with a clear understanding of the strategies, goals, and plans for the particular situation.

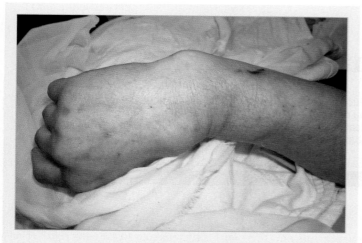

Figure B-1 This fracture is distracting but not an immediate life threat. Don't let it interfere with your initial assessment to locate the real life threats.

The team concept should not just be practised for a cardiac arrest call. Indeed, the team concept needs to be reinforced in the classroom setting with practise in numerous simulated responses. The team members and team leader will then be better prepared to respond quickly and effectively in the pre-hospital setting with real emergencies.

Practise is critically important, including practise in rotating roles and cross-training to assume various roles should the need arise. Some two person ambulance teams rotate responsibilities or roles by the call, with one being the driver/skills paramedic and the other the patient contact/assessment paramedic (team leader) who will ride in the patient compartment en route to the A&E. If the call involves more team members, they are added to this basic response and one paramedic assumes the team leader role. If only two partners are on the scene, one establishes rapport and conducts the assessment of the patient, while the other handles the on-scene skills such as obtaining vital signs, applying oxygen, and inserting an IV. Because one paramedic will drive to the A&E, he or she will most probably clean the stretcher and the back of the ambulance and prepare for the next call, while the other paramedic gives the face-to-face verbal report on arrival and completes the patient clinical record (PCR).

Is this approach the perfect strategy for all ambulance units? No, it is just one way. Other strategies might work equally well. What is essential is that the roles have been practised and worked out before arriving at the patient's side. If the team has a plan and the situation is complex, the crew has a basic starting point to adapt the response or actions to meet the challenges of the environment or situation.

Pull out the equipment, break into teams, and practise simulated responses with experienced educator/evaluators to document your actions for a post-simulation analysis. Discuss what went right and what did not, and figure out how improvements can be made to the equipment, the team members' performance, and their communication within the team, with patients and families, and with leadership. The next simulation—which could be the real thing—can flow smoothly and look as if it had been practised a hundred times.

Ambulance Equipment

When Tom Wolfe wrote *The Right Stuff* in 1979, he was describing what it took to be one of the first seven astronauts selected by NASA for the space programme. Similarly, a paramedic responding to emergency calls must carry the "right stuff"—that is, equipment that is packaged and at the patient's side when you need it. As paramedics, we always need to be prepared for the worst-case scenarios, which are threats to the patient's ABCs.

Not having equipment readily available compromises care. Consider a patient who has struck his head and has altered mental status. If he started vomiting and you did not have PPE (personal protective equipment) and a suction unit, the patient could easily aspirate.

Planning which ambulance response equipment to carry is a bit like travelling on a plane with only one piece of hand luggage that will fit in the overhead locker. You need to carry the essential items, downsize to facilitate rapid movement throughout the airport, and minimise the bulk and weight of the baggage. The essential equipment needs to be carried on every call to every patient's side. It includes the equipment to conduct the initial assessment and treat life threats you may find, as well as the cardiac monitor and defibrillator. **Table B-2** ▶ summarises this set of equipment.

The specific equipment, bags, and boxes depend on your local guidelines, the typical number of paramedic and technician responders, and the difficulty in accessing the patient.

You are the Paramedic Part 2

From your initial patient assessment, it is clear that the patient is confused, yet the rest of the initial assessment seems unremarkable. Her chief complaint seems to be medical (altered mental status), so you proceed down the patient assessment algorithm and conduct a focused history and physical examination (FHPE) of a responsive medical patient—that is, you interview the patient and obtain a history before conducting the physical examination. Your partner obtains the baseline observations while you interview the patient.

Vital Signs	Recording Time: 4 Minutes
Skin	Pale, warm, and clammy
Pulse	118 beats/min; weak; regular rate
Blood pressure	110/70 mm Hg
Respirations	24 breaths/min and normal

4. What is the value of using mnemonics such as OPQRST and SAMPLE in your assessment?
5. If the patient had been "not responsive," which steps would your focused history/physical examination involve?

Table B-2	Essential Equipment
Function	**Essential Items**
Airway control	PPE (gloves, face shield, and FFP2 mask) Oral airways, nasal airways Suction unit (electric or manual) Rigid tip Yankauer and flexible suction catheters LMA, ET tubes Laryngoscope and blades Tube check, tube restraint, tape, syringes, stylet End-tidal carbon dioxide device
Breathing	Pocket mask and one-way valve bag-valve-mask ventilation device(s) (adult and child), spare masks, reservoir bag Oxygen-delivery devices (nonrebreathing mask, cannula, extension tubing) Oxygen cylinder, regulator, transport ventilator Occlusive dressings Large-bore IV cannula for thoracic decompression Pulse oximeter
Circulation	Dressings, bandages, and tape Sphygmomanometer and stethoscope Assessment card and pen Impedance threshold device (ITD) and CPR prompt AED or manual defibrillator Drug box Glucometer Venous access supplies (IV and IO)
Disability and arrhythmia	Rigid collars Pen torch ECG monitor
Exposure	Space blanket to cover the patient Scissors or Tuffcuts

General Approach to the Patient

Your general approach to the patient entails more than simply following the standardised assessment plan. You must have a calm demeanour, look the part, act the part, and have a kind manner. For some paramedics, these details come naturally; for others, they take practise. Practising your approach is essential for ensuring that you can communicate effectively and provide the level of service patients expect to receive. Most patients are not in a position to rate your ability to conduct an accurate assessment, intubate, or insert an IV line (aside from how much it hurt or how many attempts you made), but they do gauge the quality of care in terms of the "people skills" provided and the level of compassion you showed.

Your approach to the patient should be planned in advance, in terms of which team member will do most of the talking and questioning and establish the rapport with the patient while the other team members focus on the necessary skills and equipment issues. Make sure you take in the right stuff and are ready to provide resuscitative care because confusion about equipment can unnecessarily add to the level of chaos. As the paramedic doing the assessment, you must carry on an active, concerned dialogue. Take notes—and listen to what the patient tells you!

Review of the Standardised Approach to Assessment

Throughout this book, we have emphasised using the same basic approach to the assessment of the patient. In summary, every scene is assessed to locate the hazards, recognise the MOI, and ensure you have the appropriate PPE and adequate help. The first assessment for every patient is the initial assessment, which is designed to find and deal with life threats. It includes the MS-ABC-priority elements: a check of the patient's mental status using AVPU; assessment and management of the airway, breathing, and circulation; and setting the priority as high or low for this specific patient. Next, the patient is classified as medical or trauma. Although there are some crossovers (such as an elderly patient with a broken hip who had a syncopal episode), usually a patient will have one overwhelming type of problem.

Trauma patients are further subclassified into one of two groups: those with a significant MOI and those without a significant MOI. A patient with a significant MOI will get a rapid trauma examination, with baseline vital signs and SAMPLE history being taken as you prepare the patient for transport. He or she will then get a detailed physical examination and ongoing assessment en route to the A&E department. For patients with a nonsignificant MOI, the examination focuses on the injured body part and then baseline vital signs, a SAMPLE history, and transport. These patients do not routinely receive a detailed physical examination, rather they receive an ongoing assessment en route to the A&E.

Medical patients are likewise subclassified into two groups: those who are responsive and those who are not responsive. The focus in these cases is on the chief complaint, because your line of questioning will depend on how the patient presents. In all cases, you can use the OPQRST mnemonic to remember how to elaborate on the patient's chief complaint. The patient who does not respond appropriately (is not responsive) receives the same rapid examination that the trauma patient with significant MOI would receive, but it is termed the rapid physical examination in medical cases (rather than the rapid trauma examination, as in trauma cases). Next, baseline vital signs and a SAMPLE history are obtained; for a patient who is not responsive, this history may come from bystanders and family members. All medical patients receive an ongoing assessment en route to the A&E.

A medical patient who is responsive will provide you with most of the information needed to arrive at a working diagnosis if you ask the right questions. In a responsive patient, you should elaborate on the chief complaint, obtain baseline vital signs and a SAMPLE history, and conduct a physical examination that focuses on the body system involved in the chief complaint (such as a neurological examination, a cardiopulmonary examination, or an obstetrics examination). You can then conduct the ongoing assessment en route to the A&E.

From a priority or sense of urgency perspective, some trauma patients have a significant MOI and some medical patients are not responsive; with these patients, you should take an urgent, rapid resuscitative approach. Conversely, with trauma patients without a significant MOI and medical patients who are responsive, you can take a slightly more contemplative and less rushed approach. Of course, we are still conscious of the time with some responsive medical patients (such as for a possible MI or stroke)!

This approach to the patient assessment is the same for all levels of ambulance providers.

■ Presenting the Patient

Your ability to present your patient to the next link in the chain of medical care can be a key element in ensuring continuity of care. Effective communication and transfer of the patient's assessment and management data are vital to prehospital and in-hospital providers who will ultimately be responsible for the patient. Refining this skill is important so that the right amount of the right information is presented to the right person at the right time.

An Essential Skill

The number of calls involving other typical paramedic skills (such as IV insertion or drug administration) may be minimal compared with the number of times you must present the patient to another health care provider face-to-face, over the telephone, over the radio, or in writing on the PCR. Effective presentation and communications skills are essential for continuity of care and to establish trust and credibility with the A&E doctor.

Good assessment and excellent presentation skills go hand in hand. After all, you can't report or treat anything that you haven't found! A good presentation suggests effective patient

You are the Paramedic Part 3

From your examination of the patient, you have learned that she is confused about the collision and does not remember what happened. She is not sure if she passed out, although a bystander who heard the collision states that the patient was sleepy just after they got on scene at the collision.

The patient denies having any pain but thinks she is going to miss her morning meeting with her friends. By using the SAMPLE history, you find out that the patient has medication in her pocketbook, which is a clue that she has type 2 diabetes. The patient is not sure whether she had any breakfast this morning because she was running very late for her appointment.

You decide to obtain an ECG and check her blood glucose level. Your partner inserts a cannula. Her blood glucose level is very low, which is one of many possible explanations for her altered mental state.

After receiving some oral glucose, the patient seems like a different person. She is alert and very apologetic about causing so much trouble. She says she must have forgotten to eat this morning because she was in a big rush to meet her friends. She asks you to contact her daughter who lives nearby and laughs as the police officer has her take a Breathalyser test, which is found to be negative. As you prepare to leave the scene, your patient enquires about the other woman whose car she hit. You are able to tell her that fortunately, after she was disentangled, the injuries were minor because she was wearing her seatbelt.

Vital Signs	Recording Time: 10 Minutes
Skin	Pale, warm, and clammy
Pulse	118 beats/min; weak, regular rate
Blood pressure	110/p mm Hg
Respirations	24 breaths/min; normal
Blood glucose level	3 mmol/l

6. Why might you suspect that the patient has type 2 diabetes?

7. As long as she has a gag reflex, which medication options do you have?

assessment; a poor presentation suggests poor assessment and care. The format that we use minimises rambling and disjointed presentations that cover inconsequential information but omit vital information. Most health care providers are also programmed to mentally receive a patient presentation in a specific format. The format we recommend follows the SOAP mnemonic: Subjective information, Objective information, Assessment, and Plan for treatment.

A poor presentation can compromise the patient's care because the paramedic may not be "listened to" or understood by the doctor and continuity of care could suffer as a result.

Components of an Effective Patient Presentation

The format of the radio telephone pre-alert to the receiving A&E department should include the following elements:

- **Age:** Patient's age
- **Sex:** Patient's sex
- **History:** The history of the current injury or illness to include MOI and sequence of events
- **Injuries or illness:** Provisional or suspected diagnosis including vital signs
- **Interventions:** Description of treatment so far
- **Current observations:** Heart rate, blood pressure, respiratory rate GCS, etc.
- **Estimated time of arrival** (ETA) at the A&E

Face-to-face reports are usually slightly more detailed, bringing the A&E nurse or doctor up-to-date on what has transpired during your care of the patient.

An example of a telephone pre-alert report using the ASHIICE format follows:

Ambulance crew: *Charlie eight zero one to red base, over.*
Ambulance control: *Charlie eight zero one go ahead, over.*
Ambulance crew: *Request talk-through with the Barnet accident and emergency department, over.*
Ambulance control: *Roger, stand-by over.* (Ambulance control then calls the accident and emergency department and advises they have an incoming crew wishing to pre-alert them.)
Ambulance control: *Go ahead Charlie eight zero one, you have talk through with the Barnet accident and emergency department, over.*
Ambulance crew: *Charlie eight zero one to Barnet accident and emergency department how do you receive, over.*
Barnet A&E: *Strength 5 Charlie eight zero one, go ahead over.*
Ambulance crew: *We are coming in to you with a 45-year-old male motorcyclist involved in an RTC, collided with wall; estimated speed of 30 mph. The patient is conscious and alert; has a right sided, closed chest injury, possible haemo-*

pneumothorax; with reduced air entry on that side and minimal haemoptysis. He also has an open fractured right mid-shaft of femur, which has been put into a traction splint. He currently has a tachycardia of 105 and is tachypnoeic at 33. His BP is 100 systolic and he has a GCS of 15. We have given chest needle decompression to good effect, have IV access with fluids running and given him 5 mg of IV morphine. Our ETA to you will be 12 minutes, over.

The keys to developing proficiency with a radio, telephone, or a face-to-face report are repetition and understanding the format. We suggest you use an assessment card that highlights the key areas of the report. Many pocket guides include this sample format for reference. Eventually, you will no longer need the form or pocket guide to refer to because the communication format will be second nature.

Simulations Using Common Complaints Found in the Prehospital Setting

Your paramedic programme will offer scenario-based practise in the classroom setting designed to help prepare you for the supervised practice. These simulations take place after you have learned core paramedic skills (that is, ECG, IV, drug administration) and the treatment algorithms for complaints commonly encountered in the prehospital setting. You will have the opportunity to work with the typical equipment and team members just as interactions would occur in the prehospital setting.

The goals of these simulations include practising the teamwork, team leadership, and scene choreography discussed in this appendix. You will have many opportunities to work with the equipment and practise the assessment format and skills of paramedics. Likewise, you will have a chance to work on your leadership and decision-making abilities so you can provide interventions that are based on assessment and the treatment modalities in the regional treatment guidelines and the ACLS algorithms. In addition, you will have ample opportunities to practice your verbal presentation skills and documentation using the PCR for review by your paramedic faculty.

Most simulations in the classroom setting can be carried out on well-briefed "patients" or manikins designed to allow you to use your core skills. Some paramedic programmes use highly sophisticated training simulators and classrooms that provide realistic feedback to students on a real-time basis **Figure B-2 ▶**. Video has also been incorporated as a means of reviewing the simulations.

Ideally, simulations will include scenarios that allow you to practise each of the situations in (**Table B-3 ▾**). It may be helpful to associate these scenarios with the treatment guidelines and algorithms used by your ambulance service.

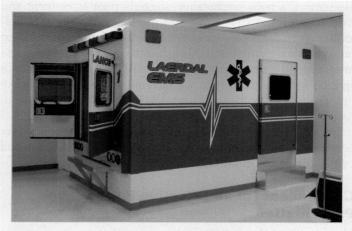

Figure B-2 This is an example of a simulations classroom used in a number of paramedic training programmes. The manikins and video can provide real-time feedback on changes in the "patient's" vital signs and reactions to your interventions.

Table B-3	Suggested Simulations		
Goals	**Scenarios**	**Goals**	**Scenarios**
Presenting Problem: **Chest pain**		**Presenting Problem:** **Cardiac arrest**	
Assess and manage	Stable with no arrhythmias Stable bradycardia Unstable bradycardia (hypotension/ chest pain) Stable supraventricular tachycardia (SVT) Unstable SVT Stable ventricular tachycardia (VT) Unstable VT Ventricular ectopy Cardiogenic shock; hypotension	Assess and manage	Trauma arrest Medical arrest Ventricular fibrillation (VF)/VT PEA/asystole Termination of resuscitation No resuscitation indicated
		Identify/differentiate	Blunt trauma with tension pneumothorax Electrocution Drowning/submersion Hypothermia
Identify/differentiate	ACS Unstable angina Aortic aneurysm Pulmonary embolism Pneumothorax Oesophageal rupture	**Abdominal pain**	
		Assess and manage	Acute abdominal pain Chronic abdominal pain
		Identify/differentiate	AMI Aortic aneurysm Renal colic Ruptured ectopic pregnancy Cholecystitis Appendicitis Hernia or intestinal obstruction
GI bleeding			
Identify/differentiate	Upper GI bleeding Lower GI bleeding		
Altered mental status			
Identify/differentiate	Alcohol overdose Drug ingestion or overdose Idiopathic convulsion disorder Hypoglycaemia or hyperglycaemia Stroke or TIA (transient ischaemic attack) Head injury	**Hazardous materials or toxicology**	
		Assess and manage	Accidental toxic ingestion or inhalation Chemical burn or contact dermatitis Chemicals in the eyes Overdose or street drug use

Table B-3	Suggested Simulations (continued)

Goals	Scenarios	Goals	Scenarios
Presenting Problem: Dyspnoea		**Presenting Problem: Trauma**	
Identify/differentiate	Emphysema or chronic bronchitis Asthma or acute bronchospasm Acute pulmonary oedema or left-sided heart failure ACS, AMI, or angina Foreign body airway obstruction Pneumonia Pulmonary embolism Spontaneous pneumothorax Hyperventilation syndrome/carpopedal spasm Smoke or toxic inhalation	Assess and manage	Isolated extremity fracture (tibia/fibula or radius/ulna) Femur fracture (hip, midshaft, supracondylar) Shoulder dislocation Clavicular fracture or AC separation Minor wounds Spinal injuries Multiple trauma, blunt Penetrating trauma Impaled object Fall of an older person Athletic injury Head injury
Syncope		Identify/differentiate	Minor wound, no sutures required Minor wound, sutures required High-risk wounds Wound with tendon and/or nerve injury Spine injury, with or without neurological deficit Concussion Subdural or extradural haematoma
Identify/differentiate	Cardiac-related (such as bradycardia, heart block, reentry SVT, VT) Vascular or volume causes (such as medication-induced, hypovolaemia, carotid sinus stimulation, postural, vasovagal) Metabolic (hypoglycaemic or hyperventilation) Neurogenic (TIA or convulsion)		
Convulsion		**Allergic reactions, bites, envenomation**	
Differentiate	Idiopathic Fever Neoplasms Infection Metabolic (such as hypoxia, hypoglycaemia, thyrotoxicosis, hypocalcaemia) Drug intoxication or withdrawal Head trauma Eclampsia Cerebral degenerative disease	Assess and manage	Bee sting or other envenomation (such as from an adder) Human bite
		Identify/differentiate	Local allergic reaction and systemic allergic reaction
		Behavioural	
		Assess and manage	Mood disorders (depression, bipolar) Schizophrenic and delusional disorders Suicidal
Environmental		**Obstetric/gynaecologic**	
Assess and manage	Hypothermia Hyperthermia Superficial or deep frostbite Thermal burns Smoke inhalation Drowning/submersion	Assess and manage	Vaginal bleeding Childbirth (normal and abnormal)
		Identify	Ectopic pregnancy
		Paediatric	
		Assess and manage	Respiratory distress, failure, and arrest Shock Cardiopulmonary failure and arrest Major trauma Fever Convulsions
		Identify/differentiate	Respiratory distress, failure, and arrest Upper airway obstruction and lower airway disease Cardiogenic vs noncardiogenic shock Major and minor trauma

You are the Paramedic Summary

1. What are some of the potential causes of a head-on collision in which the driver never hit the brakes?

Patients who suddenly lose consciousness, fall asleep at the wheel, or are highly intoxicated often veer off the road without hitting their brakes.

2. What is the significance of the MOI in this collision for your patient?

There was significant damage to the front of both vehicles, which means the patient's body may have absorbed significant energy in the form of blunt trauma. This possibility sets the tone of and priority for the assessment.

3. If it is clear that your patient was not wearing a seatbelt, how could this fact change things?

Without a seatbelt, the focus in a frontal collision is whether the patient took the up-and-over or down-and-under pathway in relationship to the dashboard and steering wheel. The up-and-over pathway is associated with head, neck, and chest injuries. The down-and-under pathway is associated with knee, leg, hip, and lower spine injuries.

4. What is the value of using mnemonics like the OPQRST and SAMPLE in your assessment?

The mnemonics help you remember key assessment questions during the focused history and physical examination. OPQRST is used to elaborate on the chief complaint. It stands for Onset; Provocation; Quality; Region, referral, or radiation; Severity; and Time. The SAMPLE history helps you obtain the patient's medical history. It stands for Signs/symptoms, Allergies, Medications, Pertinent past medical history (such as recent hospital visits, diseases, or conditions such as epilepsy, a heart condition, or diabetes), Last oral intake, and Events leading up to today's incident.

5. If the patient had been "not responsive," which steps would your focused history/physical examination (FHPE) have involved?

If your patient was not responsive, the FHPE would take a fast track that involves the rapid medical examination and the baseline vital signs. The SAMPLE history would be obtained from bystanders or family members because the patient was unable to talk. The rapid medical examination would be basically the same as the rapid trauma assessment that involves a quick hands-on examination of the head, neck, chest, abdomen, back, buttocks, and four extremities.

6. Why might you suspect that your patient has type 2 diabetes?

Because she has no obvious trauma and altered mental status, hypoglycaemia is one of several differential diagnoses you might consider. The blood glucose test is a quick way to see exactly what her blood glucose level is. In this case, with a blood glucose level less than 4 mmol/l and her oral diabetic medications, you suspect type 2 diabetes. As a general rule, people with type 1 diabetes take insulin because their pancreas does not make insulin. People with type 2 diabetes usually regulate their blood glucose levels with diet control, exercise, and oral medications.

7. As long as she has a gag reflex, which medication options do you have?

When a person with diabetes has a gag reflex and altered mental status, you can administer glucose onto the gums or a sugary drink or chocolate bar. If you have a good IV site that will not infiltrate, give glucose 10%. Glucagon is another option.

Glossary

aberrant conduction The abnormal conduction of the electrical impulse through the heart.

ABO system The antigen classification given to blood.

abortion Expulsion of the fetus, from any cause, before the 20th week of gestation.

abrasion An injury in which a portion of the body is denuded of epidermis by scraping or rubbing.

abruptio placenta A premature separation of the placenta from the wall of the uterus.

abscess A collection of pus in a sac, formed by necrotic tissues and an accumulation of white blood cells.

abscesses Areas created as a result of infection within the brain or spinal cord, in which brain cells have been attacked and tissue destroyed. The immune system erects a wall to prevent spread of the infection, which results in a pus-filled area buried in tissue.

absence convulsions The type of convulsions characterised by a brief lapse of attention in which the patient may stare and not respond; formerly known as petit mal convulsions.

absolute refractory period The early phase of cardiac repolarisation, wherein the heart muscle cannot be stimulated to depolarise.

absorption The process by which a medication's molecules are moved from the site of entry or administration into the body and into systemic circulation.

absorption (hazardous materials) A type of decontamination that is done with large pads that the hazardous materials team carry to soak up liquid and remove it from the patient.

abuse Any form of maltreatment that results in harm or loss. Maltreatment may be physical, sexual, psychological, or financial/material.

acceleration The rate of change in velocity.

acetylcholine A chemical mediator of the parasympathetic nervous system.

acholic stools Light, clay-coloured stools caused by liver failure.

acidosis A blood pH of less than 7.35.

acquired immunity A highly specific, inducible, discriminatory, and permanent method by which literally armies of cells respond to an immune stimulant.

acrocyanosis A decrease in the amount of oxygen delivered to the extremities. The hands and feet turn blue because of narrowing (constriction) of small arterioles (tiny arteries) toward the end of the arms and legs.

activation Mediators of inflammation trigger the appearance of molecules known as selectins and integrins on the surfaces of endothelial cells and PMNs, respectively.

active hyperaemia The dilation of arterioles after transient arteriolar constriction, which allows influx of blood under increased pressure.

active neglect The refusal or failure to fulfil an obligation; a conscious or intentional attempt to inflict physical or emotional stress. Examples include abandonment and denial of food or health-related services.

activities of daily living (ADLs) Normal everyday activities such as getting dressed, brushing teeth, taking out the rubbish, etc.

acute coronary syndrome Term used to describe any group of clinical symptoms consistent with acute myocardial ischaemia.

acute dystonic reaction A syndrome that may occur in patients taking typical antipsychotic agents. The patient develops muscle spasms of the neck, face, and back within a few days of starting treatment with the drug.

acute myocardial infarction (AMI) A condition present when a period of cardiac ischaemia caused by sudden narrowing or complete occlusion of a coronary artery leads to death (necrosis) of myocardial tissue.

acute radiation syndrome The clinical course that usually begins within hours of exposure to a radiation source. Symptoms include nausea, vomiting, diarrhoea, fatigue, fever, and headache. The long-term symptoms are dose-related and are haematopoietic and gastrointestinal.

acute renal failure (ARF) A sudden decrease in filtration through the glomeruli.

acute respiratory distress syndrome (ARDS) A respiratory syndrome characterised by respiratory insufficiency and hypoxaemia.

adhesion The attachment of PMNs to endothelial cells, mediated by selectins and integrins.

adipose Referring to fat tissue.

adipose tissue A connective tissue containing large amounts of lipids; fat tissue.

adolescents Individuals who are 12 to 18 years of age.

adrenal cortex The outer part of the adrenal glands that produces corticosteroids.

adrenal glands Endocrine glands located on top of the kidneys that release adrenaline when stimulated by the sympathetic nervous system.

adrenal medulla The inner part of the adrenal glands that produces catecholamines (adrenaline and noradrenaline).

adrenaline Hormone produced by the adrenal medulla that plays a vital role in the function of the sympathetic nervous system.

adrenergic Pertaining to nerves that release the neurotransmitter noradrenaline (such as adrenergic nerves, adrenergic response). The term also pertains to the receptors acted on by noradrenaline, that is, the adrenergic receptors.

adrenocorticotropic hormone (ACTH) Hormone that targets the adrenal cortex to secrete cortisol (a glucocorticoid).

adventitious A type of breath sound that occurs in addition to the normal breath sounds; examples are crackles and wheezes.

aerobic metabolism Metabolism that can proceed only in the presence of oxygen.

aetiology The cause of a disease process.

affect The outward expression of a person's mood.

afferent arteriole The structure in the kidney that supplies blood to the glomerulus.

afferent nerves The nerves that carry sensory impulses from all parts of the body to the brain.

affinity The force attraction between medications and receptors causing them to bind together.

afterdrop Continued fall in core temperature after a victim of hypothermia has been removed from a cold environment, due at least in part to the return of cold blood from the body surface to the body core.

afterload The pressure in the aorta against which the left ventricle must pump blood.

agitation Extreme restlessness and anxiety.

agnosia Inability to connect an object with its correct name.

agonal rhythm A cardiac arrhythmia seen just before the heart stops altogether; essentially asystole with occasional QRS complexes that are not associated with cardiac output.

agonists Molecules that bind to a cell's receptor and trigger a response by that cell. Agonists produce some kind of action or biological effect.

agoraphobia Literally, "fear of the marketplace"; fear of entering a public place from which escape may be impeded.

alcoholism A state of physical and psychological addiction to ethyl alcohol.

aldosterone One of the two main hormones responsible for adjustments to the final composition of urine, aldosterone increases the rate of active resorption of sodium and chloride ions into the blood and decreases resorption of potassium.

alkalosis A blood pH greater than 7.45.

allergen Any substance that causes a hypersensitivity reaction.

allergy Hypersensitivity reaction to the presence of an agent (allergen) that is intrinsically harmless.

alpha Type of energy that is emitted from a strong radiological source; it is the least harmful penetrating type of radiation and cannot travel fast or through most objects.

alveolar ridges The ridges between the teeth, which are covered with thickened connective tissue and epithelium.

alveoli Sac-like units at the end of the bronchioles where gas exchange takes place (singular: alveolus).

Alzheimer's disease A progressive organic condition in which neurons die, causing dementia.

ambulance commander (AC) The overall leader (silver) of ambulance operations, and accountable for all medical activity at the scene.

ambulance loading officer Delegated role from the ambulance commander, the person who coordinates transportation and distribution of patients to appropriate receiving hospitals.

ambulance parking officer Delegated role from the ambulance commander, the person who locates an area to store equipment and personnel and tracks ambulance arrival and deployment from the parking area.

amenorrhoea Absence of menstruation.

amnesia Loss of memory.

amniotic fluid A clear, slightly yellowish liquid that surrounds the unborn baby (fetus) during pregnancy; contained in the amniotic sac.

amniotic sac The fluid-filled, baglike membrane in which the fetus develops.

amphetamines A class of drugs that increase alertness and excitation (that is, stimulants); includes methamphetamine (crank or ice), methylenedioxyamphetamine (MDA, Adam), and methylenedioxymethamphetamine (MDMA, Eve, ecstasy).

amputation An injury in which part of the body is completely severed.

amyotrophic lateral sclerosis (ALS) Also known as Lou Gehrig's disease, this disease strikes the voluntary motor neurons, causing their death. It is characterised by fatigue and general weakness of muscle groups; eventually, the patient will not be able to walk, eat, or speak.

anaemia A lower than normal haemoglobin or erythrocyte level.

anaerobic metabolism The metabolism that takes place in the absence of oxygen; the principal product is lactic acid.

anaesthesia Lack of feeling within a body part.

anaesthetic A type of medication intended to induce a loss of sensation to touch or pain.

analgesia The absence of the sensation of pain.

analgesics A classification for medications that relieve pain, or induce analgesia.

anaphylactic shock A severe hypersensitivity reaction that involves bronchoconstriction and cardiovascular collapse.

anaphylaxis An unusual or exaggerated allergic reaction to foreign protein or other substances.

androgens Male sex hormones that regulate body changes associated with sexual development (puberty), including growth spurts, deepening of the voice, growth of facial and pubic hair, and muscle growth and strength.

aneurysm A swelling or enlargement of part of a blood vessel, resulting from weakening of the vessel wall.

anger A strong, negative emotion that may be a response to illness, and which could result in aggressive behaviour on the part of the patient.

angina pectoris The sudden pain from myocardial ischaemia, caused by diminished circulation to the cardiac muscle. The pain is usually substernal and often radiates to the arms, jaw, or abdomen and usually lasts 3 to 5 minutes and disappears with rest.

angiogenesis The growth of new blood vessels.

angio-oedema Recurrent large areas of subcutaneous oedema of sudden onset, usually disappearing within 24 hours, which is seen mainly in young women, frequently as a result of allergy to food or drugs; may cause profound swelling of the tongue and lips.

angiotensin converting enzyme (ACE) inhibitors Medications that suppress the conversion of angiotensin I to angiotensin II.

angiotensin II receptor antagonists Medications that are similar to ACE inhibitors but work by selectively blocking angiotensin II at their receptor sites.

angle of impact The angle at which an object hits another; this characterises the force vectors involved and has a bearing on patterns of energy dissipation.

anisocoria A condition in which the pupils are not of equal size.

anorexia nervosa An eating disorder in which a person diets by exerting extraordinary control over his or her eating, and loses weight to the point of jeopardising his or her health and life.

antagonist A molecule that blocks the ability of a given chemical to bind to its receptor, preventing a biological response.

antenatal The state of the pregnant woman before birth.

antepartum Before delivery.

anterior chamber The anterior area of the globe between the lens and the cornea that is filled with aqueous humour.

anterograde (post-traumatic) amnesia Loss of memory relating to events that occurred after the injury.

anthrax A deadly bacteria (Bacillus anthracis) that lays dormant in a spore (protective shell); the germ is released from the spore when exposed to the optimal temperature and moisture. The route of entry is inhalation, cutaneous, or gastrointestinal (from consuming food that contains spores).

anti-arrhythmic medications The medications used to treat and prevent cardiac rhythm disorders.

antibiotic medications The medications that fight bacterial infection by killing the bacteria or by preventing multiplication of the bacteria to allow the body's immune system to overcome them.

antibodies Proteins secreted by certain immune cells that bind antigens to make them more visible to the immune system.

anticholinergic Of or pertaining to the blocking of acetylcholine receptors, resulting in inhibition of transmission of parasympathetic nerve impulses.

anti-coagulant drugs The medications used to prevent intravascular thrombosis by preventing blood coagulation in the vascular system.

antidiuretic hormone (ADH) A hormone secreted by the posterior pituitary lobe of the pituitary gland, ADH constricts blood vessels and raises the blood pressure; also called vasopressin.

antigens Substances (usually protein) identified as foreign to the body.

anti-hypertensives The medications used to control blood pressure.

anti-neoplastic medications The medications designed to combat cancer.

anti-platelet agents The medications that interfere with the collection of platelets.

antipsychotic drugs Medications used to control psychosis.

anuria A complete stop in the production of urine.

anxiety disorder A mental disorder in which the dominant mood is fear and apprehension.

anxious avoidant attachment A bond between an infant and his or her parent or caregiver in which the infant is repeatedly rejected and develops an isolated lifestyle that does not depend upon the support and care of others.

aorta The largest artery in the body, originating from the left ventricle.

aortic valve The valve between the left ventricle and the aorta.

Apgar scoring system A scoring system for assessing the status of a newborn that assigns a number value to each of five areas of assessment.

apnoea Respiratory pause greater than or equal to 20 seconds.

apoptosis Normal, genetically programmed cell death.

apparent life-threatening event (ALTE) An unexpected sudden episode of colour change, tone change, or apnoea that required mouth-to-mouth resuscitation or vigorous stimulation.

apraxia Inability to connect an object with its proper use.

aqueous humour The clear, watery fluid in the anterior chamber of the globe.

arachnoid The middle membrane of the three meninges that enclose the brain and spinal cord.

arrhythmias Disturbances in cardiac rhythm.

arterial air embolism Air bubbles in the arterial blood vessels.

arteries The muscular, thick-walled blood vessels that carry blood away from the heart.

arteriole A small blood vessel that carries oxygenated blood, branching into yet smaller vessels called capillaries.

arteriosclerosis A pathological condition in which the arterial walls become thickened and inelastic.

arthritis Joint inflammation that causes pain, swelling, stiffness, and decreased range of motion.

Arthus reaction A localised reaction involving vascular inflammation in response to an IgG-mediated allergic response.

artifact An artificial product; in cardiology, is used to refer to noise or interference in an ECG tracing.

arytenoid cartilages One of the paired, pitcher-shaped cartilages at the back of the larynx, at the upper border of the cricoid cartilage.

ascities Abdominal oedema typically caused by liver failure.

asphyxia Condition of severely deficient supply of oxygen to the body leading to end organ damage.

asphyxiant Any gas that displaces oxygen from the atmosphere; can be deadly if exposure occurs in a confined space.

assault Unlawfully placing a person in fear of immediate bodily harm.

asthma A chronic inflammatory lower airway condition resulting in intermittent wheezing and excess mucus production.

asynchronous In CPR, when two rescuers do ventilations and compressions individually and not timed or waiting for the other rescuer to pause.

asystole The absence of ventricular contractions; a "straight-line ECG".

ataxia Inability to coordinate the muscles properly; often used to describe a staggering gait.

atelectasis Collapse of the alveolar air spaces of the lungs.

atherosclerosis A disorder in which cholesterol and calcium build up inside the walls of the blood vessels, forming plaque, which eventually leads to partial or complete blockage of blood flow.

atopic The medical term for having an allergic tendency.

atresia The process by which an oocyte dies.

atrial kick The addition to ventricular volume contributed by contraction of the atria.

atrioventricular (AV) node A specialised structure located in the AV junction that slows conduction through the AV junction.

atrioventricular (AV) valves The mitral and tricuspid valves.

atrophy A decrease in cell size due to a loss of subcellular components.

atropine A parasympathetic blocker; opposes the action of acetylcholine on the heart and elsewhere, thereby allowing the body's natural sympathetic system to speed up the heart rate.

atropine-like effects Results of some antipsychotic medications that include side effects similar to atropine, resulting in dry mouth, blurred vision, urinary retention, and cardiac arrhythmias.

auditory ossicles The bones that function in hearing and are located deep within cavities of the temporal bone.

aura Sensations experienced before an attack occurs. Common in convulsions and migraine headaches.

auricle The large outside portion of the ear through which sound waves enter the ear; also called the pinna.

auscultation The method of listening to sounds within the body with a stethoscope.

autoantibodies Antibodies directed against the patient.

autocrine hormone A hormone that acts on the cell that has secreted it.

autoimmune disorders Disorders in which the body identifies its own antigen as a foreign body and activates the inflammatory system.

autoimmunity The production of antibodies or T cells that work against the tissues of a person's own body, producing autoimmune disease or a hypersensitivity reaction.

automaticity Spontaneous initiation of depolarising electric impulses by pacemaker sites within the electric conduction system of the heart.

autonomic nervous system (ANS) The component of the peripheral nervous system that sends sensory impulses from internal structures (such as blood vessels, the heart, and organs of the chest, abdomen, and pelvis) through afferent autonomic nerves to the brain.

autoregulation An increase in mean arterial pressure to compensate for decreased cerebral perfusion pressure; compensatory response of the body to shunt blood to the brain; manifests clinically as hypertension.

autosomal dominant A pattern of inheritance that involves genes that are located on autosomes or the nonsex chromosomes. You only need to inherit a single copy of a particular form of a gene to show the trait.

autosomal recessive A pattern of inheritance that involves genes located on autosomes or the nonsex chromosomes. You must inherit two copies of a particular form of a gene to show the trait.

AV junction The atrioventricular junction; the portion of the electric conduction system of the heart located in the upper part of the interventricular septum that conducts the excitation impulse from the atria to the bundle of His.

avulsing A tearing away or forcible separation.

avulsion An injury that leaves a piece of skin or other tissue partially or completely torn away from the body.

awareness The first level of rescue training provided to all responders, with an emphasis on recognising the hazards, securing the scene, and calling for appropriate assistance. There is no actual use of rescue skills.

axon Long, slender extension of a neuron (nerve cell) that conducts electrical impulses away from the neuronal soma.

azotaemia Increased nitrogenous wastes in the blood.

bacteria Micro-organisms that reproduce by binary fission. These single-cell organisms reproduce rapidly. Some can form spores (encysted variants) when environmental conditions are harsh.

bacterial vaginosis An overgrowth of bacteria in the vagina, characterised by itching, burning, or pain, and possibly a "fishy" smelling discharge.

bandage Material used to secure a dressing in place.

barbiturates Any medications of a group of barbituric acid derivatives that act as central nervous system depressants and are used as sedatives or hypnotics.

barometric energy The energy that results from sudden changes in pressure as may occur in a diving accident or sudden decompression in an airplane.

barotrauma Injury resulting from pressure disequilibrium across body surfaces, for example from too much pressure in the lungs.

Bartholin glands The glands that secrete mucus for sexual lubrication.

basal ganglia Structures located deep within the cerebrum, diencephalon, and midbrain that have an important role in coordination of motor movements and posture.

basal metabolic rate (BMR) The heat energy produced at rest from normal body metabolic reactions, determined mostly by the liver and skeletal muscles.

base station Assembly of radio equipment consisting of at least a transmitter, receiver, and antenna connection at a fixed location.

basilar skull fractures Usually occur following diffuse impact to the head (such as falls, road traffic collisions); generally result from extension of a linear fracture to the base of the skull and can be difficult to diagnose with a radiograph (X-ray).

basophils Approximately 1% of the leucocytes, they are essential to nonspecific immune response to inflammation due to their role in releasing histamine and other chemicals that dilate blood vessels.

battery Unlawfully touching a person; this includes providing emergency care without consent.

Battle's sign Bruising over the mastoid bone behind the ear commonly seen following a basilar skull fracture; also called retroauricular bruising.

behaviour The way people act or perform, for example how they react/respond to a situation.

behavioural emergencies An emergency in which the patient's presenting problem is some disorder of mood, thought, or behaviour that interferes with their activities of daily living (ADLs).

Bell's palsy A temporary paralysis of the facial nerve (7th cranial nerve), which controls the muscles on each side of the face.

benzodiazepines Any medications of a group of psychotropic agents used as anti-anxiety, muscle relaxants, sedatives, or hypnotics.

bereavement Sadness from loss; grieving.

beta Type of energy that is emitted from a strong radiological source; is slightly more penetrating than alpha, and requires a layer of clothing to stop it.

beta-2 agonist Pharmacological agent that stimulates the beta-2 receptor sites found in smooth muscle; include common bronchodilators like salbutamol and terbutaline.

bigeminy An arrhythmia in which every other heartbeat is a premature contraction.

bioavailability The amount of a medication that is still active once it reaches its target tissue.

biological half-life The time it takes the body to eliminate half of the drug.

biomechanics The study of the physiology and mechanics of a living organism using the tools of mechanical engineering.

Biot's respirations Characterised by an irregular rate, pattern, and volume of breathing with intermittent periods of apnoea; also called ataxic respirations.

biotelemetry Transmission of physiological data, such as an ECG, from the patient to a distant point of reception (commonly referred to in the ambulance service as "telemetry").

biotransformation A process by which a medication is chemically converted to a different compound or metabolite.

bipolar mood disorder A disorder in which a person alternates between mania and depression.

blast front The leading edge of the shock wave.

blastocyst The term for an oocyte once it has been fertilised and multiplies into cells.

blood pressure The pressure exerted by the pulsatile flow of blood against the arterial walls.

blood The fluid that is pumped by the heart through the arteries, veins, and capillaries and consists of plasma and formed elements or cells, such as red blood cells, white blood cells, and platelets.

blow-by technique A method of delivering oxygen by holding a face mask or similar device near an infant's or a child's face; used when a nonrebreathing mask is not tolerated.

blowout fracture A fracture to the floor of the orbit usually caused by a blow to the eye.

blunt cardiac injury Contusion as the heart is compressed between the sternum and the spine.

blunt trauma An impact on the body by objects that cause injury without penetrating soft tissues or internal organs and cavities.

body In the context of the uterus, the portion below the fundus that begins to taper and narrow.

body holding area An area near to but separate from the casualty clearing area where the deceased can be stored prior to their removal from the scene. This area is usually guarded by a police officer and should be shielded as far as practicable from public view.

bonding The formation of a close, personal relationship.

bone marrow Specialised tissue found within bone.

borborygmi A bowel sound characterised by increased activity within the bowel.

borderline personality disorder A disorder characterised by disordered images of self, impulsive and unpredictable behaviour, marked shifts in mood, and instability in relationships with others.

botulinum Produced by bacteria, this is a very potent neurotoxin. When introduced into the body, this neurotoxin affects the nervous system's ability to function and causes muscle paralysis.

botulism Poisoning from eating food containing botulinum toxin.

bradycardia A slow heart rate, less than 60 beats/min; less than 100 beats/min in the newborn.

bradykinesia The slowing down of voluntary body movements. Found in Parkinson's disease.

brain Part of the central nervous system located within the cranium; contains billions of neurons that serve a variety of vital functions.

brain stem The area of the brain between the spinal cord and cerebrum, surrounded by the cerebellum; controls functions that are necessary for life, such as respirations.

breech presentation A delivery in which the buttocks come out first.

brisance The shattering effect of a shock wave and its ability to cause disruption of tissues and structures.

British Paramedic Association (BPA) The professional body for paramedics.

bronchial breath sounds A loud, harsh breath sound with equally long inspiratory and expiratory phases; heard over the peripheral chest (where vesicular sounds should be heard), indicating lung consolidation.

bronchiolitis A condition seen in children younger than 2 years, characterised by dyspnoea and wheezing.

bronchoconstriction Narrowing of the bronchial tubes.

bronchodilation Widening of the bronchial tubes.

bronchospasm Severe constriction of the bronchial tree.

bronze equipment officer Delegated role from the ambulance commander, the position that helps procure and stockpile equipment and supplies during an incident.

bruising Extravasation of blood under the skin to produce a "black-and-blue" mark.

bruit An abnormal "whoosh"-like sound of turbulent blood flow moving through a narrowed artery.

buboes Enlarged lymph nodes (up to the size of tennis balls) that were characteristic of people infected with the bubonic plague.

bubonic plague An epidemic that spread throughout Europe in the Middle Ages, causing over 25 million deaths, also called the Black Death, transmitted by infected fleas and characterised by acute malaise, fever, and the formation of tender, enlarged, inflamed lymph nodes that appear as lesions, called buboes.

buccal route A medication route in which medication is administered between the cheeks and gums.

buffers Molecules that modulate changes in pH to keep it in the physiological range.

bulimia nervosa An eating disorder characterised by consumption of large amounts of food, and for which the patient then sometimes compensates by using purging techniques.

bundle branch block A disturbance in electric conduction through the right or left bundle branch from the bundle of His.

bundle of His The portion of the electric conduction system in the interventricular septum that conducts the depolarising impulse from the atrioventricular junction to the right and left bundle branches.

burn shock The shock or hypoperfusion caused by a burn injury and the tremendous loss of fluids.

caladium A common houseplant that contains caladium oxalate crystals; ingestion leads to nausea, vomiting, and diarrhoea.

calcitonin The hormone secreted by the thyroid gland that helps maintain normal calcium levels in the blood.

calcium channel blockers The medications that suppress arrhythmias, provide more oxygen to the heart via coronary artery dilation, and reduce peripheral vascular resistance.

calyces (singular: calyx) Large urinary tubes that branch off the renal pelvis and connect with the renal pyramids to collect the urine draining from the collecting tubules.

capacitance vessels The smallest venules.

cape cyanosis Deep cyanosis of the face and neck and across the chest and back; associated with little or no blood flow after a large pulmonary embolism; it is particularly ominous.

capillaries Extremely narrow blood vessels composed of a single layer of cells through which oxygen and nutrients pass to the tissues. Capillaries form a network between arterioles and venules.

capillary refill time A test done on the fingers or toes by briefly squeezing the toe or finger, then evaluating the time it takes for the pink colour to return.

capsule A cylindrical gelatin container enclosing a dose of medication.

carbamates A more recent development than organophosphates, they are derivatives of carbamic acid. They are mainly used to control insect pests in agriculture and horticulture. As with organophosphates, they inhibit the action of acetylcholine at the nerve synapses.

carbon monoxide A chemical asphyxiant that results in a cellular respiratory failure; this gas has roughly a 240 times greater affinity for haemoglobin than oxygen, which leads to oxygen becoming inaccessible at cellular level.

cardiac cycle The period from one cardiac contraction to the next. Each cardiac cycle consists of ventricular contraction (systole) and relaxation (diastole).

cardiac glycosides A classification of medications that naturally occur in plant substances and that block certain ionic pumps in the heart cells' membranes, which indirectly increases calcium concentrations; an example is digoxin.

cardiac output (CO) Amount of blood pumped by the heart per minute, calculated by multiplying the stroke volume by the heart rate per minute.

cardiac tamponade Restriction of cardiac contraction, failing cardiac output, and shock, caused by the accumulation of fluid or blood in the pericardium.

cardiogenic shock A condition caused by loss of 40% or more of the functioning myocardium; the heart is no longer able to circulate sufficient blood to maintain adequate oxygen delivery.

cardiopulmonary arrest The sudden and often unexpected cessation of adequate cardiac output.

cardiovascular collapse Failure of the heart and blood vessels; shock.

cardioversion The use of a synchronised direct current (DC) electric shock to convert tachyarrhythmias (such as atrial flutter) to normal sinus rhythm.

carina Point at which the trachea bifurcates into the right and left mainstem bronchi.

carpopedal spasm Contorted position of the hand in which the fingers flex in a clawlike attitude and the thumb curls toward the palm.

castor bean A seed that contains the poison ricin; causes a variety of toxic effects: burning of the mouth and throat; nausea, vomiting, diarrhoea, and severe stomach pains; prostration; failing vision and kidney failure, which is the usual cause of death.

casualty clearing officer Delegated role from the ambulance commander, the person responsible for locating, setting up, and supervising casualty clearing station.

catatonic Lacking expression or movement, or appearing rigid.

catatonic type A type of schizophrenia in which the person displays odd motor activity, such as strange facial expression or rigidity.

catecholamines Hormones produced by the adrenal medulla (adrenaline and noradrenaline) that assist the body in coping with physical and emotional stress by increasing the heart and respiratory rates and the blood pressure.

caustics Chemicals that are acids or alkalis; cause direct chemical injury to the tissues they contact.

cavitation Cavity formation; shock waves that push tissues in front of and lateral to the projectile and may not necessarily increase the wound size or cause permanent injury but can result in cavitation.

CCBRN A mnemonic for the five types of terrorist incidents that emergency services may be confronted with in the prehospital environment.

cell-mediated immunity Immune process by which T-cell lymphocytes recognise antigens and then secrete cytokines (specifically lymphokines) that attract other cells or stimulate the production of cytotoxic cells that kill the infected cells.

cell signalling The process by which cells communicate with one another.

central cyanosis Bluish colouration of the skin due to the presence of deoxygenated haemoglobin in blood vessels near the skin surface.

central nervous system (CNS) The brain and spinal cord.

central neurogenic hyperventilation Deep, rapid respirations; similar to Kussmaul, but without an acetone breath odour; commonly seen following brain stem injury.

central shock A term that describes shock secondary to central pump failure, it includes both cardiogenic shock and obstructive shock.

central venous cannula A cannula inserted into the vena cava to permit intermittent or continuous monitoring of central venous pressure and to facilitate obtaining blood samples for chemical analysis.

central vision The visualisation of objects directly in front of you.

cerebellum The region of the brain essential in coordinating muscle movements in the body; also called the athlete's brain.

cerebral concussion Occurs when the brain is jarred around in the skull; a mild diffuse brain injury that does not result in structural damage or permanent neurological impairment.

cerebral contusion A focal brain injury in which brain tissue is bruised and damaged in a defined area.

cerebral cortex The largest portion of the cerebrum; regulates voluntary skeletal movement and one's level of awareness—a part of consciousness.

cerebral oedema Cerebral water; causes or contributes to swelling of the brain.

cerebral palsy (CP) A developmental condition in which damage is done to the brain. It presents during infancy as delays in walking or crawling, and can take on a spastic form in which muscles are in a near constant state of contraction.

cerebral perfusion pressure (CPP) The pressure of blood flow through the brain; the difference between the mean arterial pressure (MAP) and intracranial pressure (ICP).

cerebrospinal fluid (CSF) Fluid produced in the ventricles of the brain that flows in the subarachnoid space and bathes the meninges.

cerebrospinal fluid shunts Tubes that drain fluid manufactured in the ventricles of the brain from the subarachnoid space to another part of the body outside of the brain, such as the peritoneum; lowers pressure in the brain.

cerebrospinal rhinorrhoea Cerebrospinal fluid drainage from the nose.

cerebrovascular event (CVE) An interruption of blood flow to the brain that results in the loss of brain function.

cerebrum The largest portion of the brain; responsible for higher functions, such as reasoning; divided into right and left hemispheres, or halves.

cervical canal The interior of the cervix.

cervix The narrowest portion of the uterus that opens into the vagina.

chancroid A highly contagious STI caused by the bacteria Haemophilus ducreyi, which causes painful sores (ulcers), usually of the genitals.

chemical asphyxiants Substances that interfere with the utilisation of oxygen at the cellular level.

chemical energy The energy released as a result of a chemical reaction.

chemical name A description of the drug's chemical composition and molecular structure.

chemotactic factors The factors that cause cells to migrate into an area.

chemotaxins Components of the activated complement system that attract leucocytes from the circulation to help fight infections.

chemotaxis The movement of additional white blood cells to an area of inflammation in response to the release of chemical mediators, such as neutrophils, injured tissue, and monocytes.

chemotherapy The introduction of either single cytotoxic drugs or combinations of cytotoxic drugs into the body for the purpose of interrupting or eradicating malignant cellular growth.

CHEMSAFE An organisation that provides expert advice and information in the event of chemical incidents. It can be contacted via ambulance control.

Cheyne-Stokes respirations The respirations that are fast and then become slow, with intervening periods of apnoea; commonly seen following brain stem injury.

chief complaint The problem for which the patient is seeking help.

chlamydia An STI caused by the bacterium Chlamydia trachomatis.

chlorine (CL) The first chemical agent ever used in warfare. It has a distinct odour of bleach, and creates a green haze when released as a gas. Initially it produces upper airway irritation and a choking sensation.

choanal atresia A narrowing or blockage of the nasal airway by membranous or bony tissue; a congenital condition, meaning it is present at birth.

chocking Short lengths of wood that are used to stabilise vehicles.

cholestasis A common liver disease that occurs only during pregnancy, in which the flow of bile is altered resulting in acids being released into the bloodstream, causing profuse and painful itching.

cholinergic Fibres in the parasympathetic nervous system that release a chemical called acetylcholine.

chordae tendineae Fibrous strands shaped like umbrella stays that attach the free edges of the leaflets, or cusps, of the atrioventricular valves to the papillary muscles.

choroid plexus Specialised cells within the hollow areas in the ventricles of the brain that produce CSF.

chronic bronchitis Chronic inflammatory condition affecting the bronchi that is associated with excess mucous production that results from overgrowth of the mucous glands in the airways.

chronic hypertension A blood pressure that is equal to or greater than 140/90 mm Hg, which exists prior to pregnancy, occurs before the 20th week of pregnancy, or continues to persist postpartum.

chronic obstructive pulmonary disease (COPD) Illnesses that cause obstructive problems in the lower airways, including chronic bronchitis, emphysema, and sometimes asthma.

chronic renal failure (CRF) Progressive and irreversible inadequate kidney function due to permanent loss of nephrons.

chronotropic Affecting the rate of rhythmic movements, such as the heartbeat. A positive chronotropic effect would result in increasing the heart rate.

chronotropic effect The effect on the rate of contraction of the heart.

chyme The partially digested food that exits the stomach, entering the duodenum.

cilia Hairlike microtubule projections on the surface of a cell that can move materials over the cell surface.

circumferential burns A burn that encircles a particular area whose subsequent swelling may cause additional problems.

circumflex coronary artery One of the two branches of the left main coronary artery.

circumstantial thinking Situation in which a patient includes many irrelevant details in his or her account of things.

clandestine drug laboratories Locations where illegal drugs such as methamphetamine, lysergic acid diethylamide (LSD), and ecstasy are manufactured.

classic heat stroke Also called passive heat stroke, this is a serious heat illness that usually occurs during heat waves and is most likely to strike very old, very young, or bedridden people.

cleft lip An abnormal defect or fissure in the upper lip that failed to close during development. It is often associated with cleft palate.

cleft palate A fissure or hole in the palate (roof of the mouth) that forms a communicating pathway between the mouth and nasal cavities.

climacteric End phase of a woman's life menstrual cycle.

clitoris A small, cylindrical mass of erectile tissue and nerves located at the anterior junction of the labia minora, homologous to the glans penis of the male.

clonic activity Type of convulsion movement involving the contraction and relaxation of muscle groups.

closed abdominal injury An injury in which there is soft-tissue damage inside the body, but the skin remains intact.

closed-ended question A question that is specific and focused, either demanding a yes or no answer, or an answer chosen from specific options.

closed wound An injury in which damage occurs beneath the skin or mucous membrane but the surface remains intact.

clotting factors Substances in the blood that are necessary for clotting; also called coagulation factors.

CNS stimulants Any medications or agents that increase brain activity.

coagulation Clotting.

coagulation system The system that forms blood clots in the body and facilitates repairs to the vascular tree.

cochlea The shell-shaped structure within the inner ear that contains the organ of Corti.

cochlear duct A canal within the cochlea that receives vibrations from the ossicles.

coin rubbing A cultural ritual intended to treat an illness by rubbing hot coins, often on the back, which produces rounded and oblong red, patchy, flat skin lesions.

cold diuresis Secretion of large amounts of urine in response to cold exposure and the consequent shunting of blood volume to the body core.

cold protective response Phenomenon associated with cold water immersion in which reflexes in the body and a lowered metabolic rate help preserve basic body functions.

cold zone A safe area for those agencies involved in the operations; the ambulance command (AC), command post, emergency services personnel, and other support functions necessary to control the incident should be located in the cold zone.

collagen A protein that gives tensile strength to the connective tissues of the body.

collateral circulation The mesh of arteries and capillaries that furnishes blood to a segment of tissue whose original arterial supply has been obstructed.

colostomy Establishment of an opening between the colon and the surface of the body for the purpose of providing drainage of the bowel.

coma A state in which one does not respond to verbal or painful stimuli.

comedo A noninflammatory acne lesion.

communicability Describes how easily a disease spreads from one human to another human.

communication The transmission of information to another person—whether it be verbal or through body language.

compartment syndrome A condition that develops when oedema and swelling result in increased pressure within soft tissues, causing circulation to be compromised, possibly resulting in tissue necrosis.

compensated An incident, although large, which can be met from local resources.

compensated shock The early stage of shock, in which the body can still compensate for blood loss. The systolic blood pressure and brain perfusion is maintained.

complement system A group of plasma proteins whose function is to do one of three

things: attract leucocytes to sites of inflammation, activate leucocytes, and directly destroy cells.

complete abortion Expulsion of all products of conception from the uterus.

complex febrile convulsions An unusual form of convulsions that occurs in association with a rapid increase in body temperature.

complex partial convulsions Convulsions characterised by alteration of consciousness with or without complex focal motor activity.

compound incident An incident where local infrastructure has been destroyed, leading to long term recovery management (see critical infrastructure).

compulsion A repetitive action carried out to relieve the anxiety of obsessive thoughts.

computer-aided dispatch An automated computer system that processes the information received and assists the EMD with multiple functions and tasks.

concealment Protection from being seen.

concept formation Pattern of understanding based on initially obtained information.

conduction Transfer of heat to a solid object or a liquid by direct contact.

conductive deafness A curable temporary condition, caused by an injury to the eardrum.

confabulation The invention of experiences to cover gaps in memory, seen in patients with certain organic brain syndromes.

confined space A space with limited or restricted access that is not meant for continuous occupancy, such as a manhole, well, or tank.

confrontation Interviewing technique in which the interviewer points out to the patient something of interest in his/her conversation or behaviour.

confusion An impaired understanding of one's surroundings.

conjunctiva A thin, transparent membrane that covers the sclera and internal surfaces of the eyelids.

conjunctivitis An inflammation of the conjunctivae that usually is caused by bacteria, viruses, allergies, or foreign bodies; should be considered highly contagious; also called pink eye.

connective tissue Tissue that serves to bind various tissue types together.

contact and cover Technique that involves one paramedic making contact with the patient to provide care, while the second paramedic obtains patient information, gauges the level of tension, and warns his or her colleague at the first sign of trouble.

contact burn A burn produced by touching a hot object.

contact hazard A hazardous agent that gives off very little or no vapours; the skin is the primary route for this type of chemical to enter the body; also called a skin hazard.

contagious A person infected with a disease that is highly communicable.

contaminated Containing microorganisms.

contraceptive device A device used to prevent pregnancy.

contractility The strength of heart muscle contractions.

contraindications In health care, conditions or factors that increase the risk involved in using a particular drug, carrying out a medical procedure, or engaging in a particular activity.

contusion A bruise; an injury that causes bleeding beneath the skin but does not break the skin.

convection Mechanism by which body heat is picked up and carried away by moving air currents.

conventional reasoning A type of reasoning in which a child looks for approval from peers and society.

convulsion A paroxysmal alteration in neurological function, ie, behavioural and/or autonomic function.

cookbook medicine Treatment based on a guideline without adequate knowledge of the patient being treated.

cor pulmonale Heart disease that develops secondary to a chronic lung disease, usually affecting primarily the right side of the heart.

core body temperature (CBT) The temperature in the part of the body comprising the heart, lungs, brain, and abdominal viscera.

cornea The transparent anterior portion of the eye that overlies the iris and pupil.

coronal suture The point where the parietal bones join with the frontal bone.

coronary arteries The blood vessels of the heart that supply blood to its walls.

coronary artery disease (CAD) A pathological process caused by atherosclerosis that leads to progressive narrowing and eventual obstruction of the coronary arteries.

coronary sinus A large vessel in the posterior part of the coronary sulcus into which the coronary veins empty.

coronary sulcus The groove along the exterior surface of the heart that separates the atria from the ventricles.

corpus luteum The remains of a follicle after an oocyte has been released, and which secretes progesterone.

corrosives A class of chemicals with either high or low Ph levels. Exposure can cause severe soft-tissue damage.

cortex Part of the internal anatomy of the kidney; the lighter-coloured outer region closest to the capsule.

corticosteroids Hormones that regulate the body's metabolism, the balance of salt and water in the body, the immune system, and sexual function.

cortisol Hormone that stimulates most body cells to increase their energy production.

countercurrent multiplier The process in which the body produces either concentrated or diluted urine, depending on the body's needs.

coup-contrecoup injury Dual impacting of the brain into the skull; coup injury occurs at the point of impact; contrecoup injury occurs

on the opposite side of impact, as the brain rebounds.

couplet Two premature ventricular contractions occurring sequentially.

cover Obstacles that are difficult or impossible for bullets to penetrate.

covert Act in which the public safety community generally has no prior knowledge of the time, location, or nature of the attack.

crackles Abnormal breath sounds that have a fine, crackling quality; previously called rales.

cranial vault The bones that encase and protect the brain, including the parietal, temporal, frontal, occipital, sphenoid, and ethmoid bones; also called the cranium or skull.

craniofacial disjunction A Le Fort III fracture; involves a fracture of all of the midfacial bones, thus separating the entire midface from the cranium.

crepitus Crackling, grating, or grinding that is often felt or heard when two ends of bone rub together.

cribriform plate A horizontal bone perforated with numerous foramina for the passage of the olfactory nerve filaments from the nasal cavity.

cricoid cartilage Ringlike cartilage forming the lower and back part of the larynx.

cricoid pressure The application of posterior pressure to the cricoid cartilage; minimises gastric distension and the risk of vomiting and aspiration during ventilation; also referred to as the Sellick manoeuvre.

cricothyroid membrane Membrane between the cricoid and thyroid cartilages of the larynx.

crista galli A prominent bony ridge in the centre of the anterior fossa and the point of attachment of the meninges.

critical infrastructure The external foundation in communities made up of structures and services critical in the day-to-day living activities of humans: energy sources, fuel, water, sewage removal, food, hospitals, and transportation systems.

critical minimum threshold Minimum cerebral perfusion pressure required to adequately perfuse the brain; 60 mm Hg in the adult.

cross-contamination Occurs when a person is contaminated by an agent as a result of coming into contact with another contaminated person.

cross-tolerance A form of drug tolerance in which patients who take a particular medication for an extended period can build up a tolerance to other medications in the same class.

croup A childhood viral disease characterised by oedema of the upper airways with barking cough, difficult breathing, and stridor.

crown The part of the tooth that is external to the gum.

crowning The appearance of the infant's head at the vaginal opening during labour.

crush injury An injury in which the body or part of the body is crushed, preventing tissue function and, possibly, resulting in permanent tissue damage.

crush syndrome Significant metabolic derangement that can lead to renal failure and

death. It develops when crushed extremities or other body parts remain trapped for prolonged periods.

cumulative effect An effect that occurs when several successive doses of a medication are administered or when absorption of a medication occurs faster than excretion or metabolism.

cupping The cultural practice of placing warm cups on the skin to pull out illness from the body. The red, flat, rounded skin lesions are often more intensely red at the borders.

Cushing's syndrome A condition caused by an excess of cortisol production by the adrenal glands or by excessive use of cortisol or other similar steroid (glucocorticoid) hormones.

Cushing's triad Hypertension (with a widening pulse pressure), bradycardia, and irregular respirations; classic trio of findings associated with increased ICP.

cusps Points at the top of a tooth.

cutaneous Pertaining to the skin.

cyanide Agent that affects the body's ability to use oxygen. It is a colourless gas that has an odour similar to almonds. The effects begin on the cellular level and are very rapidly seen at the organ system level; exposure can occur from by-products of combustion and fires.

cyanosis Slightly bluish, greyish, slatelike, or dark purple discolouration of the skin due to hypoxia.

cystadenomas Fluid-filled cysts that form on the outer ovarian surface.

cystic fibrosis Chronic dysfunction of the endocrine system that affects multiple body systems, primarily the respiratory and digestive systems.

cytokines Products of cells that affect the function of other cells.

cytomegalovirus (CMV) A herpes virus that can produce the symptoms of prolonged high fever, chills, headache, malaise, extreme fatigue, and an enlarged spleen.

data interpretation The process of formulating a conclusion based on comparing the patient's condition with information from your training, education, and past experiences.

dead space The portion of the tidal volume that does not reach the alveoli and thus does not participate in gas exchange.

decay A natural process in which a material that is unstable attempts to stabilise itself by changing its structure.

deceleration A negative acceleration, that is, slowing down.

decerebrate (extensor) posturing Abnormal posture characterised by extension of the arms and legs; indicates pressure on the brain stem.

decompensated shock The late stage of shock, when blood pressure is falling.

decontamination The process of removing hazardous materials from the body or clothing of victims or rescuers. Includes the methods of dilution, absorption, disposal, and (in rare cases only) neutralisation.

decorticate (flexor) posturing Abnormal posture characterised by flexion of the arms and extension of the legs; indicates pressure on the brain stem.

decussation Movement of nerves from one side of the brain to the opposite side of the body.

deep fascia A dense layer of fibrous tissue below the subcutaneous tissue; composed of tough bands of tissue that ensheath muscles and other internal structures.

deep frostbite A type of frostbite in which the affected part looks white, yellow-white, or mottled blue-white and is hard, cold, and without sensation.

defibrillation The use of an unsynchronised direct current (DC) electric shock to terminate ventricular fibrillation.

degloving A traumatic injury that results in the soft tissue of the hand being drawn downward like a glove being removed.

degranulate To release granules into the surrounding tissue.

dehiscence Separation of the edges of a wound.

delirium An acute confessional state characterised by global impairment of thinking, perception, judgement, and memory.

delirium tremens (DTs) A severe withdrawal syndrome seen in people with alcoholism who are deprived of ethyl alcohol; characterised by restlessness, fever, sweating, disorientation, agitation, and convulsions; can be fatal if untreated.

delta wave The slurring of the upstroke of the first part of the QRS complex that occurs in Wolff-Parkinson-White syndrome.

delusion A fixed belief that is not shared by others of a person's culture or background and that can't be changed by reasonable argument; a false belief.

delusions of grandeur A state in which a person believes oneself to be someone of great importance.

delusions of persecution A state in which a person believes that others are plotting against him or her.

dementia The slow onset of progressive disorientation, shortened attention span, and loss of cognitive function.

demobilisation The process of "standing-down" from the emergency response of the major incident and implementing the recovery phase.

dendrites Part of the neuron that receives impulses from the axon and contains vesicles for the release of neurotransmitters.

dentine The principal mass of the tooth, which is made up of a material that is much more dense and stronger than bone.

depersonalisation A type of dissociative disorder in which a person loses his or her sense of reality, and may experience events as being "dream-like".

depolarisation The process of discharging resting cardiac muscle fibres by an electric impulse that causes them to contract.

depolarising neuromuscular blocking agents Medications designed to keep muscles in a contracted state.

depressed skull fractures Result from high-energy direct trauma to a small surface area of the head with a blunt object (such as a baseball bat to the head); commonly result in bony fragments being driven into the brain, causing injury.

depression A persistent mood of sadness, despair, and discouragement; may be a symptom of many different mental and physical disorders, or it may be a disorder on its own.

derealisation A symptom of a dissociative disorder in which objects seem to change size or shape; people may seem dead or behave like robots when viewed during a moment of acute stress.

dermal exposure Skin exposure, also known as topical exposure. Some hazardous materials may be absorbed through the skin to produce a systemic effect.

dermatomes Distinct areas of skin that correspond to specific spinal or cranial nerve levels where sensory nerves enter the CNS.

dermis The inner layer of skin containing hair follicle roots, glands, blood vessels, and nerves.

dermoid cysts Ovarian cysts containing formational tissue, such as hair and teeth.

desquamation The continuous shedding of the dead cells on the surface of the skin.

diabetes mellitus Disease characterised by the body's inability to metabolise glucose sufficiently. The condition occurs either because the pancreas doesn't produce enough insulin or the cells don't respond to the effects of the insulin that's produced.

diabetic ketoacidosis (DKA) A form of acidosis in uncontrolled diabetes in which certain acids accumulate when insulin is not available.

diaphragmatic hernia Passage of loops of bowel with or without other abdominal organs, through the diaphragm muscle; occurs as the bowel from the abdomen "herniates" upward through the diaphragm into the chest (thoracic) cavity.

diarrhoea Liquid stool.

diastole The period of ventricular relaxation during which the ventricles fill passively with blood.

dieffenbachia A common houseplant that resembles "elephant ears"; ingestion leads to burns of the mouth and tongue and, possibly, paralysis of the vocal cords and nausea and vomiting; in severe cases, may be oedema of the tongue and larynx, leading to airway compromise.

diencephalon The part of the brain between the brain stem and the cerebrum that includes the thalamus, subthalamus, and hypothalamus.

diffuse axonal injury (DAI) Diffuse brain injury that is caused by stretching, shearing, or tearing of nerve fibres with subsequent axonal damage.

diffuse brain injury Any injury that affects the entire brain.

digitalis preparations The drugs used in the treatment of congestive heart failure and certain atrial arrhythmias.

dilution A type of decontamination method that uses copious amounts of water to irrigate the contaminant from the skin or eyes.

diplopia Double vision.

dirty bomb Name given to a bomb that is used as a radiological dispersal device (RDD).

disaster management A planned, coordinated response to a disaster that involves cooperation of multiple agencies and enables effective triage and provision of care according to triage decisions.

disasters Widespread events that disrupt community resources and functions, in turn threatening public safety, lives, and property.

disease vector An animal that once infected, spreads a disease to another animal.

disorganisation A condition in which a person is characterised by uncontrolled and disconnected thought, is usually incoherent or rambling in speech, and may or may not be orientated to person and place.

disorganised symptoms Refers to erratic speech, emotional responses, and motor behaviour.

disorganised type A type of schizophrenia in which the person usually displays the wrong emotion for a particular situation, often self-absorbed.

disorientation Confusion regarding a person's sense of who one is (person), where one is (place), and at what point in time one finds oneself (time).

dispatch To send to a specific destination or to send on a task.

disposal A type of decontamination in which as much clothing and equipment as possible is disposed of to reduce the magnitude of the problem.

dissection In references to blood vessels, an aneurysm, or bulge, formed by the separation of the layers of an arterial wall.

disseminated intravascular coagulopathy (DIC) A life-threatening condition commonly found in severe trauma.

dissemination The means with which a terrorist will spread a disease, for example, by poisoning of the water supply, or aerosolising the agent into the air or ventilation system of a building.

dissociation Feelings of being detached from yourself, as if you were dreaming.

distal convoluted tubule (DCT) Connects with the kidney's collecting tubules.

distractibility The patient's attention is easily diverted.

distribution The movement and transportation of a medication throughout the bloodstream to tissues and cells of the body and, ultimately, to its target receptor.

distributive shock Occurs when there is widespread dilation of the resistance vessels (small arterioles), the capacitance vessels (small venules), or both.

diuresis Secretion of large amounts of urine by the kidney.

diuretic medications The medications designed to promote elimination of excess salt and water by the kidneys.

diuretics Chemicals that increase urinary output.

Do Not Attempt Resuscitation (DNAR) Written documentation by a general practitioner giving permission to medical personnel not to attempt resuscitation in the event of cardiac arrest.

Do Not Intubate Written documentation by a general practitioner giving permission to medical personnel not to attempt intubation.

dopaminergic receptors The receptors believed to cause dilation of the renal, coronary, and cerebral arteries.

dose effect The principle that the longer a hazardous material is in contact with the body or the greater the concentration, the greater the effect will probably be.

Down's syndrome A genetic chromosomal defect that can occur during fetal development and that results in learning difficulties as well as certain physical characteristics, such as a round head with a flat occiput and slanted, wide-set eyes.

dressing Material used to directly cover a wound.

dromotropic Relating to or influencing the conductivity of nerve fibres or cardiac muscle fibres.

dromotropic effect The effect on the velocity of conduction.

drowning The process of experiencing respiratory impairment from submersion or immersion in liquid.

drug Substance that has some therapeutic effect (such as reducing inflammation, fighting bacteria, or producing euphoria) when given in the appropriate circumstances and in the appropriate dose; any chemical compound that may be used on humans to help in diagnosis, treatment, cure, mitigation, or prevention of disease or other abnormal conditions.

drug abuse Any use of drugs that causes physical, psychological, economic, legal, or social harm to the user or others affected by the user's behaviour.

drug addiction A chronic disorder characterised by the compulsive use of a substance that results in physical, psychological, or social harm to the user who continues to use the substance despite the harm.

ductus arteriosus A duct that is present before birth that connects the pulmonary artery to the aorta in order to move unoxygenated blood back to the placenta.

ductus venosus A duct that is present before birth that connects the placenta to the heart in order to move oxygenated blood to the foetus.

duodenum The first part of the small intestine.

duplex Radio system using more than one frequency to permit simultaneous transmission and reception.

dura mater The outermost layer of the three meninges that enclose the brain and spinal cord; it is the toughest meningeal layer.

duration of action How long the medication concentration can be expected to remain above the minimum level needed to provide the intended action.

dysconjugate gaze Paralysis of gaze or lack of coordination between the movements of the two eyes.

dysmenorrhoea Painful menstruation.

dysphagia Difficulty swallowing.

dysphasia The impairment of language that affects the production or understanding of speech and the ability to read or write.

dysplasia An alteration in the size, shape, and organisation of cells.

dystonia Contractions of the body into a bizarre position.

early adults Individuals who are 19 to 40 years of age.

ecchymosis Localised bruising or blood collection within or under the skin; black-and-blue discolouration.

echolalia Meaningless echoing of the interviewer's words by the patient.

ecstasy A drug officially named methylenedioxymethamphetamine (MDMA) that is sometimes used to facilitate date rape; a methamphetamine derivative with hallucinogenic properties; street names include E, XTC, disco biscuit, rhubarb and custard, smarties, Rolex, and dolphins.

ectopic pregnancy A pregnancy in which the egg implants somewhere other than the uterine endometrium.

efferent arteriole The structure in the kidney where blood drains from the glomerulus.

efferent nerves The nerves that carry messages from the brain to the muscles and all other organs of the body.

ejection fraction The fraction of the end-diastolic volume that is ejected with each ventricle beat; it is the stroke volume divided by end-diastolic volume and is expressed as a percentage.

elastin A protein that gives the skin its elasticity.

electrical conduction system In the heart, the specialised cardiac tissue that initiates and conducts electric impulses. The system includes the SA node, internodal atrial conduction pathways, atrioventricular junction, atrioventricular node, bundle of His, and the Purkinje network.

electrical energy The energy delivered in the form of high voltage.

elixir A syrup with alcohol and flavouring added.

embryo The fetus in the earliest stages after fertilisation.

emergency medical dispatcher (EMD) A person who receives information from a call taker regarding an emergency call and dispatches the most appropriate resource to respond in a timely manner, as well as receiving incident information from ambulance crews who are travelling or already at the scene.

emotional/mental impairment Illnesses that cause a person's emotions to become out of control.

emphysema Infiltration of any tissue by air or gas; a chronic obstructive pulmonary disease characterised by distention of the alveoli and destructive changes in the lung parenchyma.

emulsion A preparation of one liquid (usually an oil) distributed in small globules in another liquid (usually water).

encoded A message is put into a code before it is transmitted.

endocardium The thin membrane lining the inside of the heart.

endocrine glands Glands that secrete or release chemicals that are used inside the body. Endocrine glands lack ducts and release hormones directly into the surrounding tissue and blood.

endocrine hormones Hormones that are carried to their target or cell group in the bloodstream.

endometriomas Ovarian cysts formed from endometrial tissue.

endometriosis A condition in which endometrial tissue grows outside the uterus.

endometritis An inflammation of the endometrium that often is associated with a bacterial infection.

endometrium The inner mucous membrane of the uterus.

endoscopy The insertion of a flexible tube into the oesophagus with the intent of visualising and repairing damage or disease.

endothelial cells Specific types of epithelial cells that serve the function of lining the blood vessels.

endotoxin A toxin released by some bacteria when they die.

end-tidal carbon dioxide The numeric partial pressure of carbon dioxide contained in the last few millilitres of the patient's exhaled air.

enhanced 999 system An emergency call-in system in which additional information such as the phone number and location of the caller is recorded automatically through sophisticated telephone technology and the EMD need only confirm the information on the screen.

enteral routes The medication administration routes in which medications are absorbed somewhere along the gastrointestinal tract.

entrapment A situation in which a patient is trapped by debris, soil, or other material and is unable to extricate himself or herself.

entry wound The point at which a penetrating object enters the body.

environmental emergencies Medical conditions caused or exacerbated by the weather, terrain, or unique atmospheric conditions such as high altitude or underwater.

eosinophils Cells that make up approximately 1% to 3% of leucocytes, which play a major role in allergic reactions and bronchoconstriction in an asthma attack.

epicardium The thin membrane lining the outside of the heart.

epidermis The outermost layer of the skin.

epigastric The right upper region of the abdomen directly inferior to the xyphoid process and superior to the umbilicus.

epiglottitis Inflammation of the epiglottis.

epimenorrhoea Menstrual blood flow that occurs more often than a 24-day interval.

episiotomy An incision in the perineal skin made to prevent tearing during childbirth.

epistaxis A nosebleed.

epithelialisation The formation of fresh epithelial tissue to heal a wound.

epithelium Type of tissue that covers all external surfaces of the body.

Erb palsy Lack of movement at the shoulder due to nerve injury resulting from the stretching of the cervical nerve roots (C5 and C6 most commonly) during delivery of the baby's head during birth. The effect is usually transient, but can be permanent

erythema Reddening of the skin.

erythrocytes Red blood cells.

escharotomy A surgical cut through the eschar or leathery covering of a burn injury to allow for swelling and minimise the potential for development of compartment syndrome in a circumferentially burned limb or the thorax.

evaluation Collection of the methods, skills, and activities necessary to determine whether a service or programme is needed, likely to be used, conducted as planned, and actually helps people.

evaporation The conversion of a liquid to a gas.

evisceration Displacement of an organ outside the body.

excretion The elimination of toxic or inactive metabolites from the body. This is primarily done by the kidneys, intestines, lungs, and assorted glands.

exertional heat stroke A serious type of heat stroke usually affecting young and fit people exercising in hot and humid conditions.

exertional hyponatraemia A condition due to prolonged exertion in hot environments coupled with excessive hypotonic fluid intake that leads to nausea, vomiting, and, in severe cases, mental status changes and convulsions.

exit wound The point at which a penetrating object leaves the body, which may or may not be in a straight line from the entry wound.

exocrine glands Glands that excrete chemicals for elimination.

exocrine hormones Hormones that are secreted through ducts into an organ or onto epithelial surfaces.

exotoxin A toxin that is secreted by living cells to aid in the death and digestion of other cells.

expressive dysphasia Damage to or loss of the ability to speak.

external auditory canal The area in which sound waves are received from the auricle (pinna) before they travel to the eardrum; also called the ear canal.

external ear One of three anatomical parts of the ear; it contains the pinna, the ear canal, and the external portion of the tympanic membrane.

external os The junction where the uterus opens into the vagina.

extract A concentrated preparation of a drug made by putting the drug into solution (in alcohol or water) and evaporating off the excess solvent to a prescribed standard.

extradural haematoma An accumulation of blood between the skull and dura.

facial nerve The seventh cranial nerve; supplies motor activity to all muscles of facial expression, the sense of taste, and anterior two thirds of the tongue and cutaneous sensation to the external ear, tongue, and palate.

facilitation An interviewing technique in which the interviewer uses noncommittal words and gestures to encourage the patient to proceed.

faeculent Smelling of faeces.

fallopian tubes The vehicles of transportation of the ova from the ovaries to the uterus; also called oviducts.

fasciotomy A surgical procedure that cuts away fascia to relieve pressure.

fear Also sometimes referred to as a phobia, this is an anxious feeling, usually about specific things or situations.

feedback inhibition Negative feedback resulting in the decrease of an action in the body.

fetus The developing, unborn infant inside the uterus.

fibrin A whitish, filamentous protein formed by the action of thrombin on fibrinogen. Fibrin is the protein that polymerises (bonds) to form the fibrous component of a blood clot.

fibrinolysis cascade The breakdown of fibrin in blood clots, and the prevention of the polymerisation of fibrin into new clots.

fibrinolytic agents The only medications available to dissolve blood clots after they have already formed; the drugs promote the digestion of fibrin.

fibrinolytic system The mechanism by which fibrin undergoes dissolution owing to the action of enzymes; clots are destroyed.

first-degree heart block A partial disruption of the conduction of the depolarising impulse from the atria to the ventricles, causing prolongation of the P-R interval.

first stage of labour The stage of labour that begins with the onset of regular labour pains, crampy abdominal pains, during which the uterus contracts and the cervix effaces.

flame burn A thermal burn caused by flames touching the skin.

flash burn An electrothermal injury caused by arcing of electric current.

flash point The temperature at which a vapour can be ignited by a spark.

flat Used to describe behaviour in which the patient doesn't seem to feel much of anything at all.

flight of ideas Accelerated thinking in which the mind skips very rapidly from one thought to the next.

fluid extract A concentrated form of a drug prepared by dissolving the crude drug in the fluid in which it is most readily soluble.

focal brain injury A specific, grossly observable brain injury.

follicle-stimulating hormone (FSH) A hormone produced by the anterior pituitary gland which is important in the menstrual cycle.

fontanelles The soft spots in the skull of a newborn and infant where the sutures of the skull have not yet grown together; usually disappear at approximately 18 months of age.

footling breech A delivery in which one or both feet dangle through the vaginal opening.

foramen magnum The large opening at the base of the skull through which the spinal cord exits the brain.

foramen ovale An opening in the septum of the heart before birth, and which closes after birth.

foramina Small natural openings, perforations, or orifices, such as in the bones of the cranial vault; plural of foramen.

forward incident officer Delegated role from the ambulance commander, the person who supervises the people working at the scene of a complex incident.

foxglove A plant that contains cardiac glycosides used in making digitalis; ingestion of leaves causes nausea, vomiting, diarrhoea, abdominal cramps, hyperkalaemia, and a variety of arrhythmias.

fractile response time A fraction (not average) of all emergency responses for the purpose of setting standards in response times.

free-flow oxygen Oxygen administered via oxygen tube and a cupped hand on patient's face.

freelancing When individual units or different organisations make independent and often inefficient decisions about the next appropriate action.

free radicals Molecules that are missing one electron in their outer shell.

frequency In radio communications, the number of cycles per second of a signal, inversely related to the wavelength.

frontal lobe The portion of the brain that is important in voluntary motor actions and personality traits.

frostbite Localised damage to tissues resulting from prolonged exposure to extreme cold.

frostnip Early frostbite, characterised by numbness and pallor without significant tissue damage.

full-thickness burn A burn that extends through the epidermis and dermis into the subcutaneous tissues beneath; previously called a third-degree burn.

fundus The dome-shaped top of the uterus.

G agents Early nerve agents that were developed by German scientists in the period after WWI and into WWII. There are three such agents: sarin, soman, and tabun.

gait Walking pattern.

galea aponeurotica Tough, tendinous layer of the scalp.

gamma (X-rays) Type of energy that is emitted from a strong radiological source that is far faster and stronger than alpha and beta

leukaemia Cancer or malignancy of the blood-forming organs, particularly affecting the WBCs that develop abnormally and/or excessively at the expense of normal blood cells.

Lewisite (L) A blistering agent that has a rapid onset of symptoms and produces immediate intense pain and discomfort on contact.

licit In relation to drugs, legalised drugs such as coffee, alcohol, and tobacco.

life expectancy The average amount of years a person can be expected to live.

ligand Any molecule that binds a receptor leading to a reaction.

limb leads The ECG leads attached to the limbs and that form the hexaxial system, dividing the heart along a coronal plane into the anterior and posterior segments.

limbic system Structures within the cerebrum and diencephalon that influence emotions, motivation, mood, and sensations of pain and pleasure.

linear skull fractures Account for 80% of skull fractures; also referred to as nondisplaced skull fractures; commonly occur in the temporal-parietal region of the skull; not associated with deformities to the skull.

liniments Liquid preparations of drugs for external use, usually to relieve some discomfort (such as pain, itching) or to protect the skin.

listening watch The placement of an ambulance at a specific geographic location in order to cover larger areas of territory and reduce response times. Also called standby.

lithium The cornerstone drug for the treatment of bipolar disorder.

local anaesthesia A type of anaesthesia that causes a loss of sensation to touch or pain at a specific isolated spot on the body where a procedure is to take place.

local effect An effect of a hazardous material on the body that is limited to the area of contact.

local effects The effects that result from the direct application of a drug to a tissue, for example when lotions are applied to the skin to relieve itching.

loop diuretics Medications that inhibit the reabsorption of sodium and calcium ions and that can cause an excessive loss of potassium.

loop of Henle The U-shaped portion of the renal tubule that extends from the proximal to the distal convoluted tubule; concentrates the filtrate and converts it to urine.

loosening of associations A situation in which the logical connection between one idea and the next becomes obscure, at least to the listener.

lordosis Inward curve of the lumbar spine just above the buttocks. An exaggerated form of lordosis results in the condition known as swayback.

lower explosive limit (LEL) The concentration of the hazardous material that can burn or explode in the air when it mixes with air.

lumen The inside diameter of an artery or other hollow structure.

Lund and Browder chart A detailed version of the rule of nines chart that takes into consideration the changes in body surface area brought on by growth.

luteinising hormone (LH) Hormone that regulates the production of both eggs and sperm, as well as production of reproductive hormones.

lymph A thin, watery fluid that bathes the tissues of the body.

lymph nodes Area of the lymphatic system where infection-fighting cells are housed.

lymphangitis Inflammation of a lymph channel.

lymphatic system A passive circulatory system that transports a plasma-like liquid called lymph, a thin fluid that bathes the tissues of the body.

lymphoblasts Lymphocytes transformed because of stimulation by an antigen.

lymphocytes The white blood cells responsible for a large part of the body's immune protection.

lymphoid system The system primarily made up of the bone marrow, lymph nodes, and spleen that participates in formation of lymphocytes and immune responses.

lymphokines Cytokines released by lymphocytes, including many of the interleukins, gamma interferon, tumour necrosis factor beta, and chemokines.

lymphomas Malignant diseases that arise within the lymphoid system; includes non-Hodgkin's and Hodgkin's lymphomas.

macrophages Cells that developed from the monocytes that provide the body's first line of defence in the inflammatory process.

major incident Any occurrence that presents serious threat to the health of the community, disruption to the service, or causes (or is likely to cause) such numbers or types of casualties as to require special arrangements to be implemented by hospitals, ambulance trusts, or primary care organisations.

malignant hyperthermia A condition that can result from common anaesthesia medications (notably suxamethonium) and present with hyperthermia, muscular rigidity, altered mental status, and a hyperdynamic state.

malocclusion Misalignment of the teeth.

malrotation A congenital anomaly of rotation of the midgut, the small bowel is found predominantly on the right side of the abdomen.

mandible The moveable lower jaw bone.

mandibular nerve A sensory and motor nerve that supplies the muscles of chewing and skin of the lower lip, chin, temporal region, and part of the external ear.

mania A mental disorder characterised by abnormally exaggerated happiness, joy, or euphoria with hyperactivity, insomnia, and grandiose ideas.

manic-depressive illness A bipolar disorder in which mood fluctuates between depression and mania. The alterations in mood are usually episodic and recurrent.

margination Loss of fluid from the blood vessels into the tissue, causing the blood left in the vessels to have an increased viscosity, which in turn slows the flow of blood and produces stasis.

marijuana The dried leaves and flower buds of the Cannabis sativa plant that are smoked to achieve a high.

mast cells The cells that resemble basophils but do not circulate in the blood. Mast cells play a role in allergic reactions, immunity, and wound healing.

mastication The process of chewing with the teeth.

mastoid process A cone-shaped section of bone at the base of the temporal bone.

maxillary nerve A sensory nerve; supplies the skin on the posterior part of the side of the nose, lower eyelid, cheek, and upper lip.

mean arterial pressure (MAP) The average (or mean) pressure against the arterial wall during a cardiac cycle.

mechanical energy The energy that results from motion (kinetic energy) or that is stored in an object (potential energy).

mechanism of action The way in which a medication produces the intended response.

mechanism of injury (MOI) The way in which traumatic injuries occur; the forces that act on the body to cause damage.

meconium A dark green faecal material that accumulates in the fetal intestines and is discharged around the time of birth.

mediastinitis Inflammation of the mediastinum, often a result of the gastric contents leaking into the thoracic cavity after oesophageal perforation.

medical ambiguity Uncertainty regarding the specific cause of the patient's condition.

medical commander (MC) A specific part of the ICS, which requires a doctor to operate in a managerial and not treatment role, alongside the AC.

medical direction Direction given to an ambulance service or provider by a medical director.

medical monitoring The process of assessing the health status of specialised team members before and after entry to a hazardous materials incident site.

medication A licensed drug taken to cure or reduce symptoms of an illness or medical condition or as an aid in the diagnosis, treatment, or prevention of a disease or other abnormal condition.

medulla Continuous inferiorly with the spinal cord; serves as a conduction pathway for ascending and descending nerve tracts; coordinates heart rate, blood vessel diameter, breathing, swallowing, vomiting, coughing, and sneezing. Also, part of the internal anatomy of the kidney; the middle layer.

medulla oblongata The inferior portion of the midbrain, which serves as a conduction pathway for both ascending and descending nerve tracts.

melaena Dark, tarry, very odourous stools caused by upper GI bleeds.

melanin The pigment that gives skin its colour.

membrane attack complex (MAC) Molecules that insert themselves into the bacterial membrane, leading to weakened areas in the membrane.

menarche The beginning phase of a woman's life cycle of menstruation.

meninges A set of three tough membranes, the dura mater, arachnoid, and pia mater, that encloses the entire brain and spinal cord.

meningitis Inflammation of the membranes of the spinal cord or brain.

menopause The ending phase of a woman's life cycle of menstruation.

menorrhagia Menstrual blood flow that lasts several days longer than it should or flow that is abnormally excessive.

menstrual cycle The entire monthly cycle of menstruation from start to finish.

menstruation Monthly flow of blood.

mental illness A generic term for a variety of illnesses that result in emotional, cognitive, or behavioural dysfunction.

mental status examination (MSE) A way of measuring the "mental vital signs" in a disturbed patient. The mnemonic COASTMAP can be used to conduct this examination, assessing consciousness, orientation, activity, speech, thought, memory, affect and mood, and perception.

mesenteries The membranes that connect organs to the abdominal wall.

mesentery A membranous double fold of tissue in the abdomen that attaches various organs to the body wall.

metaplasia A reversible, cellular adaptation in which one adult cell type is replaced by another adult cell type.

metastasis Change in location of a disease from one organ or part of the body to another. Often used to describe a cancer that has migrated to other parts of the body.

methamphetamine A highly addictive drug in the amphetamine family.

metrorrhagia Irregular but frequent vaginal bleeding.

micturition reflex A spinal reflex that causes contraction of the bladder's smooth muscles, producing the urge to void as pressure is exerted on the internal urinary sphincter.

midbrain The part of the brain that is responsible for helping to regulate level of consciousness.

middle adults Individuals who are 41 to 60 years of age.

middle ear One of three anatomical parts of the ear; it consists of the inner portion of the tympanic membrane and the ossicles.

milk In the context of pharmacology, an aqueous suspension of an insoluble drug.

miosis Bilateral pinpoint constricted pupils.

missed abortion A situation in which a fetus has died during the first 20 weeks of gestation, but has remained in utero.

missile fragmentation A primary mechanism of tissue disruption from certain rifles in which pieces of the projectile break apart, allowing the pieces to create their own separate paths through tissues.

mitochondria The metabolic centre or powerhouse of the cell. They are small and rod-shaped organelles.

mitral valve The valve located between the left atrium and the left ventricle of the heart.

mobile intensive care units (MICUs) An early title given to an ambulance-style unit.

mobile telephones Low-power portable radios that communicate through an interconnected series of repeater stations called "cells".

molar pregnancy Pregnancy in which there is a problem at the fertilisation stage, with a malfunction of the egg or sperm that results in an abnormal placenta and a fetus with an abnormal chromosome count, or which results in an empty egg.

Mongolian spots Blue-grey areas of discolouration of the skin caused by abnormal pigment, not by trauma or bruising.

monoamine oxidase inhibitors (MAOIs) Psychiatric medication used primarily to treat atypical depression by increasing noradrenaline and serotonin levels in the central nervous system.

monocytes Mononuclear phagocytic white blood cells derived from myeloid stem cells. They circulate in the bloodstream for about 24 hours and then move into tissues to mature into macrophages.

monomorphic Having one common shape of QRS complex.

mons pubis This is a rounded pad of fatty tissue that overlies the symphysis pubis and is anterior to the urethral and vaginal openings.

mood A person's sustained and pervasive emotional state.

mood disorder A group of disorders in which the disturbance of mood is accompanied by full or partial manic or depressive syndrome.

morbidity Number of nonfatally injured or disabled people. Usually expressed as a rate, meaning the number of nonfatal injuries in a certain population in a given time period divided by the size of the population.

moro reflex An infant reflex in which, when an infant is caught off guard, the infant opens his or her arms wide, spreads the fingers, and seems to grab at things.

mortality Deaths caused by injury and disease. Usually expressed as a rate, meaning the number of deaths in a certain population in a given time period divided by the size of the population.

mottling A condition of abnormal skin circulation, caused by vasoconstriction or inadequate circulation; a typical finding in states of severe protracted hypoperfusion and shock.

mucopolysaccharide gel One of the complex materials found, along with the collagen fibres and elastin fibres, in the dermis of the skin.

mucosal-associated lymphoid tissue (MALT) The lymphoid tissue associated with the skin and the respiratory, urinary, and reproductive traits as well as the tonsils.

multifocal Arising from or pertaining to many foci or locations.

multigravida A woman who has had two or more pregnancies, irrespective of the outcome.

multipara A woman who has had two or more deliveries.

multiple myeloma A disease in which an abnormal plasma cell infiltrates the bone marrow with a cancerous (neoplastic) cell, causing tumours to form inside the bones.

multiple organ dysfunction syndrome (MODS) A progressive condition usually characterised by combined failure of several organs, such as the lungs, liver, and kidney, along with some clotting mechanisms, which occurs after severe illness or injury.

multiple sclerosis (MS) An autoimmune condition in which the body attacks the myelin of the brain and spinal cord, leading to gaps in the insulation normally provided by the myelin, causing scarring.

multiplex Method by which simultaneous transmission of voice and ECG signals can be achieved over a single radio frequency.

murmur An abnormal "whoosh"-like sound heard over the heart that indicates turbulent blood flow around a cardiac valve.

muscarinic cholinergic antagonists Medications that block acetylcholine exclusively at the muscarinic receptors; an example is atropine.

muscular dystrophy (MD) A nonneurological condition of genetic origin in which defective DNA causes an error in the creation of muscle tissue, resulting in the degeneration of muscular tissue. This presents with progressive muscle weakness, delayed development of muscle motor skills, ptosis, drooling, and poor muscle tone.

muscularis The middle layer of tissue in the fallopian tubes.

mutagen Substance that mutates, damages, and changes the structures of DNA in the body's cells.

mutism The absence of speech.

myasthenia gravis An abnormal condition characterised by the chronic fatigability and weakness of muscles, especially in the face and throat. It is the result of a defect in the conduction of nerve impulses at the nerve junction. This deficit is caused by a lack of acetylcholine.

myelin An insulating-type substance present in some neurons that allows the cell to consistently send its signal along the axon without "shorting out" or losing electricity to surrounding fluids and tissues.

myocardium The cardiac muscle.

myoclonus Jerking motions of the body.

myoglobin A protein found in muscle that is released into the circulation after crush injury or other muscle damage and whose presence in the circulation may produce kidney damage.

myometrium The middle layer of tissue in the uterus.

myxoedema coma A rare condition that can occur in patients who have severe, untreated hypothyroidism.

NAAK A nerve agent antidote kit. According to the Department of Health, a NAAK should contain 2 mg atropine, 2 g pralidoxime mesylate, and 250 mg obidoxime chloride.

narcotic The generic term for opiates and opioids, drugs that act as a CNS depressant and produce insensibility or stupor.

nasal cavity The chamber inside the nose that lies between the floor of the cranium and the roof of the mouth.

nasal flaring Intermittent outward movements of the nostrils with each inspiration; indicates an increase in the work needed to breathe.

nasal septum The separation between the right and left nostrils.

nasolacrimal duct The passage through which tears drain from the lacrimal sacs into the nasal cavity.

native immunity A nonspecific cellular and humoral response that operates as the body's first line of defence against pathogens.

necrosis The death of tissue, usually caused by a cessation of its blood supply.

negative feedback The concept that once the desired effect of a process has been achieved, further action is inhibited until it is needed again; also called feedback inhibition.

negative-pressure ventilation Drawing of air into the lungs; airflow from a region of higher pressure (outside the body) to a region of lower pressure (the lungs); occurs during normal (unassisted breathing).

negative symptoms Evidence of a disease or condition, noted by lack of normal circumstances, rather than the presence of new physical evidence or a physical change; with regard to schizophrenia, refers to a lack of normal behaviour, and apathy, mutism, a flat affect, and a lack of interest in pleasure.

negative wave pulse The phase of an explosion in which pressure from the blast is less than atmospheric pressure.

neglect Refusal or failure on the part of the carer to provide life necessities, such as food, water, clothing, shelter, personal hygiene, medicine, comfort, and personal safety.

neologism An invented word that has meaning only to its inventor.

neonatal period The first month of life.

neonate Infant during the first month after birth.

neoplasms Tumours.

neoplastic cells Another term for cancerous cells.

neovascularisation Development of vessels to aid in healing an injured soft tissue.

nephrons The structural and functional units of the kidney that form urine; composed of the glomerulus, the glomerular (Bowman's) capsule, the proximal convoluted tubule (PCT), loop of Henle, and the distal convoluted tubule (DCT).

nerve agents A class of chemicals called organophosphates; they function by blocking an essential enzyme in the nervous system, which causes the body's organs to become overstimulated and burn out.

neurogenic shock Circulatory failure caused by paralysis of the nerves that control the size of the blood vessels, leading to widespread dilation; seen in spinal cord injuries.

neuroleptic malignant syndrome (NMS) A condition caused by antipsychotic and even common antiemetic medications that presents with hyperthermia, muscular rigidity, altered mental status, and a hyperdynamic state.

neuromuscular blocking agents Medications that affect the parasympathetic nervous system by inducing paralysis.

neuroneal soma The body of a neurone (nerve cell).

neurotoxins Biological agents that are the most deadly substances known to humans; they include botulinum toxin and ricin.

neurotransmission The process of chemical signalling between cells.

neurotransmitters Proteins that transmit signals between cells of the nervous system.

neutralisation A type of decontamination that uses one chemical to change the hazardous material into two less harmful substances; rarely used by specialised teams.

neutron radiation Type of energy that is emitted from a strong radiological source; neutron energy is the fastest moving and most powerful form of radiation. Neutrons easily penetrate through lead, and require several feet of concrete to stop them.

neutrophils Cells that make up approximately 55% to 70% of leucocytes responsible in large part for the body's protection against infection. They are readily attracted by foreign antigens and destroy them by phagocytosis.

newborn Infant within the first few hours after birth.

Newton's first law of motion The principle that a body at rest will remain at rest unless acted on by an outside force.

Newton's second law of motion The principle that the force that an object can exert is the product of its mass times its acceleration.

nicotinic cholinergic antagonists Medications that block the acetylcholine only at nicotinic receptors.

noise In radio communications, interference in a radio signal.

nonbarbiturate hypnotics Medications designed to sedate without the side effects of a barbiturate.

nondepolarising neuromuscular blocking agents Medications designed to cause temporary paralysis by binding in a competitive but nonstimulatory manner to part of the ACh receptor. Do not cause fasciculations.

nonopioid analgesics Medications designed to relieve pain without the side effects of opioids.

nonspecific agents Medications that produce effects on different cells through a variety of mechanisms. Generally classified by the focus of action or specific therapeutic use.

nonsteroidal anti-inflammatory drugs (NSAIDs) Medications with analgesic and fever reducing properties.

noradrenaline Hormone produced by the adrenal glands that is vital in the function of the sympathetic nervous system.

normal sinus rhythm The normal rhythm of the heart, wherein the excitation impulse arises in the SA node, travels through the internodal pathways to the atrioventricular junction, down the bundle of His, through the bundle branches, and into the Purkinje network without interference.

nuchal rigidity A stiff or painful neck; commonly associated with meningitis.

nucleus A cellular organelle that contains the genetic information. The nucleus controls the function and structure of a cell.

nullipara A woman who has never delivered.

nystagmus The rhythmic shaking of the eyes.

obesity A term used when someone's body mass index is calculated and a score of 30 or above is calculated.

objectives Specific, time-limited, and quantifiable statements that summarise an expected result of an intervention.

obsession A persistent idea that a person cannot dismiss from his or her thoughts.

obstructive shock Shock that occurs when there is a block to blood flow in the heart or great vessels, causing an insufficient blood supply to the body's tissues.

occipital condyles Articular surfaces on the occipital bone where the skull articulates with the atlas on the vertebral column.

occipital lobe The portion of the brain that is responsible for the processing of visual information.

occiput The most posterior portion of the cranium.

oculomotor nerve Third cranial nerve; innervates the muscles that cause motion of the eyeballs and upper eyelid.

oedema A condition in which excess fluid accumulates in tissues, manifested by swelling.

oestrogen One of the three major female hormones. At puberty, oestrogen brings about the secondary sex characteristics.

off-gassing The emitting of an agent after exposure, for example from a person's clothes that have been exposed to the agent.

ointment A semisolid preparation for external application to the body, usually containing a medicinal substance.

olfactory nerves Participates in the transmission of scent impulses.

oligohydramnios Decreased volume of amniotic fluid during a pregnancy; a risk factor associated with abnormalities of the urinary tract, postmaturity (birth after a prolonged pregnancy), and intrauterine growth retardation.

oliguria A decrease in urine output to the extent that total urine output drops below 500 ml/day.

onset of action The time needed for the concentration of the medication at the target tissue to reach the minimum effective level.

oocyte An egg produced from the female ovary.

open abdominal injury An injury in which there is a break in the surface of the skin or mucous membrane, exposing deeper tissue to potential contamination.

open-ended question A question that does not have a yes or no answer, and which does not give the patient specific options to choose from.

open wound An injury in which there is a break in the surface of the skin or the mucous membrane, exposing deeper tissue to potential contamination.

operations The technical rescue training level required to work in the warm zone of an incident. Training at this level allows responders to provide direct assistance to those conducting the rescue operation and to use certain rescue skills and procedures.

ophthalmic nerve A sensory nerve that supplies the skin of the forehead, the upper eyelid, and conjunctiva.

ophthalmoscope An instrument used to look into a patient's eyes and view the retina and aqueous fluid; consists of a concave mirror and a battery-powered light that is usually contained in the handle.

opiate Various alkaloids derived from the opium or poppy plant.

opioid A synthetic narcotic not derived from opium.

opioid agonist-antagonists Medications designed to relieve pain without the side effects of opioids.

opioid agonists Chemicals that are similar to or derived from the opium plant.

opioid antagonists A classification of medications that reverses the effects of opioid drugs.

opsoninisation Occurs when an antibody coats an antigen to facilitate its recognition by immune cells.

optic nerve Either of the second cranial nerves that enter the eyeball posteriorly, through the optic foramen.

orbits Bony cavities in the frontal part of the skull that enclose and protect the eyes.

organ of Corti A structure located in the cochlea that contains hairs that are stimulated by vibrations to form nerve impulses that travel to the brain and are perceived as sound.

organelles Internal cellular structures that carry out specific functions for the cell.

organic brain syndrome Temporary or permanent dysfunction of the brain, caused by a disturbance in the physical or physiological functioning of brain tissue.

organophosphates A class of chemical found in many insecticides used in agriculture and in the home.

orientation A person's sense of who one is (person), where one is (place), and at what day of the week one finds oneself (day).

oropharynx The area behind the base of the tongue between the soft palate and the upper portion of the epiglottis.

orthopnoea Severe dyspnoea experienced when lying down and relieved by sitting up.

orthostatic hypotension A drop in systolic blood pressure when moving from a sitting to a standing position. Also called postural hypotension

orthostatic vital signs Assessing vital signs in two different patient positions to determine the degree of hypovolaemia.

osmosis The movement of water down its concentration gradient across a membrane.

ossicles The three small bones in the inner ear that transmit vibrations to the cochlear duct at the oval window.

ossification centres Areas where cartilage is transformed through calcification into a new area of bone.

osteoarthritis A degenerative joint disease associated with ageing.

osteomyelitis Inflammation of the bone due to infection; a potential complication of intraosseous infusion.

osteoporosis A decrease in bone mass and density.

otoscope An instrument for examing the ear drum.

outcome (impact) objectives State the intended effect of the programme on participants or on the community in such terms as the participants' increased knowledge, changed behaviours or attitudes, or decreased injury rates.

oval window An oval opening between the middle ear and the vestibule.

ovaries Female gonads; ovaries release eggs and secrete the female hormones.

ovulation A process in which an ovum is released from a follicle.

ovum A mature oocyte.

oxygen concentrators Large, electrical devices that concentrate the oxygen in ambient air and eliminate other gases

P wave The first wave of the ECG complex, representing depolarisation of the ventricles.

pacemaker The specialised tissue within the heart that initiates excitation impulses; an electronic device used to stimulate cardiac contraction when the electric conduction system of the heart is malfunctioning, especially in complete heart block. An electronic pacemaker consists of a battery-powered pulse generator and a wire that transmits the electric impulse to the ventricles.

Paediatric Assessment Triangle (PAT) An assessment tool that allows rapid formation of a general impression of the type and level of illness or injury in an infant or child without touching him or her; consists of assessing appearance, work of breathing, and circulation to the skin.

palatine bone An irregularly shaped bone found in the posterior part of the nasal cavity.

palatine tonsils One of three sets of lymphatic organs that comprise the tonsils; located in the back of the throat, on each side of the posterior opening of the oral cavity; help protect the body from bacteria introduced into the mouth and nose.

pallor Lack of colour; paleness.

palmar grasp An infant reflex that occurs when something is placed in the infant's palm; the infant grasps the object.

palpation Physical touching for the purpose of obtaining information.

palpitations A sensation felt under the left breast of the heart "skipping a beat", usually caused by a premature ventricular contraction.

pancreas The digestive gland that secretes digestive enzymes into the duodenum through the pancreatic duct. The pancreas is considered to be both an endocrine gland and an exocrine gland.

papillary muscles Protrusions of the myocardium into the ventricular cavities to which the chordae tendineae are attached.

para The number of pregnancies a woman has carried to more than 28 weeks, regardless of whether the fetus was delivered dead or alive.

para-aminophenol derivatives Medications designed to reduce fevers and relieve pain.

paracrine hormones Hormones that diffuse through intracellular spaces to their target.

paraesthesia Sensation of tingling, numbness, or "pins and needles" in a body part.

paranasal sinuses The sinuses, or hollowed sections of bone in the front of the head, that are lined with mucous membrane and drain into the nasal cavity.

paranoid type A type of schizophrenia in which the person experiences delusions or hallucinations usually centered around a specific theme, where their cognitive functions remain intact.

paraplegia Paralysis of the lower part of the body.

parasympathetic nervous system A subdivision of the autonomic nervous system that is involved in control of involuntary, vegetative functions, mediated largely by the vagus nerve through the chemical acetylcholine.

parathyroid hormone (PTH) A hormone secreted by the parathyroid gland that acts as an antagonist to calcitonin. PTH is secreted when calcium blood levels are low.

parenchyma The functional part of an organ, rather than the supporting tissue.

parenteral exposure Entry of a hazardous material into the bloodstream, either through force of injection or through an open wound.

parenteral routes Medication routes in which medications are administered via any route other than the alimentary canal (digestive tract), skin, or mucous membranes.

parietal lobe The portion of the brain that is the site for reception and evaluation of most sensory information, except smell, hearing, and vision.

parietal pain Pain caused by inflammation of the parietal peritoneum that is generally described as steady, aching, and aggravated by movement.

parity Number of live births a woman has had.

Parkinson's disease A neurological condition in which the portion of the brain responsible for production of dopamine is damaged or overused, resulting in tremors.

Parkland formula A formula that recommends giving 4 ml of normal saline for each kilogram of body weight, multiplied by the percentage of body surface area burned; sometimes used to calculate fluid needs during lengthy transport times.

paroxysmal nocturnal dyspnoea (PND) Severe shortness of breath occurring at night after several hours of recumbency, during which fluid pools in the lungs; the person is forced to sit up to breathe. PND is caused by left heart failure or decompensation of chronic obstructive pulmonary disease.

partial-thickness burn A burn that involves the epidermis and part of the dermis, characterised by pain and blistering; previously called a second-degree burn.

passive interventions Something that offers automatic protection from injury, often without requiring any conscious change of behaviour by the individual; child-resistant bottles and airbags are some examples.

passive neglect An unintentional refusal or failure to fulfil an obligation, which results in physical or emotional distress. Examples include forgetting or isolating the person.

patch A solid medication impregnated into a membrane or adhesive that is applied to the surface of the skin.

pathological fracture A fracture that occurs when normal forces are applied to abnormal bone structures.

pathophysiology The study of how normal physiological processes are affected by disease.

pathway expansion The tissue displacement that occurs as a result of low-displacement shock waves that travel at the speed of sound in tissue.

patient history Information about the patient's chief complaint, present symptoms, and previous illnesses.

peak load A time of day or day of week in which the call volume is at its highest.

pedicle A narrow strip of tissue by which an avulsed piece of tissue remains connected to the body.

pelvic inflammatory disease (PID) An infection of the female upper organs of reproduction, specifically the uterus, ovaries, and fallopian tubes.

penetrating trauma Injury caused by objects that pierce the surface of the body, such as knives and bullets, and damage internal tissues and organs.

peptic ulcer disease (PUD) Erosion of the stomach or small intestine.

perception The way a person processes the data supplied by the five senses.

percussion Gently striking the surface of the body, typically overlying various body cavities to detect changes in the densities of the underlying structures.

percutaneous routes The medication routes of any medication absorbed through the skin or a mucous membrane.

perfusion The delivery of oxygen and nutrients to the cells, organs, and tissues of the body. Also involves the removal of waste.

pericardial tamponade Impairment of diastolic filling of the right ventricle due to significant amounts of fluid in the pericardial sac surrounding the heart, leading to a decrease in cardiac output.

pericardium The double-layered sac containing the heart and the origins of the superior vena cava, inferior vena cava, and pulmonary artery.

perimetrium The outer protective layer of tissue in the uterus.

perineum The area between the vaginal opening and the anus.

periorbital bruising Bruising under or around the orbits that is commonly seen following a basilar skull fracture; also called raccoon eyes.

peripheral nerves All of the nerves of the body extending from the brain and spinal cord.

peripheral nervous system (PNS) Consists of all nervous tissue outside of the brain and spinal cord and is subdivided into two divisions, the somatic and autonomic nervous systems.

peripheral neuropathy A group of conditions in which the nerves leaving the spinal cord are damaged, resulting in distortion of signals to or from the brain. One type is diabetic, in which the peripheral nerves are damaged as blood glucose levels rise, causing loss of sensation, numbness, burning, pain, paraesthesia, and muscle weakness.

peripheral shock A term that describes shock secondary to peripheral circulatory abnormalities—includes both hypovolaemic shock and distributive shock.

peripheral vision Visualisation of lateral objects while looking forward.

peristalsis The rhythmic contractions of the intestines and oesophagus that allow material to move.

peritoneum A membrane in the abdomen encasing the liver, spleen, diaphragm, stomach, and transverse colon.

peritonitis Inflammation of the peritoneum (the lining around the abdominal cavity) that results from either blood or hollow organ contents spilling into the abdominal cavity.

peritubular capillaries A set of capillaries unique to the kidney that branch off from the efferent arteriole; the site of tubular resorption.

periumbilical Pertaining to the area around the umbilicus.

permanent cavity The path of crushed tissue produced by a missile traversing part of the body.

permissible exposure limit (PEL) The maximum concentration of a chemical that a person may be exposed to under Health and Safety Commission regulations.

perseveration Repeating the same idea over and over again.

persistency Term used to describe how long a chemical agent will stay on a surface before it evaporates.

persistent pulmonary hypertension Delayed transition from fetal to neonatal circulation.

personal flotation device (PFD) Also commonly known as a life jacket, a PFD allows the body to float in water.

personality disorder The term used to describe a condition a person has when he or she behaves or thinks in a way that is dysfunctional or causes distress to other people.

petechiae Tiny purple or red spots that appear on the skin due to bleeding within the skin or under mucous membranes.

petechial Characterised by small purplish, nonblanching spots on the skin.

pH The measure of acidity or alkalinity of a solution.

phagocyte A kind of cell that engulfs and consumes foreign material such as microorganisms and debris.

phagocytosis Process in which a cell eats or engulfs a foreign substance to destroy it.

pharmacodynamics The branch of pharmacology that studies reactions between medications and living structures, including the processes of body responses to pharmacological, biochemical, physiological, and therapeutic effects.

pharmacokinetics The study of the metabolism and action of medications with particular emphasis on the time required for absorption, duration of action, distribution in the body, and method of excretion.

pharmacology The branch of medicine dealing with the actions of drugs in the body—therapeutic and toxic effects—and development and testing of new drugs and new uses of existing ones.

phlebitis Inflammation of the wall of a vein, sometimes caused by an IV line, manifested by tenderness, redness, and slight oedema along part of the length of the vein.

phlebotomy The withdrawal of blood from a vein.

phobia An abnormal and persistent dread of a specific object or situation.

phosgene A pulmonary agent that is a product of combustion, such as might be produced in a fire at a textile factory or house, or from metalwork or burning Freon. Phosgene is a very potent agent that has a delayed onset of symptoms, usually hours.

phosgene oxime (CX) A blistering agent that has a rapid onset of symptoms and produces immediate intense pain and discomfort on contact.

physical dependence A physiological state of adaptation to a drug, usually characterised by tolerance to the drug's effects and a withdrawal syndrome if use of the drug is stopped, especially abruptly.

physical evidence The evidence that ties a suspect or victim to a crime. It may include body materials, objects, and impressions.

physical examination The process by which quantifiable, objective information is obtained from a patient about his or her overall state of health.

physiological fracture A fracture that occurs when abnormal forces are applied to normal bone structures.

pia mater The innermost and thinnest of the three meninges that enclose the brain and spinal cord; rests directly on the brain and spinal cord.

Pierre Robin sequence A condition present at birth marked by a very small lower jaw (micrognathia). The tongue tends to fall back and downward (glossoptosis), and there is a cleft soft palate.

pill A drug shaped into a ball or oval to be swallowed; often coated to disguise an unpleasant taste.

pinna The large outside portion of the ear through which sound waves enter the ear; also called the auricle.

piriform fossa Hollow pockets on the lateral sides of the glottic opening.

pituitary gland The gland that secretes hormones that regulate the function of many other glands in the body; also called the hypophysis.

placenta The tissue attached to the uterine wall that nourishes the fetus through the umbilical cord.

placenta previa Abnormal location of the placenta in the lower part of the uterus, near or over the cervix.

plaque In cardiology, the white to yellow lesion found in atherosclerosis that is made up of lipids, cell debris, and smooth muscles cells; in older people, may also include calcium.

plasma A component of blood, made of 92% water, 6% to 7% proteins, and electrolytes, clotting factors, and glucose; this makes up 55% of the total blood volume.

plasmin A naturally occurring clot-dissolving enzyme, usually present in the body in its inactive form, plasminogen.

platelets Small cells in the blood that are essential for clot formation.

pleural effusion Excessive accumulation of fluid in the pleural space.

pneumonic plague A lung infection, also known as plague pneumonia, that is the result of inhalation of plague bacteria.

pneumonitis Inflammation of the lung. Implies lung inflammation from an irritant such as a chemical, dust, or radiation, or from aspiration. When lung inflammation is caused by an infectious agent, it would typically be called pneumonia.

podocytes Special cells in the inner membrane of the glomerulus that wrap around the capillaries in the glomerulus, forming filtration slits.

point of maximal impulse (PMI) The palpable beat of the apex of the heart against the chest wall during ventricular contraction; nor-mally palpated in the fifth left intercostal space in the midclavicular line.

poison A substance whose chemical action could damage structures or impair function when introduced into the body.

poliomyelitis A viral infection that attacks the axons, especially motor axons, and destroys them, causing weakness, paralysis, and respiratory arrest. An effective vaccine has been developed and this disease is now rare.

polycythaemia The production of more red blood cells over time, making the blood thick; a characteristic of people who have chronic lung disease and chronic hypoxia.

polyhydramnios An excessive amount of amniotic fluid. May cause preterm labour.

polymorphonuclear neutrophils (PMNs) A type of white blood cell formed by bone marrow tissue that possesses a nucleus consisting of several parts or lobes connected by fine strands; a variety of leucocyte.

polypharmacy Simultaneous use of many medications.

polyuria Frequent and plentiful urination.

pons Lies below the midbrain and above the medulla and contains numerous important nerve fibres, including those for sleep, respiration, and the medullary respiratory centre.

portal vein A large vessel created by the intersection of blood vessels from the GI system. The portal vein empties into the liver.

positive-pressure ventilation (PPV) Method for assisting ventilation (bag-valve-mask or intubated) with high-flow air or supplemental oxygen.

positive symptoms Evidence of or physical change due to a disease or condition, which can be physically noted by the patient or health care provider; with regard to schizophrenia, refers to delusions and hallucinations.

positive wave pulse The phase of the explosion in which there is a pressure front with a pressure higher than atmospheric pressure.

postconventional reasoning A type of reasoning in which a child bases decisions upon his or her conscience.

posterior chamber The posterior area of the globe between the lens and the iris.

postictal The period of time after a convulsion during which the brain is reorganising activity.

postpartum After birth.

postpolio syndrome A result of polio in which neurons break down and die, resulting in difficulty swallowing, weakness, fatigue, or breathing problems even after the patient has healed.

postrenal ARF A type of acute renal failure caused by obstruction of urine flow from the kidneys, commonly caused by a blockage of the urethra by prostate enlargement, renal calculi, or strictures.

post-term Any pregnancy that lasts more than 42 weeks.

post-traumatic stress disorder (PTSD) A severe form of anxiety that stems from a traumatic experience. PTSD is characterised by the reliving of the stress and nightmares of the original situation.

postural tremors Tremors that occur as the person holds a body part still.

posture The position of one's body.

potential energy The amount of energy stored in an object, the product of mass, gravity, and height, that is converted into kinetic energy and results in injury, such as from a fall.

potentiation In health care, the effect of increasing the potency or effectiveness of a drug or other treatment; may occur by administering two medications concurrently, and one increases the effect of the other.

powder A drug that has been ground into pulverised form.

ppb Parts per billion; an expression of concentration.

ppm Parts per million; an expression of concentration.

P-R interval The period between the beginning of the P wave (atrial depolarisation) and the onset of the QRS complex (ventricular depolarisation), signifying the time required for atrial depolarisation and passage of the excitation impulse through the atrioventricular junction.

preceptorship A period of practical experience, training, and development that is structured to facilitate learning for a trainee, whilst being overseen by an educator/trainer/coach or mentor.

preconventional reasoning A type of reasoning in which a child acts almost purely to avoid discipline to get what he or she wants.

precordial leads Another term used to describe the chest leads in an ECG.

preeclampsia A condition of late pregnancy that involves gradual onset of hypertension, headache, visual changes, and swelling of the hands and feet; also called pregnancy-induced hypertension or toxaemia of pregnancy.

preload The pressure under which the ventricle fills.

premature Underdeveloped; the condition of an infant born too soon. Refers to infants delivered before 37 weeks from the first day of the last menstrual period.

premenstrual syndrome (PMS) A cluster of all or some of the troubling symptoms that occur during a woman's menstrual phase that can include fluid retention, breast pain and tenderness, headache, severe cramping, and emotional changes, including agitation, irritability, depression, and anger.

prepuce In the anatomy of the female genitalia, a layer of skin directly above the clitoris.

prerenal ARF A type of acute renal failure that is caused by hypoperfusion of the kidneys, resulting from hypovolaemia (haemorrhage, dehydration), trauma, shock, sepsis, and heart failure (congestive heart failure, myocardial infarction); often reversible if the underlying condition can be found and perfusion restored to the kidney.

presbycusis Progressive hearing loss, particularly in the high frequencies, along with lessened ability to discriminate between a particular sound and background noise.

preschoolers Individuals who are 3 to 5 years of age.

pressure of speech Speech in which words seem to tumble out under immense emotional pressure.

preterm Used to describe an infant delivered at less than 37 completed weeks.

prevalence The number of cases of a disease in a specific population over time.

primary adrenal insufficiency Also known as Addison's disease. A rare condition in which the adrenal glands produce an insufficient amount of adrenal hormones.

primary apnoea Apnoea caused by oxygen deprivation; usually corrected with stimulation, such as drying or slapping the newborn's feet. Primary apnoea is typically preceded by an initial period of rapid breathing.

primary brain injury An injury to the brain and its associated structures that is a direct result of impact to the head.

primary contamination An exposure that occurs with direct contact with the hazardous material.

primary exit The main means of escape should violence erupt. This is usually the door you used to enter the building.

primary injury prevention Keeping an injury from occurring.

primary triage officer The person in charge of prioritising patients, whose primary duty is to ensure that every patient receives initial triage.

primigravida A woman who is pregnant for the first time.

primipara A woman who has had one delivery only.

primitive reflexes Reflex reactions such as Babinski, grasping, and sucking signs normally found in very young patients.

process objectives State how a programme will be implemented, describing the service to be provided, the nature of the service, and to whom it will be directed.

prodrome The early signs and symptoms that occur before a disease or condition fully appear, eg, dizziness before fainting.

profession A specialised set of knowledge, skills, and/or expertise.

professional A person who follows expected standards and performance parameters in a specific profession.

progesterone A hormone that influences the second phase of the menstrual cycle, when the oocyte is either fertilised or dies.

prolapsed umbilical cord When the umbilical cord presents itself outside of the uterus while the fetus is still inside; an obstetric emergency during pregnancy or labour that acutely endangers the life of the baby; can happen when the water breaks and with the gush of water the cord comes along.

pronation Turning of the lower arms in a palm-downward manner.

proprioception The ability to perceive the position and movement of one's body or limbs.

prostaglandins A group of lipids that act as chemical messengers.

protocol A treatment plan developed for a specific illness or injury.

protuberant A convex or distended shape of the abdomen. This can be caused by oedema.

proximal convoluted tubule (PCT) One of two complex sections of the nephron, the PCT includes an enlargement at the end called the glomerular capsule.

pruritus Unspecified itching.

pseudocyesis A false pregnancy that develops all the typical signs and symptoms of true pregnancy, but in which no actual pregnancy exists.

pseudomembrane A false membrane formed by a dead tissue layer. Seen in the posterior pharynx of patients with diphtheria.

psychiatric emergency An emergency in which abnormal behaviour threatens an individual's health and safety or the health and safety of another person, for example when a person becomes suicidal, homicidal, or has a psychotic episode.

psychological dependence The emotional state of craving a drug to maintain a feeling of well-being.

psychosis Breaking with common reality and existing mainly within an internal world.

psychotropic drugs Drugs that affect mood, thought, or behaviour.

ptosis Drooping of an eyelid.

public relations (PR) officer Delegated role from the ambulance commander, the person who keeps the public informed and relates any information to the press.

pulmonary artery One of two arteries that carry deoxygenated blood from the right ventricle to the lungs.

pulmonary blast injuries Pulmonary trauma resulting from short-range exposure to the detonation of high explosives.

pulmonary circulation The flow of blood from the right ventricle through the pulmonary arteries and all of their branches and capillaries in the lungs and back to the left atrium through the venules and pulmonary veins; also called the lesser circulation.

pulmonary hypertension Elevated blood pressure in the pulmonary arteries from constriction; causes problems with the blood flow in the lungs, and makes the heart work harder.

pulmonary oedema Congestion of the pulmonary air spaces with exudate and foam, often secondary to left heart failure.

pulmonary route A medication route in which medication is administered directly to the pulmonary system through inhalation or injection.

pulmonary veins The vessels that carry oxygenated blood from the lungs to the left atrium.

pulmonic valve The valve between the right ventricle and the pulmonary artery.

pulp Specialised connective tissue within the pulp cavity of a tooth.

pulse oximetry An assessment tool that measures oxygen saturation of haemoglobin in the capillary beds.

pulse pressure The difference between the systolic and diastolic pressures.

pulsus paradoxus Weakening or loss of a palpable pulse during inhalation, characteristic of cardiac tamponade and severe asthma.

puncture wound A stab injury from a pointed object, such as a nail or a knife.

pupil The circular opening in the centre of the eye through which light passes to the lens.

Purkinje fibres A system of fibres in the ventricles that conducts the excitation impulse from the bundle branches to the myocardium.

purpuric Pertaining to bruising of the skin.

purulent Full of pus; having the character of pus.

purulent exudates Discharge that contains pus.

push-to-talk Commonly abbreviated as PTT, a method for communicating on a half-duplex communications system by pushing a button on the communication device to send and releasing the button to receive.

pyelonephritis Inflammation of the kidney linings.

pylorus A circumferential muscle at the end of the stomach that acts as a valve between the stomach and duodenum.

pyrogens Chemicals or proteins that travel to the brain and affect the hypothalamus, and stimulate a rise in the body's core temperature.

QRS complex Deflections of the ECG produced by ventricular depolarisation.

quadriplegia Paralysis of all four extremities and the trunk.

raccoon eyes Bruising under or around the orbits that is commonly seen following a basilar skull fracture; also called periorbital bruising.

radioactive material Any material that emits radiation.

radiological dispersal device (RDD) Any container that is designed to disperse radioactive material.

rales Old terminology for abnormal breath sounds that have a fine, crackling quality; now called crackles.

rape Is any act of non-consensual intercourse by a man with a person; the victim can be either male or female. Intercourse can be vaginal, anal or oral. According to the Sexual Offences Act (2003) a person consents if he or she agrees by choice, and has the freedom and capacity to make that choice. The law does not require the victim to have resisted physically.

reactive airway disease A term used to describe any condition that causes hyperreactive bronchioles and bronchospasm.

recall The ability to retrieve a specific piece of stored information on demand.

recanalisation The opening up of new channels through a blocked artery.

receptive dysphasia Damage to or loss of the ability to understand speech.

receptors Specialised areas in tissues that initiate certain actions after specific stimulation.

recession Physical drawing in of the chest wall between the ribs that occurs with increased work of breathing.

recognition The ability to identify information that one has encountered before.

referred pain Pain that originates in one area of the body but is interpreted as coming from a different area of the body.

reflexes Involuntary motor responses to specific sensory stimuli, such as a tap on the knee or stroking the eyelash.

refractory period A short period immediately after depolarisation in which the myocytes are not yet repolarised and are unable to fire or conduct an impulse.

regional anaesthesia A type of anaesthesia that focuses on a particular portion of the body, such as the legs or the arms.

registration The ability to add new items to the cerebral data bank.

relative refractory period That period in the cell-firing cycle at which it is possible but difficult to restimulate the cell to fire another impulse.

renal columns Inward extensions of cortical tissue that surround the renal pyramids.

renal dialysis A technique for "filtering" the blood of its toxic wastes, removing excess fluids, and restoring the normal balance of electrolytes.

renal fascia Dense, fibrous connective tissue that anchors the kidney to the abdominal wall.

renal pelvis Part of the internal anatomy of the kidney; a flat, funnel-shaped tube filling the sinus at the level of the hilus.

renal pyramids Parallel cone-shaped bundles of urine-collecting tubules that are located in the medulla of the kidneys.

renin A hormone produced by cells in the juxtaglomerular apparatus when the blood pressure is low.

renin-angiotensin-aldosterone system (RAAS) A complex feedback mechanism responsible for the kidney's regulation of sodium in the body.

repeater Miniature transmitter that picks up a radio signal and rebroadcasts it, extending the range of a radio communications system.

reperfusion The resumption of blood flow through an artery.

resistance vessels The smallest arterioles.

respiratory arrest The absence of respirations with detectable cardiac activity.

respiratory distress A clinical state characterised by increased respiratory rate, effort, and work of breathing.

respiratory exposure Exposure of the airways and lungs to a gas or vapour.

respiratory failure A clinical state of inadequate oxygenation, ventilation, or both.

respiratory syncytial virus (RSV) A virus that commonly causes bronchiolitis; usually results in lifelong immunity following exposure.

rest tremors Tremors that occur when the body part is not in motion.

restlessness A situation in which the patient can't sit still.

retardation of thought The patient seems to take a very long time to get from one thought to the next.

retention The ability to store items in an accessible place in the mind.

reticular activating system (RAS) Located in the upper brain stem; responsible for maintenance of consciousness, specifically one's level of arousal.

reticuloendothelial system The system in the body that is primarily used to defend against infection.

retina A delicate 10-layered structure of nervous tissue located in the rear of the interior of the globe that receives light and generates nerve signals that are transmitted to the brain through the optic nerve.

retinal detachment Separation of the inner layers of the retina from the underlying choroid, the vascular membrane that nourishes the retina.

retinopathy of prematurity A disease of the eye that affects prematurely born babies, thought to be caused by disorganised growth of retinal blood vessels resulting in scarring and retinal detachment; can lead to blindness in serious cases.

retrograde amnesia Loss of memory relating to events that occurred before the injury.

retroperitoneal space The area in the abdomen containing the aorta, vena cava, pancreas, kidneys, ureters, and portions of the duodenum and large intestine.

retrosternal Situated or occurring behind the sternum.

review of systems A systematic survey of the patient's symptoms according to the major organ systems.

Rh factor A protein found on the red blood cells of most people; when a woman without this protein is impregnated by a man with this protein, the woman's body can create antibodies against the protein and attack future pregnancies.

rhabdomyolysis The destruction of muscle tissue leading to a release of potassium and myoglobin.

rhonchi (singular: rhonchus) Low-pitched wheezes also described as rattling or snoring. Caused by secretions in the larger bronchi narrowing the airways.

ribonucleic acid (RNA) Nucleic acid associated with controlling cellular activities.

ricin Neurotoxin derived from mash that is left from pressing oil from the castor bean; causes pulmonary oedema and respiratory and circulatory failure, leading to death.

right atrium The upper right chamber of the heart; receives blood from the venae cavae and supplies blood to the right ventricle.

right ventricle The lower right chamber of the heart; receives blood from the right atrium and pumps blood out through the pulmonic valve into the pulmonary artery.

risk factors Characteristics of people, behaviours, or environments that increase the chances of disease or injury. Some examples are alcohol use, poverty, or gender.

Rohypnol A benzodiazepine used to facilitate date rape and that can create memory loss; street names include roofies, roof, R2, and rocha.

rooting reflex An infant reflex that occurs when something touches an infant's cheek, and the infant instinctively turns his head toward the touch.

route of exposure Manner by which a toxic substance enters the body.

R-R interval The period between the onset of one QRS complex and the onset of the next QRS complex.

rubor Redness; one of the classic signs of inflammation.

rubs Lung sound produced by a partial loss of intrapleural integrity, when an abnormal collection of fluid has accumulated between a portion of the visceral and parietal pleura, resulting in "pleuritic" pain and a perceived rub on auscultation.

rule of nines A system that assigns percentages to sections of the body, allowing calculation of the amount of skin surface involved in the burn area.

rule of palm A system that estimates total body surface area burned by comparing the affected area with the size of the patient's palm, which is roughly equal to 1% of the patient's total body surface area.

ruptured ovarian cyst A fluid-filled sac within the ovary that bursts from internal pressure.

safety officer Delegated role from the ambulance commander, the person who gives the "go ahead" to a plan or who may stop an operation when rescuer safety is an issue.

sagittal suture The point of the skull where the parietal bones join.

salicylates Aspirin-like drugs.

sarin (GB) A nerve agent that is one of the G agents; a highly volatile colourless and odourless liquid that turns from liquid to gas within seconds to minutes at room temperature.

scald burn A burn produced by hot liquids.

scaphoid A concave shape of the abdomen. This can be caused by evisceration.

scar revision A surgical procedure to improve the appearance of a scar, reestablish function, or correct disfigurement from soft-tissue damage, surgical incision, or lesion.

school age A person who is 5 to 12 years of age.

sclera The white part of the eye.

scoliosis Sideways curvature of the spine.

search and rescue (SAR) The process of locating and removing a patient from the wilderness.

sebaceous gland The gland located in the dermis that secretes sebum.

sebum An oily substance secreted by sebaceous glands.

second stage of labour The stage of labour in which the baby's head enters the birth canal, during which contractions become more intense and more frequent.

secondary apnoea When asphyxia continues after primary apnoea, infant responds with a period of gasping respirations, falling pulse rate and falling blood pressure.

secondary brain injury The "after effects" of the primary injury; includes abnormal processes such as cerebral oedema, increased intracranial pressure, cerebral ischaemia and hypoxia, and infection; onset is often delayed following the primary brain injury.

secondary collapse A collapse that occurs following the primary collapse. This can occur in trench, excavation, and structural collapses.

secondary contamination Exposure to a hazardous material by contact with a contaminated person or object.

secondary device Additional explosives used by terrorists, which are set to explode after the initial bomb.

secondary exit Any other means of egress, including windows and rear doors.

secondary injury prevention Reducing the effects of an injury that has already happened.

secretory phase The second phase of the menstrual cycle.

secure attachment A bond between an infant and his or her parent or caregiver, in which the infant understands that his parents or caregivers will be responsive to his needs and take care of him when he needs help.

sedation An effect in which the patient experiences decreased anxiety and inhibition.

sedative-hypnotic A drug used to reduce anxiety, calm agitated patients, and help produce drowsiness and sleep (CNS depressants).

selective serotonin reuptake inhibitors (SSRIs) A class of anti-depressants that inhibit the reuptake of serotonin.

self-rescue position Position used in fast-flowing water rescue situations. The rescuer rolls into a face-up arched position with the lower back higher than the feet to avoid objects below the surface. The feet should be together and facing in the direction of travel (feet first), with arms at the sides.

Sellick manoeuvre Pressure applied over the cricoid to seal off the oesophagus and prevent reflux of gastric contents.

semilunar valves The two valves, the aortic and pulmonic, that divide the heart from the aorta and pulmonary arteries.

sensitisation Developing sensitivity to a substance that initially caused no allergic reaction.

sensorineural deafness A permanent lack of hearing caused by a lesion of or damage to the inner ear.

sepsis A disease state that results from the presence of microorganisms or their toxic products in the bloodstream.

septic abortion A life-threatening emergency in which the uterus becomes infected following any type of abortion.

septic shock This occurs as a result of widespread infection, usually bacterial. Untreated, the result is multiple organ dysfunction syndrome (MODS) and often death.

serosa The outermost layer of tissue in the fallopian tubes.

serotonin A vasoactive amine that increases vascular permeability to cause vasodilation.

serotonin syndrome An idiosyncratic complication that occurs with anti-depressant therapy in which patients have lower extremity muscle rigidity, confusion or disorientation, and/or agitation.

serous exudates Discharge that contains serum, a thin watery substance.

serum sickness A condition in which antigen antibody complexes formed in the bloodstream deposit in sites around the body, most notably in the kidney, with resultant inflammatory reactions.

sexual assault An attack against a person that is sexual in nature, the most common of which is rape.

shaken baby syndrome A syndrome seen in abused infants and children; the patient has been subjected to violent, whiplash-type shaking injuries inflicted by the abusing individual that may cause coma, convulsions, and increased intracranial pressure due to tearing of the cerebral veins with consequent bleeding into the brain.

shearing An applied force or pressure exerted against the surface and layers of the skin as tissues slide in opposite but parallel planes.

shock An abnormal state associated with inadequate oxygen and nutrient delivery to the metabolic apparatus of the cell.

shoring A method of supporting a trench wall or building components such as walls, floors, or ceilings using either hydraulic, pneumatic, or wood shoring systems. Shoring is used to prevent collapse.

shunt Situation in which a portion of the output of the right side of the heart reaches the left side of the heart without being oxygenated in the lungs; may be caused by atelectasis, pulmonary oedema, or a variety of other conditions. In haemodialysis, an anastomosis between a peripheral artery and vein.

sickle cell disease A disease that causes the RBCs to be misshapen, resulting in poor oxygen-carrying capability and potentially resulting in lodging of the RBCs in blood vessels or the spleen.

side effects Reactions that can manifest as signs or symptoms that are not desired but are expected based on how the medication works.

signs Indications of illness or injury that the examiner can see, hear, feel, smell, and so on.

simple febrile convulsions A brief, self-limited, generalised convulsion in a previously healthy child between the ages of 6 months and 6 years that is associated with the onset of or sudden increase in fever.

simple incident Incident where local infrastructure (ie, electricity supplies, water supplies, roads, hospitals, and so forth) is intact.

simple partial convulsions Focal convulsions that involve a motor or sensory abnormality in a patient who remains conscious.

simple phobia A fear that is focused on one class of objects (eg, mice, spiders, dogs) or situations (eg, high places, darkness, flying).

simplex Method of radio communication using a single frequency that enables transmission or reception of voice or an ECG signal but is incapable of simultaneous transmission and reception.

single command system A command system in which one person is in charge, generally used with small incidents that involve only one responding agency.

sinoatrial (SA) node The dominant pacemaker of the heart, located at the junction of the superior vena cava and the right atrium.

sinus arrhythmia A slight irregularity of the heart rate caused by changes in parasympathetic tone during breathing.

sinus bradycardia A sinus rhythm with a heart rate less than 60 beats/min.

sinus tachycardia A sinus rhythm with a heart rate greater than 100 beats/min.

skeletal muscle relaxants Medications that provide relief of skeletal muscle spasms.

skull The structure at the top of the axial skeleton that houses the brain and consists of 28 bones that comprise the auditory ossicles, the cranium, and the face.

slow-reacting substances of anaphylaxis (SRS-A) Biologically active compounds derived from arachidonic acid called leucotrienes.

SLUDGE A mnemonic that stands for Salivation, Lacrimation, Urination, Defecation, Gastrointestinal activity, and Emesis, which are the signs and symptoms that can be produced by exposure to organophosphate and carbamate pesticides or other nerve-stimulating agents.

small for gestational age An infant whose size and weight are considerably less than the average for babies of the same age.

smallpox A highly contagious disease; it is most contagious when blisters begin to form.

smooth muscle Nonstriated involuntary muscle found in vessel walls, glands, and the gastrointestinal tract.

sniffing position An upright position in which the patient's head and chin are thrust slightly forward to keep the airway open; appears to be sniffing the morning air.

snoring Noise made on inhalation when the upper airway is partially obstructed by the tongue.

Social Services Organisation that is responsible for the well-being, protection and care of children, elderly and disabled people and for the promotion of that well-being and protection through the use of direct services as well as their co-ordination of, and liaison with, voluntary agencies, private companies and other public authorities.

sodium channel blockers Anti-arrhythmic medications that slow conduction through the heart.

solution A liquid containing one or more chemical substances entirely dissolved, usually in water.

soman (GD) A nerve agent that is one of the G agents; twice as persistent as sarin and five times as lethal; it has a fruity odour as a result of the type of alcohol used in the agent, and is both a contact and inhalation hazard that can enter the body through skin absorption and through the respiratory tract.

somatoform disorder A condition in which a person is overly concerned with physical health and appearance to the point that it dominates his or her life; an example is hypochondria.

somnolence Sleepiness.

spacer A device that collects medication as it is released from the canister of a metered-dose inhaler, allowing more to be delivered to the lungs and less to be lost to the environment.

spalling Delaminating or breaking off into chips and pieces.

span of control The subordinate positions under the commander's direction to which the workload is distributed; the supervisor/worker ratio.

specific agents Medications that bring about an identifiable mechanism with unique receptors for the agent.

specific gravity The weight of a substance compared with water.

spina bifida A development defect in which a portion of the spinal cord or meninges may protrude outside of the vertebrae and possibly even outside of the body, usually at the lower third of the spine in the lumbar area.

spirits A preparation of a volatile substance dissolved in alcohol.

spoil pile The pile of earth that has been removed from an excavation. The pile may be unstable and prone to collapse.

spondylosis Immobility and consolidation of a vertebral joint.

spontaneous abortion Expulsion of the fetus that occurs naturally; also called miscarriage.

ST segment The interval between the end of the QRS complex and the beginning of the T wave; often elevated or depressed with respect to the isoelectric line when there is significant myocardial ischaemia.

stable angina Angina pectoris characterised by periodic pain with a predictable pattern.

state-sponsored terrorism Terrorism that is funded and/or supported by nations that hold close ties with terrorist groups.

status epilepticus A state of continuous convulsions or multiple convulsions without a return to consciousness for 30 minutes.

steam burn A burn that has been caused by direct exposure to hot steam exhaust, as from a broken pipe.

steatorrhoea Foamy, fatty stools caused by liver failure or gallbladder problems.

stem cells Cells that can develop into other types of cells in the body.

step blocks Specialised chocking assemblies made out of wood or plastic blocks in a step configuration.

stereotyped activity Repetitive movements that don't appear to serve any purpose.

stimulants An agent that increases the level of body activity.

stoma A small opening, especially an artificially created opening, such as that made by tracheostomy.

strategic (Gold) command Established during protracted major incidents, and is convened off-site, away from the actual major incident itself. It is the top tier of the Integrated Emergency Management System and comprises senior managers/directors of all emergency services and responding organisations.

strategic deployment Nominating listening watch and standby locations for ambulances to enhance the geographical coverage of emergency resources to attend 999 calls.

stratum basalis A permanent mucous membrane that makes up part of the outer endometrium.

stratum functionalis An inner mucous membrane that makes up part of the endometrium, and which is renewed following menstruation.

striae Stretch marks on the abdomen caused by size changes.

stridor Harsh, high pitched wheeze normally heard on inspiration, indicating upper airway obstruction, such as that from infection, burns, or a foreign body.

stroke volume (SV) The volume of blood pumped forward with each ventricular contraction.

subarachnoid haematoma Bleeding into the subarachnoid space, where the cerebrospinal fluid (CSF) circulates.

subarachnoid space The space located between the pia mater and the arachnoid mater.

subcutaneous Beneath the skin.

subcutaneous layer Layer of tissue located beneath the skin.

subcutaneous (SC) route A medication route in which injections are given beneath the skin into the fat or connective tissue immediately underlying it.

subdural haematoma An accumulation of blood beneath the dura but outside the brain.

subglottic space The narrowest part of the paediatric airway.

sublingual (SL) A medication route in which medication is administered under the tongue.

substance abuse Use of a substance that disrupts activities of daily living.

substance dependence Use of a substance that results in addiction and physiological dependence on the substance.

substance intoxication Use of a substance that results in impaired thinking and motor function.

substance use Use of moderate amounts of a substance without seriously affecting activities of daily living.

subthalamus The part of the diencephalon that is involved in controlling motor functions.

sucking reflex An infant reflex in which the infant starts sucking when his or her lips are stroked.

sudden unexpected death in infancy (SUDI) The abrupt and unexplained death of an apparently healthy child younger than 1 year.

suicide Any willful act designed to bring an end to one's own life.

sulphur mustard (H) A vesicant; it is a brownish-yellowish oily substance that is generally considered very persistent; has the distinct smell of garlic or mustard and, when released, it is quickly absorbed into the skin and/or mucous membranes and begins an irreversible process of damaging the cells.

summation effect The process whereby multiple medications can produce a response that the individual medications alone do not produce.

superficial burn A burn involving only the epidermis, producing very red, painful skin; previously called a first-degree burn.

superficial frostbite A type of frostbite characterised by altered sensation (numbness, tingling, or burning) and white, waxy skin that is firm to palpation, but the underlying tissues remain soft.

supine hypotensive syndrome Low blood pressure resulting from compression of the inferior vena cava by the weight of the pregnant uterus when the mother is supine.

suppository A drug mixed in a firm base that melts at body temperature and is shaped to fit the rectum.

supraglottic Located above the glottic opening, as in the upper airway structures.

suprapubic The region of the abdomen superior to the pubic bone and inferior to the umbilicus.

supraventricular tachycardia (SVT) An abnormal heart rhythm with a rapid, narrow QRS complex.

surfactant A substance formed in the lungs that helps keep the small air sacs or alveoli from collapsing and sticking together; a low level in a premature baby contributes to respiratory distress syndrome.

surveillance of syndromes The monitoring, usually by public health departments, of patients presenting to accident and emergency departments and alternative care facilities, the recording of ambulance service call volume, and the use of general-sales-list medications.

suspension A preparation of a finely divided drug intended to be (or already) incorporated in a suitable liquid.

sympathetic blocking agent An anti-hypertensive medication that decreases cardiac output and renin secretions.

sympathetic eye movement The movement of both eyes in unison.

sympathetic nervous system A subdivision of the autonomic nervous system that governs the body's fight-or-flight reactions, stimulating cardiac activity.

sympathomimetics The medications administered to stimulate the sympathetic nervous system.

symptoms The pain, discomfort, or other abnormality that the patient feels.

synapses Gaps between nerve cells across which nervous stimuli are transmitted.

synchronised cardioversion The timed delivery of energy into the myocardium to correct rapid, regular cardiac rhythms in patients who are in unstable condition.

syncope Fainting; brief loss of consciousness caused by transiently inadequate blood flow to the brain.

synergism An interaction of two or more medications that results in an effect that is greater than the sum of their effects if taken independently.

synergistic effect When two substances interact to produce an overall greater effect than either alone or combined.

syphilis An STI caused by the bacterium Treponema pallidum, which manifests in three stages—primary, secondary, and late—and is transmitted through direct contact with open sores.

syrup A drug suspended in sugar and water to improve its taste.

systemic anaesthesia A type of anaesthesia often done through the inhalation of volatile vapourised liquids and predominantly reserved for operating theatre use; also called general anaesthesia.

systemic circulation The flow of blood from the left ventricle through the aorta, to all of its branches and capillaries in the tissues, and back to the right atrium through the venules, veins, and venae cavae; also called the greater circulation.

systemic effects The effects that occur after the drug is absorbed by any route and distributed by the bloodstream; almost invariably involve more than one organ.

systole The period during which the ventricles contract.

T killer cells Cells released during a type IV allergic reaction that kill antigen-bearing target cells.

T waves The upright, flat, or inverted wave following the QRS complex of the ECG, representing ventricular repolarisation.

tablet A powdered drug that has been moulded or compressed into a small disc.

tabun (GA) A nerve agent that is one of the G agents; is 36 times more persistent than sarin and approximately half as lethal; has a fruity smell and is unique because the components used to manufacture the agent are easy to acquire and the agent is easy to manufacture.

tachycardia A rapid heart rate, more than 100 beats/min.

tachyphylaxis A condition in which the patient rapidly becomes tolerant to a medication.

tactile fremitus Vibrations in the chest as the patient breathes.

tangential thinking Leaving the current topic midconversation to talk about something else, inhibiting interpersonal communication.

target tissues Tissues to which hormones are directed to act on.

technical rescue incident (TRI) A complex rescue incident involving vehicles or machinery, water or ice, rope techniques, a trench or excavation collapse, confined spaces, a structural collapse, wilderness search and rescue, or hazardous materials, and which requires specially trained personnel and special equipment.

technical rescue team A group of rescuers specially trained in the various disciplines of technical rescue.

technician The training degree that provides a high level of competency in the various disciplines of technical or hazardous materials rescue for rescuers who will be directly involved in the rescue operation itself.

tempered glass A type of safety glass that is heat-treated so that it will break into small pieces.

temporal lobe The portion of the brain that has an important role in hearing and memory.

temporomandibular joint (TMJ) The joint between the temporal bone and the posterior condyle that allows for movements of the mandible.

tension lines The pattern of tautness of the skin, which is arranged over body structures and affects how well wounds heal.

tenting A condition in which the skin slowly retracts after being pinched and pulled away slightly from the body; a sign of dehydration.

tentorium A structure that separates the cerebral hemispheres from the cerebellum and brain stem.

term Used to describe an infant delivered at 38 to 42 weeks of gestation.

terminal drop hypothesis The theory that a person's mental function declines in the last 5 years of life.

terminal illness A sickness that the patient cannot be cured of; death may be imminent.

termination of action The amount of time after the medication's concentration falls below the minimum effective level until it is eliminated from the body.

termination of command The end of the incident command structure when an incident draws to a close.

testes Male gonads located in the scrotum that produce hormones called androgens.

testimonial evidence The verbal documentation by a witness of the facts of a criminal act.

testosterone The most important androgen in men.

thalamus The part of the diencephalon that processes most sensory input and influences mood and general body movements, especially those associated with fear or rage.

thalassaemia A type of anaemia in which not enough haemoglobin is produced, or the haemoglobin is defective.

theophylline A naturally occurring alkaloid found in a variety of plants (such as tea leaves).

therapeutic index The ratio of a drug's lethal dose for 50% (LD50) of the population to its effective dose for 50% (ED50) of the population; a medication's margin of safety.

therapeutic The desired or intended action of a medication.

thermal burn An injury caused by radiation or direct contact with a heat source on the skin.

thermogenesis The production of heat in the body.

thermolysis The liberation of heat from the body.

thermoregulation The ability of the body to maintain temperature through a combination of heat gain by metabolic processes and muscular movement and heat loss through respiration, evaporation, conduction, convection, and perspiration.

thiazides A type of diuretic medication that specifically controls the sodium and water quantities excreted by the kidneys.

third stage of labour The stage of labour in which the placenta is expelled.

thought broadcasting The belief that others can hear one's thoughts.

thought control The belief that outside forces are controlling one's thoughts.

thought insertion The belief that thoughts are being thrust into one's mind by another person.

thought withdrawal The belief that thoughts are being removed from one's mind.

threatened abortion Expulsion of the fetus that is attempting to take place but has not occurred yet; usually occurs in the first trimester.

threshold limit value (TLV) The concentration of a substance that is supposed to be safe for exposure no more than 8 hours per day and 40 hours per week.

threshold limit value ceiling exposure limit (TLV-C) The concentration that a person should never be exposed to.

threshold limit value short-term exposure limit (TLV-STEL) The concentration of a substance that a worker can be exposed to for up to 15 minutes but no more than four times per day with at least an hour between each exposure.

thrombin An enzyme that causes the conversion of fibrinogen to fibrin, which binds to the platelet plugs, forming the final mature blood clot.

thrombocytes Platelets.

thrombocytopenia Reduction in the number of platelets.

thrombolytic therapy The therapy that uses medications that act to dissolve blood clots.

thyroid Large gland located at the base of the neck that produces and excretes hormones that influence growth, development, and metabolism.

thyroid-stimulating hormone (TSH) Hormone that controls the release of thyroid hormone from the thyroid gland.

thyroid storm A rare, life-threatening condition that may occur in patients with thyrotoxicosis. The condition is usually triggered by a stressful event or increased volume of thyroid hormones in the circulation.

thyrotoxicosis A toxic condition caused by excessive levels of circulating thyroid hormone.

thyroxine The body's major metabolic hormone. Thyroxine stimulates energy production in cells, which increases the rate at which the cells consume oxygen and use carbohydrates, fats, and proteins.

tidal volume Amount of air inhaled or exhaled during normal, quiet breathing; the volume of one breath.

tincture A dilute alcoholic extract of a drug.

toddlers Individuals who are 1 to 3 years of age.

tolerance Physiological adaptation to the effects of a drug such that increasingly larger doses of the drug are required to achieve the same effect.

tonic activity Type of convulsion movement involving the constant contraction and trembling of muscle groups.

tonic/clonic convulsions Convulsions that feature rhythmic back-and-forth motion of an extremity and body stiffness.

tonicity Tension exerted on a cell due to water movement across the cell membrane.

total body surface area (TBSA) Used in the calculation of a burn injury to determine the percentage of the surface of the patient's body that has been injured. This is commonly estimated by using the rule of palm or the rule of nines.

TOXBASE An NHS information source for poisons.

toxic shock syndrome (TSS) A form of septic shock caused by *Streptococcus pyogenes* (group A strep) or *Staphylococcus aureus*; initial symptoms include syncope, myalgia, diarrhoea, vomiting, headache, fever, and sore throat.

toxicity levels Measures of the risk that a hazardous material poses to the health of an individual who comes into contact with it.

toxicological emergencies Medical emergencies caused by toxic agents such as poison.

toxidrome The syndrome-like symptoms of a poisonous agent.

toxoid A modified bacterial toxin that has been made nontoxic but retains the ability to stimulate the formation of antibodies.

tracheal transection Traumatic separation of the trachea from the larynx.

tracheostomy Surgically opening in the trachea to create an airway.

trade name The brand name registered to a specific manufacturer or owner; also called proprietary name.

transceiver A radio transmitter and receiver housed in a single unit; a two-way radio.

transdermal route A medication route generally performed by placing medication directly onto the patient's skin.

transfer of command When an incident commander turns over command to someone with more experience in a critical area.

transient ischaemic attack (TIA) A disorder of the brain in which brain cells temporarily stop working because of insufficient oxygen, causing stroke-like symptoms that resolve completely within 24 hours of onset.

transmigration (diapedesis) The PMNs permeate through the vessel wall, moving into the interstitial space.

Transport Emergency Card (TREMCARD) A document that is legally required to be carried by drivers of commercial vehicles that should provide specific information about what is carried on the vehicle.

transverse presentation A delivery in which the fetus lies crosswise in the uterus; one hand may protrude through the vagina.

trauma Acute physiological and structural change that occurs in a victim as a result of the rapid dissipation of energy delivered by an external force.

traumatic brain injury (TBI) A traumatic insult to the brain capable of producing physical, intellectual, emotional, social, and vocational changes.

trench foot A process similar to frostbite but caused by prolonged exposure to cool, wet conditions.

triage To categorise patients based on the severity of their conditions and prioritise them for care accordingly.

triage Sieve The initial categorisation of patients at the site where they are found using three parameters: mobility, respiratory rate, and circulatory status. This is sometimes referred to as primary triage.

triage Sort The categorisation of patients using three parameters: respiratory rate, systolic blood pressure, and Glasgow Coma Scale score. This is carried out in the casualty clearing station and is sometimes referred to as secondary triage.

trichomoniasis A parasitic infection.

tricuspid valve The valve between the right atrium and right ventricle of the heart.

tricyclic anti-depressants (TCAs) A group of drugs used to treat severe depression and manage pain; minimal dosing errors can cause toxic results.

trigeminal nerve Fifth cranial nerve; supplies sensation to the scalp, forehead, face, and lower jaw and innervates the muscles of mastication, the throat, and the inner ear.

trigeminy A premature complex in every third heartbeat.

tripoding An abnormal position to keep the airway open; involves leaning forward onto two arms stretched forward.

trismus The involuntary contraction of the mouth resulting in clenched teeth. Occurs during convulsions and head injuries.

trunking Sharing of radio frequencies by multiple agencies or systems.

trust and mistrust A phrase that refers to a stage of development from birth to approximately 18 months of age, during which infants gain trust of their parents or caregivers if their world is planned, organised, and routine.

tuberculosis A chronic bacterial disease caused by Mycobacterium tuberculosis that usually affects the lungs but can also affect other organs such as the brain or kidneys.

tubo-ovarian abscess An infectious mass growing within the ovaries and fallopian tubes.

tunica adventitia The outer layer of tissue of a blood vessel wall, composed of elastic and fibrous connective tissue.

tunica intima The smooth, thin, inner lining of a blood vessel.

tunica media The middle and thickest layer of tissue of a blood vessel wall, composed of elastic tissue and smooth muscle cells that allow the vessel to expand or contract in response to changes in blood pressure and tissue demand.

tunnel vision Dangerous situation when a paramedic becomes so completely involved with patient care that he or she fails to see the possibility of physical harm to the patient or other care providers.

turbinates A set of bony convolutions on the sides of the nasal cavity, also called conchae, covered with a mucous membrane to warm and humidify inspired air.

turgor Loss of elasticity in the skin.

tympanic membrane A thin membrane that separates the middle ear from the inner ear and sets up vibrations in the ossicles; also called the eardrum.

type 1 diabetes The type of diabetic disease that usually starts in childhood and requires daily injections of supplemental synthetic insulin to control blood glucose. Sometimes called juvenile or juvenile-onset diabetes.

type 2 diabetes The type of diabetic disease that usually starts in later life and often can be controlled through diet and oral medications. Sometimes called adult-onset diabetes.

U wave A small flat wave sometimes seen after the T wave and before the next P wave.

ultrahigh frequency (UHF) band The portion of the radio frequency spectrum between 300 and 3,000 mHz.

umbilical The region of the abdomen surrounding the umbilicus.

umbilical cord The conduit connecting mother to infant via the placenta; contains two arteries and one vein.

umbilical vein Blood vessel in umbilical cord used to administer emergency medications.

uncompensated Where the incident creates a demand that cannot be met from local resources.

undifferentiated type Schizophrenia that does not fit neatly into another category.

unifocal Arising from a single site.

unintentional injuries Injuries that occur without intent to harm (commonly called accidents). Some examples are road traffic accidents, poisonings, drownings, falls, and most burns.

unstable angina Angina pectoris characterised by a changing, unpredictable pattern of pain, which may signal an impending acute myocardial infarction.

upper explosive limit (UEL) The concentration of a hazardous material at which there is not enough oxygen to support the combustion in air.

uraemia Severe kidney failure resulting in the buildup of waste products within the blood. Eventually brain functions will be impaired.

uraemic frost A powdery buildup of uric acid, especially around the face.

ureterostomy The formation of an opening to allow the passage of urine.

ureters A pair of thick-walled, hollow tubes that transport urine from the kidneys to the bladder.

urethra A hollow, tubular structure that drains urine from the bladder, passing it outside of the body.

uricosuric medications The medications designed to lower the uric acid level in the blood by increasing the excretion by the kidneys into the urine.

urinary bladder A hollow, muscular sac in the midline of the lower abdominal area that stores urine until it is released from the body.

urinary tract infections (UTIs) Infections, usually of the lower urinary tract (urethra and bladder), which occur when normal flora bacteria enter the urethra and grow.

urine Liquid waste products filtered out of the body by the urinary system.

urticaria Multiple small, raised areas on the skin that may be one of the warning signs of impending anaphylaxis. Also known as hives.

uterine cavity The interior of the body of the uterus.

uterine inversion A potentially fatal complication of childbirth in which the placenta fails to detach properly and results in the uterus turning inside-out.

uterus A muscular inverted pear-shaped organ, that lies situated between the urinary bladder and the rectum.

V agent (VX) One of the G agents; it is a clear, oily agent that has no odour and looks like baby oil; over 100 times more lethal than sarin and is extremely persistent.

vaccine A suspension of whole (live or inactivated) or fractionated bacteria or viruses that have been made nonpathogenic; given to induce an immune response and prevent disease.

vagina A tubular organ lined with mucous membranes, which is the lower portion of the birth canal.

vaginal bleeding Bleeding from the vagina.

vaginal yeast infection An infection caused by the fungus, Candida albicans, in which fungi over populate the vagina.

vagus nerve The 10th cranial nerve, the chief mediator of the parasympathetic nervous system.

Valsalva manoeuvre Forced exhalation against a closed glottis, the effect of which is to stimulate the vagus nerve and, thereby, slow the heart rate.

vapour A gaseous medication form primarily used in operating room anaesthesia.

vapour density A measure that compares the hazardous material gas to air; toxic gases that are heavier than air will sink, while vapours that are lighter than air will dissipate and travel with the wind.

vapour hazard An agent that enters the body through the respiratory tract.

vapour pressure The pressure exerted by a vapour when the liquid and vapour states of a material are in equilibrium; this measure changes as a material is heated.

vasa recta A series of peritubular capillaries that surround the loop of Henle, into which water moves after passing through the descending and ascending limbs of the loop of Henle.

vasculitis An inflammation of the blood vessels.

vasoactive amines Substances such as histamine and serotonin that increase vascular permeability.

vasoconstriction Narrowing of a blood vessel, such as with hypoperfusion or cold extremities.

vasodilation Widening of the diameter of a blood vessel.

vasodilator medications The medications that work on the smooth muscles of the arterioles and/or the veins.

veins The blood vessels that carry blood to the heart (except pulmonary).

velocity The speed of an object in a given direction.

vena cavae The largest veins of the body; they return blood to the right atrium.

vena cava filter A mesh filter placed in the inferior vena cava to catch blood clots in patients who are at high risk of pulmonary embolus.

ventilation-perfusion mismatch A pathological state in which the oxygen entering the lungs is not mixing properly with the blood circulating through the lungs.

ventricles Specialised hollow areas in the brain.

venules Very small veins.

vernix A white, cheesy substance that covers the fetus' skin in utero and at birth.

very high frequency (VHF) band The portion of the radio frequency spectrum between 30 and 150 mHz.

vesicants Blister agents; the primary route of entry for vesicants is through the skin.

vestibule A cleft between the labia minora, where the urethral opening (orifice), the vaginal opening (orifice), and the hymen are located.

viral haemorrhagic fevers (VHF) A group of diseases that include the Ebola, Rift Valley, and yellow fever viruses among others. This group of viruses causes the blood in the body to seep out from the tissues and blood vessels.

virulence A measure of the disease-causing ability of a microorganism.

viruses Disease-producing micro-organisms that require a living host to multiply and survive.

visceral pain Crampy, aching pain deep within the body, the source of which is usually hard to pinpoint; common with urological problems.

visual acuity (VA) The ability or inability to see, and how well one can see.

visual cortex The area in the brain where signals from the optic nerve are converted into visual images.

vitreous humour A jellylike substance found in the posterior compartment of the eye between the lens and the retina.

volatility Term used to describe how long a chemical agent will stay on a surface before it evaporates.

Volkmann contracture Deformity of the hand, fingers, and wrist resulting from damage to forearm muscles; develops from muscle ischaemia and is associated with compartment syndrome.

vulva The female external genitalia.

Waddell triad A pattern of motor vehicle-pedestrian injuries in children and people of short stature in which (1) the bumper hits pelvis and femur, (2) the chest and abdomen hit the grille or low bonnet, and (3) the head strikes the ground.

warm zone The area located between the hot zone and the cold zone at an incident. Decontamination stations are located in the warm zone.

water reactive A property that indicates that a material will undergo a chemical reaction (for example, explosion) when mixed with water.

water soluble A property that indicates that a material can be dissolved in water.

wavelength The distance in a propagating wave from one point to the corresponding point on the next wave.

weapon of major incident (WMI) Any agent designed to bring about mass death, casualties, and/or massive damage to property and infrastructure (bridges, tunnels, airports, and seaports); also known as a weapon of mass destruction (WMD).

weapon of mass destruction (WMD) Any agent designed to bring about mass death, casualties, and/or massive damage to property and infrastructure (bridges, tunnels, airports, and seaports); also known as a weapon of major incident (WMI).

weaponisation The creation of a weapon from a biological agent generally found in nature and that causes disease; the agent is cultivated, synthesised, and/or mutated to maximise the target population's exposure to the germ.

wheezing The production of whistling sounds during expiration such as occurs in asthma and bronchiolitis.

whiplash An injury to the cervical vertebrae or their supporting ligaments and muscles, usually resulting from sudden acceleration or deceleration.

windchill factor The factor that takes into account the temperature and wind velocity in calculating the effect of a given ambient temperature on living organisms.

withdrawal syndrome A predictable set of signs and symptoms, usually involving altered central nervous system activity, that occurs after the abrupt cessation of a drug or after rapidly decreasing the usual dosage of a drug.

Wolff-Parkinson-White (WPW) syndrome A syndrome characterised by short P-R intervals, delta waves, nonspecific ST-T wave changes, and paroxysmal episodes of tachycardia caused by the presence of an accessory pathway.

xanthines A classification of medications that affect the respiratory smooth muscle and that relax bronchiole smooth muscles, stimulate cardiac muscle, and stimulate the central nervous system. absorption The process by which a medication's molecules are moved from the site of entry or administration into the body and into systemic circulation.

years of potential life lost A way of measuring and comparing the overall impact of deaths resulting from different causes. It is calculated based on a fixed age minus the age at death. Usually the fixed age is 65 or 70 or the life expectancy of the group in question.

zone of coagulation The reddened area surrounding the leathery and sometimes charred tissue that has sustained a full-thickness burn.

zone of hyperemia In a thermal burn, the area that is least affected by the burn injury.

zone of stasis The peripheral area surrounding the zone of coagulation that has decreased blood flow and inflammation. This area can undergo necrosis within 24 to 48 hours after the injury, particularly if perfusion is compromised due to burn shock.

zygomatic arch The bone that extends along the front of the skull below the orbit.

Index

Credits

Chapter 1
Opener: Courtesy of Mark Woolcock; 1-3 © National Library of Medicine; 1-4 Courtesy of Eugene L. Nagel and the Miami Fire Department.; 1-7 Courtesy of Mark Woolcock; 1-8 © John Giles/PA/AP Photos; 1-9 © Ashley Cooper/Alamy Images; 1-13 © Kevin Britland/ShutterStock, Inc.

Chapter 2
2-2 © Photos.com; 2-4 © LiquidLibrary; 2-9 Courtesy of Island Photography/U.S. Air Force; 2-11 © David Buffington/Photodisc/Getty Images; 2-13 © Hugh Van der Poorten/Alamy Images; 2-15 © Galina Barskaya/ShutterStock, Inc; 2-18 © Glen E. Ellman; 2-21 © Shout/Alamy Images; 2-25 © LM Otero/AP Photos; 2-26 Courtesy of Mark Woolcock.

Chapter 3
Opener: Courtesy of London Ambulance Service; 3-1 © Soundsnaps/ShutterStock, Inc; 3-2 © Steven Townsend/Code 3 Images; 3-3A © Ryan McVay/Photodisc/Getty Images; 3-3B © Carolyn Brule/ShutterStock, Inc; 3-4 © Steven Pepple/ShutterStock, Inc; 3-5A Courtesy of Henry Pollak; 3-5B © Vladimir Korostyshevskiy/ShutterStock, Inc; 3-5C Courtesy of Captain David Jackson, Saginaw Township Fire Department; 3-6B © Cristina Fumi/ShutterStock, Inc; 3-6C © Photos.com; 3-6D © Andreas Nilsson/ShutterStock, Inc; 3-8 © Mikael Karlsson/On Scene Photography; 3-9 © SuperStock/age fotostock; 3-10 © Shout/Alamy Images; 3-11 © Mark Humphrey/AP Photos; 3-13 Courtesy of London Ambulance Service.

Chapter 4
Opener: © Dominic Burke/Alamy Images; 4-1 © Brand X Pictures/Creatas; 4-2 © Janine Wiedel Photolibrary/Alamy Images; 4-3 © Matthew Richardson/Alamy Images; 4-4 Courtesy of London Ambulance Service.

Chapter 5
5-6 Courtesy of the MedicAlert Foundation; 5-7 © The Express Times/AP Photos.

Chapter 6
Opener: © National Cancer Institute/Photodisc/Getty Images; 6-11A&B From An Introduction to Human Disease, 7th edition. Photo courtesy of Leonard V. Crowley, MD, Century College; 6-13B Courtesy of Rocky Mountain Laboratory, NIAID, NIH; 6-16A&B; 6-19; 6-20A&B; 6-22A&B From An Introduction to Human Disease, 7th edition. Photo courtesy of Leonard V. Crowley, MD, Century College.

Chapter 7
Opener: © Photos.com; 7-2A © Stephen Aaron Rees/ShutterStock, Inc; 7-2B © Photos.com; 7-2C Courtesy of Yellowstone National Park; 7-2D Courtesy of Linda Bartlett/National Cancer Institute; 7-7 Courtesy of Schwarz Pharma AG. Used with permission.

Chapter 8
8-8; 8-9; 8-12; 8-14 Courtesy of Bob Fellows; 8-27 Courtesy of Pyng Medical Corporation; 8-28 Courtesy of VidaCare Corporation; 8-49; 8-50 Courtesy of Baxter International, Inc; 8-52 Courtesy of Wolfe Tory Medical, Inc.

Chapter 9
Opener: © Photodisc; 9-1 © Johanna Goodyear/ShutterStock, Inc; 9-5 © Scott Milless/ShutterStock, Inc; 9-6 © EML/ShutterStock, Inc; 9-7 © Maxim Bolotnikov/ShutterStock, Inc; 9-8 © GeoTrac/Alamy Images; 9-9 © Trout55/ShutterStock, Inc; 9-10 © Jamie Wilson/ShutterStock, Inc; 9-11 © SW Productions/Jupiterimages; 9-13 © Rubberball Productions; 9-14 © Photodisc; 9-15 © Blend Images/Alamy Images; 9-16; 9-20 © Photodisc.

Chapter 10
10-3 © Photofusion Picture Library/Alamy Images.

Chapter 11
11-18C The Laerdal® Suction Unit is provided courtesy of Laerdal Medical Corporation.; 11-30 The Laerdal® One Way Valve Pocket Mask provided courtesy of Laerdal Medical Corporation.; 11-33 microVENT® courtesy of Meditech (B.N.O.S. Meditech Ltd.); 11-50; 11-53; 11-54; 11-55; 11-56; 11-57A&B Courtesy of Marianne Gausche-Hill, MD, FACEP, FAAP; 11-73 © Eddie M. Sperling.

Chapter 12
12-1 © Pier Photography/Alamy Images; 12-11 © Jack Dagley Photography/ShutterStock, Inc.

Chapter 13
13-7 © Denis Pepin/ShutterStock, Inc; 13-8 © WizData, Inc/ShutterStock, Inc; 13-9 © Kenneth Chelette/ShutterStock, Inc; 13-12 Courtesy of Ronald Dieckmann, MD; 13-14 © Germán Ariel Berra/ShutterStock, Inc; 13-31 © Dr. P. Marazzi/Photo Researchers, Inc.

Chapter 14
Opener: © VStock/Alamy Images; 14-2 Courtesy of Mark Woolcock; 14-3 Courtesy of Tempe Fire Department; 14-4 © Kirsty Wigglesworth/AP Photos; 14-5 Courtesy of James Tourtellotte/U.S. Customs and Border Protection; 14-8A © Mark C. Ide; 14-8B © Corbis; 14-8D © Dan Myers; 14-8E © Jack Dagley Photography/ShutterStock, Inc; 14-8F © Larry St. Pierre/ShutterStock, Inc; 14-8G © micheal ledray/ShutterStock, Inc; 14-10 © Thinkstock/Getty Images; 14-12 © E. M. Singletary, MD. Used with permission.

Chapter 15
15-1 Courtesy of London Ambulance Service; 15-4 © Peter Willott, The St. Augustine Record/AP Photos; 15-8 © Craig Jackson/In the Dark Photography; 15-10 © fstop2/Alamy Images; 15-12 © Mark C. Ide.

Chapter 16
16-7 Courtesy of ZOLL Data Systems, Inc.

Chapter 17
Opener: Courtesy of Mark Woolcock; 17-1 © Shout Pictures/Custom Medical Stock Photo; 17-2; 17-3 © Dan Myers; 17-5 © Terry Dickson, Florida Times-Union/AP Photos; 17-6 © Dan Myers; 17-8 Courtesy of Captain David Jackson, Saginaw Township Fire Department; 17-12 © Dennis Wetherhold, Jr; 17-15 © Jack Sullivan/Alamy Images; 17-19A © Charles Stewart & Associates; 17-19B © D. Willoughby/Custom Medical Stock Photography.

Chapter 18
Opener: © Zoom 77/AP Photos; 18-4 © Mark C. Ide; 18-5 © SPL/Photo Researchers, Inc.

Chapter 19
Opener: Courtesy of Moose Jaw Police Service; 19-3 Courtesy of Rhonda Beck; 19-5A © English/Custom Medical Stock Photo; 19-7 © Custom Medical Stock Photo; 19-9 © E. M. Singletary, MD. Used with permission.; 19-10 © Mark C. Ide; 19-11 © Mike Abrahams/Alamy Images; 19-12 © Zoom 77/AP Photos; 19-14 Courtesy of Matthew J. Belan, MD; 19-17 Combat Application Tourniquet® (C-A-T®) photo courtesy of North American Rescue Products, Inc; 19-19 © E. M. Singletary, MD. Used with permission.

Chapter 20
Opener: © Glen E. Ellman; 20-1 © Dale A. Stock/ShutterStock, Inc; 20-2 © Dr. P. Marazzi/Photo Researchers, Inc; 20-6 © J. Yakwichuk/Custom Medical Stock Photo; 20-7 Courtesy of Health Resources and Services Administration, Maternal and Child Health Bureau, Emergency Medical Services for Children Program; 20-8 © Kevin Frayer/AP Photos; 20-11A&B © Charles Stewart & Associates; 20-13B © Amy Walters/ShutterStock, Inc; 20-13C © E. M. Singletary, MD. Used with permission.; 20-15 Adapted from Lund, C.C., and Browder, N.C. Surg. Gynecol. Obstet. 79 (1944): 352–358.; 20-16 Courtesy of Water-Jel® Technologies; 20-20 © Charles Stewart & Associates.

Chapter 21
Opener: © E. M. Singletary, MD. Used with permission.; 21-28 Courtesy of John T. Halgren, MD, University of Nebraska Medical Center; 21-40 © E. M. Singletary, MD. Used with permission.; 21-53 © Joe Gough/ShutterStock, Inc.

Chapter 22
22-10 Courtesy of Thomas E.M.S.; 22-14; 22-21A–C Courtesy of Mark Woolcock.

Chapter 23
Opener: © PHT/Photo Researchers, Inc; 23-1 © Shout Pictures/Custom Medical Stock Photo; 23-13 © Charles Stewart & Associates; 23-18 © SIU Bio Med Comm/Custom Medical Stock Photo.

Chapter 24
Opener: © Charles Stewart & Associates; 24-7 © David Crausby/Alamy Images; 24-9 © Dr. P. Marazzi/Photo Researchers, Inc; 24-11 © Custom Medical Stock Photo.

Chapter 25
Opener: © Charles Stewart & Associates; 25-9A&B Courtesy of International Osteoporosis Foundation; 25-19 © Charles Stewart & Associates; 25-33 © Custom Medical Stock Photo; 25-34 Courtesy of Anand M. Murthi, MD.

Chapter 26
26-3 © E. M. Singletary, MD. Used with permission.; 26-6 Courtesy of The Milton J. Dance, Jr. Head and Neck Rehabilitation Center (www.gbmc.org/voice); 26-7B © David M. Martin, MD/Photo Researchers, Inc; 26-8B © Dr. Kessel & Dr. Kardon/Tissue & Organs/Visuals Unlimited; 26-16 Courtesy of Health Resources and Services Administration, Maternal and Child Health Bureau, Emergency Medical Services for Children Program; 26-17 © Logical Images/Custom Medical Stock Photo; 26-18 © Uschi Hering/ShutterStock, Inc; 26-19B Courtesy of Stuart Mirvis, MD; 26-21 © Mediscan/Visuals Unlimited; 26-26A Courtesy of Nonin Medical, Inc; 26-27 The Masimo® Rad-ST™ Pulse CO-Oximeter™ courtesy of Masimo Corporation (www.masimo.com); 26-29 Courtesy of Marianne Gausche-Hill, MD, FACEP, FAAP; 26-30A LIFEPAK® defibrillator/monitor. Courtesy of Medtronic; 26-33B © Scott Rothstein/ShutterStock, Inc; 26-35 Courtesy of Smiths Medical. All rights reserved; 26-41 Courtesy of Respironics, Inc., Murrysville, PA. All rights reserved; 26-42 Courtesy of Airon Corporation (www.pneuton.com).

Chapter 27
27-3 © Tony Wear/ShutterStock, Inc; 27-10; 27-12, 27-24, 27-70; 27-71; 27-72; 27-73, 27-83 Adapted from 12-Lead ECG: The Art of Interpretation, courtesy of Tomas B. Garcia, MD; 27-22A–D, 27-23, 27-25; 27-26; 27-27; 27-28; 27-29; 27-31; 27-32, 27-33; 27-34; 27-35; 27-36; 27-37; 27-38; 27-39; 27-40; 27-41; 27-42; 27-44; 27-45; 27-46; 27-47; 27-48; 27-49; 27-50; 27-51; 27-52, 27-53, 27-54; 27-55; 27-56; 27-57; 27-58; 27-59; 27-60; 27-61; 27-62; 27-64; 27-65; 27-66; 27-67; 27-68; 27-69, 27-74; 27-75; 27-76; 27-77; 27-78, 27-90 Adapted from Arrhythmia Recognition: The Art of Interpretation, courtesy of Tomas B. Garcia, MD; 27-86 Reproduced from Adult Advanced Life Support Algorithm. © European Resuscitation Council; 27-87 Reproduced from Bradycardia Algorithm. © European Resuscitation Council; 27-88 Reproduced from Tachycardia Algorithm. © European Resuscitation Council.